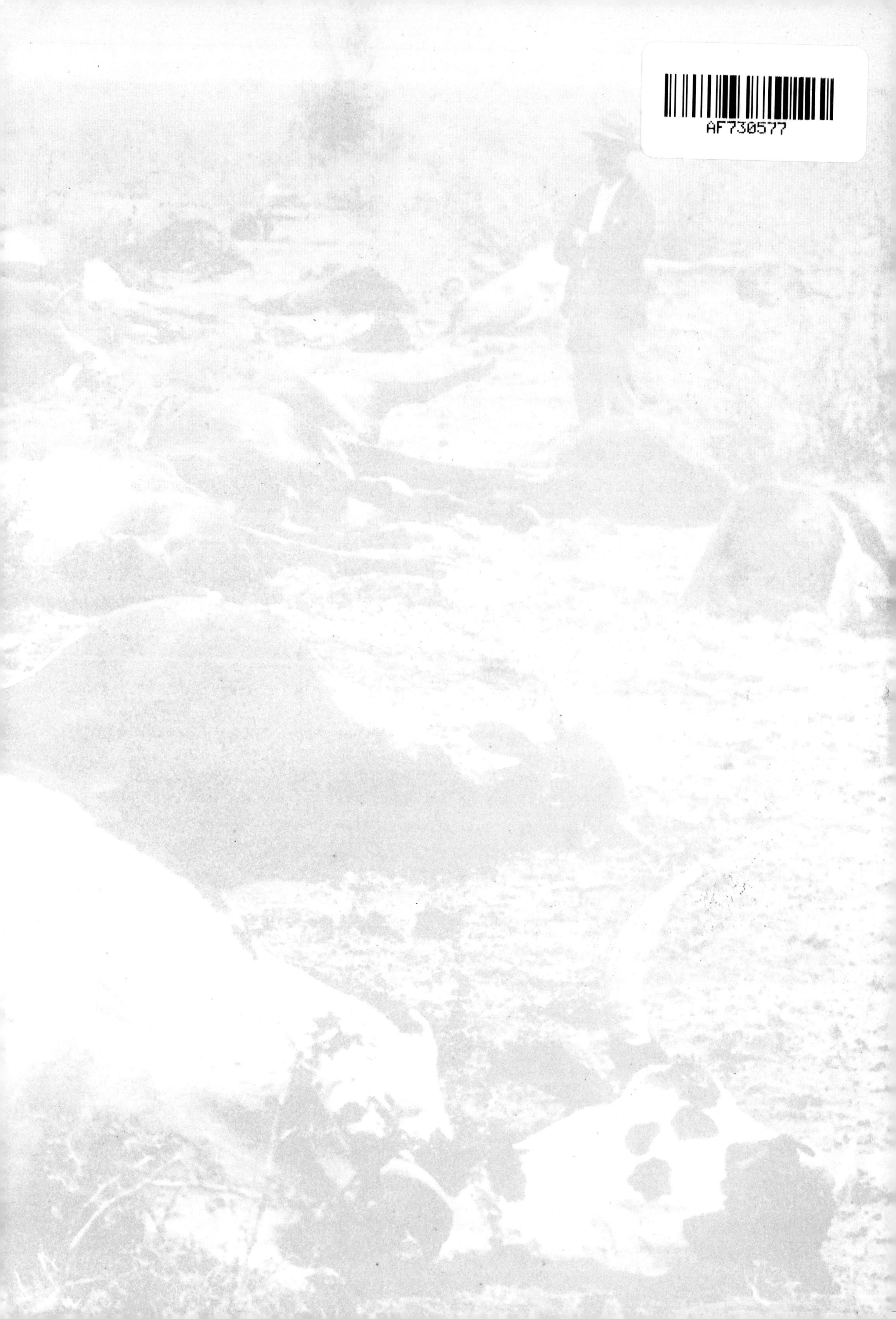

VOLUME TWO

INFECTIOUS DISEASES OF LIVESTOCK

WITH SPECIAL REFERENCE TO

Southern Africa

VOLUME TWO

INFECTIOUS DISEASES OF LIVESTOCK

WITH SPECIAL REFERENCE TO

Southern Africa

Chapters 74–193 and Index

EDITED BY

Professor J. A. W. Coetzer

Dr G. R. Thomson

Professor R. C. Tustin

ASSOCIATE EDITOR

Professor N. P. J. Kriek

CAPE TOWN OXFORD NEW YORK

OXFORD UNIVERSITY PRESS

1994

OXFORD UNIVERSITY PRESS
Walton Street, Oxford OX2 6DP, United Kingdom

Oxford New York
Athens Auckland Bangkok Bombay
Calcutta Cape Town Dar es Salaam Delhi
Florence Hong Kong Istanbul Karachi
Kuala Lumpur Madras Madrid Melbourne
Mexico City Nairobi Paris Singapore
Taipei Tokyo Toronto

and associated companies in
Berlin Ibadan

OXFORD is a trademark of Oxford University Press

INFECTIOUS DISEASES OF LIVESTOCK

STANDARD EDITION
Two volume set: ISBN 0 19 570506 8
Volume One: ISBN 0 19 570916 0
Volume Two: ISBN 0 19 570917 9

DE LUXE EDITION
Two volume set: ISBN 0 19 570551 3
Volume One: ISBN 0 19 570918 7
Volume Two: ISBN 0 19 570919 5

Editors: Susan Lawrence, Katy Cleary,
Penny Nyren, Helen Moffett
Designers: Tony Mays, Mara Singer and Mark Standley
Cover designer: Mark Standley
Cover illustrations: Chris Tugwell
Indexer: Trudie Kettley

Published by Oxford University Press Southern Africa,
Harrington House, 37 Barrack Street, Cape Town 8001,
South Africa

Set in 9.5pt on 12.5pt Palatino

Typesetting by Photoprint
Reproduction by Fotoplate, Maitland, Western Cape
Printed and bound by Clyson Printers, Maitland, Western Cape
Printed by Clyson Press, Maitland, Cape Town

This book is dedicated to the memory of the late
Professor Michiel Wilhelm Henning, author and
editor of the textbook *Animal Diseases in South Africa*,
of which editions appeared in 1932, 1949 and 1956.
His vision and dedication in producing a work
of true international acclaim gave us the
inspiration and courage to undertake
this project.

Preface

In the area of agricultural and veterinary science it is appropriate, in retrospect, to acknowledge the enormous debt owed to early authorities who in their day produced exemplary textbooks on subjects vitally important to progress in Africa. One thinks of H.O. Mönnig's monumental *Veterinary Helminthology and Entomology* which, albeit in an entirely different shape and now edited by E.J.L. Soulsby under the title *Helminths, Arthropods and Protozoa of Domesticated Animals*, is in its seventh edition. In the same category is M.W. Henning's *Animal Diseases in South Africa*, which first appeared in 1932 and which was, by popular demand, completely revised in 1949 and again in 1956.

The latter publication — which eventually concentrated on bacterial and protozoal diseases along with afflictions caused by viruses and rickettsias — has been out of print for many years, and the need for a worthy substitute had been evident for some time. Henning in fact set himself this arduous task, one which regrettably remained unfulfilled at the time of his death in 1962. Meanwhile, as has happened with many other scientific works of stature, the field originally embraced by his book has expanded well beyond the scope of one single author. Complete revision was called for in the light of the great volume of new knowledge, and the contributions of a number of authorities on different subjects were clearly necessary.

This publication focuses on the diseases of livestock in the African continent, more particularly those occurring in the southern subcontinent, but there is also considerable information on diseases in other regions of the world, tropical and otherwise, which broadens its spectrum of interest and application. Tropical and subtropical Africa, while famous for its floral and faunal wealth, is equally notorious for the number and variety of diseases which threaten its livestock. Furthermore, the roles played by game species and humans and their animals in a delicately balanced ecosystem, are additional reasons for continued concern and attention at the highest level of expertise available.

A formidable team of authors, ably guided by editors J.A.W. Coetzer, G.R. Thomson, R.C. Tustin and N.P.J. Kriek, has collated and interpreted the latest information on farm animal diseases, as well as the massive research output of many institutions (both local and international) since before the turn of the century. In this regard the Veterinary Research Institute at Onderstepoort and its adjacent Faculty of Veterinary Science of the University of Pretoria have contributed substantially, with the Institute acting as a reference laboratory for several important diseases. However, several chapters are authored by specialists working outside the borders of the subcontinent, which further broadens the appeal of the book.

The book is divided into seven sections. The first section deals with aspects influencing the occurrence of infectious diseases, with special reference to vectors, the epidemiology and control of arthropod-borne diseases, vaccines and immunization strategies, breed resistance, and the interaction of domestic animals with wildlife with respect to both spread and control. In the subsequent five sections, the diseases are grouped according to their causal agents, viz. protozoal, rickettsial and chlamydial, viral, bacterial and mycoplasmal, and mycotic and algal, while the final section covers diseases of unknown aetiology and some important disease complexes. The reader is therefore immediately impressed by a breadth of coverage which should satisfy the needs of veterinary researchers, students, and practitioners, as well as others involved in the promotion of animal health.

Both the editors and the individual authors are to be congratulated on having produced a truly definitive publication which will without doubt take its place among the other classics of southern African scientific endeavour and enterprise. In the context of a global approach to environmental protection, its contribution towards stabilizing food production on the one hand, and preserving our unique faunal heritage on the other, is assured. This is especially important now, when the African continent faces more serious challenges — in terms of predicted expectations and measurable demands — than ever before in its long and often tumultuous history.

Prof. D. M. Joubert
Former Chairman, Agricultural Research Council
Former Vice-Chancellor and Principal of the
University of Pretoria

VOLUME TWO

Contents

Section 6: Mycotic and algal diseases

Section 7: Disease complexes and diseases of unknown aetiology

Section 4

Viral diseases
(continued)

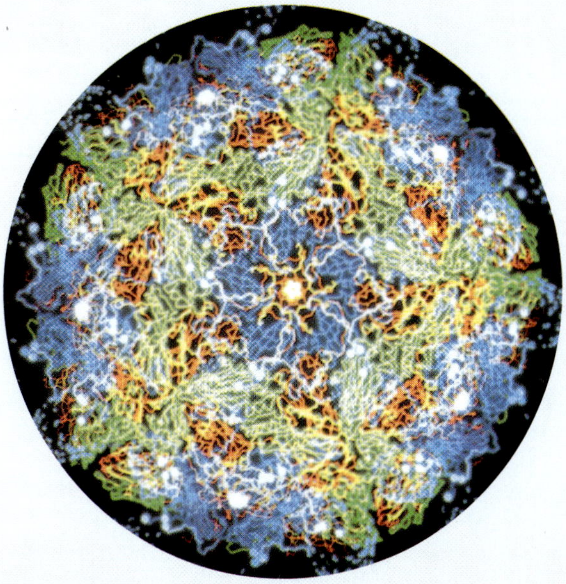

PARAMYXOVIRIDAE

The Paramyxoviridae forms one of three families included in the newly-created order Mononegavirales, and embodies two subfamilies: the Paramyxovirinae, which contains two genera (*Paramyxovirus* and *Morbillivirus*), and the Pneumovirinae, in which only one genus *(Pneumovirus)* is represented **(Table 1)**.[2]

Paramyxoviruses have relatively large (>100 nm in diameter), pleomorphic virions which generally assume a roughly spherical shape. They are surrounded by an envelope derived from the host-cell membrane. The outer surface of the envelope bears closely-packed, club-shaped projections (peplomers), 8–12 nm in length. The peplomers contain the cell fusion, haemagglutinin and neuraminidase proteins, although the latter two are not always present.

A single strand of negative-sense RNA, associated with three proteins (RNA binding protein, N; phosphoprotein, P; polymerase, L), makes up the long, contorted nucleocapsid which has helical symmetry. A small proportion of virions contains positive-sense RNA. Altogether 10–12 proteins, two or three of which are glycosylated, are contained in the virion. These proteins are encoded by seven or eight open reading frames, i.e., some are encoded by overlapping genes.[2]

Paramyxoviruses are found only in vertebrates and all are transmitted directly between infected and susceptible hosts, i.e., none are dependent on vectors for transmission. Replication occurs within the cytoplasm of cells, although viral proteins may accumulate in the nucleus after synthesis.[1]

Some of the most devastating viral diseases of humans and animals are caused by members of this family. Measles and mumps (both human), canine distemper, rinderpest and Newcastle disease have arguably caused more death and destruction than any other group of related animal viruses in recorded history. Two other viruses in this family, which have relatively recently been recognized (bovine respiratory syncytial and peste des petits ruminants viruses), are increasingly being acknowledged as important diseases of livestock. The major diseases caused by paramyxoviruses are shown in **Table 1**.

Table 1 Important human and animal viruses belonging to the Paramyxoviridae

SUBFAMILY	GENUS	VIRUS	TYPE	SPECIES AFFECTED
Paramyxovirinae	*Paramyxovirus*	Avian paramyxovirus	1–9*	Birds
		Parainfluenza virus	1	Humans, murids
			2	Canids, humans, simians
			3	Humans, cattle, sheep, simians
			4	Humans
		Mumps virus	–	Humans
	Morbillivirus	Canine distemper virus	–	Canids, mustelids
		Measles virus	–	Humans
		Phocine distemper virus	–	Phocids
		Rinderpest virus	–	Cattle, goats, sheep, pigs, some wild artiodactyles
		Peste des petits ruminants virus	–	Goats, sheep
Pneumovirinae	*Pneumovirus*	Human respiratory syncytial virus	–	Humans
		Bovine respiratory syncytial virus	–	Cattle
		Pneumonia virus of mice	–	Murids
		Turkey rhinotracheitis virus	–	Birds

* Avian paramyxovirus type 1 = Newcastle disease virus

References

1 **FENNER, F., BACHMANN, P.A., GIBBS, E.P.J., MURPHY, F.A., STUDDERT, M.J. & WHITE, D.O., 1987.** *Veterinary Virology*. Orlando, San Diego, New York: Academic Press, Inc.

2 **PRINGLE, C.R., 1991.** Paramyxoviridae. *In:* FRANCKI, R.I.B., FAUQUET, C.M., KNUDSON, D.L. & BROWN, F., (eds). Classification and nomenclature of viruses. Fifth report of the International Committee on the Taxonomy of Viruses. *Archives of Virology,* Supplementum 2. Vienna, New York:

74

Rinderpest

Synonyms: Cattle plague, la peste bovine, runderpes (Afrik.)

P.B. Rossiter

Introduction

Rinderpest is an acute to subacute contagious viral disease of cattle and other Artiodactyla characterized by necrosis and erosions in the gastrointestinal tract that result in severe diarrhoea and dehydration. Morbidity and mortality rates may exceed 90 per cent, but inapparent infections may also occur.

The decimation of cattle populations by rinderpest has influenced events in human history[86, 138, 181] and, through the eradication of cattle, wildlife and (indirectly) tsetse flies, may have altered the ecology of large areas of southern and central Africa.[284, 298] The control and eradication of rinderpest was a major factor in the establishment of the first veterinary schools in Europe during the eighteenth century, a tribute to the ravages of the disease.

It has been assumed that the disease originated in Asia since it regularly invaded Europe with armies from the Orient. A monoclonal antibody study[179] has suggested that rinderpest is the archetypal morbillivirus from which the other morbilliviruses of measles and distemper evolved some five thousand years ago, possibly in the river civilizations of south-west Asia where the domestication of cattle is believed to have occurred.[78] However, considering that the evolution of most artiodactyls, including the genus *Bos*, took place very much earlier in the late Pliocene and early Pleistocene periods, the comparative insusceptibility of European as opposed to Asian pigs, the originally restricted distribution of the related disease, peste des petits ruminants (PPR), and the recent emergence of phocine distemper, the exact origin of the disease now seems less certain.

Introductions of rinderpest into Europe, usually as a sequel to wars, were often followed by major epidemics. By the end of the nineteenth century, when mules and then motorized transport had replaced oxen as the main source of military draught power, the basic control measures of slaughter and quarantine had eradicated rinderpest from most of Europe, though a series of outbreaks occurred during and immediately after the First World War, most notably in Poland. The last reported outbreaks in Europe were in Belgium in 1920 and Rome zoo in 1949, both of which were caused by importing live infected animals from high-risk areas.[8, 51] Similarly, the only recorded outbreak in the Americas, in Brazil in 1920, and that in Australia in 1923, were due to the importation of live infected animals.[229, 230, 321]

Rinderpest is still endemic in India, where it is maintained by the vast, comparatively unconfined and inadequately vaccinated cattle population, and by goats and sheep. Neighbouring and Middle East countries are regularly infected by widespread traffic in live animals, including sheep and goats in which rinderpest is now endemic in southern Asia. The disease was, for a time, effectively controlled in the Near and Middle East, but decreased vaccination and the increased movement of cattle that has resulted from recent civil and military disturbances have led to renewed localized outbreaks in the region.[1, 13]

The history of rinderpest in Africa is often thought to have begun with the 'Great Rinderpest Pandemic' of 1889–97, though in all probability the disease had previously been introduced to North Africa, especially Egypt, and into West Africa.[59, 80, 160] The pandemic has been described by many authors, including Hutcheon,[109] Henning,[98] and Mack.[153]

The origin of the virus which started the pandemic is uncertain, as there were at least three possible sources. That most frequently quoted was the introduction of infected Indian or Arabian cattle to Massawa in Eritrea by the Italian army in either 1887, 1888 or 1889.[148, 331] The disease was helped in establishing itself by the inefficient attempts to use prophylactic and therapeutic control rather than slaughter and quarantine.[331] It was subsequently transported throughout Ethiopia and into the Nile Valley in Sudan in 1890. Alternatively, the virus may have moved slowly up the Nile from Egypt, assisted by British military campaigns which reputedly brought rinderpest to Khartoum in 1884 and 1885. Littlewood[148] also reported that, against his advice, a German military expedition brought cattle from Aden and Bombay and instigated a severe outbreak of rinderpest on the East African coast in late 1889. Virus from this outbreak could have been carried in cattle which the Maasai say were brought back to Kilimanjaro from the coast by their warriors in late 1890.

Thus this was possibly responsible for the outbreak at Oloitokitok in early 1891. Some authors[153, 250] have reported that the explorer Joseph Thompson saw rinderpest in Maasailand in 1883, but, as noted by Theiler,[298] Thompson's descriptions give a more accurate picture of contagious bovine pleuropneumonia, which was widespread in the area some six to seven years before the outbreak of rinderpest.[96]

Whatever the source, the pandemic was undoubtedly raging in Kenya, Uganda and Tanzania in 1891. Moving south in 1892 it had reached Karonga on Lake Nyasa by July and the Luapala river in Zambia by October. Very high mortality was seen not only in cattle but also in wildlife, though alcelaphines and waterbuck seem to have been relatively insusceptible. The southerly spread of the virus was halted by the Zambezi River, where the disease, which had not yet been fully confirmed as rinderpest, came to be called Zambezi cattle fever.

During this period the southerly advance of the virus may also have spread westward into Angola and Zaire, whilst further north the main western extension of the pandemic had penetrated right through sub-Saharan West Africa.

Eventually the virus was transported across the Zambezi. The disease was reported south of the river in February 1896 and appeared at Bulawayo in March, where it was confirmed by Gray and Theiler, and in the same month at Palapye in Botswana. Soon after that the Transvaal was infected via the transport routes stretching through Botswana and Mafikeng, and in October the disease rushed south through Kimberley to the Orange River in December. Here it was temporarily halted not only by the river but by a 1 600 kilometre-long fence and rigorous quarantine measures. Unfortunately, in March 1897 a drover crossed the river reputedly wearing a pair of trousers he had found in a sack containing meat. Within a few days his cattle developed rinderpest and the virus moved swiftly to the Cape. During 1897 the disease also infected Natal, Lesotho and Namibia.

Wild ungulates were, reputedly, a further factor in the spread of the disease. President Paul Kruger of the Transvaal Republic was of the opinion that game were the most important spreaders of infection, with bushbuck (*Tragelaphus scriptus*), impala (*Aepyceros melampus*) and kudu (*Tragelaphus strepsiceros*) being the primary culprits.[138]

Energetic control campaigns which included the use of newly developing prophylactic inoculations eventually contained the disease and it was briefly eradicated from South Africa in 1899. A re-introduction from Namibia in 1901 was milder and easier to control, and southern Africa was reported free of rinderpest in 1905.[305]

It was the losses incurred during the pandemic — 5,25 million cattle and innumerable wildlife south of the Zambezi — which have most dramatically illustrated the killing power of rinderpest **(Figure 74.1)**. In the Transvaal Republic alone there were 1 556 760 cattle prior to the rinderpest, of which 1 002 297 (66,5 per cent) died of or were killed as a result of the disease. A total of 205 801 (13,2 per cent) was said to have recovered from the infection, while the rest (20,3 per cent) was unaffected. The direct financial losses were estimated to total 3 006 891 pounds sterling.[138] In Natal, 46 per cent of the cattle population was lost, but the highest mortality rate in southern Africa occurred in Matabeleland (Zimbabwe), where it reached 90 per cent.[138]

The pandemic also left its mark on the continent in other ways. In East Africa the dominant cattle-keeping tribes such as the Maasai were irrevocably weakened and replaced politically and economically by agricultural tribes. Further south the disease and the stern measures employed to combat it provoked rebellions in Matabeleland and Lesotho. In South Africa not only were stock owners, both black and white, ruined financially, but the whole transport system virtually collapsed **(Figure 74.2)**. This further contributed to the impoverishment and resultant urbanization of the Afrikaners.[138]

The decimation of wildlife and cattle led to the apparent disappearance of *Glossina* spp. from many areas. The comparatively swift eradication of rinderpest from the subcontinent allowed wildlife in the region to recover their numbers and distribution, whereas the persistence of the virus further north may have contributed to anomalies such as the formation of isolated 'island' communities of species such as sable (*Hippotragus niger*) and kudu.

The pandemic also set the stage for one of the keenest competitions medical science has ever seen. The various South African states each set about finding a method of curing or preventing the disease. The race became even more significant when the Russian government offered a prize of one million roubles for the winner. Drs Arnold Theiler, of the Transvaal, and Herbert Watkins-Pitchford of Natal collaborated from October 1886 to March 1887 in developing a technique for immunizing cattle with simultaneous but separate inoculations of immune serum and infectious virus. In December 1886 Dr Robert Koch, the eminent German microbiologist, arrived at the request of the government of the Cape Colony to begin work at Kimberley. He lost no time in evaluating, amongst other things, the Boer farmers' preventive remedy of inoculating bile from dead cattle into healthy animals. Koch refined the technique to a stage where it was successful in experienced hands at the laboratory, at which point it was hastily introduced throughout the affected areas. With hindsight it is easy to criticize the bile method for being a poor way of immunizing cattle and for spreading the virus. The experiments of Theiler and Watkins-Pitchford were barely complete, while immune serum was in desperately short supply and time-consuming to produce. Undoubtedly the bile method helped to reduce the mortality in the later stages of the pandemic.

The Transvaal government also obtained the services

of the distinguished French microbiologists, Drs Jean Danyz and Jules Bordet, who arrived to begin work in January 1897. Theiler was ordered to join them, and they eventually reported jointly to the Transvaal government on the success of the serum-virus method of immunization, which then gradually replaced the bile method. Watkins-Pitchford was less fortunate: the Natal government largely ignored his results and his data were destroyed in a fire at Pietermaritzburg town hall. The million roubles were never officially awarded.

Rinderpest has persisted further north in equatorial Africa where nomadic or semi-nomadic pastoralism is common **(Figure 74.3)**. Such husbandry encourages the keeping of large herds of cattle which may range over hundreds of kilometres and are frequently inaccessible for vaccination. Southern Africa has been under constant potential threat of rinderpest from the north, but the threat has assumed real proportions on only a few occasions. Usually the danger has arisen from a southerly spread of the disease through Tanzania following natural

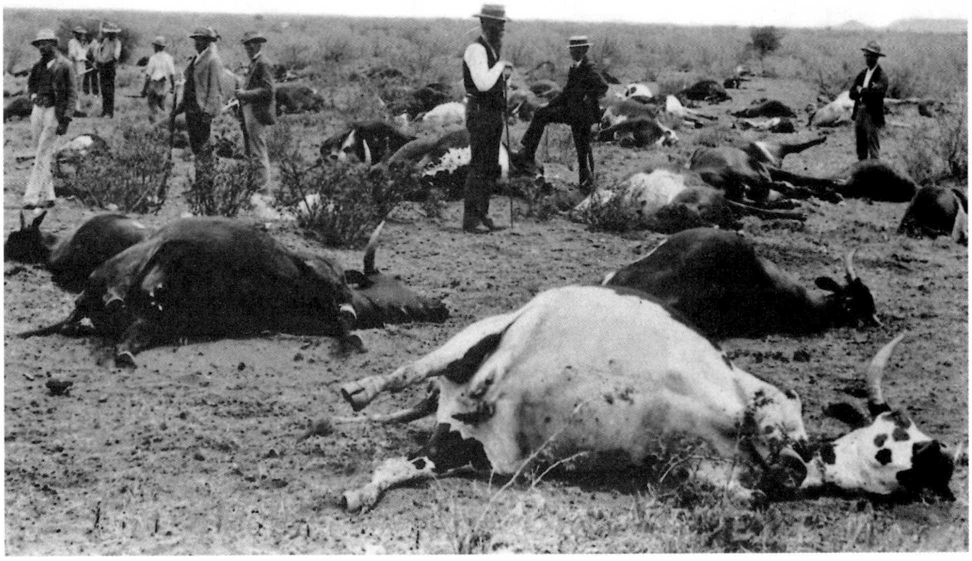

Figure 74.1 The rinderpest epidemic at the turn of the century in South Africa

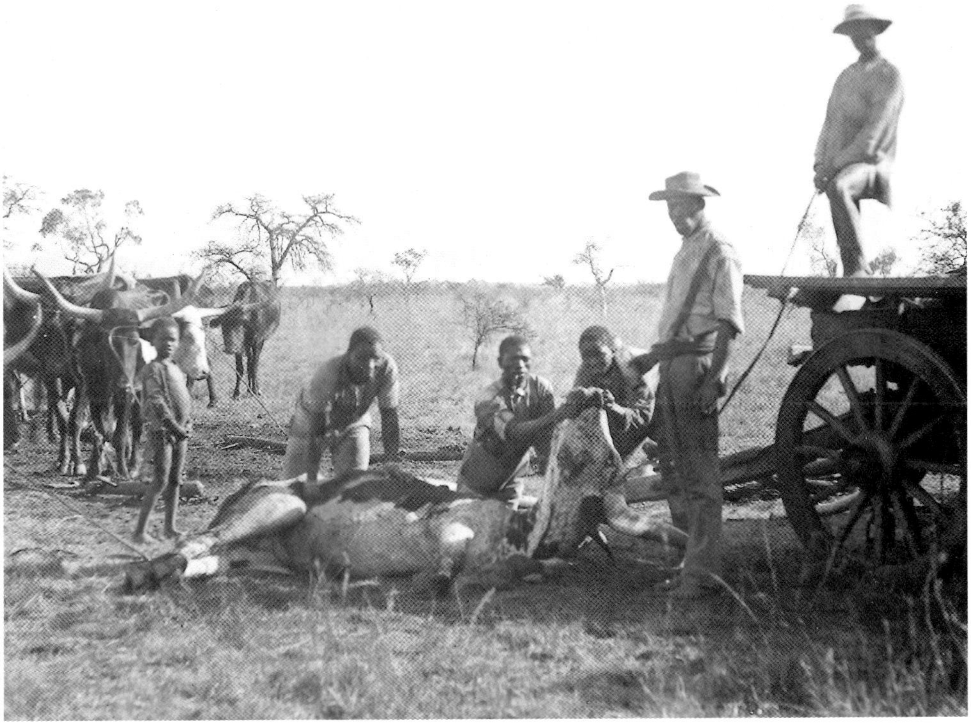

Figure 74.2 Trek oxen affected by rinderpest

stock routes towards the gap between Lakes Tanganyika and Malawi. Alarming southerly extensions occurred at the end of the First World War[61, 89] and in the years from 1937 to 1941,[35, 98, 149] but were contained by vigorous control of cattle movement and vaccination of all stock in the belt between the lakes. Implementation of a 'cordon sanitaire' involving, to varying degrees, the elimination of all stock and susceptible species of wildlife from a six- to 40-kilometre-wide strip and the erection of game-proof fencing was also carried out.[301] In 1983 and 1984, this same region was the target of co-ordinated vaccination campaigns by the governments of Tanzania, Zambia and Malawi in an attempt to generate a cordon of immune animals that would halt the passage of disease from what can now be regarded as the second Great African Pandemic. Fortunately the effectiveness of this immune belt was never tested as the virus did not spread south of the central railway line in Tanzania, and southern Africa escaped the losses and disruption experienced by less fortunate countries further north.

The progress of the second African pandemic (1979–84) attracted considerable attention, though accurate details of the origin of primary outbreaks and subsequent dissemination of the virus were often as difficult to obtain as they had been in the first pandemic 90 years before.[91, 95, 175, 177, 210, 239, 243] The underlying causes were, however, easy to discern. The outstanding success of vaccination campaigns using cell-culture attenuated rinderpest virus vaccine led to an impressive fall in the number of outbreaks of rinderpest in Africa in the mid-1970s **(Figure 74.3)**. Joint Project 15 (JP15) of the Organization of African Unity, Food and Agriculture Organization of the United Nations, and the European Economic Community, assisted by a number of individual donor countries including some African states such as Nigeria, was especially instrumental in this control.[14] The virus was eradicated throughout vast areas of the continent and by 1976 was restricted to two zones where access and animal movement control have always been difficult; one in West Africa, centred on the Mali/Mauritania border and the internal delta of the Niger; and the other in Ethiopia and Sudan **(Figure 74.3)**. When JP15 ceased in 1976 it left behind a sense of security but no funds to maintain the high levels of herd immunity it had induced. Unfortunately this coincided with a recession in the world economy, and the emergent nations, being heavily dependent on donor aid and world commodity prices, both of which were reduced, were particularly hard hit at a time when fuel prices were escalating. With rinderpest having been eradicated from many countries for over a decade, minimizing vaccination against the virus was an obvious way to save money for more pressing veterinary problems. Some countries ceased vaccination completely and others partially. Some, such as Kenya, made prudent use of available resources to try to ensure adequate herd immunity along national boundaries.

The outcome was that the proportion of susceptible cattle started to increase as soon as JP15 ceased and, despite warnings,[210, 263] the virus began to spread from its endemic strongholds. In contrast to the first pandemic, the availability of motor transport facilitated rapid spread of infection, while civil and military strife in many parts of the continent hindered control. The maps in **Figure 74.3** give a generalized resumé of this. Fortunately, in one of the most successful emergency campaigns ever seen, the second pandemic was controlled by vaccination carried out by national veterinary departments supported by international funds. In the wake of the emergency, which cost tens of millions of dollars, came renewed calls for a campaign to completely eradicate rinderpest from Africa,[12, 114, 175] and as a result the Pan African Rinderpest Campaign (PARC) was established. This European Community-funded project, advised and assisted by various other donors and executed through the Inter-African Bureau for Animal Resources of the Organization of African Unity, aims to help Africa control and possibly eradicate rinderpest within the next few years.[50, 145]

Many reviews provide details of the history of rinderpest as well as information on all other aspects of the disease and its virus.[11, 59, 98, 120, 156, 191, 260, 261, 264, 265] In order to save space, references given in this chapter have, where a large choice exists, favoured more recent studies.

Aetiology

Nicolle and Adil Bey showed in 1902 that rinderpest was caused by a filterable agent. It was grown in whole blood cultures by Boynton,[31] and Takematsu and Morimoto[290] detected increased amounts of infectivity in cultured leukocytes derived from infected animals. After earlier unsuccessful attempts to grow the agent in cell culture,[49] Plowright and Ferris[197–199] demonstrated cytopathic effects and production of infectivity in bovine-cell monolayers. Further studies revealed the close antigenic relationship of rinderpest virus (RV) to canine distemper[206, 323] and measles viruses[115, 198, 318] and led to RV being included in the measles-rinderpest-distemper subgroup of the Paramyxoviridae. This subgroup, reclassified as the genus *Morbillivirus*,[134] also includes the viruses that cause peste des petits ruminants (PPR) in sheep and goats, phocine distemper,[57, 154] and hedgehog distemper.[308]

The virus is pleomorphic and has roughly spherical (100–300 nm in diameter) or tubular forms (up to $1x10^3$ nm in length).[36, 196] Being enveloped, the virus is readily inactivated by lipid solvents and is sensitive to light, ultra-violet radiation, heat and extremes of pH.[191, 255, 256] Infectivity is destroyed by most disinfectants and chemicals such as ß-propiolactone.[119, 287, 316] Glycerol also destroys RV and must not be used in transport medium for diagnostic samples.[127, 137]

Rinderpest virus contains a negative strand of ribonucleic acid, approximately 15 kilo base pairs long, which codes for eight polypeptides.[23, 24, 74, 90, 140, 251] The virus

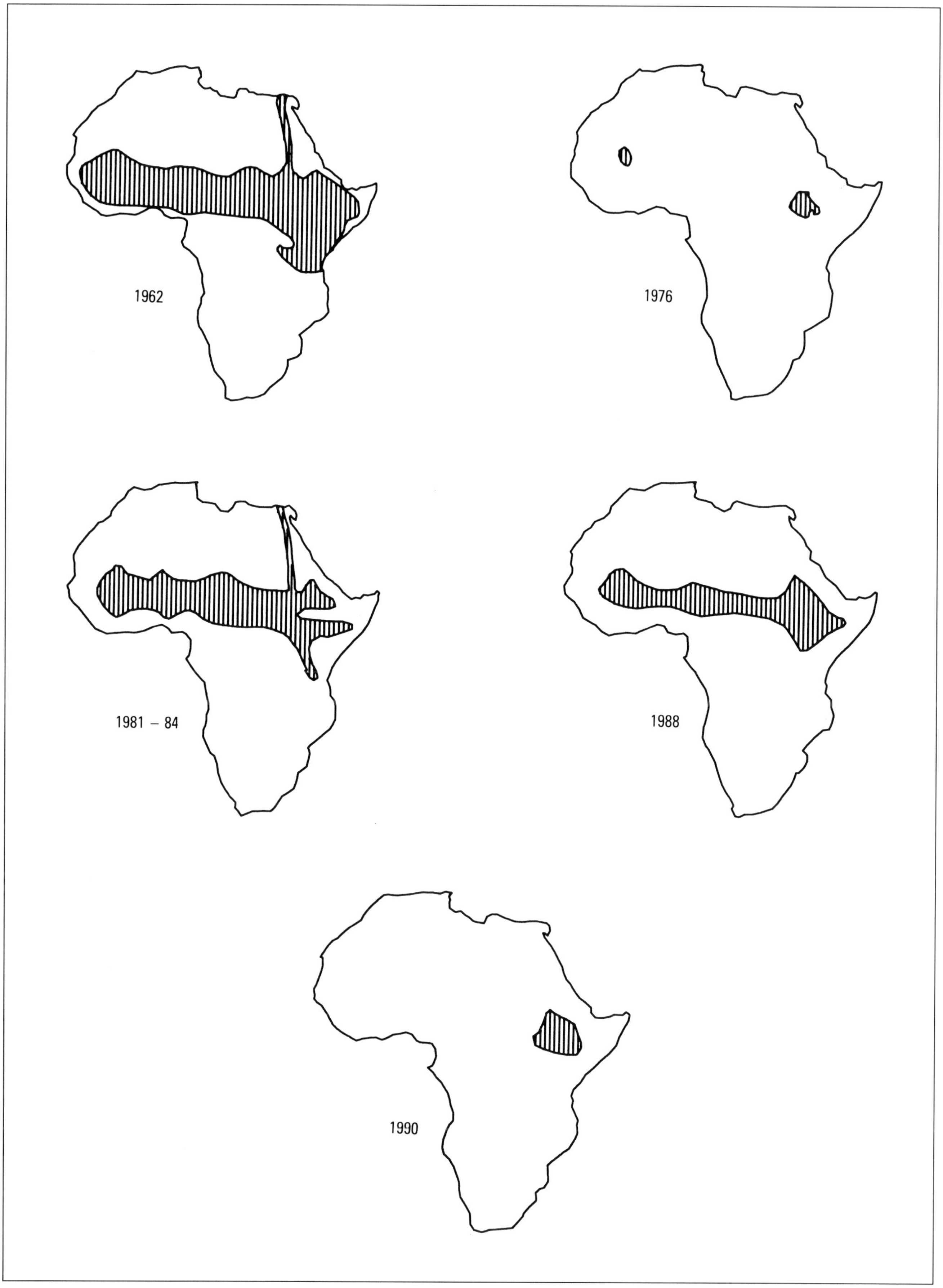

Figure 74.3 Recent distribution of rinderpest in Africa

envelope contains the H protein (a haemagglutinin in other morbilliviruses) which binds to cell receptors, and the fusion (F) protein which induces the formation of syncytia, and is underlain by the matrix (M) protein. Within the virion the RNA is protected by a nucleocapsid (N) protein. Transcription in infected cells is mediated by polymerase (L) and polymerase-associated (P) proteins. A non-structural polypeptide (C) is translated by modification from the P polypeptide mRNA.[23] The P and F genes appear to be more conserved amongst the morbilliviruses than are the other genes.

In vitro RV grows relatively slowly in cells derived from bovine tissues and in cell lines such as Hela and Vero, producing titres of cell-free virus of 10^5–10^6 (occasionally 10^7) $\log_{10}$ tissue-culture infectious doses ($TCID_{50}$) per ml of fluid.[161, 198] Cytopathic effects comprise rounding of cells which become refractive, cytomegaly, cytoplasmic stranding, the formation of small and large syncytia, and eventual degeneration of the cell sheet. In culture the virus is capable of producing plaques and induces interferon.[21, 107, 293, 330]

Individual strains of virus vary in their pathogenicity for various species. Experimentally this has best been shown by attenuation studies whereby adaptation of a strain to produce disease in one species usually brings about a concomitant reduction in the severity of clinical diseases for some but not all other species.[45] This was the basis for the production of many live vaccines.[77, 117, 123, 171, 191, 260, 286]

In contrast to measles virus, the haemagglutinin equivalent of RV does not readily agglutinate erythrocytes;[110, 255, 256] some haemagglutinating (HA) activity has been demonstrated in special circumstances,[143] but the specificity of the reaction was not established. However, since RV induces the development of antibodies which react with measles virus haemagglutinin,[30, 320] it is likely that RV bears a similar envelope antigen in a more sequestered site.

Epidemiology

Rinderpest virus infects a wide variety of vertebrates. Some of these, including rabbits, hamsters, mice, giant rats (*Cricetomys gambianus*), ferrets, and susliks (*Citellus mongoliscus ramosus*) are usually only infected experimentally, and then often only by using strains of virus adapted to them.[60, 116, 173, 191, 260, 273] In the field, only Artiodactyla are naturally infected, although dogs fed infected meat may develop antibodies to the virus, suggesting subclinical infection.[206] Amongst domestic stock, cattle and buffaloes (*Bubalus bubalus*) are especially susceptible and are more frequently infected than other species. Sheep, goats and Asiatic pigs are also susceptible and may develop clinical disease.[32, 106, 223, 253] European breeds of pig undergo subclinical infection.[69, 269] Although some early reports indicated that camels are susceptible to clinical disease,[71, 92, 147, 178] more recent experimental studies have shown only mild or subclinical disease in this species.[282, 291] Contact transmission from cattle to camels occurs under experimental conditions[290] but is probably rare in the field.[270]

Infection of wild artiodactyls with strains largely maintained in cattle causes a wide spectrum of clinical disease ranging from very severe in African buffalo (*Syncerus caffer*), giraffe (*Giraffa camelopardalis*), eland (*Taurotragus oryx*) and kudu (*Tragelaphus strepciceros, T. imberbis*) through increasingly less severe syndromes in other antelopes to mild or atypical in impala (*Aepyceros melampus*)[268] and subclinical in hippopotami (*Hippopotamus amphibius*).[202] There is also variation in susceptibility to clinical disease between breeds or races of a species, especially cattle.[101, 130, 249, 259, 306] Most European cattle breeds (*Bos taurus*) are more susceptible than *Bos indicus* breeds. African humpless cattle, such as the Ankole in East Africa, are notoriously susceptible in comparison to East African zebus.[38, 46, 55, 98, 165, 259] Because Japanese black cattle reacted so severely to goat-adapted vaccines that were sufficiently attenuated for other cattle, the virus had to be further attenuated in rabbits and embryonated chickens' eggs.[172, 173]

Infected animals excrete infectious virus in their ocular, nasal, oral and vaginal secretions and faeces.[59, 93, 102, 260] Excretion begins one or two days before the onset of fever (the first clinical sign) and continues for nine to ten days after the start of pyrexia.[81, 144] Highest titres of virus are excreted during the early stages of clinical disease when epithelial lesions, especially those in the mouth, are developing to their maximum extent. Subsequently the titres of excreted virus wane as antibody develops.[144, 267] Recovered cows may abort an infected foetus some weeks after apparent recovery, with virus excretion in their uterine and vaginal discharges.[59, 118, 311]

The fragility of the virus ensures that most infectivity survives for only a few hours outside the host, though some may persist under favourable conditions for up to two to four days.[279, 302] Carcass decomposition inactivates the virus within one to three days.[59]

Spread of RV is effected almost exclusively by contact between infected and susceptible animals. Transmission by infected aerosols probably only occurs under ideal conditions of close proximity and gentle air currents, i.e., amongst housed animals.[113] Nevertheless, experimentation has proved that airborne transmission is a theoretical possibility over several hundred metres,[112] and circumstantial evidence for such transmission occurred during the recent epidemics in Nigeria.

The high levels of antibody that are maintained in recovered animals for years after infection, usually for life, suggest persistent infection with RV. A recent preliminary study has gone some way to confirming this by demonstrating viral RNA in the peripheral blood lymphocytes of cattle for up to three months after the cessation of viraemia and recovery from clinical disease.[23] There is a handful of reports of chronic cases of rinderpest,[59, 63, 70, 88] but such cases are exceptions. As a rule, however, there is no 'carrier' state in rinderpest and recovered animals do not excrete infectious RV and are not involved in the maintenance and transmission of the disease. The virus is not transmitted by arthropods[274] and the potential for transmission through abortion[311] is limited.

Consequently, RV has a short direct cycle of infection and is spread by close contact. Even under experimental conditions regular contact transmission can be difficult to achieve.[54, 113, 295] As originally noted by Lowe,[149] the spread of rinderpest is like a bushfire; it continually moves on to new uninfected animals (unburnt bush) leaving behind dead or immune animals (burnt bush). The disease stops when it runs out of susceptibles (firebreaks) and vaccination is a technique of rendering animals non-susceptible (backburning). Therefore, rinderpest is maintained by large, heterogeneous populations of animals with a sufficient supply of susceptible animals. In Africa in recent times the endemic areas have been those with large cattle populations belonging to nomadic or semi-nomadic people, which ensures good mixing of the population, especially when restricted by the availability of water during dry seasons.

One of the most important epidemiological features of rinderpest was summarized by Huytra *et al.*:[111]

> Rinderpest causes enormous losses among cattle in regions previously free from infection and may lead to the almost complete extinction of animals in large areas. On the other hand, in permanently infected regions it may assume a milder form and cause only a slight loss.

In populations comprised mainly of susceptible animals rinderpest behaves in epidemic fashion with the virus infecting virtually all of the susceptibles and causing severe clinical disease in most age groups. Endemic rinderpest, however, is much milder and is maintained by young animals usually less than two years old that have lost their maternal immunity. Intermediate patterns also exist. Examples in Africa were the enormous losses reported in southern Africa during the Great Pandemic[98, 109] compared with the mild and frequently subclinical infections seen in endemic areas such as Maasailand later this century.[150, 189, 232] Undoubtedly the selection of resistant animals in the wake of epidemics plays a part in this.[98, 165, 259] However, selection of milder strains of the virus may be an even more important mechanism, particularly as the generation time of virus is so much shorter than that of cattle. Computer modelling provided insight as to how this might occur through selection of strains with differing transmissibility.[121, 234] The model shows that during an epidemic RV is transmitted rapidly to susceptible animals and the most transmissible strains eventually predominate. For a strain to be highly transmissible it must cause the release of large quantities of infectivity from damaged epithelia. Hence transmissibility and virulence are directly related and the selection of increasingly transmissible strains in an epidemic involves an increase in virulence. In endemic areas such highly transmissible strains tend to die out because of the lack of susceptibles. However, milder, less transmissible strains of virus which are continually produced, presumably through mutation, can persist for longer in the limited supply of susceptible individuals, thus being given the opportunity to become dominant strains.[234] When the less transmissible strain is re-introduced to an unconfined supply of susceptibles it will again transmit freely and revert to virulence. This ability of the virus to render itself less clinically obvious in endemic areas may explain those outbreaks of disease that have occurred in areas long thought to have been free of the virus.[150, 292, 296]

Other domestic species such as small ruminants play only an accessory role in the maintenance of the disease in Africa, helping it to smoulder for a while after epidemics have occurred in the cattle population.[333, 334] They are, however, insufficiently susceptible to maintain endemic strains of RV. In India this is not the case. Strains of RV, clearly distinguishable from PPR virus, have become established in sheep and goats, which can pass the disease back to bovines.[25, 67, 174, 183] The origin of such strains is unknown, though the use of insufficiently attenuated goat-adapted vaccines has been implied.[58] The appearance of such strains in Africa would greatly hinder eradication programmes. Clinical rinderpest is commonly diagnosed in pigs in southern India but it has not yet been established whether pigs maintain RV independently from cattle.[223] European pigs, which can be infected by diseased cattle and by eating contaminated meat, suffer only subclinical infection but are a potential source of infection for other pigs and cattle.[68, 269]

In Asia wildlife have been described with clinical disease, and such infected animals can transmit infection to other susceptible species, including domestic stock.[20, 63, 147, 184, 283, 307] However, the sizes and densities of wildlife populations are low and they are not considered to be involved in the maintenance of the virus in Asia.

The role of wildlife in Africa has received much closer attention. This is due to the greater population sizes and densities, the larger number of susceptible species, and the frequency with which the disease used to be reported in wildlife.[48, 56, 324] Until the 1960s a widely held view in East Africa was that wildlife, particularly the vast populations of game on the plains in Maasailand, could maintain the virus independently of cattle,[146, 149, 188, 227] though some authorities considered cattle to be the main reservoir of infection.[65, 103] However, when cell-culture attenuated vaccine led to the eradication of the disease from cattle in Maasailand in the early 1960s, clinical disease also disappeared from wildlife.[285] The absence of antibodies in wildebeest and other species born after 1963 supported this,[195, 203, 296] and as a consequence opinion changed to the view that wildlife could not maintain the virus.[193]

Subsequent events have indicated that the role of wildlife may not be so straightforward. A study of wildlife sera collected in Kenya between 1970 and 1981 detected significant levels of specific antibody to RV in 8 per cent of the samples.[240] Whilst acknowledging that these infected animals may have been sentinels for RV in nearby cattle or that other morbilliviruses might be responsible, it was suggested that certain strains of RV might be maintained independently of cattle for variable periods of time.[211, 240] Coincidentally, rinderpest was diagnosed in buffaloes in the Serengeti National Park in 1982, which was the first confirmation of the disease in Tanzania since 1965. A re-evaluation of mortalities in wildlife during the preceding two to three years in Tanzania attributed many of these to rinderpest.[180] The 1982 outbreak then expanded to involve wildlife and cattle throughout a large area of Tanzania north of the central railway line before being controlled by the vaccination of cattle in 1983 and subsequent years.

Serological surveillance showed that most of the buffalo population in the area of Kenya immediately north of the Serengeti also had high levels of antibody to RV, despite having shown no signs of clinical disease. Analysis of the birth dates of sampled animals indicated that new seroconversions had occurred during a two- to three-year period[243] but, unfortunately, no virus was recovered. Since no rinderpest was reported in cattle in this area, it appeared that the wildlife may have assisted in maintaining RV for a period of years and that the infections were inapparent or mild enough to escape notice by wildlife authorities. This has encouraged a more cautious reappraisal of the role of wildlife. At present it seems probable that wildlife do not maintain RV indefinitely, but that sufficiently large populations may occasionally maintain mild or subclinical RV for periods of a few years. In contrast to India, where RV has existed for centuries and has adapted to other hosts besides cattle, the virus is comparatively new to Africa. However, given the large number of susceptible species on the continent it may be only a matter of time before the virus adapts itself to one or more of these, unless of course it is eradicated before then.

Pathogenesis

Experimental infections can be established by all routes of parenteral inoculation and, more variably, by intranasal or conjunctival installation. Natural infection usually occurs via the upper respiratory tract following inhalation of virus-containing aerosols, or via the oropharynx after ingestion of infected material.[59, 93, 102, 190, 191, 260, 302] Primary multiplication has not been demonstrated in the invaded epithelium,[295] but following intranasal and contact challenge, virus can be recovered within 24 hours from the pharyngeal lymph nodes and tonsils and, to a lesser degree, from other lymph nodes draining the head and upper respiratory tract.[190, 295] *In vivo* infectivity is closely associated with mononuclear leukocytes and is not readily detected in plasma and other body fluids.[64, 191, 252, 302]

Following primary multiplication in draining lymph nodes, viraemia enables the virus to infect and replicate in lymphoid tissues throughout the body. This increases the viraemia, which then transports the virus to epithelial tissues, especially those of the alimentary tract. There, virus-induced cytopathic effects produce the typical lesions of the disease, some of which may also be due to infection of small lymphoid aggregates in the lamina propria.[191]

There is an inverse relationship between increasing attenuation and the degree of viral multiplication in lymph nodes of cattle.[260] Virulent strains of RV have a greater ability to infect lymphoid cells and mononuclear phagocytes and may grow to higher titres in these cells than do strains which induce mild disease.[246] The cell-culture attenuated variant of the Kabete 'O' strain of RV, which is the most commonly used vaccine, only produces low levels of infectivity in lymphoid tissues and is barely detectable in the blood.[294] These low levels of viraemia are probably one reason why attenuated and very mild strains cause so little epithelial damage. The virus has a predilection for T lymphocytes and attains higher titres in the T4 and T8 subsets of T cells than in lymphoblasts of B or null cell origin.[241, 244, 246] Rinderpest virus grows more readily than PPR virus in bovine lymphoblasts, whereas the reverse is true in sheep and goat lymphoblasts.[246]

During disease the virus is also found in non-lymphoid organs, such as the lungs, liver and kidneys.[33, 64, 144, 294, 295, 302] Immunofluorescence has shown that antigen-bearing cells in these organs are usually associated with reticuloendothelial and perivascular connective tissue.[235]

Virulent strains of RV are excreted from epithelial tissues one or two days before the appearance of fever or lesions,[144] but the amount of excreted virus increases dramatically as the lesions develop and only starts to decline when the immune response becomes detectable some four to six days after the start of fever. The virus is usually undetectable by 12–14 days after the start of fever. At the height of virus excretion, three to six days after the start of pyrexia, virus titres of up to 10^5 tissue-culture infectious doses ($TCID_{50}$)/swab and up to 10^6 $TCID_{50}$/g respectively can be found in nasal secretions and faeces from cattle infected with virulent strains.[144] This copious output of virus explains why the disease can be so contagious despite the fragility of RV. The diarrhoea and oculonasal discharge probably help to increase the transmissibility of the virus by forming infectious aerosols, and by causing greater contamination of the environment.

Infected animals mount a vigorous response against the virus. Interferon is produced within two days of infection, enabling attenuated vaccines to protect cattle very rapidly against challenge by virulent virus.[108, 319, 325] Viral antigens are produced in large amounts throughout the lymphoid tissues and affected epithelia[171, 235, 262, 267] and stimulate an effective antibody response which begins two to five days after the onset of clinical disease in virulent infections, and some six to ten days after infection with mild or avirulent strains.[124, 170, 199, 266, 314] The early response consists predominantly of IgM antibodies[7, 182] which can be detected by virus neutralization (VN), ELISA, and also, for a period of a few months, by immunoprecipitation, complement fixation and measles virus haemagglutination inhibition.[245, 272] At the same time IgG antibodies are produced, but these persist for much longer, usually for life,[194, 200, 248] and are usually measured by VN or ELISA tests.[6, 228, 236, 237, 266, 277] Generally, high titres (10^2–10^3 $\log_{10}$ VN_{50}) of neutralizing antibodies are produced within two to three weeks of infection and remain high for several months, after which they may decline slowly, but usually remain at easily detectable levels (in excess of 10^1 $\log_{10}$ VN_{50}) for the rest of the animal's life.[194, 200, 205] Rarely, neutralizing antibodies decline to very low or undetectable levels, but such animals are clinically immune, although limited replication of the virus may occur in tissues such as the tonsils before the stimulation of an anamnestic response.[194, 205, 220, 248, 332] The antibody responses of naturally infected cattle and those vaccinated with live virus vaccines are indistinguishable.

A study using ELISA showed the development of serum IgA antibodies in cattle after vaccination.[7] However, another study using indirect immunoperoxidase failed to detect IgA antibodies and, in contrast to most other studies in cattle, ascribed most of the IgG antibodies to the IgG_2 subclass.[276] Secretory antibody is found in nasal secretions of convalescent cattle[208] but its persistence is presumably limited to only a few months after recovery, and the role it plays in preventing reinfection is unknown.

The severity of the cytopathology caused by the virus before the onset of antibody development influences the course of the disease. Virulent strains cause severe lesions before being restrained by the immune response, and such animals, if sufficiently damaged, will still die despite high titres of antibody and low or undetectable amounts of virus.[255, 267] The persistence of immunity in recovered animals and those given live virus vaccines contrasts with the short-lived immunity induced by inactivated vaccines,[119, 266] thus implying that recovered animals may be continually re-stimulated immunologically by RV antigen throughout their lives.

Immunofluorescent antibody techniques have shown that the necrotic changes in the lymphoid tissues, epithelia and other organs are associated with large quantities of RV antigen.[288, 327] Cells bearing RV antigen are not only widespread in lymphoid tissues, but are also prevalent in cells in the loose connective tissue surrounding blood vessels in most tissues.[236]

Circulating or fixed immune-complexes have not been demonstrated in rinderpest but might occur, considering the rapidity with which the mass of viral antigen is eliminated by the specific humoral response. There is a transient autoimmune response in infected rabbits which produce an IgM (19S) haemagglutinin to homologous erythrocytes and an IgG (7S) anti-nuclear antibody.[83]

The massive destruction of lymphocytes causes immunosuppression. In rabbits, cell-mediated and humoral immunity are suppressed through the loss of both T and B lymphocytes.[135, 326] In cattle, lymphoid necrosis is first seen in the germinal centres which are populated with B cells.[300] However, *in vitro*, RV grows readily in bovine T and B lymphocytes. Immunosuppression in cattle therefore probably involves both cell-mediated and humoral immune responses.

Possible immunosuppression caused by the cell-culture attenuated vaccine has been investigated recently, centring on the advisability of simultaneous inoculation of RV with other immunogens against diseases such as foot-and-mouth disease and contagious bovine pleuropneumonia. Most experimental studies involving the inoculation of RV with other antigens have shown no diminished responses to RV or the other immunogens,[47, 75, 97, 128, 152, 216, 217] although doubts still linger, especially in connection with bivalent vaccines incorporating live *Mycoplasma mycoides*[122] or inactivated foot-and-mouth disease virus.[129] One report also describes the development of severe bovine virus diarrhoea (BVD) infection in cattle given live attenuated rinderpest virus in conjunction with live attenuated BVD virus.[215]

The evidence from the field, however, shows that cell-culture attenuated rinderpest vaccine does not reactivate or exacerbate other diseases and does not interfere with other immunogens. Even cattle suffering from severe non-fatal rinderpest show a rapid and full humoral response to the virus despite the changes in their lymphoid tissues. The older vaccines, including caprinized, lapinized and avianized virus, could, however, produce mild clinical signs and occasionally caused flare-ups of latent or subclinical infection,[41, 46, 259, 286] but they produced no lasting check on the growth rate of cattle[43] and did not increase the severity of a concurrent outbreak of East Coast fever in cattle being used to test lapinized virus.[9]

Rabbits inoculated with lapinized virus show depressed and delayed hypersensitivity skin responses and impaired lymphocyte responses to mitogenic stimulation.[328]

Clinical signs

The clinical signs of rinderpest have been extensively described.[18, 59, 60, 86, 98, 191, 213, 249, 262, 263] The following description gives the basic signs in the sequence in which they usually occur in severely affected cattle.

Acute natural infections and those induced by parenteral inoculation of RV have an incubation period of three to five days. Incubation periods following experimental contact infection are longer, from eight to 15 days,[144, 189, 232, 295] and there are reports of extended incubation periods in natural outbreaks.[59]

Pyrexia heralds the onset of clinical disease. The body temperature rises rapidly to 40–41,5 °C and this can be maintained for up to two weeks, though usually less, before gradually declining to normal. During the first one or two days of fever there may be depression or restlessness, a degree of inappetence and a reduction in milk yield. The visible mucosae are congested and a serous oculonasal discharge, one of the characteristic signs of rinderpest, becomes apparent. Between the second and fifth days of fever the mucosal lesions become obvious, initially as pin-point white foci on the gums and lips which spread rapidly to involve the buccal mucosa and ventral and lateral aspects of the tongue. The foci enlarge and coalesce into plaques of caseous necrotic debris which desquamate easily, leaving circumscribed erosions **(Figure 74.4)**. The halitosis is memorable. Similar lesions may be seen on the palate, posterior dorsum of the tongue, pharynx, and in the nares and vagina. Severe cases often drool foetid saliva, presumably because of discomfort in the mouth and pharynx when swallowing.

In cattle infected with strains of high virulence, diarrhoea, sometimes preceded by an absence of defecation (there are usually no signs of constipation), starts four to five days after the onset of pyrexia, usually one to three days after mouth lesions become visible. The faeces are initially thin and dark, but may progress to contain blood, mucus and shreds of necrotic epithelium. The hind quarters are fouled **(Figure 74.5)** and tenesmus with eversion of the rectal mucosa is frequent. The diarrhoea causes dehydration, weakness and prostration, and in severe cases abdominal pain is evident. Recumbent animals face their flanks in typical 'milk fever' posture. The oculonasal discharge becomes increasingly purulent during the course of the disease and conjuctivitis causes photophobia. Corneal opacity is rare in cattle, but has been recorded in some species of wildlife such as giraffe and buffalo.[275] Epiphora is evident below the medial canthus.[98]

Early descriptions of rinderpest frequently described skin lesions.[178, 249] Most recent accounts[60, 191, 260] regard these as rare, though they are sometimes present in domestic buffaloes, sheep and goats. The lesions appear as a maculo-papular rash on areas of soft skin such as the

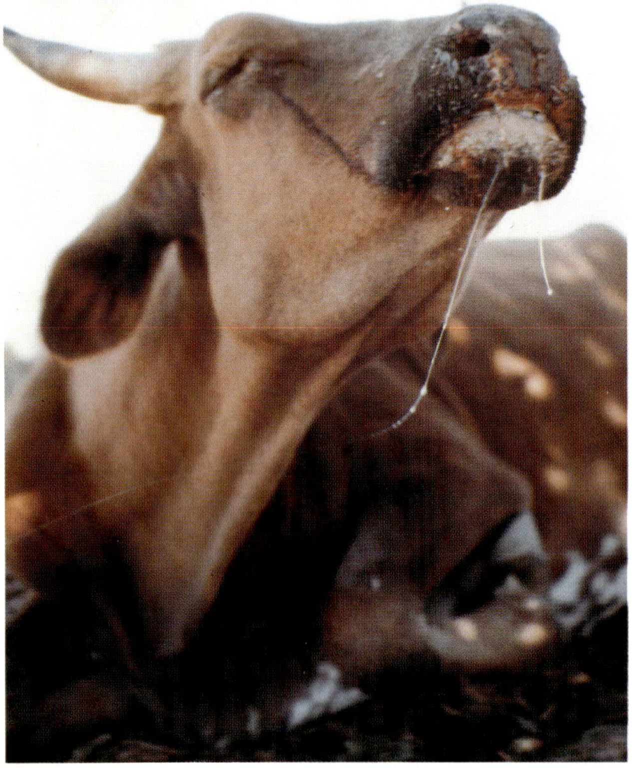

Figure 74.4 Rinderpest: note severe necrotic stomatitis, encrusted muzzle, salivation, conjunctivitis and evidence of photophobia

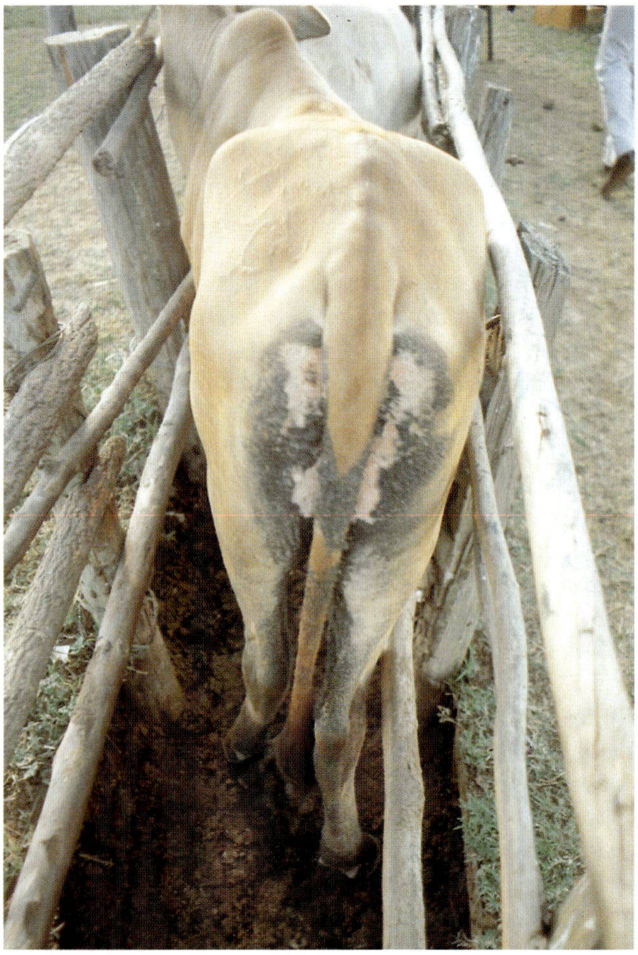

Figure 74.5 Rinderpest: severe faecal soiling of the hind quarters as a result of diarrhoea

axillae and groin, where the hair may become matted when the rash eventually becomes pustular and breaks open.[18, 59, 125, 164, 167]

Although respiration may be laboured during acute clinical disease, pulmonary lesions are uncommon and are mainly due to secondary bacterial infection. Emphysema of the lungs may occur terminally. Lymphadenopathy is not usually evident even on palpation. Milk may become watery or dry up. Pregnant animals frequently abort, sometimes weeks or months after clinical disease.[59, 118, 178, 311] Most animals that succumb to rinderpest die five to 14 days after the onset of pyrexia.

Convalescence is marked by the rapid healing, within two to six days, of mucosal lesions, starting some three to six days after their appearance. Diarrhoea diminishes more slowly and may persist in a less severe form for up to two weeks. Complete recovery from severe rinderpest takes one to two months or more, depending on how much condition the animal has lost and on the quality of subsequent nursing.

Since RV destroys lymphoid tissues, infected animals suffer from a variable degree of immunosuppression. In Africa this frequently leads to the reactivation of a variety of chronic or latent diseases, especially those caused by haemoparasites such as *Anaplasma marginale*, which, if not treated therapeutically, increase the mortality caused by RV.[59, 87, 101, 104, 214, 226, 260, 262]

In endemic areas the disease is milder than the above description.[59, 150, 189, 213, 232] Most of the signs are much reduced in severity and some may be absent. Experimental infections with such strains have shown that they may cause no deaths, no diarrhoea, transient mouth lesions in only a proportion of infected *Bos taurus* cattle, and only transient pyrexia in *Bos indicus* cattle.[189, 232, 292]

Clinical signs vary in sheep and goats. Disease was seen in sheep during the British epidemics of 1865 to 1866[249] and in the Great African Pandemic.[109] Clinical signs in naturally infected small ruminants have occasionally been reported in Africa[26, 146, 151, 253, 267, 309] but experimental infections with African strains of RV have produced only transient fever, sometimes accompanied by slight oculonasal discharges.[79, 187, 258, 309, 313] Usually sero-conversion is the only evidence that sheep and goats kept with diseased cattle have been infected.[238, 335]

Clinical rinderpest is established in sheep and goats in India. The incubation period is similar to that in cattle, with fever being the first clinical sign although its onset may be more gradual than in cattle. Diarrhoea starts two to three days later and, if severe enough, causes dehydration and death. The tail and hind quarters are soiled by faeces. Sero-mucoid, oculonasal discharges which rapidly become purulent are seen within 24 hours of fever. Mouth lesions are less obvious than in cattle. Inappetence is usual. Pneumonia is commoner in small ruminants than in cattle, but is also probably due to secondary bacterial infections.[66]

Asian pigs show pyrexia, inappetence and depression, and rapidly become prostrate.[32, 53, 106] Typical mouth lesions develop in one to two days, and diarrhoea within two to three days of the onset of fever. The diarrhoea lasts five to ten days and in severe cases leads to dehydration and death. Pregnant sows may abort. Erythematous skin lesions may be seen. Transient low fever is all that may be seen in European pigs, most infections being totally inapparent.[269]

Mouth lesions, diarrhoea[92, 147] and deaths[71] have been reported in camels, but generally, in areas where rinderpest is prevalent in other species, camels do not show clinical signs[148, 185] or develop antibodies which would indicate inapparent infection.[270] Most of the reports of clinical disease were based only on clinical evidence without other diagnostic confirmation. Experimental infection of dromedaries (*Camelus dromedarius*) with cattle strains of RV resulted in subclinical infection.[219, 291]

Disease in domestic buffalo is frequently severe, with clinical signs being the same as those in cattle, although skin lesions are reputedly more common.[18, 59]

Wild ungulates exhibit a wide range of clinical signs, from typical erosive stomatitis, gastroenteritis and death in African buffalo, eland, giraffe and warthog (*Phacochoerus aethiopicus*)[186, 301] to mild or non-specific signs in impala.[268] As a generalization, the more bovine-like species amongst the Bovidae suffer more severe clinical disease than do the caprine-like species. Corneal opacity and skin lesions have often been described for rinderpest in wildlife such as giraffe, Grant's gazelle (*Gazelle granti*) and African buffalo, though not all of these outbreaks have been confirmed in a laboratory.[193, 275, 280, 301] Affected wildlife may exhibit behavioural changes. Dehydration forces thirsty animals to migrate long distances for water, while discomfort makes them more aggressive, especially buffalo.[34, 48]

Pathology

A proportion of infected cattle shows slight lymphocytosis before the onset of pyrexia. This is followed by marked lymphopenia, caused by lymphoid necrosis, which in most cases lasts throughout the acute clinical stage of the disease.[17, 99, 158, 225, 231, 300] During convalescence, lymphocyte levels slowly return to normal over a period of days or weeks. The number of neutrophils remains relatively unaltered, though juvenile forms are not infrequent during the terminal stages of fatal infection. However, a degree of neutropenia that parallels the decline in lymphocyte levels has been reported.[300] Eosinophils may also disappear from the blood during the early stages of clinical disease, returning to normal levels some two to three weeks later. In severe cases the excessive loss of water causes haemoconcentration.[17]

Serum aspartate transaminase and blood urea nitrogen levels increase during severe cases of disease.[29, 100] Serum chloride levels fall markedly in terminal illness, and other electrolytes may decrease in absolute terms although this can be masked by haemoconcentration. Blood clotting may be impaired in severely affected animals. Serum protein levels may be lowered, especially in fatally infected animals.[59, 72, 82] In cattle recovering from experimental infections a rise in serum globulins was attributed to the specific humoral response to the virus,[82] but since the challenge material was citrated blood this may need re-interpretation in the light of known responses to heterologous tissue antigens.

The lesions of rinderpest are a direct result of virus-induced cytopathology. There are many descriptions of the gross pathology,[18, 37, 59, 86, 120, 260] but those of Maurer *et al.*[157, 158] are especially valuable. Generally, the severity of the lesions is directly related to the virulence of the strain of virus involved.[299] Complications may arise during convalescence through re-activation of latent pathogens, especially protozoa.[59, 101, 262]

The overall appearance at necropsy is similar for most species that die of typical severe rinderpest. The carcass is dehydrated, sometimes emaciated, and usually soiled with fluid faeces. The eyes are sunken and often encrusted with mucopurulent discharge and the cheeks may show signs of epiphora.

Erosions with or without necrotic material may be found throughout the mouth but predeliction sites are the gums, lips, buccal papillae, dorsal and ventral aspects of the tongue and the soft palate. The erosions often extend into the pharynx, anterior oesophagus, rumen (especially the pillars), the reticulum and omasum. Necrotic areas, some of which may penetrate the leaves of the omasum, are sometimes present.

The folds of the abomasum are congested and oedematous and often show necrosis, erosions and haemorrhage along the edges. The fundus of the abomasum may have small discrete erosions which increase in size towards the pylorus, where whole areas of mucosa may become desquamated. The early necrotic lesions are pale-greyish, whereas the erosions are often red as a result of congestion of the underlying lamina propria. Haemorrhage may occur from the raw surfaces. The abomasum is almost invariably severely affected, whereas the small intestine frequently shows less involvement. Congestion, oedema and erosions may occur on the margins of mucosal folds of the anterior duodenum and terminal ileum. The Peyer's patches, being lymphoid tissue, are severely affected and are swollen, dark red to almost black as a result of haemorrhage, and may slough completely leaving deep ulcer-like areas. Large erosions are commonly found on the ileocaecal valve. In the large intestine, marked oedema and congestion accompanied by petechiae or larger haemorrhages occur, particularly along the crests of longitudinal folds of the mucosa. This can be very striking in the colon and rectum, meriting the description 'zebra striping'. In acute cases, the gut has little content other than desquamated necrotic epithelium, blood, and fibrin exuding from exposed lamina propria.

The urinary and gall bladders are frequently congested and haemorrhagic with occasional erosions. The vaginal mucosa may be congested and have small erosions.

The mucosa of the upper respiratory tract, including the larynx, is congested and usually covered with mucopurulent exudate. Petechiae are frequent and necrotic; erosive lesions may extend from the nares to the larynx. The tracheal mucosa is frequently congested. Congestion and emphysema may be seen in the lungs, while secondary bronchopneumonia may complicate chronic cases.

Although regularly described in early reports, skin lesions are now rarely seen, although they are reputedly common in domestic buffalo. The exudative dermatitis would seem to develop from macular to pustular lesions, but the role of secondary bacterial infections such as *Dermatophilus congolensis* needs clarification.[104, 149, 167]

Although RV has a predilection for lymphoid tissues, there are usually few visible changes to the superficial and visceral lymph nodes. These may show congestion, oedema, and a few petechiae. The nodes of animals that die after a prolonged clinical course may be shrunken and may show greyish radial streaks in the cortex, presumably due to haemorrhage.[18] The spleen and haemolymph nodes appear normal or slightly enlarged.

The necropsy findings in goats inoculated with caprinized virus are similar to those in cattle, although they may be less marked.

The lymphotropism of the virus is clearly demonstrated in rabbits inoculated with lapinized virus. Although there are no observable epithelial lesions, whitish, pin-head-sized foci of necrosis are easily seen in the gut-associated lymphoid tissues.[84, 120]

Histopathological lesions become more easily detectable with increasing severity of clinical disease, implying that the pathology is directly related to the ability of a strain to multiply rapidly in the tissues.[300]

The essential histopathology of rinderpest was first described in infected rabbits.[38, 84] Widespread necrosis of lymphocytes is apparent throughout the lymphoid tissues, together with syncytia and intracytoplasmic and, less frequently, intranuclear inclusion bodies. The histology in cattle is similar,[131, 158, 299] with lytic destruction of lymphoid tissues that is most evident in the germinal centres, sometimes accompanied by an increase in the numbers of macrophages. In acute cases lymph nodes are virtually devoid of cells, with just a reticular stroma containing eosinophilic material remaining.

The early epithelial lesions in the squamous epithelium of the digestive tract are associated with the formation of syncytia and eosinophilic intracytoplasmic inclusions in the *stratum spinosum*.[132] Infected epithelial cells become necrotic and slough off, leaving clearly demarcated erosions. The erosions heal rapidly unless complicated by secondary infections which may rarely cause them to ulcerate.

Changes in other tissues are not remarkable, although Khera[133] described small foci of necrosis in the liver.

Ultrastructurally, infected cells contain large parallel arrays of tubular nucleocapsid material which are probably the intranuclear and intracytoplasmic inclusion bodies seen by light microscopy.[36, 221, 289]

Virus is released from cells by some of the tubular strands budding through the cell membrane. Similar changes were described in lymphoid cells from two Japanese black cattle infected with the virulent Fusan strain of RV,[136] and in persistently infected Vero cells.[136]

Diagnosis

Several handbooks and reports detail the diagnosis of rinderpest.[18, 22, 209, 218, 262, 272] A presumptive diagnosis of rinderpest can be made on the basis of the clinical signs and gross pathology. However, in areas where the disease is not prevalent, and especially in regions dependent on livestock exports, it is essential to obtain laboratory confirmation of the diagnosis as soon as possible. Countries where rinderpest is either endemic or a high risk should treat any syndrome resembling rinderpest as such until proven otherwise. This will allow immediate steps to be taken to control the disease and restrict losses.

The collection of adequate quantities of appropriate specimens greatly increases the chances of an accurate laboratory diagnosis. A thorough clinical examination should be made of animals in suspected herds and six or seven animals in the early acute stage of the disease with fever, mouth lesions and lachrymation should be selected for sampling. Animals that are dead, moribund or have had diarrhoea and mucopurulent discharges for more than three days are less reliable sources of virus or antigen as the levels of these decline with the onset of antibody development.[262]

Blood for serum antibody assay, blood collected in anticoagulant for virus isolation from leukocytes, a lymph-node biopsy, debris from oral lesions, and ocular and nasal swabs should be collected from each selected animal for virus isolation and antigen detection. If possible two or more animals should be killed for necropsy examination and collection of up to three universal bottles of spleen and mesenteric lymph nodes. All specimens should be collected and bottled aseptically, kept cool on ice (but not frozen) and transported as rapidly as possible to a diagnostic laboratory.[262, 272, 310] Glycerol should not be used as a preservative because it inactivates RV. The use of antiproteases increases the survival of RV antigens in tissue suspensions.[233]

At the laboratory, suspensions of solid tissues are prepared in physiological saline or cell-culture medium, the buffy coat is removed from the whole blood and the serum separated from the clotted blood. Thirty per cent tissue suspensions (w/v) for antigen detection can be prepared by most techniques, including grinding with sand in a mortar, but 10 per cent suspensions for attempted virus isolation can best be prepared in Ten Broeck or similar grinders.

The first procedure carried out is to detect viral antigen using specific rabbit hyperimmune serum against RV. The most commonly used assay is the agar-gel immunodiffusion test (AGID)[267, 322] which is simple to use, easy to read, highly specific and can be performed in the field with swabs and gum debris. A micro-version is more economical and gives results within two hours.[81] Counter-immuno-electrophoresis is quicker and more sensitive than AGID but requires more sophisticated equipment.[3, 242] Immunofluorescence and immunoperoxidase staining are very sensitive but also need more equipment than AGID.[15, 85, 208, 235, 278] Although once widely used, complement fixation and conglutinating complement absorption tests are too complicated in comparison with more recently developed tests. Various haemagglutination assays are sensitive but not yet widely applied,[20, 281] though latex bead agglutination tests have given encouraging preliminary results[162] and, if combined with monoclonal antibodies, could prove very sensitive. A positive result in any of the tests confirms rinderpest. If classically prepared rabbit hyperimmune sera[262] are unavailable, sera can be prepared using other immunizing techniques in rabbits[163, 168, 233] or in goats or cattle.[257, 271]

If cell cultures are unavailable, the specimens can be inoculated into known immune and susceptible cattle, as long as these are isolated from other susceptible animals. If cell-culture facilities are available, attempts should be made to isolate the virus. Suspensions prepared from swabs, gum debris, buffy coats or lymphoid tissues are inoculated onto growing monolayers of primary or secondary bovine kidney cells in tubes.[197, 201] Vero cells are also suitable, while culture systems such as microplates can also be used[161, 317] but may be less sensitive. After 12–24 hours adsorption the tubes are washed, refed with maintenance medium and rolled at 37 °C. Typical cytopathic effects develop within three to 14 days, occasionally longer, and consist initially of foci of round and refractile cells with cytoplasmic processes and small syncytia, followed by generalization throughout the monolayer with distinct syncytium formation. Negative test cultures should be passaged at least once. The virus can be identified by inoculating sample materials into tubes containing antiserum to RV or by examining fixed monolayers using immunofluorescent or immunoperoxidase techniques.[139, 142, 207]

If antigen detection and virus isolation are negative, then convalescent animals should be bled again two to four weeks later. Assays for serum antibodies should demonstrate a four-fold or greater increase in antibody titre in recovered cases. Virus neutralization in microplates is most commonly used for this,[5, 228, 236] although several other techniques such as measles virus haemagglutination inhibition, indirect immunofluorescence,

ELISA and counter-immuno-electrophoresis are alternatives.[126] Serum, during the early antibody response, contains significant levels of IgM to RV,[7, 182] the detection of which should confirm the diagnosis, but this approach is rarely used.

Histopathology is not sufficiently specific to confirm a diagnosis of rinderpest, but demonstration of syncytia and viral inclusions is supportive.

Nucleic acid techniques including hybridization with probes and polymerase chain reactions are capable of detecting minute quantities of RV RNA in tissues and secretions,[23] and when simplified may be the future method of choice for confirmation. Assays such as these, ELISA and latex bead agglutination should also be adapted for use beside the animal.

Differential diagnosis

All conditions that cause stomatitis and/or enteritis in domestic stock may be clinically confused with rinderpest. In cattle, difficulties arise in distinguishing rinderpest from mucosal disease (MD), malignant catarrhal fever,[298] infectious bovine rhinotracheitis (particularly when caused by strains that induce diarrhoea),[94, 95] bovine papular stomatitis,[169] Jembrana disease[297] and foot-and-mouth disease. In small ruminants, peste des petits ruminants (PPR) and Nairobi sheep disease can resemble rinderpest. Infection with *Campylobacter* spp., *Serpulina* (*Treponema*) *hyodysenteriae* and *Salmonella* serovars needs to be considered when investigating possible rinderpest in pigs.

In practice, only MD in cattle and PPR in small ruminants regularly present a problem.[44, 261] The clinical signs and gross pathology in cattle with MD can be indistinguishable from rinderpest and diagnosis requires laboratory confirmation. However, MD usually affects very few animals in a herd, whereas morbidity rates in rinderpest are much higher. Agar-gel immunodiffusion applied to tissue suspensions can rapidly differentiate the two diseases.[62] Immunohistochemical techniques can be used on frozen sections of mesenteric lymph node or on formalin-fixed tissues to distinguish between rinderpest and MD.[85] Failing this, virus isolation with subsequent virus identification must be attempted, with follow-up studies to detect rising antibody titres.

The differentiation of PPR from rinderpest is more difficult. Useful epidemiological evidence is provided by the absence of disease in cattle. The virus cross-reacts serologically with RV and is difficult to differentiate with hyperimmune polyclonal sera. Fortunately, contemporary studies have produced monoclonal antibodies and cDNA probes that clearly distinguish between PPR virus and RV, at least for the limited number of strains tested to date.[73, 159] In African countries which have previously been free of PPR it is unwise to assume that a rinderpest-like syndrome in small ruminants is not PPR.

Control

In countries to which rinderpest is exotic, confirmed outbreaks are controlled by the slaughter and disposal of all affected and in-contact animals as well as by the imposition of rigid quarantine and animal-movement controls. Such measures eradicated the only outbreak of rinderpest in Australia within two months[321] and halted the 1866 outbreak of rinderpest in Britain within six months.[305]

Virtually all outbreaks of rinderpest in virgin areas have been due to the importation of live animals.[254] Prevention in such areas is therefore largely dependent upon vigilant control of the introduction of live animals from potentially infected areas. Importation of fresh carcasses and meat products constitutes a minimal threat, although at least one epidemic has been attributed to this source[2, 52, 60] and outbreaks in endemic areas have been traced to fresh infected meat. In the Great African Pandemic the virus is reputed to have crossed the Orange River in this way. In frozen meat the virus persists for much longer than in fresh meat, and is therefore a risk to swill-fed pigs.[224, 254, 256] Infectivity disappears rapidly from adequately dried infected hides[27] and from decomposing carcasses held at ambient temperatures in tropical regions for more than two or three days.[59, 76]

Contaminated areas should be physically cleaned of all animal waste and soiled bedding and treated with disinfectant solutions of high (>10) or low (<3) pH containing solvents to destroy the virus envelope. Most disinfectants have some activity against RV, but it has been shown that solutions of caustic soda and lysol have the highest virucidal activity against virus contaminated with organic matter.[316] Such premises could be restocked after a week but the customary caution of veterinary authorities usually results in the period being longer.

Control is more difficult in endemic areas. Clinical diagnosis should be sufficient to instigate control procedures and all outbreaks of rinderpest-like disease should be treated as rinderpest until proven otherwise. Slaughter of affected and in-contact animals removes the source of virus, but may be counter-productive where owners have either a close cultural bond with their animals or are unlikely to receive compensation. In such areas, quarantine and strict movement control must be enforced immediately and the support of local cattle owners (which is usually forthcoming) is essential in this. Countries bordering high-risk zones must channel the import of domestic animals through border quarantine stations for vaccination and three weeks of observation.[146]

All susceptible animals in affected herds should be vaccinated immediately with subsequent ring vaccination of surrounding districts.

The importance of vaccination in the control of rinderpest in endemic areas cannot be overemphasized, and most early research concentrated on the development of effective vaccines.[59, 166, 260]

Following the recommendation for the inoculation of infected bile by Koch[137] in South Africa and the simultaneous administration of convalescent serum and virulent virus developed by Danyz and Bordet, Theiler and Watkins-Pitchford, and Kolle and Turner,[109] neither of which were very satisfactory, Kakizaki[127] developed a glycerol-inactivated tissue vaccine that induced a solid but short-lived immunity. This encouraged the development of many other inactivated vaccines, but these required frequent administration. Continuing research, aimed at a more permanent solution, led to the development of a series of increasingly attenuated vaccines (caprinized, lapinized, and avianized) which were produced by passage in hosts other than cattle.[77, 123, 173, 286]

Eventually, repeated passage of the virulent Kabete 'O' strain of RV in bovine kidney cells produced a totally safe and effective attenuated virus,[124, 200] which is now the principal vaccine used to combat rinderpest throughout the world. It is cheap and easy to produce and test, stable in freeze-dried form[192] and highly effective even in animals with severe infections, such as East Coast fever and trypanosomiasis.[247, 312] It induces life-long immunity. Rarely, vaccinated animals may be infected by experimental challenge, but they have not been shown to re-excrete the virus.[194] The only drawback to the vaccine is that after reconstitution it has a 'working life' of only a few hours in the high ambient temperatures common in regions where rinderpest occurs.[192, 265] There is some evidence that the vaccine ought not to be used more than one hour after reconstitution at ambient temperatures around or above 37 °C.[222] In contrast to this, however, are the strikingly successful results of the JP15 campaign, in which vaccination often produced herd antibody prevalences in excess of 90 per cent. Nevertheless, research to improve the vaccine's thermostability is now underway through the isolation of heat-resistant clones of vaccine virus and improvements in freeze-drying procedures.[141, 155, 214, 265]

Several laboratories are attempting to remove the problem of the 'cold chain' by pursuing the current trend of genetically engineered vaccine in which genes expressing RV-immunizing antigen are incorporated into vaccinia virus or some other vector.[105, 303, 304] These recombinants have proved effective against experimental challenge[28, 329] and, if approved for general use, will be a useful advance. However, the funds and efforts used to produce them could perhaps have been more valuably used to improve the 'cold chain', which is now in serious disrepair in many parts of Africa and Asia and is still needed for many veterinary products and samples. The use of freeze-dried vaccine in subcutaneous implants[42] or eye powder would do away with the 'diluent problem' in hot, isolated areas.

Prevention of rinderpest in endemic areas requires annual vaccination of all calves up to two years of age. Maternal antibodies from immune dams interfere with active immunization and may persist for nine to ten months.[39, 40] In practice, however, few animals over six months of age have antibody and it is sensible to immunize the six- to 12-month-old animals rather than only those which are over a year old (in an effort to economize on vaccine). Where vaccination is difficult, infrequent or inefficient, and where cattle populations are continually mobile, annual blanket vaccination of all cattle will produce the highest levels of herd immunity.[204, 234] In such areas some serological monitoring of herd antibody levels is also advisable. The results from this procedure indicate whether vaccination campaigns have been successful or need to be repeated. Since relatively high herd-antibody rates may be prevalent in endemic areas,[203, 234] serological monitoring can pin-point areas in which herd immunity may be too low to prevent endemic strains from establishing themselves. The successful eradication of endemic rinderpest from Maasailand in 1962 and 1963 was accomplished by very efficient vaccination campaigns which raised overall herd immunity levels to 90 per cent or more. Values in excess of this have been calculated to be necessary for the eradication of measles virus from human populations.[4]

In endemic areas sero-surveillance of unvaccinated animals such as small ruminants and wildlife is also important. These species are sentinels, since any antibody they possess must have been induced by field strains of RV or, possibly, related agents such as PPR virus. With the evidence of widespread rinderpest infection in sheep and goats in some Indian states[17] it is important that surveillance of sheep, goats and wildlife in Africa is continued in order to ensure that the establishment of similar maintenance cycles does not jeopardize the present eradication campaign.

The Pan African Rinderpest Campaign (PARC) aims to help Africa rid itself of rinderpest within ten years by implementing control programmes in endemic regions and supporting veterinary services in high- and low-risk countries.[50] Elimination of rinderpest will not only save the direct and indirect losses incurred by the disease, but will also stop its restraint on improved livestock production on the continent. Given the will, there is no obvious technical reason why PARC should not help Africa to accomplish what JP15 so narrowly failed to do.[212] Similar eradication campaigns are in progress in the Middle East and in southern Asia. If human and financial resources are enthusiastically maintained[315] the longed-for goal of worldwide eradication of rinderpest could become reality.[10, 176, 260]

References

1 **ABRAHAM, A., LEBEL, E. & DAVIDSON, M., 1984.** Virological and serological investigations on rinderpest in Israel. *Refuah Veterinarith*, 41, 112–121.

2 **ADEMOLLO, A., 1958.** A proposito di importazione di carne dai paesi infetti di peste bovina. *Veterinaria Italiana*, 9, 130–138.

3 **ALI, B. EL H. & LEES, G.E., 1979.** The application of immunoelectroprecipitation in the diagnosis of rinderpest. *Bulletin of Animal Health and Production in Africa*, 27, 1–6.

4 **ANDERSON, R.M. & MAY, R.H., 1982.** Directly transmitted infectious diseases: Control by vaccination. *Science*, 215, 1053–1060.

5 **ANDERSON, J. & ROWE, L.W., 1982.** The use of an enzyme-labelled assay as an aid to reading micro virus neutralisation tests. *Journal of Immunological Methods*, 53, 182–186.

6 **ANDERSON, J., ROWE, L.W. & TAYLOR, W.P., 1983.** Use of an enzyme-linked immunosorbent assay for the detection of IgG antibodies to rinderpest virus in epidemiological surveys. *Research in Veterinary Science*, 34, 77–81.

7 **ANDERSON, J., ROWE, L.W., TAYLOR, W.P. & CROWTHER, J.R., 1982.** An enzyme-linked immunosorbent assay for the detection of IgG, IgA and IgM antibodies to rinderpest virus in experimentally infected cattle. *Research in Veterinary Science*, 32, 242–247.

8 **ANON., 1920.** La peste bovine en Belgique. *Revue générale de Médecine Vétérinaire*, 29, 577–583.

9 **ANON., 1949.** *Rinderpest vaccines: Their production and use in the field.* FAO Agricultural Studies No. 8, Washington: Food and Agricultural Organization.

10 **ANON., 1963.** International veterinary preventive medicine. *British Veterinary Journal*, 119, 336–337.

11 **ANON., 1966.** Connaissances acquises récemment sur la peste bovine et son virus. *Revue d'Élevage et de Médecine Vétérinaire des Pays Tropicaux*, 19, 365–413.

12 **ANON., 1983.** Rinderpest in West Africa. *The Veterinary Record*, 113, 145.

13 **ATA, F.A. & SINGH, K.V., 1982.** Rinderpest in Kuwait. *Journal of the Egyptian Veterinary Medical Association*, 42, 27–32.

14 **ATANG, P.G. & PLOWRIGHT, W., 1969.** Extension of the JP-15 Rinderpest Control Campaign to eastern Africa. The epizootiological background. *Bulletin of Epizootic Diseases of Africa*, 17, 161–170.

15 **BABU, Y.H., JAMES, R.M., SREENIVAS, C.S. & KHAN, M.A., 1984.** The use of the immunoperoxidase test to the rinderpest viral antigens in infected tissue smears. *Indian Veterinary Journal*, 61, 271–275.

16 **BABU, Y.H., RAMESH, N.G. & RAJEASEKHAR, M., 1988.** Prevalence of rinderpest antibodies in sheep and goats in southern India. *The Veterinary Record*, 123, 595–597.

17 **BALDREY, F.S.H., 1906.** Some observations on normal and rinderpest blood. *Journal of Tropical Veterinary Science*, 1, 47–69.

18 **BANSAL, R.P., 1986.** *Diagnosis of Rinderpest. With Special Reference to the Application of Modern Techniques.* Mukteswar: Indian Veterinary Research Institute.

19 **BANSAL, R.P. & JOSHI, R.C., 1980.** A note on rinderpest in Gaur (*Bibos gaurus*). *Indian Veterinary Journal*, 57, 259–260.

20 **BANSAL, R.P., JOSHI, R.C., SHARMA, B. & CHANDRA, U., 1987.** Reverse phase passive haemagglutination test for the detection of rinderpest antigen. *Tropical Animal Health and Production*, 19, 53–55.

21 **BANSAL, R.P., JOSHI, R.C., TANDON, H.K.L. & KUMAR, S., 1981.** Production of interferon by rinderpest virus in calf kidney cell cultures. *Acta Virologica*, 25, 61.

22 **BANSAL, R.P., YADAV, M.P., BANDYOPADHAY, S.K., SHARMA, B. & JOSHI, R.C., 1983.** Proceedings of the Workshop on Recent Advancements in Rinderpest Diagnosis. 43pp. Mukteswar: Indian Veterinary Research Institute.

23 **BARRETT, T., 1987.** The molecular biology of the morbillivirus (measles) group. *Biochemical Society Symposia*, 53, 25–37.

24 **BARRETT, T. & UNDERWOOD, B., 1985.** Comparison of messenger RNAs induced in cells infected with each member of the morbillivirus group. *Virology*, 145, 195–199.

25 **BAWA, H.S., 1940.** Rinderpest in sheep and goats in Ajmer Merwara. *Indian Journal of Veterinary Science and Animal Husbandry*, 10, 103–112.

26 **BEATON, W.G., 1930.** Rinderpest in goats in Nigeria. *Journal of Comparative Pathology*, 43, 301–307.

27 **BEATON, W.G., 1932.** Infectivity of shade dried hides from rinderpest infected cattle. *Indian Journal of Veterinary Science and Animal Husbandry*, 2, 86–87.

28 **BELSHAM, G.J., ANDERSON, E.C., MURRAY, P.K., ANDERSON, J. & BARRETT, T., 1989.** Immune response and protection of cattle and pigs generated by a vaccinia virus recombinant expressing the F protein of rinderpest virus. *The Veterinary Record*, 124, 655–658.

29 **BHATTACHARYA, B. & CHAKRABORTY, A.K., 1979.** Serum aminotransferase activity in normal and experimentally infected Jamunapuri goats with rinderpest virus. *Indian Veterinary Journal*, 56, 435–436.

30 **BOGEL, K., RUCKLE-ENDERS, G. & PROVOST, A., 1964.** Une réaction sérologique rapide de mesure des anticorps antibovipestiques. *Comptes Rendus Hebdomadaires des Séances de l'Académie des Sciences, Paris*, 259, 482–484.

31 **BOYNTON, W.H., 1914.** A preliminary report of experiments on the cultivation of the virus of rinderpest in vitro. *Philippine Journal of Science*, (B), 9, 39–44.

32 **BOYNTON, W.H., 1916.** Rinderpest in swine with experiments upon the transmission from cattle and carabaos to swine and vice versa. *Philippine Agricultural Reviews*, 9, 288–336.

33 **BOYNTON, W.H., 1917.** Preliminary report on the virulence of certain body organs in rinderpest. *Philippine Agricultural Reviews*, 10, 410–433.

34 **BRANAGAN, D., 1966.** Behaviour of buffalo infected with rinderpest. *Bulletin of Epizootic Diseases of Africa*, 14, 341–342.

35 **BRANAGAN, D. & HAMMOND, J.A., 1965.** Rinderpest in Tanganyika: A review. *Bulletin of Epizootic Diseases of Africa*, 13, 225–246.

36 **BREESE, S.S. & DE BOER, C.J., 1963.** Electron microscopy of rinderpest virus in bovine kidney tissue culture cells. *Virology*, 19, 340–348.

37 **BRISTOWE, J.S., 1866.** Morbid anatomy of the disease. *In: Third Report of the Commissioners into the Origin and Nature etc. of the Cattle Plague.* London: Her Majesty's Stationery Office.

38 **BROTHERSTONE, J.G., 1951.** Lapinized rinderpest virus and a vaccine. Some observations in East Africa. I. Laboratory experiments. *Journal of Comparative Pathology*, 61, 263–288.

39 **BROWN, R.D., 1958.** Rinderpest immunity in calves. I. Acquisition and persistence of maternally derived antibody. *Journal of Hygiene*, Cambridge, 56, 427–434.

40 **BROWN, R.D., 1958.** Rinderpest immunity in calves. II. Active immunization. *Journal of Hygiene*, Cambridge, 56, 436–444.

41 **BROWN, R.D., 1964.** Endobronchial inoculation of cattle with various strains of *Mycoplasma mycoides* and the effects of stress. *Research in Veterinary Science*, 5, 393–404.

42 **BROWN, R.D. & GLOSSOP, W.E., 1965.** Rinderpest immunization by means of vaccine implants in tablet form. *Bulletin of Epizootic Diseases of Africa*, 13, 305–309.

43 **BROWN, R.D. & LAMPKIN, G.H., 1961.** Effect of caprinized rinderpest vaccine on the growth of weaner calves. *East African Agriculture and Forestry Journal*, 26, 156–157.

44 **BROWN, R.D. & SCOTT, G.R., 1957.** Mucosal disease complex. *The Veterinary Record*, 12, 287–298.

45 **BROWN, R.D. & SCOTT, G.R., 1960.** Vaccination of game with lapinized rinderpest virus. *The Veterinary Record*, 72, 1232–1233.

46 **BROWN, C.W., SCOTT, G.R. & BROTHERSTON, J.G., 1955.** Lapinized rinderpest vaccine: Post inoculation reactions in high-grade Guernsey cattle. *The Veterinary Record,* 67, 467–468.

47 **BROWN, R.D. & TAYLOR, W.P., 1966.** Simultaneous vaccination of cattle against rinderpest and contagious bovine pleuropneumonia. *Bulletin of Epizootic Diseases of Africa,* 14, 141–146.

48 **CARMICHAEL, J., 1938.** Rinderpest in African game. *Journal of Comparative Pathology,* 51, 264–268.

49 **CARMICHAEL, J., 1939.** Attempts to propagate the virus (rinderpest) in tissue culture. *Annual Report of the Veterinary Department, Uganda, 1938.* Entebbe: Government Printer.

50 **CHENEAU, Y., 1985.** Prevalence of rinderpest and strategy of the Pan-African Campaign. *Revue Scientifique et Technique de l'Office International des Épizooties,* 4, 415–425.

51 **CILLI, V., MAZZARACHIO, V. & ROETTI, C., 1951.** L'epidosio di peste bovina al Giardiono Zoologico di Roma. *Archivio Italiano di Scienze Mediche Tropicali e di Parassitologia,* 32, 83–94.

52 **CLAVERIE, J., 1931.** La lutte contre la peste bovine en Guinée française. *Recueil de Médecine Vétérinaire Exotique,* 4, 121–140.

53 **CONTI, P.A. & VAN DAC, N.G., 1929.** Utilisation du porcelet pour l'entretien du virus pestique servant aux pratiques d'immunisation antipestique. *Recueil de Médicine Vétérinaire Exotique,* 2, 205–215.

54 **COOPER, H., 1932.** Rinderpest: Transmission of infection by contact. *Indian Journal of Veterinary Science and Animal Husbandry,* 2, 284–392.

55 **CORNELL, R.L. & EVANS, S.A., 1937.** On the values and limitations of tissue vaccines against rinderpest. *Journal of Comparative Pathology,* 50, 122–135.

56 **CORNELL, R.L. & REID, N.R., 1934.** Rinderpest in wildebeest. *Annual report of the Department of Veterinary Science and Animal Husbandry, Tanganyika Territory, 1933.* Dar-es-Salaam: Government Printer.

57 **COSBY, S.L., McQUAID, S., DUFFY, N., LYONS, C., RIMA, B.K., ALLAN, G.M., McCULLOUGH, G.M., KENNEDY, S., SMYTH, J.A., McNEILLY, F., CRAIG, C. & ORVELL, C., 1988.** Characterisation of a seal morbillivirus. *Nature,* 336, 115–116.

58 **CRAWFORD, M., 1947.** The immunology and epidemiology of some virus diseases. *The Veterinary Record,* 59, 537–540.

59 **CURASSON, G., 1932.** *La Peste Bovine.* Paris: Vigot Frères.

60 **CURASSON, G., 1942.** La peste bovine. *In: Traité de Pathologie Exotique Vétérinaire et Comparée,* Vol. I. Paris: Vigot Frères.

61 **CURSON, H.H., 1919.** Rinderpest in the New Langenberg Province of German East Africa during 1917–1918. *Journal of Comparative Pathology and Therapeutics,* 32, 197–210.

62 **DARBYSHIRE, J.H., BROWN, R.D., SCOTT, G.R. & HUCK, R.A., 1961.** A serological differentiation of rinderpest and bovine mucosal disease by agar gel diffusion. *The Veterinary Record,* 73, 255–256.

63 **DATTA, C.A. & RAJAGOPOLAN, V.R., 1932.** An unusual case of chronic rinderpest with special reference to the carrier problem in this disease. *Indian Journal of Veterinary Science and Animal Husbandry,* 2, 357–382.

64 **DAUBNEY, R., 1928.** Observations on rinderpest. *Journal of Comparative Pathology,* 41, 228–248, 263–297.

65 **DAUBNEY, R., 1929.** Prophylactic vaccination against rinderpest. *Proceedings of the Pan-African Veterinary Conference, Pretoria.*

66 **DAUBNEY, R., 1949.** Goat-adapted virus. *In:* KESTEVEN, K.V.L. (ed.). *Rinderpest Vaccines: Their Production and Use in the Field.* FAO Agricultural Studies No. 8. Washington: Food and Agriculture Organization.

67 **D'COSTA, J. & SINGH, B., 1933.** Rinderpest: Clinical syndrome in goats in India. *Indian Journal of Veterinary Science and Animal Husbandry,* 3, 122–128.

68 **DE LAY, P.D. & BARBER, T.L., 1962.** Transmission of rinderpest virus from experimentally infected cattle to pigs. *Proceedings of the United States Livestock Sanitary Association 65th Annual Meeting,* 1961, Minneapolis.

69 **DE LAY, P.D., MOULTON, W.M. & STONE, S.S., 1962.** Survival of rinderpest virus in experimentally-infected swine. *Proceedings of the United States Livestock Sanitary Association 65th Annual Meeting,* 1961, Minneapolis.

70 **DELPY, L., 1930.** Les formes atypiques de la peste bovine et les porteurs de virus. *Revue générale de Médecine Vétérinaire,* 39, 138–141.

71 **DHILLON, S.S., 1959.** Incidence of rinderpest in camels in Hissar district. *Indian Veterinary Journal,* 36, 603–607.

72 **DHIR, R.C., DIXIT, N.K., ADAVAL, S.C. & TIWARI, G.P., 1987.** Blood biochemical changes in male buffalo calves during rinderpest infection. *Indian Journal of Animal Sciences,* 57, 177–179.

73 **DIALLO, A., BARRETT, T., BARBON, M., SUBBARAO, S.M. & TAYLOR, W.P., 1989.** Differentiation of rinderpest and peste des petits ruminants viruses using specific cDNA clones. *Journal of Virological Methods,* 23, 127–136.

74 **DIALLO, A., BARRETT, T., LEFEVRE, P.C. & TAYLOR, W.P., 1987.** Comparison of proteins induced in cells infected with rinderpest and peste des petits ruminants virus. *Journal of General Virology,* 68, 2033–2038.

75 **DOUTRE, M.P., CHAMBRON, J. & BOURDIN, P., 1972.** Valeur de l'immunité conférée par un vaccin mixte antibovipestique- antipéripneumonique lyophilisé préparé à l'aide de la souche T1 (S-R). *Revue d'Élevage et de Médecine Vétérinaire des Pays Tropicaux,* 25, 1–14.

76 **EDWARDS, J.T., 1925.** Rinderpest (etiological researches). *Report of the Imperial Bacteriological Institute, Mukteswar for 1922–23,* 30–35.

77 **EDWARDS, J.T., 1930.** The problem of rinderpest in India. *Bulletin 199 of the Imperial Institute of Agricultural Research, Pusa, Calcutta,* Government of India, Central Publications Branch.

78 **EPSTEIN, H., 1971.** *The Origin of the Domestic Animals of Africa.* New York: Africana Publishing Corporation.

79 **EVANS, S.A., 1932.** Rinderpest in goats and sheep. *Annual Report of the Department of Veterinary Science and Animal Husbandry, Tanganyika Territory, 1931.* Dar-es-Salaam: Government Printer.

80 **FLEMING, G., 1882.** *Animal Plagues: Their History, Nature and Prevention.* Vol. II. London: Baillière Tindal.

81 **FORMAN, A.J., ROWE, L.W. & TAYLOR, W.P., 1983.** Detection of rinderpest antigen by agar gel diffusion and counter-immuno-electrophoresis. *Tropical Animal Health and Production,* 15, 83–85.

82 **FRENCH, M.H., 1936.** The serum protein changes induced by rinderpest virus. *Journal of Comparative Pathology,* 49, 147–156.

83 **FUKUDA, A. & YAMANOUCHI, K., 1981.** Comparison of autoimmunity induction with virulent and attenuated virus in rabbits. *Japanese Journal of Medical Science and Biology,* 34, 149–159.

84 **FUKUSHO, K. & NAKAMURA, J., 1940.** On the experimental infection with rinderpest virus in the rabbit. II. Pathology. *Japanese Journal of Veterinary Science,* 2, 75–101.

85 **GAJENDRAGAD, M.R., SHARMA, B., PRABHUDAS, K., JOSHI, R.C. & BANSAL, R.P., 1983.** Immunoperoxidase staining of rinderpest virus antigen in formalin-fixed paraffin-embedded sections. *Indian Journal of Veterinary Pathology,* 7, 79–81.

86 **GAMGEE, J., 1866.** *The Cattle Plague.* London: Hardwick.

87 **GHAFFAR, S.A. & ATA, F.A., 1982.** Bovine virus diarrhoea in Egypt. *The Veterinary Record,* 110, 566.

88 **GIBBS, C.S., 1933.** Filterable virus carriers. *Journal of Infectious Diseases,* 53, 169–174.

89 **GRAY, C.E., 1917.** *Rinderpest in East Africa.* London: Colonial Office.

90 **GRUBMAN, M.J., MEBUS, C., DALE, B., YAMANAKA, M. & YILMA, T., 1988.** Analysis of the polypeptides synthesized in rinderpest virus-infected cells. *Virology,* 163, 261–267.

91 **GUITTIN, P., 1981.** Rinderpest epizootic in Niger. *Action Vétérinaire*, 826, 6–8.

92 **HAJI, C.S.G., 1932.** Rinderpest in camels. *Indian Veterinary Journal*, 9, 13–14.

93 **HALL, G.N., 1933.** Investigations of rinderpest immunization. D.V.M. Thesis, University of Zurich.

94 **HASSAN, A.K.M. & EL TOM, K., 1985.** Combined natural infection with infectious bovine rhinotracheitis and rinderpest viruses. *Tropical Animal Health and Production*, 17, 52.

95 **HASSAN, D.G.A., KARIM, I.A., ARAB, R.M., SABER, M.S., AMIN, M.M., OSMAN, O.A. & REDA, I.M., 1987.** Studies on rinderpest and diseases like rinderpest in Egypt. *Journal of the Egyptian Veterinary Medical Association*, 47, 399–416.

96 **HAYES, J.W., 1927.** Contagious bovine pleuropneumonia in Tanganyika Territory. *Annual Report of the Department of Veterinary Sciences and Animal Husbandry, Tanganyika Territory, 1926*. Dar-es-Salaam: Government Printer.

97 **HEDGER, R.S., TAYLOR, W.P., BARNETT, I.T.R., RIEK, R. & HARPHAM, D., 1986.** Simultaneous vaccination of cattle against foot-and-mouth disease and rinderpest. *Tropical Animal Health and Production*, 18, 21–25.

98 **HENNING, M.W., 1956.** *Animal Diseases in South Africa*. 3rd edn. Pretoria: Central News Agency.

99 **HEUSCHELE, W.P. & BARBER, T.L., 1963.** Haematologic studies of rinderpest-infected swine. *Canadian Journal of Comparative Medicine and Veterinary Science*, 27, 56–60.

100 **HEUSCHELE, W.P. & BARBER, T.L., 1966.** Changes in certain blood components of rinderpest-infected cattle. *American Journal of Veterinary Research*, 27, 1001–1006.

101 **HOLMES, J.D.E., 1904.** Some diseases complicating rinderpest among cattle in India. *Journal of Comparative Pathology*, 17, 317–326.

102 **HORNBY, H.E., 1926.** Studies in rinderpest immunity. II. Methods of infection. *The Veterinary Journal*, 82, 348–355.

103 **HORNBY, H.E., 1932.** Disease control. Rinderpest. *Annual Report of the Department of Veterinary Science and Animal Husbandry, Tanganyika Territory, 1931*. Dar-es-Salaam: Government Printer.

104 **HORNBY, H.E., 1934.** Pathogenicity of Trypanosoma theileria and Streptothricosis in cattle concurrently infected with rinderpest. *Annual Report of the Department of Veterinary Science and Animal Husbandry, Tanganyika Territory, 1933*. Dar-es-Salaam: Government Printer.

105 **HSU, D., YAMANAKA, M., MILLER, J., DALE, B., GRUBMAN, M. & YILMA, T., 1988.** Cloning of the fusion gene of rinderpest virus: Comparative sequence analysis with other morbilliviruses. *Virology*, 166, 149–153.

106 **HUDSON, J.R. & WONGSONGSARN, C., 1950.** The utilization of pigs for the production of lapinized rinderpest virus. *British Veterinary Journal*, 106, 453–472.

107 **HUSSAIN, S.F., RWEYEMAMU, M.M., KAMINJOLO, J.S., AKHTAR, A.S. & MUGERA, G.M., 1980.** Studies on viral interference induced by rinderpest virus: Interference and interferon induction by tissue culture rinderpest vaccine (TCRV) virus *in vitro*. *Zentralblatt für Veterinärmedizin*, 27B, 181–189.

108 **HUSSAIN, S.F., RWEYEMAMU, M.M., KAMINJOLO, J.S., AKHTAR, A.S. & MUGERA, G.M., 1982.** Studies on viral interference induced by rinderpest virus: IV. Induction of circulating interferon and antibodies in buffaloes following inoculation with tissue culture rinderpest vaccine (TCRV) virus. *Bulletin of Animal Health and Production in Africa*, 30, 7–10.

109 **HUTCHEON, D., 1902.** Rinderpest in South Africa. *Journal of Comparative Pathology*, 15, 300–324.

110 **HUYGELEN, C., 1960.** Failure to demonstrate agglutination of red blood cells by rinderpest virus. *Bulletin of Epizootic Diseases of Africa*, 8, 121–125.

111 **HUYTRA, F., MAREK, J. & MANNINGER, R., 1946.** Rinderpest. *In: Special Pathology and Therapeutics of the Diseases of Domestic Animals*. 5th English edn. London: Baillière, Tindall & Cox.

112 **HYSLOP, N. St. G., 1979.** Observations on the survival and infectivity of airborne rinderpest virus. *International Journal of Bioclimatology and Biometeorology*, 23, 1–7.

113 **IDNANI, J.A., 1944.** Transmission of rinderpest by expired air. *Indian Journal of Veterinary Science and Animal Husbandry*, 14, 216–220.

114 **IKEDE, B.O., 1984.** Rinderpest epidemics in Tropical Africa. *Tropical Veterinarian*, 2, 1–2.

115 **IMAGAWA, D.T., GORET, P. & ADAMS, J.M., 1960.** Immunological relationships of measles, distemper and rinderpest viruses. *Proceedings of the National Academy of Sciences*, 46, 1119–1123.

116 **INOUE, T., HARADA, S. & SHIMIZU, T., 1930.** Preliminary note on the experimental infection with rinderpest virus of susliks. Selected contributions from the Mukden Institute for infectious diseases of animals, 1, 221–222. (Abstracted in *Veterinary Bulletin*, 1, 53).

117 **ISOGAI, S., 1944.** On the rabbit-virus inoculation as an active immunization method against rinderpest for Mongolian cattle. *Japanese Journal of Veterinary Science*, 6, 388–390.

118 **JACOTOT, H., 1931.** L'infection pestique qui entraine l'ovortement peut-elle être propagée par la foetus et la femelle qui l'a expulsée. *Bulletin de la Société de Pathologie Exotique et de ses Filiales*, 24, 74–76.

119 **JACOTOT, H., 1950.** Rapport concernant le contrôle et la standardisation des sérums et vaccins contre la peste bovine. *Bulletin de l'Office International des Épizooties*, 33, 168–183.

120 **JACOTOT, H. & MORNET, P., 1967.** *La Peste Bovine*. Paris: L'Expansion Scientifique Française.

121 **JAMES, A.D. & ROSSITER, P.B., 1989.** An epidemiological model of rinderpest. I. Description of the model. *Tropical Animal Health and Production*, 21, 59–68.

122 **JEGGO, M.H., WARDLEY, R.C. & CORTEYN, A.K., 1987.** A reassessment of the dual vaccine against rinderpest and contagious bovine pleuropneumonia. *The Veterinary Record*, 120, 131–135.

123 **JENKINS, D.L. & SHOPE, R.E., 1946.** Rinderpest. VII. The attenuation of rinderpest virus for cattle by cultivation in embryonating eggs. *American Journal of Veterinary Research*, 7, 174–178.

124 **JOHNSON, R.H., 1962.** Rinderpest in tissue culture: Use of the attenuated strain as a vaccine for cattle. *British Veterinary Journal*, 118, 141–150.

125 **JOSHI, R.C., CHAUDHARY, P.G. & BANSAL, R.P., 1977.** Occurrence of cutaneous eruptions in rinderpest outbreak among bovines. *Indian Veterinary Journal*, 54, 871–873.

126 **JOSHI, R.C., SHARMA, B., BANDYOPADHAY, S.K. & BANSAL, R.P., 1984.** Detection of rinderpest antibodies. *Tropical Animal Health and Production*, 16, 167–170.

127 **KAKIZAKI, C., 1918.** Study on the glycerinated rinderpest vaccine. *Kitasato Archives of Experimental Medicine*, 2, 59–66.

128 **KAPWADI, K., 1987.** Trial of simultaneous vaccination against rinderpest and brucellosis in cattle in Zaïre. *Revue Scientifique et Technique de l'Office International des Épizooties*, 6, 1043–1049.

129 **KATHURIA, B.K., UPPAL, P.K. & KUMAR, S., 1976.** Studies on simultaneous vaccination of cattle against rinderpest and foot-and-mouth disease. *Indian Veterinary Journal*, 53, 571–576.

130 **KEYLOCK, H.E., 1933.** The control of rinderpest in a large dairy herd in Shanghai, China. *Journal of Comparative Pathology*, 46, 149–158.

131 **KHERA, K.S., 1958.** Étude histologique de la peste bovine. I. Pathogenèse du virus de la peste bovine dans les ganglions lymphatiques. *Revue d'Élevage et de Médecine Vétérinaire des Pays Tropicaux*, 11, 399–405.

132 **KHERA, K.S., 1958.** Étude histologique de la peste bovine. II. Lésions histologiques au niveau du tractus digestif. *Revue d'Élevage et de Médecine Vétérinaire des Pays Tropicaux*, 11, 406–415.

133 **KHERA, K.S., 1958.** Étude histologique de la peste bovine. III. Lésions dans les différents organes. *Revue d'Élevage et de Médecine Vétérinaire des Pays Tropicaux*, 11, 416–420.

134 **KINGSBURY, D.W., BRATT, M.A., CHOPPIN, P.W., HANSON, R.P., HOSAKA, Y., TER MEULEN, V., NORRBY, E., PLOWRIGHT, W., ROTT, R. & WUNNER, W.H., 1978.** Paramyxoviridae. *Intervirology*, 10, 137–152.

135 **KOBUNE, F., CHINO, F. & YAMANOUCHI, K., 1976.** Studies on recovery mechanism from rinderpest virus infection in rabbits. I. Effect of anti-thymocyte serum and thymectomy. *Japanese Journal of Medical Science and Biology*, 29, 265–275.

136 **KOBUNE, F., YAMANOUCHI, K., NAGASHIMA, K. & SHISHIDO, A., 1981.** Establishment of a persistently infected cell line with rinderpest virus. *Archives of Virology*, 68, 271–277.

137 **KOCH, R., 1897.** Berichte des Herrn Prof. Dr. Koch über seine in Kimberley gemachten versuche bezuglich bekämpfung der rinderpest. *Zentralblatt für Bakteriologie* 1, 21, 526–537.

138 **KOTZÉ, J.P., 1974.** Die runderpes in die Transvaal en die onmiddellike gevolge daarvan 1896–99. Magister in die Lettere en Wysbegeerte in Geskiedenis, Randse Afrikaanse Universiteit, Johannesburg, Suid-Afrika.

139 **KRISHNASWAMY, S., KESHAVAMURTHY, B.S. & SUNDARARAJAM, S., 1981.** The use of the direct immunoperoxidase test to detect the multiplication of rinderpest virus in bovine kidney cell culture. *Veterinary Microbiology*, 6, 23–29.

140 **KRISHNASWAMY, S. & VEERABHADRAPPA, G., 1982.** Intra-cellular polypeptides in the rinderpest virus infected cells. *Indian Journal of Comparative Microbiology, Immunology and Infectious Diseases*, 3, 68–71.

141 **LANGUET, B., PRECAUSTA, P., MACKOWIAK, M., DUBOURGET, P., REYLNAUD, E. & DURET, C., 1985.** Freeze-dried vaccine against rinderpest: Stability and activity study. *Journal of Comparative Immunology, Microbiology and Infectious Diseases*, 8, 285–295.

142 **LEISS, B., 1963.** Fluoreszenzserologische untersuchungen an zellkulturen nach infektion mit rinderpestvirus. *Zentralblatt für Bakteriologie*, 190, 424–444.

143 **LEISS, B., 1964.** Untersuchungen über des virus der rinderpest unter verwendung von zellkulturen. *Archives of Experimental Veterinary Medicine*, 20, 157–257.

144 **LEISS, B. & PLOWRIGHT, W., 1964.** Studies on the pathogenesis of rinderpest in experimentally infected cattle. I. Correlation of clinical signs, viraemia and virus excretion by various routes. *Journal of Hygiene*, 62, 81–100.

145 **LEPISSIER, H.E., 1983.** *Pan-African Campaign against Rinderpest. Organization and Logistics.* Nairobi: Inter-African Bureau of Animal Resources, Organization of African Unity.

146 **LIBEAU, J. & SCOTT, G.R., 1960.** Rinderpest in eastern Africa today. *Bulletin of Epizootic Diseases of Africa*, 8, 23–26.

147 **LINGARD, A., 1905.** *Report of the Imperial Institute for Bacteriology 1905–06*, 4.

148 **LITTLEWOOD, W., 1905.** Cattle plague in Egypt in 1903–04–05. *Journal of Comparative Pathology*, 18, 312–321.

149 **LOWE, H.J., 1942.** Rinderpest in Tanganyika Territory. *Empire Journal of Experimental Agriculture*, 10, 189–202.

150 **LOWE, H.J., WILDE, J.K.H., LEE, R.P. & STUTCHBERRY, H.M., 1947.** An outbreak of an aberrant type of rinderpest in Tanganyika Territory. *Journal of Comparative Pathology*, 57, 175–183.

151 **MACADAM, I., 1968.** Transmission of rinderpest from goats to cattle in Tanzania. *Bulletin of Epizootic Diseases of Africa*, 16, 53–60.

152 **MACADAM, I., EZEBUIRO, E.O. & OREFFO, V.O.C., 1964.** The response of zebu cattle to mixed bovine pleuropneumonia and tissue culture rinderpest vaccine. *Bulletin of Epizootic Diseases of Africa*, 12, 237–240.

153 **MACK, R., 1970.** The great African cattle plague epidemic of the 1890s. *Tropical Animal Health and Production*, 2, 210–219.

154 **MAHY, B.W.J., BARRETT, T., EVANS, S., ANDERSON, E.C. & BOSTOCK, C.J., 1988.** Characterization of a seal morbillivirus. *Nature*, 336, 115.

155 **MARINER, J.C., HOUSE, J.A., SOLLOD, A.E., STEM, C., VAN DEN ENDE, M. & MEBUS, C.A., 1990.** Comparison of the effect of various chemical stabilizers and lyophilization cycles on the thermostability of a Vero cell-adapted rinderpest vaccine. *Veterinary Microbiology*, 21, 195–209.

156 **MASIGA, W., HALPIN, B. & CHENEAU, Y., 1988.** Rinderpest. *In*: WILLIAMS, A.O. & MASIGA, W., (eds). *Viral Diseases of Animals in Africa*. Lagos: Scientific, Technical and Research Committee, Organization of African Unity.

157 **MAURER, F.D., JONES, T.C., EASTERDAY, B. & DE TRAY, D.E., 1955.** Pathology of rinderpest — an abstract. *Journal of the American Veterinary Medical Association*, 127, 512–514.

158 **MAURER, F.D., JONES, T.C., EASTERDAY, B. & DE TRAY, D.E., 1956.** The pathology of rinderpest. *In: Proceedings of the 92nd Annual Meeting of the American Veterinary Medical Association*, 1955, Minneapolis.

159 **McCULLOUGH, K.C., SHESHBERADARAN, H., NORRBY, E., OBI, T.U. & CROWTHER, J.R., 1986.** Monoclonal antibodies against morbilliviruses. *Revue Scientifique et Technique de l'Office International des Épizooties*, 5, 411–427.

160 **METTAM, R.W.M., 1937.** A short history of rinderpest with special reference to Africa. *The Uganda Journal*, 5, 22–26.

161 **MIRCHAMSY, H., SHAFYI, A. & BAHRAMI, S., 1970.** Use of Vero cells for titration of rinderpest virus and its neutralizing antibody. *Applied Microbiology*, 19, 545–546.

162 **MOHAMED, E.H.M., 1983.** Rapid diagnosis of rinderpest. M.Sc. Thesis, University of Reading, United Kingdom.

163 **MOHAMMED, Z.E., HAFEZ, S.M. & OZAWA, Y., 1977.** Studies on the methods of preparation of rinderpest hyperimmune serum in rabbits. *Tropical Animal Health and Production*, 9, 25–28.

164 **MOHAN, R. & BAHL, M.R., 1953.** Cutaneous eruptions of rinderpest in goats. *Indian Journal of Veterinary Science*, 23, 39–42.

165 **MORNET, P., 1948.** Schéma epizootiologique de la peste bovine en Afrique Occidentale Française. *Bulletin de la Service de l'Élevage et de l'Industrie Animal*, A.O.F., 1, 7–12.

166 **MORNET, P. & GILBERT, Y., 1958.** Les méthodes actuelles de lutte contre la peste bovine. *Les Cahiers de Médecine Vétérinaire*, 27, 1–52.

167 **MORNET, P. & GUERRET, M., 1950.** Les lésions cutanées dans la peste bovine. *Bulletin de l'Académie Vétérinaire de France*, 23, 283–285.

168 **MULLICK, S.G., RAMACHANDRAN, S.P. & RAMACHANDRAN, S., 1982.** Preparation of rinderpest precipitins using adjuvants. *Indian Veterinary Journal*, 59, 833–836.

169 **NAGINGTON, J., LANDER, I.M. & SMITH, J.S., 1967.** Bovine papular stomatitis, pseudocowpox and milker's nodules. *The Veterinary Record*, 81, 306–312.

170 **NAKAMURA, J., 1940.** On the experimental infection with rinderpest virus in the rabbit. III. Neutralization experiment. *Japanese Journal of Veterinary Science*, 2, 567–578.

171 **NAKAMURA, J., 1957.** Peste Bovine. *Bulletin de l'Office International des Épizooties*, 47, 542–554.

172 **NAKAMURA, J. & MIYAMOTO, T., 1953.** Avianisation of lapinized rinderpest virus. *American Journal of Veterinary Research*, 14, 307–317.

173 **NAKAMURA, J., WAGATUMA, S. & FUKOSHO, K., 1938.** On the experimental infection with rinderpest virus in the rabbit. I. Some fundamental experiments. *Journal of the Japanese Society of Veterinary Science*, 17, 185–204.

174 **NARAYANASWAMY, M. & RAMANI, K., 1973.** Preliminary studies on rinderpest virus isolated from outbreaks in sheep in Mysore State. *Indian Veterinary Journal*, 50, 829–832.

175 **NAWATHE, D.R. & LAMORDE, A.G., 1982.** Recurrence of rinderpest in Nigeria. *The Veterinary Record*, 11, 203.

176 **NAWATHE, D.R. & LAMORDE, A.G., 1983.** Towards global eradication of rinderpest. *Revue Scientifique et Technique, Office International des Epizooties*, 2, 997–1011.

177 **NAWATHE, D.R., LAMORDE, A.G. & KUMAR, S., 1983.** Recrudescence of rinderpest in Nigeria. *The Veterinary Record*, 113, 156–157.

178 **NOCARD, E. & LECLAINCHE, E., 1896.** Peste bovine. *In: Les Maladies Microbiennes des Animaux*. Paris: Masson.

179 **NORRBY, E., SHESBERADARAN, H., McCULLOUGH, K.C., CARPENTER, W.C. & ORVELL, C., 1985.** Is rinderpest the archvirus of the morbillivirus genus? *Intervirology*, 23, 228–232.

180 **NYANGE, J.F.C., OTARU, M.M.M. & MBISE, A.N., 1985.** Incidences of abnormal wild animal mortality in northern Tanzania, 1979–1982. *Bulletin of Animal Health and Production in Africa*, 33, 55–57.

181 **OFCANSKY, T.P., 1981.** The 1889–97 rinderpest epidemic and the rise of British and German colonialism in eastern and southern Africa. *Journal of African Studies*, 8, 31–38.

182 **OKUNA, N. & RWEYEMAMU, M.M., 1974.** Observations on the development of serum-neutralising antibodies in rinderpest infection. *Bulletin of Epizootic Diseases of Africa*, 22, 185–193.

183 **ORR, W., 1945.** Observations on rinderpest in goats imported to Malaya. *Journal of Comparative Pathology*, 55, 185–200.

184 **PEASE, H.T., 1894.** Rinderpest. Colonial Veterinary Department, Ledger Series No. 1.

185 **PÉCAUD, G., 1924.** Contribution à l'étude de la pathologie vétérinaire de la colonie du Tchad. *Bulletin de la Société de Pathologie Exotique et de ses Filiales*, 17, 196–207.

186 **PERCIVAL, A.B., 1918.** Game and disease. *Journal of the East African and Uganda Natural History Society*, 13, 302–315.

187 **PLOWRIGHT, W., 1952.** Observations on the behaviour of rinderpest virus in indigenous African sheep. *British Veterinary Journal*, 108, 450–457.

188 **PLOWRIGHT, W., 1963.** The role of game animals in the epizootiology of rinderpest and malignant catarrhal fever in East Africa. *Bulletin of Epizootic Diseases in Africa*, 11, 149–162.

189 **PLOWRIGHT, W., 1963.** Some properties of strains of rinderpest recently isolated in East Africa. *Research in Veterinary Science*, 4, 96–108.

190 **PLOWRIGHT, W., 1964.** Studies on the pathogenesis of rinderpest in experimental cattle. II. Proliferation of the virus in different tissues following intranasal infection. *Journal of Hygiene*, 62, 257–281.

191 **PLOWRIGHT, W., 1968.** Rinderpest virus. *Monographs in Virology*, 3, 25–110.

192 **PLOWRIGHT, W., 1972.** The production and use of rinderpest cell culture vaccine in developing countries. *World Animal Review*, 1, 14–18.

193 **PLOWRIGHT, W., 1982.** The effect of rinderpest and rinderpest control on wildlife in Africa. *Symposium of the Zoological Society of London*, 50, 1–28.

194 **PLOWRIGHT, W., 1984.** The duration of immunity in cattle following inoculation of rinderpest cell culture vaccine. *Journal of Hygiene*, 92, 285–296.

195 **PLOWRIGHT, W., 1987.** Investigations of rinderpest antibody in East African Wildlife, 1967–1971. *Revue Scientifique et Technique de l'Office International des Épizooties*, 6, 497–513.

196 **PLOWRIGHT, W., CRUIKSHANK, J.G. & WATERSON, A.P., 1962.** The morphology of rinderpest virus. *Virology*, 17, 118–122.

197 **PLOWRIGHT, W. & FERRIS, R.D., 1957.** Cytopathogenicity of rinderpest virus in tissue cultures. *Nature*, 179, 316.

198 **PLOWRIGHT, W. & FERRIS, R.D., 1959.** Studies with rinderpest virus. I. Growth and cytopathogenicity. *Journal of Comparative Pathology*, 69, 152–172.

199 **PLOWRIGHT, W. & FERRIS, R.D., 1959.** Studies with rinderpest virus in tissue culture. II. Pathogenicity for cattle of culture passaged virus. *Journal of Comparative Pathology*, 69, 173–184.

200 **PLOWRIGHT, W. & FERRIS, R.D., 1962.** Studies with rinderpest virus in tissue culture. The use of attenuated virus as a vaccine for cattle. *Research in Veterinary Science*, 3, 172–182.

201 **PLOWRIGHT, W. & FERRIS, R.D., 1962.** Studies with rinderpest virus in tissue culture. A technique for the detection and titration of virulent virus in cattle tissues. *Research in Veterinary Science*, 3, 94–103.

202 **PLOWRIGHT, W., LAWS, R.M. & RAMPTON, C.S., 1964.** Serological evidence for the susceptibility of the hippopotamus (*Hippopotamus amphibius* Linnaeus) to natural infection with rinderpest virus. *Journal of Hygiene, Cambridge*, 62, 329–336.

203 **PLOWRIGHT, W. & McCULLOUGH, B., 1967.** Investigations on the incidence of rinderpest virus infection in game animals of N. Tanganyika and S. Kenya 1960/1963. *Journal of Hygiene, Cambridge*, 65, 343–358.

204 **PLOWRIGHT, W., STAAK, C. & BOTTCHER, M., 1981.** The immunity following rinderpest vaccination. *In: Proceedings of the Scientific Conference, Diamond Jubilee of the National Veterinary Research Laboratory*, 1981, Vom, Nigeria.

205 **PLOWRIGHT, W. & TAYLOR, W.P., 1967.** Long-term studies of the immunity in East African cattle following inoculation with rinderpest culture vaccine. *Research in Veterinary Science*, 8, 118–128.

206 **POLDING, J.B. & SIMPSON, R.M., 1957.** A possible immunological relationship between canine distemper and rinderpest. *The Veterinary Record*, 69, 582–584.

207 **PRABHUDAS, K. & SAMBAMURTI, B., 1976.** A note on fluorescent antibody technique for rapid diagnosis of rinderpest. *Indian Journal of Animal Science*, 46, 454–457.

208 **PROVOST, A., 1970.** Observations sur les muco-anticorps nasaux des bovins. *Revue d'Élevage et de Médecine Vétérinaire des Pays Tropicaux*, 23, 283–293.

209 **PROVOST, A., 1974.** Peste bovine. *In:* BRICOUT, F., JOUBERT, L. & HURAUX, J.M., (eds). *Diagnostic Sero-Immunologique des Viruses Humaines et Animals*. Paris: Molinie.

210 **PROVOST, A., 1979.** La pérennité de la peste bovine en Afrique intertropicale. *Bulletin de l'Office International des Épizooties*, 91, 761–765.

211 **PROVOST, A., 1981.** Queries about rinderpest in African wild animals. *In*: KARSTAD, L., NESTEL, B. & GRAHAM, M., (eds). *Wildlife Disease Research and Economic Development*. Ottawa: International Development Research Centre.

212 **PROVOST, A., 1982.** Scientific and technical bases for the eradication of rinderpest in inter-tropical Africa. *Revue Scientifique et Technique de l'Office International des Épizooties*, 1, 589–665.

213 **PROVOST, A. & BORREDON, C., 1963.** Les différents aspects du diagnostic clinique et expérimental de la peste bovine. *Revue d'Élevage et de Médecine Vétérinaire des Pays Tropicaux*, 16, 445–526.

214 **PROVOST, A. & BORREDON, C., 1972.** Un vaccin mixte antibovipestique-antipéripneumonique lyophilise utilisable, sur le terrain, sans réfrigération. I. Sélection de virions bovipestiques à inactivation thermique retardée. *Revue d'Élevage et de Médecine Vétérinaire des Pays Tropicaux*, 25, 507–520.

215 **PROVOST, A. & BORREDON, C., 1972.** Note sur l'inopportunité de l'association vaccinale peste bovine–maladie des muqueuses. *Bulletin of Epizootic Diseases of Africa*, 20, 265–267.

216 **PROVOST, A., BORREDON, C. & BOCQUET, P., 1974.** Un vaccin mixte trivalent contre la peste bovine, la péripneumonie et le charbon bactéridien. *Revue d'Élevage et de Médecine Vétérinaire des Pays Tropicaux*, 27, 385–395.

217 **PROVOST, A., BORREDON, C. & QUEVAL, R., 1970.** Recherches immunologiques sur la péripneumonie. XI. Un vaccin vivant mixte antibovipestique-antipéripneumonique inoculé en un seul temps. Conception — Production — Contrôles. *Revue d'Élevage et de Médecine Vétérinaire des Pays Tropicaux*, 23, 143–162.

218 **PROVOST, A. & JOUBERT, L., 1973.** Modalités et techniques modernes du diagnostic expérimental de la peste bovine. *Revue d'Élevage et de Médecine Vétérinaire des Pays Tropicaux*, 26, 283–396.

219 **PROVOST, A., MAURICE, Y. & BORREDON, C., 1968.** Note sur la peste bovine experimentale du dromadaire. *Revue d'Élevage et de Médecine Vétérinaire des Pays Tropicaux*, 21, 293–296.

220 **PROVOST, A., MAURICE, Y. & BORREDON, C., 1969.** Comportement clinique et immunologique, lors de contamination bovipestique, de bovins vaccinés depuis plusieurs années contre la peste bovine avec des vaccins de cultures cellulaires. *Revue d'Élevage et de Médecine Vétérinaire des Pays Tropicaux*, 22, 453–464.

221 **PROVOST, A., QUEVAL, R. & BORREDON, C., 1965.** Quelques recherches fondamentales sur la virus bovipestique. *Revue d'Élevage et de Médecine Vétérinaire des Pays Tropicaux*, 18, 371–384.

222 **RAMACHANDRAN, S. & SCOTT, G.R., 1985.** Potency of reconstituted rinderpest vaccine. *Indian Veterinary Journal*, 62, 335–336.

223 **RAMANI, K., CHARLES, Y.S., SRINIVAS, R.P., NARAYANASWAMY, M. & RAMACHANDRAN, S., 1974.** Isolation of rinderpest virus from an outbreak in domestic pigs in Karnataka. *Indian Veterinary Journal*, 51, 36–41.

224 **RECEVEUR, R., 1957.** Risques de dispersion de la peste bovine par les viandes fraîches ou congelées provenant des pays contaminés? *Bulletin de l'Office International des Épizooties*, 48, 148–158.

225 **RÉFIK-BEY, 1902.** Modifications leucocytaires dans la peste bovine. *Annales de l'Institut Pasteur*, 16, 163–168.

226 **RÉFIK-BEY & RÉFIK-BEY, 1899.** La peste bovine en Turquie. Épidémiologie, formes cliniques, sérothérapie. *Annales de l'Institut Pasteur*, 13, 596–608.

227 **REID, N.R., 1949.** *Annual Report of the Department of Veterinary Science and Animal Husbandry, Tanganyika Territory 1947/1948* p. 3. Dar-es-Salaam: Government Printer.

228 **RIOCHE, M., 1969.** Adaptation en microtest de la technique de séroneutralisation par la méthode cinétique pour la recherche et le titrage des anticorps neutralisant le virus de la peste bovine. *Revue d'Élevage et de Médecine Vétérinaire des Pays Tropicaux*, 22, 465–471.

229 **ROBERTS, G.A., 1921.** Rinderpest (Peste bovina) in Brazil. *Journal of the American Veterinary Medical Association*, 13, 177–185.

230 **ROBERTSON, W.A.N., 1924.** *Rinderpest in Western Australia 1923*. Melbourne: Government Printer.

231 **ROBEY, T.O. & HALE, M.W., 1946.** Rinderpest. XI. Morphological changes in the blood of young cattle during rinderpest and after vaccination with attenuated virus vaccine. *American Journal of Veterinary Research*, 7, 222–227.

232 **ROBSON, J., ARNOLD, R.M., PLOWRIGHT, W. & SCOTT, G.R., 1959.** The isolation from an eland of a strain of virus attenuated for cattle. *Bulletin of Epizootic Diseases of Africa*, 7, 97–102.

233 **ROSSITER, P.B., 1985.** Notes on immunoprecipitation reactions with rinderpest virus. *Tropical Animal Health and Production*, 17, 55–56.

234 **ROSSITER, P.B. & JAMES, A.D., 1989.** An epidemiological model of rinderpest. II. Simulations of the behaviour of the virus in populations. *Tropical Animal Health and Production*, 21, 69–84.

235 **ROSSITER, P.B. & JESSETT, D.M., 1982.** Detection of rinderpest virus antigens *in vitro* and *in vivo* by direct immunofluorescence. *Research in Veterinary Science*, 33, 198–204.

236 **ROSSITER, P.B. & JESSETT, D.M., 1982.** Microtitre techniques for the assay of rinderpest virus and neutralising antibody. *Research in Veterinary Science*, 32, 253–256.

237 **ROSSITER, P.B., JESSETT, D.M. & HOLMES, P., 1981.** Micro-ELISA test for detecting antibodies to rinderpest virus antigens. *Tropical Animal Health and Production*, 13, 113–116.

238 **ROSSITER, P.B., JESSETT, D.M. & TAYLOR, W.P., 1982.** Neutralising antibodies to rinderpest virus in sheep and goats in western Kenya. *The Veterinary Record*, 111, 504–505.

239 **ROSSITER, P.B., JESSETT, D.M., WAFULA, J.S., KARSTAD, L., CHEMA, S., TAYLOR, W.P., ROWE, L., NYANGE, J.C., OTARU, M., MUMBALA, M. & SCOTT, G.R., 1983.** Re-emergence of rinderpest as a threat in East Africa since 1979. *The Veterinary Record*, 113, 459–461.

240 **ROSSITER, P.B., KARSTAD, L., JESSETT, D.M., YAMAMOTO, T., DARDIRI, A.H. & MUSHI, E.Z., 1982.** Neutralising antibodies to rinderpest virus in wild animal sera collected in Kenya between 1970 and 1981. *Preventive Veterinary Medicine*, 1, 257–264.

241 **ROSSITER, P.B. & MORRISON, W.I., 1988.** Unpublished results. Kenya Agricultural Research Institute, P.O. Box 32, Kikuyu, Kenya.

242 **ROSSITER, P.B. & MUSHI, E.Z., 1980.** Rapid detection of rinderpest virus antigens by counter-immuno-electrophoresis. *Tropical Animal Health and Production*, 12, 209–216.

243 **ROSSITER, P.B., TAYLOR, W.P., BWANGAMOI, B., NGEREZA, A.R.H., MOORHOUSE, P.D.S., HARESNAPE, J.M., WAFULA, J.S., NYANGE, J.F.C. & GUMM, I.D., 1987.** Continuing presence of rinderpest virus as a threat in East Africa 1983–1985. *The Veterinary Record*, 120, 59–62.

244 **ROSSITER, P.B., WAFULA, J.S., GUMM, I.D., STAGG, D.A., MOZARIA, S.P. & SHAW, M.K., 1988.** Growth of rinderpest and bovine virus diarrhoea viruses in *Theileria parva* infected cell lines. *The Veterinary Record*, 122, 491–492.

245 **ROSSITER, P.B. & WAMWAYI, H.W., 1989.** Surveillance and monitoring programmes in the control of rinderpest: A review. *Tropical Animal Health and Production*, 21, 89–99.

246 **ROSSITER, P.B. & WARDLEY, R.C., 1985.** The differential growth of virulent and avirulent strains of rinderpest virus in bovine lymphocytes and macrophages. *Journal of General Virology*, 66, 969–975.

247 **RURANGIRWA, F.R., MUSHI, E.Z., TABEL, H., TIZARD, I.R. & LOSOS, G.J., 1980.** The effect of *Trypanosoma congolense* and *T. vivax* infections on the antibody response of cattle to live rinderpest virus vaccine. *Research in Veterinary Science*, 28, 264–266.

248 **RWEYEMAMU, M.M., REID, H.W. & OKUNA, N., 1974.** Observations on the behaviour of rinderpest virus in immune animals challenged intranasally. *Bulletin of Epizootic Diseases of Africa*, 22, 1–9.

249 **SANDERSON, J.B., 1866.** Nature, propagation, progress and symptoms of the disease. *Third Report of the Commissioners into the Origin and Nature etc. of the Cattle Plague*. London: Her Majesty's Stationery Office.

250 **SANDFORD, G.R., 1920.** *An Administrative and Political History of the Masai Reserve, East African Protectorate*. London: Waterlow and Sons Ltd.

251 **SATO, T.A., HAYAMI, M. & YAMANOUCHI, K., 1981.** Analysis of structural proteins of measles, canine distemper and rinderpest viruses. *Japanese Journal of Medical Science and Biology*, 34, 355–364.

252 **SCHEIN, H., 1917.** Études sur la peste bovine. *Annales de l'Institut Pasteur*, 31, 571–592.

253 **SCOTT, G.R., 1955.** The incidence of rinderpest in sheep and goats. *Bulletin of Epizootic Diseases of Africa*, 3, 117–119.

254 **SCOTT, G.R., 1957.** The risk associated with the importation of meat from countries where rinderpest control measures are still required. *Bulletin of Epizootic Diseases of Africa*, 5, 11–13.

255 **SCOTT, G.R., 1959.** A précis of the characteristics of rinderpest virus. *Bulletin of Epizootic Diseases of Africa*, 7, 173–178.

256 **SCOTT, G.R., 1959.** Heat inactivation of rinderpest-infected bovine tissues. *Nature*, 184, 1948–49.

257 **SCOTT, G.R., 1962.** Bovine hyperimmune serum in the diagnosis of rinderpest. *The Veterinary Record*, 74, 409.

258 **SCOTT, G.R., 1962.** Experimental rinderpest in Red Maasai sheep. *Bulletin of Epizootic Diseases of Africa*, 10, 423–426.

259 **SCOTT, G.R., 1963.** Adverse reaction in cattle after vaccination with lapinized rinderpest virus. *Journal of Hygiene, Cambridge*, 61, 193–203.

260 **SCOTT, G.R., 1964.** Rinderpest. *Advances in Veterinary Science*, 9, 113–224.

261 **SCOTT, G.R., 1964.** The new pseudorinderpest. *Bulletin of Epizootic Diseases of Africa*, 12, 287–298.

262 **SCOTT, G.R., 1967.** *Diagnosis of Rinderpest*. FAO Agricultural Studies No. 71. Rome: Food and Agriculture Organization.

263 **SCOTT, G.R., 1981.** Recrudescence of rinderpest in Africa. *Transactions of the Royal Society for Tropical Medicine and Hygiene*, 75, 892.

264 **SCOTT, G.R., 1982.** Rinderpest and peste des petits ruminants. In: GIBBS, E.P.J., (ed.). *Virus Diseases of Food Animals. A World Geography of Epidemiology and Control*. Vol. II. Disease monographs. London: Academic Press.

265 **SCOTT, G.R., 1985.** Rinderpest in the 1980s. *Progress in Veterinary Microbiology*, 1, 145–174.

266 **SCOTT, G.R. & BROWN, R.D., 1958.** A neutralisation test for the detection of rinderpest antibodies. *Journal of Comparative Pathology*, 68, 303–314.

267 **SCOTT, G.R. & BROWN, R.D., 1961.** Rinderpest diagnosis with special reference to the agar gel double diffusion test. *Bulletin of Epizootic Diseases of Africa*, 9, 83–100.

268 **SCOTT, G.R., COWAN, K.M. & ELLIOT, R.T., 1960.** Rinderpest in impala. *The Veterinary Record*, 72, 787–788.

269 **SCOTT, G.R., DE TRAY, D.E. & WHITE, G., 1962.** Rinderpest in pigs of European origin. *American Journal of Veterinary Research*, 23, 452–456.

270 **SCOTT, G.R. & MACDONALD, J., 1962.** Kenya camels and rinderpest. *Bulletin of Epizootic Diseases of Africa*, 10, 495–497.

271 **SCOTT, G.R., MACLEOD, A.K. & RAMPTON, C.S., 1963.** Goats as donors of rinderpest hyperimmune serum. *The Veterinary Record*, 75, 1221–1222.

272 **SCOTT, G.R., TAYLOR, W.P. & ROSSITER, P.B., 1986.** *Manual on the Diagnosis of Rinderpest*. FAO Animal Production and Health Series No 23. Rome: Food and Agriculture Organization.

273 **SCOTT, G.R. & WITCOMB, M.A., 1958.** Rinderpest virus in laboratory animals. *Report of the East African Veterinary Research Organisation, 1957*. Nairobi: Government Printer.

274 **SEN, S.K. & SALAM, A., 1937.** Experiments on the transmission of rinderpest through the agency of *Stomoxys calcitrans* (Linnaeus). *Indian Journal of Veterinary Science and Animal Husbandry*, 7, 219–224.

275 **SHANTHIKUMAR, S.R., MALACHI, S.A. & MAJIYAGBE, K.A., 1985.** Rinderpest outbreak in free-living wildlife in Nigeria. *The Veterinary Record*, 117, 469–470.

276 **SHARMA, B., BANDYOPADHAY, S.K., JOSHI, P.C. & BANSAL, R.P., 1984.** Antibody response of cattle to rinderpest vaccine. *Veterinary Microbiology*, 10, 189–192.

277 **SHARMA, B., JOSHI, R.C., LAHIRI, D.K. & BANSAL, R.P., 1983.** Evaluation of enzyme-linked immunosorbent assay in rinderpest. *Indian Journal of Animal Science*, 53, 1292–1295.

278 **SHARMA, B., LAHIRI, D.K., JOSHI, R.C. & BANSAL, R.P., 1986.** A comparison of immunofluorescent and immunoperoxidase test for the detection of rinderpest antigen in acetone fixed smears. *Indian Journal of Animal Science*, 55, 1292–1295.

279 **SHILSTON, A.W., 1917.** The vitality of the rinderpest virus outside the body under natural conditions. *Memoirs of the Department of Agriculture in India, Veterinary Series*, 3, 1032.

280 **SIMON, N., 1962.** *Between the Sunlight and the Thunder. The Wildlife of Kenya*. London: Collins.

281 **SINGH, S.N., 1972.** A passive haemagglutination test to detect rinderpest virus in spleen and blood. *Indian Veterinary Journal*, 49, 888–889.

282 **SINGH, K.V. & ATA, F., 1967.** Experimental rinderpest in camels. A preliminary report. *Bulletin of Epizootic Diseases of Africa*, 15, 19–23.

283 **SINGH, V.P. & MURTY, D.K., 1979.** An outbreak of rinderpest in wild spotted deer (Axis axis). *Indian Veterinary Journal*, 56, 988–990.

284 **STEVENSON-HAMILTON, J., 1911.** The relation between game and tsetse flies. *Bulletin of Entomological Research*, 2, 113.

285 **STEWART, D.R.M., 1968.** Rinderpest among wild animals in Kenya, 1963–66. *Bulletin of Epizootic Diseases of Africa*, 16, 139–140.

286 **STIRLING, R.F., 1932.** Some experiments in rinderpest vaccination: Active immunization of Indian Plains cattle with goat-adapted virus alone in field conditions. *Veterinary Journal*, 88, 192–204.

287 **STONE, S.S. & DE LAY, P.D., 1961.** The inactivation of rinderpest virus by b-propriolactone and its effect on homologous complement-fixing and neutralizing antibodies. *Journal of Immunology*, 87, 464–467.

288 **TAJIMA, M. & USHIJIMA, T., 1970.** The pathogenesis of rinderpest in the lymph nodes of cattle. *American Journal of Pathology*, 62, 221–235.

289 **TAJIMA, M., USHIJIMA, T., KISHI, S. & NAKAMURA, J., 1967.** Electron microscopy of cytoplasmic inclusion bodies in cells infected with rinderpest virus. *Virology*, 31, 92–100.

290 **TAKEMATSU, M. & MORIMOTO, T., 1954.** Studies on tissue culture with rinderpest virus. *Japanese Journal of Veterinary Science*, 16, 185–193.

291 **TAYLOR, W.P., 1968.** The susceptibility of the one-humped camel (*Camelus dromedarius*) to infection with rinderpest virus. *Bulletin of Epizootic Diseases of Africa*, 16, 405–410.

292 **TAYLOR, W.P., 1986.** Epidemiology and control of rinderpest. *Revue Scientifique et Technique de l'Office International des Épizooties*, 5, 407–410.

293 **TAYLOR, W.P. & PERRY, C.T., 1970.** A plaque assay system for rinderpest virus and its use in characterising virus adsorption. *Archives of Virology*, 32, 269–282.

294 **TAYLOR, W.P. & PLOWRIGHT, W., 1965.** Studies on the pathogenesis of rinderpest in experimental cattle. III. Proliferation of an attenuated strain in various tissues following sub-cutaneous inoculation. *Journal of Hygiene, Cambridge*, 63, 263–275.

295 **TAYLOR, W.P., PLOWRIGHT, W., PILLINGER, R., RAMPTON, C.S. & STAPLE, R.F., 1965.** Studies on the pathogenesis of rinderpest in experimental cattle. IV. Proliferation of the virus following contact infection. *Journal of Hygiene, Cambridge*, 63, 497–506.

296 **TAYLOR, W.P. & WATSON, R.M., 1967.** Studies of the epizootiology of rinderpest in blue wildebeest and other game species of Northern Tanzania and Southern Kenya, 1965–1967. *Journal of Hygiene, Cambridge*, 65, 537–545.

297 **TEUSHER, E., RAMACHANDRAN, S. & HARDING, H.P., 1981.** Observations on the pathology of Jembrana disease in Bali cattle. *Zentralblatt für Veterinärmedizin*, 28A, 608–622.

298 **THEILER, A., 1909.** Notes on stock disease of German and British East Africa and Uganda, and the resolutions of the International Veterinary Congress at the Hague, Holland, 1909. *Transvaal Agricultural Journal*, 8, 183–197.

299 **THIÉRY, G., 1956.** Influence du type de virus et de l'espèce affectée sur les lésions de la peste bovine. *Revue d'Élevage et de Médecine Vétérinaire des Pays Tropicaux*, 9, 109–115.

300 **THIÉRY, G., 1956b.** Hématologie, histopathologie et histochimie de la peste bovine. Intérêt de l'étude histochimique des inclusions cellulaires de la peste bovine pour la signification générale des inclusions dans les maladies à virus. *Revue d'Élevage et de Médecine Vétérinaire des Pays Tropicaux*, 9, 117–140.

301 **THOMAS, A.D. & REID, N.R., 1944.** Rinderpest in game: A description of an outbreak and an attempt at limiting its spread by means of a bush fence. *Onderstepoort Journal of Veterinary Science and Animal Industry*, 20, 7–23.

302 **TODD, C. & WHITE, R.G., 1914.** *Experiments on Cattle Plague*. Cairo: Government Press.

303 **TSUKIYAMA, K., SUGIYAMA, M., YOSHIKAWA, Y. & YAMANOUCHI, K., 1987.** Molecular cloning and sequence

analysis of the rinderpest mRNA encoding the haemagglutinin protein. *Virology*, 163, 48–54.

304 **TSUKIYAMA, K., YOSHIKAWA, Y. & YAMANOUCHI, K., 1988.** Fusion glycoprotein (F) of rinderpest virus: Entire nucleotide sequence of the F mRNA, and several features of the F protein. *Virology*, 164, 523–530.

305 **TURNER, G., 1906.** Rinderpest: Its prevention and cure. *Report of the British Association*, 1905, 552.

306 **VARNELL, G. & PRITCHARD, W., 1866.** On the treatment of the cattle plague. *Third Report of the Commissioners into the Origin and Nature etc. of the Cattle Plague*. London: Her Majesty's Stationery Office.

307 **VITTOZ, R., 1963.** *Report of the Director of the Scientific and Technical Activities of the Office International des Épizooties*, May 1962–May 1963. Paris: O.I.E.

308 **VIZOZO, A.D. & THOMAS, W.E., 1981.** Paramyxovirus of the morbilli group in the wild hedgehog *Erinaceus europeus*. *British Journal of Experimental Pathology*, 62, 79–86.

309 **VON OSTERTAG, R., 1916.** Ueber Rinderpest. Ein beitrag zum stande und der Bekampfung der Tierseuchen in Deutsch-Ostafrika. *Zeitschrift für Infektionskrankheiten, Parasitenkund Krankheiten und Hygiene der Haustiere*, 18, 1–48.

310 **WAFULA, J.S., MIRANGI, P.K., IRERI, R.G. & MBUGUA, N., 1986.** Development and stability of rinderpest virus antigens in cattle tears and lymph nodes. *Tropical Animal Health and Production*, 18, 26–30.

311 **WAFULA, J.S., ROSSITER, P.B., WAMWAYI, H.M. & SCOTT, G.R., 1989.** Preliminary observations on rinderpest in pregnant cattle. *The Veterinary Record*, 124, 485–486.

312 **WAGNER, G.G., JESSETT, D.M., BROWN, C.G.D. & RADLEY, D.E., 1975.** Diminished antibody response to rinderpest vaccination in cattle undergoing experimental East Coast fever. *Research in Veterinary Science*, 19, 209–211.

313 **WALKER, J., 1922.** *In: Bulletin Number 4*. Department of Agriculture, Division of Veterinary Research, Kenya.

314 **WALKER, R.V.L., BAKER, J.A. & JENKINS, D.L., 1946.** Rinderpest. II. Certain immunity reactions. *American Journal of Veterinary Research*, 7, 142–144.

315 **WALSH, J., 1987.** War on cattle disease divides the troops. *Science*, 237, 1289–1291.

316 **WAMWAYI, H.M., 1989.** Efficacy of some chemicals and disinfectants against rinderpest. *Bulletin of Animal Health and Production in Africa*, In press.

317 **WAMWAYI, H.M. & WAFULA, J.S., 1987.** Microtitre technique for detection and titration of rinderpest virus in infected bovine tissue and secretions. *Bulletin of Animal Health and Production in Africa*, 35, 318–320.

318 **WARREN, J.L., 1960.** The relationships of the viruses of measles, canine distemper and rinderpest. *Advances in Virus Research*, 7, 27–60.

319 **WATANABE, M., 1970.** Rinderpest: Diagnosis and prophylaxis. *National Institute of Animal Health Quarterly*, 10, 29–43.

320 **WATERSON, A.P., ROTT, R. & RUCKLE-ENDERS, G., 1963.** The components of measles virus and their relation to rinderpest and distemper. *Zentralblatt für Naturforschung*, 18b, 377–384.

321 **WESTON, E.A., 1924.** Rinderpest in Australia. *Journal of the American Veterinary Medical Association*, 19, 337–350.

322 **WHITE, R.G., 1958.** A specific diffusible antigen of rinderpest virus demonstrated by the agar double-diffusion precipitation reactions. *Nature*, 181, 1409.

323 **WHITE, R.G., SIMPSON, R.M. & SCOTT, G.R., 1961.** An antigenic relationship between the viruses of bovine rinderpest and canine distemper. *Immunology*, 4, 203–205.

324 **WILDE, J.K.H., 1948.** Rinderpest in some African wild mammals. *Journal of Comparative Pathology*, 58, 64–72.

325 **WILDE, J.K.H. & SCOTT, G.R., 1961.** Rinderpest interference with caprinized rinderpest virus. *Journal of Comparative Pathology*, 71, 222–227.

326 **YAMANOUCHI, K., 1980.** Comparative aspects of pathogenicity of measles, canine distemper and rinderpest virus. *Japanese Journal of Medical Science and Biology*, 33, 41–66.

327 **YAMANOUCHI, K., CHINO, F., KOBUNE, F., FUKUDA, A. & YOSHIKAWA, Y., 1974.** Pathogenesis of rinderpest infection in rabbits. I. Clinical signs, immune response, histological changes and virus growth patterns. *Infection and Immunity*, 9, 199–205.

328 **YAMANOUCHI, K., FUKUDA, A., KOBUNE, F., YOSHIKAWA, Y. & CHINO, F., 1974.** Pathogenesis of rinderpest virus infection in rabbits. II. Effect of rinderpest virus on the immune function of rabbits. *Infection and Immunity*, 9, 201–211.

329 **YILMA, T., HSU, D., JONES, L., OWENS, S., GRUBMAN, M., MEBUS, C., YAMANAKA, M. & DALE, B., 1988.** Protection of cattle against rinderpest with vaccinia virus recombinants expressing the HA or F gene. *Science*, 242, 1058–1060.

330 **ZEIN, A. & SROUR, E., 1985.** Production of interferon and of plaque enhancing factor by rinderpest-virus. *Zentralblatt für Veterinärmedizin*, B, 32, 466–471.

331 **ZONCHELLO, A., 1917.** Il gultian nel Sahel. *Clinica Veterinaria*, 30, 113–132.

332 **ZWART, D. & MACADAM, I., 1966.** Resistance of two bulls against rinderpest without detectable neutralizing antibodies in their sera. *Bulletin of Epizootic Diseases of Africa*, 14, 53–54.

333 **ZWART, D. & MACADAM, I., 1967.** Transmission of rinderpest by contact from cattle to sheep and goats. *Research in Veterinary Science*, 8, 37–47.

334 **ZWART, D. & MACADAM, I., 1967.** Observations on rinderpest in sheep and goats and transmission to cattle. *Research in Veterinary Science*, 8, 53–57.

335 **ZWART, D. & ROWE, L.W., 1966.** The occurrence of rinderpest antibodies in the sera of sheep and goats in northern Nigeria. *Research in Veterinary Science*, 7, 504–511.

75

Peste des petits ruminants

Synonyms: Goat plague, pseudo-rinderpest, stomatitis-pneumoenteritis-complex, 'kata'

P.B. Rossiter and W.P. Taylor

Peste des petits ruminants (PPR) is a disease of goats, sheep and closely related wild bovidae, and is clinically and pathologically similar to rinderpest. In the areas where it occurs it is the most economically important virus disease of small ruminants.

The disease was first described in 1942 by Gargadennec and Lalanne,[33] who were investigating a syndrome in sheep and goats in Côte d'Ivoire. Because of its clinical and pathological resemblance to rinderpest ('peste bovine'), it was called peste des petits ruminants, and it was soon recognized in other French West African colonies such as Dahomey (now Benin) and Senegal.[22, 56] Over a decade later workers in Nigeria began to study a syndrome that occurred primarily in goats and was variously named stomatitis-pneumoenteritis-complex, pseudo-rinderpest or 'kata'.[69, 82] Because of its predominance in goats, as opposed to sheep in the earlier French descriptions, and because of the crusty labial lesions commonly found in convalescent cases, this syndrome was initially considered to be distinct from PPR. More detailed investigations, however, clearly showed that the two diseases were indistinguishable,[38, 42, 68, 70] and the disease is now universally referred to by its original French name.

Peste des petits ruminants is widespread in the more northerly countries of sub-Saharan Africa and has been identified in the Sudan,[30] Ethiopia,[45] and the Arabian peninsula.[10, 32, 39] However, there is no clinical or serological evidence that PPR exists south of a line from Cameroon to the Sudan, and thus it is not yet present in the southern hemisphere. The disease has been reported in India[73] and recent serological evidence indicates its presence in Jordan.[49] The chronological sequence of reports of its occurrence gives the impression that PPR has been spreading steadily eastwards, but recent molecular evidence shows that non-African isolates are quite distinct from African isolates,[79] and it may be that PPR was frequently overlooked in some areas where rinderpest and contagious caprine pleuropneumonia are common.

Although rinderpest virus can infect goats and sheep in Africa, most experimental studies have induced only mild or subclinical infection.[66, 71] It therefore seems probable that several earlier descriptions of severe rinderpest in small ruminants, particularly in West Africa, were actually PPR.[12, 43] This was demonstrated by El Hag Ali and Taylor[30] who used specific antisera and transmission studies to confirm that virus isolates originally believed to be rinderpest virus from goats were actually the first isolates of peste des petits ruminants virus in eastern Africa.

There are several reviews of the disease.[9, 19, 48, 50, 72, 76]

Aetiology

The virus responsible for PPR is a morbillivirus in the family Paramyxoviridae.[35, 36, 38, 44] Several of the original studies showed the close relationship between PPR and rinderpest viruses[36, 55, 82] and, understandably, PPR virus was for a time considered to be a host-adapted variant of rinderpest virus. Field observation, however, showed the disease to be independent of rinderpest and cattle, and serology has revealed the immunological relationship between the two viruses to be as distant as that between rinderpest and the other morbilliviruses (measles and canine distemper).[35, 38, 74, 83] Recent studies with monoclonal antibodies and nucleic acid probes have confirmed the distinction between the two viruses, and that PPR virus is a completely separate pathogen.[23, 54] It has been proposed that PPR virus must have evolved from rinderpest more recently than the divergence between rinderpest, measles and canine distemper viruses.[54] If this is the case, then, bearing in mind that the first report of PPR was not until 1942, it is implied either that PPR virus evolved after the 1889–96 African rinderpest pandemic or that rinderpest was established in Africa long before the pandemic. Alternatively, PPR might have been independently introduced into Africa with sheep and goats from Asia, much as rinderpest was introduced in cattle. However, recent molecular studies have clearly distinguished between PPR viruses isolated from Africa and those from outside Africa,[79] and it has therefore been suggested that PPR may have evolved from the adaptation of rinderpest virus to small ruminants on at least two separate occasions, in Africa and Asia. More needs to be known about the polypeptide composition and genomic variability of the morbilliviruses before such speculation can be accepted as fact.

The virus can be isolated *in vitro* in primary sheep and goat kidney and Vero cells, and, once isolated, it also grows readily in some bovine kidney cell lines.[30, 36, 47, 67, 78] The physico-chemical characteristics, morphology and cytopathic effects produced by PPR virus are similar to those of rinderpest virus, although intranuclear inclusion bodies occur more frequently.[17, 28, 35, 38]

The N polypeptide of PPR virus has a molecular weight more like those of measles and canine distemper viruses than those of rinderpest virus,[24] and it is antigenically distinct from the N polypeptide of rinderpest virus.[53] Furthermore, African isolates can be readily distinguished from non-African isolates on the basis of the electrophoretic mobility of their N polypeptides.[79]

Epidemiology

In the field, PPR virus causes disease in goats and sheep but not in cattle or pigs, although the latter can be infected subclinically by experimental inoculation.[55, 56, 57] Goats are usually considered to be more susceptible than sheep,[15] but this is not always the case.[14, 76] Mornet *et al.*[55, 56] described oral erosions in some young calves, suggesting that cattle might rarely transmit infection rather than always acting as dead-end hosts (the converse of the situation with rinderpest in cattle and small ruminants in Africa).

Infectious virus can be detected for at least seven days after the onset of pyrexia in the ocular and nasal secretions, urine and faeces of infected animals.[2, 44] The survival of infectious virus outside the body has received little attention. In one laboratory study it was shown to have a half-life of approximately two hours at 37 °C and to be destroyed within an hour at 50 °C.[48] Comparable results were obtained using the Nig 75/1 strain in liquid medium.[77] The half-life of this virus at 56, 37, 4 and -20 °C was 2,2 minutes, 3,3 hours, 9,9 days and 24,2 days respectively. Between pH 5,85 and 9,5 the virus was stable, but it was rapidly inactivated below pH 4,0 or above pH 11,0. Lymph nodes from carcasses stored at 4 °C contain viable virus for at least eight days.[48]

Transmission probably occurs predominantly by the inhalation of aerosols derived from nearby animals, or by nuzzling and licking between infected and susceptible animals. Occasionally, bedding or feed and water troughs recently used by infected animals may be a source of infection.

As with rinderpest, the underlying requirement for the maintenance of the transmission cycle of PPR virus is a regular supply of susceptible hosts plus sufficient animal movement to allow mixing of the population. However, whereas rinderpest in Africa is now mainly confined to the large populations of cattle owned by migratory and semi-migratory pastoralists, PPR virus is maintained also at the village and urban level. Goats and sheep, as a readily available source of meat, are a universal commodity in villages, towns and even cities throughout Africa, the Middle East and Asia. Their populations are maintained by their own fertility, supplemented with frequent introductions from outside. In Oman the virus is more prevalent in unconfined urban and suburban goats than in those on fenced farms or in isolated villages.[79] Whether or not the virus can be maintained in a periurban situation without periodic reinfection from outside must depend upon the size of the population. Most urban populations are probably too small to maintain the virus independently and it has been noted that PPR was particularly frequent in Kumasi, Ghana following various festivals during which large numbers of sheep, including many brought in from outside, were ritually consumed.[13] The ease with which goats and sheep are infected with PPR, as opposed to cattle with rinderpest, is a major factor in the spread of this virus.

The local, rather than overall, epidemiology of the disease requires further investigation if apparently conflicting observations on the seasonality of outbreaks and main endemic areas are to be clarified.

Direct climatic effects are referred to in many reports: the onset of the rains and the humid season has been seen as a major triggering factor,[16, 60, 82] as has the beginning of the cool and dusty 'harmattan' period in November.[64] Both are significant climatic changes that probably play a role in the development of secondary bacterial pneumonia, which is a major complication of PPR. The indirect effects of climate on husbandry may also play a role: the disease flares up after the increased marketing of goats during periods of drought in the drier northern zone of Nigeria and, conversely, following marketing of goats to protect growing crops during the rains in the southern zone.[29, 31, 64, 82] Although the disease occurs in animals of all ages, the highest incidences are found in young stock less than two years old — sometimes in animals as young as four to eight months, in which maternal immunity would have waned to unprotective levels. The seasonality of outbreaks might also be related to seasonal kidding and lambing patterns.[60]

Many authors have noted that outbreaks in Nigeria are more commonly reported from the humid forest and derived savannahs, frequently as a result of animals being introduced from the drier north.[13, 16, 26] The breeds of sheep and goats in the Sahelian regions are inherently more resistant to the disease than are the notably susceptible dwarf varieties of the southern humid zone.[16, 26] These observations might suggest that the main endemic foci for PPR are the migratory sheep and goat herds of the Sahel, but the disease is less frequently encountered there and serological surveys have not shown the infection to be more prevalent there than in the humid south.[60, 74, 75, 81] However, the morbidity and mortality rates in outbreaks in the south are often very high, suggesting sporadic epidemics rather than true endemicity. For instance, in Nigeria mortality rates ranging from 20 to over 90 per cent have frequently been reported,[8, 62, 64, 65] whilst rates of only 4 to 5 per cent were recorded in what one author considered to be a true endemic area.[52] Certainly, serological surveys have shown that infection is far more prevalent than can be assessed from clinical reports[62, 74, 75] and that many, if not most, infections are subclinical or insufficiently severe to attract veterinary attention.

Also of interest is the comparative involvement of sheep and goats. Whilst it is widely felt that goats are more susceptible to the disease than sheep,[33, 48] outbreaks have occurred with both species being equally involved,[76, 78] or mainly in sheep.[13, 73] In some cases this may simply reflect the proportions of the two species in the locality,[13] but serology indicates that both species may suffer similar attack rates with resultant disease being more obvious in one or other species. Extrapolating from rinderpest, in which species adaptation is a feature, it is possible that there are variants of PPR virus adapted to sheep or goats.[76] Sub-Sahelian sheep are comparatively insusceptible to the disease,[16] and several serological surveys have recorded higher prevalences of antibody in sheep than in goats.[60, 74, 75, 81] Perhaps higher case mortality rates in goats account for the differences in antibody prevalences. However, in view of the current interest in mild rinderpest of cattle in endemic areas, a renewed investigation of inapparently infected goats and, especially, sheep in the areas north of the humid zone might provide further insight into the epidemiology of this disease.

The single most important factor that most authors have agreed upon, however, is that virtually all outbreaks can be traced to stock movements — either migration to new areas or the introduction of new animals.

During the 1980s there was a considerable extension in the worldwide distribution of PPR. Undoubtedly this is partly due to a greater awareness of the disease encouraging its 'discovery' in new areas, but the ease with which animals incubating the disease can be transported must be a contributory factor, and a southerly spread of infection in Africa should be expected.

A natural outbreak of PPR spread through a zoo in the United Arab Emirates killing wild sheep (*Ovis orientalis laristanica*), gazelles (*Gazella dorcas*), gemsbok (*Oryx gazella*) and a Nubian ibex (*Capra ibex nubiana*).[32] Other potentially susceptible species such as Dama gazelle (*Gazella dama*), Arabian and scimitar-horned oryx (*Oryx leucoryx* and *O. tao*), red-deer (*Cervus elaphus*) and blackbuck (*Antilopa cervicapra*) were not affected. White-tailed deer (*Odocoileus virginianus*), infected experimentally, developed both acute fatal and subclinical forms of the disease.[37] It is possible that the comparative susceptibility of various species to PPR and rinderpest viruses may shed more light on the complexities of bovid taxonomy.

Fortunately the spectre of peridomestic rats, which can be infected by experimental inoculation, as maintenance hosts for the virus was removed when they failed to transmit the infection to 'in-contact' goats.[46]

Pathogenesis

The pathogenesis of PPR has not been studied but it is assumed that it is essentially similar to that of rinderpest. Infection probably occurs via the oropharynx with subsequent virus multiplication in the draining lymph nodes and then in lymphoid tissue throughout the body. The ensuing viraemia transports the virus to susceptible epithelia, where it multiplies, causing the cytopathology responsible for the development of lesions and disease.

Virus and viral antigens can be detected in blood, secretions and lymphoid organs and tissues during the early stages of clinical disease. The titres of infectivity can reach 4,0 $\log_{10}$ $TCID_{50}$ in oral, nasal, ocular and pharyngeal swabs, and 5,0 $\log_{10}$ $TCID_{50}/g$ of faeces.[2] During the later stages of disease both infectious virus and antigen are increasingly difficult to detect, probably as a result of the rising antibody levels.

Counter-immuno-electrophoresis (CIEP) can detect precipitating antibody as early as three days after infection in some animals, although most have detectable antibody only after seven or eight days.[27] Precipitating antibody detected by the use of this technique seems to persist long enough for CIEP to be considered suitable for serological monitoring of vaccinated animals.[51]

Clinical signs

After an incubation period of between two and six days the first clinical sign is a rise in temperature that reaches 40–41 °C within two or three days. This is followed by depression, inappetence and development of serous nasal and ocular discharges which gradually become purulent and more profuse. The nasal discharge may block the nares and encrust the muzzle, causing the animal to snort and sneeze, while the ocular discharge may mat the eyelids together. One or two days after the start of pyrexia the buccal mucosa becomes congested and pale areas of necrosis become visible on the gums. In severe cases these increase in size and extend to involve the cheeks, dorsum of the tongue, hard palate and dental pad **(Figure 75.1)**. The caseous epithelium easily sloughs, leaving red erosions. Diarrhoea begins two or three days after the onset of pyrexia and death may occur some three to seven days later. Less severe and mild cases also occur, in which all or some of the signs develop to a lesser degree and the mortality rate is much lower.

Two clinical signs which are frequently seen in PPR but not in rinderpest are the formation of prominent crusty scabs (sometimes referred to in early descriptions as proliferative lesions) along the outside of the lips, and the development of pneumonia during the later stages of the disease.

It has been found that a considerable proportion of PPR-affected goats are also infected with *Escherichia coli* that produce a heat-labile enterotoxin which increases the clinical severity and mortality rate of PPR.[3, 41]

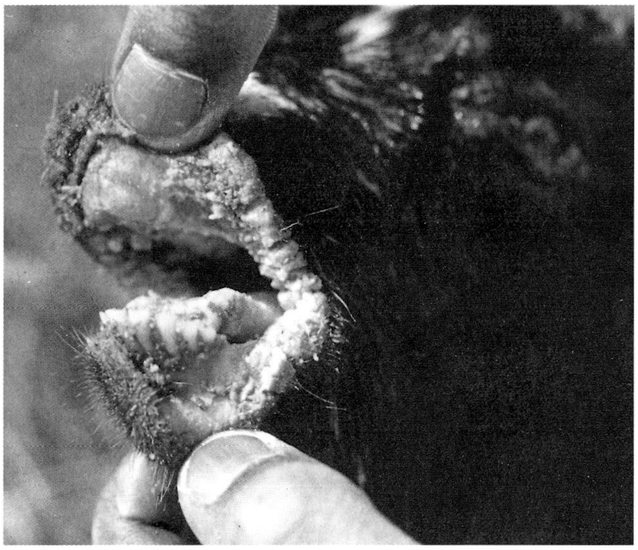

Figure 75.1
Acute necrotic stomatitis (By courtesy of Dr M. Bonniwell)

Pathology

Infected goats develop leukopenia which may correlate with the severity of clinical disease.[59, 80] Eosinopenia, monocytosis and a rise in the packed-cell volume, presumably due to haemoconcentration resulting from the diarrhoea, have also been reported.[59, 80]

The carcass is usually soiled with faeces and is frequently emaciated. Eyelids, nares and lips are usually encrusted with discharges. Erosions are found throughout the buccal cavity and pharynx, and less frequently the oesophagus. As with rinderpest, erosions in the forestomachs are not always seen, but may occasionally be found on the ruminal pillars and the leaves of the omentum.[21] The abomasum and small intestine are usually congested rather than eroded, and haemorrhages have been reported.[69, 70] Peyer's patches may be necrotic,[82] and erosions and congestion can be found on the ileocaecal valve.[55, 56] Marked congestion of the apices of the longitudinal folds of the mucosa (zebra striping) may be seen in the large intestine and rectum[21, 55, 56, 69] **(Figure 75.2)**.

The upper respiratory tract mucosa is usually congested, there may be erosions in the nares, and tracheitis has been described.[70] The lungs may be focally or diffusely congested, the affected areas appearing red and firm. Changes in the trachea and lungs are more severe if there is concurrent bacterial infection.

Peripheral and visceral lymph nodes may be oedematous and friable, but they are rarely enlarged or haemorrhagic. The spleen is often congested and firm. The female genital mucosa may be congested and show erosions.

Erosions which arise from hydropic degeneration and necrosis of epithelial cells in the *stratum granulosum* do not penetrate the underlying *stratum germinativum*.[21, 68, 69] Multinucleate giant cells, as well as eosinophilic intracytoplasmic and intranuclear inclusions are evident in the epithelium,[68] and inflammatory cells are prominent at the borders of the lesions. The 'proliferative' lesions on the lips contain necrotic debris, fibrin, mononuclear and polymorphonuclear leucocytes,[41, 69] but there is no hyperplasia or vascularization to suggest true proliferation.

Lymphoid tissues are depleted of lymphocytes. In lymph nodes the germinal centres are particularly affected. Pyknosis and karyorrhexis of lymphocytes are present in the cortex, and there is proliferation of reticuloendothelial cells along the medullary cords and in the sinuses.[21] Comparable changes are seen in the Malpighian bodies of the spleen. Necrosis throughout the Peyer's patches has been described,[82] although a mere reduction in the numbers of lymphocytes without necrosis may be all that is evident in this tissue.[69]

Isolated areas of epithelial necrosis occur in the deep glands of the abomasum, and similar but more widespread changes are seen throughout the intestine, together with atrophy of villi and accumulation of debris in the glandular crypts. The lamina propria is infiltrated with lymphocytes, macrophages and eosinophils.[41, 55, 56, 69]

Areas in the respiratory tract mucosa with both necrosis and hyperplasia have been described, and inclusion bodies can be seen in epithelial cells.[41, 69] Interstitial pneumonia involving the infiltration of lymphocytes and neutrophils, and proliferation of pneumocytes is common. A striking feature, not seen in rinderpest but characteristic of measles, is large giant cells, frequently

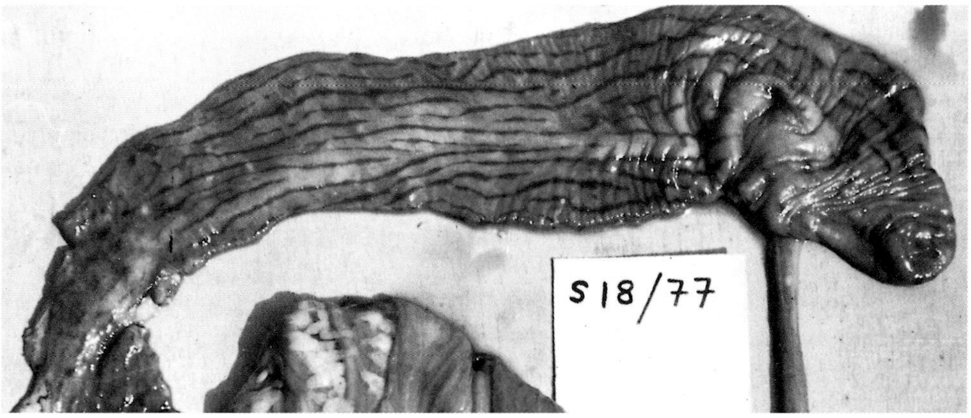

Figure 75.2 Caecum and colon manifesting streaks of congested mucosa, the so-called zebra striping (By courtesy of Dr M. Bonniwell)

containing intracytoplasmic and intranuclear viral inclusions, in the alveoli and terminal bronchioles. It seems probable that the virus is responsible for a primary pneumonia which then becomes superinfected with secondary pathogens.

Small foci of necrotic hepatocytes have been described in the liver and there may be evidence of glomerulonephritis.[56]

Paramyxovirus-like particles in degenerating cells in the lungs, particularly in alveolar macrophages, and intestinal epithelium have been described in ultrastructural studies,[41] as have intranuclear and intracytoplasmic nucleocapsids in intestinal epithelial cells, with apparent extrusion of extracellular viral particles from microvilli.[21]

Diagnosis

A presumptive diagnosis of PPR can be made from clinical signs and lesions together with epidemiological evidence such as the introduction of new and possibly diseased stock. In epidemic or virgin areas the diagnosis must be confirmed in the laboratory, either by the detection of virus-specific antigen or RNA, or by the isolation of virus in cell culture. Retrospective confirmation can be made by demonstrating a rise in antibody to PPR virus in paired sera.

Specimens should be collected from up to 10 acutely affected animals with fever and early mucosal lesions. Clotted or unclotted blood in anticoagulant as well as ocular, nasal and oral swabs should be collected from live animals. If possible two or three animals should be slaughtered and 20–30 g each of spleen, lymph nodes, lung and gut mucosa also collected. The specimens should be chilled on ice, but not frozen, and despatched to the laboratory as soon as possible.

Virus antigen in undiluted swab material or 30 per cent tissue suspensions is detected by hyperimmune serum to rinderpest virus in either immunodiffusion or counter-immuno-electrophoresis tests.[38, 51, 61, 76] Hyperimmune serum to PPR virus prepared in goats can also be used.[4] Antigen can also be detected by immunohistochemical staining of tissues.[21]

The virus is isolated by inoculating swab material, buffy coat or 10 per cent tissue suspensions onto young monolayers of primary sheep or goat kidney cells. Vero cells, some lines of primary bovine kidney and bovine T-lymphoblasts are also sensitive. Cytopathic effects develop after four days and are indistinguishable from rinderpest virus: rounding and shrinking of cells, strand formation and large flat syncytia. The identity of the virus: is confirmed as rinderpest virus or PPR virus by serological tests that use hyperimmune or convalescent sera to either virus. Distinction between the two viruses can then be made by comparative titrations against antisera to homologous and heterologous antisera, the homologous titre usually being much higher than the heterologous.[74] Alternatively the isolate can be examined with virus-specific monoclonal antibodies, or cDNA probes if these are available.[23, 54]

If cell-culture facilities are unavailable, then a pool of suspected tissue suspension should be inoculated into susceptible goats, sheep and cattle kept within suitable isolation facilities. Peste des petits ruminants usually causes severe disease in goats, milder disease in sheep and subclinical infection in cattle.[30, 76] Most African strains of rinderpest virus cause disease in cattle, but only subclinical or very mild disease in sheep and goats.

If neither antigen nor infectious virus can be detected in the test animals, survivors should be bled two to four weeks after the first sampling and the paired sera assayed for antibody levels to the virus in neutralization tests. A four-fold or greater increase in titre confirms the presumptive diagnosis.

Differential diagnosis

In India at least one strain of rinderpest virus has become adapted to sheep and goats and, therefore, investigations into PPR-like disease in south and south-west Asia and the Middle East should consider this possibility. In countries which have never reported PPR but do have rinderpest, all outbreaks of rinderpest-like disease in small ruminants should be carefully examined for both PPR and rinderpest viruses. In particular, all morbilliviruses isolated from goats or sheep should be further characterized with monoclonal antibodies, nucleic acid probes or by differential serology to reveal their true identity.[73]

The fact that the respiratory system is more frequently involved in PPR than in rinderpest increases the range of other conditions which can confuse diagnosis. Contagious caprine pleuropneumonia (CCPP) is widespread and prevalent in many parts of sub-Saharan Africa and causes high mortality in goats. In uncomplicated cases there are no mucosal lesions or diarrhoea in CCPP, and sheep are not affected. Concurrent infections with other *Mycoplasma* spp. are common and can obscure the diagnosis of PPR.[63] The frequent demonstration of intranuclear inclusions in lung tissue has suggested concurrent infection with other viruses. In particular, parainfluenza type 3 virus was thought to be involved, but serological and virological studies have not supported this.[21] Adenovirus together with PPR virus was recovered from the intestines of two goats that died of PPR in Nigeria.[34]

In East Africa PPR might be confused with Nairobi sheep disease (NSD), but oral lesions are minimal or absent in NSD, its distribution is restricted to areas infested with *Rhipicephalus appendiculatus*, and goats are rarely affected.

Peste des petits ruminants might be confused with foot-and-mouth disease or bluetongue, but these can be ruled out by closer examination of oral lesions, and the absence of diarrhoea.

Nematodiasis is a common cause of diarrhoea in sheep and goats, as is bacterial enteritis caused particularly by

E. coli and *Salmonella* serovars in kids and lambs. In convalescent goats the labial scabs can be confused with the mouth lesions of orf (contagious ecthyma), but this disease does not have the alimentary and pulmonary tract lesions seen in PPR.

Control

Affected and in-contact goats and sheep should be isolated from other stock and effective quarantine imposed until at least one month after the complete recovery of the last clinical case. Strict control of animal movement is essential for controlling the disease, but is often difficult to achieve. Goats and sheep, being more portable than cattle, are often transported long distances by bicycle and in vehicles and planes (one of the authors sat beside a man with a goat on his lap throughout a flight of several hundred kilometres in West Africa). Consequently, vaccination should be very important in the control of PPR. Regrettably, it has only been sparingly applied in most affected areas.

Since the early observations of cross-immunity between PPR and rinderpest viruses several workers have used attenuated rinderpest virus vaccine to protect sheep and goats against PPR.[1, 13–15, 18, 58, 75] This vaccine is safe in pregnant goats[6] and confers clinical immunity against challenge with virulent PPR virus for at least three years, although its longer-term duration is uncertain. Its regular use in Oman has already led to an increase in that country's small ruminant population.[79] Kids born to dams that have been immunized with rinderpest virus have heterologous colostral antibodies to PPR virus for up to three months.[11] This is shorter than the four to eight months usually described in calves with homologous maternal immunity to rinderpest virus.[20] Attenuated PPR virus vaccines which protect goats against experimental challenge have now been developed. One of these required 55–61 passages in Vero cells to achieve attenuation,[25] whereas the other[5] was still virulent at 60 passages in Vero cells and required at least 80 passages before it was suitably attenuated. Details of their efficacy in the field are being assessed at present but it seems reasonable to assume that they will induce a long, probably lifetime, immunity in small ruminants.

Infected premises should be thoroughly cleaned and disinfected with solutions containing lipid solvents, or agents with high or low pH.

There is no established therapy for affected animals. Hyperimmune serum administered during early clinical disease has been reported to help recovery,[40] but antibiotics have little effect.[7] Fluid replacement should be considered for valuable individuals with diarrhoea. Good husbandry and nursing are needed during convalescence.

References

1 **ABEGUNDE, A.A., 1983.** Problems connected with TCRV vaccination of sheep and goats. *In*: HILL, D.H., (ed.). *Peste des Petits Ruminants (PPR) in Sheep and Goats*. Proceedings of the International Workshop, Ibadan, Nigeria, 1980. 79–81. International Livestock Centre for Africa, Addis Ababa.

2 **ABEGUNDE, A.A. & ADU, F., 1977.** Excretion of the virus of peste des petits ruminants by goats. *Bulletin of Animal Health and Production in Africa*, 25, 307–311.

3 **ADETOSOYE, A.I. & OJO, M.O., 1983.** Characteristics of *Escherichia coli* isolated from goats suffering from 'peste des petits ruminants'. *Tropical Animal Health and Production*, 16, 119–122.

4 **ADU, F.D. & JOANNIS, T., 1985.** Goat hyperimmune serum for the diagnosis of peste des petits ruminants. *The Veterinary Record*, 117, 472.

5 **ADU, F.D., JOANNIS, T., NWOSUH, E. & ABEGUNDE, A.A., 1990.** Pathogenicity of attenuated peste des petits ruminants virus in sheep and goats. *Revue d'Élevage et de Médecine Vétérinaire des Pays Tropicaux*, 43, 23–26.

6 **ADU, F.D. & NAWATHE, D.R., 1981.** Safety of tissue culture rinderpest vaccine in pregnant goats. *Tropical Animal Health and Production*, 13, 166.

7 **ANENE, B.M., UGOCHUKWU, E.I. & OMAMEGBE, J.O., 1987.** The appraisal of three different pharmaceutical regimes for the treatment of naturally occurring peste des petits ruminants (PPR) in goats. *Bulletin of Animal Health and Production in Africa*, 35, 1–3.

8 **APPELL, M.J.G., GIBBS, E.P.J., MARTIN, S.J., MEULEN, V.T., RIMA, B.K., STEPHENSON, J.R. & TAYLOR, W.P., 1981.** Morbillivirus diseases of animal and man. *In*: KURSTAK, D., (ed.). *Comparative Diagnosis of Virus Diseases*. Vol. IV. New York: Academic Press.

9 **APPIAH, S.N., 1982.** Peste des petits ruminants (PPR) — A review. *Bulletin of Animal Health and Production in Africa*, 30, 179–184.

10 **ASMAR, J.A., RADWAN, A.I., ABI ASSI, H. & AL RASHEID, A., 1980.** A PPR-like disease in sheep in Central Saudi Arabia. Evidence of its immunological relation to rinderpest; prospects for a control method. *Annual Meeting of the Saudi Arabian Society of Biological Sciences*, Unpublished, 2 pp.

11 **ATA, F.A., AL SUMRY, H.S., KING, G.J., ISMAILI, S.I. & ATA, A.A., 1989.** Duration of maternal immunity to peste des petits ruminants. *The Veterinary Record*, 124, 590–591.

12 **BEATON, W.G., 1930.** Rinderpest in goats in Nigeria. *Journal of Cooperative Pathology*, 43, 301–307.

13 **BONNIWELL, M.A., 1980.** The use of tissue culture rinderpest vaccine (TCRV) to protect sheep and goats against peste des petits ruminants in the Ashanti region of Ghana. *Bulletin de l'Office International des Épizooties*, 92, 1233–1238.

14 **BONNIWELL, M.A., 1983.** The results of TCRV in Ghana. *In*: HILL, D.H., (ed.). *Peste des Petits Ruminants (PPR) in Sheep and Goats*. Proceedings of the International Workshop, Ibadan, Nigeria, 1980. 85–87. International Livestock Centre for Africa, Addis Ababa.

15 **BOURDIN, P., 1973.** La peste des petits ruminants (PPR) et sa prophylaxie au Senegal et en Afrique de l'Ouest. *Revue d'Élevage et de Médecine Vétérinaire des Pays Tropicaux*, 26, 71–74.

16 **BOURDIN, P., 1983.** History, epidemiology and economic significance of PPR in West Africa and Nigeria in particular. *In*: HILL, D.H., (ed.). *Peste des Petits Ruminants (PPR) in Sheep and Goats*. Proceedings of the International Workshop,

Ibadan, Nigeria, 1980. International Livestock Centre for Africa, Addis Ababa.

17 **BOURDIN, P. & LAURENT-VAUTIER, A., 1967.** Note sur la structure du virus de la peste des petits ruminants. *Revue d'Élevage et de Médecine Vétérinaire des Pays Tropicaux*, 20, 383–386.

18 **BOURDIN, P., RIOCHE, M. & LAURENT, A., 1970.** Emploi d'un vaccin antibovipestique produit sur cultures cellulaires dans la prophylaxie de la peste des petits ruminants au Dahomey — note preliminaire. *Revue d'Élevage et de Médecine Vétérinaire des Pays Tropicaux*, 23, 295–300.

19 **BRAIDE, V.B., 1981.** Peste des petits ruminants: A review. *World Animal Review*, 39, 25–28.

20 **BROWN, R.D., 1958.** Rinderpest immunity in calves. I. The acquisition and persistence of maternally derived antibody. *Journal of Hygiene, Cambridge*, 56, 427–434.

21 **BUNDZA, A., AFSHAR, A., DUKES, T.W., MYERS, D.J., DULAC, G.C. & BECKER, S.A.W.E., 1988.** Experimental peste des petits ruminants (goat plague) in goats and sheep. *Canadian Journal of Veterinary Research*, 52, 46–52.

22 **CATHOU, Y., 1944.** *Rapport Annuel du Service de l'Élevage au Dahomey*. Benin: Government Printer.

23 **DIALLO, A., BARRETT, T., BARBRON, M., SHAILA, M.S. & TAYLOR, W.P., 1989.** Differentiation of rinderpest and peste des petits ruminants viruses using specific cDNA clones. *Journal of Virological Methods*, 23, 127–136.

24 **DIALLO, A., BARRETT, T., LEFEVRE, P.C. & TAYLOR, W.P., 1987.** Comparison of proteins induced in cells infected with rinderpest and peste des petits ruminants virus. *Journal of General Virology*, 68, 2033–2038.

25 **DIALLO, A., TAYLOR, W.P., LEFEVRE, P.C. & PROVOST, A., 1989.** Attenuation d'une souche de virus de la peste des petits ruminants: Candidat pour un vaccin homologue vivant. *Revue d'Élevage et de Médecine Vétérinaire des Pays Tropicaux*, 42, 311–319.

26 **DUROJAIYE, O.A., 1983.** Brief notes on history, epizootiology and the economic importance of PPR in Nigeria. *In*: HILL, D.H., (ed.). *Peste des Petits Ruminants (PPR) in Sheep and Goats*. Proceedings of the International Workshop, Ibadan, Nigeria, 1980. International Livestock Centre for Africa, Addis Ababa.

27 **DUROJAIYE, O.A. & TAYLOR, W.P., 1984.** Application of countercurrent immuno-electro-osmo-phoresis to the serology of peste des petits ruminants. *Revue d'Élevage et de Médecine Vétérinarie des Pays Tropicaux*. 37, 272–276.

28 **DUROJAIYE, O.A., TAYLOR, W.P. & SMALE, C., 1985.** The ultrastructure of peste des petits ruminants virus. *Zentralblatt für Veterinärmedizin*, 32, 460–465.

29 **DURTNELL, R.E., 1972.** A disease of Sokoto goats resembling peste des petits ruminants. *Tropical Animal Health and Production*, 4, 162–164.

30 **EL HAG ALI, B. & TAYLOR, W.P., 1984.** Isolation of peste des petits ruminants virus from the Sudan. *Research in Veterinary Science*, 36, 1–4.

31 **EZEOKOLI, C.D., UMOH, J.U., CHINEME, C.N., ISITOR, G.N. & GYANG, E.O., 1986.** Clinical and epidemiological features of peste des petits ruminants in Sokoto Red goats. *Revue d'Élevage et de Médecine Vétérinaire des Pays Tropicaux*, 39, 269–273.

32 **FURLEY, C., TAYLOR, W.P. & OBI, T.U., 1987.** An outbreak of peste des petits ruminants in a zoological collection. *The Veterinary Record*, 121, 443–447.

33 **GARGADENNEC, L. & LALANNE, A., 1942.** La peste des petits ruminants. *Bulletin des Services Zootechniques et des Épizooties de l'Afrique Occidentale Française*, 5, 16–21.

34 **GIBBS, E.P.J., TAYLOR, W.P. & LAWMAN, M.J.P., 1977.** Isolation of adenoviruses from goats affected with peste des petits ruminants in Nigeria. *Research in Veterinary Science*, 23, 331–335.

35 **GIBBS, E.P.J., TAYLOR, W.P., LAWMAN, M.J.P. & BRYANT, J., 1979.** Classification of peste des petits ruminants virus as the fourth member of the genus *Morbillivirus*. *Intervirology*, 11, 268–274.

36 **GILBERT, Y. & MONNIER, J., 1962.** Adaptation du virus de la peste des petits ruminants aux cultures cellulaires — note preliminaire. *Revue d'Élevage et de Médecine Vétérinaire des Pays Tropicaux*, 15, 321–335.

37 **HAMDY, F.M. & DARDIRI, A.H., 1976.** Response of white-tailed deer to infection with 'Peste des petits ruminants' virus. *Journal of Wildlife Diseases*, 12, 191–196.

38 **HAMDY, F.M., DARDIRI, A.H., NDUAKA, O., BREESE, S.S. & IHEMELANDU, E.C., 1976.** Etiology of the stomatitis pneumoenteritis complex in Nigerian dwarf goats. *Canadian Journal of Comparative Medicine*, 40, 516–522.

39 **HEDGER, R.S., BARNETT, I.T.R. & GRAY, D.F., 1980.** Some virus diseases of domestic animals in the Sultanate of Oman. *Tropical Animal Health and Production*, 17, 83–88.

40 **IHEMELANDU, E.C., NDUAKA, O. & OJUKWU, E.M., 1985.** Hyperimmune serum in the control of peste des petits ruminants. *Tropical Animal Health and Production*, 17, 83–88.

41 **ISITOR, G.N., EZEOKOLI, C.D. & CHINEME, C.M., 1984.** A histopathological and ultrastructural study of lesions of peste des petits ruminants. *Tropical Veterinarian*, 2, 151–158.

42 **ISOUN, T.T. & MANN, E.D., 1972.** A stomatitis and pneumoenteritis complex of sheep in Nigeria. *Bulletin of Epizootic Diseases of Africa*, 20, 167–174.

43 **JOHNSON, R.H., 1958.** An outbreak of rinderpest involving cattle and sheep. *The Veterinary Record*, 70, 457–461.

44 **JOHNSON, R.H. & RITCHIE, J.S.D., 1968.** A virus associated with pseudo-rinderpest in Nigerian dwarf goats. *Bulletin of Epizootic Diseases of Africa*, 16, 411–417.

45 **KITCHING, P. & BARRETT, T., 1991.** Institute of Animal Health, Pirbright, UK. Personal communication.

46 **KOMOLAFE, O.O., UGWU, H.O. & EBIRIM, R.A., 1987.** An investigation into the possible role of peridomestic rats in the epizootiology of peste des petits ruminants in goats. *Bulletin of Animal Health and Production in Africa*, 35, 207–210.

47 **LAURENT, A., 1968.** Aspects biologiques de la multiplication du virus de la peste des petits ruminants ou PPR sur les cultures cellulaires. *Revue d'Élevage et de Médecine Vétérinaire des Pays Tropicaux*, 21, 297–308.

48 **LEFEVRE, P.C., 1987.** Peste des petits ruminants et infection bovipestique des ovins et caprins. Etudes et synthèses de l'I.E.M.V.T., nombre 5, douzième edition. Institut d'Élevage et de Médecine Vétérinaire des Pays Tropicaux, Maison Alfort, France.

49 **LEFEVRE, P.C., DIALLO, A., SCHENKEL, F., HUSSEIN, S. & STAAK, G., 1991.** Serological evidence of peste des petits ruminants in Jordan. *The Veterinary Record*, 128, 110.

50 **LOSOS, G., 1986.** Peste des petits ruminants. *In*: LOSOS, G., (ed.). *Infectious Tropical Diseases of Domestic Animals*. London: Longmans.

51 **MAJIYAGBE, K.A., NAWATHE, D.R. & ABEGUNDE, A., 1984.** Rapid diagnosis of peste des petits ruminants (PPR) infection, application of immuno-electrophoresis (IEOP) technique. *Revue d'Élevage et de Médecine Vétérinaire des Pays Tropicaux*, 37, 11–15.

52 **MATHEW, Z., 1983.** Epidemiology of PPR in Nigeria. *In*: HILL, D.H., (ed.). *Peste des Petits Ruminants (PPR) in Sheep and Goats*. Proceedings of the International Workshop, Ibadan, Nigeria, 1980. 22–23. International Livestock Centre for Africa, Addis Ababa.

53 **McCULLOUGH, K.C., OBI, T.U. & SHESHBERADARAN, H., 1991.** Identification of epitope(s) on the internal virion proteins of rinderpest virus which are absent from peste des petits ruminants virus. *Veterinary Microbiology*, 26, 313–321.

54 **McCULLOUGH, K.C., SHESHBERADARAN, H., NORRBY, E., OBI, T.U. & CROWTHER, J.R., 1986.** Monoclonal antibodies against morbilliviruses. *Revue Scientifique et Technique de l'Office International des Épizooties*, 5, 411–427.

55 **MORNET, P., ORUE, J. & GILBERT, Y., 1956.** Unicité et plasticité du virus bovipestique. A propos d'un virus naturel adapté sur petits ruminants. *Comptes Rendus Hebdomadaires des Séances de l'Académie des Sciences*, 242, 2886–2889.

56 **MORNET, P., ORUE, J., GILBERT, Y., THIERY, G. & MAMADOU, S., 1956.** La 'peste des petits ruminants' en Afrique occidentale Française. Ses rapports avec la peste bovine. *Revue d'Élevage et de Médecine Vétérinaire des Pays Tropicaux*, 9, 313–342.

57 **NAWATHE, D.R. & TAYLOR, W.P., 1979.** Experimental infection of domestic pigs with the virus of peste des petits ruminants. *Tropical Animal Health and Production*, 11, 120–122.

58 **OBI, T.U., 1983.** Results of TCRV vaccination in Nigeria. *In*: HILL, D.H., (ed.). *Peste des Petits Ruminants (PPR) in Sheep and Goats*. Proceedings of the International Workshop, Ibadan, Nigeria, 1980. 82–83. International Livestock Centre for Africa, Addis Ababa.

59 **OBI, T.U. & ODUYE, O.O., 1985.** Haematological changes in natural and experimental peste des petits ruminants virus infection in goats. *Revue d'Élevage et de Médecine Vétérinaire des Pays Tropicaux*, 39, 11–15.

60 **OBI, T.U., OJO, M.O., TAYLOR, W.P. & ROWE, L.W., 1983.** Studies on the epidemiology of peste des petits ruminants in southern Nigeria. *Tropical Veterinarian*, 1, 209–217.

61 **OBI, T.U. & PATRICK, D., 1984.** The detection of peste des petits ruminants (PPR) virus antigen by agar gel precipitation test and counter-immuno-electrophoresis. *Journal of Hygiene*, 93, 579–586.

62 **OBI, T.U., ROWE, L.W. & TAYLOR, W.P., 1984.** Serological studies with peste des petits ruminants and rinderpest viruses in Nigeria. *Tropical Animal Health and Production*, 16, 115–118.

63 **ONOVIRAN, O., MAJIYAGBE, K.A., MOLOKWU, J.U., CHIMA, J.C. & ABEGBOYE, D.S., 1984.** Experimental infection of goats with *Mycoplasma capri* and 'peste des petits ruminants' virus. *Revue d'Élevage et de Médecine Vétérinaire des Pays Tropicaux*, 37, 16–18.

64 **OPASINA, B.A., 1983.** Epidemiology of PPR in the humid forest and the dried savannah zones. *In*: HILL, D.H., (ed.). *Peste des Petits Ruminants (PPR) in Sheep and Goats*. Proceedings of the International Workshop, Ibadan, Nigeria, 1980. 14–21. International Livestock Centre for Africa, Addis Ababa.

65 **OPASINA, B.A. & PUTT, S.N.H., 1985.** Outbreaks of peste des petits ruminants in village goat flocks in Nigeria. *Tropical Animal Health and Production*, 17, 219–224.

66 **PLOWRIGHT, W., 1952.** Observations on the behaviour of rinderpest virus in indigenous African sheep. *British Veterinary Journal*, 108, 450–457.

67 **ROSSITER, P.B., JESSETT, D.M. & TAYLOR, W.P., 1985.** Microneutralization systems for use with different strains of peste des petits ruminants virus and rinderpest virus. *Tropical Animal Health and Production*, 17, 75–81.

68 **ROWLAND, A.C. & BOURDIN, P., 1970.** The histological relationship between 'peste des petits ruminants' and kata in West Africa. *Revue d'Élevage et de Médecine Vétérinaire des Pays Tropicaux*, 23, 301–307.

69 **ROWLAND, A.C., SCOTT, G.R. & HILL, H.D., 1969.** The pathology of an erosive stomatitis and enteritis in West African dwarf goats. *Journal of Pathology*, 98, 83–87.

70 **ROWLAND, A.C., SCOTT, G.R., RAMACHANDRAN, S. & HILL, H.D., 1971.** A comparative study of 'peste des petits ruminants' and 'kata' in West African dwarf goats. *Tropical Animal Health and Production*, 3, 241–247.

71 **SCOTT, G.R., 1962.** Experimental rinderpest in Red Masai sheep. *Bulletin of Epizootic Diseases of Africa*, 10, 423–426.

72 **SCOTT, G.R., 1981.** Rinderpest and peste des petits ruminants. *In*: GIBBS, E.P.J., (ed.). *Virus Diseases of Food Animals*. Vol. II. Disease monographs. 401–432. London: Academic Press.

73 **SHAILA, M.S., PURUSHOTHAMAN, V., BHAVASAR, S., VENUGOPAL, K. & VENKATESAN, R.A., 1989.** Peste des petits ruminants of sheep in India. *The Veterinary Record*, 125, 602.

74 **TAYLOR, W.P., 1979.** Serological studies with the virus of 'peste des petits ruminants' in Nigeria. *Research in Veterinary Science*, 26, 236–242.

75 **TAYLOR, W.P., 1979.** Protection of goats against 'peste des petits ruminants' with attenuated rinderpest virus. *Research in Veterinary Science*, 27, 321–324.

76 **TAYLOR, W.P., 1984.** The distribution and epidemiology of 'peste des petits ruminants'. *Preventive Veterinary Medicine*, 2, 157–166.

77 **TAYLOR, W.P., 1990.** National Project on Rinderpest Eradication, 16/15 West Extension Area, Karol Bagh, New Delhi 110005, India. Unpublished data.

78 **TAYLOR, W.P. & ABEGUNDE, A., 1979.** The isolation of peste des petits ruminants virus from Nigerian sheep and goats. *Research in Veterinary Science*, 26, 94–96.

79 **TAYLOR, W.P., AL BUSAIDY, S. & BARRETT, T., 1990.** The epidemiology of peste des petits ruminants in the Sultanate of Oman. *Veterinary Microbiology*, 22, 341–352.

80 **UGOCHUKWU, E.I., 1983.** Haematological observations in goats suffering from natural infection of pneumonia enteritis complex (peste of small ruminants virus). *Bulletin of Animal Health and Production in Africa*, 31, 337–341.

81 **WALTON, C., JEROME, C.P. & MILREE, J.M., 1977.** Prevalence of neutralizing antibodies to the virus of peste des petits ruminants (PPRV) in the sera of sheep and goats in northern Nigeria. Final report of the Royal Veterinary College, West Africa Research Team, pp. 47–54. Royal Veterinary College, London.

82 **WHITNEY, J.C., SCOTT, G.R. & HILL, D.H., 1967.** Preliminary observations on a stomatitis and enteritis of goats in southern Nigeria. *Bulletin of Epizootic Diseases of Africa*, 15, 331–341.

83 **ZWART, D. & ROWE, L.W., 1966.** The occurrence of rinderpest antibodies in the sera of sheep and goats in northern Nigeria. *Research in Veterinary Science*, 7, 504–511.

76

Parainfluenza type 3 infection

M. van Vuuren

Introduction

Parainfluenza type 3 (PI-3) virus commonly causes respiratory infection in cattle, sheep and goats with little or no clinical manifestation. However, in association with other viral and bacterial pathogens and stress-inducing situations, it causes severe pneumonia in cattle which is sometimes referred to as 'shipping fever' or enzootic pneumonia. It also infects humans. However, it is uncertain whether or not the infection can be transmitted between people and animals.

Four serotypes of parainfluenza virus have been described, but almost all infection and disease in livestock are caused by serotype 3 (PI-3). The virus was first described by Reisinger *et al.* in the USA in 1959.[20] It has a worldwide distribution in cattle, sheep and goats and is regularly isolated from clinical cases of respiratory disease in feedlot cattle. Together with other infectious agents, PI-3 virus constitutes part of the bovine respiratory disease complex[25] **(see Chapter 141: Pneumonic pasteurellosis)**. In South Africa, serological studies have shown the virus to be widespread among feedlot cattle,[2] and the virus has been isolated from cattle with clinical signs of respiratory disease.[27]

Apart from its association with disease in cattle and sheep,[13] PI-3 virus may also be involved in mild respiratory disease of goats[7] and it has been described in horses,[9] although it is not recognized as being a common or important cause of respiratory disease in that species. The virus has been isolated from an aborted bovine foetus,[22] and haemagglutination-inhibiting antibodies were found in 53 per cent of aborted foetuses in one study in the USA,[10] but the significance of these findings is unclear as PI-3 is not a common or important cause of reproductive failure.[1]

Aetiology

Parainfluenza viruses are classified in the genus *Paramyxovirus* of the family Paramyxoviridae.[15] The virions are enveloped and measure between 120 and 300 microns for the round and pleomorphic forms **(Figure 76.1)**, and up to 5 000 microns in length for filamentous forms. The single-stranded negative-sense RNA genome is unsegmented. Nucleocapsids have helical symmetry and show characteristic herring-bone patterns **(Figure 76.2)**. The envelope contains lipids and glycosylated fusion (F) and haemagglutinin-neuraminidase (HN) proteins. These proteins are responsible for cellular fusion (syncytium formation), adsorption of the virus to cell surfaces and its subsequent release.

Human, bovine and ovine PI-3 viruses are antigenically related but are not identical.[5] Differences in haemagglutinin, neuraminidase and syncytium-inducing (F protein) activities may be related to differences in pathogenicity of different isolates.[3, 23]

Epidemiology

Apart from livestock and humans, PI-3 virus has also been found in captive monkeys (*Erythrocebus patas*),[6] water buffaloes[24] and African buffaloes (*Syncerus caffer*).[14] There have also been reports of infection in deer, dogs, cats, guinea-pigs and rats,[11] indicating a wide host range. However, it is not clear whether or not these species constitute a source of infection for livestock.

The virus is shed in nasal and ocular secretions; in experimentally infected cattle shedding of the virus may continue for eight to ten days after exposure.[29] Susceptible cattle presumably become infected by means of aerosols that come into contact with the mucous membranes of the eyes, nostrils, and genital tract. Persistently infected (carrier) animals have not been reported.

The interrelationship between PI-3, other infectious agents and conditions which induce stress in the causation of the bovine respiratory complex is discussed elsewhere **(see Chapter 141: Pneumonic pasteurellosis)**.

Pathogenesis

Epithelial cells in the trachea, bronchi and alveoli are infected primarily. Necrosis of ciliated epithelium interferes with the mucociliary clearance of dust, fluid and cellular debris from the airways.

There is no evidence that PI-3 virus infection in cattle is immunosuppressive, but it does predispose lung tissue

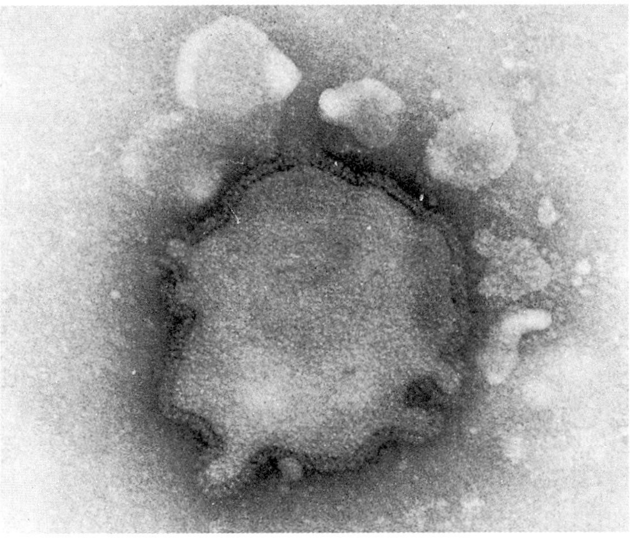

Figure 76.1 Parainfluenza type 3 virus: pleomorphic form

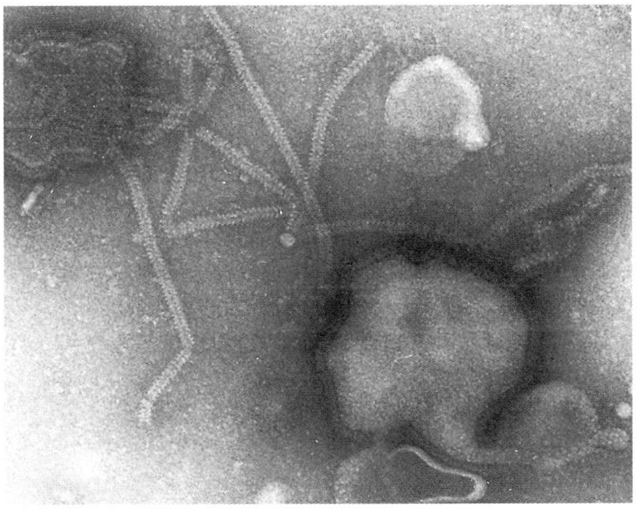

Figure 76.2 Parainfluenza type 3 virus: note herring-bone pattern of nucleocapsids

to bacterial invasion — mainly as a result of its effect on alveolar macrophages,[4, 8, 17, 18] in which it is capable of replication.[21, 26]

Clinical signs and pathology

Most PI-3 virus infections in cattle are mild or clinically inapparent. Development of clinical disease is usually dependent upon interaction with other factors, both infectious and environmental **(see Chapter 141: Pneumonic pasteurellosis)**. Where PI-3 virus expresses its pathogenic potential in combination with *Pasteurella* spp. infections, the clinical signs and lesions are typical of bovine pneumonic pasteurellosis.

After an incubation period of between 24 and 36 hours, a fever that may last six to ten days will develop in some calves. In uncomplicated cases the fever is accompanied by lachrymation, serous to mucopurulent nasal discharge, depression and dyspnoea. Recovery is the general rule, but when secondary bacterial infection occurs, coughing, dyspnoea and depression may be severe and can be fatal in three to four days.

Gross lesions in fatal cases are those of bronchopneumonia, mainly in the ventral parts of the cranial and medial lobes, and consist of areas of congestion, atelectasis and consolidation. Evidence of mucopurulent inflammation of the upper respiratory tract is also usually present.

Microscopic changes include bronchitis, bronchiolitis, atelectasis, alveolitis, interstitial pneumonia, acidophilic intracytoplasmic and, more rarely, intranuclear inclusions in nasal, bronchiolar and bronchial epithelia, and the development of syncytia in affected parts of the lungs.[12, 29]

Clinical signs in sheep and goats are characterized by nasal and ocular discharges, coughing, rapid respiration, listlessness, anorexia and fever.[7, 16]

Gross lesions in sheep and goats are similar to the lesions seen in cattle, namely consolidation of cranioventral lung lobes. Microscopically the principal features are neutrophil and macrophage accumulation in the alveoli and bronchi. Inclusions are limited to the cytoplasm of some affected epithelial cells; only bovine strains of PI-3 virus have so far been shown to produce intranuclear inclusions.[19]

Diagnosis

The diagnosis of paramyxovirus infections is dependent on virus isolation, the detection of virus antigen in tissue specimens or the demonstration of rising antibody levels.

In live animals the virus can be isolated from nasopharyngeal swabs or broncho-alveolar washings, and in dead animals from the lungs and trachea and their associated lymph nodes. The virus can be grown in a variety of primary and secondary cell cultures, such as bovine and ovine foetal lung, kidney and testis, as well as in line cells, such as MDBK and RK-13. Cytopathic effects develop, and these are characterized by syncytia, intracytoplasmic and intranuclear inclusion bodies and cell destruction. However, this does not always happen at the first passage, particularly when cell lines are employed. Virus antigen can be demonstrated in infected cell cultures by haemadsorption with bovine or guinea-pig red blood cells. Specific identification of the antigen can be achieved by haemadsorption inhibition and immunofluorescence.

Serological diagnosis is based on haemagglutination inhibition and virus neutralization or on plaque reduction tests. As a result of the presence of serum antibodies in most cattle, paired serum samples (i.e. acute and convalescent) are essential for the demonstration of seroconversion.

Parainfluenza type 3 virus antigen can be detected in tissue specimens (e.g. cryo-preserved or paraffin-embedded lung tissue) by means of immunofluorescence and immunoperoxidase staining.[28]

Control

The control of PI-3 virus infection, because of its wide distribution in cattle populations, is dependent on immunization. However, because serious disease is usually a complex condition involving interaction of PI-3 virus with other viruses, bacteria and environmental circumstances, the usual approach is to immunize cattle in those situations where respiratory disease commonly occurs (e.g. feedlots) with vaccines which contain immunogens against other agents as well. Currently two imported vaccines are used in South Africa. One contains temperature-sensitive mutants of PI-3 and infectious bovine rhinotracheitis viruses, while the other contains modified (attenuated) strains of infectious bovine rhinotracheitis, bovine virus diarrhoea, PI-3 and bovine respiratory syncitial viruses **(see Chapter 8: Vaccines, herd immunity and economics: Considerations in the control of infectious diseases)**.

The use of vaccines against PI-3 virus for the control of respiratory tract disease in sheep became popular in North America during the early 1980s, but vaccination of small ruminants is not currently practised in southern Africa.

References

1 **ANDERSON, M.L., BLANCHARD, P.C., BARR, B.C. & HOFFMAN, R.L., 1990.** A survey of causes of bovine abortion occurring in the San Joaquin Valley, California. *Journal of Veterinary Diagnostic Investigation*, 2, 283–287.

2 **BARNARD, B.J.H., 1977.** Virus diseases in feedlot cattle in South Africa. *Bulletin de l'Office International des Épizooties*, 88, 153–160.

3 **BERGMAN, R., MORENO-LOPEZ, J., MÖLLERBERG, L. & MOREIN, B., 1978.** Parainfluenza-3 virus: Difference in capacity of neuraminidase-weak and strong strains to infect young calves and to elicit cellular immune response. *Research in Veterinary Science*, 25, 193–199.

4 **BROWN, T.T. & ANANABA, G., 1988.** Effect of respiratory infections caused by bovine herpesvirus-1 or parainfluenza-3 virus on bovine alveolar macrophage functions. *American Journal of Veterinary Research*, 49, 1447–1451.

5 **BUXTON, A. & FRASER, G., 1977.** *Animal Microbiology*. London, Oxford, Edinburgh, Melbourne: Blackwell Scientific Publications.

6 **CHURCHILL, A.E., 1963.** The isolation of parainfluenza-3 virus from fatal cases of pneumonia in *Erythrocebus patas* monkeys. *British Journal of Experimental Pathology*, 45, 529–537.

7 **DAFT, B.M. & WEIDENBACH, S., 1987.** Isolation of parainfluenza type 3 virus associated with a respiratory epizootic in goats in California. *Agri-Practice*, January 1987, 35–36.

8 **DAVIES, D.H., LONG, D.L., McCARTHY, A.R. & HERCEG, M., 1986.** The effect of parainfluenza virus type 3 on the phagocytic cell response of the ovine lung to *Pasteurella haemolytica*. *Veterinary Microbiology*, 11, 125–144.

9 **DITCHFIELD, J., ZBITNEW, A. & MACPHERSON, L.W., 1963.** Association of Myxovirus parainfluenza 3 (RE 55) with upper respiratory infection of horses. *Canadian Veterinary Journal*, 4, 175.

10 **DUNNE, H.W., AJINKA, F.M., BUBASH, G.R. & GRIEL, L.C., 1973.** Parainfluenza-3 and bovine enteroviruses as possible important causative factors in bovine abortion. *American Journal of Veterinary Research*, 34, 1121–1126.

11 **FENNER, F., BACHMANN, P.A., GIBBS, E.P.J., MURPHY, F.A., STUDDERT, M.J. & WHITE, P.O., 1987.** *Veterinary Virology*. Orlando, San Diego, New York: Academic Press, Inc.

12 **FRANK, G.H. & MARSHALL, R.G., 1973.** Parainfluenza-3 virus infection of cattle. *Journal of the American Veterinary Medical Association*, 163, 858–860.

13 **GOYAL, S.M., KHAN, M.A., McPHERSON, S.W., ROBINSON, R.A. & BOYLAN, W.J., 1988.** Prevalence of antibodies to seven viruses in a flock of ewes in Minnesota. *American Journal of Veterinary Research*, 49, 464–467.

14 **HAMBLIN, C., HEDGER, R.S. & CONDY, J.B., 1980.** The isolation of parainfluenza-3 virus from free-living African buffalo (*Syncerus caffer*). *The Veterinary Record*, 107, 18.

15 **KINGSBURY, D.W., BRATT, M.A., CHOPPIN, P.W., HANSON, R.P., HOSAKA, Y., MEULEN, V., NORRBY, E., PLOWRIGHT, W., ROTT, R. & WUNNER, W.H., 1978.** Paramyxoviridae. *Intervirology*, 10, 137–152.

16 **LEHMKUHL, H.D. & CUTLIP, R.C., 1982.** Characterization of parainfluenza type 3 virus isolated from the lung of a lamb with pneumonia. *American Journal of Veterinary Research*, 43, 626–628.

17 **LIGGIT, D., HUSTON, L., SILFLOW, R., EVERMANN, J. & TRIGO, E., 1985.** Impaired function of bovine alveolar macrophages infected with parainfluenza-3 virus. *American Journal of Veterinary Research*, 46, 1740–1744.

18 **LOPEZ, A., THOMSON, R.G. & SAVAN, M., 1976.** The pulmonary clearance of *Pasteurella haemolytica* in calves infected with bovine parainfluenza-3 virus. *Canadian Journal of Comparative Medicine*, 40, 385–391.

19 **McLEAN, A.M. & DOANE, F.W., 1971.** The morphogenesis and cytopathology of bovine parainfluenza type 3 virus. *Journal of General Virology*, 12, 271–279.

20 **REISINGER, R.C., HEDDLESTON, K.I. & MANTEI, C.A., 1959.** A myxovirus (SF-4) associated with shipping fever of cattle. *Journal of the American Veterinary Medical Association*, 135, 147–152.

21 **ROSSI, C.R. & KIESEL, G.K., 1977.** Susceptibility of bovine macrophage and tracheal-ring cultures to bovine viruses. *American Journal of Veterinary Research*, 38, 1705–1708.

22 **SATTAR, S.A., BOHL, E., TRAPP, H.C. & HAMDY, A.H., 1967.** Infection of bovine fetuses with myxovirus parainfluenza-3 virus. *American Journal of Veterinary Research*, 28, 45–49.

23 **SHIBUTA, H., SUZU, S. & SHIODA, T., 1986.** Differences in bovine parainfluenza-3 virus variants studied by monoclonal antibodies against viral glycoproteins. *Virology*, 155, 688–696.

24 **SINGH, K.V. & BAZ, T.I., 1966.** Isolation of parainfluenza-3 virus from water buffalo in Egypt. *Nature*, 210, 656–657.

25 **STOTT, E.J., THOMAS, L.H., COLLINS, A.P., CROUCH, S., JEBBETT, J., SMITH, G.S., LUTHER, P.D. & CASWELL, R., 1980.** A survey of virus infections of the respiratory tract of cattle and their association with disease. *Journal of Hygiene*, 85, 257–270.

26 **TOTH, T. & HESSE, R.A., 1983.** Replication of five bovine respiratory viruses in cultured bovine alveolar macrophages. *Archives of Virology*, 75, 219–224.

27 **VAN VUUREN, M., 1991.** Unpublished results. Faculty of Veterinary Science, Medical University of South Africa.

28 **WATT, N.J., PIRIE, H.M., ALLAN, E.M., SELMAN, I.E., PETRIE, L., GIBBS, H.A. & WISEMAN, A., 1982.** Parainfluenza type 3 virus and respiratory syncytial virus antigens in paraffin-embedded sections of pneumonic lung. *Proceedings of the Twelfth World Congress on Diseases of Cattle*, Amsterdam, 1982.

29 **WOODS, G.T., 1968.** The natural history of bovine myxovirus parainfluenza-3. *Journal of the American Veterinary Medical Association*, 152, 771–777.

77

Bovine respiratory syncytial virus infection

M. van Vuuren

Introduction

Infection with bovine respiratory syncytial (BRS) virus is inapparent in the majority of animals, but in some it does cause mild to severe respiratory tract disease characterized by fever, coughing, serous nasal and ocular discharges and dyspnoea. It is one of several viruses which are primary pathogens in the bovine respiratory disease complex **(see Chapter 141: Pneumonic pasteurellosis)**. Respiratory syncytial virus also infects sheep and goats and may cause rhinitis in sheep.[11]

The virus was first isolated from cattle by Paccaud and Jacquier in Switzerland in 1970[22] and has subsequently been found in North America, Europe and Japan. Its prevalence and importance in Africa is largely unknown, although antibody to it is widespread in feedlot cattle in South Africa.[33]

A review of BRS virus has recently been published.[26]

Aetiology

The virus is classified as a member of the genus *Pneumovirus* in the family Paramyxoviridae. Virions are pleomorphic, enveloped and measure 80–500 nm in diameter for the round and pleomorphic forms **(Figure 77.1)**, and up to 5 microns in length for filamentous forms **(Figure 77.2)**. The elongated nucleocapsid is helically-coiled and tortuous and contains single-stranded RNA.

The envelope contains surface projections, but, in contrast to ortho- and paramyxoviruses, pneumoviruses lack neuraminidase and haemagglutinin. Virions mature by budding from the cytoplasmic membrane.

A wide range of cell cultures is susceptible to infection with BRS virus, including those prepared from most bovine tissue types, as well as kidney cells of pigs, hamsters, monkeys and humans.[20] Cytopathic effects are characterized by multinucleate giant cell formation, intracytoplasmic inclusions and necrosis.

Bovine respiratory syncytial virus is antigenically related to human respiratory syncytial virus,[22] but the two viruses are distinct.[28]

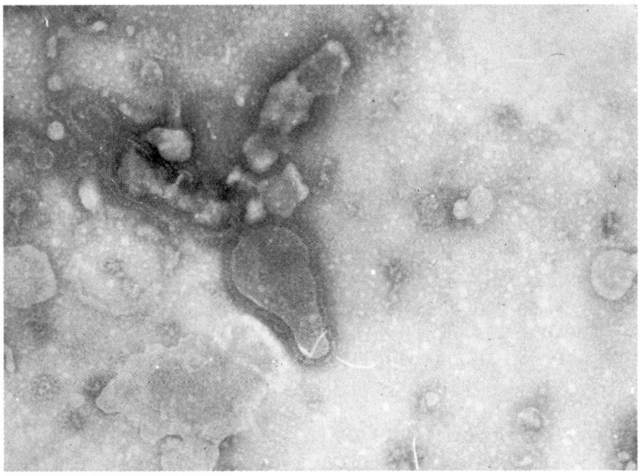

Figure 77.1 Pleomorphic form of bovine respiratory syncytial virus

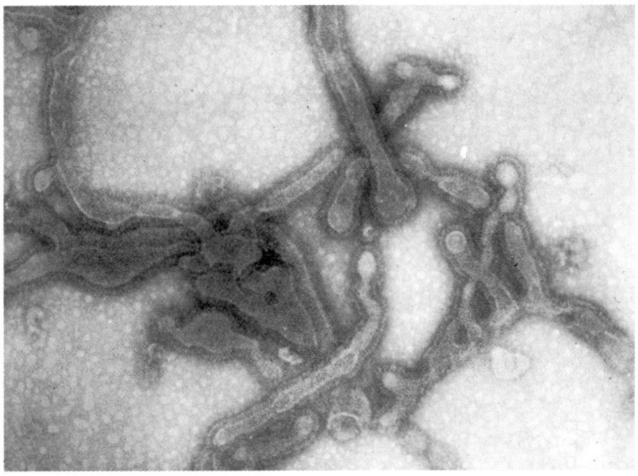

Figure 77.2 Filamentous form of bovine respiratory syncytial virus

Epidemiology

Cattle are probably the principal reservoirs of the virus. Sheep and goats may also be infected but their role in the epidemiology is not clear, and inapparent infections are common in these species.[2, 9, 10, 16, 18, 24]

Although respiratory disease caused by BRS virus infection usually occurs in three- to 12-month-old calves, it may also affect adult cattle. Infection has been reported in feedlot animals, in extensive beef farming operations, and in housed dairy calves.[8] Spread of the infection, probably by respiratory aerosols, can be rapid.

Respiratory disease in cattle in the northern hemisphere caused by BRS virus occurs during late autumn, winter and early spring.

Pathogenesis

The severity of clinical disease caused by BRS virus is dependent on the age and immune status of the calf, the route of infection, and the strain of the virus.[5] Some strains are significant primary pathogens of young cattle because, acting alone, they are able to cause severe damage to the lower respiratory tract.[7, 21, 25] However, the virus more frequently predisposes the respiratory tract of cattle to the pathogenic effects of secondary bacterial infections.[4]

The virus replicates in epithelial cells of the nasal cavity, pharynx, trachea, bronchi and bronchioli, and in type II pneumocytes and alveolar macrophages. It induces cytopathic changes characterized by loss of cilia and/or necrosis.[6] The virus also depresses opsonization and phagocytosis by alveolar macrophages.[19, 31] Depressed mucociliary clearance resulting from a loss of cilia is responsible for the accumulation of fluid and tissue debris in the airways and alveoli, which provides an ideal environment for the growth of bacterial opportunists.

The lesions which can result from BRS virus infection can be a hypersensitivity reaction in which an initial sensitizing infection induces the production of reaginic antibody (IgE), while subsequent infection induces the development of an immediate hypersensitivity reaction characterized by acute bronchiolitis, lung oedema and emphysema.[4, 13] This hypothesis has been forwarded because recently weaned calves, in particular, after showing evidence of respiratory infection, show signs of partial recovery followed, after two to three days, by severe respiratory disease. However, dietary factors cannot be ruled out as possible causes of this condition, as fasting or a change in ration early in the course of the disease may have a beneficial effect;[13] mortality is often highest in calves on a high plane of nutrition.[12]

Clinical signs

Although most infections are subclinical, some infected animals show mild to severe disease[8] after an incubation period of five to seven days. In naturally infected dairy calves, early clinical signs are characterized by fever and coughing with nasal, oral and sometimes ocular discharges followed within two to three days by rapid abdominal breathing.[13] Severely affected calves may have signs of severe respiratory distress, such as breathing through an open mouth and forced grunting expiration.[32]

Pathology

In calves that die from BRS virus infection, irregular areas of atelectasis and pneumonia, particularly of the cranioventral parts of the lungs, together with lung oedema and interstitial emphysema are usually evident. A mucopurulent exudate may be present in the bronchi of atelectatic and pneumonic areas. The interstitial emphysema may affect all the lobes of the lungs but is often more severe in the caudal lobes. Bulla formation may be prominent. Bronchial and mediastinal lymph nodes are enlarged and oedematous.[4, 23]

Microscopic changes associated with BRS virus infection are characterized by an acute necrotizing bronchiolitis with the development in many bronchioli of syncytial giant cells formed by the proliferation of epithelial cells, several of which may contain eosinophilic intracytoplasmic inclusion bodies. The lumens of the bronchioli contain neutrophils, plasma cells, macrophages, mucus and cellular debris. Evidence of atelectasis and pneumonia is present, the exudate in alveoli containing neutrophils, macrophages and cellular debris. Epithelialization may be evident in some alveoli, even with a tendency to form syncytia, some of which may possibly contain intracytoplasmic inclusion bodies.[7, 21, 32]

Diagnosis

Since respiratory infections in cattle cannot be differentiated clinically, a diagnosis of disease caused by BRS virus infection can only be made with laboratory support.

Bovine respiratory syncytial virus is labile and difficult to recover by the use of cell cultures.[7, 15, 28, 29] For this reason, primary binding assays, such as fluorescent antibody and immunoperoxidase-staining techniques applied to either cells recovered from the nasal passages or tissue sections, are considered to be more appropriate for the detection of the virus.[14, 17, 27, 30, 34, 35] Because of the close antigenic similarity between BRS and human RS viruses, enzyme immunoassays designed to identify human RS virus may be used to detect BRS virus.

When attempting virus isolation, it is imperative to use a sucrose-containing transport medium to preserve the virus if any delay during transport is anticipated, and to inoculate cell cultures as soon as possible after the specimens have been collected.[1] Tracheal washes and broncho-alveolar lavage yield cells from deeper parts of the respiratory tract than do nasopharyngeal swabs,[3] and therefore offer the possibility of more efficient detection of BRS virus. Lavage has yielded promising results in experimentally infected calves.[7]

Retrospective detection of BRS virus infections can be accomplished by antibody detection using indirect immunofluorescence, virus neutralization and complement fixation tests. However, since most infections are inapparent, care should be exercised when attributing respiratory disease in cattle to BRS virus based on serology.

Control

Treatment of both nursing and weaned calves should be based on early detection of disease and the administration of antihistamines, corticosteroids and antibiotics.[4] Some clinicians believe that a change of feed or a 48-hour fast is an important part of the early treatment of acute respiratory distress in calves.[13]

A vaccine that contains modified live BRS virus as well as modified viruses directed against three other bovine viral pathogens is imported into South Africa for use against the bovine respiratory disease complex **(see Chapter 8: Vaccines, herd immunity and economics: Considerations in the control of infectious diseases)**.

References

1 **BAKER, J.C., 1986.** What to do about bovine RSV. *Norden News*, 4–14.

2 **BAKER, J.C., AMES, T.R. & MARKHAM, R.J.F., 1985.** Serologic studies of bovine respiratory syncytial virus in Minnesota cattle. *American Journal of Veterinary Research*, 46, 891–892.

3 **BATEMAN, E.D. & AINSLIE, G.M., 1990.** Broncho-alveolar lavage — a window to the lung. *South African Medical Journal*, 77, 550–552.

4 **BOHLENDER, R.E., McCUNE, M.W. & FREY, M.L., 1982.** Bovine respiratory syncytial virus infection. *Modern Veterinary Practice*, 8, 613–618.

5 **BRYSON, D.E., McNULTY, M.S., ALLAN, G.M., CUSH, P.F. & LOGAN, E.F., 1982.** Experimental respiratory syncytial virus pneumonia in calves. *Proceedings of the Twelfth World Congress on Diseases of Cattle*. Amsterdam, 1982.

6 **CASTLEMAN, W.L., CHANDLER, S.K. & SLAUSON, D.O., 1985.** Experimental bovine respiratory syncytial virus infection in conventional calves: Ultrastructural respiratory lesions. *American Journal of Veterinary Research*, 46, 554–560.

7 **CASTLEMAN, W.L., LAY, J.C., DUBOVI, E.J. & SLAUSON, D.O., 1985.** Experimental bovine respiratory syncytial virus infection in conventional calves: Light microscopic lesions, microbiology, and studies on lavaged lung cells. *American Journal of Veterinary Research*, 46, 547–553.

8 **CASTLEMAN, W.L., TORRES-MEDINA, A., HAWKINS, K.L., DUBOVI, E.J. & ATZ, J.M., 1985.** Severe respiratory disease in dairy cattle in New York state associated with bovine respiratory syncytial virus infection. *Cornell Veterinarian*, 75, 473–483.

9 **COLLINS, J.K., TEEGARDEN, R.M., MACVEAN, D.W., SMITH, G.H. & FRANK, G.R., 1988.** Prevalence and specificity of antibodies to bovine respiratory syncytial virus in sera from feedlot and range cattle. *American Journal of Veterinary Research*, 49, 1316–1319.

10 **DUNBAR, M.R., JESSUP, D.A., EVERMANN, J.F. & FOREYT, W.J., 1985.** Seroprevalence of respiratory syncytial virus in free-ranging Bighorn sheep. *Journal of the American Veterinary Medical Association*, 187, 1173–1174.

11 **EVERMANN, J.F., LIGGIT, H.D. & PARISH, S.M., 1985.** Properties of a respiratory syncytial virus isolated from a sheep with rhinitis. *American Journal of Veterinary Research*, 46, 947–951.

12 **FENNER, F., BACHMANN, P.A., GIBBS, E.P.J., MURPHY, F.A., STUDDERT, M.J. & WHITE, D.O., 1987.** *Veterinary Virology*. Orlando, San Diego, New York: Academic Press, Inc.

13 **FREY, M.L., 1983.** Bovine respiratory syncytial virus and acute respiratory distress syndrome in cattle. *Proceedings of the Eighteenth Conference of the American Association of Bovine Practitioners*, Oklahoma City, 1983.

14 **HAINES, D.M., CLARK, E.G. & CHELACK, B.J., 1989.** The detection of bovine respiratory syncytial virus in formalin fixed bovine lung with commercially available monoclonal antibodies and avidin biotin complex immunohistochemistry. *Canadian Journal of Veterinary Research*, 53, 366–368.

15 **JACOBS, J.W. & EDINGTON, N., 1971.** Isolation of respiratory syncytial virus from cattle in Britain. *The Veterinary Record*, 88, 694.

16 **KEY, D.W. & DERBYSHIRE, J.B., 1984.** Serological studies of parainfluenza type 3 virus, bovine adenovirus type 3 and bovine respiratory syncytial virus infection in beef calves. *Veterinary Microbiology*, 9, 587–592.

17 **KIMMAN, T.G., ZIMMER, G.M., STRAVER, P.J. & DE LEEUW, P.W., 1986.** Diagnosis of bovine respiratory syncytial virus infections improved by virus detection in lung lavage samples. *American Journal of Veterinary Research*, 47, 143–147.

18 **LEHMKUHL, H.D. & GOUGH, P.M., 1977.** Investigation of causative agents of bovine respiratory tract disease in a beef cow–calf herd with an early weaning program. *American Journal of Veterinary Research*, 38, 1717–1720.

19 **LIGGIT, D., TRIGO, E. & EVERMANN, J., 1983.** The effect of parainfluenza-3 and respiratory syncytial virus on bovine alveolar macrophage function *in vitro*. *Proceedings of the Thirty-fourth Annual Meeting of the American College of Veterinary Pathologists*, San Antonio, Texas, 1983.

20 **MATUMOTO, M., INABA, Y., KUROGI, H., SATO, K., OMORI, T., GOTO, Y. & HIROSE, O., 1974.** Bovine respiratory syncytial virus: Host range in laboratory animals and cell cultures. *Archiv für die Gesamte Virusforschung*, 44, 280–290.

21 **MOHANTY, S.B., INGLING, A.L. & LILLIE, M.G., 1975.** Experimentally induced respiratory syncytial virus infection in calves. *American Journal of Veterinary Research*, 4, 417–419.

22 **PACCAUD, M.F. & JACQUIER, C., 1970.** A respiratory syncytial virus of bovine origin. *Archiv für die Gesamte Virusforschung*, 30, 327–342.

23 **PIRIE, H.M., PETRIE, L., PRINGLE, C.R., ALLAN, E.M. & KENNEDY, G.J., 1981.** Acute fatal pneumonia in calves due to respiratory syncytial virus. *The Veterinary Record*, 108, 411–416.

24 **ROSSI, C.R. & KIESEL, G.K., 1974.** Serological evidence for the association of bovine respiratory syncytial virus with respiratory tract disease in Alabama cattle. *Infection and Immunity*, 10, 293–298.

25 **SHARMA, R. & WOLDEHIWET, Z., 1990.** Pathogenesis of bovine respiratory syncytial virus in experimentally infected lambs. *Veterinary Microbiology*, 23, 267–272.

26 **SHARMA, R. & WOLDEHIWET, Z., 1991.** Bovine respiratory syncytial virus: A review. *Veterinary Bulletin*, 61, 1117–1131.

27 **SMITH, G.H., COLLINS, J.K., SANDERS, J. & ANDERSON, G., 1987.** Increased sensitivity of diagnosis of infectious bovine rhinotracheitis virus and bovine respiratory syncytial virus infection using immunoperoxidase on fixed tissue. *Agri-practice*, April 1987, 27–30.

28 **SMITH, M.H., FREY, M.L. & DIERKS, R.E., 1975.** Isolation, characterization and pathogenicity studies of a bovine respiratory syncytial virus. *Archives of Virology*, 47, 237–247.

29 **STOTT, E.J., THOMAS, L.H., COLLINS, A.P., CROUCH, S., JEBBETT, J., SMITH, G.S., LUTHER, P.D. & CASWELL, R., 1980.** A survey of virus infections of the respiratory tract of

cattle and their association with disease. *Journal of Hygiene*, 85, 257–270.

30 **THOMAS, L.H. & STOTT, E.J., 1981.** Diagnosis of respiratory syncytial virus infection in the bovine respiratory tract by immunofluorescence. *The Veterinary Record*, 108, 432–435.

31 **TOTH, T. & HESSE, R.A., 1983.** Replication of five bovine respiratory viruses in cultured bovine alveolar macrophages. *Archives of Virology*, 75, 219–224.

32 **VAN DEN INGH, T.S.G.A.M., VERHOEFF, J. & VAN NIEUWSTADT, A.P.K.M.I., 1982.** Clinical and pathological observations on spontaneous bovine respiratory syncytial virus infections in calves. *Research in Veterinary Science*, 33, 152–158.

33 **VAN VUUREN, M., 1990.** Serological studies of bovine respiratory syncytial virus in feedlot cattle in South Africa. *Journal of the South African Veterinary Association*, 61, 168–169.

34 **WATT, N.J., PIRIE, H.M., ALLAN, E.M., SELMAN, I.E., PETRIE, L., GIBBS, H.A. & WISEMAN, A., 1982.** Parainfluenza type 3 virus and respiratory syncytial virus antigens in paraffin-embedded sections of pneumonic lung. *Proceedings of the Twelfth World Congress on Diseases of Cattle*. Amsterdam, 1982.

35 **WELLEMANS, G., 1977.** Laboratory diagnosis methods for bovine respiratory syncytial virus. *Veterinary Science Communications*, 1, 179–189.

CALICIVIRIDAE

The Caliciviridae are a small and, in terms of disease-causing potential, relatively unimportant virus family. Feline calicivirus, which causes acute respiratory disease in cats, is the best known. The only virus involved in the health of domestic livestock is the serologically diverse group of viruses which cause vesicular exanthema of swine and whose presence has so far only been confirmed in the Western Hemisphere. Vesicular exanthema of swine, however, is an aberrant infection because the viruses responsible naturally infect marine animals (pinnipeds and fish) and infection of pigs only occurs when the tissues of marine animals somehow (usually in swill) come into contact with pigs.

Caliciviruses are similar in morphology to picornaviruses but are somewhat larger (35–39 nm in diameter). The virions, which are probably made up of 180 capsomeres, have 32 depressions arranged symmetrically on the surface.[1] A single strand of positive-sense RNA about 8 200 bases in length makes up the genome. The capsid is unusual in that it is comprised of only one protein.

Reference

1 **SCHAFFER, F.L., 1991.** Caliciviridae. *In:* FRANCKI, R.I.B., FAUQUET C.M., KNUDSON, D.L. & BROWN, F., (eds). Classification and nomenclature of viruses. Fifth report of the International Committee on the Taxonomy of Viruses. *Archives of Virology,* Supplementum 2. Vienna, New York: Springer-Verlag.

78

Vesicular exanthema of swine

G.R. Thomson

Introduction and aetiology

Vesicular exanthema of swine (VES) is a disease of pigs that is clinically indistinguishable from other vesicular diseases of pigs, such as foot-and-mouth disease, and is caused by an immunologically diverse group of caliciviruses whose primary hosts are marine-dwelling mammals and fish. It is almost certain that the 13 serotypes of VES virus derived from pigs, as well as a similar number of serologically distinct caliciviruses isolated from marine-dwelling mammals and opaleye fish (*Girella nigricans*) which are referred to as San Miguel sea-lion (SMS) viruses, form a single complex.[2] These viruses are distinct from feline calicivirus, but their relationship with caliciviruses isolated from a variety of reptiles, apes and cattle[9] remains to be elucidated.

The disease was first recognized in California in 1932 and became a serious problem in that state during the 1940s. In 1952 it occurred for the first time outside California, and by the end of that year had spread to 31 states in the USA. This resulted, in August 1952, in the declaration of a national state of emergency, which provided legislation for a vigorous campaign of eradication based on the slaughter-out of affected herds, with compensation, control of the movement of pork products derived from swill-fed pigs, and the prohibition of feeding uncooked swill to pigs.[1] These measures resulted in the eradication of VES in the USA by 1956. However, the disease has since reappeared sporadically on the Pacific coast of the USA and in islands in the eastern Pacific.

The last recorded outbreak of VES occurred in California in 1976.[6] Because of the wide range of sea creatures which may harbour these viruses, it must be accepted that adventitious infection of pigs that are fed untreated swill containing tissue-remnants of these hosts could result in the reappearance of VES at any time. The threat to southern Africa specifically is difficult to assess, but it is probably small, as SMS viruses have so far only been recovered from free-living animals in the eastern Pacific.

Caliciviruses are unenveloped, single-stranded RNA viruses with icosahedral symmetry (T=3) which have characteristic depressions on the virion surface. Virions have a diameter of 35–40 nm and a mass of 14–16 x 10^6 daltons. The capsid is made up of a major (Mr 60–70 k) and a minor (Mr 15–19k) polypeptide.[3] The RNA is positive-stranded with a poly A tail and covalently-linked VPg (small polypeptide), probably located at the 3′ and 5′ ends respectively.[5]

Vesicular exanthema virus replicates with the production of cytopathic effects (CPE) in a wide variety of cell cultures derived from pig tissues (such as kidney, lung, testicle and amnion), but does not usually produce CPE in cells derived from other animal species.[1] There is a direct correlation between the size of plaques produced by a strain in cell culture and its virulence for pigs.[1] In pigs, different serotypes of VES virus may differ markedly in their virulence,[1] and some strains do not produce clinical disease.

Epidemiology

Marine caliciviruses have been isolated from California sea-lions (*Zalophus californianus*), Steller sea-lions (*Eumetopias jubatus*), northern fur seals (*Callorhinus ursinus*), northern elephant seals (*Mirounga agustirostris*), captive Atlantic bottle-nosed dolphins (*Tursiops truncatus*), Pacific walruses (*Odobenus rosmarus divergens*), and opaleye fish.[2, 9, 10] A calicivirus was also isolated from a macerated liver fluke (*Zalophatrema* sp.) from a California sea-lion, and indirect evidence suggests that sea-lion lungworms, which parasitize opaleye fish as part of their life cycle, may transmit calicivirus.[6]

At least some serotypes of SMS viruses are pathogenic for California sea-lions, in which they produce vesicles on the hairless parts of the flippers and, less frequently, around the mouth and hairy regions of the body.[2] One SMS virus isolate was made from a California sea-lion with flipper lesions and which was in the process of aborting.

Antibody prevalence to SMS viruses is variable, but is sometimes high in free-living California and Steller sea-lions.[2] Up to 3 per cent of northern fur seals may be serologically positive.[4]

Apart from being found in marine animals, pigs, and mink fed on seal meat, caliciviruses (broadly classified as VES or SMS viruses) have also been recovered from or identified in snakes, toads, five species of primates, and cattle.[9] Putative caliciviruses (presumably distinct from VES and SMS viruses) have been identified in humans and in a variety of domestic and wild animals.[3] Feline caliciviruses which cause an important disease in cats[3] are distinct from the VES/SMS viruses. Antibodies to caliciviruses have been detected in the sera of feral pigs, donkeys, water buffaloes, foxes, five species of whale, and humans.[7–9] Horses and monkeys are apparently susceptible to experimental infection with VES virus,[9] although this finding conflicts with earlier reports.[1] Laboratory infection of humans with VES virus has occurred. The potential sources of infection for pigs are thus very numerous, but circumstantial evidence suggests that the primary hosts of VES virus occur in the eastern Pacific Ocean, from the Bering Sea in the north to the coast of southern California.[9]

Initial infection of pigs occurs through the consumption of untreated swill containing tissues of the primary hosts of these viruses. Whether the virus infects pigs orally or by the percutaneous route is unknown, but pigs have been experimentally infected by the application of virus suspensions to scarified skin of the snout or by intradermal inoculation.[1] Horizontal transmission between infected and susceptible pigs in direct contact with each other occurs readily, since vesicular fluid and vesicle epithelium contain large quantities of virus. However, infected pigs remain infectious for only about five days. Indirect contact between infected and susceptible pigs does not result in transmission.[1] The pig body louse (*Haematopinus suis*) may acquire the infection from viraemic pigs and transmit it, presumably mechanically, to susceptible pigs.[1]

Vesicular exanthema virus is stable in meat (even when decomposed) at a temperature of 7 °C over a two- to four-week period,[1] and is not readily inactivated at higher temperatures.[9] Heavily contaminated farm premises probably remain infectious for several months.[9]

Pathogenesis, clinical signs and pathology

The virus replicates in the Malpighian layer of the epidermis, causing hydropic and ballooning degeneration followed by necrosis and vesicle formation in squamous epithelial cells.[1, 9]

Apart from the initial rise in body temperature, the first sign of disease is usually lameness in one or more pigs in a herd as a result of vesicle formation on the heels of the feet, coronary bands and interdigital spaces. Vesicles are also often present on the snout, lips and tongue, as well as elsewhere in the mouth. Rarely, vesicles occur on the teats of sows suckling piglets. The vesicles are usually flat, blanched areas 5–30 mm in diameter, or they may be raised 10–20 mm above the surrounding unaffected epithelium. Vesicles on the snout may occasionally resemble bunches of grapes.[1, 9] The primary vesicles rupture within a day or two, but secondary vesicles may appear adjacent to those which have already ruptured. This phenomenon has resulted in the clinical signs of the disease being divided into two phases. The first phase covers the time between the initial rise in body temperature (40,6–42,2 °C) and the appearance of secondary lesions,[9] while the second phase lasts one or two days and involves rupture of the secondary vesicles, the temperature returning to normal and resumption of normal behaviour. Complete recovery is usually uneventful.

Apart from vesicular lesions, extensive necrosis of lymphocytes in lymph nodes may occur. It is not known whether the appreciable amounts of virus detectable in lymph nodes is a result of replication at that site or of drainage from other sites of replication.[9]

Diagnosis and differential diagnosis

The lesions of VES are indistinguishable from those of foot-and-mouth disease, swine vesicular disease or vesicular stomatitis. An aetiological diagnosis can only be based on identification of the virus by complement fixation, virus neutralization, or ELISA using appropriate antisera. Suspensions of virus or viral antigens may be prepared directly from vesicular epithelium or from virus cultivated in cell culture. Low levels of virus may be detectable in the blood of acutely infected pigs.[9]

Since VES is exotic to Africa, diagnosis of this disease in southern Africa would only be expected in circumstances where direct contact has occurred with pigs or pig products from outside the subcontinent.

Control

The rapid eradication of VES from the USA by the slaughter-out of affected herds, quarantine of affected premises and enforced heat treatment of swill fed to pigs demonstrates the efficacy of this approach.

References

1 **BANKOWSKI, R.A., 1965**. Vesicular exanthema. *Advances in Veterinary Science*, 10, 23–64.

2 **BERRY, E.S., SKILLING, D.E., BARLOUGH, J.E., VEDROS, N.A., GAGE, L.J. & SMITH, A.W., 1990**. New marine calicivirus infective for swine. *American Journal of Veterinary Research*, 51, 1184–1187.

3 **PEREIRA, H.G., 1989**. Caliciviruses. *In*: PORTERFIELD, J.S., (ed.) *Andrews' Viruses of Vertebrates*. London, Philadelphia: Baillière Tindall.

4 **PLOWRIGHT, W., 1988**. *Virus Transmissible Between Wild and Domestic Animals. Zoological Symposium No. 60*. London: The Zoological Society of London.

5 **SCHAFFER, F.L., BACHRACH, H.L., BROWN, F., GILLESPIE, J.H., BURROWS, J.N., MADIN, S.H., POVEY, C.R., SCOTT, F., SMITH, A.W. & STUDDERT, M.J., 1980**. Calicivirus. *Intervirology*, 14, 1–6.

6 **SMITH, A.W., 1981**. Marine reservoirs of caliciviruses. *In*: STEEL, J., (ed.). *CRC Handbook Series in Zoonoses: Viral Zoonoses*. Boca Raton, Florida: CRC Press.

7 **SMITH, A.W., AKERS, T.G. & PRATO, C.M., 1976**. Prevalence and distribution of four serotypes of SMSV serum-neutralizing antibodies in wild animal populations. *Journal of Wildlife Diseases*, 12, 326–334.

8 **SMITH, A.W. & LATHAM, A.B., 1978**. Prevalence of vesicular exanthema of swine antibodies among feral mammals associated with the southern California coastal zones. *American Journal of Veterinary Research*, 39, 291–296.

9 **SMITH, A.W. & MADIN, S.H., 1986**. Vesicular exanthema. *In*: LEMAN, A.D.L., (ed.). *Diseases of Swine*. 6th edn. Ames, Iowa: Iowa State University Press.

10 **SMITH, A.W., SKILLING, D.E. & RIDGEWAY, S., 1983**. Calicivirus-induced vesicular disease in cetaceans and probable interspecies transmission. *Journal of the American Veterinary Medical Association*, 183, 1223–1225.

RETROVIRIDAE

Following the epoch-making discoveries by Ellerman and Bang in 1908 and Peyton Rous in 1911, which eventually led to the realization that viruses are involved in the aetiology of tumours in chickens, retroviruses have been associated mainly with the ability to transform normal cells to a cancerous state.[1] Since then, a large number of retroviruses have been isolated and shown to cause leukaemias, lymphomas and sarcomas in chickens, mice, rats, cats and a variety of other animals. Only much later was it found that there are also non-oncogenic retroviruses, some apathogenic and others associated with so-called 'slow virus diseases'.

In order to accommodate the different groups, the family Retroviridae was subdivided into the three subfamilies. In the most recent (fifth) report of the International Committee on the Taxonomy of Viruses, [2] however, subfamilies within the Retroviridae are no longer recognized. This family, therefore, is now divided between seven genera and groups: the mammalian type-B oncovirus group, the mammalian type-C retrovirus group, the type-D retrovirus group, the avian type-C retrovirus group, spumaviruses, the human T-cell lymphotropic virus/bovine leukaemia virus (HTLV-BLV) group and lentiviruses. This classification was not available when Chapters 79–83 were written.

All retroviruses have certain characteristics in common. The most important of these, from which the name retrovirus is derived, is the possession of a 'reverse transcriptase' or RNA-dependent DNA polymerase as part of the viral capsid. This enzyme, which is unique to the Retroviridae, enables the virus to make a DNA copy of its RNA genome. This DNA 'provirus' can integrate into the host-cell genome, giving rise to latent infections which can escape the host's immune response. In the case of the oncogenic retroviruses the provirus can also act as a natural vector transmitting cellular oncogenes from one cell to another, which is one of the mechanisms of oncogenesis. The lentiviruses, although structurally very similar, have a completely different pathogenic effect. In all diseases associated with this group, including the human immunodeficiency virus (HIV), which causes the acquired immunodeficiency syndrome (AIDS), immunopathological changes are the primary lesions.

Table 1 shows diseases in livestock which are caused by viruses in the Retroviridae family.

Table 1 Diseases of livestock caused by members of the Retroviridae family

DISEASE	HOST ANIMAL
Jaagsiekte	Sheep (goat)*
Enzootic bovine leukosis	Cattle (sheep)*
Visna-Maedi	Sheep (goat)*
Caprine arthritis-encephalitis	Goat (sheep)*
Equine infectious anaemia	Horse, donkey

* The animals given in brackets are uncommon hosts

References

1 **GROSS, L., 1970.** *Oncogenic Viruses*. 2nd edn. Oxford: Pergamon Press.

2 **COFFIN, J.M., 1991.** Retroviridae. *In:* FRANCKI, R.I.B., FAUQUET, C.M., KNUDSON, D.L. & BROWN, F., (eds). Classification and nomenclature of viruses. Fifth report of the International Committee on the Taxonomy of Viruses. *Archives of Virology*, Supplementum 2. Vienna, New York: Springer-Verlag.

79

Enzootic bovine leukosis

Synonyms: Bovine lymphosarcoma, bovine leukaemia

D.W. Verwoerd and R.C. Tustin

Introduction

Enzootic bovine leukosis (EBL) is a retroviral infection of cattle and occasionally sheep which, following a long incubation period, may lead to the development of lymphocytosis and lymphosarcoma.

The disease is induced by an exogenous retrovirus, bovine leukaemia (BL) virus, which is the most common retroviral infection of cattle. There are three manifestations of the infection, namely covert infection characterized by seroconversion but no clinical signs, persistent B-lymphocytosis, and the development of solid lymphoid tumours.

Enzootic bovine leukosis should be distinguished from sporadic bovine leukosis (SBL), which occurs mainly in young animals aged between four months and two years and which is divided into juvenile multicentric, thymic and skin forms. Sporadic bovine leukosis is not associated with BL virus and is thought to be non-contagious. Enzootic bovine leukosis and SBL are discussed in more detail in a number of recent reviews.[5, 17] Both EBL and SBL occur in southern Africa.

Aetiology

Bovine leukaemia virus was first detected in short-term cultures of phytohaemagglutinin-treated lymphocytes derived from cattle with persistent lymphocytosis.[29] Since then several long-term cell cultures producing BL virus have been established.[13, 38] In appearance, BL virus is similar to the type-C retroviruses. Its core ranges from 40–90 nm in diameter and it possesses an outer envelope with surface spikes. The average buoyant density of virions is 1,16 g/ml. The genome consists of single-stranded RNA with a sedimentation constant of 60–70S. Two major ether-sensitive glycosylated proteins of the viral envelope have been designated gp51 and gp30, the former being the main immunogen in natural infections. As well as these, there are four internal ether-resistant structural proteins (p24, p15, p12, p10) and a reverse transcriptase requiring Mg^{++} ions for its *in vitro* activity.[11, 12, 24] Sequence analysis of these proteins has revealed a significant homology between p24 and p12 of BL virus and HTL virus-1, a human retrovirus associated with adult T-cell lymphomas.[5, 31]

Denaturation of the genome yields two subunits, each about 9,2 kilobases long. Restriction enzyme, sequence analysis and *in vitro* translation have all revealed a typical non-defective retrovirus structure, i.e. two long terminal repeats (LTR's) adjoining a sequence of gag, pol and envelope genes, coding for the internal structural proteins, reverse transcriptase, and envelope glycoproteins respectively.[10, 34]

Epidemiology

Bovine leukosis virus is distributed world-wide, but the prevalence of infection is higher in certain regions such as eastern Europe and North and South America.[4] In herds with a history of lymphosarcoma the infection rate may be 25 to 100 per cent, whereas in those herds free from tumours only 1 to 15 per cent of cattle are infected. Infected animals remain so for life and have persistent antibody responses to various BL virus antigens. Despite the presence of antibodies, about 1 per cent of infected cattle develop lymphosarcomas, whereas about 30 per cent have persistent lymphocytosis.[17]

Since BL virus is exogenous to cattle, transmission via the germ-line does not occur. However, congenital transmission from dam to offspring has been demonstrated. The mechanism whereby this occurs is not clear, but the virus may cross the placenta, or maternal blood may infect the calf during parturition. Transmission from sire to progeny has never been demonstrated. Mechanical transmission by blood-sucking insects may occur,[26] and transmission by means of milk and colostrum has been achieved experimentally.[20, 36] However, the most important transmitters of the virus are probably humans; syringes, needles and instruments contaminated with blood presumably play significant roles.

In the USA 10 to 30 per cent of dairy cattle and about 1 per cent of beef cattle are estimated to be infected with BL virus, whereas the incidence rate of lymphosarcomas in slaughtered animals is approximately 0,1 per cent.[2, 17] The situation in South Africa, based on a limited serological survey, appears to be similar to that in the USA. In dairy herds, especially those with Frieslands and Jerseys, up to 90 per cent of animals had antibody to BL virus; while in beef cattle, especially indigenous breeds, antibody prevalence was much lower.[40]

Natural transmission of BL virus to sheep is occasionally seen when the two species are kept in close contact. Virus isolated from lymphosarcomas of sheep was shown to be identical to that found in lymphosarcomas caused in cattle by BL virus.[4] Experimentally, sheep can be easily infected by inoculation of infected bovine or ovine blood, with tumours arising more often and after a much shorter incubation period (two to three years) than in cattle. High antibody titres develop in sheep, but persistent lymphocytosis has not been observed.[5] It is not certain whether goats are susceptible or not. Experimental infection, as evidenced by seroconversion, has also been reported for chimpanzees,[39], pigs,[25], rabbits, rats, guinea-pigs, dogs, cats and deer.[1] No viraemia or other changes were observed in any of these species.

Pathogenesis

The development of genomic probes from molecularly cloned BL-virus proviral DNA resulted in the elucidation of some of the mechanisms of lymphomagenesis at the molecular level. Hybridization analysis of cellular DNA proved that BL virus is not endogenous to cattle or any of the other vertebrates tested.[7] Furthermore, the complete absence of hybridization indicates the absence of V-onc equivalents to all known C-onc genes in BL virus. Similarly, no rearrangements of C-onc genes by BL virus integration could be demonstrated.[23]

All BL virus-induced tumour cells contain proviral genetic material, and less than one to four copies may integrate at many different sites. However, individual tumours are monoclonal in origin. This is in contrast to the polyclonality observed in persistent lymphocytosis.[21] Defective proviruses have been observed, with all the deletions affecting the 5′-half. It can therefore be deduced that integration of at least the 3′-half of the BL provirus is required in order to maintain the neoplastic state, but that the site of integration is not critical. In the absence of an oncogene this suggests that neoplastic transformation is effected by the activation or suppression of a cellular gene through some mediator.[17, 22]

Transcription of viral genes cannot be detected *in vivo*, although the persistent production of antibodies in infected animals suggests a limited expression of the BL virus genome, perhaps a very low level of viral replication at some obscure site. When infected lymphocytes are maintained *in vitro* for 12 to 24 hours, production of BL virus is activated. This led to the isolation of a non-immunoglobulin protein in plasma that blocked *in vivo* expression of the BL virus genome.[14] A gene product of BL virus can therefore be excluded as the mediator. Although no consistent rearrangement of chromosomes has been detected, tumour cells display a variable pattern of abnormalities in chromosomal ploidy.[15] This observation, as well as the very low transformation rate, suggests a multi-step process of lymphomagenesis in which infection with BL virus is only one of several essential factors.[5]

Clinical signs

After initial infection, no signs of viraemia, such as fever or circulating virus, are detected, but the animals develop a strong and persistent humoral response to BL virus proteins. The majority of infected animals remain healthy and no loss of production is observed. Roughly a third of them develop persistent increases in the number of circulating B-lymphocytes.[5] Only a small percentage of animals develop lymphosarcoma, usually at five to eight years of age. Lymphocytes contained in the tumours are likewise of B-cell lineage.[32] A multicentric invasion of a variety of organs and tissues leads to variable signs.

The first sign is usually the swelling of one or more lymph nodes, but in the later stages of the disease lymph node involvement may be widespread. Other manifestations, and the course of the disease, depend on the organ or organs involved, the rate of tumour growth and the extent and distribution of metastases.[3, 8] Characteristically, affected cattle lose weight, become anaemic, and show a drop in milk production. Sometimes there are signs such as exophthalmus, posterior paresis (as a result of invasion of the lumbar epidural space), evidence of cardiac failure (sudden death occurring in some animals), dysphagia or dyspnoea (if lymph nodes in the pharyngeal region are affected), or melaena. In some animals the disease may be diagnosed on rectal palpation on the basis of severely enlarged iliac lymph nodes or the involvement of the urogenital system.[19, 30]

Bovine enzootic leukosis is almost invariably fatal, death occurring several weeks or months after the onset of clinical signs in the majority of cases.[8] Death usually results from cachexia, secondary infections, anaemia and mechanical encroachment on vital organs.[28] In a small percentage of cases the course may, however, be peracute or acute, particularly if the spleen ruptures or the heart or adrenals are affected.[3]

Pathology

In some animals a leukaemic phase following bone marrow involvement may be present at some stage of the disease, and in most cases this is a terminal event.[18, 28] The presence of circulating neoplastic cells, however, is not necessarily reflected in the total lymphocyte count.[17] In addition, anaemia, which is generally normocytic and normochromic, may develop in as many as 55 per cent of cases.[28] Haemoglobin values decline steadily during the course of the disease, with values below 5 g/100 ml being not unusual. Haematocrit values parallel haemoglobin levels.[28] The anaemia is due to a reduction in erythrocyte production after invasion of the bone marrow by neoplastic cells resulting in a reduction in haemopoietic tissue.[28] In some animals blood loss from, for example, a haemorrhaging tumour in the abomasum, may contribute to the anaemia.

Elevation of levels of serum uric acid, aspartate transaminase (SGOT) and lactate dehydrogenase (LDH) may be present, but other chemical pathological findings are not remarkable, or only appear in the terminal stages.[28]

Enzootic bovine leukosis is characterized by a proliferation of neoplastic lymphocytes that results in the formation of discrete solid neoplasms and/or the diffuse infiltration of such cells into various tissues and organs.[8, 35] In most animals the neoplastic process becomes widespread. Lymph nodes are most prominently and frequently affected, the number varying from a few to many, if not all. Organs or tissues such as the abomasum, intestines, myocardium, kidneys, liver, epidural tissue or uterus are commonly involved.[28] Neoplasms appear to originate from lymphoid tissue, or from tissues with lymphoid potential, at any site in the body.[28] They may commence at one or many foci simultaneously and then metastasize. At death the lesions are usually so widely disseminated that it is impossible to determine the primary site(s) of origin.[28] The discrete nodular lesions consist of greyish-white to yellowish or pinkish uniform masses of soft to moderately firm consistency which, if large, may contain areas of haemorrhage and/or necrosis. Diffuse, infiltrative lesions produce greatly enlarged, pale, soft or friable organs without marked changes in shape.[27, 28] Tumours in the epidural space of the spinal cord are most frequently present in the lumbar region and may vary from a few millimetres in diameter to large masses which completely encircle the spinal cord. Lesions in the myocardium occur particularly in the right atrium and often result in evidence of central venous congestion, while those in the abomasum produce a diffusely thickened submucosa, ulceration and haemorrhage.

Microscopically lymphosarcomatous tissue is made up of fairly uniform sheets of closely packed cells, many of which are in mitosis. There is no architectural arrangement and the stroma is scanty.[27] In a survey involving 59 cattle, two basic tumour types were found; in one the majority of cells present were lymphocytes, while in the other they were mostly lymphoblastoid.[28] In all tumours both cell types were represented but one predominated, the cellular pattern being consistent for all organs involved.[28] In another study of lymphosarcomas in cattle, an attempt was made to classify the tumours according to cell size, nuclear cleavage and histological architecture.[37] It was found that the majority of tumours in the cattle were diffuse, composed of small and medium-sized cells, and contained non-cleaved nuclei.

Neoplastic cells not only insinuate themselves between normal cells of the organ or tissue concerned and eventually displace them, but they also invade adjacent tissue, such as serosal surfaces, organ capsules and blood-vessel walls. Neoplastic emboli may be found in blood and lymphatic vessels and in sinusoids.[28]

Diagnosis

A diagnosis of EBL can often be made on the clinical signs, but should be confirmed histologically.

Bovine leukosis virus infection can be detected in cell cultures by transmission electron microscopy, reverse transcriptase assay, hybridization and haemagglutination or syncytium induction.[5, 22] Proviral DNA can also be detected in peripheral lymphocytes by using the polymerase chain reaction (PCR).[6] Two types of syncytia occur: early polykaryocytosis is found in virus-transformed cells a few hours after infection by co-cultivation, while late polykaryocytosis is found in appropriate indicator cells four to eight days after infection. The latter has been developed into a quantitative assay.[9]

Antibodies to BL virus can be detected by various serological tests including immunodiffusion, immunofluorescence, complement fixation, radio-immuno-assay, ELISA and neutralization tests.[4, 16, 17, 33] Antibodies to all the BL virus structural proteins occur, but the titres in infected cattle and sheep are usually highest against the gp51 surface antigen. As sheep are normally seronegative but rapidly develop high titres after infection, a common approach to BL virus identification is to inoculate sheep with blood from affected cattle and test for seroconversion by means of one of these tests.

Differential diagnosis

Few conditions in cattle are likely to be confused with EBL, although lymphoid hyperplasia in lymph nodes and the spleen as a result of chronic inflammation may be. In isolated organs, such as the kidneys, lymphoid accumulations which appear as circumscribed whitish foci also occur in East Coast fever and malignant catarrhal fever. However, these diseases are, in general, quite distinct from EBL.

Control

Eradication of EBL is desirable and has been successfully achieved in some western European countries.[5] Although losses due to lymphosarcoma can sometimes be high, the major reason for eradication is the restriction it places on exports to countries free of the disease. The recent demonstration of a relationship between BL virus and the human retrovirus, HTL virus-1, has added impetus to the attempts to eradicate the disease, although many studies have failed to reveal any hazard to human health associated with BL virus.

In some countries in the European Economic Community, the disease was eradicated by testing all animals in an infected herd for gp51 antibodies at three- to six-month intervals, and eliminating seropositive animals until the herd was free of reactors. Such an approach is also feasible in individual herds in endemic areas, but would be difficult to justify on a national scale in southern Africa.

Since antibodies to BL virus gp51 neutralize virus infectivity and also have complement-dependent cytotoxic activity, a vaccine against gp51 should be protective. So far, experimental vaccines, based mainly on inactivated virus, have proved ineffective.[17] However, fixed infected cells and purified gp51 has produced short-term protection to BL virus infection, suggesting that it may prove possible to develop an effective vaccine by the genetic manipulation of the antigenic sequences of gp51.[5] Effective synthetic vaccines or recombinant live vaccines are also possible. Subunit vaccines would have the added advantage that they would enable a distinction to be made between vaccinated and naturally infected animals, including colostrum-fed calves (which acquire passive immunity for six to eight months) from infected mothers. There is enough evidence available to be able to predict that an effective vaccine will soon be available and that the disease can then be eradicated.

References

1 **BAUMGARTENER, L.E. & OLSON, C., 1982.** Host range of bovine leukosis virus: Preliminary report. *Current Topics in Veterinary Medicine and Animal Research*, 15, 338–347.

2 **BAUMGARTENER, L.E., OLSON, C., MILLER, J.M. & VAN DER MAATEN, M.J., 1975.** Survey for antibodies to leukemia (C-type) virus in cattle. *Journal of the American Veterinary Medical Association*, 166, 249–258.

3 **BENDIXEN, H.J., 1965.** Bovine enzootic leukosis. *In*: BRADLEY, C.A. & CORNELIUS, C.E., (eds). *Advances in Veterinary Science*, 10, 129–204. New York: Academic Press.

4 **BURNY, A., BRUCK, C., CHANTRENNE, H., CLEUTER, Y., DEKEGEL, D., GHYSDAEL, J., KETTMANN, R., LECLERCQ, M., LEUNEN, J., MAMMERICKX, M. & PORTETELLE, D., 1980.** Bovine leukaemia virus: Molecular biology and epidemiology. *In*: KLEIN, G., (ed.). *Viral Oncology*. New York: Raven Press.

5 **BURNY, A., BRUCK, C., CLEUTER, Y., COUEZ, D., DESCHAMPS, J., GREGOIRE, T., GHYSDAEL, J., KETTMANN, R., MAMMERICKX, M., MARBAIX, G. & PORTETELLE, D., 1985.** Bovine leukaemia virus and enzootic bovine leukosis. *Onderstepoort Journal of Veterinary Research*, 52, 133–144.

6 **COCKERELL, G.L. & ROVNATE, J., 1988.** The correlation between the direct and indirect detection of bovine leukaemia virus infection in cattle. *Leukaemia Research*, 12, 465–469.

7 **DESCHAMPS, J., KETTMANN, R. & BURNY, A., 1981.** Experiments with cloned complete tumour-derived bovine leukaemia virus information prove that the virus is totally exogenous to its target animal species. *Journal of Virology*, 40, 605–609.

8 **FERRER, J.F., 1980.** Bovine lymphosarcoma. *Advances in Veterinary Science and Comparative Medicine*, 24, 1–68.

9 **FERRER, J.F. & DIGLIO, C.A., 1976.** Development of an *in vitro* infectivity assay for the C-type bovine leukaemia virus. *Cancer Research*, 36, 1068–1073.

10 **GHYSDAEL, J., KETTMANN, R. & BURNY, A., 1979.** Translation of BLV virion RNAs in heterologous protein synthesizing systems. *Journal of Virology*, 29, 1087–1098.

11 **GILDEN, R.V., LONG, C.W., HANSON, M., TONI, R., CHARMAN, H.P., OROSZLAN, S., MILLER, J.M. & VAN DER MAATEN, M.J., 1975.** Characteristics of the major internal protein and DNA-dependent DNA polymerase of bovine leukaemia virus. *Journal of General Virology*, 29, 305–314.

12 **GRAVES, D.C., DIGLIO, C.A. & FERRER, J.F., 1977.** A reverse transcriptase assay for detection of bovine leukaemia virus. *American Journal of Veterinary Research*, 38, 1739–1744.

13 **GRAVES, D.C. & FERRER, J.F., 1976.** *In vitro* transmission and propagation of the bovine leukaemia virus in monolayer cell cultures. *Cancer Research*, 36, 4152–4159.

14 **GUPTA, P. & FERRER, J.F., 1982.** Expression of bovine leukaemia virus genome is blocked by a non-immunoglobulin protein in plasma from infected cattle. *Science*, 215, 405–407.

15 **HARE, W.C.D., YANG, T.J. & McFEELY, R.A., 1967.** A survey of chromosome findings in 47 cases of bovine lymphosarcoma (leukaemia). *Journal of the National Cancer Institute*, 38, 383–387.

16 **HOFF-JORGENSEN, R., 1989.** An international comparison of different laboratory tests for the diagnosis of bovine leukosis: Suggestions for international standardization. *Veterinary Immunology and Immunopathology*, 22, 293–297.

17 **JACOBS, R.M., 1985.** Bovine lymphoma. *In*: OLSEN, R.G., KRAKOWA, S. & BLAKESLEE, J.R., (eds). *Comparative Pathology of Viral Diseases*, Vol. II. Boca Raton: CRC Press.

18 **JARRETT, W.F.H., CRIGHTON, G.W. & DALTON, R.G., 1966.** Leukaemia and lymphosarcoma in animals and man. I. Lymphosarcoma or leukaemia in the domestic animal. *The Veterinary Record*, 79, 693–699.

19 **JUBB, K.V., KENNEDY, P.C. & PALMER, N., 1985.** *Pathology of Domestic Animals*. 3rd edn. New York: Academic Press.

20 **KENYON, S.J., GUPTA, P. & FERRER, J.F., 1982.** Presence of the bovine leukaemia virus (BLV) in milk of naturally infected cows. *Current Topics on Veterinary Medicine and Animal Science*, 15, 289–297.

21 **KETTMANN, R., CLEUTER, Y., MAMMERICKX, M., MEUNIER-ROTIVAL, M., BERNARDI, G., BURNY, A. & CHANTRENNE, H., 1980.** Genomic integration of bovine leukaemia pro-virus: Comparison of persistent lymphocytosis with lymph node tumour form of enzootic bovine leukosis. *Proceedings of the National Academy of Science*, 77, 2577–2581.

22 **KETTMANN, R., DESCHAMPS, J., CLEUTER, Y., COUEZ, D., BURNY, A. & MARBAIX, G., 1982.** Leukemogenesis by bovine leukaemia virus: Proviral DNA integration and lack of RNA expression of viral long terminal repeat and 3′ proximate cellular sequences. *Proceedings of the National Academy of Science*, 79, 2465–2469.

23 **KETTMANN, R., DESCHAMPS, J., COUEZ, D., CLAUSTRIAUX, J.J., PALM, R. & BURNY, A., 1983.** Chromosome integration domain for bovine leukaemia provirus in tumours. *Journal of Virology*, 47, 146–150.

24 **KETTMANN, R., PORTETELLE, D., MAMMERICKX, M., CLEUTER, Y., DEKEGEL, D., GALOUX, M., GHYSDAEL, J., BURNY, A. & CHANTRENNE, H., 1976.** Bovine leukaemia virus: An exogenous RNA oncogenic virus. *Proceedings of the National Academy of Science*, 73, 1014–1018.

25 **MAMMERICKX, M., PORTETELLE, D. & BURNY, A., 1981.** Experimental cross-transmissions of bovine leukaemia virus (BLV) between several animal species. *Zentralblatt für Veterinärmedizin*, (B), 28, 69–81.

26 **MARIN, C., DE LOPEZ, N., DE ALVAREZ, M., CASTANOS, H., ESPANA, W., LEON, A. & BELLO, A., 1982.** Humoral spontaneous response to bovine leukaemia virus infection in zebu, sheep, buffalo and capybara. *Current Topics in Veterinary Medicine and Animal Science*, 15, 310–320.

27 **MARSHAK, R.R., 1968.** Criteria for the determination of the normal and leukotic state in cattle. *Journal of the National Cancer Institute*, 41, 243–263.

28 **MARSHAK, R.R., CORIELL, L.L., LAWRENCE, W.C., CROSHAW, J.E., SCHRYVER, H.F., ALTEA, K.P. & NICHOLS, W.W., 1962.** Studies on bovine lymphosarcoma. I. Clinical aspects, pathological alterations and herd studies. *Cancer Research*, 22, 202–216.

29 **MILLER, J.M., MILLER, L.D., OLSON, C. & GILLETTE, K.G., 1969.** Virus-like particles in phytohaemagglutinin-stimulated lymphocyte culture with reference to bovine lymphosarcoma. *Journal of the National Cancer Institute*, 43, 1297–1305.

30 **MOULTON, J.E., 1978.** *Tumours in Domestic Animals*. 2nd edn. Berkeley: University of California Press.

31 **OROSZLAN, S., SARNGADHARAN, M.G., COPELAND, T.D., KALYANARAMAN, V.S., GILDEN, R.V. & GALLO, R.C., 1982.** Primary structure analysis of the major internal protein p24 of human type-C T-cell leukaemia virus. *Proceedings of the National Academy of Science*, 79, 1291–1294.

32 **PARODI, A.L., MIALOT, M., CRESPEAU, F., LEVY, D., SALMON, H., NOGUES, G. & GERARD-MARCHAND, R., 1982.** Attempt for a new cytological and cytoimmunological classification of bovine malignant lymphoma (BML) (lymphosarcoma). *Current Topics in Veterinary Medicine and Animal Sciences*, 15, 561–572.

33 **PORTETELLE, D., BRUCK, C., MAMMERICKX, M. & BURNY, A., 1983.** In animals infected by bovine leukaemia virus (BLV) antibodies to envelope glycoprotein gp51 are directed against the carbohydrate moiety. *Virology*, 105, 223–233.

34 **SHIH, T.Y. & SCOLNICK, E.M., 1980.** Molecular biology of mammalian sarcoma viruses. *In*: KLEIN, G., (ed.). *Viral Oncology*. New York: Raven Press.

35 **SMITH, H.A., 1965.** The pathology of malignant lymphoma in cattle. *Pathologica Veterinaria*, 2, 68–76.

36 **STRAUB, O., 1982.** Transmission studies from leukaemic cattle to sheep using secretions, excretions, breath and skin scrapings. *Current Topics in Veterinary Science and Animal Science*, 15, 299–308.

37 **VALLI, V.E., McSHERRY, B.J., DUNHAM, B.M., JACOBS, R.M. & LUMSDEN, J.H., 1981.** Histocytology of lymphoid tumors in the dog, cat and cow. *Veterinary Pathology*, 18, 494–512.

38 **VAN DER MAATEN, M.J. & MILLER, J.M., 1976.** Replication of bovine leukaemia virus in monolayer cell cultures. *Bibliography of Haematology*, 43, 360–362.

39 **VAN DER MAATEN, M.J. & MILLER, J.M., 1976.** Serological evidence of transmission of bovine leukaemia virus to chimpanzees. *Veterinary Microbiology*, 1, 351–357.

40 **VERWOERD, D.W., 1990.** Veterinary Research Institute, Onderstepoort, South Africa. Unpublished data.

80

Jaagsiekte

Synonyms: Ovine pulmonary adenomatosis, ovine pulmonary carcinomatosis

D.W. Verwoerd, R.C. Tustin and A-L. Williamson

Introduction

Jaagsiekte is a contagious neoplasm which affects the lungs of sheep. It was first recognized in South Africa more than a century ago,[56, 60] when a detailed description of its clinical signs and macroscopic pathology was published by Hutcheon in 1891, along with evidence of its infectivity and an account of attempts to control it.[20] This was followed by reports from England,[21] Germany[15] and France.[1] The disease is now known to have an almost world-wide distribution and to have considerable economic impact in those countries which have substantial sheep populations. In South Africa a survey over a 40-year period indicated that jaagsiekte is by far the most common neoplasm reported in sheep (64 per cent).[3]

In the early literature the disease was often confused with other lung conditions of sheep. The most important of these is maedi, which is caused by a lentivirus and characterized by chronic, non-neoplastic inflammatory lesions.[36] Today it is known that the two diseases are closely associated in many countries and are often present as co-infections in the same animal, which adds to the existing confusion.[8, 20, 24, 41, 51]

Aetiology

Even though jaagsiekte was known to be contagious long before its neoplastic nature had been elucidated, many years of research in various countries failed to reveal its causal agent, though filtration experiments suggested a viral aetiology. The first successful experimental transmission of the disease by co-habitation was reported by De Kock,[6] yielding results that were to be confirmed in Iceland nine years later.[13] An ovine herpesvirus was the first candidate virus isolated,[5, 9, 22, 23] but transmission and molecular hybridization experiments proved that this virus is a passenger and not directly involved in the aetiology of the disease.[10]

The possibility of a retroviral aetiology was first suggested by the observation in Israel of typical retrovirus particles in adenomatous lesions.[44] Retroviruses were also found in cell cultures established from jaagsiekte lungs[23] and reverse transcriptase activity in extracts of tumour tissue.[45] However, no transmission studies were done and the results were difficult to interpret in view of the possible presence of maedi-visna lentivirus in the material studied. Transmission of jaagsiekte with lung extracts containing reverse transcriptase activity was first reported by Martin, Scott and Sharp[26] and later confirmed by Perk[42] and Herring, Sharp, Scott and Angus.[16] The most convincing evidence that a retrovirus, which was designated jaagsiekte retrovirus (JSRV), is indeed the aetiological agent of jaagsiekte was obtained by means of serial transmissions in new-born lambs. Concentrated and partially purified lung-rinse material was used for intra-tracheal inoculation. That the disease can be transmitted experimentally by means of a retrovirus[63] was proved by an inverse relationship between the incubation period of the disease and the concentration of reverse transcriptase in the density-gradient fraction used.

All attempts to cultivate significant quantities of the virus *in vitro* have failed so far, severely hampering its characterization and attempts to develop a vaccine. Some viral properties have been determined by using partially purified preparations from lung washes or tumour extracts.[61] It was demonstrated, however, that the virus isolated in this way consists mainly of immune complexes with IgA, which could affect some of the properties reported.[61]

Mature virions have an average diameter of 110 nm and, when negatively-stained **(Figure 80.1)**, appear as pleomorphic, enveloped particles with spikes on the surface, typical of most retroviruses. The morphology of positively-stained JSRV is distinct from that of any other retrovirus **(Figure 80.2)**. It possesses a slightly eccentric nucleoid with an electron-dense perinucleoidal space.[39] The virus has a density of 1,17–1,18 g/ml, similar to that of mouse mammary tumour (MMT) virus, and Mason-Pfizer monkey (MPM) virus, respectively type B and type D retroviruses. The viral genome consists of single-stranded RNA with a sedimentation constant of 60–70S.

Replicating jaagsiekte retrovirus particles are occasionally seen in tumour cells. Immature particles, 75 nm in diameter, assemble in the cytoplasm **(Figure 80.3)** and are then transported to the cell membrane, where budding of

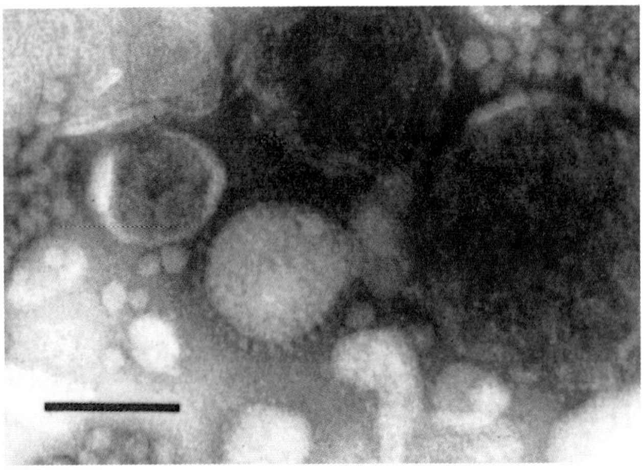

Figure 80.1 Jaagsiekte retrovirus particle with surface projections surrounded by disrupted particles. This preparation was purified from a jaagsiekte lung wash, fixed with osmium tetroxide and negatively-stained with phosphotungstic acid. Bar = 100 nm

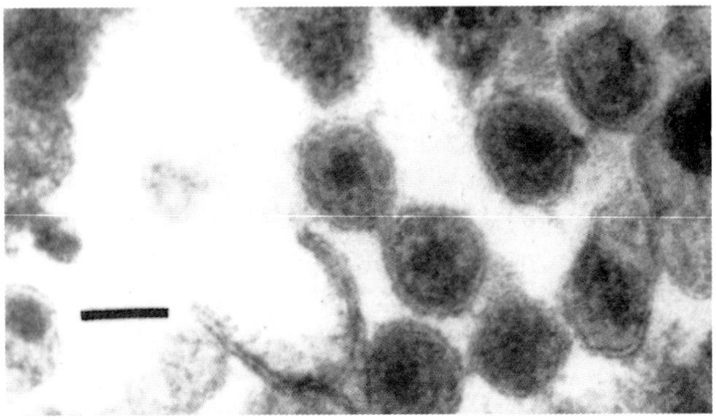

Figure 80.2 Positively-stained jaagsiekte retrovirus particles purified from a jaagsiekte lung wash. Bar = 100 nm

mature particles takes place **(Figure 80.4)**. The morphogenesis is similar to that of type B and D retroviruses, but is quite distinct from that of type C oncoviruses (bovine leukaemia virus) and lentiviruses (maedi-visna virus), where the virions are assembled at the cell membrane in a crescent shape before budding as an immature particle.[39]

In addition to the similarities in morphology, morphogenesis and density, JSRV also shares a common antigenic determinant[49] and a preference by its reverse transcriptase for Mg^{++} ions[63] with MPM virus (type D) and MMT virus (type B) oncoviruses. In contrast, both type C oncovirus and lentivirus enzymes prefer Mn^{++} and no serological cross-reactions can be demonstrated with these viruses. Molecular hybridization experiments also fail to reveal any significant homology between the genome of JSRV and any other retrovirus tested.[11] However, anti-MPM virus p27 serum has been used successfully to localize the related JSRV p29 antigen by using immunocytochemical techniques in sections of jaagsiekte lung lesions.[40]

It can be concluded, therefore, that the aetiological agent of jaagsiekte is an oncovirus belonging to the family Retroviridae, distantly related to type B and D oncoviruses.

Epidemiology

Jaagsiekte occurs in sheep as a sporadic or endemic disease in all continents of the world except Australia.[2, 4, 7, 27, 34, 46, 52, 53, 55, 56, 64] Natural disease with a low prevalence does occur in goats in some countries, but it has not been diagnosed in this species in southern Africa. It has,

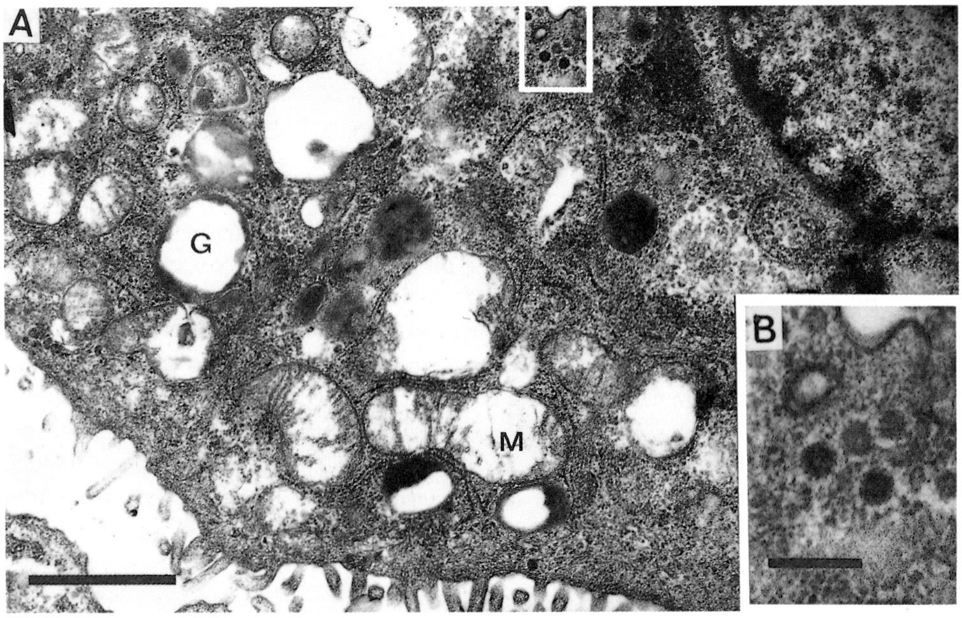

Figure 80.3 A jaagsiekte tumour cell (A). Note the secret ory granules (G), mitochondria (M) as well as intracytoplasmic jaagsiekte retrovirus particles (rectangle). Bar = 1 µm. Intracytoplasmic jaagsiekte retrovirus particles (B). Bar = 200 nm

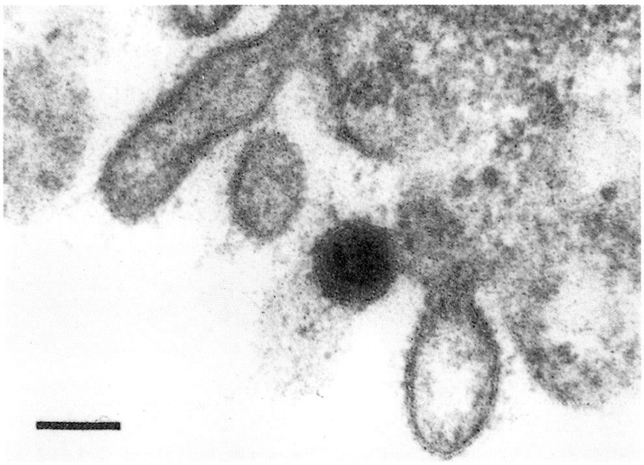

Figure 80.4 Jaagsiekte retrovirus particle budding from a tumour cell into an alveolar lumen. Bar = 100 nm

however, been experimentally transmitted to kids in South Africa.[58]

It would appear that goats are less susceptible to infection by JSRV than are sheep, because in one experiment a viral dose that produced extensive lesions in more than 90 per cent of new-born lambs after two to three months[62] produced only small circumscribed lesions in two out of five kids after nine to 13 months.[58] Transmission studies in Europe have provided similar results.[48] Apart from the low prevalence of the natural disease in goats, this view is supported by the fact that in Iceland during the epidemic of jaagsiekte in the 1930s and 1940s, jaagsiekte was not seen in goats despite close contact between them and sheep suffering from the disease.[13]

Jaagsiekte is endemic throughout South Africa and Namibia.[56] Observations suggest that more animals die as a result of the disease during winter[56] or after a sudden drop in environmental temperature,[14] possibly as a result of secondary bacterial pneumonia. This gives a false impression of a greater prevalence during the colder months.

Outbreaks of jaagsiekte occur when affected sheep are introduced into clean flocks. In Iceland, where the disease was eradicated in 1952,[50] it was observed that approximately five-and-a-half to eight months elapsed between the introduction of affected sheep and the appearance of new cases[14] in a highly susceptible population where the animals are closely confined during winter. In South Africa several years may elapse between the introduction of an infected animal into a 'clean' flock and the realization by the farmer that something is seriously amiss.[56]

It seems that there are breed differences in susceptibility. In a major epidemic of jaagsiekte in Iceland it was found that Gottorp sheep were far more susceptible than were the Adalbol breed.[12] In the United Kingdom, the fact that the disease has a higher prevalence in Scotland than in England also suggests that there are breed differences in susceptibility.[49] In South Africa, Merino and Karakul sheep and their cross-breeds are possibly more susceptible than English breeds.[59] In addition, it was found in Iceland that offspring of different rams varied greatly in their susceptibility to the disease.[12] When these genetic differences in susceptibility were recognized, farmers were urged to breed from resistant families and breeds and this led to a decrease in the prevalence of the disease.

In a survey in South Africa the annual mortality due to jaagsiekte in infected flocks varied from less than 1 to 24 per cent, with an average of 3,6 per cent.[56] The sex of the animal does not seem to play a role in its susceptibility.[56]

It is assumed that all sheep with lung lesions, however small, may excrete the virus. In most affected animals the tumour probably grows slowly and clinical signs are only manifested when the lesions are relatively well advanced and have therefore been present for some considerable time.[56] Examination of the lungs of sheep from infected flocks which have been slaughtered out *in toto* suggests that some animals possess lung lesions which are static or, at most, progress very slowly.[56]

Although sheep of all ages are susceptible to infection, neonatal lambs are more susceptible than are lambs more than a few days old.[47, 62] It is likely, therefore, that affected sheep contract the disease at a very early age from infected dams, some of which are asymptomatic.

Experimental results suggest that intra-uterine transmission does not occur.[37, 56] If this is so, embryo transfer has a potentially important role in creating 'clean' flocks, while enabling the introduction of new genes.[37]

Pathogenesis

Experimental transmission of jaagsiekte suggests that the respiratory system is the natural route of infection.[56, 64]

The primary lesion in jaagsiekte is neoplastic transformation of type II secretory epithelial cells and possibly also of the non-ciliated terminal bronchiolar epithelial (Clara) cells. Transformed cells, in which replication of the virus has been observed,[39] proliferate and form clusters that invade and eventually obliterate the alveolar lumen, resulting in death due to hypoxia. The transformed cells retain their secretory function, producing large amounts of surfactant-containing, clear, viscous fluid which accumulates in the air passages and aggravates respiratory distress. It also leads to coughing and the formation of aerosol droplets containing the virus or tumour cells, which can infect other animals.

Natural cases of jaagsiekte are often complicated by secondary infections, most commonly pasteurellosis. In such cases the immediate cause of death is usually an acute or chronic pneumonia.

A characteristic histological feature of jaagsiekte is the presence of large numbers of macrophages, usually in the areas adjacent to the adenomatous lesions. Various studies of their possible role in the pathogenesis of the disease have failed to provide a clear-cut answer. On the one hand, it has been clearly demonstrated that jaagsiekte tumour cells produce a chemotactic factor which stimulates proliferation of macrophages,[30] while on the other hand, activated alveolar macrophages produce substances which stimulate the proliferation of type II cells. After chemotactic stimulation, macrophages have even been shown to produce both growth-stimulatory and inhibitory factors, depending on their interaction with other lymphoid cells.[31]

Another factor in the pathogenesis of jaagsiekte about which little is known is the apparently close association of the disease with lentivirus infections.[7, 41] Lentiviruses remain latent in alveolar macrophages and replicate only after these cells are activated.[32] The presence of large numbers of activated macrophages in jaagsiekte lungs may therefore create ideal conditions for lentivirus replication, possibly aided by an immunosuppressive activity of the jaagsiekte retrovirus. On the other hand, it was recently demonstrated that the South African lentivirus isolate causes mild immunosuppression in sheep, the degree of which correlates well with the latent period before the appearance of jaagsiekte signs in co-infected animals. It is possible that the lentivirus, in addition to causing a mild interstitial pneumonia, may also predispose animals to secondary infections, including jaagsiekte.[29]

All attempts at demonstrating circulating antibodies against JSRV in natural or experimental cases of jaagsiekte have failed, even in animals from which relatively large amounts of virus have been isolated from lung washes. However, large amounts of JSRV-specific IgA as well as some IgG can be isolated from affected lungs, proving that the virus is immunogenic and that there is an efficient local immune response. In fact, all the virus isolated from the lungs has been shown to be complexed with immunoglobulins.[61] Thus, the failure to detect circulating antibodies may simply be due to the use of what were in effect immune complexes rather than unfettered virus in the serological techniques applied. Alternatively, the formation of immune complexes, localized in the lungs, may preclude the formation of circulating antibodies. The existence of JSRV in immune complexes could also explain its low infectivity as well as its stability upon fluorocarbon treatment.[62]

No evidence for cellular immunity has yet been found, and attempts to demonstrate cytotoxic activity of the alveolar macrophages against tumour cells have been unsuccessful.

Clinical signs

The incubation period varies from about nine months to two or three years. Clinical disease is therefore rarely seen in lambs under the age of nine months.[12] Experimentally, however, because of the large number of lesions induced, the incubation period in lambs can be reduced to as little as three weeks by inoculation of concentrated lung-rinse material containing the aetiological agent in high concentrations. In these animals the course of the disease is acute, with death often intervening within a few days of the first signs of the disease.[59]

The onset of clinical signs is insidious in natural cases. Initially, while the habitus is normal and the condition of the animal good, the respiratory rate is more rapid than normal after an animal has been driven. As the disease progresses, affected animals have reduced appetite, lose body weight and lag behind the flock when it is driven. Marked respiratory distress is evident on exercise, the respiratory movements being short and jerky. Tachypnoea and dyspnoea eventually become evident even at rest. Spasmodic bouts of coughing occur and there is a great increase in the amount of secretion from the lungs. This is regarded as almost pathognomonic for jaagsiekte.[12, 28, 57] Moist rales are heard on auscultation of the thorax, sometimes even without the aid of a stethoscope.

There is generally no fever, but pyrexia may occur as a result of pneumonia following secondary bacterial infection.

The duration of the clinical disease varies considerably and depends largely on factors such as the presence, nature and extent of secondary bacterial pneumonia and on the environmental conditions under which the animal is kept. Sheep may survive for a few weeks or months, and cases are on record where affected animals have survived for more than a year.[12] Results of a field survey indicate that the average duration of clinical disease is two months, with a range of a few days to six months.[56] Once clinical signs manifest, the disease is irreversible.[63]

Pathology

No consistent haematological abnormalities have been reported in animals suffering from jaagsiekte. However, increased blood levels of IgG occur in cases with advanced lesions,[18, 42] and these have been ascribed to the presence of numerous plasma cells in the lungs.[17]

The extent and nature of the lung lesions depends to a large extent on the duration of the disease and whether or not secondary infection by organisms such as *Actinomyces pyogenes* and *Pasteurella* spp. has occurred. The presence of secondary lesions in the lungs often obscures those due to the primary condition and makes tenuous the diagnosis of the disease on gross pathological evidence alone.

In advanced cases of jaagsiekte the lungs are three or more times their normal weight and almost fill the thoracic cavity. They do not collapse when the thorax is opened. Both lungs are usually involved, but not necessarily to the same extent. The cranial and middle lobes and the cranial part of the caudal lobes are commonly affected, but any part of the lung may be involved. Nodules and areas of diseased tissue of various sizes (the smallest being less than one millimetre in diameter) are sometimes scattered throughout the normal lung tissue. The larger lesions consist of very dense tumorous tissue with a relatively firm consistency, and may protrude slightly above unaffected lung tissue **(Figure 80.5)**.

The distribution of lesions suggests that the primary lesion or lesions grow by expansion. Intrapulmonary spread of the infection with the development of new foci probably occurs both aerogenously and via the lymph and blood streams. Each new focus is seen grossly as a small greyish-white, semi-transparent nodule which at first is barely visible to the naked eye. As it expands it may coalesce with neighbouring nodules and, in this way, large lesions eventually develop. The lesions of experimentally induced cases tend to be more multicentric than those resulting from natural infection.

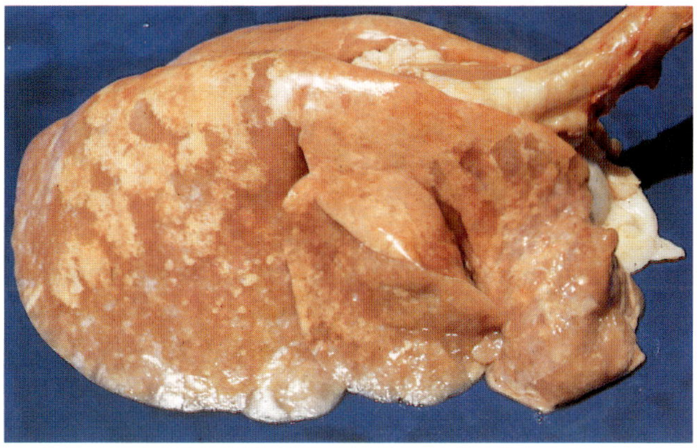

Figure 80.5 Macroscopic appearance of the lungs in an uncomplicated case of jaagsiekte. Note the enlargement of the affected lung as well as the darker colour and consolidated appearance of the ventral part of the lung

Intra- and extrathoracic metastasis of the tumour may occur.[1, 56] In South Africa extrapulmonary metastasis is rare, whereas it frequently occurs in Awassi or fat-tailed sheep in Israel, where metastasis both within and outside the thorax may be found in 30–50 per cent of cases.[35, 43] The most frequent metastatic sites are the bronchial and mediastinal lymph nodes, peritoneum, skeletal musculature, liver, spleen, kidneys, heart and mesenteric lymph nodes.[35, 56, 57, 64] Spread to the visceral and parietal pleura may also occur.[56, 57]

Apparently healthy sheep may, when slaughtered, reveal the presence of one or more isolated lesions, some of which are associated with fairly extensive fibroplasia. These lesions appear to be long-standing and give the impression that they grow very slowly.[56]

Histopathologically, jaagsiekte lesions have been classified as bronchiolo-alveolar adenocarcinomas.[54] The earliest lesions are found particularly in the epithelium of the alveoli, but also in the terminal and respiratory bronchioles. Very early lesions consist of a small number of neoplastic cuboidal to columnar epithelial cells which proliferate to form acinus-like structures which resemble glandular tissue **(Figure 80.6)**. The acinus-like structures are generally lined by a single layer of well-differentiated tumour cells which are mainly cuboidal in shape, have large nuclei with several nucleoli, and often have a vacuolated cytoplasm. These cells stain intensely with the

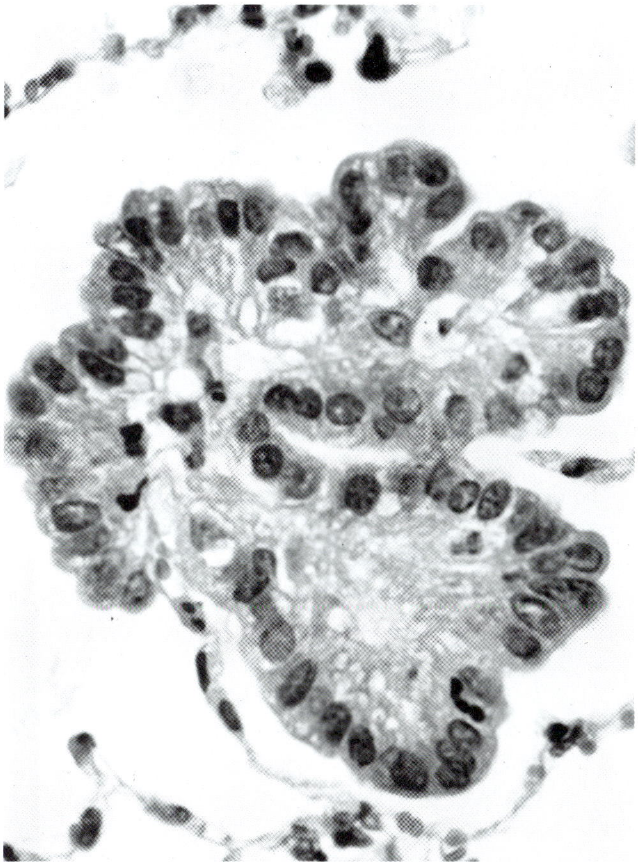

Figure 80.6 Early histopathological lesion in jaagsiekte consisting of a nodule of proliferated cuboidal to columnar epithelial cells

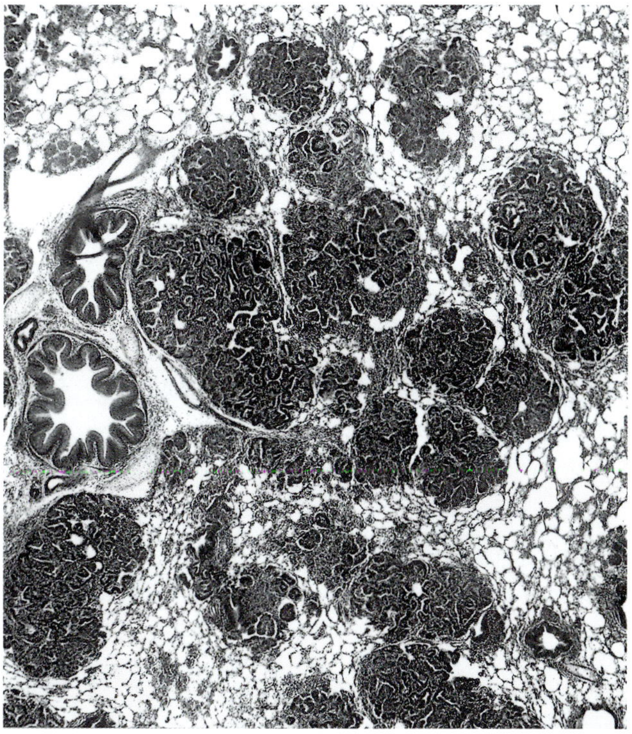

Figure 80.7 Multiple neoplastic foci scattered throughout the parenchyma of the lung

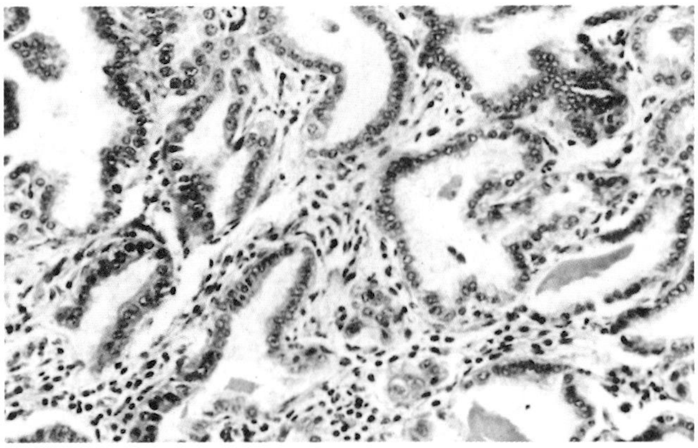

Figure 80.8 Advanced jaagsiekte case showing moderate fibrosis between tumour acini

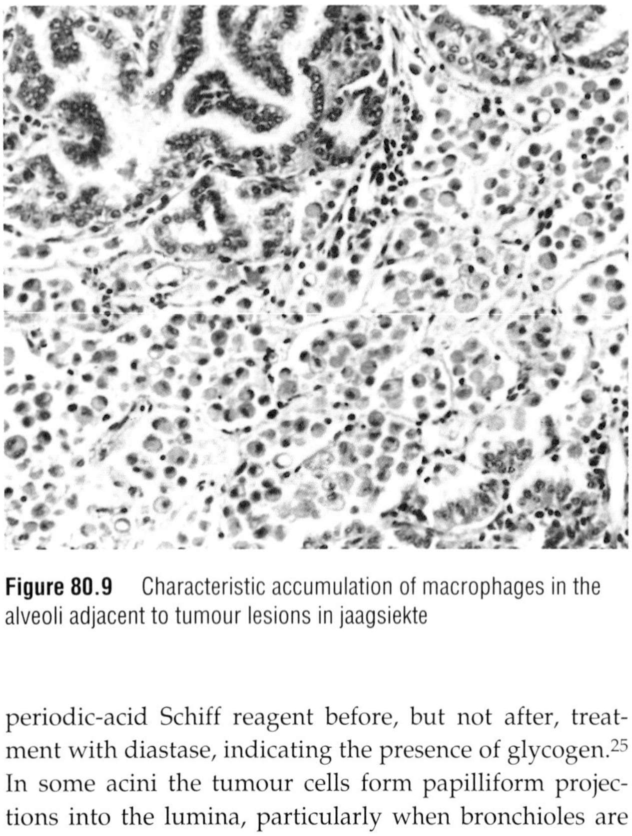

Figure 80.9 Characteristic accumulation of macrophages in the alveoli adjacent to tumour lesions in jaagsiekte

periodic-acid Schiff reagent before, but not after, treatment with diastase, indicating the presence of glycogen.[25] In some acini the tumour cells form papilliform projections into the lumina, particularly when bronchioles are involved. Neoplastic foci are scattered throughout the parenchyma **(Figure 80.7)**.

In some cases the connective tissue stroma is very prominent and may proliferate to form thick layers between the tumour acini or beneath the pleura. It generally consists of mature collagen, but occasionally may appear myxomatous **(Figure 80.8)**.

A conspicuous feature of the lesions in animals with extensive disease is the alveolar macrophage response. These cells may be present within the lumens of the tumour acini, but are more prominent in the alveoli of the lung tissue adjacent to the neoplasm **(Figure 80.9)**. Macrophages are not prominent in early lesions. Also conspicuous in some animals are perivascular, peribronchial and peribronchiolar lymphoid hyperplasia and increased numbers of plasma cells.

Evidence of exudative pneumonia due to secondary invaders is almost invariably present to a greater or lesser degree in and around the neoplastic lesions. This is generally represented by varying amounts of a fibrinous or purulent inflammatory reaction which may obscure the underlying primary lesion. Abscesses and pleuritis may be present.

Ultrastructural studies of jaagsiekte lesions[4, 17, 33, 38, 44, 65] indicate that most neoplastic cells originate from granular (type II) pneumocytes. The cells on the periphery of the lesion are usually well differentiated, contain many free polysomes and show nucleolar margination, indicating that they are in a state of rapid protein synthesis and cell division. Intracytoplasmic JSRV particles, when seen, are often associated with centrioles, suggesting that the virus replicates in actively dividing cells.[39] As is the case in most malignant cells, the nuclei and mitochondria are often abnormal. Numerous secretory granules, containing varying amounts of osmiophilic material and myelinoid bodies, are present in the cytoplasm. These granules are associated with surfactant production and are responsible for the large amount of lung secretion characteristic of jaagsiekte.

Scanning electron microscopy reveals that the surface of the neoplastic cells is usually covered by abundant microvilli, in stark contrast to the smooth surface of normal alveolar epithelial cells **(Figure 80.10)**. A single transformed cell first proliferates to form a single layer lining the alveolar lumen, which then develops into a grape-like cluster with papilliform projections eventually filling the alveolar space and spreading to adjacent alveoli **(Figure 80.11)**. The most common non-malignant cells, found mainly in advanced lesions, are macrophages. They have an 'angry' appearance, being large and possessing a highly ruffled surface **(Figure 80.12)**, indicating that they are in an activated state.

Diagnosis

The clinical diagnosis of jaagsiekte cannot be made with certainty, especially in the first case to be encountered in a flock. A history of long-standing, progressively worsening respiratory distress syndrome in a flock, coupled with the results of clinical examination of affected animals, should alert one to the possible presence of jaagsiekte. Up-ending an affected animal by its hind legs (often called 'wheelbarrow' test) may, in cases with extensive lung pathology, induce the flow of a clear viscous fluid from the nostrils, supporting a diagnosis of jaagsiekte.[12, 28] In considering the diagnosis, it must be borne in mind that the course and clinical signs may be complicated by secondary pneumonia.

The diagnosis of jaagsiekte must, at least initially, be confirmed by histopathological examination of the lung lesions. Lung neoplasia may be obscured, both macroscopically and microscopically, by secondary pneumonia. For this reason, several specimens of diseased tissue

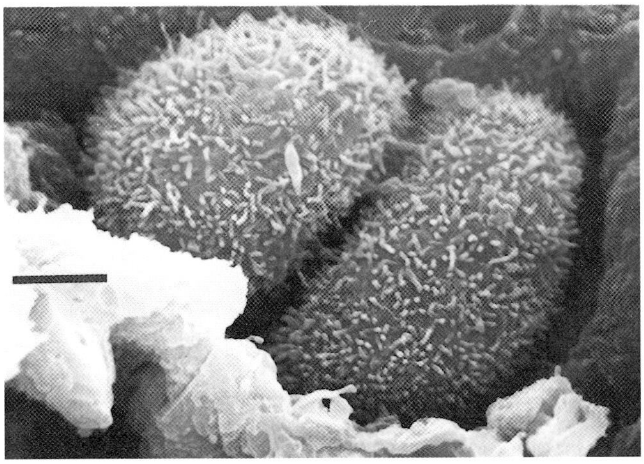

Figure 80.10 A scanning electron micrograph of jaagsiekte tumour cells. Note the microvilli on the surface of the cells. Bar = 1 μm

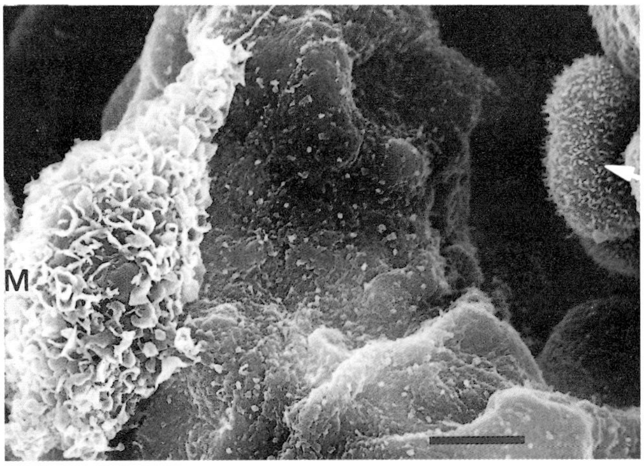

Figure 80.12 A scanning electron micrograph of an activated macrophage (M) with a highly ruffled surface and jaagsiekte tumour cells (arrow) in an adjacent alveolus. Bar = 5 μm

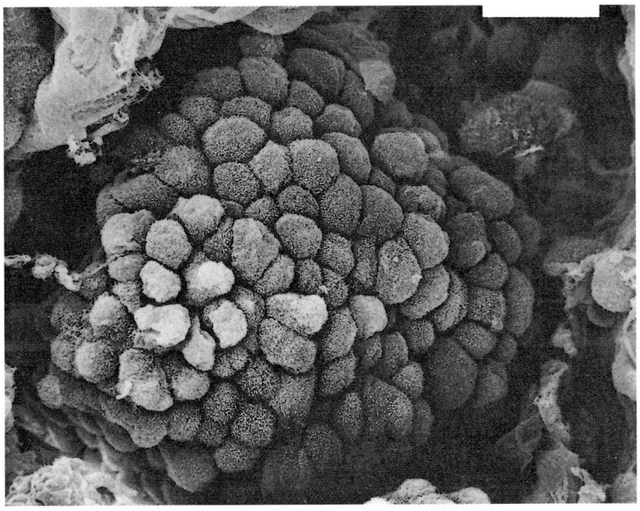

Figure 80.11 A scanning electron micrograph of a grape-like cluster of jaagsiekte tumour cells. Bar = 15 μm

should be collected for histopathological examination and reliance should not be placed on the results of the examination of a single specimen.

Attempts at developing a serum-based assay for the detection of circulating antibodies in affected animals have failed. An ELISA test for detecting viral antigens and immune complexes in lung-rinse fluid has been developed, but its use is impractical because of the problem of sample collection.[62]

Differential diagnosis

Clinically and pathologically, jaagsiekte can be confused with various forms of chronic pneumonia. In South Africa, pasteurellosis is the most commonly encountered lung condition in sheep, and is also the most common secondary complication in cases of jaagsiekte. In countries where it occurs, maedi must also be differentiated from jaagsiekte. Other organisms causing lung lesions include *Actinomyces pyogenes, Corynebacterium pseudotuberculosis, Mycoplasma* spp., and lungworm.

Histologically, advanced jaagsiekte lesions are so characteristic that a typical case should not be confused with any other disease. However, very early lesions may be difficult to distinguish from epithelialization of the alveoli, which tends to occur in chronic interstitial pneumonias caused by lungworm infestations and lentivirus infections. Co-infection with JSRV and lentivirus may give rise to 'mixed lesions'. These lesions consist of the proliferative changes typical of jaagsiekte as well as interstitial cell infiltration and collagen deposition characteristic of maedi.[57, 59]

Control

Jaagsiekte has been successfully eradicated from Iceland but this entailed the slaughter of the entire sheep population except in one isolated area.[50] However, unless a sensitive diagnostic test for detecting carriers is developed, eradication will not be economically feasible in other countries. The alternative option of establishing and maintaining closed flocks free from infection is also hampered by the lack of techniques for determining whether or not an animal is free from infection. Under southern African conditions the prevalence in a flock can be reduced to less than 1 per cent by strict isolation and removal of animals showing early clinical signs. Furthermore, susceptibility to infection decreases rapidly after birth and lambs four to six months old are almost completely resistant to experimental infection. Therefore, if the lambs of infected ewes are eliminated together with their dams, the prevalence of jaagsiekte can be further reduced. The probability that the aetiological agent does not cross the placental barrier enhances the possibility of building up a 'clean' flock by either embryo transfer or by removing lambs from their dams by caesarian section or immediately after birth and subsequently raising them in a disease-free environment.[37, 56] As natural infection by droplet inhalation requires close contact and retroviruses are relatively unstable when the atmosphere is dry and temperatures high, good management practices can contribute considerably to the control of the disease.

Apart from an age resistance in sheep to jaagsiekte, circumstantial evidence exists for acquired resistance to infection, and for differences in breed susceptibility. In Iceland, initial losses in flocks first exposed to jaagsiekte were high (50–60 per cent), but gradually declined to 5–10 per cent. English breeds were found to be less susceptible in South Africa than were the Merino, Karakul and cross-breeds which make up the bulk of the sheep population. There is no evidence that this resistance is immunological.

Retroviruses integrated into the cell genome may be transmitted vertically, although this has yet to be demonstrated for jaagsiekte. In this way these viruses can escape immune defences and it is therefore unlikely that control of jaagsiekte by immunization will be possible. On the other hand, the localized secretory IgA-mediated immune response in the lung may suffice to prevent initial infection. Attempts will therefore continue to be made to develop a vaccine, for example, by using biotechnology to overcome the inability to cultivate the virus in cell cultures.

References

1 **AYNAUD, M., 1926.** Origine vermineuse du cancer pulmonaire de la brebis. *Comptes Rendus des Séances de la Société de Biologie*, Paris, 95, 1540.

2 **BASSETT, H.F. & SHEEHAN, P., 1989.** Outbreak of sheep adenomatosis in the Irish Republic. *The Veterinary Record*, 124, 46–47.

3 **BASTIANELLO, S.S., 1982.** A survey on neoplasia in domestic species over a 40-year period from 1935 to 1974 in the Republic of South Africa. II. Tumours occurring in sheep. *Onderstepoort Journal of Veterinary Research*, 49, 205–209.

4 **CUTLIP, R.C. & YOUNG, S., 1982.** Sheep pulmonary adenomatosis (jaagsiekte) in the United States. *American Journal of Veterinary Research*, 43, 2108–2113.

5 **CVJETANOVIC, V., FORSEK, Z., NEVJESTIC, A. & RUKANVIA, L.J., 1972.** Isolation of the sheep pulmonary adenomatosis (SPA) virus. *Veterinaria*, 21, 493–496.

6 **DE KOCK, G., 1929.** Further observations on the aetiology of jaagsiekte in sheep. *Fifteenth Annual Report, Director of Veterinary Services, Union of South Africa*, 1169–1183.

7 **DEMARTINI, J.C., ROSADIO, R.H. & LAIRMORE, M.D., 1988.** The etiology and pathogenesis of ovine pulmonary carcinoma (sheep pulmonary adenomatosis). *Veterinary Microbiology*, 17, 219–236.

8 **DEMARTINI, J.C., ROSADIO, R.H., SHARP, J.M., RUSSEL, H.I. & LAIRMORE, M.D., 1987.** Experimental co-induction of type D retrovirus-associated pulmonary carcinoma and lentivirus-associated lymphoid interstitial pneumonia in lambs. *Journal of the National Cancer Institute*, 79, 167–177.

9 **DE VILLIERS, E-M., ELS, H.J. & VERWOERD, D.W., 1975.** Characteristics of an ovine herpes virus associated with pulmonary adenomatosis (jaagsiekte) in sheep. *South African Journal of Medical Science*, 40, 165–175.

10 **DE VILLIERS, E-M. & VERWOERD, D.W., 1980.** Presence of *Herpesvirus ovis* DNA sequences in cellular DNA from sheep lungs affected with jaagsiekte (pulmonary adenomatosis). *Onderstepoort Journal of Veterinary Research*, 47, 109–112.

11 **DE VILLIERS, E-M., VERWOERD, D.W. & PAYNE, A., 1983.** Comparative studies on ovine retroviruses. *European Economic Community Symposium on Slow Virus Diseases of Sheep and Goats*, Edinburgh, Scotland.

12 **DUNGAL, N., 1938.** Epizootic adenomatosis of the lungs of sheep in relation to verminous pneumonia and jaagsiekte. *Proceedings of the Royal Society of Medicine*, 31, 497–505.

13 **DUNGAL, N., 1946.** Experiments with jaagsiekte. *American Journal of Pathology*, 22, 737–759.

14 **DUNGAL, N., GISLASON, G. & TAYLOR, E.L., 1938.** Epizootic adenomatosis in the lungs of sheep — comparisons with jaagsiekte, verminous pneumonia and progressive pneumonia. *Journal of Comparative Pathology and Therapeutics*, 51, 46–68.

15 **EBER, A., 1899.** Uber multiple adenombildung in den Lungen der Schafe. *Zeitschrift für Tiermedizin*, 3, 161–165.

16 **HERRING, A.J., SHARP, J.M., SCOTT, F.M.M. & ANGUS, K.W., 1983.** Further evidence for a retrovirus as the aetiological agent of sheep pulmonary adenomatosis (jaagsiekte). *Veterinary Microbiology*, 8, 237–249.

17 **HOD, I., HERZ, A. & ZIMBER, A., 1977.** Pulmonary carcinoma (jaagsiekte) of sheep. Ultrastructural study of early and advanced tumour lesions. *American Journal of Pathology*, 86, 545–558.

18 **HOD, I., ZIMBER, A., KLOPFER, U., HELDER, A.W., NOBEL, T.A. & PERK, K., 1974.** Pulmonary carcinoma (jaagsiekte) of sheep: Pathologic findings and comparison in multiple-case and case-free herds. *Journal of the National Cancer Institute*, 53, 103–110.

19 **HOUWERS, D.J. & TERPSTRA, C., 1984.** Sheep pulmonary adenomatosis. *The Veterinary Record*, 114, 23.

20 **HUTCHEON, D., 1891.** Reply to query no. 191 about jagziekte or chronic catarrhal pneumonia. *Agricultural Journal of the Cape of Good Hope*, 4, 87–89.

21 **MACFADYEAN, J., 1894.** Verminous pneumonia in the sheep. *Journal of Comparative Pathology and Therapeutics*, 7, 31–39.

22 **MACKAY, J.M.K., 1969.** Tissue culture studies of sheep pulmonary adenomatosis (jaagsiekte). II. Transmission of cytopathic effects to normal cultures. *Journal of Comparative Pathology*, 79, 147–154.

23 **MALMQUIST, W.A., KRAUSS, H.H., MOULTON, J.E. & WANDERA, J.G., 1972.** Morphologic study of virus-infected lung cell cultures from sheep pulmonary adenomatosis (jaagsiekte). *Laboratory Investigation*, 26, 528–533.

24 **MARKSON, L.M., SPENCE, J.B. & DAWSON, M., 1983.** Investigation of a flock heavily infected with maedi-visna virus. *The Veterinary Record*, 112, 267–271.

25 **MARKSON, L.M. & TERLECKI, S., 1964.** The experimental transmission of ovine pulmonary adenomatosis. *Pathologica Veterinaria*, 1, 269–288.

26 **MARTIN, W.B., SCOTT, M.M., SHARP, G.M., ANGUS, K.W. & NORVAL, M., 1976.** Experimental production of sheep pulmonary adenomatosis (jaagsiekte). *Nature*, 264, 1976–77.

27 **McCULLOUGH, S.J., MALONE, F.E. & GREENE, J.A., 1985.** Sheep pulmonary adenomatosis in Ireland. *The Veterinary Record*, 116, 470.

28 **MITCHELL, D.T., 1915.** Investigation into jagziekte or

chronic catarrhal-pneumonia of sheep. *Report of the Director Veterinary Research, Union of South Africa*, 314, 585–614.
29 **MYER, M.S., HUCHZERMEYER, H.F.A.K., YORK, D.F., HUNTER, P., VERWOERD, D.W. & GARNETT, H.M., 1988.** The possible involvement of immunosuppression caused by a lentivirus in the aetiology of jaagsiekte and pasteurellosis in sheep. *Onderstepoort Journal of Veterinary Research*, 55, 127–133.
30 **MYER, M.S., VERWOERD, D.W. & GARNETT, H.M., 1987.** Production of a macrophage chemotactic factor by cultured jaagsiekte tumour cells. *Onderstepoort Journal of Veterinary Research*, 54, 9–15.
31 **MYER, M.S., VERWOERD, D.W. & GARNETT, H.M., 1987.** Demonstration of growth-inhibitory as well as growth-stimulatory factors in medium conditioned by lung-lavage cells stimulated with a chemotactic factor secreted by jaagsiekte tumour cells. *Onderstepoort Journal of Veterinary Research*, 54, 123–130.
32 **NARAYAN, O., WOLINSKY, J.S., CLEMENTS, J.E., STRANDBERG, J.D., GRIFFIN, D.E. & CORK, L.C., 1982.** Slow virus replication: The role of macrophages in the persistence and expression of visna viruses of sheep and goats. *Journal of General Virology*, 59, 345–356.
33 **NISBET, D.I., MACKAY, J.M.K., SMITH, N. & GRAY, E.W., 1971.** Ultrastructure of sheep pulmonary adenomatosis (jaagsiekte). *Journal of Pathology*, 103, 157–162.
34 **NOBEL, T.A., 1958.** Pulmonary adenomatosis (jaagsiekte) in sheep with special reference to its occurrence in Israel. *Refuah Veterinarith* (Israel), 15, 98–101.
35 **NOBEL, T.A., NEUMANN, F. & KLOPFER, U., 1969.** Histological patterns of the metastases in pulmonary adenomatosis of sheep (jaagsiekte). *Journal of Comparative Pathology*, 79, 537–540.
36 **PALSSON, P.A., 1976.** Maedi and visna in sheep. *In*: KIMBERLIN, R.H., (ed.). *Slow Virus Diseases of Animals and Man*. Amsterdam: North-Holland Publishing Company.
37 **PARKER, B.W.J., WRATHALL, A.E., SAUNDERS, R.W., DAWSON, M., DONE, S.H. & BRADLEY, R., 1989.** Outbreak of sheep pulmonary adenomatosis in the Irish Republic. *The Veterinary Record*, 177.
38 **PAYNE, A-L., & VERWOERD, D.W., 1984.** A scanning and transmission electron microscopy study of jaagsiekte lesions. *Onderstepoort Journal of Veterinary Research*, 51, 1–13.
39 **PAYNE, A-L., VERWOERD, D.W. & GARNETT, H.M., 1983.** The morphology and morphogenesis of jaagsiekte retrovirus (JSRV). *Onderstepoort Journal of Veterinary Research*, 50, 317–322.
40 **PAYNE, A-L., VERWOERD, D.W. & GARNETT, H.M., 1986.** The localization of a Mason-Pfizer monkey virus-related antigen in jaagsiekte tumour tissue and cell lines. *Onderstepoort Journal of Veterinary Research*, 53, 87–91.
41 **PAYNE, A-L., YORK, D.F., DE VILLIERS, E-M., VERWOERD, D.W., QUERAT, G., BARBAN, V., SAUZE, N. & VIGNE, R., 1986.** Isolation and identification of a South African lentivirus from jaagsiekte lungs. *Onderstepoort Journal of Veterinary Research*, 53, 55–62.
42 **PERK, K., 1982.** Slow virus infections of ovine lung. *Advances in Veterinary Science and Comparative Medicine*, 26, 267–287.
43 **PERK, K., 1988.** Koret School of Veterinary Medicine. The Hebrew University of Jerusalem. Personal communication.
44 **PERK, K., HOD, I. & NOBEL, T.A., 1971.** Pulmonary adenomatosis of sheep (jaagsiekte). I. Ultrastructure of the tumour. *Journal of the National Cancer Institute*, 46, 525–537.
45 **PERK, K., MICHALIDES, R., SPIEGELMAN, S. & SCHLOM, J., 1974.** Biochemical and morphologic evidence for the presence of an RNA tumour virus in pulmonary carcinoma of sheep (jaagsiekte). *Journal of the National Cancer Institute*, 53, 131–135.
46 **RAJYA, B.S. & SINGH, C.M., 1964.** The pathology of pneumonia and associated respiratory disease of sheep and goats. I. Occurrence of jaagsiekte and maedi in sheep and goats in India. *American Journal of Veterinary Research*, 25, 61–67.
47 **ROSADIO, R.H., LAIRMORE, M.D., RUSSEL, H.I. & DEMARTINI, J.C., 1988.** Retrovirus-associated ovine pulmonary carcinoma (sheep pulmonary adenomatosis) and lymphoid interstitial pneumonia. I. Lesion development and age susceptibility. *Veterinary Pathology*, 25, 475–483.
48 **SHARP, J.M., ANGUS, K.W., JASSIM, F.A. & SCOTT, F.M.M., 1986.** Experimental transmission of sheep pulmonary adenomatosis to a goat. *The Veterinary Record*, 119, 245.
49 **SHARP, J.M. & HERRING, A.J., 1983.** Sheep pulmonary adenomatosis: Demonstration of a protein which cross-reacts with the major core proteins of Mason-Pfizer monkey virus and mouse mammary tumour virus. *Journal of General Virology*, 64, 2323–2327.
50 **SIGURDSSON, B., 1958.** Adenomatosis of sheep's lungs. Experimental transmission. *Archiv der Gesamte Virusforschung*, 8, 51–58.
51 **SNYDER, S.P., DEMARTINI, J.C., AMEGHINO, E. & CALETTI, E., 1983.** Coexistence of pulmonary adenomatosis and progressive pneumonia in sheep in the central sierra of Peru. *American Journal of Veterinary Research*, 44, 1334–1338.
52 **STEFANOU, D., TSANGARIS, T.H. & LEKKAS, S.T., 1975.** Pulmonary adenomatosis in the goats in the District of Pieria (Greece). *In: Twentieth World Veterinary Congress Summaries*, Vol. 1, Thessaloniki, Greece.
53 **STEVENSON, R.G. & REHMTULLA, A.J., 1980.** Pulmonary adenomatosis (jaagsiekte) in sheep in Canada. *Canadian Veterinary Journal*, 21, 267.
54 **STUNZI, H., HEAD, K.W. & NIELSEN, S.W., 1974.** Tumours of the lung. *Bulletin of the World Health Organization*, 50, 9–19.
55 **TOUMAZOS, P., 1989.** First report of sheep pulmonary adenomatosis in Cyprus. *British Veterinary Journal*, 145, 299–290.
56 **TUSTIN, R.C., 1969.** Ovine jaagsiekte. *Journal of the South African Veterinary Medical Association*, 40, 3–23.
57 **TUSTIN, R.C., 1989.** Faculty of Veterinary Science, University of Pretoria. Personal observation.
58 **TUSTIN, R.C., WILLIAMSON, A.L., YORK, D.F. & VERWOERD, D.W., 1988.** Experimental transmission of jaagsiekte (ovine pulmonary adenomatosis) to goats. *Onderstepoort Journal of Veterinary Research*, 55, 27–32.
59 **VERWOERD, D.W., 1985–89.** Veterinary Research Institute, Onderstepoort. Unpublished data.
60 **VERWOERD, D.W., 1990.** Jaagsiekte (ovine pulmonary adenomatosis). *In*: DINTER, Z. & MOREIN, B., (eds). *Virus Infections of Ruminants*. Amsterdam: Elsevier.
61 **VERWOERD, D.W., PAYNE, A.-L., YORK, D.F. & MYER, M.S., 1983.** Isolation and preliminary characterization of the jaagsiekte retrovirus (JSRV). *Onderstepoort Journal of Veterinary Research*, 50, 309–316.
62 **VERWOERD, D.W., TUSTIN, R.C. & PAYNE, A-L., 1985.** Jaagsiekte: An infectious pulmonary adenomatosis of sheep. *In*: OLSEN, G., KRAKOWKA, S. & BLAKESLEE, J.R., (eds). *Comparative Pathobiology of Viral Diseases*. Vol. II. Boca Raton, Florida: CRC Press, Inc.
63 **VERWOERD, D.W., WILLIAMSON, A.L. & DE VILLIERS, E.-M., 1980.** Aetiology of jaagsiekte: Transmission by means of subcellular fractions and evidence for the involvement of a retrovirus. *Onderstepoort Journal of Veterinary Research*, 47, 275–280.
64 **WANDERA, J.G., 1971.** Sheep pulmonary adenomatosis. *In*: BRANDLEY, C.A. & CORNELIUS, C.E., (eds). *Advances in Veterinary Science and Comparative Medicine*, 15, 251–283. New York, London: Academic Press, Inc.
65 **WANDERA, J.G. & KRAUSS, H., 1971.** The ultrastructure of sheep pulmonary adenomatosis. *Zentralblatt für Veterinärmedizin*, 18, 325–334.

81

Maedi-visna

Synonyms: Ovine progressive pneumonia, Montana sheep disease, zwoegersiekte, Graaff-Reinet disease, la bouhite

D.W. Verwoerd, R.C. Tustin and A-L. Williamson

Introduction

Maedi-visna, one of the so-called 'slow virus diseases' of sheep, is caused by a non-oncogenic lentivirus. The Icelandic name denotes the two most common forms of the disease, maedi (dyspnoea) referring to the progressive interstitial pneumonia, and visna (wasting) to the chronic encephalitic form. Arthritis and chronic mastitis are more rarely seen. The disease is also known as ovine progressive pneumonia or Montana sheep disease in the USA, zwoegersiekte in the Netherlands, la bouhite in France and Graaff-Reinet disease in South Africa.[5, 7]

It was first described in South Africa by Mitchell,[18] who regarded the condition as an aberrant form of jaagsiekte, and then followed by reports from Montana.[1, 17] The confusion with pulmonary adenomatosis (jaagsiekte) caused by Mitchell's report was resolved by De Kock,[9] who was the first to realize that he was dealing with two distinct diseases, often co-existing in the same animal. The chronic pneumonia was named Graaff-Reinet disease after the experimental station from which the diseased animals were obtained.

After these initial reports the disease seemed to disappear, however, and South Africa was thought to be free of maedi-visna until a lentivirus was isolated in 1986 from the lungs of sheep suffering from jaagsiekte.[24] A preliminary serological survey revealed a wide distribution of the virus but it seems to have lost its pathogenicity, which may explain its 'disappearance' during the intervening years. Alternatively, the present isolate may represent a later introduction.

In Iceland, the introduction of maedi-visna virus was traced to the importation in 1933 of Karakul rams from Germany, one of which carried both maedi-visna and jaagsiekte viruses.[23] Most of the early work on maedi-visna was done in Iceland, where it was initially considered to be two separate diseases.[25]

Aetiology

The virulent maedi-visna (MV) virus isolated in Iceland is the prototype of a large group of lentiviruses that have been recovered from sheep in various parts of the world. All, including isolates from ovine progressive pneumonia (OPP virus) in the USA, the South African ovine maedi-visna isolate (SA-OMV virus) and caprine arthritis-encephalitis (CAE) virus are serologically related, but there is considerable variation in their biological properties, including their pathogenicity. All strains give rise to the formation of syncytia in cell cultures, but they vary in their ability to induce cell lysis.[27]

The morphogenesis and morphology of the viral particles are quite distinct from those of jaagsiekte and other retroviruses.[14, 24] Virions bud with a crescent-shaped core and have no intermediate space between core and envelope. The immature particles thus formed have an electron-dense layer immediately below the viral envelope. Mature virions are 80–100 nm in diameter, are membrane-bound and have eccentric cores, sometimes surrounded by a clear intermediate layer. Negatively-stained particles sometimes show short surface projections, but usually the surface is smooth.

The buoyant density of MV virus is 1,15 g/ml, which is similar to that of most type C oncogenic retroviruses but different from jaagsiekte retrovirus (JSR virus) and type D viruses, which are denser (1,18 g/ml). The polypeptide compositions of all the ovine lentiviruses are very similar, with four major viral proteins named gp135 (envelope), p3O(28), p16 and p14. The different lentivirus isolates cannot be distinguished serologically by conventional techniques such as immunodiffusion (which mainly detects the gp135 antigen), immunofluorescence, or ELISA. However, using a western-blot technique, MV virus strains were found to share both the p30 and p16 antigens, whereas CAE virus antiserum only cross-reacts with the p30 of MV virus and can therefore be distinguished from it.[24] There is no serological relationship between lentiviruses and JSR virus or other retroviruses.

A significant genetic divergence was demonstrated between MV, CAE and SA-OMV viruses by means of endonuclease restriction analysis, nucleic acid hybridization techniques and nucleotide sequence studies.[24–27] Hybridization results demonstrated that the SA-OMV virus genome is only 16,5–27,4 per cent homologous to

MV virus and 8,3–15 per cent to CAE virus, indicating that it is more closely related to MV virus than to CAE virus, but sufficiently distinct to be regarded as a separate subgroup. Based on these results the three lentivirus groups were classified as types I, II and III.[27] A phylogenetic history, based on the divergence of nucleotide sequences, suggested that the two ovine lentiviruses have been evolving independently for at least 42 years.[26]

Epidemiology

With the exception of Australasia, ovine lentiviruses have been isolated from all the major sheep-producing countries, and are often closely associated with jaagsiekte. They also occur in areas with a very low prevalence of jaagsiekte, such as the USA,[2] and they were responsible for large-scale sheep mortalities in Iceland after the eradication of jaagsiekte.[23] In South Africa, SA-OMV virus was isolated from jaagsiekte cases from various parts of the country and a limited serological survey revealed widespread prevalence of antibodies to the virus.[24]

Differences in breed susceptibility to SA-OMV virus have not been found in South Africa, but have been reported elsewhere for MV virus.[7] Goats are also susceptible to infection with MV virus and SA-OMV virus, and natural cases of maedi-visna in goats have been reported in various countries. However, no distinction was made between infection with MV and CAE viruses in the majority of cases and therefore this information is unreliable.

Transmission of the disease occurs under conditions of close contact. Droplet infection via the respiratory route has therefore been implicated, especially between adult animals.[23] Transmission from ewe to lamb has been shown to occur mainly through the colostrum[8] — presumably by means of infected monocytes.[21] Transmission by blood-sucking insects could also play a role. Transplacental transmission is possible but rare. Semen has never been implicated as a source of infection; nor has any evidence been published of indirect transmission by excretions or fomites.

The virus is able to persist latently, generally in the presence of high antibody titres, and infected animals are therefore carriers for life. Latent virus, in the form of integrated or non-integrated provirus, may be activated at any stage, providing stimulation for the immune system and an explanation for the slow development of the disease. Antigenic drift has been proposed as a mechanism for the evasion of the immune response.[13, 20] Most infected sheep in fact show little or no sign of disease, but remain carriers and can transmit the infection to others. No sex or age predilection has been found in the susceptibility of animals to infection.

Pathogenesis

The primary target cells for lentivirus infections are thought to be leukocytes. In the case of maedi-visna, monocytes are primarily involved. After initial viral replication at the site of infection the host animal mounts an immune response which effectively eliminates cell-free virus but is unable to destroy infected cells in which the viral genome is latent, i.e. in which viral proteins are not expressed. In this form the virus can continue to circulate or spread to all tissues of the body, from which it can be recovered by *in vitro* techniques. Restriction of viral replication *in vivo* has been shown to be mediated by a non-immunoglobulin protein factor in the serum which blocks viral RNA synthesis. Explants from many different organs will produce cell cultures in which the restriction is lifted and the virus can replicate to high titres, indicating that the latent virus is not defective. Virus replication is induced when monocytes mature into macrophages *in vitro*,[21] but this process is inhibited *in vivo* by a unique interferon, LV-IFN.[30] The occasional induction of *in vivo* replication presumably results in a sustained stimulation of the inflammatory response,[15] lesions in maedi-visna essentially consisting of chronic inflammatory changes.

The discovery of the human immune deficiency (AIDS) virus with its strong immunosuppressive action prompted an investigation of the possibility that SA-OMV virus may also induce immunopathological lesions. It was shown that this virus causes mild immunosuppression by affecting macrophage activity, an effect which may play a role in predisposing infected animals to secondary infections.[19]

Clinical signs

The onset of clinical disease is insidious and loss of condition is usually the first clinical sign recognized in both the maedi and visna syndromes. Clinical signs of maedi are rarely seen in animals before the age of three or four years. Dyspnoea is common, at first following exercise, but later also at rest. A dry cough may develop, but nasal discharges are typically absent in uncomplicated cases. In the absence of secondary infections there is no fever and the animal eventually dies from weakness and hypoxia six to 12 months after the appearance of clinical signs. Secondary bacterial pneumonia, often associated with *Pasteurella* spp. infection, is commonly the cause of death in field cases.

Clinical evidence of visna, characterized by nervous signs, is much less common, even though the incubation period is shorter than in maedi. Unsteady gait, particularly affecting the hind limbs, stumbling and falling, trembling of facial muscles and inability to extend the fetlock may be early signs of the disease. Gradual progression leads to paresis and eventually to total paralysis, accompanied by loss of condition, although the appetite is usually unaffected. Fever is absent and the animal remains alert throughout the course of the disease. The clinical course may last up to a year, but there is no recovery once clinical signs are manifested.[7, 13] Other clinical signs reported, especially for ovine progressive pneumonia, include swollen joints and mastitis which results in induration of the mammary gland.[5]

Pathology

In MV virus infections, the lungs and regional lymph nodes, brain, joints, and mammary glands can be affected to a greater or lesser extent; all or any of these tissues may be involved in a single sheep.[5] Hyperplasia of lymphoid tissue that may develop into lymphoid nodules, some with germinal centres, constitutes the basic lesion, but primary degenerative changes occur in the brain, joints, and walls of blood vessels.[5, 15]

In advanced cases of maedi, the lungs do not collapse fully when the thoracic cavity is opened, and the impressions of the ribs may be retained. The lungs are enlarged, may be two to four times their normal weight, have a firm rubbery consistency, lack normal crepitations, and are greyish in colour. The cut surface is dry, and the exudate typical of jaagsiekte is absent. Secondary bacterial pneumonia may be evident. The bronchial and mediastinal lymph nodes are usually grossly enlarged, may be three to five times their normal size, and, on cut section have a whitish, homogenous appearance.[5, 7, 11–13]

The most characteristic histopathological feature in the lungs is diffuse, often pronounced, thickening of the alveolar septa caused by infiltration of mononuclear cells, mainly lymphocytes and monocytes, and hyperplasia of smooth muscle cells. These changes may, in parts, lead to complete or partial obliteration of alveoli. Fibrosis is not a prominent feature, but perivascular, peribronchial and peribronchiolar lymphoid hyperplasia, sometimes with development of lymphoid follicles, is a consistent and conspicuous change. Transformation of some alveolar epithelial cells to cuboidal cells, which could be confused with early jaagsiekte lesions, may be present. Intra-alveolar exudate is generally inconspicuous and consists mainly of alveolar macrophages and some cellular debris, unless secondary bacterial pneumonia is also present.[11, 12] In South Africa, mild interstitial pneumonia caused by SA-OMV virus has so far only been detected by histological examination.

Visna has been characterized as a chronic demyelinating encephalomyelitis.[28] It commences in the ependyma of the ventricles of the brain and central canal of the spinal cord, and spreads to involve particularly the white matter of the brain and grey matter of the spinal cord. The lesions may be widespread but patchy in distribution. In brains taken from advanced cases, lesions consisted basically of lymphocytic choroiditis with, in some places, necrosis and fragmentation of the ependyma. A lymphocyte infiltration, which may be extensive and show evidence of lymphoid follicle formation, and prominent perivascular infiltrations in the nervous tissues, composed of lymphocytes, macrophages and plasma cells, are characteristic lesions. The number of cells, chiefly lymphocytes, in the cerebrospinal fluid may increase in some animals to 1 000/ml^3 or more.[16] Demyelination, foci of necrosis and gliosis in the white matter (that of the cerebrum and cerebellum often being most severely affected), and mild to severe lymphocytic meningitis are usually present.[11, 22] In the spinal cord, lesions occur along almost its entire length but vary in intensity. There is a nonsuppurative poliomyelitis, patchy demyelination and gliosis of white matter, and a lymphocytic meningitis and choroiditis. Cellular exudate may be present in the central canal.[11]

When arthritis is present, it is usually the carpal and tarsal joints which are affected, but more commonly the former.[6, 30] The lesion is characterized by hyperplasia and necrosis of the synovial membrane, necrosis and erosions of articular cartilage, necrosis and fibrosis of subchondral bone, and extensive periarticular fibrosis. Some affected joints may contain a small amount of fibrin, but no pus. The inflammatory reaction, which is prominent, is chiefly lymphocytic.

The mastitis which some infected sheep develop is characterized by interstitial accumulations of lymphocytes, the formation of periductal lymphoid nodules, and necrosis at the site of these nodules.[3, 10] Vascular lesions have also been reported in some cases of MV virus infection. These are most frequently associated with lesions in other organs and comprise intramural oedema and haemorrhage, mononuclear cell infiltration, and fibrinoid necrosis of the media of arteries. Thrombosis may be present.[4]

Diagnosis

A tentative diagnosis can be based on clinical signs and serological results. Confirmation by means of histopathology is essential, however, as the clinical signs are not specific and clinical disease can occur in the absence of antibodies. Virus isolation provides supportive evidence but, in view of the persistent nature of the infection, a positive result may only be indicative of subclinical infection.

Various serological methods have been used for the detection of MV virus and OPP virus antibodies, including neutralization, complement fixation, immunofluorescence, agar-gel immunodiffusion (AGID) and ELISA tests. The latter is the most sensitive technique, but the detection of precipitating antibodies to the gp135 antigen remains the method of choice for routine screening because of its simplicity and reproducibility. A western-blot technique has been used to distinguish between SA-OMV and CAE viruses.[24]

Virus isolation from live animals can be achieved by *in vitro* cultivation of macrophages from peripheral blood or milk, with or without the addition of indicator cells. Most ovine cell cultures are suitable for this purpose, but sheep choroid plexus cells are most often used. After the death of an animal, virus is most readily isolated by explanting affected tissues, such as lung, choroid plexus, synovial membrane or udder. Cytopathic effects develop slowly (over several weeks) and include the appearance of refractile stellate cells and syncytia. The presence of virus can be detected by reverse transcriptase assay, electron microscopy or immunolabelling techniques.[7]

Differential diagnosis

The respiratory signs of maedi-visna are basically those associated with chronic pneumonia. Pneumonia caused by bacteria and other viral infections is usually more acute and accompanied by fever, but such secondary infections often occur in maedi and complicate the diagnosis. Proliferative interstitial pneumonia,[29] shown to be associated with *Mycoplasma ovipneumoniae,* closely resembles maedi, as does the bronchopneumonia associated with *Dictyocaulus filaria* infestation. Typical cases of jaagsiekte and maedi are easy to distinguish by means of the presence or absence of lung exudate, but it is not always so straightforward, especially when secondary infection is present. Wasting and nervous signs may resemble those caused by scrapie, internal parasites, and vitamin E/selenium deficiency (white muscle disease).

Control

Except for symptomatic medication, there is no specific treatment for maedi-visna and the outcome of the disease is invariably fatal. Successful vaccination has not yet been achieved, leaving eradication of the disease as the only viable option. This has been achieved on a national basis in Iceland by the implementation of a drastic slaughter-out policy. It can be eradicated from a flock, or its incidence reduced to an insignificant level, by test and removal. Such programmes have been in operation for many years in several European countries, resulting in successful control. A nucleus of disease-free animals can be established in a short time by isolating lambs at birth and rearing them artificially.[5,7,25]

References

1 **COWDRY, E.V. & MARSH, H., 1927.** Comparative pathology of South African jaagsiekte and Montana progressive pneumonia of sheep. *Journal of Experimental Medicine,* 45, 571–585.

2 **CUTLIP, R.C., JACKSON, T.A. & LAIRD, G.A., 1977.** Prevalence of ovine progressive pneumonia in a sampling of cull sheep from western and midwestern United States. *American Journal of Veterinary Research,* 38, 2091–2093.

3 **CUTLIP, R.C., LEHMKUHL, H.D., BROGDEN, K.A. & BOLIN, S.R., 1985.** Mastitis associated with ovine progressive pneumonia virus infection in sheep. *American Journal of Veterinary Research,* 46, 326–328.

4 **CUTLIP, R.C., LEHMKUHL, H.D., BROGDEN, K.A. & McCLURKIN, A.W., 1985.** Vasculitis associated with ovine progressive pneumonia infection in sheep. *American Journal of Veterinary Research,* 46, 61–64.

5 **CUTLIP, R.C., LEHMKUHL, H.D., SCHMERR, M.F. & BROGDEN, K.A., 1988.** Ovine progressive pneumonia (maedi-visna) in sheep. *Veterinary Microbiology* 17, 237–250.

6 **CUTLIP, R.C., LEHMKUHL, H.D., WOOD, R.L. & BROGDEN, K.A., 1985.** Arthritis associated with ovine progressive pneumonia. *American Journal of Veterinary Research,* 46, 65–68.

7 **DAWSON, M., 1980.** Maedi-visna: A review. *The Veterinary Record,* 106, 212–216.

8 **DE BOER, G.F., 1970.** Zwoegerziekte, een persisterende virus infection bij schapen. Ph.D Thesis, University of Utrecht, The Netherlands.

9 **DE KOCK, G., 1929.** Are the lesions of jaagsiekte in sheep of the nature of a neoplasm? *Fifteenth Annual Report of the Director of Veterinary Services, Union of South Africa,* 611–641.

10 **DENG, P., CUTLIP, R.C., LEHMKUHL, H.D. & BROGDEN, K.A., 1986.** Ultrastructure and frequency of mastitis caused by ovine progressive pneumonia virus infection in sheep. *Veterinary Pathology,* 23, 184–189.

11 **GEORGSSON, G., NATHANSON, N., PALSSON, P.A. & PETURSSON, G., 1976.** The pathology of visna and maedi in sheep. *In*: KIMBERLIN, R.H., (ed.). *Slow Virus Diseases of Animals and Man.* Amsterdam: North Holland Publishing Company.

12 **GEORGSSON, G. & PALSSON, P.A., 1971.** The histopathology of maedi. A slow, viral pneumonia of sheep. *Veterinary Pathology,* 8, 63–80.

13 **GUDNADOTTIR, M., 1974.** Visna-maedi in sheep. *Progress in Medical Virology,* 18, 336–349.

14 **HAASE, A.T., 1975.** The slow infection caused by visna virus. *Current Topics in Microbiology and Immunology,* 72, 102–156.

15 **HAASE, A.T., 1986.** Pathogenesis of lentivirus infections. *Nature,* 322, 130–136.

16 **JUBB, K.V.F., KENNEDY, P.C. & PALMER, N., 1985.** *Pathology of Domestic Animals.* Vol. II, 3rd edn. Orlando: Academic Press, Inc.

17 **MARSH, D.T., 1923.** Progressive pneumonia in sheep. *Journal of the American Veterinary Association,* 62, 458–473.

18 **MITCHELL, D.T., 1915.** Investigations into Jaagsiekte. *Third and Fourth Reports of the Director of Veterinary Research, Union of South Africa,* 585–614.

19 **MYER, M.S., HUCHZERMEYER, H.F.A.K., YORK, D.F. HUNTER, P., VERWOERD, D.W. & GARNETT, H.M., 1988.** The possible involvement of immunosuppression caused by a lentivirus in the aetiology of jaagsiekte and pasteurellosis in sheep. *Onderstepoort Journal of Veterinary Research,* 55, 127–133.

20 **NARAYAN, O., GRIFFIN, D.E. & CHASE, J., 1977.** Antigenic shift of visna virus in persistently infected sheep. *Science,* 197, 376–378.

21 **NARAYAN, O., WOLINSKY, J.S., CLEMENTS, J.E., STRANDBERG, J.D., GRIFFIN, D.E. & CORK, L.C., 1982.** Slow virus replication: The role of macrophages in the persistence and expression of visna viruses of sheep and goats. *Journal of General Virology,* 345–356.

22 **OLIVER, R.E., GORHAM, J.R., PARISH, S.F., HADLOW, W.J. & NARAYAN, O., 1981.** Ovine progressive pneumonia: Pathologic and virologic studies on the naturally occurring disease. *American Journal of Veterinary Research,* 42, 1554–1559.

23 **PALSSON, P.A., 1976.** Maedi and visna in sheep. *In*: KIMBERLIN, R.H., (ed.). *Slow Virus Diseases of Animals and Man.* Amsterdam: North Holland Publishing Company.

24 **PAYNE, A-L., YORK, D.F., DE VILLIERS, E-M., VERWOERD, D.W., QUERAT, G., BARBAN, V., SAUZE, N. & VIGNE, R., 1986.** Isolation and identification of a South

African lentivirus from jaagsiekte. *Onderstepoort Journal of Veterinary Research*, 53, 55–62.

25 **PETURSSON, G. & HOFF-JORGENSEN, R., 1990.** *Maedi-visna and Related Diseases*. Dordrecht: Kluwer Academic Publishers.

26 **QUERAT, G., AUDOLY, G., SONIGO, P. & VIGNE, R., 1990.** Nucleotide sequence analysis of SA-OMV virus, a visna-related ovine lentivirus: Phylogenetic history of lentiviruses. *Virology*, 175, 434–447.

27 **QUERAT, G., BARBAN, V., SAUZE, N., VIGNE, R., PAYNE, A-L., YORK, D.F., DE VILLIERS, E-M. & VERWOERD, D.W., 1987.** Characteristics of a novel lentivirus from South African sheep with pulmonary adenocarcinoma (jaagsiekte). *Virology*, 158, 158–167.

28 **SIGURDSSON, B. & PALSSON, P.A., 1958.** Visna of sheep. A slow, demyelinating infection. *British Journal of Experimental Pathology*, 39, 519–528.

29 **SULLIVAN, N.D., ST. GEORGE, T.D. & HORSFALL, N., 1973.** A proliferative interstitial pneumonia of sheep associated with mycoplasma infection. *Australian Veterinary Journal*, 49, 57–62.

30 **ZINK, M.C., NARAYAN, O., KENNEDY, P.G.E. & CLEMENTS, T.E., 1987.** Pathogenesis of visna-maedi and caprine arthritis-encephalitis: New leads in the mechanism of restricted virus replication and persistent inflammation. *Veterinary Immunology and Immunopathology*, 15, 167–180.

82

Caprine arthritis-encephalitis

D.W. Verwoerd and R.C. Tustin

Introduction

Caprine arthritis-encephalitis (CAE) is a multisystemic, inflammatory syndrome of goats caused by a lentivirus. In young kids it is characterized by leukoencephalomyelitis, whereas older animals usually present with slowly progressing arthritis and occasionally progressive interstitial pneumonia or chronic mastitis.

The disease has not yet been diagnosed in South Africa, and a limited serological survey of 200 serum samples from 10 different sites in South Africa showed all as being negative for antibodies to CAE virus.[1]

Aetiology

Caprine arthritis-encephalitis is caused by a lentivirus (CAE virus) which is morphologically and physically indistinguishable from the maedi-visna (MV) virus. Conflicting results on the serological relationship between CAE virus and MV virus have been reported, depending on the techniques used and the strains studied. In an immunoblot assay CAE virus antiserum cross-reacted with the p30 antigens of both prototype MV virus and the South African ovine isolate (SA-OMV virus), but not with the p16 antigen of either strain.[12] A clear distinction could thus be made between CAE virus and MV virus. The use of an immunoprecipitation technique demonstrated cross-reactivity between all eight major viral proteins of CAE virus, MV virus and isolates of MV virus derived from the USA called ovine progressive pneumonia (OPP) virus.[7] The genetic relatedness of these three lentivirus groups was studied by means of a DNA/RNA hybridization assay. Whereas 70 per cent hybridization occurred within the groups, only 20 per cent hybridization was obtained between CAE virus and MV virus, 30 per cent between CAE virus and OPP virus, and 45 per cent between OPP virus and MV virus.[6] Endonuclease restriction analysis confirmed that there are significant genetic differences between MV virus and CAE virus.[12, 14] It is clear, therefore, that CAE virus is closely related to, but genetically distinct from, the ovine lentiviruses. It has been calculated from the respective nucleotide sequences that there has been a time lapse of 93 years since the divergence between ovine and caprine lentiviruses.[13]

Epidemiology

Chronic arthritis in goats was first reported in Switzerland[18] and subsequently in Germany[16] and Japan.[9] The encephalitic form was also recognized by Stavrou *et al.*[16] and reported in the USA[2] before the retroviral aetiology was discovered.[4, 10] Virus was later isolated from affected goats of milk producers in various European countries, Australia[15] and New Zealand. A global serological survey confirmed the almost worldwide distribution of the disease, the only exceptions being Somalia, Sudan and South Africa. In Kenya infection was limited to imported dairy goats.[1] All the evidence therefore suggests a European origin for the disease and international movement of dairy goats as the major mechanism of its dissemination.

Transmission of CAE virus is mainly through colostrum, but the respiratory and other routes cannot be excluded. Sheep can be infected experimentally with CAE virus and, depending on the virulence of the strain, do develop typical clinical signs. Infected animals acquire antibodies against viral core proteins but remain carriers of the virus for life. There is restricted virus replication *in vivo*, and integration of the viral genome into the host-cell DNA also occurs. This, the lack of neutralizing antibodies, and antigenic drift are probably responsible for the failure of the immune response to clear infection.[11]

Pathogenesis

The pathogenesis of CAE is very similar to that of maedi-visna except for the preponderance of arthritic lesions, which may be due to host-specific factors. Limited viral production occurs in latently infected target cells, which are likely to be leukocytes, in the presence of high antibody titres. The chronic inflammatory response, which is the primary pathological lesion, probably results from sustained low-level stimulation of the immune system.

Clinical signs

Generally the first clinical signs in adult animals are swelling of the carpal joints and lameness. Swelling and signs of joint pain usually increase gradually and may involve other joints and bursae as the disease progresses. The affected animals lose condition and eventually become recumbent, developing secondary lesions such as dermatitis, abscessation, and osteomyelitis. The rarer encephalitic form of the disease is usually seen in kids less than four months old, but occasionally also in old, arthritic goats. It is characterized by nervous signs such as tremors, 'star gazing' and paralysis. The rate at which both forms of the disease progress is highly variable.[3] Mastitis and pneumonic signs, such as a chronic cough and weight loss, are occasionally seen in affected animals.

Pathology

Evidence of both the arthritic and encephalitic forms of the disease may occur in the same animal, but generally one form tends to predominate.[8] Interstitial pneumonia and/or mastitis may also be present.

The virus affects all synovial membranes, including those of joints, tendon sheaths and bursae. The carpal, tarsal and stifle joints, and the atlantal and supraspinous bursae are most frequently involved.[8] There is often gross enlargement of the affected joints, with thickening of tissue around joints and of joint capsules, and marked proliferation of synovial villi and hyperplasia of synovial membranes. Acute inflammation is accompanied by distension of joint capsules, tendon sheaths and bursae with excessive synovial fluid which is serous in nature, dark yellow or blood-tinged, and often contains small free-floating pieces of fibrin or synovial membrane, lymphocytes and macrophages. In more acute cases, the articular cartilage remains intact until the later stages of the disease.[5, 8] In chronic cases, the synovial fluid may appear normal, but degeneration, which progresses to necrosis and mineralization, occurs in the periarticular collagenous tissues, joint capsules, tendons, tendon sheaths and bursae.[5] Degenerative joint disease, manifested by erosions and loss of articular cartilage, and periarticular osteophyte development may also be present.[8] Severe and long-standing disease sometimes results in axial or lateral deviation of a limb, joint deformation, rupture of tendons or collapse of osseous structures.[5] Severely affected joints may show fibrous ankylosis, and fibrinous material may fill severely enlarged and distended atlantal and supraspinous bursae and tendon sheaths.[4, 5] Histopathologically, the synovitis is characterized by infiltration of lymphocytes, macrophages and plasma cells, and there is lymphoid follicle formation in synovial membranes.[5, 8]

The lesions in the encephalitic form of the disease have been characterized as demyelinating encephalomyelitis, resembling, and having the same distribution as, those of visna in sheep.[5, 8] The changes in the lungs and mammary gland are similar to those of maedi.[8]

Diagnosis

The diagnosis of CAE is complicated by the variability of clinical signs and the fact that not all animals infected with CAE virus develop clinical signs. Various serological techniques such as gel diffusion, fluorescent antibody staining and ELISA can be used to detect inapparent infection and carrier animals.

Because of the persistence of infection, virus isolation is easily achieved by explant cultures of various tissues, preferably synovial membrane or choroid plexus. Cytopathological changes in cell cultures are the same as those produced by MV virus.

Seropositivity combined with the history, clinical signs and pathological lesions form the basis of a positive diagnosis, but other causes of arthritis should be excluded.[3]

Differential diagnosis

Arthritis in goats can also be caused by bacteria, mycoplasms and chlamydiae. Bacterial and mycoplasmal arthritis are usually acute, suppurative or fibrinous in nature, and accompanied by fever. Positive reaction to antibiotic treatment and isolation of the causative agent suffice to distinguish these causes from CAE virus. Polyarthritis caused by *Chlamydia psittaci* (which usually affects young animals) can be treated with tetracyclines in the early stage.[17] The differential diagnosis in the case of central nervous system involvement or pneumonia is the same as for maedi-visna.

Control

Southern Africa so far seems to be free of CAE, and control therefore depends on the strict regulation of imports, especially of European dairy breeds. In Kenya the disease has apparently been eradicated by the elimination of all seropositive goats.[1] In countries where the disease has a high prevalence, it should be feasible to reduce and eventually eliminate losses by a test-and-removal scheme similar to that followed in the case of maedi-visna. There is no treatment for the disease other than symptomatic relief.

References

1 **ADAMS, D.S., OLIVER, R.E., AMEGHINO, E., DE MARTINI, J.C., VERWOERD, D.W., HOUWERS, D.J., WAGHELA, S., GORHAM, J.R., HYLLSETH, B., DAWSON, M., TRIGO, F.J. & McGUIRE, T.C., 1984.** Global survey of serological evidence of caprine arthritis-encephalitis virus infection. *The Veterinary Record*, 115, 493–495.

2 **CORK, L.C., HADLOW, W.J., CRAWFORD, T.B., GORHAM, J.R. & PIPER, R.C., 1974.** Infectious leukoencephalomyelitis of young goats. *Journal of Infectious Diseases*, 129, 134–141.

3 **CRAWFORD, T.B. & ADAMS, D.S., 1981.** Caprine arthritis-encephalitis: Clinical features and presence of antibody in selected goat populations. *Journal of the American Veterinary Medical Association*, 178, 713–719.

4 **CRAWFORD, T.B., ADAMS, D.S., CHEEVERS, W.P. & CORK, L.C., 1980.** Chronic arthritis in goats caused by a retrovirus. *Science*, 207, 997–999.

5 **CRAWFORD, T.B., ADAMS, D.S., SANDE, R.D., CORHAM, J.R. & HENSON, J.B., 1980.** The connective tissue component of the caprine arthritis-encephalitis syndrome. *American Journal of Pathology*, 100, 443–450.

6 **GAZIT, A., YANIV, A., DVIR, M., PERK, K., IRVING, S.R. & DAHLBERG, J.E., 1983.** The caprine arthritis-encephalitis virus is a distinct virus within the lentivirus group. *Virology*, 124, 192–195.

7 **GOGOLEWSKI, R.P., ADAMS, D.S., McGUIRE, T.C., BANKS, K.L. & CHEEVERS, W.P., 1985.** Antigenic cross-reactivity between caprine arthritis-encephalitis, visna and progressive pneumonia viruses involves all virion-associated proteins and glycoproteins. *Journal of General Virology*, 66, 1233–1240.

8 **KNIGHT, A.P. & JONKINEN, M.P., 1982.** Caprine arthritis-encephalitis. *The Compendium on Continuing Education*, 4, S263–S269.

9 **NAKAGAWA, M., MOTOI, Y., IIZUKA, M. & AZUMA, R., 1971.** Histopathology of enzootic chronic polyarthritis of goats in Japan. *National Institute of Animal Health Quarterly*, 11, 191–200.

10 **NARAYAN, O., CLEMENTS, J.E., STRANDBERG, J.D., CORK, L.C. & GRIFFIN, D.E., 1980.** Biological characterization of the virus causing leukoencephalomyelitis and arthritis in goats. *Journal of General Virology*, 41, 343–352.

11 **NARAYAN, O., SHEFFER, D., GRIFFIN, D.E., CLEMENTS, J. & HESS, J., 1984.** Lack of neutralizing antibodies to caprine arthritis-encephalitis lentivirus in persistently infected goats can be overcome by immunization with inactivated *Mycobacterium tuberculosis*. *Journal of Virology*, 49, 349–355.

12 **PAYNE, A.-L., YORK, D.F., DE VILLIERS, E-M., VERWOERD, D.W., QUERAT, G., BARBAN, V., SAUZE, N. & VIGNE, R., 1986.** Isolation and identification of a South African lentivirus from jaagsiekte lungs. *Onderstepoort Journal of Veterinary Research*, 53, 55–62.

13 **QUERAT, G., AUDOLY, G., SONIGO, P. & VIGNE, R., 1990.** Nucleotide sequence analysis of SA-OMV virus, a visna-related ovine lentivirus: Phylogenetic history of lentiviruses. *Virology*, 175, 434–447.

14 **QUERAT, G., BARBAN, V., SAUZE, N., VIGNE, R., PAYNE, A-L., YORK, D.F., DE VILLIERS, E-M. & VERWOERD, D.W., 1987.** Characteristics of a novel lentivirus derived from South African sheep with pulmonary adenocarcinoma (jaagsiekte). *Virology*, 158, 158–167.

15 **ROBINSON, W.F. & ELLIS, T.M., 1986.** Caprine arthritis-encephalitis virus infection: From recognition to eradication. *Australian Veterinary Journal*, 63, 237–241.

16 **STAVROU, D., DEUTSCHLANDER, N. & DAHME, E., 1969.** Granulomatous encephalomyelitis in goats. *Journal of Comparative Pathology*, 79, 393–396.

17 **STORZ, J., 1971.** *Chlamydia and Chlamydia-induced Diseases*. Springfield: Charles C. Thomas.

18 **STUNZI, V.H., BUCHI, H.F., LEROY, H.L. & LEEMANN, W., 1964.** Endemische arthritis chronica bei Ziegen. *Schweizer Archiv für Tierheilkunde*, 106, 778–788.

83

Equine infectious anaemia

Synonym: Swamp fever

D.W. Verwoerd and R.C. Tustin

Introduction

Equine infectious anaemia (EIA) is an acute or chronic lentiviral infection of horses and other Equidae, characterized by intermittent fever, anaemia, progressive weakness, loss of weight and life-long persistence of the virus.

The disease has been recognized in Europe since 1843 and in the USA, where it is known as swamp fever, since 1896. In South Africa the disease was described by De Kock in 1920,[4] based on symptomatology and pathology, but all subsequent attempts to demonstrate antibodies or to isolate the virus failed. Whether the early diagnoses were incorrect or whether the virus has since disappeared is uncertain, but it is generally accepted today that southern Africa is free from the disease.

Aetiology

The morphology, morphogenesis and physicochemical characteristics of the virus causing EIA are typical of lentiviruses **(see Chapter 81: Maedi-visna)**.[3, 14, 16] It is found primarily in macrophages in infected horses, in which it persists for life. The virus may be detected in blood or in a variety of other tissues, as is the case with the other lentiviruses.[7] Its ability to persist in the presence of high antibody levels is due, in part, to its sequestration from antibody when latent in macrophages, and to antigenic variation.

Different isolates of EIA virus do not cross-neutralize, and immunization of horses with a cell-culture attenuated virus conferred homologous, but not heterologous, protection.[11] When two horses were infected with the same virus it was demonstrated by peptide analysis and oligonucleotide mapping that each of nine isolates, made at various intervals after infection from both animals, was different.[13, 15] Thus, although EIA virus isolates possess a common group-specific internal antigen that can be detected by immunoprecipitation, the envelope glycoproteins are highly variable, leading to the generation of random, non-cumulative immunogenic variants.

Nucleotide sequencing of EIA virus proviral DNA revealed significant structural similarities to maedi-visna virus and the human immunodeficiency virus (HIV), but little sequence homology in the envelope genes of these viruses.[10, 17]

Epidemiology

Equine infectious anaemia has been experimentally transmitted to susceptible horses by the inoculation of blood as well as by milk, semen and urine from infected animals. There is some evidence that foals from infected mares can be infected *in utero*, during birth or by colostrum. The most common mode of transmission, however, is by infected blood. Contaminated instruments and equipment used for restraint, such as twitches, bridles and gags are sometimes responsible, but blood-sucking insects are probably the most important transmitters in nature.[8] The prevalence of the disease in low-lying, humid and swampy areas, particularly during summer when insects abound, supports this contention. The fact that outbreaks often occur at places where large numbers of horses are present, such as race tracks, may also reflect the presence of large populations of biting flies or inadequate sterilization of instruments.

Antigenic variability of the causal agent and its persistence in infected animals are important factors in the maintenance of the infection. Apparently recovered animals remain carriers for life, and circulating virus is present in low concentration during the periods between clinical episodes, mainly in the form of immune complexes.[12]

Pathogenesis

As is the case for other lentiviruses, the persistence of EIA virus in the host's leukocytes is central to the pathogenesis of the disease. Primary infection is followed by rapid spread of the virus throughout the body and consequent vigorous immune response. High antibody levels in the first phase of the disease give rise to circulating immune complexes which are primarily responsible for the glomerulonephritis. The intermittent nature of the febrile episodes suggests recurrent activation of latent virus.[6]

Two mechanisms have been implicated in the development of the anaemia characteristic of EIA. The most important is haemolysis, caused by the reaction of viral antigens on the erythrocyte surface with antibody and complement.[18] Bone-marrow suppression, possibly caused by depletion of iron, has also been demonstrated.[1, 7] Chronic inflammatory changes, such as the infiltration of mononuclear cells into various tissues, play a relatively minor part in the pathogenesis of EIA. This is in contrast to maedi-visna, where they form the major pathogenic mechanism.

Clinical signs

The incubation period can vary from five days to months, but clinical signs usually develop some seven to 12 days after infection. The clinical course of EIA is also variable, with four interchanging syndromes being recognized.[5] Acute cases develop a high fever for one to three weeks until death occurs in most cases. Severe anaemia, icterus, petechial haemorrhages in the mucosae, and weight loss are commonly seen. Animals which survive the acute form pass into the subacute form with continuing moderate fever. This may be followed by chronic disease with signs varying from failure to thrive to persistent or episodic fever, cachexia and ventral oedema. Inapparent infection may follow any of the above forms and persist for life, or subsequently revert to clinical disease.

Pathology

Gross lesions that are commonly seen include anaemia, emaciation, lymphadenopathy, and accentuation of the lobulation of the liver. Splenomegaly, serosal haemorrhages and kidneys which are darker than normal are less frequently seen.

Microscopically, erythrophagocytosis is often observed in lymphoid tissues, while haemosiderosis is common in macrophages, both in the circulation and in organs such as the liver, kidneys and bone marrow. Lymphoproliferative changes consisting of lymphocytic and histiocytic infiltration occur in most organs in chronic cases, whereas lymphoid necrosis is more marked than hyperplasia in acute cases. Glomerular lesions consist of increased cellularity, infiltration by neutrophils and thickening of the glomerular tufts.[7]

A decrease in the platelet count, coincident with fever, is the most consistent haematological feature in horses experimentally infected with EIA virus. Decreased erythrocyte counts and packed cell volumes commonly occur during the recurring febrile episodes. Leukocyte numbers may be decreased and differential white cell counts mostly reflect an increase in the proportion of monocytes.[9]

Diagnosis

The diagnosis of EIA is usually based on clinical signs, pathological lesions and serology. Virus isolation in horse leukocyte or other equine cell cultures or sub-inoculation of blood into susceptible horses can be used for confirmation, but is rarely necessary. Haematological examinations, such as total and differential white cell counts, haematocrit, and haemoglobin determination, can be useful.

The agar-gel immunodiffusion test is the most commonly used serological technique because of its simplicity and accuracy, although ELISA is slightly more sensitive.[2]

Differential diagnosis

Chronic splenic or abdominal abscesses can resemble EIA in that they cause intermittent fever and weight loss. Differential leukocyte counts would, however, indicate neutrophilia in such cases. In babesiosis, which also causes fever, anaemia, icterus and hepatic lesions, the parasites are readily identifiable in blood smears examined microscopically.

Control

There is no specific treatment for EIA and the disease can therefore only be controlled by preventive measures. Transmission can be reduced by eliminating carriers, controlling biting arthropods, and preventing the mechanical transfer of infected blood by means of contaminated instruments.

Negative serological tests are required in most countries for the importation of all Equidae, and similar regulations often apply to the movement of horses within an endemic country. Test-and-removal schemes could eventually lead to eradication of the disease.

No effective vaccine is currently available for EIA.

References

1 **CHEEVERS, W.P. & McGUIRE, T.C., 1985.** Equine infectious anemia: Immunopathogenesis and persistence. *Review of Infectious Diseases*, 7, 83–88.

2 **COGGINS, L., NORCROSS, N.L. & NUSSBAUM, S.R., 1972.** Diagnosis of equine infectious anemia by immunodiffusion test. *American Journal of Veterinary Research*, 33, 11–18.

3 **CRAWFORD, T.B. & ARCHER, B.G., 1978.** Demonstration of RNA-dependent DNA polymerase in EIA virus. *In:* BRYANS, J.T. & GERBER, H., (eds). *Equine Infectious Diseases*. IV. Basel: S. Karger.

4 **DE KOCK, G.v.d.W., 1920.** Further observations on the disease equine pernicious anaemia. *Report of the Director of Veterinary Research*, 13, 587–636.

5 **FENNER, F., BACHMANN, P.A., GIBBS, E.P.J., MURPHY, F.A., STUDDERT, M.J. & WHITE, D.O., 1987.** *Veterinary Virology.* Orlando, San Diego, New York: Academic Press, Inc.

6 **HAASE, A.T., 1986.** Pathogenesis of lentivirus infections. *Nature,* 322, 130–136.

7 **HENSON, J.B. & McGUIRE, T.C., 1974.** Equine infectious anaemia. *Progress in Medical Virology,* 18, 143–159.

8 **ISHII, S., 1963.** Equine infectious anaemia or swamp fever. *Advances in Veterinary Science and Comparative Medicine,* 8, 263–298.

9 **ISSEL, C.J. & COGGINS, L., 1979.** Equine infectious anaemia: Current knowledge. *Journal of the American Veterinary Medical Association,* 174, 727–733.

10 **KAWAKAMI, T., SHERMAN, L., DAHLBERG, T., GAZIT, A., YANIV, A., TRONICK, S.R. & AARONSON, S.A., 1987.** Nucleotide sequence analysis of equine infectious anaemia virus. *Virology,* 158, 300–312.

11 **KONO, Y., KOBAYASHI, K. & FUKUNAGA, Y., 1971.** Immunization of horses against equine infectious anaemia (EIA) with an attenuated EIA virus. *National Institute of Animal Health Quarterly,* 10, 113–122.

12 **McGUIRE, T.C., CRAWFORD, T.B. & HENSON, J.B., 1972.** Equine infectious anaemia: Detection of infectious virus-antibody complexes in the serum. *Immunological Communications,* 1, 545–551.

13 **McGUIRE, T.C., O'ROURKE, K. & CHEEVERS, W.P., 1987.** A review of antigenic variation by the equine infectious anaemia virus. *Contributions to Microbiology and Immunology,* 8, 77–89.

14 **NAKAJIMA, H., 1973.** Physicochemical and biological characteristics of equine infectious anemia virus. *In:* BRYANS, J.T. & GERBER, H. (eds). *Equine Infectious Diseases.* III. Basel: S. Karger.

15 **PAYNE, S.L., SALINOVICH, O., NAUMAN, S.M., ISSEL, C.J. & MONTELARO, R.C., 1987.** Course and extent of variation of EIAV during parallel persistent infection. *Journal of Virology,* 61, 1266–1270.

16 **ROBERTS, D.H. & LUCAS, M.H., 1987.** Equine infectious anaemia. *Veterinary Annual,* 27, 147–150.

17 **RUSHLOW, K., OLSEN, K., STIEGLER, G., PAYNE, S.L., MONTELARO, R.C. & ISSEL, C.J., 1986.** Lentivirus genome organization: The complete nucleotide sequence of the env-gene region of equine infectious anaemia virus. *Virology,* 155, 309–321.

18 **SENTSUI, H. & KONO, Y., 1987.** Complement-mediated hemolysis of horse erythrocytes treated with equine infectious anaemia virus. *Archives of Virology,* 95, 53–66.

PAPOVAVIRIDAE

The family Papovaviridae (the name is derived from the sigla: papilloma, polyoma and vacuolating agent (the early name for the virus SV40)) contains only two genera, *Papillomavirus* and *Polyomavirus*, both of whose members may be oncogenic under some circumstances. The virions are unenveloped and have icosahedral symmetry. Papillomaviruses are slightly larger (55 nm in diameter) than polyomaviruses (45 nm). Both genera have genomes consisting of supercoiled, double-stranded, circular DNA, but those of papillomaviruses are larger than the genomes of polyomaviruses (7–8 versus 5 kilobase pairs).

Papillomaviruses produce warts (papillomas) and occasionally other tumours in a wide range of animals including many species of mammals and some reptiles and birds.[2] Polyomaviruses, on the other hand, do not cause disease in their natural hosts but may be oncogenic when inoculated into new-born rodents.[1] Cattle and pigs have been found to be infected by polyomaviruses, but these are not discussed in the following chapter since they are not pathogenic.

Both papilloma- and polyomaviruses may have long latent periods (the period between infection of the cell and appearance of progeny virus), but while polyomaviruses are able to replicate in cell culture (they usually transform cells which do not support their replication), this is not so for papillomaviruses.

Replication of both polyoma- and papillomaviruses occurs in the nucleus of the cell; polyomavirus DNA may be integrated into the host-cell DNA but that of papillomaviruses remains episomal.

References

1 **FENNER, F., BACHMANN, P.A., GIBBS, E.P.J., MURPHY, F.A., STUDDERT, M.J. & WHITE, D.O., 1987.** *Veterinary Virology*. Orlando, San Diego, New York: Academic Press, Inc.

2 **FRISQUE, R., 1991.** Papovaviridae. *In:* FRANCKI, R.I.B., FAUQUET, C.M., KNUDSON, D.L. & BROWN, F., (eds). Classification and nomenclature of viruses. Fifth report of the International Committee on the Taxonomy of Viruses. *Archives of Virology*, Supplementum 2. Vienna, New York: Springer-Verlag.

84

Papillomavirus infections

S.S. Bastianello and G.R. Thomson

Introduction

Papillomas (warts) are benign neoplastic growths of the skin and mucous membranes of a variety of animal species. They are caused by species-specific papillomaviruses, which have also been associated with the development of squamous cell carcinomas.[55]

Cattle are more commonly afflicted by this condition than any of the other domestic species; six types of bovine papillomavirus having been identified. With the exception of humans, where 56 papillomavirus types are recognized, and cattle, only one virus type has so far been identified in each of the other species affected. In addition to being generally species-specific, papillomaviruses infect specific cell types.

Aetiology and epidemiology

Papillomaviruses are classified within the family Papovaviridae. The virions are 55 nm in diameter, spherical with icosahedral symmetry, and have 72 capsomeres composed of at least three proteins.[7] The genome consists of circular DNA comprising approximately eight kilobase pairs.[26]

Transmission of papillomaviruses between animals usually occurs via abrasions or microlesions of the skin and genital mucosa, but iatrogenic transmission through rectal examination has also been reported.[52] Ropes, grooming equipment and contaminated instruments may transmit the infection between animals, and mechanical transmission by arthropods is possible.[26, 38] Cows with teat papillomas may transfer the virus through the milk to their offspring.[27]

As is the case in humans,[8] papillomaviruses of other species are probably widely distributed and so animals are usually exposed at an early age. Papillomatosis is therefore predominantly an affliction of the young; older animals tend to be immune because of exposure early in life.

Papillomaviruses are highly resistant to mild forms of denaturation and dessication, and this promotes contamination of the environment.

Because lesions may recur after surgery or appear *de novo* in animals which have been immunosuppressed,[3] it is probable that papillomaviruses have the capacity to remain latent and later recrudesce. However, the mechanism by which this occurs is not yet clear.

Cattle

Bovine papillomaviruses are divided into two groups (subgroups A and B) on the basis of their biological behaviour and the molecular biological composition of their genomes. Subgroup A cause fibropapillomas and subgroup B squamous (true epithelial) papillomas **(Table 84.1)**.[3, 4] Immunity to bovine papillomaviruses appears to be type-specific.[18]

Although squamous papillomas and fibropapillomas are common skin tumours, particularly of the head and neck in cattle, other epithelial surfaces such as those of the forestomachs and genitals (and in particular the penis and prepuce) can also be affected. Variation in the sites affected can probably be ascribed to different forms of management.[16] For example, in the USA, genital lesions in cattle are rarely seen in herds in which artificial insemination is practised.[44] Lesions generally occur during the first two years of life and there is no breed predilection.

The incubation period for the development of papillomas is approximately three-and-a-half to four months, although it can be as short as 30 days in experimental cases. Papillomas do not usually persist for longer than five-and-a-half months.[16]

Squamous cell carcinomas occur in the less pigmented or unpigmented areas of the eyes, vulva and horn core, and in the oesophagus. Bovine papillomaviruses, together with cellular and other co-factors such as high intensity sunlight, are probably associated with the development of these lesions on exposed areas.[12] Virus particles have been demonstrated in the precursor lesions[12] and the viral genome in the carcinomas themselves.[43]

Prolonged and regular ingestion of bracken fern (*Pteridium aquilinum*) has been associated with oesophageal carcinomas in Scotland and Brazil. These tumours are often accompanied by adenomas and adenocarcinomas of the intestines and neoplasms of the urinary bladder. Bovine papillomavirus 2 has been identified in

Table 84.1 Papillomavirus infections of livestock

VIRUS	SPECIES	DISEASE	REFERENCE
Bovine papillomavirus			3, 4
Subgroup A:			
BPV-1	Cattle	Penile fibropapilloma	4
		Teat frond fibropapilloma	4
		Cutaneous fibropapilloma	4
	Horses	Sarcoid	22
BPV-2	Cattle	Cutaneous fibropapilloma	3
		Alimentary tract fibropapilloma*	3
	Horses	Sarcoid	22
BPV-5	Cattle	'Rice grain' fibropapilloma	4
Subgroup B:			
BPV-3	Cattle	Cutaneous papilloma	22
BPV-4		Alimentary tract papilloma*	22
BPV-6		Teat frond papilloma	3
?		Ocular squamous cell carcinoma**	12
?		Vulvar squamous cell carcinoma**	43
Equine papillomavirus	Horses	Cutaneous papilloma	31
Ovine papillomavirus	Sheep	Cutaneous fibropapilloma	13, 53, 54
?		Cutaneous squamous cell carcinoma (head)**	15, 51, 54
?		Vulvar squamous cell carcinoma**	54
Caprine papillomavirus	Goats	Cutaneous papilloma	50
?	Pigs	Genital papilloma	44

* tend to become malignant
** malignant

the latter.[3] Although a mutagen, quercitin, has been isolated,[36] the carcinogen in bracken fern is still unknown but seems to develop only in certain soil conditions.[32] Bovine papillomavirus 4 has been implicated in the aetiology of squamous cell carcinoma of the alimentary tract in cattle.[22]

Horses, donkeys and mules

Papillomas are common in horses and mules, occurring mostly in the skin of the muzzle and limbs, on the mucous membranes of the prepuce, vulva and conjunctiva, and on the cornea.[20] Animals develop papillomas during the first two years of life and congenital infections are common. Complete immunity follows infection.[49] Recently a papillomavirus isolated from a cutaneous lesion was characterized,[31] and when used as a probe, enabled viruses to be identified in papillomas from other anatomical sites. The indications are that these are related but not identical viruses. As yet, no papillomaviruses have been incriminated in squamous cell carcinomas of horses.

Equine sarcoid is one of the most common neoplasms in horses,[2, 45] mules and donkeys, and there is no breed, age or sex predilection in horses.[44] Bovine papillomaviruses 1 and 2 and possibly a third papillomavirus have been demonstrated in the fibroblasts in sarcoids of horses,[1, 23] and in cell lines derived from such tumours.[23] Equine papillomavirus has not been demonstrated in these growths.

Sheep

Papillomavirus particles have been detected in papillomatous lesions of the face, keratinized horn on the ears[53] and hyperkeratotic scales of the perineum.[54] These lesions are prevalent in ageing sheep.

In both Australia and South Africa there is a high prevalence of squamous cell carcinomas of the vulva and perineum in sheep following the radical Mules operation or short docking of tails.[15, 51, 54] This practice results in the exposure of these areas to sunlight, which probably acts as a co-factor in the development of squamous cell carcinomas. Papillomaviruses have been detected in these neoplasms.[54]

Goats

Although papillomas occur more commonly on the skin of the mammary gland, lesions may arise in the skin and mucous membranes elsewhere.[11, 50] Mammary gland papillomas in goats that lack pigmentation and are exposed to actinic radiation are prone to progress to squamous cell carcinomas. The indications are that a papillomavirus occurs in these neoplasms.[50]

Pigs

Papilloma-like structures are normal anatomical features on the border of the tongue of new-born piglets.[40] Genital papillomas occur rarely in pigs and neither papilloma viral antigens nor DNA have been demonstrated in them.[44]

Other species

Apart from farm animals, papillomatosis afflicts a variety of other animals including dogs,[6, 47] where papillomavirus-specific antigens have also been detected in spontaneous squamous cell carcinomas of the vulva, African grey parrots (*Psittacus erithacus*),[44] Indian elephants (*Elephas maximus*),[48] impala (*Aepyceros melampus*), giraffe (*Giraffa camelopardalis*),[21] multimammate mice (*Praomys* or *Mastomys natalensis*),[29] domestic rabbits (*Oryctolagus cuniculus*) and cottontail rabbits (*Sylvilagus floridanus*).[10, 30]

Other papillomatous conditions, for example in domestic cats and rhinoceros, have been reported, but there is as yet no evidence for their association with papillomaviruses.

Pathogenesis

After the initial infection of cells in the basal layer of the skin, where the early genes[5] code for products involved in cellular transformation[24, 41, 42] and viral replication,[25] the late genes code for the production of capsid proteins.[9] Mature virions are only formed in the keratinized layers of the skin, and this requirement for cell differentiation has made it impossible so far to develop an *in vitro* cell culture system for the propagation of papillomaviruses.

Malignant transformation may occur in the basal cell layer; the papillomavirus genome and early proteins can be demonstrated in these transformed cells, but late proteins are not found. It has been postulated that papillomaviruses alone do not induce malignant transformation and that co-factors as well as cellular factors[39] are also required.[55]

Papillomaviruses may produce malignant tumours in animals other than the definitive host, an example being bovine papillomavirus 1 in hamsters. It has been shown that a live vaccine for oral papillomatosis in dogs resulted in cutaneous sarcoma when the vaccine was inoculated subcutaneously.[46]

Clinical signs and pathology

Squamous (true epithelial) papillomas are benign neoplasms of the skin and mucous membranes. They are usually multiple and generally occur on the face and neck or in the mouth **(Figure 84.1)**. These papillomas may vary markedly in size, usually have a dry or crusty surface, and are often pedunculated. The affected epithelium is hyperplastic, with excessive folding which leads to the formation of proliferative outgrowths. The epithelial hyperplasia is characterized by marked acanthosis and para- and hyperkeratosis, with elongation of the rete ridges which extend deeply into the underlying dermal connective tissue which in turn is mildly hyperplastic **(Figures 84.2 and 84.3)**.[19, 28]

Fibropapillomas are benign neoplasms of the skin and mucous membranes and are usually present as firm, white, fibrous outgrowths which, unlike true papillomas,

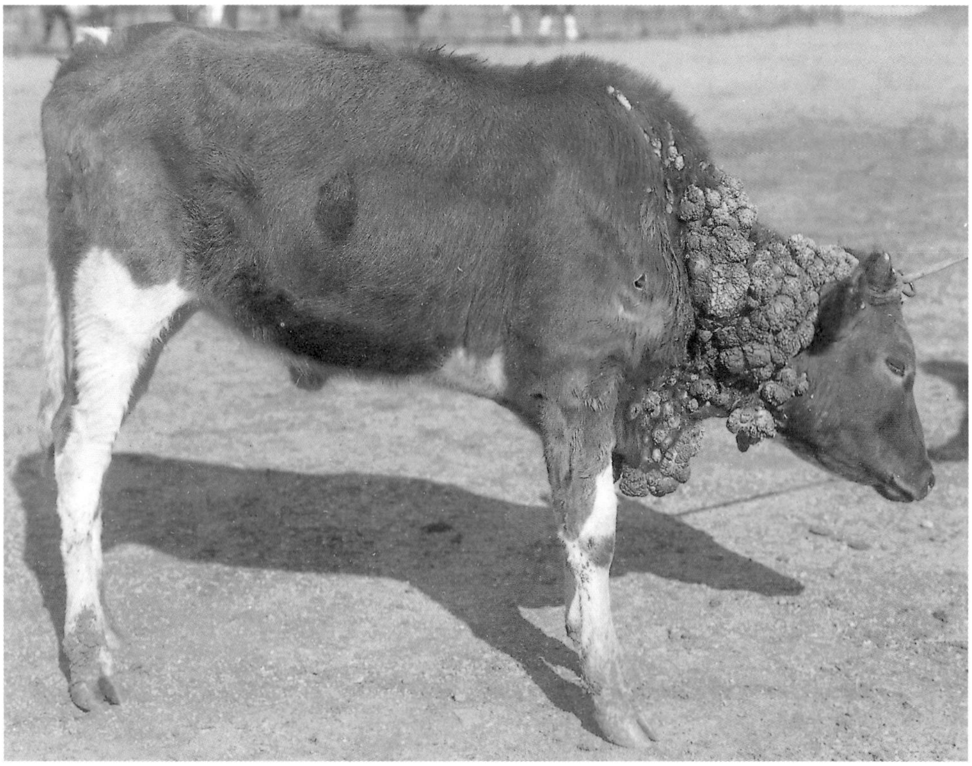

Figure 84.1 A calf suffering from severe papillomatosis. Note the numerous confluent warts on its neck

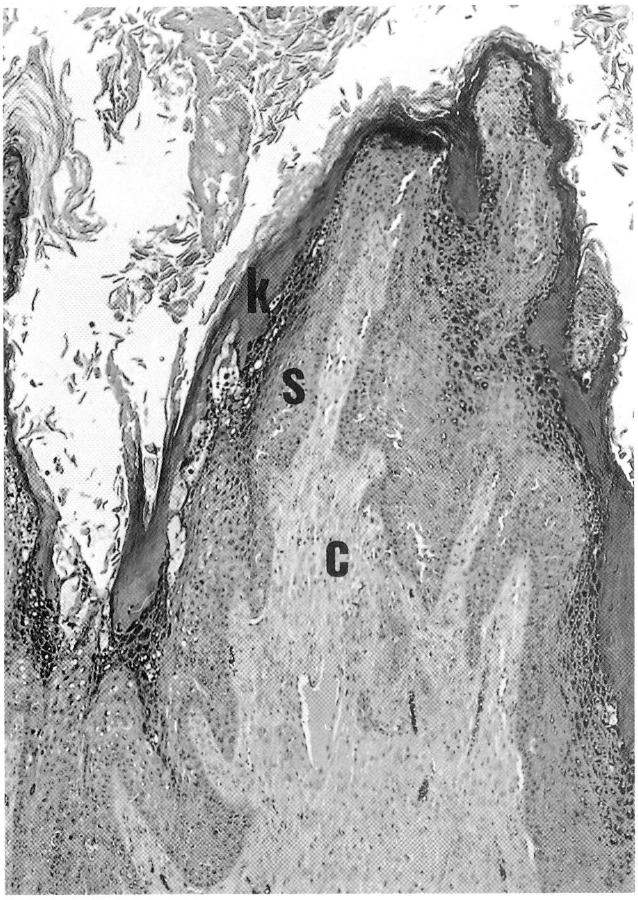

Figure 84.2 Squamous papilloma in a goat. Papillary outgrowth composed of squamous epithelium (s), thick *stratum corneum* (k), and a supportive connective tissue stalk (c)

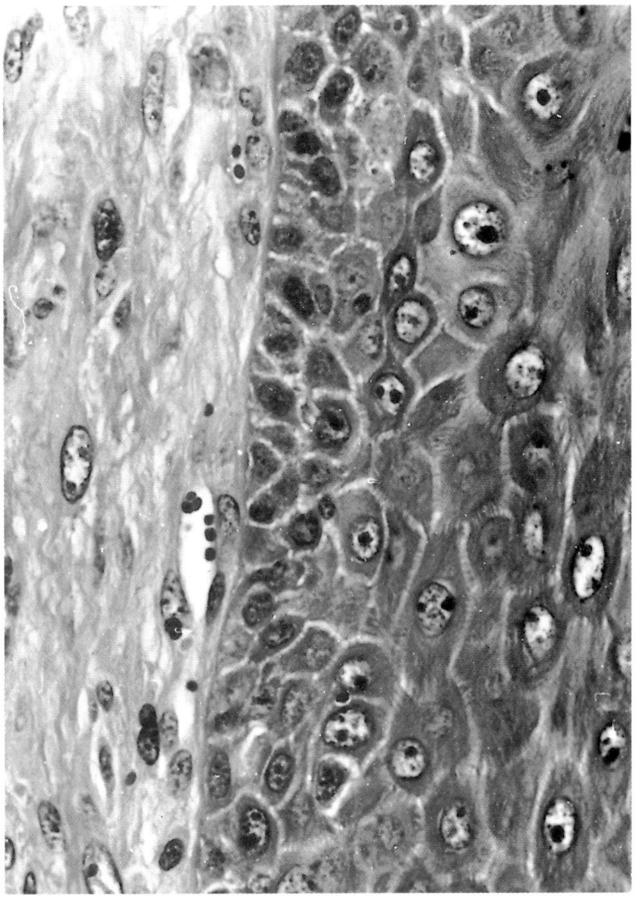

Figure 84.3 Squamous papilloma in a goat. Note the connective tissue stroma and well-differentiated epithelium containing intercellular bridges

are generally broad-based. In contrast to squamous papillomas, the connective tissue component of the growth is neoplastic and strands of epithelium may penetrate the connective tissue. There may be acanthosis and hyperkeratosis, but this is much less marked than in squamous papillomas. Microscopically, the connective tissue appears as densely packed, interwoven or whorled bundles of fibroblasts and collagen fibres. In young animals, these neoplasms tend to be largely cellular (fibroblastic), in contrast to the more collagenous types in older animals.[28]

Sarcoids are usually multiple, crusty and wart-like or large, firm, fibrous growths, often having ulcerated surfaces. They occur particularly on the head and legs. Although sarcoids are generally benign neoplasms, they may be extensive and invasive and have the ability to recur following surgical excision. They are biphasic (i.e. both the epithelial and connective tissue components are neoplastic), although in long-standing sarcoids the epithelial component is often absent as a result of ulceration. The epithelial component shows acanthosis and hyperkeratosis and may extend deeply into the underlying connective tissue as pseudoepitheliomatous cords **(Figure 84.4)**. The mass of the neoplasm is composed of fibroblasts and varying quantities of collagen fibres arranged in bundles or whorls **(Figure 84.5)**. A distinctive feature is the perpendicular orientation of the nuclei of the fibroblasts to the bordering basal layer of the epidermis.[19]

Squamous cell carcinomas are cauliflower-like, malignant neoplasms of the skin and mucous membranes. They are invasive and are often associated with ulceration and inflammation. The neoplastic cells may be well-differentiated squamous epithelial cells or may be highly anaplastic. The presence of keratin pearls and intercellular bridges are characteristic diagnostic features.

Diagnosis and differential diagnosis

Infectious and non-infectious granulomas and various neoplasms can be confused macroscopically with papillomas or fibropapillomas in livestock. However, these growths and lesions can usually be differentiated by their microscopic features.

Proliferative, crusty lesions often occur in and around the mouth, on the face, ears and lower parts of the legs in lambs and kids affected by orf, and these lesions may also be found on the udders of their dams. Although the macro- and microscopic lesions of orf and papillomas may be very similar, the conditions can be

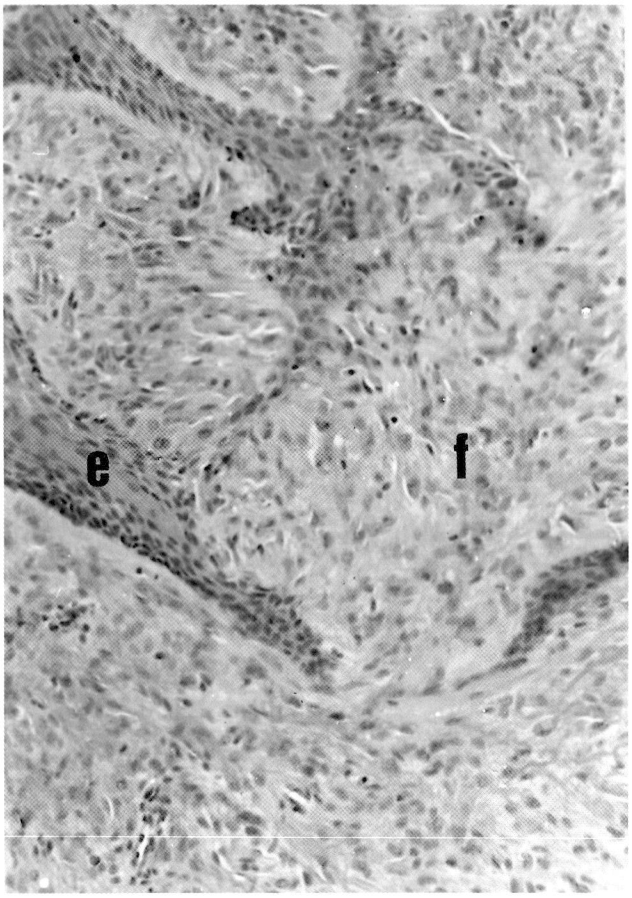

Figure 84.4 Equine sarcoid. Pseudoepitheliomatous hyperplasia causing branching rete pegs (e) to penetrate the neoplastic fibrous connective tissue (f)

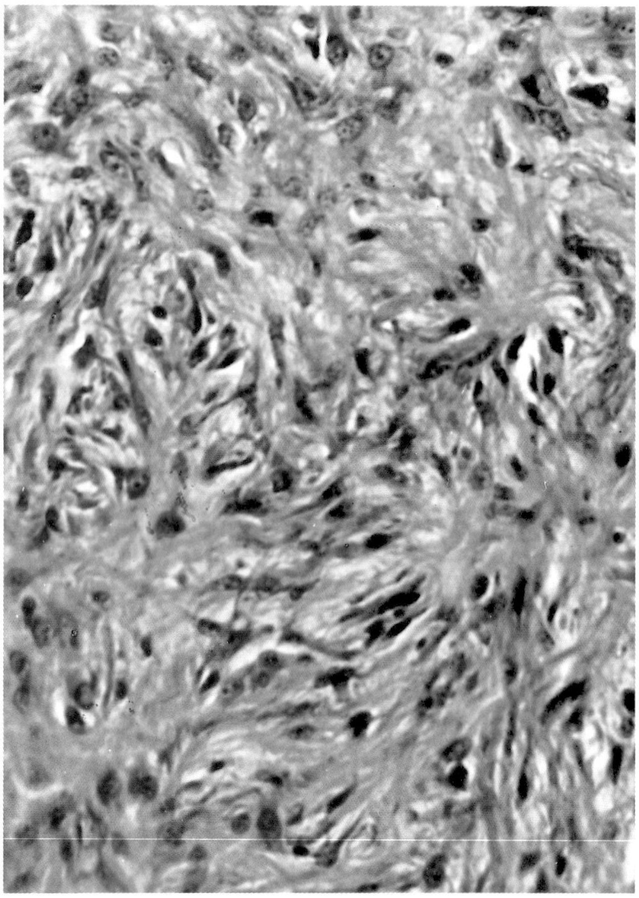

Figure 84.5 Equine sarcoid. Note the haphazard arrangement of neoplastic fibroblasts to create a whorl formation

differentiated by demonstrating poxviruses in negatively-stained preparations made from the lesions of orf.

The gross lesions caused by dermatophytes and *Dermatophilus congolensis* (particularly in sheep but also in cattle) may occasionally be mistaken for warts. Bacteriological, mycological and histopathological examinations of the lesions are helpful in distinguishing them from each other.

In Equidae, sarcoids, especially the larger growths, are frequently confused macroscopically with granulation tissue (so-called proud flesh), but they can be differentiated histopathologically. Fibromas and fibrosarcomas may also grossly resemble sarcoids. Microscopically, the biphasic nature of sarcoids and the characteristic appearance of the epithelial and connective tissue components of sarcoids differentiate them from fibromas and fibrosarcomas.

In some instances it may be difficult to distinguish fibromas from fibropapillomas in cattle histologically.

Control

Papillomatosis is generally a mild, self-limiting disease and therefore neither prevention nor treatment is usually necessary. Occasionally, however, epidemics in young cattle do occur, and some individuals may be so severely affected that their growth is retarded. In such circumstances a variety of treatments have been tried, but there is a lack of unanimity, not to mention reliable evidence, as to the efficacy of these treatments.

A commonly used treatment is the excision or, alternatively, crushing of a number of warts on the animal; the theory being that virus liberated in the process will somehow enter the blood stream and thereby induce a heightened immune response — or that the inflammatory reaction which results will have the same effect. Immunotherapy involving the use of immunopotentiators such as levamizole or BCG (bacillus Calmette-Guerin) has its adherents, but no reliable proof of efficacy has been produced.

In South Africa, sarcoids are treated by surgical excision which should include as complete a rim of surrounding unaffected skin as is possible, or surgical excision in combination with the implantation of radioactive gold-seed in the wound. Results obtained are generally favourable but when the sarcoids are large, tumour regrowth or defective wound-healing frequently occur.

Sarcoids that are small or present in inoperable or difficult sites, such as the eyelids, have been treated by the weekly injection into the tumour of Rubrigen (a non-specific immune-stimulator similar to BCG) until it has disappeared or is small enough to be excised. Injection of BCG into the tumour has also been attempted with some success.[14]

The use of formalinized autogenous vaccines or, alternatively, controlled infection using extracts of warts obtained from animals on the affected property, has been applied,[16, 33–35, 37] but evidence for its efficacy is lacking. However, type-specific immunity to purified virus resulting in resistance to severe experimental challenge has been demonstrated recently.[18] It appears that prophylactic immunity may be induced by viral structural proteins but not by tumour-specific antigens.[17]

References

1 **ANTMANN, E. & WAYSS, K., 1987.** Papillomaviruses and carcinogenic progression. II. The *Mastomys natalensis* papillomavirus. *In*: SALZMAN, N.P. & HOWLEY, P.M., (eds). *The Papovaviridae. II. The Papillomaviruses.* New York: Plenum Press.

2 **BAKER, J.R. & LEYLAND, A., 1975.** Histological survey of tumours of the horse, with particular reference to those of the skin. *The Veterinary Record* 96, 419–422.

3 **CAMPO, M.S. & JARRETT, W.F.H., 1987.** Papillomaviruses and disease. *In: SGM40, Molecular Basis of Virus Disease.* Cambridge: Cambridge University Press.

4 **CAMPO, M.S., MOAR, M.H., LAIRD, H.M. & JARRETT, W.F.H., 1981.** Molecular heterogeneity and lesion site specificity of cutaneous bovine papillomaviruses. *Virology,* 113, 323–325.

5 **CHEN, E.Y., HOWLEY, P.M., LEVINSON, A.D. & SEEBURG, P.H., 1982.** The primary structure and genetic organization of bovine papillomavirus type 1 genome. *Nature,* 299, 529–534.

6 **DAVIS, P.W., HUXTABLE, C.R.R. & SABINE, M., 1975.** Virus papilloma in the racing greyhound. *In*: JONES, O.G., (ed.). *The Racing Greyhound.* Vol. 1. London: World Greyhound Racing Federation.

7 **DELLA TORRE, G., MUTTINI, M., BALLINARI, D., FERRARI, G., PIEROTTI, M.A. & DELLA PORTA, G., 1988.** Characterization of papillomavirus polypeptides from bovine cutaneous fibropapillomas. *Journal of General Virology,* 69, 2919–2924.

8 **DE VILLIERS, E-M., WAGNER, S.A., WESCH, M.H., WAHRENDORF, J., PAPENDICK, U. & ZUR HAUSEN, H., 1987.** Human papillomavirus infection in women with and without abnormal cervical cytology. *The Lancet,* 2, 703–706.

9 **ENGEL, L.W., HEILMAN, C.A. & HOWLEY, P.M., 1983.** Transcriptional organization of bovine papillomavirus type 1. *Journal of Virology,* 47, 516–528.

10 **FENNER, F., BACHMANN, P.A., GIBBS, E.P.J., MURPHY, F.A., STUDDERT, M.J. & WHITE, D.O., 1987.** *Veterinary Virology.* Orlando, London, Sydney, Tokyo: Academic Press.

11 **FICKEN, M.D., ANDREWS, J.J. & ENGELTES, I., 1983.** Papillomasquamous cell carcinoma of the udder of a saanen goat. *Journal of the American Veterinary Medical Association,* 183, 467.

12 **FORD, J.N., JENNINGS, P.A., SPRADBROW, P.B. & FRANCIS, J., 1982.** Evidence for papillomaviruses in ocular lesions in cattle. *Research in Veterinary Science,* 32, 257–259.

13 **GIBBS, E.P.J., SMALE, C.J. & LAWMAN, M.J.P., 1975.** Warts in sheep. Identification of a papillomavirus and transmission of infection to sheep. *Journal of Comparative Pathology,* 85, 327–334.

14 **GOTTSCHALK, R.D., 1990.** Department of Surgery, Faculty of Veterinary Science, University of Pretoria, Onderstepoort, South Africa. Personal communication.

15 **HAWKINS, C.D., SWAN, R.A. & CHAPMAN, H.M., 1981.** The epidemiology of squamous cell carcinoma of the perineal region of sheep. *Australian Veterinary Journal,* 57, 455–457.

16 **HUCK, R.A., 1965.** Bovine papillomatosis. *Veterinary Bulletin,* 35, 475–478.

17 **JARRETT, W.F.H., O'NEIL, B.W., GAUKROGER, J.M., LAIRD, H.M., SMITH, K.T. & CAMPO, M.S., 1990.** Studies on vaccination against papillomaviruses: A comparison of purified virus, tumour extract and transformed cells in prophylactic vaccination. *The Veterinary Record,* 126, 449–452.

18 **JARRETT, W.F.H., O'NEIL, B.W., GAUKROGER, J.M., SMITH, K.T., LAIRD, H.M. & CAMPO, M.S., 1990.** Studies on vaccination against papillomaviruses: The immunity after infection and vaccination with bovine papillomaviruses of different types. *The Veterinary Record,* 126, 473–475.

19 **JUBB, K.V.F., KENNEDY, P.C. & PALMER, N., 1985.** *Pathology of Domestic Animals.* Vol. 1. 3rd edn. Orlando: Academic Press, Inc.

20 **JUNGE, R.E., SUNDBERG, J.P. & LANCASTER, W.D., 1984.** Papillomas and squamous cell carcinomas of horses. *Journal of the American Veterinary Medical Association,* 185, 656–659.

21 **KARSTAD, L. & KAMINJOLO, J.S., 1978.** Skin papillomas in an impala (*Aepyceros melampus*) and a giraffe (*Giraffa camelopardalis*). *Journal of Wildlife Diseases,* 14, 309–313.

22 **LANCASTER, W.D. & OLSON, C., 1982.** Animal papillomaviruses. *Microbiological Reviews,* 46, 191–207.

23 **LANCASTER, W.D., OLSON, C. & MEINKE, W., 1977.** Bovine papillomavirus: Presence of virus-specific DNA sequences in naturally occurring equine tumors. *Proceedings of the National Academy of Sciences, USA,* 74, 524–528.

24 **LOWY, D.R., DVORETZKY, I., SHOBER, R., LAW, M.F., ENGEL, L. & HOWLEY, P.M., 1980.** *In vitro* tumorigenic transformation by a defined sub-genomic fragment of bovine papillomavirus DNA. *Nature,* 287, 72–74.

25 **LUSKY, M. & BOTCHAN, M.R., 1986.** Transient replication of bovine papillomavirus type 1 plasmids: cis and trans requirements. *Proceedings of the National Academy of Sciences, USA,* 83, 3609–3613.

26 **MATHEWS, R.E.F., 1982.** Classification and nomenclature of viruses. Fourth Report of the International Committee on Taxonomy of Viruses. *Intervirology,* 17, 1–99.

27 **MEISCHKE, H.R.C., 1979.** Experimental transmission of bovine papillomavirus (BPV) extracted from morphologically distinct teat and cutaneous lesions and the effects of inoculation of BPV transformed fetal bovine cells. *The Veterinary Record,* 104, 360–366.

28 **MOULTON, J.E., 1985.** *Tumours in Domestic Animals.* 2nd edn. Berkley: University of California Press.

29 **MÜLLER, H. & GISSMANN, L., 1978.** *Mastomys natalensis* papillomavirus (MnPV), the causative agent of epithelial proliferations: Characterization of the virus particle. *Journal of General Virology,* 41, 315–323.

30 **O'BANION, M.K., CIALKOWSKI, M.E., REICHMANN, M.E. & SUNDBERG, J.P., 1988.** Cloning and molecular characterization of an oral papillomavirus of domestic rabbits. *Virology,* 162, 221–231.

31 **O'BANION, M.K., REICHMANN, M.E. & SUNDBERG, J.P., 1986.** Cloning and characterization of an equine cutaneous papillomavirus. *Virology,* 152, 100–109.

32 **OLSON, C., 1987.** Animal papillomas. Historical perspectives. *In*: SALZMAN, N.P. & HOWLEY, P.M., (eds). *The*

Papovaviridae II. The Papillomaviruses. New York: Plenum Press.

33 **OLSON, C., SERGE, D. & SKIDMORE, L.V., 1959.** Immunity to bovine cutaneous papillomatosis produced by vaccine homologous to the challenge agent. *Journal of the American Veterinary Association,* 135, 499–502.

34 **OLSON, C., SERGE, D. & SKIDMORE, L.V., 1960.** Further observations on immunity to bovine cutaneous papillomatosis. *American Journal of Veterinary Research,* 21, 233–242.

35 **OLSON, C. & SKIDMORE, L.V., 1959.** Therapy of experimentally produced bovine cutaneous papillomatosis with vaccines and excision. *Journal of the American Veterinary Medical Association,* 135, 339–343.

36 **PAMUCKU, A.M., YALCINIER, J.F. & BRYAN, G.T., 1980.** Quercitin, a rat intestinal and bladder carcinogen present in bracken fern *(Pteridium aquilinum). Cancer Research,* 40, 1468–1472.

37 **PEARSON, J.K.L., KERR, W.R., McCARTNEY, W.D.J. & STEELE, T.H.J., 1958.** Tissue vaccines in the treatment of bovine papillomas. *The Veterinary Record,* 70, 971–973.

38 **PULLEY, L.T., SHIVELY, J.N. & PAWLICKI, J.J., 1974.** An outbreak of bovine cutaneous fibropapillomas following dehorning. *Cornell Veterinarian,* 64, 427–434.

39 **RÖSL, F., DÜRST, M. & ZUR HAUSEN, H., 1988.** Selective suppression of human papillomavirus transcription in nontumorogenic cells by 5–azacytidine. *The EMBO Journal,* 7, 1321–1328.

40 **SACK, W.O., 1982.** *Essentials of Pig Anatomy.* Ithaca, New York: Veterinary Textbooks.

41 **SARVER, N., RABSON, M.S., YANG, Y., BYRNE, J.C. & HOWLEY, P.M. 1984.** Localization and analysis of bovine papillomavirus type 1 transforming functions. *Journal of Virology,* 52, 377–388.

42 **SCHILLER, J.T., VOSS, W.C., VOUSDEM, K.H. & LOWY, D.R., 1986.** E5 open reading frame of bovine papillomavirus type 1 encodes a transforming gene. *Journal of Virology,* 57, 1–6.

43 **SPRADBROW, P.B., 1987.** Immune response to papillomavirus infection. *In*: SYRJÄNEN, K., GISSMANN, L. & KOSS, L.G., (eds). *Papillomaviruses and Human Disease.* Heidelberg, New York: Springer Verlag.

44 **SUNDBERG, J.P., 1987.** Papillomavirus infections in animals. *In*: SYRJÄNEN, K., GISSMANN, L. & KOSS, L.G., (eds). *Papillomaviruses and Human Disease.* Heidelberg, New York: Springer Verlag.

45 **SUNDBERG, J.P., BURNSTEIN, T., PAGE, E.H., KIRKHAM, W.W. & ROBINSON, F.R., 1977.** Neoplasms of equidae. *Journal of the American Veterinary Medical Association,* 170, 150–152.

46 **SUNDBERG, J.P., JUNGE, R.E. & LANCASTER, W.D., 1984.** Immunoperoxidase localization of papillomaviruses in hyperplastic and neoplastic epithelial lesions of animals. *American Journal of Veterinary Research,* 45, 1441–1446.

47 **SUNDBERG, J.P., O'BANION, M.K., SCHMIDT-DIDIER, REICHMANN, M.E., 1986.** Cloning and characterization of a canine oral papillomavirus. *American Journal of Veterinary Research,* 47, 1142–1144.

48 **SUNDBERG, J.P., RUSSELL, W. & LANCASTER, W.D., 1981.** Papillomatosis in Indian elephants, *Elephas maximus. Journal of the American Veterinary Medical Association,* 179, 1247–1248.

49 **SUNDBERG, J.P., TODD, K.S. & DIPIETRO, J.A., 1985.** Equine papillomatosis: Is partial resection of lesions an effective treatment? *Veterinary Medicine,* 80, 71–74.

50 **THEILEN, G., WHEELDON, E.B., EAST, N., MADEWELL, B., LANCASTER, W.D. & MUNN, R., 1985.** Goat papillomatosis. *American Journal of Veterinary Research,* 46, 2519–2526.

51 **TUSTIN, R.C., THORNTON, D.J. & McNAUGHTON, H., 1982.** High incidence of squamous cell carcinoma of the vulva in Merino ewes on a South African farm. *Journal of the South African Veterinary Association,* 53, 141–143.

52 **TWEDDLE, N.E. & WHITE, W.E., 1977.** An outbreak of fibropapillomatosis in cows following rectal examinations. *Australian Veterinary Journal,* 53, 492–495.

53 **VANSELOW, B.A. & SPRADBROW, P.B., 1982.** Papillomaviruses, papillomas and squamous cell carcinomas in sheep. *The Veterinary Record,* 110, 561–562.

54 **VANSELOW, B.A. & SPRADBROW, P.B., 1983.** Squamous cell carcinoma of the vulva, hyperkeratosis and papillomaviruses in an ewe. *Australian Veterinary Journal,* 60, 194–195.

55 **ZUR HAUSEN, H., 1986.** Intracellular surveillance of persisting viral infections. *The Lancet,* 2, 489–491.

PICORNAVIRIDAE

The Picornaviridae are a large family of small (30 nm in diameter) RNA viruses. 'Picorna' apparently has two derivations: 1) pico = small and rna = ribonucleic acid; and 2) sigla for polio, insensitivity to ether, coxsackievirus, orphan virus, rhinovirus and ribonucleic acid (the two rs being contracted to one).[1, 3]

Apart from their small size and icosahedral symmetry (T=1), the virions are almost featureless; there is no envelope. The capsid is comprised of 60 protomers, each consisting of four polypeptides derived by cleavage from a single polyprotein. A small protein (VPg) is covalently linked to the 5′ end of the single-stranded RNA genome of positive-sense which is between 7,5 and 8,5 kilobases in length. Replication occurs in the cytoplasm of infected cells. The distinguishing features of the five genera (*Enterovirus, Cardiovirus, Rhinovirus, Aphthovirus* and *Hepatovirus*) which comprise the family are shown in **Table 1**. The genus *Hepatovirus* is the most recently created, to make provision for human and simian hepatitis A viruses which were formerly regarded as enteroviruses.

Many of the viruses classified as enteroviruses, rhinoviruses and aphthoviruses have a remarkable variety of immunological variants which do not induce effective cross-immunity. Prime examples are enteroviruses of humans (polioviruses, coxsackieviruses, echoviruses), monkeys and pigs, and human rhinoviruses, of which there are at least 100 serotypes.[3] Antigenic variation is

Table 1 The distinguishing features of genera within the Picornaviridae and the infections they produce in domestic livestock (adapted from Minor[3])

Genus	Buoyant density of virions in CsCl (g/ml)	Stability at acid pH (+ = stable)	Presence of a poly (C) tract in the 5' non-coding region of the genome	Species in which they occur	Number of serotypes in domestic animals	Diseases caused in domestic animals
Aphthovirus	1,43–1,45	–	+	Cloven-hoofed animals	7 – many subtypes	Foot-and-mouth disease
Cardiovirus	1,33–1,34	–	+	Mice (pigs)	1	Encephalomyocarditis
Enterovirus	1,30–1,34	+	–	Humans, pigs, cattle	Pigs – 9*	Swine vesicular disease Polioencephalomyelitis (SMEDI syndrome)
					Cattle – >2**	Subclinical
Hepatovirus	1,32–1,34	+	–	Humans, monkeys	–	–
Rhinovirus	1,38–1,42	–	–	Humans, cattle, horses***	Cattle – 2 Horses – 2	Rhinitis Rhinitis

* Eight of these viruses are classified as porcine enteroviruses, while the ninth, swine vesicular disease (SVD), also has the characteristics of an enterovirus but induces a distinct disease. SVD virus is closely related to, or perhaps the same virus as, coxsackie B5 virus, which is an infection of humans

** Evidence of more than two serotypes has recently been published [2]

*** Equine rhinoviruses have not yet been accepted by the International Committee on the Taxonomy of Viruses as proven rhinoviruses. Furthermore, the so-called acid-stable picornavirus identified in horses has characteristics of both entero- and rhinoviruses[3, 4]

SMEDI Stillbirth, mummification, embryonic death and infertility

( ) Indicates uncommon events

even more pronounced among aphthoviruses because although there are only seven types, there is wide intratypic variation, particularly within the types O, A, SAT-1 and SAT-2.

Picornaviruses are generally transmitted horizontally from infected to susceptible individuals. Most are host-specific, the exceptions being coxsackie B5 virus, encephalomyocarditis virus and aphthoviruses (foot-and-mouth disease viruses).

With the noteworthy exception of foot-and-mouth disease (and swine vesicular disease, which is only important because it clinically resembles foot-and-mouth disease), picornaviruses do not cause economically important diseases of livestock **(Table 1)**. In humans, however, a number of enteroviruses are of great importance, with polio, hepatitis A, and the many serotypes of human rhinovirus that cause the common cold being prime examples.

References

1 **FENNER, F., BACHMANN, P.A., GIBBS, E.P.J., MURPHY, F.A., STUDDERT, M.J. & WHITE, W.O., 1987.** *Veterinary Virology*. Orlando, San Diego, New York: Academic Press, Inc.

2 **HÖFNER, M.C., CARPENTER, W.C., LYONS, S.A. & HAMBLIN, C., 1993.** An indirect sandwich ELISA for the identificfation of bovine enteroviruses. *Journal of Virological Methods*, 41, 239–244.

3 **MINOR, P., 1991.** Picornaviridae. *In:* FRANCKI, R.I.B., FAUQUET, C.M., KNUDSON, D.L. & BROWN, F., (eds). Classification and nomenclature of viruses. Fifth report of the International Committee on the Taxonomy of Viruses. *Archives of Virology*, Supplementum 2. Vienna, New York: Springer-Verlag.

4 **MUMFORD, J.A. & THOMSON, G.R., 1978.** Studies on picornaviruses isolated from the respiratory tract of horses. *In:* BRYANS, J.T. & GERBER, H., (eds). *Equine Infectious Diseases*, Vol. IV. *Proceedings of the Fourth International Conference on Equine Infectious Diseases.* Lyon, France, 24–27 September 1976. Princeton: Veterinary Publications Inc.

85

Teschen, Talfan and reproductive disorders of pigs caused by porcine enteroviruses

Synonyms: Porcine polioencephalomyelitis, SMEDI infections, enteric cytopathic porcine orphan (ECPO) virus infection

G.R. Thomson

Introduction

Most infections with porcine enteroviruses, which are ubiquitous in pig populations, cause no apparent disease, but some strains are capable of causing polio-encephalomyelitis (Teschen and Talfan), reproductive disorders (stillbirths, foetal mummification, embryonic death and infertility — known collectively by the acronym SMEDI) and, less commonly, pneumonia or pericarditis and myocarditis.

Swine vesicular disease, caused by a virus which is either a distinct serotype of porcine enterovirus or a coxsackie B5 virus of human origin, is discussed in a separate chapter **(see Chapter 86: Swine vesicular disease)**.

Teschen and Talfan are names given to porcine encephalomyelitis caused by serotype 1 strains of porcine enterovirus. Teschen is the more severe form and was first recognized in 1930 in Czechoslovakia. It is now endemic in Central Europe, southern Zaïre and Madagascar.[27] Talfan, also known in Denmark as benign enzootic paresis, is a milder disease which has occurred in North America, France, Belgium, Britain, Ireland, Denmark, Greece and Australia as well as in parts of north-eastern Europe.[17, 27] The other serotypes of porcine enterovirus, of which there are at least 12, and whose disease-causing potential is not as clearly understood, are thought to be ubiquitous and can safely be presumed to occur in southern Africa,[5, 9, 16, 17] although serological evidence has been obtained for the existence of only four serotypes (1, 2, 3 and 8) in South Africa and Zimbabwe.[31] The prevalence of serotypes has not been determined except in the United Kingdom between 1973 and 1980, when serotypes 8 and 9 were most often isolated from pig faeces.[16]

The relative importance of porcine enteroviruses in the causation of the SMEDI syndrome is unclear, because when the syndrome was first associated with these viruses in the 1960s[7] it was not known that porcine parvovirus is also an important cause. Furthermore, porcine parvovirus is widespread in pig populations and commonly contaminates cell cultures in which its presence cannot easily be detected **(see Chapter 99: Porcine parvovirus infection)**. It is therefore possible that some of the early experimental work on the enteroviruses of pigs was confounded by the presence of porcine parvovirus. Since porcine parvovirus' role in reproductive disease of pigs has been identified, only one study has found porcine enteroviruses to be a more common cause of foetal and early neonatal death than porcine parvovirus.[15] In an abattoir survey conducted in the USA, almost 90 per cent of dead embryos and foetuses collected from 1 787 sows were believed to have died as a result of porcine parvovirus infection.[24] There is a danger, however, in taking this finding at face value because porcine parvovirus, and particularly its haemagglutinating antigens, are more resistant to the effects of decomposition than are porcine enteroviruses, and this makes it more difficult to identify enteroviruses in foetuses which have been dead for more than two weeks.[4] Nevertheless, the balance of evidence presently available indicates that porcine parvovirus is a more common cause of the SMEDI syndrome than are porcine enteroviruses.

Aetiology

The genus *Enterovirus* is one of five in the family Picornaviridae, the others being *Cardiovirus, Rhinovirus, Hepatovirus,* and *Aphthovirus*. General properties of the Picornaviridae are given in **Chapter 89: Foot-and-mouth disease**, and the distinguishing features of four genera are summarized by Pereira.[29] Essentially, enteroviruses are characterized by a buoyant density of 1,34 g/ml in CsCl, stability at pH 3,0 and the absence of a poly (c) tract at the 5′ end of the single-stranded RNA which comprises approximately 7 500 nucleotides.

All porcine enteroviruses can be cultivated *in vitro* in pig kidney primary or secondary cultures as well as IB-RS-2 cells (pig kidney cell line). However, different serotypes vary not only in their ability to replicate in baby hamster kidney (BHK21), Vero and Hela cell lines, but also in the cytopathic effects they induce in different cell lines.[5, 9, 18, 32]

Isolates of porcine enteroviruses which have been made over many years in different parts of the world have a bewildering nomenclature with much duplication.[8, 26] The system of identifying serotypes has now been considerably simplified — the serotypes are now numbered 1–11.[16] A table has been published that clearly lists the currently accepted serotypes and their synonyms.[5] However, because, apart from swine vesicular disease virus which is arguably the twelfth serotype of porcine enterovirus, a number of isolates do not fit into the existing 11 groups based on cross-neutralization and complement fixation tests, it is clear that at least one additional serotype exists but probably more.[16]

The ability of some common disinfectants to neutralize the infectivity of porcine enteroviruses has been evaluated.[6]

Epidemiology

In general, porcine enteroviruses are probably transmitted by the oral–faecal route. These viruses have also been found in semen, which makes venereal transmission a possibility,[30] although it appears that the viruses do not productively infect early embryos (blastomeres).

Most piglets are protected from infection for the first four to nine weeks of life by lactogenic immunity provided by antibodies in the milk of nursing sows.[33] Thereafter young animals are infected, probably sequentially, by the serotypes of porcine enterovirus present in the environment. Individual animals excrete these viruses for between one and several weeks,[2, 25] the levels of excretion being highest (up to $10^{6,5}$ plaque-forming units per gram of faeces) soon after infection.[33]

There is no apparent seasonality in infections with these viruses, although it has been found that reproductive problems associated with them are less common in summer than at other times of the year.[7]

Pathogenesis

Initial replication of porcine enteroviruses following oral infection occurs in the tonsils and the intestinal tract and associated lymph nodes;[1, 11, 12] the ileum and colon being more frequently infected than the proximal small intestine.[5] The cells in which replication occurs have not been established, but epithelial cell destruction in the intestine is not a feature of these infections.[5]

Viraemia occurs in Teschen disease as well as in other virulent type 1 infections,[13, 34, 36] and it is assumed that virus in the blood is the source of virus which enters the central nervous system as well as that which crosses the placenta to infect foetuses in cases of reproductive disease. In the central nervous system, the virus multiplies in neurones in ganglia as well as in capillary endothelial and glial cells.[19] In transplacental infections, when one foetus has been infected, transmission to other foetuses may occur by intra-uterine spread.[4, 35] There is evidence of virus replicates in the adrenals of experimentally infected piglets and that it causes necrosis of cells in the adrenal cortex.[11]

Experimental intra-uterine inoculation of porcine enteroviruses into sows on the fifteenth day of gestation did not always result in embryonic death; pathogenicity appears to depend on the serotype involved and thus, as with polioencephalomyelitis, it seems that not all porcine enteroviruses are equally pathogenic for porcine embryos and foetuses.[12] This observation is supported by the fact that natural infection of gilts at times close to mating or in mid-gestation apparently failed to infect the embryos and foetuses.[28] Foetuses do not easily become infected with porcine enteroviruses after the first four to six weeks of gestation,[35] and by about 68 days of gestation foetuses are capable of mounting an antibody response.[35] However, even in foetuses of 68 days or older, experimental infection resulted in widespread replication of the virus in foetal tissues — the lungs and intestine yielding the most virus.[35]

Myocarditis is occasionally associated with Teschen disease, and a particular strain of porcine enterovirus (O2B) consistently produced non-lethal serofibrinous pericarditis in addition to encephalomyelitis in young germ-free piglets to which the virus was fed.[20] It was not clear whether the myocardial involvement, which consisted of the formation of contraction bands and occasional necrosis of myocytes, was due to the direct effects of the virus or to secondary metabolic changes. Similarly, some porcine enteroviruses are thought to be capable of causing pneumonia in pigs following inhalation.[25]

Clinical signs

Most infections with porcine enteroviruses are clinically inapparent. In Teschen disease, which is characterized in piggeries by high morbidity and mortality, the most obvious sign is locomotor ataxia, which may be accompanied by nystagmus, convulsions and opisthotonus. In severe cases, the ataxia progresses to paralysis and death within three or four days of the onset of clinical signs.[5] The paralysis is usually flaccid but may later become spastic.[21] In the acute stage, more general signs of systemic infection such as elevated body temperature and listlessness are evident and there may also be diarrhoea.[11, 19, 21] Animals which survive the acute stage of the disease regain their appetite and general habitus, but the paralysis is usually permanent and atrophy of the affected muscle groups occurs.[5]

In Talfan disease, in which piglets are predominantly affected and morbidity and mortality rates low, a range of signs may be evident that extend from only a fever to loss of spinal reflexes and ataxia. Paralysis rarely occurs.

Gilts and sows afflicted by the SMEDI syndrome rarely show any clinical signs at the time when infection occurs; only the subsequent birth of dead, often mummified, foetuses, and of small litters, or failure of sows to farrow after apparent conception and repeat breeding are indicative of infection.[7] The syndrome is described in more detail in **Chapter 99: Porcine parvovirus infection**.

Pathology

In pigs suffering from polioencephalomyelitis there are no lesions visible macroscopically other than in paralysed animals, where muscle wasting may be evident in one or more limbs.[11]

Experimental studies with a serotype 2 virus administered orally[11] have identified the brain stem, lumbar spinal cord (especially the ventral horn) and associated dorsal root ganglia as the sites where the first microscopically visible lesions developed. These lesions were present in animals killed seven or more days after experimental infection. The most pronounced lesions were disseminated in the grey matter of the spinal cord and adjacent dorsal root ganglia, followed by the medulla oblongata and pons and then the diencephalon and mesencephalon. Lesions were also present in cerebellum but were not extensive, and were rare in the cerebral cortex.

Histologically, the lesions consist of diffuse chromatolysis progressing to ganglion cell necrosis with diffuse infiltration of microglia and monocytes. Perivascular cuffing with mononuclear cells is also evident.[11] Lymphocytic meningitis may be prominent, especially over the cerebellum in cases in which the course was not acute.[14]

Electron microscopic studies[19] showed that detachment of ribosomes from endoplasmic reticulum and disappearance of ribosomal clusters were the earliest ultrastructural lesions in ganglion cells. Thereafter dilation of endoplasmic reticular cisternae occurred that led to vesiculation and cellular necrosis. Viral crystals were seen in capillary endothelial cells and in astrocytic processes near capillaries and neuronal membranes.

Lung lesions have been described in pigs that have been infected naturally with porcine enteroviruses, and intranasal installation of a virus into specific pathogen-free piglets led to the development of chronic interstitial pneumonitis characterized by the infiltration of inflammatory cells, primarily lymphocytes, and areas of alveolar collapse.[25, 32]

Serofibrinous pericarditis, in addition to polioencephalomyelitis, has been observed in piglets infected experimentally. A cloudy pericardial effusion containing predominantly mesothelial cells early in the course of the disease, and neutrophils later, occurred ten or more days after exposure.[20] Focal myocardial necrosis with cellular infiltration was evident in some animals.

Diagnosis

Infections with these viruses have not yet been shown to be important in southern Africa, so diagnosis of either enteroviral polioencephalomyelitis or SMEDI-type disease depends on virus isolation as other techniques have not been developed. The diagnosis of polioencephalomyelitis does not constitute a problem because, in acute cases, porcine enteroviruses can be recovered from the central nervous system using cell culture techniques. On the other hand, in the SMEDI syndrome, the viruses do not survive for more than about 14 days after foetal death, which makes it difficult, if not impossible, to recover the virus from mummified foetuses even when it is responsible for foetal death.[4, 7] It must be borne in mind that porcine enteroviruses are recoverable from the intestines of normal pigs and therefore the possibility of contamination of other tissues by intestinal contents during necropsy must be excluded if a reliable diagnosis is to be ensured. Detecting antibody to porcine enteroviruses in the sera of stillborn piglets or those deprived of colostrum, particularly in litters which are smaller in number than normal, may be used to incriminate porcine enterovirus as a probable cause of foetal death.[3]

The efficacy of antigen detection using direct immunofluorescence staining of tissues obtained from experimentally infected porcine foetuses has been demonstrated,[35] but it is unlikely that this approach would be effective on decomposing tissues. Techniques such as the polymerase chain reaction, which enable the identification of the genomes of these viruses, may be useful in such instances, but the paucity of nucleotide sequence data and information on sequence conservation between porcine enteroviruses precludes this at present. In one instance a tentative diagnosis of porcine enterovirus infection was made on the basis of it being possible to identify picornavirus-like particles electron microscopically in pig tissue suspensions centrifuged to a density of 1,34 g/ml in CsCl gradients.[23] This, however, is too tedious and equivocal a technique to be used routinely.

Serological diagnosis of these infections other than in stillborn or colostrum-deprived piglets is inappropriate because of the wide distribution of the viruses in pig populations and the large number of serotypes.

Differential diagnosis

Diseases which could be confused with porcine polioencephalomyelitis are rabies, pseudorabies, hog cholera, Japanese B encephalitis, and haemagglutinating encephalomyelitis and porcine adenovirus type 4 infections.[23]

The SMEDI syndrome may be caused by porcine parvovirus infection. Hog cholera and pseudorabies, apart from their other features, may result in reproductive failure superficially similar to that of the SMEDI syndrome.

Control

Both attenuated and inactivated vaccines produced in cell culture have been used to immunize pigs against Teschen disease but vaccines have not been developed for the less virulent causes of porcine polioencephalomyelitis.[5, 10] Similarly, no vaccines against the SMEDI syndrome caused by porcine enteroviruses have been evaluated.

In pig slurry, which is widely used to fertilize fields in Europe, the rate of inactivation of porcine enteroviruses has been shown to be enhanced by aeration.[22]

References

1 **BABA, S.P., BOHL, E.H. & MEYER, R.C., 1966.** Infection of germ-free pigs with a porcine enterovirus. *Cornell Veterinarian*, 56, 386–394.

2 **CARTWRIGHT, S.F. & HUCK, R.A., 1963.** Studies on enterovirus of swine. Isolation in tissue culture of a strain (FS_{55}) of the Teschen group of viruses. *The Journal of Comparative Pathology and Therapeutics*, 73, 27–38.

3 **CROPPER, M., DUNNE, H.W., LEMAN, A.D., STARKEY, L. & HOEFLING, D.C., 1976.** Prevalence of antibody to porcine enteroviruses and porcine parvovirus in body fluids of fetal pigs from small vs large litters. *Journal of the American Veterinary Medical Association*, 168, 233–235.

4 **DE MEURICHY, W., PENSAERT, M. & BONTE, P., 1976.** Het SMEDI-syndrome bij het varken: Rol van de enterovirussen en het parvovirus. *Vlaamse Diergeneeskundige Tijdschrift*, 45, 241-261.

5 **DERBYSHIRE, J.B., 1986.** Porcine enterovirus infection. *In*: EMAN, A.D., SHAW, B., GLOCK, R.D., MENGELING, W.L., PENNY, R.H.C. & SCHOLL, E., (eds). *Diseases of Swine*. 6th edn. Ames, Iowa: Iowa State University Press.

6 **DERBYSHIRE, J.B. & ARKELL, S., 1971.** The activity of some chemical disinfectants against Talfan virus and porcine adenovirus type 2. *British Veterinary Journal*, 127, 137–142.

7 **DUNNE, H.W., GOBBLE, J.L., HOKANSON, J.F., KRADEL, D.C. & BUBASH, G.R., 1965.** *American Journal of Veterinary Research*, 26,1284–1297.

8 **DUNNE, H.W., KRADEL, D.C., CLARK, C.D., BUBASH, G.R. & AMMERMAN, E., 1967.** Porcine enteroviruses: A serologic comparison of thirty-eight Pennsylvania isolates with other reported North American strains, Teschen, Talfan, and T80 serums — a progress report. *American Journal of Veterinary Research*, 27, 557–568.

9 **DUNNE, H.W., WANG, J.T. & AMMERMAN, E.H., 1971.** Classification of North American porcine enteroviruses: A comparison with European and Japanese strains. *Infection and Immunity*, 4, 619–631.

10 **HAZLETT, D.T.G. & DERBYSHIRE, J.B., 1977.** The protective effect of two porcine enterovirus vaccines in swine. *Canadian Journal of Comparative Medicine*, 41, 264–273.

11 **HOLMAN, J.E., KOESTNER, A. & KASZA, L., 1966.** Histopathogenesis of porcine polioencephalomyelitis in the germ-free pig. *Pathologia Veterinaria*, 3, 633–651.

12 **HUANG, J., GENTRY, R.F. & ZARKOWER, A., 1980.** Experimental infection of pregnant sows with porcine enteroviruses. *American Journal of Veterinary Research*, 41, 469–473.

13 **IZAWA, H., HOWORTH, J.A. & BANKOWSKI, R.A., 1962.** Porcine enteroviruses. II. Pathogenesis of viral agents isolated from the intestinal tract of swine. *American Journal of Veterinary Research*, 23, 1142–1149.

14 **JUBB, K.V.F., KENNEDY, P.C. & PALMER, N., 1985.** *Pathology of Domestic Animals*. 3rd edn. Orlando, Florida: Academic Press, Inc.

15 **KIRKBRIDE, C.A. & McADARAGH, J.P., 1978.** Infectious agents associated with fetal and early neonatal death and abortion in swine. *Journal of the American Veterinary Medical Association*, 172, 480–483.

16 **KNOWLES, N.J., 1983.** Isolation and identification of porcine enteroviruses in Great Britain, 1979 to 1980. *British Veterinary Journal*, 139, 19–22.

17 **KNOWLES, N.J. & BUCKLEY, L.S., 1980.** Differentiation of porcine enterovirus serotypes by complement fixation. *Research in Veterinary Science*, 29, 113–115.

18 **KNOWLES, N.J., BUCKLEY, L.S. & PEREIRA, H.G., 1979.** Classification of porcine enteroviruses by antigenic analysis and cytopathic effects in tissue culture: Description of three new serotypes. *Archives of Virology*, 62, 201–208.

19 **KOESTNER, A., KASZA, L. & HOLMMAN, J.E., 1966.** Electron microscopic evaluation of the pathogenesis of porcine polioencephalomyelitis. *American Journal of Pathology*, 49, 325–337.

20 **LONG, J.F., KASZA, L. & KOESTNER, A., 1969.** Pericarditis and myocarditis in germ-free and colostrum-deprived pigs experimentally infected with a porcine polioencephalomyelitis virus. *The Journal of Infectious Diseases*, 120, 245–249.

21 **LONG, J.F., KOESTNER, A. & KASZA, L., 1966.** Infectivity of three porcine polioencephalomyelitis viruses for germ-free and pathogen-free pigs. *American Journal of Veterinary Research*, 27, 274–279.

22 **LUND, E. & NISSEN, B., 1983.** The survival of enterovirus in aerated and unaerated cattle and pig slurry. *Agricultural Wastes*, 7, 221–233.

23 **LYNCH, J.A., BINNINGTON, B.D. & HOOVER, D.M., 1984.** Virus isolation studies in an outbreak of porcine encephalomyelitis. *Canadian Journal of Comparative Medicine*, 48, 233–235.

24 **MENGELING, W.L., 1978.** Prevalence of porcine parvovirus-induced reproductive failure: An abattoir study. *Journal of the American Veterinary Medical Association*, 172, 1291–1294.

25 **MEYER, R.C., WOODS, G.T. & SIMON, J., 1966.** Pneumonitis in an enterovirus infection in swine. *Journal of Comparative Pathology*, 76, 397–405.

26 **MORIMOTO, T., DUNNE, H.W. & WANG, J.T., 1968.** Serologic comparison of North American and Japanese porcine picornaviruses. *American Journal of Veterinary Research*, 29, 2275–2280.

27 **ODEND'HAL, S., 1983.** *The Geographical Distribution of Animal Viral Diseases*. New York, London: Academic Press, Inc.

28 **PARKER, B.N.J., WRATHALL, A.E. & CARTWRIGHT, S.F., 1981.** Accidental introduction of porcine parvovirus and Talfan virus into a group of minimal-disease gilts and their effects on reproduction. *British Veterinary Journal*, 137, 262–267.

29 **PEREIRA, H.G., 1989.** *In*: PORTERFIELD, J.S., (ed.). *Andrews' Viruses of Vertebrates*. 5th edn. London, Philadelphia: Baillière Tindall.

30 **PHILLIPS, R.M., FOLEY, C.W. & LUKERT, P.D., 1972.** Isolation and characterization of viruses from semen and the reproductive tract of male swine. *Journal of the American Veterinary Medical Association*, 161, 1306–1316.

31 **PINI, A. & SMIT, G., 1973.** Incidence and distribution of neutralizing antibodies to porcine enteroviruses in southern Africa. *Journal of the South African Veterinary Association*, 44, 247–250.

32 **SIBALIN, M. & LANNEK, N., 1960.** An enteric porcine virus producing encephalomyelitis and pneumonitis in baby pigs. *Archiv für die Gesamte Virusforschung*, X, 31–45.

33 **SINGH, K.V. & BOHL, E.H., 1972.** The pattern of enteroviral infections in a herd of swine. *Canadian Journal of Comparative Medicine*, 36, 243–248.

34 **SINGH, K.V., McCONNELL, S.J., BOHL, E.H. & BIRKLAND, J.M., 1960.** Faecal excretion of porcine enteroviruses following experimental infection of pigs. *Virology*, 12, 139–141.

35 **WANG, J.T., DUNNE, H.W., GRIEL, L.C., HOKANSON, J.F. & MURPHY, D.M., 1973.** Mortality, antibody development, and viral persistence in porcine fetuses inoculated *in utero* with SMEDI (entero-) virus. *American Journal of Veterinary Research*, 34, 785–791.

36 **YAMANOUCHI, K., BANKOWSKI, R.A. & HOWORTH, J.A., 1964.** Pathogenicity of E1 and E4 strains of porcine enteroviruses in specific pathogen-free pigs. *Journal of Infectious Diseases*, 144, 450–457.

86

Swine vesicular disease

G.R. Thomson

Introduction

Swine vesicular disease (SVD) is a contagious virus disease of pigs that is characterized by the formation of vesicular lesions in the mouth and on the feet and lower legs. Laboratory infection of humans with SVD has been recorded.[3, 10]

The disease was first recognized in Italy in 1966, appearing in Hong Kong in 1971 and in Britain, Austria and Poland in 1972. Since then the disease has occurred in a number of other European countries and also in Japan and Taiwan.[28] It has not been diagnosed in southern Africa and all indications are that it is exotic to the subcontinent.

Between November 1986 and November 1987, 2 846 pig sera originating from 300 different farms in the Transvaal, Natal and the western Cape Province were found to be negative for antibody to SVD virus, using an indirect ELISA technique.[9] Although not exhaustive, this survey supports the contention that SVD virus is not present in South Africa.

Swine vesicular disease is a relatively mild and unimportant disease, but because it is clinically indistinguishable from foot-and-mouth disease, each occurrence must be considered as foot-and-mouth disease until proved otherwise. This necessitates expensive and disruptive zoosanitary measures as well as laboratory investigation, thus making outbreaks of SVD very disruptive for countries with large and sophisticated pig industries; most therefore strive either to eradicate the disease or to maintain their infection-free status. Diagnosis and control of SVD is further hampered by the fact that many infections are subclinical.[16, 21]

Aetiology

Swine vesicular disease virus is classified in the genus *Enterovirus*, family Picornaviridae. It is a typical picornavirus **(see Chapter 89: Foot-and-mouth disease)** and is serologically related to coxsackie B5 virus, an enteroviral infection of humans.[3]

Comparison of the RNA genome sequences of an SVD virus with coxsackie B1, B3 and B4 and polio viruses revealed homologies of approximately 90 per cent with the coxsackie viruses and 60 per cent with poliovirus.[14] However, because attempted infection of pigs with human coxsackie B5 has provided equivocal results, it is not clear whether SVD virus should be considered to be the twelfth serogroup of the porcine enteroviruses or a porcine strain of coxsackie B5 virus.[15] There are also immunological and structural differences in the viral polypeptides between SVD virus isolates.[11]

Like other enteroviruses, SVD virus is stable over a wide pH range (3,9–9,1 for up to 38 days at 5 °C).[12] It is also stable in faeces and infected tissue kept at ambient or higher temperatures for four months or more.[8, 24]

The disinfectant of choice for SVD virus varies with the prevailing circumstances, but for long-term disinfection in the presence of organic matter, alkalis such as 1 per cent sodium hydroxide, which combine a detergent action with inactivation, are ideal.[12]

Epidemiology

Although most enterovirus infections are transmitted by the faecal–oral route, this does not appear to be so for SVD, as more than 200 000 plaque-forming units (pfu) of virus installed by the oral, nasal or ocular routes failed to infect pigs. Infection by these routes was only achieved by $10^{5,5-6,8}$ pfu.[21, 22] On the other hand, placing the virus on abraded skin achieved infection with 1 500 times less virus than would have been the case with oral infection. Attempts at isolating SVD virus from the intestinal tract of acutely infected pigs were unsuccessful, as were searches for viral antigen in intestinal tissue.[7, 22] Nevertheless, up to $10^{3,5}$ pfu/g of faeces were recovered from pigs infected experimentally by adding large quantities of virus to their feed. This probably represented 'survivor' virus rather than virus which had replicated in the gut.[21]

Lesions on the feet and in the mouth are the major sources of virus in infected animals;[27] the virus content of vesicular epithelium may exceed 10^9 pfu/g.[6] The fact that lesions are the major source of virus explains the observation that subclinically infected pigs are usually unable to transmit the infection.

The feeding of swill containing pig tissues to susceptible pigs is considered to have been important in maintaining and spreading the infection in Britain,[1, 20] and this method of spread probably accounts for many of the new introductions of the virus into previously uninfected countries.

Contact with diseased pigs, either direct or indirect, is necessary for disease transmission, as there is no evidence for air-borne spread,[20, 27] and spread from one pen to another on the same farm may not occur in the absence of a common drainage system or movement of pigs between the pens.[20] In Britain, movement of pigs and contaminated vehicles have been the most common source of infection.[20]

There is no evidence that pigs become carriers when they recover from infection.

Sheep may be susceptible to infection but this is probably not important in the spread and maintenance of the virus.[4]

Pathogenesis, clinical signs and pathology

Swine vesicular disease virus has an affinity for, and replicates in, the epithelium of the coronary band, tongue, snout and lips (where it affects principally the cells of the *stratum spinosum*), as well as the myocardium, the tonsils and the brain stem.[7, 19] In experimental cases the tonsils appear to be the most consistently infected tissue irrespective of the route of infection.[7, 22]

The incubation period of SVD is usually three to five days, but varies with the weight of infection.[28] Many infections are subclinical or mild.[21, 28]

There may initially be a temperature rise to 41 °C but this reverts to normal within two to three days. In severe cases, which are more common in young animals, the lesions are indistinguishable from those of foot-and-mouth disease. Vesicles, which soon rupture, develop on the coronary bands, particularly at the bulbs of the heels and supernumary digits, and less frequently on the snout, lips, tongue and teats. Lesions may also develop over bony prominences on the lower legs.[20] The lesions on the coronary bands may enlarge and involve the interdigital area before progressing to an extensive necrotizing dermatitis.[7]

The lesions may result in initial anorexia as well as lameness. Vesicles soon rupture to leave shallow erosions which usually heal uneventfully within two to three weeks unless they have become secondarily infected.

Nervous signs are not a feature of the disease, despite the fact that microscopic lesions in the central nervous system are a constant finding.

Morbidity rates generally range from 25 to 65 per cent on affected farms, but in individual pens they may exceed 90 per cent.[21] Mortality is negligible.[28]

Reproductive disorders in affected herds have been ascribed to the effects of SVD virus, but experimental investigation has provided no support for this contention.[5]

Microscopically, the early vesicular lesions (which may be multilocular) appear as intra-epidermal vesicles in the *stratum spinosum*.[7] The epidermis at the periphery of lesions is markedly hyperplastic, while foci of intracellular and intercellular oedema coalesce with neighbouring lesions to form macroscopically visible vesicles. Micro-abscesses may also be present. Healing of the lesions commences within eight days of their appearance.[18]

The lesions in the central nervous system, which are only evident microscopically, comprise non-suppurative meningitis and encephalomyelitis, and principally affect the olfactory bulbs as well as the mid- and fore-brain.[18, 19] Ganglioneuritis and the presence of intranuclear inclusion bodies in perineuronal amphicytes have been reported as a feature of experimental cases. Spinal radiculitis and optic neuritis are also sometimes present in acute cases.[19]

Small foci of necrotic myocytes may be scattered in the myocardium,[7, 18] with mild lymphocytic infiltration.[7]

Diagnosis and differential diagnosis

Swine vesicular disease, vesicular stomatitis, vesicular exanthema of swine, and foot-and-mouth disease are clinically indistinguishable. For this reason, and because of the potentially serious consequences of foot-and-mouth disease outbreaks in pigs, any suspect vesicular disease (and particularly if both the feet and the mouth are affected) must be further investigated using laboratory methods to determine which, if any, of these viruses is involved.

Porcine parvovirus may also produce lesions difficult to distinguish from those caused by the above viruses,[17] as may phototoxins produced by green vegetables contaminated with the fungus *Sclerotinia sclerotiorium*.[26] The radiomimetic effect of *Stachybotrys* spp. fungi may cause necrotic lesions in the mouth and the skin of the teats, snout and feet of pigs when they are exposed to contaminated bedding or feed.[13]

The diagnosis of SVD should involve the isolation and identification of the virus or viral antigens in the epithelium covering vesicles as well as detection of antibody in diseased or recovered pigs. The virus replicates readily and rapidly in swine kidney and IB-RS-2 (a transformed pig kidney cell line) cells and also in the brains of newborn mice. Viral antigens can be rapidly identified in direct complement fixation and ELISA tests. Antibody detection can be effected by a variety of methods, including ELISA, virus neutralization, counter-immuno-electro-osmophoresis, and immuno-diffusion.[2, 20]

Control

Since SVD is exotic to southern Africa, control is presently confined to ensuring that the disease is not introduced into the subcontinent. Breeding stock should preferably be acquired from countries where the disease is not active, but, because of the possibility of importing the disease in inapparently or mildly infected pigs, appropriate quarantine and serological testing must still be applied.

Processed and unprocessed pork products are a potential source of infection; and swill derived from kitchen wastes of aircraft and ships is particularly dangerous in this regard.[23–25]

Should SVD be introduced to a country or region formerly free of the disease, slaughter-out of the affected herds is essential. The carcasses should either be incinerated or buried on the affected premises. The farm buildings or enclosures involved should then be cleaned and disinfected under supervision on at least two occasions 14 days apart. Limited restocking should be delayed until eight weeks after the final disinfection. If the newly introduced stock is disease-free three weeks after its introduction, full re-stocking can be permitted.[20]

References

1 **ANON., 1980.** Swine vesicular disease 1972–1979. *The Veterinary Record*, 106, 323.

2 **ARMSTRONG, R.M. & BARNETT, I.T.R., 1989.** An enzyme-linked immuno-sorbent assay (ELISA) for the detection and quantification of antibodies against swine vesicular disease virus (SVD). *Journal of Virological Methods*, 25, 71–80.

3 **BROWN, F., GOODRIDGE, D. & BURROWS, R., 1976.** Infection of man by swine vesicular disease virus. *Journal of Comparative Pathology*, 86, 409–414.

4 **BURROWS, R., MANN, J.A., GOODRIDGE, D. & CHAPMAN, W.G., 1974.** Swine vesicular disease: Attempts to transmit infection to cattle and sheep. *Journal of Hygiene*, 73, 101–107.

5 **BURROWS, R., MANN, J.A., GOODRIDGE, D., WRATHALL, A.E. & DONE, J.T., 1977.** Swine vesicular disease — studies in pregnant sows. *Zentralblatt für Veterinärmedizin*, B, 24, 177–182.

6 **CHAPMAN, W.G. & BURROWS, R., 1973.** Rapid identification of swine vesicular disease virus in epithelium using the fluorescent antibody technique. *Research in Veterinary Science*, 15, 397–399.

7 **CHU, R.M., MOORE, D.M. & CONROY, J.D., 1979.** Experimental swine vesicular disease, pathology and immunofluorescence studies. *Canadian Journal of Comparative Medicine*, 43, 29–30.

8 **DAWE, P.S., 1974.** Viability of swine vesicular disease in carcasses and faeces. *The Veterinary Record*, 94, 430.

9 **ESTERHUYSEN, J.J. & THOMSON, G.R., 1988.** Veterinary Research Institute, Onderstepoort, South Africa. Unpublished data.

10 **GRAVES, J.H., 1973.** Serological relationship of swine vesicular disease virus and coxsackie B5 virus. *Nature*, 245, 314.

11 **HARRIS, T.J.R., UNDERWOOD, B.O., KNOWLES, N.J., CROWTHER, J.R. & BROWN, F., 1979.** Molecular approach to the epidemiology of swine vesicular disease: Correlation of variation in the virus structural polypeptides with serological properties. *Infection and Immunity*, 24, 593–599.

12 **HERNIMAN, K.A.J., MEDHURST, P.M., WILSON, J.N. & SELLERS, R.F., 1973.** The action of heat, chemicals and disinfectants on swine vesicular disease virus. *The Veterinary Record*, 93, 620–625.

13 **HINTIKKA, E-L., 1978.** Stachybotryotoxicosis in swine. *In*: WYLIE, T.D. & MOOREHOUSE, L.G., (eds). *Mycotoxic Fungi, Mycotoxins, Mycotoxicoses. An Encyclopedic Handbook*. Vol. 2. New York & Basel: Marcel Dekker, Inc.

14 **INOUE, T., SUZUKI, T. & SEKIGUCHI, K., 1989.** The complete nucleotide sequence of swine vesicular disease virus. *Journal of General Virology*, 70, 919–934.

15 **KNOWLES, N.J., BUCKLEY, L.S. & PEREIRA, H.G., 1979.** Classification of porcine enteroviruses by antigenic analysis and cytopathic effects in tissue culture: Description of three new serotypes. *Archives of Virology*, 62, 201–208.

16 **KODAMA, M., OGANA, T., SAITO, T., TOKUDA, G., SASAHARA, J. & KUMAGAI, T., 1980.** Swine vesicular disease virus isolated from healthy pigs in non-epizootic period: 1. Isolation and identification. *National Institute of Animal Health Quarterly*, 20, 1–10.

17 **KRESSE, J.I., TAYLOR, W.D., STEWART, W.W. & EERNISSE, K.A., 1985.** Parvovirus infection in pigs with necrotic and vesicle-like lesions. *Veterinary Microbiology*, 10, 525–531.

18 **LAI, S.S., McKERCHER, P.D., MOORE, D.M. & GILLESPIE, J.H., 1979.** Pathogenesis of swine vesicular disease in pigs. *American Journal of Veterinary Research*, 40, 463–468.

19 **LENGHAUS, C., MANN, J.A., DONE, J.T. & BRADLEY, R., 1976.** Neuropathology of experimental swine vesicular disease in pigs. *Research in Veterinary Science*, 21, 19–27.

20 **LOXAM, J.G. & HEDGER, R.S., 1983.** Swine vesicular disease: Clinical signs, diagnosis, epidemiology and control. *Revue Scientifique et Technique: International Office of Epizootics*, 2, 11–24.

21 **MANN, J.A., BURROWS, R. & GOODRIDGE, D., 1975.** Mild and subclinical infections with swine vesicular disease virus. *Bulletin de l'Office International des Épizooties*, 83, 117–122.

22 **MANN, J.A. & HUTCHINGS, G.H., 1980.** Swine vesicular disease: Pathways of infections. *Journal of Hygiene*, 84, 355–363.

23 **McKERCHER, P.D., BLACKWELL, J.H., MURPHY, R., CALLIS, J.J., PANINA, G.F., CIVARDI, A., BUGNETTI, M., DE SIMONE, F. & SCATOZIA, F., 1985.** Survival of swine vesicular disease virus in 'Prosciutto di Parma' (Parma Ham). *Canadian Journal of Food Science and Technology*, 18, 163–167.

24 **McKERCHER, P.D., GRAVES, J.H., CALLIS, J.J. & CARMICHAEL, F., 1974.** Swine vesicular disease: Virus survival in pork products. *Proceedings of the 78th Annual Meeting of the United States Animal Health Association*, 213a–g.

25 **McKERCHER, P.D., HESS, W.R. & HAMDY, F., 1978.** Residual viruses in pork products. *Applied and Environmental Microbiology*, 35, 142–145.

26 **MONTGOMERY, J.F., OLIVER, R.E., POOLE, W.S.H. & JULIAN, A.F., 1987.** A vesiculo-bullous disease in pigs resembling foot-and-mouth disease. II. Experimental production of the lesion. *New Zealand Veterinary Journal*, 35, 27–30.

27 **SELLERS, F.R. & HERNIMAN, K.A.J., 1974.** The airborne excretion by pigs of swine vesicular disease virus. *Journal of Hygiene*, 72, 61–65.

28 **WATSON, W.A., 1981.** Swine vesicular disease in Great Britain. *Canadian Veterinary Journal*, 22, 195–208.

87

Equine rhinovirus infections

J.A. Mumford

Introduction

Equine rhinoviruses (ERV) frequently infect the upper respiratory tract of horses but their role in the causation of disease is uncertain.

Experimental infections indicate that ERV-1 is capable of causing upper respiratory disease although field evidence suggests that many infections are subclinical. The pathogenic potential of ERV-2 and ERV-3 and the acid-stable picornavirus (ASPV) is uncertain. There is no information on the occurrence of these infections in horses in southern Africa.

Aetiology

Several picornaviruses have been isolated from horses in different parts of the world.[4–6, 8–10, 15, 18, 21, 22] The majority of isolates have the properties of rhinoviruses and have been recovered from the respiratory tract, the oral cavity, and, on occasions, from blood and faeces. On the basis of serological cross-reactivities and physicochemical properties, isolates have been classified as ERV-1, -2 or -3. A virus with properties of both rhinoviruses and enteroviruses, referred to as acid-stable picornavirus (ASPV), has been recovered from the upper respiratory tract of Thoroughbreds.[15]

Equine rhinoviruses 1, 2 and 3 have the basic characteristics of viruses belonging to the genus *Rhinovirus*, family Picornaviridae. They are small, non-enveloped, and resistant to ether and chloroform and acid-labile, and contain RNA.[15, 21]

Equine rhinoviruses 1 and 2 have been further characterized and have minor differences in their physicochemical properties.[16] Both viruses sediment at approximately 160S, but co-centrifugation of the two viruses in a sucrose gradient revealed minor differences, and they also have different buoyant densities. Equine rhinovirus 1 has a precise density of 1,45 g/ml in CsCl, whereas ERV-2 is more heterogeneous, with a density range of 1,41–1,45 g/ml.[17] The relative sedimentation coefficients for the RNA's are 35S for ERV-1 and 37S for ERV-2. Both viruses contain four polypeptides (VP1–4), although migrational patterns on polyacrylamide gels are distinguishable. No detailed physicochemical data is available for ERV-3.

All three equine rhinoviruses can be distinguished on the basis of their distinctive serology.

A fourth equine picornavirus has been identified which has some of the properties of both rhinoviruses and enteroviruses.[15] In common with equine rhinoviruses, ASPV is a small (22 nm diameter), isometric, non-enveloped, RNA virus. It has a high buoyant density (1,45 g/ml in CsCl) and, in common with ERV-2 but not ERV-1, it is stabilized at 50 °C by $MgCl_2$. Unlike both ERV-1 and ERV-2, it is stable at pH3,6, a property normally associated with enteroviruses. Serologically, it can be distinguished by virus neutralization tests from ERV-1, ERV-2 and ERV-3.[15]

Epidemiology

Serological surveys indicate that ERV-1 has a worldwide distribution and it is probable that the other equine picornaviruses share this widespread distribution.[1–3, 8, 10, 12, 20, 22]

Serological monitoring of infection in foals, yearlings and adult Thoroughbred horses in the United Kingdom has shown that most foals and yearlings are seronegative to ERV-1 and that first infection usually occurs in two- and three-year-old horses in training. In individual stables most seroconversions occur within a short period of time (four to six weeks), with or without clinical signs of respiratory disease.[20, 23] Similar observations have been made in the USA[12] and Switzerland.[11] The majority of horses of four years and older have experienced infection with ERV-1.

There is little information about reinfection with ERV-1, as most serosurveys have measured virus neutralizing antibody which is stimulated to high levels after first infection and persists for many months. Surveys using the complement fixation test indicate that older horses may experience reinfection with this virus.[14]

Although persistent neutralizing antibody levels to ERV-1 could indicate a long-term carrier state, no evidence of persistence for more than a month after infection has been obtained.[7, 19]

The epidemiology of ERV-2 is somewhat different. Foals usually experience first infection at four to six months of age and may experience two infections within the first year of life.[7, 12, 23] These infections are seldom associated with clinical signs of respiratory disease. There is a high prevalence of antibody in adult horses in most of the populations studied in the USA, Europe and New Zealand.[2, 12, 13, 21] Seroconversion of groups of animals over a short period of time is seldom observed.

Infections with ERV-2 and ASPV differ from those caused by ERV-1 in that the virus neutralizing antibody responses are ephemeral and some recovered animals continue to carry virus for long periods. They are a source of infection for other horses.[10] There is no information on ERV-3.

Although no investigations have been reported, it is presumed that these viruses are transmitted directly between the respiratory tracts of horses shedding the viruses and those of susceptible animals.

Clinical signs and pathology

Equine rhinovirus 1 was first isolated from faeces of horses with fever and respiratory disease.[18] When the isolate was used to infect seronegative horses experimentally via the respiratory tract, the recipients developed pyrexia (up to 40 °C) during the viraemic phase, which persisted for up to five days, and a serous nasal discharge which became mucopurulent three to eight days after infection. This was accompanied by swelling of the pharyngeal lymph nodes, anorexia for four to five days and a moist cough.[19] Similar clinical signs have been observed during natural infection, although it is well recognized that many infections are asymptomatic.[9, 11, 22]

Both natural and experimental infections with ERV-2 are usually subclinical.[15] However, ERV-2 can cause fever and mild respiratory signs in young horses and this may be complicated by bacterial infection.[21]

There is no information available on the pathogenic potential of ERV-3.

The ASPV has been isolated from horses showing clinical signs of upper respiratory tract disease, but it has more frequently been recovered from healthy animals. It failed to induce clinical signs when a seronegative gnotobiotic foal was infected with it,[15] and thus its clinical significance remains obscure.

Diagnosis and differential diagnosis

Equine picornaviruses have been cultured from nasopharyngeal and oral secretions, blood and faeces.

Monkey kidney, rabbit kidney (RK13) and equine foetal cells (lung and kidney) support viral replication. Infected cells become highly refractile, rounded and dense, and detach from the monolayer. Cytopathic effects develop fastest in rapidly dividing cells. Viruses are identified in neutralization assays using specific antisera.

Both virus neutralization and complement fixation tests have been used to measure antibody to equine picornaviruses.[5, 12, 15] Four-fold increases in antibody titre develop two weeks after infection with ERV-1. Antibody responses to ERV-2 may be slower.[7]

Infection with these viruses should be borne in mind in the differential diagnosis of acute upper respiratory tract disease in horses **(see Chapters 90: Equine influenza, and 102: Equid herpesvirus 1 and 4 infections)**.

Control

No control is required because these infections are rarely involved in clinical disease, and even when this does occur it is not serious. Although no vaccines are produced commercially, immunization with inactivated virus has been shown to stimulate virus neutralizing antibody and to provide protection against experimental infection.[7]

References

1 **BECKER, W., KELLER, S. & TEUFEL, P., 1974.** Rhinovirus infections in horses. *Berliner und Münchener Tierärztliche Wochenschrift*, 87, 305–308.

2 **BOER, G.F., OSTERHAUS, A.D.M.E. & WEMMENHOVE, R., 1978.** Prevalence of antibody to equine viruses in the Netherlands. *In*: BRYANS, J.T. & GERBER, H., (eds). *Equine Infectious Diseases. IV*. Princetown, New Jersey: Veterinary Publications Inc.

3 **BRION, A., 1971.** La rhinovirose équine. *Recueil de Médecine Vétérinaire de l' École d'Alfort*, 147, 481–487.

4 **BURROWS, R., 1968.** Some observations on the viral aetiology of upper respiratory disease of British horses, 1956–65. *Bulletin de l'Office International des Épizooties*, 181–196.

5 **BURROWS, R., 1968.** Laboratory diagnoses of some virus infections of the upper respiratory tract of the horse. *Equine Veterinary Journal*, 1, 32–38.

6 **BURROWS, R., 1970.** Equine rhinoviruses. *In*: BRYANS, J.T. & GERBER, H., (eds). *Equine Infectious Diseases. II*. Basel, München, New York: S. Karger.

7 **BURROWS, R., 1979.** Equine rhinovirus and adenovirus infections. *Proceedings of the Twenty-fourth Annual Convention of the American Association of Equine Practitioners*, December 1978, St. Louis, Missouri.

8 **DITCHFIELD, J. & MACPHERSON, L.W., 1965.** The properties and classification of two new rhinoviruses recovered from horses in Toronto, Canada. *Cornell Veterinarian*, 55, 181–189.

9 **FLAMMINI, C.F. & ALLEGRI, G., 1970.** Rhinovirus strain as a possible cause of equine respiratory infection. *Archivio Veterinario Italiano*, 21, 309–316.

10 **FUKUNAGA, Y., KUMANOMIDO, T., KAMADA, M. & WADA, R., 1983.** Equine picornavirus. Isolation of virus from the oral cavity of healthy horses. *Bulletin of the Equine Research Institute*, 20, 103–109.

11 **HOFER, B., STECK, F., GERBER, H., LOHRER, J., NICOLET, J. & PACCAUD, M.F., 1973.** An investigation of the etiology of viral respiratory disease in a remount depot. *In*: BRYANS, J.T. & GERBER, H., (eds). *Equine Infectious Diseases. III*. Basel, München: S. Karger.

12 **HOLMES, D.F., KEMEN, M.J. & COGGINS, L., 1978.** Equine rhinovirus infection — Serological evidence of infection in selected United States horse populations. *In*: BRYANS, J.T. & GERBER, H., (eds). *Equine Infectious Diseases. IV*. Princeton, New Jersey: Veterinary Publications Inc.

13 **JOLLY, P.D., ZHEN, F.F. & ROBINSON, A.J., 1986.** Viruses associated with respiratory disease of horses in New Zealand: An update. *New Zealand Veterinary Journal*, 34, 46–50.

14 **MUMFORD, J.A., 1990.** The Animal Health Trust, P.O. Box 5, Newmarket, Suffolk CB8 FDW, UK. Unpublished data.

15 **MUMFORD, J.A. & THOMSON, G.R., 1978.** Studies on picornaviruses isolated from the respiratory tract of horses. *In*: BRYANS, J.T. & GERBER, H., (eds). *Equine Infectious Diseases. IV*. Princeton, New Jersey: Veterinary Publications Inc.

16 **NEWMAN, J.F.E., ROWLANDS, D.J. & BROWN, F., 1973.** A physicochemical subgrouping of mammalian picornaviruses. *Journal of General Virology*, 18, 171–180.

17 **NEWMAN, J.F.E., ROWLANDS, D.J., BROWN, F., GOODRIDGE, D., BURROWS, R. & STECK, F., 1977.** Physicochemical characterization of two serologically unrelated equine rhinoviruses. *Intervirology*, 8, 145–154.

18 **PLUMMER, G., 1962.** An equine respiratory virus with enterovirus properties. *Nature*, 195, 519–520.

19 **PLUMMER, G. & KERRY, J.B., 1962.** Studies on an equine respiratory virus. *The Veterinary Record*, 74, 967–970.

20 **POWELL, D.G., BURROWS, R. & GOODRIDGE, D., 1974.** Respiratory viral infections among Thoroughbred horses in training during 1972. *Equine Veterinary Journal*, 6, 19–24.

21 **STECK, F., HOFER, B., SCHAEREN, B., NICOLET, J. & GERBER, H., 1978.** Equine rhinoviruses: New serotypes. *In*: BRYANS, J.T. & GERBER, H., (eds). *Equine Infectious Diseases. IV*. Princetown, New Jersey: Veterinary Publications Inc.

22 **STUDDERT, M.J. & GLEESON, L.J., 1978.** Isolation and characterization of an equine rhinovirus. *Zentralblatt für Veterinärmedizin*, 25, 225–237.

23 **THOMSON, G.R., 1978.** The role of equid herpesvirus 1 in acute respiratory disease of horses and the use of inactivated antigens to immunize against the infection. Ph.D. thesis, University of London.

88

Bovine rhinovirus infection

G.R. Thomson

Introduction and aetiology

Bovine rhinovirus infection is probably ubiquitous in cattle populations, but its association with disease is uncertain.

The virus was first identified in Germany by Bögel and Böhm in 1962, and it has subsequently been found in England, the USA, Japan and Sudan. Three serotypes (1, 2 and 3) have been identified.[3, 8, 10]

Apart from their typical picornavirus morphology and physico-chemical characteristics,[4, 6] bovine rhinoviruses have features common to all rhinoviruses — instability at pH 3,0–3,6, optimal replication in slightly acidic or neutral medium at 30–34 °C, resistance to treatment with ether and chloroform, and lack of stabilization by 1M $MgCl_2$ when heated to 50 °C for 60 minutes.[3, 4, 7, 9, 10]

There are conflicting reports about the ease with which bovine rhinoviruses can be cultivated in cell cultures, the variation probably being due to differences inherent in different viruses.[7] One virus isolation was only achieved after eight passages in calf tracheal organ cultures, whereafter the virus was adapted to growth in monolayers of primary bovine kidney cells.[7] In other cases isolation, usually in bovine kidney cultures, has been achieved without difficulty,[2, 4, 9] although it may take up to nine days for cytopathic effects to develop on primary isolation. The rolling of cell cultures may be advantageous to viral replication and the production of cytopathic effects.[4, 9]

Epidemiology, clinical signs, pathogenesis, pathology, diagnosis and control

It is presumed that bovine rhinoviruses are transmitted directly between the upper respiratory tracts of cattle because viral isolations have been made only from the nasal and tracheal secretions of infected cattle. The quantities of virus present in the nasal secretions of acutely infected animals are probably low, as dilution of specimens often results in their failure to yield virus in culture.[3] Attempts to isolate the virus from blood and faeces have failed.[3]

The prevalence of infection in cattle populations is largely unknown, but 48 per cent of cattle in one study in Maryland (USA) were found to contain neutralizing antibody to the virus.[5] Many infections do not produce obvious disease.[5, 8] Experimental infection has provided evidence that at least some bovine rhinoviruses are able to cause acute rhinitis in calves[1, 2] which is accompanied by fever, depression, inappetence, lachrymation, conjunctivitis and serous nasal discharge.[8] Whether these viruses may also cause lower respiratory tract disease accompanied by coughing and dyspnoea is uncertain because although lung consolidation, collapse and emphysema have been associated with bovine rhinovirus infection,[5] there is no unequivocal proof that bovine rhinovirus was the cause. These lesions were characterized microscopically as interstitial pneumonia.[1, 2]

It is possible that bovine rhinovirus may interact with other infectious agents to cause respiratory disease, but there is no categorical evidence for this.[3]

The diagnosis of bovine rhinovirus infection can at present only be made on the basis of isolation of the virus from the upper respiratory tract of cattle using kidney cell cultures of bovine origin, or foetal or calf tracheal organ cultures. However, because some viruses are apparently poorly adaptable to growth *in vitro* and the quantities of virus in upper respiratory tract secretions are low, this may not always be possible.[3, 7]

Serological diagnosis is usually performed using neutralization tests[3] but may be complicated by the low levels of antibody induced by these viruses.[5]

Other infectious agents which may be associated with acute upper respiratory tract disease in cattle include bovine respiratory syncytial virus, parainfluenza virus 3, infectious bovine rhinotracheitis (bovine herpesvirus 1), adenoviruses, *Chlamydia psittaci* and *Pasteurella* spp.

No control of this infection has so far been deemed necessary.[5]

References

1 **BETTS, O.A., EDINGTON, N., JENNINGS, A.R. & REED, S.E., 1971.** Studies on a rhinovirus (EC11) derived from a calf. II. Disease in calves. *Journal of Comparative Pathology*, 81, 41–48.

2 **IDE, P.R. & DARBYSHIRE, J.H., 1972.** Studies with a rhinovirus of bovine origin. III. The pathogenesis and pathology of infection with strain RS 3x in calves. *Archiv für die Gesamte Virusforschung*, 36, 335–342.

3 **KUROGI, H., INABA, Y., GOTO, Y., TAKAHASHI, A., SATO, K., OMORI, T. & MATUMOTO, M., 1974.** Isolation of rhinovirus from cattle in outbreaks of acute respiratory disease. *Archiv für die Gesamte Virusforschung*, 44, 215–226.

4 **LUPTON, H.W., SMITH, M.H. & FREY, M.L., 1980.** Identification and characterization of a bovine rhinovirus from Iowa cattle with acute respiratory tract disease. *American Journal of Veterinary Research*, 41, 1029–1034.

5 **MOHANTY, S.B., 1973.** New herpesviral and rhinoviral respiratory infections. *Journal of the American Veterinary Medical Association*, 163, 855–857.

6 **PEREIRA, H.G., 1989.** Picornaviridae. *In*: PORTERFELD, J.S., (ed.). *Andrew's Viruses of Vertebrates*. 5th edn. London, Philadelphia: Baillière Tindall.

7 **RHEED, S.E., TYRRELL, D.A.J., BETTS, O.A. & WATT, R.G., 1971.** Studies on a rhinovirus (EC11) derived from a calf. I. Isolation in calf tracheal organ cultures and characterization of the virus. *Journal of Comparative Pathology*, 81, 33–40.

8 **SELLERS, R.F., 1990.** Bovine rhinoviruses. *In*: DINTER, Z. & MOREIN, B., (eds). *Virus Infections of Ruminants*. Amsterdam: Elsevier Science Publishers B.V.

9 **SHIMIZU, Y., NARITA, M. & MURASE, N., 1974.** Isolation of bovine rhinovirus from calves with respiratory disease. *National Institute of Animal Health Quarterly*, 14, 35–41.

10 **YAMASHITA, H., AKASHI, H. & INABA, Y., 1985.** Isolation of a new serotype of bovine rhinovirus from cattle. *Archives of Virology*, 83, 113–116.

89

Foot-and-mouth disease

Synonyms: Aphthous fever, fièvre aphteuse (Fr.), fiebre aftosa (Sp.), Maul- und Klauenseuche (Ger.), bek-en-klouseer (Afrik.)

G.R. Thomson

Introduction

Foot-and-mouth disease (FMD) is a highly contagious acute viral infection, almost exclusively of ruminants and pigs. It is characterized in livestock by high morbidity, low mortality, and by vesicles and erosions in the mucosa of the mouth and skin of the interdigital spaces and coronary bands.

In northern Europe, North America and elsewhere where the effects of the disease have historically been great, vast sums of money have been spent either to eradicate the infection or to reduce its incidence to acceptably low levels.[176, 196] This was because in the second half of the nineteenth and first half of the twentieth centuries repeated epidemics of rapidly spreading disease resulted in serious losses, predominantly amongst high-producing livestock raised under increasingly intensive systems. Countries which have been successful in controlling FMD are therefore wary of re-importing the disease, particularly from regions where exotic types of virus occur, and have instituted measures to prevent this, including embargoes on agricultural imports from countries where efficient control is not practised or where the epidemiological situation with respect to FMD has not been accurately established.

As an example of the direct and indirect losses that may result from an outbreak in an FMD-free country, Krystynak[145] recorded those which occurred in Canada in 1951. The costs of eradication amounted to one million dollars, while 70 million dollars was spent on supporting cattle prices, which had dropped dramatically; the cash inventory value of livestock fell by 654 million dollars in the three-month period following the outbreak. Blackwell[25] quotes a study which indicated that direct and indirect losses resulting from an FMD outbreak in the USA would amount to four and 40 billion dollars respectively in the first year.

Since Botswana, South Africa and Zimbabwe rely heavily on agricultural exports of animal origin, the uncontrolled presence of FMD in any of these countries could be disastrous for agricultural exports. The widespread outbreaks in Zimbabwe in 1989 resulted in beef exports to the European Economic Community, worth 100 million Zimbabwean dollars annually, being suspended for at least two years. In South Africa it is estimated that a widespread outbreak would affect approximately R2 billion-worth of agricultural products annually.[143] Foot-and-mouth disease is therefore the most economically important disease of livestock in southern Africa. This is despite the fact that most endemic areas in the region are located in areas where subsistence agriculture or extensive cattle farming is practised. In these areas FMD is usually a comparatively mild disease, although the effect on draught animals may be crippling.

It is unlikely that countries in southern Africa will eradicate FMD in the foreseeable future, because the African buffalo (*Syncerus caffer*) is a maintenance host for the SAT-types of FMD virus,[118] and large herds of infected buffalo are present in all the larger countries of the subcontinent. While there has been a concerted effort in Zimbabwe to eliminate buffaloes from areas other than game reserves, the wholesale eradication of buffalo populations is aesthetically, ecologically and, arguably, economically undesirable. Hence healthy agricultural activity in southern Africa is dependent upon the effective control of FMD, rather than its eradication.

Foot-and-mouth disease is probably not an ancient disease; the first identifiable description was that of Hieronymus Francastorius in 1546, who described an outbreak in cattle in what is now Italy.[127] However, probably because of the prevalence of other major animal plagues such as rinderpest in Europe during the nineteenth century, relatively little mention of FMD was made prior to 1886.[34] After that FMD became increasingly important, and a number of FMD institutes to counter the ravages of the disease were established in Europe and South America in the first quarter of the twentieth century.

Foot-and-mouth disease virus was the first filterable agent to be identified. Prior to this discovery by Loeffler and Frosch in 1898, no known microorganism was capable of passing through Berkfeld filters. This finding led Loeffler and Frosch to deduce that the agent of FMD was beyond the resolution of the light microscope.[194]

The early history of FMD in southern Africa, as described by Henning,[127] is excellent and is therefore quoted in full:

In 1780 le Vaillant[151] described a disorder in cattle, 'klowsiekte', which 'attacked the feet of oxen causing them to swell prodigiously, and often producing suppuration; sometimes the hoofs dropped off. It was not attended with any danger and generally terminated in a fortnight'. Gordon Cumming[57] also reported serious losses among his oxen from the 'tongue or hoof sickness', along the Vaal River. He was detained for several days and was forced to purchase or barter fresh oxen from Mahura and his tribe. From enquiries made by him it appeared that the disease was well known to his Hottentot servants. In 1858 General S.J.P. Kruger[144] reported on the campaign against Mahura along the Harts River, stating, 'By this time our bullocks suffered much from the tongue and claw sickness'. According to information obtained from some of the oldest inhabitants of the Transvaal and Free State, a disease resembling foot-and-mouth disease had been prevalent for a considerable time before it was recognized officially. On the other hand, there seems to be very little doubt that some forms of bluetongue have been mistaken for foot-and-mouth disease in the past.[19]

The first official record of foot-and-mouth disease in South Africa was made by Hutcheon in 1892,[134] when an outbreak occurred in Griqualand West. Although the source of the infection could not be traced, Hutcheon[134] stated that the disease was first reported in parts of Mashonaland (Southern Rhodesia), from whence it was considered to have spread along the traffic routes through Bechuanaland into Griqualand West, the Transvaal, the Orange Free State and Natal. Otto Henning,[126] who investigated the outbreak, found the disease to be identical with the European disorder. The scourge was well known to several farmers and, according to information obtained from some of the older inhabitants, it had been prevalent in South Africa for many years before this outbreak was reported. Although over 75 per cent of the in-contact cattle contracted the disease, the mortality in adult animals did not exceed 3 per cent; but the losses in calves were reported to be considerably greater. At first attempts were made to confine the disease from the north to the south of the river; but this was not possible, and as soon as Hutcheon[135] realized that outbreaks were occurring in several districts south of the river, he withdrew the restrictions. In the two following years mild epizootics occurred in different parts of the country;[136] but the disease never assumed serious proportions, and no further outbreaks were reported after 1895. The advent of rinderpest in 1896 completely eclipsed foot-and-mouth disease in importance, and it may be that the devastation of the cattle population by that plague was responsible for its disappearance.

In April 1903[183] foot-and-mouth disease reappeared in South Africa. The infection was introduced into the Cape Peninsula by means of shipments of cattle from the Argentine. Fortunately the disease was confined to two places only, a farm where the imported cattle were kept and a local dairy that harboured a runaway heifer from the Argentine shipment. Both areas were immediately placed under strict quarantine; the affected animals were dressed with antiseptic lotions and kept under as hygienic conditions as circumstances permitted; and the premises were thoroughly disinfected. Although several of the Argentine animals succumbed to the secondary infection that resulted from their exposure to dirty, muddy surroundings, no deaths occurred in the local dairy herd. At about the end of July of the same year there was no further evidence of the disease, and the quarantine restrictions were raised.

Apart from the 1903 incident, FMD disappeared from the subcontinent with the advent of the rinderpest pandemic in 1896 and did not reappear until April 1931, when it occurred on Nuanetsi Ranch in what is now Zimbabwe. The reappearance of the disease was a source of great consternation at the time as the ability of buffalo to provide a reservoir of infection was unknown and many people believed that the infection had been re-introduced by imported animals or animal products, although no evidence for this could be found.[82]

Foot-and-mouth disease has occurred regularly in most southern African countries since 1931, during which time the cost of control has undoubtedly eclipsed that of any other viral disease.

It is impossible to cover all aspects of the disease in this chapter. Other reviews with different emphases[12, 13, 34, 37, 138, 173, 176] should therefore also be consulted.

Aetiology

Foot-and-mouth disease virus belongs to the family Picornaviridae, and is the only member of the genus *Aphthovirus*. The seven serological types, A, O, C, SAT-1, SAT-2, SAT-3 and Asia 1, are distinguished from members of other picornavirus genera by their lability at pH below 5–6, relatively high density in CsCl (1,41–1,45g/ml), cross-reactive antigens, and their ability to produce FMD in susceptible species.[2, 176, 221]

In common with other picornaviruses, FMD virions have a dry diameter of 27–28 nm, are spherical in shape and exhibit icosahedral symmetry.[180, 190] The virion consists of approximately 70 per cent protein and 30 per cent RNA, as well as a small quantity of lipid.[16, 47] It has a relative molecular mass of about $8{,}5 \times 10^6$,[190] with a sedimentation constant of 146S.[36] This characteristic sedimentation rate in sucrose gradients is widely used in vaccine manufacture to determine the mass of intact virions present in culture harvests because disintegration of virus particles results in loss of immunogenicity.

The viral RNA consists of a single plus (messenger-sense) strand, approximately 8 450 nucleotides long, which is polyadenylated (poly (A)) at the 3′ end and

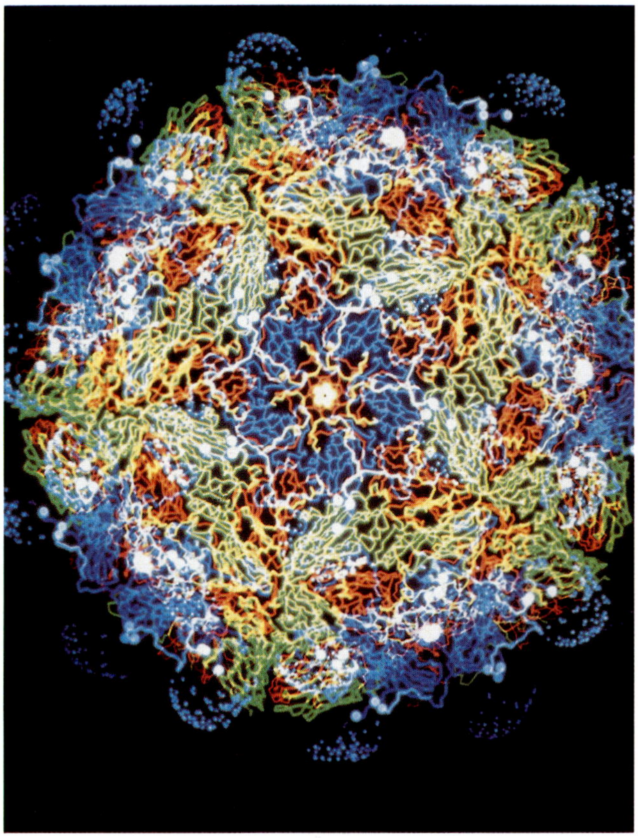

Figure 89.1 (a) Representation of a foot-and-mouth disease virion at 2,9Å resolution showing the relative position of the four structural proteins.

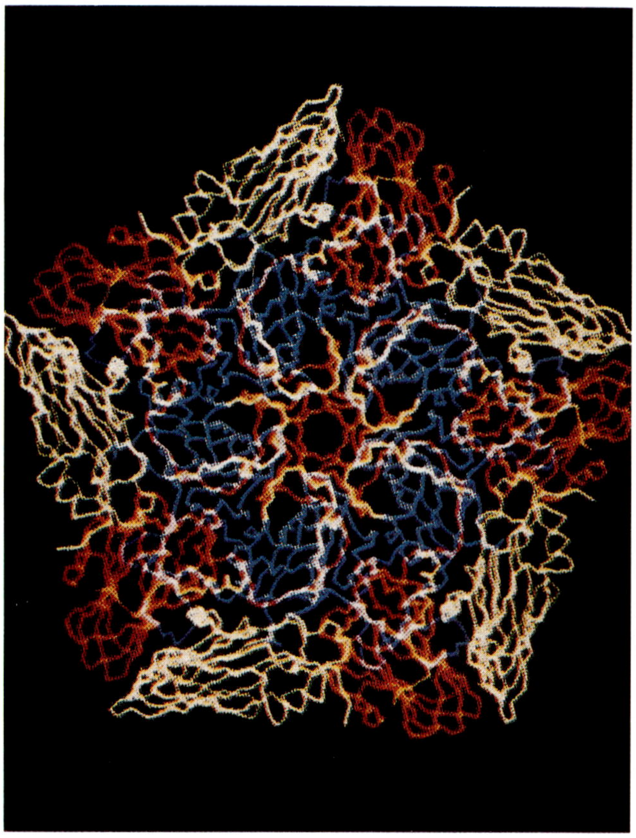

Figure 89.1 (b) A pentamer comprising five protomers showing the relative positions of the four structural proteins. View down the five-fold axis: blue = VP1, green = VP2, red = VP3, yellow = VP4. Source: Acharya *et al.*[2]

contains a 50–200 polycytodylic (poly (C)) tract 150–500 nucleotides from the 5′ end within the noncoding region.[92, 160] The function of the poly (A) and poly (C) tracts is not known, although most eukaryotic messenger RNAs are polyadenylated, and attenuated FMD strains show shortening of the poly (C) tract.[115] Both the single-stranded, positive-sense 35S RNA and the double-stranded, replicative form are infectious.[20]

Sixty subunits termed protomers (poorly defined capsomeres), the majority of which contain one molecule of each of the four structural proteins (VP1, VP2, VP3 and VP4), make up the virion capsid. A few protomers within each capsid are immature and contain VP0 instead of VP2 and VP4; VP0 being the uncleaved precursor of VP2 and VP4.[36, 194] Each virion, on average, also contains one molecule of RNA polymerase, sometimes referred to as virion infection-associated antigen (VIA).[36]

Some cell culture harvests contain virus particles that lack RNA, and their protomers do not contain VP2 and VP4, as the VP0 is uncleaved. These particles have a sedimentation rate of 75S and are referred to as 'empty particles'.

When the virion is disassembled by mild denaturation (such as heat or acid treatment), subviral particles comprising five protomers (known as pentamers) with a sedimentation coefficient of 12S **(Figure 89.1)** result.[36, 194] These 12S particles are not associated with RNA or VP4, showing that the latter two elements have a loose internal arrangement inside the virion.[36]

The precise topography of the four structural proteins with respect to one another and their configuration, particularly at the surface of the virion and with respect to neutralization and attachment sites, is presently a subject of intensive study.[2, 155, 190–192] Recent x-ray diffraction studies have elucidated the tertiary structure of the four structural proteins and their topographic relationships. An apparently unique feature of FMD virus is that the most immunogenic region of VP1, which is also involved in cell attachment, (amino acid residues 135–158) forms disordered protrusions on the surface of the virion **(Figure 89.1)**.[2]

Mechanisms of viral attachment, penetration and uncoating, as well as the biochemical events involved in the replication of FMD virus in infected cells, are detailed elsewhere.[180, 194, 198] However, the basic features need to be appreciated if one is to have an effective understanding of the pathogenesis, epidemiology and immunology of FMD.

Attachment of virions to cells is effected by electrostatic affinity between specific viral receptors, which appears to be determined largely by VP1, and in particular by the 133–158 loop,[2] and 'antireceptors' located in the plasmalemma of the cell. The chemical configuration of these complementary sites is unknown but, because attachment of virus alone can be damaging to the cell, the 'antireceptors' obviously have other biological functions.[194] There is evidence to suggest the conservation of receptor sites among picornaviruses in general but, on the other hand, closely associated neutralization sites tend to be variable in their amino acid composition. It is postulated that this situation ensures access to cells by viruses but, at the same time, enables them to elude the immune response of the host.[191, 192] In this regard FMD virus differs from other picornaviruses in that the pit or canyon on the surface of the virion is absent.[2] After attachment, virions gain entry to the cytoplasm of the cell by pinocytosis, during which process VP4 is lost and the viral RNA liberated from the capsid.

Viral RNA is translated into a large polyprotein which is sequentially cleaved by proteases into the structural and non-structural proteins.[228] Progeny RNA, produced through a complementary minus (negative-sense) strand, and the structural proteins are then assembled into new virions which are released by infection-mediated disintegration of the host cell.[88, 194] In cell cultures the time between infection and the liberation of new virus can be as short as six hours.

Shortly after infection, cellular protein and RNA synthesis are inhibited, whereas viral RNA synthesis in the cytoplasm proceeds rapidly to give rise to a pool of structural and non-structural proteins. Thus, apart from eventual cell disintegration, the functional physiology of infected cells is altered profoundly within a few minutes of infection.

The genomes of RNA viruses have high mutation rates as a result of nucleotide substitution or deletion as well as of phenomena such as genetic recombination and reassortment in the case of segmented genomes. This, coupled with short generation times, results in RNA evolution rates that can be a million-fold greater than the rates in the DNA of their hosts.[129, 211] Conversely, there are selective forces, such as the need to conserve protein structure and function, which tend to stabilize virus populations.[213] Thus, RNA virus populations are a dynamic equilibrium with mutants arising at a high rate on the one hand, and being selected against on the other.[213] It has been argued that factors which alter the intensity of selection may ultimately determine the rate of variation in the field.[211] A population equilibrium model for RNA genomes[69] predicts that RNA virus populations are complex and indeterminate mixtures of variants, each of which is kept in low concentration by competition unless endowed with a selective advantage. The finding that each FMD virus isolate is genetically unique, even when sequential isolates are made from the same animal, accords with the above theories.[103] Despite this considerable and continuous antigenic variation between FMD virus isolates, all can be grouped into one of the seven serological types.

Under conditions of severe challenge, such as when virus is inoculated into the epithelium of the tongue of cattle (intradermalingual inoculation), there is no cross-protection between virus types.[34] Likewise, a single dose of a monotypic vaccine fails to protect against heterotypic challenge.[46] Some cross-protection between A, O and C types has, however, been encountered in experiments involving contact exposure[34] and, at the level of the secondary humoral immune response, antigenic similarities between the above types have been demonstrated,[46] as is the case with SAT-1 and SAT-2.[226]

On the basis of RNA hybridization studies, it would appear that the A, O, C and Asia 1 types on the one hand and the three SAT types on the other form two distinct groups. Within these groups there is 60–70 per cent genome-sequence homology, while between the groups homology falls to 25–40 per cent.[185]

The occurrence and range of intratypic variation (i.e. subtypes) differs between FMD virus types. For instance, while the A and O types have a number of more or less identifiable subtypes (A_5, A_{24}, O_1, O_5, etc.),[174, 184] it is difficult to identify specific subtypes within the SAT-1 and SAT-2 types despite the fact that there is a wide range of variation.[84] The C, Asia 1 and SAT-3 types, on the other hand, exhibit relatively little intratypic variation.[175]

Conventionally, subtyping is based on cross-neutralization or complement fixation (CF) tests which generally show good correlation with cross-protection *in vivo*.[174] However, the latter technique has waned in popularity as the CF reaction is not exclusively dependent on antigens that are relevant to immunological protection.[170–172]

Clear rules were recognized at one time for establishing the immunological relationships of FMD virus isolates, but practical problems resulted in modified proposals being advanced periodically.[174] More recently, the concept of a continuous spectrum of intratypic antigenic variation (without there necessarily being a clear distinction between variants)[174] has become established.

The relationship of an uncharacterized virus (call it B) to a reference isolate (say A), which in practice is usually a vaccine strain, is normally expressed as r (which may be either r_1 or r_2) or R values. These values are derived from the results of serological tests (preferably virus neutralization) using antisera to one or both viruses (called *a* and *b*: viz. antiserum *a* is derived from animals either infected with virus A or immunized with vaccine virus A) and are determined as follows:[162]

$$r_1 = \frac{\text{titre of antiserum } a \text{ against virus B}}{\text{titre of antiserum } a \text{ against virus A}}$$

$$r_2 = \frac{\text{titre of antiserum } b \text{ against virus A}}{\text{titre of antiserum } b \text{ against virus B}}$$

$$R = 100\sqrt{r_1 \times r_2}$$

R is thus a composite value expressed as a percentage but, because asymmetric relationships are common, R is often misleading.[172] Since the ability of a vaccine strain to induce an immune response which protects against the 'new' virus is what is important in practice, r_1 values provide the most valuable information. However it has been suggested that for two isolates to be considered different subtypes, the r value must be <0,25 in both directions.[174]

Newer techniques[56] such as enzyme-linked immunosorbent assay (ELISA),[1, 167] radio-immuno-assay[55] and the use of monoclonal antibodies are being adapted to the testing of intratypic relationships between FMD viruses, but the criteria for the routine application of these methods have yet to be established. Although it does not provide a direct measure of immunological relationships, sequencing part of the 1D gene of FMD viruses is increasingly being used to establish intratypic variation of FMD viruses and has, for example, been used successfully in differentiating SAT-2 outbreak viruses in southern Africa. Two SAT-2 outbreaks in Zimbabwe which occurred within a few days of each other in 1989 (one at Mutorashanga and the other around Gweru) were shown by these techniques to be caused by different viruses. Furthermore, these viruses were distinct from SAT-2 viruses which caused outbreaks in impala in the Kruger National Park (South Africa) and in cattle in the Caprivi strip (Namibia) in 1989 **(Figure 89.2)**.

Epidemiology

With the exception of North America, Australia and islands such as Greenland, New Zealand and Ireland, FMD has essentially a worldwide distribution. However, the incidence of FMD in most of the northern European countries has decreased to such an extent over the last 10–20 years that it is now a rare condition there[235] and, in the recent past, the majority of outbreaks can be traced to improperly inactivated vaccine or to escapes from laboratories.[214] The disease is now considered exotic to countries which comprise the European Economic Community.

The geographic distribution of the seven virus types is heterogeneous. Types A, O and C are prevalent in South America, Europe, Africa and the Middle and Far East. Asia 1 is confined to the Far and Middle East and the Balkans.[58, 176, 196] The three SAT types are restricted to sub-Saharan Africa, although there have been incursions of SAT-1 into North Africa and the Middle East.[176]

The occurrence of FMD in cattle in the larger southern African countries since 1850 is given in **Table 89.1**. Other species are excluded because in southern Africa the disease (as opposed to the infection) is far more prevalent in cattle than in the other domestic species, and, with the exception of buffalo, infection of other species, both wild and domestic, is infrequent.

SAT-1, 2 and 3 viruses have caused the overwhelming majority (84 per cent) of identifiable outbreaks in cattle in southern Africa. It is likely that outbreaks caused by type A, O and C viruses have either spread southward from countries in central or eastern Africa where they are

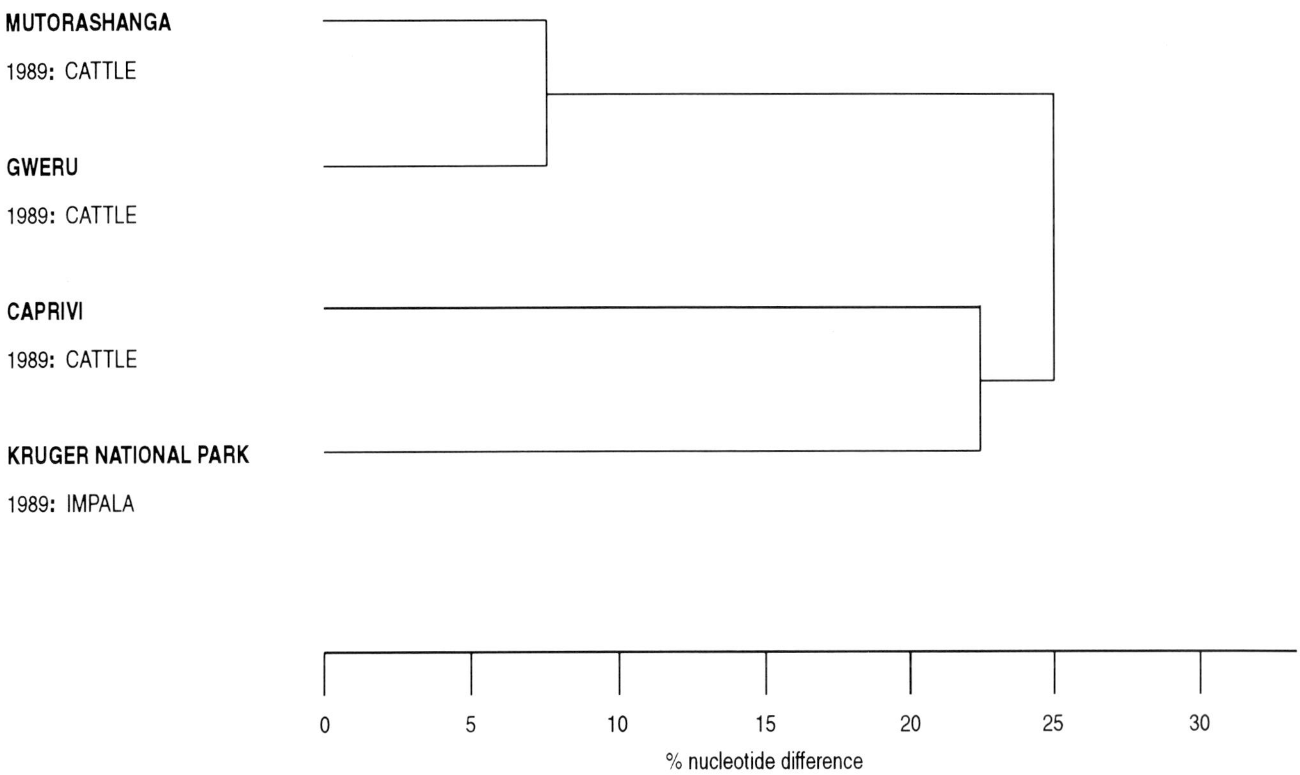

Figure 89.2 Dendogram depicting the relationships between SAT-2 isolates from outbreaks which occurred in southern Africa during 1989. (The percentage nucleotide difference between two isolates is inferred by the position of the node connecting the isolates.) Source: reference 31

Table 89.1 The annual prevalence[w] of FMD in domestic cattle in some southern African countries between 1850 and 1987. (The information was derived from references 7, 10, 11, 48, 58, 60, 63, 73, 86, 127, 176, 177, 199 and 239.)

YEAR	COUNTRY							
	South Africa[X]	Zimbabwe[X]	Namibia[X]	Botswana[X]	Zambia[X]	Mozambique[Y]	Angola[Y]	Malawi[Y]
1850–99	Prevalent	Prevalent	Situation unknown	Prevalent	Situation unknown	Situation unknown	Situation unknown	Situation unknown
1900–29	1903–* (originated from imported Argentinian cattle)	Undetected	Undetected	Undetected	Undetected	Undetected	Undetected	
1930								
1931		2a						
1932								
1933	* (x2)			*	*			
1934		3	*	*	* (x2)			
1935					*			
1936		* (x2)			*			
1937	*	1		*		*		
1938	*	*						
1939	* (x2)							
1940		*						
1941				*				
1942				*	*			
1943		*						
1944	* (x3)	*		*	*			
1945	* (x3)	*	*					
1946			*		*			
1947		2			*			
1948				1	2 (x2)			
1949			1		2			
1950		2		1	2			
1951	2 (x2)	2				2		
1952		2 (x2)						
1953		1 (x2) 2 3			1		2	
1954	* (x3)	2 3 (x2)			1			
1955	1	2 (x3)			1	1		
1956			2		2			
1957	1 (x4)	1 (x2) 2		1	2			0
1958	1 3	1 2	A	3	2	2	A	
1959	1 2	1 2				3	A	2
1960	2 (x3)	1 (x2)	2	1 3	2	2		
1961	1 2 3	2 (x2)	1	1 3			A	
1962		1 2	A 1				A	0
1963				3			A	
1964		2	1	3	2	1 2	0	
1965	1	2		3	2	1 2	2	
1966		1 2 (x3)		3		1	A	A
1967	1	2	A			1	A	A
1968	1 (x3)		2	1			A 2	
1969	2		2		2	2	A 2	
1970		2	2		2	2	A	1

Table 89.1 (continued)

YEAR	COUNTRY							
	South Africa[X]	Zimbabwe[X]	Namibia[X]	Botswana[X]	Zambia[X]	Mozambique[Y]	Angola[Y]	Malawi[Y]
1971	1	2	2			1 2	A	1
1972		1 2 (x3)				2	A 1	
1973	1 2	2			1		A O C	A 2
1974	1 2	1 2 3			1	O 1 2 3	A O C 1 2	A O 1 2
1975	1 2	1 2 3 (x2)	2		2	1	A O C 1 2	2
1976		1 2 3			O	1	A O C 1 2	3
1977	2	1 2 3		1 2 *		1 2 (x2)	A O C 1 2	
1978	2	1 2 3	2	1 2		1 (x5) 2 (x6)	A O C 1 2	
1979	1 2 3	1 2		1 2	1	* 2 (x6)		
1980	1 3	1 2	1	2	1	O 1 2 (x4)		
1981	2	1 (x2) 2		2	1 2	* 1 2 (x3)		A
1982					O 2	* (x2) 2		A
1983	2	2 3 (x2)			O	2 (x5)		O
1984		3			O 2	2		O
1985						*		O
1986								O
1987		2 (x2)						

w In some cases the source material does not differentiate between separate outbreaks and in others does not give the duration of individual outbreaks
X Reliable data
Y Data may be incomplete

a 1 SAT-2 outbreak in Zimbabwe in 1931
* Outbreaks where virological confirmation was not obtained
1 SAT-1
2 SAT-2
3 SAT-3
A Type A
O Type O
C Type C
(x2) 2 separate outbreaks with that virus type

endemic or have entered the region with imported cattle,[60, 176] since, unlike the SAT types, A, O and C viruses are not, as far as is known, established in wildlife populations.[123] It is therefore reasonable to assume that they are exotic to southern Africa, although their regular occurrence in some countries in recent years **(Table 89.1)** suggests that they are becoming endemic in cattle in some parts of the subcontinent.

Of the three SAT types, SAT-2 has had the highest incidence in domestic animals in this century (48 per cent of SAT-type outbreaks), followed by SAT-1 (36 per cent) and SAT-3 (16 per cent). SAT-3 has a more restricted distribution than the other two SAT types and has never been diagnosed in domestic species outside southern Africa. It has, however, been found in buffalo in East Africa.[123]

The regions of southern Africa historically associated with FMD in domestic stock are shown in **Figure 89.3**. It is, however, impossible to be accurate as to the present distribution of the disease in the subcontinent because of the inconsistent reporting by various countries.[153] The widespread use of vaccines and other control measures probably masks the real situation, and the continually changing and poorly documented distribution and population densities of wildlife, especially buffalo, make it difficult to know where potential reservoir hosts occur and where they do not.

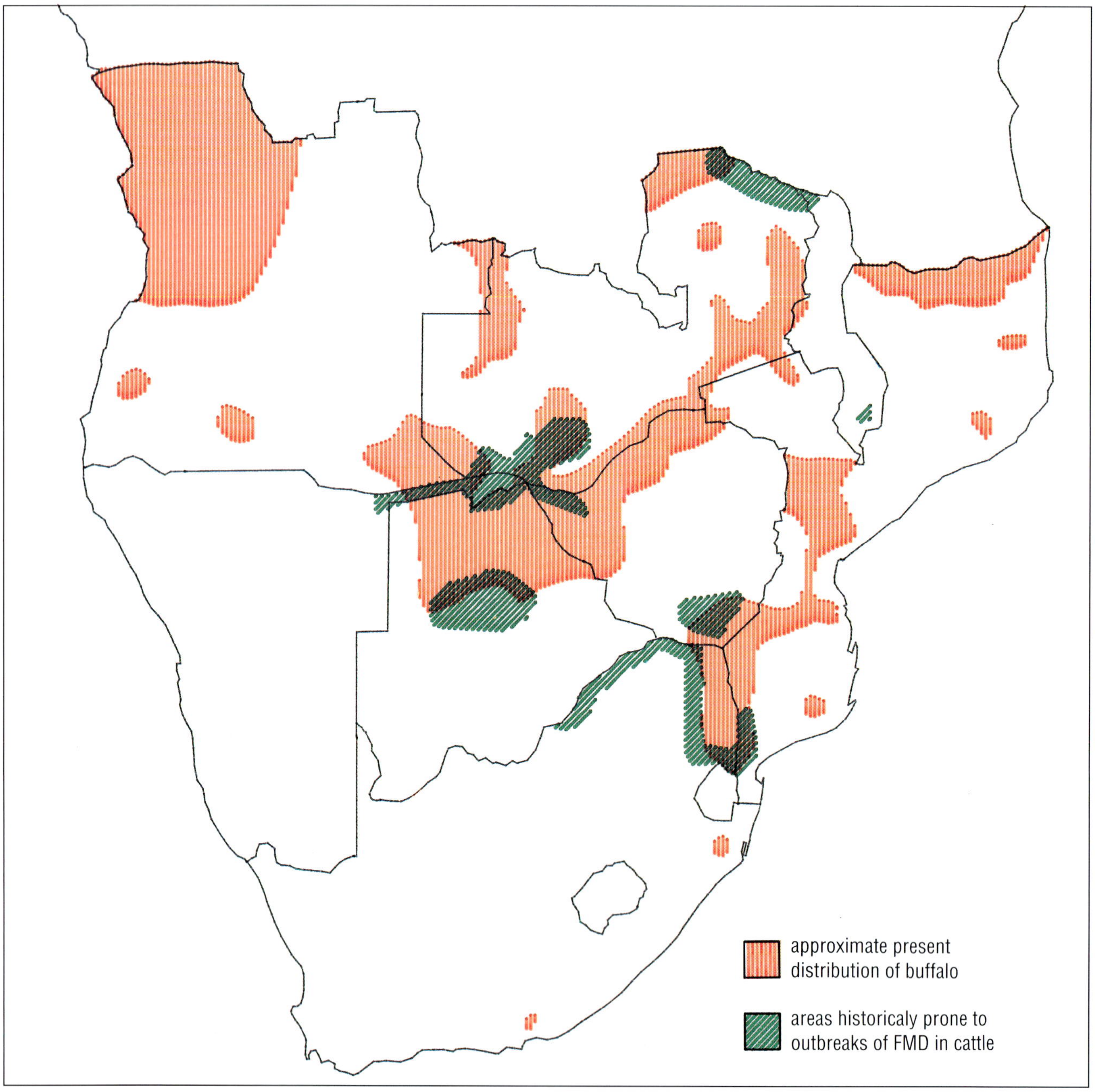

Figure 89.3 The approximate present distribution of African buffalo in southern Africa and areas historically prone to foot-and-mouth disease outbreaks in domestic cattle

Changes in the distribution of FMD outbreaks have occurred in South Africa over the last 20–40 years. In the farming area south of the Kruger National Park (Barberton and Nelspruit districts) outbreaks were common **(Figure 89.3)** before cattle numbers declined as a result of the introduction of sugarcane plantations in the 1960s. Similarly, in the period 1930–1960, outbreaks occurred regularly along the Botswana and Zimbabwe borders with South Africa, but in more recent times this has ceased, no doubt due to the more efficient control of FMD in those countries and to border fencing.

The prevalence of FMD in cattle in southern Africa for the first two decades after its reappearance in 1931 was relatively low **(Table 89.1)**. A sharp increase occurred in the 1950s and again in the 1970s. Although only eight years of the 1980s have been assessed, it would appear that the prevalence dropped in the 1980s **(Table 89.1)**. The reason for this pattern can, at present, only be speculated upon. Possible reasons include changes in control strategies, such as immunization versus aphthization ('firing'),[86] climatic changes, changing cattle and wildlife distributions, changing population densities and military conflict in the region. The effects of these factors are likely to have varied between countries of the subcontinent, and an overall assessment is therefore impossible.

It is commonly held that water scarcity, such as that due to drought or seasonal variation, is conducive to the occurrence of FMD outbreaks as it results in the congregation of both domestic and wild animals at water points.[59, 131, 132, 152] This contention is, however, not supported by an association of disease incidence in cattle in South Africa with dry periods of the quasi 18-year oscillation in rainfall[228] **(Table 89.2)**. The opposite may be the case. Similarly, for southern Africa as a whole, there was no appreciable difference in the prevalence of FMD between 1950–59, which were generally wet years, and 1968–73, which was a generally dry period,[228] **(Table 89.1)**. There is also no evidence for seasonality in the occurrence of FMD in livestock in South Africa,[224] Zimbabwe,[48, 60] Namibia[199] or Zambia,[239] which generally have dry winters. However, between 1957 and 1975, seven out of eight FMD outbreaks in Malawi began in winter.[59]

The African buffalo is the only free-living species known to be capable of sustaining FMD infections for indefinite periods,[118] although in the field the vast majority of infections are clinically inapparent.[223] In individual animals the virus may persist in the pharyngeal region for at least five years.[51] A variety of other wildlife species becomes infected periodically,[52, 62, 63, 118, 146, 152, 189] but there is little evidence to suggest that they are important for viral maintenance or transmission to cattle. Impala (*Aepyceros melampus*) in the Kruger National Park (KNP) in South Africa are a possible exception, as regular epidemics, sometimes characterized by the development of severe disease, occur in this species.[224] However, due to a lack of congruity between the virus type and the timing of epidemics in cattle and impala, it appears likely that FMD outbreaks in cattle in areas adjacent to the KNP have only rarely originated from impala.[159, 224] This is despite the fact that experiments have shown that it is possible for FMD to be transmitted from acutely infected impala to cattle in close contact with them.[223] These experiments indicated that, although impala are highly susceptible to low doses of virus in inspired aerosols, infected animals excrete relatively small quantities of virus for short periods.[101] Serological surveillance in the KNP has also shown that FMD viruses do not persist in the impala population in interepidemic periods.[223]

That buffalo are the major source of infection for cattle in southern Africa is indicated by the fact that buffalo occur in or adjacent to all endemic FMD areas in the subcontinent, although there are at least two buffalo populations which are not infected with FMD viruses — those in the northern Natal game parks and the National Addo Elephant Park in South Africa **(Figure 89.3)**.[85] Furthermore, infection rates in buffalo populations are high[52, 87, 117, 119] **(Table 89.3)**, first infection occurs early in life[50] **(Table 89.3)**, and acutely infected buffalo excrete SAT-type viruses in approximately the same quantities, by the same routes and for roughly the same period of

Table 89.2 The association between outbreaks of FMD within the borders of South Africa and wet and dry rainfall periods. Source: reference 228

WET/DRY PERIOD	DURATION	NO. OF FMD OUTBREAKS
WET	1933/4 – 1943/4	6
DRY	1944/5 – 1952/3	8
WET	1953/4 – 1961/2	18
DRY	1962/3 – 1970/1	7
WET	1971/2 – 1980/1	11
DRY	1981/2 – 1986/7 (incomplete)	4

Table 89.3 Age-related seropositivity to SAT-type viruses in buffalo sampled in the Kruger National Park

Year	Type of test	No. of sera tested	Age of animals (months)	Percentage of sera positive SAT-1	SAT-2	SAT-3
1984/5	SVN	33	≤6	70	24	27
1984/5	SVN	25	7 – 12	56	40	40
1984/5	SVN	24	13 – 18	46	42	42
1984/5	SVN	50	19 – 30	88	84	54
1984/5	SVN	16	31 – 42	94	63	56
1984/5	SVN	23	43 – 54	91	78	52
1984/5	SVN	106	≥55	97	77	75
1987	ELISA	44	≤6	93	66	39
1987	ELISA	22	7 – 12	86	68	55
1987	ELISA	25	13 – 18	96	100	88
1987	ELISA	36	19 – 30	94	89	89
1987	ELISA	9	31 – 42	100	100	100
1987	ELISA	4	34 – 54	100	100	100
1987	ELISA	81	≥55	100	96	85

Table 89.4 Maximum virus levels and the time over which FMD virus has been recorded in secretions and excretions of domestic animals commonly affected by FMD

Species	Secretion or excretion	Maximum titre recorded ($\log_{10}$)	Maximum duration of virus presence (days)*	References
Cattle	Expired air	2,2/min. (2,4/min)	5 (4)	72, 100
	Saliva	8,5/ml (6,4/ml)	14 (6)	100, 137, 138, 120
	Nasal secretion	7,7/g (5,6/specimen)	7 (6)	53, 100, 120
	Oesophago-pharyngeal secretion	7,7/ml	>530	34, 66, 103, 157, 217
	Lachrymal secretion	7,6/ml (4,0/specimen)	>3 (5)	100, 217
	Milk	5,5/ml (7,0/ml[a])	9 (49[a])	26, 44, 53, 122
	Preputial secretion	(6,5/specimen)	(6)	100
	Semen	6,2/ml	10	53, 204
	Vaginal secretion	3,3/specimen	NAFA	42
	Urine	4,9/ml (0,9/ml)	7 (2)	53, 54, 100
	Faeces	2,0/g (5,5/g[b])(1,7/g)	15 (1)	100, 169, 204
	Lesion material:			
	vesicular fluid	10,0/ml		138, 166, 120
	epithelium	9,9/g		
Pig	Expired air	5,4/min (4,3/min)	5 (5)	72, 100
	Saliva	7,0/ml or specimen[c]	>9 (5)	65, 100
	Nasal secretion	(5,4/specimen)	(5)	100
	Oesophago-pharyngeal secretion	NAFA		34, 65
	Lachrymal secretion	(2,0/specimen)	(3)	100
	Semen	NAFA		182
	Preputial secretion	(7,0/specimen)	(4)	100
	Urine	(0,9/ml)	(1)	100
	Faeces	2,9/g (1,8/g)	(1)	100, 202
	Lesion material: foot epithelium	9,6/g		202
Sheep	Expired air	2,2/min	5	72, 202
	Saliva	3,8/specimen	6	206
	Nasal secretion	6,1/specimen	>7	206
	Oesophago-pharyngeal fluid	4,5/ml	365	53, 106, 206, 215
	Lachrymal secretion	3,1/specimen	6	206
	Urine	2,6/ml	3	206
	Faeces	3,2/g	4	83, 206
Goat	Nasal secretion	5,4/ml	7	4
	Oesophago-pharyngeal	4,0/ml[d]	30	4, 53
	Faeces	Trace	2	4

* ( ) results obtained with SAT-type viruses[100]
a Data derived by direct inoculation of virus into the teat canal
b Faeces collected from the floor of a contaminated isolation stable
c The sample was a swab of the oral cavity including the pharynx
d It is not clear whether this represents the whole specimen or a portion thereof
NAFA No accurate figure available

time as cattle.[102] Efficient surveillance and control measures in South Africa, Botswana and Zimbabwe preclude the possibility that most outbreaks in cattle are merely an extension of undetected infection in cattle or other domestic species.

Precisely how SAT-type viruses are transmitted from buffalo to cattle populations is a subject of debate. One theory suggests that they are perpetuated in buffalo populations by periodic epidemics among juveniles and that at such times buffalo herds transmit the infection to other species, including cattle, in the immediate vicinity.[21, 117] This is supported by the fact that buffalo in southern Africa breed seasonally (most calves are born in mid-summer, although a few are born at other times throughout the year[178, 209]), which has the effect of synchronizing the recruitment of susceptible animals into the population. It is presumed that during the infection episodes large numbers of juveniles (more than 10 per cent of breeding herds that may number above 1 000 animals) become infected more-or-less simultaneously, and that the resultant environmental contamination provides a source of infection for other species in the immediate vicinity.

An alternative theory is that persistently infected (carrier) buffalo are the usual source of infection for cattle. Evidence for this has been advanced[120] but, because many more attempts at demonstrating this have failed,[5, 49, 102] it is unlikely that this possibility could account for more than a small minority of FMD outbreaks in cattle.[5, 118, 196] It is, however, likely that persistently infected buffalo maintain the infection in inter-epidemic periods.

An important aspect with respect to wildlife and FMD is that unusual and unexpected eventualities are possible. A recent good example of this was the very high mortality among mountain gazelles (*Gazella gazella*) caused by type O virus in a nature reserve in Israel.[207]

Foot-and-mouth disease virus may spread by either direct or indirect contact.[138, 196, 202] Most commonly, it occurs by direct contact between animals excreting virus and susceptible individuals.[233] On rare occasions, indirect transmission is effected by objects or materials contaminated with virus containing secretions, excretions or tissues, or by animal products, such as milk, or by air currents in which virus-containing aerosols are suspended. Humans, animals, vehicles, and birds may serve as mechanical transmitters of the infection,[202] although doubt has been expressed about birds.[187]

While strong circumstantial and theoretical evidence for long-distance (greater than 1 km) airborne transmission of FMD outbreaks in northern Europe has been reported,[71, 91, 107, 137] no convincing evidence for its involvement in FMD incidents in southern Africa has been advanced. Little attention has, however, been paid to mechanisms of transmission in the subcontinent in recent times.[22, 82, 233]

As is the case with other directly transmitted infectious agents, there are three factors which determine the characteristics of FMD transmission: the quantity, duration and means by which virus is liberated into the environment; the ability of the agent to survive outside the animal body; and the quantities of virus required to initiate infection at the primary infection sites.

With the exception of oesophago-pharyngeal secretions, measurable quantities of FMD virus are present in animal secretions and excretions for less than two weeks after infection.[110] In viraemic animals FMD virus is present in most physiological fluids and hence potentially in nearly all secretions and excretions.[138] There are, however, differences in this respect between virus strains, host species and different secretions and excretions[72] **(Table 89.4)**. Nevertheless, the fact that FMD in southern Africa has often spread more slowly than would be expected in Europe[82, 86, 149] is not due to the SAT virus types being excreted at lower rates than is the case for the 'European' types **(Table 89.4)**.

Significant excretion may occur up to four days, or perhaps longer, before the appearance of lesions, so that apparently healthy animals can be an important source of infection.[44, 138] In this regard milk is of particular importance because of the high virus content, rapid dispersal of the product and the movement of bulk tankers between farms.

Domestic pigs are the most efficient excreters of FMD virus; individual pigs may excrete more than 1 500 times as much virus into the atmosphere in 24 hours as individual cattle or sheep.[72] Since pigs are often intensively farmed, the disease in piggeries can result in an enormous multiplication of infectivity. Airborne spread of infection from primary outbreaks in Europe has rarely occurred, except where pigs were the predominant source of infection.[73] The fact that pigs are generally not raised in significant numbers in FMD-prone areas in southern Africa **(Figure 89.3)** is probably a major reason why airborne transmission has not presented a problem in the subregion so far.

Virus-containing aerosols are probably derived from the upper respiratory tract[77] as they are present in the breath of pigs. The particle size of such aerosols ranges in diameter from about 3–10 µm, the majority being greater than 5 µm.[195] Most infectivity is associated with droplets larger than 6 µm.[79] Because aerosols are subject to evaporation and may coalesce, the particle-size structure is not static,[195] and it may be that aerosols smaller than 3 µm are rapidly destroyed by atmospheric conditions.[205] Should meteorological factors be suitable for virus survival in aerosols, their fall-rate is such that they remain airborne long enough to be conveyed at least 10 km from the source by air currents.[195]

Of all the secretions and excretions in acutely infected animals (certainly in cattle and pigs) saliva contains the highest concentrations of virus **(Table 89.4)**. Hyslop pointed out that when virus levels in saliva exceed 10^7/ml it could contribute to virus-containing aerosols as well as causing gross contamination of the immediate environment.[137, 138] There is a non-specific viral inhibitor (dialysable inactivating factor) in the saliva of cattle which limits virus survival outside the body[72, 76] but this aspect has not been quantified.

Other secretions which contain appreciable quantities of virus are those of the nasal passages, the oesophago-pharyngeal region and the urogenital tract as well as milk **(Table 89.4)**. Semen, which in bulls may attain virus levels of up to $10^{4,7}$ MLD_{50}/ml prior to the development of visible lesions, is also a potential source of infection in both cattle and pigs.[203] Artificial insemination is thus a possible avenue of transmission. The possibility of FMD transmission occurring during embryo transfer remains to be elucidated, because although the virus does not appear to penetrate the *zona pellucida*, it may be capable of infecting hatched bovine embryos.[210]

The importance of urine and faeces in the transmission of FMD is uncertain. Both excretions have been claimed to contain high levels of virus — in the case of urine for prolonged periods as a result of supposed persistent kidney infection.[128, 169, 232] However, a recent investigation, admittedly on a small scale, failed to reveal virus levels greater than 10 MLD_{50}/ml in the urine of either cattle or pigs **(Table 89.4)**. The fact that urogenital secretions, particularly those of the preputium, may contain high virus levels **(Table 89.4)** presents the possibility that virus in urine may be derived largely from such secretions. Similarly, a number of investigators have found little or no virus in faeces,[53, 100, 138] and it is probable that virus found in faeces in some investigations was predominantly due to environmental contamination after defecation.[169]

An aspect which is still unresolved after 80 years of speculation[138] is the ability of carriers to transmit the infection.[41] These carriers are recovered animals in which FMD virus persists in the mucosa of the soft palate, pharynx and cranial oesophagus. Persistent infection occurs in cattle, sheep, goats, buffaloes **(Table 89.4)**, and other wildlife species, but not in pigs.[34, 103, 119, 138, 231]

In cattle, as in buffalo,[5] virus levels in the oesophago-pharyngeal region begin to decline soon after initial infection[41, 79] and they may fluctuate.[103, 231] By six months after infection, the presence of persistent virus becomes erratic[103, 231] but virus may persist in up to 20 per cent of cattle for a year[116] and in some animals for as long as two years.[116] Viral persistence occurs despite the occurrence of antibody in oesophago-pharyngeal secretions.[94] Super-infection with other virus strains also occurs.[158, 231]

Circumstantial evidence indicates that persistently infected cattle are able to transmit FMD virus occasionally,[138, 231] but this has not been proven conclusively.[41, 216, 231, 233] In many of the FMD outbreaks which have occurred in cattle in southern Africa over the last 50 years **(Table 89.1)**, aphthization or 'firing' (the deliberate infection of all animals present within the outbreak focus) was practised. Aphthized cattle were often allowed to move to disease-free areas within a few months of the end of the outbreak. Despite this, FMD control in South Africa, Botswana and Zimbabwe has historically been successful, indicating that persistently infected cattle are not a common source of infection.[86] On the other hand, circumstantial evidence from the study of recent FMD outbreaks in Zimbabwe suggests that persistently infected (carrier) cattle may have been responsible for inter-epidemic persistence of the infection.

In vitro studies have shown that viral persistence possibly involves co-evolution of both the infecting virus and the host cells.[64] A similar situation may obtain in the pharyngeal mucosa. Because every virus isolate is a fleeting representative of a continuously evolving population,[103] and such transmission only rarely occurs, it is possible that infection derived from persistently infected cattle (or other species) provides a mechanism whereby dominant virus populations are periodically replaced.[103]

Foot-and-mouth disease virus is very labile in even mildly acid solutions. At pH 6,0 the rate of inactivation is 90 per cent per minute, while at pH 5,0 it is 90 per cent per second.[12] In mildly acidic conditions FMD virions disintegrate into their constituent 12S subunits (pentamers), liberating RNA. Although the latter is infectious, environmental ribonucleases will normally rapidly inactivate naked RNA.[13] The virus is also labile in alkaline solutions; at pH 10 its loss of infectivity is 90 per cent every 14 hours.[12] For this reason, 2 per cent NaOH or KOH and 4 per cent Na_2C0_3 are used as cheap and effective disinfectants. They are generally more effective than acid solutions because they are not as easily neutralized by organic material such as faeces and blood.

Lactic acid formation in skeletal muscle after slaughter, where the pH usually drops to pH 5,5–6,0 within 48 hours at 4 °C, renders meat free of infectious virus.[54] However, in lymph nodes, which are not subject to acid formation, the virus can persist for at least 120 days at 4 °C.[53] The same applies to bone marrow and blood in large blood vessels. Details of the occurrence and persistence of FMD viruses in meat and meat products has been published elsewhere.[9, 24, 25]

There is variation between virus strains so far as their lability at low or high pH is concerned. Although inactivation is rapid at first, a residuum of infectivity may remain after exposure to extreme pH.[13, 14] Foot-and-mouth disease virus may also be protected from the effects of pH by chemical agents,[12] and in dairy products by the association of the virus with a variety of cell structures and casein micelles.[25] In milk from FMD-infected cows, the virus survives in casein after iso-electric precipitation from skim milk at pH 4,6, in butter ripened with lactic acid cultures at pH 4,6, in cheese at pH 5,1 and in sweet whey at pH 5,2.[25]

In contrast to the effects of pH, FMD virus is relatively resistant to heat inactivation, although there is considerable variation between virus types and strains.[13, 68] In the case of primarily infected milk this resistance is extreme.[234] The reason for this is at least partly the association of the virus with cell and fat structures.[25] The virus can only be inactivated with certainty by exposure of milk to low-temperature pasteurization for periods in excess of 20 minutes, while 2,5 seconds is sufficient at 148 °C.[234] At 37 °C 146S particles lose 90 per cent of their infectivity within eight hours.[39] Foot-and-mouth disease virus in infected ground-beef products survived cooking to an internal temperature of up to 72 °C, but not 79,4 °C.[25, 156]

Foot-and-mouth disease virus in various dairy products subjected to heat and chemical treatments has generally resulted in the survival of only a small fraction of the original infectivity; highly artificial means have been required to demonstrate it. There is, therefore, some doubt as to the necessity for the disruption of international trade which these results occasioned.[73]

In general, denaturation of protomer proteins is relatively rapid at temperatures above 43 °C,[12] while virus inactivated by prolonged incubation at 37 °C apparently loses infectivity through disruption of the RNA without damage to the protein coat.[13, 39]

At temperatures of 55 and 61 °C, type A virus in cell culture fluid showed initial first-order inactivation followed by 'tailing', indicating the presence of a small thermal-resistant fraction.[14] Hence the common practice in southern Africa of heating sera and other products to 56 °C for 30 minutes in order to render them free of FMD virus has the disadvantage that a small fraction of infectivity may remain after such treatment.

Normal ambient temperatures have relatively little effect on the survival of FMD virus in aerosols; at 27 °C high recoveries were achieved between 30 and 60 minutes after the formation of the aerosols.[72]

As is the case for most non-enveloped viruses, FMD virus survives best in aerosols and microdroplets under conditions where relative humidity exceeds 60 per cent. There is a critical relative humidity range of 55–60 per cent below which virus survival is poor,[17, 70, 195] although the reason for this is not clearly understood.[75] The fact that most regions in southern Africa where FMD is prevalent **(Figure 89.3)** are relatively dry is probably another explanation as to why long-distance airborne transmission of FMD virus appears not to occur in the subcontinent.

The nature of the suspending fluid is important as far as FMD virus survival in aerosols is concerned. Survival of virus in aerosols generated from saliva was much poorer than in those generated from milk, nasal fluid or faeces.[72] This was ascribed to an organic antiviral molecule in saliva that is inactivated within three hours at 70 °C, but not at 60 °C.[72]

Detailed studies conducted earlier this century[40] indicated that the long-term survival of FMD virus on the surface of hay and bran, but not on other materials tested, was possible under conditions of relative dryness and absence of light. An unidentified rehydrating agent extractable from hay and bran was held to be responsible for this effect.

There is an ingrained belief in southern Africa that, because of the susceptibility of FMD virus to ultraviolet light, FMD is less easily transmitted here than, for example, in northern Europe. Available evidence, however, suggests that this is not the case, because FMD virus has been found to be photoresistant to the ultraviolet levels in sunlight — albeit northern European sunlight.[74]

More detail on the interaction of FMD virus with chemicals and disinfectants is available from review articles[12, 201] and Simm's[208] bibliography.

In cattle, infection with FMD virus by the respiratory route can be achieved with as little as 25 cell culture infective doses[80] and with as few as 10 doses in sheep.[105] Conversely, from comparative titrations conducted by intradermalingual inoculation of sheep and cattle with five different viruses (four of them SAT types), sheep appeared to be less susceptible than cattle.[104]

Since infection by the oral route in cattle requires at least 10 000 times as much virus as by the respiratory route,[43, 202] the respiratory tract appears to be the virus' usual portal of entry in cattle (and probably also in sheep and goats). Most infectivity in aerosols is associated with larger droplets[79] which are likely to be predominantly trapped in the upper respiratory tract.

Cattle are efficient samplers of infected air because of their relatively large inspiratory volume (86–167 m^3 per day for adults),[202] and they therefore serve as the most efficient indicators of the presence of infection among domestic host species. Presumably for this reason the attack rate in the 1967–68 FMD epidemic in Britain increased with the density of the cattle population.[133] The relatively low stocking rate in southern Africa, particularly in FMD prone regions **(Figure 89.3)**, is another explanation as to why long-distance airborne transmission has so far not been reported in the subcontinent.

For pigs the situation is probably different in that the minimal infectious doses by both the oral and respiratory routes are relatively high; c.10^5 and 10^2 MLD_{50} respectively.[202, 220] Furthermore, circumstantial evidence suggests that, in Western Europe at least, infection in pigs usually results from the feeding of contaminated and untreated swill.[214]

Little is known about the role sheep and goats play in the epidemiology of FMD in southern Africa. Sheep are highly susceptible to infection[105] and both species excrete significant quantities of virus when acutely infected **(Table 89.4)**. Although infection has occurred in these species during epidemics in the subcontinent,[7] cattle are far more important than sheep and goats in the spread of infection. This is probably due to a combination of their relatively small inspiratory volume[202] and generally lower rates of virus excretion **(Table 89.4)**. In East Africa also, goats and sheep appear to have little importance in the epidemiology of FMD.[4] Conversely, both sheep and goats have been considered epidemiologically important in some European and Turkish outbreaks and this, together with their tendency to develop mild or even inapparent infection, makes them a potentially dangerous source of infection.[173]

Coitus or artificial insemination as methods of transmission by infected bulls are possible,[203] but the minimal infectious dose for cattle by this route is high, viz. $10^{3,4}$ MLD_{50}. Sellers[203] states without corroborating evidence that this route does not appear possible for sows and nanny goats.

Other routes of viral entry are also possible. For example, infection of cattle was achieved with as little as 100 infective doses inoculated onto the conjunctiva.[217] This suggested that face flies (*Musca* spp.) could possibly transmit the virus mechanically, but a preliminary investigation into this possibility failed to substantiate it.[227] Arthropods in general probably play no part in FMD virus transmission.[111, 138, 225]

Small rodents and hedgehogs (family Erinaceidae) in Europe[138] and capybaras (*Hydrochoerus hydrochoeris*) in South America[108] have been implicated in spreading FMD, but as yet there is no evidence that similar animals are important in this respect in southern Africa.

The immune response of domestic animals to FMD viruses is characteristically ephemeral and this, together with the wide immunological diversity present within this group of viruses, often results in poor herd immunity.

Although the responses of very young piglets and calves differ from those of more mature animals, they are immunologically competent to FMD virus from an early age.[96, 165, 197] The poor responses of calves and piglets to immunization are probably due more to immunological interference by maternally-derived antibody[96, 164] than to immunological immaturity. Maternally-derived antibody (MDA) disappears before pigs and cattle attain the age of six months,[95, 164] the half-life being 21,5 days in cattle.[197] In pigs the half-life varies with the class of immunoglobulin which predominates in the colostrum. The half-life of IgM is four to eight days, while that of IgG is seven to 21 days.[95] For this reason it has been recommended that sows not be vaccinated or revaccinated within 30 days of farrowing since this will elevate the IgM level with its short half-life.[93]

Cattle are immune to re-infection with homologous virus for one to three years, and occasionally for up to four-and-a-half years.[12, 34] Circumstantial evidence suggests that the duration of immunity after infection with SAT-type viruses may be shorter. The duration of immunity in other domestic species is largely unknown, but it is probably shorter than in cattle.[12] That there is considerable species variation has been shown by serological studies in wildlife.[121]

Since recovery from infection with FMD virus is the rule, little attention has been paid to the immunological mechanisms involved in recovery, although interferon levels and the 'opsono-phagocytic' activity of peripheral blood leukocytes have been examined in acutely infected animals.[3] Conversely, since it is clear that the level of neutralizing antibody in the circulation correlates with resistance to infection or re-infection in immunized and recovered animals respectively,[154, 170, 218] the humoral immune response and the antigens which are able to induce it have been extensively studied. The relationship between neutralizing antibody level and the degree of resistance to infection is, however, not simple and depends on the virus type as well as, in immunized animals, the period between immunization and exposure to infection.[230]

Neutralization of the FMD virion can occur at several sites.[155, 222, 237] The major immunogenic site is composed of a complex arrangement of two regions of VP1 (amino acid residues 140–160 and 200–213) in addition to contributions from at least one of the other surface proteins, VP2 or VP3.[36, 163, 237] The 140–160 region of VP1 seems to be the major determinant involved in neutralization,[193] and amino acid residues 133–158 of VP1 form disordered protrusions on the virion surface.[2] VP1 is the only structural protein of FMD virus which is at all immunogenic in isolation.[15, 147]

The antibody response to FMD virus is T-cell dependent.[97] Since different species recognize different determinants as T-cell recognition sites, not all FMD virus antigens are equally immunogenic in different species.[36] This has presented problems in the development of synthetic vaccines.

Because the usual route of infection in FMD is the respiratory tract, local immunity may be important as far as resistance to infection is concerned, but the extent to which this is so with respect to overall immunity remains to be established. Neutralizing activity occurs in the secretions of the upper respiratory tract in cattle and pigs recovered from FMD. In cattle it reaches a peak within one week of infection achieved by inoculation of virus into the epithelium of the tongue.[94, 98] The major constituent of the local response in cattle is IgA, although IgM is also present in appreciable amounts for approximately the first ten days.[98]

Pathogenesis

The respiratory tract is the usual route of infection in species other than pigs. In cattle and sheep initial viral replication occurs in the mucosa and possibly the lymphoid tissues of the pharynx, particularly in the tonsillar region and soft palate.[41–43] These regions are exposed directly to virus which enters the body either by inspiration or orally, as well as indirectly to virus cleared by the mucocilliary mechanisms from both the nasal passages and the lungs, and from ingested virus regurgitated during rumination.[43]

In domestic ruminants and buffaloes the pharynx and dorsal soft palate are predilection sites for FMD virus replication. Not only does initial viral replication occur at these sites, but virus persists there for prolonged periods **(Table 89.4)**. The initially high virus levels (>$10^{6,0}$ MLD_{50}/ml) which occur in the secretions of the pharyngeal region in cattle fall sharply during the following eight weeks,[79] so that in persistently infected cattle the quantities of virus usually recoverable from pharyngeal secretions are low.[41]

The fact that high levels of virus could be recovered from retropharyngeal, mandibular and parotid lymph nodes in more than 50 per cent of cattle in the pre-viraemic stage of infection suggests that spread from the initial replication site usually occurs via the lymphoid system.[43] The fact that these high levels are reached in lymph nodes suggests that replication may occur in lymphoid tissue, although it has not been established whether FMD virus is capable of replicating in macrophages or lymphocytes. Alternatively, it may be that such levels of virus merely occur in lymph nodes draining sites of efficient viral replication.

The liberation of virus into the efferent lymphatic system results in an initial viraemia whereby virus reaches a wide variety of organs and tissues. Further replication occurs in many of these, giving rise at some sites to lesions characteristic of FMD.[43, 53] High virus levels may occur in organs and tissues which do not generally develop gross changes referable to FMD virus replication, such as lymph nodes, adrenals, myocardium, pancreas, thyroid and mammary glands,[27, 43, 53] and skin of unaffected areas.[99] In mammary tissue and myocardium, however, viral replication in secretory epithelial cells of the alveoli or myocytes may result in clear microscopic lesions[27, 28, 78] and it is therefore possible that this situation also occurs in other organs and tissues.

Viral replication, other than in the mucosa of the pharyngeal region, does not persist for longer than 14 days in infected animals **(Table 89.4)**, while in the vast majority of experimental infections with SAT-type viruses in cattle and pigs, virus could not be isolated for longer than seven days.[100] Detectable viraemias resulting from SAT-type infections in cattle and pigs do not last longer than three days.[100]

Development of characteristic vesicular lesions in FMD is dependent on two factors — infection of squamous epithelium and persistent local irritation or friction.[179] In transplantation studies in guinea-pigs it was shown that epithelium from predilection sites grafted to other body areas lost that predilection and vice versa. This explains why the mouth, feet and teats are predilection sites for the development of lesions, and why pigs often develop lesions on the dorsum of the snout, as a result of 'snuffling'. Similarly, warthogs, which often 'kneel' on their carpal joints while feeding, tend to develop lesions on their 'knees'.

Epithelial lesions in FMD are initiated by infection of single cells in the *stratum spinosum*.[238] The virus is probably carried to this avascular site by mononuclear cells from the underlying dermis.[238] Following infection of these cells bullae may develop by lysis of swollen cells and the release of intracellular fluid, or by the formation of areas of focal intercellular oedema. The bullae then rupture or, rarely, the fluid seeps away resulting in desiccation of the lesion.[238]

Clinical signs and pathology

All cloven-hoofed species including camels are susceptible to infection with FMD virus, although the resulting disease varies with the level of immunity, the virus dose and strain, host species and even between individuals of a given species. For example, there are virus strains with a predilection for individual species.[33, 138] Goats, particularly those indigenous to East and South Africa, generally suffer inapparent infection.[4, 100] In adult animals of all species mortality rates are low, although instances of rates as high as 30 per cent have been recorded in cattle.[138] In southern Africa outbreaks involving indigenous or *Bos indicus*-type cattle are often mild and difficult to recognize.[86, 139]

Foot-and-mouth disease is characteristically a rapidly spreading infection.[109] The incubation period is generally short, ranging from two to eight days, but may last up to 11–13 days. In most outbreaks the morbidity rate approaches 100 per cent. However, an important observation in southern Africa, dating from the earliest investigations,[82] is that spread between cattle may be surprisingly slow, so that morbidity rates may be as low as 0,2 per cent — a situation referred to as the 'occult form' of FMD.[86]

Although, as its name implies, FMD is characterized by the development of lesions in the mouth and on the feet, the earliest clinical signs are those of a nonspecific infectious illness and include fever, dullness, inappetence, a fall in milk yield and the cessation of rumination. Because the disease is usually rapid in onset and development, these signs are superseded within a few hours by signs more obviously referable to the development of lesions. These include lameness, a disinclination to stand, salivation and other signs of discomfort in the mouth, such as smacking of the lips and grinding of the teeth. There is often a concomitant serous nasal discharge which becomes mucopurulent over the next two to three days.

The young of domestic species susceptible to FMD may die suddenly without premonitory signs, as a result of myocarditis (sometimes referred to as 'tiger-heart disease' because of the macroscopic appearance of the myocardium). In some animals myocardial lesions may only be discernible microscopically. This has been a feature of recent outbreaks in Europe.

Lesions in cattle are usually present in the mouth, particularly at the tip and on the dorsal surface of the tongue, and on all four feet. However, this is not invariable and lesions may be absent from the mouth or one or more feet.[86, 109]

Lesions in the mouth are first visible as small, blanched foci which may occur anywhere except on the ventral

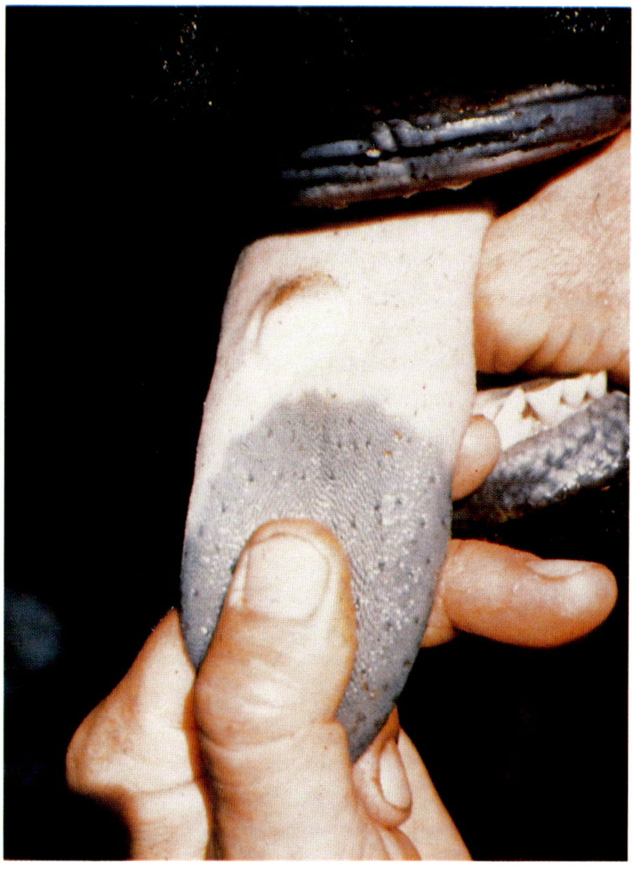

Figure 89.4 Vesicle on the tongue of an ox

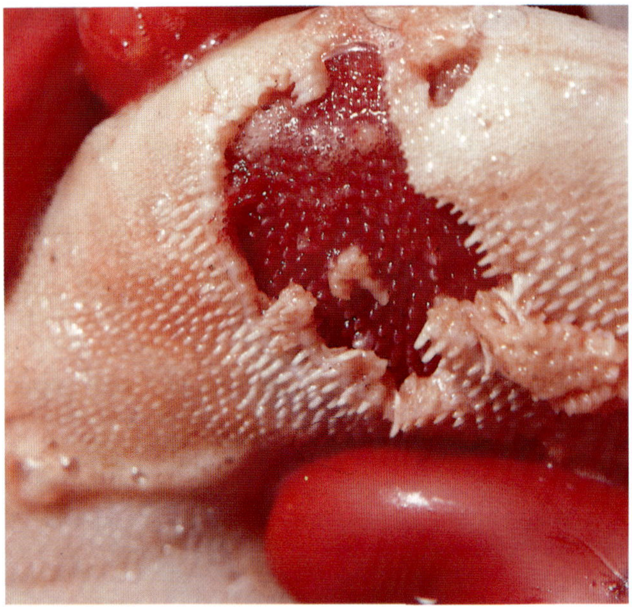

Figure 89.5 Ruptured vesicle on the tongue of an ox

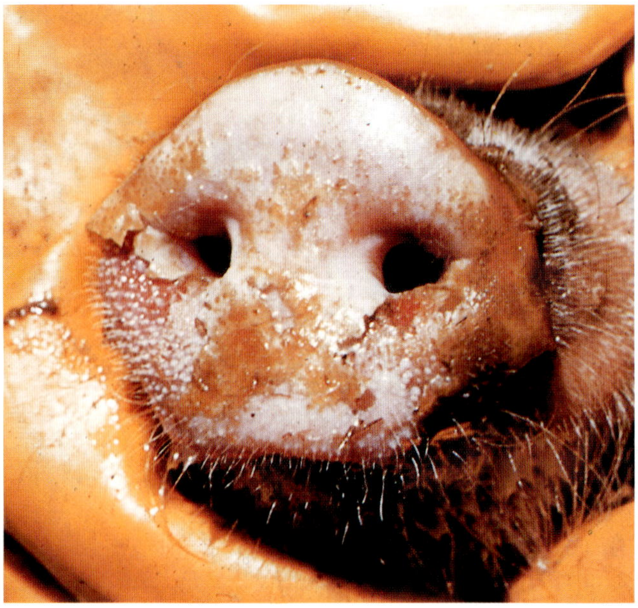

Figure 89.6 Erosions on the snout of a pig following rupture of vesicles

aspect of the tongue. These foci rapidly increase in size and develop into vesicles containing serous fluid **(Figure 89.4)** which rupture easily. For this reason unruptured vesicles are not often seen during the examination of field cases. In acute cases approximately circular erosions with shreds of epithelium adhering to the edges of the lesion are the common finding. Other than on the dorsal surface of the tongue, these lesions are usually less than 20 mm in diameter, but on the tongue they may be more than 60 mm in diameter. Rarely, the epithelium of a large part of the dorsal surface of the tongue desquamates during examination, leaving a raw and bleeding surface **(Figure 89.5)**.

Mouth lesions are less common and less pronounced in other species such as sheep and pigs[12, 104, 127, 173] and may proceed directly from epithelial necrosis to erosion without vesicle formation.[73, 104] In sheep and other small ruminants, lesions commonly occur on the dental pad, where they may be difficult to detect.

In pigs, lesions may occur on the snout **(Figure 89.6)** but in other species lesions on the muzzle are rare, although they have been described in the mucous membrane of the nostrils and even in the conjunctiva of cattle.[127]

In all species foot lesions develop in the interdigital space **(Figure 89.7)**, at the bulbs of the heel and around the coronet.[109] In cattle, lesions predominate at the two former sites, while coronary band lesions are more common in smaller species. In severe cases, lesions are usually present at all three sites and may be so severe that the horn of the hoof is lost completely. Pigs often develop lesions at the base of the supernumary digits.

The skin covering intact or recently ruptured vesicles is pale and in the course of the one or two days following vesicle development becomes necrotic and friable **(Figure 89.8)**. In less severe cases, fluid liberated from small vesicles becomes mixed with soil particles to form brown scabs or crusts.

Secondary bacterial infection of foot lesions occurs frequently, particularly where animals are kept in muddy, unhygienic conditions. The severity of this varies, but it may result in suppuration extending into the joints, tendon sheaths and even the bones of the foot, with crippling consequences.

Healing of mouth lesions is far more rapid than is the case with foot lesions. In cattle, mouth lesions that are more than one or two weeks old are often only discernible as circumscribed areas with poorly developed papillae **(Figure 89.9)**, and can be easily missed. By contrast, foot lesions at two weeks are usually still clearly visible, being covered by necrotic epithelium or scabs, or they may occur as raw areas where the epithelium or scabs have been brushed off.

Particularly on the bulbs of the heel in cattle, but also elsewhere along the coronet, the break in continuity between skin and the horn of the hoof becomes more marked in severe cases after seven to ten days and the horn begins to separate from the underlying tissues. As new horn grows down inside the old it may appear as if the animal is wearing 'slippers'. The end result is a fault in the hoof which is a valuable aid in ageing the lesion as it grows down **(Figure 89.10)**. In pigs, the rate of growth has been estimated at 1 mm/week beginning one week after the development of the lesion — the number of millimetres of new horn growth plus one will give the age of the lesion in weeks.[125]

Cows may develop vesicles on the teats and udder, and the udder may be turgid and hard as a result of viral-induced mastitis, which is frequently complicated by secondary infections.[34] Milk production is often lost for

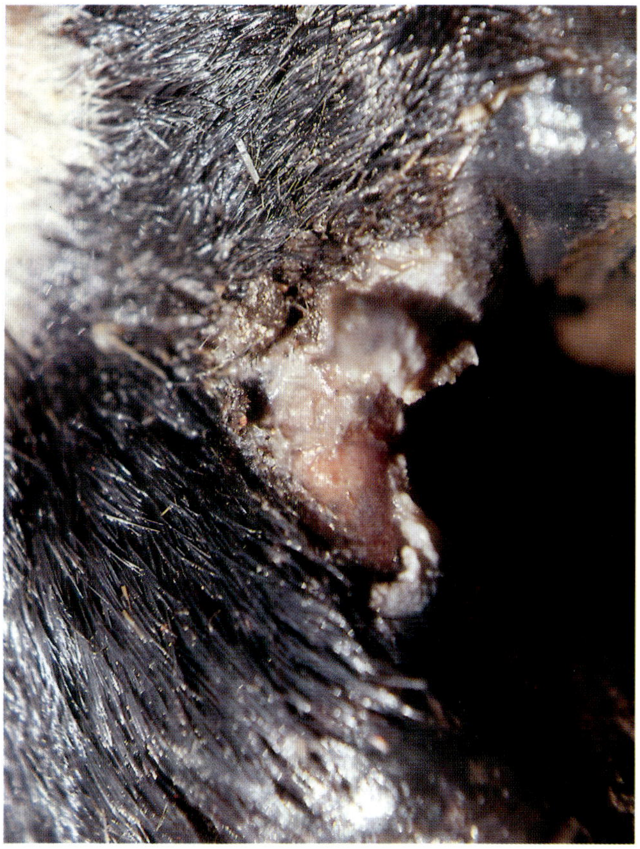

Figure 89.7 Interdigital erosion following rupture of a vesicle

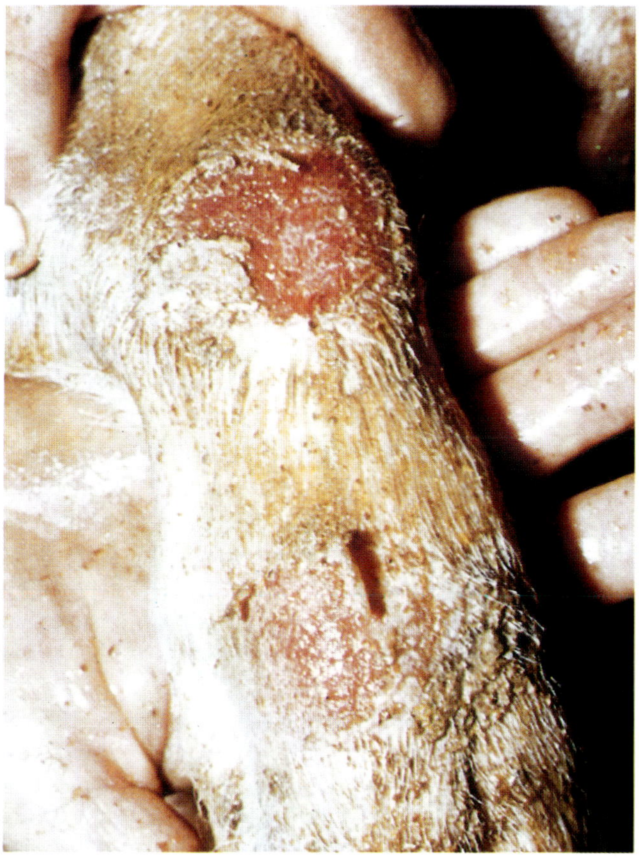

Figure 89.8 Erosive dermatitis affecting the carpal and metacarpal skin of a pig

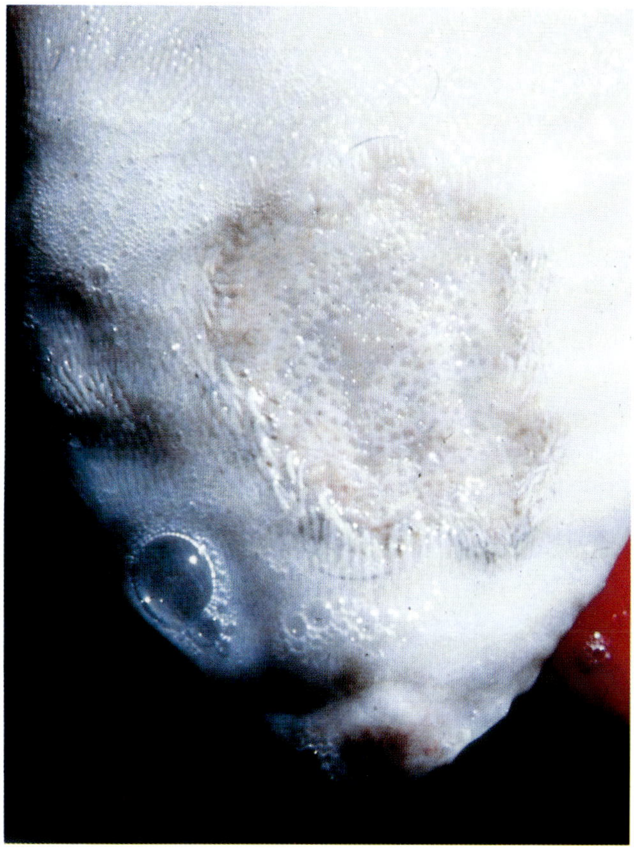

Figure 89.9 Healing lesion on the dorsal surface of the tongue of an ox

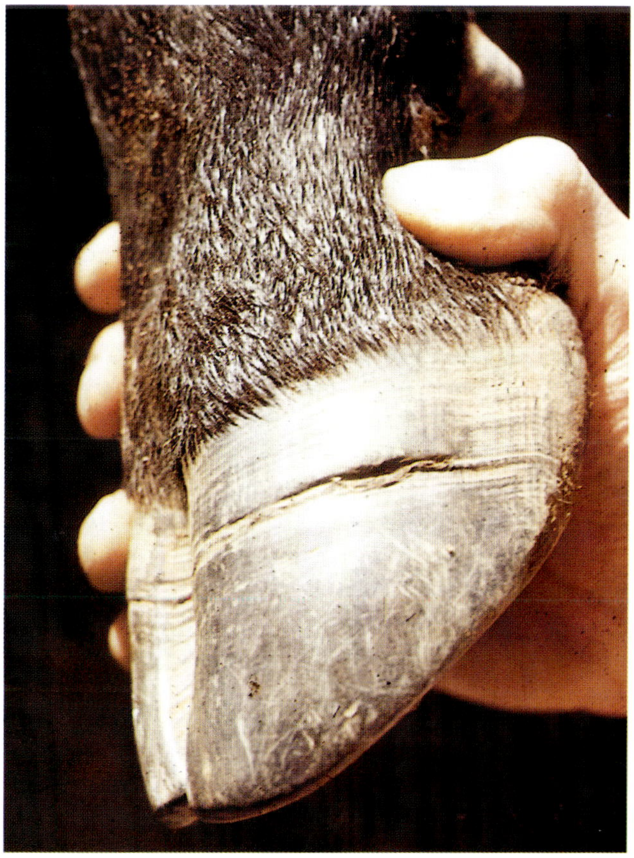

Figure 89.10 Fault in the hoof of an ox that has recovered from foot-and-mouth disease

the remainder of the lactation and FMD in a dairy herd may result in a reduction of more than 25 per cent of milk production over a period of several months.[88]

On rare occasions cows may abort, while a syndrome in cattle characterized by dyspnoea, long, rough coat and poor condition may occur in isolated individuals six to eight weeks after the vesicles have healed.[60, 104]

A booklet of quality photographs of FMD lesions in cattle, sheep, goats and pigs was published in Britain in 1986.[8]

Diagnosis

The ability to diagnose FMD rapidly and accurately is a prerequisite for efficient animal production as well as for the support of export-oriented agricultural economies in large parts of the world, including countries where FMD does not occur.

Because of the renowned ability of FMD virus to spread rapidly, the handling of this virus, including procedures involved in diagnosis, is restricted to high-security laboratories.

The diagnosis of FMD in domestic animals is dependent upon clinical assessment, identification of FMD virus or viral antigens in the early stages of infection, and serology if the condition has been in progress for longer than two weeks. The diagnosis of persistently infected or carrier animals is effected by the isolation of virus from oesophago-pharyngeal secretions, although the use of nucleic acid probes for this purpose is a possibility for the near future.[188]

Since both the fluid contained in and the epithelium covering vesicles usually contain high concentrations of FMD virus ($>10^{6,0}$ infectious doses/ml), these are the specimens of choice in acute cases of FMD. The fluid is easily aspirated from unruptured vesicles using a needle and syringe, while epithelial fragments may simply be cut free from the edges of lesions with scissors. Epithelial specimens from mouth and foot lesions contain detectable quantities of live virus for four and seven days respectively after the appearance of the lesions.[166]

It is essential to add a transport medium buffered between pH 7 and 8 to specimens collected for laboratory examination, to prevent dessication and changes in pH during transport. Phosphate-buffered saline (PBS), at pH 7,4 is ideal, and is the medium usually recommended. The molarity of such solutions is not as important as the pH, but should be close to normal.

If suspect specimens can be kept cool (4–10 °C) and reach a suitable laboratory within about 12 hours, no further preservative is needed. If this cannot be achieved, an equal volume of glycerol and antibiotics may be added to the PBS in which epithelial specimens are suspended, to prevent putrefaction.[141] Glycerol should not be added to specimens of vesicular fluid because it is toxic to cell cultures. There is no practical way to separate vesicular fluid from the glycerol except by dilution, which could hamper the isolation of virus present in small quantities. Glycerol can be removed from epithelial specimens by washing in PBS. Detailed instructions for the collection, packaging, and dispatch of FMD specimens have been published.[141] The collection of probang specimens from animals persistently infected with FMD virus has likewise been described.[124]

Until recently, and in some laboratories it is still the case, the rapid identification and typing of FMD viruses was generally done by microplate complement fixation (CF) tests which incorporate short fixation times. Thus, if good specimens from vesicular lesions are available, typing can be achieved in less than a day.[23] In those specimens where direct typing by CF is not possible, such as when the viral antigens are present in quantities too low for detection or because of the anticomplementary activity of the specimen, it is necessary to culture the virus before repeating the CF test using the cell culture fluid. Fortunately, FMD viruses usually grow quickly and produce rapid cytopathic effects in a wide variety of cell cultures, the most commonly used being primary or secondary calf thyroid cells and IB-RS-2 or BHK21 cell lines. Cell culture supernatants often contain sufficient virus to enable CF typing within 24 hours of cell culture inoculation.[130, 212]

Where virus isolation of minimal quantities of FMD virus is necessary, such as in the detection of virus in oesophago-pharyngeal secretions of carrier animals, the culture system of choice is primary calf thyroid cells, as this is the most sensitive system known.[212]

Recently, enzyme-linked immunosorbent assay (ELISA) has been applied to FMD virus typing, and is finding increasing favour because it is more sensitive than CF while also being able to provide rapid results.[90, 186, 236]

In cases where fresh epithelial specimens are not available, blood and, particularly, saliva which contain high concentrations of FMD virus in acute cases **(Table 89.4)** are useful specimens. Blood, collected in anticoagulant or merely allowed to clot to provide serum, should be submitted chilled. Saliva should also be submitted chilled and be diluted approximately 1:10 in PBS to lower the pH (in the case of ruminants) and to dilute antiviral factors. In practice, if saliva is not easily obtainable, the mouth of the animal can be rinsed with PBS and the recovered fluid submitted for laboratory examination.

It is imperative that measures should be taken during the collection and dispatch of specimens to ensure that the process itself does not disseminate infective virus. Instruments and other equipment, the outer surfaces of specimen containers, clothing and exposed skin surfaces of the people involved should be thoroughly decontaminated. For this purpose a 4 per cent solution of sodium carbonate (washing soda) in cold water is ideal. However, any solution which ensures a pH of less than three or greater than 11 is suitable. The specimens must also be packed in such a manner that no virus leakage is possible, even if the parcel were to be mishandled. Details of how to pack specimens are available elsewhere.[143]

Serum antibody to FMD viruses is conventionally measured by microplate virus neutralization (VN)[102] or, increasingly, by ELISA techniques.[112–114] The latter has the advantages of offering economy of consumables, providing results which are more reproducible, and of being amenable to large-scale application.

Distinction between antibody to FMD viruses that has developed as a result of infection and that which develops following immunization presents a problem. Since all FMD vaccines currently in use are inactivated, antibody to the viral infection-associated (viral polymerase) antigen (VIA) has been suggested as being useful for this purpose — because vaccine virus does not replicate it was held that antibodies directed against VIA would only be detectable following active infection and not immunization.[157] However, it has since transpired that animals which have been vaccinated, particularly if vaccinated repeatedly, may develop antibody to VIA, presumably because this protein is present in vaccine-culture harvests.[61, 89]

In addition to detecting the presence of FMD virus it is usually essential to determine the origin of the virus involved. Hence, once the virus is typed it is important to establish the relationship of this virus to vaccine strains and others known to have been previously present in the vicinity. This can be done by conventional subtyping or by newer techniques such as one- or two-dimensional electrophoresis of viral RNA fragments generated by ribonuclease T1 treatment (T1 mapping),[6, 148] iso-electric focusing of viral structural proteins[140] or nucleotide sequencing of viral RNA.[18] The latter technique is becoming increasingly popular **(Figure 89.2)**.

Differential diagnosis

Vesicular stomatitis, swine vesicular disease and vesicular exanthema of pigs all produce lesions in cattle or pigs which are clinically indistinguishable from FMD.[45, 88] The definitive hosts of swine vesicular disease virus are either fish or sea lions (family Otariidae), so that pigs only become infected by contact with these animals or their tissues. None of these diseases has ever occurred in southern Africa.

Conditions which produce erosions or ulceration in the mouth or on the muzzle of cattle, goats, sheep or pigs and which need to be differentiated from FMD include bovine viral diarrhoea/mucosal disease, rinderpest, bluetongue, malignant catarrhal fever, lumpy skin disease, bovine papular stomatitis, infectious bovine rhinotracheitis and orf (contagious pustular dermatitis). None of these diseases except bluetongue and orf and, rarely, malignant catarrhal fever produce foot lesions.

Foot lesions caused by bacteria and fungi in animals housed in unhygienic, wet and crowded conditions, such as foot rot, may produce lesions that are difficult to differentiate from those of FMD which have progressed beyond the vesicle stage. The absence of mouth lesions in such cases usually obviates confusion with FMD.

Furocoumarins contained in celery and parsnips, particularly if infected with the fungus *Sclerotinia sclerotiorum*, and which interact with ultraviolet rays in sunlight, are capable of producing both snout and foot lesions in white-skinned pigs.[161, 162]

Control

Two separate but overlapping patterns of FMD incidence occur in southern Africa — (i) disease associated with the presence of buffalo and SAT-type viruses, and (ii) that which arises due to transhumance or other cross-border movement of livestock.[58] The latter situation frequently involves the A, O and C virus types, particularly in countries such as Angola, Malawi and Zambia. Control areas in southern Africa are therefore generally confined to regions where buffalo occur **(Figure 89.3)** and to international borders.[58, 177]

Control strategies in these localities are aimed at preventing the unrestrained movement of all susceptible animals and their products out of endemic areas, and the immunization of cattle and other domestic ruminants which occur either in or adjacent to these areas.

Separation of endemic and FMD-free areas is effected by the use of both cattle and game fences and by movement control. Thus the boundaries of the Kruger National Park as well as the entire northern border of South Africa are game-fenced to prevent the migration of game and domestic animals. Similarly, in Zimbabwe fences isolate buffalo and associated cattle populations in the north-western and south-eastern parts of the country.[219] In Botswana cattle fences have been used extensively to compartmentalize the country,[153] and a game fence separates the large buffalo populations of the Okavango Delta from domestic ruminants to the south and east.

The use of fencing for FMD control is controversial.[219] Apart from its effect on wild animal migration, especially during droughts, a major criticism has been that fences are unlikely to stop an infection that can be conveyed on air currents. It must be borne in mind, however, that long-distance airborne transmission has never been documented or even suspected in southern Africa. Experimental and field observations support the contention that fences are effective in preventing the spread of FMD.[82, 86, 102, 149]

Movement control of domestic animals is only effective if it can be enforced and monitored. Therefore, the use of legally binding movement permits, the maintenance of accurate census figures, and adequate quarantine and inspection prior to movement out of endemic areas are essential. Movement permits not only regulate animal movement, but also allow a record to be kept which, in the event of an outbreak, can be used to trace the movement of potentially infected animals.

Domestic animals in or adjacent to endemic areas should be regularly inspected so that outbreaks which occur can be rapidly detected and the necessary measures taken to control spread. To this end, cattle 'behind the red line' in South Africa are inspected every seven days, while those in the 'second and third zones' are inspected at 14- and 28-day intervals respectively.

Regular immunization aimed at maintaining a high degree of herd immunity is an essential feature of FMD control in southern Africa. There are, however, logistical problems in this respect because the vaccines in current use do not provide a long-lasting immunity and require continuous refrigeration up to the time of inoculation. In addition it is necessary to ensure that the virus strains incorporated into the vaccine will immunize adequately against the virus strains in circulation in the field. In relation to herd immunity the interplay between the duration of immunity and challenge-virus subtype has been graphically illustrated.[170–172] Essentially this implies that animals whose immunity is starting to wane, some three to four months after immunization, may be susceptible to challenge with virus subtypes distantly related to those incorporated into the vaccine, while still being immune to subtypes closely related to the vaccine strain.

Establishing which vaccine strains are appropriate to southern African countries is problematic. Unlike most other regions, where it is relatively easy to establish the immunological characteristics of viruses in circulation because they only occur in farm animals, in southern Africa they are often confined to buffalo populations. This makes obtaining representative virus strains difficult and dangerous. However, other approaches are also possible. For example, some strains appear to have an inherently wider immunogenicity than others and therefore may generate good 'broad-spectrum' responses.[25, 30, 168] Alternatively, mixing different subtypes in a vaccine sometimes results in synergism and a consequent broadening of the immune response.[84]

Currently all the FMD vaccines in use in southern Africa consist of inactivated virus grown in cell or surviving-tongue-epithelium (Frenkel) cultures which are adsorbed onto alhydrogel (aluminium hydroxide). The latter and saponin constitute the adjuvant which potentiates the immune response. These vaccines have a shelf-life of one year, as long as they are stored between 4 and 10 °C.

International agreement[29] has laid down a minimum potency of three cattle-protective doses 50 (PD_{50}) for FMD vaccine, although it is recommended that in practice at least 6 PD_{50} should be attained.

Because FMD vaccines are inactivated they should ideally be administered as a primary and secondary dose two to eight weeks apart to establish basic immunity, with booster doses at four- or six-monthly intervals.[170] However, due to the practical difficulties of implementing this policy, most countries in southern Africa immunize all cattle (with the exception of calves under six months of age) in control areas every six months. Despite the fact that this practice will not produce optimal basic immunity, available evidence indicates that animals which have been inoculated repeatedly in this way develop an effective immunity which lasts at least six months. Whether the proportion of immunized animals and the population turnover in endemic areas are generally such that a significant proportion of the animal population is protected throughout the year is a moot point. Nevertheless, over the years this policy has proved to be generally effective.

The approach in other species such as sheep and goats is variable, with no known scientific basis. In South Africa, for example, these animals are only immunized annually at present. The poor response of goats to presently formulated vaccine[100] and the rapid population turnover in small stock leads one to wonder whether the level of herd immunity likely to be achieved by annual immunization is cost-effective.

Pigs are not immunized, mainly because they are not farmed in appreciable numbers in endemic areas in southern Africa. Pigs in any case respond poorly to vaccines formulated with alhydrogel — only oil-adjuvanted vaccines are effective in pigs[35] — and have a very rapid population turnover. Attaining satisfactory levels of herd immunity in pigs is consequently problematic.

In both cattle and pigs replication of virus in the oesophago-pharyngeal region may occur in immunized animals that are exposed to infection, even though they are clinically protected.[65, 80] For this reason, vaccinated animals may be a potential source of infection. It would appear, however, that only cattle within three weeks of primary inoculation are potentially capable of transmitting FMD.[80, 81] The position with regard to pigs is less certain.[65]

Considerable effort and expenditure are being directed towards producing improved vaccines for FMD and it appears likely that synthetic or genetically engineered vaccines will become available in the foreseeable future.[32, 38, 67, 142, 193]

The actual and potential problems confronting southern African countries where vaccines are either ineffective or impossible to administer regularly have been outlined.[150]

Outbreaks of FMD in any animal species outside endemic or declared FMD control areas require special procedures. The rapid identification and elimination of such foci of infection is of the utmost importance for countries with developed agricultural economies, and even more particularly if access to export markets is to be maintained. Even within endemic areas the general approach to the control of FMD outbreaks in domestic animals should follow the procedure set out below.

The first step in such an event is to confirm the clinical diagnosis by laboratory tests which include typing of the virus involved. A quarantine area should immediately be

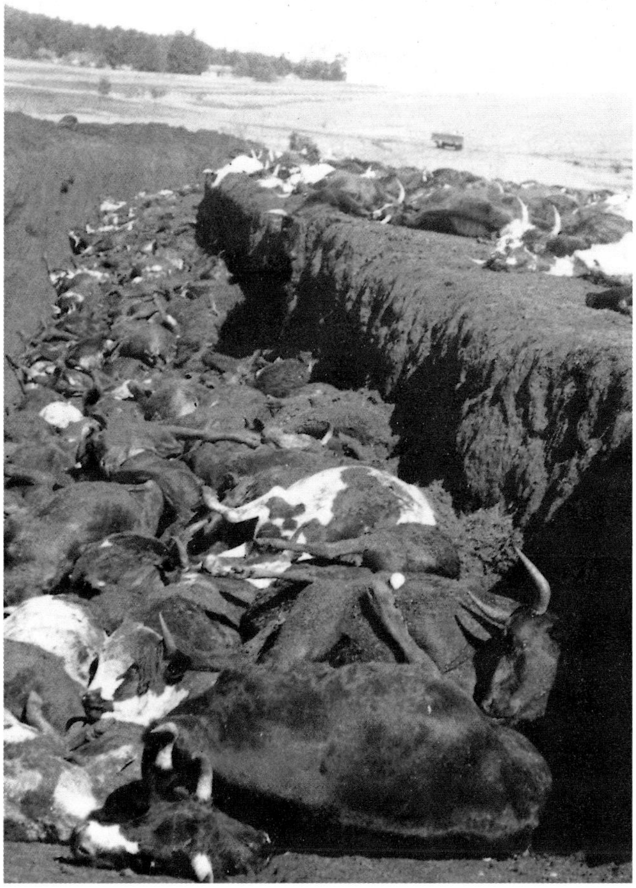

Figure 89.11 Slaughter and disposal of cattle infected with foot-and-mouth disease at Hectorspruit during the 1930s

declared and enforced around the affected area. In South Africa this is usually applied initially to a magisterial district but, if the situation later allows, this area may be reduced in size. In Europe such quarantine areas are often relatively small, and may be no more than about 10 km in diameter.

Thereafter it is important to establish the exact extent of spread by inspecting all herds within the quarantine area. It is important to ensure that inspectors do not themselves spread the infection. Thus, in South Africa, it is the policy to ensure strict separation of personnel working inside the affected area and those inspecting areas considered to be 'clean'. For this reason it is advisable that inspection should start at the periphery of the quarantined area and progress inwards towards the infection focus. Once the size of the outbreak has been ascertained, the extent of the quarantine area can be reassessed. However, continuing inspection both inside and outside the focus is essential in order to establish the clinical end-point and any subsequent transmission to previously uninfected localities.

In southern Africa it is traditional to erect around the infected area a cordon that makes use of natural physical barriers such as rivers, as well as fences which may have to be erected specifically for this purpose. It is necessary that the cordon be staffed along its entire length (not only at road entrances) to prevent unauthorized movement of people, animals and animal products in and out of the control area. In particularly dangerous localities a double cordon may be advisable.

Ideally, an animal-free zone outside the cordon, between infected and 'clean' areas, should be established to prevent contact between infected and non-infected animals. However, this is not always possible under the conditions which prevail in southern Africa.

Early in the eradication campaign a study of permits relating to animal movements into and out of the affected area before the imposition of control measures should be made. This might reveal the likely source of infection as well as possible movement of infected animals out of the affected area.

As soon as the extent of the infected focus has been established, immunization with vaccine containing appropriate virus strains should commence, both within the infection focus to immunize animals not already infected, and in the rest of the quarantine area. Different teams for the infected and 'clean' areas should be utilized for this purpose to ensure that vaccinators do not spread the infection. A second inoculation should be administered to all ruminants two or three weeks later, but pigs should only be immunized if oil-adjuvanted vaccines are available. Booster immunizations should be given to all animals every three months for the duration of the outbreak.

If no spread has occurred in the quarantine area within three months of the clinical end-point, the control measures may be lifted, preferably gradually. Precisely what should be allowed regarding the subsequent movement of potential carriers is a matter over which disagreement exists. Strictly speaking they are a potential source of infection for up to two years or perhaps even longer.

It is important that all the people involved in, and affected by, the control measures be fully informed as to what the rules are and why they are necessary. Unless the co-operation of these people can be gained, effective control is unlikely to be achieved.

Outside endemic areas, particularly where the focus of infection is small, it may be decided to 'slaughter-out' infected cattle, sheep and goats and susceptible animals in direct contact with them rather than to use cordons, quarantine and immunization to control spread of the infection. In such cases the approach is usually to shoot all the animals on the farm and to bury or burn the carcasses *in situ*. Some of the outbreaks in the 1930s in South Africa were controlled in this way **(Figure 89.11)**. Where carcasses are buried it is vital to ensure that the trench is sufficiently deep to prevent scavengers from digging the trench open, and also to cover the carcasses with washing soda to ensure that any flooding which may occur does not result in 'run-off' containing live virus. Because pigs are a potent source of infection and oil-adjuvanted vaccines are required to produce an adequate immune response in this species, the approach to the control of FMD outbreaks involving pigs is usually to 'slaughter-out' all the pigs in the infected area and those in direct contact with them. However, if large pig units containing many thousands of animals are involved, 'slaughter-out' (often also referred to as 'stamping-out') may be impossible for logistical reasons.

Whatever the FMD status of a country, it is essential to preclude the importation of FMD viruses — if only to make certain that 'foreign' virus types and subtypes are not introduced. It is therefore necessary to control and monitor the import of susceptible animals and their products and to ensure that all access routes into a country are covered — road, rail, air and sea. The proper testing and quarantining of all imported cloven-hoofed animals from potentially infected regions is absolutely essential. It is also important that waste from ships, aeroplanes and trains be decontaminated immediately and not used as swill for pigs.

References

1 **ABU ELZEIN, E.M.E. & CROWTHER, J.R., 1982.** Differentiation of foot-and-mouth disease virus strains using a competition enzyme-linked immunosorbent assay. *Journal of Virological Methods*, 3, 355–365.

2 **ACHARYA, R., FRY, E., STUART, D., FOX, D., ROWLANDS, D. & BROWN, F., 1989.** The three-dimensional structure of foot-and-mouth disease virus at 2.9A revolution. *Nature*, 337, 709–716.

3 **AMADORI, M. & MELEGARI, M., 1987.** Humoral and cellular parameters of experimental foot-and-mouth disease in heifers. *Journal of Veterinary Medicine*, B34, 480–488.

4 **ANDERSON, E.C., DOUGHTY, W.J. & ANDERSON, J., 1976.** The role of sheep and goats in the epizootiology of foot-and-mouth disease in Kenya. *Journal of Hygiene*, 76, 395–402.

5 **ANDERSON, E.C., DOUGHTY, W.J., ANDERSON, J. & PALING, R., 1979.** The pathogenesis of foot-and-mouth disease in the African buffalo (*Syncerus caffer*) and the role of this species in the epidemiology of the disease in Kenya. *Journal of Comparative Pathology*, 89, 541–549.

6 **ANDERSON, E.C., UNDERWOOD, B.O., BROWN, F. & NGICHABE, C.K., 1985.** Variation in foot-and-mouth disease virus isolates in Kenya: An examination of field isolates by T1 oligonucleotide fingerprinting. *Veterinary Microbiology*, 10, 409–423.

7 **ANON., 1972–86,** *FAO-WHO-OIE Animal Health Year Books*. BELLVER-GALLENT, M., (ed.). International Office of Epizootics, Food and Agriculture Organization of the United Nations, World Health Organization.

8 **ANON., 1986.** *Foot and Mouth Disease: Ageing of Lesions*. London: HMSO Publications Centre.

9 **ANON., 1986.** *Investigation on the Possible Effect of Electrical Stimulation on pH and Survival of Foot-and-mouth Disease Virus in Meat and Offals from Experimentally Infected Animals*. Agriculture, Report EUR 10048 en. Luxembourg: Commission of the European Communities.

10 **ANON., 1987.** Directorate of Animal Health, Department of Agricultural Economy, South Africa. Unpublished data.

11 **ANON., 1988.** Information leaflet distributed by the Direçao Nacional de Pecuária, Ministério da Agricultura, Republica Popular de Moçambique.

12 **BACHRACH, H.L., 1968.** Foot-and-mouth disease. *Annual Review of Microbiology*, 22, 201–244.

13 **BACHRACH, H.L., 1977.** Foot-and-mouth disease virus: Properties, molecular biology and immunogenicity. In: ROMBERGER, J.A., (ed.). *Beltsville Symposia in Agricultural Research. I. Virology in Agriculture*. Montclair: Allanheld, Osmun & Co.

14 **BACHRACH, H.L., BREESE, S.S., CALLIS, J.J., HESS, W.R. & PATTY, R.E., 1957.** Inactivation of foot-and-mouth disease virus by pH and temperature changes and by formaldehyde. *Proceedings of the Society of Experimental Biology and Medicine*, 95, 147–152.

15 **BACHRACH, H.L. MOORE, D.M., McKERCHER, P.D. & POLATNICK, J., 1975.** Immune and antibody responses to an isolated capsid protein of foot and mouth disease virus. *Journal of Immunology*, 115, 1635–1641.

16 **BACHRACH, H.L., TRAUTMAN, R. & BREESE, S.S., 1964.** Chemical and physical properties of virtually pure foot-and-mouth disease virus. *American Journal of Veterinary Research*, 25, 333–342.

17 **BARLOW, D.F., 1972.** The aerosol stability of a strain of foot-and-mouth disease virus and the effects on its stability of precipitation with ammonium sulphate or other chemicals. *General Virology*, 15, 17–24.

18 **BECK, E. & STROHMAIER, K., 1986.** Subtyping of European FMDV outbreak strains by nucleotide sequence determination. Paper presented at the 17th Conference of the O.I.E. Foot-and-mouth Disease Commission, Paris, 1–3 October, 1986.

19 **BEKKER, J.G., DE KOCK, G. & QUINLAN, J.B., 1934.** The occurrence and identification of bluetongue in cattle and the so-called pseudo-foot-and-mouth disease in South Africa. *Onderstepoort Journal of Veterinary Research*, 2, 393–507.

20 **BELSHAM, G.J. & BOSTOCK, C.J., 1988.** Studies on the infectivity of foot-and-mouth disease virus RNA using microinjection. *Journal of General Virology*, 69, 265–274.

21 **BENGIS, R.G., THOMSON, G.R., HEDGER, R.S., DE VOS, V. & PINI, A., 1986.** Foot-and-mouth disease and the African buffalo (*Syncerus caffer*). I. Carriers as a source of infection for cattle. *Onderstepoort Journal of Veterinary Research*, 53, 69–73.

22 **BEVAN, L.E.W., 1932.** Foot-and-mouth disease in Southern Rhodesia and a method of emergency inoculation. *Transactions of the Royal Society of Tropical Medicine and Hygiene*, 26, 89–93.

23 **BLACKBURN, N.K., 1982.** Foot-and-mouth disease typing and serology in Zimbabwe. *Tropical Animal Health and Production*, 14, 101–103.

24 **BLACKWELL, J.H., 1980.** Internationalism and the survival of foot-and-mouth disease in cattle and food products. *Journal of Dairy Science*, 63, 1019–1030.

25 **BLACKWELL, J.H., 1984.** Foreign animal disease agent survival in animal products: Present developments. *Journal of the American Veterinary Association*, 184, 674–679.

26 **BLACKWELL, J.H., McKERCHER, P.D., KOSIKOWSKI, F.V., CARMICHAEL, L.E. & GOREWIT, R.C., 1982.** Concentration of foot-and-mouth disease virus in milk of cows infected under simulated field conditions. *Journal of Dairy Science*, 65, 1624–1631.

27 **BLACKWELL, J.H., McKERCHER, P.D., KOSIKOWSKI, F.V., CARMICHAEL, L.E. & GOREWIT, R.C., 1983.** Histological and histochemical characterisation of mammary gland tissue of cows infected with foot-and-mouth disease by contact exposure. *Research in Veterinary Science*, 35, 106–113.

28 **BLACKWELL, J.H., WOOL, S. & KOSIKOWSKI, F.V., 1981.** Vesicular exocytosis of foot-and-mouth disease virus from mammary gland secretory epithelium of infected cows.

Journal of General Virology, 56, 207–212.

29 **BOLDRINI, G.M., 1978.** Vaccination and the control of foot-and-mouth disease. *The Veterinary Record*, 102, 194–198.

30 **BOLWELL, C., PARRY, N.R., ROWLANDS, D.J., BROWN, F. & OULDRIDGE, E., 1986.** Foot-and-mouth disease virus variants with broad and narrow antigenic spectra. In: BROWN, F., (ed.). *New Approaches to Immunization.* Cold Spring Harbour Laboratory.

31 **BOSCH, W., 1990.** Veterinary Research Institute, Onderstepoort, South Africa. Unpublished data.

32 **BROEKHUIJSEN, M.P., VAN RIJN, J.A.M., BLOM, A.J.M., PONWELS, P.H., ENGER-VALK, B.E., BROWN, F. & FRANCIS, J.M., 1987.** Fusion proteins with multiple copies of the major antigenic determinant of foot-and-mouth disease virus protect both natural and laboratory animals. *Journal of General Virology*, 68, 3137–3143.

33 **BROOKSBY, J.B., 1950.** Strains of the virus of foot-and-mouth disease showing natural adaption to swine. *Journal of Hygiene*, 47, 184–195.

34 **BROOKSBY, J.B., 1982.** Portraits of viruses: Foot-and-mouth disease virus. *Intervirology*, 18, 1–23.

35 **BROWN, F., 1972.** Comments on immunology of foot-and-mouth disease in swine. *Journal of the American Veterinary Association*, 160, 526–527.

36 **BROWN, F., 1985.** Antigenic structure of foot-and-mouth disease virus. In: VAN REGENMORTEL, M.H.V. & NEURATH, A.R., (eds). *Immunochemistry of Viruses. The Basis for Serodiagnosis and Vaccines.* Elsevier Scientific Publishers B.V. (Biomedical Division).

37 **BROWN, F., 1986.** Foot-and-mouth disease: One of the remaining great plagues. *Proceedings of the Royal Society*, London, B229, 215–226.

38 **BROWN, F., 1988.** Use of peptides for immunization against foot-and-mouth disease. *Vaccine*, 6, 180–182.

39 **BROWN, F. & WILD, T.F., 1966.** The effect of heat on the structure of foot-and-mouth disease virus and the viral ribonucleic acid. *Biochemica et Biophysica Acta*, 119, 301–308.

40 **BURBURY, Y.M., 1928.** VII. Survival of foot-and-mouth disease virus when dried upon various materials. *Third Progress Report of the Foot-and-mouth Disease Research Committee.* London: His Majesty's Stationery Office.

41 **BURROWS, R., 1966.** Studies on the carrier state of cattle exposed to foot-and-mouth disease virus. *Journal of Hygiene*, 64, 81–90.

42 **BURROWS, R., 1968.** Excretion of foot-and-mouth disease virus prior to the development of lesions. *The Veterinary Record*, 82, 387–388.

43 **BURROWS, R., MANN, J.A., GARLAND, A.J.M., GRIEG, A. & GOODRIDGE, D., 1981.** The pathogenesis of natural and simulated natural foot-and-mouth disease infection in cattle. *Journal of Comparative Pathology*, 91, 599–609.

44 **BURROWS, R., MANN, J.A., GRIEG, A., CHAPMAN, W.G. & GOODRIDGE, D., 1971.** The growth and persistence of foot-and-mouth disease virus in the bovine mammary gland. *Journal of Hygiene*, 69, 307–321.

45 **CALLIS, J.J., 1984.** Foot-and-mouth disease. *In: Foreign Animal Diseases: Their Prevention, Diagnosis and Control.* Richmond, Viurginia: Committee on Foreign Animal Diseases of the United States Animal Health Association.

46 **CARTWRIGHT, B., CHAPMAN, W.G. & SHARPE, R.T., 1982.** Stimulation of heterotypic antigens of foot-and-mouth disease virus antibodies in vaccinated cattle. *Research in Veterinary Science*, 32, 338–342.

47 **CHOW, M., NEWMAN, J.F.E., FILMAN, D., HOGLE, J.M., ROWLANDS, D.J. & BROWN, F., 1987.** Myristylation of picornavirus capsid protein VP4 and its structural significance. *Nature*, 327, 482–486.

48 **CONDY, J.B., 1979.** A history of foot and mouth disease in Rhodesia. *Rhodesian Veterinary Journal*, 10, 2–10.

49 **CONDY, J.B. & HEDGER, R.S., 1974.** The survival of foot-and-mouth disease virus in African buffalo with non-transferance of infection to domestic cattle. *Research in Veterinary Science*, 16, 182–185.

50 **CONDY, J.B. & HEDGER, R.S., 1978.** Experiences in the establishment of a herd of foot-and-mouth disease-free African buffalo (*Syncerus caffer*). *South African Journal of Wildlife Research*, 8, 87–89.

51 **CONDY, J.B., HEDGER, R.S., HAMBLIN, C. & BARNETT, I.T.R., 1985.** The duration of the foot-and-mouth disease virus carrier state in African buffalo (i) in the individual animal and (ii) in a free-living herd. *Comparative Immunology, Microbiology and Infectious Diseases*, 8, 257–265.

52 **CONDY, J.B., HERNIMAN, K.A.J. & HEDGER, R.S., 1969.** Foot-and-mouth disease in wildlife in Rhodesia and other African territories. *Journal of Comparative Pathology*, 79, 27–31.

53 **COTTRAL, G.E., 1969.** Persistence of foot-and-mouth disease virus in animals, their products and the environment. *Bulletin de l'Office International des Épizooties*, 71, 549–568.

54 **COTTRAL, G.E., COX, B.F. & BALDWIN, D.E., 1960.** The survival of foot-and-mouth disease virus in cured and uncured meat. *American Journal of Veterinary Research*, 21, 288–297.

55 **CROWTHER, J.R., 1977.** Examination of differences between foot-and-mouth disease virus strains using a radio-immunoassay technique. *Developments in Biological Standardization*, 35, 185–193.

56 **CROWTHER, J.R., 1978.** Subtyping of FMD virus. New Approaches. *Bulletin de l'Office International des Épizooties*, 89, 831–850.

57 **CUMMING, R.G., 1850.** *Five Years of a Humbert's Life in South Africa.* Vol. II. London: Murray.

58 **DABORN, C.J., 1982.** Foot-and-mouth disease control in the Songwe Valley, Malawi — a review. *Tropical Animal Health and Production*, 14, 185–188.

59 **DAWE, P.S., 1978.** Seasonal foot and mouth disease and its control in Malawi. *British Veterinary Journal*, 134, 249–257.

60 **DAWE, P.S., 1987–9.** Veterinary Research Institute, Harare, Zimbabwe. Personal communication.

61 **DAWE, P.S. & PINTO, A.A., 1978.** Antibody responses to type-specific and 'virus-infection-associated' antigens in cattle vaccinated with inactivated polyvalent foot-and-mouth disease virus in North Malawi. *British Veterinary Journal*, 134, 504–511.

62 **DE KOCK, G., 1938.** Wild animals as carriers of infection. *South African Medical Journal*, 1–15.

63 **DE KOCK, G., 1946.** Problems of game conservation in southern Africa. *South African Journal of Science*, 62, 162–171.

64 **DE LA TORRE, J.C., MARTINEZ-SALAS, E., DIEZ, J., VILLAVERDE, F., GEBAUER, F., ROCHA, E., DAVILA, M. & DOMINGO, E., 1980.** Co-evolution of cells and viruses in a persistent infection of foot-and-mouth disease virus in cell culture. *Journal of Virology*, 62, 2050–2058.

65 **DE LEEUW, P.W., TIESSINK, J.W.A. & VAN BEKKUM, J.G., 1979.** The challenge of vaccinated pigs with foot-and-mouth disease virus. *Zentralblatt für Veterinärmedizin*, Reihe B, 26, 98–109.

66 **DE LEEUW, P.W., VAN BEKKUM, J.G. & TIESSINK, J.W.A., 1978.** Excretion of foot-and-mouth disease virus in oesophageal-pharyngeal fluid and milk of cattle after intranasal infection. *Journal of Hygiene*, 81, 415–425.

67 **DEVANEY, M.A., 1988.** New approaches to animal vaccines utilizing genetic engineering. *Critical Reviews in Microbiology*, 15, 269–295.

68 **DOEL, T.R. & BACCARINI, P.J., 1981.** Thermal stability of foot-and-mouth disease virus. *Archives of Virology*, 70, 21–32.

69 **DOMINGO, E. & HOLLAND, J.J., 1988.** High error rates, population equilibrium and evolution of RNA replication systems. *In*: DOMINGO, E., HOLLAND, J.J. & AHLQUIST, P., (eds). *RNA Genetics*, Vol. III. Boca Raton, Florida: CRC Press, Inc.

70 **DONALDSON, A.I., 1972.** Influence of relative humidity on the aerosol stability of different strains of foot-and-mouth disease virus suspended in saliva. *Journal of General Virology*, 15, 25–33.

71 **DONALDSON, A.I., 1979.** Airborne foot-and-mouth disease. *The Veterinary Bulletin*, 49, 653–659.

72 **DONALDSON, A.I., 1983.** Quantitative data on airborne foot-and-mouth disease virus: Its production, carriage and deposition. *Philosophical Transactions of the Royal Society, London*, B302, 529–534.

73 **DONALDSON, A.I., 1986–8.** Institute for Animal Health, Purbright, Surrey. Personal communications.

74 **DONALDSON, A.I. & FERRIS, N.P., 1975.** The survival of foot-and-mouth disease virus in open-air conditions. *Journal of Hygiene*, 74, 409–416.

75 **DONALDSON, A.I. & FERRIS, N.P., 1976.** The survival of some airborne animal viruses in relation to relative humidity. *Veterinary Microbiology*, 1, 413–420.

76 **DONALDSON, A.I. & FERRIS, N.P., 1978.** The influence of inhibitors and antibody on the airborne survival of foot-and-mouth disease virus. *Proceedings of the First International Conference on Aerobiology*. Berlin: Schmidt Verlag.

77 **DONALDSON, A.I. & FERRIS, N.P., 1980.** Sites of release of airborne foot-and-mouth disease from infected pigs. *Research in Veterinary Science*, 29, 315–319.

78 **DONALDSON, A.I., FERRIS, N.P. & WELLS, G.A.H., 1984.** Experimental foot-and-mouth disease in fattening pigs, sows and piglets in relation to outbreaks in the field. *The Veterinary Record*, 115, 509–512.

79 **DONALDSON, A.I., GARLAND, A.J.M., FERRIS, N.P. & COLLEN, T., 1981.** The 1975 foot-and-mouth disease epidemic in Malta. I. Experimental studies with the causal virus strain O1 Malta. *British Veterinary Journal*, 137, 300–307.

80 **DONALDSON, A.I., GIBSON, C.F., OLIVER, R., HAMBLIN, C. & KITCHING, R.P., 1987.** Infection of cattle by airborne foot-and-mouth disease virus: Minimal doses with O1 and SAT-2 strains. *Research in Veterinary Science*, 43, 339–346.

81 **DONALDSON, A.I. & KITCHING, R.P., 1989.** Transmission of foot-and-mouth disease by vaccinated cattle following natural challenge. *Research in Veterinary Science*, 46, 9–14.

82 **DU TOIT, P.J., 1932.** Foot-and-mouth disease in Southern Rhodesia. *Journal of the South African Veterinary Medical Association*, 3, 26–37.

83 **EISNER, R.J. & McVICAR, J.N., 1980.** Foot-and-mouth disease virus on wool of infected sheep. *Bulletin de l'Office International des Épizooties*, 92, 29–36.

84 **ESTERHUYSEN, J.J., THOMSON, G.R., ASHFORD, W.A., LENTZ, D.W., GAINARU, M.D., SAYER, A.J., MEREDITH, C.D., VAN RENSBURG, D.J. & PINI, A., 1988.** The suitability of a rolled BHK21 monolayer system for the production of vaccines against the SAT types of foot-and-mouth disease virus. 1. Adaptation of virus isolates to the system, immunogen yields achieved and assessment of serotype cross-reactivity. *Onderstepoort Journal of Veterinary Research*, 55, 77–84.

85 **ESTERHUYSEN, J.J., THOMSON, G.R., FLAMMAND, J.R.B. & BENGIS, R.G., 1985.** Buffalo in the northern Natal game parks show no serological evidence of infection with foot-and-mouth disease. *Onderstepoort Journal of Veterinary Research*, 52, 63–66.

86 **FALCONER, J., 1972.** The epizootiology and control of foot-and-mouth disease in Botswana. *The Veterinary Record*, 91, 354–359.

87 **FALCONER, J. & CHILD, G., 1975.** A survey of foot-and-mouth disease in wildlife in Botswana. *Mammalia*, 39, 518–520.

88 **FENNER, F., BACHMANN, P.A., GIBBS, E.P.J., MURPHY, F.A., STUDDART, M.J. & WHITE, D.O., 1987.** *Veterinary Virology*. Orlando, New York, London, Sydney, Tokyo, Toronto: Academic Press Inc.

89 **FERNANDEZ, A.A., DE MELLO, P.A., GOMES, I. & ROSENBERG, F., 1975.** The use of virus-infection-associated antigen (VIA) in the detection of cattle exposed to foot-and-mouth disease virus. *Bulletin Centro Panamericano Fiebre Aftosa*, 17&18, 17–22.

90 **FERRIS, N.P. & DAWSON, M., 1988.** Routine application of enzyme-linked immunosorbent assay in comparison with complement fixation for the diagnosis of foot-and-mouth and swine vesicular diseases. *Veterinary Microbiology*, 16, 201–209.

91 **FOGEDBY, E.G., MALINQUIST, W.A., OSTEEN, O.L. & JOHNSON, M.L., 1960.** Airborne transmission of foot-and-mouth disease virus. *Nordisk Veterinaermedicin*, 12, 490–498.

92 **FORSS, S., STREBEL, K., BECK, E. & SCHALLER, H., 1984.** Nucleotide sequence and genome organisation of foot-and-mouth disease virus. *Nucleic Acids Research*, 12, 6587–6601.

93 **FRANCIS, M.J., 1986.** The humoral immune response of young animals to foot-and-mouth disease vaccination. *Foot and Mouth Disease Bulletin*, 23, 1–44. Purbright: Coopers Animal Health Ltd.

94 **FRANCIS, M.J. & BLACK, L., 1983.** Antibody response in nasal fluid and serum following foot-and-mouth disease infection or vaccination. *Journal of Hygiene*, 91, 329–334.

95 **FRANCIS, M.J. & BLACK, L., 1984.** The effect of vaccination regimen on the transfer of foot and mouth disease antibodies from the sow to her piglets. *Journal of Hygiene*, 93, 123–131.

96 **FRANCIS, M.J. & BLACK, L., 1986.** Response of young pigs to foot-and-mouth disease oil-emulsion vaccine in the presence and absence of maternally derived neutralizing antibodies. *Research in Veterinary Science*, 41, 33–39.

97 **FRANCIS, M.J., HASTINGS, G.Z., SYRED, A.D., McGINN, B., BROWN, F. & ROWLANDS, D.J., 1987.** Non-responsiveness to a foot-and-mouth disease virus peptide overcome by addition of foreign helper T-cell determinants. *Nature*, 300, 168–170.

98 **FRANCIS, M.J., OULDRIDGE, E.J. & BLACK, L., 1983.** Antibody response in bovine pharyngeal fluid following foot-and-mouth disease vaccination and/or exposure to live virus. *Research in Veterinary Science*, 35, 206–210.

99 **GAILIUNAS, P. & COTTRAL, G.E., 1966.** Presence and persistence of foot-and-mouth disease virus in bovine skin. *Journal of Bacteriology*, 91, 2333–2338.

100 **GAINARU, M.D., 1988.** Veterinary Research Institute, Onderstepoort, South Africa. Unpublished data.

101 **GAINARU, M.D. & THOMSON, G.R., 1987.** Veterinary Research Institute, Onderstepoort, South Africa. Unpublished data.

102 **GAINARU, M.D., THOMSON, G.R., BENGIS, R.G., ESTERHUYSEN, J.J., BRUCE, W. & PINI, A., 1986.** Foot-and-mouth disease and the African buffalo (*Syncerus caffer*). II. Virus transmission and excretion during acute infection. *Onderstepoort Journal of Veterinary Research*, 53, 75–85.

103 **GEBAUER, F., DE LA TORRE, J.C., GOMES, I., MATEN, M.G., BARAHONA, H., TIRABOSCHI, B., BERGMANN, I., DE MELLO, P.A. & DOMINGO, E., 1988.** Rapid selection of genetic and antigenic variants of foot-and-mouth disease during persistence in cattle. *Virology*, 62, 2041–2049.

104 **GEERING, W.A., 1967.** Foot-and-mouth disease in sheep. *Australian Veterinary Journal*, 43, 485–489.

105 **GIBSON, C.F. & DONALDSON, A.I., 1986.** Exposure of sheep to natural aerosols of foot-and-mouth disease virus. *Research in Veterinary Science*, 41, 45–49.

106 **GIBSON, C.F., DONALDSON, A.I. & FERRIS, N.P., 1984.** Response of sheep vaccinated with large doses of vaccine to challenge by airborne foot-and-mouth disease virus. *Vaccine*, 2, 157–161.

107 **GLOSTER, J., SELLERS, R.F. & DONALDSON, A.I., 1982.** Long distance transport of foot-and-mouth disease virus over the sea. *The Veterinary Record*, 110, 47–52.

108 **GOMES, I. & ROSENBERG, F.J., 1984/85.** A possible role of capybaras (*Hydrochoerus hydrochoeris hydrochoeris*) in foot-and-mouth disease (FMD) endemicity. *Preventive Veterinary Medicine*, 3, 197–205.

109 **GRAHAM, A.M., 1967.** Foot-and-mouth disease. *The Veterinary Record*, (Special Issue — Information Supplement), 84, 25–30.

110 **GRAVES, J.H., McVICAR, J.W., SUTMOLLER, P. &**

TRAUTMAN, R., 1971. Contact transmission of foot-and-mouth disease from infected to susceptible cattle. *Journal of Infectious Diseases*, 123, 386–391.
111 **GREENBERG, B., 1973.** *In: Flies and Disease. Biology and Disease Transmission.* Vol. II. New Jersey, USA: Princeton University Press.
112 **HAMBLIN, C., BARNETT, I.T.R. & CROWTHER, J.R., 1986.** A new enzyme-linked immunosorbent assay (ELISA) for the detection of antibodies against foot-and-mouth disease virus. II. Application. *Journal of Immunological Methods*, 93, 123–129.
113 **HAMBLIN, C., BARNETT, I.T.R. & HEDGER, R.S., 1986.** A new enzyme-linked immunosorbent assay (ELISA) for the detection of antibodies against foot-and-mouth disease virus. I. Development and method of ELISA. *Journal of Immunological Methods*, 93, 115–121.
114 **HAMBLIN, C., KITCHING, R.P., DONALDSON, A.I., CROWTHER, J.R. & BARNETT, I.T.R., 1987.** Enzyme-linked immunosorbent assay (ELISA) for the detection of antibodies against foot-and-mouth disease virus. III. Evaluation of antibodies after infection and vaccination. *Epidemiology and Infection*, 99, 733–744.
115 **HARRIS, T.R. & BROWN, F., 1977.** Biochemical analysis of a virulent and an avirulent strain of foot-and-mouth disease virus. *Journal of General Virology*, 34, 87–105.
116 **HEDGER, R.S., 1968.** The isolation and characterization of foot-and-mouth disease virus from clinically normal herds of cattle in Botswana. *Journal of Hygiene*, 66, 27–36.
117 **HEDGER, R.S., 1972.** Foot-and-mouth disease and the African buffalo (*Syncerus caffer*). *Journal of Comparative Pathology*, 82, 19–28.
118 **HEDGER, R.S., 1976.** Foot-and-mouth disease in wildlife with particular reference to the African buffalo (*Syncerus caffer*). *In:* PAGE, A.L., (ed.). *Wildlife Diseases*. New York: Plenum Publishing Corporation.
119 **HEDGER, R.S., 1976.** The maintenance of foot-and-mouth disease in Africa. Ph.D. thesis, London School of Hygiene and Tropical Medicine, University of London.
120 **HEDGER, R.S. & CONDY, J.B., 1985.** Transmission of foot-and-mouth disease from African buffalo virus carriers to bovines. *The Veterinary Record*, 117, 205.
121 **HEDGER, R.S., CONDY, J.B. & GOLDING, S.M., 1972.** Infection of some species of African wildlife with foot-and-mouth disease virus. *Journal of Comparative Pathology*, 82, 455–461.
122 **HEDGER, R.S. & DAWSON, P.S., 1970.** Foot-and-mouth disease virus in milk: An epidemiological study. *The Veterinary Record*, 87, 186–188; 213.
123 **HEDGER, R.S., FORMAN, A.J. & WOODFORD, M.H., 1973.** Foot-and-mouth disease in East African buffalo. *Bulletin of Epizootic Diseases of Africa*, 21, 99–101.
124 **HEDGER, R.S. & STUBBINS, A.G.J., 1971.** The carrier state in foot-and-mouth disease, and the probang test. *State Veterinary Journal (UK)*, 26, 45–50.
125 **HENDERSON, W.M., 1947.** Vesicular lesions in farm animals. *The Veterinary Record*, 59, 497–498.
126 **HENNING, O., 1892.** *Annual Report of the Colonial Veterinary Surgeon for 1892*, 15.
127 **HENNING, M.W., 1956.** Foot-and-mouth disease, Mond-en-Klouseer. *In: Diseases in South Africa*. Pretoria: Central News Agency.
128 **HESS, W.R., BACHRACH, H.L. & CALLIS, J.J., 1960.** Persistence of foot-and-mouth disease virus in bovine kidneys and blood as related to the occurrence of antibodies. *American Journal of Veterinary Research*, 21, 1104–1108.
129 **HOLLAND, J., SPINDLER, K., HORODYSKI, F., GRABOU, E., NICOL, S. & VAN DE POL, S., 1982.** Rapid evolution of RNA genomes. *Science*, 215, 1577–1585.
130 **HOUSE, J.A. & YEDLOUTSCHNIG, R.J., 1982.** Sensitivity of seven different types of cell cultures to three serotypes of foot-and-mouth disease virus. *Canadian Journal of Comparative Medicine*, 46, 186–189.
131 **HOWELL, P.G., 1984.** Foot and mouth disease as a limiting factor in game farming. *Acta Zoologica Fennica*, 172, 227–229.
132 **HOWELL, P.G. & MANSVELT, P.R., 1972.** The epizootiology of foot-and-mouth disease in the Republic of South Africa. *Bulletin de l'Office International des Épizooties*, 77, 629–634.
133 **HUGH-JONES, M.E., 1972.** Epidemiological studies on the 1967–68 foot-and-mouth epidemic: Attack rates and cattle density. *Research in Veterinary Science*, 13, 411–417.
134 **HUTCHEON, D., 1892.** *Annual Report of the Colonial Veterinary Surgeon, 1892*, 9.
135 **HUTCHEON, D., 1893.** *Annual Report of the Colonial Veterinary Surgeon, 1893*, 10.
136 **HUTCHEON, D., 1894.** *Annual Report of the Colonial Veterinary Surgeon, 1894*, 8.
137 **HYSLOP, N. St.G., 1965.** Airborne infection with the virus of foot-and-mouth disease. *Journal of Comparative Pathology*, 75, 119–126.
138 **HYSLOP, N. St.G., 1970.** The epizootiology and epidemiology of foot and mouth disease. *Advances in Veterinary Science*, 14, 261–307.
139 **KENNEDY, D.J., JACKSON, R.B. & RAMSAY, G.C., 1984.** Difficulties experienced in recognizing foot-and-mouth disease in an outbreak in Zimbabwe. *Australian Veterinary Journal*, 61, 163–164.
140 **KING, A.M.Q., UNDERWOOD, B.O., McCAHON, D., NEWMAN, J.W.I. & BROWN, F., 1981.** Biochemical identification of viruses causing the 1981 outbreaks of foot and mouth disease in the UK. *Nature*, 293, 479–480.
141 **KITCHING, R.P. & DONALDSON, A.I., 1987.** Collection and transportation of specimens for vesicular virus investigation. *Revue Scientifique et Technique*, 6, 263–272.
142 **KLEID, D.G., YANSURA, D.Y., DOWBENKO, D., WEDDELL, G.N., HOATLIN, M.E., CLAYTON, N., SHIRE, S.J., BOCK, L.A., OGEZ, J., BUILDER, S. & PATZER, J., 1984.** Cloned viral protein for control of foot-and-mouth disease. *Developments in Industrial Microbiology*, 25, 317–325.
143 **KRIGE, J., 1988.** Directorate of Veterinary Services, Pretoria. Personal communication.
144 **KRUGER, S.J.P., 1858.** Quoted from 'Staats Cocarant' No. 43, November 19th, 1858. Bloemhof Blue Book. Evidence taken in connection with the diamond fields arbitration, 1871, 313.
145 **KRYSTYNAK, R.H.E., 1987.** Canada's experience with foot-and-mouth disease. *Canadian Veterinary Journal*, 28, 540–542.
146 **LAMPRECHTS, M.C., BUHR, W.H.B. & VAN DER MERWE, J.P., 1956.** Observations on the transmission of foot-and-mouth disease to game and controlled transmission of the disease from game to cattle and vice versa by means of contact. *Journal of the South African Veterinary Medical Association*, 27, 133–137.
147 **LAPORTE, J., GROSCLAUDE, J., WONTYGEM, J., BERNARD, S. & RONZE, P., 1973.** Neutralisation en culture cellulaire du ponvoir infectieux du virus de la fièvre aphteuse des sérums provenants de porcs immunisés à l'aide d'une protéine virale purifiée. *Compte Rendu Hebdomadaire des Séances de l'Académie des Sciences*, 276D, 3399–3402.
148 **LA TORRE, J.L., UNDERWOOD, B.O., LEBENDIKER, M., GORMAN, B.M. & BROWN, F., 1982.** Application of RNase T1 one- and two-dimensional analyses to the rapid identification of foot-and-mouth disease viruses. *Infection and Immunity*, 36, 142–147.
149 **LAWRENCE, D.A., 1935.** Foot-and-mouth disease in Southern Rhodesia. *Journal of the South African Veterinary Medical Association*, 6, 253–262.
150 **LAWRENCE, J.A., FOGGIN, C.M. & NORVAL, R.A.I., 1980.** The effects of war on the control of diseases of livestock in Rhodesia (Zimbabwe). *The Veterinary Record*, 107, 82–85.
151 **LE VAILLANT, M., 1795.** *Travels into the Interior Parts of Africa*, Vol. II. 1780–1785.
152 **MACAULAY, J.W., 1963.** Foot-and-mouth disease in non-domestic animals. *Bulletin of Epizootic Diseases of Africa*, 11, 143–146.

153 **MANNATHOKO, M.M., 1986.** *Epidemiology: FMD Situation in Africa 1982–86*. Working document of the 17th OIE Foot-and-mouth Disease Commission, 1–3 October, 1986, Paris.

154 **MARTIN, W.B. & CHAPMAN, W.G., 1961.** The tissue culture colour test for assaying the virus and neutralizing antibody of foot-and-mouth disease and its application to the measurement of immunity in cattle. *Research in Veterinary Science*, 2, 53–61.

155 **McCULLOUGH, K.C., CROWTHER, J.W., CARPENTER, W.C., BROCCHI, E., CAPUCCI, L., DE SIMONE, F., XIE, Q. & McCAHON, D., 1987.** Epitopes on foot-and-mouth disease particles. I. Topology. *Virology*, 157, 516–525.

156 **McKERCHER, P.D., MORGAN, D.O., McVICAR, J.W. & SHNOT, N.J., 1980.** Thermal processing to inactivate viruses in meat products. *Proceedings of the 84th Annual Meeting of the United States Health Association*, San Diego, California, 320–328.

157 **McVICAR, J.W. & SUTMÖLLER, P., 1970.** Foot-and-mouth disease: The agar gel diffusion precipitation test for antibody to virus-infection-associated (VIA) antigen as a tool for epizootiology surveys. *American Journal of Epidemiology*, 92, 273–278.

158 **McVICAR, J.W. & SUTMÖLLER, P., 1976.** Growth of foot-and-mouth disease virus in the upper respiratory tract of non-immunized, vaccinated, and recovered cattle after intranasal inoculation. *Journal of Hygiene*, 76, 467–481.

159 **MEESER, M.J.A., 1962.** Foot-and-mouth disease in game animals with special reference to the impala (*Aepyceros melampus*). *Journal of the South African Veterinary Medical Association*, 33, 351–355.

160 **MELLOR, E.J.C., BROWN, F. & HARRIS, T.J.R., 1985.** Analysis of the secondary structure of the poly(C) tract in foot-and-mouth disease virus RNAs. *Journal of General Virology*, 66, 1919–1929.

161 **MONTGOMERY, J.F., OLIVER, R.E. & POOLE, W.S.H., 1987.** A vesiculo-bullous disease in pigs resembling foot-and-mouth disease. I. Field codes. *New Zealand Veterinary Journal*, 35, 21–26.

162 **MONTGOMERY, J.F., OLIVER, R.E., POOLE, W.S.H. & JULIAN, A.F., 1987.** A vesiculo-bullous disease in pigs resembling foot-and-mouth disease. II. Experimental reproduction of the lesions. *New Zealand Veterinary Journal*, 35, 27–30.

163 **MORRELL, D.J., MELLOR, E.J.C., ROWLANDS, D.J. & BROWN, F., 1987.** Surface structure and RNA-protein interactions of foot-and-mouth disease virus. *Journal of General Virology*, 68, 1649–1658.

164 **NICHOLLS, M.J., BLACK, L. & RWEYEMAMU, M.M., 1984.** The effect of maternally derived antibodies on the response of calves to vaccination against foot-and-mouth disease. *Journal of Hygiene*, 92, 105–116.

165 **NICHOLLS, M.J., BLACK, L., RWEYEMAMU, M.M. & GRADWELL, D.V., 1985.** Effect of age on response of cattle to vaccination against foot-and-mouth disease. *British Veterinary Journal*, 141, 17–26.

166 **OLIVER, R.E., DONALDSON, A.I., GIBSON, C.F., ROEDER, P.L., LE BLANC SMITH, P.M. & HAMBLIN, C., 1988.** Detection of foot-and-mouth disease antigen in bovine epithelial samples: Comparison of sites of sample collection by an enzyme linked immunosorbent assay (ELISA) and complement fixation test. *Research in Veterinary Science*, 44, 315–319.

167 **OULDRIDGE, E.J., BARNETT, P., HINGLEY, P., HEAD, M. & RWEYEMAMU, M.M., 1982.** The use of an indirect sandwich ELISA assay for the differentiation of FMD virus strains. *The Eliza*, 22, 152–160.

168 **OULDRIDGE, E.J. & ROWLANDS, D.J., 1986.** New approaches to the epidemiology of foot-and-mouth disease. *Outlook on Agriculture*, 15, 40–45.

169 **PARKER, J., 1971.** Presence and inactivation of foot-and-mouth disease virus in animal faeces. *The Veterinary Record*, 88, 659–662.

170 **PAY, T.W.F., 1983.** Variation in foot-and-mouth disease: Application to vaccination. *Revue Scientifique et Technique*, 2, 701–723.

171 **PAY, T.W.F., 1985.** Factors influencing the performance of foot-and-mouth disease vaccines under field conditions. *In:* DELLA-PORTA, A.J., (ed.). *Veterinary Viral Diseases: Their Significance in South-East Asia and the Western Pacific*. Sydney, New York, London: Academic Press Inc.

172 **PAY, T.W.F., 1985.** The comparison of the antigenic relationship of a vaccine strain with a new field isolate of foot-and-mouth disease virus. *Foot-and-mouth Disease Bulletin*, 23, 1–6.

173 **PAY, T.W.F., 1988.** Foot-and-mouth disease in sheep and goats: A review. *Foot-and-mouth Disease Bulletin*, 26, 2–13.

174 **PEREIRA, H.G., 1977.** Subtyping of foot-and-mouth disease virus. *Developments in Biological Standardization*, 35, 167–174.

175 **PEREIRA, H.G., 1978.** Antigenic variation in relation to epidemiology and control of foot and mouth disease. *British Veterinary Journal*, 134, 58–62.

176 **PEREIRA, H.G., 1981.** Foot-and-mouth disease. *In:* GIBBS, E.P.J., (ed.). *Virus Diseases of Food Animals*. Vol. II. Disease Monographs. London, New York: Academic Press Inc.

177 **PERRY, B.D. & HEDGER, R.S., 1984.** History and epidemiology of foot-and-mouth disease in Zambia: A review. *Tropical Animal Health and Production*, 16, 107–114.

178 **PIENAAR, U. DE V., 1969.** Observations on the developmental biology, growth and some aspects of the population ecology of African buffalo (*Syncerus caffer* Sparrman) in the Kruger National Park. *Koedoe*, 12, 29–52.

179 **PLATT, H., 1960.** The localization of lesions in experimental foot-and-mouth disease. *British Journal of Experimental Pathology*, 41, 150–159.

180 **PUTNAK, J.R. & PHILLIPS, B.A., 1981.** Picornaviral structure and assembly. *Microbiological Reviews*, 45, 287–315.

181 **RICHMOND, J.Y., 1978.** Preabsorption of boar serum with kaolin: Increased efficiency of foot-and-mouth disease virus detection. *American Journal of Veterinary Research*, 39, 1612–1616.

182 **RICHMOND, J.Y., McVICAR, J.W. & EISNER, R.J., 1978.** Problems in the development of protocols for detecting foot-and-mouth and swine vesicular disease viruses in boar semen. *Proceedings of the 21st Annual Meeting of the American Association of Veterinary Laboratory Diagnosticians*, 319–330.

183 **ROBERTSON, W., 1903.** *Annual Report of the Colonial Veterinary Surgeon*, 42.

184 **ROBSON, K.J.H., CROWTHER, J.R., KING, A.M.Q. & BROWN, F., 1979.** Comparative biochemical and serological analysis of five isolates of a single serotype of foot-and-mouth disease virus. *Journal of General Virology*, 45, 579–590.

185 **ROBSON, K.J.H., HARRIS, T.J.R. & BROWN, F., 1977.** An assessment by competition hybridization of the sequence homology between the RNAs of the seven serotypes of FMDV. *Journal of General Virology*, 37, 271–276.

186 **ROEDER, P.L. & LE BLANC SMITH, P.M., 1987.** Detection and typing of foot-and-mouth disease virus by enzyme-linked immunosorbent assay: A sensitive, rapid and reliable technique for primary diagnosis. *Research in Veterinary Science*, 43, 225–232.

187 **ROHRER, H., 1983.** Differential significance of epizootiological factors in the control of foot-and-mouth disease. A brief review. *Acta Virologica*, 27, 371–375.

188 **ROSSI, M.S., SADIR, A.M., SCHUDEL, A.A. & PALMA, E.L., 1988.** Detection of foot-and-mouth disease virus with DNA probes in bovine esophageal-pharyngeal fluids. *Archives of Virology*, 99, 67–74.

189 **ROSSITER, L.W. & ALBERTYN, A.A.L., 1947.** Foot-and-mouth disease in game. *Journal of the South African Veterinary Medical Association*, 18, 16–19.

190 **ROSSMAN, M.G., ARNOLD, E., ERICSON, J.W., FRANKENBERGER, E.A., GRIFFITH, J.P., HECHT, H-J., JOHNSON, J.E., KAMER, G., LUO, M., MOSSER, A.G., RUECKERT, R.R., SHERRY, B. & VRIEND, G., 1985.** Structure of human common cold virus and functional

relationship to other picornaviruses. *Nature*, 317, 145–153.

191 **ROSSMAN, M.G. & PALMENBERG, A.A., 1988.** Conservation of the putative receptor attachment site in picornaviruses. *Virology*, 164, 373–382.

192 **ROSSMAN, M.G. & RUECKERT, R.R., 1987.** What does the molecular structure of viruses tell us about viral functions? *Microbiological Sciences*, 4, 206–214.

193 **ROWLANDS, D.J., 1985.** Novel approaches to foot-and-mouth disease vaccination. *Vaccine*, 3, 37–38.

194 **RUECKERT, R.R., 1985.** Picornaviruses and their replication. *In:* FIELDS, B.N., KNIPE, D.M., MELNICK, J.L., CHANOCK, R.M., ROIZMAN, R. & SHOPE, R.E., (eds). *Virology*. New York: Raven Press.

195 **RUMNEY, R.P., 1986.** Meteorological influences on the spread of foot-and-mouth disease. *Journal of Applied Bacteriology*, Symposium Supplement 1986, 105S–114S.

196 **RWEYEMAMU, M.M., PAY, T.W.F. & SIMMS, M.J., 1982.** The control of foot-and-mouth disease by vaccination. *Veterinary Annual*, 22, 63–80.

197 **SADIR, A.M., SCHUDEL, A.A. & LAPORTE, O., 1988.** Response of foot-and-mouth disease vaccines in newborn calves. Influence of age, colostral antibodies and adjuvants. *Epidemiology and Infection*, 100, 135–144.

198 **SANGER, D.V., 1979.** The replication of picornaviruses. *Journal of General Virology*, 45, 1–13.

199 **SCHNEIDER, H., 1977.** *Analyse der Tiergesundheits-situation in Südwestafrika/Namibia*. Inaugural-Dissertation. Justus Liebig-Universität zu Giessen (Institut für Tropische Veterinärmedizin).

200 **SCOTT, F.W., COTTRAL, G.E. & GAILIUNAS, P., 1966.** Resistance of foot-and-mouth disease virus in external lesions and saliva of experimentally infected cattle. *American Journal of Veterinary Research*, 27, 1531–1536.

201 **SELLERS, R.F., 1968.** The inactivation of foot-and-mouth disease virus by chemicals and inactivants. *The Veterinary Record*, 83, 504–506.

202 **SELLERS, R.F., 1971.** Quantitative aspects of the spread of foot-and-mouth disease. *The Veterinary Bulletin*, 41, 431–439.

203 **SELLERS, R.F., 1983.** Transmission of viruses by artificial breeding techniques: A review. *Journal of the Royal Society of Medicine*, 76, 772–775.

204 **SELLERS, R.F., BURROWS, R., MANN, J.A. & DAWE, P.S., 1968.** Recovery of virus from bulls affected with foot-and-mouth disease. *The Veterinary Record*, 83, 303.

205 **SELLERS, R.F. & PARKER, J., 1969.** Airborne excretion of foot-and-mouth disease virus. *Journal of Hygiene*, 67, 671–677.

206 **SHARMA, S.K. & MURTY, D.K., 1981.** Foot-and-mouth disease in sheep. Pattern of virus excretion and distribution in experimentally infected animals. *Indian Journal of Animal Science*, 51, 61–66.

207 **SHIMSHONY, A., ORGAD, U., BAHARAV, D., PRUDOVSKY, S., YAKOBSON, B., BAR MOSHE, B. & DAGAN, D., 1986.** Malignant foot-and-mouth disease in mountain gazelles. *The Veterinary Record*, 119, 175–176.

208 **SIMMS, M.J., 1969.** Inactivation of foot-and-mouth disease virus. *Foot-and-mouth Disease Bulletin*: Supplement No. 2. The Wellcome Research Laboratories, Beckenham, Kent. 12.

209 **SINCLAIR, A.R.E., 1977.** *The African Buffalo*. Chicago, London: University of Chicago Press.

210 **SINGH, E., 1984.** *Proceedings of the 10th International Congress on Animal Reproduction and Artificial Insemination*, 10–14 June 1984, Urbana Ill. (USA).

211 **SMITH, D.B. & INGLIS, S.C., 1987.** The mutation rate and variability of eukaryotic viruses: An analytical review. *Journal of General Virology*, 68, 2729–2740.

212 **SNOWDON, W.A., 1966.** Growth of foot-and-mouth disease virus in monolayer cultures of calf thyroid cells. *Nature*, 210, 1079–1080.

213 **STEINHAUER, D.A. & HOLLAND, J.J., 1987.** Rapid evolution of RNA viruses. *Annual Review of Microbiology*, 41, 409–433.

214 **STROHMAIER, K., 1987.** Die Maul- und Klauenseuche. III. Erfahrungen und Folgerungen aus 20 Jahren Bekämpfung der Maul- und Klauenseuche. *Tierärztliche Umschau*, 5, 417–422.

215 **SUTMÖLLER, P., 1971.** Persistent foot-and-mouth disease virus infections. *In:* SAUNDERS, M., (ed.). *Viruses Affecting Man and Animals*. St. Louis: Warren H. Green, Inc.

216 **SUTMÖLLER, P. & McVICAR, J.W., 1972.** The epizootiological importance of foot-and-mouth disease carriers. III. Exposure of pigs to bovine carriers. *Archiv für die Gesamte Virusforschung*, 37, 78–84.

217 **SUTMÖLLER, P. & McVICAR, J.W., 1973.** Foot-and-mouth disease: Growth of virus after conjunctival inoculation of cattle. *Archiv für die gesamte Virusforschung*, 43, 284–287.

218 **SUTMÖLLER, P. & VIERIRA, A., 1980.** The relationship of neutralizing antibody titres for foot-and-mouth disease virus and the protection of cattle. *Bulletin Centro Panamericano Fiebre Aftosa*, 39–40, 57–62.

219 **TAYLOR, R.D. & MARTIN, R.B., 1987.** Effects of veterinary fences on wildlife conservation in Zimbabwe. *Environmental Management*, 11, 327–334.

220 **TERPSTRA, C., 1972.** Pathogenesis of foot-and-mouth disease in experimentally infected pigs. *Bulletin de l'Office International des Épizooties*, 77, 859–874.

221 **TERRY, G.M., CLARK, R.P. & RWEYEMAMU, M.M., 1982.** Variations in the buoyant density of foot-and-mouth virus disease strains. *Archives of Virology*, 71, 333–341.

222 **THOMAS, A.A.M., WOORTMEIJER, R.J., BARTELING, S.J. & HELOEN, R.H., 1988.** Evidence for more than one important neutralizing site on foot-and-mouth disease virus. *Archives of Virology*, 99, 237–242.

223 **THOMSON, G.R. & BENGIS, R.G., 1987–88.** Veterinary Research Institute, Onderstepoort, South Africa. Unpublished data.

224 **THOMSON, G.R., BENGIS, R.G., ESTERHUYSEN, J.J. & PINI, A., 1984.** Maintenance mechanisms for foot-and-mouth disease virus in the Kruger National Park and potential avenues for its escape into domestic animal populations. *Proceedings of the XIIIth World Congress on Diseases of Cattle*. Vol. I. September 1984. Durban, South Africa.

225 **THOMSON, G.R., DOUBE, B.M., BRAAK, L.F.O., GAINARU, M.D. & BENGIS, R.G., 1988.** Failure of *Haematobia thirouxi potans* (Bezzi) to transmit foot-and-mouth disease virus mechanically between viraemic and susceptible cattle. *Onderstepoort Journal of Veterinary Research*, 55, 121–122.

226 **THOMSON, G.R., ESTERHUYSEN, J.J., GAINARU, M.D., BRUCE, W. & BENGIS, R.G., 1985.** Transmission of foot-and-mouth disease virus to cattle by the African buffalo. *In:* DELLA-PORTA, A.J., (ed.). *Veterinary Viral Diseases*. Sydney, Orlando, San Diego, New York, London: Academic Press, Inc.

227 **THOMSON, G.R. & NEVILL, E.M., 1988.** Unpublished data.

228 **TYSON, P.D., 1986.** *Climatic Change and Variability in Southern Africa*. Cape Town: Oxford University Press Southern Africa.

229 **VAKHARIA, V.N., DAVANEY, M.A., MOORE, D.M., DUNNAND, J.J. & GRUBMAN, M.J., 1987.** Proteolytic processing of foot-and-mouth disease virus polyproteins expressed in a cell-free system from clone-derived transcripts. *Journal of Virology*, 61, 3199–3207.

230 **VAN BEKKUM, J.G., FISH, R.C. & NATHAUS, I., 1969.** Immunologic responses in Dutch cattle vaccinated with foot-and-mouth disease vaccines under field conditions: Neutralizing antibody responses and immunity to O, A and C types. *American Journal of Veterinary Research*, 30, 2125–2129.

231 **VAN BEKKUM, J.G., FRENKEL, H.S., FREDERIKS, H.H.J. & FRENKEL, S., 1959.** Observations on the carrier state of cattle exposed to foot-and-mouth disease virus. *Tijdschrift voor Dieregeneeskunde*, 84, 1159–1164.

232 **WALDMAN, O., TRAUTWEIN, K. & PYL, F., 1931.** Die Persistenz des Maul und Klauenseuche virus im korper durchgeseuchter Fiere und Seine Ausscheidung. *Zentralblatt für Bakteriologie, Parasitenkunde, Infektionskrankheiten und Hygiene*, Abteiling I Originale, 121, 1932.

233 **WALKER, J., 1934.** Some observations on foot-and-mouth disease in the Bechuanaland Protectorate. *Journal of the South African Veterinary Medical Association*, 5, 73–91.

234 **WALKER, J.S., DE LEEUW, P.W., CALLIS, J.J. & VAN BEKKUM, J.G., 1984.** The thermal death time curve of foot-and-mouth disease virus contained in primarily infected milk. *Journal of Biological Standardization*, 12, 185–189.

235 **WATSON, W.A., 1981.** Vesicular diseases: Recent advances and concepts of control. *Canadian Veterinary Journal*, 22, 311–320.

236 **WESTBURY, H.A., DOUGHTY, W.J., FORMAN, A.J., TANGCHAITRONG, S. & KONGTHON, A., 1988.** A comparison of enzyme-linked immunosorbent assay, complement fixation and virus isolation for foot-and-mouth disease diagnosis. *Veterinary Microbiology*, 17, 21–28.

237 **XIE, Q-C., McCAHON, D., CROWTHER, J.R., BELSHAM, G.J. & McCULLOUGH, K.C., 1987.** Neutralization of foot-and-mouth disease virus can be mediated through any of at least three separate antigenic sites. *Journal of General Virology*, 68, 1637–1647.

238 **YILMA, T., 1980.** Morphogenesis of vesiculation in foot-and-mouth disease. *American Journal of Veterinary Research*, 41, 1537–1542.

239 **ZYAMBO, G.C.N., 1975.** Foot-and-mouth disease outbreaks in Zambia. *Bulletin de l'Office International des Épizooties*, 83, 19–25.

ORTHOMYXOVIRIDAE

The family Orthomyxoviridae (influenza viruses) embodies three genera (A/B, C and D) which, at one time, were considered to be four groups (A, B, C and D).[1] Influenza virus D comprises tick-borne viruses, e.g. Dhori and Thogoto, that differ biologically from A, B and C viruses which are transmitted directly, usually by respiratory aerosols.

Virions are medium-sized (20–120 nm in diameter), pleomorphic, but usually roughly spherical. Filamentous forms may be up to several micrometres in length. They are surrounded by a host cell-derived envelope through which project 'spikes' formed by the glycoproteins of the haemagglutinin and neuraminidase in a ratio of 4:1 or 5:1. The genome consists of 6–8 single-stranded segments of negative-sense RNA (total length about 13,6 kilobases), the number depending on the genus, as is the case for the structural proteins.[1]

Both the nucleus and cytoplasm of infected cells are involved in the replicative cycle of these viruses, although viral-protein synthesis occurs only in the cytoplasm of host cells. Newly formed virions bud from the plasmalemma. During replication, gene reassortment may occur in mixed infections with viruses of the same but not different species, resulting in antigenic shift. True recombination has also been demonstrated.[1]

Humans are infected by all four groups of influenza viruses (A, B, C and D), although only Group A viruses produce epidemic disease. In animals, too, only A-group influenza viruses are important. Amongst domestic animals, severe and costly epidemics caused by influenza A viruses occur particularly in horses, and also in pigs and poultry. Natural infection with Group A viruses has also been detected in seals, whales and mink.

Reference

1 **KLENK, H.-D., 1991.** Orthomyxoviridae. *In:* FRANCKI, R.I.B., FAUQUET, C.M., KNUDSON, D.L. & BROWN, F., (eds). Classification and nomenclature of viruses. Fifth report of the International Committee on the Taxonomy of Viruses. *Archives of Virology*, Supplementum 2. Vienna, New York: Springer-Verlag.

90

Equine influenza

Synonyms: Equine or horse flu, perdegriep (Afrik.)

J.A. Mumford

Introduction

Equine influenza is an acute and highly contagious respiratory disease of horses caused by infection with type A influenza viruses.

Epidemics of acute respiratory disease in horses have been reported for several centuries,[14, 35] but it was only in 1956 during a widespread epidemic among horses in eastern Europe,[34] that the first isolate of equine influenza virus was recovered. The virus was characterized as H7N7, and designated as influenza A/equine-1/Prague/56 (sometimes referred to as subtype 1). It caused epidemics during the 1960s and 1970s,[11] but in the early spring of 1963 a major epidemic occurred in the USA which was caused by an influenza A virus of a different antigenic subtype, H3N8.[40] This virus, designated as influenza A/equine-2/Miami/63 (or subtype 2), was introduced into the equine population of Florida by the importation of horses from Argentina. Isolation of an H3N8 virus was also made from South American horses in 1963.[32] A/equine-2/Miami/63 was subsequently introduced into France towards the end of 1964,[4, 5, 12] spreading rapidly throughout Europe in the late winter and spring of 1965.[11]

A/equine-2 was repeatedly isolated from horses involved in the 1965 epidemic that spread throughout the USA and Canada.[6] In the same year, horses in England experienced influenza, but this was caused by a virus similar to the A/equine-1/Prague/56 virus.[11] However, two years later horses in Europe were to be affected by the A/equine-2/Miami/63 virus. Subsequently there have been numerous reports of outbreaks of equine influenza in Europe, the USA and other countries.[7, 19, 36, 38]

Until 1986 there was no evidence that equine influenza had affected the southern African equine population,[9] but in that year virus A/equine-2/Johannesburg/86 (H3N8)[23] was introduced into South Africa by horses incubating the diseases that were imported from the USA. Comparison of the nucleotide sequence of the H genes demonstrated that A/equine-2/Johannesburg/86 virus is very similar to recent equine-2 influenza A viruses isolated in the USA, especially A/equine-2/Tennessee/86.[23] The disease spread explosively in the susceptible population in South Africa and resulted in severe economic losses, particularly to the racing industry.[9] The widespread use of vaccine against the disease has stabilized the situation in southern Africa.

Aetiology

Influenza viruses are pleomorphic, spherical or filamentous virions with a diameter of 80–120 nm and have a segmented, single-stranded RNA genome of negative sense. The eight gene segments code for two surface glycoproteins, the haemagglutinin (H) and neuraminidase (N), the internal matrix protein and nucleoprotein, and other structural and non-structural proteins involved in virus replication. The RNA segments are closely associated with the nucleoprotein and are surrounded by the matrix protein, which is itself closely associated with the lipid envelope containing the two surface glycoproteins.[18] The haemagglutinin is the major surface glycoprotein, making up approximately 25 per cent of the virus protein as compared with 5 per cent for the neuraminidase.

There are three types of influenza viruses, A, B and C, which are all classified within the Orthomyxovirus group, the virus type being determined by the antigenic character of the nucleoprotein and matrix proteins. All the equine influenza viruses which have been identified from horses are type A. Subtypes within a virus type are defined by the antigenic character of the haemagglutinin and neuraminidase.

Among influenza viruses, 12 different haemagglutinins (H) and nine neuraminidases (N) have been identified.[31] However, only two combinations have so far occurred in horses, viz. H7N7 and H3N8. Minor antigenic drift has been identified within the H7N7 subtype (subtype 1),[13] while among H3N8 viruses (subtype 2) more extensive antigenic drift has been detected, to the extent that variants have been identified, represented by A/Kentucky/81 and A/Fontainebleau/79.[20]

Antigenic drift occurs when mutations in the gene sequence result in amino acid substitutions, particularly in the haemagglutinin. It is thought to be influenced by immunological pressure brought about, for example, by vaccination during inter-epidemic periods.

Major or subtype changes in the surface glycoproteins occur as a result of recombinational events with other influenza viruses and are called antigenic shifts. Antigenic shift gives rise to new viruses which result in pandemics in susceptible populations.

Influenza is an enveloped virus and, as such, is not infectious for long periods outside the host. It is rapidly inactivated by sunlight and disinfectants.

Epidemiology

Equine influenza has been reported in North and South America, the West Indies, Europe, the former USSR, North Africa, the Middle East, India, Singapore, Japan, and Mongolia. The introduction of equine influenza into South Africa in 1986 was another milestone in the spread of this virus throughout the world. Australia and New Zealand are the only large countries currently free of the infection.[41]

There are many different factors that influence the epidemiology of equine influenza. Some relate to the intrinsic properties of the virus; some to the pathogenesis of the disease, the immune system of the horse and, not least, to the equine population structure and workings of the equine industry.

A key factor in the spread of equine influenza in the last two decades has been the rapid transportation of horses over long distances by air. Horses incubating the disease, or which are clinically or subclinically infected, can introduce the infection into a susceptible population if they are not quarantined adequately. In some areas of the world quarantining is virtually ignored in order to facilitate the international movement of horses for racing and breeding purposes. In addition, inadequate vaccination may lead to horses with partial immunity and result in the suppression of clinical signs. This may make infections unrecognizable while still allowing virus excretion.[29] Such horses probably play an important role in the maintenance and spread of equine influenza.

Equine influenza is a highly contagious disease which is characterized by rapid spread in susceptible populations. Morbidity rates are consequently high. In a study conducted during 1965, only 11 out of 634 susceptible horses resisted the disease, giving a morbidity rate of 98,2 per cent.[11]

Influenza viruses in horses infect the epithelium of the upper and lower respiratory tract and produce a frequent and harsh cough. This cough is an efficient way of spreading the virus in aerosols[12] — over distances of up to 32 metres or more.[25] The infection is believed to be transmitted almost exclusively by direct contact between horses, although recent evidence from the South African outbreak indicates that the virus can be transmitted indirectly by people and contaminated vehicles.[9] Virus excretion in fully susceptible horses lasts between seven and ten days, although infected animals are rarely infectious beyond seven days. However, coughing may persist for longer. The short incubation period also contributes to the rapid spread of infection.

Although long-term carriers have been postulated as being an important element in the epidemiology of equine influenza, this has not been unequivocally proven[2].

Immunity to equine influenza is short-lived, with clinical immunity lasting little more than a year. Immunity to infection may be even more short-lived, allowing reinfection without clinical signs to occur within a matter of months after a previous exposure.[17]

There is no evidence that variation in the prevalence of equine influenza is influenced by climatic conditions. Outbreaks of disease, particularly in the USA, are primarily related to the movement of horses and to the introduction of young stock onto race tracks where the infection is often endemic.

The widespread epidemic that was caused by a variant of the H3N8 subtype in the USA and Europe during 1979–80[20] raised the possibility that antigenic drift could be playing a major role in the epidemiology of equine influenza. Retrospective studies on the antigenic character of H3N8, however, demonstrated that Miami/63- and Kentucky/81-like viruses had been co-circulating in the equine population for some years.

The features of the disease are similar in other equids such as donkeys, mules and zebras[9, 37] although a high mortality rate has been reported in donkeys.[30] Indigenous equids are likely to be important reservoirs for equine influenza viruses in regions where widespread vaccination is impractical.

Pathogenesis

Influenza virus infects epithelial cells in the mucosae of both the upper and lower airways after attaching to the cilia. The haemagglutinin mediates the attachment of virus to host cells. Antigenically, the haemagglutinin is of prime importance, as antibodies which react with it can neutralize the virus. There are four antigenic sites on the haemagglutinin molecule, and amino acid changes in all four sites result in antigenic drift of significant epidemic potential.[33]

The function of the neuraminidase is not fully understood, but it is known that its catalytic activity allows transport of virus through mucin and destroys haemagglutinin receptors, thus allowing elution of progeny virus from infected cells[39] and release of virus particles. Antibody to neuraminidase inhibits cell-to-cell spread of virus.

Viral replication is rapid, viral antigen appearing in cells within two hours,[10] and complete deciliation of the epithelium of the trachea occurring within four days of infection.[3]

Clinical signs

The clinical features of equine influenza have been reviewed.[11]

In controlled studies the incubation period usually varied between one and three days, with a range of 18 hours to five days. The length of the incubation period is inversely related to the virus dose.[27]

Coughing and fever are the most common clinical signs of equine influenza, the cough being dry, harsh and initially non-productive. It is frequent during the first week of infection, and in uncomplicated cases, given sufficient rest, will disappear within one to three weeks. There is usually a mild rhinitis but no obvious swelling of the submaxillary lymph nodes. The nasal discharge is serous, becoming mucoid later.

In general, subtype 2 infections produce more severe clinical disease with higher and more prolonged pyrexia[24] than subtype 1. They also appear to be more pneumotropic. Peak temperatures recorded in subtype 1 and 2 infections were 40,4 and 41,2 °C respectively.[11] The fever reaction may be biphasic during the purely viral phase of the disease, and the height and duration of pyrexia may relate not only to the subtype involved but also to the challenge dose received.[27] Continuous fever beyond four or five days accompanied by pronounced mucopurulent nasal discharge is indicative of secondary bacterial infection.

Other signs of influenza infection include anorexia, dyspnoea and myalgia, and there may be icterus in severe cases. Cardiac damage has been encountered, particularly in older animals and in those which have been worked during the acute phase of the disease.[11]

Mortality rates are usually very low in uncomplicated cases, except for young foals which have no maternal immunity. Foal deaths occurred during the A/equine-2 outbreaks in Britain in 1965[25] and in the A/equine-2 epidemic in South Africa in 1986.[9] Deaths occurred particularly in young foals which were born at the time their dams were suffering acute disease. They develop a very high temperature (41–42 °C), stop suckling and show elevated pulse rates and signs of severe respiratory distress, including polypnoea (80–90 respirations per minute) and soft gurgling sounds. Pneumonia develops soon afterwards and foals become weak, with death ensuing in seven to ten days.

Mortality also occurs in donkeys and mules after influenza infections.[30] Necropsies performed on donkeys affected in the 1969 British outbreak of A/equine-2 revealed acute bronchopneumonia complicated by secondary bacterial infection.[30]

Secondary complications and sequelae to equine influenza are common in stressed or neglected animals. Bacterial infections (including *Streptococcus equisimilis, S. zooepidemicus, Escherichia coli, Staphylococcus* spp., *Pseudomonas* spp., *Pasteurella* spp., *Aerobacter* spp., *Actinobacillus equuli* and *Bordetella bronchiseptica*) result in purulent nasal discharges, pharyngitis, conjunctivitis, and, in some instances, bronchopneumonia. Strangles and purpura haemorrhagica have also occurred in association with influenza.

Chronic pulmonary disease following uncomplicated influenza or secondary bacterial infection were common after the 1965 pandemic. Horses showed signs of asthmatic bronchitis combined with bronchiolitis for months after the acute infection. Such sequelae have been attributed to horses being worked during the acute infection, and to early resumption of hard work. Poor environmental conditions and inadequate antibacterial therapy contribute to the development of sequelae.

Pathology

Haematological changes during infections with equine influenza viruses are non-specific and variable. Anaemia, leukopenia and lymphopenia are often observed in the first three to seven days, with an increased neutrophil : lymphocyte ratio in the first two or three days after infection.[1, 11] A monocytosis may also be observed during early convalescence from about day seven.

The most important changes associated with infection of horses with influenza A/equine-1 (H7N7) and A/equine-2 (H3N8) viruses occur in the lower respiratory tract and include bronchitis, bronchiolitis, and interstitial pneumonia accompanied by congestion, oedema and neutrophil infiltration. Laryngitis and tracheitis have been associated particularly with A/equine-1 infections.[11, 22, 24]

Secondary infections or other complications may result in conjunctivitis, pharyngitis, purulent bronchopneumonia, chronic pulmonary disease, guttural pouch infections, purpura haemorrhagica and strangles.

Diagnosis

The characteristic features of equine influenza in susceptible animals (harsh cough, high temperature, and rapid spread) are sufficient to permit a tentative clinical diagnosis. However, in animals that have previously experienced the infection or which have a waning vaccinal immunity it is difficult to differentiate influenza from other viruses involved in the respiratory disease complex. In such situations, or where equine influenza has not occurred in the locality in the recent past, laboratory diagnosis by virus isolation/detection or serology is required.

Specimens for virus isolation should be collected as soon as possible after the onset of pyrexia and coughing, since in primed animals the period of virus excretion may be as short as one to two days. Virus may be cultured from nasopharyngeal secretions collected into virus transport medium by suction or by swabbing, or from tracheal washes. As with all samples for virus isolation, those for influenza isolation should be maintained on ice while being transported to the laboratory as quickly as possible.

Influenza virus can be cultured in embryonated hens' eggs or in susceptible mammalian cells such as Madin-Darby canine kidney (MDCK). Embryonated hens' eggs are inoculated via the amniotic (six- to eight-day-old embryos) or allantoic (eight- to 12-day-old embryos) routes. Amniotic and allantoic fluids harvested after incubation for 48–72 hours at 34 °C are examined for haemagglutinating activity using chick erythrocytes.

For isolation of virus in mammalian cell culture (MDCK cells), specimens must be collected in virus transport medium which does not contain foetal calf serum. The specimens are inoculated onto the cell culture in the presence of trypsin and the absence of serum. The presence of virus, which may not cause obvious cytopathic effect, is detected by assay of culture fluid for haemagglutinating activity after four to seven days' incubation at 34 °C. Two or three passages may be required in order to isolate infectious virus. Virus is subtyped using haemagglutination inhibition (HI) tests with sera specific for the H3N8 or H7N7 subtypes.

Submission of specimens in a good state of preservation to laboratories for virus isolation may not be practical when the distances are great or the temperatures are unfavourable for maintaining viability. However, a diagnosis may still be achieved by the detection of nucleoprotein in nasal secretions in the absence of infectious virus.[8] Subtyping of the virus does, however, require the examination of serological responses, as the nucleoprotein is antigenically similar in all influenza A viruses. This assay is therefore not able to differentiate between H3N8 and H7N7 subtypes.

Antibody to influenza virus may be detected by its ability to inhibit the agglutination of chick erythrocytes mediated by the viral haemagglutinin. Haemagglutination inhibition is subtype-specific.

The HI test is much more sensitive for antibody to H7 viruses than it is to H3 virus antibody when whole virus is used in the assay. The sensitivity of the test for antibody to the H3 viruses may be enhanced by disruption of the virus with detergent.[21] In HI tests a four-fold or greater increase in antibody titre between acute- and convalescent-phase sera is regarded as significant and indicative of infection.

Subclinical infections may occur in vaccinated horses, but they do not necessarily stimulate a four-fold increase in HI antibody. Nevertheless, such animals may be a source of infection to others. Significant increases in antibody may be detected in such animals using the single radial haemolysis test. This assay is based on the ability of antibody to the haemagglutinin to lyse sheep erythrocytes that have been sensitized with virus in the presence of complement.[42] The reproducibility of the assay allows the identification of infections which stimulate no more than a two-fold increase in antibody.

Serological diagnosis of infection in a vaccinated population is complicated by the presence of vaccine-induced antibody. Most vaccines are bivalent, containing representative strains of the H7N7 and H3N8 viruses, and vaccination usually stimulates significant increases in antibody to both subtypes, whereas antibody to infection is subtype-specific. Nevertheless, good vaccination records are required by laboratories in order to interpret the significance of serological responses in vaccinated horses.

Differential diagnosis

Equine influenza must be differentiated from acute respiratory diseases caused by both infectious and non-infectious agents. Viral infections which should be considered are equid herpesvirus 1 (subtypes 1 and 2), equine rhinoviruses, and equine viral arteritis. Bacterial infections produced by *Streptococcus equi* (strangles), *Rhodococcus equi* and others may produce similar disease.

Control

Because direct transmission from acutely infected to susceptible horses is the usual mode of transmission, the most effective means of control in the face of an outbreak are vaccination and restriction of the movement of horses. Vaccination programmes are most successful when the majority of horses which are travelling and mixing for competition or breeding purposes are vaccinated. This can best be achieved by instituting mandatory vaccination policies, and such systems operate in many European countries. It is usually not possible to impose or monitor vaccination of indigenous equine species which neither take an active part in competition nor travel nationally or internationally. Nevertheless, mandatory vaccination of the high-risk group has reduced the prevalence of equine influenza in Europe in the past decade.

Vaccines against equine influenza are usually inactivated, whole-virus vaccines containing at least one representative of each subtype (H7N7 and H3N8). Many vaccines include two strains of the H3N8 virus representing Miami/63- and Kentucky/81-like viruses.

Most equine influenza vaccines contain an aluminium-based adjuvant, although polymer and oil adjuvants are also used. Aqueous non-adjuvanted vaccines are available in some countries. Influenza vaccines can be obtained in combination with vaccines such as those for tetanus and equid herpesvirus 1.

Since the 1979 subtype 2 epidemic in Europe, in which there was clear evidence of vaccine breakdown, there have been extensive studies on the efficacy of equine influenza vaccines, particularly with respect to their HA content,[43] ability to stimulate antibody,[29, 42] and protective efficacy.[28] The failure of inactivated vaccines to perform adequately in the 1979 influenza epidemic has been largely attributed to low potency and unrealistic vaccination schedules, although antigenic differences between the A/equine-2/Miami/63 prototype virus contained in the vaccines and the A/Fontainebleau/79 variant may have contributed. A clear relationship has been demonstrated between the haemagglutinin content of vaccines, the antibody level to haemagglutinin stimulated in horses measured by the single radial haemolysis test, and protection against infection in experimental and field challenges.[28, 29, 42]

Vaccine manufacturers recommend the primary course of immunization to include two doses four to eight weeks apart, followed by a third dose at approximately six months. Thereafter, different manufacturers recommend six-, nine- or 12-monthly booster doses, with additional vaccination in high-risk situations, such as in the event of an epidemic.

These recommendations should be regarded as a minimum, since antibody stimulated after the second dose of vaccine may persist for less than eight weeks after vaccination with aqueous products, or 12–14 weeks after immunization with adjuvanted vaccines. Challenge studies using A/equine-2 virus have demonstrated that the majority of vaccinated horses are susceptible to infection six months after the primary course of two doses. This rapid decline in circulating antibody also occurs after the third dose of vaccine, and antibody levels may decline below that required for protection within three to four months.[26]

On the other hand, serological surveillance of vaccinated animals indicates that repeated vaccination with inactivated vaccines eventually results in durable antibody responses to the extent that annual revaccination is adequate for the provision of a solid immunity. For example, brood mares vaccinated in the month prior to parturition usually maintain high levels of HA antibody throughout the year.

The frequency of vaccination of mares also affects the level and duration of maternal immunity provided to their foals. This in turn affects the response of foals to primary immunization, since maternally-derived antibody may inhibit the foals' antibody response. For this reason, vaccine manufacturers recommend initiating influenza vaccination programmes in foals at three months of age. However, much younger foals are capable of mounting an immune response, and in cases where mares have little or no influenza antibody, earlier vaccination may be indicated. This approach was adopted during the epidemic of A/equine-2 in South Africa in 1986. Conversely, passively-acquired antibody in foals from dams vaccinated repeatedly may persist for four to six months or longer, and vaccination of such foals at three months of age may fail to stimulate an antibody response even after two doses of vaccine.

Foals born of sero-negative mares during an influenza outbreak may be protected by the administration of immune plasma with antibiotic cover to minimize the risk of secondary bacterial infection.

Antibody responses to equine influenza are highly variable among individual horses. More than 5 per cent of horses may fail to produce an adequate antibody response after two doses of vaccine, and even after three doses a small number of individuals fail to respond. Thus protection of individual animals in high-risk situations may require vaccination based on the results of antibody determinations.

An anamnestic response can be detected in primed animals four days after vaccination,[17] with significant levels of antibody developing seven to ten days later.

The mechanisms involved in immunity induced by vaccination and by previous infection are apparently different. While parenteral inoculation with inactivated vaccines stimulates locally produced antibody in the respiratory tract[16] and cytotoxic T-cells,[15] protection correlates most closely with HI antibody in serum. In vaccinated animals which do become infected, the suppression of clinical signs (duration of pyrexia and coughing), and the suppression of virus excretion in terms of titre and duration, is inversely proportional to the level of circulating HI antibody.

In horses that have been previously exposed to infection, immunity to re-infection only occurs in the presence of high levels of HI antibody. However, clinical protection (suppression of pyrexia and coughing), has been observed in the absence of circulating antibody,[17] and this suggests that infection is more effective than vaccination at stimulating other mechanisms of immunity such as local antibody or cell-mediated responses. Immunity capable of resisting infection may persist for only three to six months, whereas immunity to disease persists for 12–18 months.

During the febrile stage of the disease horses may be treated with non-steroidal anti-inflammatory drugs, while antibiotics such as penicillin may be useful to combat secondary infections. Horses recovering from equine influenza, even after mild or subclinical disease, should be given adequate rest before training is resumed, in order to avoid subsequent chronic respiratory disease. As a guide, the number of weeks' rest recommended is the number of days of pyrexia, with a minimum of two weeks rest, and slow resumption of work thereafter.

References

1 **ALLEN, B.V. & FRANK, C.J., 1982.** Haematological changes in two ponies before and during an infection with equine influenza. *Equine Veterinary Journal*, 14, 171–172.

2 **BEVERIDGE, W.I.B., 1968.** Influenza du cheval. *Bulletin de l'Office International des Épizooties*, 70, 305.

3 **BLUNDEN, A.S., 1988.** Animal Health Trust, Newmarket. Unpublished data.

4 **BRION, A., 1968.** La grippe et la rhinopneumonie du cheval en France. *Bulletin de l'Office International des Épizooties*, 70, 300.

5 **BRION, A., FONTAINE, M., FONTAINE, M.P. & MORAILLON, R., 1966.** Grippe du cheval: Enzooties en 1965 en France. *Recueil de Médecine Vétérinaire*, 12, 269.

6 **BRYANS, J.T., DOLL, E.R., WILSON, J.C. & ZENT, W.W., 1967.** Epizootiologic features of disease caused by Myxovirus

influenza A equine. *American Journal of Veterinary Research*, 28, 9–17.

7 **BURROWS, R., DENYER, M., GOODRIDGE, D. & HAMILTON, F., 1981.** Field and laboratory studies of equine influenza viruses isolated in 1979. *The Veterinary Record*, 109, 353–356.

8 **COOK, R.F., SINCLAIR, R. & MUMFORD, J.A., 1988.** Detection of influenza nucleoprotein antigen in nasal secretions from horses infected with A/equine influenza H3N8 viruses. *Journal of Virological Methods*, 20, 1–12.

9 **ERASMUS, B.J., 1986.** Veterinary Research Institute, Onderstepoort, South Africa. Unpublished data.

10 **FENNER, F., BACHMANN, P.A., GIBBS, E.P.J., MURPHY, F.A., STUDDERT, M.J. & WHITE, D.O., 1987.** *Veterinary Virology*. Orlando, New York, London, Sydney, Tokyo, Toronto: Academic Press, Inc.

11 **GERBER, H., 1970.** Clinical features, sequelae and epidemiology of equine influenza. *In*: BRYANS, J.T. & GERBER, H., (eds). *Second International Conference on Equine Infectious Disease*. Basel, München, New York: Karger.

12 **GERBER, H., BURKI, F., LOHRER, J. & PACCAUD, M.F., 1965.** Influenza A/equi-2 in der Schweiz. II. Epizootologie. *Zentralblatt für Veterinärmedicin*, 13, 427.

13 **GIBSON, C.A., DANIELS, R.S., McCAULEY, J.W. & SCHILD, G.C., 1988.** Haemagglutinin gene sequencing studies of equine-1 influenza A viruses. *Proceedings of the Fifth International Conference on Equine Infectious Diseases*. Kentucky: Kentucky University Press.

14 **GIBSON, W., 1751.** *A new Treatise on the Diseases of the Horse*. London: A. Minar.

15 **HANNANT, D., 1987.** Animal Health Trust, England. Unpublished data.

16 **HANNANT, D., JESSETT, D.M., O'NEILL, T., SUNDQUIST, B. & MUMFORD, J.A., 1988.** Nasopharyngeal, tracheobronchial and systemic immune responses to vaccination and aerosol infection with equine-2 influenza A virus (H3N8). *Proceedings of the Fifth International Conference on Equine Infectious Diseases*. Kentucky: Kentucky University Press.

17 **HANNANT, D., MUMFORD, J.A. & JESSETT, D.M., 1988.** Duration of circulating antibody and immunity following infection with equine influenza virus. *The Veterinary Record*, 122, 125–128.

18 **HAY, A.H. & SKEHEL, J.J., 1982.** The structure and replication of influenza virus. *In*: BEARE, A.S., (ed.). *Basic and Applied Influenza Research*. Boca Raton, Florida: CRC Press, Inc.

19 **HIGGINS, W.P., GILLESPIE, J.H., HOLMES, D.F. & ROBSON, D.S., 1987.** Surveys of equine influenza outbreaks during 1983 and 1984. *Equine Veterinary Science*, 6, 15–19.

20 **HINSHAW, V.S., NAEVE, C.W., WEBSTER, R.G., DOUGLAS, A., SKEHEL, J.J. & BRYANS, J., 1983.** Analysis of antigenic variation in equine-2 influenza A viruses. *Bulletin of the World Health Organization*, 61, 153–158.

21 **JOHN, T.J. & FULGINITI, V.A., 1966.** Parainfluenza-2 virus. Increase in haemagglutinin titre on treatment with tween-80 and ether. *Proceedings of the Society for Experimental Biology and Medicine*, 212, 109–111.

22 **JUBB, K.V., KENNEDY, P.C. & PALMER, C., 1985.** *In: Pathology of Domestic Animals*. Orlando, Florida: Academic Press, Inc.

23 **KAWAOKA, Y., BEAN, W.J. & WEBSTER, R.G., 1988.** Origin of the A/equine/Johannesburg/86 (H3N8) virus: Antigenic and genetic analyses of equine-2 influenza A haemagglutinins. *Proceedings of the Fifth International Conference of Equine Infectious Diseases*. Kentucky: Kentucky University Press.

24 **LUCAM, F., FEDIDA, M., DANNACHER, G., COUDERT, M. & PEILLON, M., 1974.** La grippe equine. Caracters de la maladie expérimentale et de l'immunité post-vaccinal. *Revue de Médecine Vétérinaire*, 125, 1273–1393.

25 **MILLER, W.M.C., 1965.** Equine influenza. Further observations on the 'coughing' outbreak 1965. *The Veterinary Record*, 77, 455–456.

26 **MUMFORD, J.A., 1985.** Animal Health Trust, England. Unpublished data.

27 **MUMFORD, J.A., HANNANT, D. & JESSETT, D., 1990.** Experimental infections of ponies with equine influenza (H3N8) virus by intranasal inoculation or exposure to aerosols. *Equine Veterinary Journal*, 22, 93–98.

28 **MUMFORD, J.A., WOOD, J.M., FOLKERS, C. & SCHILD, G.C., 1988.** Protection against experimental infection with influenza virus A/equine/Miami/63 (H3N8) provided by inactivated whole-virus vaccines containing homologous virus. *Epidemiology and Infection*, 100, 501–510.

29 **MUMFORD, J.A., WOOD, J.M., SCOTT, A.M., FOLKERS, C. & SCHILD, G.C., 1983.** Studies with inactivated equine influenza vaccine. II. Protection against experimental infection with influenza virus A/equine/Newmarket/79 (H3N8). *Journal of Hygiene*, 90, 385–395.

30 **ROSE, M.A., ROUND, M.C. & BEVERIDGE, W.I., 1970.** Influenza in horses and donkeys in Britain, 1969. *The Veterinary Record*, 86, 768–769.

31 **SCHILD, G.C., NEWMAN, R.W., WEBSTER, R.G., MAJOR, D. & HINSHAW, V.S., 1980.** Antigenic analysis of influenza A virus surface antigens: Considerations for the nomenclature of influenza virus. *Archives of Virology*, 63, 171–184.

32 **SCHOLTENS, R.G. & STEELE, J.H., 1964.** US epizootic of equine influenza 1963. *Epizootiology Public Health Report Washington*, 79, 393.

33 **SKEHEL, J.J., DOUGLAS, A.R., WILSON, I.A. & WILEY, D.C., 1982.** *In*: *Virus Resistance Symposium 33*. Society for General Microbiology Ltd., Cambridge University Press.

34 **SOVINOVA, O., TUMOVA, B., POUSKA, F. & NEMEC, J., 1958.** Isolation of a virus causing respiratory disease in horses. *Acta Virologica*, 2, 52–61.

35 **TAPLIN, W., 1796.** *The Gentleman's Stable Dictionary*. London: G.G. & J. Robinson.

36 **THOMSON, G.R., MUMFORD, J.A., SPOONER, P.R., BURROWS, R. & POWELL, D.G., 1977.** The outbreak of equine influenza in England January 1976. *The Veterinary Record*, 100, 465–468.

37 **UPPAL, P., 1987.** National Equine Centre, India. Unpublished data.

38 **VAN OIRSCHOT, J.T., MASSUREL, N., HUFFELS, A.D. & ANKER, W.J.J., 1981.** Equine influenza in the Netherlands during the winter of 1978–79: Antigenic drift of the A equi-2 virus. *The Veterinary Quarterly*, 3, 80–84.

39 **VARGHESE, J.N., LAVER, W.G. & COLMAN, P.M., 1983.** Structure of the influenza virus glycoprotein antigen neuraminidase at 2.9 °A resolution. *Nature*, 303, 35–40.

40 **WADDELL, G.H., TEIGLAND, M.B. & SIGEL, M.M., 1963.** A new influenza virus associated with equine respiratory disease. *Journal of the American Veterinary Medical Association*, 143, 587–590.

41 **WEBSTER, R.G., 1985.** WHO Influenza Centre, Memphis. Personal communication.

42 **WOOD, J.M., MUMFORD, J.A., FOLKERS, C., SCOTT, A.M. & SCHILD, G.C., 1983.** Studies with inactivated equine influenza vaccine. I. Serological responses of ponies to graded doses of vaccine. *Journal of Hygiene*, 90, 371–384.

43 **WOOD, J.M., SCHILD, G.C., FOLKERS, C., MUMFORD, J.A. & NEWMAN, R.W., 1983.** The standardisation of inactivated equine influenza vaccines by single radial immunodiffusion. *Journal of Biological Standardisation*, 11, 133–136.

91

Swine influenza

Synonyms: Pig flu, swine flu, hog flu

G.R. Thomson

Introduction and aetiology

Swine influenza is a highly contagious, acute, but generally non-fatal, respiratory disease of pigs caused by type A orthomyxoviruses. However, not all infections with these viruses result in clinical disease.

The disease was first recognized in Illinois, USA in August 1918 and described by Dr. J.S. Koen.[9, 31] The appearance of swine influenza coincided with the 1918–19 pandemic of 'Spanish flu' in humans which resulted in the death of approximately 20 million people worldwide. There is little doubt that the same virus infected both humans and pigs in the USA at that time. Whether humans or pigs were primarily infected will probably never be known because influenza viruses from pigs and people were not isolated until 1930[30] and 1933 respectively.

In pigs, infection with influenza viruses appears to be almost exclusively confined to those with the haemagglutinin (H)/neuraminidase (N) configuration H1N1 or H3N2, although infection with H1N2 viruses — probably reassortants resulting from co-infection of pigs with H1N1 and H3N2 viruses of either human or porcine origin — have been reported from Japan and China.[33, 38]

Swine influenza virus with the antigenic configuration H1N1 has persisted in the USA, particularly the Midwest, since the disease was first recognized, and has apparently since spread to such other parts of the world as Hong Kong, Italy and Japan.[4, 26] Other H1N1 viruses, which are antigenically more like avian H1N1 isolates, have recently caused widespread infection in western Europe,[14] where the disease appears to be a more serious problem than in the USA.[13]

Infection of pigs with H3N2 viruses, antigenically similar to the so-called Hong Kong influenza virus of humans which appeared in 1968 (A/Hong Kong/68), was first recognized in 1970 in Taiwan[16] and has since been demonstrated in many parts of the world. Since 1984 a variant related to the human A/Port Chalmers/1/73 strain has been associated with clinical episodes of respiratory disease in pigs: prior to 1984 H3N2 infections were only rarely associated with disease.[4]

Porcine infections with type C influenza virus have been described from Japan and China,[12, 39] but at present it appears that such infections are rare.

In southern Africa infection of pigs with swine influenza viruses has not been recognized, although it has been reported in Kenya.[28] The source of the information claiming that the infection occurs both in South Africa and Namibia *(FAO Animal Health Year Book, 1979–80)* cannot be traced and should therefore be ignored.[21]

The general characteristics of type A influenza viruses are described in **Chapter 90: Equine influenza**.

Epidemiology

Swine influenza is common in North America and western Europe and has also been identified in many countries outside those regions (i.e. China, Taiwan, Japan, Hong Kong, Israel, Thailand, Czechoslovakia, Poland, the former USSR, Brazil, Columbia, Iran, Singapore, Cuba, Mexico, India, Malaysia and Egypt).[1, 3, 4, 8, 10, 11, 17, 22, 29, 32]

Although overt disease usually has a seasonal occurrence (autumn, winter or early spring) in the USA,[11, 24] infections (as opposed to disease) occur throughout the year.[19] There is therefore no reason to postulate the existence of intermediate hosts such as lungworms or earthworms to perpetuate the infection in inter-epidemic periods.[11]

Transmission of the virus is generally by direct contact between infected pigs and susceptible individuals, although fomites may also be capable of transmitting the virus. Short distance transmission by aerosols suspended in air currents may also be possible.[34] There are no reliable data on the quantities of virus excreted by acutely infected pigs or on the duration of virus excretion, although experimental studies suggest that excretion may continue intermittently for as long as four months.[5] In other studies excretion did not occur for more than four weeks.[35] Evidence for the existence of carriers has been presented but not proved.[19]

Circumstantial evidence indicates that pigs play an important intermediary role in the transmission of influenza A viruses from birds to humans, i.e. viruses with haemagglutinins and/or neuraminidases novel to the human population (antigenic shifts — **see Chapter 90: Equine influenza**). There is a vast reservoir of influenza A viruses in both wild and domestic birds[1] but, in general, it appears that avian viruses are not directly transmissible to humans. However, in some cases pigs are susceptible to infection with at least some of these viruses of avian origin, and vice versa.[2] In birds, influenza viruses cause infection not only of the respiratory tract but also of the intestinal tract, and are excreted in the faeces. In South-east Asia it has historically been the practice to farm pigs and poultry together in close association with humans and, particularly where ponds are available, to have domestic water-fowl which may mix with wild species on the water. In such circumstances it is thought that pigs may act as 'mixing vessels' from which reassortant viruses arise following their simultaneous infection with two different viruses, and that, albeit rarely, these new viruses infect humans. In this way potentially pandemic viruses arise.[20, 40]

Although influenza A viruses replicate primarily in tissues of the respiratory tract of mammals, the finding that some viruses also replicate in the intestinal tract of ferrets resulted in this aspect being investigated in pigs.[15] However, only a human isolate (A/Hong Kong/1/68–H3N2) was excreted in the faeces — neither of the two pig isolates tested showed evidence of replication in the intestinal tract.

Pathogenesis

Virus-specific antigen has been detected in epithelial cells of the respiratory tract within two hours of experimental infection, and virions were seen budding from the surface of type II pneumocytes within five hours.[4] At 24 hours, occasional type I pneumocytes contained both intracytoplasmic and intranuclear inclusions.[36] From this observation it has been inferred that viral replication interferes not only with surfactant production and release in type II pneumocytes but also with regeneration of type I pneumocytes.[36]

The acuteness of swine influenza is illustrated by the presence in the lungs of dark red areas of consolidation less than 100 mm^2 scattered throughout the parenchymal tissue within five to 24 hours of experimental infection.[36] The fact that, at least in the USA, swine influenza occurs generally in late autumn, winter and early spring, while infections occur throughout the year, indicates that weather conditions influence the occurrence of disease, but precisely how remains to be established.

Virus levels attained in lung tissue within 24 hours of infection may be greater than 10^8 egg-infective $doses_{50}/g$ of tissue.[13]

Clinical signs

Acute onset of respiratory disease with high morbidity (approaching 100 per cent) characterizes outbreaks of swine influenza in piggeries. Affected animals usually have high body temperatures (up to 42,8 °C),[25, 34] lie huddled together and are disinclined to move even when disturbed. Severe cases may suffer from apparent muscular weakness and prostration. Respiration is jerky and abdominal and affected pigs often cough paroxysmally, especially when disturbed. During coughing they adopt a typical kyphotic posture.[4] Serous oculonasal discharges are frequent and there may be erythema of the skin, particularly in the perineal area.[11] Diarrhoea and vomiting have also been described.[24]

The course of the disease typically lasts three to seven days, with the speed of recovery being as rapid as the onset, although severely affected individuals may take some weeks to regain their previous condition, as severe tissue-wasting accompanies the acute disease. Mortality rates are usually less than 1 per cent, but secondary bacterial infections may increase the severity and mortality rate of the disease.[24, 25]

A severe proliferating and necrotizing pneumonia in pigs, in which influenza infection may be involved, has recently been described in Canada.[18] There is uncertainty as to whether swine influenza is capable of causing pre- and perinatal mortality subsequent to intra-uterine infection as experimental investigations have produced conflicting results.[7, 37] However, bearing in mind the features of type A influenza infections in other species, this seems unlikely.

Pathology

In severe cases the mucosa of the nasal turbinates, pharynx, larynx, trachea and large bronchi may be hyperaemic, swollen and covered by a tenacious exudate.[11] Some of the smaller bronchi and bronchioles may even be distended and occluded by the exudate, which results in lobular atelectasis of the lungs.[4] Gross lung lesions appear as sharply demarcated dark red or purple areas of consolidation, mainly in the cranioventral parts.[4] Lung oedema may be present. Alveolar epithelial necrosis with sloughing of necrotic cells occurs between 24 and 96 hours after experimental infection and is associated with alveolar oedema and diffuse interstitial pneumonia (initially neutrophilic, but subsequently histiocytic) which increase the air–blood tissue barrier by 85 per cent within 96 hours of infection.[36] Peribronchial and perivascular neutrophil and mononuclear cell infiltration have also been observed, as well as numerous polymorphonuclear granulocytes in septal capillaries,[4, 36] and platelet aggregates in septal capillaries associated with sites of endothelial swelling and detachment.[36]

Diagnosis and differential diagnosis

Swine influenza should be suspected whenever there is sudden-onset respiratory disease with high morbidity in a piggery. However, an aetiological diagnosis requires laboratory assistance because subclinical infections may occur and clinical signs are not always typical.[19]

Virus isolation and serological techniques for the diagnosis of swine influenza are essentially identical to those described for equine influenza[23] **(see Chapter 90: Equine influenza)**.

Conditions which may be confused with swine influenza are porcine pleuropneumonia, pasteurellosis, enzootic pneumonia, inclusion body rhinitis and, in mature pigs, pseudorabies (where mortality rates are lower than in immature animals). Classical swine fever, African swine fever and septicaemic bacterial infections (e.g. erysipelas and salmonellosis) should be considered when skin erythema is evident.

Control

Inactivated vaccines are used to control swine influenza in western Europe,[13] but the disease is not considered serious enough to warrant the use of vaccine in the USA.[6]

Because swine influenza viruses are potentially transmissible from pigs to humans, the ability of the virus to survive in the tissues of slaughtered pigs suffering from experimental infection has been investigated.[27] This showed that, although the virus may be present in pork, it does not survive for more than two to three weeks in deep-frozen or refrigerated storage.

References

1 **ALEXANDER, D.J., 1982.** Ecological aspects of influenza A viruses in animals and their relationship to human influenza: A review. *Journal of the Royal Society of Medicine*, 75, 799–811.

2 **ANDRAL, B., TOQUIN, D., MADEX, F., AYMARD, M., GOURREAU, J.-M., KAISER, C., FONTAINE, M. & METZ, M.-H., 1985.** Disease in turkeys associated with H1N1 influenza virus following an outbreak of the disease in pigs. *The Veterinary Record*, 116, 617–618.

3 **ANDRIES, K., PANSAERT, M. & VAN DE PUTTE, J., 1981.** Virological examination of pigs with acute respiratory disorders. *Vlaams Diergeneeskundïge Tijdschrift*, 50, 236–241.

4 **BACHMANN, P.A., 1989.** Swine influenza virus. *In:* PENSAERT, M.B., (ed.). *Virus Infections of Porcines*. Amsterdam: Elsevier Science Publishers B.V.

5 **BLASKOVIC, D., JAMRICHOVA, O., RATHOVA, V., KOCISKOVA, D. & KAPLAN, M.M., 1970.** Experimental infection of weanling pigs with A/Swine influenza virus. *Bulletin of the World Health Organization*, 42, 767–770.

6 **BOFFY, P.M., 1976.** Swine flu campaign: Should we vaccinate the pigs? *Science*, 192, 870–871.

7 **BROWN, T.T., MENGLING, W.L. & PIRTLE, E., 1982.** Failure of swine influenza virus to cause transplacental infection of porcine fetuses. *American Journal of Veterinary Research*, 43, 817–819.

8 **DAS, K.P. & MALLICK, B.B., 1981.** Note on the prevalence of influenza antibodies in swine. *Indian Journal of Animal Science*, 51, 907–908.

9 **DORSET, M., McBRYDE, C.N. & NILES, W.B., 1922.** Remarks on 'hog flu'. *Journal of the American Veterinary Medical Association*, 62, 162–171.

10 **EASTERDAY, B.C., 1975.** Swine influenza. *In:* DUNNE, H.W. & LEMAN, A.D., (eds). *Diseases of Swine*. 4th edn. Ames, Iowa: Iowa State University Press.

11 **EASTERDAY, B.C., 1986.** Swine Influenza. *In*: LEMAN, A.D., STRAW, B., GLOCL, R.D., MENGELING, W.L., PENNY, R.H.G. & SCHOLL, E., (eds). *Diseases of Swine*. 6th edn. Ames, Iowa: Iowa State University Press.

12 **GUO, Y., JIN, F., WANG, P., WANG, M. & ZHU, J., 1983.** Isolation of influenza C virus from pigs and experimental infection of pigs with influenza C virus. *Journal of General Virology*, 64, 177–182.

13 **HAESEBROUCK, F. & PENSAERT, M.B., 1986.** Effect of intratracheal challenge of fattening pigs previously immunised with an inactivated influenza H1N1 vaccine. *Veterinary Microbiology*, 11, 239–249.

14 **HINSHAW, V.S., ALEXANDER, D.J., AYMARD, M., BACHMANN, P.A., EASTERDAY, B.C., HANNDUN, C., KIDA, H., LIPKIND, M., MACKENZIE, J.S., NEROME, K., SCHILD, G.C., SCHOLTISSER, C., SENNE, D.A., SHORTRIDGE, K.F., SKEHEL, J.J. & WEBSTER, R.G., 1984.** Antigenic comparisons of swine-influenza-like H1N1 isolates from pigs, birds and humans: An international collaborative study. *Bulletin of the World Health Organization*, 62, 871–878.

15 **KAWAOKA, Y., BORDWELL, E. & WEBSTER, R.G., 1987.** Intestinal replication of influenza A viruses in two mammalian species. *Archives of Virology*, 93, 303–308.

16 **KUNDIN, W.D., 1970.** Hong Kong A_2 influenza virus infection among swine during a human epidemic in Taiwan. *Nature*, 228, 857.

17 **KUPRADINUM, S., PAENPIJT, P., BHODHIKOSOOM, C., YOSHIOKA, Y., ENDO, A. & NEROME, K., 1991.** The first isolation of swine H1N1 influenza viruses from pigs in Thailand. *Archives of Virology*, 118, 289–297.

18 **MORIN, M., GIRARD, C., EL AZHARY, Y., FAJARDO, R., DROLET, R. & LAGACÉ, A., 1990.** Severe proliferative and necrotizing pneumonia in pigs: A newly recognized disease. *Canadian Veterinary Journal*, 31, 837–839.

19 **NAKAMURA, R.M., EASTERDAY, B.C., PAWLISCH, R. & WALKER, G.L., 1972.** Swine influenza: Epizootiological and serological studies. *Bulletin of the World Health Organization*, 47, 481–487.

20 **NAYLOR, E. & SCHOLTISSEK, C., 1989.** A potential human health hazard in integrated aquaculture-agriculture systems which include both pigs and poultry. *Pig News and Information*, 10, 17–18.

21 **ODEND'HAL, S., 1983.** *The Geographical Distribution of Animal Viral Diseases*. New York, London: Academic Press, Inc.

22 **OTTIS, K., SIDOLI, L., BACHMANN, P.A., WEBSTER, R.G. & KAPLAN, M.M., 1982.** Human influenza A viruses in pigs: Isolation of a H3N2 strain antigenically related to A/England/42/72 and evidence for continuous circulation of human viruses in the pig population. *Archives of Virology*, 73, 103–108.

23 **PALMER, D.F., DOWDLE, W.R., COLEMAN, M.T. & SCHILD, G.C., 1975.** *Advanced Laboratory Techniques for Influenza Diagnosis*. United States Department of Health, Education and Welfare. Immunology Series No. 6.

24 **POTGIETER, L.N.D., STAIR, E.L., MORTON, R.J. & WHITENACK, D.L., 1977.** Isolation of swine influenza virus in Oklahoma. *Journal of the American Veterinary Medical Association*, 171, 758–760.

25 **PRITCHARD, G.C., DICK, I.G.C., ROBERTS, D.H. & WIBBERLEY, G., 1987.** Porcine influenza outbreak in East Anglia due to influenza A virus (H3N2). *The Veterinary Record*, 121, 548.

26 **ROBERTS, D.H., 1989.** Pigs and influenza. *Veterinary Annual*, 29, 110–114.

27 **ROMIJN, P.C., SWALLOW, C. & EDWARDS, S., 1989.** Survival of influenza virus in pig tissues after slaughter. *The Veterinary Record*, 124, 163–166.

28 **SCOTT, G.R., 1957.** Notes on animal diseases. XI. Virus disease of pigs. *East African Agricultural Journal*, 22, 168–174.

29 **SHALABY, M.A., NAFI, B.M., SABER, M.S. & HOSNEY, A.H., 1981.** Serological studies on swine influenza in Egypt. *International Journal of Zoonoses*, 8, 100–106.

30 **SHOPE, R.E., 1931.** Swine influenza. III. Filtration, experiments and aetiology. *Journal of Experimental Medicine*, 54, 373–385.

31 **SHOPE, R.E., 1964.** Swine influenza. *In*: DUNNE, H.W., (ed.). *Diseases of Swine*. 2nd edn. Ames, Iowa: Iowa State University Press.

32 **SHORTRIDGE, K.F. & WEBSTER, R.G., 1979.** Geographic distribution of swine (Hsw1N1) and Hong Kong (H3N3) influenza virus variants in pigs in South-east Asia. *Intervirology*, 11, 9–15.

33 **SUGIMURA, T., YONEMOCHI, H., OGAWA, T., TANAKA, Y. & KUMAGAI, T., 1980.** Isolation of a recombinant influenza virus (Hsw1N2) from swine in Japan. *Archives of Virology*, 66, 271–274.

34 **TOFTS, S.W., 1986.** Porcine influenza outbreak. *The Veterinary Record*, 119, 22.

35 **VANNIER, P., GOURREAU, J.M. & KAISER, C., 1985.** Infection expérimentale de porcs exempts d'organismes pathogènes spécifiques avec une souche du virus de la grippe porcine (HSW_1N_1) et étude de la durée d'excrétion virale. *The Canadian Veterinary Journal*, 26, 138–143.

36 **WINKLER, G.C. & CHEVILLE, N.F., 1986.** Ultrastructural morphometric investigation of early lesions in the pulmonary alveolar region of pigs during experimental swine influenza infection. *American Journal of Pathology*, 122, 541–552.

37 **WOODS, G.T. & MANSFIELD, M.E., 1974.** Transplacental migration of swine influenza virus in gilts exposed experimentally. *Research Communication in Chemical Pathology and Pharmacology*, 7, 629–632.

38 **XING SHAN LI, CUI YENG ZHAO, HUI MING GAO, YU QI ZHANG, MASATOSHI ISHIDA, YUMI KANEGAE, ATSUSHI ENDO, REIKO NEROME, KATSUHIKO OMOE & KUNIAKI NEROME, 1992.** Origin and evolutionary characteristics of antigenic reassortant influenza A (H1N2) viruses isolated from man in China. *Journal of General Virology*, 73, 1329–1337.

39 **YAMAOKA, M., HOTTA, H., ITOH, M. & HOMMA, M., 1991.** Prevalence of antibody to influenza C virus among pigs in Hyoqo Prefecture, Japan. *Journal of General Virology*, 72, 711–714.

40 **YASUDA, J., SHORTRIDGE, K.F., SHIMIZU, Y. & KIDA, H., 1991.** Molecular evidence for a role of domestic ducks in the introduction of avian H3 influenza viruses to pigs in southern China, where the A/Hong Kong/68 (H3N2) strain emerged. *Journal of General Virology*, 72, 2007–2010.

CORONAVIRIDAE

Coronaviruses (so named because large, club-shaped peplomeres project from the envelope, giving the particles the appearance of a solar corona) infect the gastro-intestinal and respiratory tracts of mammals and birds. They are generally species-specific and are transmitted directly by the oral-faecal and respiratory routes.

In pigs, coronaviruses cause three distinct diseases: transmissible gastroenteritis (TGE), porcine epidemic diarrhoea, and haemagglutinating encephalomyelitis (vomiting and wasting disease). Transmissible gastro-enteritis is widely recognized as being one of the most economically important diseases of pigs.

In 1984/5 a variant of TGE virus emerged in Europe with pronounced tropism for the respiratory system. This is referred to as porcine respiratory coronavirus (PRC). Comparative studies on TGE virus and PRC have shown that PRC is probably a deletion mutant of TGE virus, but the epidemiological and pathological features of these two infections are so different that they can be considered to be separate diseases.

A bovine coronavirus has been associated with neonatal diarrhoea in calves and winter dysentery in older cattle. Putative coronaviruses have also been recognized by electron microscopy in the faeces of foals and sheep with diarrhoea, but these viruses have not yet been isolated and are not recognized in the latest (fifth) report of the International Committee on Taxonomy of Viruses.[1]

Reference

1 **FRANCKI, R.I.B., FAUQUET, C.M., KNUDSON, D.L. & BROWN, F., 1991.** Classification and nomenclature of viruses. Fifth report of the International Committee on the Taxonomy of Viruses. *Archives of Virology*, Supplementum 2, 234–236.

92

Transmissible gastroenteritis

M.B. Pensaert and P. Callebaut

Introduction

Transmissible gastroenteritis (TGE) is a highly contagious disease of piglets less than two weeks old that is characterized by vomiting, diarrhoea and high mortality. It is caused by a coronavirus infection.

The TGE virus was first isolated in the USA in 1946 from outbreaks of acute diarrhoea with high mortality in baby pigs.[6] Since then it has been reported in most parts of the world where intensive pig farming is practised, including Europe, Asia (Japan, Korea, Malaysia, Taiwan), America (North, Central and South) and Africa (Zaïre, Ghana). Until recently, it was a major cause of disease and death in piglets in the USA, Europe and elsewhere, notwithstanding the widespread application of vaccines. However, the disease has never been diagnosed in southern Africa. Since the emergence and rapid spread throughout Europe of porcine respiratory coronavirus (PRC),[14] a large proportion of the pig population has acquired immunity to PRC and, consequently, also to TGE virus. The endemicity of PRC has thus markedly decreased the clinical and economic importance of TGE **(see Chapter 93: Porcine respiratory coronavirus infection)**.

Aetiology

Transmissible gastroenteritis virus is a member of the family Coronaviridae. Virions are roughly spherical (diameter of 60–160 nm) with a fringe of widely-spaced, club-shaped projections 12–25 nm in length.[17]

The genome consists of single-stranded RNA. The virions are composed of three structural proteins: the nucleocapsid protein (N), a small membrane glycoprotein (M or E1), and a large glycoprotein constituting the viral projections (S or E2). The S glycoprotein bears the epitope responsible for inducing neutralizing antibodies as well as several epitopes that induce non-neutralizing antibodies.[5]

There is only one serotype of TGE virus, although some antigenic variation exists between field strains with different geographical origins, and between virulent and attenuated strains. Transmissible gastroenteritis virus is antigenically closely related to canine coronavirus and feline infectious peritonitis coronavirus,[10] and is distantly related to human coronavirus 229E.[16]

The virus is sensitive to lipid solvents and to various disinfectants such as formaldehyde, sodium hypochloride, iodine and quaternary ammonium compounds. It is inactivated within a few days at 37 °C and within a few hours when exposed to sunlight. Most strains of TGE virus are moderately sensitive to trypsin and are stable at pH 3. Further details on the physicochemical properties of TGE virus are given by Saif and Bohl[18] and Bohl.[2]

Transmissible gastroenteritis virus can be propagated in primary cultures of porcine kidney and thyroid cells. A continuous swine testis (ST) cell line permits the replication of most field strains. Viruses adapted to cell culture can also be grown in the continuous pig kidney cell line SK6, which is often used in serological testing. Cytopathic effects comprise syncytium formation and rounding of affected cells.[12]

Epidemiology

Pigs are the only animals for which TGE virus is pathogenic. Other non-porcine hosts such as dogs, cats and foxes have been infected experimentally, but they do not show signs of illness and the possibility that such species could be a source of infection for pigs is doubtful.

Transmission of TGE virus occurs either directly, when pigs excreting the virus come into contact with susceptible individuals, or indirectly, by contact with virus contained in faecal material or contaminated fomites. Pigs infected with TGE virus excrete the virus in their faeces for about 14 days. Even though TGE virus also replicates in the respiratory tract, spread of the virus by aerosols does not seem to occur.

On isolated small farms, the infection is self-limiting because a high level of herd immunity soon develops. Conversely, on large farms (more than 200 sows) with a continuous farrowing system, TGE virus can become endemic after the primary outbreak. Subsequent groups of pigs become infected after weaning when their maternal immunity wanes, and they in turn pass on the virus to other groups. The only clinical evidence of infection in these groups is mild diarrhoea at weaning. Typical TGE in young piglets that is associated with high mortality therefore only occurs when gilts or sows fail to provide passive protection in the form of antibodies in the colostrum and milk to their offspring.

Generally, outbreaks of TGE occur in winter. It is not known how the virus survives the summer, but viral persistence on endemically-infected farms is probably responsible.[18] The existence of long-term carrier pigs has been suggested and there are reports of virus persistence for periods of up to 104 days,[19] but this is the exception rather than the rule.

Since the emergence of PRC, typical and severe outbreaks of TGE with high mortality in new-born piglets have become rare in many European countries.

Pathogenesis

The pathogenesis of TGE in the gastrointestinal tract has been studied in detail[8, 15] and has served as a model for coronaviral diarrhoea in other animal species, such as cattle and dogs.

After ingestion, the virus passes unharmed through the stomach and replicates in the enterocytes of villous tips throughout the small intestine, resulting in rapid and massive epithelial cell necrosis, marked villous shortening or atrophy (reduction of villous length:crypt depth ratio from 7:1 to 1:1) **(Figure 92.1)**, malabsorption and diarrhoea. Vomiting is a consequence of the upper jejunum being affected. Dehydration is severe, especially in pigs up to one week of age, and is frequently the immediate cause of death. As crypt epithelium is not affected, the epithelium of affected villi begins to regenerate early in the course of the disease. The lower mortality rate which results after the infection of older pigs is possibly due either to the enterocytes being less

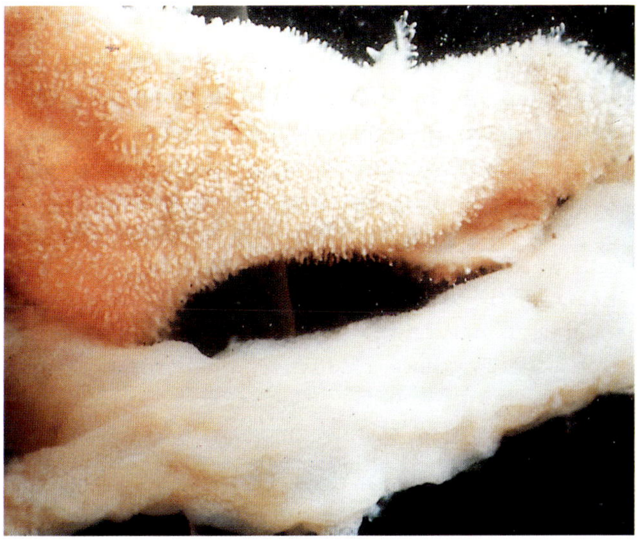

Figure 92.1 Note the marked villous atrophy in the intestine of a pig affected by transmissible gastroenteritis (lower section) compared to the villi in a healthy pig (upper section)

susceptible to infection or to their having greater regenerative capacity, or because older pigs are better able to compensate for the physiological effects of dehydration. In pigs partially protected by lactogenic immunity, the proximal jejunum is usually spared from villous atrophy, and this explains the milder course of the disease.

The effect of TGE virus on the tissues of the respiratory tract is poorly understood, but replication of TGE virus in tissues of the respiratory system does not result in manifestation of clinical disease.

Mixed infection with TGE virus and other enteric viruses or bacteria seldom occurs in neonatal piglets.

Pigs that recover from enteric infections with TGE virus develop immunity that is manifested by the appearance of antibodies of all isotypes in the circulation and IgA antibodies in intestinal secretions. It is the antibodies in the intestinal secretions and not those in the circulation which provide protection. There is complete protection against enteric reinfection for at least six months after primary infection. Thereafter, if reinfection occurs, its effects are of short duration and usually subclinical. The role of cell-mediated immunity in either recovery or protection against reinfection is still not clear.

During intestinal infection of sows, lymphocytes stimulated by viral antigens apparently migrate to the mammary gland (gut/mammary link), become plasma cells, and produce IgA antibodies against TGE virus which are then excreted in the sow's milk throughout the lactation. Piglets which ingest milk from an immune mother are protected against TGE for as long as they continue to ingest such milk regularly, and for as long as the virus doses to which they are exposed are not abnormally high. Complete passive (lactogenic) protection is afforded only if the sow has undergone intestinal infection, as viral antigens inoculated parenterally induce little or no IgA in milk.[4] This mechanism which protects pigs from enteric infections is therefore different from that which operates in cattle.

Clinical signs

The clinical signs of TGE in fully susceptible pigs (epidemic situation) differ from those observed in endemically infected herds.

In the epidemic situation, TGE is a rapidly spreading disease that is characterized by the sudden onset of acute diarrhoea in pigs of all ages, with neonatal animals being most severely affected. After an incubation period of 24 hours, the pigs may first vomit and then develop very watery faeces. Young piglets are thirsty and continue to suckle, but soon become dehydrated. They die after two or three days. In piglets infected during the first week of life, the mortality rate is high and may approach 100 per cent, but this rate decreases to almost nil in pigs that are older than two weeks of age. Usually all the litters in the farrowing house become affected within two days. Sows may be subclinically infected, may be merely anorectic, or may develop diarrhoea and agalactia. In growing and finishing pigs, a watery diarrhoea develops that lasts five to seven days. Transmissible gastroenteritis in its epidemic form spreads rapidly throughout the herd, all the animals becoming infected within a week unless special precautions are taken to prevent transmission of the virus.

Sows in the endemic situation show no signs of illness because they are immune. Piglets are also protected by antibodies in their mother's milk. The advent of weaning results in the cessation of antibody uptake from the milk, and the pig's intestine becomes susceptible to infection, which usually occurs within two to three weeks of weaning. Infection in such animals is manifested by the development of diarrhoea and the spread of the virus to subsequent groups of recently weaned pigs. In the endemic situation, diarrhoea may occasionally develop in three- to eight-day-old piglets born to non-immune or partially immune sows or gilts. The mortality rate in partially protected piglets is variable.

Pathology

The gross lesions in pigs that die of TGE are essentially those of dehydration. Histologically, villous atrophy is the main lesion, and the shortened villi are usually covered with flat to cuboidal epithelium **(Figure 92.2)**, with the number of mitotic cells in the crypts markedly increased.[9] In typical cases, these lesions are present throughout the small intestine except for the first few centimetres of the duodenum. Lymphocyte infiltration is marked in the lamina propria and between the epithelial cells of the villi during recovery, when regeneration of the villous epithelium is evident.

Diagnosis

The diagnosis of TGE in neonatal piglets is best achieved by the detection of viral antigens in enterocytes by the use of immunofluorescence on cryostat sections or mucosal impression smears of the small intestine. Ideally, specimens should be collected from pigs killed soon after the onset of diarrhoea, preferably before severe dehydration occurs.

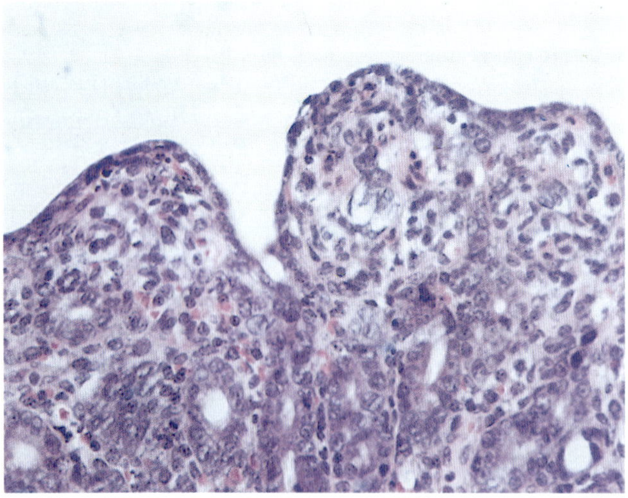

Figure 92.2 Atrophied small intestinal villi covered by cuboidal epithelial cells in a pig that died naturally of transmissible gastroenteritis

Demonstration of the virus in the faeces of pigs with diarrhoea is not always successful. The continuous pig testis cell line ST is generally the most sensitive system for virus isolation.[12] Virus replication is indicated by the presence of cytopathic effects or immunofluorescence which is aimed at the detection of viral antigen, but one or two passages may be necessary to overcome the toxicity in the original inoculum and to increase viral replication. Coronaviral particles can be detected in negatively-stained preparations of faeces from piglets with diarrhoea by transmission electron microscopy. This technique is cumbersome and time-consuming, and TGE and porcine endemic diarrhoea (PED) viruses cannot be differentiated unless immuno-electron microscopy is employed.

Viral antigens can be demonstrated by ELISA in the faeces of infected animals. Ideally, faecal samples collected from several animals at an early stage in the course of the disease should be examined.[1]

Serological diagnosis of TGE is often useful in older animals. The serum neutralization test in microtitre plates is routinely applied, and is very reliable. Cell lines, such as ST and SK6, used in conjunction with well-adapted virus strains, enable the test to be read on the basis of the presence or absence of cytopathic effects. Susceptible animals seroconvert within 14 days of primary infection.[20]

In countries where both TGE virus and PRC occur, the serodiagnosis of TGE requires the use of an ELISA system that differentiates between the two **(see Chapter 93: Porcine respiratory coronavirus infection)**.

Differential diagnosis

Typical epidemics of TGE are unlikely to be confused with outbreaks of diarrhoea caused by other enteropathogens (e.g. rotavirus and *Escherichia coli*) which are limited to suckling or recently weaned pigs. In contrast with TGE virus, none of the other enteropathogens is capable of causing mortality approaching 100 per cent in all litters of neonatal piglets, and none spreads as quickly as TGE virus on affected premises.

Although weaned pigs are predominantly affected in outbreaks of diarrhoea due to *E. coli*, rotavirus, PED virus and coccidiosis, endemic TGE cannot be clinically differentiated from them,[13] and laboratory tests are required to confirm the diagnosis.

Control

A variety of methods for immunizing sows with the aim of inducing lactogenic immunity and consequent protection of neonatal piglets has been attempted.[3, 11, 20] Intramuscular or intramammary inoculation of sows with live, inactivated or subunit vaccines during pregnancy has not resulted in complete protection, although it has achieved decreased mortality rates. Vaccination of pregnant sows with live attenuated TGE virus has provided variable results, but complete lactogenic protection is not achieved. Attenuated virus apparently does not stimulate the gut/mammary link sufficiently for the induction of lactogenic immunity similar to that following natural intestinal infection with virulent virus. Feeding virulent virus to sows is effective in this respect, but it also propagates the disease on the farm unless all the sows are immunized. This practice results in the rapid development of immunity in pregnant sows (particularly in those due to farrow two weeks or more after the start of the outbreak) and so minimizes losses in new-born piglets. It may also result in dissemination of the virus to adjacent herds.

Elimination of endemic TGE in a herd can be attempted by deliberately infecting all the sows and weaned pigs simultaneously with virulent virus. If this is done, no weaning of piglets should occur during the following three to four weeks, so that there are no susceptible animals present in the herd while TGE virus circulates on the farm.

Treatment of clinically affected new-born piglets with electrolyte/glucose solutions is usually ineffective in field situations, but may reduce mortality in piglets which are one week or older.

Precautions should be taken to prevent the introduction of TGE virus to susceptible herds by avoiding the introduction of animals that excrete the virus, contaminated vehicles and fomites.

Countries which are free of TGE, such as those in southern Africa, should apply stringent measures to prevent the importation of the disease. This applies not only to the importation of live animals, but also, as has recently been shown, to the tissues of slaughtered animals.[7]

References

1 **BERNARD, S., LANTIER, I., LAUDE, H. & AYNAUD, J.M., 1986.** Detection of transmissible gastroenteritis coronavirus antigens by a sandwich enzyme-linked immunosorbent assay technique. *American Journal of Veterinary Research*, 47, 2441–2444.

2 **BOHL, E.H., 1989.** Transmissible gastroenteritis virus (Classical Enteric Variant). *In*: PENSAERT, M.B., (ed.). *Virus Infections of Porcines*. Amsterdam, Oxford, New York, Tokyo: Elsevier Science Publishers.

3 **BOHL, E.H., FREDERICK, G.T. & SAIF, L.J., 1975.** Passive immunity in transmissible gastroenteritis of swine: Intramuscular injection of pregnant swine with a modified live virus vaccine. *American Journal of Veterinary Research*, 36, 267–271.

4 **BOHL, E.H. & SAIF, L.J., 1975.** Passive immunity in transmissible gastroenteritis of swine: Immunoglobulin characteristics of antibodies in milk after inoculating virus by different routes. *Infection and Immunity*, 11, 23–32.

5 **DELMAS, B., GELFI, J. & LAUDE, H., 1986.** Antigenic structure of transmissible gastroenteritis virus. II. Domains of the peplomer glycoprotein. *Journal of General Virology*, 67, 1405–1418.

6 **DOYLE, L.P. & HUTCHINGS, L.M., 1946.** A transmissible gastroenteritis in pigs. *Journal of the American Veterinary Medical Association*, 108, 257–259.

7 **FORMAN, A.J., 1991.** Infection of pigs with transmissible gastroenteritis virus from contaminated carcases. *Australian Veterinary Journal*, 68, 25–27.

8 **HAELTERMAN, E.O., 1972.** On the pathogenesis of TGE of swine. *Journal of the American Veterinary Medical Association*, 160, 534–540.

9 **HOOPER, B.E. & HAELTERMAN, E.O., 1969.** Lesions of the gastrointestinal tract of pigs infected with transmissible gastroenteritis. *Canadian Journal of Comparative Medicine*, 33, 29–36.

10 **HORZINEK, M.C., LUTZ, H. & PEDERSEN, N.C., 1982.** Antigenic relationships among homologous structural polypeptides of porcine, feline, and canine coronaviruses. *Infection and Immunity*, 37, 1148–1155.

11 **KAJI, T. & SHIMIZU, Y., 1978.** Passive immunization against transmissible gastroenteritis virus in piglets in ingestion of milk of sows inoculated with attenuated virus. *National Institute of Animal Health Quarterly*, 18, 43–52.

12 **McCLURKIN, A.W. & NORMAN, J.O., 1966.** Studies on transmissible gastroenteritis in swine. II. Selected characteristics of a cytopathogenic virus common to five isolates from transmissible gastroenteritis. *Canadian Journal of Comparative Medicine*, 30, 190–198.

13 **MORIN, M., TURGEON, D., JOLETTE, J., ROBINSON, Y., PHANEUF, J.B., SAUVAGEAU, R., BEAUREGARD, M., TEUSCHER, E., HIGGINGS, R. & LARIVERE, S., 1983.** Neonatal diarrhoea of pigs in Quebec: Infectious causes of significant outbreaks. *Canadian Journal of Comparative Medicine*, 47, 11–17.

14 **PENSAERT, M.B., CALLEBAUT, P. & VERGOTE, J., 1986.** Isolation of a porcine respiratory nonenteric coronavirus related to transmissible gastroenteritis. *Veterinary Quarterly*, 8, 257–260.

15 **PENSAERT, M.B., HAELTERMAN, E.O. & BURNSTEIN, T., 1970.** Transmissible gastroenteritis of swine: Virus–intestinal cell interactions. I. Immunofluorescence, histopathology and virus production in the small intestine through the course of infection. *Archives für die Gesamte Virusforschung*, 31, 321–334.

16 **PEREIRA, H.G., 1989.** Coronaviridae. *In*: PORTERFIELD, J.S., (ed.). *Andrew's Viruses of Vertebrates*. 5th edn. London, Philadelphia: Baillière Tindall.

17 **PHILLIP, J.I.H., CARTWRIGHT, S.F. & SCOTT, A.C., 1971.** The size and morphology of TGE and vomiting and wasting disease viruses in pigs. *The Veterinary Record*, 88, 311–312.

18 **SAIF, L.J. & BOHL, E.H., 1986.** Transmissible gastroenteritis. *In*: LEMAN, A.D., STRAW, B., GLOCK, R.D., MENGELING, W.L., PENNY, R.H. & SCHOLL, E., (eds). *Diseases of Swine*. 6th edn. Ames, Iowa: Iowa State University Press.

19 **UNDERDAHL, N.R., MEBUS, C.A. & TORRES-MEDINA, A., 1975.** Recovery of transmissible gastroenteritis virus from chronically infected experimental pigs. *American Journal of Veterinary Research*, 236, 1473–1476.

20 **VOETS, M.T., PENSAERT, M.B. & RONDHUIS, P.R., 1980.** Vaccination of pregnant sows against transmissible gastroenteritis with two attenuated virus strains and different inoculation routes. *Veterinary Quarterly*, 2, 211–219.

93

Porcine respiratory coronavirus infection

M.B. Pensaert and P. Callebaut

Introduction

Porcine respiratory coronavirus predominantly infects the respiratory tract of pigs, but it is unclear whether or not it is a pathogen of any significance under natural conditions.

In 1984, a virus that was antigenically closely related to transmissible gastroenteritis (TGE) virus appeared in the pig population of Belgium and subsequently spread rapidly to all other European countries. Unlike TGE virus, this variant does not cause an enteropathogenic infection, but it does replicate to high levels in the respiratory tract of piglets. The virus was therefore designated porcine respiratory coronavirus (PRC).[9]

Aetiology

The virions in infected cell-culture fluid have the typical morphology of coronaviruses. Infectivity is completely neutralized by antisera prepared against TGE virus and vice versa. However, an epitope which induces non-neutralizing antibodies, and which is located in the S glycoprotein of TGE virus, is absent in PRC.[1] It is most probably a natural-deletion mutant of TGE virus, the deletion being in the gene encoding the S glycoprotein.[10] It is clear that PRC is not a TGE virus vaccine strain, as all vaccine strains so far examined have the TGE virus epitope.

The virus can be cultured in primary pig kidney cells, producing discrete cytopathic effects. Porcine kidney (PD5) and, particularly, swine testis (ST) cell lines are most suitable for propagation of the virus. In these cells it causes marked cytopathic effects, notably the formation of large syncytia and the destruction of the monolayer.

Epidemiology

After its first appearance in Belgium in 1984, PRC spread rapidly in western Europe, with the result that by 1987 nearly all piggeries were infected.

Transmission of PRC occurs by respiratory aerosols containing the virus, which may be wind-borne between farms situated several kilometres apart.

In Belgium and other European countries regular episodes of infection and reinfection occur on closed breeding and breeding–fattening farms, particularly during winter and early spring. The virus probably persists on these farms by pigs between five and ten weeks of age becoming infected, at which time their maternally-derived immunity is waning. Sows may be reinfected with PRC during these waves of infection. The virus may temporarily disappear from closed herds, particularly during summer and autumn, resulting in a seronegative status of feeder and fattening pigs. However, the infection may reappear after a few months.[9] It is not known whether the virus is reintroduced from outside the herd or whether virus carriers exist.

The spread of PRC in Europe has altered the epidemiology of transmissible gastroenteritis **(see Chapter 92: Transmissible gastroenteritis)**.

Pathogenesis

Exposure of week-old piglets, delivered by hysterotomy and deprived of colostrum, to infected aerosols results in the virus replicating to high titre (up to $10^{8.3}$ $TCID_{50}$/g lung tissue) in the respiratory tract.[3] Replication occurs mainly in alveolar epithelial cells, but it also occurs in epithelial cells of nasal, tracheal, bronchial and bronchiolar pathways. Viral antigen is also present in alveolar macrophages and in tonsillar tissue. After replication at these sites, viraemia occurs and virus can be isolated from lymph nodes and parenchymal organs such as liver and spleen.[3]

Porcine respiratory coronavirus replicates to a limited degree in enterocytes located on the villi or in the crypts of the small intestine in one-week-old piglets. Infection is first detectable in the ileum and then spreads within two days to the duodenum. The infection, however, remains limited to a few cells located in or underneath the epithelial layer. This differs from TGE, where nearly all the enterocytes of the small intestine are infected. Infection of pigs by inoculation of PRC directly into the intestinal lumen can only be achieved if quantities $\geq 10^3$ $TCID_{50}$ are administered. Infectious virus is found subsequently in the faeces at low levels for between four and ten days.[4]

In six-week-old pigs aerosol infection results in high

virus titres in lung tissue, but intestinal replication cannot be demonstrated in these or in older pigs.[5]

Clinical signs

It is not clear whether or not PRC causes respiratory disease. Most field infections in pigs aged between five and ten weeks are subclinical.[9] There is, however, one report of an outbreak of respiratory disease (fever, anorexia and coughing) which was attributed to PRC infection.[7] Inoculation of pigs with PRC may result in no clinical evidence of disease,[9] in mild disease with hyperthermia, dyspnoea and growth retardation,[6] or in severe respiratory disease with laboured jerky respiration and mortality.[11] It is unclear what factors determine these different outcomes.

No clinical evidence of disease involving the gastro-intestinal tract has been observed after experimental infection with PRC of pigs of different ages.[9]

Pathology

Lobular pneumonia in the cranial and medial lobes has been observed two to three days after aerosol infection of week-old piglets which were hysterotomy derived and deprived of colostrum. These lesions may be disseminated throughout the lungs by six days after infection.[3] Similar lung lesions were also observed in older pigs after experimental inoculation.[11] Histopathologically, broncho-interstitial pneumonia and degeneration of the alveolar and bronchiolar epithelium are usually evident. Macrophages, fibrin and cellular debris are present in the lumens of bronchi and bronchioli, and in alveoli.[11]

Diagnosis and differential diagnosis

The diagnosis of PRC infections can be achieved by isolation of the virus in cell cultures from nasopharyngeal swabs or lung-tissue homogenates.

In experimental animals, PRC antigens can be demonstrated by immunofluorescence in frozen sections of lung tissue and in smears of nasal cells.[3, 8]

Serodiagnosis of PRC infection by the demonstration of neutralizing antibodies against TGE virus is only presumptive for PRC if there is no diarrhoea or history of TGE on the farm. For confirmation, the absence of antibodies directed against the differential epitope on TGE virus (see aetiology) must be demonstrated by the use of a blocking ELISA. The test necessitates the use of a monoclonal antibody specific for that epitope.[2]

Infections with organisms which, on their own or mixed with other pathogens, cause respiratory tract disease in fattening pigs include porcine influenza virus, pseudorabies virus, *Mycoplasma hyopneumoniae, Bordetella bronchiseptica, Pasteurella multocida* and *Actinobacillus (Haemophilus) pleuropneumoniae.*

Control

The role of PRC as a cause of respiratory tract disease under field conditions is still uncertain, and therefore immunoprophylaxis is presently not applied. Vaccination may be useful if additional evidence can be obtained to show that the infection can play a role in respiratory disease in fattening pigs, possibly as a contributor to a multifactorial aetiology.

References

1 **CALLEBAUT, P., CORREA, I., PENSAERT, M.B., JIMENEZ, G. & ENJUANES, L., 1988.** Antigenic differentiation between transmissible gastroenteritis virus of swine and a related porcine respiratory coronavirus. *Journal of General Virology*, 69, 1725–1730.

2 **CALLEBAUT, P., PENSAERT, M.B. & HOOYBERGHS, J., 1989.** A competitive inhibition ELISA for the differentiation of serum antibodies from pigs infected with transmissible gastroenteritis virus (TGEV) or with the TGEV-related porcine respiratory coronavirus. *Veterinary Microbiology*, 20, 9–19.

3 **COX, E., HOOYBERGHS, J. & PENSAERT, M.B., 1990.** Sites of replication of a porcine respiratory coronavirus related to transmissible gastroenteritis virus. *Research in Veterinary Science*, 48, 165–169.

4 **COX, E., PENSAERT, M.B., CALLEBAUT, P. & VAN DEUN, K., 1990.** Intestinal replication of a porcine respiratory coronavirus closely related antigenically to the enteric transmissible gastroenteritis virus. *Veterinary Microbiology*, 23, 237–243.

5 **COX, E., PENSAERT, M.B., HOOYBERGHS, J. & VAN DEUN, K., 1990.** Sites of replication of a porcine respiratory coronavirus in five-week-old pigs with or without maternal antibodies. *In*: CAVANAGH, D. & BROWN, T.D.K., (eds). *Coronaviruses and their Diseases*. New York: Plenum Publishing Corporation.

6 **DURET, C., BRUN, A., GUILMOTO, H. & DAUVERGNE, M., 1988.** Isolement, identification, et pouvoir pathogène chez le porc d'un coronavirus apparenté au virus de la gastro-enterite transmissible. *Recueil de Médecine Vétérinaire*, 164, 221–226.

7 **JESTIN, A., LE FORBAN, Y., VANNIER, P., MADDEC, F. & GOURREAU, J., 1987.** Un nouveau coronavirus porcin. Études séro-épidémiologiques rétrospectives dans les élevages de Bretagne. *Recueil de Médecine Vétérinaire*, 163, 567–571.

8 **ONNO, M., JESTIN, A., CARIOLET, R. & VANNIER, P., 1989.** Rapid diagnosis of TGEV-like coronavirus in fattened pigs by indirect immunofluorescence labelling in nasal cells. *Journal of Veterinary Medicine, series B*, 36, 629–634.

9 **PENSAERT, M.B., CALLEBAUT, P. & VERGOTE, J., 1986.** Isolation of a porcine respiratory, nonenteric coronavirus related to transmissible gastroenteritis. *Veterinary Quarterly*, 8, 257– 261.

10 **RASSCHAERT, D., DUARTE, M. & LAUDE, H., 1990.** Porcine respiratory coronavirus differs from transmissible gastroenteritis virus by a few genomic deletions. *Journal of General Virology*, 71, 2599–2607.

11 **VAN NIEUWSTADT, A.P. & POL, J.M.A., 1989.** Isolation of a TGE virus-related respiratory coronavirus causing fatal pneumonia in pigs. *The Veterinary Record*, 124, 43–44.

94

Porcine epidemic diarrhoea

M.B. Pensaert and P. Callebaut

Introduction

Porcine epidemic diarrhoea is a frequent cause of non-fatal diarrhoea in weaner, fattening and adult pigs in Europe and Asia. It is caused by a coronavirus.

Outbreaks of diarrhoea similar to transmissible gastroenteritis (TGE), but without the involvement of sucking piglets, and caused by a coronavirus distinct from TGE virus, were reported in England in 1972.[9] A coronavirus unrelated to the other porcine coronaviruses was isolated in 1978 and was named porcine epidemic diarrhoea (PED) virus.[10, 11, 15] The occurrence of specific PED virus antibodies in pigs has been reported from many countries in Europe (Belgium, England, Germany, France, the Netherlands, Switzerland, Hungary, Bulgaria) and Asia (Taiwan, China), but not from the Americas, Australia or Africa.

Aetiology

Morphologically, the virions of PED virus in faecal material have the typical appearance of coronaviruses. They are nearly spherical or pleomorphic and have a mean overall diameter of 130 nm with a fringe of club-shaped projections with a mean length of 20 nm[11] **(Figure 94.1)**.

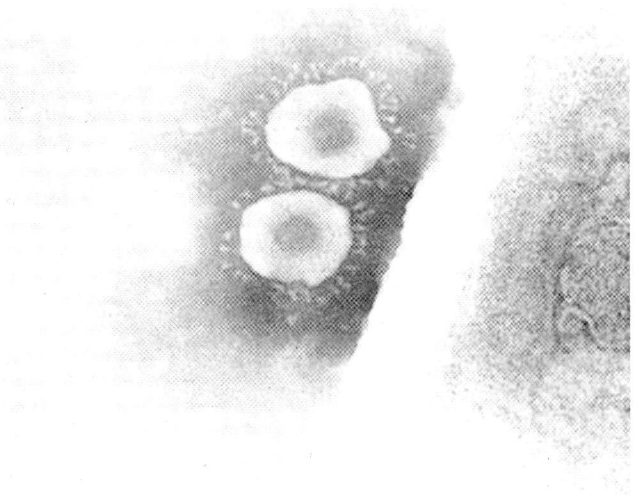

Figure 94.1 Negatively-stained porcine epidemic diarrhoea virus particles covered by typical surface projections, x 84 000

The virus has three structural proteins: an RNA-binding nucleocapsid protein, a small glycosylated membrane protein, and a large glycosylated protein that constitutes the surface projections.[6]

Porcine epidemic diarrhoea virus is antigenically related to the coronavirus which causes feline infectious peritonitis, the common antigenic determinants being located on the nucleocapsid protein.[16] Antigenic relationships to other members of the family Coronaviridae have not been found, and there are no indications that different serotypes of PED virus exist.

The virus is sensitive to ether and chloroform. It loses its infectivity when heated at 60 °C for 30 minutes, but is moderately stable at 50 °C. The virus is stable between pH 5 and 9 at 4 °C.

A strain of PED virus has been serially cultured in Vero cells treated with trypsin and maintained in serum-free medium. Cytopathic effects comprise cell vacuolation and syncytium formation.[7]

Epidemiology

Pigs appear to be the only species which are naturally infected by PED virus. Although information on the prevalence of the virus in pig populations worldwide is not available, a serological survey in Belgium showed that antibodies to it were present in fattening pigs in approximately half of the 31 farms tested.[12]

After the infection has been introduced onto breeding farms, it may either disappear or become endemic. In the latter case, subsequent groups of weaned pigs or recently introduced susceptible animals become infected by the faecal–oral route and the virus is maintained in this way. Porcine epidemic diarrhoea then becomes a regular cause of post-weaning diarrhoea on the farm.[2]

Porcine epidemic diarrhoea in its epidemic form spreads more slowly than TGE virus in a piggery, and it may take four to five weeks before animals housed in different units become infected. Some groups may even escape infection.

Pathogenesis

The pathogenesis of PED resembles that of TGE except that the colon is also involved and the lesions are less severe.[4] Why the intestines of baby piglets are less susceptible to infection with PED virus than those of older and adult pigs is unknown. Porcine epidemic diarrhoea virus replicates in the enterocytes which cover the villi in the small intestine and colon, and it causes cell necrosis and desquamation with consequent malabsorption. The virus has not been detected in organs other than the intestine. Other enteropathogens may act synergistically with PED virus in the causation of diarrhoea.

Clinical signs

On farms on which PED virus is endemic, pigs develop a watery diarrhoea within two to three weeks of weaning. Although the diarrhoea does not lead to mortality, it may retard the growth of affected animals. In situations where feeder pigs are gathered from different sources in fattening units, PED virus may similarly be a common cause of diarrhoea. The diarrhoea usually appears one to two weeks after grouping.

The introduction of PED virus onto previously uninfected farms causes diarrhoea in animals older than four to five weeks. Sucking piglets usually remain healthy even if their dams are suffering from diarrhoea. Agalactia of sows as a result of PED, with consequent poor nutrition of the piglets, may render the piglets more susceptible to other enteropathogens.

Fattening pigs reaching the end of the fattening period and adults are most severely affected. They are reluctant to stand, appear to have abdominal pain and develop watery diarrhoea. Recovery occurs after seven to ten days of illness. Mortality in adult animals may reach 1 to 2 per cent and is mainly observed in those breeds which are more sensitive to stress. Such animals die, usually during the early stages of the disease.

Pathology

Apart from the necrosis of the back muscles that is found in stress-sensitive breeds, no gross lesions are usually evident in animals that die during the acute stages of the disease. Microscopic lesions are characterized by degeneration and necrosis of enterocytes on the villi of the small intestine during the acute stage of diarrhoea, and by villous atrophy (the villi are reduced to approximately half their normal size) once the animals have been ill for two to three days.[5, 13] These lesions in the small intestine are not specific for PED and are similar to those which occur in TGE. Lesions in the colon have not been described.

Diagnosis and differential diagnosis

A clinical diagnosis of PED is difficult, if not impossible, but on breeding farms, the occurrence of severe diarrhoea of sudden onset in pigs from weaning age and older, usually in the absence of clinical signs in baby piglets, is indicative of the disease. On closed breeding–fattening farms where the sow population is immune as a result of previous infection, the disease may be limited to the fattening pigs.

An aetiological diagnosis can be made in the laboratory by demonstrating PED virus and/or its antigens in faeces, or by the detection of serum antibodies. So far, field strains of PED virus from diarrhoeic faeces cannot be routinely cultivated in cell culture. For this reason, direct immunofluorescence on frozen sections of small intestine of pigs sacrificed during the acute stage of the disease is the method of choice for the diagnosis of PED.[3] As this technique requires the sacrifice of an affected animal, it is infrequently used in older pigs. Coronaviral particles can be demonstrated by electron microscopy of negatively-stained preparations of diarrhoeic faeces. Immuno-electron microscopy is useful in differentiating PED from other coronavirus infections, especially TGE, particularly in field outbreaks.

An ELISA system is frequently used to detect PED virus antigens in faecal material of older pigs. The assay is more sensitive than electron microscopy and is very reliable if faeces are collected within three days of the onset of diarrhoea.[1]

Serological diagnosis can be effected by the use of either an indirect immunofluorescence or an immunofluorescence-blocking test applied to frozen sections of pig intestine containing PED virus antigens. A blocking ELISA may also be performed using viral antigens derived from faecal and intestinal material from pigs infected artificially, or produced in Vero cell cultures. Virus neutralization in Vero cell cultures is, however, not applicable for serum-antibody detection as the virus cannot be grown in the presence of serum. Recently, a sensitive indirect ELISA for the demonstration of antibodies has been developed, which uses PED virus produced in cell cultures.[8]

For serological testing, paired serum specimens should be collected at an interval of at least four weeks.[14] Serological diagnosis is, however, difficult in pigs which develop PED virus-induced diarrhoea shortly after weaning in the presence of circulating maternal antibodies, since in such cases clear-cut seroconversion may not be evident.

Rotavirus and *Escherichia coli* infections may mimic PED.

Control

No vaccine is available against PED. Vaccine development has been hampered by the difficulty of culturing the virus *in vitro*.

Good management practices which are generally applied to prevent the introduction of infectious agents onto farms are successful in preventing PED virus from being introduced. However, animal and human traffic cannot be avoided when feeder pigs from many breeding farms are grouped at fattening units. When an acute PED outbreak occurs in susceptible fattening pigs, it is advisable to treat affected animals symptomatically. This includes the temporary withholding of feed and the provision of an adequate supply of drinking water.

References

1 **CALLEBAUT, P., DEBOUCK, P. & PENSAERT, M.B., 1982.** Enzyme-linked immunosorbent assay for the detection of the coronavirus-like agent and its antibodies in pigs with porcine epidemic diarrhoea. *Veterinary Microbiology*, 7, 295–306.

2 **CALLEBAUT, P., PENSAERT, M.B., MIRY, C., HAESEBROUCK, F. & VERGOTE, J., 1986.** Prevalence of influenza-Aujeszky, transmissible gastroenteritis and porcine epizootic diarrhoea virus infections in feeder pigs. *Proceedings of the Ninth International Congress of the Pig Veterinary Society*, Barcelona.

3 **DEBOUCK, P., CALLEBAUT, P. & PENSAERT, M.B., 1981.** The diagnosis of coronavirus-like agent (CVLA) diarrhoea in suckling pigs. *Current Topics in Veterinary Medicine and Animal Science*, 13, 59–61.

4 **DEBOUCK, P., PENSAERT, M.B. & COUSSEMENT, W., 1981.** The pathogenesis of an enteric infection in pigs experimentally induced by the coronavirus-like agent CV777. *Veterinary Microbiology*, 6, 157–165.

5 **DUCATELLE, R., COUSSEMENT, W., PENSAERT, M.B., DEBOUCK, P. & HOORENS, J., 1982.** Pathology of experimental CV777 coronavirus enteritis in piglets. I. Histological and histochemical study. *Veterinary Pathology*, 19, 46–56.

6 **EGBERINK, H.F., EDERVEEN, J., CALLEBAUT, P. & HORZINEK, M.C., 1988.** Characterization of the structural proteins of porcine epizootic diarrhoea virus, strain CV777. *American Journal of Veterinary Research*, 49, 1320–1324.

7 **HOFMANN, M. & WYLER, R., 1988.** Propagation of the virus of porcine epidemic diarrhoea in cell culture. *Journal of Clinical Microbiology*, 26, 2235–2239.

8 **HOFMANN, W. & WYLER, R., 1990.** Enzyme-linked immunosorbent assay for the detection of porcine epidemic diarrhoea coronavirus antibodies in swine sera. *Veterinary Microbiology*, 21, 263–273.

9 **OLDHAM, J., 1972.** *Pig farming: Supplement*, October 1972, 72–73.

10 **PENSAERT, M.B., CALLEBAUT, P. & DEBOUCK, P., 1982.** Porcine epidemic diarrhoea (PED) caused by a coronavirus: Present knowledge. *Proceedings of the Seventh International Congress of the Pig Veterinary Society*, Mexico City.

11 **PENSAERT, M.B. & DEBOUCK, P., 1978.** A new coronavirus-like particle associated with diarrhoea in swine. *Archives of Virology*, 58, 243–247.

12 **PENSAERT, M.B. & HOUDART, P., 1990.** State University Ghent. Unpublished data.

13 **POSPISCHIL, A., HESS, R.G. & BACHMANN, P.A., 1981.** Light microscopy and ultrahistology of intestinal changes in pigs infected with enzootic diarrhoea virus (EVD): Comparison with transmissible gastroenteritis (TGE) virus and porcine rotavirus infections. *Zentralblatt für Veterinärmedizin, Reihe B*, 28, 564–577.

14 **WITTE, K.H. & PRAGER, D., 1987.** Der Nachweis von Antikörpern gegen das Virus der Epizootischen Virusdiarrhoe (EVD) des Schweines mit dem Immunofluoreszenzblockadetest (IFBT). *Tierärtzliche Umschau*, 42, 817–820.

15 **WOOD, E.N., 1977.** An apparently new syndrome of porcine epidemic diarrhoea. *The Veterinary Record*, 100, 243–244.

16 **YALING, R., EDERVEEN, K., EGBERINK, H., PENSAERT, M.B. & HORZINEK, M.C., 1988.** Porcine epidemic diarrhoea virus (CV777) and feline infectious peritonitis virus (FIPV) are antigenically related. *Archives of Virology*, 102, 63–71.

95

Haemagglutinating encephalomyelitis virus infection

M.B. Pensaert and P. Callebaut

Introduction

Infection with haemagglutinating encephalomyelitis (HE) virus is usually inapparent in adult pigs, but in piglets it may cause either encephalomyelitis or a condition that is characterized by vomiting and wasting.

The virus was first isolated in Canada in 1962 from the brains of very young piglets suffering from disorders of the central nervous system.[9] Because of its ability to haemagglutinate the erythrocytes of a variety of animals, and its neurotropic characteristics, the virus was called haemagglutinating encephalomyelitis virus. Subsequently, the same virus was isolated in England from pigs affected with a disease called 'vomiting and wasting disease'.

The virus has a worldwide prevalence, although the infection is often not recognized as many infections are subclinical. For this reason the infection is not economically important.

Aetiology

Haemagglutinating encephalomyelitis virus is a coronavirus with typical morphology.[14] Virus particles are spherical, with a diameter of 120 nm. They are covered by a double-layered fringe of club-shaped projections about 20 nm long **(Figure 95.1)**.

The virus contains four structural proteins, only one of which — the nucleocapsid protein — is not glycosylated. The three glycosylated proteins constitute the surface projections, the haemagglutinin and the membrane. There is only one serotype, but HE virus is antigenically related to several other coronaviruses, including human respiratory coronavirus OC43, bovine coronavirus, turkey coronavirus and mouse hepatitis virus.[7, 15]

Primary cultures of pig kidney or thyroid cells are the most sensitive system for primary isolation. Syncytium formation characterizes the cytopathic effect. The virus also replicates in several continuous porcine cell lines, such as PK15, SK6, IB-RS-2 and RPD.[3] It agglutinates erythrocytes of chicken, mouse, rat and several other animal species. Haemadsorption of the same spectrum of erythrocytes occurs on HE virus-infected cells.[13]

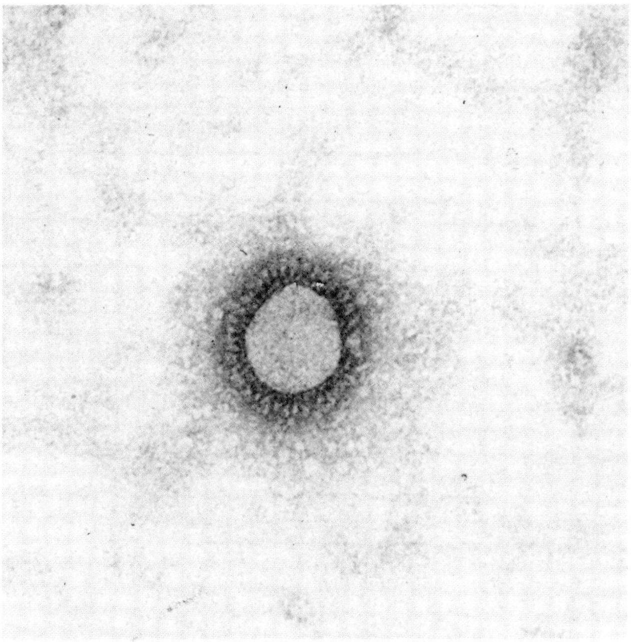

Figure 95.1 Negatively stained haemagglutinating encephalomyelitis virus particle with the characteristic double-layered fringe of surface projections

Haemagglutinating encephalomyelitis virus is sensitive to lipid solvents, including sodium deoxycholate. Infectivity is lost when heated to 56 °C for 30 minutes, but is only slightly reduced after seven days at 4 °C. The virus is stable between pH 4 and 10.

Epidemiology

Pigs are the only natural hosts of HE virus, which is endemic in most pig populations, including those in South Africa.[8] It is also prevalent in regions or countries with relatively low pig population densities. Serological surveys have shown that between 43 and 98 per cent of pigs are serologically positive in infected regions.[2]

Virus spread occurs by respiratory aerosols.

The virus is only pathogenic for pigs under two to three weeks of age, and because of its high prevalence in pig populations, most sows have experienced infection prior to parturition. Their offspring are protected by colostral antibodies which remain detectable in piglets for two to three months on average.[11] By the time natural infection occurs at four to five weeks of age, age-related resistance to the disease has developed. Passively acquired colostral immunity is thus superseded by active immunity without the occurrence of overt disease.[2, 12] The disease is therefore self-limiting, because once all the sows and gilts have become infected, maternal immunity will protect their new-born litters. This usually occurs within two to three weeks of the start of an outbreak.

Pathogenesis

The pathogenesis of HE virus infection has been studied experimentally in colostrum deprived piglets following oronasal inoculation.[4, 5] Initial infection occurs in the respiratory tract (nasal mucosa and lungs), tonsils and in a few cells whose identity has not, as yet, been determined, but which are located between the epithelial cells in the small intestine. The virus spreads from the tonsillar and respiratory sites of entry along the trigeminal and vagal nerves and their respective ganglia to the corresponding sensory nuclei in the brain stem **(Figure 95.2)**. From the intestinal plexi, it spreads neurally via local sensory ganglia to the spinal cord. Virus dissemination follows within the spinal cord and brain. Spread of virus from the primary sites of replication to neural tissues is efficiently halted by circulating antibodies.

Vomiting in the acute stage of the disease appears to be induced by viral replication in the vagal sensory ganglion, while wasting is probably the result of delayed emptying of the stomach due to virus-induced lesions in the intramural nervous plexi. Virus replication in the respiratory tract does not result in respiratory disease, but is responsible for the dissemination of virus in respiratory aerosols.

Clinical signs

There are two clinical syndromes which are caused by infection with HE virus: acute encephalomyelitis, and so-called vomiting and wasting disease. Because clinical signs only occur in piglets under three weeks of age which have failed to receive colostral antibodies from their dams, disease may be present only in the litters of non-immune gilts, while the litters of older (immune) sows in the same unit remain healthy.

Vomiting and wasting disease has an incubation period of four to seven days. The piglets continue to suckle but soon withdraw from the sow and vomit. Initially, there are no other clinical signs except for some depression and constipation. As the disease progresses, vomiting occurs after each intake of milk and results in dehydration, loss of condition and often death. Piglets which survive several days or weeks of persistent vomition become emaciated and have markedly distended abdomens. This chronic or 'wasting' syndrome lasts several weeks and leads to starvation and death. Mortality approaches 100 per cent in some litters and survivors remain stunted.

The encephalomyelitic form only occurs in piglets that are more than three days old. Initially there may be vomition, but that is soon followed by motor disorders such as muscle tremors and hyperaesthesia. As the disease progresses, signs include walking backwards, sitting dog-like, and paddling movements of the legs, or piglets may develop opisthotonus and become blind. Finally, the animals become paralysed, at which time they are often dyspnoeic. Mortality is 100 per cent in pigs that are infected

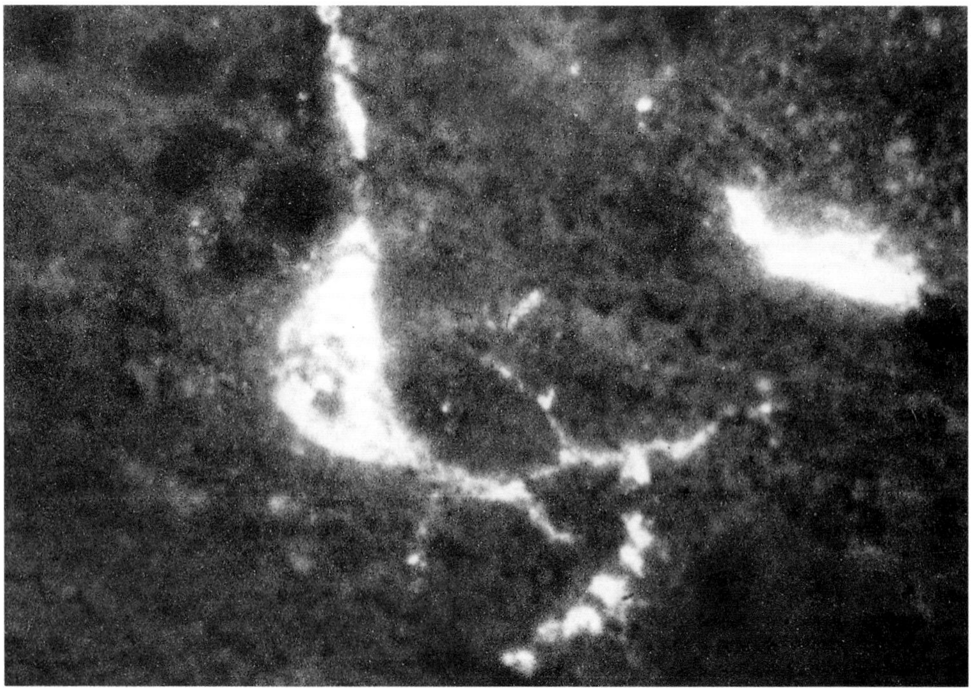

Figure 95.2 Fluorescence in the brain stem of a piglet inoculated with haemagglutinating encephalomyelitis virus

within a few days of birth. Older piglets may recover after a transient illness characterized by posterior paralysis.

Both clinical syndromes may occur on the same farm. Vomiting and wasting disease was most frequently observed in Europe[6] when HE virus was introduced during the early 1970s, while the encephalomyelitic form appears to have been predominant in North America.[17]

Pathology

The only significant gross changes are cachexia and distension of the stomach by gas in chronically affected or wasted pigs. Microscopic lesions are present mainly in the central nervous system in both clinical syndromes, and these consist of a non-suppurative encephalomyelitis characterized by perivascular cuffing, gliosis and neuronal degeneration. Lesions are most pronounced in the grey matter of the pons, the medulla oblongata and in the dorsal horns of the upper spinal cord.[1, 10]

Diagnosis and differential diagnosis

Frequent and persistent vomition in litters of piglets between four days and three weeks of age is suggestive of HE virus infection, whether or not it is accompanied by motor disorders. A definitive diagnosis requires laboratory confirmation.

Haemagglutinating encephalomyelitis virus can be isolated from suspensions of the tonsils, brain stem and lungs of piglets sacrificed in the early stages of the disease. Apart from the appearance of cytopathic effects, the presence of the virus in cell cultures can be demonstrated by haemadsorption and haemagglutination tests. Direct immunofluorescent staining of frozen sections of the brain stem has been useful for the demonstration of HE virus antigens during pathogenesis studies and may therefore be helpful in diagnosis.

Antibody determination in the sera of pigs is usually achieved by virus neutralization or haemagglutination inhibition tests.[16] Since antibodies may be detectable in the sera of piglets within six days of the start of disease, and because antibody titres in older pigs are usually the result of subclinical infection, the serological results require careful interpretation.

Pseudorabies (Aujeszky's disease) may also cause neurological disease in young piglets, but pseudorabies progresses more rapidly than HE virus infection and death usually occurs within 36 to 48 hours of the first signs of illness. In pseudorabies, furthermore, older pigs may exhibit neurological and respiratory signs and sows may abort. An outbreak of the encephalomyelitic form of porcine enterovirus (Teschen-Talfan) infection may start, as does HE virus infection, with vomition commencing four to seven days after birth. After two to three days of vomition, however, piglets will exhibit various combinations of nervous signs characterized by tremor, hyperaesthesia, paddling limb movements and paralysis leading to 100 per cent mortality during the acute phase of disease.

Control

Gilts should ideally be exposed to the virus before the first farrowing. Their offspring will then be protected by antibodies which they acquire in the colostrum. Seronegative sows may be present on small farms where the virus has not persisted or on farms where, for some reason, infection has not occurred before. For this reason, breeding animals should not be isolated from the rest of the population while growing up.

When an outbreak occurs, new-born piglets can be protected at birth by the inoculation of pooled serum collected from several sows in the slaughterhouse, since the chances are good that such pooled serum will contain specific antibodies. This procedure should be continued for litters born up to three weeks after the start of the outbreak. Thereafter, natural immunity will have developed in pregnant sows.

References

1 **ALEXANDER, T.J.L., 1962.** Viral encephalomyelitis of swine in Ontario. Experimental and natural transmission. *American Journal of Veterinary Research*, 32, 756–762.2 **ANDRIES, K., 1989.** Haemagglutinating encephalomyelitis virus. *In*: PENSAERT, M.B., (ed.). *Virus Infections of Porcines*. Amsterdam, Oxford, New York, Tokyo: Elsevier Scientific Publishers.

3 **ANDRIES, K. & PENSAERT, M.B., 1980.** Propagation of haemagglutinating encephalomyelitis virus in porcine cell cultures. *Zentralblatt für Veterinärmedizin, Reihe B*, 27, 280–290.

4 **ANDRIES, K. & PENSAERT, M.B., 1980.** Immunofluorescence studies on the pathogenesis of haemagglutinating encephalomyelitis virus after oronasal inoculation. *American Journal of Veterinary Research*, 41, 1372–1378.

5 **ANDRIES, K. & PENSAERT, M.B., 1980.** Virus isolation and immunofluorescence in different organs of pigs infected with haemagglutinating encephalomyelitis virus. *American Journal of Veterinary Research*, 41, 215–218.

6 **CARTWRIGHT, S.E. & LUCAS, M., 1970.** Vomiting and wasting disease in piglets. *The Veterinary Record*, 86, 278–280.

7 **DEA, S. & TIJSEN, P., 1989.** Detection of turkey enteric coronavirus by enzyme-linked immunosorbent assay and differentiation from other coronaviruses. *American Journal of Veterinary Research*, 50, 226–231.

8 **ESTERHUYSEN, J.J. & THOMSON, G.R., 1985.** Unpublished data. Veterinary Research Institute, Onderstepoort.

9 **GREIG, A.S., MITCHELL, D., CORNER, A.H., BANNISTER, G.L., MEADS, E.B. & JULIAN, R.J., 1962.** A haemagglutinating virus producing encephalomyelitis in baby pigs. *Canadian Journal of Comparative Medicine*, 26, 49–56.

10 **HOORENS, J., THOONEN, H., GHEYLE, M. & VAN

BUYTEN, A., 1977. Braakziekte bij biggen. *Vlaams Diergeneeskundig Tijdschrift*, 46, 209–224.

11 **PAUL, P.S. & MENGELING, W.L., 1984.** Persistence of passively acquired antibodies to haemagglutinating encephalomyelitis virus in swine. *American Journal of Veterinary Research*, 45, 932–934.

12 **PENSAERT, M.B., ANDRIES, K. & CALLEBAUT, P., 1980.** A seroepizootiologic study of vomiting and wasting disease virus in pigs. *Veterinary Quarterly*, 2, 142–148.

13 **PENSAERT, M.B. & CALLEBAUT, P., 1974.** Characteristics of a coronavirus causing vomiting and wasting in pigs. *Archives für die Gesamte Virusforschung*, 44, 35–50.

14 **PHILLIP, J.I.H., CARTWRIGHT, S.F. & SCOTT, A.C., 1971.** The size and morphology of T.G.E. and vomiting and wasting disease viruses in pigs. *The Veterinary Record*, 88, 311–312.

15 **SATO, K., INABA, Y. & MATUMOTO, M., 1980.** Serological relation between calf diarrhoea coronavirus and haemagglutinating encephalomyelitis virus. *Archives of Virology*, 66, 157–159.

16 **SATO, K., INABA, Y., MIURA, Y., TPKUHISA, S. & MATUMOTO, M., 1983.** Inducement of cytopathic changes and plaque formation by porcine haemagglutinating encephalomyelitis virus. *Veterinary Microbiology*, 8, 521–530.

17 **WERDIN, R.E., SORENSEN, D.K. & STEWART, W.C., 1976.** Porcine encephalomyelitis caused by haemagglutinating encephalomyelitis virus. *Journal of the American Veterinary Medical Association*, 168, 240–246.

96

Bovine coronavirus infection

M.B. Pensaert and P. Callebaut

Introduction

Infection with bovine coronavirus (BCV) causes neonatal diarrhoea and respiratory tract disease in calves and winter dysentery in older cattle.

A coronavirus associated with diarrhoea in three- to four-week-old calves was first reported in 1972 in the USA.[20] Since then there have been numerous reports of similar enteric coronavirus infections in calves.[29] This virus appears to have a tropism for the intestinal and respiratory tracts, although respiratory disease, if it occurs, is mild.

'Winter dysentery' involves diarrhoea in young mature cattle and has been ascribed to infection with a coronavirus which is antigenically similar, if not identical, to neonatal-calf diarrhoea coronavirus.

Aetiology

Bovine coronavirus is a typical member of the family Coronaviridae.[5] Negatively-stained virions are almost spherical but vary in size, with a mean diameter of 120 nm. Virions have a double-layered fringe of widely spaced, petal-shaped projections, approximately 20 nm in length.[32]

Virions have a buoyant density of 1,18–1,21 g/ml in sucrose and 1,24 g/ml in CsCl. In common with some other coronaviruses, BCV agglutinates chicken, mouse, rat and hamster erythrocytes. Haemadsorption of erythrocytes from these species occurs in infected cell cultures.[4]

The RNA genome has a molecular weight of $6{,}8 \times 10^6$ dalton. As with other coronaviruses, various subgenomic RNA species with molecular weights between $0{,}6 \times 10^6$ and $3{,}3 \times 10^6$ dalton are synthesized during virus replication. Virions are comprised of four structural proteins. The proteins constituting the projections, the haemagglutinin and the matrix are glycosylated and have molecular weights of 100, 124 and 25 kilodaltons respectively, while the nucleocapsid protein is unglycosylated and has a molecular weight of 53 kilodaltons.[9] Using monoclonal antibodies, it has been shown that the glycoproteins which form the projections and the haemagglutinin induce the formation of antibodies which neutralize BCV *in vitro* and protect against villous atrophy in intestinal loops of calves.[8]

There is no indication that more than one serotype of BCV exists, although some variation between strains has been demonstrated by the use of monoclonal antibodies.[12] There is close antigenic similarity between BCV isolates obtained from calves and those isolated from cattle with winter dysentery,[1] and BCV isolates derived from the intestinal and respiratory tracts of calves are probably identical.[27–29] Bovine coronavirus has close antigenic relationships with several other coronaviruses, including human coronavirus OC43, porcine haemagglutinating encephalomyelitis virus and turkey enteric coronavirus.[6, 31]

Bovine coronavirus can be grown with difficulty in primary cultures of calf and bovine foetal kidney cells. Following serial passage, it induces a discrete cytopathic effect that involves the formation of syncytia. Growth of BCV from intestinal contents has also been achieved in bovine tracheal-organ cultures and in continuous cell lines, including Vero, Madin-Darby bovine kidney (MDBK) and porcine kidney (PK15) cells. Once it has been adapted to cell culture, BCV can be cultivated in a wide variety of primary and continuous bovine cell types and in a human rectal-adenocarcinoma cell line (HRT 18). The addition of trypsin to cell-culture medium has been found to enhance virus multiplication and syncytium formation in most cell types. Trypsin appears to activate viral infectivity through proteolytic cleavage of the viral glycoprotein of the petal-shaped projections.[3]

The virus is enveloped and is therefore sensitive to lipid solvents. It is inactivated by treatment with 0,02 per cent formalin at 37 °C for 24 hours, and by heating to 50 °C for one hour, but it is stabilized in the presence of $MgCl_2$. It is stable at pH 3.

Epidemiology

Bovine coronavirus has a worldwide distribution and infects both cattle and water buffaloes (*Babalus babalis*). Antibodies to BCV have been demonstrated in sheep, but it is not known whether these antibodies are induced by BCV or by a related ovine coronavirus.

Infections and reinfections appear to occur throughout the year. Although few studies have been conducted, it is probable that in most cases initial infection occurs in calves which are less than three months of age and that in older cattle serological evidence of infection is almost universal.[13] Older calves may apparently suffer recurrent respiratory infections.[15]

Bovine coronavirus infection in calves frequently occurs during the first few days or weeks after birth, and may result in diarrhoea, particularly if it occurs in association with concomitant infections due to other enteropathogens, such as bovine rotavirus (and possibly other viruses whose enteropathogenicity under field conditions remains to be determined), *Escherichia coli*, or *Cryptosporidium* spp. The development of diarrhoea is also dependent on management practices and level of hygiene, but many, if not most, infections are subclinical. Since enteric disease mainly occurs in calves, diarrhoea due to BCV infection is generally confined to the calving season.

Bovine coronavirus is transmitted largely by the oro–faecal route, but as the virus is excreted in nasal secretions, it may also be spread via respiratory aerosols. Following experimental infection, virus excretion in faeces and nasal secretions of calves lasts for periods that range from three to 14 days.[18, 27, 29] Persistent virus excretion in the faeces has not been reported, although the virus has been detected in the faeces of healthy cows at parturition.

Outbreaks of winter dysentery are generally considered to be caused by BCV, but other factors, including sudden decreases in temperature and changes in atmospheric pressure, are also involved in the aetiology of this syndrome.[11]

Pathogenesis

It has been shown that colostrum-deprived calves inoculated orally or intranasally with a faecal isolate of BCV excreted virus in both nasal secretions and faeces.[29] All the calves developed diarrhoea, but none showed signs of respiratory disease.

Intestinal infection is characterized by virus replication in epithelial cells of the villi of the small intestine, particularly in the ileum, and in the villous and crypt epithelium of the colon. Virus replication causes necrosis resulting in loss of enterocytes, villous atrophy, and consequent malabsorption and diarrhoea. Since secretion of fluids and electrolytes in the crypts of the small intestine continues and water absorption in the colon is impaired, dehydration is inevitable. Death is a consequence of dehydration, hypoglycaemia, lactic acidaemia and hyperkalaemia.[26]

Virus replication in respiratory infection occurs in nasal epithelium, and sometimes viral antigens are also found in epithelial cells of the trachea and lungs. It has been suggested that the ability of BCV to infect the lungs and to cause pneumonic lesions may depend on the virus strain, infective dose and variation in host susceptibility.[18, 29]

As with other enteropathogenic viruses, circulating antibodies do not protect the calf's intestines against BCV infection but, when present in large numbers, serum antibodies reduce the extent of neonatal respiratory infection and possibly enteric infection. Protection of the intestine is dependent upon frequent and regular ingestion of antibodies to BCV in milk. Since such antibodies do not persist in the cow's milk for more than three days after parturition, intestinal infection and diarrhoea are often observed in suckling calves.

In animals which have recovered from infection, a local mucosal immunity develops in the intestine, but it does not persist for more than a few months and therefore reinfections (in which the course is usually subclinical) do occur. Such reinfections are thought to be responsible for the persistence of BCV in cattle populations.

Clinical signs

The incubation period in calves that have been infected experimentally is 24–48 hours. Under field conditions, particularly when new-born calves are held in close proximity to infected animals and when the antibody concentration in the cow's milk is low or absent, diarrhoea occurs at three to four days of age. Diseased calves are depressed and pass watery, yellowish faeces. Rectal temperatures are normal or may be slightly increased (up to 39,8 °C). Within two to three days of the commencement of diarrhoea the faeces contains mucus and curds but usually no blood. Severely affected calves are dehydrated, frequently unable to stand, and become comatose. Morbidity is variable but may reach 100 per cent when calves are born into a highly contaminated environment. Mortality rates are variable and are influenced by the severity of dehydration.

Respiratory tract infection resulting from BCV may occur prior to, concomitantly with, or following enteric infection in calves. However, respiratory disease does not occur in new-born animals or in calves which receive maternal antibodies. Rhinitis and coughing in animals between two and four months of age have been reported, while cattle between five and 13 months of age may develop bronchopneumonia after BCV infection in association with parainfluenza 3 virus.[21]

Winter dysentery has an incubation period of three to seven days and is characterized by the acute onset of profuse diarrhoea lasting three to six days. The liquid faeces are dark green to black, may contain blood, and have a foetid odour. Oculonasal discharges and coughing are sometimes present and faeces may be expelled during the act of coughing. The morbidity rate is variable; initially it may be 10–20 per cent but this may increase after one to two weeks to 100 per cent. Although death rarely occurs, milk production can be reduced by up to 50 per cent and the animals may temporarily lose weight.[14]

Pathology

Macroscopic lesions, except those associated with dehydration, are not found in calves that die from diarrhoea. Respiratory infection with BCV may result in the presence of small pneumonic lesions.

Microscopic lesions in the intestines depend upon the severity of the disease and the stage at which examination is performed.[10, 17, 19] Loss of enterocytes, denudation and atrophy of villi (villous length is reduced to 200–250 nm and the villous-length:crypt-depth ratio may be only 1:3) occur particularly in the distal small intestine and are most prominent during the initial stage of diarrhoea. Adjacent villi may fuse and undifferentiated cuboidal epithelial cells cover the villi. Once the villi approach their normal length (about one week after infection), immature regenerative cells become functional and numerous lymphocytes infiltrate the lamina propria and between the villous epithelial cells. The lesions observed in the small intestine as a result of BCV infection are similar to those which occur in other coronavirus infections, such as transmissible gastroenteritis and epidemic diarrhoea in pigs. Atrophy of the colonic ridges has been observed in the spiral colon.[19]

Respiratory infection with BCV results in necrosis of the pseudostratified columnar epithelial cells of the nasal cavity, of a few ciliated columnar cells in the cranial trachea, and of cuboidal cells in the mid- and caudal trachea. Histologically, parenchymal collapse and small amounts of purulent exudate may occur in some bronchioli.[28]

The lesions in the intestines of cattle with winter dysentery show some similarity to those described for calfhood coronavirus infection, but there is usually greater damage to the epithelium in the crypts of the colon.[33]

Diagnosis

Demonstration of BCV antigens in enterocytes by direct immunofluorescence staining of intestinal frozen sections is the most reliable diagnostic technique. For this purpose sections from the distal small intestine and the middle of the spiral colon should be collected from calves killed within four days of the onset of diarrhoea. Antigens of BCV can also be detected in nasal epithelial cells, and this provides a rapid and sensitive method for diagnosing upper respiratory tract infection.[15]

Coronavirus virions can be demonstrated in preparations of diarrhoeal faecal material by transmission electron microscopy. The probability of finding viral particles is increased if specimens from several animals are examined. However, recognition of coronaviral particles by this method is often difficult if their structure, in particular the fringe of surface projections, is not preserved. In addition, diarrhoeic faeces often contains fringed particles which resemble coronaviruses in morphology. In order to identify BCV particles specifically, immuno-electron microscopy should be applied.

Coronaviral antigens can be demonstrated by ELISA in faeces. The test is reliable and more sensitive than electron microscopy and has the advantage that it is suitable for handling a large number of specimens.[16]

Demonstration of infectious BCV in diarrhoeal faeces by virus isolation in cell cultures is not reliable and is not routinely performed. Cultures of primary calf kidney cells and of the continuous cell lines Vero, MDBK, PK15 and HRT 18 have been used. Virus replication is monitored by immunofluorescent staining.

Several methods can be used for the detection of antibodies to BCV. Virus-neutralization (VN) tests can be performed in cultures of a variety of continuous cell lines, including the bovine embryonic-kidney cell line (BEK-1), MDBK and HRT 18. The haemagglutination-inhibition test is performed with chicken erythrocytes, and titres generally correlate well with those obtained by VN tests.[30] Examination of paired sera (acute and convalescent phase) is necessary to make a serological diagnosis, because of the high prevalence of antibody in healthy cattle populations. Even then, some calves possessing high levels of circulating maternal antibodies at the time of infection may not show a clear rise in antibody titre. This limits the usefulness of serological diagnoses.

Differential diagnosis

A number of enteric viruses are associated with diarrhoea in calves. While the pathogenicities of BCV, bovine rotaviruses and Bredavirus (a bovine torovirus) have been established, those of Astrovirus, calici-like virus, and possibly others, are less clear. As these viral and bacterial (especially *E. coli*) infections causing diarrhoea cannot be differentiated on clinical grounds, and because mixed infections are common, definitive diagnosis requires the application of laboratory methods.

Control

Control of neonatal viral diarrhoea in calves is difficult because the aetiology is often complex, the clinical signs appear shortly after birth, and the disease has a rapid course. Oral vaccination of new-born calves with a combined vaccine containing attenuated bovine rotavirus and coronavirus induces active intestinal immunity under experimental circumstances. In the field, such vaccination has to be performed as soon as possible after birth, but antibodies to BCV in colostrum frequently neutralize the vaccine virus in the lumen of the intestine and thereby inhibit the development of active intestinal immunity. Oral immunization of calves has not, therefore, been successful.[7]

Control of BCV-induced diarrhoea in neonatal calves can only be effected by the repeated ingestion of antibodies in milk.[25] Since most cows are immune to BCV, antibodies to the virus occur regularly in colostrum. However, lactogenic protection ceases once the antibodies in the milk of cows have decreased in concentration or disappeared, which occurs at approximately three days after parturition. For this reason, feeding first-day colostrum to calves during the first eight to ten days of life is sometimes useful in controlling this neonatal disease. A colostrum bank can be made by freezing or acidifying colostrum. Feeding of stored colostrum must be done as regularly as possible so that protection of the intestine is constant.

In experimental studies, feeding calves artificial colostrum containing gamma globulins and colostral whey in which anti-BCV antibodies were present resulted in the prevention of diarrhoea upon challenge.[24]

Vaccination of cows appears to be a more efficient method of controlling BCV infections in calves.[2, 22] Immunization of cows, particularly with inactivated virus, increases the amount of antibody in colostrum and milk.[23] Neonatal diarrhoea due to BCV is either controlled or markedly reduced in severity when calves are fed the colostrum of vaccinated cows on a continuous basis. Lactogenic immunity is insufficiently potent to consistently protect calves when kept under natural conditions in the presence of a relatively high degree of virus exposure.[22]

Even when effective levels of lactogenic immunity can be achieved, calves should be born into a clean environment to minimize exposure to high concentrations of virus immediately after birth. Calves which are removed from their mothers should be individually housed and not allowed direct contact with older animals. Colostrum containing antibodies from vaccinated cows should be fed to calves on a routine basis, using containers with artificial teats for at least the first ten days of life.

The treatment of severely affected calves is aimed at minimizing dehydration. Parenteral administration of rehydrating solutions should supplement oral administration in very dehydrated calves.

References

1 **BENFIELD, D.A. & SAIF, L.J., 1990.** Cell culture propagation of a coronavirus isolated from cows with winter dysentery. *Journal of Clinical Microbiology*, 28, 1454–1457.

2 **BÜRKI, F., MÖSTL, K., SPIEGL, E., HORVATH, E. & SZELELY, H., 1986.** Reduction of rotavirus, coronavirus and *Escherichia coli* associated calf diarrhoeas in a large-size dairy herd by means of dam vaccination with a triple vaccine. *Journal for Veterinary Medicine Series B*, 33, 241–252.

3 **CYR-COATS, K.S., STORZ, J., HUSSAIN, K.A. & SCHNORR, K.L., 1988.** Structural proteins of bovine coronavirus strain L9: Effects of the host cell and trypsin treatment. *Archives of Virology*, 103, 35–46.

4 **DEA, S., ROY, R.S. & BEGIN, M.E., 1980.** Physicochemical and biological properties of neonatal calf diarrhoea coronaviruses isolated in Quebec and comparison with the Nebraska calf coronavirus. *American Journal of Veterinary Research*, 41, 23–39.

5 **DEA, S., ROY, R.S. & ELAZHARY, M.A.S.Y., 1981.** La diarrhée néonatale due au coronavirus de veau. Une revue de la littérature. *Journal of the Canadian Veterinary Journal*, 22, 51–58.

6 **DEA, S., VERBEEK, A.J. & TIJSSEN, P., 1990.** Antigenic and genomic relationships among turkey and bovine enteric coronaviruses. *Journal of Virology*, 64, 3112–3118.

7 **DE LEEUW, P.W. & TIESSINK, J.W.A., 1985.** Laboratory experiments on oral vaccination of calves against rotavirus or coronavirus induced diarrhoea. *Zentralblatt für Veterinärmedizin, Reihe B*, 32, 55–64.

8 **DEREGT, D., GIFFORD, G.A., IJAZ, M.K., WATTS, T.C., GILCHRIST, J.E., HAINES, D.M. & BABIUK, L.A., 1989.** Monoclonal antibodies to bovine coronavirus glycoproteins E2 and E3: demonstrations of *in vivo* virus-neutralizing activity. *Journal of General Virology*, 70, 993–998.

9 **DEREGT, D., SABARA, M. & BABIUK, L.A., 1987.** Structural proteins of bovine coronavirus and their intracellular processing. *Journal of General Virology*, 68, 2863–2867.

10 **DOUGHRI, A.M. & STORZ, J., 1977.** Light and ultrastructural pathologic changes in intestinal coronavirus infection of newborn calves. *Zentralblatt für Veterinärmedizin*, 24, 367–385.

11 **DURHAM, P.J.K., HASSARD, L.E., ARMSTRONG, K.R. & NAYLOR, J.M., 1989.** Coronavirus-associated diarrhoea (winter dysentery) in adult cattle. *Canadian Veterinary Journal*, 30, 825–827.

12 **EL GHORR, A.A., SNODGRASS, D.R., SCOTT, F.M.N. & CAMPBELL, I.A., 1989.** Serological comparison of bovine coronavirus strains. *Archives of Virology*, 104, 241–248.

13 **ELLENS, D.J., DE LEEUW, P. & STRAVER, P.J., 1979.** Recurrent rotavirus and coronavirus infections in cattle. *Les Colloques de l'INSERM, Viral Enteritis*, 90, 355–360.

14 **ESPINASSE, J., SAVEY, M. & VISO, M., 1990.** Winter dysentery of adult cattle virus. *In*: DINTER, Z. & MOREIN, B., (eds). *Virus Infections in Vertebrates*. Amsterdam, Oxford, New York, Tokyo: Elsevier Science Publishers.

15 **HECKERT, R.A., SAIF, L.J., HOBLET, K.H. & AGNES, A.G., 1990.** A longitudinal study of bovine coronavirus enteric and respiratory infections in dairy calves in two herds in Ohio. *Veterinary Microbiology*, 22, 187–201.

16 **HECKERT, R.A., SAIF, L.J. & MYERS, G.W., 1989.** Development of protein A-gold immunoelectron microscopy for detection of bovine coronavirus in calves: Comparison with ELISA and direct immunofluorescence of nasal epithelial cells. *Veterinary Microbiology*, 19, 217–231.

17 **LANGPAP, T.J., BERGELAND, M.E. & REED, D.E., 1979.** Coronaviral enteritis of young calves: Virologic and pathologic findings in naturally occurring infections. *American Journal of Veterinary Research*, 40, 1476–1478.

18 **McNULTY, M.S., BRYSON, D.G., ALLAN, G.M. & LOGAN, E.F., 1984.** Coronavirus infection of the bovine respiratory tract. *Veterinary Microbiology*, 9, 425–434.

19 **MEBUS, C.A., NEWMAN, L.E. & STAIR, E.L. Jr., 1975.** Scanning electron microscopy, light microscopy and immunofluorescent microscopy of intestine of gnotobiotic calf infected with calf diarrhoeal coronavirus. *American Journal of Veterinary Research*, 36, 1719–1725.

20 **MEBUS, C.A., STAIR, E.L., RHODES, M.B. & TWIEHAUS, M.J., 1973.** Pathology of neonatal calf diarrhoea induced by a corona-like agent. *Veterinary Pathology*, 10, 45–64.

21 **MÖSTL, K. & BÜRKI, F., 1988.** Ursächliche Beteilung boviner Coronaviren an respiratorischen Krankheistaus briichen bei Kälbern und pathogenetisch-immunologische Überlegungen hierzu. *Deutsche Tierärtzliche Wochenschrift*, 95, 19–22.

22 **MÖSTL, K. & BÜRKI, F., 1988.** Incidence of diarrhoea and of rotavirus and coronavirus shedding in calves whose dams had been vaccinated with experimental oil-adjuvanted vaccine containing bovine rotavirus and bovine coronavirus. *Journal for Veterinary Medicine Series B*, 35, 186–196.

23 **MURAKAMI, T., HIRANO, N., INOUE, A., CHITOSE, K.I., TSUCHIYA, K., ONO, K. & NAITO, Y., 1985.** Transfer of antibodies against viruses of calf diarrhoea from cows to their offspring via colostrum. *Japanese Journal of Veterinary Science*, 47, 507–510.

24 **MURAKAMI, T., HIRANO, N., INOUE, A., CHITOSE, K.I., TSUCHIYA, K., ONO, K., NAITO, Y. & YANAGIHARA, T., 1986.** Protective effect of orally administered immunoglobulins against experimental calf diarrhoea. *Japanese Journal of Veterinary Science*, 48, 237–246.

25 **MYERS, L.L. & SNODGRASS, D.R., 1982.** Colostral and milk antibody titres in cows vaccinated with a modified live-rotavirus-coronavirus vaccine. *Journal of the American Veterinary Medical Association*, 181, 486–488.

26 **PHILLIPS, R.W. & CASE, E.L., 1980.** Altered metabolism, acute shock and therapeutic response in a calf with severe coronavirus-induced diarrhoea. *American Journal of Veterinary Research*, 41, 1039–1044.

27 **REYNOLDS, D.J., 1983.** Coronavirus replication in the intestinal and respiratory tracts during infection of calves. *Annales de Recherches Vétérinaires*, 14, 445–446.

28 **REYNOLDS, D.J., DEBNEY, T.G., HALL, G.A., THOMAS, L.H. & PARSONS, K.R., 1985.** Studies on the relationship between coronaviruses from the intestinal and respiratory tracts of calves. *Archives of Virology*, 85, 71–83.

29 **SAIF, L.J., REDMAN, D.R., MOORHEAD, P.D. & THEIL, K.W., 1986.** Experimentally induced coronavirus infections in calves: Viral replication in the respiratory and intestinal tracts. *American Journal of Veterinary Research*, 47, 1426–1432.

30 **SATO, K., INABA, Y., KUROGI, H., TAKAHASHI, E., SATODA, K., OMORI, T. & MATUMOTO, M., 1977.** Haemagglutination by calf diarrhoea coronavirus. *Veterinary Microbiology*, 2, 83–87.

31 **SATO, K., INABA, Y. & MATUMOTO, M., 1980.** Serological relationship between calf diarrhoea coronavirus and haemagglutinating encephalomyelitis virus. *Archives of Virology*, 66, 157–160.

32 **STAIR, E.L., RHODES, M.B., WHITE, R.G. & MEBUS, C.A., 1972.** Neonatal calf diarrhoea: Purification and electron microscopy of a coronavirus-like agent. *American Journal of Veterinary Research*, 33, 1147–1156.

33 **VAN KRUININGEN, H.J., KHAIRALLAH, L.H., SASSEVILLE, V.G., WYAND, M.S. & POST, J.E., 1987.** Calfhood coronavirus enterocolitis: A clue to the aetiology of winter dysentery. *Veterinary Pathology*, 24, 564–567.

97

Ovine coronavirus infection

M.B. Pensaert and P. Callebaut

Virus particles that morphologically resemble coronaviruses have been detected in the faeces of sheep in Australia.[4, 5] So far, however, there is no direct evidence that these infections are associated with disease. There is also serological evidence that the infection occurs in sheep in the USA and Germany.[1–3]

It still needs to be established whether coronavirus infections of sheep are caused by a distinct coronavirus or by bovine coronavirus.

References

1 **CHENGPING, L.U., 1985.** Isolierung, Charakterisierung und Epizootiologie boviner Coronaviren. Veterinär-Medizin Dissertation, München, Germany.

2 **HARP, J.A., MYERS, L.L., RICH, J.E. & GATES, N.L., 1981.** Role of *Salmonella arizonae* and other infective agents in enteric disease of lambs. *American Journal of Veterinary Research*, 42, 596–599.

3 **LIEBERMANN, H.G. & HEROLD, M., 1986.** Coronavirus-infektionen bei schafen (Kurzmitteilung). *Monatshefte für Veterinär-Medizin*, 41, 814–815.

4 **PASS, D.A., PENHALE, W.J., WILCOX, G.E. & BATEY, R.G., 1982.** Intestinal coronavirus-like particles in sheep with diarrhoea. *The Veterinary Record*, 111, 106–107.

5 **TZIPORI, S., SMITH, M., MAKIN, T. & McCAUGHAN, C., 1978.** Enteric coronavirus-like particles in sheep. *Australian Veterinary Journal*, 54, 320–321.

98

Equine coronavirus infection

M.B. Pensaert and P. Callebaut

A virus designated as a coronavirus on the basis of its morphology was observed in the faeces of diarrhoeic foals in 1975 in the USA and named foal enteritis coronavirus.[1] This virus has neither been cultured nor definitely classified as a separate member of the family Coronaviridae. All the reports related to the equine coronavirus are based on the detection of coronavirus-like particles by electron microscopy.

It seems to have been established that there is an association between coronavirus infection and diarrhoea in foals.[5, 6] The disease is characterized by profuse watery diarrhoea, fever, extensive lymphatic involvement and a high mortality rate. In one case, coronavirus infection was detected in a four-week-old Arabian colt with combined immunodeficiency syndrome which was showing profuse watery diarrhoea.[4]

In nearly all the investigations into equine coronavirus infection, disease was observed in foals during the first week of life. According to one, however, a coronavirus-like agent was detected in mature horses suffering from acute diarrhoea.[3] There is some doubt about the morphology of the particles which, in the authors' opinion, represented fringed particles often found in remnants of cells (probably representing pieces of fused cell membrane).

A coronavirus was detected in homogenized lung tissue from an aborted equine foetus of five-and-a-half months' gestation.[2] The stable to which the mare belonged had had a severe problem with chronic diarrhoea. However, a causative relationship between the diarrhoea and the abortion was not established and the significance of the coronavirus in the aborted foetus is unclear.

References

1 **BASS, E.P. & SHARPEE, R.L., 1975.** Coronavirus and gastroenteritis in foals. *The Lancet*, 2, 822.

2 **EUGSTER, A.K. & JONES, L.P., 1980.** Coronavirus in an aborted equine foetus. *The Southwestern Veterinarian*, 33, 12.

3 **HUANG, J.C.M., WRIGHT, S.L. & SHIPLEY, W.D., 1983.** Isolation of coronavirus-like agent from horses suffering from acute equine diarrhoea syndrome. *The Veterinary Record*, 113, 262–263.

4 **MAIR, T.S., TAYLOR, R.G.R., HARBOUR, D.A. & PEARSON, G.R., 1990.** Concurrent cryptosporidium and coronavirus infections in an Arabian foal with combined immuno-deficiency syndrome. *The Veterinary Record*, 126, 127–130.

5 **TRAUB-DARGATZ, J.L., GAY, C.C., EVERMANN, J.F., WARD, A.C.S., ZEGLEN, M.E., GALLINA, M.D. & SALMAN, M.D., 1988.** Epidemiologic survey of diarrhoea in foals. *Journal of the American Veterinary Medical Association*, 192, 1553–1556.

6 **WARD, A.C.S., EVERMANN, J.F. & REED, S.M., 1983.** Presence of coronavirus in diarrhoeic foals. *Veterinary Medicine*, 78, 563–565.

PARVOVIRIDAE

Members of the family Parvoviridae (*parvus* = small in Latin) are the smallest viruses (18–22 nm in diameter) which infect vertebrates. They are remarkably resistant to a range of environmental conditions that most other viruses are unable to survive, e.g. lipid solvents, pH 3–9, and heating to 56 °C for 60 minutes.[1]

Virions are isometric with icosahedral symmetry, the capsid being comprised of three (four in the case of densoviruses) polypeptides derived from a common sequence. The genome comprises a molecule of single-stranded DNA, mostly of negative sense, although some virions may contain a positive-sense molecule.[1]

Three genera *(Parvovirus, Dependovirus* and *Densovirus)* make up the family Parvoviridae. The latter are infections of insects (Diptera, Lepidoptera and Orthoptera), while the genus *Dependovirus* is more commonly known as the adeno-associated virus group. These viruses are defective since they require the presence of an adenovirus in the host cell to enable them to replicate. Adeno-associated viruses occur usually in the pharyngeal area of humans, cattle, dogs and birds, and probably also in horses and sheep. However, none so far have been shown to be pathogenic.

Parvoviruses replicate preferentially in the nuclei of rapidly dividing cells in which they frequently produce large eosinophilic or amphiphilic inclusion bodies.

Members of the genus *Parvovirus* infect a wide range of mammals and birds, the most common amongst domestic livestock being porcine and bovine parvoviruses. Porcine parvovirus is an important cause of reproductive failure in gilts and young sows throughout the world. The pathogenic potential of bovine parvovirus is less well understood. Feline parvovirus (feline panleukopenia virus) causes a devastating disease of cats, and variants of this virus are pathogenic in a number of other carnivore species, such as dogs (canine parvovirus), mink (mink enteritis virus) and raccoons (raccoon parvovirus).

Reference

1 **SIEGL, G., 1991.** Parvoviridae. *In:* FRANCKI, R.I.B., FAUQUET, C.M., KNUDSON, D.L. & BROWN, F., (eds). Classification and nomenclature of viruses. Fifth report of the International Committee on the Taxonomy of Viruses. *Archives of Virology,* Supplementum 2. Vienna, New York: Springer-Verlag.

99

Porcine parvovirus infection

G.R. Thomson and L. Prozesky

Introduction

Porcine parvovirus (PPV) is a common cause of reproductive failure — principally foetal death and mummification — in pigs.

The association between PPV and porcine infertility was first demonstrated by Cartwright and Huck in 1967,[7] although the virus had previously been identified in stocks of hog cholera (classical swine fever) virus grown in cell culture.[25] Subsequent investigation showed that PPV is widespread in all pig populations but that it is non-pathogenic in pigs infected after birth. In pregnant animals, however, the virus is able to cross the placental barrier and infect embryos and foetuses. In foetuses younger than approximately 60–70 days of gestation, infection is usually fatal. The ability of older foetuses to withstand infection appears to be associated with the onset of immunological competence.

Porcine parvovirus is probably the most important infectious cause of reproductive failure in pigs throughout the world and is undoubtedly a more important cause of the SMEDI (S = stillbirth, M = mummification, ED = embryonic death, I = infertility) syndrome than the porcine enteroviruses with which it was first associated. When the virus encounters a fully susceptible breeding herd it can have a devastating effect.[13, 45] It is periodically a cause of reproductive failure in pigs in southern Africa.[54, 63]

Aetiology

The genus *Parvovirus* is one of the three genera classified in the family Parvoviridae.

Virions of PPV are 18–26 nm in diameter, unenveloped and cubic in shape, and have icosahedral symmetry. Infectious virions have a buoyant density of 1,39–1,42 g/ml in CsCl,[1] while 'empty' (DNA-deficient) particles have a lower density (1,30 g/ml).[41]

The genome of PPV, as in other members of this virus family, comprises a single linear strand of DNA made up of approximately 5 000 bases[43] with Mr about 1,5–1,8 x 10^6.[53] During viral replication, the single-stranded DNA is converted to a double-stranded replicative form which serves both as a template for viral-messenger RNA synthesis and as an intermediate for the generation of progeny genomic DNA. It has been inferred that single DNA strands with negative (minus) polarity are encapsulated.[42] Genomic DNA has terminal hairpin structures at both ends as a result of palindromic (inverted repeat) sequences[42, 58, 67] and two open reading frames, the left encoding the structural polypeptides and the right the non-structural polypeptide NS1.[58] Complete nucleotide sequences of infectious clones of PPV are available.[58, 61, 67]

Three structural polypeptides (VP1, VP2 and VP3 with Mr values of 83 000, 64 000 and 60 000 respectively) and at least one non-structural polypeptide (NS1 of Mr 8 400) are encoded by the genome, VP3 being the most abundant structural protein.[41, 43] The three structural polypeptides have similar amino acid sequences and therefore, as is the case with other Parvoviridae, the lower molecular weight polypeptides are thought to be subsets of the largest polypeptide, probably derived from a common precursor.[42, 53]

Porcine parvovirus has a predilection for rapidly proliferating cells both *in vivo* and *in vitro* and there is a requirement that one or more cellular functions be associated with the late S or early G phase of the cell cycle.[53] During replication, viral proteins accumulate and are packaged in the nucleus with the formation of intranuclear inclusion bodies, margination of the chromatin and slight swelling of the nucleoli.[1] Staining with haematoxylin and eosin is usually employed to make these changes evident microscopically. In cell cultures the cytopathic effects (CPE) of viral replication develop slowly and are rarely pronounced. They eventually become evident as granulation, rounding and finally lysis of the cells. For this reason, CPE in unstained preparations are difficult to detect or to differentiate from non-specific cell degeneration.

Primary and secondary cultures of pig tissues and organs are susceptible to infection, the most commonly employed being kidney or thyroid cell cultures. Most cell lines of porcine origin have low sensitivity to PPV infection, as is the case for cells derived from animals other than pigs,[25, 55] but at least three porcine cell lines, two derived from lung tissue and one from kidney, have been shown to be suitable for the propagation of vaccine virus.[14, 57]

Intact virions of PPV agglutinate erythrocytes from a variety of species including guinea-pigs, rats, humans (type O), monkeys, mice, fowls and cats but not those of cattle, sheep or pigs.[25] Haemagglutination is most efficient at 4 °C[18, 31] and, because of the close association between haemagglutinating and virus neutralizing antibody, it is possible that a common antigen(s) is responsible for the induction of both antibody types.[25] On the other hand, animals inoculated with experimental vaccines which induce protection against foetal infection on challenge may fail to induce the development of significant haemagglutination inhibiting antibody.[14] Haemagglutinating activity is not destroyed by heating, ultraviolet irradiation or treatments with inactivants such as 0,5 per cent formalin or 0,2 per cent propiolactone which destroy infectivity.[8, 25]

A striking overall DNA homology (approximately 63 per cent) between minute virus of mice, canine parvovirus and PPV has been reported, and in the left open reading frame encoding NS1 this is even more marked (70 per cent).[58] Homologies with human parvovirus B19 and bovine parvovirus are much lower (approximately 20 per cent). Despite this genetic relationship, there are only minor antigenic similarities between porcine parvovirus and canine and feline parvoviruses.[34]

No significant antigenic heterogeneity between PPV isolates has been detected.[8, 19, 20, 44, 60]

Porcine parvovirus is extraordinarily resistant to environmental conditions and can, for example, survive heating to 56 °C for 48 hours or 70 °C for two hours, but not to 80 °C for five minutes.[8] It survives pH values between 3 and 9 for 18 hours.[44] Sodium hypochlorite (1:16 or 1:32) is an effective and safe disinfectant and destroys $10^{5,5}$ $TCID_{50}$ within five minutes.[5] Five per cent sodium hydroxide is equally effective but is less desirable because of its caustic and toxic properties.[5] Other agents such as formaldehyde solution or gas, gluteraldehyde and ultraviolet irradiation have also been evaluated but are less practical disinfectants than is sodium hypochlorite.[5]

Epidemiology

Infection with PPV is widespread in pig populations throughout the world, including those of southern Africa.[1, 7, 19, 32, 54, 60, 66] The result is that only a small proportion of herds (probably less than 5 per cent) contain exclusively seronegative individuals, usually as a consequence of a closed-herd policy.[22] Most herds consist of adults with high antibody prevalence rates (77 per cent)[46] and animals less than 12 months of age with lower rates of active immunity.[22] In South Africa and Zimbabwe, Pini[54] found herd infection rates of 90 and 50 per cent respectively, based on a serological survey of herds with a history of reproductive failure. Of the 310 sera tested (presumably from adult animals), 84 and 39 per cent had detectable antibody to PPV.

The antibody level in the colostrum of a sow may exceed that in her serum by a five- to 100-fold factor.[22] Most piglets born to multiparous sows acquire antibodies, and consequently resistance, to PPV within the first few hours of life, when they ingest colostrum. Thereafter, levels of circulating antibody in piglets decline progressively, the half-life being approximately 20 days.[52] In practice, maternally-acquired antibody levels have declined below protective levels by the time pigs are between 12 and 26 weeks of age,[21, 30, 52, 65] although protection may persist for up to 36 weeks in a small proportion.[22] Thus pigs become susceptible to infection at approximately the time when gilts are first bred (24 to 30 weeks of age).[57]

After becoming infected, pigs excrete the virus in faeces and oral secretions for about two weeks,[22, 38, 51] but the quantities of virus excreted have not so far been determined. Persistent virus-shedding has been suggested as a possibility in those pigs which survive intra-uterine infection prior to the onset of immunological competence, i.e. in immunologically tolerant animals.[20–22] The existence of such animals remains to be unequivocally proven and seems unlikely.

Infection is presumed to occur via the oronasal route, most frequently when susceptible animals encounter individuals actively excreting the virus. However, because PPV is very resistant to environmental conditions, premises which have housed infected pigs may continue to be a source of infection for four months or more.[22, 38] Gilt pens, as might be expected, are more heavily contaminated than other housing on pig farms.[22] Contaminated fomites are also likely to be infectious for protracted periods, and personnel are probably able to transfer the infection unless effectively decontaminated.[25]

Transmission of PPV from infected boars to susceptible sows and gilts may occur during mating, since it has been shown by DNA hybridization that PPV binds 'tightly' to the spermatozoa of experimentally infected boars, with 0,01–0,32 genome copies of PPV per spermatozoon being detectable.[15] However, isolation of PPV from the semen of infected boars has usually been unsuccessful,[62] and in one experiment, even when large quantities of PPV were mixed with semen and introduced artificially into the uteri of five seropositive gilts, only mild lesions were evident and four of the gilts conceived normally and contained uninfected embryos when killed 10–20 days later.[71] This supports the finding that PPV is incapable of penetrating the *zona pellucida*,[3, 70] but, on the other hand, as PPV may adhere to the surface of the *zona pellucida*, embryo transfer to susceptible sows may result in transmission of the virus.[71] Likewise, susceptible boars may acquire the infection by serving sows with PPV present in the vaginal mucus.[29]

Antibody to PPV, detected by haemagglutination inhibition tests, has been reported in 1 to 18 per cent of sera of warthogs (*Phacochoerus aethiopicus*) tested in South Africa, Zimbabwe and Namibia.[64] The pathogenic potential of PPV for warthogs, however, remains to be determined.

It has been suggested that rats may act as vectors of PPV,[25] but subsequent investigation has shown that this is unlikely to be important in practice.[10]

Pathogenesis and clinical signs

Although PPV has been reported as being associated with a variety of post-natal conditions, such as respiratory disease,[8, 31] and with a vesicular disease-like condition of pigs in mid-western states of the USA,[27] it is probably only important in the causation of embryonic and foetal death and the signs associated therewith. Abortion, although it has been ascribed to PPV infection,[56] is not usually a feature of foetal death caused by PPV.[9, 16]

In a large number of experiments and field observations designed to assess the effect of PPV on embryos (up to 30 days after conception) and foetuses (more than 30 days after conception) of different ages, the consensus is that if infection occurs at less than approximately 60–70 days, the conceptus is usually severely affected and is likely to die.[2, 3, 11, 12, 17, 21, 23, 28, 35, 39, 40, 47, 56, 71] Older foetuses, although they frequently still develop lesions and occasionally succumb, are less severely affected and respond immunologically to infection.[17, 23, 36, 47, 56, 66] Experimentally induced infection of one-day-old and six-week-old piglets produced no discernible ill effects,[6, 11] although PPV was present in all the tissues tested, particularly in lymphoid tissues.[11] The numbers of T and B cells are unaffected by infection, as are their responses to mitogens.[6]

In six- to seven-week-old pigs infected experimentally, PPV has been recovered from, or antigen detected in, a wide variety of tissues and organs (lymph nodes, salivary glands, tonsils, thymus, lungs, spleen, nasal turbinates and blood), indicating that in acutely infected pigs the virus is widely distributed in the body of the animal but the quantities of virus present have not, as yet, been accurately determined.[49, 51]

Porcine parvovirus is able to replicate in peripheral blood lymphocytes (T, B and null cells), but only if they are stimulated to proliferate by mitogens. Monocytes and peritoneal macrophages are able to phagocytose the virus, but no replication in them occurs.[50]

The association between the onset of immunological competence and increasing resistance to the effects of infection with PPV has resulted in the assumption that the ability of foetuses to mount humoral responses after approximately 55 days of conception[4] accounts for the decreased pathogenicity of PPV for older foetuses and piglets, although there is no direct proof of this.[47]

The stage of gestation at which infection of gilts or sows occurs determines the particular signs of reproductive failure that become apparent. Frequently the first sign of PPV infection in a herd is an increase in the number of gilts or sows returning to oestrus three to eight weeks after service or artificial insemination, i.e. 'repeat breeders'. This is caused by infection of embryos and young foetuses, which die and are rapidly resorbed. Such sows may show a slight vaginal discharge.[66] Experimentally, it has been shown that it takes 23–32 days for PPV to cross the placenta following oral infection; intramuscular inoculation of the virus reduces this period to 15 days.[23]

Older foetuses in which ossification has occurred are not easily resorbed and tend to be retained and become mummified. If all the foetuses are so affected, sows or gilts that were apparently pregnant lose abdominal girth and do not farrow. They are infertile and do not return to oestrus. The cause of the infertility generally only becomes apparent when they are examined after slaughter. More frequently, only a proportion of foetuses become infected and, at farrowing, smaller than normal litters are produced in which there are often one or more mummified foetuses, a characteristic feature of PPV infection.[10] In addition, there may be piglets which are smaller than normal, stillborn piglets, or even weak individuals which do not survive, but this is uncommon.

The precise mechanism whereby transplacental infection occurs remains to be determined, but the source of virus is presumably the low-grade viraemia which persists for one to six days.[1, 25, 47] However, not all foetuses are infected transplacentally; a variable proportion are infected by intra-uterine spread from adjacent infected foetuses.[1, 25, 47] This explains why foetuses frequently die at different stages of development.[33]

The virus may also affect the uterus directly and contribute to foetal loss due to placental insufficiency.[28, 40, 56] Hormonal effects, such as the failure of oestrone sulphate values to increase in sows infected experimentally during early pregnancy, may lower endometrial activity, with similar consequences.[40] Nevertheless, there is general consensus that the direct cytolytic effects of PPV on embryos and foetuses is far more important than uterine insufficiency in the causation of reproductive failure.

Pathology

Lesions in foetuses infected before they become immunologically competent include various degrees of stunting, widespread haemorrhages with the accumulation of serosanguineous fluid in body cavities, and eventually foetal death with resorption or mummification. Microscopic changes are characterized by widespread necrosis, sometimes accompanied by mineralization, and the presence of intranuclear inclusions in various organs including the liver, lungs, kidneys, brain and mesenteric and mediastinal lymph nodes.[24, 28, 35, 36, 59]

Macroscopic changes do not usually occur in foetuses infected after approximately 70 days of gestation, but in one experiment piglets which survived into the neonatal period following infection with PPV showed multifocal hepatic necrosis, accumulation of fluid in the body cavities and myocarditis.[66] Microscopically there was little damage to the myocytes in the heart, but a round cell infiltration was present. There was also perivascular cuffing in the cerebral cortex, brain stem and cerebellum. Direct proof that these lesions were caused by PPV was, however, not obtained.

Microscopic changes have been reported in foetuses exposed to PPV during the second half of gestation.[12, 37] These have varied in extent and included perivascular infiltration of mononuclear cells (lymphocytes, lymphoblasts and plasma cells) in various tissues including the meninges, brain and kidneys, accompanied by endothelial hypertrophy and hyperplasia of small blood vessels.[12, 17, 37, 56]

Uterine lesions in seropositive dams infected by transuterine inoculation of virus during either the first or second half of gestation comprised focal accumulation of mononuclear cells in the mucosa and perivascular cuffing of endometrial and myometrial vessels.[17, 56] Seronegative gilts infected at 70 days of gestation had, in addition to the lesions described in the uteri of seropositive dams, perivascular cuffs of plasma cells and lymphocytes in the brain, spinal cord and choroid of the eyes.[17, 28]

Diagnosis

A sudden increase in the number of repeat breeders followed some months later by a decrease in average litter size and litters with increased numbers of mummified foetuses is characteristic of PPV infection. Delayed returns to oestrus are, however, uncommon.[9] The initial sign of repeat breeding is sometimes missed by the farmer, with the result that the first indication of a problem is a sudden increase in the number of mummified foetuses and apparently infertile sows or gilts. Because a number of viruses which are common causes of foetal death in pigs do not occur in southern Africa, reproductive problems of this nature in pigs justify a provisional diagnosis of PPV infection. Confirmation requires laboratory support.

Foetuses which have died and become mummified before the onset of immunological competence (less than approximately 160 mm in length) are usually rich in PPV antigens, although live virus is often no longer recoverable.[25] The antigens can be demonstrated in foetal tissue suspensions (lungs, liver and kidneys) by their ability to agglutinate guinea-pig erythrocytes (the specificity of the reaction can be proved by inhibition with PPV antiserum) or by direct or indirect immunofluorescence on the same foetal organs.[12, 23, 24] In older (larger) foetuses, virus and viral antigens may be masked by the presence of antibody. However, if antibody to PPV can be demonstrated in the blood of foetuses (the chambers of the heart are the best source of blood) which are not too autolysed, in tissue suspensions prepared from decomposing foetuses, or in neonatal piglets which have not ingested colostrum, it is a good indication that infection occurred *in utero*.

Isolation of PPV from infected foetuses and piglets is not an efficient method for diagnosing the infection because it may take up to 21 days to recover the virus.[25] In addition, not only is virus recovery from foetuses which are autolysed inefficient,[25] but primary cell cultures vary in their sensitivity.[14, 57]

Serological diagnosis of infection in gilts or sows with unequivocal association with disease is usually difficult to achieve because the infection is ubiquitous. For this reason, paired sera (acute and convalescent phase) are essential, but acute phase sera are almost impossible to obtain because the acute phase of the infection is usually past by the time infection is suspected. On the other hand, finding sows or gilts that are serologically negative to PPV after suffering reproductive failure would preclude the possibility of PPV being the cause of such failure.

The conventional serological test for PPV is haemagglutination inhibition, which is unusually sensitive, and titres of over 1:100 000 are common. However, in this system relatively high titres (e.g. over 1:256) are necessary to be sure of the specificity of the reaction.[25] High haemagglutination inhibition titres develop and persist for four years or longer after the initial infection.[25] A competition ELISA test which is equally sensitive but amenable to automation has been developed.[68]

Differential diagnosis

Infection with hog cholera, pseudorabies and porcine picornaviruses may all cause the SMEDI syndrome, although other signs usually also occur in the former two infections. Fortunately, neither hog cholera nor pseudorabies occurs in southern Africa. The role of porcine picornaviruses in the SMEDI syndrome in southern Africa is unknown, as it has never been reliably determined.

A number of other infections cause reproductive failure in pigs, but these are usually associated with abortion or the birth of weak piglets, e.g. *Brucella suis*, Japanese encephalitis virus (a flavivirus confined to South-East Asia) and *Leptospira* spp. Abortion can also be caused by an array of factors, such as endotoxaemia or hormonal dysfunction, which may result in maternal failure to maintain the pregnancy.[69] Because PPV infection rarely causes abortion it should not be difficult to differentiate it from these conditions.

Control

There are basically two approaches to the control of disease caused by PPV. The first involves ensuring that the virus is actively maintained in breeding herds so that gilts are infected, and become immune, before first mating. Alternatively, gilts can be immunized prior to breeding and the immunity maintained by booster inoculations.

Since the virus is present in most large breeding herds, infection of gilts prior to first service can be promoted by enabling contact between gilts and as many other age groups as possible on the farm, particularly those aged between three and eight months. The rationale is that pigs in the latter age category are likely to have the highest infection rate. Promoting transmission on the farm can also be achieved by spreading small amounts of dung between pens — this is simpler than moving the pigs themselves. The disadvantage of this approach is that it also promotes the transmission of other infections which may not be desirable. Furthermore, one cannot ensure that all gilts become infected in the period between the waning of maternal immunity (12–26 weeks) and the time of mating (six to seven months of age). To increase the likelihood of infection prior to mating it is sometimes recommended that gilts not be bred until they are at least eight months old. This might have important economic consequences on large breeding units and is of doubtful value since in the United Kingdom it has been found that approximately 20 per cent of multiparous sows are susceptible to infection.[46]

Immunization is a more effective way of ensuring immunity in sows and gilts. Both live attenuated and inactivated vaccines are produced, but, presumably because they are safer, inactivated products are more widely used. Only inactivated vaccine is imported into South Africa **(see Chapter 8: Vaccines, herd immunity and economics: Considerations in the control of infectious diseases)**.

A PPV, designated NADL-2, which has undergone 54 passages in cell culture has been shown to be immunogenic when as little as 100 median cell culture infective doses are administered intramuscularly to seronegative pigs. The virus is apparently incapable of crossing the placenta to infect embryos and foetuses, but if inoculated directly into the fluids surrounding foetuses, replication of the virus and foetal death occurs.[48, 49] The virus is excreted in the faeces of vaccinated pigs and is able to infect susceptible animals. Oral administration of this virus is inefficient in stimulating immunity when compared to that obtained following intramuscular inoculation.[49]

Vaccines containing inactivated PPV derived from suspensions prepared from infected foetuses,[14, 72] primary porcine cell cultures[26, 33] or continuous porcine line cells[14, 57] have been shown to be effective and safe. The latter have considerable advantages with respect to characterization for microbial purity and achievement of reproducible yields.[57] A variety of inactivants encompassing aziridine compounds, formalin and ß-propiolactone are effective, as are both aluminium hydroxide and water-in-oil adjuvants.[14, 57]

Efficient application of a vaccination programme should greatly reduce the rate of circulation of PPV on large farms, and for that reason immunization of both gilts and sows according to the vaccine manufacturers' instructions is vital when a vaccination programme is instituted.

References

1 **BACHMAN, P.A., HOGAN, M.D., KURSTAK, E., MELNICK, J.L., PEREIRA, H.G., TATTERSAL, P. & VAGO, C., 1979.** Parvoviridae: Second report. *Intervirology*, 11, 248–254.

2 **BANE, D.P., JAMES, J.E., GRADIL, C.M. & MOLITOR, T.W., 1990.** *In vitro* exposure of preimplantation porcine embryos to porcine parvovirus. *Theriogenology*, 33, 553–561.

3 **BOLIN, D.R., TUREK, J.J., RUNNELS, L.J. & GUSTAFSON, D.O., 1983.** Pseudorabies virus, porcine parvovirus and porcine enterovirus interactions with the *zona pellucida* of the porcine embryo. *American Journal of Veterinary Research*, 44, 1036–1039.

4 **BOURNE, F.J., CURTIS, J., JOHNSON, R.H. & COLLINGS, D.F., 1974.** Antibody formation in porcine foetuses. *Research in Veterinary Science*, 16, 223–227.

5 **BROWN, T.T., 1981.** Laboratory evaluation of selected disinfectants as virucidal agents for porcine parvovirus, pseudorabies virus, and transmissible gastroenteritis virus. *American Journal of Veterinary Research*, 42, 1033–1036.

6 **BROWN, T.T., PAUL, P.S. & MENGLING, W.L., 1980.** Response of conventionally raised weanling pigs to experimental infection with a virulent strain of porcine parvovirus. *American Journal of Veterinary Research*, 41, 1221–1224.

7 **CARTWRIGHT, S.F. & HUCK, R.A., 1967.** Virus isolated in association with herd infertility, abortions and stillbirths in pigs. *The Veterinary Record*, 81, 196–197.

8 **CARTWRIGHT, S.F., LUCAS, M. & HUCK, R.A., 1969.** A small haemagglutinating porcine DNA virus. I. Isolation and properties. *Journal of Comparative Pathology*, 79, 371–377.

9 **CUTLER, R.S., MOLITOR, T.W., LEMAN, A.D. & WERDIN, R.E., 1983.** Farm studies on porcine parvovirus infection. *Journal of the American Veterinary Medical Association*, 182, 592–594.

10 **CUTLER, R.S., MOLITOR, T.W., SAUBER, T.E. & LEMAN, A.D., 1982.** Role of the rat in transmission of porcine parvovirus. *American Journal of Veterinary Research*, 43, 493–496.

11 **CUTLIP, R.C. & MENGLING, W.A., 1975.** Experimentally induced infection of neonatal swine with porcine parvovirus. *American Journal of Veterinary Research*, 36, 1179–1182.

12 **CUTLIP, R.C. & MENGLING, W.A., 1975.** Pathogenesis of *in utero* infection: Experimental infection of eight- and ten-week-old porcine foetuses with porcine parvovirus. *American Journal of Veterinary Research*, 36, 1751–1754.

13 **DONALDSON-WOOD, C.R., JOO, H.S. & JOHNSON, R.H., 1977.** The effect on reproductive performance of porcine parvovirus infection in a susceptible pig herd. *The Veterinary Record*, 100, 237–239.

14 **EDWARDS, K.R., EMMERSON, M.A., LUFF, P.R., WELLS, D.E., MUSKETT, J.C., WARTHALL, A.E., RICHARDSON, C., PARKER, B.N.J. & THORNTON, D.H., 1986.** Efficacy of porcine parvovirus vaccines. *The Veterinary Record*, 119, 203–205.

15 **GARDIL, C., MOLITOR, T., HARDING, M. & CRABO, B., 1990.** Excretion of porcine parvovirus through the genital tract of boars. *American Journal of Veterinary Research*, 51, 359–362.

16 **GILLICK, J.C., 1977.** An outbreak of swine foetal mummification associated with porcine parvovirus. *Australian Veterinary Journal*, 53, 105–106.

17 **HOGG, G.G., LENGHAUS, C. & FORMAN, A.J., 1977.** Experimental porcine parvovirus infection of foetal pigs resulting in abortion, histological lesions, and antibody

formation. *Journal of Comparative Pathology*, 87, 539–549.

18 **HUYGELEN, C. & PEETERMANS, J., 1967.** Isolation of a haemagglutinating picornavirus from a primary swine kidney-cell culture. *Archiv des Gesamte Virusforschung*, 20, 260–262.

19 **JOHNSON, R.H., 1973.** Isolation of swine parvovirus in Queensland. *Australian Veterinary Journal*, 49, 157–159.

20 **JOHNSON, R.H. & COLLINGS, D.F., 1969.** Experimental infection of piglets and pregnant gilts with a parvovirus. *The Veterinary Record*, 85, 446–447.

21 **JOHNSON, R.H. & COLLINGS, D.F., 1971.** Transplacental infection of piglets with a porcine parvovirus. *Research in Veterinary Science*, 12, 570–572.

22 **JOHNSON, R.H., DONALDSON-WOOD, C.R., JOO, H.S. & ALLENDER, U., 1976.** Observations on the epidemiology of porcine parvovirus. *Australian Veterinary Journal*, 52, 80–84.

23 **JOO, H.S., DONALDSON-WOOD, C.R. & JOHNSON, R.H., 1976.** Observations on the pathogenesis of porcine parvovirus. *Archives of Virology*, 51, 123–129.

24 **JOO, H.S., DONALDSON-WOOD, C.R., JOHNSON, R.H. & CAMPBELL, R.S.F., 1977.** Pathogenesis of porcine parvovirus infection: Pathology and immunofluorescence in the foetus. *Journal of Comparative Pathology*, 87, 383–391.

25 **JOO, H.S. & JOHNSON, R.H., 1976.** Porcine parvovirus: A review. *The Veterinary Bulletin*, 46, 653–660.

26 **JOO, H.S. & JOHNSON, R.H., 1977.** Serological responses in pigs vaccinated with inactivated porcine parvovirus. *Australian Veterinary Journal*, 53, 560–562.

27 **KRESSE, J.I., TAYLOR, W.D., STEINART, W.W. & EERNISSE, K.A., 1985.** Parvovirus infection in pigs with necrotic and vesicle-like lesions. *Veterinary Microbiology*, 10, 525–531.

28 **LENGHAUS, C., FORMAN, A.J. & HALL, C.J., 1978.** Experimental infection of 35-, 50- and 60-day old pig foetuses with porcine parvovirus. *Australian Veterinary Journal*, 54, 418–422.

29 **LUCAS, M.H., CARTWRIGHT, S.F. & WRATHALL, A.E., 1974.** Genital infection of pigs with porcine parvovirus. *Journal of Comparative Pathology*, 84, 347–350.

30 **McCORMICK, B.M., DRIESEN, S.J., CONNAUGHTON, I.D. & MONCKTON, R.P., 1986.** Prevalence of enteroviral and parvoviral antibodies in pig sera. *Research in Veterinary Science*, 41, 397–401.

31 **MENGLING, W.L., 1972.** Porcine parvovirus: Properties and prevalence of a strain isolated in the United States. *American Journal of Veterinary Research*, 33, 2239–2248.

32 **MENGLING, W.L., 1978.** Prevalence of porcine parvovirus-induced reproductive failure: An abattoir study. *Journal of the American Veterinary Medical Association*, 172, 1291–1294.

33 **MENGLING, W.L., BROWN, T.T., PAUL, P.S. & GUTEKUNST, D.E., 1979.** Efficacy of an inactivated virus vaccine for prevention of porcine parvovirus-induced reproductive failure. *American Journal of Veterinary Research*, 40, 204–208.

34 **MENGLING, W.L., BUNN, T.O. & PAUL, P.S., 1983.** Antigenic relationship between porcine and canine parvoviruses. *American Journal of Veterinary Research*, 44, 865–867.

35 **MENGLING, W.L. & CUTLIP, R.C., 1975.** Pathogenesis of *in utero* infection: Experimental infection of five-week-old porcine foetuses with porcine parvovirus. *American Journal of Veterinary Research*, 36, 1173–1177.

36 **MENGLING, W.L. & CUTLIP, R.C., 1976.** Reproductive disease experimentally induced by exposing pregnant gilts to porcine parvovirus. *American Journal of Veterinary Research*, 57, 1393–1400.

37 **MENGLING, W.L., CUTLIP, R.C., WILSON, R.A., PARKS, J.B. & MARSHALL, R.F., 1975.** Foetal mummification associated with porcine parvovirus infection. *Journal of the American Veterinary Medical Association*, 166, 993–995.

38 **MENGLING, W.L. & PAUL, P.S., 1986.** Interepizootic survival of porcine parvovirus. *Journal of the American Veterinary Medical Association*, 188, 1293–1295.

39 **MENGLING, W.L., PAUL, P.S. & BROWN, T.T., 1980.** Transplacental infection and embryonic death following maternal exposure to porcine parvovirus near the time of conception. *Archives of Virology*, 65, 55–62.

40 **MEYERS, P.J., LIPTRAP, R.M., MILLER, R.B. & THORSEN, J., 1987.** Hormonal changes in sows after induced porcine parvovirus infection in early pregnancy. *American Journal of Veterinary Research*, 48, 621–626.

41 **MOLITOR, T.W., JOO, H.S. & COLLETT, M.S., 1983.** Porcine parvovirus: Virus purification and structural and antigenic properties of virion polypeptides. *Journal of Virology*, 45, 842–854.

42 **MOLITOR, T.W., JOO, H.S. & COLLETT, M.S., 1984.** Porcine parvovirus DNA: Characterization of the genomic and replicative form DNA of two virus isolates. *Virology*, 137, 241–254.

43 **MOLITOR, T.W., JOO, H.S. & COLLETT, M.S., 1985.** KBSH parvovirus: Comparison with porcine parvovirus. *Journal of Virology*, 55, 257–263.

44 **MORIMOTO, T., FUTSAKI, Y., ITO, Y. & TANAKA, Y., 1972.** Biological and physiochemical properties of porcine parvovirus recovered from stillborn piglets. *The National Institute of Animal Health Quarterly*, 12, 137–144.

45 **MORRISON, R.R. & JOO, H.S., 1984.** Acute reproductive losses due to porcine parvovirus infection in a swine herd: Herd observations and economic analysis of the losses. *Preventive Veterinary Medicine*, 2, 699–706.

46 **NASH, W.A., 1990.** Porcine parvovirus survey. *The Veterinary Record*, 126, 175–176.

47 **NIELSON, L., RONSHOLT, L. & SORENSON, K.J., 1991.** Experimental *in utero* infection of pig foetuses with porcine parvovirus (PPV). *Veterinary Microbiology*, 28, 1–11.

48 **PAUL, P.S. & MENGLING, W.L., 1980.** Evaluation of a modified live virus vaccine for the prevention of porcine parvovirus-induced reproductive disease in swine. *American Journal of Veterinary Research*, 41, 2007–2011.

49 **PAUL, P.S. & MENGLING, W.L., 1984.** Oronasal and intramuscular vaccination of swine with a modified live porcine parvovirus vaccine: Multiplication and transmission of the vaccine virus. *American Journal of Veterinary Research*, 45, 2481–2485.

50 **PAUL, P.S., MENGLING, W.L. & BROWN, T.T., 1979.** Replication of porcine parvovirus in peripheral blood lymphocytes, monocytes, and peritoneal macrophages. *Infection and Immunity*, 25, 1003–1007.

51 **PAUL, P.S., MENGLING, W.L. & BROWN, T.T., 1980.** Effect of vaccinal and passive immunity on experimental infection of pigs with porcine parvovirus. *American Journal of Veterinary Research*, 41, 1368–1371.

52 **PAUL, P.S., MENGLING, W.L. & PIRTLE, E.C., 1982.** Duration and biological half-life of passively acquired colostral antibodies to porcine parvovirus. *American Journal of Veterinary Research*, 43, 1376–1379.

53 **PEREIRA, M.S., 1989.** Parvoviridae. *In*: PORTERFIELD, J.E., (ed.). *Andrew's Viruses of Vertebrates*. London, Philadelphia: Baillière Tindall.

54 **PINI, A., 1975.** Porcine parvovirus in pig herds in southern Africa. *Journal of the South African Veterinary Association*, 46, 241–244.

55 **PRITLE, E.C., 1974.** Titration of two porcine respiratory viruses in mammalian cell cultures by direct fluorescent antibody staining. *American Journal of Veterinary Research*, 35, 249–250.

56 **PROZESKY, L., THOMSON, G.R., GAINARU, M.D., HERR, S. & KRITZINGER, L.J., 1980.** Lesions resulting from inoculation of porcine foetuses with porcine parvovirus. *Onderstepoort Journal of Veterinary Research*, 47, 269–274.

57 **PYE, D., BATES, J., EDWARDS, S.J. & HOLLINGWORTH, J., 1990.** Development of a vaccine preventing parvovirus-induced reproductive failure in pigs. *Australian Veterinary Journal*, 67, 179–182.

58 **RANZ, A.I., MANCLUS, J.J., DIAZ-AROCA, E. & CASAL, J.I., 1989.** Porcine parvovirus: DNA sequence and genome organization. *Journal of General Virology*, 70, 2541–2553.

59 **RODEFFER, H.E., LEMAN, A.D., DUNNE, H.W., CROPPER, M. & SPRECHER, D.J., 1975.** Reproductive failure in swine associated with maternal seroconversion for porcine parvovirus. *Journal of the American Veterinary Medical Association*, 166, 991–992.

60 **RUCKERBAUER, G.M., DULAC, G.C. & BOULANGER, P., 1978.** Demonstration of parvovirus in Canadian swine and antigenic relationships with isolates from other countries. *Canadian Journal of Comparative Medicine*, 42, 278–285.

61 **SAKURAI, M., NISHIMORI, T., USHIMI, C. & NAKAJIMA, H., 1989.** Nucleotide sequence of capsid protein gene of porcine parvovirus. *Virus Research*, 13, 79–86.

62 **THACKER, B.J., JOO, H.S., WINKELMAN, N.L., LEMAN, A.D. & BARNES, D.M., 1987.** Clinical, virologic and histopathologic observations of induced porcine parvovirus infection in boars. *American Journal of Veterinary Research*, 48, 763–767.

63 **THOMSON, G.R., 1981.** Veterinary Research Institute, Onderstepoort 0110, South Africa. Unpublished observations.

64 **THOMSON, G.R. & PEENZ, I., 1980.** Antibody to porcine parvovirus in warthog (*Phacochoerus aethiopicus*). *Onderstepoort Journal of Veterinary Research*, 47, 45–46.

65 **TOO, H.L. & LOVE, R.J., 1985.** Persistence of passive immunity to porcine parvovirus. *Australian Veterinary Journal*, 62, 282–284.

66 **VAN LEENGOED, L.A., VOS, J., GRUYS, E., RONDHUIS, P. & BRAND, A., 1983.** Porcine parvovirus infection: Review and diagnosis in a sow herd with reproductive failure. *The Veterinary Quarterly*, 5, 131–141.

67 **VASUDEVACHARYA, J., BASAK, S., SRINVAS, R.V. & COMPANS, R.W., 1990.** The complete nucleotide sequence of an infectious clone of porcine parvovirus, strain NADL-2. *Virology*, 178, 611–616.

68 **WESTENBRINK, F., VELDHUIS, M.A. & BRINKHOF, J.M.A., 1989.** An enzyme-linked immunosorbent assay for detection of antibodies to porcine parvovirus. *Journal of Virological Methods*, 23, 169–178.

69 **WRATHALL, A.E., 1977.** Reproductive failure in the pig: Diagnosis and control. *The Veterinary Record*, 100, 230–237.

70 **WRATHALL, A.E. & MENGLING, W.L., 1979.** Effect of porcine parvovirus on development of fertilized pig eggs *in vitro*. *British Veterinary Journal*, 135, 249–254.

71 **WRATHALL, A.E. & MENGLING, W.L., 1979.** Effect of transferring parvovirus-infected fertilized pig eggs into seronegative gilts. *British Veterinary Journal*, 135, 255–261.

72 **WRATHALL, A.E., WELLS, D.E., CARTWRIGHT, S.F. & FRERICHS, E.N., 1984.** An inactivated, oil-emulsion vaccine for the prevention of porcine parvovirus-induced reproductive failure. *Research in Veterinary Science*, 36, 136–143.

100

Bovine parvovirus infection

Synonym: HADEN virus infection

G.R. Thomson

Introduction and aetiology

Six isolates of a previously unidentified virus were made from the faeces of clinically healthy calves on widely separated farms in Maryland (USA) in 1959.[1] This virus was initially named HADEN in view of its haemadsorbing abilities and location (HaemADsorbing, ENteric virus). It was subsequently shown that HADEN virus is a typical autonomous parvovirus (genus *Parvovirus*) and it was then named bovine parvovirus (BPV).[2, 17, 22]

Limited epidemiological investigation and studies into the pathogenesis of BPV infection have been conducted and there is uncertainty as to its pathogenic potential in cattle. There is no information on the presence of the agent in southern Africa, although it is possibly ubiquitous.[16]

Bovine parvovirus has most features that are common to other viruses within the genus *Parvovirus*[17] **(see Chapter 99: Porcine parvovirus infection)**, but there are apparent differences between the structural proteins of BPV and those of most other autonomous parvoviruses. Mature virions of BPV are made up of four, as opposed to three, structural proteins and there are also small differences in molecular mass.[15] However, the fourth protein of BPV appears to exist merely as the result of enzymatic cleavage of VP3.[15]

Antigenic similarities between the viral proteins of a wide variety of autonomous parvoviruses have been demonstrated, but those of BPV and goose parvovirus show no such homology either with other parvoviruses or each other.[14, 15] It is also possible that there may be two antigenic variants of BPV, namely types 1 and 2.[9]

The complete nucleotide sequence of the BPV genome shows it to comprise 5 491 nucleotides with terminal regions containing non-identical, imperfect palindromic sequences of 150 and 121 nucleotides.[6] As might be expected from the lack of antigenic similarity between BPV and other parvoviruses, the overall DNA homology between BPV and other members of the genus is low, although several small regions of high homology occur in the left and right open reading frames.[6]

Bovine parvovirus replicates in a wide variety of bovine and buffalo (*Babalus babalus*) cell types *in vitro*, but foetal lung and spleen cells appear to be most suitable for diagnostic purposes.[4, 5, 11] Continuous cell lines are generally ineffective. Plaque titration has been achieved,[7] despite the fact that the cytopathic effect produced in cell cultures is often difficult to distinguish from cell degeneration. The use of serum to induce parasynchrony of cells in primary cultures apparently improves virus isolation.[21]

The presence of the virus in tissues and organs can be detected and measured by haemadsorption and haemagglutination. The haemagglutinin is mainly cell-associated[19] and erythrocytes of horses, sheep, goats, guinea-pigs, hamsters, ducks, geese, rhesus monkeys and humans are agglutinated, but not those of mice, rabbits, chickens and cattle.[1, 8]

Epidemiology

Serological studies show that BPV infection is widespread in the USA,[1, 3, 5, 18, 20] with an antibody prevalence rate of between 14 and 100 per cent in infected herds.[20] The infection has also been identified in Japan and Algeria.[8, 21]

Although not proven, it can be assumed that infection is transmitted predominantly by the faecal-oral route. The virus has, however, also been isolated from nasal swabs[18] and from conjunctival secretions and the tonsils of infected cattle.[21] It has been isolated intermittently from the faeces of calves which have antibodies to the virus in their sera,[19, 21] indicating the possibility of there having been prolonged excretion.

Antibody to BPV has been detected in the sera of pigs and humans but this has been ascribed to ingestion of bovine milk or milk products containing the virus.[12, 13] Presumably calves can also be infected in this way.

Pathogenesis, clinical signs and pathology

Viraemia, associated particularly with the leukocyte fraction of blood, lasting four to six days, has been detected in calves infected experimentally by both oral and intravenous routes.[19, 23] Thereafter, BPV and its antigens were found in a wide range of tissues,[21] particularly lymphoid tissues, the adrenals and throughout the intestinal tract, especially the jejunum and ileum. In the intestine, a variety of cell types is infected, antigen having been shown in the epithelium as well as in the lamina propria. In the epithelium, cells at the tips, bases and transition zones of the villi, as well as at the crypts of Lieberkühn, all fluoresced in experimentally infected calves.[19] Infection of enterocytes appears to be cytocidal.[19, 21]

Diarrhoea in both naturally and experimentally infected calves has been reported,[5, 18, 21] and in one instance the diarrhoea was followed by apparent poor growth in some of the calves.[21] On the other hand, the virus has been recovered from clinically normal animals.[1] Other potentially pathogenic agents were also present in some animals where diarrhoea was associated with this infection.[8, 18]

The detection of antibody to BPV in bovine foetal serum as well as in foetuses after the experimental inoculation of pregnant cows has shown that the virus is able to cross the placental barrier.[23] Experimental studies suggest that foetuses are most susceptible during the first and second trimesters of gestation. Infection has been detected in the lymphatic tissues, heart muscle, liver and kidneys of foetuses and this apparently resulted, at least in some cases, in foetal death.[23] Bovine foetuses are capable of responding immunologically to the virus by the 93rd day of gestation[23] and there is no evidence for a reduction in immunological responsiveness of foetuses that have been inoculated experimentally during the third trimester of gestation.[10] It remains to be established with certainty whether BPV is a significant cause of bovine infertility.

Diagnosis and differential diagnosis

The involvement of BPV should be considered in cases of diarrhoea in young cattle and also in herds in which repeat breeding and abortion in cows is a problem.

Isolation of the virus can be achieved by the use of cell culture techniques with the presence of the virus being indicated by haemadsorption or haemagglutination.[1, 8, 19, 21] Inhibition of these reactions with specific antisera will enable identification of the virus.

Control

No studies on the control of this infection have been conducted as its pathogenicity is uncertain.

References

1 **ABINANTI, F.R. & WARFIELD, M.S., 1961.** Recovery of a hemadsorbing virus (HADEN) from the gastrointestinal tract of calves. *Virology*, 14, 228–289.

2 **BACHMANN, P.A., 1971.** Properties of a bovine parvovirus. *Zentralblatt für Veterinärmedizin*, Reihe B, 18, 80–85.

3 **BARNES, M.A., WRIGHT, R.E., BODINE, B. & ALBERTY, C.F., 1982.** Frequency of bluetongue and bovine parvovirus infection in cattle in South Carolina dairy herds. *American Journal of Veterinary Research*, 43, 1078–1080.

4 **BATES, R.C. & STORZ, J., 1973.** Host cell range and growth characteristics of bovine parvoviruses. *Infection and Immunity*, 7, 398–402.

5 **BATES, R.C., STORZ, J. & REED, D.E., 1972.** Isolation and comparison of bovine parvoviruses. *The Journal of Infectious Diseases*, 126, 531–536.

6 **CHEN, K.C., SHULL, B.C., MOSES, E.Z., LEDERMAN, M., STOUT, E.R. & BATES, R.C., 1986.** Complete nucleotide sequence and genome organization of bovine parvovirus. *Journal of Virology*, 60, 1085–1097.

7 **DURHAM, P.J.K. & JOHNSON, R.H., 1984.** Plaque titration and inhibition tests for bovine parvovirus. *Journal of General Virology*, 65, 1425–1429.

8 **INABA, Y., KUROGI, H., TAKAHASHI, E., SATO, K., TANAKA, Y., GOTO, Y., OMORI, T. & MATUMOTO, M., 1973.** Isolation and properties of bovine parvovirus type 1 from Japanese calves. *Archiv für die Gesamte Virusforschung*, 42, 42–54.

9 **INABA, Y., OMORI, T., KONO, M., ISHII, S. & MATUMOTO, M., 1973.** A new serotype of bovine parvovirus. *Japanese Journal of Microbiology*, 17, 85–86.

10 **LIGGITT, H.D., DEMARTINI, J.C. & PEARSON, L.D., 1982.** Immunologic responses of the bovine fetus to parvovirus infection. *American Journal of Veterinary Research*, 43, 1355–1359.

11 **LUBECK, M.D. & JOHNSON, F.B., 1976.** Multiplication of bovine parvovirus in two cell strains. *Infection and Immunity*, 13, 1289–1292.

12 **MENGELING, W.L. & MATTHEWS, P.J., 1990.** Antibodies to bovine parvovirus acquired by neonatal pigs through ingestion of virus and antibody in the diet. *American Journal of Veterinary Research*, 51, 632–635.

13 **MENGELING, W.L. & PAUL, P.S., 1986.** Antibodies for autonomous parvoviruses of lower animals detected in human serum. *Archives of Virology*, 88, 127–133.

14 **MENGELING, W.L., PAUL, P.S., BUNN, T.O. & RIDPATH, J.F., 1986.** Antigenic relationships among autonomous parvoviruses. *Journal of General Virology*, 67, 2839–2844.

15 **MENGELING, W.L., RIDPATH, J.F. & VORWALD, A.C., 1988.** Size and antigenic comparisons among the structural proteins of selected autonomous parvoviruses. *Journal of General Virology*, 69, 825–837.

16 **PEREIRA, M.S., 1989.** Parvoviridae. *In*: PORTERFIELD, J.S., (ed.). *Andrews' Viruses of Vertebrates*. London, Philadelphia, Toronto: Baillière Tindall.

17 **SIEGL, G., BATES, R.C., BERNS, K.I., CARTER, B.J., KELLY, D.C., KURSTAK, E. & TATTERSALL, P., 1985.** Characteristics and taxonomy of parvoviridae. *Intervirology*, 23, 61–73.

18 **SPAHN, G.J., MOHANTY, S.B. & HETRICK, F.M., 1966.** Experimental infection of calves with hemadsorbing enteric (HADEN) virus. *Cornell Veterinarian*, 56, 377–386.

19 **STORZ, J. & BATES, R.C., 1973.** Parvovirus infections in calves. *Journal of the American Veterinary Medical Association*, 163, 884–886.

20 **STORZ, J., BATES, R.C., WARREN, G.S. & HOWARD, T.H., 1972.** Distribution of antibodies against bovine parvovirus 1 in cattle and other animal species. *American Journal of Veterinary Research*, 33, 269–272.

21 **STORZ, J., LEARY, J.J., CARLSON, J.H. & BATES, R.C., 1978.** Parvoviruses associated with diarrhea in calves. *Journal of the American Veterinary Medical Association,* 163, 624–627.

22 **STORZ, J. & WARREN, G.S., 1970.** Effect of antimetabolites and actinomycin D on the replication of HADEN, a bovine parvovirus. *Archiv für die Gesamte Virusforschung,* 30, 271–274.

23 **STORZ, J., YOUNG, S., CARROL, E.J., BATES, R.C., BOWEN, R.A. & KENY, D.A., 1978.** Parvovirus infection of the bovine fetus: Distribution of infection antibody response, and age-related susceptibility. *American Journal of Veterinary Research,* 39, 1099–1102.

ADENOVIRIDAE

The family Adenoviridae, so named because the first isolates were made from adenoidal tissues of humans, is divided into two genera: *Mastadenovirus* (mast: from *mastos*, the Greek word for breast) and *Aviadenovirus*. Members of the former infect mammals, while those of the latter infect birds.[19]

There are at least 100 serotypes within the genus *Mastadenovirus*, most of which infect humans and other primates. Relatively few serotypes have been found in association with domestic livestock: ten in cattle, six in sheep, four in pigs, one in goats, and one or possibly two in horses.[13, 19, 20] Serotypes are generally species-specific, although some may infect animals closely related to the definitive host. Sheep, for example, have been shown to be infected naturally with bovine adenoviruses[2] and bovine adenovirus serotypes (bos 3, 4 and 8) have been isolated from African buffaloes *(Syncerus caffer)* in the Zambezi Valley in Zimbabwe.[4] Human serotypes have been divided among six subgenera, distinguished by the letters A–F, on the basis of their structural, biochemical, biological and antigenic characteristics.[19] The human serotypes are indicated by the letter 'h', while those infecting other species are designated by a three-letter code, e.g. 'bos' for cattle, 'ovi' for sheep, 'sus' for pigs, 'cap' for goats and 'equ' for horses. The serotypes that infect each species are indicated by sequential numbers following the three-letter code, e.g. bos 5.[19] However, other systems of nomenclature are still often used, e.g. bovine adenovirus 5 (BAV 5) for bos 5.

Adenovirus infections of the respiratory and gastrointestinal tracts are common in domestic livestock, but their role in the causation of disease is often uncertain. Apart from equ 1 infection of Arabian foals suffering from severe combined immune deficiency, no clearly defined disease syndrome of livestock has been shown unequivocally to be caused by an adenovirus. Adenovirus infections are common in humans suffering from immune deficiencies, such as those resulting from chemotherapy for cancer, following organ transplantation surgery, or due to human immunodeficiency virus (HIV) infection.[12] Adenovirus infections may therefore be pathogenic in other species under similar circumstances.

Mastadenoviruses are frequently recovered from the pharyngeal lymphoid tissue of apparently healthy animals, indicating that prolonged excretion is a strategy used by them to ensure their transmission.[11] Some, at least, are also transmitted transplacentally.[5, 7, 17]

Most adenoviruses can be cultivated in cell cultures, most commonly kidney or thyroid, from the homologous species. Some, however, differ in this respect: those that produce enteric infection may not replicate readily in conventional cell cultures, and bovine subgroup 2 adenoviruses are difficult to culture other than in bovine testis cells.[8]

Members of the genus *Mastadenovirus* have a group-specific (hexon) antigen, although in subgroup 2 bovine adenoviruses (bos 4–8 and 10) this antigen is difficult to detect.[3] Aviadenoviruses, however, have no such group antigen.[15] Serotypes are defined by virus neutralization with antisera produced against each serotype in species (usually rabbits or chickens) other than the definitive host. Distinct serotypes must show homologous-to-heterologous titre ratios of greater than 16 in both directions. If this ratio is between eight and 16, other factors such as cross-haemagglutination-inhibition reactions and biophysical or biochemical differences between the DNAs (e.g. restriction endonuclease patterns) are considered.[1] The ability of different adenoviruses to agglutinate erythrocytes of various animal species has also been used to distinguish isolates. For example, bos 2 isolates have been divided into two subtypes, A and B.[6] Subtype A viruses infect only cattle, agglutinate bovine erythrocytes, and have DNA restriction patterns similar to the bos 2 prototype. Subtype B isolates, on the other hand, infect both cattle and sheep, agglutinate only rat erythrocytes, and have distinct DNA restriction profiles. Analysis of genetic variation between adenoviruses by electrophoresis of restriction endonuclease-generated DNA fragments is being used increasingly because this technique reflects variation over a greater proportion of the genome than that produced by serology.[21]

Because, like poxviruses, adenoviruses have a relatively large, double-stranded DNA genome, there is considerable interest in producing recombinants between adenoviruses and foreign genes which can be incorporated into the adenovirus genome. In this way adenoviruses can be used as vectors for potentially beneficial genes. For example, the rabies glycoprotein gene has been inserted into the deleted E3 region of a human adenovirus (h5)[18] which could possibly be used to immunize either people or animals against rabies.

It has been known for many years that adenoviruses (particularly those in the (human) A and B subgenera) are able to transform cells in culture and cause tumours in new-born hamsters and other rodents. However, these viruses are not oncogenic in humans, and the same applies to adenoviruses of domestic livestock.[16]

Adeno-associated viruses (AAVs), which are parvoviruses classified in the genus *Dependovirus,* are sometimes identified as contaminants of adenovirus isolates. The reason for this is that AAVs are dependent on co-infection of the cell with an adenovirus in order to be able to replicate. Apart from AAVs of humans, dogs and birds, AAVs have been recovered from cattle, sheep and horses.[9, 10, 14, 19] No AAV has so far been associated with disease.

References

1 **ADAIR, B.M., McFERRAN, J.B. & McKILLOP, E.R., 1982.** A sixth species of ovine adenovirus isolated from lambs in New Zealand. *Archives of Virology,* 74, 269–275.

2 **ADAIR, B.M., McKILLOP, E.R. & COAKLEY, B.H., 1986.** Serological identification of an Australian adenovirus isolate from sheep. *Australian Veterinary Journal,* 63, 162.

3 **ADAIR, B.M., McKILLIP, E.R., McFERRAN, J.B. & TODD, D., 1983.** Studies on the antigenic relationship between bovine subgroup 2 and conventional mammalian adenoviruses using immunofluorescence. *Veterinary Microbiology,* 8, 121–128.

4 **BARBER, D.J. & CONDY, J.B., 1981.** Isolation and characterisation of bovine adenoviruses types 3, 4 and 8 from free-living African buffalo *(Syncerus caffer). Research in Veterinary Science,* 31, 69–75.

5 **BARTHA, A. & MATE, S., 1983.** Transplacental transmission of bovine adenoviruses. *Comparative Immunology and Microbiology of Infectious Diseases,* 6, 189–192.

6 **BELAK, S., BERENCSI, G., RUSVAY, M., LUKACS, K. & NASI, I., 1983.** DNA structure and haemagglutination properties of bovine adenovirus type 2 strains which bypass species specificity. *Archives of Virology,* 77, 181–194.

7 **BELAK, S. & RUSVAI, M., 1986.** *In utero* adenoviral infection of sheep. *Veterinary Microbiology,* 12, 87–91.

8 **BENKÖ, M., BARTHA, A., MÖSTL, K. & BÜRKI, F., 1989.** A heteroploid permanent cell line originating from embryonic calf thyroid supporting the replication of all known bovine adenovirus serotypes. *Veterinary Microbiology,* 19, 317–324.

9 **CLARK, J.K., McFERRAN, J.R., McKILLOP, E.R. & CURRAN, W.L., 1979.** Isolation of an adeno-associated virus from sheep. *Archives of Virology,* 60, 171–176.

10 **DUTTA, S.K., 1975.** Isolation and characterization of an adenovirus and isolation of its adenovirus-associated virus in cell culture from foals with respiratory tract disease. *American Journal of Veterinary Research,* 36, 247–250.

11 **FENNER, F., BACHMANN, P.A., GIBBS, E.P.J., MURPHY, F.A., STUDDERT, M.J. & WHITE, D.O., 1987.** *Veterinary Virology.* Orlando, San Diego, New York: Academic Press, Inc.

12 **HIERHOLZER, J.C., WIGAND, R., ANDERSON, L.J., ADRIAN, T. & GOLD, J.W.M., 1988.** Adenovirus from patients with AIDS: A plethora of serotypes and a description of five new serotypes of subgenus D (Types 43–47). *The Journal of Infectious Diseases,* 158, 804–813.

13 **HORNER, G.W. & HUNTER, R., 1982.** Isolation of two serotypes of equine adenovirus from horses in New Zealand. *New Zealand Veterinary Journal,* 30, 62–64.

14 **LUCHSINGER, E., STROBBE, R., WELLEMANS, G., DEKEGEL, D. & SPRECHER-GOLDBERGER, S., 1970.** Haemagglutinating adeno-associated virus (AAV) in association with bovine adenovirus type 1. *Archiv für die Gesamte Virusforschung,* 31, 390–392.

15 **MAUTNER, V., 1989.** Adenoviridae. *In:* PORTERFIELD, J.S., (ed.). *Andrew's Viruses of Vertebrates.* 5th edn. London, Philadelphia: Baillière Tindall.

16 **MOHANTY, S.B., 1971.** Comparative study of bovine adenoviruses. *American Journal of Veterinary Research,* 32, 1899–1905.

17 **NARITHA, M., 1985.** Pathologic changes caused by transplacental infection with an adenovirus-like agent in pigs. *American Journal of Veterinary Research,* 46, 1126–1129.

18 **PREVEC, L., CHRISSTIE, B.S., BELBECK, L. & GRAHAM, F.L., 1990.** A recombinant human adenovirus vaccine against rabies. *Journal of Infectious Diseases,* 161, 27–30.

19 **RUSSELL, W.C., 1991.** Adenoviridae. *In:* FRANCK, R.I.B., FAUQUET, C.M., KNUDSON, D.L. & BROWN, F., (eds). Classification and nomenclature of viruses. Fifth report of the International Committee on the Taxonomy of Viruses. *Archives of Virology,* Supplementum 2. Vienna, New York: Springer-Verlag.

20 **STUDDERT, M.J. & BLACKNEY, M.H., 1982.** Isolation of an adenovirus antigenically distinct from equine adenovirus type 1 from diarrhoeic foal faeces. *American Journal of Veterinary Research,* 43, 543–544.

21 **WADELL, G., HAMMARSKJÖLD, M-L., WINBERG, G., VARSANYI, T.M. & SUNDELL, G., 1980.** Genetic variability of adenoviruses. *Annals of the New York Academy of Science,* 354, 16–24.

101

Adenovirus infections

G.R. Thomson

ADENOVIRUS INFECTIONS OF CATTLE

Introduction

Adenovirus infections of cattle probably occur universally, although most are subclinical. Bovine adenovirus infections have been associated with a variety of respiratory and alimentary tract diseases, but their role in the causation of these diseases remains uncertain.

Aetiology

Adenovirus virions are 70–90 nm in diameter (i.e. a medium-sized virus), non-enveloped and have icosahedral symmetry. They have a buoyant density of 1,32–1,35 g/ml in CsCl. Each virion is made up of 252 capsomeres which are 8–9 nm in diameter. The capsomeres at the 12 vertices of the virion (also known as vertex capsomeres or penton bases) differ from the other 240 (known as hexons) in that each penton base carries one (*Mastadenovirus*) or two (*Aviadenovirus*) glycoprotein projections with terminal knobs, known as fibers, each of which is 10–50 nm in length (the length being characteristic for each serotype).[40, 82, 99]

The genome comprises a linear molecule of double-stranded DNA, to the 5′-end of which a viral-coded protein with a molecular weight (MW) of about 55 kilodaltons is covalently linked. The genomes of viruses in the genus *Mastadenovirus* are smaller (MW = 20–25 x 10^6) than aviadenoviruses (c. 30 x 10^6) and there are also differences in G + C content — 48–61 per cent for *Mastadenovirus* and 54–55 per cent for *Aviadenovirus*. Inverted terminal repetitions (50–200 base-pairs) of the type abc–c′b′a′[48] have been found in all adenoviruses so far sequenced.[82, 99] The DNA is tightly bound to protein VII and is also associated with four other proteins. This complex (DNA-proteins) makes up the viral core.[67]

In addition to the 55k protein linked to the 5′-end of the DNA, virions contain at least 10 polypeptides with MWs varying between 5 and 120 kilodaltons. Each fiber polypeptide, the only glycosylated structural protein, contains two molecules of N-acetylglucosamine. Hexons have been shown by x-ray crystallography to have a pseudohexagonal base and a triangular top and to consist of three molecules of polypeptide II, while penton bases are pentamers or trimers of polypeptide III.[67]

Adenoviruses attach to specific cell receptors by the fibers and are probably internalized by endocytosis. The viral core enters the cell nucleus, where transcription, DNA replication and virus assembly occur. Host-cell DNA synthesis is shut off early during replication and RNA and protein synthesis at a late stage. DNA replication occurs by strand displacement, using viral-coded DNA polymerase and terminal protein priming.[82] As adenoviruses are being assembled in the nucleus they form crystalline arrays which appear as basophilic or amphiphilic intranuclear inclusions when examined by light microscopy.[34]

The ten recognized serotypes of bovine adenovirus (bos 1–10)[45] are divided into two subgroups, 1 and 2. Subgroup 1 consists of bos 1, 2, 3 and 9, while the others make up subgroup 2. Viruses in serotype 2 have been further divided into two subtypes, A and B **(see Adenoviridae: Introduction).**

Epidemiology

Although the limited number and extent of serological studies so far undertaken have failed to give an accurate indication of the prevalence rates of infections with adenovirus serotypes in cattle in different geographic locations and in various sex and age classes, it is probably safe to presume that infection with adenoviruses is widespread in cattle populations.[15, 17, 62, 88] For example, 76 and 59 per cent of calf sera collected at two Austrian abattoirs had virus neutralizing antibodies against selected serotypes.[15, 73] In a group of 29 heifers monitored serologically in Idaho (USA) from birth to 24 months of age, there were 28 bos 3 and 33 bos 7 infections (representatives of subgroups 1 and 2 respectively), some of which occurred in the presence of maternally-derived antibody.[88]

It is presumed that most infections occur by close, direct respiratory transmission or by the faecal-oral route.

Table 101.1 Some associations reported between adenovirus infections and health status in cattle

CLINICAL SYNDROME	TYPE AND AGE OF CATTLE	SEROTYPE	REFERENCE
None	Heifers: 0–24 months	Bos 3, 7	88
	Calves	Various	91
	Cow	Bos 2 (WBR1)	32
	Cow	NS	53
	Calf	NS	54
Keratoconjunctivitis	NS	Various	100, 101
Respiratory disease	Bull calves	Various (esp. subtype A)	17
	Calves	Bos 3	62
	Feedlot cattle	Bos 3	61
	Calf	Bos 7	80
	Calves	Bos 3	65
Lachrymation, nasal discharge, tympanites, colic, diarrhoea	New-born calves	Bos 3	64
Weak calf syndrome	Calves	Bos 5	24
	Calves	Bos 5	19
	Calves	Bos 7	90
Reduced dietary nitrogen digestibility	Beef calves	Bos 3	18
Enteritis	10-month-old bullock	Not determined	87
	7 to 18 month-old cattle	NS	41
	Calves: 2 weeks	NS	14
	Calves/steer	Bos 3	95
	3-week-old calf	NS	76
	Calves	Bos 4	84
Systemic infection	Yearling heifer	Bos 10	46
Pyrexia	Feeder calves	Bos 3	65

NS Not stated

The virus has been detected for up to eight days in the respiratory secretions and rectal swabs of experimentally infected calves.[74] Transplacental transmission has also been shown,[5] but how common this is remains uncertain.

Apart from evidence of infection in sheep and African buffaloes *(Syncerus caffer)*, antibodies to bos 3 and 7 have been detected in the sera of pronghorn antelope *(Antilocapra americana)* in Idaho (USA).[89] However, it is not clear whether this was cross-reacting antibody or antibody specific to these two serotypes.

Pathogenesis, clinical signs and pathology

Although most adenovirus isolations have been made from cattle that were apparently healthy,[32, 53, 54, 91] a variety of conditions, most of which involve the respiratory or alimentary tract, have been associated with adenovirus infections **(Table 101.1)**. The two most comprehensive studies on the association between adenoviruses and disease in cattle, both conducted in Britain, reached conflicting conclusions. One, based on the isolation of viruses from nearly 1 600 diseased and healthy calves over a period of 43 months, found that adenoviruses played no significant part in the causation of respiratory illness.[91] The other, based on serological monitoring of young bulls over a period of 18 months, demonstrated a statistically significant association between serological responses to adenovirus infections, especially those caused by subgroup 1 viruses, and the occurrence of clinical disease.[17]

Similarly, experimental infection of calves with a variety of bovine serotypes has resulted in either no obvious ill effect or a variety of non-lethal respiratory or enteric conditions.[74] The lungs of experimentally infected calves that developed lesions have necrotizing and proliferative bronchiolitis, and sometimes bronchopneumonia, with intranuclear inclusions in bronchiolar epithelial cells. However, these lesions rarely occur in natural cases.[35, 74]

Enteric lesions are probably the result of endothelial necrosis (the cells often contain typical large intranuclear inclusions) in the vessels of the lamina propria and submucosa, and may occur anywhere in the gastrointestinal tract from the rumen to the colon, but especially over the Peyer's patches.[3] These lesions result in the development of thrombi with resultant ischaemic necrosis of the dependent epithelium. Ulceration is a frequent consequence and a fibrinocellular exudate often covers the mucosal surface.[3]

Intranuclear inclusions may also occur in endothelial cells in the adrenals, mesenteric lymph nodes, liver, spleen, glomeruli and the capillaries in the interstitial tissues of the kidneys and the mucosa of the urinary bladder.[3]

Diagnosis and differential diagnosis

Adenoviruses produce characteristic intranuclear inclusion bodies with margination of the chromatin. These may be recognized on histological examination of affected tissues.[47, 77] Examination of such inclusions by electron microscopy may reveal the characteristic adenovirus structure in virion arrays that make up the inclusions.[47, 77]

Bovine adenoviruses can readily be isolated, when present, from nasal and conjunctival swabs or faeces in either bovine kidney, testis or thyroid cell cultures — subgroup 2 viruses favour testis cultures.[7] A bovine thyroid cell line has been shown to support the replication of nine of the ten bovine serotypes.[11] It may be necessary to passage the material submitted for virus isolation several times before a cytopathic effect is obtained.

Serological tests usually rely on virus neutralization reactions or haemagglutination-inhibition (HI). The erythrocytes used in HI tests depend on the serotype involved; those obtained from rats are most commonly used.

Control

Vaccines against bovine adenoviruses have been produced,[4, 15, 66] but as the role of adenoviruses in cattle disease remains unclear, there is little justification for their use. However, a case has been made for the use of vaccine against subgroup 1 viruses.[91] A beneficial effect was demonstrated when an inactivated, aluminium hydroxide-adjuvanted vaccine was used in a herd in which pneumonia associated with bos 3 infection had been a severe problem.[66]

ADENOVIRUS INFECTIONS OF SHEEP

Introduction and aetiology

Infection of sheep with adenoviruses is probably ubiquitous. Most are subclinical, although a variety of clinical conditions have been associated with such infections. However, there is a stronger body of evidence implicating adenoviruses in the causation of respiratory tract disease in sheep than in cattle. In combination with other infectious agents, particularly *Pasteurella haemolytica*, they sometimes cause bronchopneumonia.

Six ovine serotypes are recognized.[1] The general characteristics of adenoviruses are described in the section on adenovirus infections in cattle.

Epidemiology

There is little information on the prevalence of adenovirus infections of sheep in different geographic locations or in various sex and age classes. Adenoviruses have been isolated from sheep in Northern Ireland, Britain, Turkey, New Zealand, Australia, Hungary and the USA.[59, 77] However, not all sheep isolates are ovine adenoviruses, as some from Hungary, Australia and New Zealand have been shown to be closely related, if not identical, to bos 2 and 7.[2, 8, 77] A serological study conducted primarily in Iowa (USA) found that 95 per cent of ram lambs between one and four months of age had been infected with ovi 5 and 42 per cent with ovi 6 viruses.[60]

Adenovirus has been detected in the secretions of the upper respiratory tract of experimentally infected lambs for at least eight days after infection,[58] and such virus-laden secretions probably transmit the infection during close contact between infected and susceptible individuals. The faecal-oral route is probably also important,[71] although no virus could be detected in faeces in some experimental infections.[58, 59] Excretion lasting at least 80 days has been claimed.[85] Transplacental transmission has been demonstrated.[10]

Pathogenesis

Several studies indicate that ovine adenoviruses (in addition to other viral infections of the respiratory tract, such as respiratory syncytial virus and parainfluenza type 3) act synergistically with *P. haemolytica* to cause serious bronchopneumonia.[9, 23, 56, 59] The consensus appears to be that adenovirus infections are relatively mild but that they predispose to colonization of the lungs by *P. haemolytica* as they impair the bacterial clearance mechanisms.

It appears that adenoviruses replicate in the epithelial cells of the airways, except possibly the alveolar epithelium.[22] In an experimental model in which a human adenovirus (h5) was used to induce respiratory disease in cotton rats (*Sigmodon hispidus*), it was shown that type II alveolar cells supported only an incomplete replicative cycle of the virus.[79]

Clinical signs and pathology

Most adenovirus infections in sheep are subclinical.[6, 25, 27, 59, 71] Serious respiratory disease, particularly bronchopneumonia, has been ascribed to adenoviruses, usually in association with other viral and secondary bacterial infections.[9, 23, 26, 56, 57] Lung lesions, as in cattle, are characterized by proliferative and necrotizing bronchiolitis, with some epithelial cells containing typical intranuclear inclusions. Some of the cells bearing inclusions have markedly enlarged nuclei and cytoplasm.[35]

An unusual outbreak of liver haemorrhage and hepatocyte necrosis associated with adenovirus infection in Merino wethers and ewes was described in Australia.[77] However, these animals also had lesions consistent with cycad poisoning. In a number of independent experimental infections no virus was found in the liver,[58, 59] except for one instance.[81]

Two outbreaks of pneumo-enteritis associated with adenovirus infection were described among lambs on large-scale farms in Germany.[9] Numerous adenovirus isolates were made from affected lambs which also showed rises in virus neutralizing antibody titres between acute and convalescent phase sera. Vaccine produced from one of the viruses involved provided measurable protection against experimental and field challenge. Focal interstitial pneumonia, affecting mainly the ventral parts of the cranial, medial and accessory lobes, characterized infections that were not accompanied by secondary bacterial infection. Secondary infection induced croupous or chronic catarrhal pneumonia. Some bronchi showed epithelial hyperplasia. Pathological changes in the kidneys and lymph nodes of the respiratory tract were also described.[9]

A consistent finding in experimentally induced respiratory disease caused by adenoviruses has been proliferative bronchiolitis, which may progress to bronchopneumonia. Basophilic intranuclear inclusion bodies were sometimes visible in swollen epithelial cells, while cytomegaly and karyomegaly occurred in some cells containing inclusions.[22, 23, 25, 26, 97]

Diagnosis and control

The diagnosis of adenovirus infections of sheep is similar to that described for cattle; sheep cell cultures (kidney or thyroid) are usually used for virus isolation.

The routine use of vaccines against ovine adenovirus infections has not been described, but specially formulated vaccine may be beneficial in particular problem situations.[4, 9]

ADENOVIRUS INFECTIONS OF PIGS

Introduction and aetiology

Most adenovirus infections of pigs are subclinical, but some strains may cause enteric or respiratory disease and, in rare instances, meningoencephalitis. The pathogenicity of porcine adenovirus infection may be increased by co-infection with other agents.

Four serotypes are recognized, but there may be others.[30, 82] The general characteristics of adenoviruses are described in the section on adenovirus infections in cattle.

Epidemiology

Adenovirus infections of pigs are probably ubiquitous — they have been identified in the United Kingdom, Belgium, Germany, Australia, Canada, Japan and the USA.[12, 29, 42, 50, 52, 55, 75, 83]

Infection rates may be high (seropositivity rates of up to 50 per cent have been observed)[12] and infection may occur in piglets less than three weeks of age,[83] and therefore possibly in the presence of maternally derived antibody. However, infection may be acquired transplacentally prior to the acquisition of maternal antibody by piglets,[52, 75] but the frequency with which this occurs is unknown.

Horizontal transmission between pigs presumably occurs by the faecal-oral route or by the transfer of virus-containing oronasal secretions during close contact, because both respiratory and enteric infections have been reproduced in these ways experimentally.[21, 83] Adenovirus inclusion bodies have been shown to persist for at least 15 days in enterocytes of the lower small intestine, and it is possible that alimentary excretion of porcine adenoviruses occurs for longer than is usual with other viruses that infect the porcine gastrointestinal tract.[33] Excretion in faeces is probably heaviest in pigs for a short while after weaning; adults rarely excrete adenoviruses in their faeces.[31]

Pathogenesis, clinical signs and pathology

Transplacental infection in porcine foetuses may result in widespread infection of the endothelial cells of the capillaries and small blood vessels throughout the body,[75] leading to cyanosis of the skin and oedema of the subcutaneous tissues at birth. Inclusions in the nuclei of endothelial cells of the infected piglets are most plentiful in the liver, spleen, kidneys and lymph nodes.[75] Adenovirus infection has also been implicated on rare occasions as a cause of porcine abortion.[52]

More commonly, porcine adenoviruses have been associated with the respiratory and/or gastrointestinal tracts of pigs infected after birth, but their involvement in the causation of disease is problematic as they can frequently be recovered from healthy animals.[13, 28, 83] However, some porcine adenoviruses regularly cause respiratory and enteric disease when administered to susceptible pigs.[21, 33] At least one porcine adenovirus has been shown to be a cause of meningoencephalitis in piglets.[37, 50]

The intestine is probably the primary site of infection; the tonsils, for example, being infected more sporadically and at a later stage than the intestine, probably following viraemic spread.[33] Both villus and crypt enterocytes, as well as goblet cells, are infected in villi that are severely shortened. There is a predilection for the enterocytes that cover the short villi of the terminal parts of the jejunum and ileum, particularly those that cover lymphocytic aggregates. Typical adenovirus intranuclear inclusions occur in enterocytes;[13, 21] this differs from the situation in cattle, where the inclusions occur in endothelial cells of vessels in the lamina propria and submucosa.[3]

Porcine adenoviruses appear to have less affinity for pulmonary epithelium than is the case with bovine or ovine adenoviruses, but where obvious lesions do result, interstitial pneumonia is the primary lesion.[35]

As is the case with adenovirus infections in sheep and cattle, it is likely that co-infection with other agents increases the pathogenicity of adenoviruses. Such synergistic action has been demonstrated between sus 4 and *Mycoplasma hyopneumoniae*,[51] although not between sus 4 and *Pasteurella septica*.[86]

Diagnosis and control

The diagnosis of porcine adenovirus infections is similar to that described for cattle. Porcine thyroid cells are appropriate for virus isolation.[28]

There are no reports of attempts to control adenovirus infections in pigs.

ADENOVIRUS INFECTIONS OF HORSES

Introduction and aetiology

The vast majority of equine adenovirus infections are clinically inapparent, although association with respiratory disease has been claimed. In Arabian foals suffering from the inherited combined immune deficiency syndrome, pneumonia caused by adenovirus infection is usually the immediate cause of death.

Although the original studies on the possible antigenic diversity of equine adenovirus isolates found little variation,[16, 39, 93] subsequent studies have indicated that there are at least two serotypes.[44, 92] The existence of two equine adenovirus serotypes has, however, not yet been officially recognized by the International Committee on the Taxonomy of Viruses.[82]

The general characteristics of adenoviruses are described in the section on adenovirus infections in cattle.

Epidemiology

Antibodies to equine adenoviruses have been identified in horse sera in many countries in Europe, Asia and North America as well as in Australia and New Zealand, indicating that they are probably ubiquitous.[43] Lack of reports on their prevalence in African countries merely reflects failure to look for them. Not only is the geographic distribution of equine adenoviruses wide, but antibodies against them have been found in all the horse breeds in which a significant number of animals have been serologically tested.[43] Prevalence rates are usually higher than 70 per cent in adult horses,[43, 93] although in some groups of horses under the age of one year, 50 per cent or more are seronegative.[93]

The observation has been made that equine adenovirus infection was able to persist in a small pony herd which was maintained in relative isolation.[16] This indicates that prolonged, possibly intermittent, virus excretion occurs. Transmission is presumably dependent upon direct contact with the respiratory secretions, or perhaps faeces, of infected horses.

Pathogenesis, clinical signs and pathology

Most equine adenovirus infections are inapparent and it is generally accepted that they are not important as a cause of upper respiratory tract disease in racehorses.[78] They may, however, cause mild upper respiratory tract disease in foals,[36, 49, 70] especially, it is postulated, in the presence of other infectious agents.[16] They have also been associated with diarrhoea in foals[20, 92] and cauda equina neuritis.[38]

The most commonly reported clinical condition associated with equine adenovirus infection is pneumonia, which occurs in young (ten days to three months of age) Arabian foals afflicted with the combined immune deficiency syndrome.[69, 70, 72, 94] This syndrome is inherited via a simple recessive autosomal gene, and the inability of affected animals to withstand infection invariably leads to a fatal outcome.[94] It is diagnosed in about 2 per cent of Arabian foals.[98]

Clinically, affected foals have fever which may be intermittent, mucopurulent nasal and ocular discharges, dyspnoea, bronchial râles and sometimes a cough. Because the course of the disease is between 13 and 42 days, foals in the advanced stages of the disease may be in poor condition.[68, 70, 94] They may also suffer from dermatitis due to dermatophilosis and other concurrent infections.[94]

B-lymphocyte deficiency in these foals is indicated by an absolute lymphopenia, hypogammaglobulinaemia in which IgM and IgA are usually undetectable while IgG and IgG(T) are present in lower-than-normal concentration, and absence of germinal centres in the spleen and lymph nodes.[72] T-lymphocyte deficiency is shown by the absence of thymus tissue and peri-arteriolar lymphocytic sheaths in the spleen.[72] The lymph nodes are smaller than normal.[69] Neutropenia also occurs.[68]

Macroscopically, the lungs have lesions consistent with atelectasis and pneumonia, while microscopically there is swelling, hyperplasia and necrosis of the respiratory epithelium throughout the respiratory tract, and some cells contain typical intranuclear inclusion bodies.[69, 70] In some instances the pneumonia has been described as interstitial, and secondary bacterial infection has resulted in the development of bronchopneumonia.[72]

Epithelial lesions similar to those of the respiratory tract have also been observed microscopically in the transitional epithelium of the renal pelvis, ureters, bladder and urethra as well as conjunctival epithelium, ductal and parenchymatous epithelium of the lachrymal glands, salivary glands, pancreas and tubuloacinar glands. In a minority of cases, small groups of epithelial cells in the intestinal tract may be swollen, contain intranuclear inclusion bodies and undergo necrosis.[69]

Diagnosis and control

Apart from primary and low-passage kidney cells, equine adenoviruses can be cultured in MDCK (canine kidney), MDBK (bovine kidney)[48] and BS-c-1[96] cells. In general the diagnosis of equine adenovirus infection is similar to that described for bovine adenovirus infections.

Because equine adenoviruses are not important in the causation of disease in horses that are unaffected by the combined immune deficiency syndrome, no specific control measures have so far been deemed necessary. The production of an experimental vaccine containing virus inactivated by application of a combination of ultraviolet radiation and ß-propiolactone has been described.[63] This vaccine induced the development of high antibody levels in foals inoculated with it.

Although adenoviral infection that complicates the combined immune deficiency syndrome in Arabian foals is almost invariably fatal, beneficial effects have been obtained in affected animals by administering antisera or whole blood with high antibody levels against equine adenovirus, and antibiotics.[69]

References

1 **ADAIR, B.M., McFERRAN, J.B. & McKILLOP, E.R., 1982.** A sixth species of ovine adenovirus isolated from lambs in New Zealand. *Archives of Virology*, 74, 269–275.

2 **ADAIR, B.M., McKILLOP, E.R. & COACKLEY, B.H., 1986.** Serological identification of an Australian adenovirus isolate from sheep. *Australian Veterinary Journal*, 63, 162.

3 **BAKER, I.K., VAN DREUMEL, A.A. & PALMER, N., 1993.** The alimentary system. *In:* JUBB, K.V.F., KENNEDY, P.C. & PALMER, N., (eds). *Pathology of Domestic Animals*. 4th edn. Vol. II. San Diego, New York: Academic Press, Inc.

4 **BARTHA, A., 1974.** Immunization of cattle with a polyvalent bovine adenovirus vaccine. Thirteenth International Congress of LABS, Budapest; Part B: Selected Veterinary Vaccines. *Development of Biological Standardization*, 26, 15–18.

5 **BARTHA, A. & MATE, S., 1983.** Transplacental transmission of bovine adenoviruses. *Comparative Immunology and Microbiology of Infectious Diseases*, 6, 189–192.

6 **BAUER, K., MÜLLER, H. & GÜRTÜRK, S., 1975.** Isolierung eines virus von schafen und seine einordnung als neuer serotyp oviner adenoviren. *Zentralblatt für Veterinärmedizin*, Reihe B, 22, 656–665.

7 **BELAK, S., BERENCSI, G.Y., RUSVAY, M., LUKACS, K. & NASZ, I., 1983.** DNA structure and hemagglutination properties of bovine adenovirus type 2 strains which bypass species specificity. *Archives of Virology*, 77, 181–194.

8 **BELAK, S. & PALFI, V., 1974.** An adenovirus isolated from sheep and its relationship to type 2 bovine adenovirus. *Archiv für die Gesamte Virusforschung*, 46, 366–369.

9 **BELAK, S., PALFI, V. & PALYA, V., 1976.** Adenovirus infection in lambs. I. Epizootiology of the disease. *Zentralblatt für Veterinärmedizin*, Reihe B, 23, 320–330.

10 **BELAK, S. & RUSVAI, M., 1986.** *In utero* adenoviral infection of sheep. *Veterinary Microbiology*, 12, 87–91.

11 **BENKÖ, M., BARTHA, A., MÖSTL, K. & BÜRKI, F., 1989.** A heteroploid permanent cell line originating from embryonic calf thyroid supporting the replication of all known bovine adenovirus serotypes. *Veterinary Microbiology*, 19, 317–324.

12 **BIBRACK, B., 1970.** Vorkommen und verbreitung von adenoviren bei gesunden und an enzootischer pneumonie erkrankten schweinen. *Zentralblatt für Veterinärmedizin*, Reihe B, 17, 195–199.

13 **BULLER, C.R. & MOXLEY, R.A., 1988.** Natural infection of porcine Ileal Dome M cells with rotavirus and enteric adenovirus. *Veterinary Pathology*, 25, 516–517.

14 **BULMER, W.S., TSAI, K. & LITTLE, P.B., 1975.** Adenovirus infection in two calves. *Journal of the American Veterinary Medical Association*, 166, 233–238.

15 **BÜRKI, F., 1973.** Experimental adenovirus vaccines in cattle. *Journal of the American Veterinary Medical Association*, 163, 897–900.

16 **BURROWS, R., 1979.** Equine rhinovirus and adenovirus infections. *Proceedings of the Twenty-fourth Annual Convention of the American Association of Equine Practitioners*, December 1978, St Louis, Missouri.

17 **CALDOW, G.L., EDWARDS, S., NIXON, P. & PETERS, A.R., 1988.** Associations between viral infection and respiratory disease in young beef bulls. *The Veterinary Record*, 122, 529–531.

18 **COLE, N.A., DELANEY, D.D., CUMMINS, J.M. & HUTCHESON, D.P., 1986.** Nitrogen metabolism of calves inoculated with bovine adenovirus 3 or with infectious bovine rhinotracheitis virus. *American Journal of Veterinary Research*, 47, 1160–1164.

19 **CORIA, M.F., McCLURKIN, A.W., CUTLIP, R.C. & RITCHIE A.E., 1975.** Isolation and characterization of bovine adenovirus type 5 associated with weak calf syndrome. *Archives of Virology*, 47, 309–317.

20 **CORRIER, D.E., MONTGOMERY, D. & SCUTCHFIELD, W.L., 1982.** Adenovirus in the intestinal epithelium of a foal with prolonged diarrhea. *Veterinary Pathology*, 19, 564–567.

21 **COUSSEMENT, W., DUCATELLE, R., CHARLIER, G. & HOORENS, J., 1981.** Adenovirus enteritis in pigs. *American Journal of Veterinary Research*, 42, 1905–1911.

22 **CUTLIP, R.C. & LEHMKUHL, H.D., 1983.** Experimental infection of lambs with ovine adenovirus isolate RTS-151: lesions. *American Journal of Veterinary Research*, 44, 2395–2402.

23 **CUTLIP, R.C. & LEHMKUHL, H.D., 1986.** Pulmonary lesions in lambs experimentally infected with ovine adenovirus 5 strain RTS-42. *Veterinary Pathology*, 23, 589–593.

24 **CUTLIP, R.C. & McCLURKIN, A.W., 1975.** Lesions and pathogenesis of disease in young calves experimentally induced by a bovine adenovirus type 5 isolated from a calf with weak calf syndrome. *American Journal of Veterinary Research*, 36, 1095–1098.

25 **DAVIES, D.H., DUNGWORTH, D.L. & MARLASSY, A.T., 1981.** Experimental adenovirus infection of lambs. *Veterinary Microbiology*, 6, 113–128.

26 **DAVIES, D.H., HERCEG, M. & THURLEY, D.C., 1982.** Experimental infection of lambs with an adenovirus followed by *Pasteurella haemolytica*. *Veterinary Microbiology*, 7, 369–381.

27 **DAVIES, D.H. & HUMPHREYS, S., 1977.** Characterization of two strains of adenovirus isolated from New Zealand sheep. *Veterinary Microbiology*, 2, 97–107.

28 **DEA, S. & ELAZHARY, M.A.S.Y., 1984.** Cultivation of a porcine adenovirus in porcine thyroid cell cultures. *Cornell Veterinarian*, 74, 208–271.

29 **DEA, S. & ELAZHARY, M.A.S.Y., 1984.** Prevalence of antibodies to porcine adenovirus in swine by indirect fluorescent antibody test. *American Journal of Veterinary Research*, 45, 2109–2112.

30 **DERBYSHIRE, J.B., CLARKE, M.C. & COLLING, A.P., 1975.** Serological and pathogenicity studies with some unclassified porcine adenoviruses. *Journal of Comparative Pathology*, 85, 437–443.

31 **DERBYSHIRE, J.B., CLARKE, M.C. & JESSETT, D.M., 1966.** Observations on the faecal excretions of adenoviruses and enteroviruses in conventional and minimal disease pigs. *The Veterinary Record*, 21, 595–599.

32 **DERBYSHIRE, J.H., DAWSON, P.S. & LAMONT, P.H., 1965.** A new adenovirus serotype of bovine origin. *Journal of Comparative Pathology*, 75, 327–330.

33 **DUCATELLE, R., COUSSEMENT, W. & HOORENS, J., 1982.** Sequential pathological study of experimental porcine adenovirus enteritis. *Veterinary Pathology*, 19, 179–189.

34 **DUCATELLE, R., THOONEN, H., COUSSEMENT, W. & HOORENS, J., 1981.** Pathology of natural canine adenovirus pneumonia. *Research in Veterinary Science*, 31, 207–212.

35 **DUNGWORTH, D.L., 1993.** The respiratory system. *In:* JUBB, K.V.F., KENNEDY, P.C. & PALMER, N., (eds). *Pathology of Domestic Animals*. 4th edn. Vol. II. San Diego, New York: Academic Press, Inc.

36 **DUTTA, S.K., 1975.** Isolation and characterization of an adenovirus and isolation of its adenovirus-associated virus in cell culture from foals with respiratory tract disease. *American Journal of Veterinary Research*, 36, 247–250.

37 **EDINGTON, N., KASZA, L. & CHRISTOFINIS, G.J., 1972.** Meningo-encephalitis in gnotobiotic pigs inoculated intranasally and orally with porcine adenovirus 4. *Research in Veterinary Science*, 13, 289–291.

38 **EDINGTON, N., WRIGHT, J.A., PATEL, J.R., EDWARDS, G.B. & GRIFFITHS, L., 1984.** Equine adenovirus 1 isolated from cauda equina neuritis. *Research in Veterinary Science*, 37, 252–254.

39 **FATEMIE-NAINIE, S. & MARUSYK, R., 1979.** Biophysical and serologic comparison of four equine adenovirus isolates. *American Journal of Veterinary Research*, 40, 521–528.

40 **FENNER, F., BACHMANN, P.A., GIBBS, E.P.J., MURPHY, F.A., STUDDERT, M.J. & WHITE, D.O., 1987.** *Veterinary Virology*. Orlando, San Diego, New York: Academic Press, Inc.

41 **FUJIWARA, H. & KONNO, S., 1968.** Histopathology of an enzootic diarrheal disease in cattle. *National Institute of Animal Health Quarterly*, 8, 16–25.

42 **HAIG, D.A. & CLARKE, M.C., 1964.** Isolation of an adenovirus from a pig. *Journal of Comparative Pathology*, 74, 81–84.

43 **HARASAWA, R., KONISHI, S-I. & OGATA, M., 1977.** Detection of antibody against adenovirus in horses imported into Japan. *Japanese Journal of Veterinary Science*, 39, 451–454.

44 **HORNER, G.W. & HUNTER, R., 1982.** Isolation of two serotypes of equine adenovirus from horses in New Zealand. *New Zealand Veterinary Journal*, 30, 62–64.

45 **HORNER, G.W., HUNTER, R., BARTHA, A. & BENKÖ, M., 1989.** A new subgroup 2 bovine adenovirus proposed as the prototype strain 10. *Archives of Virology*, 109, 121–124.

46 **HORNER, G.W., HUNTER, R. & THOMPSON, E.J., 1980.** Isolation and characterization of a new adenovirus serotype from a yearling heifer with systemic infection. *New Zealand Veterinary Journal*, 28, 165–167.

47 **HORNER, G.W. & REED, D.H., 1982.** Presumptive adenoviral bronchiolitis in a red deer (*Cervus elaphus*). *Journal of Comparative Pathology*, 92, 631–634.

48 **ISHIYAMA, T., SHINAGAWA, M., SATO, G., FUJINAGA, K. & PADMANABHAN, R., 1986.** Generation of packaging-defective DNA molecules of equine adenovirus. *Virology*, 151, 66–76.

49 **JOLLY, P.D., FU, Z.F. & ROBINSON, A.J., 1986.** Viruses associated with respiratory disease of horses in New Zealand: An update. *New Zealand Veterinary Journal*, 34, 46–50.

50 **KASZA, L., 1966.** Isolation of an adenovirus from the brain of a pig. *American Journal of Veterinary Research*, 27, 751–758.

51 **KASZA, L., HODGES, R.T., BETTS, A.O. & TREXLER, P.C., 1969.** Pneumonia in gnotobiotic pigs produced by simultaneous inoculation of a swine adenovirus and *Mycoplasma hyopneumoniae*. *The Veterinary Record*, 84, 262–267.

52 **KIRKBRIDE, C.A. & McADARAG, J.P., 1978.** Infectious agents associated with fetal and early neonatal death and abortion in swine. *Journal of the American Veterinary Medical Association*, 172, 480–483.

53 **KLEIN, M., EARLEY, E. & ZELLAT, J., 1959.** Isolation from cattle of a virus related to human adenovirus. *Proceedings of the Society for Experimental Biology and Medicine*, 102, 1–4.

54 **KLEIN, M., ZELLAT, J. & MICHAELSON, T.C., 1960.** A new bovine adenovirus related to human adenovirus. *Proceedings of the Society for Experimental Biology and Medicine*, 105, 340–342.

55 **KWON, H.J. & SPRADBROW, P.B., 1971.** The isolation of a porcine adenovirus in Queensland. *Australian Veterinary Journal*, 47, 54–56.

56 **LEAMASTER, B.R., EVERMANN, J.F. & LEHMKUHL, H.D., 1987.** Identification of ovine adenovirus types 5 and 6 in an epizootic of respiratory tract disease in recently weaned lambs. *Journal of the American Veterinary Medical Association*, 12, 1545–1547.

57 **LEHMKUHL, H.D., CONTRERAS, J.A., CUTLIP, R.C. & BROGDEN, K.A., 1989.** Clinical and microbiologic findings in lambs inoculated with *Pasteurella haemolytica* after infection with ovine adenovirus type 6. *American Journal of Veterinary Research*, 50, 671– 675.

58 **LEHMKUHL, H.D. & CUTLIP, R.C., 1984.** Experimental infection of lambs with ovine adenovirus isolate RTS-151: Clinical, microbiological, and serologic responses. *American Journal of Veterinary Research*, 45, 260–262.

59 **LEHMKUHL, H.D. & CUTLIP, R.C., 1986.** Inoculation of lambs with ovine adenovirus 5 (Mastadenovirus ovi 5) strain RTS-42. *American Journal of Veterinary Research*, 47, 724–726.

60 **LEHMKUHL, H.D., CUTLIP, R.C., BOLIN, S. & BROGDEN, K.A., 1985.** Seroepidemiologic survey of antibodies to selected viruses in the respiratory tract of lambs. *American Journal of Veterinary Research*, 46, 2601–2604.

61 **LEHMKUHL, H.D., SMITH, M.H. & DIERKS, R.E., 1975.** A bovine adenovirus type 3: Isolation, characterization, and experimental infection in calves. *Archives of Virology*, 48, 39–46.

62 **LEHMKUHL, H.D., SMITH, M.H. & GOUGH, P.M., 1979.** Neutralizing antibody to bovine adenovirus serotype 3 in healthy cattle and cattle with respiratory tract disease. *American Journal of Veterinary Research*, 40, 580–583.

63 **LEW, A.M., SMITH, H.V. & STUDDERT, M.J., 1979.** Development and preliminary testing of an inactivated equine adenovirus vaccine. *American Journal of Veterinary Research*, 40, 1707–1712.

64 **MATTSON, D.E., 1973.** Naturally occurring infection of calves with a bovine adenovirus. *American Journal of Veterinary Research*, 34, 623–629.

65 **MATTSON, D.E., NORMAN, B.B. & DUNBAR, J.R., 1988.** Bovine adenovirus type-3 infection in feedlot calves. *American Journal of Veterinary Research*, 49, 67–69.

66 **MATTSON, D.E., WANGELIN, J.R. & SWEAT, R.L., 1987.** Vaccination of dairy calves with bovine adenovirus type 3. *Cornell Veterinarian,* 77, 351–361.

67 **MAUTNER, V., 1989.** Adenoviridae. *In:* PORTERFIELD, J.S. (ed.) *Andrew's Viruses of Vertebrates.* 5th edn. London, Philadelphia, Toronto, Sydney, Tokyo: Baillière Tindall.

68 **McCHESNEY, A.E., ENGLAND, J.J., ADCOCK, J.L., STACKHOUSE, L.L. & CHOW, T.L., 1970.** Adenoviral infection in suckling Arabian foals. *Pathologia Veterinaria,* 7, 547–565.

69 **McCHESNEY, A.E., ENGLAND, J.J. & RICH, L.J., 1973.** Adenoviral infection in foals. *Journal of the American Veterinary Medical Association,* 162, 545–549.

70 **McCHESNEY, A.E., ENGLAND, J.J., WHITEMAN, C.E., ADCOCK, J.L., RICH, L.J. & CHOW, T.L., 1974.** Experimental transmission of equine adenovirus in Arabian and non-Arabian foals. *American Journal of Veterinary Research,* 35, 1015–1023.

71 **McFERRAN, J.B., NELSON, R. & KNOX, E.R., 1971.** Isolation and characterisation of sheep adenoviruses. *Archiv für die Gesamte Virusforschung,* 35, 232–241.

72 **McGUIRE, T.C. & POPPIE, M., 1973.** Hypogammaglobulinemia and thymic hypoplasia in horses: A primary combined immunodeficiency disorder. *Infection and Immunity,* 8, 272–277.

73 **MESSNER, A., HINAIDY, B. & BÜRKI, F., 1983.** Bovine adenoviruses V. Diagnostic efficiency of dual-antigen immuno-diffusion test using two different group-reactive antigens in parallel. *Zentralblatt für Veterinärmedizin,* Reihe B, 30, 762–774.

74 **MOHANTY, S., 1971.** Comparative study of bovine adenoviruses. *American Journal of Veterinary Research,* 32, 1899–1905.

75 **NARITA, M., IMADA, T. & FUKUSHO, A., 1985.** Pathologic changes caused by transplacental infection with an adenovirus-like agent in pigs. *American Journal of Veterinary Research,* 46, 1126–1129.

76 **ORR, J.P., 1984.** Necrotizing enteritis in a calf infected with adenovirus. *Canadian Veterinary Journal,* 25, 72–74.

77 **PEET, R.L., COACKLEY, W., PURCELL, D.A., ROBERTSON, C.W. & MICKE, B.M., 1983**. Adenovirus inclusions in sheep liver. *Australian Veterinary Journal,* 60, 307–308.

78 **POWELL, D.G., BURROWS, R., SPOONER, P.R., GOODRIDGE, D., THOMSON, G.R. & MUMFORD, J., 1978.** A study of infectious respiratory disease among horses in Great Britain, 1971–76. *In: Equine Infectious Diseases.* IV. Proceedings of the Fourth International Conference on Equine Infectious Disease, Lyon, 24–27 September 1976. Princeton, New Jersey: Veterinary Publications, Inc.

79 **PRINCE, G.A., PORTER, D.D., BENNETT JENSON, A., HORSWOOD, R.L., CHANOCK, R.M. & GINSBERG, H.S., 1993.** Pathogenesis of adenovirus type 5 pneumonia in cotton rats (*Sigmodon hispidus*). *Journal of Virology,* 67, 101–111.

80 **REED, D.E., WHEEL, J.G., LUPTON, H.W., 1978.** Isolation of bovine adenovirus type 7 from calves with pneumonia and enteritis. *American Journal of Veterinary Research,* 39, 1968–1971.

81 **RUSHTON, B. & SHARP, J.M., 1977.** Pathology of ovine adenovirus type 4 infection in SPF lambs: Pulmonary and hepatic lesions. *Journal of Pathology,* 121, 163–167.

82 **RUSSELL, W.C., 1991.** Adenoviridae. *In:* FRANCKI, R.I.B., FAUQUET, C.M., KNUDSON, D.L. & BROWN, F. (eds). *Classification and Nomenclature of Viruses,* Fifth Report of the International Committee on the Taxonomy of Viruses. *Archives of Virology,* Supplementum 2. Vienna, New York: Springer-Verlag.

83 **SANFORD, S.E. & HOOVER, D.M., 1983.** Enteric adenovirus infection in pigs. *Canadian Journal of Comparative Medicine,* 47, 396–400.

84 **SCANZIANI, E., SIRONI, G., FINAZZI, M. & LUINI, M., 1989.** Adenoviral fibrinous enteritis in calves. *Deutsche Tierärztliche Wochenschrift,* 96, 165–168.

85 **SHARP, J.M., 1983.** Acute respiratory virus infections. *In:* MARTIN, W.B. (ed.). *Diseases of Sheep.* Edinburgh: Blackwell Scientific Publications.

86 **SMITH, I.M., BETTS, A.O., WATT, R.G. & HAYWARD, A.H.S., 1973.** Experimental infections with *Pasteurella septica* (serogroup A) and an adeno- or enterovirus in gnotobiotic piglets. *Journal of Comparative Pathology,* 83, 1–12.

87 **SMYTH, J.A., CUSH, P.F., ADAIR, B.M. & YOUNG, J.A., 1986.** Adenovirus-associated enterocolitis in a bullock. *The Veterinary Record,* 119, 574–576.

88 **STAUBER, E.H., ABINANTI, F.R. & WHITBECK, G.D., 1986.** Seroepizootiology of types 3 and 7 adenoviruses and bovine viral diarrhea virus infections of beef cattle from birth to first parturition. *American Journal of Veterinary Research,* 47, 774–776.

89 **STAUBER, E.H., AUTENRIETH, R., MARKHAM, O.D. & WHITBECK, V., 1980.** A seroepidemiologic survey of three pronghorn (*Antilocapra americana*) populations in south-eastern Idaho, 1975–77. *Journal of Wildlife Diseases,* 16, 109–113.

90 **STAUBER, E.H., RENSHAW, H.W., BORO, C., MATTSON, D. & FRANK, F.W., 1976.** Isolation of a subgroup 2 adenovirus from a calf with weak calf syndrome. *Canadian Journal of Comparative Medicine,* 40, 98–103.

91 **STOTT, E.J., THOMAS, L.H., COLLINS, A.P., CROUCH, S., JEBBETT, J., SMITH, G.S., LUTHER, P.D. & CASWELL, R., 1980.** A survey of virus infections of the respiratory tract of cattle and their association with disease. *Journal of Hygiene (Cambridge),* 85, 257–270.

92 **STUDDERT, M.J. & BLACKNEY, M.H., 1982.** Isolation of an adenovirus antigenically distinct from equine adenovirus type 1 from diarrheic foal faeces. *American Journal of Veterinary Research,* 43, 543–544.

93 **STUDDERT, M.J., WILKS, C.R. & COGGINS, L., 1974.** Antigenic comparison and serologic survey of equine adenoviruses. *American Journal of Veterinary Research,* 35, 693–699.

94 **THOMPSON, D.B., STUDDERT, M.J., BEILHARZ, R.G. & LITTLEJOHNS, I.R., 1975.** Inheritance of a lethal immunodeficiency disease of Arabian foals. *Australian Veterinary Journal,* 51, 109–113.

95 **THOMPSON, K.G., THOMSON, G.W. & HENRY, J.N., 1981.** Alimentary tract manifestations of bovine adenovirus infections. *Canadian Veterinary Journal,* 22, 68–71.

96 **TODD, J.D., 1969.** Comments on rhinoviruses and parainfluenza viruses of horses. *Journal of the American Veterinary Medical Association,* 155, 387–390.

97 **ULLRICH, N.A., MATTSON, D.E. & SCHMITZ, J.A., 1982.** Preliminary report on the isolation and pathogenicity of two ovine adenoviruses. *Twenty-fifth Annual Proceedings of the American Association of Veterinary Laboratory Diagnosticians.* 185–196.

98 **VALLI, V.E.O. & PARRY, B.W., 1993.** The hematopoietic system. *In:* JUBB, K.V.F., KENNEDY, P.C. & PALMER, N. (eds) *Pathology of Domestic Animals.* 4th edn. Vol. III. San Diego, New York: Academic Press, Inc.

99 **WIGAND, R., BARTHA, A., DREIZIN, R.S., ESCHE, H., GINSBERG, H.S., GREEN, M., HIERHOLZER, J.C., KALTER, S.S., McFERRAN, J.B., PETTERSSON, U.P., RUSSELL, W.C. & WADELL, G., 1982.** Adenoviridae: Second report. *Intervirology,* 18, 169–176.

100 **WILCOX, G.E., 1969.** Isolation of adenoviruses from cattle with conjunctivitis and keratoconjunctivitis. *Australian Veterinary Journal,* 45, 265–270.

101 **WILCOX, G.E., 1970.** The aetiology of infectious bovine keratoconjunctivitis in Queensland. II. Adenovirus. *Australian Veterinary Journal,* 46, 415–420.

HERPESVIRIDAE

The family Herpesviridae is made up of a group of at least 112 viruses which infect mammals, birds, reptiles, amphibians and fish.[5] Many of these viruses produce no known disease, but some are the cause of important afflictions of both humans and animals. Cattle, sheep, goats, horses, donkeys and pigs are susceptible to a variety of infections caused by one or more different herpesviruses in each species **(Table 1)**. These infections, some of which result in economically important diseases of livestock, are described in the following chapters.

The nomenclature of herpesviruses, and particularly of those that infect ruminants, is complicated and somewhat confused. For example, bovine (or bovid) herpesvirus 3 (BHV-3) has been used to refer not only to the wildebeest-associated virus which causes malignant catarrhal fever (now known as alcelaphine herpesvirus 1), but also to bovine herpesvirus 4 (BHV-4), which in turn has variously been labelled Movar-type bovine herpesvirus, bovine orphan herpesvirus and bovine herpesvirus 5.[1, 4, 5] The designation BHV-3 is now considered redundant and therefore bovine herpesviruses are currently numbered 1, 2, 4, and 5.[5] This complexity and confusion is due on the one hand to the wide variety of hosts and biological properties these viruses have and,

Table 1 Members of the Herpesviridae that infect domestic livestock

VIRUS	COMMONLY APPLIED SYNONYMS	SUBFAMILY	DISEASE CAUSED IN DOMESTIC LIVESTOCK
Bovine herpesvirus 1	Infectious bovine rhinotracheitis (IBR) virus	α	Infectious bovine rhinotracheitis, infectious pustular vulvovaginitis, infectious balanoposthitis and other syndromes
Bovine herpesvirus 2	Bovine mammillitis virus, Allerton virus, pseudo-lumpy skin disease virus	α	Pseudo-lumpy skin disease/bovine herpes mammillitis
Bovine herpesvirus 4	BHV-3, BHV-5, bovine orphan herpesvirus, Movar-type herpesvirus	γ	?
Bovine herpesvirus 5	IBR virus, BHV-1, BHV-1.3, bovine encephalitis herpesvirus	α	Meningoencephalitis
Caprine herpesvirus 1	Goat herpesvirus, BHV-6	α	Gastroenteritis, pustular vulvovaginitis
Ovine herpesvirus 1	Herpesvirus ovis, BHV-4, BHV-5, caprine herpesvirus 1	u	?
Ovine herpesvirus 2	Sheep-associated malignant catarrhal fever virus	γ	Malignant catarrhal fever (snotsiekte)
Alcelaphine herpesvirus 1	Malignant catarrhal fever virus, wildebeest herpesvirus	γ	Malignant catarrhal fever (snotsiekte)
Alcelaphine herpesvirus 2	Hartebeest herpesvirus	γ	?
Equid herpesvirus 1	Equid herpesvirus 1 subtype 1, equine herpesvirus 1, equine abortion virus	α	Neonatal deaths, abortion, rhinopneumonitis, meningoencephalomyelitis
Equid herpesvirus 2	Equine herpesvirus 2, equine cytomegalovirus	β	?
Equid herpesvirus 3	Equine herpesvirus 3, coital exanthema virus	α	Coital exanthema
Equid herpesvirus 4	Equine herpesvirus 4, equid herpesvirus 1 subtype 2	α	Rhinopneumonitis
Equid herpesvirus 5	Equine herpesvirus 5	β	?
Equid herpesvirus 6	Asinine herpesvirus 1	α	Vesicular and erosive lesions on muzzle, genitalia and udder
Equid herpesvirus 7	Asinine herpesvirus 2	β	?
Equid herpesvirus 8	Asinine herpesvirus 3	α	Rhinitis
Suid herpesvirus 1	Pseudorabies virus, Aujeszky's disease virus	α	Pseudorabies (Aujeszky's disease)
Suid herpesvirus 2	Inclusion body rhinitis virus, porcine cytomegalovirus	β	Inclusion body rhinitis

α Alphaherpesvirinae   β Betaherpesvirinae   ? Role in disease uncertain
γ Gammaherpesvirinae   u As yet unplaced

on the other, to differences in the recommendations made by successive study groups of the International Committee on the Taxonomy of Viruses (ICTV) as well as to proposals offered by unofficial groups and individuals.[1, 3–5]

Based on biological properties (host range, duration of reproductive cycle, cytopathology and characteristics of latent infection), herpesviruses that have been well studied have been placed in three subfamilies — Alphaherpesvirinae, Betaherpesvirinae and Gammaherpesvirinae.[2, 4, 5]

In an alternative approach, variation in genome size, G+C content and the arrangement of tandemly repeated sequences have been used to identify five groups of herpesviruses (labelled A to E).[4, 5] These criteria, together with serological relationships and, where possible, sequence homology, have been used to propose classification into genera, but so far few herpesviruses of veterinary importance have been assigned to a genus.[4, 5] Therefore, herpesviruses are at present generally referred to only by their specific name, e.g. bovine herpesvirus 2 (BHV-2).

The ICTV study group[4, 5] has proposed that herpesviruses should be named after the taxonomic unit — family or subfamily — to which their primary natural host belongs. When family names are used, the word should end in id (e.g. equid or suid) but when subfamily names are used (as in the case of primates and Bovidae), the name should end in ine (e.g. bovine or caprine). The exceptions to this rule are viruses which infect humans, where 'human' is used, e.g. human herpesvirus 1.

In the following chapters an endeavour has been made to abide by the recommendations of the latest ICTV study group of Roizman *et al.*,[5] **(Table 1)** although most chapters were written before the recommendations became available. Viruses of veterinary importance which have been renamed in the latest report of the Herpesvirus Study Group of the ICTV[5] are: equid herpesvirus 4 [replaces EHV-1 subtype 2 **(see Chapter 102)**], equid herpesvirus 5 [previously part of EHV-2 **(see Chapter 103)**], bovine herpesvirus 5 [previously part of BHV-1 **(see Chapter 105)**], ovine herpesvirus 1 [replaces caprine herpesvirus 1 **(see Chapter 110)**], ovine herpesvirus 2 [previously referred to as the cause of sheep-associated malignant catarrhal fever **(see Chapter 107)**], equid herpesvirus 6 [instead of asinine herpesvirus 1 **(see Chapter 110)**], equid herpesvirus 7 [instead of asinine herpesvirus 2 **(see Chapter 110)**], and equid herpesvirus 8 [instead of asinine herpesvirus 3 **(see Chapter 110)**].

References

1 **BARTHA, A., FADOL, A.M., WEBERMAN, H.** ***et al.***, 1987. Problems concerning the taxonomy of 'Movar-type' bovine herpesviruses. *Intervirology*, 28, 1–7.

2 **HONESS, R.W., 1984.** Herpes simplex and 'the herpes complex'. Diverse observations and a unifying hypothesis. *Journal of General Virology*, 65, 2077–2107.

3 **ROIZMAN, B., BARTHA, A., BIGGS, M.P., CARMICHAEL, L.E., GRANOFF, A., HAMPAR, B., KAPLAN, A.S., MELENDEZ, L.V., MUNK, K., NAHMIAS, A.J., PLUMMER, G., RAJCANI, J., TERNI, M., de-THE, G., WATSON, P.H. & WILDY, P., 1973.** Provisional labels for herpesviruses. *Journal of General Virology*, 20, 417–419.

4 **ROIZMAN, B., CARMICHAEL, L.E., DEINHART, F., de-THE, G., NAHMIAS, A.J., PLOWRIGHT, W., RAPP, F., SHELDRICK, P., TAKAHASHI, M. & WOLF, K., 1981.** Herpesviridae. Definition, provisional nomenclature and taxonomy. *Intervirology*, 16, 201–217.

5 **ROIZMAN, B., DESROSIERS, R.C., FLECKENSTEIN, B., LOPEZ, C., MINSON, A.C. & STUDDERT, M.J., 1992.** The family Herpesviridae: An update. *Archives of Virology*, 123, 425–449.

102

Equid herpesvirus 1 and 4 infections

Synonyms: Equine rhinopneumonitis, equine viral abortions

J.A. Mumford

Introduction

Equid herpesvirus 1 (EHV-1) is a directly transmitted cause of four distinct syndromes in horses: respiratory disease (rhinopneumonitis), abortion, neonatal foal disease and, more rarely, paresis or paralysis. Like herpesviruses, EHV-1 can establish latent infections. Furthermore, immunity is short-lived and horses experience repeated infections throughout life as a result of re-exposure[136] or reactivation of latent virus.[32, 61] In older animals, these infections are often subclinical.

The virus exists as two subtypes which are distinguishable on the basis of their genetic and antigenic characteristics and the disease syndromes they induce. Subtype 1 virus is a cause of respiratory disease, multiple abortions, neonatal foal death, and paresis and paralysis, while subtype 2 virus is associated mainly with respiratory disease, but has occasionally been isolated from individual aborted foetuses.[118] On just one occasion subtype 2 was isolated from the spinal cord of a horse with a nervous disorder.[96]

The magnitude of genetic differences between subtype 1 and subtype 2 viruses led Studdert to propose that they should be reclassified as EHV-1 and EHV-4 respectively.[132] This has been widely accepted.

A group of respiratory diseases in horses was known to veterinary practitioners during the early years of this century as 'equine influenza'.[81] Equid herpesvirus 1 was eventually recognized as being one of the aetiological agents involved.[54] The first reported case of equine abortion resulting from a possible viral infection was in 1932 by Dimock and Edwards,[44–46] who noted that abortion occurred late in gestation and that the breeding capacity of mares which had aborted was not subsequently impaired. This syndrome became known as enzootic abortion. Their clinical and pathological observations were confirmed in subsequent studies.[84, 143] In 1942, the virus was propagated in hamsters, in which intranuclear inclusion bodies in hepatocytes were observed.[11] This work was soon followed by culture of the virus in a wide range of *in vitro* cell systems.[124]

The relationship between enzootic abortion and respiratory disease was not appreciated for several years. Jones *et al.*[81] isolated a virus from horses suffering from respiratory disease thought to be equine influenza, and in 1954 Doll and Kintner[54] demonstrated that this 'equine influenza virus' was identical to equine abortion virus, now known as EHV-1 subtype 1.

The first evidence for an association between EHV-1 infection and neurological disease was reported by Saxegaard in 1966, when he isolated EHV-1 from the brain and spinal cord of a paralysed horse in Norway.

The fourth clinically recognizable disease syndrome associated with EHV-1 is neonatal foal disease, which was recognized in the USA in 1977[24] and Australia in 1979.[74]

Both subtypes of EHV-1 are widely distributed throughout the world. Respiratory disease, abortion, neonatal foal disease, and paresis and paralysis caused by EHV-1 have been reported in South Africa.[14, 64, 68, 133]

Outbreaks of disease caused by EHV-1 are a major cause of economic loss to the racing and breeding industries as they result in poor racing performance, mortality, closure or quarantine of stud farms following cases of abortion, and restrictions on the movement of horses.

Aetiology

Equid herpesvirus 1 is a typical herpesvirus.[103, 112] In the early years of research on equine abortion virus all EHV-1 isolates were thought to be antigenically homologous, belonging to a single serotype and having the same disease potential.[28] However, evidence has accumulated over more than 25 years which indicates the existence of antigenic differences within EHV-1 isolates.

Cross-neutralization studies and serological surveys have demonstrated that there are two antigenic subtypes; subtype 1 represented by strains KyD, Army 183 and RACH,[26, 55, 81, 93] and subtype 2 represented by H45 and H46.[83, 84, 90, 124]

Correlation between viral subtype and the anatomical site of isolation was first demonstrated by Burrows and Goodridge,[29] who showed that all the viruses isolated from the respiratory tract were antigenically similar, as were all the reference foetal strains tested. Thus, although there were detectable cross-reactions between the two groups of viruses, they formed two more or less distinct groups. It is now recognized however, that it is not unusual for subtype 1 virus to be isolated from horses with respiratory tract infection, and rarely, for subtype 2 virus to be isolated from aborted foetuses.

Equid herpesvirus subtype 1 isolates replicate in a wider range of cell cultures, multiply more prolifically and produce larger plaques than do subtype 2 viruses.[29, 131] Furthermore, subtype 1 isolates are recoverable from the buffy coat (subtype 2 only rarely so) fraction of blood, and they induce higher levels of neutralizing antibody than do subtype 2 isolates. After direct intra-uterine inoculation of pregnant mares, subtype 1 virus grows to a higher titre in the foetal tissue than do subtype 2 viruses,[29, 30] indicating that the pathogenicity of subtype 1 viruses for the foetus is greater than that of subtype 2 isolates.

Despite the existence of two subtypes, the degree of difference between them was not fully appreciated until the genomes were compared by restriction endonuclease analysis. Sabine, Robertson and Whalley[119] compared the restriction profiles of respiratory (subtype 2), foetal (subtype 1) and neonatal (subtype 1) isolates, using a number of restriction enzymes, and demonstrated a lack of common cleavage sites between the subtypes. This contrasted with the restriction profiles within each viral subtype, which were closely related. Similar observations were reported independently by two other groups.[132, 141]

Virions of EHV-1 have four major structural components; the internal DNA core, the icosahedral capsid (which, together with the core, makes up the nucleocapsid), the tegument and the outer envelope. The core is an electron-dense structure with a less electron-dense central cylinder around which the linear genome is wound.[108] This is surrounded by a capsid consisting of 162 capsomeres arranged to form an icosadeltahedron approximately 100 nm in diameter.[102] The most abundant nucleocapsid protein is a Mr 140k phosphoprotein (VP9) and is present as 800 copies per virion. This accounts for more than 80 per cent of the total protein content of the virus capsid.[103] The tegument is an ill-defined region around the capsid which contains at least eight proteins of unknown structure or function.[139] In turn, the tegument is enclosed by a triple-layered membranous envelope which is acquired as the nucleocapsid buds through the nuclear membrane of the host cell. The envelope contains glycoproteins, phosphoproteins and lipid.[1, 101]

Equid herpesvirus 1 virions are made up of at least 28 structural proteins.[139, 140] Six major glycoproteins (gp2, 10 13, 14, 18 and 22a) and six or seven minor glycoproteins have been identified as being components of the virus envelope. Six non-glycosylated polypeptides occur in the nucleocapsid and eight to nine non-glycosylated polypeptides in the tegument. In a study of the glycoproteins that used monoclonal antibodies, an antigenic relationship was demonstrated as existing between the minor gp17 and the major gp18, and also between minor gp21 and major gp22a which resulted in the redesignation of the six major glycoproteins (gp2, 10, 13, 14, 17/18 and 21/22a).[6]

Glycoprotein 2 of EHV-1 possesses epitopes which are predominantly subtype cross-reactive.[139] Non-neutralizing monoclonal antibodies directed against this glycoprotein inhibit the growth of plaques, suggesting that it plays a role in the cell-to-cell spread of virus.[60] Glycoprotein 10 also has epitopes that are mainly subtype cross-reactive.[139] Glycoprotein 13 of EHV-1 is the structural homologue of gC-like glycoproteins within the Alphaherpesvirinae[4] and carries both subtype-specific and subtype cross-reactive epitopes.[8, 126]

The role of gp13 in the virus-host interaction and, in particular, its importance in stimulating protective immune responses in the equine host is unknown. However, some monoclonal antibodies directed against gp13 neutralize viral infectivity,[8, 123, 126] and monoclonal antibodies against gp13 have been identified which passively protect hamsters against respiratory and lethal EHV-1 infection.[125, 130] Hamsters immunized with recombinant gp13 (expressed by a vaccinia virus vector) are protected against lethal challenge.[72]

Glycoprotein 14 of EHV-1 is the structural homologue of gB-like glycoproteins within the Alphaherpesvirinae.[117, 143] The mature glycosylated protein consists of two subunits linked by disulphide bonds.[95] Common epitopes have been identified on gp14 of both EHV-1 subtypes,[128] and common amino acid sequences have been described.[144]

The role of gp14 in the virus-host interaction and its importance in stimulating host immunity is largely unknown, but it has been established that it is a major target for antibodies in convalescent horse sera.[2] Some monoclonal antibodies directed against gp14 neutralize viral infectivity,[123] and some are able to passively protect hamsters against a self-limiting EHV-1 infection.[130]

Glycoproteins 17/18 possess mainly subtype-specific epitopes,[139] whereas gp21/22 possess mainly subtype cross-reactive epitopes.[3]

Variation in the neutralizing activity of polyclonal antisera against different EHV-1 strains is common.[29, 136, 141] It is, however, possible that the innate variability of the assays accounts for such variation, since measurement of the rate of neutralization of different viral strains by polyclonal antisera has failed to detect differences between either subtype 1 or subtype 2 strains.[139]

In contrast, analysis of isolates using monoclonal antibodies has clearly demonstrated antigenic variants in the virus population. Extensive variation has been identified in subtype 1 gp13 of isolates from the USA,[8] with 16 different binding patterns (representing different epitopes) having been identified with 42 monoclonal antibodies among 72 virus isolates. No correlation has been found with disease manifestation.

The genome of subtype 1 virus has been studied in more detail than that of subtype 2. It consists of a linear double-stranded molecule of DNA with an approximate Mr of 90–94 x 10^6 and forms 9 per cent of the particle dry weight. It has a buoyant density of 1,1716 g/ml and a G+C content of 57 moles per cent.[42, 102, 129] There is only 17 per cent nucleotide homology between the two subtypes.[5]

Restriction endonuclease analysis of viral DNA is a highly specific method for the detection of genetic variation and has been applied to subtype 1 and subtype 2 isolates.[9, 36] The effect of *in vitro* and *in vivo* serial passage on the genetic stability of the genome has revealed that no changes occur in the restriction profiles of DNA within 100 passages in an equine cell line, but that passage in a non-equine cell or in hamsters quickly gives rise to alterations.[7] A high degree of genetic homogeneity has been demonstrated in the USA among subtype 1 isolates propagated in equine cells, with only 16 distinct strains being identified among 148 epidemiologically unrelated subtype 1 isolates using five different restriction enzymes. Two subtype 1 strains were identified which accounted for over 90 per cent of the non-vaccine-related abortions that occurred in the Kentucky area in the period between 1960 and 1983. These were designated electropherotypes IP (prototype) and IB. Type IP dominated the period between 1960 and 1979 and IB the period between 1982 and 1983.

The degree of genetic diversity observed in subtype 2 isolates is greater than that for subtype 1 isolates. Thirteen distinct strains have been identified from 21 epidemiologically unrelated outbreaks. In contrast to subtype 1 outbreaks, there were no dominant strains — the most prevalent accounting for only 33 per cent of outbreaks.[10]

Epidemiology

The epidemiology of EHV-1 infections has been reviewed.[3, 51]

Serological surveys have demonstrated the worldwide distribution of this virus.[90] The respiratory syndrome of the disease is common to all horse populations,[13, 27, 58, 65, 113] whereas the prevalence of the abortigenic and neurological syndromes of the disease varies in different geographical areas. Abortions are common in the USA and parts of Europe, but are less frequent in other countries, including Britain, Australia, Japan and South Africa.[68, 75] In Australia, abortion storms were unknown before 1977, when EHV-1 subtype 1 was isolated for the first time.[48, 74] Prior to that time, only EHV-1 subtype 2 viruses had been recovered from individual sporadic abortions.[107, 118, 131]

The prevalence of the neurological syndrome also varies between countries. Confirmed cases have occurred in Europe,[18, 36, 39, 40, 47, 71, 109, 120] North America[35, 87] and India.[80] The syndrome has also been diagnosed in South Africa,[68] but not in Australia or New Zealand.

Identifying the source of infection in EHV-1 outbreaks is a difficult task because many infections are subclinical, and the problem is further complicated by the existence of latent infections which may be reactivated many months or years after primary infection.[19, 32, 61]

In primary infections, virus is shed from the nasopharynx for seven to 14 days, whereas virus excretion is usually transient (two to four days) after re-infection. Virus is also shed in saliva and ocular discharges, and subtype 1 virus may be recovered from faeces.[106] Cell-associated viraemias may persist for weeks or months in subtype 1 infections,[97] but it has not been established whether animals with such infections can infect susceptible cohorts.

Virus is transmitted by the inhalation of infectious aerosols, by direct contact of the respiratory mucosa with infected fomites, and possibly by ingestion of contaminated feed and water.[64] While spread of virus among a group of housed animals, particularly those sharing a common airspace, may be rapid, the spread among groups of horses at pasture is much slower, taking a number of weeks, and is dependent on contact between infected and susceptible animals.[100]

Equid herpesvirus 1 is readily inactivated by a wide range of disinfectants but it may persist in the environment for one or two weeks if it is protected in nasal secretions.[12]

As with equine influenza, seasonality in the occurrence of outbreaks of respiratory disease caused by EHV-1 tends to reflect management practices within the equine industry which expose young horses to infection, particularly in stressful circumstances such as weaning, mixing of groups from diverse backgrounds, transport, and castration.[3, 31, 66, 122] Thoroughbred foals on stud farms are often weaned in groups and assembled into new social groups in the autumn, creating ideal circumstances for the initiation of respiratory infections. In the autumn, yearlings are assembled for sales and sent to breaking and training yards, ready for careers in racing as two- and three-year-olds. Rhinopneumonitis is therefore common among young animals in the autumn. Since natural immunity is short-lived and repeated infections may occur among the same animals within a matter of months, some foals will experience more than one infection in the first year of life.[3, 135] Clinical respiratory disease is rarely recognized in older animals; subclinical respiratory infections continue throughout life.

Apart from outbreaks of respiratory disease caused by EHV-1 among groups of animals, sero-surveillance of young animals in training has demonstrated repeated infection/recrudescence throughout the year. These individual seroconversions are rarely associated with clinical signs, but affected animals may act as a source of infection to other animals when natural immunity wanes.[113]

Circumstantial evidence has frequently been highly suggestive of EHV-1 existing in a latent form in the population and being reactivated in situations of stress.[32] Reactivation of both EHV-1 subtypes has also been achieved by the administration of corticosteroids to previously infected horses.[19, 61] The genomes of both subtype 1 and subtype 2 have been shown to be present in lymph nodes of the respiratory tract of about 80 per cent of horses in Britain.[142]

Reactivation of latent virus is an important aspect of the epidemiology of EHV-1, but the proportion of latently infected horses which experience reactivation during their lifetime is unknown.

Historically, it was assumed that respiratory disease in young foals was the source of abortigenic virus for mares on studs where respiratory disease prevailed. However, respiratory disease in young animals can be caused by both subtypes of EHV-1; the relative prevalence of subtype 1 and 2 infections varies both geographically and temporally. For example, during a three-year survey of foals on studs in the UK between 1977 and 1979, all EHV-1 respiratory disease episodes were attributed to subtype 2. During this period no abortions occurred as a result of EHV-1 on the studs under surveillance.[135] Similarly, a serological study in Kentucky attributed the majority of respiratory infections in young horses to subtype 2.[3] In contrast, during the period 1980–84 the majority of EHV-1 viruses isolated from outbreaks of respiratory disease among young horses in Britain were identified as being of subtype 1. These observations followed the first recognized occurrence of the neurological form of EHV-1 in Britain.[71] It is possible that a more virulent subtype 1 strain was introduced in 1979 into the equine population of Britain, which had little natural immunity to this subtype.

For many years it was thought that the majority of primary EHV-1 infections occur in foals after weaning. Sero-epidemiological studies on stud farms, however, have shown that foals can experience their first infection under the cover of maternal antibody.[135] If a high level of antibody to EHV-1 is transferred in the colostrum, the infection may be subclinical even though large quantities of virus are shed from the respiratory tract.[100] On the other hand, if transfer of maternal antibody is poor, foals are highly susceptible to infection and disease.[3, 100]

The ability of one subtype to stimulate immunity to reinfection of the respiratory tract with the heterologous subtype was studied experimentally in seronegative foals.[3] Primary infection with one subtype was sufficient to stimulate immunity to challenge four weeks later with the homologous subtype. However, immunity to infection with the heterologous subtype was acquired only after repeated infections.[3, 59]

In the general horse population, the sporadic occurrence of respiratory disease caused by EHV-1 is not of great significance. On the other hand, in specific populations, such as racehorses in training, it may lead to loss of performance,[99] and in horses at stud it may cause more serious sequelae (abortion, neonatal and neurological disease).

The majority (95 per cent) of abortions occur in the last four months of gestation,[49, 50] although EHV-1-infected foetuses have been identified from as early as the fourth month. Abortions due to EHV-1 may occur as single events or as epidemics (abortion storms).

The initial source of virus in a group of pregnant mares may be the introduction of an infected mare who is shedding virus, the recrudescence of latent virus in a resident mare, or contact with young horses actively excreting the virus. Heavy losses have been recorded in some outbreaks of abortion, particularly where large numbers of pregnant mares are housed in big barns with a common airspace.[25, 100] There may be no indication of spread of the virus in the group because infection is often subclinical in older mares, and abortion is the first indication of the presence of the infection. In this case little can be done to limit the ensuing losses.

Abortions do not usually occur in the same mares in consecutive years, and outbreaks of abortion can rarely be traced to animals involved in outbreaks in the previous breeding season. There is no clear relationship between the age or antibody status of individual mares and their likelihood of aborting,[100] but putative factors contributing to the occurrence of abortigenic diseases are the immune status of groups of animals, overcrowding, and stress, such as that which occurs when mares in late pregnancy are transported long distances to stud farms so that, after foaling, they may be covered there during the foaling and subsequent heat periods.

Neurological disease as a result of EHV-1 subtype 1 infection is most commonly observed in mares soon after normal foaling or concurrently with abortion, although barren mares, geldings, stallions and foals may also be affected.[39, 71] The proportion of animals which develop clinical manifestations within a group of horses varies from single sporadic cases to 90 per cent of animals.[71] The source of infection has often been ascribed to aborted foetuses. Several individuals are usually affected on a property over a period of several weeks and neurological disease may occur in waves.[71] Experimental studies have shown that neurological signs usually develop seven to ten days after respiratory infection.[106]

Why the neurological syndrome is a rare occurrence is presently unknown. Two hypotheses have been advanced. The first is that there exists a strain of EHV-1 that is inherently predisposed to cause neurological disease and this infects restricted numbers of individuals in a horse population. The second is that there are individuals which are predisposed to the development of neurological disease following infection with 'normal' subtype 1 strains.

Pathogenesis

Following the inhalation of infectious aerosols or contact with contaminated secretions, the virus replicates in, and causes cytopathic changes in, epithelial cells of the nasal passages, corneal conjunctiva, pharynx, trachea and bronchi as well as in macrophages in the respiratory tract.

Subsequently, it is disseminated to the regional lymph nodes of the pharynx and lower respiratory tract. In young animals with no maternal or natural immunity, virus may also replicate in the lungs, causing bronchopneumonia.

Subtype 2 (respiratory) strains are usually cleared from the respiratory tract within seven to 20 days after the first infection and within two to seven days following subsequent infections. This subtype rarely infects circulating leukocytes, although it is presumed that occasionally this must occur in animals which abort foetuses infected with subtype 2.

Although classical cases of rhinopneumonitis do occur, with profuse watery nasal discharges which later become mucopurulent, primary damage to the respiratory tract caused by the virus may be sufficiently limited for the acute phase of the infection to go unnoticed, and it may only become clinically apparent following secondary bacterial infection.[138] If horses are not treated and rested adequately, a chronic inflammatory condition may ensue.

Following respiratory infections caused by subtype 1 viruses, animals develop a cell-associated viraemia which is detectable two to four days after infection. As a result of the presence of a viraemia the animals may develop other syndromes of the disease (abortion, neonatal disease and neurological disorders).

The pathogenesis of abortion is not fully understood.[23] The blood stream is presumed to be the route by which the cell-associated virus reaches the foeto-maternal junction.[3] However, the likelihood of abortion cannot be predicted from either the number of circulating virus-infected leukocytes or the duration of viraemia. The presence of a marked lymphocytic vasculitis in the endometrium of pregnant mares infected experimentally indicates that EHV-1 subtype 1 may cross from the endometrial to the allantochorial vessels as a latent leukocyte-associated infection protected from high levels of neutralizing antibody in the blood and interstitial fluid.[3] Certainly, EHV-1 has been shown to replicate in monocytes[41] and lymphocytes.[121] An alternative hypothesis involves thrombosis of infected endometrial vessels, necrosis of the local stroma and leakage of free virus from lysed endothelial cells.[63]

In horses suffering from the neurological disorder, virus may be found in the lymph nodes of the upper respiratory tract as early as 12 hours after infection, and in circulating lymphocytes after two to three days. The virus is thought to spread from circulating mononuclear cells to vascular endothelium without an extracellular phase,[34, 79] and along blood vessel walls by cell-to-cell spread, thus avoiding the often-high level of neutralizing antibody in the blood. Infection of the vessel wall results in vasculitis and thrombosis with secondary ischaemic necrosis of the neuropil. Viral antigen may be difficult to detect in neural tissue despite marked vasculitis and it is thought that the vascular lesion may represent an Arthus reaction, i.e. that this syndrome is a form of immune complex-induced disease, initiated by the presence of high levels of neutralizing antibody.[79, 111] Circulating immune complexes have been identified in horses with experimental EHV-1 myeloencephalopathy.[62] The neurological signs are ascribable to vasculitis and localized ischaemia in the cerebrum and spinal cord (particularly the lumbar and sacral parts). There is no immunohistological evidence of infection of neurones or neurophagia — in contrast to encephalitis in other animal species that is caused by alphaherpesviruses, e.g. herpes simplex in humans, infectious bovine rhinotracheitis in calves and pseudorabies in pigs, in which virus multiplication occurs in neurones and latency may be established in sensory ganglia.[34, 86]

As with other herpesviruses, both cellular and humoral immune responses appear to contribute to the protection of the host, although attempts to correlate the immune status of animals with the results of *in vitro* assays have, in general, been unsuccessful. Horses with high levels of neutralizing antibodies have been found to be resistant to respiratory disease and abortion,[21] whereas other researchers have reported both abortion and respiratory disease in horses with high levels of neutralizing antibody.[33, 100] Similarly, Pachciarz and Bryans[104] reported higher levels of cell-mediated immunity (CMI) (assessed by lymphocyte stimulation) and greater protection from abortion in immunized pregnant mares. Conversely, in a natural outbreak of EHV-1 abortion, no differences in levels of CMI were detected between mares which aborted and those which foaled normally.[56] Thus the relative importance of both types of immunity has still to be determined.

There is evidence to suggest that EHV-1 infection may result in depression of CMI responses, since cell-associated viraemia occurs in parallel with a decrease in the white blood cell count, and a reduction in lymphocyte proliferation following stimulation with phytohaemagglutinin.[104]

While antigen-specific T-cell responses develop progressively in ponies after infection with EHV-1, there is a marked depression of non-specific T-cell function which lasts for up to 74 days after infection.[73] These results suggest that, although specific immune responses to EHV-1 develop in horses after infection, the immune responses to other infectious agents or vaccines may be compromised for some weeks.

The fact that cell-mediated immunity is depressed during pregnancy, with maximal suppression occurring during the last three months of pregnancy,[67, 82] possibly contributes to the high incidence of EHV-1 abortion during this period.[52]

Attempts to identify the site(s) of viral latency for EHV-1 have revealed that, unlike herpes simplex virus, EHV-1 appears to be non-neurotropic. The majority of attempts to isolate the virus from cranial, cervical and sensory ganglia[3, 32, 61] have been unsuccessful. The fact that EHV-1 resides in the buffy coat of blood but can only be isolated from it[20, 32, 70] after co-cultivation with cells susceptible to the virus, has led to the proposition that the cell-associated viraemia of EHV-1 is tantamount to the reactivation of latent infection in leukocytes.[121]

Clinical signs

Respiratory syndrome

Clinical signs associated with respiratory infection are variable and the infecting subtype of the virus cannot be identified on the basis of the clinical signs. The severity of 'rhinopneumonitis' is influenced by the age and level of immunity of the animal, the dose of virus[114] and the subtype of the virus involved.[106] The incubation period ranges from two days to two weeks. Infections may be subclinical with either subtype, even in unprimed animals. Alternatively, infection may induce acute clinical illness characterized by rhinopharyngitis and tracheobronchitis. In its most severe form, pyrexia (40,6–41,1 °C) is usually biphasic and serous nasal and ocular discharges occur, which become mucoid or mucopurulent. Anorexia and depression, enlargement of the submandibular and parapharyngeal lymph nodes, coughing and hyperaemia and congestion of the nasal mucosa may also be evident. More rarely, weight loss, icterus, chronic lower respiratory tract disease and loss of performance are observed.[20, 22, 99, 114] Acute clinical signs may persist for one to ten days, although secondary bacterial involvement may prolong the duration of disease. In foals which experience respiratory infection with neurological strains of EHV-1, transient uveitis is a common feature, and there may be pneumonia, diarrhoea and colic with associated intussusception.[97, 106]

Abortion and neonatal syndromes

Mares which abort as a result of EHV-1 infection usually display no signs of respiratory disease and no premonitory signs of abortion. The incubation period may last from ten days to four months, with most abortions occurring in the last three months of gestation. The abortion is sudden and the placenta, which is often grossly normal, or occasionally oedematous with a few small haemorrhages, is usually delivered with the foetus.[43, 114] The foetus is frequently alive when the abortion occurs, but dies of suffocation during expulsion. Thus foetal carcasses rarely show any evidence of post-mortem changes, the exception being foetuses that are aborted early in the gestation period and which may be severely autolysed. When near-term foals are infected *in utero*, they may be born alive, but are weak, have a high body temperature, are sometimes icteric, and suffer severe respiratory distress as a result of pneumonia. Most are severely leukopenic and show an absolute neutropenia.[48] They are highly susceptible to secondary bacterial infection and usually succumb within the first week of life.

Mares which abort as a result of EHV-1 infection recover as quickly as mares that follow normal, uncomplicated parturition. Virus may be recovered from the genital and respiratory tracts of mares for several days, but the reproductive efficiency is not compromised, and they may be successfully covered during the foaling heat.

Neurological syndrome

Clinical signs of this form of the disease are highly variable and depend on the location and extent of the neurological lesions. Signs may include ataxia of the hind limbs, weakness, swaying of the hind quarters, dragging of the hind feet, stumbling or falling, difficulty in turning and reluctance to move. Paresis or paralysis occurs most commonly in the hind limbs although quadriplegia has been reported. Some animals assume a 'dog-sitting position' or complete recumbency. Paralysis or atony of the urinary bladder, urinary incontinence with dribbling of urine, subcutaneous oedema of the limbs, loss of sensation and sensory reflexes of the skin of the legs, tail and perineum, slackness of the vulval lips, prolapse of the penis and scrotal oedema may also be evident.[3, 35, 39, 71, 78]

Prior to the onset of ataxia, infected animals usually experience pyrexia, a slight nasal discharge and oedema of the limbs, but these signs may have regressed by the time neurological signs are evident. The signs of neurological disorder are often most severe during the first three to four days, and many horses improve progressively after that time, provided that they do not become recumbent.

Death may ensue as a result of pulmonary congestion, pneumonia, bowel atony and intussusception or rupture of the urinary bladder. The mortality rate varies considerably and may reach 40 per cent.[3] Animals that remain recumbent for more than two days rarely recover fully. Those that do survive neurological disease may recover completely in a matter of days[87] or may require three months or longer for full recovery.[71] Alternatively, slight but permanent incoordination may persist. Chronic cystitis, with spread of the inflammatory process to the retroperitoneal area resulting in adhesions between the bladder, uterus and ovaries, and subsequent reduced fertility, has been observed.[37]

Pathology

Neutropenia primarily, but also lymphopenia, may accompany subtype 1 infections.[20]

Respiratory syndrome

Owing to the low mortality of uncomplicated respiratory disease, the pathology of field cases has been poorly studied. Foals infected experimentally with EHV-1 show hyperaemia, vesiculation, degeneration, necrosis and ulceration of the mucosa of the upper respiratory tract, and miliary dark-red foci in the lungs.[114]

The histopathology of lung lesions is characterized by hyperaemia, terminal bronchiolitis with neutrophilic infiltration of the walls of the bronchioles, peribronchiolar and perivascular infiltration of mononuclear cells, and the presence of a serofibrinous exudate in the alveoli. The pharyngeal lymphoid follicles may show hyperplasia and foci of necrosis of lymphoid cells and numerous herpetic inclusion bodies.[114] Intranuclear inclusions may be present in the respiratory tract epithelium as well as in the germinal centres of the mandibular, pharyngeal and bronchial lymph nodes.[114]

Abortion and neonatal syndromes

Gross lesions are usually not discernible in the uterus of mares which have aborted as a result of EHV-1 infection. Histologically, the endometrium of some infected mares prior to abortion may reveal no changes, while that of others may show a low-grade perivascular infiltration of eosinophils in the interglandular connective tissues.[78, 114] Following abortion, there is marked perivascular cuffing by lymphocytes and plasma cells in the deep endometrium. Immunohistochemical studies have demonstrated infection of endothelial cells, as well as lymphocytic vasculitis and thrombosis of some of the blood vessels in the endometrium.[63, 145] Viral antigen may also be located in the endothelial cells of the allantochorion and umbilical cord.

Generally, foetuses aborted after the sixth month of gestation show no post-mortem autolysis. Foot pads and amniotic fluids are often discoloured orange-yellow as a result of foetal stress and passage of meconium *in utero*. The foetus **(Figures 102.1 and 102.2)** usually shows small haemorrhages in the lungs, moderate to severe pulmonary oedema, severe hydrothorax, mild ascites, variable icterus, petechiation of serosal surfaces and mucous membranes, subcutaneous and perirenal oedema, enlarged adrenals which may contain a few small cortical haemorrhages, slight splenomegaly with prominent lymphoid follicles, lymphadenopathy, moderate hepatomegaly and a few petechiae and pin-point-sized foci of necrosis in the liver.[37] Foetuses aborted earlier in pregnancy (at four to five months of gestation) are often severely autolysed.

Microscopically, the lesions in foetuses aborted late in pregnancy consist of bronchiolitis, pneumonitis, pyknosis and karyorrhexis of lymphocytes in the spleen, lymph nodes and thymus, and foci of necrosis in the liver and adrenals.[114] Typical herpetic intranuclear inclusions may be found in affected bronchiolar and pulmonary alveolar epithelial cells and hepatocytes, but they may also be present in affected cells in the thymus, lymphoid tissue and adrenal cortex. In some cases the inclusions may be difficult to find.

Foetuses which are aborted as a result of EHV subtype 2 infection may exhibit very mild or sparse lesions, rendering a histopathological diagnosis difficult.

Neurological syndrome

The gross lesions in horses affected by this syndrome are often unremarkable. Occasionally small, focal haemorrhages distributed throughout the meninges and parenchyma of the spinal cord and brain may be present.[35, 79, 111] Petechiae may also be evident in the mucosa of the nasal passages, guttural pouches, trachea and in the lung parenchyma.

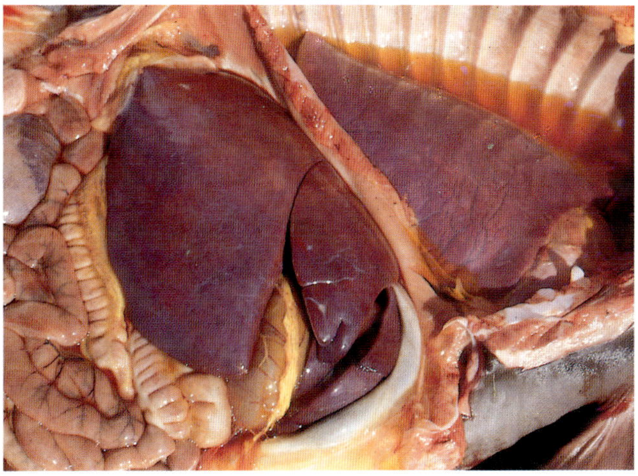

Figure 102.1 Aborted equine foetus. Note severe hydrothorax, moderately enlarged liver and mild icterus

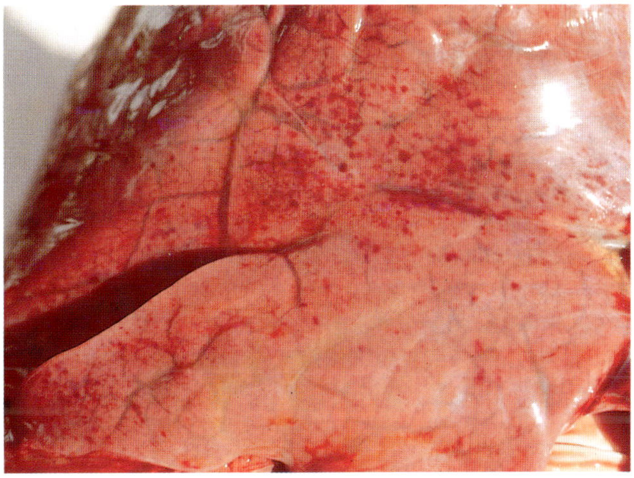

Figure 102.2 Numerous petechiae in the lung of an equine foetus

The severity of histopathological lesions is variable. Lesions may be found in the brain, but are more common in the lumbar and sacral regions of the spinal cord, and range from mild non-purulent meningitis to severe disseminated foci of necrosis and haemorrhages.[35, 78, 79, 111, 134] There is usually multifocal lymphocytic vasculitis in the brain, spinal cord, meninges and nerve sheaths. Haemorrhages, perivascular oedema, thrombosis and ischaemic necrosis of the neuropil is sometimes associated with affected blood vessels.[62, 111]

The presence of vasculitis has also been described in the respiratory tract, small intestine and other tissues.[106]

Diagnosis

Diagnosis of EHV-1 infections is complicated and, at the clinical level, requires recognition of the different syndromes. Because the clinical signs can be highly variable, even within a single outbreak, laboratory investigations are essential if one is to make a specific diagnosis.

Equid herpesvirus 1 may be isolated, with variable success, from nasal and ocular secretions, the leukocyte fraction (buffy coat) of blood, foetal tissues and fluids, and tissues (nasal turbinate, pharynx, respiratory tract lymph nodes, spleen, brain and spinal cord) of adult horses which suffered from the neurological syndrome of the disease.[39] Subtype 1 viruses grow in a wide range of cell cultures, including equine foetal kidney and lung, pig kidney and rabbit kidney (RK-13). Subtype 2 viruses are more host-restricted, preferring cells of equine origin. Equine foetal kidney and lung cells are particularly sensitive for primary isolations.

In horses suffering from respiratory tract infection, nasopharyngeal swabs should be taken within a day or two of the onset of pyrexia. In subtype 1 infections, primary replication in the respiratory tract is followed by cell-associated viraemia which may persist for several weeks after infection. The virus can only be recovered from the buffy coat by co-cultivation with permissive cells, as infection of leukocytes is not productive and the virus cannot be recovered from cell extracts. Isolation of EHV-1 from blood collected in heparin is particularly useful in establishing whether it is the cause of ataxia following nervous involvement, when the clinical signs develop eight to ten days after respiratory infection and shedding from the respiratory tract may have ceased. It is particularly difficult, although possible in some cases, to recover virus from tissues taken at necropsy from fatal cases of the neurological syndrome. This is probably because by the time paralysis has developed, so too has a very strong antibody response which may neutralize virus and prevent isolation. Foetal tissues are usually a rich source of virus, with lungs, liver, spleen, thymus and adrenals being the organs of choice.

In cases where EHV-1 has caused abortion late in gestation, a rapid diagnosis can often be achieved by examination of frozen sections of liver and lungs for characteristic lesions and Cowdry type A inclusion bodies. Viral antigen can usually be detected by immunohistochemical staining of foetal endothelial cells, hepatocytes, bronchiolar epithelium, reticular cells of the spleen and thymus, and cells of the adrenal cortex close to areas of necrosis.[69, 127] Type-specific monoclonal antibodies permit the direct identification of EHV-1 subtypes in pathological material.[60, 147]

In horses with neurological disease, vasculitis with associated thrombosis and ischaemic lesions in the spinal cord and brain are highly suggestive of myeloencephalopathy caused by EHV-1.[86] It is sometimes difficult to achieve a specific diagnosis by immunohistochemical staining for viral antigen in endothelial cells of the central nervous system, particularly when the duration of recumbency has been longer than 24 hours.

When an outbreak of respiratory disease occurs as a result of EHV-1 infection it is important to determine the subtype of virus in order to assess the potential dangers to horses in contact with index cases. This is particularly important on stud farms, where the virus causing respiratory disease may have abortigenic potential. Historically, host-range characteristics of viruses have been used to differentiate isolates, and viruses recovered from the blood of aborted foetuses were assumed to be subtype 1. The use of restriction endonuclease analysis of viral DNA has provided a definitive subtyping system.[119]

The production of subtype-specific monoclonal antibodies[147] has simplified the differentiation of the two subtypes of EHV-1 by enzyme immunofiltration assay, or immunohistochemical staining of infected cell cultures.[60] The infecting subtype can also be identified in frozen sections of foetal tissues using pools of directly conjugated monoclonal antibodies.[125]

Serological diagnosis of EHV-1 is complicated by a number of factors. Most horses are exposed to EHV-1 in the first year of life and suffer repeated exposures or reactivation of latent virus thereafter. Neutralizing antibody stimulated by infection persists for months, particularly in older animals, and most animals of two years and older have antibody to EHV-1.[26] Thus limited information can be gained from measurement of neutralizing antibody in single serum samples. However, antibody measured by complement fixation tests is less durable following infection, and high complement fixing (CF) antibody titres in single serum samples can provide an indication of recent infection.[136] Ideally, acute and convalescent samples should be taken, with at least a two-week interval between sampling. However, initial infections with subtype 2 viruses often fail to stimulate strong antibody responses, and a third sample four to six weeks after the acute phase is sometimes required before a significant rise in antibody is detected.[135]

Antibody stimulated by infection with one subtype may or may not cross-react with the other subtype, depending on the specificity of the individual animal's response; thus no reliable information on the pathogenic potential of the circulating virus can be obtained from serological investigations.

Measurement of antibody is an important aspect of diagnosing the neurological syndrome caused by EHV-1. Neurological signs usually develop eight to ten days after infection, by which time exceptionally high CF and virus neutralizing (VN) antibody titres are present.[98] If CF antibody levels are high, further serological investigations and virus isolation attempts from affected or in-contact animals may establish a diagnosis of EHV-1. On present experience, if an ataxic horse has low levels of CF antibody, EHV-1 can be excluded as the cause of the nervous disorder.[97]

A number of ELISA tests have been described for the diagnosis of EHV-1 infection,[3, 57, 76] but none of these offer the advantages of the CF test, which can provide an indication of recent infection based on measurement of antibody in a single sample.[136] The most urgent requirement in the serological diagnosis of EHV-1 is an assay with subtype-specificity, but, paradoxically, the antigens recognized most strongly by horses are those with cross-reactive antigenic sites.[125]

Differential diagnosis

Infection with EHV-1 causes a variety of clinical syndromes, each of which should be differentiated from a number of similar conditions. Submission of suitable specimens to a laboratory is essential to confirm the diagnosis.

Apart from EHV-1, signs of respiratory system involvement may result from other viral (e.g. influenza, rhino-, reo-, adeno-, and equine viral arteritis viruses) and bacterial (e.g. *Streptococcus equi* and *Rhodococcus equi*) infections.

When not caused by EHV-1, abortion in horses may follow infection with certain other viruses (e.g. equine encephalosis and equine viral arteritis viruses) and infections by bacteria (e.g. *Streptococcus zooepidemicus, Klebsiella* spp. and *Borrelia burgdorferi*), rickettsiae (*Coxiella burnetti* and *Chlamydia psittaci*), and protozoa (e.g. *Babesia equi* and *Toxoplasma gondii*). In southern Africa, equine babesiosis is a relatively common cause of abortion and the lesions in the foetus (icterus, splenomegaly, hepatomegaly, scattered haemorrhages) ascribed to it are very similar to those caused by EHV-1 infections.[37] In both infections abortion usually occurs in the last two or three months of gestation. However, whereas the aborted foetuses in the case of EHV-1 infections are usually very fresh, babesia-infected foetuses are usually moderately autolysed. An easy and fast method of confirming a diagnosis of babesiosis in an aborted foetus is to make an impression smear of the spleen, staining it with Giemsa or Diff-Quick and demonstrating the babesia parasites in red blood cells, of which 80–90 per cent in the spleen are parasitized.[37]

Neonatal deaths may also be caused by infection with certain bacteria (e.g. *Actinobacillus equuli, Streptococcus zooepidemicus, Klebsiella* spp., *Salmonella* serovars, *Escherichia coli*) and with *Babesia equi*, or they may follow iso-immune haemolytic erythrolysis.

The clinical signs associated with the neurological syndrome caused by EHV-1 infection are variable and may be confused with those observed in wobblers and in cases suffering from equine encephalosis, *Fusarium moniliforme* poisoning (the cause of leukoencephalomalacia or mouldy corn disease) or botulism.

Control

There are two established approaches to the control of disease caused by EHV-1: immunization of susceptible animals, and management practices which minimize the chances of infection or the effects thereof.

During the past 25 years, repeated attempts have been made to develop either live attenuated or inactivated vaccines for the control of EHV-1, but, at best, these attempts have been only partially successful. In some cases, vaccines have actually been implicated in the causation of outbreaks of disease.

The observation that mares rarely abort as a result of EHV-1 infection in consecutive seasons was ascribed to natural immunity following abortigenic infection. Based on this conclusion, a planned-infection programme was introduced on stud farms in Kentucky in which, each year, mares were infected early in gestation, with a hamster-adapted live virus which was partially attenuated. Abortion rates were reduced from 30 per cent in unvaccinated animals to 1,5 per cent or less in the treated group.[52, 53] This method of immunization was used extensively prior to 1972.[110] The hamster-adapted virus was, however, not fully attenuated and its inoculation sometimes resulted in respiratory disease and abortion. It became clear that further attenuation of the vaccine virus was required.

As a result of these observations, a number of vaccines containing viruses which were more attenuated were developed in the USA and Europe using cell culture passage as the means of attenuation. A modified live-virus vaccine (Rhinomune) was introduced in the USA in 1973.[15, 16] This virus was derived from a hamster-adapted EHV-1 strain (Rac-H), which had been attenuated further by passage in equine cell cultures, and could be differentiated from field viruses on the basis of the plaque morphology when grown on cell culture.[77] It was subsequently shown to have a unique DNA restriction profile.[10] The vaccine was administered in two doses, four to eight weeks apart, followed by booster doses at six-monthly intervals because the immunity induced was short-lived. Field data suggested that abortion rates were lower in pregnant mares vaccinated with this vaccine than in mares immunized by the planned-infection programme.[15, 92] Initially, the vaccine appeared to be safe, as the virus was not spread by contact, but it was subsequently shown to possess the potential for causing abortion when a virus indistinguishable from the vaccine strain was isolated from a number of aborted foetuses.[10] This resulted in the use of the vaccine being discontinued on stud farms, but it is still used in attempts to control respiratory disease.[146]

A similar live attenuated virus vaccine (Prevaccinol) was developed and used in Europe. It was derived from the same hamster-adapted virus (Rac-H), which was further passaged in pig-kidney cells.[92, 94] The vaccine was claimed to be highly immunogenic, but non-pathogenic and non-infectious to foals and mares in contact with vaccinated horses. It was used widely in Europe for several years, although subsequent studies demonstrated its potential for causing abortion after direct intra-uterine inoculation into pregnant mares.[31]

The difficulty of attenuating EHV-1 by cell culture passage was clearly demonstrated by experiences with a vaccine prepared by virus passage in Vero cells. Initial studies indicated that the virus was not transmitted between horses, as it was not recovered from the pharynx after vaccination.[115, 116] It did, however, cause viraemia. In challenge studies, the vaccine provided good protection, but when used in the field it caused neurological disease.[88] Thus a satisfactory live vaccine against EHV-1 has not yet been developed.

Because of the difficulties surrounding the production and evaluation of a safe live vaccine for EHV-1, there has been a substantial research effort to produce an effective killed-virus vaccine. Studies in hamsters have demonstrated that protective antigens reside in the envelope component of the virus as opposed to the nucleocapsid.[105] The principal of vaccination with inactivated antigens of EHV-1 was established by Thomson, Mumford and Plowright,[137] who demonstrated that it is possible to protect against infection with EHV-1 provided that the inactivated virus is delivered in combination with Freund's complete adjuvant which, unfortunately, causes local reactions too severe to permit commercial exploitation. This vaccine stimulated higher levels of neutralizing antibody and CMI responses (lymphocyte stimulation) than did infection with live virus. Other adjuvants suitable for use in horses, such as Adjuvant 65 and alhydrogel (aluminium hydroxide-based), were less effective in stimulating both neutralizing antibody and CMI responses and were only capable of reducing levels of virus excretion and clinical signs following challenge.[138] Attempts by Kawakami and Shimizu[85] to develop an inactivated vaccine for control of respiratory disease demonstrated that inactivated antigens failed to stimulate strong antibody responses in young animals with no history of previous infection. However, vaccine-induced responses were enhanced when vaccine was administered after a primary infection.

In 1980, the first licensed vaccine containing inactivated whole virus was introduced into the state of Kentucky and vaccination with it replaced the planned-infection programme then in use. The vaccine (Pneumobort K) contained EHV-1 strain Army 183 grown in equine cells, inactivated with formaldehyde and combined with an oil adjuvant. In experimental challenge studies completed prior to licensing, this vaccine prevented abortion in pregnant mares when administered at 60-day intervals during the fifth, seventh and ninth months of gestation.[21] In contrast, when the commercial product was evaluated in a challenge study using an isolate which causes paralysis, it was found that the vaccine failed to prevent abortion.[33] Nevertheless, introduction of the vaccine on a wide scale (over 65 per cent of mares have been vaccinated since 1982) in Kentucky has more than halved the number of abortions recorded per 1 000 mares. Field evidence would suggest that the vaccine reduces the number of abortion storms, even though vaccinated individuals may still abort. There have been notable exceptions to this observation, among them a major abortion storm which occurred in vaccinated mares in South Africa in 1989/90.[68]

Attempts to produce subunit vaccines have also been made. An envelope preparation in combination with an oil adjuvant is now available in Europe,[89] and an experimental ISCOM (immune-stimulating complex) vaccine has been evaluated in hamsters.[38] The efficacy of both these approaches remains to be confirmed.

While vaccination may limit the spread of infection, it does not prevent abortion in individual mares, and there is no evidence that it protects against the neurological syndrome of the disease. Thus, because of the ever-present possibility of reactivation of latent virus, management practices should be designed to minimize stress and reduce mixing of different groups of animals. Pregnant mares should be kept separate from young stock as far as possible, and new animals arriving on stud farms should be isolated for two to three weeks before being introduced into the main herd.

When an abortion occurs, the foetus and placenta should be removed immediately and, after specimens have been collected for pathological and virological examination, incinerated, and the mare isolated from her cohorts. The housing area and bedding should be saturated with disinfectant (e.g. an iodophore) and left for 24 hours before the bedding is removed and burned.

Mares which abort do not shed virus from the reproductive tract for more than two or three days, but they may still be viraemic and shed virus from the respiratory tract for several days longer. Separate personnel should, therefore, be assigned to the care of mares which have recently aborted. Such mares may be covered at the second heat without risk.

Serological screening for EHV-1 antibody is a useful tool to employ in the limitation of abortion storms. Testing mares which have been in contact with abortion cases for CF antibody will reveal whether respiratory spread has occurred prior to the first abortion or whether the aborted foetus is likely to be the index case. In the latter situation, prompt separation and isolation of in-contact animals into small groups is an effective way of limiting the spread of infection. If mares have been recently vaccinated, it will not be possible to differentiate between vaccine- and infection-induced antibody.

To prevent the spread of infection between premises, the movement of mares should be stopped until at least 30 days after the last abortion. Even so, abortions may occasionally occur at intervals greater than 30 days. Where the accommodation is available, mares which have aborted an infected foetus should be maintained and foaled in isolation in the subsequent season, as abortions in consecutive years have been recorded occasionally for some mares.[97]

During outbreaks of EHV-1 abortion, stallions should be observed closely for signs of respiratory disease or loss of libido. If infected, they may pass infection to visiting mares via the respiratory route.

In cases which show neurological disorders, the differential diagnosis is complicated and it is important to establish as quickly as possible whether the cause is infectious. Where possible, movement onto and off premises should cease until EHV-1 has been excluded and, where practical, affected animals have been isolated. Blood specimens from affected animals should be sent to a laboratory immediately for measurement of CF antibody to EHV-1.

Treatment is rarely necessary in the acute phase of respiratory infections caused by EHV-1. Antibiotics may be used to treat or limit secondary infections. Most of the secondary bacterial infections are caused by Gram-positive microorganisms, so procaine penicillin G once or twice daily at 20 000 IU/kg by intramuscular injection should be sufficient.[17] In refractile cases an appropriate antibiotic can be selected after bacterial isolation and performance of an antibiogram. Mucolytics, nebulization and bronchodilators are rarely indicated.

For horses suffering from the neurological syndrome, good nursing care with catheterization of the urinary bladder, if necessary, is most important for a successful outcome. In the acute phase, glucocorticosteroids may be used to treat the immune-mediated vasculitis. Prednisolone at 0,5–2 mg/kg or dexamethasone at 0,1–0,25 mg/kg should be administered twice daily for the first three days.[91] To prevent secondary bacterial cystitis an appropriate antibiotic or antimicrobial that will be excreted in the urine is also indicated. Trimethoprim-sulphonamide can be used intravenously or orally. The combination is usually dosed at 15 mg/kg of sulphonamide, administered twice a day.

The use of slings and stocks lined with bales of straw has been successfully employed to support paretic horses suffering from the neurological syndrome while standing, and slings attached to tractors have been used to assist animals to walk and graze during the recovery phase. In this way, recumbency may be avoided and horses have been saved to breed successfully in following years.

References

1 **ABODEELY, R.A., PALMER, E., LAWSON, L.A. & RANDALL, C.C., 1971.** The proteins of enveloped and de-enveloped equine abortion (herpes) virus and the separated envelope. *Virology*, 44, 146–152.

2 **ALLEN, G.P., 1989.** Characterisation of EHV-1 glycoprotein B as an antigen for stimulating antibody production by the horse. *Equine Virology Research Foundation Report*, Newmarket, October 1989.

3 **ALLEN, G.P. & BRYANS, J.T., 1986.** Molecular epizootiology, pathogenesis, and prophylaxis of equine herpesvirus-1 infections. *Progress in Veterinary Microbiology and Immunology*, 1, 78–144.

4 **ALLEN, G.P. & COOGLE, L.D., 1988.** Characterisation of an equine herpesvirus type 1 gene encoding a glycoprotein (gp13) with homology to herpes simplex virus glycoprotein C. *Journal of Virology*, 62, 2850–2858.

5 **ALLEN, G.P. & TURTINEN, L.W., 1982.** Assessment of the base sequence homology between the two subtypes of equine herpesvirus 1. *Journal of Virology*, 44, 249–255.

6 **ALLEN, G.P. & YEARGAN, M.R., 1987.** Use of gp11 and monoclonal antibodies to map the genes for the six major glycoproteins of equine herpesvirus 1. *Journal of Virology*, 61, 2454–2461.

7 **ALLEN, G.P., YEARGAN, M.R. & BRYANS, J.T., 1983.** Alterations in the genome of equine herpesvirus 1 after *in vitro* and *in vivo* virus passage. *Infection and Immunity*, 40, 436–439.

8 **ALLEN, G.P., YEARGAN, M.R. & COOGLE, L.D., 1988.** Equid herpesvirus-1 glycoprotein 13 (gp13); epitope analysis, gene structure, and expression in *E. coli*. *In*: POWELL, D.G., (ed.). *Equine Infectious Diseases*. I. Lexington, Kentucky: The University Press of Kentucky.

9 **ALLEN, G.P., YEARGAN, M.R., TURTINEN, L.W. & BRYANS, J.T., 1985.** A new field strain of equine abortion virus (equine herpesvirus 1) among Kentucky horses. *American Journal of Veterinary Research*, 46, 138–140.

10 **ALLEN, G.P., YEARGAN, M.R., TURTINEN, L.W., BRYANS, J.T. & McCOLLUM, W.H., 1983.** Molecular epizootiologic studies of equine herpesvirus 1 infections by restriction endonuclease fingerprinting of viral DNA. *American Journal of Veterinary Research*, 44, 263–271.

11 **ANDERSON, K. & GOODPASTURE, E.W., 1942.** Infection of newborn Syrian hamsters with the virus of mare abortion. *American Journal of Pathology*, 18, 555–561.

12 **ANONYMOUS, 1961.** Equine virus rhinopneumonitis: Influenza-like respiratory infections: 'Equine virus abortion'. *The Veterinary Record*, 73, 604–606.

13 **BAGUST, T.J. & PASCOE, R.R., 1968.** Isolation of equine rhinopneumonitis virus from acute respiratory disease in a horse in Queensland. *Australian Veterinary Journal*, 44, 296.

14 **BAKER, B., 1990.** P.O. Box 787, Hillcrest 3650, South Africa. Unpublished observations.

15 **BASS, E.P., 1978.** Immunisation with a modified live-virus equine rhinopneumonitis vaccine and an aluminium-hydroxide-absorbed equine influenza vaccine. *Proceedings of the American Association of Equine Practitioners*, 24, 65–74.

16 **BECKENHAUER, W.H. & BASS, E.P., 1973.** A modified live-virus vaccine for equine rhinopneumonitis. *Journal of the American Veterinary Medical Association*, 163, 1182.

17 **BEECH, J., 1987.** Drug therapy of respiratory disorders. *Veterinary Clinics of North America: Equine Practice*, 3, 59–80.

18 **BITSCH, V. & DAM, A., 1971.** Nervous disturbances in horses in relation to infection with equine pneumonitis virus. *Acta Veterinaria Scandinavica*, 12, 134–136.

19 **BROWNING, G.F., BULACH, D.M., FICORILLI, N., ROY, E.A., THORP, B.H. & STUDDERT, M.J., 1988.** Latency of equine herpesvirus 4 (equine rhinopneumonitis virus). *The Veterinary Record*, 123, 518–519.

20 **BRYANS, J.T., 1969.** On immunity to disease caused by equine herpesvirus 1. *Journal of the American Veterinary Medical Association*, 155, 294–300.

21 **BRYANS, J.T., 1978.** Immunisation of pregnant mares with an inactivated equine herpesvirus vaccine. *In*: BRYANS, J.T. & GERBER, H., (eds). *Equine Infectious Diseases*, IV. Princeton, New Jersey: Veterinary Publications, Inc.

22 **BRYANS, J.T., 1980.** Application of management procedures and prophylactic immunization to the control of equine pneumonitis. *Proceedings of the American Association of Equine Practitioners*, 26, 259–272.

23 **BRYANS, J.T. & PRICKETT, M.E., 1972.** A consideration of the pathogenesis of abortigenic disease caused by equine

herpesvirus 1. *In*: BRYANS, J.T. & GERBER, H., (eds). *Equine Infectious Diseases*, III. Basel, Munchen, Paris, London: S. Karger.

24 **BRYANS, J.T., SWERCZEK, T.W., DARLINGTON, R.W. & CROWE, M.W., 1977.** Neonatal foal disease associated with perinatal infection by equine herpesvirus 1. *Journal of Equine Medicine and Surgery*, 1, 20–26.

25 **BURKI, V.F., NOWOTNY, N., HINAIDY, B. & PALLAN, C., 1984.** Die atiologie der Lippizanerseuche in Piber 1983: Equines herpesvirus 1. *Wiener Tierärztliche Monatsschrift*, 11, 312–320.

26 **BURROWS, R., 1966.** Rhinopneumonitis virus-neutralizing antibody levels in British Thoroughbred mares. *In*: BRYANS, J.T. & GERBER, H., (eds). *Proceedings of the First International Conference on Equine Infectious Diseases*, Stresa, Italy: 11–13 July 1966. Lexington, Kentucky: Grayson Foundation Inc.

27 **BURROWS, R., 1968.** Laboratory diagnosis of some virus infections of the upper respiratory tract of the horse. *Equine Veterinary Journal*, 1, 32–36.

28 **BURROWS, R., 1970.** The general virology of the herpesvirus group. *In*: BRYANS, J.T. & GERBER, H., (eds). *Equine Infectious Diseases*, II. Basel, Munchen, New York: S. Karger.

29 **BURROWS, R. & GOODRIDGE, D., 1973.** *In vivo* and *in vitro* studies of equine rhinopneumonitis strains. *In*: BRYANS, J.T. & GERBER, H., (eds). *Equine Infectious Diseases*, III. Basel, Munchen, New York: S. Karger.

30 **BURROWS, R. & GOODRIDGE, D., 1975.** Experimental studies on equine herpesvirus type 1 infections. *Journal of Reproduction and Fertility*, Suppl. 23, 611–615.

31 **BURROWS, R. & GOODRIDGE, D., 1978.** Observations of picornavirus, adenovirus and equine herpesvirus infections in the Pirbright pony herd. *In*: BRYANS, J.T. & GERBER, H., (eds). *Equine Infectious Diseases*, IV. Princeton, New Jersey: Veterinary Publications, Inc.

32 **BURROWS, R. & GOODRIDGE, D., 1984.** Studies of persistent and latent equine herpesvirus 1 and herpesvirus 3 infections in the Pirbright pony herd. *In*: WITTMANN, G., GASKELL, R.M. & RZIHA, H.J., (eds). *Latent Herpesvirus Infections in Veterinary Medicine*. Boston: Nijhoff.

33 **BURROWS, R., GOODRIDGE, D. & DENYER, M.S., 1984.** Trials of an inactivated equid herpesvirus 1 vaccine: Challenge with a subtype 1 virus. *The Veterinary Record*, 114, 369–374.

34 **CAMPBELL, T.M. & STUDDERT, M.J., 1983.** Equine herpesvirus type 1 (EHV-1). *Veterinary Bulletin*, 53, 135–146.

35 **CHARLTON, K.M., MITCHELL, D., GIRARD, A. & CORNER, A.H., 1976.** Meningoencephalomyelitis in horses associated with equine herpesvirus 1 infection. *Veterinary Pathology*, 13, 56–68.

36 **CHOWDURY, S.I., KUBIN, G. & LUDWIG, H., 1986.** Equine herpesvirus type 1 (EHV-1) induced abortions and paralysis in a Lipizzaner stud: A contribution to the classification of equine herpesvirus. *Archives of Virology*, 90, 273–288.

37 **COETZER, J.A.W., 1989.** Faculty of Veterinary Science, University of Pretoria, Pretoria. Unpublished observations.

38 **COOK, R.F., O'NEILL, T., STRACHEN, E., SUNDQUIST, B. & MUMFORD, J.A., 1990.** Protection against lethal equine herpesvirus type 1 (subtype) infection in hamsters by immune-stimulating complexes (ISCOMS) containing the major viral glycoproteins. *Vaccine*, 8, 491–496.

39 **CROWHURST, F.A., DICKINSON, G. & BURROWS, R., 1981.** An outbreak of paresis in mares and geldings associated with equid herpesvirus 1. *The Veterinary Record*, 109, 527–528.

40 **DALSGAARD, H., 1970.** Enzootic paresis in horses in association with an outbreak of pneumonitis (virus abortion). *Medlemsblad for den danske DyrlaegeForening*, 53, 71–76.

41 **DARLINGTON, R.W., 1978.** The role of equine macrophages in resistance or susceptibility to infection by equine herpesvirus 1. *In*: BRYANS, J.T. & GERBER, H., (eds). *Equine Infectious Diseases*. IV. Princeton, New Jersey: Veterinary Publications, Inc.

42 **DARLINGTON, R.W. & RANDALL, C.C., 1963.** The nucleic acid content of equine abortion virus. *Virology*, 19, 332–337.

43 **DIMOCK, W.W., 1940.** The diagnosis of virus abortion in mares. *Journal of the American Veterinary Medical Association*, 96, 665–666.

44 **DIMOCK, W.W. & EDWARDS, P.R., 1932.** Infections of foetuses and foals. *Kentucky Agricultural Station, Bulletin*, 333, 665–666.

45 **DIMOCK, W.W. & EDWARDS, P.R., 1933.** Is there a filterable virus of abortion in mares? *Kentucky Agricultural Station, Bulletin*, 333, 297–301.

46 **DIMOCK, W.W. & EDWARDS, P.R., 1936.** The differential diagnosis of equine abortion with special references to a hitherto undescribed form of epizootic abortion in mares. *Cornell Veterinarian*, 26, 231–240.

47 **DINTER, Z. & KLINGEBORN, B., 1976.** Serological study of an outbreak of paresis due to equine herpesvirus (EHV1). *The Veterinary Record*, 99, 10–12.

48 **DIXON, R.J., HARTLEY, W.J., HUTCHINS, R.D., LEPHERD, E.E., FEILEN, C., JONES, R.F., LOVE, D.N., SABINE, M. & WELLS, A.L., 1978.** Perinatal foal mortality associated with a herpesvirus. *Australian Veterinary Journal*, 54, 103–105.

49 **DOLL, E.R., 1952.** Seasonal incidence and fetal age in equine virus abortion. *Cornell Veterinarian*, 42, 505–509.

50 **DOLL, E.R. & BRYANS, J.T., 1962.** Incubation periods for abortion in equine viral pneumonitis. *Journal of the American Veterinary Medical Association*, 141, 351–354.

51 **DOLL, E.R. & BRYANS, J.T., 1963.** Epizootiology of equine viral pneumonitis. *Journal of the American Veterinary Medical Association*, 142, 31–37.

52 **DOLL, E.R. & BRYANS, J.T., 1963.** A planned infection program for immunising mares against viral pneumonitis. *Cornell Veterinarian*, 53, 249–262.

53 **DOLL, E.R. & BRYANS, J.T., 1963.** Immunisation against viral pneumonitis of horses with live virus propagated in hamsters. *Journal of the American Veterinary Medical Association*, 139, 1324–1330.

54 **DOLL, E.R. & KINTER, J.H., 1954.** A comparative study of the equine abortion and equine influenza viruses. *Cornell Veterinarian*, 44, 355–367.

55 **DOLL, E.R., WALLACE, M.E. & RICHARDS, M.G., 1954.** Thermal, haematological and serological responses of weaning horses following inoculation with equine abortion virus; its similarity to equine influenza. *Cornell Veterinarian*, 44, 181–190.

56 **DUTTA, S.K. & CAMPBELL, D.L., 1977.** Cell-mediated immunity in equine herpesvirus type 1 infection. I. *In vitro* lymphocyte blastogenesis and serum-neutralisation antibody in normal paturient and aborting mares. *Canadian Journal of Comparative Medicine*, 41, 404–408.

57 **DUTTA, S.K., TALBOT, N.C. & MURPHY, A.C., 1983.** Detection of equine herpesvirus 1 antigen and the specific antibody by enzyme-linked immunosorbent assay. *American Journal of Veterinary Research*, 44, 1930–1934.

58 **DUXBURY, A.E. & OXER, D.T., 1968.** Isolation of equine rhinopneumonitis virus from an epidemic of acute respiratory disease in horses. *Australian Veterinary Journal*, 44, 58–63.

59 **EDINGTON, N. & BRIDGES, C.G., 1990.** One-way protection between equid herpesvirus 1 and 4 *in vivo*. *Research in Veterinary Science*, 48, 235–239.

60 **EDINGTON, N., BRIDGES, C.G. & BROAD, S.C., 1987.** Rapid diagnosis and characterisation of equid herpesvirus 1 using monoclonal antibodies. *Tierärztliche Praxis*, Supplement 2, 37–40.

61 **EDINGTON, N., BRIDGES, C.G. & HUCKLE, A., 1985.** Experimental reactivation of equid herpesvirus 1 (EHV-1) following the administration of corticosteroids. *Equine Veterinary Journal*, 17, 369–372.

62 **EDINGTON, N., BRIDGES, C.G. & PATEL, J.R., 1986.** Endothelial cell infection and thrombosis in paralysis caused

by equid herpesvirus-1: Equine stroke. *Archives of Virology*, 90, 111–124.

63 **EDINGTON, N., SMYTH, B. & GRIFFITH, L., 1991.** The role of endothelial cell infection in the endometrium, placenta and foetus of equid herpesvirus 1 abortions. *Journal of Comparative Pathology*, 104, 379–387.

64 **ERASMUS, B.J., 1963.** Equine viral rhinopneumonitis (1963). *Journal of the South African Veterinary Medical Association*, 34, 461–469.

65 **ERASMUS, B.J., 1965.** Viruses as etiological agents in equine respiratory disease. *Journal of the South African Veterinary Medical Association*, 36, 209–216.

66 **ERASMUS, B.J., 1966.** The activation of herpesvirus infections of the respiratory tract in horses by immunization against horse sickness. *Proceedings of the First International Conference on Equine Infectious Diseases*, Stresa, Italy, 11–13 July 1966, 117–121.

67 **GERBER, J.D., MARRON, A.E., BASS, E.P. & BECKENHAUER, W.H., 1977.** Effect of age and pregnancy on the antibody and cell-mediated immune responses of horses to equine herpesvirus 1. *Canadian Journal of Comparative Medicine*, 41, 471–478.

68 **GERDES, T., COETZER, J.A.W. & VAN DEN BERG, J., 1989.** Veterinary Research Institute, Onderstepoort. Unpublished data.

69 **GIMENO, E.J., NOSETTO, E.O., MARTIN, A.A., GALOSI, C.M., ANDO, Y. & ETCHEVERRIGARRAY, M.E., 1987.** Demonstration of equine herpesvirus 1 (EHV-1) in histological sections and tissue cultures by the peroxidase-antiperoxidase (PAP) technique. *Journal of Veterinary Medicine*, 68, 740–742.

70 **GLEESON, L.J. & COGGINS, L., 1980.** Response of pregnant mares to equine herpesvirus 1 (EHV-1). *Cornell Veterinarian*, 70, 391–400.

71 **GREENWOOD, R.E.S. & SIMSON, A.R.B., 1980.** Clinical report of a paralytic syndrome affecting stallions, mares and foals on a Thoroughbred stud farm. *Equine Veterinary Journal*, 12, 113–117.

72 **GUO, P., GOEBEL, S., DAVIS, S., PERKUS, M.E., LANQUET, B., DESMETTRE, P., ALLEN, G. & PAOLETTI, E., 1989.** Expression in recombinant vaccinia virus of the equine herpesvirus 1 gene encoding glycoprotein gp13 and protection of immunised animals. *Journal of Virology*, 63, 4189–4198.

73 **HANNANT, D., O'NEILL, T., JESSETT, D.M. & MUMFORD, J.A., 1991.** Evidence for non-specific immunosuppression during the development of immune responses to Equid herpesvirus-1. *Equine Veterinary Journal*, Suppl. 11, 41–45.

74 **HARTLEY, W.J. & DIXON, R.J., 1979.** An outbreak of foal perinatal mortality due to equine herpesvirus type 1; pathological observations. *Equine Veterinary Journal*, 11, 215–218.

75 **HENNING, M.W., 1946.** On the etiology of epizootic or infectious equine abortion. *Onderstepoort Journal of Veterinary Science*, 21, 17–40.

76 **HOHDATSU, T., EIKI, T., IDE, S. & YAMAGISHI, H., 1986.** Enzyme-linked immunosorbent assay for the detection of antibodies to equid herpesvirus type 1 (EHV-1). *Japanese Journal of Veterinary Science*, 48, 1045–1048.

77 **HOLMES, D.F., KEMEN, M.J. & JOUBERT, J., 1978.** Differentiation of field strains and a vaccine strain of equine herpesvirus 1, using plaque characteristics. *American Journal of Veterinary Research*, 40, 305–306.

78 **JACKSON, T. & KENDRICK, J.W., 1971.** Paralysis of horses associated with equine herpesvirus 1 infection. *Journal of the American Veterinary Medical Association*, 158, 1351–1357.

79 **JACKSON, T.A., OSBURN, B.I., CORDY, D.R. & KENDRICK, J.W., 1977.** Equine herpesvirus 1 infection of horses: Studies on the experimentally induced neurologic disease. *Journal of the American Veterinary Medical Association*, 38, 709–719.

80 **JAIN, N.C., BATRA, S.K. & RAM, G.C., 1981.** Isolation of equine herpesvirus 1 from paralysis and encephalitis cases in equines. *Indian Journal of Microbiology*, 21, 337–339.

81 **JONES, T.C., GLEISER, C.A., MAURER, F.D., HALE, M.W. & ROBY, T.O., 1948.** Transmission and immunisation studies on equine influenza. *American Journal of Veterinary Research*, 9, 243–253.

82 **KASAKURA, S., 1971.** A factor in maternal plasma during pregnancy that suppresses the reactivity of mixed leukocyte cultures. *Journal of Immunology*, 107, 1296–1301.

83 **KAWAKAMI, Y., KAJI, T., ISHIZAKI, R., SHIMIZU, T. & MATUMOTO, M., 1962.** Etiologic study on an outbreak of acute respiratory disease among colts due to equine pneumonitis virus. *Japanese Journal of Experimental Medicine*, 32, 211–229.

84 **KAWAKAMI, Y., KAJI, T., SUGIMURA, K., ISHITANI, R., SHIMIZU, T. & MATUMOTO, M., 1959.** Histopathological study of aborted foetuses naturally infected with equine abortion virus and some epidemiological findings. *Japanese Journal of Experimental Medicine*, 29, 635–641.

85 **KAWAKAMI, Y. & SHIMIZU, T., 1978.** Combined immunising effects of live and inactivated equine herpesvirus 1 horses. *In*: BRYANS, J.T. & GERBER, H., (eds). *Equine Infectious Diseases*. IV. Princeton, New Jersey: Veterinary Publications, Inc.

86 **KOHN, C.W. & FENNER, W.R., 1987.** Equine herpesvirus myeloencephalopathy neurologic diseases. *Veterinary Clinics of North America: Equine Practice*, 3, 405–419.

87 **LITTLE, P.B. & THORSEN, J., 1976.** Disseminated necrotizing myeloencephalitis: A herpes-associated neurological disease of horses. *Veterinary Pathology*, 13, 161–171.

88 **LIU, I. & CASTLEMAN, W., 1977.** Equine posterior paresis associated with equine herpesvirus 1 vaccine in California: A preliminary report. *Journal of Equine Medicine and Surgery*, 12, 397–401.

89 **MACKOVIAK, M., DURET, C., DEVAUX, B., FARGEAUD, D., BRUN, A. & SAINT GERAND, A.L., 1990.** Study of a purified, inactivated, oil-adjuvant vaccine against equine influenza and rhinopneumonitis. *Bulletin Mensuel de la Société Vétérinaire Pratique de France*, 74, 193–208.

90 **MATUMOTO, M., ISHIZAKI, R. & SHIMIZU, T., 1965.** Serological survey of equine pneumonitis virus infection among horses in various countries. *Archiv des gesamte Virusforschung*, 50, 609–623.

91 **MAYHEW, I.G., 1989.** Tetraparesis, paraparesis and ataxia of the limbs, and episodic weakness. *Large Animal Neurology — A Handbook for Veterinary Clinicians*. Philadelphia: Lea & Febiger.

92 **MAYR, A., 1970.** Vaccination of horses against equine herpesvirus 1 infection. *In*: BRYANS, J.T. & GERBER, H., (eds). *Equine Infectious Diseases*. II. Basel, Munchen, New York: S. Karger.

93 **MAYR, A., BOHM, H.O., BRILL, J. & WOYCIECHOWSKA, S., 1965.** Charakteridierung eines Stutenabortvirus aus Polen und Vergleich mit bekannten Rhinopneumonitisvirus-Stammen des Pferdes. *Archiv für Virusforschung*, 16, 216–230.

94 **MAYR, A., THEIN, P. & SCHEID, R., 1968.** Utersuchungen zur entwicklung eines Lebendimpfstoffes gegen die Rhinopneumonitis (stutenabort) der Pferde. *Zentralblatt für Veterinärmedizin*, 15B, 406–418.

95 **MEREDITH, D.M., STOCKS, J.M., WHITTACKER, I.W., HALLIBURTON, I., SNOWDEN, B.W. & KILLINGTON, R., 1989.** Identification of the gB homologues of equine herpesvirus types 1 and 4 as disulphide-linked heterodimers and their characterisation using monoclonal antibodies. *Journal of General Virology*, 70, 1161–1172.

96 **MEYER, H., THEIN, P. & HUBERT, P., 1987.** Characterisation of two equine herpesvirus (EHV) isolates associated with neurological disorders in horses. *Journal of Veterinary Medicine*, B34 545–548.

97 **MUMFORD, J.A., 1979–91.** The Animal Health Trust, P O Box 5, Newmarket, Suffolk CB8 FDW, UK. Unpublished data.

98 **MUMFORD, J.A. & EDINGTON, N., 1980.** EHV-1 and equine paresis. *The Veterinary Record*, 106, 277.

99 **MUMFORD, J.A. & ROSSDALE, P.D., 1980.** Virus and its relationship to the 'poor performance' syndrome. *Equine Veterinary Journal*, 12, 3–9.

100 **MUMFORD, J.A., ROSSDALE, P.D., JESSETT, D.M., GANN, S.J., OUSEY, J. & COOK, R.F., 1987.** Serological and virological investigation of an equid herpesvirus 1 (EHV-1) abortion storm on a stud farm in 1985. *Journal of Reproduction and Fertility*, Suppl. 35, 509–518.

101 **O'CALLAGHAN, D.J., ALLEN, G.P. & RANDALL, C.C., 1978.** Structure and replication of the equine herpesvirus. *In*: BRYANS, J.T. & GERBER, H., (eds). *Equine Infectious Diseases*. IV. Princeton, New Jersey: Veterinary Publications, Inc.

102 **O'CALLAGHAN, D.J., GENTRY, G.A. & RANDALL, C.C., 1983.** The equine herpesvirus. *In*: ROIZMAN, B., (ed.). *The Herpesviruses*. Vol. 2. New York: Plenum Press.

103 **O'CALLAGHAN, D.J. & RANDALL, C.C., 1976.** Molecular anatomy of herpesviruses: Recent studies. *Progress in Medical Virology*, 22, 152–210.

104 **PACHCIARZ, J.A & BRYANS, J.T., 1978.** Cellular immunity to equine pneumonitis virus in pregnant mares. *In*: BRYANS, J.T. & GERBER, H., (eds). *Equine Infectious Diseases*. IV. Princeton, New Jersey: Veterinary Publications, Inc.

105 **PAPP-VID, G. & DERBYSHIRE, J.B., 1978.** The protective antigens of equine herpesvirus type 1. *Canadian Journal of Comparative Medicine*, 42, 219–226.

106 **PATEL, J.R., EDINGTON, N. & MUMFORD, J.A., 1982.** Variation in cellular tropism between isolates of equine herpesvirus 1 in foals. *Archives of Virology*, 74, 41–51.

107 **PEET, P.L., COACKLEY, W., SMITH, V. & MAIN, C., 1978.** Equine abortion associated with a herpesvirus. *Australian Veterinary Journal*, 54, 151.

108 **PERDUE, M.L., COHEN, J.C., KEMP, M.C., RANDALL, C.C. & O'CALLAGHAN, D.J., 1975.** Characteristics of three species of nucleocapsids of equine herpesvirus type 1 (EHV-1). *Virology*, 64, 187–204.

109 **PETZOLDT, K., LUTTMAN, U., POHLENZ, J. & TEICHERT, U., 1972.** Virologische Untersuchungen des Zentralnervensystems von Pferdenfeten und Befunde bei Zentralvervos erkrankten Stuten nach Aborten durch das equine herpesvirus 1. *Schweizer Archiv für Tierheilkunde*, 114, 129–139.

110 **PIERSON, R.H., 1973.** Clinical observations on planned infection and preventive vaccination for control of equine pneumonitis. *Proceedings of the American Association of Equine Practitioners*, 19, 69–72.

111 **PLATT, H., SINGH, H. & WHITWELL, K.E., 1980.** Pathological observations on an outbreak of paralysis in brood mares. *Equine Veterinary Journal*, 12, 118–126.

112 **PLUMMER, G. & WATERSON, A.P., 1963.** Equine herpesviruses. *Virology*, 19, 412–416.

113 **POWELL, D.G., BURROWS, R., SPOONER, P.R., GOODRIDGE, D., THOMSON, G.R. & MUMFORD, J.A., 1978.** A study of infectious respiratory disease among horses in Great Britain, 1971 to 1976. *In*: BRYANS, J.T. & GERBER, H., (eds). *Equine Infectious Diseases*. IV. Princeton, New Jersey: Veterinary Publications Inc.

114 **PRICKETT, M.E., 1970.** The pathology of disease caused by equine herpesvirus 1. *In*: BRYANS, J.T. & GERBER, H., (eds). *Equine Infectious Diseases*. II. Basel, Munchen, New York: S. Karger.

115 **PURDY, C.W., FORD, S.J. & PORTER, R.C. 1977.** Equine pneumonitis vaccine: Immunogenicity and safety in adult horses, including pregnant mares. *American Journal of Veterinary Research*, 39, 377–383.

116 **PURDY, C.W., PORTER, R.C. & FORD, J.F., 1978.** Equine rhinopneumonitis vaccine: Immunogenicity and safety in foals. *American Journal of Veterinary Research*, 39, 745–752.

117 **RIGGIO, M.P., CULLINANE, A. & ONIONS, D.E., 1989.** Identification and nucleotide sequence of glycoprotein gB gene of equine herpesvirus 4. *Journal of Virology*, 63, 1123–1133.

118 **SABINE, M., FEILEN, C., HERBERT, L., JONES, R., LOMAS, S., LOVE, D. & WILD, J., 1983.** Equine herpesvirus abortion in Australia (1977–1982). *Equine Veterinary Journal*, 15, 366–370.

119 **SABINE, M., ROBERTSON, G.R. & WHALLEY, J.M., 1981.** Differentiation of subtypes of equine herpesvirus 1 by restriction endonuclcase analysis. *Australian Veterinary Journal*, 57, 148–149.

120 **SAXEGAARD, F., 1966.** Isolation and identification of equine pneumonitis virus (equine abortion virus) from cases of abortion and paralysis. *Nordisk Veterinaermedicin*, 18, 504–516.

121 **SCOTT, J.C., DUTTA, S.K & MYRUP, A.C., 1983.** *In vivo* harbouring of equine herpesvirus 1 in leukocyte populations and subpopulations and their quantitation from experimentally infected ponies. *American Journal of Veterinary Research*, 44, 1344–1348.

122 **SHERMAN, J., MITCHELL, W.R., MARTIN, S.W., THORSEN, J. & INGRAM, D.G., 1979.** Epidemiology of equine upper respiratory tract disease on standardbred racetracks. *Canadian Journal of Comparative Medicine*, 43, 1–9.

123 **SHIMIZU, M., SATOU, K. & NISHIOKA, N., 1989.** Monoclonal antibodies with neutralising activity to equine herpesvirus 1. *Archives of Virology*, 104, 169–174.

124 **SHIMIZU, M., ISHIZAKI, R., ISHII, S., KAWAKAMI, Y., KAJI, R., SUGIMURA, K. & MATUMOTO, M., 1959.** Isolation of equine abortion virus from natural cases of equine abortion in horse kidney cell culture. *Japanese Journal of Experimental Medicine*, 29, 643–649.

125 **SINCLAIR, R.S., 1991.** Equid herpesvirus type-1: Antigenic analysis and diagnosis of infection using monoclonal antibodies. Ph.D. Thesis, University of London.

126 **SINCLAIR, R.S., COOK, R.F. & MUMFORD, J.A., 1989.** The characterisation of neutralising and non-neutralising monoclonal antibodies against equid herpesvirus 1. *Journal of General Virology*, 70, 455–459.

127 **SMITH, I.M., GIRAND, A., CORNER, A.H. & MITCHELL, D., 1972.** The fluorescent antibody technique in the abortion. *Canadian Journal of Comparative Medicine*, 36, 303–308.

128 **SNOWDEN, B.W. & HALLIBURTON, I.W., 1985.** Identification of cross-reacting glycoproteins of four herpesviruses by western blotting. *Journal of General Virology*, 66, 2039–2044.

129 **SOEHNER, R.L., GENTRY, G.A. & RANDALL, C.C., 1965.** Some physicochemical characteristics of equine abortion virus nucleic acid. *Virology*, 26, 394–405.

130 **STOKES, A., ALLEN, G.P., PULLEN, L.A. & MURRAY, P.K., 1989.** A hamster model of equine herpesvirus 1 (EHV-1) infection: Passive protection by monoclonal antibodies to EHV-1 glycoproteins 13, 14 and 17/18. *Journal of General Virology*, 70, 1173–1183.

131 **STUDDERT, M.J. & BLAKENEY, M.H., 1979.** Equine herpesviruses: On differentiation of respiratory from foetal strains of type 1. *Australian Veterinary Journal*, 55, 488–492.

132 **STUDDERT, M.J., SIMPSON, T. & ROIZMAN, B., 1981.** Differentiation of respiratory and abortigenic isolates of equine herpesvirus 1 by restriction endonucleases. *Science*, 214, 562–564.

133 **THEIN, P., 1981.** Infection of the central nervous system of horses with equine herpesvirus serotype 1. *Journal of the South African Veterinary Association*, 52, 239–241.

134 **THOMPSON, G.W., McCREADY, R., SANFORD, E. & GAGNON, A., 1979.** An outbreak of herpesvirus myeloencephalitis in vaccinated horses. *Canadian Veterinary Journal*, 20, 22–25.

135 **THOMSON, G.R., 1978.** The role of Equid herpesvirus 1 in acute respiratory disease of horses and the use of inactivated antigens to immunise against the infection. Ph.D. Thesis, University of London.

136 **THOMSON, G.R., MUMFORD, J.A., CAMPBELL, J., GRIFFITHS, L. & CLAPMAN, P., 1976.** Serological detection

of equid herpesvirus 1 infection of the respiratory tract. *Equine Veterinary Journal*, 8, 58–65.

137 **THOMSON, G.R., MUMFORD, J.A. & PLOWRIGHT, W., 1978.** Immunological responses of conventional and gnotobiotic foals to infectious and inactivated antigens of equine herpesvirus 1. *In*: BRYANS, J.T. & GERBER, H., (eds). *Equine Infectious Diseases*. IV. Princeton, New Jersey: Veterinary Publications, Inc.

138 **THOMSON, G.R., MUMFORD, J.A. & SMITH, I.M., 1979.** Experimental immunisation against respiratory disease due to equid herpesvirus 1 infection (pneumonitis) using formalin-inactivated virus with various adjuvants. *Veterinary Microbiology*, 4, 209–222.

139 **TURTINEN, L.W., 1983.** Studies on the antigenic and genetic variation between the two subtypes of equine herpesvirus 1. Ph.D. dissertation. University of Kentucky.

140 **TURTINEN, L.W. & ALLEN, G.P., 1982.** Identification of the envelope surface glycoproteins of equine herpesvirus type 1. *Journal of General Virology*, 63, 481–485.

141 **TURTINEN, L.W., ALLEN, G.P., DARLINGTON, R.W. & BRYANS, J.T., 1981.** Serological and molecular comparisons of several equine herpesvirus type 1 strains. *American Journal of Veterinary Research*, 42, 2099–2104.

142 **WELCH, H.M., BRIDGES, C.G., LYON, A.M., GRIFFITHS, L. & EDINGTON, N., 1992.** Latent equid herpesviruses 1 and 4: Detection and distinction using the polymerase chain reaction and cocultivation from lymphoid tissues. In press.

143 **WESTERFIELD, C. & DIMOCK, W.W., 1946.** The pathology of equine virus abortion. *Journal of the American Veterinary Medical Association*, 109, 101–111.

144 **WHALLEY, J.M., ROBERTSON, G.R., SCOTT, N.A., HUDSON, G.C., BELL, C.W. & WOODWORTH, L.M., 1989.** Identification and nucleotide sequence of a gene in EHV-1 analogous to the herpes simplex virus gene encoding the major envelope glycoprotein gB. *Journal of General Virology*, 70, 383–394.

145 **WHITWELL, K.E. & MUMFORD, J.A., 1988.** The Animal Health Trust, P.O. Box 5, Newmarket, Suffolk CB8 FDW, UK. Unpublished data.

146 **WITHERSPOON, D.M., 1984.** A modified vaccination schedule for prevention of equine herpesvirus 1 infection. *Norden News*, 59, 34–36.

147 **YEARGAN, M.R., ALLEN, G.P. & BRYANS, J.T., 1985.** Rapid subtyping of equine herpesvirus 1 isolates with monoclonal antibodies. *Journal of Clinical Microbiology*, 21, 694–697.

103

Equid herpesvirus 2 infection

Synonyms: Equine cytomegalovirus, slowly cytopathic equine herpesvirus

J.A. Mumford

Introduction and aetiology

Equid herpesvirus 2 (EHV-2) infection of horses is ubiquitous, but the association of the virus with disease is equivocal because isolations are commonly made from both healthy and diseased animals.

Equid herpesvirus 2 was first isolated in 1963[18] and since then has been recovered from nasal, ocular, and vaginal secretions, leukocytes and a variety of tissues of horses.[1, 6, 9, 13, 14, 18, 22]

The virus has provisionally been included among the betaherpesviruses.[19] Its genome has a molecular weight of approximately 126 MDa, which is at least 35 per cent greater than the genomes of the highly cytocidal equid herpesviruses (EHV-1, EHV-3 and EHV-4).[5] Only about 3 per cent of EHV-2 DNA sequences are shared with those of EHV-1, EHV-3 and EHV-4, and unlike EHV-1, there is marked heterogeneity in the DNA restriction endonuclease profiles of EHV-2 isolates, which fall broadly into two groups.[4] One group has similar restriction endonuclease patterns to the prototype strain LK, which has been characterized as having a genome of about 190 kilobase pairs,[24] while the second group has a significantly smaller genome of approximately 148 kilobase pairs.

The nucleocapsids are made up of nine proteins whose average molecular weights (Mr) range from 18 to 148K. The 148K protein represents 47,3 per cent of the total protein, and is therefore the major capsid protein. At least 37 proteins have been identified in purified virions (Mrs 200–14K), of which three are major glycoproteins (83K, 78K, 73,5K) and four minor.[5]

The protein composition of EHV-2 differs substantially from those of EHV-1 and EHV-3, and no cross-reactivity between the nucleocapsid proteins of these viruses has been detected with rabbit antisera.[5]

Equid herpesvirus 2 has many of the properties associated with cytomegaloviruses, including persistent infection of its natural host, replication in leukocytes, a growth cycle characterized by a long eclipse period (24–48 hours), relatively low yield of virus (much of which remains cell-associated[19]), and cytopathic effects which often manifest as cytomegaly and syncytia.[10, 16, 20, 24]

There are differences in biological (plaque size and host cell range) and antigenic properties[11] between some EHV-2 isolates, but the epidemiological significance of these remain to be established.

Epidemiology

Equid herpesvirus 2 has a worldwide distribution.

Horses are exposed to EHV-2 early in life and acquire the infection, probably via the respiratory tract, either from their dams or from other young foals.[25] Foals are born without antibody, but acquire high levels from colostrum.[25] They may shed the virus in respiratory secretions for many months or even years, initially in the presence of maternal antibody, and, later, actively produced antibody.[12, 23]

The complexity of EHV-2 transmission has been demonstrated by identifying multiple, concurrent infections with EHV-2 viruses with different restriction endonuclease profiles in individual horses.[4] These viruses may be shed, possibly continuously, for periods of at least 54 days, or this may become latent and recrudesce months later.[3] However, the virus is unable to cross the placenta.[8]

Pathogenesis and pathology

Cell-associated viraemia is established early in life and may persist for years. The virus replicates in cells at mucosal surfaces such as the respiratory tract, conjunctiva and genital tract.[4] Because EHV-2 can be cultured regularly from leukocytes by co-cultivation with permissive cells such as equine foetal kidney and rabbit kidney (RK13) cells, it has been concluded that leukocytes are persistently or latently infected.[7]

Although EHV-2 has been isolated from horses with ulcerative pharyngitis, from outbreaks of conjunctivitis in foals,[22] and from foals and young horses suffering from respiratory disease,[17] its causative role in equine diseases remains in doubt because it may also be isolated from a high proportion of healthy animals. Most experimental studies have failed to prove the pathogenic potential of EHV-2, although Blakeslee *et al.*[2] reported observing chronic pharyngitis in two young foals inoculated with EHV-2, and Thein[22] described the development of keratoconjunctivitis following experimental infection of horses with EHV-2.

Diagnosis

Equid herpesvirus 2 can be cultured on cells of both equine and non-equine origin. Equine cells vary in sensitivity depending on the organ from which they are derived, with equine foetal kidney cells being more sensitive than equine foetal lung cells, which in turn are more sensitive than equine dermal cells. In general, non-equine cells such as RK13 and green monkey kidney (Vero) cells are less sensitive than equine cells.

Equid herpesvirus 2 is slow-growing *in vitro* and cytopathic effects (CPE) often only become obvious after two or three passages. The CPE is usually focal, with syncytial formation being a feature in some cell types (e.g. RK13 cells). Exceptionally, some isolates may produce CPE within 48 hours, particularly in sensitive cells, such as equine foetal kidney.[15]

Since EHV-2 can be isolated from the respiratory tract, genital tract and blood, it is essential to have a reliable means of differentiating EHV-2 from other equine herpesviruses with known pathogenicities.

Virus neutralization tests are not suitable for the identification of EHV-2 virus because a high degree of heterogeneity has been identified within EHV-2 isolates.[15] Immunofluorescence using hyperimmune rabbit sera is more suitable, as this technique detects antigens common to a wide range of EHV-2 isolates, while distinguishing EHV-2 from other herpesviruses of equine, bovine and human origin.[15] Alternatively, EHV-2 isolates can be identified by agar-gel immunodiffusion, using infected cell extracts and suitable antisera.[21]

Antibody to EHV-2 may be detected by complement fixation, immunofluorescence and neutralization tests.[15] However, the interpretation of results is difficult. Many infections do not stimulate strong neutralizing antibody responses, and so this test is not a sensitive indicator of exposure. High levels of antibody that are detectable by complement fixation or immunofluorescence may only represent exposure which occurred some months previously. As a result of these problems, serological diagnosis of EHV-2 infections is rarely used.

References

1 **BELAK, S., PALFI, V. TUBOLY, S. & BARTHA, L., 1980.** Passive immunization of foals to prevent respiratory disease caused by equine herpesvirus type 2. *Zentralblatt für Veterinärmedizin*, 27, 826–830.

2 **BLAKESLEE, J.E. Jr., OLSEN, R.G., McALLISTER, E.S., FASBENDER, J. & DENNIS, R., 1975.** Evidence of respiratory tract infection induced by equine herpesvirus, type 2, in the horse. *Canadian Journal of Microbiology*, 21, 1940–1946.

3 **BROWNING, G.F. & STUDDERT, M.J., 1986.** Epidemiology of equine herpesvirus 2 (equine cytomegalovirus). *Journal of Clinical Microbiology*, 25, 13–16.

4 **BROWNING, G.F. & STUDDERT, M.J., 1987.** Genomic heterogeneity of equine betaherpesviruses. *Journal of General Virology*, 68, 1441–1447.

5 **CAUGHMAN, G.B., STACZEK, J. & O'CALLAGHAN, D.J., 1984.** Equine cytomegalovirus: Structural proteins and virions and nucleocapsides. *Virology*, 134, 184–195.

6 **ERASMUS, B.J., 1970.** Equine cytomegaloviruses. *In: Proceedings of the Second International Conference on Equine Infectious Diseases*, Paris, 1969. Basel: S. Karger.

7 **GLEESON, L.J. & COGGINS, L., 1985.** Equine herpesvirus type 2: Cell–virus relationship during persistent cell-associated viraemia. *American Journal of Veterinary Research*, 46, 19–23.

8 **GLEESON, L.J. & STUDDERT, M.J., 1977.** Equine herpesvirus: Experimental infection of a foetus with type 2. *Australian Veterinary Journal*, 53, 360–362.

9 **HARDEN, T.J., BAGUST, T.J., PASCOE, R.R. & SPRADBROW, P.B., 1974.** Studies on equine herpesvirus. 5. Isolation and characterization of slowly cytopathic equine herpesviruses in Queensland. *Australian Veterinary Journal*, 50, 483–488.

10 **HSUING, G.D., FISCHMAN, H.R., FONG, C.K.Y. & GREEN, R.H., 1969.** Characterization of a cytomegalo-like virus isolated from spontaneously degenerated equine kidney cell culture. *Proceedings of the Society for Experimental Biology and Medicine*, 130, 80–84.

11 **KARPAS, A., 1966.** Characterization of a new herpesvirus-like virus isolated from foal kidney. *Annales de l'Institut Pasteur*, 110, 688–696.

12 **KEMENY, L. & PEARSON, J.E., 1970.** Isolation of herpesvirus from equine leukocytes: Comparison with equine rhinopneumonitis virus. *Canadian Journal of Comparative Medicine*, 34, 59–65.

13 **KONO, Y. & KOBAYASHI, K., 1964.** Cytopathogenic equine orphan (CEO) virus in horse kidney cell culture. I. Isolation and properties. *National Institute of Animal Health Quarterly*, 4, 10–20.

14 **KONO, Y. & KOBAYASHI, K., 1964.** Cytopathogenic equine orphan (CEO) virus in horse kidney cell culture. II. Immunological studies of CEO virus. *National Institute of Animal Health Quarterly*, 4, 21–27.

15 **MUMFORD, J.A. & THOMSON, G.R., 1978.** Serological methods for identification of slowly growing herpesviruses isolated from the respiratory tract of horses. *In*: BRYANS, J.T. & GERBER, H., (eds). *Equine Infectious Diseases*. Vol. IV. Princeton: Veterinary Publications, Inc.

16 **O'CALLAGHAN, D.J., GENTRY, G.A. & RANDALL, C.C., 1983.** The equine herpesviruses. *In*: FRAENKEL-CONRAT, H. & WAGNER, R.R., (eds). *The Herpesviruses*. Vol. II. New York: Plenum Press.

17 **PALFI, V., BELAK, S. & MOLNAR, T., 1978.** Isolation of equine herpesvirus type 2 from foals showing respiratory symptoms. *Zentralblatt für Veterinärmedizin, Reihe B*, 25, 165–167.

18 **PLUMMER, G. & WATERSON, A.P., 1963.** Equine herpesviruses. *Virology*, 19, 412–416.

19 **ROIZMAN, B., 1982.** The family Herpesviridae: General description, taxonomy and classification. *In*: ROIZMAN, B., (ed.). *The Herpesviruses*. New York: Plenum Press.

20 **STACZEK, J., ATHERTON, S.S. & O'CALLAGHAN, D.J., 1984.** Genetic relatedness of the genomes of equine herpesvirus type 1, 2 and 3. *Journal of Virology*, 45, 855–858.

21 **SUGIURA, T., FUKUZAWA, Y., KAMADA, M., ANDO, Y.**

& HIRASAWA, K., 1983. Isolation of equine herpesvirus type 2 from foals with pneumonitis. *Bulletin of the Equine Research Institute*, 20, 148–153.

22 **THEIN, P., 1978.** The association of EHV-2 infection with keratitis and research on the occurrences of equine coital exanthema (EHV-3) of horses in Germany. *In*: BRYANS, J.T. & GERBER, H., (eds). *Equine Infectious Diseases*. Vol. IV. Princeton: Veterinary Publications, Inc.

23 **TURNER, A.J. & STUDDERT, M.J., 1970.** Equine herpesvirus. III. Isolation and epizootiology of slowly cytopathic viruses and the serological incidence of equine rhinopneumonitis. *Australian Veterinary Journal*, 46, 581–586.

24 **WHARTON, J.H., HENRY, B.E. & O'CALLAGHAN, D.J., 1981.** Equine cytomegalovirus: Cultural characteristics and properties of viral DNA. *Virology*, 109, 106–119.

25 **WILKS, C.R. & STUDDERT, M.J., 1974.** Equine herpes-viruses. V. Epizootiology of slowly cytopathic viruses in foals. *Australian Veterinary Journal*, 50, 438–442.

104

Equine coital exanthema

Synonym: Equid herpesvirus 3 infection

J.A. Mumford

Introduction

Equine coital exanthema is an acute, highly contagious, relatively mild disease characterized by the formation of vesicles, pustules and ulcers on the genitalia of mares and stallions.

The disease has been recognized for many years,[8, 10] but it was not until 1968 that a herpesvirus distinguished from EHV-1 and EHV-2 was isolated from clinical cases.[3, 12, 21] The infection is endemic throughout the world,[3, 12, 16, 21] and is occasionally clinically diagnosed by veterinarians in South Africa.[18]

Equine coital exanthema has not been associated with abortions, but breeding of stallions and mares may be affected as a result of the inability to cover or the enforced sexual rest that is often necessary to prevent spread of the disease.

Aetiology

Equid (equine) herpesvirus 3 is an alphaherpesvirus antigenically distinct from EHV-1 and EHV-2 in cross-neutralization tests, although antigens common to EHV-1 and EHV-3 have been demonstrated in immunofluorescence, immunoprecipitation and complement fixation tests.[14, 19] Antigenic variation is not a feature of EHV-3 isolates.[5]

The density and base composition of the DNA of EHV-3 differ from those of EHV-1 and 2.[17] No genetic variation has been identified,[2] but differences in restriction profiles have been associated with small and large plaque variants derived from the same isolate.[15]

Epidemiology

Venereal transmission is the usual means of transmission, and coital exanthema therefore usually occurs during the breeding season. The disease may, however, occur in horses which have had no sexual contact.[16] Iatrogenic transmission during vaginal or rectal examination or by the use of contaminated instruments, as well as transmission through grooming,[11] have been suggested. Infection of the respiratory tract has been reported.[9]

Foals acquire maternal antibody, which may persist for four to six months, from colostrum. However, apart from passively-acquired antibody in young foals, antibody is rarely detected before the age of sexual maturity. After two years of age the proportion of seropositives increases, reaching a maximum of 50 per cent in animals of eight or more years old.[1] Not all infections result in clinical disease, and inapparently infected horses may transmit the infection.[7]

Re-infections and/or recrudescence of latent virus play a significant role in the epidemiology of coital exanthema, but so far the virus has only been isolated from animals when lesions were evident. Disease may recur repeatedly in some mares, usually during the terminal period of pregnancy, or immediately after foaling; recrudescence is particularly common in aged broodmares, but also occurs in stallions. Clinical episodes have been recorded in consecutive years in both mares and stallions,[16] but, on the other hand, it may take up to five years for infection introduced into a herd to become clinically evident.[7]

Virus neutralizing antibody titres stimulated by infection or recrudescence return to pre-exposure levels 15–20 weeks after infection, and remain at low levels for variable periods ranging from one to six months.[7]

Pathogenesis

Following infection of the mucous membrane or skin of the genitalia, localized lesions (initially vesicles, which progress to pustules, erosions and ulcers) are formed as a result of the cytocidal effect of EHV-3 on epithelial cells. Generally these lesions heal without scar formation. No viraemia is detectable during the course of the disease, and except in complicated cases fever is absent.[12]

Clinical signs and pathology

Pock-like lesions are found particularly at or near the mucocutaneous junctions of the vulva and orifice of the prepuce, in the mucosa of the vagina and vestibule, and on the prepuce (mostly at reflection) and body of the penis.[12, 16, 20, 21] The skin of the perineum (especially in mares), ventral aspects of the tail, udder, teats, prepuce, scrotum, inner thighs and belly, and occasionally also the lips, muzzle, respiratory tract and conjunctiva may also be affected.[16, 18]

Early lesions comprise small (2–3 mm) vesicles which are not often noticed. These vesicular lesions develop into greyish pustules, followed by scab formation. Beneath the scabs, sharply defined erosions or ulcers, 5–10 mm in diameter, are formed, the number and severity of lesions increasing over a five-day period. Acutely affected animals may show evidence of pain and frequent micturition.[21] Once healed, the lesions leave white areas of depigmentation. In uncomplicated cases, healing takes place within two or three weeks, after which stallions may be returned to service.

Systemic responses such as fever and depression are rarely evident unless secondary bacterial infections are present, and in these animals fever is accompanied by a mucopurulent discharge and oedema of the genitalia.[21] Severely affected stallions may develop a necrotizing balanitis and phimosis. The libido of stallions with severe lesions may be reduced.[20]

Horses with respiratory tract involvement may show ulcerated lesions as well as conjunctivitis.[16]

Microscopically, there is ballooning, lysis and sloughing of surface epithelial cells. Characteristic herpesvirus intranuclear inclusion bodies are present in the epithelial cells at the margin of the lesions. Intense mononuclear and polymorphonuclear leukocyte infiltrations are found in the tissue immediately adjacent to the lesions.[5, 22]

Under natural conditions EHV-3 has not been implicated as a cause of abortion, although inoculation has resulted in infection and abortion of a foetus.[13] Generally, there is no reduction in fertility in infected horses.[20]

Diagnosis and differential diagnosis

Equid herpesvirus 3 may be isolated in the acute phase of the disease from swabs or scrapings taken from the edges of lesions or from ocular or nasal secretions.[4, 6] For this purpose equine cell cultures are required; unlike EHV-1 and EHV-2, EHV-3 only replicates in equine cells (e.g. horse kidney cells). Cytopathic effects consist initially (after approximately 24 hours) of foci of rounded refractile cells and some greatly enlarged cells. The entire monolayer is usually destroyed within 48 hours of infection. Stained cultures reveal, in addition to necrotic cells, extensive syncytia containing up to 150 nuclei and large Cowdry type A intranuclear inclusion bodies.[16, 21] Virus isolates may be differentiated from EHV-1 and EHV-2 by virus neutralization or immunofluorescence tests using specific antisera.[19]

Complement fixation and virus neutralization tests have been used to demonstrate increase in antibody to EHV-3 in convalescent sera. Antibody responses are relatively short-lived, and titres return to pre-infection levels within three to six months.[7] Subclinical infections or recrudescence may be detected by sequential serum sampling in the absence of virus isolation, but elevated levels of neutralizing antibody are often already present by the time clinical signs are apparent, and it is therefore not always possible to demonstrate clear increases in antibody between acute and convalescent phase sera.

Clinically, the lesions on the genitalia of mares and stallions suffering from coital exanthema are quite indicative of the disease. However, dourine, caused by *Trypanosoma equiperdum*, should also be considered in the case of those stallions which reveal severe oedema of the sheath and scrotum.

Control

Enforced sexual rest of acutely affected animals for three to four weeks is essential if the spread of this highly contagious disease is to be prevented. Antibiotic therapy is useful for the control of secondary bacterial infections.

Contaminated stables, gear or instruments should be disinfected properly, and special precautions should be taken by veterinarians to prevent iatrogenic transmission.

References

1 **BAGUST, T.J., PASCOE, R.R. & HARDEN, T.J., 1972.** Studies on equine herpesvirus-3. The incidence in Queensland of three different equine herpesvirus infections. *Australian Veterinary Journal*, 847–853.

2 **BOUCHEY, D., EVERMANN, J. & JACOB, R.J., 1987.** Molecular pathogenesis of equine coital exanthema (ECE): Temperature-sensitive (TS) and restriction endonuclease (RE) fragment profiles of several field isolates. *Archives of Virology*, 92, 293–299.

3 **BRYANS, J.T., 1968.** The herpesviruses in disease of the horse. *Proceedings of the American Association of Equine Practitioners*, Philadelphia, 1968, 119–125.

4 **BRYANS, J.T., 1980.** Herpesviral diseases affecting reproduction in the horse. *Symposium on Equine Reproduction. Veterinary Clinics of North America: Large Animal Practice*, 2, 303–312.

5 **BRYANS, J.T. & ALLEN, G.P., 1973.** *In vitro* and *in vivo* studies of equine coital exanthema. *In:* BRYANS, J. & GERBER, H., (eds). *Equine Infectious Diseases*. Vol. III. Basel: S. Karger.

6 **BURKI, F., LORN, D., SIBALIN, M., RUTHER, O. & ARBENTER, K., 1974.** Experimentelle genitale und nasal Infektion von Pferde mit dem Virusae equinem coital exanthema. *Zentralblatt für Veterinärmedizin*, 21, 362–375.

7 **BURROWS, R. & GOODRIDGE, D., 1984.** Studies of persistent and latent equine herpesvirus 1 and herpesvirus 3 infections in the Pirbright pony herd. *In*: WITTMAN, G., (ed.). *Latent Herpesvirus Infections in Veterinary Medicine*. Boston: Martinus Nijhoff.

8 **CRAIG, J.F. & KEHOE, D., 1921.** Horse pox and coital exanthema. *Journal of Comparative Pathology*, 34, 126–129.

9 **CRANDELL, R. & DAVIS, E.R., 1985.** Isolation of equine coital exanthema virus (equine herpesvirus 3) from the nostril of a foal. *Journal of the American Veterinary Medical Association*, 187, 503–504.

10 **DAY, F.T., 1957.** The veterinary clinician's approach to breeding problems in mares. *The Veterinary Record*, 69, 1258–1264.

11 **GIBBS, E.P.J., ROBERTS, M.C. & MORRIS, J.M., 1972.** Equine coital exanthema in the United Kingdom. *Equine Veterinarian*, 4, 74–80.

12 **GIRARD, A., GRIEG, A.S. & MITCHELL, D., 1968.** A virus associated with vulvitis and balanitis in the horse. A preliminary report. *Canadian Journal of Comparative Medicine*, 32, 603–604.

13 **GLEESON, L.J., SULLIVAN, N.D. & STUDDERT, M.J., 1976.** Equine herpesvirus Type 3 as an abortigenic agent. *Australian Veterinary Journal*, 52, 349–354.

14 **GUTEKUNST, D.E., MALMQUIST, W.A. & BECVER, C.S., 1978.** Antigenic relatedness of equine herpesvirus Type 1 and 3. *Archives of Virology*, 56, 33–45.

15 **KAMADA, M. & STUDDERT, M.J., 1983.** Analysis of small and large plaque variants of equine herpesvirus Type 3 by restriction endonuclease. *Archives of Virology*, 77, 259–264.

16 **KROGSRUD, J. & OUSTAD, O., 1971.** Equine coital exanthema — isolation of a virus and transmission experiments. *Acta Veterinaria Scandinavica*, 12, 1–14.

17 **LUDWIG, H., BISWAL, N., BRYANS, J.T. & McCOMBS, R.M., 1971.** Some properties of the DNA from a new equine herpesvirus. *Virology*, 45, 534–547.

18 **MARLOW, C.H.B., 1990.** P.O. Box 138, Cradock, South Africa. Unpublished data.

19 **MUMFORD, J.A. & THOMSON, G.R., 1978.** Serological methods for identification of slowly-growing herpesvirus isolated from the respiratory tract of horses. *In:* BRYANS, J. & GERBER, H., (eds). *Equine Infectious Diseases*. Vol. IV. Princeton: Veterinary Publications, Inc.

20 **PASCOE, R.R., 1981.** The effect of equine coital exanthema on the fertility of mares covered by stallions exhibiting the clinical disease. *Australian Veterinary Journal*, 57, 111–114.

21 **PASCOE, R.R., SPADBROW, P.B. & BAGUST, T.J., 1969.** An equine genital infection resembling coital exanthema associated with a virus. *Australian Veterinary Journal*, 45, 166–170.

22 **STUDDERT, M.J., 1974.** Comparative aspects of equine herpesviruses. *Cornell Veterinarian*, 64, 94–122.

105

Infectious bovine rhinotracheitis/ infectious pustular vulvovaginitis

Synonym: Bovine (bovid) herpesvirus 1 infection

B.J.H. Barnard and M.G. Collett

Introduction

In cattle, bovine (bovid) herpesvirus 1 (BHV-1) is the cause of a variety of syndromes, of which infectious bovine rhinotracheitis (IBR), infectious pustular vulvovaginitis (IPV) and infectious (pustular) balanoposthitis (IBP) are the most common.[97] It may also cause conjunctivitis, meningoencephalomyelitis, digestive tract disease, abortion, and generalized infections in neonates.[31, 54, 118]

During the last century a venereally transmitted vesicular disease, known as Bläschenausschlag, was described in cattle in Germany,[131] while a similar disease was reported in North America in 1900, although it was thought to be caused by a bacterium.[86] In 1913 the infectivity of vaginal discharges was demonstrated,[133] and in 1928 the agent was shown to be filterable.[93] A virus was isolated in cell culture in 1958 by Kendrick *et al.*,[59] who referred to the syndrome associated with it as infectious pustular vulvovaginitis, a name which replaced various terms (Bläschenausschlag, vesicular venereal disease, vesicular vaginitis and coital vesicular exanthema) used in other countries. This virus was shown to be identical to that isolated from cases of IBR by Madin *et al* in 1956.[65] It has become customary to refer to these two syndromes as IBR and IPV/IBP, and the virus is now named bovine (bovid) herpesvirus 1.[31, 68]

In both eastern and southern Africa a condition previously known as 'epivag' has long been recognized,[22, 123] the term being derived from an amalgamation of 'epididymitis' and 'vaginitis', but the condition later became known as infectious bovine infertility.[41] The aetiology of this syndrome has not been unequivocally determined, but BHV-1 and BHV-4 as well as other microorganisms have been isolated from affected animals[40, 56, 66, 117, 120] **(see Chapter 192: Epivag)**.

Although it had been shown earlier that BHV-1 isolated from South African cattle suffering from IPV could cause respiratory disease,[40] IBR was only recognized in South Africa after the establishment of feedlots.[6] This is not surprising, since IBR is most severe under conditions of intensification and is responsible for severe economic losses in feedlots in North America.[67, 114]

Apart from respiratory and genital disease, none of the other syndromes associated with BHV-1 have been reported in southern Africa, although Hellig[40] showed that BHV-1 isolated from natural cases of IPV could cause encephalitis and keratoconjunctivitis in cattle infected experimentally. Infectious balanoposthitis has only rarely been encountered in southern Africa.

Aetiology

Bovine herpesvirus 1 is a typical alphaherpesvirus consisting of an enveloped capsid of 162 capsomeres arranged in icosahedral symmetry containing double-stranded DNA.[19, 30, 31, 78, 127] The nucleocapsid develops within the nucleus of the host cell and acquires the envelope on budding through the cell membranes.[48, 107] The virus has a relatively short replication cycle of about 12 hours and produces Cowdry type A intranuclear inclusions in infected cells.[18, 78]

In common with other herpesviruses, BHV-1 is ether-sensitive, labile at low pH, and sensitive to heat.[109] It is inactivated within 10 days at 37 °C and is stable for at least a month at 4 °C.[109] The virus is rapidly inactivated by various disinfectants, including 0,5 per cent sodium hydroxide, 0,1 per cent mercuric chloride, 1 per cent chlorinated lime, 1 per cent phenolic derivatives, 1 per cent quaternary ammonium bases, and 10 per cent Lugol's iodine. Five per cent formalin solution inactivates the virus within one minute,[113] whereas live virus can still be detected in a 0,8 per cent solution after one hour.[36]

With the exception of caprine herpesvirus,[25] no cross neutralization has been detected between BHV-1 and herpesviruses of other domestic species.[50, 92] In addition, BHV-1 does not cross-react with other herpesviruses which infect cattle[91] (including BHV-4, the Movar-type virus[62]).

Although isolates of BHV-1 from cases of IBR and IPV were initially found to be biologically and immunologically indistinguishable,[32] they may be differentiated on the basis of electrophoretic patterns produced by restriction endonuclease-generated DNA fragments.[26, 73, 125] However, findings in this respect have not been unanimous.[77, 105] Viral isolates from cases of meningoencephalitis have also been reported to produce restriction endonuclease patterns distinct from those of IBR and IPV.[12, 73] Genome variation, demonstrated by changes in electrophoretic patterns of restriction endonuclease-treated viral DNA, has been shown to occur within a single passage *in vivo* after the inoculation of cloned virus, and also after reactivation in latently infected animals.[125] However, the extent of this variation is limited, since BHV-1 isolates from diverse clinical conditions including IBR, IPV, meningoencephalomyelitis, and aborted foetuses showed 95 per cent genome homology.[105] It therefore appears that subtypes of BHV-1 can be differentiated on the basis of restriction endonuclease patterns, but that individual strains cannot be identified in this way.[125]

Epidemiology

Cattle are the principal hosts of BHV-1, although goats,[79] pigs, water buffalo[112] and several African game species — in particular Cape buffalo (*Syncerus caffer*), eland (*Taurotragus oryx*) and black and blue wildebeest (*Connochaetes* spp.) — may also be susceptible.[57, 90] The significance of antibody prevalence in wildlife species is unknown, because although buffalo, eland and wildebeest populations may have a high proportion of seropositive animals,[39] the recent finding of herpesviruses specific to wildlife species but serologically indistinguishable from BHV-1, makes interpretation of earlier serological surveys difficult.[90] The virus is widely distributed among cattle in southern Africa.[29, 40, 117] Carrier cattle are important in maintaining the infection in inter-epidemic periods.

Infectious bovine rhinotracheitis

The rarity and apparent mildness of IBR in range cattle as compared to cattle in feedlots may be due to the quantity of virus to which individual animals are exposed,[13] although other factors peculiar to feedlots and intensive farming systems may play an important role **(see Chapter 141: Pneumonic pasteurellosis in cattle)**. For example, cattle entering feedlots are usually of an age when passively acquired immunity is low; and high population densities and a continuous throughput of cattle from diverse backgrounds (in terms of susceptibility and disease or carrier status) facilitate transmission of the virus.

The virus survives well enough in aerosol droplets for airborne transmission to occur.[20, 27] Under experimental conditions, doses of BHV-1 between $10^{3,6}$–$10^{5,4}$ tissue culture infective doses administered intranasally were adequate to produce typical IBR.[103]

Calves recovered from infection and subsequently treated with dexamethasone may excrete up to $10^{6,8}$–$10^{8,5}$ plaque-forming units/ml in nasal mucus.[88] This demonstrates that stress factors may precipitate the excretion of BHV-1 by latently infected (carrier) animals.

The role of primary BHV-1 infection in the bovine respiratory disease complex is not well understood because, although a number of other viruses, including bovine respiratory syncytial, bovine virus diarrhoea, para-influenza-3, adeno-, rhino-, and reoviruses may also sometimes be involved, only BHV-1 regularly causes disease after experimental inoculation.[115] The interaction between BHV-1 and bacteria such as *Pasteurella* spp. in the causation of pneumonia has also not been accurately established.[132]

Uncomplicated cases of IBR in feedlots in South Africa are rare and, conversely, BHV-1 is not always involved in respiratory infections in feedlots in South Africa.[7]

Infectious pustular vulvovaginitis/balanoposthitis

Introduction and spread of IPV/IBP into a herd usually results from either venereal transmission between infected bulls or cows and susceptible animals, or the use of infected semen in artificial insemination.[16, 126] As IPV has been recorded in virgin heifers,[74] non-venereal mechanisms of transmission must occur. Mechanical transmission of the virus by flies has been suspected.[17]

Virus strains associated with IBR can cause IPV and vice versa,[40, 47] but outbreaks of IBR and IPV/IBP rarely occur concurrently,[47] although one such instance has been reported.[55] Similarly, BHV-1 isolated from cases of meningoencephalomyelitis may produce both IBR and IPV experimentally. However, outbreaks of meningoencephalomyelitis usually occur in the absence of other BHV-1-associated syndromes.[9, 51] These observations need to be re-evaluated in the light of more recent findings which show that there are consistent differences in the genomes of BHV-1 isolates made in different clinical conditions.

Pathogenesis

In IBR the virus multiplies in the upper respiratory tract[72] and may spread throughout the respiratory system.[134] Virus may also be carried from the nasal cavity, via the lachrymal ducts, to the ocular tissues to establish a secondary site of replication. Viraemia is rare, but virus has been recovered from the brain, kidneys, mesenteric lymph nodes and peritoneal fluid. This distribution is ascribed to small numbers of infected monocytes and lymphocytes in the blood which carry virus from the initial foci of infection to other sites, including the placenta.[72, 85] Systemic disease is seldom observed, except in foetuses and neonatal calves.[31]

Experimental infection in calves with BHV-1 resulted in alveolar macrophages being unable to produce chemotactic factors, and these cells also show reduced complement receptor activity and phagocytosis,[28, 69] which may predispose to secondary bacterial infection.

In IPV and IBP viral replication is restricted to the epithelium of the vulva, vagina, penis and prepuce,[38, 110] and viraemia probably does not occur. The virus can easily be isolated from pustules which form approximately 48 hours after infection. The development of latent infections is indicated by the intermittent excretion of virus for periods of up to 578 days.[110]

In cases of meningoencephalomyelitis the virus has been shown to spread directly to the brain from the nasal, tonsillar and pharyngeal regions, probably by way of the maxillary and mandibular branches of the trigeminal nerve.[5]

Following initial infection, BHV-1 usually becomes latent in the neurones of the trigeminal and sacral ganglia in IBR and IPV respectively.[1, 2, 45, 83, 89] Virus persists in the neurones as episomal DNA (i.e. circles of viral DNA in the cell cytoplasm) and, although some transcription to mRNA may occur, there is little or no translation of mRNA into viral proteins.[44] Periodically latent infections recrudesce, involving the virus moving down the sensory nerves and replicating in the epithelium served by the nerves involved. Recrudescence of infection does not necessarily result in recrudescence of the disease, but it may explain the occurrence of outbreaks of IBR in the absence of known sources of infection, and it provides the virus with a mechanism for surviving inter-epidemic periods.

Latent virus can be reactivated by the administration of corticosteroids, and this has been used to demonstrate inapparent infection.[23, 82] Reactivated BHV-1 is most frequently isolated from secretions and tissues of the respiratory tract.[10]

Humoral antibodies against BHV-1, as measured by virus neutralization,[71, 101, 109] have been used as an indicator of the immune status of cattle. However, latency occurs in the presence of strong antibody responses[63] and, consequently, most cattle with humoral antibody are latently infected.[23]

Cell-mediated immune responses play an important role in the defence against the disease. Inactivated virus and viral proteins are weak antigens so far as the stimulation of cell-mediated immune responses are concerned,[100] which may explain why inactivated IBR vaccine is considered to be less effective than live-virus vaccines.[102] The severity of the disease in individual animals is dependent upon the level of local immunity as well as on the non-specific defence mechanisms.[70]

Clinical signs

Infectious bovine rhinotracheitis

The incubation period of IBR varies from one to two days in experimentally induced cases, and from two to 20 days in cattle introduced into feedlots.[54, 64] The course of the disease may be as long as two weeks in uncomplicated cases.[31, 110] Clinical signs are believed to be influenced by the age of the animal, dose of virus, route of infection and concurrent infections with other pathogens.[54]

In epidemics the morbidity rate may be as high as 100 per cent. The case fatality rate is approximately 1 per cent, but on rare occasions may be as high as 7 per cent.[54, 129, 132] Mortality is usually higher in feedlot cattle than in dairy animals, probably because cattle in feedlots are subjected to greater degrees of stress.[98]

The usual signs are pyrexia (as high as 42 °C), tachypnoea, hyperpnoea, reduced appetite, variable cough (which may be sharp and explosive), lachrymation, serous to mucopurulent nasal discharge, halitosis, a drop in milk production in dairy cattle, and weight loss.[31, 54, 55, 130] Less common signs include severe hyperaemia and focal necrosis of the nasal mucosa. As the disease progresses, a diphtheritic pseudomembrane may cover the nasal mucosa, in severe cases the muzzle becomes hyperaemic, and the epithelium becomes necrotic and encrusted by exudate. The underlying tissues are hyperaemic, hence the name 'red nose'.[31, 55] Partial blockage of air passages may result in open-mouthed breathing with protrusion of the tongue.[54] Excessive salivation, which may be due to a reluctance to swallow, and diarrhoea are sometimes observed.[130] Pneumonia is generally not a feature of IBR, so when râles are heard on auscultation, complications or an alternative diagnosis should be considered.[54] Sudden deaths associated with uncomplicated IBR have been recorded.[21]

Conjunctivitis, either uni- or bilateral, associated with profuse lachrymation and photophobia may be seen in cattle with typical IBR, although it may occur in the absence of other signs of BHV-1 infection.[31, 111]

Some authors maintain that BHV-1 does not influence fertility,[4, 87] while others have shown that experimentally-induced IBR can cause failure of conception, early embryonic death and prolonged oestrus cycles.[75, 76] Abortions, usually at between four and seven months of gestation, have been associated with outbreaks of IBR.[116, 128] They may coincide with respiratory signs or may occur up to 100 days later. Abortion is the result of foetal infection and death[31] and may result even when the cows show no obvious signs of respiratory involvement.[54] The foetus is usually autolysed and the placenta often retained.[31] In southern Africa, however, there is no clear proof that BHV-1 has ever been the cause of abortion in cattle.

Although rare, IBR has been recorded in neonates. Calves may be healthy at birth and only develop typical signs when three or four days old,[99, 121] showing fever, anorexia, ptyalism, rhinitis and uni- or bilateral conjunctivitis.[42]

Infectious pustular vulvovaginitis/balanoposthitis

Acute IPV usually develops one to three days after service and is initially characterized by restlessness, frequent micturition and tail swishing.[17] In typical cases the mucosa of the vulva and vagina is oedematous and hyperaemic, and small pustules, 1–2 mm in diameter, are disseminated in the mucosal surface **(Figure 105.1)**. The pustules often coalesce, giving rise to a yellowish-white membrane which is easily detached to leave a raw surface.[31, 66] The lesions usually heal in 10 to 14 days, but in some animals a purulent discharge from the vulva persists for several weeks.

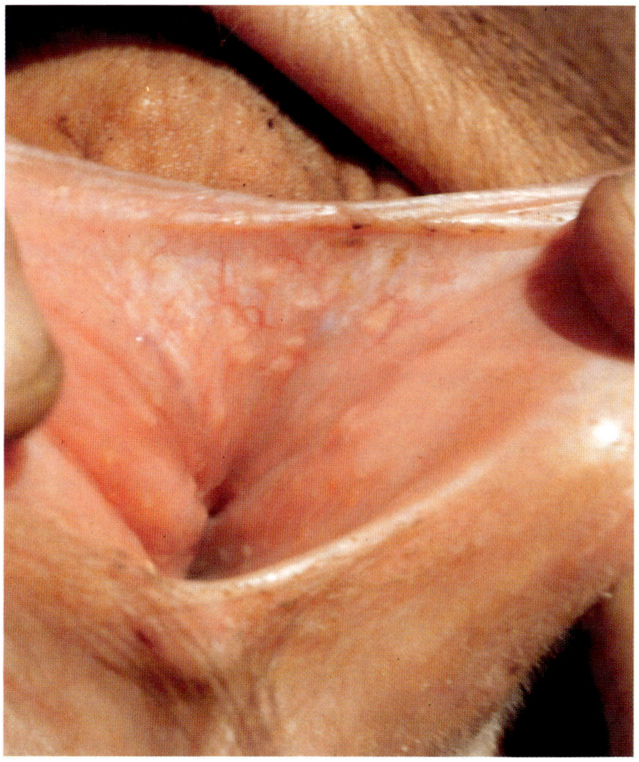

Figure 105.1 Hyperaemia and focally disseminated small pustules in the vaginal mucosa of a cow suffering from infectious pustular vulvovaginitis

Infectious balanoposthitis also develops after an incubation period of one to three days. The presence of disease is rarely obvious externally, although the prepuce may be swollen, and a bloody or mucopurulent discharge may occur. Lesions in most bulls are only obvious after extrusion of the penis. Penoposthitis may be a better description of the condition, as lesions similar to those in the vulva and vagina of cows are usually widespread over the penis and prepuce and not confined to the glans.[17, 46] Secondary infection is usual and scar tissue may form, resulting in adhesions, annular constriction and penile distortions. Some bulls lose their libido or find erection and ejaculation painful. It may take several weeks before regular service is resumed. Mild or subclinical forms of IPV and IBP are common.[31]

There is disagreement as to whether or not infertility occurs after IPV or IBP.[11, 17, 19, 46]

Nervous syndrome

Affected cattle may vary from two weeks[8] to three years[9] in age, and may show slight incoordination progressing to ataxia, depression or excitement, opisthotonus, convulsions and amaurosis. Other signs, including ptyalism, bellowing, aggressive behaviour, tenesmus, aimless wandering, head-pressing, flaccid paralysis, and intense local pruritis, have also occurred.[51] Coma and death usually follow three to four days after the onset of signs. Recovered animals may be blind.[8, 31] Although cases are usually isolated,[8] an outbreak in Australia was recorded where the morbidity rate was 50 per cent and the mortality rate close to 100 per cent.[51]

Digestive tract syndrome

Bovine herpesvirus 1 has been isolated from the faeces of adult cattle with enteritis.[124] In young calves diarrhoea is a feature of systemic BHV-1 infection, which is often fatal.[20] Diarrhoea associated with ulceration of the mucosa of the mouth, oesophagus and forestomach was a prominent sign in an outbreak with high mortality in adult cattle.[95]

Other syndromes

Bovine herpesvirus 1 has been isolated from skin scrapings of the perineum of bulls with chronic perineal dermatitis,[14] from cases of ocular carcinoma (cancer eye),[31] and from cows with mastitis.[33, 35, 94] The virus, probably a recrudescent infection, has also been recovered from vesicular lesions on the udder and teats of a cachectic cow.[37]

Pathology

Infectious bovine rhinotracheitis

Initially, a serous rhinitis with hyperaemia and oedema of the nasal mucosa is present. In severe or complicated cases lesions extend to involve the trachea and sinuses. In these animals, fibrinous to mucopurulent exudates producing a pseudomembrane cover ulcerated areas in the mucosa of the nasal cavity and trachea. Laryngeal oedema and intense tracheal hyperaemia with haemorrhages may progress to a purulent laryngotracheitis.The lower respiratory tract is not usually affected, although in fulminating infections acute necrotizing and obstructive bronchitis, bronchiolitis, pulmonary emphysema and pneumonia may occur.[21] Bacteria, particularly *Pasteurella* spp., *Fusobacterium necrophorum*, and *Mycoplasma* spp., contribute to the severity of lesions.[3, 17, 31, 52, 54, 96]

Since 1980 some outbreaks of IBR in Europe and Australia have produced more severe lesions than those previously recorded. These have included acute necrotizing rhinitis, severe necrotizing laryngotracheitis with extensive pseudomembrane formation, pulmonary oedema, pulmonary thrombosis, severe pneumonia and pulmonary emphysema. Abomasal ulcers and renal infarction were also evident.[3]

Other lesions of IBR may include marked hyperaemia and oedema of the conjunctivae[129] or serous to purulent conjunctivitis with multifocal white plaques 1–2 mm in diameter, consisting of hyperplastic lymphoid aggregates, on the palpebral or bulbar conjunctiva.[52]

Histologically, lesions in the mucosa of the upper respiratory tract range from acute catarrhal changes in uncomplicated cases to severe pseudomembranous and ulcerative lesions as a result of secondary bacterial infection.[31] Acidophilic Cowdry type A intranuclear inclusions may be evident in stratified squamous and pseudostratified columnar epithelial cells of the upper respiratory tract adjacent to necrotic foci, as well as in macrophages and alveolar septal cells in the lungs.[18, 49] Fixation of tissues in Bouin's or Zenker's fluid favours the detection of these inclusions.[18]

Chronic pulmonary changes include purulent bronchitis and bronchiolitis obliterans with epithelialization of the alveolar epithelium.[96]

Necrotic foci associated with intranuclear inclusions may be seen in the adrenal cortices.[75] Trigeminal ganglionitis and encephalitis have also been reported.[83]

Transmission electron microscopic studies have concentrated on aspects of viral morphology.[17, 119, 120, 130] Examination of the tracheal mucosa under the scanning electron microscope reveals extensive loss of cilia, with resulting exposure of microvilli of epithelial cells.[129]

Infectious pustular vulvovaginitis/balanoposthitis

In the acute stage the mucosa of the vulvovagina and penis/prepuce are hyperaemic and petechiae occur in the submucosal lymphoid follicles. The petechiae are later replaced by small, elevated, pock-like lesions which are pale yellow and friable. The epithelium overlying these lesions is desquamated within a few days and adjacent lesions coalesce to produce ulcers.[59] The lesions usually regress in about eight days.[31]

Microscopically, ballooning degeneration and intranuclear inclusions occur in affected epithelium.[80] The outline of hyperplastic lymphoid follicles in the submucosa becomes obscured by the infiltration of numerous lymphocytes and plasma cells.

Artificial insemination with BHV-1-contaminated semen has been associated with IPV, necrotizing endometritis, suppurative salpingitis, and cystic corpora lutea and intranuclear inclusions in the epithelium of the uterus.[60] Similarly, endometritis, oophoritis, cystic and necrotic corpora lutea and follicles have been described in experimental BHV-1 infection.[75]

Aborted foetuses

The foetus is usually autolysed but neither the foetus nor the placenta show characteristic macroscopic changes. Icterus is occasionally observed. Microscopically, necrotic foci and small haemorrhages may occur in the liver, spleen, adrenal cortices, brain, kidneys and lymph nodes. Intranuclear inclusions may be visible in these organs.[31]

Meningoencephalomyelitis syndrome

The lesions are exclusively microscopic. They comprise multifocal non-suppurative leptomeningitis and encephalomyelitis characterized by perivascular oedema and lymphocytic cuffing with areas of necrosis, demyelination and haemorrhage. Intranuclear inclusions may be evident in astrocytes and neurones.[31, 43, 51, 81]

Digestive tract syndrome

In young calves, BHV-1 may cause catarrhal enteritis which is particularly evident over the Peyer's patches. Erosions of the pillars of the rumen, ulceration of the abomasal mucosa and multifocal necrosis of the liver and associated lymph nodes may also occur. Upper respiratory tract lesions, when present, resemble those of IBR.[31] In adult cattle, multifocal necrosis and ulceration in the mouth (dental pad, gums, buccal mucosa, palate and tongue), oesophagus, and forestomachs, accompanied by necrotic lymphadenitis of draining lymph nodes has been described.[98] This condition has been associated with high mortality.[95]

Systemic neonatal syndrome

This syndrome is characterized by the development in most calves of necrotic pharyngitis and laryngitis, multifocal necrotizing bronchiolitis, multiple pin-point necrotic foci in the liver, adrenal cortices, spleen and kidneys, and a non-suppurative meningoencephalomyelitis. Intranuclear inclusions may be found in association with the lesions.[8, 42]

Diagnosis

Infectious bovine rhinotracheitis appears to be overdiagnosed, as there is a tendency to regard most cattle with nasal discharges, polypnoea and fever as suffering from IBR.[54] Care must be taken in the diagnosis of cases of bovine respiratory disease in the field, as several other viruses, *Mycoplasma* spp., chlamydiae and bacteria may be involved **(see Chapter 141: Pneumonic pasteurellosis in cattle)**.

A definitive diagnosis is dependent upon laboratory procedures — demonstration of virus or viral antigens and antibody. Virus can be readily isolated from tissues collected during the acute stage of IBR, maximum viral excretion occurring three to six days after infection, when fever and serous oculonasal discharges are present. In cases of suspected IBR, cotton wool swabs should be used for the collection of serous (rather than mucopurulent) ocular and nasal discharges for virus isolation. Calcium alginate swabs used for bacterial isolation inactivate the virus,[24] so cotton wool swabs should be used when virus recovery is attempted. Vaginal and preputial swabs are the best specimens for virus isolation from cases where genital infection is present.

In aborted foetuses and neonatal calves which have succumbed to systemic infection, blood, liver, spleen, adrenal, kidney, brain and lung tissue are good sources of virus, although it is unlikely that virus will be found in autolysed tissues.[116] Despite being less sensitive and specific than virus isolation, immunofluorescence can be used for the rapid detection of viral antigens.[84]

Great care is essential in the identification of viral isolates, as BHV-1, BHV-2 and BHV-4 have many similarities, and the two latter viruses can also cause IBR/IPV-like lesions in cattle.[66, 108, 120]

Neutralizing antibodies to BHV-1 increase more rapidly and reach higher levels after IBR than they do after genital infection, and so serology may not always reveal cattle that have recovered from IPV or IBP. This underlies the importance of examining animals for lesions and testing bull semen for the presence of viruses, rather than relying solely on serological screening methods.[56] Antibody titre may rise after the recrudescence of latent virus.[43]

Differential diagnosis

Infectious bovine rhinotracheitis may be confused (particularly clinically and pathologically) with diseases that also affect the respiratory system, such as bovine malignant catarrhal fever, and most of the conditions that are part of the bovine respiratory disease complex **(see Chapter 141: Pneumonic pasteurellosis in cattle)**, but especially with pneumonic pasteurellosis. Similarly, IPV/IBP should be distinguished from conditions such as infectious bovine infertility ('epivag'), granular vaginitis and posthitis (hyperplastic submucosal lymphoid follicles of unknown cause), and BHV-4 infection.[119, 120]

Signs and lesions that are sometimes associated with BHV-1 infection (such as necrosis and crusting of the muzzle) may resemble changes which are sometimes seen in necrotic laryngopharyngitis or calf diphtheria caused by *Fusobacterium necrophorum*. The conjunctival form of the disease must be differentiated from other causes of conjunctivitis **(see Chapter 120: *Moraxella* spp. infections)**, and particularly from *Moraxella bovis* infection. The necrotic foci in the liver and other organs of animals suffering from the neonatal systemic infection of the virus are very similar to those seen in salmonellosis and listeriosis, and virus isolation and/or the detection of intranuclear inclusion bodies may be useful in distinguishing BHV-1-induced encephalitis from that associated with bovine malignant catarrhal fever, rabies, heartwater, sporadic bovine encephalomyelitis, listeriosis, thrombotic meningoencephalitis and other non-infectious causes of central nervous system disorders in cattle.[58]

Control

Most control measures are based on the use of BHV-1 vaccines. Vaccines prepared from inactivated virus do not stimulate adequate protection against respiratory tract infection although they are safe.[53, 102, 106] This is because this type of vaccine is unable to induce local immunity, which is important in the defence of the respiratory tract against infection.

Intranasal immunization with attenuated virus stimulates the production of interferon, local antibody and cell-mediated immunity, and provides protection as soon as 72 hours after application.[34, 61, 70, 122] However, the use of attenuated virus vaccines in breeding stock is unsafe, as abortion may occur in pregnant females, and latency of vaccine virus may be induced.

These disadvantages have been overcome by the development of vaccines incorporating temperature-sensitive mutants. The mutant virus is able to replicate in the cooler upper respiratory tract where it is localized, thereby preventing vaccine-induced abortion. Temperature-sensitive mutants can also be differentiated from field viruses.[15]

A general recommendation is that the choice of vaccine should be evaluated in the light of the local situation. In breeding cattle it is advisable to use only vaccines that will not cause latency or abortion.[54] Heifers and cows kept for breeding should be immunized with inactivated vaccine, preferably more than once, before their first conception.[54] However, vaccination of bulls is not recommended where purchasers of either bulls or their semen discriminate against seropositive animals.[104]

Local immunity of the respiratory tract is essential, especially in feedlot cattle, which have the highest prevalence of IBR. Consequently, attenuated virus vaccine is recommended for intranasal application. Cattle should be vaccinated at least 72 hours before admission to a feedlot,[54] using a vaccine containing attenuated virus for use in feedlot cattle which is available in South Africa. Immunization of cattle kept under extensive farming conditions is usually not necessary.

Treatment is supportive and is directed at the prevention of secondary bacterial infections.[54] The use of corticosteroids in the treatment of bronchopneumonia in cattle is contraindicated, as latent infection can be reactivated.[129, 130]

References

1 **ACKERMANN, M., PETERHANS, E. & WYLER, R., 1982.** DNA of bovine herpesvirus type 1 in trigeminal ganglia of latently infected calves. *American Journal of Veterinary Research*, 43, 36–40.

2 **ACKERMANN, M. & WYLER, R., 1984.** The DNA of an IPV strain of bovid herpesvirus 1 in sacral ganglia during latency after intravaginal infection. *Veterinary Microbiology*, 9, 53–63.

3 **ALLAN, E.M., PIRIE, H.M., MSOLLA, P.M., SELMAN, I.E. & WISEMAN, A., 1980.** The pathological features of severe cases of infectious bovine rhinotracheitis. *The Veterinary Record*, 107, 441–445.

4 **ALLAN, P.J., DENNETT, D.P. & JOHNSON, R.H., 1975.** Studies on the effects of infectious bovine rhinotracheitis virus on reproduction in heifers. *Australian Veterinary Journal*, 51, 370–373.

5 **BAGUST, T.J. & CLARK, L., 1972.** Pathogenesis of meningo-encephalitis produced in calves by infectious bovine rhinotracheitis. *Journal of Comparative Pathology*, 82, 375–383.

6 **BARNARD, B.J.H., 1977.** Virus diseases in feedlot cattle in South Africa. *Bulletin de l'Office International des Épizooties*, 88, 153–160.

7 **BARNARD, B.J.H., 1984.** Veterinary Research Institute, Onderstepoort, South Africa. Unpublished data.

8 **BAXTER, G.M., 1984.** Neonatal meningoencephalitis

associated with infectious bovine rhinotracheitis virus. *Bovine Practitioner*, 19, 41–44.

9 **BECK, B.E., 1975.** Infectious bovine rhinotracheitis encephalomyelitis in cattle and its differential diagnosis. *Canadian Veterinary Journal*, 16, 269–271.

10 **BITSCH, V., 1973.** Infectious bovine rhinotracheitis virus infection in bulls, with special reference to preputial infection. *Applied Microbiology*, 26, 337–343.

11 **BOECKX, M., IBRAHIM, M. & BOUTERS, R., 1968.** Die invloed van een acute IPV/IBR infectie op de bevrugtingsresultaten van K.I. stieren. *Vlaams Diergeneeskundige Tijdschrift*, 37, 177–188.

12 **BRAKE, F. & STUDDERT, M.J., 1985.** Molecular epidemiology and pathogenesis of ruminant herpesviruses including bovine and caprine herpesvirus 2 and bovine encephalitis herpesvirus. *Australian Veterinary Journal*, 62, 331–334.

13 **BURROUGHS, A.H., 1967.** Viral respiratory infection in commercial feedlot cattle. *American Journal of Veterinary Research*, 28, 365–371.

14 **BWANGAMOI, O. & KAMINJOLO, J.S., 1971.** Isolation of IBR/IPV virus from the semen and skin lesions of bulls at Kabete, Kenya. *Zentralblatt für Veterinärmedizin*, 18B, 262–269.

15 **CARRELL, J.K., WHITE, R.G. & BECKENHAUER, W.H., 1978.** Evaluation of the safety and efficacy of an intranasal vaccine containing a temperature-sensitive strain of infectious bovine rhinotracheitis virus. *American Journal of Veterinary Research*, 39, 607–610.

16 **CHAPMAN, M.S., LUCAS, M.H., HERBERT, C.N. & GOODEY, R.G., 1979.** Survival of infectious bovine rhinotracheitis virus in stored bovine semen. *Veterinary Science Communications*, 3, 137–139.

17 **COLLINGS, D.F., GIBBS, E.P.J. & STAFFORD, L.D., 1972.** Concurrent respiratory and genital disease associated with infectious bovine rhinotracheitis/infectious pustular vulvovaginitis (IBR/IPV) virus in a dairy herd in the United Kingdom. *The Veterinary Record*, 91, 214–219.

18 **CRANDELL, R.A., CHEATHAM, W.J. & MAURER, F.D., 1959.** Infectious bovine rhinotracheitis — the occurrence of intranuclear inclusion bodies in experimentally infected animals. *American Journal of Veterinary Research*, 20, 505–509.

19 **CRUICKSHANK, J.G. & BERRY, A.M., 1965.** Morphology of infectious bovine rhinotracheitis virus. *Virology*, 25, 481–482.

20 **CURTIS, R.A., VAN DREUMEL, A.A. & DITCHFIELD, J., 1966.** Infectious bovine rhinotracheitis — clinical pathological and virological aspects. *Canadian Veterinary Journal*, 7, 161–168.

21 **CURTIS, R.A., VAN DREUMEL, A.A. & DITCHFIELD, J., 1966.** Infectious bovine rhinotracheitis — sudden death in feedlot cattle. *Canadian Veterinary Journal*, 7, 208–209.

22 **DAUBNEY, R., HUDSON, J.R. & ANDERSON, J., 1938.** Preliminary description of a form of sterility in cattle associated with vaginitis in female stock and with chronic changes in the epididymis and in the testicles of bulls. *East African Agricultural Journal*, 4, 31–34.

23 **DAVIES, D.H. & DUNCAN, J.H., 1974.** The pathogenesis of recurrent infections with infectious bovine rhinotracheitis virus induced in calves by treatment with corticosteroids. *Cornell Veterinarian*, 64, 340–366.

24 **DOHERTY, P.C., SIMMONS, G.C. & PAYNE, E., 1967.** Inactivation of infectious bovine rhinotracheitis virus by calcium alginate wool swabs. *Australian Veterinary Journal*, 43, 257–260.

25 **ENGELS, M., GELDERBLOM, H., DARAI, C. & LUDWIG, H., 1983.** Goat herpes viruses: Biological and physiochemical properties. *Journal of General Virology*, 64, 2237–2247.

26 **ENGELS, M., STECK, F. & WYLER, R., 1981.** Comparison of the genomes of infectious bovine rhinotracheitis and infectious pustular vulvovaginitis virus strains by restriction endonuclease analysis. *Archives of Virology*, 67, 169–174.

27 **ELAZHARY, M. & DERBYSHIRE, J.B., 1979.** Effect of temperature, relative humidity and medium on the aerosol stability of infectious bovine rhinotracheitis. *Canadian Journal of Comparative Medicine*, 43, 158–167.

28 **FORMAN, A.J. & BABIUK, L.A., 1982.** Effect of infectious bovine rhinotracheitis virus infection on bovine alveolar macrophage function. *Infection and Immunity*, 35, 1041–1047.

29 **GEIGER, R., MUNZ, E., HÜBSCHLE, O.J.B. & REIMANN, M., 1992.** Seroepizootiologische Untersuchen über die Verbreitung von Bovinum Herpesvirus Typ 1 und 2 (BHV1, BHV2) in Namibia. *Journal of Veterinary Medicine*. In press.

30 **GIBBS, E.P.J., JOHNSON, R.H. & VOYLE, C.A., 1970.** Differential diagnosis of virus infections of the bovine teat skin by electron microscopy. *Journal of Comparative Pathology*, 80, 455–463.

31 **GIBBS, E.P.J. & RWEYEMANU, M.M., 1977.** Bovine herpesviruses. Part I. Bovine herpesviruses 1. *The Veterinary Bulletin*, 47, 317–343.

32 **GILLESPIE, M.H., McENTEE, K., KENDRICK, J.W. & WAGNER, W.C., 1959.** Comparison of infectious pustular vaginitis virus with infectious bovine rhinotracheitis virus. *Cornell Veterinarian*, 49, 228–297.

33 **GOURLAY, R.N., STOTT, E.J., ESPINASSE, J. & BARLE, C., 1974.** Isolation of *Mycoplasma agalactiae* var. *bovis* and infectious bovine rhinotracheitis virus from an outbreak of mastitis in France. *The Veterinary Record*, 95, 534–535.

34 **GREGERSON, J.P. & WAGNER, K., 1985.** Persistent infection of the genital tract and excretion of the vaccine strain after live virus immunization with bovine herpesvirus 1 (IBR/IPV virus). *Zentralblatt für Veterinärmedizin*, B32, 354–360.

35 **GREIG, A.S. & BANNISTER, G.L., 1965.** Infection of the bovine udder with bovine herpesviruses. *Canadian Journal of Comparative Medicine*, 29, 57–62.

36 **GRIFFIN, T.P., HOWELLS, M.V., CRANDELL, R.A. & MAURER, F.D., 1958.** Stability of the virus of infectious rhinotracheitis. *American Journal of Veterinary Research*, 19, 990–992.

37 **GUY, J.S., POTGIETER, L.N.D., McCRACKEN, M. & MARTIN, W., 1984.** Isolation of bovine herpesvirus-1 from vesicular lesions of the bovine udder. *American Journal of Veterinary Research*, 45, 783–785.

38 **HAIG, D.A., 1957.** Lumpy skin disease. *Bulletin of Epizootic Diseases of Africa*, 9, 421–430.

39 **HEDGER, R.S. & HAMBLIN, C., 1978.** Neutralizing antibodies to bovid herpesvirus 1 (infectious bovine rhinotracheitis/infectious pustular vulvovaginitis) in African wildlife with special reference to the Cape buffalo (*Syncerus caffer*). *Journal of Comparative Pathology*, 88, 211–218.

40 **HELLIG, H., 1965.** Investigation into natural outbreaks of infectious pustular vulvovaginitis in cattle in South Africa. *Journal of the South African Veterinary Medical Association*, 36, 219–226.

41 **HENNING, M.W., 1956.** *Animal Disease in South Africa*. 3rd edn. Pretoria: Central News Agency.

42 **HIGGINS, R.J. & EDWARDS, S., 1986.** Systemic neonatal infectious bovine rhinotracheitis virus infection in suckler calves. *The Veterinary Record*, 119, 177–178.

43 **HILL, B.D., HILL, M.W.M., CHUNG, Y.S. & WHITTLE, R.J., 1984.** Meningoencephalitis in calves due to bovine herpesvirus type 1 infection. *Australian Veterinary Journal*, 61, 242–243.

44 **HILL, T.J., 1985.** Mechanisms of herpes virus latency and reactivation with particular reference to immune response. *In*: PASTORET, P.P., THIRY, E. & SALIKI, J., (eds). *Immunity to Herpesvirus Infection of Domestic Animals*. Luxemburg: Office for Official Publications of the European Communities.

45 **HOMAN, E.J. & EASTERDAY, B.D., 1980.** Isolation of bovine herpesvirus-1 from trigeminal ganglia of clinically normal cattle. *American Journal of Veterinary Research*, 41, 1212–1213.

46 **HUCK, R.A., MILLAR, P.G., EVANS, D.H., STABLES, J.W. & ROSS, A., 1971.** Penoposthitis associated with infectious bovine rhinotracheitis/infectious pustular vulvovaginitis

(IBR/IPV) virus in a stud of bulls. *The Veterinary Record*, 88, 292–297.

47 **HYNE, R.H.J. & JOHNSTON, K.G., 1964.** An outbreak of infectious pustular vulvovaginitis in dairy cattle in New South Wales. *Australian Veterinary Journal*, 40, 385–386.

48 **JASTY, V. & CHANG, P.W., 1972.** Release of infectious bovine rhinotracheitis virus from productively infected bovine kidney cells: An electronmicroscopic study. *Journal of Ultrastructure Research*, 38, 433–443.

49 **JERICHO, K.W.F. & DARCEL, C. LE Q., 1978.** Response of the respiratory tract of calves kept at controlled climatic conditions to bovine herpesvirus-1 in aerosol. *Canadian Journal of Comparative Medicine*, 42, 156–167.

50 **JOHNSON, R.H. & THOMAS, R.G., 1966.** Feline viral rhinotracheitis in Britain. *The Veterinary Record*, 79, 188–190.

51 **JOHNSTON, L.A.Y., SIMMONS, G.C. & McGAVIN, M.D., 1962.** A viral meningoencephalitis of calves. *Australian Veterinary Journal*, 38, 207–215.

52 **JUBB, K.V.F., KENNEDY, P.C. & PALMER, N., 1985.** *Pathology of Domestic Animals*. 3rd edn. New York: Academic Press, Inc.

53 **KAHRS, R.F., 1974.** Rational basis for an immunization program against the common diseases of the bovine respiratory tract. *Canadian Veterinary Journal*, 15, 251–256.

54 **KAHRS, R.F., 1977.** Infectious bovine rhinotracheitis: A review and update. *Journal of the American Veterinary Medical Association*, 171, 1055–1064.

55 **KAHRS, R.F. & SMITH, R.S., 1965.** Infectious bovine rhinotracheitis, infectious pustular vulvovaginitis and abortion in a New York dairy herd. *Journal of the American Veterinary Medical Association*, 146, 217–220.

56 **KAMINJOLO, J.S., NYAGA, P.N., OMUSE, J.K. & MUTIGA, E.R., 1975.** Infectious bovine rhinotracheitis/infectious pustular vulvovaginitis viral isolates from cattle with epididymitis and vaginitis. *American Journal of Veterinary Research*, 36, 123–125.

57 **KARSTAD, L., 1978.** Parasites, wild animals and animal production. *In*: FALLIS, A.M., (ed.). *Parasites, Their World and Ours. Proceedings of the 18th Symposium of the Royal Society of Canada, 1977*. Ottawa: Royal Society of Canada.

58 **KELLERMAN, T.S., COETZER, J.A.W. & NAUDÉ, T.W., 1987.** *Plant Poisonings and Mycotoxicoses of Livestock in Southern Africa*. Cape Town: Oxford University Press Southern Africa.

59 **KENDRICK, J.W., GILLESPIE, J.H. & McENTEE, K., 1958.** Infectious pustular vulvovaginitis of cattle. *Cornell Veterinarian*, 48, 458–495.

60 **KENDRICK, J.W. & McENTEE, K., 1967.** The effects of artificial insemination with semen contaminated with IBR-IPV virus. *Cornell Veterinarian*, 57, 3–11.

61 **KUCERA, C.J., WHITE, R.G. & BECKENHAUER, W.H., 1978.** Evaluation of the safety and efficacy of an intranasal vaccine containing a temperature-sensitive strain of infectious bovine rhinotracheitis virus. *American Journal of Veterinary Research*, 39, 607–610,

62 **LUDWIG, H., 1983.** Bovine herpesviruses. *In*: ROIZMAN, B., (ed.). *The Herpesviruses*. Vol. II. New York, London: Plenum Press.

63 **LUDWIG, H. & GREGERSEN, J.P., 1986.** Infectious bovine rhinotracheitis/infectious pustular vulvovaginitis: HBV-1 infections. *Revue Scientifique et Technique*, 5, 869–878.

64 **LUPTON, H.W. & REED, D.E., 1980.** Clearance and shedding of infectious bovine rhinotracheitis virus from the nasal mucosa of immune and non-immune calves. *American Journal of Veterinary Research*, 41, 117–119.

65 **MADIN, S.H., YORK, C.J. & McKERCHER, D.G., 1956.** Isolation of the infectious bovine rhinotracheitis virus. *Science*, 124, 721–722.

66 **MARÉ, C.J. & VAN RENSBURG, S.J., 1961.** The isolation of viruses associated with infertility in cattle: A preliminary report. *Journal of the South African Veterinary Medical Association*, 32, 201–210.

67 **MARTIN, S.W. & BOHNE, J.C., 1986.** The association between serological titres in infectious bovine rhinotracheitis virus, bovine viral diarrhoea virus, parainfluenza-3 virus, respiratory syncytial virus and treatment for respiratory disease in Ontario feedlot calves. *Canadian Journal of Veterinary Research*, 50, 351–358.

68 **MATHEWS, R.E.F., 1982.** Classification and nomenclature of viruses. *Intervirology*, 17, 28–199.

69 **McGUIRE, R.L. & BABIUK, L.A., 1984.** Evidence for defective neutrophil function in lungs of calves exposed to infectious bovine rhinotracheitis virus. *Veterinary Immunology and Immunopathology*, 5, 259–271.

70 **McKERCHER, D.G. & GRENSHAW, G.L., 1971.** Comparative efficacy of intranasally and parenterally administered infectious rhinotracheitis vaccine. *Journal of the American Veterinary Medical Association*, 159, 1362–1369.

71 **McKERCHER, D.G. & SAITO, J.K., 1965.** The serologic diagnosis of infectious bovine rhinotracheitis. *Proceedings of the US Livestock Sanitary Association*, 68, 518–524.

72 **McKERCHER, D.G. & THEILEN, G.H., 1963.** New manifestations of disease associated with the virus which causes Bläschenausschlag. *Proceedings of the 17th World Veterinary Congress*, Hanover, 1, 625–630.

73 **METZLER, A.E., MATILE, H., GASSMANN, U., ENGELS, M. & WYLER, R., 1985.** European isolates of bovine herpesvirus 1: A comparison of restriction endonuclease sites, polypeptides and reactivity with monoclonal antibodies. *Archives of Virology*, 85, 57–69.

74 **MILLAR, P.G., 1955.** Viral infertility in cattle. *British Veterinary Journal*, 111, 309–315.

75 **MILLER, J.M. & VAN DER MAATEN, M.J., 1987.** Early embryonic death in heifers after inoculation with bovine herpesvirus-1 and reactivation of latent virus in reproductive tissues. *American Journal of Veterinary Research*, 48, 1555–1558.

76 **MISRA, P.K. & MISHRA, A., 1987.** Infectious bovine rhinotracheitis virus infection and infertility in cows, heifers and bulls. *Indian Journal of Animal Sciences*, 57, 267–271.

77 **MISRA, V., BABIUK, L.A. & DARCEL, C. LE Q., 1983.** Analysis of bovine herpes virus-type 1 isolates by restriction endonuclease fingerprinting. *Archives of Virology*, 76, 341–354.

78 **MOHANTY, S.B., 1978.** Bovine respiratory viruses. *Advances in Veterinary Science and Comparative Medicine*, 22, 83–109.

79 **MOHANTY, S.B., LILLI, M.G., CORSELIUS, N.P. & BECK, J.D., 1972.** Natural infection with infectious bovine rhinotracheitis virus in goats. *Journal of the American Veterinary Medical Association*, 160, 879–880.

80 **MOORTHY, A.R.S., 1985.** Outbreak of balanoposthitis in breeding bulls. *The Veterinary Record*, 116, 98.

81 **NARITA, M., INUI, S., NANBA, K. & SHIMIZU, Y., 1976.** Trigeminal ganglionitis and encephalitis in calves intranasally inoculated with infectious bovine rhinotracheitis virus. *Journal of Comparative Pathology*, 86, 93–100.

82 **NARITA, M., INUI, S., NANBA, K. & SHIMIZU, Y., 1981.** Recrudescence of infectious bovine rhinotracheitis virus and associated neural changes in calves treated with dexamethasone. *American Journal of Veterinary Research*, 42, 1192–1197.

83 **NARITA, M., INUI, S., NANBA, K. & SHIMIZU, Y., 1983.** Detection of virus particles in trigeminal ganglion cells in a calf recurrently infected with infectious bovine rhinotracheitis virus. *Japanese Journal of Veterinary Science*, 45, 691–693.

84 **NETTLETON, P.F., 1986.** The diagnosis of bovine rhinotracheitis. *Veterinary Annual*, 26, 90–99.

85 **NYAGA, P.N. & McKERCHER, D.G., 1979.** Pathogenesis of bovine herpesvirus-1 (BHV-1) infections: Interactions of the virus with peripheral bovine blood cellular components. *Comparative Immunology, Microbiology and Infectious Diseases*, 2, 587–602.

86 **PARKER, J.W., 1900.** A bacillus from an infectious vulval disease of cattle. *American Veterinary Review*, *XXIV*, 682.

87 **PARSONSON, I.M. & SNOWDON, W.A., 1975.** The effect of natural and artificial breeding using bulls infected with, or

semen contaminated with, infectious bovine rhinotracheitis virus. *Australian Veterinary Journal*, 51, 365–369.

88 **PASTORET, P.-P., BABIUK, L.A., MISRA, V. & GRIEBEL, P., 1980.** Reactivation of temperature-sensitive and non-temperature-sensitive infectious bovine rhinotracheitis vaccine virus with dexamethasone. *Infection and Immunity*, 29, 483–488.

89 **PASTORET, P.-P., THIRY, E., BROCHIER, B. & DERBOVEN, G., 1982.** Bovid herpesvirus. I. Infection of cattle: Pathogenesis, latency, consequences of latency. *Annales de Recherches Vétérinaires*, 13, 221–235.

90 **PASTORET, P.-P., THIRY, E., BROCHIER, B., SCHWERS, A., THOMAS, I. & DUBUISSON, J., 1988.** Diseases of wild animals transmissible to domestic animals. *Revue Scientifique et Technique*, 7, 705–736.

91 **PLOWRIGHT, W., MACADAM, R.F. & ARMSTRONG, J.A., 1965.** Growth and characterization of the virus of bovine malignant catarrhal fever in East Africa. *Journal of General Microbiology*, 39, 253–266.

92 **POSTE, G., 1972.** Characterization of a new canine herpesvirus. *Archive für die Gesamte Virusforschung*, 36, 147–157.

93 **REISINGER, L. & REIMANN, H., 1928.** Beitrag zur Ätiologie des Bläschenausschlag des Rindes. *Wiener Tierärztliche Monatschrift*, 15, 435.

94 **ROBERTS, A.W., CARTER, G.R. & CARTER, F.A., 1974.** Infectious bovine rhinotracheitis virus recovered from the milk of a cow with mastitis. *Journal of the American Veterinary Medical Association*, 164, 413.

95 **ROGERS, R.J., KNOTT, S.G., EAVES, F.W. & CLAGUE, R.C., 1978.** Bovine herpesvirus 1 — infection of the upper alimentary tract of cattle and its association with a severe mortality. *Australian Veterinary Journal*, 54, 562–565.

96 **ROGERS, R.J., McCUBBIN, I.K., McKENZIE, R.A., CHUNG, Y.S. & ROSENFELD, L.E., 1980.** Severe rhinotracheitis and pneumonia of feedlot cattle due to bovine herpesvirus type 1 infection. *Australian Veterinary Journal*, 56, 147–148.

97 **ROIZMANN, B., CARMICHAEL, L.E., DEINHARDT, F., DE THÉ, G., NAHMIAS, A.J., PLOWRIGHT, W., RAPP, F., SHELDRICK, P., TAKAHASHI, M. & WOLFF, K., 1981.** Herpes viridiae: Definition, provisional nomenclature and taxonomy. *Intervirology*, 16, 201–217.

98 **ROSNER, R.F., 1968.** Infectious bovine rhinotracheitis: Clinical review, immunity and control. *Journal of the American Veterinary Medical Association*, 153, 1631–1638.

99 **ROSS, H.M., HUNTER, A.R., MASSON, A.G. & NETTLETON, P.F., 1983.** Fatal infection of neonatal calves by infectious bovine rhinotracheitis virus. *The Veterinary Record*, 113, 217–218.

100 **ROUSE, B.T., 1984.** Cell-mediated immune mechanisms: *In*: ROUSE, B.T. & LOPEZ, C., (eds). *Immunology of Herpes Simplex Infection*. Boca Raton, Florida: CRC Press.

101 **RÜSCH, P., ENGELS, M., BERCHTOLD, M. & WYLER, R., 1981.** Untersuchungen über den Titerverlaug virusneutralisierender Antikorper nach akuter IBR. *Schweizer Archiv für Tierheilkunde*, 123, 419–427.

102 **SCHIPPER, I.A. & KELLING, C.L., 1975.** Evaluation of inactivated infectious bovine rhinotracheitis vaccines. *Canadian Journal of Comparative Medicine*, 39, 402–405.

103 **SCHROYER, E.L. & EASTERDAY, B.C., 1968.** Studies on the pathogenesis of infectious bovine rhinotracheitis following aerosol exposure. *Cornell Veterinarian*, 58, 442–461.

104 **SCHULTZ, R.D., HALL, C.E., SHEFFY, B.E., KAHRS, R.F. & BEAN, B.H., 1976.** Current status of IBR/IPV infection in bulls. *Proceedings of the 80th Annual Meeting of the United States Health Association*, 80, 159–168.

105 **SEAL, B.S., ST. JEOR, S.C. & TAYLOR, R.E.L., 1985.** Restriction endonuclease analysis of bovine herpesvirus 1 DNA and nucleic acid homology between isolates. *Journal of General Virology*, 66, 2787–2792.

106 **SHEFFY, B.E. & RODNAN, S., 1973.** Activation of local infectious bovine rhinotracheitis infection. *Journal of the American Veterinary Medical Association*, 163, 850–851.

107 **SILVA, R.F., AMBORSKI, R.L., WHITE, M.R. & AMBORSKI, G.F., 1973.** An electronmicroscopic study of single-cycle infection of Madin-Darby bovine kidney cells by infectious bovine rhinotracheitis virus. *Journal of Comparative Pathology*, 83, 167–172.

108 **SMITH, P.C., 1976.** The bovine herpesvirus: An overview. *Proceedings of the 80th Annual Meeting of the United States Animal Health Association*, 80, 149–158.

109 **SNOWDON, W.A., 1964.** Infectious bovine rhinotracheitis and infectious pustular vulvovaginitis in Australian cattle. *Australian Veterinary Journal*, 40, 277–288.

110 **SNOWDON, W.A., 1965.** The IBR/IPV virus: Reaction to infection and intermittent recovery of virus from experimentally infected cattle. *Australian Veterinary Journal*, 41, 135–142.

111 **ST. GEORGE, T.D., 1965.** Keratoconjunctivitis associated with infectious bovine rhinotracheitis infection in Victorian cattle. *Australian Veterinary Journal*, 41, 222–223.

112 **ST. GEORGE, T.D. & PHILPOT, M., 1972.** Isolation of IBR virus from the prepuce of water buffalo bulls in Australia. *Australian Veterinary Journal*, 48, 126.

113 **STRAUB, O.C., 1965.** *In vitro*-untersuchungen über die Wirkung einiger Desinfectionsmittel auf ein zur Herpesgruppe gehorendes virus die IBR-IPV-Virusgruppe. *Tierärtztliche Umschau*, 20, 568–573.

114 **STRAUB, O.C., 1978.** Bovine respiratory viruses. *Advances in Veterinary Science and Comparative Medicine*, 22, 83–109.

115 **STRAUB, O.C., 1978.** The role of viruses as aetiological agents for respiratory disease in cattle. *In*: MARTIN, W.B. (ed.). *Respiratory Diseases in Cattle*. The Hague: Martinus Nijhoff, 241–247.

116 **STUBBINGS, D.P. & CAMERON, I.R.D., 1981.** Bovine abortion associated with infectious bovine rhinotracheitis virus infection. *The Veterinary Record*, 108, 101–102.

117 **SWANEPOEL, R. & CHRISTIE, G.J., 1972.** A survey of infectious bovine rhinotracheitis in Rhodesian cattle. *Rhodesian Veterinary Journal*, 3, 20–25.

118 **TANYI, J., BAJMOCY, E., FAZEKAS, B. & KASZANYITZKY, E.J., 1983.** Mass abortion caused by infectious rhinotracheitis (IBR/IPV) virus in a beef cattle herd. *Acta Veterinaria Hungarica*, 31, 135–143.

119 **THEODORIDIS, A., 1978.** Preliminary characterization of viruses isolated from cases of epididymitis and vaginitis in cattle. *Onderstepoort Journal of Veterinary Research*, 45, 187–195.

120 **THEODORIDIS, A., 1985.** Studies on bovine herpesviruses. Part I. Isolation and characterization of viruses isolated from the genital tract of cattle. *Onderstepoort Journal of Veterinary Research*, 52, 239–254.

121 **THIRY, E., DETILLEUX, P., DE VRIESE, A., PIRAK, M. & PASTORET, P.-P., 1984.** Infectious bovine rhinotracheitis in the neonatal period: A review and a case report. *Annales de Médecine Vétérinaire*, 128, 33–40.

122 **TODD, J.D., 1973.** Immune response to parenteral and intranasal vaccinations. *Journal of the American Veterinary Medical Association*, 163, 807–809.

123 **VAN RENSBURG, S.W.J., 1949.** Contagious epididymitis and vaginitis in cattle. *Farming in South Africa*, 366.

124 **WELLEMANS, G., LEUNEN, J., LOMBA, F. & GOUFFAUX, M., 1974.** Le tropisme digestif du virus IBR. *Annales de Médecine Vétérinaire*, 118, 175–183.

125 **WHETSTONE, C.A., MILLER, J.M., BORTNER, D.M. & VAN DER MAATEN, M.J., 1989.** Changes in the bovine herpesvirus 1 genome during acute infection, after reactivation from latency, and after superinfection in the host animal. *Archives of Virology*, 106, 261–279.

126 **WHITE, M.B. & SNOWDON, W.A., 1973.** The breeding record of cows inseminated with a batch of semen contaminated with infectious bovine rhinotracheitis virus. *Australian Veterinary Journal*, 49, 501–506.

127 **WILDY, P., 1986.** Herpesvirus. *Intervirology*, 25, 117–140.

128 **WILSON, T.E., 1974.** Observations and comments on two outbreaks of abortion associated with IBR virus infection. *Canadian Veterinary Journal*, 15, 227–229.

129 **WISEMAN, A., ALLAN, E.M. & SELMAN, I.E., 1984.** A study of the respiratory diseases of adult cattle in Britain. 4. Infectious bovine rhinotracheitis. *Irish Veterinary Journal*, 38, 145–151.

130 **WISEMAN, A., MSOLLA, P.M., SELMAN, I.E., ALLAN, E.M., CORNWELL, H.J.C., PIRIE, H.M. & IMRAY, W.S., 1978.** An acute severe outbreak of infectious bovine rhinotracheitis: Clinical epidemiological, microbiological and pathological aspects. *The Veterinary Record*, 103, 391–397.

131 **WITTE, J., 1933.** Untersuchungen über den Bläschenausschlag (exanthema pustulosum coitale) des Rindes. *Zeitschrift für Infektionskrankheit Parasitäre Krankheiten und Hygiene der Haustiere*, 44, 163.

132 **YATES, W.D.G., 1982.** A review of infectious bovine rhinotracheitis, shipping fever pneumonia and viral-bacterial synergism in respiratory disease in cattle. *Canadian Journal of Comparative Medicine*, 46, 225–263.

133 **ZWICK, P. & GMINDER, D., 1913.** Untersuchungen über den Bläschenausschlag (Exanthema visiculosum coitale) der Rinder. *Berliner Tierärztliche Wochenschrift*, 29, 637–640.

134 **ZYGRAICH, N., VASOBOINIC, F.E. & HUYGELEN, C., 1974.** Replication of a temperature-sensitive mutant of infectious bovine rhinotracheitis virus in the tissues of inoculated calves. *Zentralblatt für Veterinärmedizin*, 21B, 138–144.

106

Pseudo-lumpy skin disease/ bovine herpes mammillitis

Synonyms: Bovine (bovid) herpesvirus 2 infection, Allerton disease

B.J.H. Barnard

Introduction

Bovine herpesvirus 2 (BHV-2) infection is the cause of at least two well-recognized clinical entities; pseudo-lumpy skin disease (PLSD), a nodular skin disease almost exclusively confined to southern Africa, and bovine herpes mammillitis (BHM), an ulcerative dermatitis of the teats and udders of cows, with a more widespread distribution.

Pseudo-lumpy skin disease was first described in South Africa, where it is a common disease, following the isolation of a herpesvirus from cattle with skin lesions similar to lumpy skin disease (LSD).[1] To distinguish this benign disease from LSD it was initially named Allerton disease, and the virus Allerton virus. Pseudo-lumpy skin disease has also been reported in Kenya[25] and Minnesota, where a generalized infection occurred together with BHM.[47] Bovine herpes mammillitis has been described in the UK,[10, 30, 33] the USA,[47] Australia,[44] Italy[6] and Bulgaria[18] but not in South Africa.

Bovine herpes mammillitis occurs predominantly in dairy cows, but also in heifers about to calve. Outbreaks may reduce the yield of saleable milk as a result of milking difficulties, spoilage of milk or intercurrent mastitis.[18, 22]

Aetiology

Bovine herpesvirus 2 possesses the general characteristics of viruses in the herpes group,[3, 4, 18] and it has been classified as a member of the subfamily Alphaherpesvirinae.[35]

Cross-neutralization, gel-diffusion, ferretin-tagging, and fluorescent antibody techniques demonstrate that all BHV-2 isolates are closely related antigenically.[2, 27, 32, 38, 47]

Primary cell cultures of bovine origin are particularly susceptible to infection and are generally used for virus isolation and propagation.[32, 37] Cytopathic changes caused by BHV-2 are characterized by the formation of large syncytial masses. Isolated foci of infected cells usually enlarge by lateral spread into prominent syncytial bands and may involve almost all of the monolayer before the cell sheet disintegrates.[1, 11, 37] Syncytia may contain up to a thousand nuclei, most of which contain large inclusion bodies which may stain either basophilic or eosinophilic according to their age.

Sheep, goats and pigs, but not humans, are susceptible to experimental infection,[5, 8] as are laboratory animals such as mice,[1, 30, 46, 47] rats and Chinese hamsters[41] as well as rabbits[20] and guinea-pigs.[41]

Bovine herpesvirus 2 is moderately resistant to environmental conditions outside its hosts. After eight days at 37 °C the infectivity titre fell from $10^{8,4}$ to $10^{3,5}$ $TCID_{50}$/ml, and to $10^{2,5}$ $TCID_{50}$/ml when virus was kept at room temperature for 105 days.[32, 37] Freezing and thawing do not significantly lower the titre of the virus.[37] It is inactivated at pH 3,[33, 36] is sensitive to ether and chloroform, and is inactivated by iodophor disinfectants and less effectively by hypochlorite solutions.[28]

Epidemiology

The incidence of PLSD peaks in summer and the disease occurs commonly in moist, low-lying areas.[19, 46] This, and the observation that transmission does not occur after mere contact between diseased and susceptible cattle housed together in insect-proof accommodation, has led to the assumption that arthropods are involved in transmission. The virus was isolated from *Musca confiscata* found on cattle in the acute stage of PLSD, but attempts at experimental transmission with this species were unsuccessful.[46]

Bovine herpes mammillitis, like PLSD, often occurs on farms in sheltered valleys. Two epidemiological patterns exist: in some outbreaks most of the herd is affected, while in others the disease is confined to cows which have just produced their first calves,[40] suggesting that older cows have been immunized by previous infection. Circumstantial evidence from the United Kingdom and Australia also incriminates insects as vectors of BHM,[16, 40, 45] although attempts at transmitting the virus to cattle by using stable flies (*Stomoxys calcitrans*) were unsuccessful.[15, 17]

Antibodies to BHV-2 are common in East African cattle while clinical disease is not, suggesting that BHV-2 infections are usually subclinical.[26, 34]

Pathogenesis

In PLSD a primary focus of infection (such as an insect bite) probably initiates a viraemia followed by the development of multifocal nodular skin lesions. In experimental infections with the Allerton strain, focal lesions developed within three days of inoculation, while secondary lesions became obvious in six to eight days in approximately 50 per cent of animals.[5, 46] Virus can be recovered from skin lesions for up to 10 days from when they first appear and for shorter periods in low concentrations from blood, semen, saliva, faeces, and urine. Pseudo-lumpy skin disease develops in cattle inoculated either intravenously, intradermally or subcutaneously.[46]

In BHM, on the other hand, detectable viraemia does not occur and the virus apparently spreads by local extension.[14, 29, 36] The teats develop raised, focal lesions with or without vesication of the skin, followed by erosions and scab formation. The scabs detach without scar formation. Primiparous cows inoculated into the dermis of the teat soon after calving developed severe lesions at the inoculation sites. These then spread to invade the rest of the skin of the teat and to the skin of the udder and escutcheon.[17]

Local skin temperature appears to play a role in the pathogenesis of BHM.[24] Lesions in skin which has a temperature lower than the rest of the body generally appear sooner after inoculation, are larger and deeper, persist for longer, and contain more infective virus and interferon. This may explain why lesions are usually restricted to the skin of the udder and teats of cows and why outbreaks of the disease occur mostly in the cooler months.

Intramuscular or intradermal inoculation of BHM virus into the neck and flanks of cattle produced localized, necrotic lesions at the site of inoculation.[7, 13, 29, 42] Similarly, inoculation of BHV-2 into the tongue and muzzle produced only localized lesions.[14]

Latency with recrudescence of lesions and the excretion of virus after corticosteroid treatment has been observed several months after the primary lesions had healed.[31, 43]

In natural infection, antibody develops rapidly and persists for more than two years,[16, 36] but does not last as long as this after experimental inoculation.[23, 39] Passive immunity resulting from colostral antibody may last for several months, depending on the level of maternal antibody at the time of calving.[36]

Clinical signs and pathology

Pseudo-lumpy skin disease is characterized by a mild febrile reaction and the sudden appearance of a variable number of skin nodules after an incubation period of between six and eight days.[46] Firm circular nodules, approximately 10 mm in diameter, may develop in the skin over the entire body but are most prevalent on the face, neck, thorax and perineum. In mildly affected animals only a few scattered nodules are seen, but in severe cases several hundred may be present. The nodules have a characteristic flat surface with a slightly depressed centre and some may coalesce to form large irregularly-shaped lesions. After about two weeks the lesions dry up and slough, taking with them the superficial layer of skin, including the hair. Healing, without scar formation and with regrowth of hair, is complete within a few weeks.

Bovine herpes mammillitis is characterized by the sudden appearance of multiple, thickened, raised oedematous plaques 10–20 mm in diameter in the skin of the teats, udder and sometimes the perineum.[10, 13, 30, 33] General signs of illness are usually absent but cattle occasionally develop a fever which coincides with the appearance of the skin lesions. The lesions may merge and involve a large part of the surface of the teat. Vesicle development in the affected skin is rare. Lesions on teats progress rapidly to form clearly delineated erosions covered with dark brown or black scabs made up of tissue debris. On the udder and perineum the lesions tend to be more diffuse and superficial. Mastitis frequently follows BHM, especially if the tips of the teats are involved. Healing of the skin lesions takes place by regrowth of epithelium without scarring. Damage caused by milking slows down the healing process.

Calves suckling affected cows may develop ulcers on the muzzle and in the oral cavity.[13, 14, 21]

Microscopically the lesions of PLSD and BHM are similar,[7, 29, 46] and are characterized by severe intercellular oedema of the germinal cells of the epidermis. Perivascular infiltration with mononuclear cells, including lymphocytes, is prominent in the dermis. Eosinophilic intranuclear inclusion bodies may be present in some epidermal cells.

Diagnosis and differential diagnosis

A tentative diagnosis of PLSD or BHM is based on the presence of characteristic lesions in the skin of the body or udder. However, the differentiation between PLSD and early or mild cases of LSD may be difficult, and laboratory confirmation is essential.[46] The benign nature of PLSD, the generally superficial lesions in the skin and the shorter course of the disease are helpful in differentiating it from LSD **(see Chapter 52: Lumpy skin disease)**.

Bovine herpes mammillitis must be differentiated from pseudocowpox and cowpox, although the latter has not been reported in southern Africa. The fully developed lesions in these infections are often similar. Dual infections with BHV-2 and pseudocowpox virus may occur.

A presumptive diagnosis of BHV-2 infection can be confirmed by virus isolation or demonstration of the virus by electron microscopy in skin biopsies collected during the peak of the infection,[9] as well as from scab material.[12]

Control

Inactivated vaccines are insufficiently immunogenic to be protective.[39] Conversely, unattenuated live virus administered intramuscularly provides an immunity that persists for at least eight months.[13] However, no commercial vaccine is available for the protection of cattle against BHM or PLSD.

References

1 **ALEXANDER, R.A., PLOWRIGHT, W. & HAIG, D.A., 1957.** Cytopathogenic agents associated with lumpy skin disease of cattle. *Bulletin of Epizootic Diseases of Africa*, 5, 489–492.

2 **BREEZE, S.S. & DARDIRI, A.H., 1972.** Electron microscopic characterization of a bovine herpesvirus from Minnesota. *Journal of General Virology*, 15, 69–72.

3 **BUCHMAN, T.G. & ROIZMAN, B., 1978.** Anatomy of bovine herpes mammillitis DNA. II. Size and arrangements of the deoxynucleotide sequences. *Journal of Virology*, 27, 239–254.

4 **BUCHMAN, T.G. & ROIZMAN, B., 1978.** Anatomy of bovine mammillitis virus DNA. Restriction endonuclease map of four populations of molecules that differ in the relative orientation of their long and short components. *Journal of Virology*, 25, 395–407.

5 **CAPSTICK, P.B., 1959.** Lumpy skin disease — experimental infection. *Bulletin of Epizootic Diseases of Africa*, 7, 51–62.

6 **CASTRUCCI, G., 1975.** Bovid herpesvirus 2 infection of cattle in Italy. *Proceedings of the 20th World Veterinary Congress*, Thessaloniki, 2, 1303–1308.

7 **CASTRUCCI, G., DI ANTONIO, E., RAMPICHINI, L., SEVERINI, M., PEDINI, B. & VALENTE, C. 1972.** Study of the pathogenesis of skin lesions produced in calf by intradermal inoculation with 69/1 LD strain of bovine herpes mammillitis virus. *Archivio Veterinario Italiano*, 23, 83–92.

8 **DARDIRI, A.H., 1975.** Similarities of bovine dermopathic herpesviruses from Africa, Europe and USA. *Proceedings of the 20th World Veterinary Congress*, Thessaloniki, 2, 1312–1315.

9 **DAVIES, F.G., KRAUSS, H., LUND, L.J. & TAYLOR, M., 1971.** The laboratory diagnosis of lumpy skin disease. *Research in Veterinary Science*, 12, 123–127.

10 **DEAS, D.W. & JOHNSTON, W.S., 1966.** An outbreak of an ulcerative skin condition of the udder and teats of dairy cattle in the East of Scotland. *The Veterinary Record*, 78, 828–829.

11 **DILOVSKI, M., 1974.** Plaque characteristics of bovine herpes mammillitis virus. *Veterinärnomeditsiuski Medicine*, Nauki, Sofia, 12, 44–50.

12 **GERDES, T.G., 1986.** Veterinary Research Institute, Onderstepoort, South Africa. Unpublished data.

13 **GIBBS, E.P.J., 1970.** A study on virus infections of the skin of the bovine teat. Ph.D. Thesis, University of Bristol.

14 **GIBBS, E.P.J. & COLLINGS, D.F., 1972.** Observations on bovine herpes mammillitis (BHM) virus infections of heavily pregnant heifers and young calves. *The Veterinary Record*, 90, 66–68.

15 **GIBBS, E.P.J., JOHNSON, R.H. & OSBORNE, A.D., 1970.** The differential diagnosis of viral skin infections of the bovine teat. *The Veterinary Record*, 87, 602–609.

16 **GIBBS, E.P.J., JOHNSON, R.H. & OSBORNE, A.D., 1972.** Field observations on the epidemiology of bovine herpes mammillitis. *The Veterinary Record*, 91, 395–401.

17 **GIBBS, E.P.J., JOHNSON, R.H. & OSBORNE, A.D., 1973.** Experimental studies of the epidemiology of bovine herpes mammillitis. *Research in Veterinary Science*, 14, 139–144.

18 **GIBBS, E.P.J. & RWEYEMAMU, M.M., 1977.** Bovine herpesviruses. II. Bovine herpesvirus 2 and 3. *The Veterinary Bulletin*, 6, 411–425.

19 **HAIG, D.A., 1957.** Lumpy skin disease. *Bulletin of Epizootic Diseases of Africa*, 5, 421–430.

20 **HUYGELEN, C., THIENPONT, D., DEKEYSER, P.J. & VANDERVELDEN, M., 1960.** Allerton virus, a cytopathogenic agent associated with lumpy skin disease. II. Inoculation of animals with tissue culture passaged virus. *Zentralblatt für Veterinärmedizin*, 7, 754–760.

21 **HUYGELEN, C., THIENPONT, D. & VANDERVELDEN, M., 1960.** Isolation of a cytopathogenic agent from skin lesions of cattle. *Nature*, 186, 979–980.

22 **JOHNSTON, W.S., WRAY, C. & SCOTT, J.A., 1971.** An outbreak of bovine herpes mammillitis in a suckler herd. *The Veterinary Record*, 88, 372.

23 **KALUNDA, M. & PLOWRIGHT, W., 1972.** Pathogenicity for cattle of Allerton-type herpesvirus isolated from a Tanzanian buffalo (*Syncerus caffer*). *Journal of Comparative Pathology*, 82, 65–72.

24 **LETCHWORTH, G.J. & CARMICHAEL, L.E., 1984.** Local tissue temperature: A critical factor in the pathogenesis of bovid herpesvirus 2. *Infection and Immunity*, 43, 1072–1079.

25 **MACCOWAN, K.D.S., 1961.** *Annals of the Republic of Kenya Veterinary Department*, 45.

26 **MARTIN, W.B. & GWYNNE, M., 1968.** Antibodies to the group II lumpy skin disease viruses in the sera of cattle in Kenya. *Bulletin of Epizootic Diseases of Africa*, 16, 217–222.

27 **MARTIN, W.B., HAY, D., CRAWFORD, L.V., LE BOUVIER, G.L. & CRAWFORD, E.M., 1966.** Characteristics of bovine mammillitis virus. *Journal of General Microbiology*, 45, 325–332.

28 **MARTIN, W.B. & JAMES, Z.H., 1969.** Inactivation of the bovine mammillitis herpesvirus by disinfectants. *The Veterinary Record*, 85, 100.

29 **MARTIN, W.B., JAMES, Z.H., LAUDER, I.M., MURRAY, M. & PIRIE, H.M., 1969.** Pathogenesis of bovine mammillitis virus infection in cattle. *American Journal of Veterinary Research*, 30, 2151–2166.

30 **MARTIN, W.B., MARTIN, B., HAY, D. & LAUDER, I.M., 1966.** Bovine ulcerative mammillitis caused by a herpesvirus. *The Veterinary Record*, 78, 494–497.

31 **MARTIN, W.B., WELLS, P.W., LAUDER, I.M. & MARTIN, B., 1975.** Features of the epidemiology of bovine mammillitis in Britain. *Proceedings of the 20th World Veterinary Congress*, Thessaloniki, 2, 1307–1311.

32 **MUSHI, E.Z. & RWEYEMAMU, M.M., 1975.** A comparison of some *in vitro* properties of Allerton-type (herpesvirus bovis 2) virus isolates. *Bulletin of Animal Health and Production of Africa*, 23, 235–248.

33 **PEPPER, T.A., STAFFORD, L.P., JOHNSON, R.H. & OSBORNE, A.D., 1966.** Bovine ulcerative mammillitis caused by a herpesvirus. *The Veterinary Record*, 78, 569–570.

34 **PLOWRIGHT, W. & JESSETT, D.M., 1971.** Investigations of Allerton-type herpesvirus infection in East African game animals and cattle. *Journal of Hygiene*, 69, 209–222.

35 **ROIZMAN, B., CARMICHAEL, L.E., DEINHARDT, F., DE THÉ, G., NAHMIAS, A.J., PLOWRIGHT, W., RAPP, F., SHELDRICK, P., TAKAHASHI, M. & WOLF, K., 1981.** Herpesviridae. Definition, provisional nomenclature, and taxonomy. *Intervirology*, 16, 201–217.

36 **RWEYEMAMU, M.M., 1968.** Studies on bovine herpes mammillitis. Ph.D. Thesis, University of Bristol.

37 **RWEYEMAMU, M.M. & JOHNSON, R.H., 1967.** Bovine

herpes mammillitis virus. I. *In vitro* behaviour of the virus. *British Veterinary Journal*, 123, 482–491.

38 **RWEYEMAMU, M.M. & JOHNSON, R.H., 1968.** Bovine herpes mammillitis virus. II. Standardization of an *in vitro* serum-neutralization test. *British Veterinary Journal*, 124, 9–15.

39 **RWEYEMAMU, M.M. & JOHNSON, R.H., 1969.** A serological comparison of seven strains of bovine herpes mammillitis virus. *Research in Veterinary Science*, 10, 102–104.

40 **RWEYEMAMU, M.M., JOHNSON, R.H. & LAURILLARD, R.E., 1969.** Serological findings in bovine herpes mammillitis. *British Veterinary Journal*, 125, 317–325.

41 **RWEYEMAMU, M.M., JOHNSON, R.H. & McCREA, M.R., 1968.** Bovine herpes mammillitis virus: Observations on experimental infection. *British Veterinary Journal*, 124, 317–324.

42 **RWEYEMAMU, M.M., OSBORNE, A.D. & JOHNSON, R.H., 1969.** Observations on the histopathology of bovine herpes mammillitis. *Research in Veterinary Science*, 10, 203–207.

43 **SCOTT, F.M.M., GILMORE, J.S. & MARTIN, W.B., 1984.** Recovery of BHV2 from the nervous system of experimentally infected calves. *In*: WITTMANN, G., GASKELL, R. & RZIHA, H.G., (eds). *Latent Herpesvirus Infections in Veterinary Medicine*. The Hague: Martinus Nijhoff Publishers.

44 **TURNER, A.J., KOVESDY, L., CIANTER, M.S., NICHOLLS, W.A. & CHATHAM, R.O., 1974.** Isolation of bovine herpes mammillitis virus from dairy cattle in Victoria. *Australian Veterinary Journal*, 50, 578–579.

45 **TURNER, A.J., MORGAN, I.R., SYKES, W.E. & NICHOLLS, W.A., 1976.** Bovine herpes mammillitis of dairy cattle in Victoria. *Australian Veterinary Journal*, 52, 170–173.

46 **WEISS, K.E., 1963.** Lumpy skin disease. *FAO Handbook: Emerging Diseases of Animals.* FAO Agricultural Studies, No. 61, 177–201.

47 **YEDLOUTSCHNIG, R.J., BREEZE, S.S. Jr., HESS, W.R., DARDIRI, A.H., TAYLOR, W.D., BARNES, D.M., PAGE, R.W. & RUEBKE, H.J., 1970.** Bovine herpes mammillitis-like disease diagnosed in the USA. *Proceedings of the USA Animal Health Association*, 74, 208–212.

107

Malignant catarrhal fever

Synonym: Snotsiekte (Afrik.)

B.J.H. Barnard, J.J. van der Lugt and E.Z. Mushi

Introduction

Malignant catarrhal fever (MCF) is a sporadic but almost invariably fatal viral disease of cattle and deer characterized in cattle by profuse mucopurulent nasal and ocular discharges, keratoconjunctivitis with corneal opacity, and enlargement of peripheral lymph nodes.

The disease has a worldwide distribution. Outside Africa it is usually associated with contact between sheep and susceptible species (principally cattle),[61] although in New Zealand MCF commonly occurs in farmed deer where no sheep are present on the property.[57] Sheep-associated malignant catarrhal fever (SA MCF) is also encountered in southern Africa,[21] but is less common than the wildebeest-derived (WD) form which is predominantly associated with blue wildebeest (*Connochaetes taurinus*) but also occasionally with black wildebeest (*C. gnou*). Wildebeest-derived malignant catarrhal fever is caused by a herpesvirus and, although serological evidence suggests that sheep harbour a virus antigenically related to the herpesvirus of wildebeest, the aetiological agent of SA MCF has not yet been isolated.

Sheep-associated malignant catarrhal fever was first recognized in Europe more than a century ago,[18] while WD MCF was occasionally encountered by hunters and Voortrekkers who penetrated the interior of southern Africa during the 18th century.[19] They referred colloquially to the disease as 'snotsiekte', which means snotting sickness. The first investigation into the disease in South Africa was conducted by Mettam in 1920.[49] In 1904 a farmer attempted to raise black wildebeest calves using Friesian cows as foster-dams, but some of the cows contracted snotsiekte. The owner, realizing the danger of keeping cattle and wildebeest together, then separated the two species. Another outbreak on this farm occurred in 1920, when the owner allowed cattle into the camp containing the wildebeest. Further early outbreaks of the disease in South Africa were recorded in 1938[23] and 1950.[21]

In 1906 a disease with clinical signs recognizable as MCF was described in Kenya,[1] although WD MCF had historically occurred annually (and still occurs) in the Maasai Reserve of Kenya and Tanzania[20] where the Maasai tribesmen, realizing the connection between wildebeest and MCF, used the same word for wildebeest and the disease in cattle. In Zimbabwe several outbreaks were recorded between 1932 and 1936,[3] while in Zambia MCF was first reported in 1932.[2]

With the decline in the number of game animals, including wildebeest, in the farming areas of South Africa during the first half of this century, the disease was less frequently diagnosed. Consequently little attention was paid to MCF until game farming became an economic proposition in the 1970s. The increase in game farming, together with the greater awareness of the need to conserve wildlife which has arisen over the past two decades, has resulted in an increase in the prevalence of WD MCF. Recently losses due to the disease reached alarming proportions in some localities, such as the north-western Transvaal, causing the death of up to 34 per cent of animals in individual herds adjacent to game farms.[9] In Tanzania WD MCF annually causes the death of 3 to 12 per cent of cattle in Maasailand.[44]

The disease has also increased in importance in zoological gardens where increasing numbers of susceptible species are kept, as well as on farms adjoining zoological collections.[38] To prevent losses among exotic animals, wildebeest are no longer exhibited in the National Zoological Garden in Pretoria.[24]

Malignant catarrhal fever is a major disease of farmed deer in New Zealand and was the cause of 43 per cent of the deaths of these animals in 1980.[10]

Aetiology

Wildebeest-derived malignant catarrhal fever virus has been classified as Alcelaphine (Alcelaphid) herpesvirus 1 (AHV-1).[81] The virions are approximately 109–220 nm in diameter, depending on the number of envelopes present. Like other herpesviruses, they have icosahedral symmetry and comprise a DNA core enclosed in a capsid approximately 100 nm in diameter. The nucleocapsid matures in the nucleus of infected cells, and envelopment occurs at the nuclear and cytoplasmic membranes. Virions egress from cells by budding from the plasmalemma, or through channels of either the Golgi apparatus or the endoplasmic reticulum.[15, 16]

The genome of 155–165 kilo base pairs (kbp) has a G+C content of 50 per cent and comprises a region of unique DNA of approximately 130 kbp and approximately 30 kbp of additional tandem direct repeat sequences with a G+C content of 72 per cent.[12] Based on similarities between the genomic organization of AHV-1 and T-lymphotropic viruses as well as similarities between WD MCF infection and those produced by members of the Gammaherpesvirinae, it has been suggested that AHV-1 is a member of the latter virus subfamily.[12]

Closely related herpesviruses have also been isolated from free-living Jimela topi (*Damaliscus lunatus jimela*)[53] and red hartebeest (*Alcelaphus buselaphus*)[53] in East Africa, the latter provisionally classified as AHV-2, and also from captive red hartebeest and Jimela topi in the USA.[36] Although AHV-2 recovered from a hartebeest was able to produce atypical MCF in cattle after experimental infection, natural transmission could not be established.[80]

In vitro multiplication of AHV-1 was obtained and the cytopathology studied in primary and secondary cell cultures prepared from bovine thyroid tissue.[70] However, difficulty in producing adequate quantities of these cells led to the use of serially passaged foetal calf kidney cells, of which only some lines sustained optimal viral multiplication,[65] but cytopathic foci in these cells are inclined to regress or even disappear. Calf testis cells[59, 60] were later shown to be sensitive for the detection and assay of infectivity in animal tissue. Cytopathic effects in calf testis cells are more easily detected than in foetal calf kidney cells, as syncytia exhibit long refractile processes and generalization occurs more readily.

A variety of other culture systems have been adapted to the growth of AHV-1. These range from cell types such as foetal lamb kidney[7] and Vero cells[86] to cultivation at reduced temperature (32–34 °C),[31] and fusion of infected leukocytes with culture cells using polyethylene glycol.[16, 17] Even the use of specific breeds of sheep as a source of foetal lamb kidney cells has been advocated.[34, 35]

In bovine tissues at least, AHV-1 is highly cell-associated and can be recovered only from living cells. Initial virus isolation therefore requires the co-cultivation of dispersed tissues from infected cattle and susceptible cells.

Although the virus of SA MCF has not yet been isolated, it is well known that mixing sheep with cattle may result in MCF.[21, 27, 96] Some attempts at transmitting MCF of sheep origin between cattle by the subinoculation of blood have been successful.[64] In general, however, the success rate has been far lower than that experienced with WD MCF. There is increasing evidence that SA MCF is caused by a herpesvirus related to AHV-1; indirect immunofluorescent antibody titres against AHV-1 in sheep and in wildebeest are comparable,[82] and rising antibody titres to AHV-1 have been detected in cattle suffering from SA MCF.[30] Similar results were obtained with western blotting, where it was shown that sheep antisera reacted with the same viral proteins as wildebeest antisera.[73] Furthermore, low titre, virus neutralizing antibodies to AHV-1 are frequently found in species of the subfamily Caprinae, which includes domestic sheep and goats.[73]

Epidemiology

The involvement of wildebeest in the epidemiology of MCF was demonstrated when blood from black[49] and blue wildebeest[20] **(Figure 107.1)** was inoculated into cattle, leading to the subsequent development of signs typical of MCF, as well as by the recovery of AHV-1 from five of 35 wildebeest in Kenya in 1959.[70] There is also evidence of infection with a related virus or viruses in several other African wildlife species, especially those of the subfamilies Alcelaphinae and Hippotraginae **(Table 107.1)**.

Neutralizing antibodies against AHV-1 have been demonstrated in a number of species of wildlife in South Africa **(Table 107.2)**, but there is no indication that species other than wildebeest are able to transmit the disease in natural circumstances.

Most free-living adult wildebeest are persistently infected with AHV-1 **(Table 107.2)**,[5, 66] but adult wildebeest probably only excrete virus under conditions

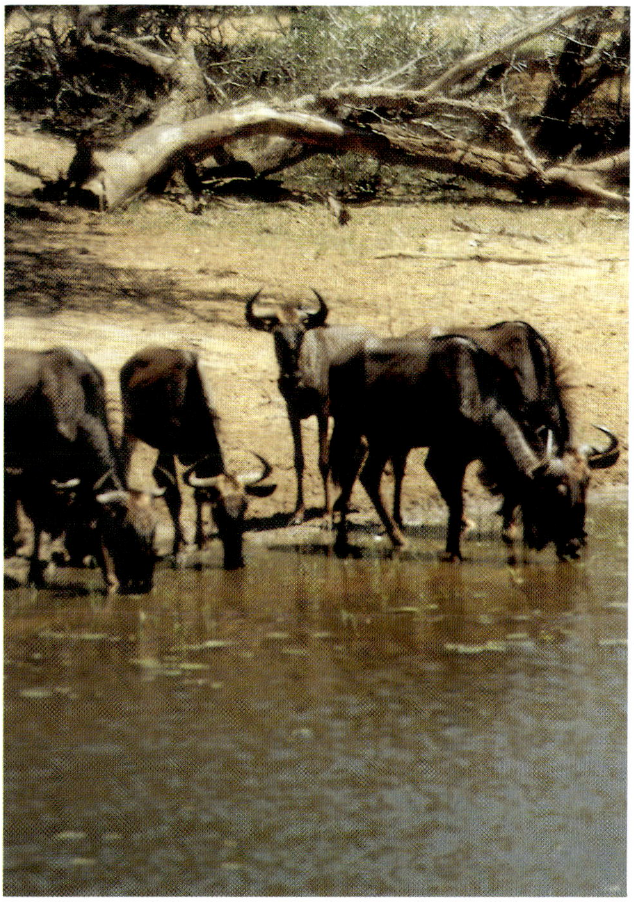

Figure 107.1 Blue wildebeest *(Connochaetes taurinus)*

Table 107.1 Reservoirs and potential reservoirs of Alcelaphine herpesvirus 1

WILDLIFE SPECIES			REFERENCES			
SUBFAMILY	GENUS	COMMON NAME	SEROLOGY		VIRUS ISOLATION	
			FIELD	ZOO	FIELD	ZOO
Alcelaphinae	*Connochaetes taurinus*	Blue wildebeest	5, 66, 79, 80, 88	29, 36, 73	5, 7, 66	36
	Connochaetes gnou	Black wildebeest	5	7, 36	7	36
	Alcelaphus buselaphus	Red hartebeest	5, 7, 79, 80	36, 66	80	36
	Damaliscus korrigum	Topi	66	29, 36	53	
	Damaliscus lunatus	Tsessebe	7	29, 36		
	Damaliscus lunatus jimela	Jimela topi		36		36
	Damaliscus dorcas	Blesbok		36		
Hippotraginae	*Oryx gazella beisa*	Fringe-eared or Beisa oryx	51, 79	7, 36		
	Oryx gazella gazella	Scimitar-horned oryx		7, 36		
	Oryx lenconyx	Arabian oryx		36		
	Oryx gazella	Gemsbok	5	7, 36		
	Hippotragus equinus	Roan antelope	7	7, 36		
	Hippotragus niger	Sable antelope	5	7, 36		
	Adenota kob	Uganda kob		36		
	Addax nasomaculatus	Defassa waterbuck		7, 36		
Reduncinae	*Redunca arundinum*	Reedbuck		29		
	Kobus defasa	Waterbuck		29, 36		
	Kobus ellipsiprymnus	Waterbuck		29		
Atelopinae	Various species			36		
Other				36		

of severe stress such as during captivity and exposure to high environmental temperatures.[69, 93] There is no convincing evidence that wildebeest ever manifest signs of clinical disease, although it has been suggested that the vasculitis observed histologically in tissues of yearling or adult wildebeest is similar to that of MCF.[17] No wildebeest populations have been conclusively shown to be free of AHV-1 infection, despite rumours to the contrary.

Viraemia has been demonstrated in pregnant blue wildebeest cows that were near full-term.[65, 72] Blue wildebeest calves may become infected *in utero* or they may contract the infection shortly after birth by horizontal spread from other calves despite the presence of maternally-derived antibody.[16, 70] AHV-1 may thus persist in small groups of wildebeest kept in isolation.

Blue wildebeest calves up to four months of age are important in the transmission of MCF as they excrete non-cell-associated virus in their nasal and ocular secretions.[37, 54] In calves aged between six and eight weeks the level of virus in these secretions may reach $10^{3,2}$ $TCID_{50}$/ml.[55] The excreted virus is probably derived from sites of replication in the cornea and turbinate mucosa.[55] After three months of age, shedding of virus declines, coinciding with the appearance of specific antibody, predominantly IgA, in the nasal cavity.[50, 91] Approximately 40 per cent of calves may be viraemic.[65]

Maasai herdsmen apparently believe that cattle contract MCF when they come into contact with wildebeest placentas or with the hair of juvenile wildebeest shed when the calves are three to four months of age.[20] Recent studies have, however, failed to demonstrate infective AHV-1 in placentas.[84]

In Kenya MCF usually occurs between April and July, following the wildebeest calving season in February to April.[65] In South Africa two peaks in the incidence of MCF are encountered; one in January to May, following the wildebeest calving season in December to February, and a second, where the incidence is higher, from September to November. At the latter time wildebeest calves are nine to 11 months old.[5, 8, 9]

Although close contact is generally regarded as necessary for the transmission of WD MCF to cattle, there are several accounts in South Africa of transmission across fences, even at distances of up to several hundred metres.[5, 8, 9] Wildebeest-derived MCF usually occurs sporadically, despite the fact that cattle at risk are sometimes exposed for prolonged periods of time. There are, however, instances of a number of deaths due to MCF being observed within a short period on farms in South Africa.

In South Africa, cases encountered between January and May are usually amongst cattle that share grazing and watering places with wildebeest, whereas most cases occurring during September to November are in cattle which are not in direct contact with wildebeest.[9]

The route of natural infection for cattle is unknown. However, it has been shown that intranasal instillation of cell-free viral suspensions can produce infection in both cattle and rabbits.[56] Hence, transfer by virus-containing aerosols from young wildebeest to cattle may be possible, but it is unlikely that aerosol infection can occur over distances as great as several hundred metres, since nasal

Table 107.2 Virus neutralizing antibody titres to AHV-1 in some species of wildlife in South Africa

WILDLIFE SPECIES		NUMBER OF ANIMALS WITH OR WITHOUT NEUTRALIZING ANTIBODY TITRE							
GENUS	COMMON NAME	NEGATIVE	8	16	32	64	128	256	PERCENTAGE WITH TITRES
Aepyceros melampus	Impala	37							0
Diceros bicornis	Black rhinoceros	14							0
Ceratotherium simum	White rhinoceros	9							0
Equus spp.	Zebra	17							0
Giraffa camelopardalis	Giraffe	6							0
Sylvicapra grimmia	Duiker	2							0
Oreotragus oreotragus	Klipspringer	3							0
Phacochoerus aethiopicus	Warthog	23							0
Syncerus caffer	African buffalo	4							0
Antidorcas marsupialis	Springbok	15							0
Taurotragus oryx	Eland	3							0
Tragelaphus strepsiceros	Kudu	24							0
Tragelaphus angasi	Nyala	8	2						25
Redunca fulvorufula	Mountain reedbuck	16	1		1				13
Hippotragus equinus	Roan antelope	3	1		1				40
Hippotragus niger	Sable antelope	2	1	1	1	1			66
Damaliscus lunatus	Tsessebe	5	2	0	2	1			50
Kobus ellipsiprymnus	Waterbuck	2	1	1			1		60
Oryx gazella	Gemsbok	7	3	5	4	1	1		66
Alcelaphus buselaphus	Red hartebeest	1		1	3	1	2	1	88
Connochaetes gnou	Black wildebeest	5	1	10	8	2	2	2	83
Connochaetes taurinus	Blue wildebeest	7	2	8	16	22	28	17	93

secretions contain at most only $10^{3.2}$ $TCID_{50}$/ml of virus.[54] In cases where transmission occurs over several hundred metres a vector may be involved.[9]

The epidemiology of SA MCF is essentially the same as that of WD MCF. As with wildebeest, sheep do not show any clinico-pathological evidence of infection, although suspected MCF in sheep has been reported.[94] In South Africa the incidence of SA MCF is low and is not seasonal,[5] whereas in countries outside Africa a seasonal incidence has been reported;[32, 75] cattle being most likely to develop the disease during the lambing season.[39] In an outbreak in the north-western Cape Province where only karakul sheep could have been the source of infection, a farmer lost 75 cattle over a period of three years as a result of MCF. The mortalities stopped when the sheep, which had been housed overnight in the same building as the cattle, were removed to other stabling facilities.[7]

Cattle of all breeds and ages and domestic buffaloes (*Bubalus bubalus*) are susceptible to both WD and SA MCF, although yearling beef cattle in New Zealand appear to suffer a higher incidence of SA MCF than do cattle of other ages.[32] In South Africa the incidence of WD MCF in cows just before and after calving is significantly higher than in other groups.[9]

Transmission of AHV-1 between cattle either does not occur or is very rare.[20, 21, 67] A probable explanation for this is that although ocular and nasal secretions of infected cattle do contain AHV-1, the virus levels are low as well as being cell-associated.[42, 54, 55]

The number of species known to be potentially susceptible to MCF is increasing continuously. Cases encountered in zoological collections indicate that the species most susceptible to AHV-1 are probably Asiatic cattle,[33] including banteng (*Bos javanicus*), Indian gaur (*Bos gaurus*), as well as bison species (*Bison bison* and *B. bonasus*) and the Asian nilgai (*Boselaphus tragocamelus*). Confirmed cases in African game species have been restricted to kudu (*Tragelaphus strepsiceros*), sitatunga (*Tragelaphus spekei*), eland (*Taurotragus oryx*)[65] and roan antelope (*Hippotragus equinus*).[28] It must be stressed, however, that MCF has never been reported in free-living animals although herds of wildebeest and other species are sometimes closely associated in game reserves and on game farms.

Experimental inoculation of AHV-1 resulted in MCF-like clinical signs in five of 19 sheep.[42] An MCF-like condition was also produced in sheep foetuses by the inoculation of material derived from deer with MCF.[14]

Members of the Cervidae — red deer (*Cervus elaphus*), axis deer (*C. axis*), Siku deer (*C. nippon*), Rusa deer (*C. timorensis*), Roe deer (*Capreolus capreolus*), Pere David deer (*Elaphus davidianus*), white-tailed deer (*Odocoileus virginianus*) and black-tailed deer (*O. hemionus columbianus*) — appear to be more susceptible than cattle to both WD and SA MCF.[10, 33, 39, 41, 74] African buffalo (*Syncerus caffer*) are probably susceptible to SA MCF, as two young animals died of MCF at the Veterinary Research Institute, Onderstepoort after having been in contact with sheep.[97]

Rabbits can be easily infected with AHV-1 by intraperitoneal or intravenous inoculation of cells derived from lymphoid tissues or leukocytes of infected cattle.[62, 67] In contrast, transmission of SA MCF to rabbits has only been successful on a few occasions.[13, 21, 58, 99] However, once established in rabbits, even the SA MCF agent can readily be transferred between rabbits by the inoculation of blood or lymph node suspensions containing at least 10 viable cells.[78] The incubation period ranges from 12 days to several weeks. The clinical signs, pathology, and probably the pathogenesis of the infection in rabbits are similar to WD and SA MCF in cattle.[78] Syrian hamsters[78] and guinea-pigs[43] may also be susceptible.

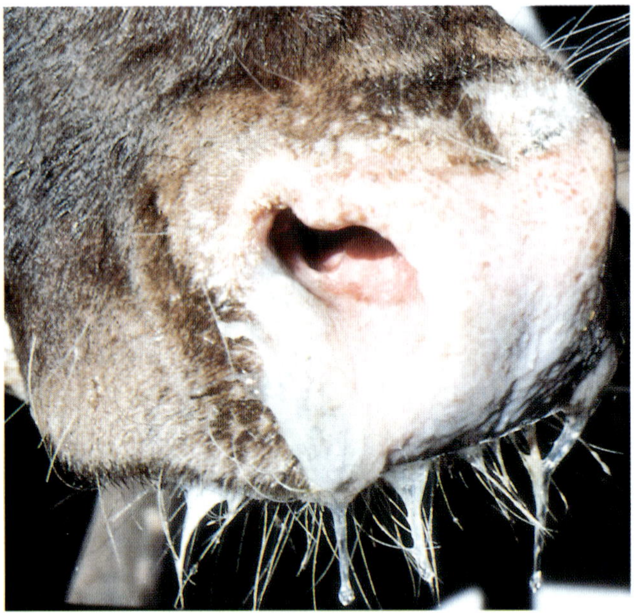

Figure 107.2 Voluminous mucopurulent nasal discharge

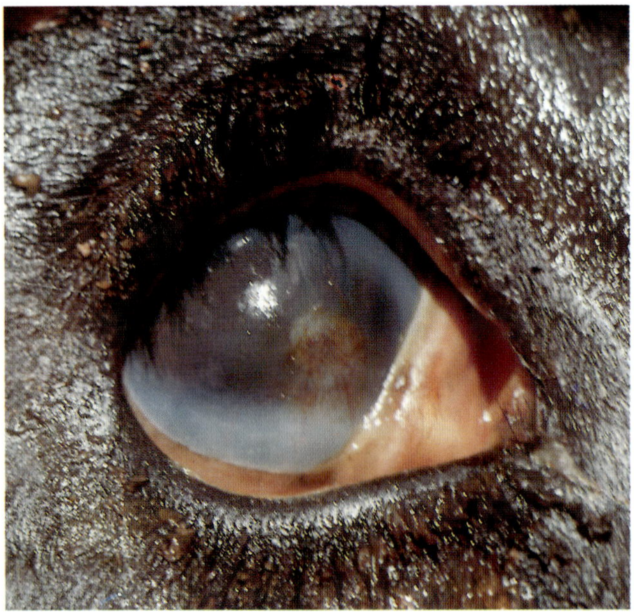

Figure 107.3 Peripheral keratitis

Pathogenesis

The pathogenesis of MCF is clearly unique but, at the same time, poorly understood and the process therefore remains speculative.

Plowright[69] gives three essential components in the pathogenesis of MCF:

- destruction of smaller lymphocytes, particularly in the germinal follicles of lymph and haemolymph nodes and the thymus;
- proliferation and infiltration in many tissues of large, granular lymphoblastoid cells, particularly around blood vessels and in T-cell-dependent areas in lymph nodes and the spleen;
- an irregular segmental angiitis, predominantly of medium-sized arteries, which affects all components of the walls of arteries and veins.

A peculiarity of MCF is that the virus is not detectable in the lesions produced by the disease,[76] although antigen-bearing cells, detectable by immunofluorescence, occur in a small proportion ($1/10^6$ cells) of small or medium lymphocytes in cattle, and particularly rabbits, infected with AHV-1.[85] This, as well as the extended but variable incubation period and the long prepatent viraemia associated with lymphocytes are taken as evidence that the changes in MCF are primarily cell-mediated immunopathological events.[6, 25, 45, 47, 68, 69, 74, 75, 85]

Large, granular lymphocytes with T-cell surface antigens and natural killer activity have been cultured from cases of SA MCF in rabbits, deer and cattle.[76] Such cells normally also have suppressor T-cell activity.[76] Since as few as 100 of these cells may transmit the disease to rabbits that have been parenterally inoculated but at the same time do not contain detectable virus or result in antibody development to AHV-1 in inoculated rabbits, it has been hypothesized that large, granular lymphocytes become latently infected with the viral genome, which is possibly located episomally. The desuppression of the T-cell response and the nonspecific natural killer activity then result in the production of the lesions typical of MCF.[76, 85] However, the inhibition of lymphoid proliferation in experimentally infected rabbits by cyclosporin-A treatment does not change the fatal course of the disease or prevent the development of vasculitis.[46]

Clinical signs

Following an incubation period of three to seven weeks or sometimes longer, the onset of MCF is heralded by a sudden sharp rise in body temperature, reaching a peak of about 41,6 °C by the third or fourth day of the disease. A minority of cattle infected experimentally with AHV-1 show a biphasic temperature reaction.[69] Occasionally enlargement of the peripheral lymph nodes may occur prior to pyrexia.[20, 61, 63, 65, 74]

A bilateral nasal discharge is a consistent sign in cattle suffering from the disease. At first serous, it then

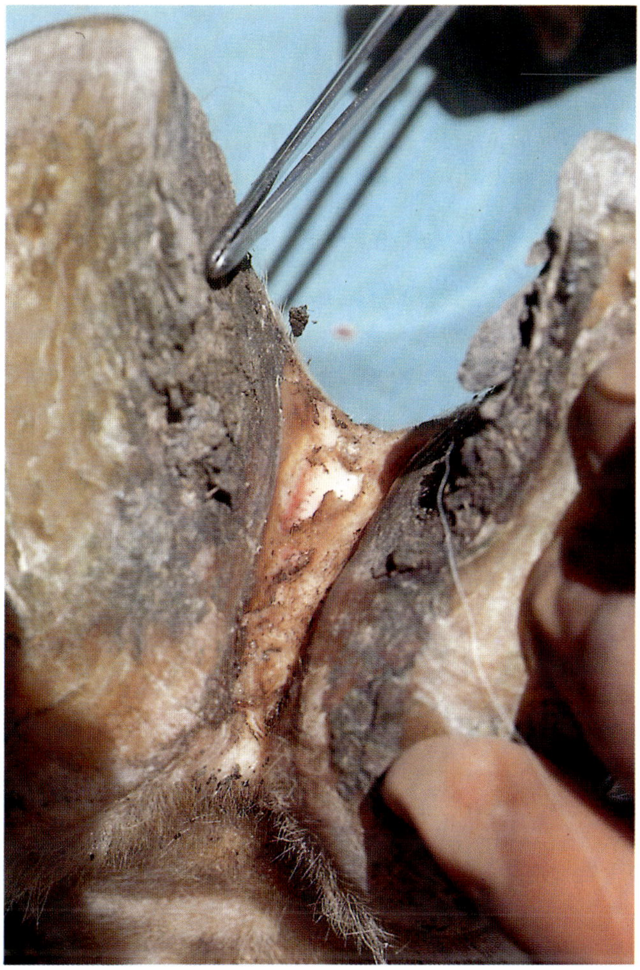

Figure 107.4 Erosive to ulcerative interdigital dermatitis

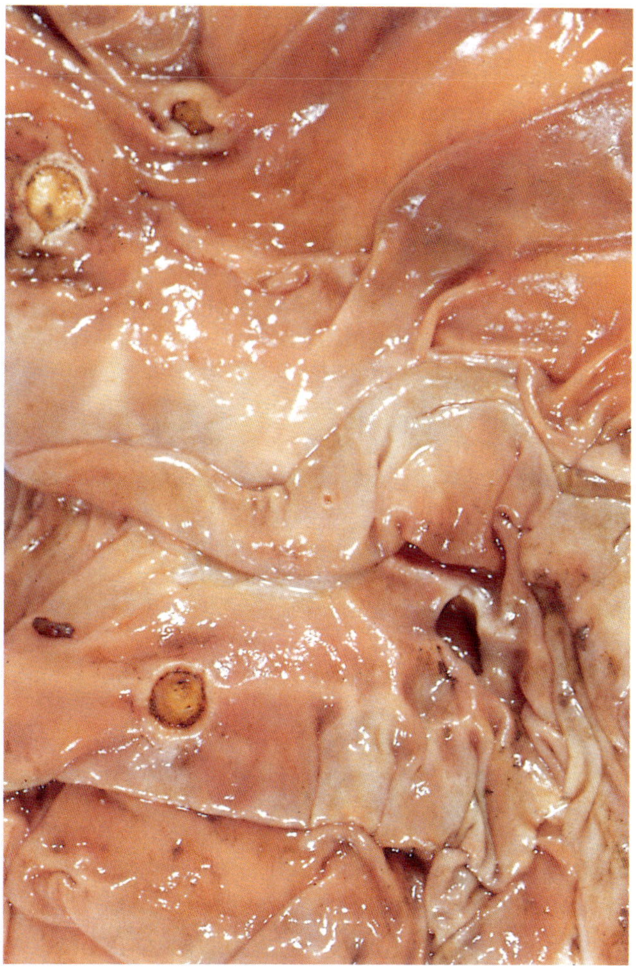

Figure 107.6 Focally disseminated ulcerative abomasitis

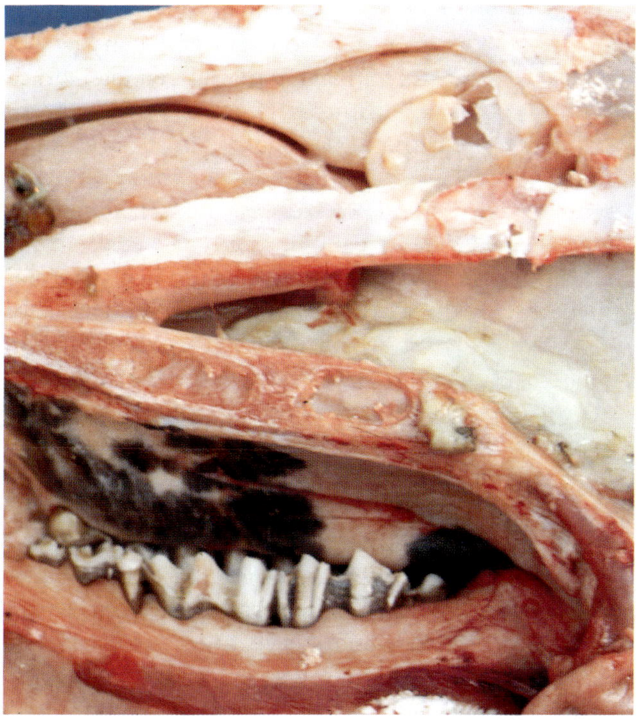

Figure 107.5 Large volume of a mucopurulent exudate in the nasopharynx

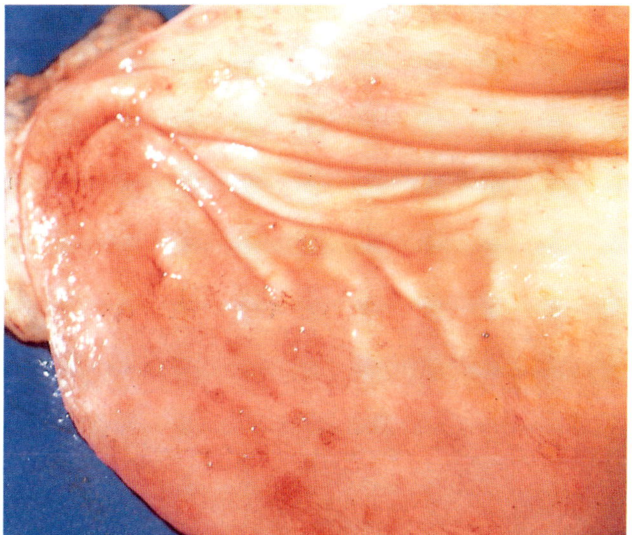

Figure 107.7 Urinary bladder: acute erosive cystitis

becomes mucoid before changing into a thick, copious mucopurulent discharge **(Figure 107.2)**. The discharge accumulates and encrusts around the nostrils and on the muzzle, and sometimes obstructs the nasal passages and causes dyspnoea.[49, 65]

Congestion, erosion and necrosis of the nasal and oral mucosae and the muzzle occur in most cases of WD MCF from about the sixth day of the fever.[42, 63, 65] These changes are less frequent and less severe in animals suffering from SA MCF.[22, 40, 77] Generally speaking, the longer the survival time, the more severe the lesions.

Ocular lesions are characteristic of MCF. Congestion and sometimes oedema of the conjunctivae and sclerae are accompanied by serous or seromucoid discharges which quickly become mucopurulent. Bilateral corneal opacity, caused by oedema, starts at the limbus **(Figure 107.3)** and progresses centripetally to eventually cause impaired vision or total blindness. Affected animals are often photophobic.

Diarrhoea is rarely observed in WD MCF[65] but is more common in SA MCF.

An exudative dermatitis characterized by congestion and sloughing of the superficial layers of the skin occurs sometimes at the base of the horns and the dew claws, in the interdigital space **(Figure 107.4)**, and on the flanks. Skin lesions are more common in SA MCF than in WD MCF.[20, 22, 49, 58]

Nervous signs such as muscle tremors, incoordination, twitching of the ears, torticollis, and nystagmus, as well as aggressive behaviour have been reported in the majority of species affected by MCF.[65]

Cattle with MCF usually die within four to five days of obvious clinical signs developing, although the course of the disease may be considerably longer — up to 21 days for WD MCF and even more for SA MCF.

The clinical signs of the disease in deer differ from those in cattle, and common signs include sudden death, diarrhoea and dysentery as well as anorexia and depression.[57]

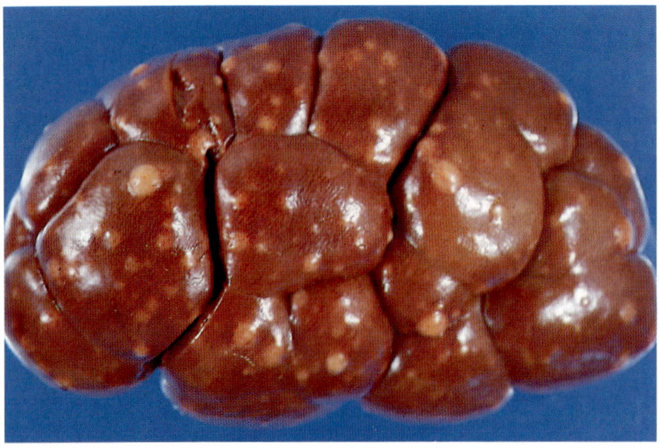

Figure 107.8 Multifocal lymphoid infiltration in the renal cortex

Pathology

The lesions produced by SA and WD MCF in cattle are similar. The upper respiratory and digestive tracts, lymph nodes, brain, eyes, liver, kidneys and urinary bladder are most consistently affected.[4, 11, 20, 48, 49, 65, 95]

In animals where the course of the disease is prolonged, the carcass is emaciated and dehydrated. Apart from the lesions of the eyes, muzzle, external nasal orifices and skin, which are clinically discernible, the mucous membranes of the nasal septum, turbinates, larynx, pharynx, trachea and bronchi are congested and sometimes oedematous, and may also show small haemorrhages, multifocal necrosis of the epithelium, erosions and ulcerations. The mucosa of the affected parts is frequently covered by a serous to mucopurulent exudate **(Figure 107.5)** or occasionally a pseudomembrane. The lungs are often mildly oedematous and emphysematous and may show evidence of secondary bacterial bronchopneumonia.[20, 65]

Similar mucosal lesions are found in the oral cavity, the anterior third of the oesophagus, forestomachs, abomasum **(Figure 107.6)**, and along the ridges of the mucosal folds in the caecum, the ileocaecal valve, the anterior colon and the terminal portion of the rectum.[11, 65] The contents of the large intestine may be dry and covered by mucus, or blood-stained and watery.

All lymph nodes, but particularly those of the head and neck, and the haemolymph nodes are usually enlarged as a result of lymphoid hyperplasia, congestion and oedema. These nodes may also show multifocal haemorrhages and necrosis. In most cases there is mild to moderate splenomegaly and the white pulp is prominent. The palatine tonsils are often enlarged and congested, and the crypts sometimes contain a mucopurulent exudate.[65]

The liver is slightly enlarged and finely mottled as a result of accentuation of the portal tracts. Haemorrhages and a few erosions occur occasionally in the mucosa of the gall bladder.

The cortices of the kidneys frequently contain multiple greyish-white foci, 1–5 mm in diameter **(Figure 107.8)**, and in some cases small haemorrhagic foci are also evident. In most animals the mucosa of the urinary bladder shows oedema, small haemorrhages, erosions and ulcerations **(Figure 107.7)**. Haematuria may be present.[11]

The principal microscopic changes comprise lymphoid hyperplasia and widespread vascular and epithelial lesions which are associated with the infiltration of cells, mostly of the lymphocytic series, and in which the presence of lymphoblasts is prominent. The severity of the epithelial changes seem to correlate with the severity of the cellular infiltration into the epithelium, lamina propria or dermis.[47]

The arterial and venous lesions are characterized by a fibrinoid vasculitis and the infiltration of lymphoblasts, lymphocytes and macrophages into the walls and adventitia of the vessels and perivascular spaces[11, 46, 48, 95]

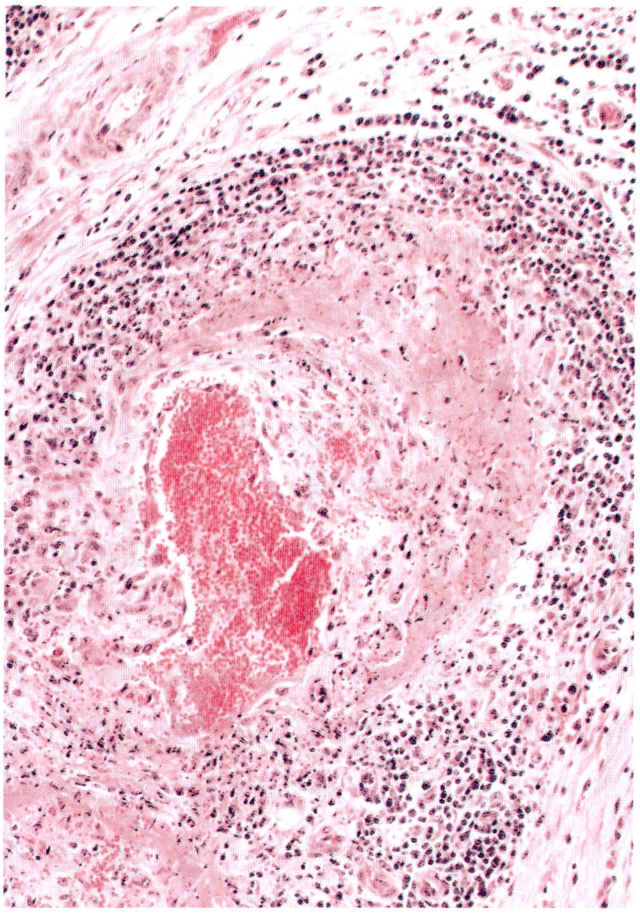

Figure 107.9
Acute arteritis manifesting segmental fibrinoid changes

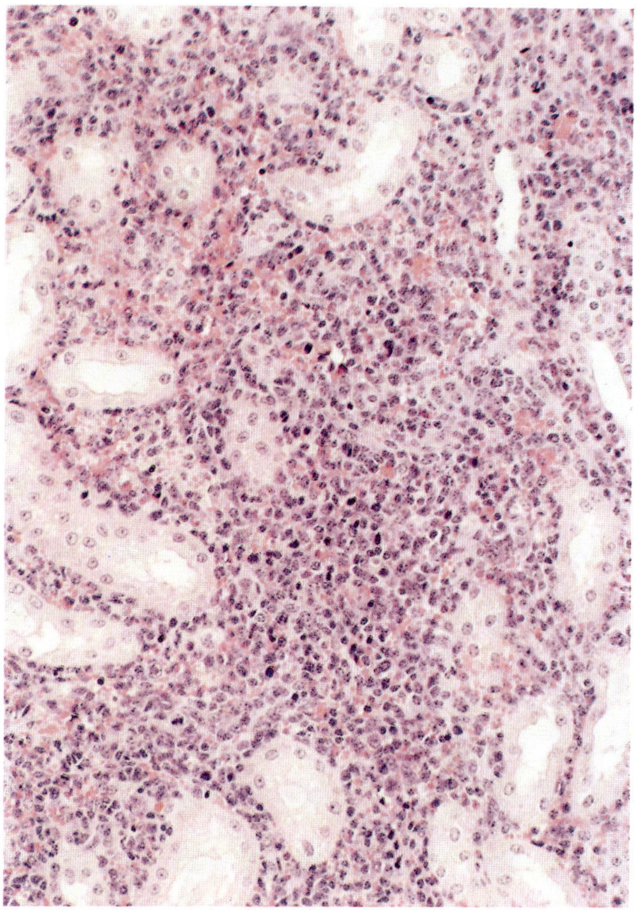

Figure 107.10
Perivascular and intertubular lymphocytic infiltrates

(Figure 107.9). Thrombosis is rare. The vascular lesions may occur throughout the body, but are most pronounced in the brain and meninges, carotid rete, liver, kidneys, lungs, capsule and medulla of the adrenals, as well as areas of the skin and alimentary tract which are grossly affected.

Marked hyperplasia of lymphocytes and reticuloendothelial cells occur in lymphoid tissues. Focal necrosis associated with vasculitis may be evident in the cortex and medulla of the lymph nodes.

Large numbers of lymphocytic cells, mainly lymphoblasts, and some macrophages are found in the portal triads of the liver, and multifocally in the interstitium of the cortices of the kidneys in particular **(Figure 107.10)**. Occasionally thrombosis of arcuate or interlobular arteries gives rise to small renal infarcts.[95]

Consistent ocular findings include keratitis, uveitis, and vasculitis in most structures of the eyes.[100] Oedema, neovascularization, and mononuclear cell infiltration of the cornea arise at the limbus and spread centripetally. Erosion of the cornea may occur. The uveitis is frequently accompanied by the accumulation of fibrin, neutrophils and mononuclear cells in the anterior chamber and vitreous body.

In deer which have died of MCF, acute mesenteric lymphadenitis and acute haemorrhagic colitis and typhlitis are common.[57, 76]

Diagnosis

A presumptive diagnosis of MCF can be made on the herd history, clinical signs and pathology. In most outbreaks in Africa there is evidence of recent close contact between cattle and either wildebeest or (rarely) sheep. Confirmation of the diagnosis of WD MCF requires either isolation of the virus from tissues of the affected animal(s) or demonstration of specific antibody in the serum. Since infectivity in the tissues of cattle suffering from SA MCF cannot be detected by regular means, diagnosis is dependent upon the history, clinical signs and pathology.

As infectivity in WD MCF is associated with viable cells, blood should be collected in anticoagulant (EDTA or heparin), preferably before death, and organs collected as soon as possible after death. To retain viability of lymph node and spleen cells, specimens from these tissues should be dispersed by being cut into small fragments in cell culture medium containing 5 to 10 per cent serum and diluted (i.e. titrated to dilute out the effect of inhibitory and toxic substances).[67, 68] All specimens should be kept at 4 °C and inoculated into rabbits or cell cultures as soon as possible, preferably on the day of collection. If this is not possible, specimens may be stored at –70 °C provided that a cryoprotectant such as glycerol or 10 per cent DMSO is used. Some loss of infectivity can, however, be expected.[67, 68] For virus isolation in cell cultures, washed leukocytes and dilutions of lymphoid tissues are co-cultivated with susceptible cells and the culture examined for the development of cytopathic effects typical of AHV-1. Identification of the virus is effected by neutralization tests using antisera specific to AHV-1 that has been prepared in cattle or rabbits.[51]

Serology is of limited value in the diagnosis of WD MCF, as only a small proportion of cattle develop humoral antibody responses late in the course of the disease. This, together with the serological cross-reactions which occur between herpesviruses and the fact that even where antibody is produced in measurable quantities, it is present in low concentration,[34, 36, 89] makes interpretation difficult.

Serology may on the other hand be useful in establishing the prevalence of AHV-1 or related viruses in wildlife.[5, 29, 35, 52] Here virus neutralization is preferred because of its specificity, but indirect immunofluorescence, enzyme-linked immunosorbent assay (ELISA), and immunoperoxidase have also been used.[87, 89, 90, 98]

Differential diagnosis

The sporadic occurrence and very high mortality rate of MCF is helpful in distinguishing it from other diseases of cattle.

Nasal discharge, erosions and ulcers in the oral cavity and upper respiratory tract, keratitis and conjunctivitis, and diarrhoea also occur in bovine viral diarrhoea/mucosal disease, rinderpest and infectious bovine rhinotracheitis, but the eye lesions and nasal discharges in cattle with MCF are generally more severe than in those suffering from these diseases. Erosions and ulcerations in the mouth, usually in the absence of diarrhoea, are also features of foot-and-mouth disease, bovine papular stomatitis and lumpy skin disease, but the other presenting signs and epidemiologies of these diseases are often sufficiently specific to enable them to be differentiated from MCF. Laboratory procedures, including histopathology of tissue specimens, are necessary before a specific diagnosis of MCF can be made.

The intestinal haemorrhage in peracute MCF of deer may resemble yersiniosis.[76]

Control

It is often stated that MCF can be avoided in susceptible species by the prevention of close contact with wildebeest or sheep, especially at times when the latter are producing offspring.[69] However, in South Africa it has become clear that close contact is not essential for the transfer of WD MCF virus to cattle, and that transmission can occur over distances of up to several hundred metres.[5, 8] Consequently separation of wildebeest and cattle by at least 1 000 metres is regarded as necessary to prevent the infection of cattle.

Until 1993 MCF was a controlled disease in South Africa and the movement of wildebeest was restricted by regulation. All farms and nature reserves harbouring wildebeest in South Africa had to be registered with the Directorate of Animal Health, and wildebeest could only be moved to and from registered properties. These regulations have now been lifted.

Attempts to develop attenuated or inactivated vaccines by conventional methods have so far been unsuccessful, in spite of the production of high levels of virus neutralizing antibodies in vaccinated rabbits and cattle.[6, 26, 67, 71, 80, 83, 85, 92]

References

1 **ANON., 1910.** Annual report, 1909–1910. Department of Agriculture, British East Africa.

2 **ANON., 1933.** Department of Health annual report for the year 1933. Government Printer, Livingstone.

3 **ANON., 1933–38.** Report of the Veterinary Surgeon, Salisbury, Southern Rhodesia. Government Printer.

4 **BARKER, I.K. & VAN DREUMEL, A.A., 1985.** The alimentary system. In: JUBB, K.V.F., KENNEDY, P.D. & PALMER, N., (eds). *Pathology of Domestic Animals*. 3rd edn. Orlando, San Diego: Academic Press, Inc.

5 **BARNARD, B.J.H., 1984.** Transmitters and potential transmitters of malignant catarrhal fever. *Proceedings of the XIII World Congress on Diseases of Cattle*. World Buiatrics Association, September 1984. Durban, South Africa.

6 **BARNARD, B.J.H., 1984.** Increased susceptibility of rabbits to malignant catarrhal fever virus after vaccination. *Proceedings of the XIII World Congress on Diseases of Cattle*. World Buiatrics Association, September 1984. Durban, South Africa.

7 **BARNARD, B.J.H., 1986.** Veterinary Research Institute, Onderstepoort, South Africa. Unpublished data.

8 **BARNARD, B.J.H. & VAN DE PYPEKAMP, H.E., 1988.** Wildebeest-derived malignant catarrhal fever: Unusual epidemiology in South Africa. *Onderstepoort Journal of Veterinary Research*, 55, 69–71.

9 **BARNARD, B.J.H., VAN DE PYPEKAMP, H.E. & GRIESSEL, M.D., 1989.** Epizootiology of wildebeest-derived malignant catarrhal fever in an outbreak in the north-western Transvaal: Indications of an intermediate host. *Onderstepoort Journal of Veterinary Research*, 56, 135–139.

10 **BEATSON, N.S., 1984.** Malignant catarrhal fever — field progress. *Proceedings of a Deer Course for Veterinarians*, Palmerston North, 1985. Deer Branch Course No. 1. Wellington, New Zealand. New Zealand Veterinary Association, 117–121.

11 **BERKMAN, R.N., BARNER, R.D., MORRILL, C.C. & LANGHAM, R.F., 1960.** Bovine malignant catarrhal fever in Michigan. II. Pathology. *American Journal of Veterinary Research*, 21, 1015–1026.

12 **BRIDGEN, A., HERRING, A.J., INFLIS, N.F. & REID, H.W., 1989.** Preliminary characterization of the alcelaphine herpesvirus 1 genome. *Journal of General Virology*, 70, 1141–1150.

13 **BUXTON, D. & REID, H.W., 1980.** Transmission of malignant catarrhal fever to rabbits. *The Veterinary Record*, 106, 243–245.

14 **BUXTON, D., REID, H.W., FINLAYSON, J., POW, I. & BERRIE, E., 1985.** Transmission of malignant catarrhal fever-like syndrome to sheep: Preliminary experiment. *Research in Veterinary Science*, 38, 22–29.

15 **CASTRO, A.E., DALEY, G.G., ZIMMER, M.A., WHITENACK, D.L. & JENSEN, J., 1982.** Malignant catarrhal fever in Indian gaur and greater kudu: Experimental transmission, isolation and identification of a herpesvirus. *American Journal of Veterinary Research*, 42, 5–11.

16 **CASTRO, A.E., RAMSAY, E.C., DOTSON, J.F., SCHRAMKE, M.L., KOCAN, A.A. & WHITENACK, D.L., 1984.** Characteristics of the herpesvirus of malignant catarrhal fever isolated from captive wildebeest calves. *American Journal of Veterinary Research*, 45, 409–415.

17 **CASTRO, A.E., SCHRAMKE, M.L., RAMSAY, E.C., WHITENACK, D.L. & DOTSON, J.F., 1983.** A diagnostic approach in the identification of malignant catarrhal fever virus from inapparent carriers in a wildebeest herd. *Proceedings of the Third International Symposium of Veterinary Laboratory Diagnosticians*, June 1983, Ames, Iowa, USA. Vol. 2. 715–721.

18 **COLSON, M., 1930.** Contribution a l'étude du coryza gangréneux des bovidés. *Dissertation École Nationale Vétérinaire*. Alfort.

19 **CUMMING, G.R., 1850.** *Five Years of a Hunter's Life in the Interior of South Africa*. London: John Murray.

20 **DAUBNEY, R. & HUDSON, J.R., 1936.** Transmission experiments with bovine malignant catarrhal fever. *Journal of Comparative Pathology*, 49, 63–89.

21 **DE KOCK, G. & NEITZ, W.O., 1950.** Sheep as a reservoir host of snotsiekte (or malignant catarrhal fever in cattle) in South Africa. *South African Journal of Science*, 46, 176–180.

22 **DENHOLM, L.J. & WESTBURY, H.A., 1982.** Malignant catarrhal fever in farmed Rusa deer (*Cervus timorensis*). I. Clinicopathological observation. *Australian Veterinary Journal*, 58, 81–87.

23 **DU TOIT, P.J. & ALEXANDER, R.A., 1938.** Malignant catarrhal fever and similar diseases. *Congress Manual of the XIIIth International Veterinary Congress*, Zürich 1938. 15–21.

24 **EBEDES, H., 1986.** Zoological Gardens, Pretoria. Personal communication.

25 **EDINGTON, N., PATEL, J., RUSSEL, P.H. & PLOWRIGHT, W., 1979.** The nature of acute lymphoid proliferation in rabbits infected with herpes virus of bovine malignant catarrhal fever. *European Journal of Cancer*, 15, 1515–1522.

26 **EDINGTON, N. & PLOWRIGHT, W., 1980.** The protection of rabbits against the herpes virus of malignant catarrhal fever by inactivated vaccines. *Research in Veterinary Science*, 28, 384–386.

27 **GÖTZE, R. & LIESS, J., 1930.** Untersuchungen über das bosartige Katarrhalfieber des Rindes. II. Schafe als Ubertrager. *Deutsche Tierärtzliche Wochenschrift*, 38, 194–200.

28 **GULLAND, F.M.D., REID, H.W., BUXTON, D., LEWIS, J.C.M., KOCK, R.A. & KIRKWOOD, J.K., 1989.** Malignant catarrhal fever in a roan antelope (*Hippotragus equinus*) at Regent's Park. *The Veterinary Record*, 14, 42–43.

29 **HAMBLIN, C. & HEDGER, R.S., 1984.** Neutralizing antibodies to wildebeest-derived malignant catarrhal fever virus in African wildlife. *Comparative Immunology and Microbiology of Infectious Diseases*, 7, 195–199.

30 **HARKNESS, J., 1985.** Bovine malignant catarrhal fever in the United Kingdom. *State Veterinary Journal*, 39, 60–64.

31 **HARKNESS, J.W. & JESSETT, D.M., 1981.** Influence of temperature on the growth in cell culture of malignant catarrhal fever virus. *Research in Veterinary Science*, 31, 164–168.

32 **HARRIS, R.E., CHRISTIANSEN, K.H. & BLUNT, M.H., 1978.** Observations on the epidemiology of malignant catarrhal fever. *New Zealand Veterinary Journal*, 26, 86–87.

33 **HEUSCHELE, W.P., 1982.** Malignant catarrhal fever virus in wild ruminants — A review and current status report. *Proceedings of the 86th Annual Meeting of the United States Animal Health Association*, November 1982, San Diego, USA. 552–572.

34 **HEUSCHELE, W.P., 1983.** Diagnosis of malignant catarrhal fever due to alcelaphine herpesvirus 1. *Proceedings of the Third International Symposium of Veterinary Laboratory Diagnosticians*, June 1983, Iowa, USA. Vol. 2. 707–713.

35 **HEUSCHELE, W.P. & FLETCHER, H.R., 1984.** Improved methods for the diagnosis of malignant catarrhal fever. *27th Annual Proceedings of the American Association of Veterinary Laboratory Diagnosticians*, San Diego, USA. 137–150.

36 **HEUSCHELE, W.P., FLETCHER, H.R., OOSTERHUIS, J., JANSSEN, D. & ROBINSON, P.T., 1984.** Epidemiological aspects of malignant catarrhal fever in the USA. *Proceedings of the 88th Annual Meeting of the US Animal Health Association*, October 1984, San Diego, USA, 640–651.

37 **HEUSCHELE, W.P., NIELSON, N.O., OOSTERHUIS, I.E. & CASTRO, A.E., 1985.** Dexamethasone-induced recrudescence of malignant catarrhal fever and associated lymphosarcoma and granulomatous disease in a Formosan sika deer (*Cervus nippon taiouanus*). *American Journal of Veterinary Research*, 46, 1578–1583.

38 **HEUSCHELE, W.P., SWANSEN, M. & FLETCHER, H.R., 1982.** Malignant catarrhal fever in wild ruminants — A review and current status. *Annual Proceedings of the American Association of Zoo Veterinarians*, 1982, 67–72.

39 **HUCK, R.A., SHAND, A., ALLSOP, P.J. & PATERSON, A.B., 1961.** Malignant catarrh of deer. *The Veterinary Record*, 73, 457–465.

40 **JAMES, M.P., NIELSON, F.L.A. & STEWART, W.J., 1975.** An epizootic of malignant catarrhal fever. I. Clinical and pathological observations. *New Zealand Veterinary Journal*, 23, 7–12.

41 **JESSUP, D.A., 1985.** Malignant catarrhal fever in free-ranging black-tailed deer (*Odocoilens hemiorus columbiansis*) in California. *Journal of Wildlife Diseases*, 21, 167–169.

42 **KALUNDA, M., DARDIRI, A.H. & LEE, K.M., 1981.** Malignant catarrhal fever. I. Response of American cattle to malignant catarrhal fever isolated in Kenya. *Canadian Journal of Comparative Medicine*, 45, 70–76.

43 **KALUNDA, M., FERRIS, D.H., DARDIRI, A.H. & LEE, M., 1981.** Malignant catarrhal fever. III. Experimental infection of sheep, domestic rabbits and laboratory animals with malignant catarrhal fever virus. *Canadian Journal of Comparative Medicine*, 45, 310–314.

44 **KALUNDA, M., SHAKA, S., HENRIKSON, K., KALAYE, J. & SEMUGURUKA, W., 1982.** An epizootic of bovine malignant catarrhal fever in Northern Tanzania in 1976. *Bulletin of Animal Health and Production in Africa*, 30, 229–234.

45 **LIGGITT, H.C., 1978.** Studies on the pathology and pathogenesis of experimental bovine malignant catarrhal fever. Ph.D Thesis, Colorado State University, Fort Collins, Colorado, USA.

46 **LIGGITT, H.C. & DE MARTINI, J.C., 1980.** The pathomorphology of malignant catarrhal fever. I. Generalised lymphoid vasculitis. *Veterinary Pathology*, 17, 59–73.

47 **LIGGITT, H.C. & DE MARTINI, J.C., 1980.** The pathomorphology of malignant catarrhal fever. II. Multisystemic epithelial lesions. *Veterinary Pathology*, 17, 74–78.

48 **LIGGITT, H.C., DE MARTINI, J.C., McCHESNEY, A.E., PIERSON, R.E. & STORZ, J., 1978.** Experimental transmission of malignant catarrhal fever in cattle: Gross and histopathologic changes. *American Journal of Veterinary Research*, 39, 1249–1257.

49 **METTAM, R.W.M., 1923.** Snotsiekte in cattle. *Ninth and Tenth Reports of the Director of Veterinary Services, Education and Research, Union of South Africa*, 395–430.

50 **MUSHI, E.Z., JESSETT, D.M., RURANGIRWA, F.R., ROSSITER, P.B. & KARSTAD, L., 1981.** Neutralising antibodies to malignant catarrhal fever herpesvirus in wildebeest

nasal secretions. *Tropical Animal Health Production*, 13, 55–56.

51 **MUSHI, E.Z. & KARSTAD, L., 1981.** Prevalence of virus-neutralizing antibodies to malignant catarrhal fever virus in oryx (*Oryx beissa*). *Journal of Wildlife Diseases*, 17, 467–470.

52 **MUSHI, E.Z. & PLOWRIGHT, W., 1979.** A microtitre technique for assay of malignant catarrhal fever virus and neutralizing antibody. *Research in Veterinary Science*, 27, 230–232.

53 **MUSHI, E.Z., ROSSITER, P.B., JESSETT, D.M. & KARSTAD, L., 1981.** Isolation and characterization of a herpesvirus from topi (*Damaliscus korrigum, Ogilby*). *Journal of Comparative Pathology*, 91, 63–68.

54 **MUSHI, E.Z. & RURANGIRWA, F.R., 1981.** Epidemiology of malignant catarrhal fever: A review. *Veterinary Research Communications*, 5, 127–142.

55 **MUSHI, E.Z. & RURANGIRWA, F.R., 1981.** Malignant catarrhal fever virus-shedding by infected cattle. *Bulletin of Animal Health and Production of Africa*, 29, 111–112.

56 **MUSHI, E.Z. & WAFULA, J.A., 1983.** Infectivity of cell-free malignant catarrhal fever virus in rabbits and cattle. *Veterinary Research Communications*, 6, 153–155.

57 **OLIVER, R., 1985.** Malignant catarrhal fever of red deer. In: DELLA-PORTA, A.J., (ed.). *Veterinary Viral Diseases: Their Significance in South-East Asia and the Western Pacific.* Sydney: Academic Press.

58 **OLIVER, R.E., BEATSON, N.S., CATHCART, A. & POOLE, W.S., 1983.** Experimental transmission of malignant catarrhal fever of red deer (*Cervus claphus*). *New Zealand Veterinary Journal*, 31, 209–212.

59 **PATEL, J.R. & EDINGTON, N., 1980.** The detection of the herpes virus of bovine malignant catarrhal fever in rabbit lymphocytes *in vivo* and *in vitro*. *Journal of General Virology*, 48, 437–444.

60 **PATEL, J.R. & EDINGTON, N., 1981.** The detection and behaviour of the herpesvirus of malignant catarrhal fever in bovine lymphocytes. *Archives of Virology*, 68, 321–326.

61 **PIERCY, S.E., 1952.** Studies in bovine malignant catarrh. I. Experimental infection in cattle. *British Veterinary Journal*, 108, 35–47.

62 **PIERCY, S.E., 1955.** Studies in bovine malignant catarrhal fever. VI. Adaptation to rabbits. *British Veterinary Journal*, 110, 87–96.

63 **PIERSON, R.E., HAMDY, F.M., DARDIRI, A.H., FERRIS, D.H. & SCHLOER, G.M., 1979.** Comparison of African and American forms of malignant catarrhal fever: Transmission and clinical signs. *American Journal of Veterinary Research*, 40, 1091–1095.

64 **PIERSON, R.E., STORZ, J., McCHESNEY, A.E. & THAKES, D., 1974.** Experimental transmission of malignant catarrhal fever. *American Journal of Veterinary Research*, 35, 523–525.

65 **PLOWRIGHT, W., 1964.** Studies on bovine malignant catarrhal fever of cattle. DVSc Thesis, University of Pretoria, South Africa.

66 **PLOWRIGHT, W., 1967.** Malignant catarrhal fever in East Africa. III. Neutralising antibody in free-living wildebeest. *Research in Veterinary Science*, 8, 129–136.

67 **PLOWRIGHT, W., 1968.** Malignant catarrhal fever. *Journal of the American Veterinary Medical Association*, 152, 795–804.

68 **PLOWRIGHT, W., 1984.** Malignant catarrhal fever virus: A lymphotropic herpesvirus of ruminants. In: WITTMAN, G., GASKELL, R.M. & RZIHA, H.-J. (eds). *Latent Herpesvirus Infections in Veterinary Medicine.* Martinus Nijhoff for the Commission of the European Community. 279–305.

69 **PLOWRIGHT, W., 1986.** Malignant catarrhal fever. *Revue Scientifique et Technique*, 5, 897–918.

70 **PLOWRIGHT, W., FERRIS, R.D. & SCOTT, G.R., 1960.** Blue wildebeest and the aetiological agent of bovine malignant catarrhal fever. *Nature*, 188, 1167–1169.

71 **PLOWRIGHT, W., HERNIMAN, K.A.J., JESSETT, D.M., KALUNDA, M. & RAMPTON, C.S., 1975.** Immunisation of cattle against the herpesvirus of malignant catarrhal fever: Failure of inactivated culture vaccines with adjuvant. *Research in Veterinary Science*, 19, 159–166.

72 **PLOWRIGHT, W., KALUNDA, M., JESSETT, D.M. & HERNIMAN, K.A.J., 1972.** Congenital infection of cattle with the herpesvirus causing malignant catarrhal fever. *Research in Veterinary Science*, 13, 37–45.

73 **RAMSAY, E.C., CASTRO, A.E. & BURMEISTER, B.M., 1982.** Investigation of malignant catarrhal fever at the Oklahoma City Zoo. *Proceedings of the 86th Annual Meeting of the US Animal Health Association*, November 1982, San Diego, USA, 571–582.

74 **REID, H.W. & BUXTON, D., 1984.** Malignant catarrhal fever of deer. *Proceedings of the Royal Society of Edinburgh*, 82b, 261–273.

75 **REID, H.W. & BUXTON, D., 1985.** Immunity and pathogenesis of malignant catarrhal fever. In: PASTORET, P.P., THIRY, E. & SALIKI, J., (eds). *Immunity to Herpesvirus Infections of Domestic Animals.* Report EUR 9737 En., Commission of the European Communities.

76 **REID, H.W., BUXTON, D., BERRIE, E., POW, I. & FINLAYSON, J., 1984.** Malignant catarrhal fever. *The Veterinary Record*, 114, 582–584.

77 **REID, H.W., BUXTON, D., CORRIGAL, W., HUNTER, A.R., McMARTIN, D.A. & RUSHTON, R., 1979.** An outbreak of malignant catarrhal fever in red deer (*Cervus elaphus*). *The Veterinary Record*, 104, 120–123.

78 **REID, H.W., BUXTON, D., POW, I., FINLAYSON, J., 1986.** Malignant catarrhal fever: Experimental transmission of the 'sheep-associated' form of the disease from cattle and deer to cattle, deer, rabbits and hamsters. *Research in Veterinary Science*, 41, 76–81.

79 **REID, H.W., PLOWRIGHT, W. & ROWE, L., 1975.** Neutralizing antibody to herpesviruses derived from wildebeest and hartebeest in wild animals in East Africa. *Research in Veterinary Science*, 18, 269–273.

80 **REID, H.W. & ROWE, L., 1973.** The attenuation of a herpesvirus (malignant catarrhal fever virus) isolated from hartebeest (*Alcelaphus buselaphus cohei* Gunther). *Research in Veterinary Science*, 15, 144–146.

81 **ROIZMANN, B., CARMICHAEL, L.E., DEINHARDT, F., DE THE, G., NAHMIAS, A.J., PLOWRIGHT, W., RAPP, F., SHELDRICK, P., TAKAHASHI, M. & WOLFF, K., 1981.** Herpesviridae; definition, provisional nomenclature and taxonomy. *Intervirology*, 16, 201–217.

82 **ROSSITER, P.B., 1981.** Antibodies to malignant catarrhal fever in sheep sera. *Journal of Comparative Pathology*, 91, 303–311.

83 **ROSSITER, P.B., 1982.** Attempts to protect rabbits against challenge with virulent, cell-associated malignant catarrhal fever virus. *Veterinary Microbiology*, 7, 419–425.

84 **ROSSITER, P.B., 1983.** Role of wildebeest fetal membranes and fluids in the transmission of malignant catarrhal fever virus. *The Veterinary Record*, 113,150–152.

85 **ROSSITER, P.B., 1985.** Immunology and immunopathology of malignant catarrhal fever. *Progressive Veterinary Microbiology and Immunology*, 1, 121–144.

86 **ROSSITER, P.B., GUMM, I.D. & WAMWAYI, H.M., 1987.** Use of vero cells for the isolation and propagation of malignant catarrhal fever virus. *Tropical Animal Health Production*, 19, 77–81.

87 **ROSSITER, P.B., JESSET, D.M. & MUSHI, E.Z., 1980.** Antibodies to malignant catarrhal fever virus antigens in the sera of normal and naturally infected cattle in Kenya. *Research in Veterinary Science*, 29, 235–239.

88 **ROSSITER, P.B., JESSET, D.M., MUSHI, E.Z. & KARSTAD, L., 1983.** Antibodies in carrier wildebeest to the lymphoproliferative herpesvirus of malignant catarrhal fever. *Comparative Immunology and Microbiology of Infectious Diseases*, 6, 39–43.

89 **ROSSITER, P.B., MUSHI, E.Z. & PLOWRIGHT, W., 1977.** The development of antibodies in rabbits and cattle infected experimentally with an African strain of MCF virus. *Veterinary Microbiology*, 2, 57–66.

90 **ROSSITER, P.B., MUSHI, E.Z. & PLOWRIGHT, W., 1978.** The antibody response in cattle and rabbits to early antigens of malignant catarrhal fever virus in cultured cells. *Research in Veterinary Science*, 25, 207–210.

91 **RURANGIRWA, F.R., MUSHI, E.Z. & KARSTAD, L., 1982.** Malignant catarrhal fever virus specific secretory IgA in nasal secretions of wildebeest calves. *Comparative Immunology and Microbiology of Infectious Diseases*, 5, 429–436.

92 **RUSSEL, P.H., 1980.** Malignant catarrhal fever in rabbits — reproduction of clinical disease by cell-free virus and partial protection against such disease by vaccination with inactivated virus. *Veterinary Microbiology*, 5, 161–163.

93 **RWEYEMAMU, M.M., KARSTAD, L., MUSHI, E.Z., OTEMA, J.C., JESSETT, D.M., ROWE, L., DREVEMO, S. & GROOTENHUIS, J., 1974.** Malignant catarrhal fever virus in nasal secretions of wildebeest: A probable mechanism for virus transmission. *Journal of Wildlife Diseases*, 10, 478–487.

94 **SCHMITZ, J.A. & GRUMBEIN, S.L., 1981.** Two possible cases of malignant catarrhal fever in sheep. *24th Annual Proceedings of the American Association for Veterinary Diagnosticians*, October 1981, Oregon, USA, 61–66.

95 **SELMAN, I.E., WISEMAN, A., MURRAY, M. & WRIGHT, N.G., 1974.** A clinico-pathological study of bovine malignant catarrhal fever in Great Britain. *The Veterinary Record*, 94, 483–490.

96 **SNOWDON, W.A., 1972.** Bovine malignant catarrh. *Annual Report*, Division of Animal Health CSIRO, Australia, 16.

97 **TUSTIN, R., 1989.** Faculty of Veterinary Science, University of Pretoria. Unpublished observation.

98 **WAN, S. & CASTRO, A.E., 1984.** Development of an enzyme-linked immunosorbent assay (ELISA) for the detection of antibodies to MCF (malignant catarrhal fever) virus. *Proceedings of the 65th Annual Meeting of the Conference of Research Workers in Animal Diseases*, 12–13 November, Chicago, Illinois, USA. Abstract No. 13.

99 **WESTBURY, H.A.I. & DENHOLM, L.J., 1982.** Malignant catarrhal fever in farmed Russa deer (*Cervus timorensis*). II. Animal transmission and virological studies. *Australian Veterinary Journal*, 58, 88–92.

100 **WHITELEY, H.E., YOUNG, S., LIGGITT, H.D. & DE MARTINI, J.C., 1985.** Ocular lesions of bovine malignant catarrhal fever. *Veterinary Pathology*, 22, 219–225.

108

Aujeszky's disease

Synonyms: Pseudorabies, mad itch

C. J. Maré

Introduction

Pseudorabies is a severe, frequently fatal disease of new-born pigs caused by suid herpesvirus 1. In weanling and adult pigs pseudorabies may also be fatal, but is more often a mild or subclinical infection which may result in abortions or stillbirths in pregnant sows. Infection of sheep, dogs and cats appears to be invariably fatal.[32, 34, 40] However, in cattle recovery may be more frequent than was previously suspected.[19]

The disease was first described by Aujeszky in Hungary in 1902,[3] but there is evidence[21] that the disease, known as 'mad itch', was present in the USA during the nineteenth century. In the first half of the twentieth century pseudorabies in the USA was considered to be a sporadic but acute disease of new-born piglets. However, in the 1960s and 1970s[23, 26, 36] the disease became more prevalent, and severe infection of adult pigs, as experienced in Europe, became a regular feature of pseudorabies outbreaks.

Pseudorabies is widespread in eastern and western Europe, where it is an economically important disease of both pigs and cattle. It is also widespread in the USA and Latin America and has been reported from India, Korea, Taiwan, Vietnam, Iran, Japan and New Zealand. It appears to be absent from Australia.[17] The prevalence of pseudorabies in sub-Saharan Africa remains obscure, although on one occasion the virus was isolated from specimens submitted from Zaïre for African swine fever diagnosis.[38]

In spite of the importation of pigs for breeding purposes from pseudorabies endemic areas of Europe and the USA over many years, the disease does not appear to have become established in southern Africa, and no outbreaks have been confirmed. A serological survey of sows in several pig-breeding establishments in South Africa was conducted in 1977–78, but no animals with neutralizing antibodies to pseudorabies virus were encountered.[39]

Aetiology

Pseudorabies is caused by a herpesvirus of the subfamily Alphaherpesvirinae.[29] The virus is officially designated suid herpesvirus l (SHV-l), but it is also commonly referred to as pseudorabies virus or Aujeszky's disease virus.

Suid herpesvirus 1 possesses a double-stranded DNA genome with molecular weight 91 x 10^6 daltons, and a G+C ratio of 74 per cent. Its icosahedral capsid consists of 162 tubular capsomeres enclosed in a lipoprotein envelope.[20]

In common with other herpesviruses, SHV-1 is sensitive to lipid solvents such as ether and chloroform, heat (destroyed by 56 °C within 30 minutes),[10] enzymes (trypsin and pronase),[4] acid pH, desiccation, ultraviolet light,[10] and all commonly used antiviral disinfectants.

Suid herpesvirus 1 can be propagated in a wide range of cell culture systems: kidney cells derived from cattle, pigs, dogs, cats, rabbits, or monkeys are commonly used. The virus causes a rapid cytopathic effect, characterized by rounding and eventual destruction of the cells. Appropriately stained SHV-1-infected cells contain large eosinophilic intranuclear inclusions typical of herpesviruses.

Suid herpesvirus 1 and bovine herpesvirus 1 (infectious bovine rhinotracheitis virus) have been shown to be biochemically[16] and immunologically similar,[7] as well as genetically related by DNA-RNA hybridization.[6]

Epidemiology

Suid herpesvirus 1 has an extremely wide host range. Species such as pigs, cattle, sheep, goats, dogs, cats and at least eight species of wild animals have contracted the disease under natural conditions. In addition, a wide variety of domestic and wild animals and birds are susceptible to the virus by experimental inoculation.[17] Unconfirmed human infections with pruritis have been reported from Europe.

Infected pigs are by far the most important source of infection for pigs as well as other species. While the existence of other maintenance species, including wild animals, has been suspected, none have so far been shown to be significant in the spread of the disease, although raccoons (*Procyon lotor*) possibly play a minor role in the USA.[14, 46]

Acutely infected pigs excrete virus in nasal discharges, aerosols, saliva and semen. Susceptible pigs are infected by inhalation of virus-containing aerosols or by contact with contaminated feed and water. Close contact is considered a prerequisite for virus spread, but there are indications that air-borne transmission between farms is possible.[13] Coital transmission can occur in pigs.

Pigs, dogs, cats and wildlife can become infected by ingestion of infected tissues and foetuses. Cattle and sheep acquire the infection by being nuzzled or nipped by infected pigs. While spread of the infection between cattle and sheep has been reported, pigs are the primary source of infection.

Pigs which have either recovered from pseudorabies or have been vaccinated and subsequently exposed to wild SHV-1 may become asymptomatic carriers. As such they can transmit the wild virus to susceptible animals with which they come into contact.[31, 35, 45] Carrier pigs may transmit SHV-1 to their offspring either *in utero*[28] or after birth.

Pathogenesis

Following inhalation or ingestion of virus, viral replication takes place in the tonsils and epithelium of the upper respiratory tract and olfactory parts of the nasal cavity,[17] from whence it spreads via the cerebrospinal fluid to the central nervous system and via the blood and lymph to the liver, kidneys and adrenals.

When the virus enters the host through the skin (such as when the host is bitten by an infected pig), the virus first multiplies at the inoculation site and then spreads centripetally along the peripheral nerve to the central nervous system, in which the infection becomes generalized.[30] The transfer of virus along peripheral nerves is rapid, and there is evidence that a retrograde flow in the axoplasm is responsible for this movement.[12, 30]

Clinical signs

The clinical signs in pigs vary from asymptomatic to acutely lethal depending on the age of the animal and the strain of virus involved. Although the clinical signs may be highly variable they mainly relate to the respiratory and alimentary tracts as well as to the central nervous system.[27]

Piglets up to three weeks of age suffer the most acute disease, characterized by an incubation period of one or two days, fever, anorexia, respiratory distress, nasal and oral discharge, occasional vomiting and diarrhoea, trembling and ataxia, depression, occasional convulsions and death within one to two days of the appearance of the first clinical signs. Mortality in fully susceptible new-born piglets is usually close to 100 per cent.

In pigs three weeks to five months of age the disease causes much lower mortality and is also more protracted than in very young piglets. After an incubation period of 36–48 hours there is a febrile response, together with respiratory signs (sneezing, coughing, nasal discharge), anorexia, diarrhoea or constipation, salivation and occasional vomition. Central nervous system involvement is manifested initially by depression and listlessness, followed by trembling, incoordination, muscle spasms (especially of the hind legs), and convulsions. Death usually occurs between three and eight days after the first clinical signs. Mortality rates decline progressively with increasing age and are only about 5 per cent at five months of age. Blindness is a common sequel in recovered pigs.

In mature pigs SHV-1 infection is frequently subclinical, but severe clinical disease with a mortality rate of up to 25 per cent can occur occasionally. The incubation period and clinical features are similar to those of three-week to five-month-old pigs, with the exception that constipation is common and severe pruritis manifested by continuous rubbing on objects may occur. Nasal and vaginal discharges may been seen in sows. Blindness in one or both eyes may occur in recovered animals.

In pregnant sows, transplacental infection may result in resorption of early embryos, abortion, the farrowing of mummified foetuses or of a mixture of normal piglets and mummified foetuses.[26]

Piglets infected with SHV-1 *in utero* may show clinical signs of myoclonia congenita immediately after birth.[28] The uncontrollable shaking and spontaneous clonic convulsions characteristic of this condition are usually followed by the death of the affected piglets within three to five days.

Sows and boars that have recovered from SHV-1 infection may be sterile or suffer reduced fertility.

Cattle and sheep characteristically show severe pruritis at the site of exposure (often a bite in the perineal region by an infected pig). The disease is almost always fatal and is usually preceded by rabies-like signs such as anorexia, salivation, incoordination, and aggression, followed by convulsions, coma and death.

Horses are rarely affected.

The clinical signs in dogs, cats and wild carnivores are fever, depression, salivation, occasional hyperexcitability, recumbency, coma and death.[14, 34]

Pathology

Although there are no specific gross lesions in pseudorabies,[24] the mucosae of the turbinates, epiglottis, trachea and bronchi are usually hyperaemic, haemorrhagic, and often ulcerated.[9, 26] Tonsillitis is frequently evident and may be severe **(Figure 108.1)**. The nasal mucosa may be covered by a thick, fibrinopurulent exudate. Haemorrhage and congestion of the retropharyngeal lymph nodes is common, and ulcers may be present on the gingivae. In acute cases petechiae are evident in the cortex of the kidneys and small necrotic foci may be distributed throughout the liver. Congestion of the meninges is commonly seen.

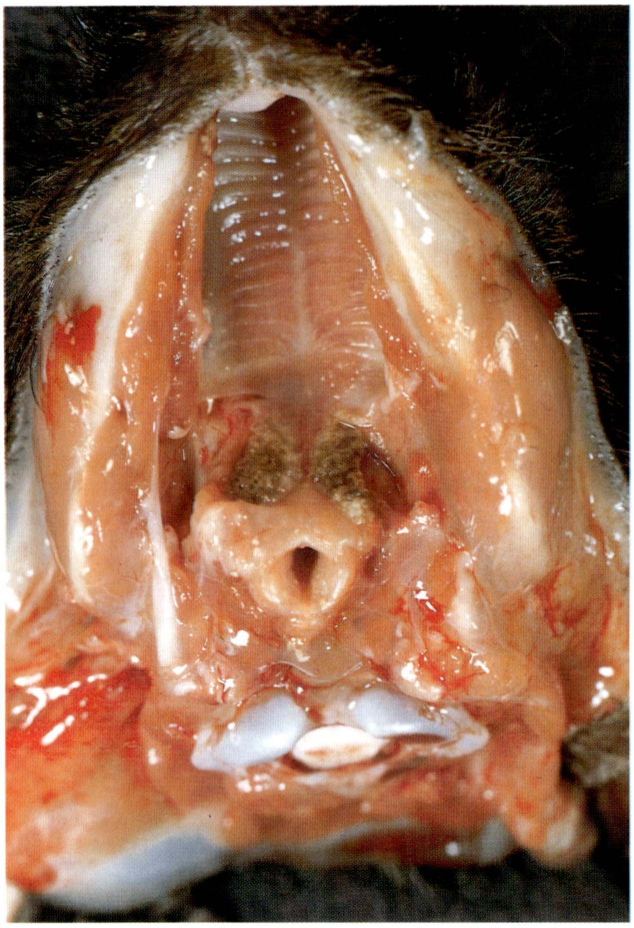

Figure 108.1 Severe tonsillitis in a pig

The most prominent microscopic lesions of pseudorabies occur in the central nervous system, particularly in the cerebral cortex, although death may supervene before there are any lesions in the brain. Ganglioneuritis of the paravertebral ganglia and diffuse non-suppurative meningoencephalitis characterized by perivascular infiltration of mononuclear cells, glial nodules, focal malacia, and neuronal degeneration have been reported.[24, 26] Extensive pyknosis and karyorrhexis of the perivascular inflammatory cells may be evident. Lesions in the mucosae of the upper respiratory tract include ulcers covered by diphtheritic membranes, necrosis of the lymphoid tissues, hyperplasia of the reticuloendothelial cells in the submucosa, and squamous metaplasia of the mucosal epithelium. Purulent bronchitis and bronchopneumonia may be present, as may necrosis and abscessation of the tonsils and retropharyngeal lymph nodes. Focal disseminate necrosis of the adrenal cortex, liver and spleen are often present in piglets,[8, 24] and focal interstitial nephritis has been reported. Intranuclear inclusions typical of herpesvirus infections may occur in the epithelial cells of the nasopharyngeal mucosae, in neurones and astrocytes in the central nervous system, and in epithelial cells of the adrenal cortex, but are not consistently present. The inclusions are more clearly discernible in tissues that have been fixed in a mercurial fixative than in those fixed in formalin.

Lesions have not been observed in the uterus or foetal membranes of sows that have aborted.[26] In aborted foetuses and stillborn piglets focal necrosis may be evident in the liver and other parenchymatous tissues as well as in the bronchioles in addition to interstitial pneumonia.[24]

Diagnosis

The clinical signs, gross and microscopic lesions, and (in the case of dogs, cats, cattle and sheep) the association of the disease with pigs should suggest pseudorabies.

In the absence of virological and serological laboratory facilities the diagnosis can be confirmed by inoculation of rabbits. A suspension of tonsil or brain from an infected animal inoculated subcutaneously into a rabbit will result in severe pruritis at the site of inoculation in one to three days, and death in less than five.

Virus isolation from fresh tonsillar or brain specimens can be readily accomplished using a wide variety of primary cell cultures (usually pig or bovine kidney) or established cell lines (such as Vero, PK15, MDBK). Characteristic cytopathic effects are usually observed within 48–72 hours. Neutralization of the cytopathic effects with anti-SHV-1 serum confirms the identity of the virus. The virus in cell cultures can also be rapidly identified by a variety of immunochemical techniques, including immunoperoxidase plaque staining.[1]

Rapid diagnosis of SHV-1 infection can be achieved by direct immunofluorescence of infected tissue, tonsils being especially useful in this respect.[22]

Serum antibodies to SHV-1 can be demonstrated by a variety of procedures. These include virus neutralization, enzyme-linked immunosorbent assay (ELISA), agar-gel immunodiffusion and reverse immunodiffusion enzyme assay.[11, 15, 18] Recently an ELISA which is able to differentiate between SHV-1 antibodies resulting from natural infection and postvaccinal antibodies has been described.[43]

Differential diagnosis

Pseudorabies in new-born piglets can easily be confused with transmissible gastroenteritis, colibacillosis or hog cholera.

In older pigs, pseudorabies may resemble rabies, salmonellosis, oedema disease, hog cholera, African swine fever, streptococcal meningitis, Teschen disease or salt poisoning.

In cattle, rabies and lead poisoning may resemble pseudorabies; while in sheep, severe pruritis is characteristic of scrapie.

Isolation and identification of SHV-1 readily differentiates pseudorabies from the above diseases.

Control

In view of the devastating effect pseudorabies may have on pig industries, countries free of the disease should endeavour to prevent its introduction. This, in essence, involves prohibiting the importation of pigs and potentially infectious pig products from countries where the disease occurs. When pigs with desired genetic characteristics have to be imported from these countries, strict and appropriate screening and quarantine must be implemented.

In countries where the disease is already present, control strategies depend on a variety of factors such as the size and importance of the pig industry, husbandry practices, and the infrastructure and financial resources available to support control programmes.

Pseudorabies control and eradication strategies range from the strict 'detect and slaughter' policy presently employed in Great Britain[44] to the mixed approach used in the USA[47] and France,[41] where control methods include widespread vaccination, 'test and removal', 'offspring segregation', and 'depopulation and repopulation'. An economic analysis of the various eradication options[2] used in pilot projects in the USA reveals that the extent of the herd involvement together with the regional status of pseudorabies will dictate the most economic and/or effective approach.

Vaccination of pigs should be a last resort. Both live attenuated and inactivated virus vaccines have been used in the USA and Europe.[27] While these vaccines have been useful in preventing losses in the face of pseudorabies outbreaks, none of them have prevented the infection of pigs. Furthermore, vaccinated pigs exposed to virulent SHV-1 may become carriers,[33, 45] thus constituting potential reservoirs of the disease.

The new generation of genetically engineered vaccines now emerging[25, 37] may be the answer to the 'carrier pig' problem, but until this has been established, vaccine should only be used when a decision has been made to 'live with the disease'.

Species which are not known to become 'carriers' can be vaccinated. This has been done extensively in Europe with cattle[5, 42] and dogs.[34]

References

1 **AFSHAR, A. & DULAC, G.C., 1986.** Immunoperoxidase plaque staining for detection of pseudorabies virus. *Canadian Journal of Veterinary Research*, 50, 118–119.

2 **ALDERINK, F.J., 1986.** Summary of the economic studies of the pseudorabies pilot projects. *Proceedings of the United States Animal Health Association*, 90, 311–329.

3 **AUJESZKY, A., 1902.** Über eine neue Infektionskrankheit bei Haustieren. *Zentralblatt für Bakteriologie* (Orig), 32, 353–357.

4 **BEN-PORAT, T. & KAPLAN, A.S., 1973.** *The Herpesviruses*. New York: Academic Press.

5 **BIRONT, P., VANDEPUTTE, J., PENSAERT, M.B. & LEUNEN, J., 1982.** Vaccination of cattle against pseudorabies (Aujeszky's disease) with homologous virus (herpes suis) and heterologous virus (herpes bovis 1). *American Journal of Veterinary Research*, 43, 760–763.

6 **BRONSON, D.L., GRAHAM, B.J. & LUDWIG, H., 1972.** Studies on the relatedness of herpesviruses through DNA-RNA hybridization. *Biochemica et Biophysica Acta*, 259, 24–34.

7 **BUSH, C.E. & PRITCHETT, R.F., 1986.** Immunologic comparison of the proteins of pseudorabies (Aujeszky's disease) virus and bovine herpesvirus-l. *American Journal of Veterinary Research*, 47, 1708–1712.

8 **CORNER, A.H., 1965.** Pathology of experimental Aujeszky's disease in piglets. *Research in Veterinary Science*, 6, 337–343.

9 **CSONTOS, L. & SZÉKY, A., 1966.** Macro- and microscopic lesions in the nasopharyngeal cavity of pigs affected by Aujeszky's disease. *Magyar Allatarvosok Lapja*, 21, 53–56.

10 **DAVIES, E.B. & BERAN, G.W., 1981.** Influence of environmental factors upon the survival of Aujeszky's disease virus. *Research in Veterinary Science*, 31, 32–36.

11 **DURHAM, P.J.K., SILLARS, J.M. & HOBBS, I.F., 1985.** Comparison of enzyme-linked immunosorbent assay (ELISA) and serum neutralization test for serodiagnosis of Aujeszky's disease. *New Zealand Veterinary Journal*, 33, 132–135.

12 **FIELD, H.J. & HILL, T.J., 1975.** The pathogenesis of pseudorabies in mice: Virus replication at the inoculation site and axonal uptake. *Journal of General Virology*, 26, 145–148.

13 **GLOSTER, J., DONALDSON, A.I. & HOUGH, M.N., 1984.** Analysis of a series of outbreaks of Aujeszky's disease in Yorkshire in 1981–82: The possibility of airborne disease spread. *The Veterinary Record*, 114, 234–239.

14 **GOYAL, S.M., DROLET, R. & KING, P., 1986.** Pseudorabies in free-ranging raccoons. *Journal of the American Veterinary Medical Association*, 189, 1163–1164.

15 **GOYAL, S.M., HAN SOO JOO, MOURNING, J.R., McPHERSON, J.R. & GOYAL, K., 1987.** Comparison of three serotests for detection of pseudorabies antibodies in pigs. *Comparative Immunology, Microbiology and Infectious Diseases*, 10, 167–171.

16 **GRAHAM, B.J, LUDWIG, H. & BRONSON, D.L., 1972.** Physicochemical properties of the DNA of herpesvirus. *Biochemica et Biophysica Acta*, 259, 13–23.

17 **GUSTAFSON, D.P., 1986.** Pseudorabies. In: LEMAN, A.D., STRAW, B., GLOCK, R.D., MENGELING, W.L., PENNY, R.H.C. & SCHOLL, E., (eds). *Diseases of Swine*. 6th edn. Ames, Iowa: Iowa State University Press.

18 **GUTEKUNST, D.E., PIRTLE, E.C. & MENGELING, W.L., 1978.** Development and evolution of a microimmunodiffusion test for detection of antibodies to pseudorabies virus in swine serum. *American Journal of Veterinary Research*, 39, 207–210.

19 **HAGEMOSER, W.A. & MOSS, E.W., 1978.** Nonfatal pseudorabies in cattle; clinical reports. *Journal of the American Veterinary Medical Association*, 173, 205–206.

20 **HAMPL, H., BEN-PORAT, T., EHRLICHER, L., HABERMEHL, K.O. & KAPLAN, A.S., 1984.** Characterization of the envelope proteins of pseudorabies virus. *Journal of Virology*, 52, 583–590.

21 **HANSON, R.P., 1954.** The history of pseudorabies in the United States. *Journal of the American Veterinary Medical Association*, 124, 259–261.

22 **HILL, H.T., CRANDELL, R.A., KANITZ, C.L., McADARAGH, J.P., SEAWRIGHT, G.L., SOLORZANO, R.F. & STEWART, W.C., 1977.** Recommended minimum standards for diagnostic tests employed in the diagnosis of pseudorabies (Aujeszky's disease). *Proceedings of the 20th Annual Meeting, American Association of Veterinary Laboratory Diagnosticians*, 375–390.

23 **HOWARTH, J.A. & DEPAOLI, A., 1968.** An epizootic of pseudorabies in swine in California. *Journal of the American Veterinary Medical Association*, 152, 1114–1118.

24 **JUBB, K.V.F., KENNEDY, P.C. & PALMER, N., 1985.** *Pathology of Domestic Animals*. 3rd edn. Vol. I. Orlando, San Diego,

New York, London: Academic Press, Inc.

25 **KIT, S., SHEPPARD, M., ICHIMURA, J. & KIT, M., 1987.** Second generation pseudorabies virus vaccine with deletions in the thymidine kinase and glycoprotein genes. *American Journal of Veterinary Research*, 48, 780–793.

26 **KLUGE, J.P. & MARÉ, C.J., 1974.** Swine pseudorabies: Abortion, clinical disease and lesions in pregnant gilts infected with pseudorabies virus. *American Journal of Veterinary Research*, 35, 911–915.

27 **LEE, J.Y.S. & WILSON, M.R., 1979.** A review of pseudorabies (Aujeszky's disease) in pigs. *Canadian Veterinary Journal*, 20, 65–69.

28 **MARÉ, C.J. & KLUGE, J.P., 1974.** Pseudorabies virus and myoclonia congenita in pigs. *Journal of the American Veterinary Medical Association*, 164, 309–310.

29 **MATTHEWS, R.E.F., 1982.** Classification and nomenclature of viruses. Fourth report of the International Committee on the Taxonomy of Viruses. *Intervirology*, 17, 1–99.

30 **McCRACKEN, R.M., McFERRAN, J.B. & DOW, C., 1973.** The neural spread of pseudorabies virus in calves. *Journal of General Virology*, 20, 17–28.

31 **McFARLANE, R.G., THAWLEY, D.G. & SOLORZANO, R.F., 1986.** Detection of latent pseudorabies virus in porcine tissue using a DNA hybridization dot-blot assay. *American Journal of Veterinary Research*, 47, 2329–2336.

32 **McFERRAN, J.B. & DOW, C., 1964.** The distribution of the virus of Aujeszky's disease in experimentally infected sheep. *Research in Veterinary Science*, 5, 143–148.

33 **MOCK, R.E., CRANDELL, R.A. & MESFIN, G.M., 1981.** Induced latency in pseudorabies-vaccinated pigs. *Canadian Journal of Comparative Medicine*, 45, 56–59.

34 **PENSAERT, M.B., COMMEYNE, S. & ANDRIES, K., 1980.** Vaccination of dogs against pseudorabies (Aujeszky's disease) using an inactivated virus vaccine. *American Journal of Veterinary Research*, 41, 2016–2019.

35 **SABO, A. & RAJCANI, J., 1976.** Latent pseudorabies virus infection in pigs. *Acta Virologica*, 20, 208–214.

36 **SAUNDERS, R.J., GUSTAFSON, D.P. & OLANDER, H.J., 1964.** An unusual outbreak of Aujeszky's disease in swine. *Proceedings of the 67th Annual Meeting of the US Livestock Sanitary Association*, New Mexico, 15–18 October 1963, 331–346.

37 **SHIMIZU, M., 1986.** Effect of subunit vaccine prepared from virus-infected cell membrane on Aujeszky's disease in pigs. *Japan Agricultural Research Quarterly*, 20, 68–71.

38 **THOMSON, G.R., 1979.** Veterinary Research Institute, Onderstepoort, South Africa. Unpublished data.

39 **THOMSON, G.R. & SPENCER, B.T., 1978.** Veterinary Research Institute, Onderstepoort, South Africa. Unpublished data.

40 **VANDEPUTTE, J. & PENSAERT, M.B., 1979.** Virusexcretie bij katten met die ziekte van Aujeszky en hun rol in die virusoverdracht naar biggen. *Vlaamse Diergeneeskundige Tijdschrift*, 48, 140–150.

41 **VANNIER, 1987.** Aujeszky's disease: Principal characteristics of the control campaign in France. *Point Vétérinaire*, 19, 335–340.

42 **VAN OIRSCHOT, J.T., DE LEEW, P.W. & TIESSINK, J.W.A., 1985.** Vaccination confers protection against Aujeszky's disease in cattle. *Zeitschrift für Veterinärmedicin*, Reihe B., 32, 173–180.

43 **VAN OIRSCHOT, J.T. & DE WAAL, 1987.** An ELISA to distinguish between Aujeszky's disease-vaccinated and -infected pigs. *The Veterinary Record*, 121, 305–306.

44 **WATSON, W.A., 1986.** Epidemiology and control of Aujeszky's disease. *State Veterinary Journal*, 40, 3–18.

45 **WITTMAN, G., OHLINGER, V. & RZIHA, H.J., 1983.** Occurrence and reactivation of latent Aujeszky's disease virus following challenge in previously vaccinated pigs. *Archives of Virology*, 75, 29–41.

46 **WRIGHT, J.C. & THAWLEY, D.G., 1980.** Role of the raccoon in the transmission of pseudorabies. A field and laboratory investigation. *American Journal of Veterinary Research*, 41, 581–583.

47 **WRIGHT, J.C., THAWLEY, D.G. & SOLORZANO, R.F., 1982.** Field evaluation of test-and-removal and vaccination as control measures for pseudorabies in Missouri swine. *Canadian Journal of Comparative Medicine*, 46, 420–425.

109

Suid herpesvirus 2 infection

Synonyms: Porcine cytomegalovirus infection, inclusion body rhinitis

N. Edington

Introduction

Suid herpesvirus 2 (SHV-2) infection, also called porcine cytomegalovirus (PCMV) infection, may cause foetal or neonatal deaths and is associated with runting, rhinitis and pneumonia in piglets less than three weeks of age, and rhinitis in growing pigs.

Suid herpesvirus 2 was first identified by Done[6] as a cause of cytomegalic cells with characteristic basophilic intranuclear inclusion bodies in the nasal mucosal glands of turbinates of pigs. Restriction of viral replication to pigs, localization of the virus in the nasal mucosa, lachrymal and salivary glands, and occasionally in renal tubular epithelium, as well as ultrastructural studies,[8, 23] indicated that this was a cytomegalovirus of the pig similar to those described for some other species.[18, 20, 25] These viruses usually cause clinically silent infections in healthy adults but often induce severe, generalized infections in young animals. Virus may also cross the placenta. Like other herpesviruses, SHV-2 induces latent infection. A cell-associated viraemia can occur in the presence of circulating antibody.

In herds where good management is applied, and in which the virus is endemic, there may be no clinical signs or economic loss.

Since SHV-2 is an ubiquitous infection it can be presumed to occur in southern Africa, although this remains to be proved.

Aetiology

Suid herpesvirus 2 is a gammaherpesvirus, with an 80–100 nm icosahedral capsid surrounded by an envelope making the complete virion 120–150 nm in diameter. The 45–70 nm core is usually elongated and may be oval, rectangular or dumb-bell shaped.[8, 23] The DNA is double-stranded, but has not been further characterized. The virus is sensitive to chloroform and ether.[2]

Watt[24] found pulmonary macrophage cultures derived from three- to five-week-old pigs to be the most sensitive system for both primary isolation and propagation of virus. Cytomegaly and intranuclear inclusions develop 11–14 days after inoculation **(Figure 109.1)** and infectivity titres of up to $10^{5,5}$ $TCID_{50}$ may occur. This culture system has limitations because of the fastidiousness and variability of the cells, and because of residual adventitious viruses. Primary pig lung cells[15] and a cell line derived from porcine Fallopian tube[3] also support viral replication. Suid herpesvirus 2 appears to be host-specific both *in vivo* and *in vitro*.

In cultures, infected cells enlarge by up to six times and their mitochondria, endoplasmic reticulum, and Golgi apparatus swell.[8] The large intranuclear inclusions contain the nuclear capsids, often in crystalline array.[22] The capsids acquire an electron-dense coat in the nucleus, the envelope derives from the inner nuclear membrane, and the virions come to lie free inside intracytoplasmic cisternae.

Epidemiology

Suid herpesvirus 2 has been detected wherever it has been sought. In the UK a serological survey indicated that over 95 per cent of herds had been exposed to the virus.[17] The ubiquity of the infection and the possibility of transplacental infection indicate that even hysterotomy-derived litters may be infected.

After neonatal pigs have been infected, the virus is shed predominantly in nasal secretions, but also in urine and ocular secretions.[11, 17] Levels of passive antibody fall initially during the period of virus excretion, but rise when the pigs are between eight and 11 weeks as a result of active production. They continue to increase until at least 23 weeks after infection. Susceptible sows show a similar pattern of excretion but, in addition, shedding of virus from the cervix occurs in some pregnant sows.

Recovery of virus from lung macrophages of apparently healthy pigs suggests that the virus either persists at this site or may establish a true latent infection. Infection may be reactivated after the administration of corticosteroids.[11]

Pathogenesis

The mucous glands of the nasal mucosa are the primary site of viral replication. Thereafter a cell-associated

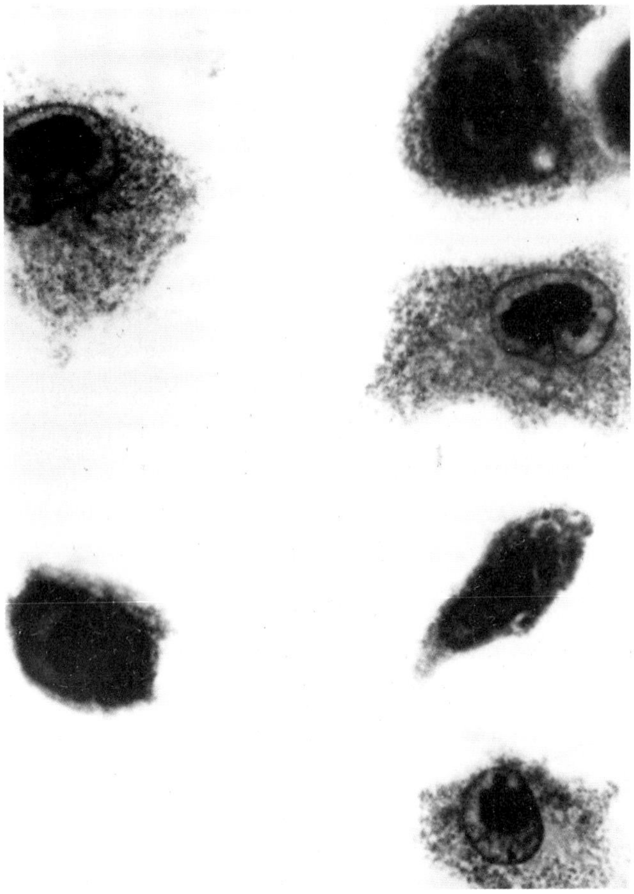

Figure 109.1 Infected porcine alveolar macrophages show cytomegaly and distinctive basophilic intranuclear inclusion bodies at 11 days after infection. May-Grunewald Giemsa (Courtesy of R.G. Watt)

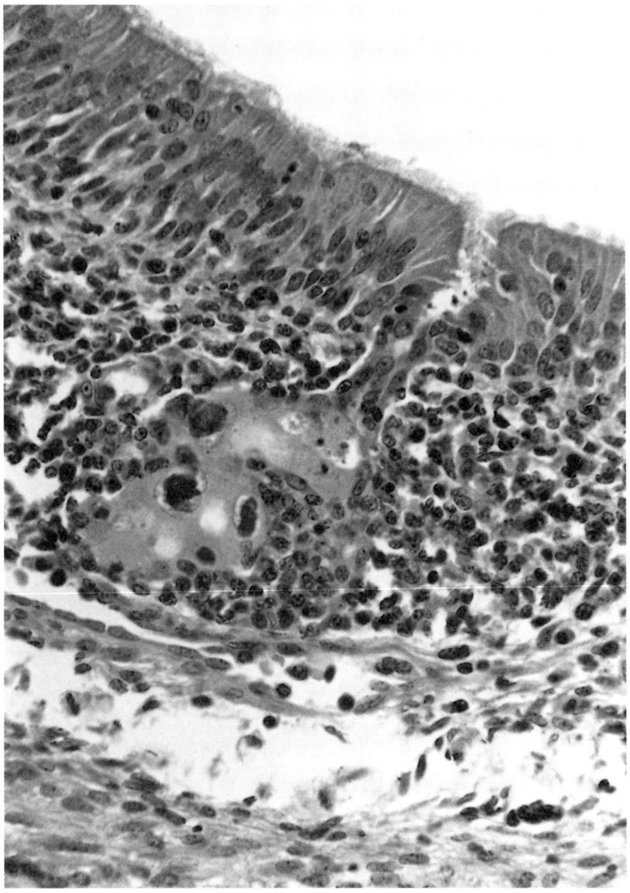

Figure 109.2 Foci of cytomegaly and intranuclear inclusions are most commonly seen in the mucous glands of the nasal mucosa. A periglandular infiltration of lymphocytes, plasma cells and occasional macrophages is also a prominent feature by 18 days after infection

viraemia develops which is detectable 14–16 days after infection in pigs older than three weeks, and from five to 19 days after infection in neonatal pigs.[11]

In animals older than three weeks, the virus occurs most commonly in the glands of the nasal mucosa but it may also be present in the Harderian and lachrymal glands and in the renal tubules. On rare occasions it is found in the mucous glands of the oesophagus and duodenal epithelium. In foetuses or neonates, the virus has a predilection for reticuloendothelial cells. Inclusions occur in capillary endothelium, the sinus and sinusoidal lining cells of lymphoid tissues, and in macrophages.

In susceptible sows, isolation of the virus from cervical fluids 30–35 days after infection corresponds with the time when viral replication occurs in foetuses. Foetal death generally occurs 60–80 days after infection, suggesting that secondary spread of virus within the uterus may occur.[12] Congenitally infected animals may be born alive but die within seven to 14 days of birth.

Semen from infected boars has not been shown to yield virus, but nasal secretions and urine are possible sources of infection for susceptible sows.

Clinical signs

Suid herpesvirus 2 infection in foetuses or neonates less than three weeks old results in a generalized disease which may be fatal. In neonates the clinical signs comprise subcutaneous oedema, pallor, dyspnoea, and generalized weakness. Field outbreaks involving litters of piglets are characterized by shivering, sneezing and respiratory distress.[4, 5] Up to 25 per cent of the litter may die and the remaining pigs show poor weight gain. Uncomplicated infection in pigs older than three weeks is usually not clinically apparent, although rhinitis may ensue and subsequent secondary bacterial infection can result in the development of atrophic rhinitis.[10]

Pregnant sows may be listless and anorectic during the period when viraemia is present, 14–21 days after infection, but do not show pyrexia or any other clinical abnormality during pregnancy. However, transplacental infection is associated with the SMEDI syndrome (stillbirths, mummification, embryonic death and infertility) as well as neonatal deaths and runt piglets.[4, 5, 12, 16, 19]

Pathology

Lesions in pigs older than three weeks are restricted to epithelial tissues and are scattered. In neonates and foetuses infection is generalized but restricted to reticulo-endothelial tissues.[9]

Macroscopic lesions are not usually seen in animals with disseminated infections. Histologically the characteristic cytomegaly and intranuclear inclusion bodies may be seen in the nasal mucous glands **(Figure 109.2)** as well as in the acini of the Harderian and lachrymal glands, and renal tubular epithelium. Infiltrates of lymphocytes and plasma cells may eventually obliterate the acini. In field infections, secondary bacterial infection with *Bordetella bronchiseptica* or *Pasteurella multocida* may induce lesions of atrophic rhinitis; these changes are not seen in pigs experimentally infected with SHV-2 alone.[10] Interstitial nephritis may be a sequel to the infection.[14]

In generalized infections, petechiae and oedema may be widespread. The oedema in neonatal pigs manifests most commonly as an interlobular oedema of the lungs, hydrothorax, ascites, or occasionally anasarca. Subcutaneous oedema is most marked around the throat and tarsal joints. Petechiae are found particularly in lymph nodes but also occur in the kidneys, where subcapsular haemorrhages may result, resembling those associated with hog cholera and African swine fever.

Intranuclear inclusions are found in capillary endothelium and in sinusoidal cells, particularly in lymph nodes, the spleen, lungs, renal glomeruli, choroid plexus, cerebellum and olfactory lobes. [21] Monocytes in the lungs may also contain inclusions.

Infection of the foetus does not produce characteristic macroscopic lesions and the foetuses are often autolysed.

Diagnosis and differential diagnosis

Both an indirect immunofluorescence and an ELISA test have been described for the serological detection of SHV-2 antibody.[1, 17] Neutralizing antibody has been detected, but serum titres are rarely greater than one log. However, association of positive serological results with disease may be difficult because the infection is ubiquitous.

Isolation of virus is difficult because of the problems of obtaining and maintaining sensitive cell lines. Detection of virus may be effected by applying either indirect immunofluorescent antibody or special techniques to nasal swabs or scrapings of older pigs,[7] or alternatively to tissues such as the lungs, liver and central nervous system of aborted foetuses and neonates.[12, 13] The characteristic cytomegaly and inclusion bodies may be demonstrated in histological sections of foetal or neonatal tissues.

It is only in the area of reproductive losses that confusion arises. Infections with porcine parvovirus, suid herpesvirus-1 (Aujeszky's disease), hog cholera virus, and *Leptospira* spp. are all associated with reproductive losses.

Control

Outbreaks of reproductive losses and rhinitis which have been associated with SHV-2 have generally been self-limiting.[4, 5] Concurrent bacterial infections may be controlled by the use of antibiotics. Virus-free herds can be established by hysterotomy, but the ability of SHV-2 to cross the placenta must always be considered, and offspring should be monitored serologically for at least 70 days after birth to ensure freedom from this infection.

References

1 **ASSAF, R., BOUILLANT, A.M. & DI FRANCO, E., 1982.** Enzyme-linked immunosorbent assay (ELISA) for the detection of antibodies to porcine cytomegalovirus. *Canadian Journal of Comparative Medicine*, 46, 183–185.

2 **BOOTH, J.C., GOODWIN, R.F.W. & WHITTLESTONE, P., 1967.** Inclusion-body rhinitis of pigs: Attempts to grow the causal agent in tissue cultures. *Research in Veterinary Science*, 8, 338–345.

3 **BOUILLANT, A.M., DULAC, G., WILLIS, N., GIRARD, A., GREIG, A.S. & BOULANGER, P., 1975.** Viral susceptibility of a cell line derived from the pig oviduct. *Canadian Journal of Comparative Medicine*, 39, 450–456.

4 **CAMERON-STEPHEN, I.D., 1961.** Inclusion-body rhinitis of swine. *Australian Veterinary Journal*, 37, 87–91.

5 **CORNER, A.H., MITCHELL, D., JULIAN, R.J. & MEADS, E.B., 1964.** A generalised disease in piglets associated with the presence of cytomegalic inclusions. *Journal of Comparative Pathology*, 74, 192–199.

6 **DONE, J.T., 1955.** An 'inclusion body' rhinitis of pigs. *The Veterinary Record*, 67, 525–527.

7 **DONE, J.T., 1958.** Inclusion-body rhinitis of swine; nasal scrapings as an aid to diagnosis. *The Veterinary Record*, 70, 877–878.

8 **DUNCAN, J.R., RAMSEY, F.K. & SWITZER, W.P., 1965.** Electron microscopy of cytomegalic inclusion disease of swine (inclusion body rhinitis). *American Journal of Veterinary Research*, 26, 939–946.

9 **EDINGTON, N., PLOWRIGHT, W. & WATT, R.G., 1976.** Generalised cytomegalic inclusion disease: Distribution of cytomegalic cells and virus. *Journal of Comparative Pathology*, 86, 191–202.

10 **EDINGTON, N., SMITH, I.M., PLOWRIGHT, W. & WATT, R.G., 1976.** Relationship of porcine cytomegalovirus and *B. bronchiseptica* to atrophic rhinitis in gnotobiotic piglets. *The Veterinary Record*, 98, 42–45.

11 **EDINGTON, N., WATT, R.G. & PLOWRIGHT, W., 1976.** Cytomegalovirus excretion in gnotobiotic pigs. *Journal of Hygiene*, 77, 283–290.

12 **EDINGTON, N., WATT, R.G., PLOWRIGHT, W., WRATHALL, A.E. & DONE, J.T., 1977.** Experimental transmission of porcine cytomegalovirus. *Journal of Hygiene*, 78, 243–251.

13 **EDINGTON, N., WRATHALL, A.E. & DONE, J.T., 1988.** Porcine cytomegalovirus in early gestation. *Veterinary Microbiology*, 17, 117–128.

14 **KELLY, D.F., 1967.** Pathology of extranasal lesions in experimental inclusion body rhinitis of pigs. *Research in Veterinary Science*, 8, 472–478.

15 **L'ECUYER, C. & CORNER, A.H., 1966.** Propagation of porcine cytomegalic inclusion disease virus in cell cultures. Preliminary report. *Canadian Journal of Comparative Medicine*, 30, 321–326.

16 **L'ECUYER, C., CORNER, A.H. & RANDALL, G.C.B., 1972.** Porcine cytomegalic inclusion disease. Transplacental transmission. *Proceedings of the 2nd International Congress of the Pig Veterinary Society*, Hanover.

17 **PLOWRIGHT, W., EDINGTON, N. & WATT, R.G., 1976.** The behaviour of porcine cytomegalovirus in commercial pig herds. *Journal of Hygiene*, 75, 125–135.

18 **PLUMMER, G., 1973.** Cytomegaloviruses of man and animals. *Progress in Medical Virology*, 15, 92–125.

19 **RAC, R., 1961.** Infectious rhinitis in pigs: Laboratory aspects. *Australian Veterinary Journal*, 37, 91–93.

20 **SMITH, M.G., 1959.** The salivary gland viruses of man and animals. *Progress in Medical Virology*, 2, 171–202.

21 **STEPHANO HORNEDO, A. & EDINGTON, N., 1987.** Encefalitis experimental por citomegalovirus porcino en cerdos gnotobióticos: Estudio histopatológico. *Veterinaria Mexico*, 18, 189–202.

22 **VALICEK, L., SMID, B. & MEUSIK, J., 1973.** Electron microscopy of porcine cytomegalovirus. *Archiv für die Gesamte Virusforschung*, 41, 344–353.

23 **VALICEK, L., SMID, B., PLEVAV & MEUSIK, J., 1970.** Porcine cytomegalic inclusion disease virus. Electron microscopic study of the nasal mucosa. *Archiv für die Gesamte Virusforschung*, 32, 19–30.

24 **WATT, R.G., PLOWRIGHT, W., SABO, A. & EDINGTON, N., 1973.** A sensitive cell-culture system for the virus of porcine inclusion body rhinitis (cytomegalic inclusion disease). *Research in Veterinary Science*, 14, 119–121.

25 **WELLER, T.H., HANSHAW, J.B. & SCOTT, D.E., 1960.** Serologic differentiation of viruses responsible for cytomegalic inclusion disease. *Virology*, 12, 130–132.

110

Other herpesvirus infections

G.R. Thomson

There are a number of herpesviruses that infect domestic livestock which either produce no known disease or are only rarely implicated in disease. These are grouped together in this chapter.

BOVINE HERPESVIRUS 4 INFECTION

Synonyms: Bovine herpesvirus 3 (BHV-3), BHV-5, bovine orphan herpesvirus, 'Movar-type' bovine herpesvirus, bovine cytomegalovirus infections.

Introduction

Infection with bovine herpesvirus 4 (BHV-4) occurs in most (probably all) cattle populations but its association with disease is tenuous because it can regularly be recovered from healthy animals as well as from those suffering from a wide variety of clinical conditions.

One of the earliest descriptions of BHV-4 was by scientists working in East and South Africa.[1]

The nomenclature of this virus is confusing, as is evident from the large number of synonyms. Bovine herpesvirus 4 is most commonly used in recent publications, following the recommendations of Bartha *et al.*[2] and the latest report of the Herpesvirus Study Group of the International Committee on the Taxonomy of Viruses.[40]

Aetiology

The typical enveloped herpesvirus nucleocapsid of BHV-4[27, 50] contains a double-stranded DNA genome comprising 144 ± 6 kilobase pairs (kbp). A large region of unique DNA (approximately 110 kbp in length) is flanked at both ends by multiple (usually 15) tandem copies of a 1,5–3 kbp polyrepetitive region.[52, 56] Gel electrophoresis profiles of restriction endonuclease-generated DNA fragments of BHV-4 isolates distinguish this virus from other herpesvirus infections of ruminants.[27] Two basic restriction endonuclease patterns are recognized for BHV-4 isolates — Movar 33/63-like and DN 599-like — these being reference strains originating from Europe and the USA respectively.[5]

Of the 29 structural proteins that have so far been shown to make up the capsid, 10 are glycosylated. There are two glycoprotein complexes at the surface of the capsid which contain epitopes involved in neutralization; there are three domains in the 150K/120K/51K glycoprotein complex and two in the 120K/16,5K complex.[52] The neutralizing domains are clearly complex because monoclonal antibodies are usually only capable of effecting neutralization if used in pairs.[11]

The thymidine kinase of BHV-4 isolates is distinguishable from that of other herpesviruses because it lacks iododeoxycytidine-phosphorylating activity.[24]

The antigenic similarity of different isolates of BHV-4 has been shown by the ability of polyclonal sera to cross-react with heterologous isolates.[13, 36, 50] However, serological comparison of different isolates has been hampered by the generally poor antigenicity of these viruses.[27]

Recent studies have shown clear genetic and antigenic similarities between BHV-4 and members of the subfamily Gammaherpesvirinae, such as alcelaphine herpesvirus 1 and saimirine herpesvirus 2 (herpesvirus saimiri),[4, 41] and BHV-4 is presently considered to belong to this subfamily.[18] Previously, based on biological characteristics, BHV-4 had been assigned to the Betaherpesvirinae, and sometimes referred to as bovine cytomegalovirus.[15, 53]

Bovine herpesvirus 4 is capable of replication in a wide range of unestablished cell cultures derived from bovine, sheep, goat, dog, cat, rabbit, pig and chicken kidneys as well as the MDBK (bovine) cell line.[19] Optimum growth requires actively dividing cells, and plaque production[27] is promoted by the inclusion of protamine in the overlay.[38, 42]

Production of cytopathic effects (CPE) typically requires three to ten days for primary isolates, but on passage the CPE may appear within 48 hours and high virus levels (up to $10^{8,5}$ $TCID_{50}$/ml) may be attained.[19, 28] The CPE initially consist of the appearance of isolated rounded cells which progress to clumps of rounded, degenerated cells. In stained preparations these cells frequently contain Cowdry type A intranuclear inclusions.

Gradually the entire cell-sheet is affected and the degenerated cells are linked by intercellular cytoplasmic strands which may be long.[19]

Characteristically, isolates of BHV-4 do not produce syncytia in cell culture,[1, 50] although these have been observed in some cases.[20] An isolate named Pennsylvania 47, which produces syncytia but which also cross-reacts serologically with BHV-4, was advanced as a putative 'new' herpesvirus of cattle,[36] but this has apparently not been formally approved.

The serological cross-relationship demonstrated between BHV-4 isolates and alcelaphine herpesvirus 1 (AHV-1, the cause of wildebeest associated malignant catarrhal fever) is interesting — especially in view of the preliminary finding that some cattle hyperimmunized with BHV-4 are able to withstand challenge with AHV-1.[41]

Epidemiology, pathogenesis and pathology

The natural host of BHV-4 is almost certainly cattle, but the virus has also been recovered from American bison (*Bison bison*),[53] African buffalo (*Syncerus caffer*),[41] sheep[55] and domestic cats. In the latter context, felid herpesvirus 2 (FHV-2) has been shown to be a strain of BHV-4,[24] although it remains uncertain whether FHV-2 really has a non-feline origin or not: it could possibly have infected cats via foetal calf serum used in the manufacture of feline viral vaccines.[51] However, an attempt to infect cats experimentally by intranasal or intravenous inoculation with the Movar 33/63 strain failed.[51] Similarly, a herpesvirus isolate from an owl monkey (*Aotus trivirgatus*) is also apparently in reality BHV-4.[5]

Rabbits are susceptible to experimental inoculation with BHV-4, and this species provides a useful model to study the behaviour of BHV-4 in cattle.[48] Restriction endonuclease patterns of DNA obtained from BHV-4 isolates derived from species other than cattle show either the Movar 33/63 or DN-599 pattern, indicating that other species probably do not harbour distinct viruses.[52]

Bovine herpesvirus 4 has been identified as an infection of cattle in Africa,[1, 42] Europe, North America and Australia.[19] Few investigations into sero-prevalence rates have been conducted, probably because BHV-4 infection induces only poor and ephemeral neutralizing antibody responses although, if complement is included in the neutralization reaction, the measurable response is improved.[12, 14] Antibody responses measured by immunofluorescence may exceed titres of 1:1 000 and persist for more than three months following experimental infection.[12] An ELISA system developed for the detection of antibody to BHV-4 showed that high antibody levels prevailed after the experimental infection of calves and that most reactivity resided in IgG_1.[14] Antibody prevalence rates of 17 per cent or less were found in cattle in East Africa and the USA,[33, 41] but in herds in the USA with a history of 'reproductive disorders', prevalence rates were between 36 and 88 per cent.[33] Similarly, in Belgium the seroprevalence rate in cattle with chronic metritis is higher than the rate in the national herd, which is in the order of 34 per cent.[54, 58] Antibody prevalence rates of over 90 per cent were reported in East African buffalo, but in the same study only a low proportion of blue wildebeest (*Connachaetes taurinus*) sera had antibody, while none was detected in the sera of three species of tragelaphine antelope.[41] Wild ruminant species from western Europe apparently have no serological evidence of infection with BHV-4.[52]

It is presumed that BHV-4 is transmitted directly between cattle through contact with respiratory or genital secretions.[52] However, since there is evidence that the virus is able to cross the placental barrier it is possible that at least a proportion of animals is infected *in utero*.[23, 33] Bovine herpesvirus 4 has been associated with abortion in cattle but this remains to be proved.[23, 39, 52] It has also been isolated from diarrhoeic faeces.[17]

Following multiplication at the primary infection site, the virus is transported to all parts of the animal's body by mononuclear cells.[34] It is probable, based on experiments performed in rabbits, that the primary replication site in cattle is the spleen,[35, 37] and that the primary target cells are splenic macrophages.[37] The virus becomes latent in mononuclear cells present in the circulation, and for that reason BHV-4 can be isolated from virtually all organs and tissues. Latency also occurs in neural ganglia — especially the trigeminal.[52] Isolation of BHV-4 virus latent in blood mononuclear cells of both cattle and African buffalo can be achieved by cocultivation with susceptible cells,[12, 34, 41] but it is not known whether the continuous presence of BHV-4 in blood mononuclear cells is due to persistent infection of stem cells in the bone marrow or immortalization of latently infected cells in the circulation.[52]

Recrudescence of latent infection *in vivo* can be achieved by treatment of animals with dexamethasone[12, 26] and the virus can then be detected in nasal and conjunctival secretions.[12] A 'booster' antibody response measured by immunofluorescence may be detected in animals in which the infection has been induced to recrudesce with dexamethasone, but no increase in neutralizing activity occurs.[12] Other diseases which involve inflammatory processes appear to induce recrudescence,[27] as may parturition.[52] Experimental evidence suggests that BHV-4 may induce postpartum metritis with prolonged excretion of the virus (as cited by Thiry *et al.*[52]). In South Africa, experimental infection of cows resulted in the development of mild vaginitis accompanied by a mucous discharge and enlarged vaginal lymphoid follicles. The vaginitis was more severe when a pool of BHV-4 and BHV-1 viruses was administered, resulting in a copious mucopurulent discharge.[49] Other experimental infections have produced variable responses in the animals inoculated; some have resulted in respiratory disease,[6, 31, 47] but most have produced no untoward effect.[48]

Apart from possible association with the diseases already mentioned, a variety of other clinical conditions have been associated with BHV-4 infection, viz. orchitis, 'skin afflictions', 'altered lymph nodes', lymphosarcoma, and tumours of the urinary bladder.[27, 51] These disease associations are tenuous, however, because of the ease with which BHV-4 can be isolated from the organs and blood of latently infected cattle.

Diagnosis and control

The presence of the infection can readily be ascertained by inoculation of a wide range of cell cultures with tissue suspensions obtained from infected cattle. Alternatively, leukocytes from blood collected in an anticoagulant from latently infected cattle and cocultivated with susceptible cell cultures may reveal the presence of the virus. The CPE, which may develop within three to ten days, are reasonably characteristic, but the virus is best identified by restriction endonuclease treatment of viral DNA and subsequent analysis by gel electrophoresis.[27]

Control of BHV-4 infection has not been investigated because its importance in the health of cattle still requires to be established.

CAPRINE HERPESVIRUS 1 INFECTION

Synonyms: Bovine herpesvirus 6, goat herpesvirus infection

Introduction and aetiology

Herpesviruses have been isolated from goats with respiratory, gastrointestinal and genital infections, as well as from clinically healthy goats in the USA, Switzerland, New Zealand and Norway.[21, 25, 27, 32, 43] All but the first of these virus isolates[32] have been shown to be antigenically related to, but distinguishable from, bovine herpesvirus 1 (BHV-1) which is the cause of infectious bovine rhinotracheitis and infectious pustular vulvovaginitis/balanoposthitis in cattle.

Caprine herpesvirus 1 (CHV-1) and BHV-1 are very similar, certainly as far as their genome size and composition are concerned; both have a buoyant density of 1,7295 g/ml, G+C percentage of 71–72 and molecular weights of approximately 90 x 10^6, corresponding to a genome of about 140 kilobase pairs.[16] However, the fragments generated by restriction endonuclease treatment of the DNAs of CHV-1 and BHV-1 are very different; CHV-1 has an unusual cleavage pattern which has only one recognition site for each of the restriction endonucleases *Eco* R1 and *Hind* III.[16]

Like BHV-1, CHV-1 multiplies to high titre in a wide variety of cell types *in vitro*[16, 43] and fulfils the criteria for the subfamily Alphaherpesvirinae.[40]

Antigenically, one-way cross neutralization between CHV-1 and BHV-1 has been shown — BHV-1-specific antisera neutralize BHV-1 to a greater extent than the converse.[16] Nevertheless, the two viruses are antigenically distinct.[43]

Epidemiology, pathogenesis, clinical signs and pathology

Although antibodies to CHV-1 have been demonstrated in goats in a number of countries (Norway, Northern Ireland, Spain, Italy, Greece, Turkey and Syria[25]) it is not clear how universal this infection is in goat populations. A diagnosis of probable CHV-1 infection (based on typical gastrointestinal tract lesions) in kids on a farm in South Africa was made in 1984.[7] Unfortunately the tissues submitted for diagnosis were fixed in formalin and so virus isolation was not attempted.

Infection rates in excess of 90 per cent have been found in individual goat herds without obvious ill effect on the herd.[25] It appears that transmission may be associated with breeding,[25] although there is no information on the mechanism(s) involved. Kids born to sero-positive dams have colostral antibody for approximately the first four months of life.[25]

The first association of CHV-1 with disease in goats was a gastrointestinal condition with a high mortality rate in young kids, most of which were approximately one week old.[43] The animals had necrosis and ulceration in the rumen, caecum and colon, with lesions most pronounced in the caecum and anterior colon. Inclusion bodies were present in the nuclei and cytoplasm of 'epithelial and connective tissue cells' of affected tissues.[43] Experimental infection by intranasal or intravenous administration of virus resulted in abortion of nanny goats without other clinical signs.[43] Intravenous inoculation of the virus into kids resulted in a fatal generalized infection. Lambs and calves, although they became infected by virus administered intranasally or intravenously, showed no clinical ill effect.[43]

Similar high mortality in kids which showed conjunctivitis, rhinitis, erosions in the mouth and, in some cases, petechiae in the skin prior to death, has been described.[27] Gross lesions at necropsy were predominantly in the gastrointestinal tract and comprised ulcerations and necrosis of the mucosae of the rumen, abomasum, caecum and colon. Lung lesions that consist of thickening of the interstitium and round-cell infiltration were evident microscopically.[27]

Transient vulvovaginitis in a herd of Saanen goats soon after mating was ascribed to CHV-1 in New Zealand.[21]

Diagnosis and control

Caprine herpesvirus 1, like other alphaherpesviruses, can readily be recovered from infected tissues by inoculation of a wide range of cell cultures with tissue suspensions from infected animals. Restriction endonuclease treatment of viral DNA followed by gel electrophoresis will readily distinguish CHV-1 from other herpesviruses.[27]

Methods of controlling CHV-1 have not yet been investigated.

OVINE HERPESVIRUS 1 INFECTION

Synonyms: Herpesvirus ovis, bovine herpesvirus 4, bovine herpesvirus 5, caprine herpesvirus 1 infections

Introduction

Ovine herpesvirus 1 (OHV-1) was for a time thought to be the cause of jaagsiekte (pulmonary adenomatosis) in sheep because it can regularly be isolated from the lungs of sheep suffering from that disease.[9, 29, 30] However, failure of experimentally infected lambs to develop lesions characteristic of jaagsiekte,[9] the inability to demonstrate the presence of the viral genome in all tumours[10] and the identification of an oncovirus which is considered to be the cause of jaagsiekte **(see Chapter 80: Jaagsiekte)** make it unlikely that OHV-1 is involved in the pathogenesis of jaagsiekte.

Infection with this virus is widespread in sheep in South Africa and Namibia.

Aetiology

The South African isolate of OHV-1 can be cultured *in vitro* in lung fibroblasts derived from sheep foetuses or in foetal sheep kidney cells,[9] while an isolate from Scotland seems to have a predilection for ovine alveolar macrophages.[45]

Ovine herpesvirus 1 is highly cell-associated in cell culture.[9] The viral DNA has a buoyant density of 1,706 ± 001 g/ml, a sedimentation constant of 47,5 ± 1,5S and molecular weight of 67,3 ± 5,4 x 10^6. The G+C content of the DNA is 47 per cent.[8] Although no serological differences have been demonstrated between the South African and the Scottish isolates, they can be distinguished by restriction endonuclease analysis of their genomic DNA.[46]

Epidemiology

Using immunofluorescence and neutralization tests, antibodies have been detected in up to 76 per cent of healthy adult sheep in South Africa and Namibia.[57] The breed of sheep does not seem to influence the infection rate. Antibodies to OHV-1 have also been detected in sheep from Great Britain, Northern Ireland, the USA, Australia and New Zealand.[44]

Pathogenesis, clinical signs and pathology

Ovine herpesvirus 1 has been shown to be capable of inducing fatal interstitial pneumonia in immunosuppressed lambs during the first few weeks of life, but not in untreated lambs. Older lambs, even when immunosuppressed, did not develop obvious illness or lesions following experimental infection.[9] However, Scott *et al.*[45] found pulmonary changes in 17 of 18 lambs infected experimentally with a Scottish isolate.

Young lambs often possess high antibody titres against OHV-1 but lose this passively acquired immunity within the first few months of life. It is not known at what age infection usually occurs and, similarly, the routes of virus excretion and infection have yet to be established. The presence of the virus in peripheral blood leukocytes and nasal swabs up to 34 days after experimental infection has been demonstrated.[45]

As occurs after infection with other herpesviruses, OHV-1 induces latent infection, and isolation of the virus is possible from animals treated with corticosteriods several weeks after primary infection.[45]

HERPESVIRUS INFECTIONS OF DONKEYS

There are at least three herpesvirus infections of donkeys,[3] although very little is known about their pathogenic potential.

The first isolation was made from vesicular and erosive lesions on the muzzle of a foal and the external genitalia and udder of its dam.[3] This virus was originally called asinine herpesvirus 1 but is now officially designated equid herpesvirus 6 (EHV-6).[40] Although the lesions in these donkeys were reminiscent of coital exanthema (caused by EHV-3), restriction endonuclease and hybridization studies showed that EHV-6 and EHV-3 are distinct viruses.[22]

A slowly cytopathic herpesvirus was isolated from the leukocytes of an apparently healthy donkey in Australia.[3] This virus (originally called asinine herpesvirus 2) has features in common with slowly cytopathic herpesviruses of horses (EHV-2 and EHV-5), but was shown by Southern blot cross-hybridization analysis to be different from both EHV-2 and EHV-5. It is now designated EHV-7.[40]

Treatment of three healthy donkeys that had antibody to equid herpesvirus 1 with corticosteroids resulted in a rapidly cytopathic virus appearing in the nasal secretions of the animals eight days after commencement of the steroid treatment.[3] Direct nose-to-nose swabbing from the animals with this virus in their nasal secretions to two naïve donkeys resulted in an afebrile rhinitis occurring in the recipient animals.[3] This virus was originally named asinine herpesvirus 3, but is now designated EHV-8.[40]

Browning *et al.*[3] have proposed a hierarchy of relationships between the known alphaherpesviruses of Equidae (EHV-1, EHV-3, EHV-4, EHV-6, EHV-8). On this basis they raise the possibility that EHV-1 may have been derived from either a donkey herpesvirus or from a herpesvirus of one of the Equidae more closely related to donkeys than horses.

References

1 **ALEXANDER, R.A., PLOWRIGHT, W. & HAIG, D.A., 1957.** Cytopathogenic agents associated with lumpy skin disease of cattle. *Bulletin of Epizootic Diseases in Africa*, 5, 489–492.

2 **BARTHA, A., FADOL, A.M., LIEBERMANN, H., LUDWIG, H., MOHANTI, S.B., OSARIO, F.A., REED, D.E., STORZ, J., STRAUB, O., VAN DER MAATEN, M.J. & WELLEMANS, G., 1987.** Problems concerning the taxonomy of the 'Movar-type' bovine herpesviruses. *Intervirology*, 28, 1–7.

3 **BROWNING, G.F., FICORILLI, N. & STUDDERT, M.J., 1988.** Asinine herpesvirus genomes: Comparison with those of the equine herpesviruses. *Archives of Virology*, 101, 183–190.

4 **BUBLOT, M., LOMONTE, P., LEQUARRE, A.-S., ALBRECHT, J.-C., NICHOLAS, J., FLECKENSTEIN, B., PASTORET, P.-P. & THIRY, E., 1992.** Genetic relationships between bovine herpesvirus 4 and the gammaherpesviruses Epstein-Barr virus and herpesvirus saimiri. *Virology*, 190, 654–665.

5 **BUBLOT, M., WELLEMANS, G., VAN BRESSEM, M.F., DUBUISSON, J., PASTORET, P.P. & THIRY, E., 1991.** Genomic diversity among bovine herpesvirus 4 field isolates. *Archives of Virology*, 116, 1–8.

6 **CASTRUCCI, G., FRIGER, F., FERRARI, M., RANUCCI, S., ALDROVANDI, V., CILLI, V., RAMPICHINIL, L. & GATTI, R., 1987.** Experimental infection of calves with strains of bovid herpesvirus 4. *Comparative Immunology and Microbiology of Infectious Diseases*, 10, 41–49.

7 **COETZER, J.A.W., 1984.** Faculty of Veterinary Science, University of Pretoria, South Africa. Unpublished data.

8 **DE VILLIERS, E-M., 1979.** Purification of the JS-3 isolate of *Herpesvirus ovis* (Bovid Herpesvirus 4) and some properties of its DNA. *Journal of Virology*, 32, 705–709.

9 **DE VILLIERS, E-M., ELS, H.J. & VERWOERD, D.W., 1975.** Characteristics of an ovine herpesvirus associated with pulmonary adenomatosis (jaagsiekte) in sheep. *South African Journal of Medical Sciences*, 40, 165–175.

10 **DE VILLIERS, E-M. & VERWOERD, D.W., 1980.** Presence of *Herpesvirus ovis* DNA sequences in cellular DNA from sheep lungs affected with jaagsiekte (pulmonary adenomatosis). *Onderstepoort Journal of Veterinary Research*, 47, 109–112.

11 **DUBUISSON, J., GUILLAUME, J., BOULANGER, D., THIRY, E., BUBLOT, M. & PASTORET, P.-P., 1990.** Neutralization of bovine herpesvirus type 4 by pairs of monoclonal antibodies raised against two glycoproteins and identification of antigenic determinants involved in neutralization. *Journal of General Virology*, 71, 647–653.

12 **DUBUISSON, J., THIRY, E., BUBLOT, M., THOMAS, I., VAN BRESSEM, M.F., COIGNOUL, F. & PASTORET, P.-P., 1989.** Experimental infection of bulls with a genital isolate of bovine herpesvirus 4 and reactivation of latent virus with dexamethasone. *Veterinary Microbiology*, 21, 97–114.

13 **DUBUISSON, J., THIRY, E., THALASSO, F., BUBLOT, M. & PASTORET, P.-P., 1988.** Biological and biochemical comparison of bovid herpesvirus 4 strains. *Veterinary Microbiology*, 16, 339–349.

14 **EDWARDS, S. & NEWMAN, R.H., 1984/85.** Detection of antibodies to bovid herpesvirus 4 by ELISA. *Veterinary Microbiology*, 10, 149–154.

15 **EHLERS, B., BUHK, H.-J. & LUDWIG, H., 1985.** Analysis of bovine cytomegalovirus genome structure: Cloning and mapping of the monomeric polyrepetitive DNA unit, and comparison of European and American strains. *Journal of General Virology*, 66, 55–68.

16 **ENGELS, M., GELDERBLOM, H., DARAI, G. & LUDWIGH, H., 1983.** Goat herpesviruses: Biological and physicochemical properties. *Journal of General Virology*, 64, 2237–2247.

17 **EUGESTER, A.K., 1978/79.** Isolation of bovine herpesvirus III from diarrhoeic faeces. *Veterinary Microbiology*, 3, 199–204.

18 **FRANCKI, R.I.B., FAUQUET, C.M., KNUDSON, D.L. & BROWN, F., 1991.** Classification and nomenclature of viruses. Fifth report of the International Committee on the Taxonomy of viruses. *Archives of Virology*, Supplementum 2, 216–233.

19 **GIBBS, E.P.J. & RWEYEMAMU, M.M., 1977.** Bovine herpesviruses. Part I. Bovine herpesviruses 2 and 3. *Veterinary Bulletin*, 47, 411–425.

20 **HENRY, B.E., OTA, R. & EVERMANN, J.F., 1986.** Genetic relatedness of disease-associated field isolates of bovid herpesvirus type 4. *American Journal of Veterinary Research*, 47, 2242–2246.

21 **HORNER, G.W., HUNTER, R. & DAY, A.M., 1982.** An outbreak of vulvovaginitis in goats caused by a caprine herpesvirus. *New Zealand Veterinary Journal*, 30, 150–152.

22 **JACOB, R.J., COHEN, D., BOUCHY, D., DAVIS, T. & BORCHELT, J., 1988.** Molecular pathogenesis of equine coital exanthema (ECE): Identification of a new equine herpesvirus (dky) isolated from lesions reminiscent of coital exanthema in a donkey. *In*: POWELL, D., (ed.). *Equine Infectious Diseases*. Vol. V. Lexington, Kentucky: The University Press of Kentucky.

23 **KENDRICK, J.W., OSBURN, B.I. & KRONLUND, N., 1976.** Pathogenicity studies on a bovine herpesvirus. *Theriogenology*, 6, 447–453.

24 **KIT, S., KIT, M., ICHIMURA, H., CRANDELL, R. & McDONNELL, S., 1986.** Induction of thymidine kinase activity by viruses with group B DN genomes: Bovine cytomegalovirus (bovine herpesvirus 4). *Virus Research*, 4, 197–212.

25 **KOPTOPOULOS, G., PAPANASTASOPOULOU, M., PAPADOPOULOS, D. & LUDWIG, H., 1988.** Epizootiology of caprine herpesvirus (BHV-6) infections in goat populations in Greece. *Comparative Immunology and Microbiology of Infectious Diseases*, 11, 199–205.

26 **KROGMAN, L.A. & McADARAGH, J.P., 1982.** Recrudescence of bovine herpesvirus 5 in experimentally infected calves. *American Journal of Veterinary Research*, 43, 336–338.

27 **LUDWIG, H., 1983.** Bovine herpesviruses. *In*: ROIZMAN, B., (ed.). *The Herpesviruses*. Vol. 2. New York, London: Plenum Press.

28 **LUTHER, P.D., BRADLEY, P.G. & HAIG, D.A., 1971.** The isolation and characterization of a herpesvirus from calf kidney cultures. *Research in Veterinary Science*, 12, 496–498.

29 **MACKAY, J.M.K., 1969.** Tissue culture studies of sheep pulmonary adenomatosis (jaagsiekte). II. Transmission of cytopathic effects to normal cultures. *Journal of Comparative Pathology*, 79, 147–154.

30 **MALMQUIST, W.A., KRAUSS, H.H., MOULTON, J.E. & WANDERA, J.G., 1972.** Morphologic study of virus-infected lung-cell cultures from sheep pulmonary adenomatosis (jaagsiekte). *Laboratory Investigation*, 26, 528–533.

31 **MOHANTY, S.B., HAMMOND, R.C. & LILLIE, M.G., 1971.** A new bovine herpesvirus and its effect on experimentally infected calves. *Archiv für die Gesamte Virusforschung*, 34, 394–395.

32 **MOHANTY, S.B., LILLIE, M.G., CORSELIUS, N.P. & BECK, J., 1972.** Natural infection with bovine rhinotracheitis virus in goats. *Journal of the American Veterinary Medical Association*, 160, 879–880.

33 **NAEEM, K., GOYAL, S.M. & WERDIN, R.E., 1989.** Prevalence of bovid herpesvirus 4 and its antibody in cattle in Minnesota. *American Journal of Veterinary Research*, 50, 1931–1935.

34 **OSORIO, F.A. & REED, D.E., 1983.** Experimental inoculation of cattle with bovine herpesvirus 4: Evidence for a lymphoid-associated persistent infection. *American Journal of Veterinary Research*, 44, 975–980.

35 **OSORIO, F.A., REED, D.E. & ROCK, D.L., 1982.** Experimental infection of rabbits with bovine herpesvirus 4: Acute and persistent infection. *Veterinary Microbiology*, 7, 503–513.

36 **OSORIO, F.A., REED, D.E., VAN DER MAATEN, M.J. &**

METZ, C.A., 1985. Comparison of the herpesviruses of cattle by DNA restriction endonuclease analysis and serologic analysis. *American Journal of Veterinary Research*, 46, 2104–2109.

37 **OSORIO, F.A., ROCK, D.L. & REED, D.E., 1985.** Studies on the pathogenesis of a bovine cytomegalovirus-like virus in an experimental host. *Journal of General Virology*, 66, 1941–1951.

38 **POTGIETER, L.N.D. & MARÉ, E.J., 1974.** Assay and antigenic relationships of the recently isolated bovine herpesviruses, DN599, FTC and V11. *Archiv für die Gesamte Virusforschung*, 46, 238–247.

39 **REED, D.E., LANGPAP, T.J. & BERGELAND, M.E., 1979.** Bovine abortion associated with mixed Movar 33/63 type herpesvirus and bovine viral diarrhoea virus infection. *Cornell Veterinarian*, 69, 54–66.

40 **ROIZMAN, B., DESROSIERS, R.C., FLECKENSTEIN, B., LOPEZ, C., MINSON, A.C. & STUDDERT, M.J., 1992.** The family Herpesviridae: An update. *Archives of Virology*, 123, 425–449.

41 **ROSSITER, P.B., GUMM, I.D., STAGG, D.A., CONRAD, P.A., MUKOGWE, S., DAVIES, F.G. & WHITE, H., 1989.** Isolation of bovine herpesvirus 3 from African buffaloes *(Syncerus caffer)*. *Research in Veterinary Science*, 46, 337–343.

42 **RWEYEMAMU, M.M. & LORETU, K., 1973.** Isolation of non-syncitia forming herpesviruses from cattle in Tanzania. *Journal of Comparative Pathology*, 83, 377–386.

43 **SAITO, J.K., GRIBBLE, D.H., BERRIOS, P.E., KNIGHT, H.D. & McKERCHER, D.G., 1974.** A new herpesvirus isolate from goats: Preliminary report. *American Journal of Veterinary Research*, 35, 847–848.

44 **SCOTT, F.M.M., 1985.** Caprine herpesvirus 1 infection of sheep. *In*: SHARP, J.M. & HOFF-JORGENSON, R., (eds). *Slow Viruses in Sheep, Goats and Cattle*. Luxembourg: CEC Report EUR 8076EN.

45 **SCOTT, F.M.M., SHARP, J.M., ANGUS, K.W. & GRAY, E.W., 1984.** Infection of specific-pathogen free lambs with a herpesvirus isolated from pulmonary adenomatosis. *Archives of Virology*, 80, 147–162.

46 **SHARP, J.M., 1987.** Sheep pulmonary adenomatosis: A contagious tumour and its cause. *Cancer Surveys*, 6, 73–83.

47 **SMITH, P.C., CUTLIP, R.C., RITCHIE, A.E. & YOUNG, J.K., 1972.** A bovine herpesvirus associated with a disease of the upper respiratory tract of feedlot cattle. *Journal of the American Veterinary Medical Association*, 161, 1134–1141.

48 **STACZEK, J., 1990.** Animal cytomegaloviruses. *Microbiological Reviews*, 54, 247–265.

49 **THEODORIDIS, A., 1981.** The pathogenicity of some herpesviruses in the genital tract of cattle. D.V.Sc. Thesis, University of Pretoria.

50 **THEODORIDIS, A., 1985.** Studies on bovine herpesviruses. Part 1. Isolation and characterization of viruses isolated from the genital tract of cattle. *Onderstepoort Journal of Veterinary Research*, 52, 239–254.

51 **THIRY, E., CHAPPUIS, G., BUBLOT, M., VAN BRESSEM, M.F., DUBUISSON, J. & PASTORET, P.-P., 1991.** Failure to infect cats with bovine herpesvirus type 4 strain Movar 33/63. *The Veterinary Record*, 128, 614–615.

52 **THIRY, E., DUBUISSON, J., BUBLOT, M., VAN BRESSEM, M.F. & PASTORET, P.-P., 1990.** The biology of bovine herpesvirus 4 infection of cattle. *Deutsche Tierärztliche Wochenschrift*, 97, 72–77.

53 **TODD, W.J. & STORZ, J., 1983.** Morphogenesis of a cytomegalovirus from an American bison affected with malignant catarrhal fever. *Journal of General Virology*, 64, 1025–1030.

54 **VAN MALDEREN, G., VAN OPDENBOSCH, E. & WELLMANS, G., 1987.** Bovine herpesvirus 1 and 4: A seroepidemiological survey of the Belgian cattle population. *Vlaamse Diergeneeskundige Tijdschrift*, 56, 364–371.

55 **VAN OPDENBOSCH, E.G., WELLMANS, G. & OUDEWATER, J., 1986.** Toevallige isolatic van het boviene herpesvirus 4 uit de long van een schaap. *Vlaamse Diergeneeskundige Tijdschrift*, 55, 432–433.

56 **VAN STANTEN, V.L. & CHANG, L-Y., 1992.** Cloning and mapping of *Eco*R1, *Hind* III and *Pst*1 fragments of bovine herpesvirus 4 (DN-599) genome. *Intervirology*, 34, 44–52.

57 **VERWOERD, D.W., MEYER-SCHARRER, E., BROEKMAN, J. & DE VILLIERS, E-M., 1979.** The serological relationship of *Herpesvirus ovis* to other herpesviruses and its possible involvement in the aetiology of jaagsiekte. *Onderstepoort Journal of Veterinary Research*, 46, 61–63.

58 **WELLMANS, G., BROES, A.H., CHARLIER, G. & VAN OPDENBOSCH, E., 1984.** Cited by BUBLOT, M., DUBUISSON, J., VAN BRESSEM, M.-F., DANYI, S., PASTORET, P.-P. & THIRY, E., 1991. Antigenic and genomic identity between simian herpesvirus aotus type 2 and bovine herpesvirus type 4. *Journal of General Virology*, 72, 715–719.

UNCLASSIFIED VIRUSES AND VIRUS-LIKE AGENTS

Two diseases of the central nervous system — scrapie and Borna disease — are discussed in the following chapters. Although scrapie was briefly imported into South Africa in the 1960s, it was subsequently eradicated. Neither of these diseases occurs in southern Africa at present.

Scrapie is not a virus infection but it has features in common with slow virus diseases, which have long incubation periods, are slowly progressive and are almost invariably fatal. There is a group of diseases related to scrapie in which spongiform encephalopathy in the absence of a clear inflammatory response is the principal lesion. These are mink encephalopathy, wasting disease of deer and elk, and kuru and Creutzfeldt-Jacob disease in humans. Recently, bovine spongiform encephalopathy (BSE), also known as mad cow disease, has been added to this list. There is epidemiological evidence indicating that BSE in cattle approximates scrapie in sheep.

In the case of Borna disease, the agent is known to be a virus. It was listed as 'unclassified' in the fourth report of the International Committee on the Taxonomy of Viruses,[2] but it is not mentioned in the fifth report.[1]

African swine fever virus **(see Chapter 51: African swine fever)** is another unclassified agent which does not appear in the fifth report of the International Committee on the Taxonomy of Viruses.[1] It is not included here, however, because when the layout of this book was planned, African swine fever virus was classified as a member of the family Iridoviridae.[2]

References

1 **FRANKI, R.I.B., FAUQUET, C.M., KNUDSON, D.L. & BROWN, F. (eds), 1991**. Classification and nomenclature of viruses. Fifth report of the International Committee on the Taxonomy of Viruses. *Archives of Virology*, Supplementum 2. Vienna, New York: Springer-Verlag.

2 **MATHEWS, R.E.F., 1982**. Classification and nomenclature of viruses. Fourth report of the International Committee on the Taxonomy of Viruses. *Intervirology*, 17, 1–199.

111

Scrapie

D.W. Verwoerd

Introduction

Scrapie is a slow virus disease, predominantly of sheep, characterized by pruritus and ataxia. The primary lesion is a spongiform degeneration of the brain and the disease is invariably fatal. Its aetiological agent, the biochemical nature of which remains obscure, is not a conventional virus. It also occasionally causes natural disease in goats and possibly cattle,[42] and has been transmitted experimentally to mice,[6] rats,[7] hamsters,[44] mink,[20] and non-human primates.[16]

The disease has attracted considerable attention during the past two decades both because of the uniqueness of its aetiological agent and because of its similarity to the spongiform encephalopathies of man, including kuru, Creutzfeldt-Jacob disease and the Gerstmann-Straussler syndrome. Transmissible mink encephalopathy and chronic wasting disease of elk and mule deer are also characterized by similar neuropathology, an exceptionally long incubation period and the absence of a demonstrable virus.[25, 31]

Scrapie has been known for many years in most of the old-world countries, including China. It has also been diagnosed more recently in the USA, Canada and New Zealand. The disease was introduced to South Africa on one occasion. The first suspected case was found in Natal in 1966, and the diagnosis confirmed by histopathology. Subsequently scrapie was diagnosed in a total of 11 sheep on nine farms in Natal, the eastern Cape Province and the Orange Free State. All cases were first or second generation progeny of a group of Hampshire Down sheep imported from England. A strict slaughter-out policy was applied and no new cases have been identified in South Africa since 1972, indicating successful eradication of the disease.[11, 41]

Aetiology

The infective agent causing scrapie can be recovered in relatively high concentrations from the brain and the spleen of infected animals, and can be transmitted by intracerebral inoculation. No viral particles can be demonstrated in this material, however, and the intensive search over two decades for a scrapie-specific nucleic acid has failed.

Early studies indicated that the agent is resistant to ultraviolet inactivation,[1] but a subsequent comparison of its inactivation kinetics after ionizing radiation with that of several other viruses suggested that scrapie could be caused by a conventional virus with a very small genome.[38] Separate studies postulated a small, non-coding nucleic acid, protected by host proteins, called a 'virino'.[13]

More recently, however, methods have been developed to obtain purified preparations of the infectious agent, which has been shown to resist various treatments which inactivate a range of viruses and viroids. These treatments include irradiation, hydrolysis by nucleases or bivalent cations, and shearing by ultrasonification.[2, 3] Although these experiments do not totally exclude the possible presence of a small polynucleotide, they do indicate the existence of a unique class of agent.

Highly purified infective material was subsequently found to contain rod-like structures consisting of a single polypeptide with an apparent molecular weight of 27–30 kilodaltons. The infectivity of the preparation was destroyed by protein-specific reagents but not by nucleases.[33–35] It was suggested that the agent might be a self-replicating protein and the term 'prion' (proteinaceous infectious particle) was coined for it. N-terminal sequencing of the prion protein, PrP 27–30, led to the construction of a synthetic probe and the isolation of cDNA clones from scrapie-infected brains of hamsters[32] and mice.[8] Using these clones as probes, it could be demonstrated that PrP 27–30 is encoded by a cellular gene which is present in the genomes of many vertebrates and some invertebrates.[14] This gene is expressed in both normal and scrapie-infected sheep brain as well as in other tissues. The PrPs from normal and infected tissues are not identical, however, and several isoforms are found. Post-translational modifications, such as glycosylation, could explain some of these differences, leading to speculation that the prion protein could possibly stimulate its own production in the infected cell by modification of the cellular protein, in an autocatalytic way rather than by self-replication.[37]

Prion rods observed *in vitro* are probably artifacts of the purification procedure, but antibodies to PrP react with filamentous structures observed in thin sections of scrapie-infected hamster brains.[4] These structures also stain with Congo Red, suggesting that they are identical to the amyloid plaques which are seen extracellularly in several encephalopathies. It is less clear whether PrP is also identical to the scrapie-associated fibrils (SAF) which are consistently found in alkaline extracts of infected brains.[30] Antiserum to PrP does react with SAF preparations, but more particularly with material surrounding the fibrils.[29] Furthermore, the fibrils do not stain with Congo Red, and SAF protein was shown to be absent from the spleens of infected animals.[9]

The main argument against the prion hypothesis is the fact that there are many distinct strains of scrapie agent with stable characteristics, such as their incubation periods.[27] Bruce and Dickenson[5] also demonstrated that strains can be changed in a predictable way by altered passage strategy, suggesting mutation of a nucleic acid genome. It has been argued, however, that there are other ways in which a strain could transmit specific information.[14] Cell membranes are known to act as their own templates, i.e. the structure of new membranes is determined by signals and receptors on existing membranes. The amino acid sequence of PrP is consistent with that of a membrane-bound protein and *in vitro* studies suggest that PrP spans the membrane bi-layer twice.[21] Hay *et al.*[21] also found that during *in vitro* synthesis of PrP it is glycosylated only in the presence of membranes. It is thus conceivable that when the scrapie form of PrP is integrated into a membrane after infection, a change in the membrane results which is both pathogenic and self-perpetuating. This 'membrane' hypothesis of scrapie infectivity in essence corroborates a model proposed by Hunter *et al.* as long ago as 1968.[23]

Epidemiology

Although the infectious agent has not been finally characterized, the disease can be transmitted by infected ewes to their lambs both *in utero* and postnatally. Transmission between adults is only possible under conditions of close contact. Overt disease only develops when the central nervous system is affected, and infected animals may remain carriers without ever developing clinical disease. The long incubation period, the variability of clinical signs and the fact that there is no means of detecting infection in the absence of clinical disease has resulted in a paucity of epidemiological data.

Recent outbreaks of a disease called bovine spongiform encephalopathy (BSE) in cattle in Great Britain have been linked to the presence of ruminant derived protein in their feed. By analogy to the transmission of kuru in man by cannibalism, it has been suggested that BSE could be scrapie transmitted to cattle by means of sheep brain tissue in the feeds.[42]

Clinical signs

Between infection and the appearance of clinical signs, there is an incubation period which is usually longer than a year and can exceed the productive life-span of the animal.

The more specific signs of scrapie are often preceded by a gradual decline in condition and wasting, as well as behavioural changes such as lagging behind a driven flock. This can progress to incoordination, stumbling, an exaggerated high-stepping action of the fore legs, or ataxia of the hind quarters with an inability to stand. The most characteristic signs, however, are loss of wool and self-inflicted wounds, which are caused by generalized pruritus resulting in the animal rubbing itself against objects and fences. Nibbling of wool is also commonly seen, and some animals show an exaggerated nibbling reflex when handled. These signs are progressive and may last for weeks to months, but invariably lead to death.[12, 26, 40]

Pathology

There are no gross changes characteristic of scrapie, and microscopic lesions are confined to the central nervous system.[15] The most important lesion is single or multiple vacuoles in neurones in the medulla oblongata, pons, midbrain and spinal cord, with the medulla oblongata being most consistently affected. Spongy changes in the neuropil are commonly seen, as well as a non-specific hypertrophy of astrocytes.[19, 22, 43] A cerebrovascular amyloidosis occurs in many cases of scrapie,[18] whereas inflammatory lesions and demyelination do not.

Diagnosis

The scrapie agent does not elicit a specific immune response. Although it can be transmitted to rodents, the efficiency of primary isolation is so low and the incubation period so long that it is of little diagnostic use. The agent has been successfully passaged in cell culture,[36] but again a very small proportion of cells are infected and cytopathic effects are not usually seen. Diagnosis of the disease therefore depends on recognizing the clinical signs and on histopathological confirmation. In a minority of cases, however, very little or no neuronal vacuolation occurs, necessitating the development of additional diagnostic criteria to improve diagnosis and control of the disease. A histochemical technique for the detection of enzymic inclusions in neurones has been developed[28] but is not widely used. The electron microscopic detection of SAF in aqueous extracts of brain material has been well studied[17, 30, 39] and shown to be specific.[10] Immunological methods to detect SAF are also being developed.

Differential diagnosis

Pruritus with rubbing and loss of wool can be caused by ectoparasites, particularly in southern Africa by *Psoroptes ovis*, the cause of mange or brandsiekte. Viral infections such as rabies and pseudorabies (Aujeszky's disease) may produce local pruritus, although the latter has not yet been diagnosed in southern Africa. Apart from pruritus, similar nervous signs could also be the result of a variety of plant poisonings such as cynanchosis, and krimpsiekte.[24] These conditions are not, in most instances, chronic and progressive, as is the case with scrapie.

Control

There is no treatment for the disease and no basis for the development of a vaccine. The only effective control therefore consists of strict quarantine measures to prevent spread of the disease and a slaughter-out policy to eliminate foci of infection. The application of these measures resulted in the eradication of the only recorded outbreak of scrapie in southern Africa. Stringent control of animal imports from endemic areas is obviously essential.

References

1 **ALPER, T., HAIG, D.A. & CLARKE, M.C., 1978.** The scrapie agent: Evidence against its dependence for replication on intrinsic nucleic acid. *Journal of General Virology*, 41, 503–516.

2 **BELLINGER-KAWAHARA, C., CLEAVER, J.E., DIENER, T.O. & PRUSINER, S.B., 1987.** Purified scrapie prions resist inactivation by UV irradiation. *Journal of Virology*, 61, 159–166.

3 **BELLINGER-KAWAHARA, C., DIENER, T.O., McKINLEY, M.P., GROTH, D.F., SMITH, D.R. & PRUSINER, S.B., 1987.** Purified scrapie prions resist inactivation by procedures that hydrolyze, modify or shear nucleic acids. *Virology*, 160, 271–274.

4 **BENDHEIM, P.E., BARRY, R.A., DAARMOND, S.J., STITES, D.P. & PRUSINER, S.B., 1984.** Antibodies to a scrapie prion protein. *Nature*, 310, 418–421.

5 **BRUCE, M.E. & DICKENSON, A.G., 1987.** Biological evidence that scrapie agent has an independent genome. *Journal of General Virology*, 68, 79–89.

6 **CHANDLER, R.L., 1961.** Encephalopathy in mice produced by inoculation with scrapie brain material. *Lancet* i, 1378–1379.

7 **CHANDLER, R.L. & FISHER, J., 1963.** Experimental transmission of scrapie to rats. *Lancet* ii, 1165.

8 **CHESEBRO, B., RACE, R.E., WEHRLY, K., NISHIO, J., BLOOM, M., LECHNER, D., BERGSTROM, S., ROBBINS, K., MAYER, L., KEITH, J., GARON, C. & HAASE, A., 1985.** Identification of scrapie prion protein-specific mRNA in scrapie-infected and uninfected brain. *Nature*, 315, 331–333.

9 **CZUB, M., BRAIG, H.R. & DIRINGER, H., 1986.** Pathogenesis of scrapie: Study of the temporal development of clinical symptoms, of infectivity titres and scrapie-associated fibrils in brains of hamsters infected intraperitoneally. *Journal of General Virology*, 67, 2005–2009.

10 **DAWSON, M., MANSLEY, L.M., HUNTER, A.R., STACK, M.J. & SCOTT, A.C., 1987.** Comparison of scrapie-associated fibril detection and histology in the diagnosis of natural sheep scrapie. *The Veterinary Record*, 121, 591.

11 **DENT, G.C. & SAYER, A.J., 1988.** 1002 Shangri-la, Doonside, Amanzimtoti, South Africa 4125. Personal communication.

12 **DICKENSON, A.G., 1976.** Scrapie in sheep and goats. In: KIMBERLIN, R.H., (ed.). *Slow Virus Diseases of Animals and Man*. Amsterdam: North-Holland.

13 **DICKENSON, A.G. & OUTRAM, G., 1979.** The scrapie replication-site hypothesis and its implications for pathogenesis. In: PRUSINER, S.B. & HADLOW, W.J., (eds). *Slow Transmissible Diseases of the Nervous System*. Vol. II. New York: Academic Press.

14 **DIENER, T.O., 1987.** PrP and the nature of the scrapie agent. *Cell*, 49, 719–712.

15 **FRASER, H., 1976.** The pathology of natural and experimental scrapie. In: KIMBERLIN, R.H., (ed.). *Slow Virus Diseases of Animals and Man*. Amsterdam: North-Holland.

16 **GIBBS, C.J., GAJDUSEK, D.C. & AMYX, H., 1979.** Strain variation in the viruses of Creutzfeldt-Jakob disease and kuru. In: PRUSINER, S.B. & HADLOW, W.J., (eds). *Slow Transmissible Diseases of the Nervous System*. New York: Academic Press.

17 **GIBSON, P.H., SOMERVILLE, R.A., FRASER, H., FOSTER, J.D. & KIMBERLIN, R.H., 1987.** Scrapie-associated fibrils in the diagnosis of scrapie in sheep. *The Veterinary Record*, 120, 125–127.

18 **GILMOUR, J., BRUCE, M.E. & McKELLAR, A., 1986.** Cerebrovascular amyloidosis in scrapie-affected sheep. *Neuropathology and Applied Neurobiology*, 12, 173–183.

19 **HADLOW, W.J. & RACE, R.E., 1986.** Cerebrocortical degeneration in goats inoculated with mink-passaged scrapie virus. *Veterinary Pathology*, 23, 543–549.

20 **HANSON, R.P., ECKROADE, R.J., MARSH, R.F., ZURHEIN, G.M., KARITZ, C.L. & GUSTAFSON, D.P., 1971.** Susceptibility of mink to sheep scrapie. *Science*, 172, 859–861.

21 **HAY, B., BARRY, R.A., LIEBERBURG, I., PRUSINER, S.B. & LINGAPPA, V.R., 1987.** Biogenesis and transmembrane orientation of the cellular isoform of the scrapie prion protein. *Molecular and Cellular Biology*, 7, 914–920.

22 **HOLMAN, H. & PATTISON, I.H., 1943.** Further evidence on the significance of vacuolated nerve cells in the medulla oblongata of sheep affected with scrapie. *Journal of Comparative Pathology*, 53, 231–236.

23 **HUNTER, G.D., KIMBERLIN, R.H. & GIBBONS, R.A., 1968.** Scrapie: A modified membrane hypothesis. *Journal of Theoretical Biology*, 20, 355–357.

24 **KELLERMAN, T.S., COETZER, J.A.W. & NAUDÉ, T.W., 1988.** *Plant Poisonings and Mycotoxicoses of Livestock in Southern Africa*. Cape Town: Oxford University Press Southern Africa.

25 **KIMBERLIN, R.H., 1976.** *Slow Virus Diseases of Animals and Man*. Amsterdam: North-Holland.

26 **KIMBERLIN, R.H., 1981.** Scrapie. *British Veterinary Journal*, 137, 105–112.

27 **KIMBERLIN, R.H. & WALKER, C.A., 1978.** Evidence that the transmission of one source of scrapie agent to hamsters involves separation of agent strains from a mixture. *Journal of General Virology*, 39, 487–496.

28 **MACKENZIE, A., 1984.** Intraneuronal enzymic inclusions in the histological diagnosis of scrapie. *Journal of Comparative Pathology*, 94, 9–24.

29 **MERZ, P.A., KOSCSAK, R.J., RUBINSTEIN, R., CARP, R.I. & WISNIEWSKI, H.M., 1987.** Antisera to scrapie-associated fibril protein and prion protein decorate scrapie-associated fibrils. *Journal of Virology*, 61, 42–49.

30 **MERZ, P.A., SOMERVILLE, R.A., WISNIEWSKI, H.M. & IQBAL, K., 1981.** Abnormal fibrils from scrapie-infected brain. *Acta Neuropathologica*, 54, 63–74.

31 **NARANG, H.K., 1987.** Scrapie, an unconventional virus: The current views. *Proceedings of the Society for Experimental Biology and Medicine*, England, 1987. 184, 375–388.

32 **OESCH, B., WESTAWAY, D., WÄLCHLI, M., McKINLEY, M.P., KENT, S.B.H., AEBERSOLD, R., BARRY, R.A., TEMPST, P., TEPLOW, D.B., HOOD, L.E., PRUSINER, S.B. & WEISSMANN, C., 1985.** A cellular gene encodes scrapie PrP 27–30 protein. *Cell*, 40, 735–746.

33 **PRUSINER, S.B., 1982.** Novel proteinaceous infectious particles cause scrapie. *Science*, 216, 136–144.

34 **PRUSINER, S.B., GROTH, D.F., BOLTON, D.C., KENT, S.B. & HOOD, L.E., 1984.** Purification and structural studies of a major scrapie prion protein. *Cell*, 38, 127–134.

35 **PRUSINER, S.B., McKINLEY, M.P., BOWMAN, K.A., BOLTON, D.C., BENDHEIM, P.E., GROTH, D.F. & GLENNER, G.G., 1983.** Scrapie prions aggregate to form amyloid-like birefringent rods. *Cell*, 35, 349–358.

36 **RACE, R.E., FADNESS, L.H. & CHESEBRO, B., 1987.** Characterization of scrapie infection in mouse neuroblastoma cells. *Journal of General Virology*, 68, 1391–1399.

37 **ROBERTSON, H.D., BRANCH, A.D. & DAHLBERG, J.E., 1985.** Focussing on the nature of the scrapie agent. *Cell*, 40, 725–727.

38 **ROHWER, R.G., 1984.** Scrapie infectious agent is virus-like in size and susceptibility to inactivation. *Nature*, 308, 658–662.

39 **SCOTT, A.C., DONE, S.H., VENABLES, C. & DAWSON, M., 1987.** Detection of scrapie-associated fibrils as an aid to the diagnosis of natural sheep scrapie. *The Veterinary Record*, 120, 280–281.

40 **STAMP, J.T., 1962.** Scrapie: A transmissible disease of sheep. *The Veterinary Record*, 74, 357–362.

41 **VEENSTRA, T., 1968.** Scrapie — a new disease among South African sheep. *Farming in South Africa*, 305, 1–2.

42 **WILESMITH, J.W., WELLS, G.A.H., CRANWELL, M.P. & RYAN, J.B.M., 1988.** Bovine spongiform encephalopathy: Epidemiological studies. *The Veterinary Record*, 123, 638–644.

43 **ZLOTNIK, I.M., 1958.** The histopathology of the brain stem of sheep affected with natural scrapie. *Journal of Comparative Pathology*, 68, 148–165.

44 **ZLOTNIK, I.M. & RENNIE, J.C., 1965.** Experimental transmission of mouse passaged scrapie to goats, sheep, rats and hamsters. *Journal of Comparative Pathology*, 75, 147–157.

112

Borna disease

R. Rott and S. Herzog

Introduction

Borna disease is a slowly progressive viral polioencephalomyelitis predominantly affecting horses and donkeys, more rarely other Equidae and sheep and, exceptionally, a variety of other species. After an incubation period lasting a few weeks to many months, the infection causes locomotor and sensory dysfunctions followed by paralysis and death. Infection may not be apparent.[5, 24]

In Germany, where Borna disease is endemic in certain areas, the disease has been known for more than 250 years. The commonly used name, 'Borna'sche Krankheit', originated from the frequent outbreaks of the disease in the district of Borna (Saxony) between 1894 and 1896. In 1976 Borna disease was described in Switzerland for the first time.[14] It is uncertain whether clinically similar cases of equine encephalitis in France, Rumania, Libya, and the Near East were Borna disease. There is, however, no reason to believe that Borna disease is confined to Germanic countries. The disease has not been diagnosed in southern Africa.

Detailed studies on the pathology of Borna disease were conducted during the first decade of this century.[9] Some years later Zwick and co-workers[25] established its viral aetiology by reproducing the disease with bacteria-free filtrates. More recently a soluble, virus-specific, intranuclear antigen has been shown to exist in brain material from infected animals,[4, 22, 23] the virus has been propagated in cell cultures,[7, 13] and aspects of the pathogenesis of the disease elucidated.[16]

Aetiology

Although the viral aetiology of the disease was demonstrated as long ago as 1927,[25] and despite strenuous efforts to characterize it, no details of the biochemical or structural properties of the virus have been established and it therefore remains unclassified. It has an estimated diameter of 100 nm and is sensitive to lipid solvents, which suggests that it is enveloped. All isolates seem to be serologically identical.[2] However, antibodies which occur in the serum and cerebrospinal fluid of infected animals do not neutralize infectivity.[16]

Embryonic brain cells can be infected, and cocultivation of infected brain cells with continuous cell lines of diverse origin may result in cell cultures that slowly but continuously produce virus without the production of cytopathic effects. Initially virus produced in such cultures is cell associated and spreads by cell-to-cell contact. Later, the virus produced by co-cultivation is capable of infecting 'clean cultures' of the cell line concerned without further co-cultivation.[7]

No virus-like structures have been observed in persistently infected cells, but virus-specific antigen can be demonstrated, mainly in the nuclei of infected cells, by immunofluorescence with antibodies obtained from infected animals.

Epidemiology

The large spectrum of animals and types of cell culture that can be infected experimentally suggests that natural infections occur more frequently and in a wider range of animal species than was previously believed. In addition to Equidae and sheep, natural infections have also been reported in cattle, goats, deer and rabbits.[5] Recently Borna disease virus-specific antibodies have been demonstrated in sera and cerebrospinal fluid from human patients suffering from psychiatric disorders.[20]

Many species of animals, ranging from chickens to rhesus monkeys, can be infected by intracerebral or intranasal inoculation of brain homogenates or cerebrospinal fluid from diseased animals. Rabbits are the most sensitive laboratory species. The manifestation of the experimental disease differs between species and is dependent on the virus strain used. The disease may not be apparent (hamster, mouse), or it may produce alterations in the behaviour of the animal (tree shrew, rat), or cause obesity, disturbances in fertility and blindness, or paralysis followed by death.[16, 19, 24]

In the regions of Germany where Borna disease is endemic, it occurs predominantly in spring. Recent sero-epidemiological studies have shown that the infection in horses is more widely distributed in Germany than was previously thought.[10] The discrepancy between the number of infected animals and those that show clinical signs may be due to the infection being largely subclinical, particularly in sheep.[5] It is possible that the age of animals at the time of infection might affect the course of the disease.

The mode of transmission is unknown, but the presence of the virus in nasal secretions, saliva and urine suggests that dissemination occurs either by direct contact or through fomites and food. Vertical transmission has not been demonstrated. No free-living reservoirs of the virus have been identified, although it is suspected that rats may be involved. Arthropod vectors have never been convincingly incriminated.[5]

Pathogenesis

The understanding of the pathogenesis of Borna disease is based mainly on studies of rats.

In natural infections the virus apparently enters the body through the olfactory epithelium, from whence it migrates intra-axonally via the olfactory bulb to other parts of the brain.[1, 15] Virus replication in adult animals takes place exclusively in neurones, from where the virus migrates along the axons to occur eventually in nerve cells in all the body tissues. In contrast to adult rats, viral antigen can be found in all organs of infected new-born animals,[6] and although they do not manifest clinical signs, they shed virus persistently.

The mechanism of cell damage produced by this virus is undetermined. However, since experimental infection of immunocompetent rats invariably results in clinical signs, whereas immuno-incompetent rats do not show pathological alterations despite the high levels of virus in the central nervous system (CNS),[16] it is likely that Borna disease is the result of an immunopathological reaction. Although antibody transfer to immunosuppressed animals does not initiate the development of the disease, adoptive transfer of immune cells from the spleen or from lymph nodes at various intervals after infection has been shown to be effective in the induction of encephalitis and clinical manifestation in immunologically competent recipients.[8, 16, 17] There is, furthermore, evidence that T helper/inducer (CD4) cells are responsible for the immunopathological effect which leads to Borna disease.[18] It therefore seems that the pathogenesis is based on a delayed hypersensitivity-type reaction.

Clinical signs

Typical cases are characterized by signs of meningitis and encephalitis which become apparent after a long incubation period lasting several weeks to months. This extended incubation period distinguishes Borna disease from the other forms of viral encephalitis in horses.[5] Frequently an elevated body temperature, icterus, digestive disturbances and a general uneasiness accompany the signs referable to meningitis and encephalitis. Variable and often uncharacteristic clinical signs may, however, occur during the course of the disease.

During the early stages of the disease these are reduced appetite, difficulty in swallowing, a fluctuating body temperature, and disturbed sensory functions. As the disease progresses, animals show hyperaesthesia, unco-ordinated movements, unnatural body positions, ataxia, and periods of excitement. Epilepsy and amaurosis often occur, and relapse of the disease in apparently recovered animals is a feature of Borna disease.[5] Increasing paresis and paralysis develop during the final stages of the disease, and death usually occurs one to three weeks after the onset of clinical signs. The mortality rate varies from 37 to 94 per cent.[5]

In sheep, disturbances of sensory functions are more pronounced than the paralysis that develops in horses. In addition there are frequently disorders of vision and delayed pupillary reflexes.

In both sheep and horses, clinical signs do not always occur in the same sequence and not all signs are manifested in milder cases.

Pathology

There are no gross lesions in the brain and, according to Joest and Degen.[9] and Seifried and Spatz,[21] the histopathology of spontaneous Borna disease is characterized by a non-purulent polioencephalomyelitis comprising perivascular infiltrations of mononuclear cells and lesser infiltrations of the neuropil by similar cells. The lesions are mostly located in the olfactory bulbs, basal cortex, nucleus caudatus and hippocampus, implying that primarily the limbic system is involved. Degeneration of nerve cells and neuronophagia are not prominent but there is a clear astrocytosis. There is no evidence of demyelination. In neurones, and less frequently in glial cells, eosinophilic intranuclear and sometimes intracytoplasmic inclusion bodies (Joest-Degen bodies) may occur. Inflammatory changes are also present in the periventricular areas of the diencephalon and the midbrain, and to a lesser extent in the medulla oblongata. The cerebellum, spinal cord, spinal nerves and the retina are only rarely involved, while the peripheral nervous system is unaffected.[3]

Diagnosis and differential diagnosis

The clinical signs, which are inconsistently present, and intranuclear Joest-Degen bodies, if present in the neurones, are useful in making a provisional diagnosis of Borna disease. The diagnosis can only be confirmed by serological and/or virological methods.

Borna disease-specific antibodies are present in the serum and cerebrospinal fluid of diseased animals[11, 12] and can be detected by indirect immunofluorescence using persistently infected cell cultures.[7] Monoclonal antibodies are available for the demonstration of viral antigen in formalin fixed, paraffin embedded brain

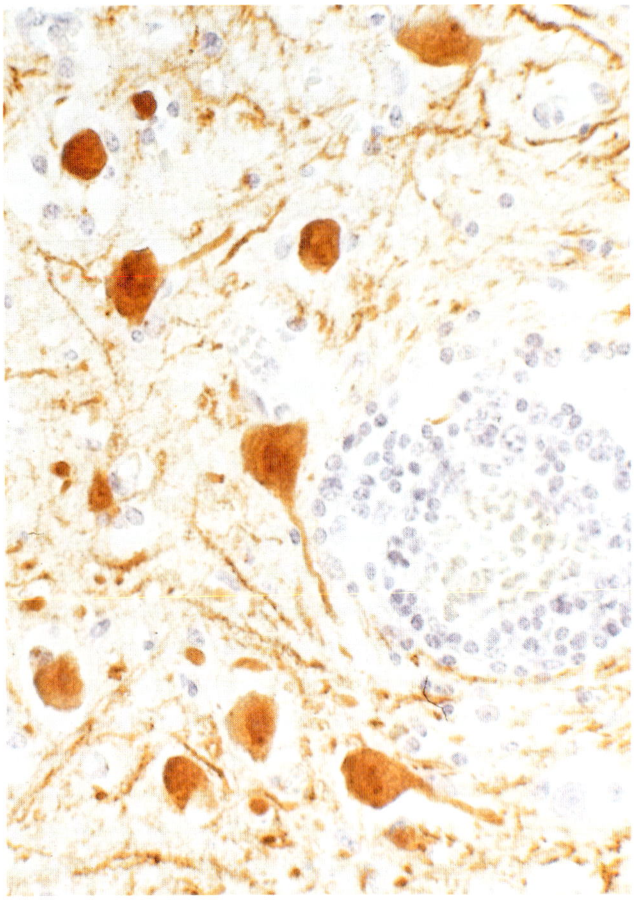

Figure 112.1 Section of the hippocampus of a horse with spontaneous Borna disease. Note the mononuclear cells in the perivascular area and viral antigen in numerous neurones (PAP method, using monoclonal antibodies against a 38/39 kd virus-specific antigen). (By courtesy of Dr K. Frese)

sections **(Figure 112.1)**. The virus can also be demonstrated in homogenates of infected brain or in cerebrospinal fluid by infection of appropriate cell cultures derived from embryonic rabbit or rat brain, or by the intracerebral inoculation of rabbits. The latter is the most sensitive method for the detection of small amounts of virus; in positive cases rabbits become ill three to four weeks after inoculation.

Neurological signs of Borna disease in horses need to be distinguished from those resulting from rabies, equid herpesvirus 1, equine encephalosis and Venezuelan, eastern and western equine encephalitis infections, as well as equine leukoencephalomalacia caused by the ingestion of maize contaminated by *Fusarium moniliforme*.

Control

There is no rational basis for therapy and no satisfactory vaccine exists. A protective immunity can only be induced experimentally by inoculating animals with live virus.[2] However, such a practice would pose the unacceptable risk of viral dissemination. In Germany, Borna disease is a notifiable disease and the disease is controlled by a slaughter-out policy.

References

1 **CARBONE, K., DUCHALA, C.S., GRIFFIN, J.W., KINCAID, H.L. & NARAYAN, O., 1987.** Pathogenesis of Borna disease in rats: Evidence that intra-axonal spread is the major route of virus dissemination and for disease incubation. *Journal of Virology*, 61, 3431–3440.

2 **DANNER, K., 1982.** *Borna-Virus und Borna-Infektion: Vom Miasma zum Modell.* Stuttgart: Ferdinand Enke Verlag.

3 **GOSZTONYI, G. & LUDWIG, H., 1984.** Neurotransmitter receptors and viral neurotropism. *Neuropsichiatria Clinical*, 3, 107–114.

4 **HAAS, B., BECHT, H. & ROTT, R., 1986.** Purification and properties of an intranuclear virus-specific antigen from tissue infected with Borna disease virus. *Journal of General Virology*, 67, 235–241.

5 **HEINIG, H., 1969.** Die Borna'sche Krankheit der Pferde und Schafe. *In*: ROHRER, H., (ed.) *Handbuch der Virusinfektionen bei Tieren*, Vol. IV. Jena: VEB Gustav Fischer Verlag.

6 **HERZOG, S., KOMPTER, S.C., FRESE, K. & ROTT, R., 1984.** Replication of Borna disease virus in rats: Age-dependent differences in tissue distribution. *Medical Microbiology and Immunology*, 173, 171–177.

7 **HERZOG, S. & ROTT, R., 1980.** Replication of Borna disease virus in cell cultures. *Medical Microbiology and Immunology*, 168, 153–158.

8 **HERZOG, S., WONIGEIT, K., FRESE, K., HEDRICH, H.J. & ROTT, R., 1985.** Effect of Borna disease virus infection on athymic rats. *Journal of General Virology*, 66, 503–508.

9 **JOEST, E. & DEGEN, H., 1911.** Untersuchungen über die pathologische Histologie, Pathogenese und postmortale Diagnose der seuchenhaften Gehirnrückenmarkentzündung (Borna'sche Krankheit) der Pferde. *Zeitschrift für Infektionskrankheiten, Parasitäre Krankheiten und Hygiene der Haustiere*, 9, 1–98.

10 **LANGE, H., HERZOG, S., HERBST, W. & SCHLIESSER, T., 1987.** Seroepidemiologische Untersuchungen zur Borna'sche Krankheit (ansteckende Gehirnrückenmarkentzündung) der Pferde. *Tierärztliche Umschau*, 42, 938–946.

11 **LUDWIG, H., KOESTER, U., PAULI, G. & ROTT, R., 1977.** The cerebrospinal fluid of rabbits infected with Borna disease virus. *Archives of Virology*, 55, 209–223.

12 **LUDWIG, H. & THEIN, P., 1977.** Demonstration of specific antibodies in the central nervous system of horses naturally infected with Borna disease virus. *Medical Microbiology and Immunology*, 163, 215–226.

13 **MAYR, A. & DANNER, K., 1972.** In vitro-Kultivierung von Bornavirus über Gehirn-Explantate infizierter Tiere. *Zentralblatt für Veterinärmedizin*, B19, 785–800.

14 **METZLER, A., MINDER, H.-P., WEGEMANN, Ch. & ZINDEL, W., 1979.** Die Borna'sche Krankheit, ein veterinärmedizinisches Problem von regionaler Bedeutung. *Schweizer Archiv für Tierheilkunde*, 121, 207–213.

15 **MORALES, J.A., HERZOG, S., KOMPTER, C., FRESE, K. & ROTT, R., 1988.** Axonal transport of Borna disease virus along olfactory pathways in spontaneously and experimentally

infected rats. *Medical Microbiology and Immunology*, 177, (in press).

16 **NARAYAN, O., HERZOG, S., FRESE, K., SCHEEFERS, H. & ROTT, R., 1983.** Pathogenesis of Borna disease in rats: Immune-mediated viral ophthalmoencephalopathy causing blindness and behavioural abnormalities. *Journal of Infectious Diseases*, 148, 305–315.

17 **RHEINBABEN, F.V., STITZ, L. & ROTT, R., 1985.** Influence of interferon on persistent infection caused by Borna disease virus. *Journal of General Virology*, 66, 2777–2780.

18 **RICHT, J.A., STITZ, L., WEKERLE, H. & ROTT, R., 1988.** Borna disease, a progressive meningoencephalitis as a model for CD4+T cell-mediated immunopathology in the brain. *Journal of Experimental Medicine*, 170, 1045–1050.

19 **ROTT, R. & HERZOG, S., 1987.** Institut für Virologie, Frankfurterstrasse 107, D-6300 Giessen, West Germany. Unpublished data.

20 **ROTT, R., HERZOG, S., FLEISCHER, B., WINOKUR, A., AMSTERDAM, J., DYSON, W. & KOPROWSKI, H., 1985.** Detection of serum antibodies to Borna disease virus in patients with psychiatric disorders. *Science*, 228, 755–756.

21 **SEIFRIED, O. & SPATZ, H., 1930.** Die Ausbreitung der encephalitischen Reaktion bei der Bornaschen Krankheit der Pferde und deren Beziehungen zur Encephalitis epidemica, der Heine-Medinschen Krankheit und der Lyssa des Menschen. Eine vergleichende pathologische Studie. *Zeitschrift für Neurologie*, 124, 317–382.

22 **SPROCKHOFF, H.V. & NITZSCHKE, E., 1955.** Untersuchungen über das komplementbindende Antigen in Gehirnen Bornavirus-infizierter Kaninchen. 1. Nachweis eines loslichen Antigens. *Zentralblatt für Veterinärmedizin*, 2, 185–192.

23 **WAGNER, K., LUDWIG, H. & PAULSEN, J., 1968.** Fluoreszenzserologischer Nachweis von Borna-Virus Antigen. *Berliner und Münchener Tierärztliche Wochenschrift*, 81, 395–396.

24 **ZWICK, W., 1939.** Borna'sche Krankheit und Encephalomyelitis der Tiere. *In*: GILDEMEISTER, E., HAAGEN, E. & WALDMANN, O., (eds). *Handbuch der Viruskrankheiten*. Vol. II. Jena: Gustav Fischer Verlag.

25 **ZWICK, W., SEIFRIED, O. & WITTE, J., 1927.** Experimentelle Untersuchungen über die Gehirnrückenmarkentzündung der Pferde (Borna'sche Krankheit). *Zeitschrift für Infektionskrankheiten, Parasitäre Krankheiten und Hygiene der Haustiere*, 30, 42–136.

Section 5

Bacterial and mycoplasmal diseases

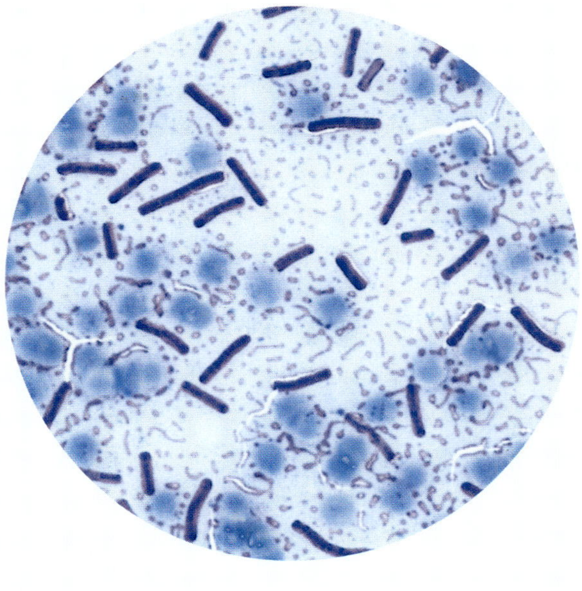

SPIROCHAETES

Members of the order Spirochaetales are helical, motile, unicellular bacteria 0,1–3,0 x 5,0–250 μm in size. Spirochaetes have periplasmic flagella (ranging from two to more than 100 per cell) which are encased in an outer sheath and are responsible for their typical motility. The lack of free flagella distinguishes the spirochaetes from other motile bacteria. The spirochaetes are propelled along by rotating on their longitudinal axis and by flexing motions which are elicited by the action of the sheathed flagella.[1]

The order Spirochaetales contains two families, the Spirochaetacaea and the Leptospiracaea, both of which have members that are pathogenic. The family Spirochaetacaea embodies two genera (*Treponema* and *Borrelia*) of veterinary importance. The genus *Treponema* has recently been reclassified as *Serpulina*.[2] The family Leptospiracaea has only a single genus, *Leptospira*, which is an important pathogen of both animals and humans.[1]

The members of the genus *Serpulina* (*Treponema*) frequent the oral cavities as well as the genital and intestinal tracts of humans and animals.[1] *Serpulina (Treponema) hyodysenteriae* is the only species within the genus that is known to be a pathogen of veterinary importance; in pigs it causes swine dysentery, which occurs wherever pigs are farmed.[2]

Borrelia spp. are actively motile, Gram-negative bacteria which are pathogenic to humans, other mammals and birds. They are usually transmitted by ticks or lice that have been infected with them. Borreliosis in animals occurs throughout the world and is caused by a number of *Borrelia* spp. which initiate diverse disease conditions in a variety of animal species. *Borrelia theileri* infection has been associated with anaemia, lymph node enlargement and petechiation of the mucous membranes in horses, cattle and sheep, while *Borrelia suilla* has been isolated from necrogranulomatous skin lesions in pigs. Infection by both these species has been recognized in South Africa but it is rarely diagnosed. Recently *Borrelia burgdorferi* has been incriminated as cause of fever, lymphadenopathy, lymphocytic proliferative synovitis, arthralgia, recurrent lameness and encephalitis in horses, dogs and humans. It may also cause abortion in mares. It is not known whether it occurs in southern Africa.

Among the Leptospiracaea, only serovars of *Leptospira interrogans* are pathogenic, and these infect mammals, amphibians and reptiles. The bacteria are characteristically transmitted by carriers. Infections in various animal species (cattle and pigs in particular) are caused by serovars which are more or less host-specific **(see Chapter 116: Leptospirosis: Table 116.1)**. These infections are associated with a number of syndromes, including haemolytic crisis, chronic interstitial nephritis, mastitis, abortion and, in horses, periodic ophthalmia. In southern Africa the occurrence of leptospirosis is restricted, and it is only rarely responsible for economically important disease outbreaks in pigs and cattle.

References

1 **CANALE-PAROLA, E., 1984.** The spirochaetes. *In*: KRIEG, N.R. & HOLT, J.G., (eds) *Bergey's Manual of Systematic Bacteriology*. Vol. I. Baltimore, London: Williams & Wilkins.

2 **STANTON, D., 1992.** Proposal to change the genus *Serpula* to *Serpulina* gen. nov. containing the species *Serpulina hyodysenteriae* comb. nov. and *Serpulina innocens* comb. nov. *Journal of Systematic Bacteriology*, 42, 189–190.

113

Swine dysentery

Synonyms: Bloody diarrhoea, black scours, vark disenterie (Afrik.)

R.K. Loveday

Introduction

Swine dysentery (SD), also known as bloody diarrhoea or black scours, is a peracute to chronic infectious enteric disease characterized by diarrhoea (caused by typhlocolitis, with the presence in the faeces of mucus, blood, necrotic material and fibrin), loss of weight and dehydration. Young growing pigs of six to 12 weeks of age are particularly susceptible, but animals of all ages may be affected. It results in severe economic losses, mainly due to reduced growth rates, and its presence may result in a 15 per cent increase in production costs. Recovered animals may remain carriers of the disease for up to 90 days.[62]

Swine dysentery was first reported from Indiana in 1921 as a disease of unknown cause.[67] Fifty years later, the primary aetiologic agent was identified as an anaerobic spirochaete initially referred to as *Borrelia hyodysenteriae* and later named *Treponema hyodysenteriae*.[26] It has recently been renamed *Serpulina hyodysenteriae*.This organism is capable of initiating the disease on its own, but various Gram-negative anaerobes resident in the large intestine may contribute to the development of the lesions.[62]

The disease occurs worldwide and has a prevalence of 20 – 40 per cent in many countries.[52] It was first recognized in South Africa in 1964,[40] and four subsequent outbreaks have been reported.[18] Swine dysentery is believed to have a prevalence of 20–30 per cent among herds participating in the South African National Pig Health Scheme.[59] This estimate correlates well with the results of a recent Australian survey using ELISA testing of blood samples, where approximately one third of the herds tested showed evidence of infection.[22]

Aetiology

Serpulina hyodysenteriae is a large, Gram-negative, oxygen-tolerant, anaerobic spirochaete, 6–10 µm in length and 320–380 nm in diameter. It is loosely coiled, motile, strongly haemolytic and indole-positive, and has a characteristic API-ZYM profile.[21] It contains seven to nine periplasmic fibrils which are inserted at each end of the cell, and it is surrounded by an envelope.[27] Electron microscopically, various strains of *S. hyodysenteriae* manifest a distinct morphological heterogeneity, varying in length and width and also in the number of flagella inserted at each end. Poorly haemolytic, non-pathogenic strains possess fewer polar flagella but have a lattice-like substructure covering the ends of the cells.[28]

The organisms grow on blood agar in atmospheres containing 5 per cent carbon dioxide and 95 per cent hydrogen and form colonies surrounded by beta-haemolysis after 48 hours' incubation.[62] Selective media such as trypticase soy agar containing 5 per cent pig faeces extract and antimicrobial agents inhibit the growth of contaminant faecal flora.[37] Various additional growth substrates and combinations of antimicrobials are also advantageous.[60,61]

In addition to the initial seven serotypes of *S. hyodysenteriae* identified (based on lipopolysaccharide components), an additional two serotypes have been added.[39] Serotypes are either designated 1–9[39] or A–I.[21, 22] Typing is done on the basis of reaction patterns of its lipopolysaccharides, employing slide-agglutination tests, an agarose-gel double-diffusion precipitation test,[22] using its reaction to various lectins,[5] sodium dodecyl sulphate electrophoresis and immunoblot analysis.[56] Strains from the USA, Great Britain and Australia typed by immunoblotting manifest a marked heterogeneity in their lipopolysaccharide composition.[56]

Distinct from *S. hyodysenteriae*, a group of weakly haemolytic spirochaetes, some of which have been named *T. innocens*,[35] has been isolated from pigs with diarrhoea and from rodents. Certain members of this group are regarded as non-pathogenic, while others are capable of causing colitis.[29, 34, 36] All these organisms may be distinguished from *S. hyodysenteriae* on ultrastructural, biochemical or antigenic grounds,[56] which include immunoblotting,[56] multilocus enzyme electrophoresis and DNA restriction endonuclease analysis, the latter being the most sensitive test.[42]

Serpulina hyodysenteriae is sensitive to drying, heat, and an acid pH of less than six, is readily destroyed within minutes by phenol and hypochlorite disinfectants, but can survive in moist organic matter for days or weeks.

Epidemiology

Domesticated pigs appear to be the only animals to become clinically ill following infection by *S. hyodysenteriae*. Wild pigs in Europe,[16] mice, rats, dogs, birds and flies may also become infected.

Initial infection in susceptible stock on a farm is generally derived from introduced carrier weaners or breeding stock. The organism may also be introduced onto farms by contaminated clothing, footwear, and workers' utensils. Mice and rats may also play a role in the epidemiology of the disease. They may carry the organisms as part of their caecal and colonic flora for months.[8] Experimentally infected mice shed bacteria in their faeces for up to six months,[32] while rats do so for two months[12] and dogs for 13 days. Similar serotypes occur in both pigs and rats on the same property.[22] It has been suggested that these rodents may be the primary natural reservoir of the organism and that SD develops after the extension of the host range of *S. hyodysenteriae* to include pigs.[8] Susceptible pigs are infected by the ingestion of faecal-contaminated food or water.

The disease occurs throughout the year without any specific seasonal pattern.[17] All pig breeds appear to be susceptible and all age groups may be infected, although there is a peak occurrence of the disease in weaners from six to 12 weeks of age as a result of the waning of maternally-derived immunity. It is uncommon in suckling pigs and in breeding stock. Recovered pigs are immune but some may become re-infected, while others may be asymptomatic but shed the organism in their faeces for at least 70 days.[58] Animals treated during the early stages of disease are not generally regarded as immune.

In the external environment, the bacteria only survive for any length of time in moist environments and at low temperatures. For example, at temperatures of 4–6 °C the bacteria will remain alive for up to two months, whereas at ambient temperatures of 15–38 °C the bacteria in soil and in clean pig pens die within one week. Dilution of contaminated faeces with tap water at a ratio of up to 1:10 will enhance survival.[13] *Serpulina hyodysenteriae* occurs particularly in liquid faeces and also in water from anaerobic lagoons.[25]

Pathogenesis

Treponemes are present in the colon within two days of oral infection. The reason for their localization in the large intestine is not known, but the bacteria first occur in goblet cells in the depth of the colonic crypts. Hyperplasia of the colonic mucosa develops within four days of infection, at which time goblet cells appear to increase towards the luminal surface of the mucosa.[50] Vascular congestion and dilatation develop, followed by oedema of the lamina propria, separation of epithelial cells at the crypt shoulders, necrosis and desquamation of the epithelial cells, and subsequent haemorrhage. Numerous spirochaetes are found under and between necrotic cells, while they also enter unaffected enterocytes and multiply intracytoplasmically. Penetration of epithelial cells only occurs at their lateral borders.[1]

Two toxins, a lipopolysaccharide and a haemolysin, elaborated by the treponemes, may be involved in the cellular damage. The haemolysin is a potent cytotoxin which experimentally has been shown to cause severe degeneration and necrosis of the differentiated epithelial cells of intercrypt spaces, resulting in lesions similar to those occurring in natural cases.[43] Members of the large intestinal bacterial flora may, in addition, be involved in the development of the lesions.[62] Deficiency of selenium, which plays a complex role in mucosal defence mechanisms, appears to potentiate the effects of *S. hyodysenteriae*.[64]

The colonic mucosal damage causes a failure of the ability of the epithelial cells to reabsorb chloride and sodium ions, which results in ion and fluid loss and the production of a mucohaemorrhagic diarrhoea. Death is the consequence of dehydration and electrolyte loss.[3] The mechanism of the failure in absorption remains to be elucidated, but appears not to be associated with increased levels of intracellular cyclic adenosine monophosphate.[3]

Serum antibody is demonstrable within seven to ten days of the clinical onset of the disease and IgG antibody may reduce the rate of mucosal colonization. Sows' milk has been shown to contain IgA antibody to envelope antigens and is probably responsible for the protection of suckling pigs.[62]

Clinical signs

The incubation period in field outbreaks may be as long as two months, but is usually between seven and 14 days in experimentally infected animals. In natural cases, animals may only show signs of the disease 30 or more days after being in contact with diseased pigs.[17] Some affected animals have an inconsistently elevated body temperature, but in most cases it is usually normal. An outbreak of SD is usually characterized by the development of an acute mucohaemorrhagic diarrhoea, listlessness, anorexia and emaciation in a group of animals.[67] The disease spreads rapidly and may involve 75 per cent of a herd within a short time. The severity and course of the disease can, however, be categorized into peracute, acute, subacute and chronic. Animals that die peracutely are found dead without having been seen to be ill, although most that die do show signs of diarrhoea.

Animals that suffer from the acute disease are anorectic, lose weight and show signs of abdominal discomfort and diarrhoea. The diarrhoea develops early in the course of the disease and is characterized by faeces that are yellowish to grey in colour, watery and foetid, and which may contain mucus, blood and, later in the course of the disease, shreds of fibrin or necrotic material. The animal's hind legs are soiled and faecal material may ooze from the anus. Animals also become increasingly thirsty. They then become recumbent after a few days as a result of progressive dehydration and weakness. In acutely affected animals the disease does not usually last for more than a week; in subacute and chronic cases it may persist for much longer. Subacutely affected animals become unthrifty and lose weight. Signs of diarrhoea may be absent, but if they do develop are usually manifested late in the course of the disease, often only after the animals have been ill for a week. In chronically affected animals, the diarrhoea is consistent, the faecal material very fluid and containing necrotic material which imparts a so-called 'rice-water' appearance. This may persist for weeks and cause a progressive emaciation and dehydration.[17]

Pathology

The clinical pathological changes are non-specific but reflect the effects of the diarrhoea and dehydration, causing blood electrolyte depletion and marked metabolic acidosis. Terminal hyperkalaemia, together with the acidosis, may be a significant cause of death.[20]

Except for those animals that have suffered from the peracute disease, the carcasses at necropsy show signs of emaciation and dehydration. Intestinal lesions are confined to the large intestine. The serosal surface of the spiral colon is oedematous and hyperaemic. Regional lymph nodes are enlarged and reactive. The contents of the large intestine are generally fluid, foul-smelling and dark grey in colour, sometimes slightly blood-stained, and reflect the nature of the inflammatory reaction, which varies from catarrhal to haemorrhagic or fibrinonecrotic; frank haemorrhagic enteritis is rarely seen. The mucosal surface shows diffuse congestion, petechial haemorrhages, erosion and ulceration, and it may have large amounts of mucus adhering to it. In more chronic cases the mucosa of the caecum and colon may be covered by a yellowish, diphtheritic exudate.[40, 41] Enlarged submucosal glands are often visible as white, raised nodular structures beneath the colonic serosa.[27]

Histologic lesions are consistent with the gross pathological changes and essentially involve the upper (luminal) third of the mucosa. Congestion and exudation characterize the early lesions and accompany goblet cell hyperplasia and secretion of large amounts of mucus. Subsequently, epithelial cells become necrotic and separated from the lamina propria, and this exposes capillaries and results in focal haemorrhages and the development of fibrinous pseudomembranes, erosions and ulcers. Crypts may be dilated and contain necrotic material. Spirochaetes may be demonstrated in the lumen and crypts of affected parts of the large intestines in Warthin-Starry-stained histological sections and are particularly numerous in the acute phase of infection.[27]

Diagnosis

Swine dysentery may only be distinguished from other enteric diseases after consideration of the clinical signs, the nature and distribution of the intestinal lesions, and the isolation and positive identification of *S. hyodysenteriae* from affected pigs. Examination of direct mucosal or faecal wet-mount smears will reveal the presence of treponemes, but neither this method nor the use of electron microscopy makes it possible to distinguish *T. innocens* from *S. hyodysenteriae*. The accuracy of isolation procedures has been increased by the development of a selective isolation medium incorporating spectinomycin[36] but it appears, in general, that neither rectal smears nor culturing techniques, alone or in combination, are sufficient for confirmation of the diagnosis.[48] Cultural and conventional biochemical methods appear to lack the sensitivity to distinguish between *S. hyodysenteriae* and *T. innocens*.[4] The demonstration of the bacteria by silver-impregnation techniques is highly suggestive, but not specific enough to confirm a diagnosis of SD.

Recent developments in molecular biological diagnostic techniques offer more reliable and sensitive diagnoses. Oligodeoxynucleotide[31] and whole chromosomal[15] probes have been developed and appear to be highly specific. With these techniques, nanogram amounts of specific DNA can be detected in specimens and there are no cross-reactions between *S. hyodysenteriae* and *T. innocens* or a variety of other treponemes.[31] Improved serological tests may also be used to detect and monitor the presence of *S. hyodysenteriae* in pig herds. A combination of a microplate ELISA and immunoblotting used for the detection of IgG is a very sensitive test and also allows identification of serotypes of *S. hyodysenteriae* on the basis of antibodies against serotype-specific anti-lipopolysaccharide antibodies.[55]

Differential diagnosis

Several enteric diseases, including salmonellosis, post-weaning colibacillosis, trichuriasis, and possibly gastric ulceration and porcine haemorrhagic enteropathy, may be confused clinically. The last two conditions may present with blood-stained faeces but are easily differentiated at necropsy.[65]

Salmonellosis may cause lesions in the small intestine as well as in the large bowel, which may be accompanied by haemorrhages, and foci of necrosis in parenchymatous organs and lymph nodes. Intestinal adenomatosis and haemorrhagic enteropathy involve distinct proliferative changes of the ileal mucosa and may be confirmed by the presence of *Campylobacter* organisms in the cytoplasm of ileal epithelial cells in silver-stained histopathological tissue sections.

Swine dysentery must also be distinguished from so-called 'grower scour and non-specific colitis' in weaner pigs which has recently been described in the UK, and in which large intestinal lesions very similar to those of SD occur. Some of the agents cited as possibly causative in this condition, which may well be occurring largely unrecognized in southern Africa, are enterotoxigenic *Clostridium perfringens* type A, campylobacters, cryptosporidia and non-hyodysenteriae treponemes. These last-named organisms have in some cases been found to form a mat of attached spirochaetes visible in haematoxylin and eosin-stained intestinal sections.[19, 57, 63]

Control

Small outbreaks of SD may be controlled by adding chemotherapeutic drugs to the drinking water or feed, or by a single intramuscular injection of tiamulin at 10 mg/kg body weight given to individual animals. Drinking water medication is preferred, but few local piggeries are properly equipped with header tanks for this purpose. Water-soluble and feed-premix presentations of dimetridazole (1,5 kg/tonne of feed or in 2 400 litres of the drinking water for 21 days),[46] tiamulin, tylosin and a combination of lincomycin and spectinomycin are available in South Africa, while injectable preparations of tiamulin, tylosin, and a combination of lincomycin and spectinomycin are also used. Depending upon the therapeutic compound, feed or water medication programmes should be continued for seven to 14 days for satisfactory results. Thereafter, in-feed subtherapeutic levels of medication are applied as a prophylactic measure for between four and six weeks, accompanied by thorough cleaning, disinfection and rodent control programmes. Such programmes, plus blanket medication of the whole herd (to eliminate carriers among the breeding stock) have been successfully employed to control the disease on farms in South Africa.[66]

Sodium arsanilate (220 ppm in feed) may precipitate the development of clinical cases in herds previously infected[49] and may be used to identify carrier animals. Resistance to sodium arsanilate, lincomycin and tylosin has been reported for some strains of *S. hyodysenteriae*,[35] and recurrence of the disease, apparently due to the presence of resistant strains, may occur within three months of treatment.[10]

Although monensin is not registered for this purpose in South Africa, its continuous administration from weaning until slaughter is also effective in the prevention of the disease and, at initial levels of 100 ppm in the feed, causes significant improvement in average daily weight gain and feed-conversion ratio. Similar effects are attained if monensin is administered after the disease has been established.[38]

Sodium hypochlorite added to drinking water at a concentration of 15 ml of a 15 per cent solution/litre of water, reduces the number of clinically affected pigs, but does not fully eliminate the disease. It is cheap, however, and does reduce the amount of antibiotic medication required. Premises should be disinfected with sodium hypochlorite at concentrations of 100 ml of 15 per cent solution in 15 litres of water.[11]

Eradication of the disease from a region or country appears to be possible only when it is dealt with as a notifiable disease. In such a scheme the movement of pigs should be controlled, all infected herds treated with an effective antimicrobial drug, and effective cleaning, disinfection and rodent control programmes applied.[7] In planning herd eradication programmes of this nature, drug resistance must also be taken into account.[7]

One such scheme was instituted in the German Democratic Republic in 1977 with the intention of eradicating SD by the systematic treatment of clinically affected herds, using intensive medication and hygiene control programmes. Due to the application of these methods, the last outbreak of the disease occurred in 1983, despite the continued isolation of the pathogen from pigs submitted for necropsy.[9] The chance of success of such a programme combining treatment and disinfection has been estimated to vary from 50 to 90 per cent. The cost of such programmes, which may be substantial, can be recovered within 12 months as a result of the improved feed conversion ratios and live-weight gains, and the reduction in veterinary costs in such herds. The actual improvement is due not only to the reduction of clinical disease, but also, more importantly, to the elimination of subclinical disease.[68]

Several vaccination programmes have been described. In the UK the administration of an adjuvanted, killed, virulent strain of *S. hyodysenteriae* by intramuscular injection, combined with an oral sensitization programme using an avirulent strain of *S. hyodysenteriae* has been claimed to provide good protection.[45] In Australia, a killed, whole-cell, adjuvanted vaccine has been submitted to extensive trials involving over 20 000 post-weaned pigs over a period of three years. It is claimed that this method of immunization provides protection against clinical disease in more than 90 per cent of the animals and that economic losses are reduced significantly following its use.[14]

References

1 **ALBASSAM, M.A., OLANDER, H.J., THACKER, H.L. & TUREK, J.J., 1985.** Ultrastructural characterization of colonic lesions in pigs inoculated with *Treponema hyodysenteriae*. *Canadian Journal of Comparative Medicine*, 49, 384–390.

2 **AMTSBERG, G. & MERKT, M., 1986.** Swine dysentery: Pathogenesis, epidemiology and detection. *Praktische Tierärzt*, 67, 584–591.

3 **ARGENZIO, R.A., 1985.** Pathophysiology of swine dysentery. *In*: PFEIFFER, C.J., (ed.) *Animal Models for Intestinal Disease*. Boca Raton, Florida: CRC Press, Inc.

4 **BECKMANN, G., 1990.** Vergleichende biochemiesche und serologische Untersuchungen an Treponemen-isolaten aus dem Darmkanal von Schweinen, Hunden, Mausen und Ratten. Inaugural dissertation, Tierärztliche Hochschule,

Hannover, Germany.

5 **BECKMANN, G. & AMTSBERG, G., 1990.** Lectin agglutination for differentiating intestinal *Treponema* isolates from various animal species. *Berliner und Münchener Tierärztliche Wochenschrift*, 103, 266–273.

6 **BLAHA, T., 1983.** Significance of small rodents in the epidemiology of swine dysentery. *Monatshefte für Veterinärmedizin*, 38, 606–608.

7 **BLAHA, T., ERLER, W. & BURCH, D.G.S., 1987.** Swine dysentery control in the German Democratic Republic and the suitability of injections of tiamulin for the programme. *The Veterinary Record*, 121, 416–419.

8 **BLAHA, T., GUNTHER, H., FLOSSMANN, K-D. & ERLER, W., 1984.** Epidemiological basis of swine dysentery. *Zentralblatt für Veterinärmedizin*, B31, 541–565.

9 **BLAHA, T., STAHL, U., GAREISS, G. & KIELSTEIN, P., 1991.** Eradication of swine dysentery. *Praktische Tierärzt*, 72, 324–336.

10 **BRIGGS, I.M., 1989.** An outbreak of swine dysentery and an attempt to eradicate it by medication. *Pig Veterinary Journal*, 22, 127–137.

11 **BUKH, K., 1988.** Use of chlorine in experiments on controlling swine dysentery. *Dansk Veterinaertidsskrift*, 71, 1278–1286.

12 **CHIA, S.P., 1977.** Studies of the survival of *Treponema hyodysenteriae* and the epidemiology of swine dysentery. M.V.M. dissertation, University of Glasgow, Scotland.

13 **CHIA, S.P. & TAYLOR, D.J., 1978.** Factors affecting the survival of *Treponema hyodysenteriae* in dysenteric pig faeces. *The Veterinary Record*, 103, 68–70.

14 **COLOE, P.J. & GERRATY, N.L., 1988.** The use of vaccination against swine dysentery to improve health status and productivity in intensively housed pigs. *Proceedings of the Tenth Congress of the International Pig Veterinary Society*, Rio de Janeiro, Brazil, August 14–17, page 123.

15 **COMBS, B.G. & HAMPSON, D.J., 1991.** The use of a whole chromosomal probe for identification of *Treponema hyodysenteriae*. *Research in Veterinary Science*, 50, 286–289.

16 **DEDEK, J. LOEPELMANN, H. & BLAHA, T., 1985.** Epidemiological importance of wild boar for swine dysentery. *Monatshefte für Veterinärmedizin*, 40, 834–835.

17 **DOYLE, L.P., 1945.** Enteritis in swine. *Cornell Veterinarian*, 35, 103–109.

18 **DUCASSE, F.B.W. & NIXON, R.C., 1967.** Investigations into swine dysentery in Natal. *Journal of the South African Veterinary Medical Association*, 38, 205–209.

19 **DUNCAN, A.L. & LYSONS, R.J., 1987.** The diagnosis of colitis. *The Veterinary Record*, 121, 430.

20 **GLOCK, R.D., 1971.** Studies on the etiology, hematology and pathology of swine dysentery. Ph.D. thesis, Iowa State University.

21 **HAMPSON, D.J., 1990.** New serogroups of *Treponema hyodysenteriae* (G, H and I). *The Veterinary Record*, 127, 524.

22 **HAMPSON, D.J., 1991.** Slide agglutination for rapid serological typing of *Treponema hyodysenteriae*. *Epidemiology and Infection*, 106, 541–547.

23 **HAMPSON, D.J., 1991.** New developments in research on swine dysentery and spirochaetal colitis. *Pig News and Information*, 12, 233–235.

24 **HAMPSON, D.J., COMBS, B.G., HARDERS, S.J., CONNAUGHTON, I.D. & FAHY, V.A., 1991.** Isolation of *Treponema hyodysenteriae* from a wild rat living in a piggery. *Australian Veterinary Journal*, 68, 308.

25 **HARRIS, D.L., 1984.** The epidemiology of swine dysentery as it relates to the eradication of the disease. *Compendium on Continuing Education for the Practising Veterinarian*, 6, S83–S88.

26 **HARRIS, D.L., GLOCK, R.D., CHRISTENSEN, C.R. & KINYON, J.M., 1972.** Swine dysentery. I. Inoculation of pigs with *Treponema hyodysenteriae* (new species) and reproduction of the disease. *Veterinary Medicine/Small Animal Clinician*, 67, 61–64.

27 **HARRIS, D.L. & GLOCK, R.D., 1986.** Swine Dysentery. *In*: LEMAN, A.D., STRAW, B., GLOCK, R.D., MENGELING, W.L., PENNY, R.H.C. & SCHOLL, E., (eds). *Diseases of Swine*. 6th edn. Ames, Iowa: Iowa State University Press.

28 **HOVIND-HOUGEN, K., HOGH, P. & BIRCH-ANDERSEN, A., 1990.** Morphological heterogeneity among spiroachetes isolated from cases of swine dysentery. *Zentralblatt für Bakteriologie*, 274, 1–15.

29 **HUDSON, M.J., ALEXANDER, T.T.L. & LYSONS, R.J., 1976.** Diagnosis of swine dysentery: Spirochaetes which may be confused with *Treponema hyodysenteriae*. *The Veterinary Record*, 99, 498–500.

30 **IVANYI, T.S., 1985.** Experiences on pathogenesis and control of swine dysentery in Hungary. *Wiener Tierärztliche Monatschrift*, 72, 33–36; 38.

31 **JENSEN, N.S., CASEY, T.A. & STANTON, T.B., 1990.** Detection and identification of *Treponema hyodysenteriae* by using oligodeoxynucleotide probes complementary to 16S rRNA. *Journal of Clinical Microbiology*, 28, 2717–2721.

32 **JOENS, L.A., 1980.** Experimental transmission of *Treponema hyodysenteriae* from mice to pigs. *American Journal of Veterinary Research*, 41, 1225–1226.

33 **JOENS, L.A., DE YOUNG, D.W., GLOCK, R.D., MAPOTHER, M.E., CRAMER, J.D. & WILCOX, H.E., 1985.** Passive protection of segmented swine colonic loops against swine dysentery. *American Journal of Veterinary Research*, 46, 2369–2371.

34 **JOENS, L.A., SONGER, J.G. & HARRIS, D.L., 1979.** Comparison of selective culture and serologic agglutination of *Treponema hyodysenteriae* for diagnosis of swine dysentery. *The Veterinary Record*, 105, 463–465.

35 **KINYON, J.M. & HARRIS, D.L., 1979.** *Treponema innocens*, a new species of intestinal bacteria, and amended description of the type strain of *Treponema hyodysenteriae* Harris *et al*. *International Journal of Systematic Bacteriology*, 29, 102–109.

36 **KINYON, J.M., SONGER, J.G., JANC, M. & HARRIS, D.L., 1976.** Isolation and identification of *Treponema hyodysenteriae*: Aid to the diagnosis and treatment of swine dysentery. *Nineteenth Annual Proceedings of the American Association of Veterinary Laboratory Diagnosticians*, 65–74.

37 **KUNKLE, R.A. & KINYON, J.M., 1988.** Improved selective medium for the isolation of *Treponema hyodysenteriae*. *Journal of Clinical Microbiology*, 26, 2357–2360.

38 **KYRIAKIS, S.C., 1989.** The effect of monensin against swine dysentery. *British Veterinary Journal*, 145, 373–377.

39 **LI, Z., BELANGER, M. & JACQUES, M., 1991.** Serotyping of Canadian isolates of *Treponema hyodysenteriae* and description of two new serotypes. *Journal of Clinical Microbiology*, 29, 2794–2797.

40 **LOVEDAY, R.K., 1964.** Swine dysentery in South Africa — report of an outbreak. *Journal of the South African Veterinary Medical Association*, 35, 51–55.

41 **LUSIER, G., 1962.** Vibrionic dysentery in swine in Ontario. I. Clinical aspects and pathology. *Canadian Veterinary Journal*, 3, 228–237.

42 **LYMBERY, A.J., HAMPSON, D.J., HOPKINS, R.M., COMBS, B. & MHOMA, J.R.L., 1990.** Multilocus enzyme electrophoresis for identification and typing of *Treponema hyodysenteriae* and related spirochaetes. *Veterinary Microbiology*, 22, 89–99.

43 **LYSONS, R.J., KENT, K.A., BLAND, A.P., SELLWOOD, R., ROBINSON, W.F. & FROST, A.J., 1991.** A cytotoxic haemolysin from *Treponema hyodysenteriae* — a probable virulence determinant in swine dysentery. *Journal of Medical Microbiology*, 34, 97–102.

44 **LYSONS, R.J., LEMCKE, R.M., BEW, J., BURROWS, M.R. & ALEXANDER, T.J.L., 1982.** An avirulent strain of *Treponema hyodysenteriae* isolated from herds free of swine dysentery. *Proceedings of the Seventh International Congress of the Pig Veterinary Society*, Mexico City, Mexico, July 26–31, 33.

45 **LYSONS, R.J., BURROWS, M.R., JONES, P.W. &**

COLLINS, P., 1987. Swine dysentery: A new and effective vaccine. *The Pig Veterinary Society Proceedings*, 18, 87–91.

46 **MEIER, C., 1988.** Practical experience with dimetridazole against swine dysentery. *Praktische Tierärzt*, 69, 52–54.

47 **OLSON, D., 1986.** Probable elimination of swine dysentery after feeding romidazole, carbadox or lincomycin and verification by feeding sodium arsanilate. *Canadian Journal of Veterinary Research*, 50, 365–368.

48 **OLSON, L.D. & FALES, W.H., 1983.** Comparison of stained smears and culturing for identification of *Treponema hyodysenteriae*. *Journal of Clinical Microbiology*, 18, 950–955.

49 **OLSON, L.D. & RODABAUGHM, D.E., 1986.** Feeding sodium arsanilate for exciting diarrhea and identifying carriers of swine dysentery. *Canadian Journal of Veterinary Research*, 50, 359–364.

50 **POHLENZ, J.F.L., WHIPP, S.C. & ROBINSON, I.M., 1983.** Pathogenesis of swine dysentery caused by *Treponema hyodysenteriae*. *Deutsche Tierärztliche Wochenschrift*, 90, 363–367.

51 **PROHASZKA, L. & LUKACS, K., 1984.** Influence of the diet on the antibacterial effect of volatile fatty acids and on the development of swine dysentery. *Zentralblatt für Veterinärmedizin*, B31, 779–785.

52 **RONCALLI, R.A. & LEANING, W.H.D., 1976.** Geographical distribution of swine dysentery. *Proceedings of the Fourth Congress of the International Pig Veterinary Society*, Iowa, U.S.A., June 22–24, L17.

53 **SATO, H., YAMAGUCHI, H. & MIWA, A., 1988.** Studies on swine dysentery. Tiamulin injection for the treatment of swine dysentery. *Bulletin of the Faculty of Agriculture, Kagoshima University*, No. 38.

54 **SCHRARER, E., 1986.** Pathophysiology of diarrhoea. *Praktische Tierärzt*, 67, 373–376; 378–379.

55 **SMITH, S.C., BARRETT, L.M., MUIR, T., CHRISTOPHER, W.L. & COLOE, P.J., 1991.** Application and evaluation of enzyme-linked immunosorbent assay and immunoblotting for detection of antibodies to *Treponema hyodysenteriae* in swine. *Epidemiology and Infection*, 107, 285–296.

56 **SMITH, S.C., RODDICK, F., LING, S., GERRATY, N.L. & COLOE, P.J., 1990.** Biochemical and immunochemical characterization of strains of *Treponema hyodysenteriae*. *Veterinary Microbiology*, 24, 29–41.

57 **SMITH, W.J. & NELSON, E.P., 1987.** Grower scour and non-specific colitis. *The Veterinary Record*, 121, 334.

58 **SONGER, J.G. & HARRIS, D.L., 1978.** Transmission of swine dysentery by carrier pigs. *American Journal of Veterinary Research*, 39, 913–916.

59 **SPENCER, B.T., 1976.** Personal communication.

60 **STANTON, T.B. & LEBO, D.F., 1988.** *Treponema hyodysenteriae* growth under various culture conditions. *Veterinary Microbiology*, 18, 177–190.

61 **SZYNKIEWICZ, Z.M. & BINEK, M., 1986.** Evaluation of selective media for primary isolation of *Treponema hyodysenteriae* and *Treponema innocens*. *Comparative Immunology, Microbiology and Infectious Diseases*, 9, 71–77.

62 **TAYLOR, D.J., 1986.** *Pig Diseases*. 4th edn. Published by author, University of Glasgow, 98–105.

63 **TAYLOR, D.J., CORREA, A.E. & ROA, P.P., 1987.** Grower scour and non-specific colitis. *The Veterinary Record*, 121, 479.

64 **TEIGE, J., LARSEN, H.J. & TOLLERSRUD, S., 1984.** Swine dysentery: The influence of dietary selenium on clinical and pathological effects of *Treponema hyodysenteriae* infection. *Acta Veterinaria Scandinavica*, 25, 1–9.

65 **TUBBS, R.C., 1987.** Four causes of mucohaemorrhagic diarrhoea you should recognize. *Veterinary Medicine*, 82, 89–94.

66 **WELLINGTON, A.C. & AUCOCK, H.W., 1977.** The use of dimetridazole in the sow herd for swine dysentery control: A preliminary field report. *Journal of the South African Veterinary Association*, 48, 193–194.

67 **WHITING, R.A., DOYLE, L.P. & SPRAY, R.S., 1921.** Swine dysentery. *Purdue University Agricultural Experimental Station Bulletin*, 257, 3–15.

68 **WOOD, E.N. & LYSONS, R.J., 1988.** Financial benefit from the eradication of swine dysentery. *The Veterinary Record*, 122, 277–279.

114

Borrelia theileri *infection*

G.C. Bishop

Introduction

According to Canham,[8] *Borrelia theileri* was first found in 1902 in the blood of cattle, sheep and a horse in South Africa by Theiler, and causes a benign disease with a very low mortality.[4] Borreliosis has been reported from many countries in Africa,[1, 11, 15, 18, 19, 24] South America,[9] and Europe,[10] and from Australia,[7] Mauritius[3] and Madagascar.[23] The disease, although fairly widespread and common,[11, 18] is of little economic importance, and few deaths have been reported.

Aetiology and epidemiology

Borrelia theileri (synonyms *Treponema theileri, Spirochaeta theileri*) varies somewhat in length, being slightly shorter in solipeds than in cattle, sheep, goats and antelope.[7] Most reports give its width as 0,25–0,30 µm and its length as 9–18 µm,[7] but some maintain that most are 20–30 µm long.[6] Although the organism appears shorter in solipeds, transmission from equine animals to cattle has been successful.[11] *Borrelia* spp. are difficult to culture, and specific media such as Barbour-Stoener-Kelly are required for this purpose.[16]

Several tick species have been listed as vectors of *B. theileri*, including *Rhipicephalus evertsi evertsi, Boophilus decoloratus, B. australis, B. microplus* and *B. annulatus*.[2, 6, 7, 18, 19, 21, 22] The nymphal and adult stages of these ticks are more infective than the larvae, and the parasite is passed from the parents via the eggs to their progeny.[21] Infection by *B. theileri* is often associated with infection by *Babesia* spp., which has led some workers to believe that *B. theileri* may be of secondary importance.[11, 24]

Pathogenesis and clinical signs

Following a prepatent period of two to three weeks,[7, 17, 20] spirochaetes are usually found in the peripheral blood at the onset of the febrile attack. This is followed by anorexia, listlessness, depression and pyrexia.[5, 7, 20, 24] Anaemia occurs occasionally in splenectomized calves. A

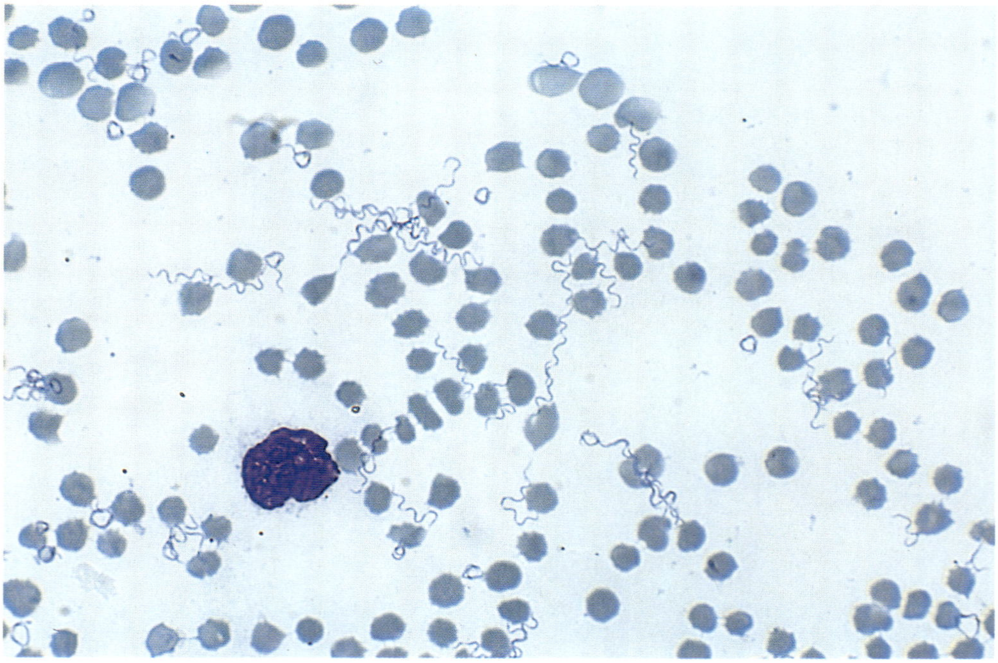

Figure 114.1 Blood smear: *Borrelia theileri*

Borrelia-like organism was found in the tick *Ornithodorus coriaceus*, and it was postulated that it might be a cause of bovine epizootic abortion.[14] Spleen smears made from aborted bovine foetuses in South Africa have revealed *Borrelia*-like spirochaetes which may be the cause of sporadic bovine abortions.[13]

Pathology

A few non-specific lesions including slight lymph node enlargement and petechiae in pale mucous membranes have been described.[12]

Diagnosis, differential diagnosis and control

Spirochaetes are easily seen in blood smears and stain well with aniline dyes **(Figure 114.1)**.[6] Clinically, borreliosis may be confused with mild cases of babesiosis, anaplasmosis and East Coast fever.[4, 12] Concomitant infections by *Babesia* spp. often complicate the diagnosis.

Control of the disease can be accomplished by controlling the tick population.[19] It has been shown in Zimbabwe that the prevalence of borreliosis increases when the frequency of dipping is reduced.

References

1 **ASSOKU, R.K.G., 1979.** A study of the incidence of blood-borne parasites of livestock in southern Ghana. *Bulletin of Animal Health and Production in Africa*, 27, 29–39.

2 **BARBOUR, A.G. & HAYES, S.F., 1986.** Biology of *Borrelia* species. *Microbiological Reviews*, 381–400.

3 **BARRÉ, N. & MOREL, P.C., 1983.** Ticks (Acarina, Ixodoidea) of the Mascarene Islands and tick-borne diseases. *Revue d'Élevage et de Médecine Vétérinaire des Pays Tropicaux*, 36, 371–377.

4 **BRUNER, D.W. & GILLESPIE, J.H., 1973.** *Hagan's Infectious Diseases of Domestic Animals*. London: Cornell University Press.

5 **BRYSON, R.W. & WELLS, G.E., 1963.** Spirochaetosis (Borreliosis) in a horse. *Journal of the South African Veterinary Medical Association*, 34, 103–104.

6 **BUCHANAN, R.E. & GIBBONS, N.E., 1974.** *Bergey's Manual of Determinative Bacteriology*. 8th edn. Baltimore: Williams & Wilkins.

7 **CALLOW, L.L., 1967.** Observations on tick-transmitted spirochaetes of cattle in Australia and South Africa. *British Veterinary Journal*, 123, 492–496.

8 **CANHAM, A.S., 1947.** Spirochaetosis in pigs. *Journal of the South African Veterinary Medical Association*, 18, 32–38.

9 **GUGLIELMONE, A.A., AGUIRRE, D.H., MANGOLD, A.J. & GAIDO, A.B., 1987.** *Borrelia* sp. in *Boophilus microplus*, the common tick of cattle, in Tucaman (Argentina). *Veterinaria Argentina*, 4, 248–249.

10 **HOVMARK, A., ASBRINK, E., SCHWAN, O., HENDERSTEDT, B. & CHRISTENSSON, D., 1986.** Antibodies to *Borrelia spirochaetes* in sera from Swedish cattle and sheep. *Acta Veterinaria Scandinavica*, 27, 479–485.

11 **KASCHULA, V.R., 1948.** *Treponema theileri* of a donkey and its transmission to a calf. *Journal of the South African Veterinary Medical Association*, 19, 100–102.

12 **KIPTOON, J.C., MARIBEI, J.M., KAMUA, L.L.W. & THUO, P., 1979.** Bovine borreliosis in Kenya: *Borrelia theileri* associated with bovine anaemia. *Kenyan Veterinarian*, 3,11–12.

13 **KITCHING, J.P. & BISHOP, G.C., 1980–87.** Allerton Regional Veterinary Laboratory, Pietermaritzburg, South Africa. Unpublished data.

14 **LANE, R.S., BURDORFER, W., HAYES, S.F. & BARBOUR, A.G., 1985.** Isolation of a spirochaete from the soft tick *Ornithodorus coriaceus*: A possible agent of epizootic bovine abortion. *Science, USA*, 230, 85–87.

15 **LEEFLANG, R., 1978.** Prevalence and significance of tick-borne diseases of domestic animals in northern Nigeria. *In:* WILDE, J.K.H., (ed.) *Tick-borne Diseases*. Scotland: Edinburgh University Press.

16 **MADIGAN, J.E. & TEITLER, J., 1988.** *Borrelia burgdorferi* borreliosis. *Journal of the American Veterinary Medical Association*, 192, 892–896.

17 **NEITZ, W.O., 1935.** The transmission of *Spirochaeta theileri* to a blesbuck (*Damaliscus albifrons*). *Onderstepoort Journal of Veterinary Science and Animal Industry*, 5, 7.

18 **NEITZ, W.O., 1965.** A check-list and host-list of the zoonoses in mammals and birds in South and South West Africa. *Onderstepoort Journal of Veterinary Science*, 32, 189–355.

19 **NORVAL, N.I.A., 1979.** Tick infestations and tick-borne diseases in Zimbabwe–Rhodesia. *Journal of the South African Veterinary Association*, 50, 289–292.

20 **SMITH, R.D., 1985.** *Borrelia theileri*: Isolation from ticks (*Boophilus microplus*) and tick-borne transmission from splenectomized calves. *American Journal of Veterinary Research*, 46, 1396–1398.

21 **SMITH, R.D., BRENER, J., OSBORNO, M. & RISTIC, M., 1978.** Pathobiology of *Borrelia theileri* in the tropical cattle tick, *Boophilus microplus*. *Journal of Invertebrate Pathology*, 32, 182–190.

22 **TREES, A.J., 1978.** The transmission of *Borrelia theileri* by *Boophilus annulatus*. *Tropical Animal Health and Production*, 10, 93–94.

23 **UILENBERG, G., 1971.** Studies of cowdriosis in Madagascar. Part 1. *Revue d'Élevage et de Médecine Vétérinaire des Pays Tropicaux*, 24, 239–249.

24 **VAN HEERDEN, J., 1984.** *Borrelia* sp. infection in a horse. *Journal of the South African Veterinary Association*, 55, 41–43.

115

Borrelia suilla *infection*

G.C. Bishop

Introduction

According to Henning,[6] spirochaetosis in pigs was first described in South Africa by Dodd in 1906. The disease, which is frequently associated with conditions of poor hygiene, is also known as porcine ulcerative granuloma, and has been reported in New Zealand, Australia, the USA and the UK.[1, 6] It is seen infrequently today and in South Africa it is not considered to be of any economic importance.

Aetiology and epidemiology

Borrelia suilla is 9–12 µm in length and has between two and six spirals. According to Canham,[4] Neitz believed that the spirochaete was definitely not identical to *B. theileri*. The bacteria stain readily with Giemsa, May-Grünwald, Gram's stain and 1 per cent carbol fuchsin, and using dark-field microscopy and fresh specimens they may be observed as actively motile spirochaetes.

The primary role of *B. suilla* (synonym *Spirochaeta suilla*) in the ulcerative granuloma syndrome is uncertain. *Borrelia suilla* has never been cultured on artificial media[1] and it is almost always to be found together with other bacteria in the lesions. The bacterium is not accorded species status in the eighth edition of *Bergey's Manual of Determinative Bacteriology*.[3]

Osborne[8] reproduced typical lesions by subcutaneous

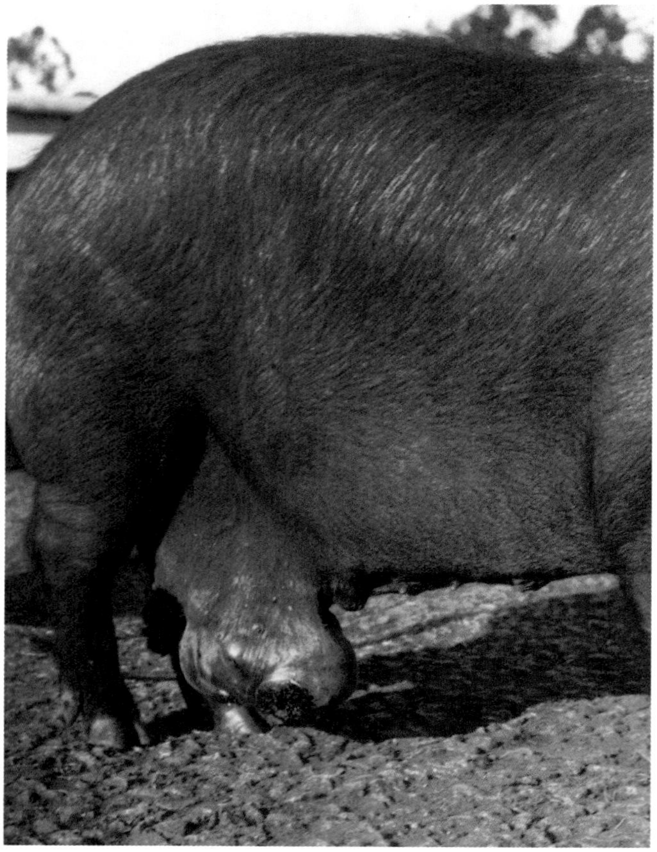

Figure 115.1 Ulcerative granuloma of the mammary gland of a sow

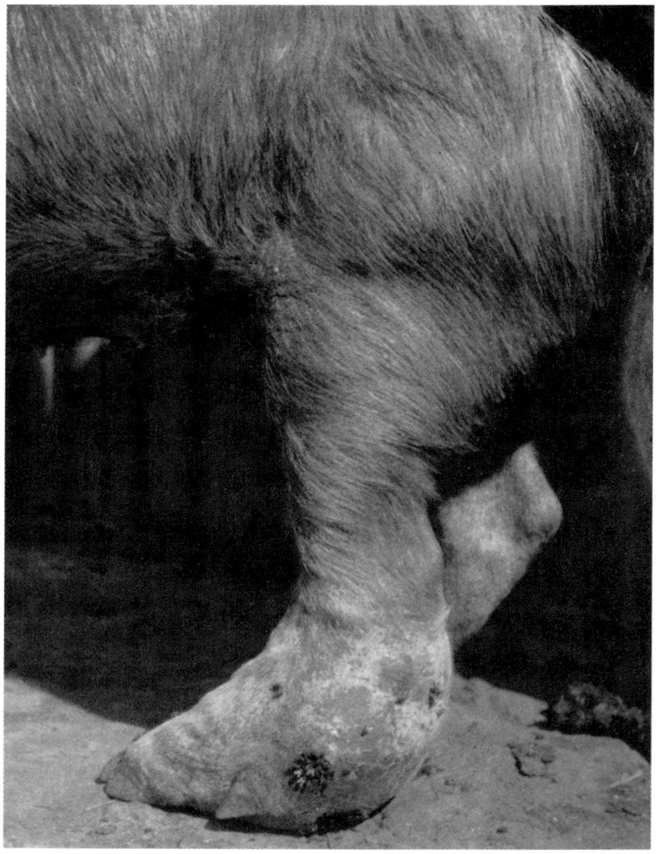

Figure 115.2 Ulcerative granuloma affecting the hind leg of a pig

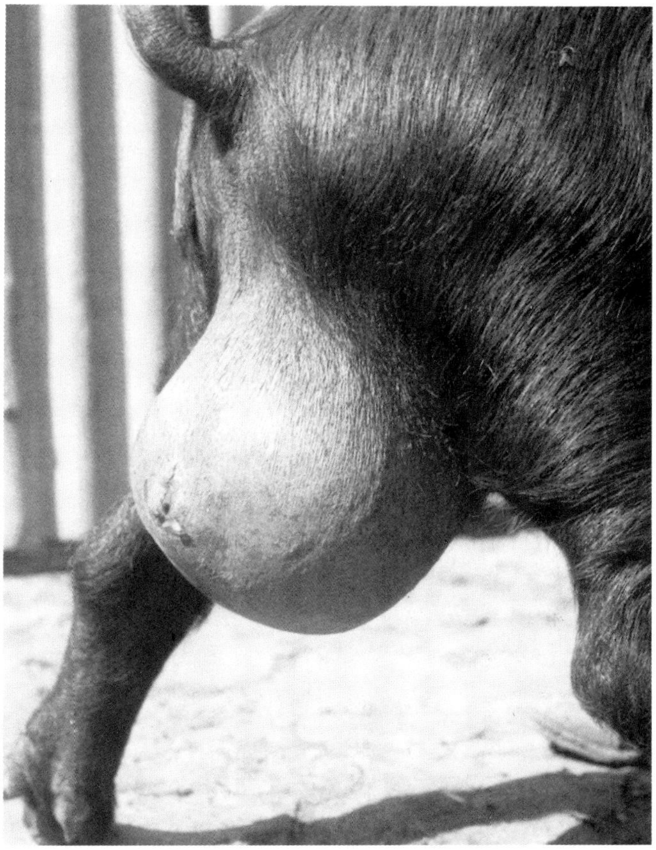

Figure 115.3 Granulomatous orchitis in a pig

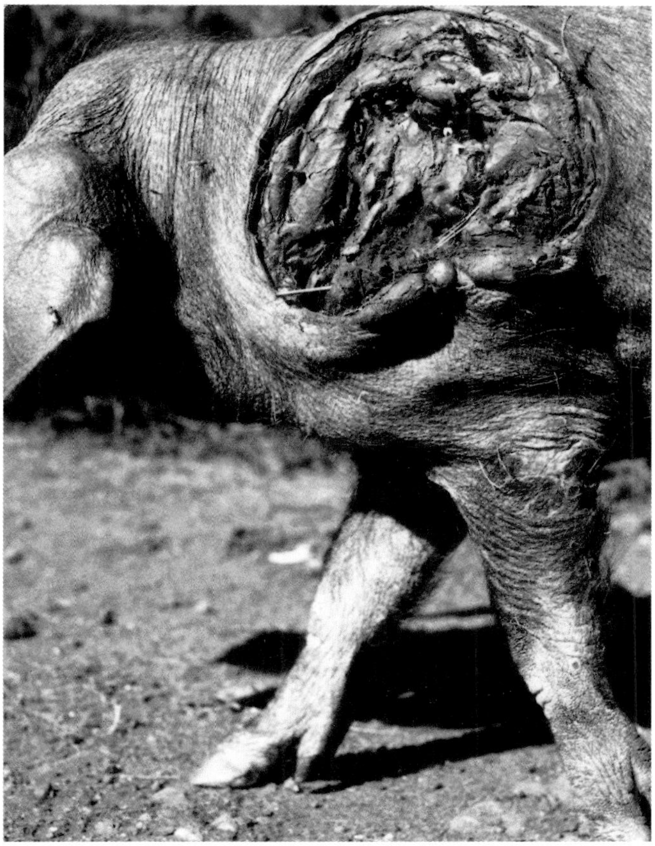

Figure 115.4 Severe ulcerative lesion affecting the shoulder of a pig

injection of material from natural cases, which also contained actively motile spirochaetes, into healthy pigs. Although it has not yet been proved,[5] some workers believe that predisposing factors (such as trauma due to biting, or self-trauma due to the irritation caused by mange or flea infestations) are prerequisites for infection and that the spirochaete may not be the primary pathogen.

Spirochaetosis was commonly seen in pigs of six to ten weeks of age, especially following castration.[6] Generally, less severe lesions were seen in older pigs.[1, 5]

Pathogenesis, clinical signs and pathology

The spirochaetes usually enter the body through superficial wounds and provoke the formation of abscesses or ulcerative lesions of varying severity in the subcutaneous tissues.[6] Lesions may occur on the face of sucking pigs, the ventral abdominal wall of sows **(Figure 115.1)**,[2] the legs **(Figure 115.2)**, which may result in varying degrees of lameness, or in the testes **(Figure 115.3)**.[1, 4] Lesions confined mainly to the ears, lips, gums, tongue and larynx have been reported in pigs in Britain.[1] Superficial abscesses may attain considerable dimensions and, on rupturing, may leave open wounds which persistently discharge necrotic material.[6] The surrounding skin, and sometimes the underlying tissues, may slough **(Figure 115.4)**.

Lesions vary widely in appearance.[7] Chronic ulcerations, accompanied by considerable fibrosis of the surrounding tissue, may develop. Histologically, numerous spirochaetes may be found in the necrotic tissue and the active margins of the ulcers.

Diagnosis, differential diagnosis and control

The demonstration of spirochaetes in tissue specimens by dark-field microscopy, or in tissue sections using the usual stains, supports the diagnosis.[6] In young pigs, lesions should be differentiated from necrotic lesions due to snout-rubbing, ear-biting, and self-trauma resulting from mange infestation.[2]

Potassium iodide administered orally, penicillin injections, or topical tetracycline treatment have been used successfully.[2, 5] Prevention of the condition by improvement of hygiene, disinfection and treatment of skin wounds should reduce its occurrence in affected piggeries.

References

1 **BLANDFORD, T.B., BYGRAVE, A.C., HARDING, D.J. & LITTLE, T.W.A., 1972.** Suspected porcine ulcerative spirochaetosis in England. *The Veterinary Record*, 90, 15.

2 **BLOOD, D.C., RADOSTITS, O.M. & HENDERSON, J.A., 1983.** *Veterinary Medicine*. 6th edn. London: Baillière Tindall.

3 **BUCHANAN, R.E. & GIBBONS, N.E., 1974.** *Bergey's Manual of Determinative Bacteriology*. 8th edn. Baltimore: Williams & Wilkins.

4 **CANHAM, A.S., 1947.** Spirochaetosis in pigs. *Journal of the South African Veterinary Medical Association*, 18, 32–38.

5 **HARCOURT, R.A., 1973.** Porcine ulcerative spirochaetosis. *The Veterinary Record*, 92, 647–648.

6 **HENNING, M.W., 1956.** *Animal Diseases in South Africa*. 3rd edn. Pretoria: Central News Agency Ltd.

7 **JUBB, K.F.E. & KENNEDY, P.C., 1970.** *Pathology of Domestic Animals*. 2nd edn. Vol. II. New York: Academic Press.

8 **OSBORNE, H.G., 1955.** Some aspects of the pathology, aetiology and therapeutics of footrot in pigs. *New Zealand Veterinary Journal*, 3, 91–99.

116

Leptospirosis

P. Hunter and S. Herr

Introduction

Leptospirosis in livestock is caused by spirochaetes of the genus *Leptospira* and is manifested by different syndromes including a haemolytic crisis, chronic interstitial nephritis and mastitis. Leptospirosis is also an important worldwide cause of abortions, stillbirths and reproductive failure in cattle and pigs in particular, and there is an increasing prevalence of leptospirosis in humans resulting from contact with infected stock. 'Periodic ophthalmia' in horses is associated with leptospiral infections.

Leptospirosis was first recognized in humans in 1886 by Weil,[132] who described it as an infectious disease characterized by icterus. The responsible organism was simultaneously isolated and reported in 1916 by two independent groups of researchers,[72, 126] and shortly afterwards, rats, from which *Leptospira icterohaemorrhagiae* was isolated, were shown to be a source of infection for humans.[71] Subsequently, *Leptospira* have been isolated from a variety of animal species and from humans manifesting various clinical syndromes such as 'mud fever' and 'swineherd's disease'.[12, 50, 84, 120]

In South Africa, leptospirosis is of importance in the pig and, to a lesser extent, cattle industries. *Leptospira pomona* is present in piggeries throughout the country, while the prevalence of *L. hardjo* is increasing on cattle farms. The latter organism is also being found increasingly in humans.[7]

Aetiology

Leptospira spp. belong to the family Leptospiraceae. They differ from members of the family Spirochaetaceae in that they have hooked ends, are obligate aerobes and use fatty acids or alcohols as carbon and energy sources.[74]

Leptospires are helical, motile bacteria, consisting of a cell body or protoplasmic cylinder enclosed by a membrane or outer envelope. Depending on the serovar and cultural conditions, the length of leptospires ranges from 3–20 µm. The cells are usually 0,1 µm in width and the helix has a wavelength of approximately 0,5 µm.[68] The organism's unique method of locomotion is effected by rotation about its longitudinal axis and by a flexing action. This is made possible by two periplasmic flagella wound around the length of the cell, one of which is inserted at the end of the helix.[75]

The genus *Leptospira* contains two species: *L. biflexa*, which, although it may on occasion be isolated from animals, is a free-living, non-pathogenic saprophyte found in moist environments; and *L. interrogans*, whose serovars are pathogens. The two species are morphologically indistinguishable but can be differentiated biochemically and by their growth characteristics.[76] In addition, based on DNA homology, three genetic groups are recognized within the genus *Leptospira*.[16]

Antigenically-related serovars of *L. interrogans* are placed in serogroups **(see Table 116.1)**. Thus the Icterohaemorrhagiae serogroup contains, amongst others, the serovars *icterohaemorrhagiae, copenhageni, birkini, budapest* and *dakota*. Roughly 180 different serovars have been isolated.[13]

Table 116.1 Serogroups and important serovars of leptospires (adapted from Faine[41])

SEROGROUP	IMPORTANT SEROVARS
Australis	*Australis, bratislava, muenchen*
Autumnalis	*Autumnalis*
Ballum	*Ballum*
Bataviae	*Bataviae*
Butembo	*Butembo*
Canicola	*Canicola*
Celledoni	*Celledoni*
Cynopteri	*Cynopteri*
Djasiman	*Djasiman*
Grippotyphosa	*Grippotyphosa*
Hebdomadis	*Georgia, hebdomadis, mini,* * *szwajizak**
Icterohaemorrhagiae	*Copenhageni, icterohaemorrhagiae*
Javanica	*Javanica*
Panama	*Panama*
Pomona	*Pomona*
Pyrogenes	*Pyrogenes*
Sejroe	*Balcanica,**** hardjo,** polonica,**** saxkoebing,*** sejroe,**** wolffi,***
Shermani	*Shermani*
Tarassovi	*Tarassovi*

* Serogroup Mini
** Subgroup Wolffi
*** Subgroup Saxkoebing
**** Subgroup Sejroe

Serovars are distinguished on the basis of their antigenic composition, which is determined by agglutination and cross-agglutinin absorption tests. Biochemical tests are of no value in distinguishing between serovars, but differences in aminopeptidase activity are useful in serovar identification.[98] Restriction endonuclease digests of leptospiral DNA promise a means of specific differentiation between serovars.[124]

The *in vitro* cultivation of leptospires requires the supplementation of growth media with long-chain fatty acids and with vitamins B_1 and B_{12}. Fatty acids are supplied by the addition of serum to growth media or, alternatively, an albumin-polysorbate 80 medium can be used. Another suitable medium, the EMJH medium,[28] is available commercially or can be prepared in-house. Protein-free media containing charcoal-detoxified polysorbates are popular — especially for vaccine production.[13, 23]

Liquid, semi-solid or solid media can be used for cultivation. Most laboratories employ semi-solid media for initial isolation and maintenance of cultures, and liquid media for antigen production. For isolation of leptospires from most sources, it is essential to add 5-fluorouracil[77] or a combination of several antibiotics[2] in order to inhibit the growth of contaminating bacteria which may hamper isolation. It is essential to use specimens of fresh organs and body fluids for isolation in order to lessen the detrimental effects of other bacteria and products of autolysis on leptospires. In addition, tissue samples and urine may have to be diluted to minimize these effects. Leptospires in culture grow at an optimal temperature of 29–30 °C. Samples may have to be incubated for long periods before organisms can be detected, and cultures should not be discarded before they have been incubated for at least six weeks.

The survival of *Leptospira* in the environment is dependent on variations in temperature and humidity. Drying and pH values below six or exceeding eight are detrimental to their survival outside hosts. Bacteria can survive for at least 183 days in wet soil, whereas they live for less than 30 minutes in air-dried soil. Stagnant water also remains contaminated by live leptospires for prolonged periods. The survival time in acid soils with a low moisture content may be as long as 24 days.[61]

Epidemiology

Leptospira interrogans has been isolated from a wide range of hosts including a large number of free-living mammals,[128] domestic animals and poikilothermic vertebrates such as amphibians and reptiles.[94] In many countries where leptospirosis occurs, wild animals such as rats, mice, jackals, foxes, mongoose, skunks, raccoons, wild boar and deer[128] are carriers of specific serovars and act as sources of infection for domestic animals.

The various serovars of *L. interrogans* have differing affinities for animal hosts, of which two distinct categories (maintenance and accidental hosts) are recognized.[14]

Maintenance hosts serve as sources of infection for accidental hosts.[58] They are easily infected but they develop mild or no clinical signs. Localization occurs in the kidneys without the concurrent development of renal lesions once organisms have been cleared from the circulation after the initial infection. Transmission occurs readily to members within the same maintenance host species. Rats (*Rattus norvegicus*), for example, are readily infected by a low dose of the serovar *L. icterohaemorrhagiae*, after which large numbers of organisms are shed in their urine — in some instances for the rest of their lives. Many wildlife species such as bat, mongoose, jackal, fox, opossum and raccoon are maintenance hosts for *Leptospira* serovars which infect accidental hosts such as humans and domestic animals. Domestic livestock species have also become effective maintenance hosts for certain serovars, such as pigs for *L. pomona*, and cattle for *L. hardjo*. Although there is wide-spread serological evidence of infection in horses in many countries, this species does not appear to act as a maintenance host for any specific serovar[60] — except for *L. bratislava*, which may be adapted to and maintained by horses in Northern Ireland.

Few wild animal reservoirs of leptospiral organisms have been found in Africa, despite their high prevalence in domestic stock.[95] A few isolates, all from rodents such as the grass mice (*Arvicanthis niloticus*) in the Nile Delta[89] and (*A. abyssinicus*) in Zaïre, and gerbils (*Tatera robusta vicinia*) in Kenya,[8] have been made from free-living animals in Africa.[127] No leptospires have been found in wild species in Uganda[8] and Ethiopia.[95] A survey conducted in South Africa, in which leptospiral isolation was attempted from the kidneys of 879 rodents representing 19 different species, yielded negative results.[110] Serology on 416 rodents of 14 different species produced only a single positive titre to *L. grippotyphosa* in a wild mouse (*Mastomys* sp.) from the eastern Transvaal.[110] Sera of free-living game in the northern Natal game parks contained antibody to *L. mini* in a reedbuck (*Redunca* sp.), a bushpig (*Potamachoerus porcus*), a black wildebeest (*Connochaetes gnu*), and to *L. tarassovi* in a nyala (*Tragelaphus angasii*). Two black rhino (*Diceros bicornis*) had multi-serovar titres to *L. mini*, *L. hardjo*, *L. tarassovi*, *L. copenhageni* and *L. pomona*.[69]

Accidental hosts are fairly resistant to infection, but once infected, they exhibit severe clinical signs. In these hosts the renal phase is short and inter-species transmission is inefficient.

Transmission of leptospirosis depends on conditions favouring the survival of the organism in the environment, on the number of carrier animals in a population, and on the length of time for which carrier animals shed leptospires.

Leptospirosis is transmitted most effectively from the urine of carrier animals to susceptible ones via water-borne wastes such as slurry or run-off water from infected animal houses.[41] Organisms shed in the urine survive only under favourable conditions such as adequate moisture and a neutral to slightly alkaline pH.[48, 82] Salinity, run-off caused by heavy rainfall, and high levels of other species of bacteria further reduce the chances of survival. Adsorption of leptospires onto the surface of clay-like soils reduces the chances of contact with a suitable host.[48]

Leptospires may be transmitted venereally, transplacentally, or via the cutaneous, oral, respiratory or conjunctival routes.[5] Oral infection of cattle has failed experimentally, but it is suspected that it does occur naturally.[5] Carnivores could be successfully infected by consuming contaminated food.[104] Aerosol transmission has been achieved experimentally,[105] and is thought to be an important method of spread, as a fine spray of droplets is produced during urination — especially in animals such as dairy cattle or pigs confined to buildings with cement floors. Transmission is also possible through coitus or by artificial insemination.[107, 112] Pathogenic serovars of *Leptospira* are well preserved in semen and in media used for its dilution.[80]

Leptospirosis in cattle in South Africa occurs mostly in relatively high-rainfall areas — the eastern Transvaal, Natal and the coastal area of the Cape Province (from Port Elizabeth in the east to the western Cape area). However, it has also been diagnosed in the dry northern and north-western Transvaal.[62] Serovars *L. pomona*, *L. mini*, *L. canicola* and *L. hardjo* have been isolated from cattle in South Africa.[63, 121] It appears that *L. hardjo* is the most important cause of bovine leptospirosis in South Africa, and that *L. pomona* causes sporadic infections. During 1986–87, 27,9 per cent of bovine serum samples tested at the Veterinary Research Institute, Onderstepoort, were positive for *L. tarassovi*, 25,5 per cent for *L. mini* and 20,8 per cent for *L. hardjo*.[7] As none of the multivalent leptospiral bacterins used in South Africa contain either *L. tarassovi* or *L. mini*, significant antibody levels against these serovars as a consequence of immunization are not possible and cattle are probably exposed to these strains from as yet unidentified sources. *Leptospira mini* has been reported as a cause of abortion in cattle[46] but, at present, the role of *L. tarassovi* as a cause of bovine infertility is unknown.[85] In Zimbabwe positive titres in 27 per cent of cattle have been recorded,[44] the most common reactions being against *L. sejroe* and *L. tarassovi*. In Botswana *L. pomona* has been isolated from cattle with a history of abortions.[64]

Leptospirosis in pigs in South Africa is widespread; *L. pomona*, in particular, has been incriminated as a cause of abortions, stillbirths, perinatal deaths, and chronic interstitial nephritis.[70] *Leptospira canicola* and *L. icterohaemorrhagiae* have also been isolated from pigs in infected herds.[130]

In South Africa serological investigations have indicated that *L. pomona* infection caused an outbreak of leptospirosis in sheep, where the source was an infected piggery.[26] Leptospirosis has not yet been described in goats in South Africa.

Infection of horses with leptospirosis has been reported from Australia,[119] North America,[56] Egypt,[9] and Great Britain.[60] Twenty-seven per cent of all sera from horses tested in South Africa in 1986–87 were positive for *L. pomona*, but no clinical disease has been recorded yet in this species.[7]

Pathogenesis

The disease is transmitted indirectly by water or mud contaminated with infected urine, particularly when the skin is abraded[123] or softened by prolonged immersion in water.[51] Following infection, leptospires enter the blood stream and localize in the liver, where primary replication takes place. From here the organisms are released into the blood, resulting in a leptospiraemia which coincides with the development of a febrile reaction and malaise. Thereafter organisms localize in the lungs, brain, kidneys, eyes or the pregnant uterus.[51] Clinical signs (which are seen after an incubation period of two to 16 days) are dependent on the site of localization.

It is thought that some of the lesions of leptospirosis are caused by bacterial toxins. A cytotoxic sphingomyelinase[20] produced during the replication of the organism may be responsible for hepatocellular damage and haemorrhages in the lungs, mucous membranes, and kidneys.[51] Certain serovars produce a haemolysin which causes haemolytic anaemia and subsequent haemoglobinuria, icterus, and also hepatocellular and bile duct necrosis. Agalactia may also be caused by this cytotoxin.[51]

Leptospires localizing in the brain may persist there for long periods, giving rise, in some cases, to nervous signs.[41] Localization in the proximal tubules of the kidneys in maintenance hosts may cause a mild, chronic, inter-stitial nephritis and long-term leptospiruria.[123]

Foetal infection as a result of leptospires crossing the placenta varies in outcome, depending on the age of the foetus. Abortion may result or the foetus may produce antibodies and survive, or it may be born weak and be latently infected.[42, 43]

The pathogenesis of the ophthalmia in horses is still unknown, but it is probably a combination of an ocular leptospiral infection and the effects of immunopathological mechanisms. There is a close antigenic relationship between certain leptospiral antigens of the *interrogans, hardjo, icterohaemorrhagiae, tarassovi* and *pomona* serovars and the cornea of horses which appears to contribute to the development of corneal opacity in infected horses.[102]

Clinical signs

The clinical signs of leptospirosis vary from severe to inapparent and differ according to the specific syndrome.

Cattle

Most serovars of *Leptospira* which infect cattle cause acute, subacute or inapparent leptospirosis.[127]

Leptospira pomona is the most common cause of acute leptospirosis,[35] which is characterized by fever, anorexia, malaise, leptospiruria and haemoglobinuria, followed by icterus and anaemia.[87] Affected calves may also have diarrhoea.[99] The fever which accompanies the leptospiruria may last from one to five days and relapses occur recurrently for up to 53 days in 80 per cent of infected animals.[36] Calves tend to die within one to seven days.[78]

Cows infected with *L. pomona* have a reduced milk yield and may abort,[5] while calves born following this infection are weak and some are immature.[36, 122] Cows that abort during the acute phase manifest only mild clinical signs; 'mastitis' and an accompanying agalactia (referred to as the 'milk-drop' or the 'flabby-bag' syndrome) however, occur consistently.[122] All quarters of the udder become flaccid, the milk is thick and yellowish resembling colostrum and is California milk-ring test positive.[103] The alagactia resolves within a week and its course is not affected by treatment. It appears not to be a true mastitis as the affected udder lacks an inflammatory response, though leptospires can be isolated from the milk and udder tissue.[103]

Subacute cases manifest fever, mild haemoglobinuria and 'mastitis', which is characterized by the secretion of reduced amounts of thick, blood-stained milk.[5] Subclinical or inapparent infections are detected only when they result in abortions or during serological surveillance. *Leptospira pomona* infection in South African cattle has been the cause of abortion storms.[1, 63]

Leptospires of the Hebdomadis serogroup, and in particular the serovar *hardjo*, have been recognized worldwide as being a cause of bovine abortion, infertility and mastitis.[52, 65, 86, 117] Infection with *L. hardjo* causes fever of up to 41 °C which lasts from one to five days in some cases,[38] depression, listlessness,[122] a precipitous drop in milk production, and abortions or the birth of weak, sometimes premature, calves depending on the stage of pregnancy when infection occurred.[38, 65, 103, 122] 'Mastitis' occurs consistently in cows that calve,[122] varying in severity; in some animals the udder is just flaccid, while in others there is a severe 'mastitis' characterized by thick, cream-coloured milk with a pasty consistency, or by bloody milk with a normal consistency which varies in colour from pale pink to dark red.

Low conception rates often occur in *L. hardjo*-infected herds.[52] In such herds *L. hardjo* can be isolated from the genital tract of non-pregnant cows.[40] Animals with subclinical *L. hardjo* infections are serologically positive[38] and may have a leptospiruria which can persist for up to 450 days or longer.[27, 122] In all instances these animals suffer from a subclinical, mild, focal, interstitial nephritis.[122]

Pigs

Leptospirosis in pigs is predominantly a chronic, asymptomatic disease which may go unnoticed in a herd for a long time. When it manifests itself, it is characterized primarily by the occurrence of abortions, infertility and the birth of premature and weak piglets. Abortion may occur from as early as six week' gestation, although it mostly occurs towards term; many litters reach term and are either all stillborn or are a mixture of stillborn and live, weak piglets.[33] Serovars of the Pomona and Tarassovi serogroups are recognized as being the major causes of infertility in pigs. However, serogroups like Canicola, Hebdomadis, Icterohaemorrhagiae, Autumnalis and Autralis have also been implicated.[33] Acute systemic disease characterized by a haemolytic crisis and death is rarely encountered, but may be caused by *L. icterohaemorrhagiae*.[78]

Leptospira pomona, which is the most important cause of porcine leptospirosis in South Africa, usually causes only mild or inapparent infections.[53] The *pomona* serovar also causes an asymptomatic chronic interstitial nephritis which is usually only identified at slaughter.

Natural and experimental infections by *L. canicola* cause abortions, mummification, stillbirths, neonatal mortality and low conception rates.[92] Serovars of the Australis serogroup are similarly associated with infertility,[59] and have been isolated from the genital tracts of sows and boars.[34]

Sheep and goats

Leptospirosis of sheep manifests as two distinct clinical syndromes: an acute and often fatal systemic disease, and genital disease.

Leptospira hardjo infections in sheep cause agalactia,[90] abortion, stillbirths, and the birth of weak lambs.[30] Abortion rates of up to 20 per cent have been recorded[6] — abortions being caused largely by the Hebdomadis, Australis and Pomona serogroups.[30] Ewes manifesting 'agalactia' clinically show only a partial or total loss in milk production, which resolves itself without treatment within three to four days. The syndrome is usually only noticed when lambs with a normal birth weight die of malnutrition.[90] *Leptospira hardjo* has also been isolated from the kidneys of infected wethers suffering from a subclinical, chronic, interstitial nephritis.[32, 47]

The acute systemic disease in lambs is characterized by icterus, haemoglobinaemia, haemoglobinuria, fever and death, and has been associated with infections by the Pomona serogroup in particular, but also by the Hebdomadis, Ballum and Grippotyphosa serogroups.[30] Adult animals have also been reported as succumbing to a similar infection.[10] This fatal haemolytic disease may kill up to 5 per cent of the lamb crop,[108, 113] losses being experienced in two- to four-month-old lambs, which are reluctant to move, become depressed and stand off by themselves. If not closely observed, lambs may not be found until they are dead or are seen straggling behind the flock when they are moved over a distance; at these times lambs may be seen passing red urine.[108] Haemolytic disease causing icterus, haemoglobinuria and high mortality, and abortion caused by *L. pomona* infection have also been recorded.[67] In this type of infection, even mildly affected animals manifest haemolysis, haemoglobinaemia and haemoglobinuria, as well as mild impairment of the renal tubular and glomerular function.[93]

Goats are susceptible to infection by the *grippotyphosa* serovar, which causes an acute disease characterized by haemoglobinuria, anaemia, icterus, and death in severe cases.[78] Experimental *hardjo* and *pomona* infections in goats cause only mild clinical signs, fever, and a drop in milk production in some animals.[125] Serovars *pomona, sejroe, icterohaemorrhagiae* and *grippotyphosa* have been associated with outbreaks of abortion in goats.

Horses

Most infections of horses by *Leptospira* are subclinical.[58] Knowledge of the role of the specific serovars as a cause of disease in horses is limited,[60] but the recognized clinical syndromes include abortions between six months and term, stillbirth, and premature live birth;[31] fever and icterus;[54] and death from interstitial nephritis.[54, 78, 83]

Leptospiral infections in horses are more commonly associated with the development of ophthalmia, often referred to as 'periodic ophthalmia, equine recurrent uveitis, recurrent iridocyclitis or endogenous uveitis'. Involvement of the eyes is considered to be a sequel to equine leptospirosis. It develops some time (sometimes years[25]) after the animal initially became infected, and manifests as a painful keratitis or ophthalmitis.[118] It is recurrent, uni- or bilateral and characterized clinically by miosis, congestion of the sclera, photophobia, severe lachrymation and sometimes blindness.[25, 114]

Pathology

Cattle

The pathology of leptospirosis in cattle varies according to the respective syndrome.

In the acute systemic disease the macroscopic lesions are characteristic of a haemolytic crisis and septicaemia, and they include icterus, anaemia, splenomegaly, and subcutaneous and mucosal haemorrhages.[78, 99] Pulmonary oedema, hepatomegaly and nephritis are also typical of acute leptospirosis. The microscopic lesions in the liver and kidneys are those associated with a haemolytic crisis.[78]

Macroscopically the renal lesions, which may be as small as 1–2 mm in diameter, may be restricted to the cortex or also extend into the medulla. These lesions are sometimes accompanied by a few haemorrhages and small pitted areas. The renal capsule is adherent to the cortex over the affected areas.[122] Vaccination does not prevent the development of interstitial nephritis as a consequence of leptospiral infection, but the lesions in these animals are less common and less severe.[81] Histologically there is a mild, focally disseminated, interstitial, lymphoplasmacytic nephritis. The infiltrate in the affected kidneys occurs primarily in the interstitial tissue and around the glomeruli[99] and consists mostly of lymphocytes and plasma cells; a few neutrophils and eosinophils may also be seen.[81] Leptospiral organisms are not necessarily associated with lesions in the kidneys.[36] Other lesions in the kidneys include degeneration, necrosis and atrophy of the tubular epithelium, few cellular and hyaline casts, and the development later of mild fibrosis. Glomeruli may show swelling of the tuft, an accumulation of protein in the urinary space, and fibrosis of Bowman's capsule. Focal areas of calcification may occur in the cortex and in the medulla.[81]

Leptospires may be detected histologically in the tissues of affected animals by the application of silver staining or immunogold staining techniques.[111] Certain modifications of the Warthin-Starry stain give reliable results.[91] In calves, the organisms may be demonstrated in various tissues, including the kidneys, liver and lungs; and organisms are seen in the kidneys, placenta, cotyledons, and the liver of some affected cows.[122] The presence of leptospires in the kidneys does not necessarily induce a nephritis[111] and there is often no correlation between the severity of the renal lesions and the isolation of leptospires from the respective tissues.

Few specific lesions occur in the placenta of animals that have aborted. The intercotyledonary tissue may be oedematous while the cotyledons may be fawn-coloured and atonic. Hydropic degeneration and focal necrosis of the epithelial cells in the cotyledons occur in the affected placentas. The degree of change varies between animals and also between the cotyledons of the same animal.[36]

Aborted foetuses may be quite fresh,[36] oedematous or autolysed at the time of abortion. No characteristic features are seen except that organisms may be found in the organs, and that foci of tubular necrosis, sometimes associated with the early stages of an interstitial nephritis, occur.[36, 78] Few lesions are seen in weak, live-born calves. However, haemorrhages may occur in the urinary bladder, lungs and kidneys — or the kidneys may be only oedematous.[122]

Sheep and goats

Few lesions are seen in sheep with leptospirosis. The only macroscopic lesions in cases due to *L. pomona* are acute nephritis and concurrent haemorrhage.[96, 113] *Leptospira hardjo* infections cause focal, chronic, interstitial nephritis, a multifocal, acute hepatitis or chronic cholangiohepatitis.[47]

Infection by the *hardjo* and *pomona* serovars also causes a fatal haemolytic syndrome in lambs, which is characterized by severe icterus, anaemia, haemoglobinuria, and pale brown[113] to dark red or blackish kidneys.[67, 108] On cut surface the kidneys manifest dark brown streaks and the focal white spots of an interstitial nephritis. Cell swelling and necrosis of a few hepatocytes are seen histologically in these animals, while haemosiderin

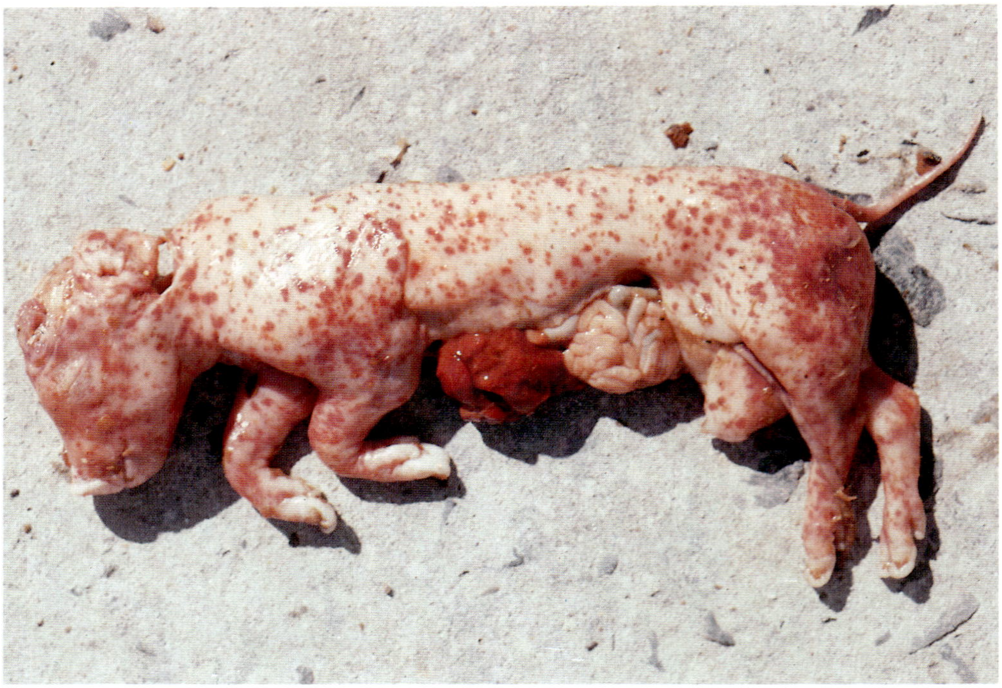

Figure 116.1 Numerous cutaneous haemorrhages in a pig foetus aborted as a result of leptospirosis

pigmentation of the tubular epithelium and clumps of leptospires, hyaline casts, haemoglobin and cellular debris also occur in the kidneys.[113]

Leptospires have been detected by immunoperoxidase in the tissues of aborted or stillborn foetuses.[30]

Pigs

With the exception of multiple haemorrhages **(Figure 116.1)**, no specific lesions occur in piglets which die soon after birth, in foetuses, or in stillborn piglets. In acute, fatal leptospirosis, splenomegaly, hepatomegaly, haemorrhages, and focal necrosis of the liver may occur.[78] Histologically, acute hepatitis, lymphocytic myocarditis and interstitial nephritis are seen in these cases.

Chronic interstitial nephritis is frequently found in slaughter pigs infected with leptospires.[66, 70] These lesions are seen as greyish foci, a few millimetres to centimetres in diameter, in the cortex and medulla.[53] Advanced lesions become fibrosed.[55]

Histologically the lesions in the kidneys vary according to the stage of their development. Acute lesions are characterized by hyperaemia, oedema and degeneration of the tubular epithelium, but when they become subacute, they are characterized by the presence of monocytes and macrophages which are replaced at a later stage by plasma cells and lymphocytes. Even serovars of low virulence cause lesions in the kidneys. Leptospires occur in affected kidneys at all stages of the development of the lesions. Initially they are present in all the structures, including blood vessels, but as the lesions progress in age they are restricted to the lumens of the renal tubules **(Figures 116.2 and 116.3)**.[22]

Leptospiral organisms in tissues of affected animals may be detected in 10 per cent suspensions of fresh tissues examined by dark-field microscopy, or by applying the indirect fluorescent antibody technique to frozen tissue sections.[73]

Horses

The sequestration of leptospires in the eyes causes a progressive uveitis, thought to be the consequence of a hypersensitivity reaction. The anterior uveitis which is seen initially progresses during repeated attacks to involve the posterior uvea, cornea, retina and optic nerve, with resulting blindness.

Lesions are rarely seen in aborted foetuses, even though the infection may be diagnosed by immunofluorescence or by isolation of the organism.[31] Detection of the organism by immunofluorescence is most successful in the kidneys and the liver. Histologically no changes other than those caused by autolysis are seen in aborted foetuses. Rarely, dissociation of the hepatocytes, necrosis of individual hepatocytes, and confluent and multiple areas of necrosis can be seen. Non-specific lesions include degeneration of the renal tubules and perivascular haemorrhages in the kidneys and the brain.[31] Concurrent infections such as equid herpesvirus 1 cause more severe lesions in the affected organs. In these cases, inclusions are present in the affected cells and serve to confirm the diagnosis.[29]

Diagnosis

The history and clinical signs in affected animals may indicate leptospirosis, but the diagnosis should be confirmed by laboratory tests.

Serology on paired serum samples collected during the acute and convalescent phases of the disease is useful in confirming a diagnosis of leptospirosis.[35] A rising titre to a specific serovar indicates infection with that specific serovar, but cross-reactions between different serovars may occur. Factors which limit the usefulness of serology in individual animals are the administration of antibiotics which suppress the development of antibodies, previous vaccination which hampers the interpretation of serological results, and the prevalence of significant antibody levels in endemic areas.

Serological tests are useful for screening herds with a history of abortions or reproductive problems. The antibody levels in the dam sometimes decline shortly after abortion. In addition, some mature animals do not respond serologically despite being infected.[41] The microscopic agglutination test (MAT) with live antigens is the standard serological test, but its main disadvantage is that it requires the maintenance of live cultures of *Leptospira*, which exposes staff to infection, and alone it is insufficient for the routine diagnosis of leptospirosis in individual animals. However, it is effective on a herd basis.[62, 131] The ELISA test has also been used with success in the diagnosis of leptospirosis in some species,[3, 24] particularly in differentiating between acute and chronic infections.[57] It is an acceptable alternative to the MAT

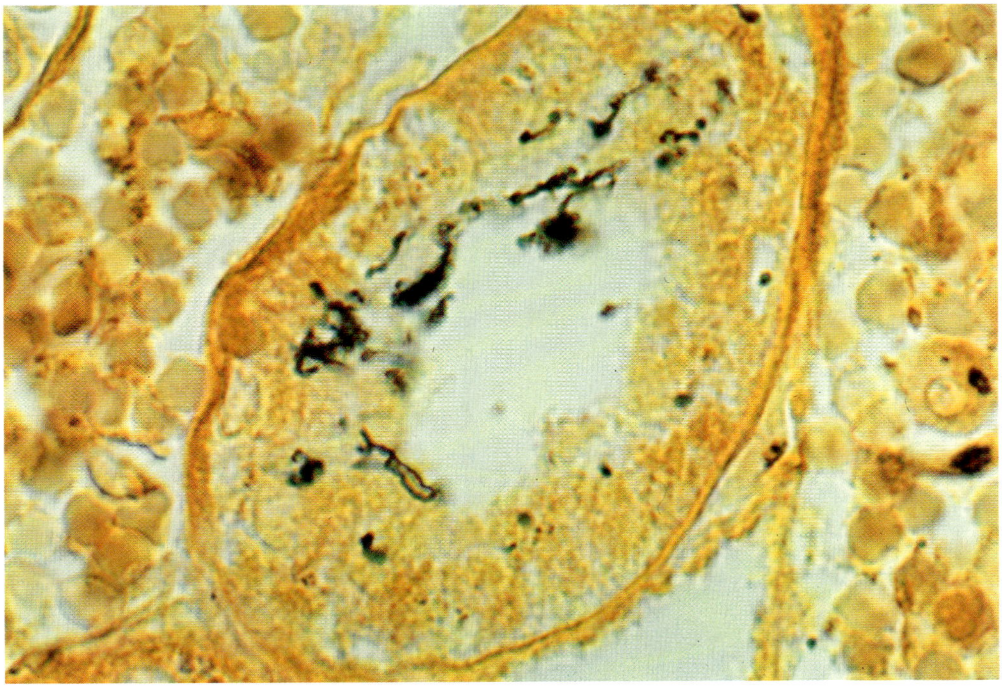

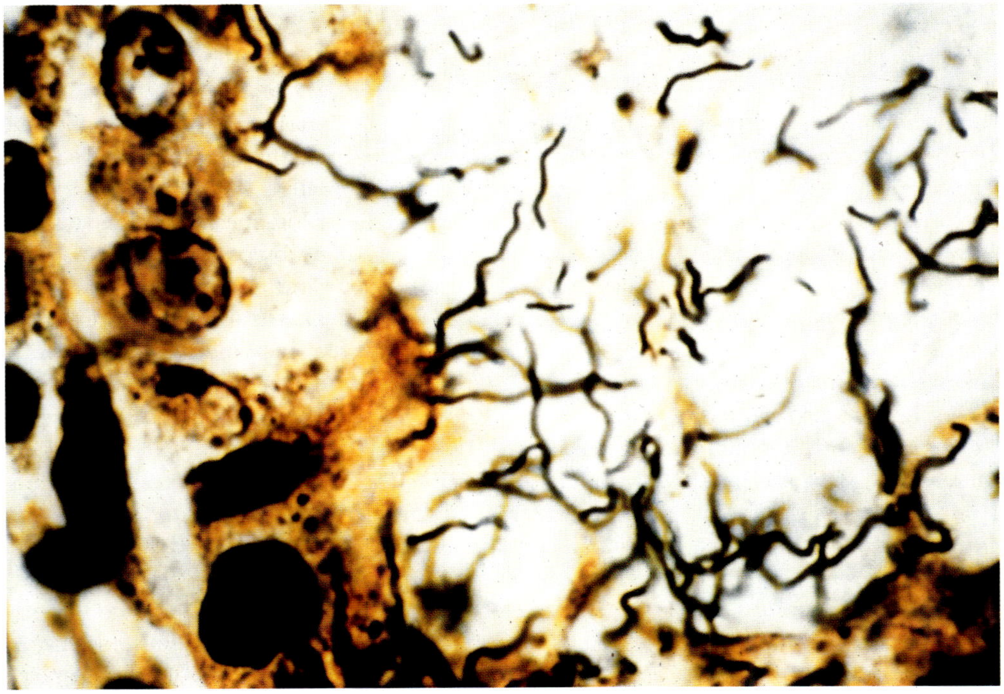

Figures 116.2 (above) and 116.3 (below)
Histological sections showing numerous leptospires entwined in microvilli and free in lumen of renal tubule (Warthin-Starry stain)

even though it reacts positively at a later stage after infection (25 as opposed to 10 days),[11] and it is useful for screening large numbers of sera.[3] In horses, the acute stage of leptospirosis is characterized by high titres and a predominantly IgM response. Cross-reactions are more likely to develop at this time than during the chronic stage when IgG is the predominant antibody.[21] The high prevalence of leptospiral titres in healthy horses necessitates the demonstration of rising titres in blood samples and the isolation of the organism for confirmation of the diagnosis.[60]

Isolation of leptospires from blood, cerebrospinal fluid and milk can be attempted in acute cases. Cultures from urine samples can also be made from clinically affected or suspected carrier animals.[15] The administration of diuretics such as furosamide to aid in the collection of urine samples has been successfully employed.[100] At necropsy, specimens should be taken from the kidneys, liver, lungs, brain and body fluids of foetuses and neonates and of adult animals that die in the acute phase. The kidneys are the organs of choice in chronically infected or carrier animals. All samples submitted for isolation of leptospires must be kept at 4 °C and must reach the laboratory with minimal delay. Inoculation of media with samples collected immediately after slaughter will increase the chances of leptospires being isolated from kidneys.[49, 70] A delay of less than three hours[101] is beneficial but leptospires have been isolated from cooled and frozen (-15 °C) specimens.[66, 111]

Fluorescent antibody tests on infected organs are especially useful for the examination of foetuses, as they are less time-consuming. An immunoperoxidase staining technique employing rabbit antileptospiral antibody has been described for use in formalin-fixed, paraffin-embedded tissues of pigs.[39] The technique is easy to perform and is serovar-specific.[37]

Dark-field examination of blood and urine samples for the detection of live leptospires has been advocated.[106] As there are numerous protoplasmic threads and fibrin strands in blood and urine which can easily be confused with leptospires, the technique is not recommended for general use, unless it is performed by experienced workers.[41] Polymerase chain reaction assays appear to be more reliable and give positive results when urine samples contain few leptospires.[129]

Silver impregnation techniques such as the modifications of the Warthin-Starry method[19, 134] for the demonstration of spirochaetes in tissue sections are of greater value in acute than chronic cases. The infecting serovar cannot be identified by this technique and it should therefore be conducted in conjunction with bacterial isolation.

Intradermal testing with leptospiral antigen has been performed with variable results in pigs.[109]

Serology is a poor diagnostic tool for confirming the role of leptospires in specific cases of 'periodic ophthalmia' in horses. Positive serological titres are more common than the occurrence of uveitis, and many serologically positive horses are clinically normal. Antibodies, however, appear also to be synthesized intra-ocularly — particularly during the active stages of 'periodic ophthalmia', as their levels in the aqueous humor may exceed those in the serum.[133] For diagnosing 'periodic ophthalmia', antibody levels in aqueous humor obtained by paracentesis which are in excess of those in the blood are considered to be diagnostic.[25]

Differential diagnosis

In cattle the haemolytic syndrome of leptospirosis should be differentiated from babesiosis and anaplasmosis, as well as from other causes of a haemolytic anaemia.

Other causes of abortion, stillbirths, neonatal deaths and/or infertility in cattle include brucellosis, campylobacteriosis, chlamydiosis and trichomoniasis and should be differentiated.

The abortions, stillbirths and mummification caused by porcine parvovirus and other viral infections can be confused with leptospirosis. The multifocal, subacute to chronic nephritis in cases of leptospiral infection in pigs is similar to that caused by other bacteria such as *Escherichia coli*, *Streptococcus* spp., *Actinomyces (Corynebacterium) pyogenes*, and by the mycotoxins (ochratoxin A, citrinin and others) produced by *Aspergillus* and *Penicillium* spp.[79]

Control

Clinically ill animals can be treated successfully with 25 mg/kg of dihydrostreptomycin administered intramuscularly for three to five days.[41] Supportive and symptomatic treatment may be needed.

Abortion storms in cows and sows, as well as the renal carrier state in these species, may be arrested by a single treatment of 25 mg/kg dihydrostreptomycin when the infection is due to *L. pomona*.[45, 88, 115, 116] The same treatment, however, has failed to clear renal and genital tissue of infection with *L. hardjo* in cattle. Medication of the feed with chlortetracycline at 400 – 800g/ 1 016 kg for 10 days reduces the number of carriers on infected premises, but does not necessarily eliminate all carriers and should thus be done in conjunction with vaccination.[41] New stock brought onto clean premises must be held in isolation for two weeks and should be given a single parenteral treatment with dihydrostreptomycin in order to eliminate a possible renal carrier state.[116]

Vaccination is the only reliable means of controlling leptospirosis in all species. A wide range of bacterins are available for use in farm animals. These are mostly multivalent, as immunity is serovar-specific,[4] and species-specific vaccines are produced which include the important serovars for each species. It appears that, because of variation in potency, some vaccines do not prevent renal colonization and leptospiruria despite protection against clinical disease and abortion. Some vaccines may promote the development of carriers.[18, 81, 97]

The recommendations of the vaccine manufacturer should be followed, as they vary for the different vaccines. Some general guidelines for effective vaccination can be given, however. Pigs inoculated for the first time should receive two injections four to six weeks apart. Breeding sows should be vaccinated six weeks before breeding and revaccinated four to six weeks later. A booster should be given four weeks before each subsequent farrowing. Boars should be vaccinated every six months. Colostral antibodies from vaccinated sows protect piglets from leptospiral infection for approximately three months.[5] Piglets of vaccinated sows should therefore be vaccinated at the age of three months, when passive immunity is waning. Inoculation of piglets less than one month old has been shown to be ineffective.[17] Under South African conditions, bacterins used in pig units should contain *L. pomona, L. icterohaemorrhagiae* and *L. canicola*.

Previously unvaccinated cattle should receive two inoculations one month apart. An annual booster is recommended by most manufacturers. It has been suggested that cattle should be vaccinated up to three times annually in order to prevent abortion and infertility.[13] Bacterins used for cattle under South African conditions should contain serovars *L. hardjo, L. pomona, L. icterohaemorrhagiae* and *L. canicola*.

Rats may be carriers of *L. icterohaemorrhagiae* and must be controlled. No other wild reservoir of leptospirosis has been identified as yet in South Africa.

Infected premises can be disinfected with products containing sodium hypochlorite. The addition of 0,1 per cent of calcium chloride or 0,1 per cent sodium hydroxide to infected drinking water will render it usable.[127]

References

1 **ABREY, A., 1981.** Abortions in the Natal Midlands due to leptospirosis. *Veterinary Clinician*, 7–9.

2 **ADLER, B., FAINE, S. & CHAPPEL, R.J., 1986.** Development of improved selective medium for isolation of leptospires from clinical material. *Veterinary Microbiology*, 12, 377–381.

3 **ADLER, B., FAINE, S. & GORDON, L.M., 1981.** The enzyme-linked immunosorbent assay (ELISA) as a serological test for detecting antibodies against *Leptospira interrogans* serovar *hardjo* in sheep. *Australian Veterinary Journal*, 57, 414–417.

4 **ALEXANDER, A.D., 1976.** Immunity in leptospirosis. *In*: JOHNSON, R.C., (ed.) *The Biology of Parasitic Spirochaetes*. New York, San Francisco, London: Academic Press, Inc.

5 **AMATREDJO, A. & CAMPBELL, R.S.F., 1975.** Bovine leptospirosis. *Veterinary Bulletin*, 43, 875–891.

6 **ANDREANI, E., SANTARELLI, E. & DILIGENTI, R., 1974.** Leptospirosi delgi ovi. Infezione naturale de serotype hardjo. *Annali della Facolta di Medicina Veterinaria Universita di Pisa*, 27, 33.

7 **ANON., 1986–1987.** Bacteriology and reproduction 1986–87. *Annual Report of the Veterinary Research Institute, Onderstepoort*.

8 **BALL, M.G., 1966.** Animal hosts of leptospires in Kenya and Uganda. *American Journal of Tropical Medicine and Hygiene*, 15, 523–530.

9 **BARSOUM, I.S., BOTROS, B.A.B. & MORCOS, M.B., 1978.** Equine leptospirosis with some clinical observations. *Annales de Recherche Vétérinaire*, 9, 115–118.

10 **BEAMER, P.D., HARDENBROOK, H. & MORRILL, CC., 1953.** Studies on leptospirosis in domestic animals. I. Leptospirosis in sheep. *Veterinary Medicine*, 48, 365–366.

11 **BERCOVICH, Z., TAAIJKE, R. & BOKHOUT, B.A., 1990.** Evaluation of an ELISA for the diagnosis of experimentally induced and naturally occurring *Leptospira* infections in cattle. *Veterinary Microbiology*, 21, 255–262.

12 **BERNKOPF, H., 1946.** Experimental work on leptospirosis in man and cattle in Palestine. *Refuah Vet*, 3, 49.

13 **BEY, R.F. & JOHNSON, R.C., 1986.** Current status of lepto vaccines. *In*: PANDY, R., (ed.). *Progressive Veterinary Microbiology and Immunology*. Basel: S. Karger.

14 **BLACKMORE, D.K. & HATHAWAY, S.C., 1979.** The nodality of zoonoses. *Proceedings of the Second International Symposium on Veterinary Epidemiology and Economics*, Canberra.

15 **BOLIN, C.A., ZUERNER, R.L. & TRUEBA, G., 1989.** Comparison of three techniques to detect *Leptospira interrogans* serotype *hardjo* var. *hardjo-bovis* in bovine urine. *American Journal of Veterinary Research*, 50, 1001–1003.

16 **BRENDLE, J.J., ROGUL, M. & ALEXANDER, A.D., 1974.** Deoxyribonucleic acid hybridization among selected leptospiral serotypes. *International Journal of Systematic Bacteriology*. 24, 205–212.

17 **CACCHIONE, R.A., CASCELLI, E.S., SARAVI, M.A. & MARTINEZ, E.S., 1981.** Evaluacion de una vacuna trivalente antileptospira en bovina y porcinos de la Argentina. *Revista de Medicina Veterinaria Argentina*, 62, 24–31.

18 **CARGILL, C.F. & DAVOS, D.E., 1981.** Renal leptospirosis in vaccinated pigs. *Australian Veterinary Journal*, 57, 236–238.

19 **CARLETON, H.M. & DRURY, R.A.B., 1957.** *Histological Technique*. 3rd edn. London: Oxford University Press.

20 **CHAPERON, K.M., DAVIS, R.B. & MILLER, N.G., 1979.** Effect of a plasma factor in leptospirosis on platelets *in vivo*. *Thrombosis Research*, 14, 975–980.

21 **CHERHUKCHA, Y.G., SHISHKINA, Z.S., BARYSHEV, P.M. & KOKOVIN, I.L., 1976.** *Zentralblatt für Bakteriologie*, Abteilung 1, 236, 336.

22 **CHEVILLE, N.F., HUHN, R. & CUTLIP, R.C., 1980.** Ultrastructure of renal lesions in pigs with acute leptospirosis caused by *Leptospira pomona*. *Veterinary Pathology*, 17, 338–351.

23 **CHRISTOPHER, W., ADLER, B. & FAINE, S., 1982.** Immunogenicity of leptospiral vaccines grown in protein-free medium. *Journal of Medical Microbiology*, 15, 493–501.

24 **COUSINS, D.V. & ROBERTSON, G.M., 1986.** Use of enzyme immuno assay in a serological survey of leptospirosis in sheep. *Australian Veterinary Journal*, 63, 36–39.

25 **DAVIDSON, M.G., NASISSE, M.P. & ROBERTS, S.M., 1987.** Immunodiagnosis of leptospiral uveitis in two horses. *Equine Veterinary Journal*, 19, 155–157.

26 **DE LANGE, J.F., GUMMOW, B., TURNER, G.V. & REDMAN, A.R., 1987.** The isolation of *Leptospira interrogans* serovar *pomona* and related serological findings associated with a mixed farming unit in the Transvaal. *Onderstepoort Journal of Veterinary Research*, 54, 119–121.

27 **DOHERTY, P.C., 1967.** Bovine *Leptospira pomona* infection: The disease in cattle infected during an experimental outbreak. *Queensland Journal of Agriculture and Animal Science*, 24, 351–364.

28 **ELLINGHAUSEN, H.C. & McCULLOUGH, W.C., 1965.** Nutrition of *Leptospira pomona* and growth of 13 other serotypes. Fractionation of oleic albumin complex and a medium of bovine albumin and polysorbate 90. *American Journal of Veterinary Research*, 26, 45–51.

29 **ELLIS, T.M., BRYSON, D.G. & McFERRAN, J.B., 1983.** Abortion associated with mixed leptospira/equid herpesvirus 1 infection. *The Veterinary Record*, 98, 218–219.

30 **ELLIS, W.A., BRYSON, D.G., NEILL, S.D., McPARLAND, P.J. & MALONE, F.E., 1983.** Possible involvement of leptospires in abortion, stillbirths and neonatal deaths in sheep. *The Veterinary Record*, 112, 291–293.

31 **ELLIS, W.A., BRYSON, D.G., O'BRIEN, J.J. & NEILL, S.D., 1983.** Leptospiral infection in aborted equine foetuses. *Equine Veterinary Journal*, 15, 321–324.

32 **ELLIS, W.A., HUSTAS, L., ROBERTSON, G.M. & MAYBERRY, C., 1984.** Kidney disease of sheep infected by lepto-spires of the Serjoe serogroup. *Australian Veterinary Journal*, 61, 304–305.

33 **ELLIS, W.A., McPARLAND, P.J., BRYSON, D.G. & CASSELLS, J.A., 1986.** Prevalence of *Leptospira* infection in aborted pigs in Northern Ireland. *The Veterinary Record*, 118, 63–65.

34 **ELLIS, W.A., McPARLAND, P.J., BRYSON, D.G. & McNULTY, M.S., 1985.** Leptospires in pig urogenital tracts and foetuses. *The Veterinary Record*, 117, 66–67.

35 **ELLIS, W.A. & MICHNA, S.W., 1976.** Bovine leptospirosis: A serological and clinical study. *The Veterinary Record*, 99, 387–391.

36 **ELLIS, W.A. & MICHNA, S.W., 1977.** Bovine leptospirosis: Experimental infection of pregnant heifers with a strain belonging to the Hebdomadis serogroup. *Research in Veterinary Science*, 22, 229–236.

37 **ELLIS, W.A., O'BRIEN, J.J., NEILL, S.D., FURGUSON, H.W. & HANNA, J., 1982.** Bovine leptospirosis: Microbiological and serological findings in aborted foetuses. *The Veterinary Record*, 110, 147–150.

38 **ELLIS, W.A., O'BRIEN, J.J., PEARSON, J.K.L. & COLLINS, D.S., 1976.** Bovine leptospirosis: Infection by the Hebdomadis serogroup and mastitis. *The Veterinary Record*, 99, 368–370.

39 **ELLIS, R.M., ROBERTSON, G.M., HUSTAS, L. & KIRBY, M., 1983.** Detection of leptospires in tissue using an immunoperoxidase staining procedure. *Australian Veterinary Journal*, 60, 364–367.

40 **ELLIS, W.A., SONGER, J.G., MONTGOMERY, J. & CASSELLS, J.A., 1986.** Prevalence of *Leptospira interrogans* serovar *hardjo* in the genital and urinary tracts of non-pregnant cattle. *The Veterinary Record*, 118, 11–13.

41 **FAINE, S., 1982.** *Guidelines for the Control of Leptospirosis.* WHO offset publication No. 67. Geneva: World Health Organization.

42 **FENNESTAD, K.L. & BORG-PETERSEN, C., 1958.** Fetal leptospirosis and abortion in cattle. *Journal of Infectious Diseases*, 102, 227–236.

43 **FENNESTAD, K.L. & BORG-PETERSEN, C., 1962.** Antibody and plasma cells in bovine fetuses infected with *Leptospira saxkoebing*. *Journal of Infectious Diseases*, 110, 63–69.

44 **FERESU, S.B., 1987.** Serological survey of leptospiral antibodies in cattle in Zimbabwe. *Tropical Animal Health and Production*, 19, 209–214.

45 **FERGUSON, L.C., LOCOCO, S., SMITH, H.R. & HAMDY, A.H., 1956.** The control and treatment of swine leptospirosis during a naturally occurring outbreak. *Journal of the American Veterinary Medical Association*, 129, 263.

46 **GLOSSER, J.W., SULZER, C.R., REYNOLDS, G.C. & WHITTSETT, D.K., 1975.** Isolation of leptospiral serotype *szwajizak* from dairy cattle in Oregon. *Proceedings of the 78th Annual Meeting of the United States Animal Health Association, 1974*, 78, 119–125.

47 **GORDON, L.M., 1980.** Isolation of *Leptospira interrogans hardjo* from sheep. *Australian Veterinary Journal*, 56, 348–349.

48 **GORDON SMITH, C.E. & TURNER, L.H., 1961.** The effect of pH on the survival of leptospires in water. *Bulletin of the World Health Organization*, 24, 35–43.

49 **GRÉGOIRE, N., HIGGINS, R. & ROBINSON, Y., 1987.** Isolation of leptospires from nephritic kidneys of beef cattle at slaughter. *American Journal of Veterinary Research*, 48, 370–371.

50 **GSELL, O., 1944.** The history of leptospirosis: 100 years. *Zentralblatt für Bakteriologische und Mikrobiologische Hygiene*, 257, 473–478.

51 **HANSON, L.E., 1976.** Pathogenesis of leptospirosis. *In*: JOHNSON, R.C., (ed.). *The Biology of Parasitic Spirochaetes.* New York: Academic Press, Inc.

52 **HANSON, L.E. & BRODIE, B.O., 1967.** *Leptospira hardjo* infections in cattle. *Proceedings of the 71st Annual Meeting of the United States Livestock Sanitary Association 1967*, 71, 210–215.

53 **HANSON, L.E. & FERGUSON, L.C., 1975.** Leptospirosis. *In*: DUNNE, H.W. & LEMAN, A.D., (eds). *Diseases of Swine.* Ames, Iowa: Iowa State University Press.

54 **HANSON, L.E., MARTIN, R.J., GIBBONS, R.N. & SCHAURRENBERGER, P.R., 1969.** Equine leptospirosis. *Proceedings of the 79th Annual Meeting of the United States Animal Health Association.*

55 **HANSON, L.E. & TRIPATHY, D.N., 1981.** *In*: LEMAN, A.D., GLOCK, R.D., MENGELING, W.L., PENNEY, R.H.C., SCHOLL, E. & STRAW, B., (eds). *Diseases of Swine.* 5th edn. Ames, Iowa: Iowa State University Press.

56 **HARRINGTON, R., 1975.** Leptospiral antibodies in serum from cattle, swine, horses, deer, sheep and goats: 1973–74. *American Journal of Veterinary Research*, 36, 1367–1370.

57 **HARTMAN, E.G., 1986.** Detection of leptospira antibodies by the solid phase ELISA. *In*: ELLIS, W.A. & LITTLE, T.W.A., (eds). *The Present State of Leptospirosis Diagnosis and Control.* Netherlands: Martinus Nijhoff Publishers.

58 **HATHAWAY, S.C., 1981.** Leptospirosis in New Zealand: An ecological view. *New Zealand Veterinary Journal*, 27, 109–112.

59 **HATHAWAY, S.C. & LITTLE, T.W.A., 1981.** Prevalence and clinical significance of leptospiral antibodies in pigs in England. *The Veterinary Record*, 108, 224–228.

60 **HATHAWAY, S.C., LITTLE, T.W.A., FINCH, S.M. & STEVENS, A.E., 1981.** Leptospiral infection in horses in England: A serological study. *The Veterinary Record*, 108, 396–398.

61 **HELLSTROM, J.B. & MARSHALL, R.B., 1978.** Survival of *Leptospira interrogans* serovar *pomona* in an acidic soil under simulated New Zealand field conditions. *Research Veterinary Science*, 25, 29–33.

62 **HERR, S., 1987.** Veterinary Research Institute, Onderstepoort. Unpublished data.

63 **HERR, S., RILEY, A.E., NESER, J.A., ROUX, D. & DE LANGE, J.F., 1982.** *Leptospira pomona* associated with abortion in cattle. *Onderstepoort Journal of Veterinary Research*, 49, 57–62.

64 **HERR, S. & WINNEN, G.M., 1983.** The first isolation of *Leptospira interrogans* serovar *pomona* from cattle in Botswana. *Journal of the South African Veterinary Association*, 54, 83–84.

65 **HIGGINS, R.J., HARBOURNE, J.F., LITTLE, T.W.A. & STEVENS, A.E., 1980.** Mastitis and abortion in dairy cattle associated with *Leptospira* of the serotype *hardjo*. *The Veterinary Record*, 107, 307–310.

66 **HO, H.F. & BLACKMORE, D.K., 1979.** Effects of chilling and freezing on *Leptospira interrogans* serovar *pomona* in naturally infected pig kidneys. *New Zealand Veterinary Journal*, 27, 121–123.

67 **HODGES, R.T., 1974.** Some observations on experimental *Leptospira* serotype *pomona* infection in sheep. *New Zealand Veterinary Journal*, 22, 151–154.

68 **HOUVIND-HOUGEN, K., 1986.** Morphology of leptospires: Electron microscopic studies in relation to the classification of *Leptospira*. *In*: ELLIS, W.A. & LITTLE, T.W.A., (eds). *Present State of Leptospirosis Diagnosis and Control.* Netherlands: Martinus Nijhoff Publishers.

69 **HUNTER, P., FLAMAND, J.R.B., MYBURGH, J. & VAN DER MERWE, S.M., 1988.** Serological reactions to *Leptospira*

species in game animals of northern Natal. *Onderstepoort Journal of Veterinary Research*, 55, 191–192.

70 **HUNTER, P., VAN DER VYVER, F.H., SELMER-OLSEN, A., HENTON, M.M., HERR, S. & DE LANGE, J.F., 1987.** Leptospirosis as a cause of 'white spot' kidneys in South African pig abattoirs. *Onderstepoort Journal of Veterinary Research*, 54, 59–62.

71 **IDO, Y., HOKI, R., ITO, H. & WANI, H., 1917.** The rat as a carrier of spirochaeta icterohaemorrhagiae. The causative agent of Weil's disease. *Journal of Experimental Medicine*, 26, 341–353.

72 **INADA, R., IDO, Y., HOKI, R., KANEKO, R. & ITO, H., 1916.** The aetiology, mode of infection and specific therapy of Weil's disease (Spirochaetosis icterohaemorrhagica). *Journal of Experimental Medicine*, 23, 377–401.

73 **INZANA, T.J. & DAWE, D.L., 1979.** Experimentally induced *Leptospira interrogans autumnalis* infections in young swine. *American Journal of Veterinary Research*, 40, 1355–1358.

74 **JOHNSON, R.C., 1976.** Comparative spirochaete physiology and cellular composition. *In*: JOHNSON, R.C., (ed.) *Biology of Parasitic Spirochaetes*. New York, San Francisco, London: Academic Press, Inc.

75 **JOHNSON, R.C. & FAINE, S., 1986.** *Bergey's Manual of Systematic Bacteriology*. Vol. I. Baltimore, London: Krieg, Holt, Williams & Wilkins.

76 **JOHNSON, R.C. & ROGERS, P., 1964.** Differentiation of pathogenic and saprophytic leptospires with 5–azaguanidine. *Journal of Bacteriology*, 88, 1618–1623.

77 **JOHNSON, R.C. & ROGERS, P., 1964.** 5–Fluorouracil as a selective agent for growth of leptospirae. *Journal of Bacteriology*, 87, 422–426.

78 **JUBB, K.V.F., KENNEDY, P.C. & PALMER, N., 1985.** *Pathology of Domestic Animals*. 3rd edn. New York: Academic Press.

79 **KELLERMAN, T.S., COETZER, J.A.W. & NAUDÉ, T.W., 1988.** *Plant Poisonings and Mycotoxicoses of Livestock in Southern Africa*. Cape Town: Oxford University Press Southern Africa.

80 **KIKTENKO, V.S., BALASHOV, N.G. & RODINA, V.N., 1976.** Leptospirosis infection through insemination of animals. *Journal of Hygiene, Epidemiology, Microbiology and Immunology*, 20, 207–213.

81 **KILLINGER, A.H., TAYLOR, P.L., HUHN, R.G., HANSON, L.E. & MANSFIELD, M.E., 1976.** Immunity to leptospirosis: Renal changes in vaccinated cattle given challenge inoculum. *American Journal of Veterinary Research*, 37, 93–94.

82 **KIRSCHNER, L. & MAGUIRE, T., 1957.** Survival of *Leptospira* outside their hosts. *New Zealand Medical Journal*, 56, 385–391.

83 **KITSON-PIGGOT, A.W. & PRESCOTT, J.F., 1987.** Leptospirosis in horses in Ontario. *Canadian Journal of Veterinary Research*, 51, 448–451.

84 **KLARENBEEK, A. & SCHUFFNER, W., 1933.** Het voorkomen van een afwykend Leptospiras in Nederland. *Geneeskunde, Nederlandse Tijdschriften*, 77, 4271–4276.

85 **LAUERMAN, L.H., KISER, D.D. & LONG, I.R., 1983.** *Leptospira tarassovi* in Alabama cattle: Serologic evidence. *Proceedings of the 87th Annual Meeting of the United States Animal Health Association*, 87, 193–198.

86 **LITTLE, T.W.A., RICHARDS, M.S., HUSSAINI, S.N. & JONES, T.D., 1980.** The significance of leptospiral antibodies in calving and aborting cattle in south-west England. *The Veterinary Record*, 106, 221–224.

87 **LITTLE, T.W.A. & SALT, G.F.H., 1976.** Isolation of a leptospira of the *pomona* serogroup from a field vole. *The Veterinary Record*, 97, 56.

88 **LOCOCO, S., BOHL, E.H. & SMITH, H.R., 1958.** Treatment of porcine leptospiruria. *Journal of the American Veterinary Medical Association*, 132, 251–253.

89 **McGUIRE, C.D. & MEYERS, D.M., 1957.** Leptospirosis in Egypt. *American Journal of Tropical Medicine and Hygiene*, 6, 532–539.

90 **McKEOWN, J.D. & ELLIS, W.A., 1986.** *Leptospira hardjo* agalactia in sheep. *The Veterinary Record*, 118, 482.

91 **MERCY, A.R., PEET, R.L. & HUSTAS, L., 1988.** Macroscopic kidney lesions in slaughtered pigs as an indication of current leptospiral infections. *Australian Veterinary Journal*, 65, 35–36.

92 **MICHNA, S.W., 1965.** Further observations on abortion of the sow due to infections by *Leptospira canicola*. *The Veterinary Record*, 77, 802–810.

93 **MILLAR, K.R., HODGES, R.T., SHEPPARD, A.D. & HAMMINGTON, M.W., 1977.** Clinical and biochemical changes in sheep inoculated with *Leptospira interrogans* serotype *pomona*. *New Zealand Veterinary Journal*, 25, 203–207.

94 **MINETTE, H.P., 1983.** Leptospirosis in poikilothermic vertebrates: A review. *International Journal of Zoonoses*, 10, 111–121.

95 **MOCH, R.W., EBNER, E.E., BARSOUM, I.S. & BOTROS, A.M., 1975.** Leptospirosis in Ethiopia: A serological survey in domestic and wild animals. *Journal of Tropical Medicine and Hygiene*, 78, 38–42.

96 **MORSE, E.V., MORTER, R.L., LANGHAM, R.F., LUNDBERG, A. & ULLREY, E., 1957.** Experimental ovine leptospirosis: *Leptospira pomona* infection. *Journal of Infectious Diseases*, 101, 129–136.

97 **MORSI, H.M., SHIBLEY, G.F. & STROTHER, H.L., 1973.** Renal leptospirosis: Challenge exposure of vaccinated and non-vaccinated cattle to *Leptospira icterohaemorrhagiae* and *Leptospira canicola*. *American Journal of Veterinary Research*, 34, 175–179.

98 **NEIL, S.D., REID, R.L., WEATHERUP, S.T.C. & ELLIS, W.A., 1986.** The use of aminopeptidase activity in leptospira identification. *In*: ELLIS, W.A. & LITTLE, T.W.A., (eds). *The Present State of Leptospirosis Diagnosis and Control*. Netherlands: Martinus Nijhoff Publishers.

99 **NERVIG, R.M., CHEVILLE, N.F. & BAETZ, A.L., 1978.** Experimental infection of calves with *Leptospira interrogans* serotype *szwajizak*. *American Journal of Veterinary Research*, 39, 523–525.

100 **NERVIG, R.M. & GARRETT, L.A., 1979.** Use of furosemide to obtain bovine urine samples for leptospiral isolation. *American Journal of Veterinary Research*, 40, 1197–1200.

101 **ORR, H.S. & LITTLE, T.W.S., 1979.** Isolation of leptospira of the serotype *hardjo* from bovine kidneys. *Research in Veterinary Science*, 27, 343–346.

102 **PARMA, A.E., SANTISTEBAN, C.G., VILLALBA, J.S. & BOWDEN, R.A., 1985.** Experimental demonstration of an antigenic relationship between *Leptospira* and equine cornea. *Veterinary Immunology and Immunopathology*, 10, 215–224.

103 **PEARSON, J.K.L., MACKIE, D.P. & ELLIS, W.A., 1980.** Milk-drop syndrome resulting from *Leptospira hardjo*. *The Veterinary Record*, 106, 135–136.

104 **REILLY, J.R., HANSON, L.E. & SIMON, J., 1970.** Experimentally induced predator-chain transmission of *Leptospira grippotyphosa* from rodents to wild marsupialia and carnivora. *American Journal of Veterinary Research*, 31, 1443–1448.

105 **RINGEN, L.M. & BRACKEN, F.K., 1956.** Studies on bovine leptospirosis. *Journal of the American Veterinary Medical Association*, 129, 266–271.

106 **RIS, D.R. & HAMEL, K.L., 1978.** The detection of leptospirae in cattle urine. *New Zealand Veterinary Journal*, 26, 246, 255–256.

107 **ROBERTS, S.J., 1958.** A study of leptospirosis in a large artificial insemination stud. *Cornell Veterinarian*, 48, 363–371.

108 **SCHMITZ, J.A., COLES, B.M. & SHIRES, G.M., 1981.** Fatal haemolytic disease in sheep attributed to *Leptospira interrogans* serotype *hardjo* infection. *Cornell Veterinarian*, 71, 175–182.

109 **SCHONBERG, A., 1986.** Application of skin test and other diagnostic tests. *In*: ELLIS, W.A. & LITTLE, T.W.A., (eds). *Present State of Leptospirosis Diagnosis and Control*. Netherlands: Martinus Nijhoff Publishers.

110 **SHEPHERD, A.J. & LEMAN, P.A., 1985.** Bacterial surveillance of South African rodents. *South African Journal of Science*, 81, 302–308.

111 **SKILBECK, N.W., FORSYTH, W.M. & DOHNT, M., 1988.** Bovine leptospirosis: Microbiological and histological findings

in cattle at slaughter. *Australian Veterinary Journal*, 65, 73–75.

112 **SLEIGHT, S.D. & WILLIAMS, J.A., 1961.** Transmission of bovine leptospirosis by coition and artificial insemination. *Journal of the American Veterinary Medical Association*, 138, 151–152.

113 **SMITH, B.P. & ARMSTRONG, J.M., 1975.** Fatal haemolytic anemia attributed to leptospirosis in lambs. *Journal of the American Veterinary Medical Association*, 167, 739–741.

114 **SMITH, A.S., JONES, T.C. & HUNT, R.D., 1972.** *Veterinary Pathology*. Philadelphia: Lea and Febiger.

115 **SOUTH, P.J. & STOERNER, H.G., 1974.** The control of outbreaks of leptospirosis in beef cattle by simultaneous vaccination and treatment with dihydrostreptomycin. *Proceedings of the 78th Annual Meeting of the United States Animal Health Association*, 78, 126–130.

116 **STALHEIM, O.H.V., 1972.** Swine leptospirosis certification: A proposal. *Journal of the American Veterinary Medical Association*, 161, 1244–1247.

117 **SULLIVAN, N.D. & CALLAN, D.P., 1970.** Isolation of *Leptospira hardjo* from cows with mastitis. *Australian Veterinary Journal*, 46, 123–125.

118 **SWAN, R.A., WILLIAMS, E.S. & TAYLOR, E.G., 1981.** Clinical and serological observations on horses with suspected leptospirosis. *Australian Veterinary Journal*, 57, 528–529.

119 **SWART, K.S., CALVERT, K. & MENERY, C., 1982.** The prevalence of antibodies to serovars of *Leptospira interrogans* in horses. *Australian Veterinary Journal*, 59, 25–27.

120 **TARASSOFF, S., 1928.** Traits éclosions d'épidémie de fièvre aquatique du *Leptospirosis grippotyphosa* aquatilis en URSS. *Bulletin de l'Office International d'Hygiène*, 27, 928.

121 **TE BRUGGE, L.A. & DREYER, T., 1985.** *Leptospira interrogans* serovar *hardjo* associated with bovine abortion in South Africa. *Onderstepoort Journal of Veterinary Research*, 52, 51–52.

122 **THIERMANN, A.B., 1982.** Experimental leptospiral infections in pregnant cattle with organisms of the Hebdomadis group. *American Journal of Veterinary Research*, 43, 780–784.

123 **THIERMANN, A.B., 1984.** Leptospirosis: Current development and trends. *Journal of the American Veterinary Medical Association*, 184, 722–725.

124 **THIERMANN, A.B. & ELLIS, W.A., 1986.** Identification of leptospires of veterinary importance by restriction endonuclease analysis. *In*: ELLIS, W.A. & LITTLE, T.W.A., (eds). *The Present State of Leptospirosis Diagnosis and Control*. Netherlands: Martinus Nijhoff Publishers.

125 **TRIPATHY, D.N., HANSON, L.E., MANSFIELD, M.E. & THILSTED, J.P., 1985.** Experimental infection of lactating goats with *Leptospira interrogans* serovars *pomona* and *hardjo*. *American Journal of Veterinary Research*, 46, 2512–2514.

126 **UHLENHUTH, P. & FROMME, W., 1916.** Untersuchungen über die Aetiologie, Immunität und specifische Behandlung der Weilsche Krankheit (Icterus Infectiousus). *Zeitschrift für Immunitätsforschung*, 25, 317.

127 **VAN DER HOEDEN, J., 1958.** *Leptospira canicola* in cattle. *Journal of Comparative Pathology*, 65, 278–283.

128 **VAN DER HOEDEN, J., 1964.** *Zoonoses*. Elsevier Publishing Company.

129 **VAN EYS, G.J., GRAVENKAMP, C., GERRITSEN, M.J., QUINT, W., CORNELISSEN, M.T., SHEGGET, J.T. & TERPSTRA, W.J., 1989.** Detection of leptospires in urine by polymerase chain reaction. *Journal of Clinical Microbiology*, 27, 2258–2262.

130 **VAN RENSBURG, W.J.J., 1973.** Isolasie van *Leptospira canicola* by varke en honde in Suid-Afrika. *Journal of the South African Veterinary Association*, 44, 435–436.

131 **WANYANGU, S.W., PALMER, M.F., ZOCHOVSKI, W.J. & WAITKENS, S.A., 1987.** Comparison of the DIFCO and Patoc 1 slide antigens in the screening of leptospirosis. *Comparative Immunology and Microbial Infectious Diseases*, 10, 155–161.

132 **WEIL, A., 1886.** Uber eine eigentumliche mit Miltztumor, Ikterus und Nephritis einhergehende akute Infektionskrankheit. *Deutches Archiv für Klinische Medicin*, 39, 209.

133 **WITNER, R.H., 1954.** Periodic ophthalmia in horses. *American Journal of Ophthalmology*, 37, 961–967.

134 **YOUNG, B.J., 1969.** A reliable method for demonstrating spirochaetes in tissue sections. *Journal of Medical Laboratory Technology*, 26, 248–252.

UNCLASSIFIED AEROBIC/ MICROAEROPHILIC, MOTILE, HELICAL/ VIBROID GRAM-NEGATIVE BACTERIA

This group of Gram-negative aerobic or microaerophilic bacteria, which are currently unclassified, characteristically have helical or vibroid cell forms with anything from less-than-one to many complete helical turns. They are all motile in broth cultures by virtue of the action of their polar flagella. They move in straight lines with a characteristic corkscrew-like motion.[1]

Of the large number of genera in the group, the genus *Campylobacter* is the most important in humans and animals. In livestock, *Campylobacter* spp. are usually found in the oral cavity, intestinal tract and reproductive organs. Certain *Campylobacter* spp. are commonly associated with infertility in cattle, sporadic abortions in cattle and sheep, and the porcine intestinal adenomatosis complex (which includes four different enteropathic syndromes) (**Table 1**). Infertility in cattle and the intestinal adenomatosis complex in pigs are both economically important syndromes in herds in which the infections occur. Infection in cattle with *Campylobacter jejuni* is associated with enteritis and the organism has been alleged to be the cause of 'winter dysentery', a syndrome which is now considered to be caused by a coronavirus. It is also responsible for enteritis in humans.

Two other pathogenic members of this group are *'Spirillum minus'* and *'Spirillum pulli'*, but they do not actually belong to the genus *Spirillum* and are described by Krieg as being *Species Incertae Sedis*.[1] *Spirillum minus* infection occurs rarely in humans and is the cause of a form of rat-bite fever, while *Spirillum pulli* is responsible for a disease associated with diphtheroid stomatitis in chickens.

Table 1 Common pathogenic *Campylobacter* spp. that cause disease in livestock

CAMPYLOBACTER SPP.	DISEASE	ANIMAL SPECIES AFFECTED
C. fetus venerealis	Infertility (embryonic loss)	Cattle
C. fetus fetus	Abortions	Cattle and sheep
C. hyointestinalis	Porcine intestinal adenomatosis complex	Pigs
C. mucosalis	Porcine intestinal adenomatosis complex	Pigs
C. jejuni	Winter dysentery	Cattle and sheep
	Mastitis	Cattle
	Abortions	Cattle, sheep and goats

Reference

1 **KRIEG, N.R., 1984.** Aerobic/microaerophilic, motile, helical/vibroid Gram-negative bacteria. *In*: KRIEG, N.R. & HOLT, J.G., (eds). *Bergey's Manual of Systematic Bacteriology*. Vol. I. Baltimore, London: Williams & Wilkins.

117

Genital campylobacteriosis in cattle

Synonyms: Vibriosis, vibriose (Afrik.)

A.P. Schutte, M.L. van der Walt and G.C. Bishop

Introduction

Campylobacteriosis (vibriosis) is a genital disease of cattle caused by *Campylobacter fetus venerealis* and is regarded as one of the most important infectious causes of poor calving crops in southern Africa. It is a venereal disease causing embryonic mortality and resorption, aberrant oestrus cycles, delayed conception, reduced fertility and (on rare occasions) abortions. Bulls are transiently or permanently infected; younger bulls lose the infection, but those older than three years may remain permanently infected and carry the infection from one breeding season to the next. Heifers and cows of all ages are susceptible. Females develop an incomplete and transient immunity after exposure.

Campylobacter fetus venerealis occurs more frequently than *C. fetus fetus* in cattle in southern Africa. The latter is generally associated with sporadic abortions in cattle, but may also cause abortion in sheep. *Campylobacter sputorum bubulus*, a saprophytic inhabitant of the prepuce of bulls, is encountered mainly in direct cultures of preputial samples and must be differentiated from the pathogenic subspecies of *C. fetus*.

Campylobacter fetus was first described as a cause of abortion by MacFadyan and Stockman[57] in 1913, but the bacterium received little attention until it was incriminated as an important cause of abortion and 'temporary sterility' in cattle in the USA.[63, 66] Terpstra and Eisma[88] presented evidence that the same organism was responsible for 'enzootische steriliteit' in cattle in the Netherlands. The suggestion by Snyman[85] in 1931 and Canham[18] in 1948 that *C. fetus* could be responsible for bovine infertility in southern Africa was confirmed by Van Rensburg[92] and expanded by others.[4, 70, 73, 79]

Campylobacteriosis is probably widespread in nearly all countries where cattle are raised.[23, 26, 32, 36, 51, 86, 93, 94] In southern Africa it has been reported in beef and dairy breeds.[73, 79]

Aetiology

More than one variety of *Campylobacter* can be isolated from the genital tracts of cattle. Akkermans *et al.*[2] first reported a catalase-positive and weak H_2S-positive isolate which differed from the other campylobacters in that it was associated with abortion. Two varieties within the same species, namely *Vibrio fetus* var. *venerealis* (*C. fetus venerealis*) and *Vibrio fetus* var. *intestinalis* (*C. fetus fetus*) were subsequently established.[33]

Until the early 1960s, all the micro-aerophilic vibrios isolated from cattle and sheep were classified under the genus *Vibrio*. However, based on genotypic and phenotypic differences, these organisms were reclassified as *C. fetus*,[95] but because uniform nomenclature for *C. fetus* did not exist at that time, confusing classifications followed. In **Table 117.1**, an attempt is made to clarify the situation by comparing the current nomenclature with the different classifications and nomenclature used during the period 1953 to 1984.

Currently, *Campylobacter* is a well-defined genus, although taxonomic problems still exist at the species level.[84] The organisms are slender, curved, Gram-negative rods, 0,01 to 0,08 µm in diameter and 0,5 to 0,8 µm in length. They may have one or more spirals, or appear to be S- or gull-wing-shaped. In culture, two or more organisms joined at their ends form a spiral chain. In older cultures, coccoid forms may be present. *Campylobacter* organisms are motile and are propelled by a single polar flagellum at one or both ends of the cells. They have a characteristic darting, corkscrew motion. They are best examined under phase-contrast illumination, where they are recognized by their typical morphology and motion.

Colonies on blood agar attain a diameter of 1–2 mm, and are convex and raised. They are colourless to grey, and are non-haemolytic. On moist media, growth may spread along the line of inoculation.

Campylobacter fetus is micro-aerophilic and will only grow on solid media in an atmosphere with a reduced (10 per cent) oxygen and increased (4–8 per cent) CO_2 tension. In semi-solid media, growth occurs under aerobic conditions. A suitable micro-aerophilic atmosphere can be achieved by the use of specially designed gas-incubators, by gas-generating kits used in anaerobic jars, or through the evacuation of air from anaerobic jars

Table 117.1 A compilation of various nomenclatures pertaining to *Campylobacter* spp. isolated from the bovine genital tract

Date	*Campylobacter fetus* subsp. *venerealis*	*Campylobacter fetus* subsp. *fetus*	*Campylobacter jejuni*	*Campylobacter sputorum* subsp. *bubulus*	Reference
1953	Serotype 3 Serotype 5, 3	Serotype 5, 3 Serotype 2			55
1956	Serotype 1 Serotype 3				2
1958	Serotype 1	Serotype 2			58
1959	Serotype A	Serotype B		*Vibrio bubulus*	60
1959	*Vibrio fetus* var. *venerealis*	*Vibrio fetus* var. *intestinalis*		*Vibrio bubulus*	33
1962	Serotype 1 Serotype 3, 2				59
1962	Serotype 1 Serotype sub-1	Serotype 2			15
1964	Serotype 1 Serotype 2				67
1971	Serotype A-1 Serotype A-1	Serotype A-2 Serotype B	Serotype C		5
1973	*Campylobacter fetus* subsp. *venerealis*	*Campylobacter fetus* subsp. *fetus*	*Campylobacter jejuni*	*Campylobacter sputorum* subsp. *bubulus*	95
1974	*Campylobacter fetus* subsp. *fetus*	*Campylobacter fetus* subsp. *intestinalis*	*Campylobacter fetus* subsp. *jejuni*	*Campylobacter sputorum* subsp. *bubulus*	83
1980	*Campylobacter* subsp. *venerealis*	*Campylobacter fetus* subsp. *fetus*	*Campylobacter jejuni*		82
1984	*Campylobacter fetus* subsp. *venerealis*	*Campylobacter fetus* subsp. *fetus*	*Campylobacter jejuni*	*Campylobacter sputorum* subsp. *bubulus*	84

and its replacement with a mixture of inert gases. The optimal growth temperature is 37 °C, but *C. fetus* can also grow at 25 °C. Cultures should be examined for growth after two to three days.

The biochemical properties of *C. fetus* are well documented. Both *C. fetus venerealis* and *C. fetus fetus* are catalase- and oxidase-positive, reduce nitrates and do not ferment carbohydrates. The latter is also tolerant to 1 per cent glycine and produces H_2S.[7, 9, 27, 31, 53, 54, 83, 84]

Campylobacter fetus has two types of surface antigens. A heat-stable O-antigen (somatic) is incorporated in the lipopolysaccharide cell wall structure. The subspecies *C. fetus fetus* contains the heat-stable antigens B and A-2, while antigens A and A-1 are limited to biovars of *C. fetus venerealis*. *Campylobacter jejuni* carries the heat-stable C antigen. There is no cross-reaction between antigens A, B or C.[84]

Seven heat-labile antigens (of which up to five may be present in a single strain) have been identified.[5] They are antiphagocytic[56] and undergo structural changes in the animal which enable the organisms to overcome or escape the immune response.[24, 74]

Epidemiology

There is a distinct difference in the diseases caused by the two subspecies of *C. fetus* and by *C. jejuni*, the latter being described in **Chapter 119: *Campylobacter jejuni* infection**.

Campylobacter fetus venerealis is spread by coitus and by the use of infected semen in artificial insemination. Although there is little doubt that venereal contact is the most important means of transmission, there are indications that bulls can become infected in other ways, such as by contact with contaminated bedding.[1, 76] Heifers can be easily infected intravaginally with *C. fetus venerealis*-contaminated semen or with preputial washings.[91]

Bulls may be either transiently or permanently infected. Younger bulls lose the infection, whereas bulls older than three years usually remain permanently infected. The reason for this is unclear,[29] but it may be associated with the increased number and depth of the crypts in the preputial and penile mucosa that occur as bulls grow older.[72] Additionally, as the organisms remain restricted to the epithelial surfaces of the penis and prepuce during infection, the lack of both sufficient antigenic stimulation and of antigenic variation of the organism during infection may explain the absence of appreciable antibody formation and the prolonged survival of these organisms in the prepuce.[6, 43] The greatest concentration of *C. fetus venerealis* is found in the fornix of the prepuce and on the penis.[43] The antibody response is weak and localized.[89]

Pathogenesis

Following coitus, *C. fetus venerealis* bacteria localize in the vagina of susceptible females. After five to seven days the organisms migrate through the cervix into the uterine body and then continue to spread during the following weeks. In 25 per cent of cases the organisms also spread to the oviducts.[91]

Campylobacter fetus venerealis produces a subacute to chronic superficial endometritis.[98] The inflammatory reaction causes an unfavourable environment for embryonic survival. The lowered oxygen tensions caused by the bacteria[95] may be an additional cause of early embryonic death.[96]

Colonization of the uterus stimulates a local immune response in which IgG, IgM and IgA are produced.[90] Uterine secretions contain IgG, whereas IgA is found primarily in the cervico-vaginal mucus.[24] IgG acts as an opsonin, thus aiding neutrophils and macrophages in the phagocytosis of the organisms, while IgA is capable only of immobilizing the organism. This could be the reason why, in the carrier state in females, *C. fetus venerealis* organisms persist in the cervix.

As a result of embryonic death, a large percentage of infected heifers and cows undergo prolonged oestrus cycles of 24 to 40 days or more. The infection is generally self-limiting. In most cases, if lesions are not severe, heifers which overcome the infection are subsequently fertile.[98] Bilateral salpingitis can, however, result in permanent sterility. A few animals may remain permanently infected and are sources of infection during the following breeding season.

In contrast to *C. fetus venerealis*, sporadic abortions caused by *C. fetus fetus* are the result of a bacteraemia following the dissemination of organisms from the intestine or gall bladder after ingestion of infected material. The pathogenesis of the sporadic abortions is not fully understood. It is suggested that foetal disease after maternal infection may result in the premature decline of blood progesterone level. Whether the decline of progesterone levels represents a generalized hormonal failure or whether it is due to an interaction between hormones and endotoxin produced by *Campylobacter* remains to be determined. The susceptibility of the foetus may be attributable to foetal immunological incompetence.[62]

Abortions in sheep are caused by *C. jejuni* and occasionally by *C. fetus fetus* following ingestion of infected material. They generally occur as a sudden outbreak, with abortion rates varying from 5 to 70 per cent. Outbreaks stop abruptly and only rarely occur in successive seasons.[80] *Campylobacter jejuni* is mainly associated with enteric disturbances and abortions in humans.[8, 16, 48]

Clinical signs

Irregular oestrus cycles, delayed conception and sporadic abortions are the main clinical manifestations of *C. fetus venerealis* infection. A number of females returning to the bull at irregular intervals is usually the first sign of the disease in a herd. Animals believed to be in calf suddenly return to oestrus. When served, they may or may not conceive, and the conception rate in a herd is sometimes less than 20 per cent.[91]

A scant mucopurulent vaginal exudate may be present and, apart from mild hyperaemia of the mucosa near the cervix, very few changes are observed. There may be an increased flow of mucus from the vagina; in cases that are secondarily infected the discharge may be copious and purulent.

Infertility is usually temporary, and conception is merely delayed. Sometimes a heifer is served repeatedly before conception supervenes. In due course the animals develop a degree of immunity and return to normal breeding.[91]

When an infected bull is introduced into a clean herd, conception rates will be low at first, but eventually the majority of cows will conceive and calve normally. The infection seems to be more persistent in heifers, which therefore take longer to recover.

No signs of infection are evident in bulls.[91] The semen remains normal and fertile and the bull's breeding ability is unaffected. However, because of cows returning to oestrus, bulls may be overworked.

Pathology

Campylobacter fetus venerealis causes no macroscopic lesions in the genital organs of bulls. Only mild changes, consisting of a diffuse infiltration of lymphocytes and plasma cells within the lamina propria of the preputial mucosa, are encountered histologically.[6] Plasma cells are generally located in clusters at the apex of dermal papillae.

More severe changes occur in the female genital tract.[28] *Campylobacter fetus venerealis* can produce a diffuse, subacute to chronic, superficial endometritis.[98] The major changes in the endometrium are marked degeneration and mild hyperplasia of the surface epithelium and a moderate to marked neutrophil and lymphocyte infiltration into the stroma. Periglandular and perivascular cuffs of lymphocytes are prominent, while exudate may also accumulate in the lumen of the uterine glands.[30] The stratum compacta is infiltrated by neutrophils and lymphocytes. Experimentally these changes are first observed five days after intravaginal inoculation of *C. fetus*, and they reach a peak between the 30th and the 60th day. Thereafter lesions of a lesser degree persist for at least 120 days.[28] *Campylobacter fetus venerealis* can be isolated from cervical mucus for up to 122 days post-infection.

The effect of *C. fetus fetus* infection in the foetus and placenta after the seventh month of gestation is that a fibrinous peritonitis and pleuritis, hepatitis, and necrotic placentitis develop.[62]

In abortions due to *C. jejuni* in sheep, macroscopic lesions in the foetus are confined to the liver **(Figure 117.1)**. Numerous focal, circular, and tannish-orange areas, 5–15 mm in diameter, are randomly scattered throughout the liver. Microscopically, the foci are poorly circumscribed areas of necrotizing hepatitis. There is also a mild to moderate fibrinopurulent bronchopneumonia. Necrotic placentitis occurs inconsistently; neutrophils occur in the necrotic cotyledons.[80]

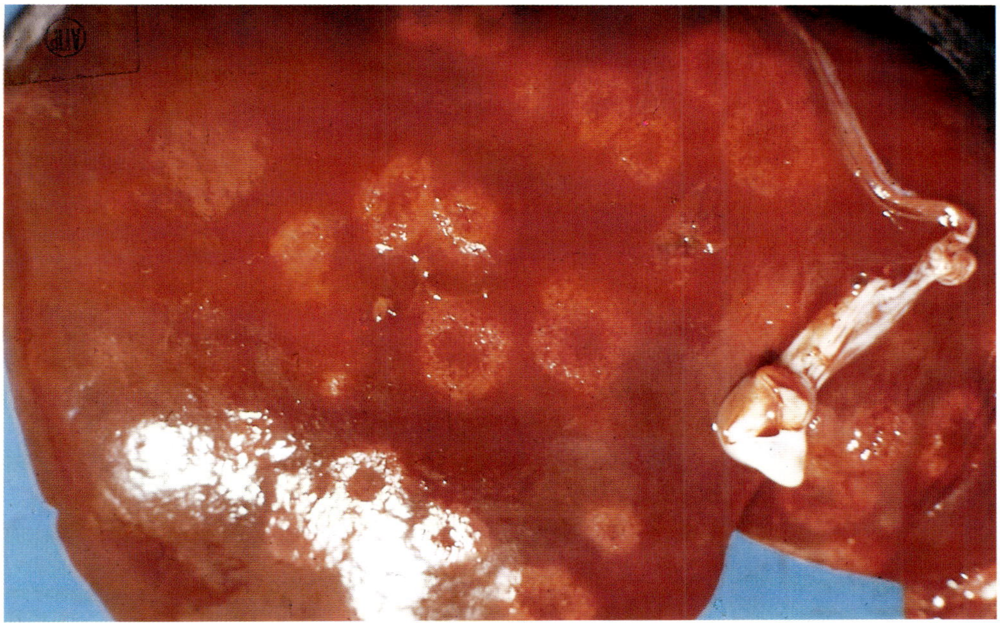

Figure 117.1 *Campylobacter jejuni* infection: circular, umbilicated necrotic foci in the liver of an aborted ovine foetus. (By courtesy of Dr W.J. Hartley, Jaranga Zoo, Mosman, NSW, Australia)

Diagnosis

The diagnosis of *C. fetus* infection is based on a reliable herd history, clinical signs, isolation and identification of the organism, and the demonstration of species-specific antibodies.

Earlier attempts to isolate *Campylobacter* spp. from bulls' preputial material were not usually successful. Overgrowth by contaminating saprophytes and the fastidious growth requirements of *C. fetus* proved to be the major obstacles. However, since the advent of millipore filtration and selective media, the organism can be isolated with greater confidence.[26, 33, 45, 47, 65, 68]

Campylobacter fetus can be cultivated from foetal and placental tissue by filtration and by using selective media. For this purpose, the tissues are homogenized and filtered through a membrane filter with a 0,65 µm pore size. The filtrate is then inoculated into both non-selective and selective media. Several specially formulated media for campylobacter isolation are commercially available.

Bulls are most important when making a diagnosis of campylobacteriosis on a herd basis, as the chance of a positive diagnosis in them is far greater than in cows. Preferably all the bulls in a herd, or a selection of the older bulls, should be examined for infection immediately after the breeding season or while they are running with the cows. Fluorescent antibody techniques complemented by specific cultural methods using preputial material for the diagnosis of *C. fetus venerealis* infection in bulls[39, 100] are presently the methods of choice in identifying infected bulls.[25, 37, 38, 51, 86] The accuracy of these diagnostic methods has been confirmed by Schutte.[76]

The quality of samples submitted for examination affects the accuracy of the diagnosis, and preputial material should be collected correctly. For this purpose 50 ml buffered-saline is run into the preputial cavity of the bull with a sterilized glass funnel and rubber tube. With the tube still *in situ*, the preputial orifice is ensnared and the prepuce vigorously massaged for a few minutes. The sheath washing, which should be milky and cloudy in appearance, is siphoned back into the bottle. *Campylobacter fetus venerealis* does not remain viable for more than six to eight hours in preputial washings. Samples should therefore reach the laboratory and be cultured within this period. If this period is to be exceeded, a transport medium should be used instead.[38]

Specimens of genital secretions of cows or heifers are collected directly from the vagina, and various methods for the collection of such material have been described.[1, 60, 91] To ensure adequate numbers of organisms, vaginal material should be taken during or close to oestrus.

The serological diagnosis of *C. fetus venerealis* infection in cattle is of limited value, since genital infection does not produce measurable serum antibody titres.[100] The vaginal mucus agglutination test is a more convenient and accurate method for diagnosing the infection in a herd.[46, 50, 63] The best results are obtained when mucus is collected during anoestrus, as the excessive amounts present during oestrus dilute the agglutinins and false-negative results may be recorded. It is not considered to be a reliable test in individual animals.

An enzyme-linked immunosorbent assay (ELISA) has been developed which is believed to be more sensitive than the vaginal mucus agglutination test, and antibodies present during the earlier stage of infection may be detected in mucus.[40] Since false-negative reactions may be encountered, it has value as a herd test only.

Differential diagnosis

Trichomonas foetus infection can simulate campylobacteriosis very closely. The causative agent should therefore be isolated from, and identified in, the vaginal mucus or preputial material, either by direct microscopy or by culture. In countries where brucellosis is endemic, this should be considered in the differential diagnosis, particularly in chronically infected herds. *Brucella abortus*, however, can readily be demonstrated by serological or biological tests. Infectious infertility ('epivag') is associated with vaginitis and epididymitis in cattle. It usually causes complete sterility of the bull, but a certain number of infected cows can become fertile again. Abortions have not been associated with 'epivag'.

Nutritional or functional infertility are non-infectious, and usually follow specific physiological disturbances.

Control

In most of the earlier reports on campylobacteriosis, the treatment of *C. fetus*-infected animals or *C. fetus*-contaminated semen is emphasized.[51, 67, 69, 76, 81] Acridine derivatives[91] and antibiotics, including streptomycin administered locally and/or systemically at 22 mg/kg,[81] are very effective for the treatment of *C. fetus*-infected bulls, as long as measures are instituted to prevent reinfection.[76]

Campylobacter fetus venerealis can be rendered inactive by incorporating antibiotics into fresh ejaculates and semen diluents.[1, 3, 44, 67, 77, 87] Although this method is effective, a sounder policy is to ensure that bulls are free of the disease prior to their introduction into a herd or an artificial insemination centre.

Individual females may be treated successfully by intrauterine antibiotic infusion.[1] The need to treat females is questioned, however, as infection in the female is self-limiting, and the most effective method is simply to postpone breeding for a period of 60 to 90 days. During this period the infected females will acquire an immunity which should be sufficient to protect them against reinfection.

Several researchers have studied the value of *C. fetus* vaccines in the prevention of abortion and the improvement of breeding efficiency in cows and heifers,[10, 11, 35, 41, 42, 52, 64, 97] but all commercially available vaccines are equally effective.[13, 14, 61] The efficacy of the vaccine depends on the type of adjuvant used, the concentration of antigen, the antigenicity of the specific strain present and the time interval between vaccination and breeding. To obtain optimal results, the recommendations of the manufacturers should be strictly adhered to. The trivalent vaccine, consisting of two *C. fetus fetus* strains (A-2 and B) and one *C. fetus venerealis* strain (A-1) in an oil adjuvant,[17] produced at the Veterinary Research Institute, Onderstepoort, has been used with great success. Data supplied by the Regional Diagnostic Laboratories in South Africa and the Veterinary Research Institute, where two to three thousand specimens for *C. fetus* identification are processed annually, indicate a dramatic drop in the prevalence of infection since the vaccine became available.[73, 78]

It is recommended that initial vaccination should consist of two injections prior to breeding. Annual booster vaccinations close to the breeding time will assure a high degree of immunity during the breeding season.[21, 22, 43, 75]

A bacterin containing high concentrations of antigen can be curative in bulls,[12, 19, 20–22, 71, 78, 94] but the mechanism by which the vaccine exerts its curative and preventive effect is not clear.[49, 99] It could, however, be associated with IgG, IgM or IgA preputial antibodies, which may play a role in clearing the infection.[89] No significant correlation between intrapreputial immunoglobulin concentration, histological findings, and age or vaccination status of the bulls has been found.[34]

References

1 **ADLER, H.C., 1957.** Genital vibriosis in the bovine. Thesis, A/S Card Fn. Montensen, Copenhagen.

2 **AKKERMANS, J.P., TERPSTRA, J.I. & VAN WAVEREN, H.G., 1956.** Over de betekenis van verschillende vibrionen voor de steriliteit van het rund. *Tijdschrift voor Diergeneeskunde*, 81, 430 – 435.

3 **AL-MASHAT, R.R. & TAYLOR, D.J., 1983.** *In vitro* sensitivity of 28 bovine isolates of *Campylobacter* to some commonly used antimicrobials. *The Veterinary Record*, 113, 89.

4 **BARNARD, B.J.H., 1968.** Die diagnose van vibriose by beeste. *Journal of the South African Veterinary Medical Association*, 39, 75–78.

5 **BERG, R.L., JULITA, J.W. & FIREHAMMER, B.D., 1971.** A revised classification of *Vibrio fetus*. *American Journal of Veterinary Research*, 32, 11–22.

6 **BIER, P.J., HALL, C.E., DUNCAN, J.R. & WINTER, A.J., 1977.** Experimental infections with *Campylobacter fetus* in bulls of different ages. *Veterinary Microbiology*, 2, 12–27.

7 **BLASSER, M.J., MOSS, C.W. & WEAVER, R.E., 1980.** Cellular fatty acid composition of *Campylobacter fetus*. *Journal of Clinical Microbiology*, 11, 448–451.

8 **BOKKENHEUSER, V.D., BRYNER, J.H., SCHUTTE, A.P., ROUX, D.J. & KOORNHOF, H.J., 1979.** Detection of enteric campylobacteriosis in children. *Journal of Clinical Microbiology*, 9, 227–232.

9 **BOLTON, F.J., HOLT, A.V. & HUTCHINSON, D.N., 1984.** *Campylobacter* biotyping scheme of epidemiological value. *Journal of Clinical Pathology*, 37, 677–681.

10 **BORDER, M.M. & FIREHAMMER, B.D., 1980.** Antigens of *Campylobacter fetus* subsp. *fetus* eliciting vaccinal immunity in heifers. *American Journal of Veterinary Research*, 41, 746–750.

11 **BOUTERS, R., DE KEYSER, J., VANDEPLASSCHE, M. & VAN AERT, A., 1976.** Weerstand tegen infectie en vruchtbaarheid van vaarzen na vaccinatie tegen *Vibrio fetus*. *Vlaams Diergeneeskundig Tijdschrift*, 45, 207–211.

12 **BOUTERS, R., DE KEYSER, J., VANDEPLASSCHE, M., VAN AERT, A., BRONE, E. & BONTE, P., 1973.** *Vibrio fetus* infection in bulls: Curative and preventative vaccination. *British Veterinary Journal*, 129, 52–57.

13 **BRYNER, J.H., FOLEY, J.W., HUBBERT, W.T. & MATHEWS, P.J., 1978.** Pregnant guinea-pig model for testing efficacy of *Campylobacter fetus* vaccines. *American Journal*

of *Veterinary Research*, 39, 119–121.

14 **BRYNER, J.H., FOLEY, J.W. & THOMPSON, B.A., 1979.** Comparative efficacy of ten commercial *Campylobacter fetus* vaccines in the pregnant guinea-pig: Challenge with *Campylobacter fetus* serotype A. *American Journal of Veterinary Research*, 40, 433–435.

15 **BRYNER, J.H., FRANK, A.H. & O'BERRY, P.A., 1962.** Dissociation studies of vibriosis from the bovine genital tract. *American Journal of Veterinary Research*, 23, 32–41.

16 **BUTZLER, J.P., 1984.** *Campylobacter Infection in Man and Animals*. Boca Raton, Florida: CRC Press, Inc.

17 **CAMERON, C.M., 1982.** Antibody response of guinea-pigs and cattle to a *Campylobacter fetus* oil emulsion vaccine. *Onderstepoort Journal of Veterinary Research*, 49, 177–179.

18 **CANHAM, A.S., 1948.** *Vibrio fetus* infection in cattle. *Journal of the South African Veterinary Medical Association*, 19, 103–104.

19 **CLARK, B.L. & DUFTY, J.H., 1982.** The duration of protection against infection with *Campylobacter fetus* subsp. *venerealis* in immunized bulls. *Australian Veterinary Journal*, 58, 220.

20 **CLARK, B.L., DUFTY, J.H. & MONSBOURGH, M.J., 1968.** Vaccination of bulls against bovine vibriosis. *Australian Veterinary Journal*, 44, 530.

21 **CLARK, B.L., DUFTY, J.H., MONSBOURGH, M.J. & PARSONSON, I.M., 1974.** Immunisation against bovine vibriosis. *Australian Veterinary Journal*, 50, 407–409.

22 **CLARK, B.L., DUFTY, J.H., MONSBOURGH, M.J. & PARSONSON, I.M., 1975.** Studies on venereal transmission of *Campylobacter fetus* by immunised bulls. *Australian Veterinary Journal*, 51, 531–532.

23 **COLLINS, J.D., AL-NASSIR, H.S., O'MAHONEY, H. & HANNAN, J., 1985.** Campylobacteriosis and *Campylobacter* in animals: Diagnostic aspects. *In*: LANDER, K.P., (ed.) *Campylobacter*. Luxemburg: Commission of the European Communities.

24 **CORBEIL, L.B., DUNCAN, J.R., SCHURIG, G.G.D., HALL, C.E. & WINTER, Q.J., 1974.** Bovine venereal vibriosis: Variations in immunoglobulin class of antibodies in genital secretions and serum. *Infection and Immunity*, 10, 1084–1090.

25 **DAWSON, L.L., 1986.** Diagnosis, prevention, and control of campylobacteriosis and trichomoniasis. *The Bovine Practitioner*, 21, 180–183.

26 **DE KEYSER, P.J., 1984.** Bovine genital campylobacteriosis. *In*: BUTZLER, J.P. (ed.) *Campylobacter Infection in Man and Animals*. Boca Raton, Florida: CRC Press, Inc.

27 **DE KEYSER, P.J., 1985.** The genus *Campylobacter*: Classification, nomenclature, habitat and pathogenicity. *In*: LANDER, K.P., (ed.) *Campylobacter*. Luxemburg: Commission of the European Communities.

28 **DOZZA, L., OLSON, N.O. & CAMPBELL, A., 1960.** The uterine biopsy technique for following the histologic changes caused by *Vibrio fetus* in the uterine mucosa. *American Journal of Veterinary Research*, 21, 878–883.

29 **DUFTY, J.H., CLARK, B.L. & MONSBOURGH, M.J., 1975.** The influence of age on the susceptibility of bulls to *Campylobacter fetus* subsp. *venerealis*. *Australian Veterinary Journal*, 51, 294–297.

30 **ESTES, P.C., BRYNER, J.H. & O'BERRY, P.A., 1966.** Histopathology of bovine vibriosis and the effects of *Vibrio fetus* extracts on the female genital tract. *Cornell Veterinarian*, 56, 610–622.

31 **FERGUSON, D.A. & LAMBE, D.W., 1984.** Differentiation of *Campylobacter* species by protein banding patterns in polyacrylamide slab gels. *Journal of Clinical Microbiology*, 20, 453–460.

32 **FISCHERLEITNER, F., BRANDL, G. & WEBER, A., 1984.** Klinisch-spermatologische Befunde nach Impfung gegen Campylobakteriose unter Berücksichtigung verschiedener Antibiotikatherapien. *Tierärztliche Umschau*, 39, 627–630.

33 **FLORENT, A., 1959.** Le Dex vibriosis genitales: La vibriose due à IV. *fetus venerealis* at la bivriose d'origine intestinale due à IV. *fetus intestinalis*. Mededelinge Veearts School, Ghent, 3, 1–60.

34 **FLOWER, J.P., LADDS, P.W., THOMAS, A.D. & WATSON, D.L., 1983.** An immunopathologic study of the bovine prepuce. *Veterinary Pathology*, 20, 189.

35 **FRANK, A.H., BRYNER, J.A. & O'BERRY, P.A., 1967.** The effect of *Vibrio fetus* vaccination on the breeding efficiency of cows bred to *Vibrio fetus*–infected bulls. *American Journal of Veterinary Research*, 28, 1237–1242.

36 **GALASSI, J.F., 1985.** Trichomoniasis y vibriosis genital bovina en la provincia del Chaco. *Veterinaria Argentina*, 2, 568–569.

37 **GARCIA, M.M., EAGLESOME, M.D. & RIGBY, C., 1983.** Campylobacters important in veterinary medicine. *Veterinary Bulletin*, 53, 793–818.

38 **GARCIA, M.M., RUCKERBAUER, G.M., EAGLESOME, M.D. & BOISCLAIR, W.E., 1983.** Detection of *Campylobacter fetus* in artificial insemination bulls with a transport enrichment medium. *Canadian Journal of Comparative Medicine*, 47, 336–340.

39 **HERSCHLER, R.C., 1963.** The diagnosis of *Vibrio fetus* in the bovine. Thesis, University of Minnesota, St. Paul.

40 **HEWSON, P.I., LANDER, K.P. & GILL, K.P.W., 1985.** Enzyme-linked immunosorbent assay for antibodies to *Campylobacter fetus* in bovine vaginal mucus. *Research in Veterinary Science*, 38, 41–45.

41 **HOERLEIN, A.B. & CARROLL, E.J., 1970.** Duration of immunity to bovine genital vibriosis. *Journal of the American Veterinary Medical Association*, 156, 775–778.

42 **HOERLEIN, A.B., CARROLL, E.J., KRAMER, T. & BECKENHAUER, W.H., 1965.** Bovine vibriosis immunisation. *Journal of the American Veterinary Medical Association*, 146, 828–835.

43 **HOFFER, M.A., 1981.** Bovine campylobacteriosis: A review. *The Canadian Veterinary Journal*, 22, 327–330.

44 **HOWARD, T.H., VASQUEZ, L.A. & AMANN, R.P., 1982.** Antibiotic control of *Campylobacter fetus* by three extenders of bovine semen. *Journal of Dairy Science*, 65, 1596–1600.

45 **JORGENSEN, K., 1985.** Identification methods for campylobacters. *In*: LANDER, K.P., (ed.) *Campylobacter*. Luxemburg: Commission of the European Communities.

46 **KENDRICK, J.A., 1967.** The vaginal mucus agglutination test for bovine vibriosis. *Journal of the American Veterinary Medical Association*, 150, 495–498.

47 **KIGGENS, E.M. & PLASTRIDGE, W.N., 1956.** Effect of gaseous environment on growth and catalase content of *Vibrio fetus* cultures of bovine origin. *Journal of Bacteriology*, 72, 397–401.

48 **KING, E.O., 1962.** The laboratory recognition of *Vibrio fetus* and closely related *Vibrio* isolated from cases of human vibriosis. *Annals of the New York Academy of Science*, 98, 700–711.

49 **LADDS, P.W., FLOWER, P.J. & McCOLL, C.J., 1981.** Campylobacteriosis, trichomoniasis and immune mechanisms in the bovine prepuce. *Australian Veterinary Association Yearbook*, 180–181.

50 **LAING, J.A., 1960.** *Vibrio fetus* infection in cattle. *Food and Agricultural Organization Agricultural Studies*, 51, 21–25, 32–35.

51 **LEIN, D., ERICKSON, I., WINTER, A.J. & McENTEE, K., 1968.** Diagnosis, treatment and control of vibriosis in an artificial insemination centre. *Journal of the American Veterinary Medical Association*, 153, 1574–1580.

52 **LINCOLN, G.J. & TROUT, K.J., 1967.** Evaluation of a new trivalent bovine vibriosis bacterin. *Veterinary Medicine/Small Animal Clinician*, 46, 561–564.

53 **LIOR, H., 1984.** New extended biotyping scheme for *Campylobacter jejuni*, *Campylobacter coli* and *Campylobacter laridis*. *Journal of Clinical Microbiology*, 20, 636–640.

54 **LUECHTEFELD, N.W. & WANG, W.L.L., 1982.** Hippurate hydrolysis by and triphenyltetrazolium tolerance of *Campylobacter fetus*. *Journal of Clinical Microbiology*, 15, 137–140.

55 **MARSH, H. & FIREHAMMER, B.D., 1953.** Serological relationships of 23 ovine and three bovine strains of *Vibrio fetus*.

American Journal of Veterinary Research, 14, 396–398.

56 **McCOY, E.C., DOYLE, D., BURDA, K., CORBEIL, L.B. & WINTER, A.J., 1975.** Superficial antigens of *Campylobacter (Vibrio) fetus*: Characterization of an antiphagocytic component. *Infection and Immunity*, 11, 517–525.

57 **McFADYEN, J. & STOCKMAN, S., 1913.** Report of Departmental Committee on Epizootic Abortions. Board of Agriculture and Fisheries, Great Britain.

58 **MITSCHERLICH, E. & LIESS, B., 1958.** Die serologische differenzierung von *V. fetus* stammen. *Deutsche Tierärztliche Wochenschrift*, 65, 2–7.

59 **MOHANTY, S.B., PLUMER, G.J. & FABER, J.E., 1962.** Biochemical and colonial characteristics of some bovine vibrios. *American Journal of Veterinary Research*, 23, 554–557.

60 **MORGAN, W.J.B., 1959.** Studies on the antigenic structure of *Vibrio fetus*. *Journal of Comparative Pathology*, 69, 125–140.

61 **NEWHALL, J.H., 1966.** Results of field trials and controlled laboratory studies on bovine vibriosis bacterins. *Journal of the American Veterinary Medical Association*, 149, 1643–1646.

62 **OSBURN, B.I. & HOSKINS, R.K., 1971.** Infection with *Vibrio fetus* in the immunologically immature fetal calf. *The Journal of Infectious Diseases*, 123, 32–40.

63 **PLASTRIDGE, W.N., EASTERBROOKS, H.L. & WILLIAMS, L.F., 1953.** The tampon method of collection and the examination of cervicovaginal mucus for *Vibrio fetus* agglutinins. *Journal of the American Veterinary Medical Association*, 123, 516–520.

64 **PLASTRIDGE, W.N., KERSTING, E.J. & WILLIAMS, M.S., 1966.** Resistance of vaccinated heifers to vibriosis. *American Journal of Veterinary Research*, 27, 186–190.

65 **PLASTRIDGE, W.N., KOTHS, M.E. & WILLIAMS, L.F., 1961.** Antibiotic mediums for the isolation of vibrios from semen. *American Journal of Veterinary Research*, 22, 867–871.

66 **PLASTRIDGE, W.N. & WILLIAMS, L.F., 1943.** Observations on *Vibrio fetus* infection in cattle. *Journal of the American Veterinary Medical Association*, 102, 89–95.

67 **PLASTRIDGE, W.N., WILLIAMS, L.F. & TROWBRIDGE, D.G., 1964.** Antibiotic sensitivity of physiological groups of micro-aerophilic vibrios. *American Journal of Veterinary Research*, 25, 1295–1299.

68 **PLUMER, G.J., DUVAL, W.C. & SHEPLER, V.R., 1962.** A preliminary report on a new technique for the isolation of *Vibrio fetus* from carrier bulls. *Cornell Veterinarian*, 52, 110.

69 **PRIER, J.E., 1951.** The *in vitro* effect of several antibiotics against *Vibrio fetus*. *Veterinary Medicine*, 46, 358–365.

70 **RETIEF, G.P., SCHUTTE, A.P. & COUBROUGH, R.I., 1975.** The herd approach to bovine reproduction disorders part I: The diagnosis and management of infectious infertility. *Journal of the South African Veterinary Medical Association*, 47, 19–22.

71 **ROSLANOWSKI, K., SZPRYNGIEL, I. & WYSZANOWSKI, J., 1980.** Studies on the efficacy of the vaccine against campylobacteriosis (vibriosis) in bulls. *Bulletin of the Veterinary Institute in Pulawy*, 24, 1–5.

72 **SAMUELSON, J.D. & WINTER, A.J., 1966.** Bovine vibriosis: The nature of the carrier state in the bull. *Journal of Infectious Diseases*, 116, 581–585.

73 **SCHMIDT-DUMONT, A.M.A., 1984.** The incidence of *Campylobacter fetus* and *Tritrichomonas foetus* in cattle in South West Africa/Namibia. *Proceedings of the Tenth International Congress on Animal Reproduction and Artificial Insemination*, June 10–14 1984, Urbana Champaign, Illinois.

74 **SCHURIG, G.D., HALL, C.E., BURDA, K., CORBEIL, L.B., DUNCAN, J.R. & WINTER, A.J., 1973.** Persistent genital tract infection with *Vibrio fetus intestinalis* associated with serotypic alteration of the infecting strain. *American Journal of Veterinary Research*, 34, 1399–1403.

75 **SCHURIG, G.D., HALL, C.E. & CORBEIL, L.B., 1975.** Bovine venereal vibriosis: Cure of genital infections in females by systemic immunization. *Infection and Immunity*, 11, 245–251.

76 **SCHUTTE, A.P., 1969.** Some aspects of *Vibrio fetus* infection in bulls. Thesis, University of Ghent.

77 **SCHUTTE, A.P., 1970.** *Vibrio fetus* infektion bei Bullen. *Zuchthygiene*, 5, 36–37.

78 **SCHUTTE, A.P., 1975.** Vibriose van beeste en die waarde van entstowwe teen die siekte. *In*: LOTTER, L., (ed.) *Boerdery Keur*. Johannesburg: Promedia Uitgewers.

79 **SCHUTTE, A.P., 1977.** Ondersoek na onvrugbaarheid by beeste. *Journal of the South African Veterinary Association*, 48, 173–175.

80 **SCHUTTE, A.P., McCONNELL, E.E. & BOSMAN, P.P., 1971.** Vibrionic abortion in ewes in South Africa: Preliminary report. *Journal of the South African Veterinary Medical Association*, 42, 223–225.

81 **SEGER, C.L., LANK, R.B. & LEVY, H.E., 1966.** Dihydrostreptomycin for treatment of genital vibriosis in the bull. *Journal of the American Veterinary Medical Association*, 149, 1634–1639.

82 **SKERMAN, V.B.D., McGOWAN, V. & SNEATJ, P.H.A., 1980.** Approval lists of bacterial names. *International Journal of Systematic Bacteriology*, 30, 225–420.

83 **SMIBERT, R.M., 1974.** *Campylobacter*. *In*: BUCHANAN, R.E. & GIBBONS, N.E., (eds). *Bergey's Manual of Determinative Bacteriology*, 8th edn. Baltimore, London: Williams & Wilkins.

84 **SMIBERT, R.M., 1984.** *Campylobacter*. *In*: KRIEG, N.R. & HOLT, J.G., (eds). *Bergey's Manual of Systematic Bacteriology*. Baltimore, London: Williams & Wilkins.

85 **SNYMAN, P.S., 1931.** *Vibrio fetus* as a cause of bovine abortion in South Africa. *Seventeenth Report of the Department of Veterinary Services, Union of South Africa*, 1, 197, 201.

86 **STADTFELD, H., NITZSCHKE, E., HAHN, W. & KONZ, A., 1982.** Zum kulturellen Nachweis von *Campylobacter fetus* subspecies *fetus* in Präputialspülproben von Besamungs- und Deckbullen. *Berliner und Münchener Tierärztliche Wochenschrift*, 95, 393–397.

87 **SULLIVAN, J.J., ELLIOT, F.I., BARTLETT, D.E., MURPHY, D.M. & KUZDAS, C.D., 1966.** Further studies on use of polymyxin B sulphate with dihydrostreptomycin and penicillin for control of *Vibrio fetus* in frozen semen process. *Journal of Dairy Science*, 49, 1569–1571.

88 **TERPSTRA, L.I. & EISMA, W.A., 1951.** *Vibrio fetus* infection in cattle and enzootic infertility. *Tijdschrift voor Diergeneeskunde*, 76, 433–447.

89 **VAN AERT, A., DE KEYSER, P., BRONE, E., BOUTERS, R. & VANDEPLASSCHE, M., 1976.** Nature of antibodies to *Campylobacter fetus* in preputial secretions from a vaccinated bull. *British Veterinary Journal*, 132, 615–620.

90 **VAN AERT, A., DE KEYSER, P., FLORENT, A.F., BOUTERS, R., VANDEPLASSCHE, M. & BRONE, E., 1977.** Nature of *Campylobacter fetus* agglutinins in vaginal mucus from experimentally infected heifers. *British Veterinary Journal*, 133, 88–94.

91 **VANDEPLASSCHE, M., FLORENT, A., BOUTERS, R., HUYSMAN, A., BRONE, E. & DE KEYSER, P., 1963.** The pathogenesis, epidemiology and treatment of *Vibrio fetus* infection in cattle. *I.W.O.N.L. Verslagen over Navorsing*, No. 29, University of Ghent.

92 **VAN RENSBURG, S.W.J., 1954.** Vibriosis as a cause of herd infertility in South Africa. *Journal of the South African Veterinary Medical Association*, 25, 25–35.

93 **VASQUEZ, L.A., AVILA, J.D., ROSSANIGO, C.E. & SAGER, R.L., 1984.** Trichomoniasis y campylobacteriosis en la region semiarida Central Argentina. *Veterinaria Argentina*, 1, 940, 942–947.

94 **VASQUEZ, L.A., BALL, L., BENNETT, B.W., RUPP, G.P., ELLIS, R., OLSON, J.D. & HUFFMAN, M.H., 1983.** Bovine genital campylobacteriosis (vibriosis): Vaccination of experimentally infected bulls. *American Journal of Veterinary Research*, 44, 1553–1557.

95 **VERON, M. & CHATELEIN, R., 1973.** Taxonomic study of the genus *Campylobacter* Sebald and Veron and designation of the neotype strain of the type species, *Campylobacter fetus* (Smith and Taylor) Sebald and Veron. *International Journal of*

Systematic Bacteriology, 23, 122–134.

96 **WARE, D.A., 1980.** Pathogenicity of *Campylobacter fetus* subsp. *venerealis* in causing infertility in cattle. *British Veterinary Journal*, 136, 501–503.

97 **WHITFORD, H.W., BROWN, L.N. & BRYNER, J.H., 1977.** The isolation of *Campylobacter fetus* subspecies *intestinalis* and other vibrios from aborted bovine fetuses. *Proceedings of the Annual Meeting of the American Association of Veterinary Laboratory Diagnosticians*, 20, 55–68.

98 **WILLS, F.K., 1965.** Response of the bovine uterus to several infectious agents. Thesis, University of Connecticut.

99 **WINTER, A.J., CLARK, B.L., PARSONSON, I.M., DUNCAN, J.R. & BIER, P.J., 1981.** Nature of immunity in the male bovine reproductive tract based upon responses to *Campylobacter fetus* on *Trichomonas fetus*. *Advances in Experimental and Medical Biology*, 137, 745–752.

100 **WINTER, A.J., SAMUELSON, J.D. & ELKANA, M., 1967.** A comparison of immunofluorescence and cultural techniques for demonstration of *Vibrio fetus*. *Journal of the American Veterinary Medical Association*, 150, 499–502.

118

The porcine intestinal adenomatosis complex

M.C. Williams and M.L. van der Walt

Introduction

The porcine intestinal adenomatosis complex is associated with the presence of intracellular bacteria of the genus *Campylobacter*, and is made up of four different enteropathy syndromes: porcine intestinal adenomatosis (PIA), [also known as porcine proliferative enteritis (PPE)], proliferative haemorrhagic enteropathy (PHE), regional (terminal) ileitis (RI) and necrotic enteritis (NE).[44] Marked hyperplasia of immature intestinal epithelium, particularly affecting the ileal and caecal mucosa, is the underlying lesion in all four syndromes.

Porcine intestinal adenomatosis was first recorded in North America in 1931 as 'intestinal adenoma in swine',[1] but the aetiology and significance of the lesion has been clarified to some extent only in the last decade and a half.

The PIA complex has been recorded in many countries and has a worldwide distribution. The disease has probably been present in southern Africa for many decades, and a local museum specimen of the ileum of a pig dating from the 1950s clearly manifests classic RI. In 1978 an outbreak of PHE in sows in a large commercial piggery in the Orange Free State was investigated,[55] and outbreaks of PHE were also diagnosed in piggeries in the south-western Cape Province.[57] In South Africa, and probably elsewhere in southern Africa, PIA complex most commonly manifests as PHE in large, intensive, commercial units, but no detailed investigations of its prevalence have been reported.

Aetiology

Campylobacter spp. are most consistently isolated from clinical cases suffering from the PIA complex. Intestinal specimens of PIA cases yielded the first isolates of *C. mucosalis*[16] and of *C. hyointestinalis*.[9] *Campylobacter jejuni* and *C. coli* in conjunction with either *C. mucosalis* or *C. hyointestinalis* are sometimes isolated from animals with PIA, but the former two species are not believed to be involved in disease in pigs.[51] *Campylobacter mucosalis* and *C. hyointestinalis* are clearly not the sole aetiological agents involved in the disease, as dosing animals with these organisms alone does not initiate disease,[3, 29, 37, 38] whereas scrapings of affected mucosa which may contain additional unidentified organisms are effective in reproducing the disease.[26, 27, 41] Viruses do not appear to be involved.[16]

Campylobacter hyointestinalis and *C. mucosalis* are morphologically similar, both being Gram-negative, short, irregular rods, 0,25 μm wide and 0,92–2,8 μm long. Sea-gull, spiral, comma and coccoid forms occur. The organisms are motile by means of a single polar flagellum. The bacteria are free in the cytoplasm of epithelial cells, while in stained sections of the intestine they are surrounded by a narrow, unstained halo.[12, 43] Ultrastructurally they are elongated and curved with rounded ends and measure 2–3 x 0,3 μm.[12, 25, 43] They have a distinct cell wall and a dense, osmiophilic internal structure.[12, 43] The organisms are micro-aerophiles and require 5 per cent oxygen levels for optimum growth. This 5 per cent level is essential for the growth of *C. mucosalis* and stimulatory for *C. hyointestinalis*. The fastidious organisms are cultivated on suitable media in anaerobic jars which are evacuated and filled with a gas mixture to give a satisfactory atmosphere.[53, 54] Colonies are 1–1,5 mm in diameter. Those of *C. mucosalis* are distinctly yellow,[16] while *C. hyointestinalis* colonies are beige[10] and those of *C. coli* are pink. *Campylobacter mucosalis* is catalase-negative, while *C. hyointestinalis* and *C. coli* are catalase-positive. Biochemical tests are used for further differentiation.[53, 54]

Campylobacter hyointestinalis appears to be antigenically distinct,[5] while *C. mucosalis* comprises three groups of serotypes (A, B and C) on the basis of distinct, heat-labile surface antigens, serotypes A and B having a common, heat-stable antigen.[17] Serotype A is the most prevalent, while serotype B is rare. It does not appear as if serotype C is a cause of clinical disease.[14] Only serotype A has been isolated in South Africa.[54] Although antigenic variation of the infecting population's antigens does apparently occur,[20] it does not seem that any particular antigenic type is involved with PIA, NE, RI or PHE.

Epidemiology

Little is known of the epidemiology of the PIA complex, except that *C. mucosalis* is only present intracellularly in the intestinal epithelium of clinically affected pigs, and that the organism may be isolated from the oral cavity but not the intestine of apparently healthy pigs in herds which have histories of being infected.[18, 54] *Campylobacter hyointestinalis* has a wider distribution in nature, but it is only in cases of PIA that it occurs intracellularly.[4] It can be isolated from the faeces of healthy animals or from those with enteric disease.[10] Syndromes of the PIA complex occur in pigs of all ages, although suckling piglets appear to be less susceptible. There is a period after weaning when agglutinating antibodies are low and animals are highly susceptible, and this usually coincides with the time when most animals are clinically affected.[5]

Pathogenesis

Because of the difficulty of producing the disease experimentally, the pathogenesis of the syndromes in the PIA complex remains speculative. It appears that PIA is the essential lesion and that PHE, NE and RI are variations arising from complications that follow on the initial adenomatous change. The invasion of mucosal epithelial cells by *C. mucosalis* or *C. hyointestinalis*, or both, is the initial event in the pathogenesis of PIA. This invasion appears to be mediated by various factors, including the age and/or weight of the pig, herd of origin, and other unknown environmental 'stressors'.[27, 37, 38, 41] It is not known whether the morphological changes in the epithelial cells are caused by the invading organisms or by other factors which predispose to bacterial invasion.[13, 19, 44] Although there is no evidence to support the supposition, it may be that the intracellular bacteria cause the infected cells to multiply more rapidly, giving rise to an adenomatous mucosa.

Porcine haemorrhagic enteropathy appears to be an acute hypersensitivity phenomenon, judging from the finding of eosinophils, mast cells and thrombosed blood vessels in the affected mucosa.[21, 23, 32, 33, 35] It has been suggested that the relevant antigens that cause the hypersensitivity may be released from degenerating epithelial cells in sensitized hosts.[23]

Necrotic enteritis is characterized not only by necrosis but also by inflammation of the affected mucosa. It has been speculated that this occurs because the immature epithelium, without its protective mucus coat, is more susceptible to damage by the gut flora than is the mature epithelium.[44]

Regional ileitis seems to be the most protracted form of the disease, judging by the often chronic, granulomatous inflammation which involves virtually the full thickness of the intestinal wall. The cause of the marked hypertrophy of the muscular layers is unknown, but it may be in response to the chronic inflammatory process which causes a narrowing of the lumen and so necessitates an increased force to move the ingesta along.

Despite the convincing association that has been found between *C. mucosalis* and/or *C. hyointestinalis* and the syndromes of the PIA complex, experimental reproduction of the disease is not easy. In conventional suckling piglets exposed to *C. mucosalis* and *C. hyointestinalis* cultures, the organisms do not extensively colonize the alimentary chyme, they are only irregularly associated with intestinal mucosa, and no adenomatous change develops.[37] Weaned pigs are even more resistant to infection, and it is only after treatment with the anticholinergic drug, benzetimide, that low levels of infection become established.[38] However, *C. mucosalis* remained in the oral cavity of neonatal pigs for weeks.[39]

In studies which used gnotobiotic pigs, both *C. hyointestinalis* and *C. mucosalis* colonized the gut mucosal surface when dosed orally, but did not induce adenomatous change.[3, 29] When mucosal scrapings from affected pigs were dosed to caesarian-derived, colostrum deprived piglets, gross and/or microscopic lesions of proliferative enteritis were observed and *C. mucosalis* was isolated.[22]

Colonization of the intestine is a frequent feature when animals are dosed with *Campylobacter* cultures,[29, 37] but the lesions indicative of PIA are seldom observed.[3, 22] However, limited experiments have shown that the dosing of scrapings of macroscopically affected tissue successfully reproduces clinical PIA.[26, 27, 41] These results suggest that although the *Campylobacter* spp. may be responsible for the proliferative type of lesion, another factor, present in PIA lesions, may be involved in initiating the disease. Additional factors, such as the age of the animal and its immune status, may also be important in the induction of the disease.[27]

Seroconversion has been shown to occur during the course of the clinical stage of PHE, providing additional evidence that *C. hyointestinalis* and *C. mucosalis* are involved in that condition, despite the difficulty experienced in the recovery of *C. mucosalis* from PHE-affected tissue.[25] Pigs with confirmed lesions of PIA have been shown to have no or low serum antibody titres to both *C. hyointestinalis* and *C. mucosalis*.[5]

Clinical signs

The PIA complex, because of its varied syndromes, does not present a uniform set of clinical signs. Since PIA probably represents the uncomplicated disease, NE, RI and PHE may be regarded as variants or, more probably, complications of PIA.

Uncomplicated PIA does not usually result in death. In the majority of cases, signs of the disease are mild or absent,[7, 40] but if they do appear, they are observed almost exclusively in post-weaning pigs.[13, 40, 43] Affected animals often show decreased appetite and a reduced weight gain.[40, 43, 49] In more severe cases, an initial period during which there may be a protracted, mild diarrhoea may be followed by wasting, anaemia, the appearance of a roughened hair coat and even emaciation.[1, 6, 13, 40, 43] Most of the clinically affected animals recover within six weeks after a remarkably sudden return of appetite.[43, 49]

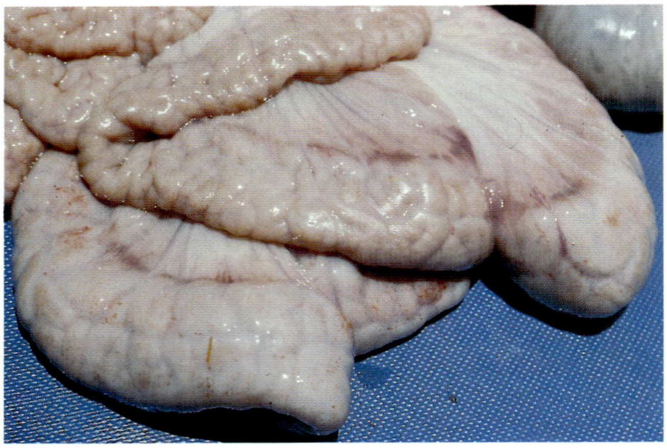

Figure 118.1 Terminal small intestine of a pig suffering from porcine intestinal adenomatosis. Note the convoluted, thickened mucosa as seen from the serosal surface

Cases of NE occur sporadically in weaned pigs, mostly between the ages of three and six months.[1, 2] Affected animals usually show mild to moderate diarrhoea that lasts several weeks,[1, 2, 6] and pieces of pseudomembrane reminiscent of those seen in chronic salmonellosis may be observed in the stools.[12] The pigs gradually lose weight, become emaciated and eventually die.[1, 2]

Regional ileitis is a chronic manifestation of the disease and occurs only in weaned pigs. It is generally asymptomatic and found incidentally in baconers at slaughter.[7] Those that are clinically affected may show mild anorexia, weight loss and either diarrhoea or constipation.[7, 8, 28, 30] In a small proportion of cases perforation of the ileum may supervene, leading to peritonitis and sudden death.[7, 8, 30] These animals show sudden and complete anorexia together with excessive thirst, dullness, hind quarter weakness and a disinclination to get up. They may have a hunched appearance, wobbly gait and vomit repeatedly.

Porcine haemorrhagic enteropathy is the most serious syndrome in the PIA complex, as it usually occurs as explosive outbreaks in weaned and/or adult pigs.[32, 33] Occasionally, sudden death occurs without premonitory signs.[25] Most animals that develop PHE become anorexic, show mucosal pallor and a profuse, watery, black and foul-smelling diarrhoea (melaena).[25, 31, 32, 35, 49] Some animals vomit, have laboured breathing, and pregnant sows may abort.[25, 32, 49] A few pigs are pyrexic but most have normal to subnormal temperatures.[25, 32, 35, 49] The mortality rate in affected pigs is between 10 and 40 per cent. Animals that recover often show poor appetite and weight gain.[49]

Pathology

The carcasses of animals affected by uncomplicated PIA are usually in good condition,[42] but there may be varying degrees of wasting and even emaciation in a minority of cases.[13] The most characteristic lesion invariably occurs in the mucosa of the terminal ileum,[6, 13] and less often in the caecum and proximal colon.[1, 13] In a few cases just the large intestine, including the distal colon, is affected.[1, 36] The affected mucosa is markedly thickened and thrown into interconnecting longitudinal and transverse folds up to 5 mm wide and 4 mm high **(Figure 118.1)**.[6, 13] This thickening is usually diffuse, but may have a nodular pattern.[13] The nodules are 2–15 mm in diameter, raised above the adjacent mucosal surface, and in some cases resemble polyps, as they are often wider at the surface than at the base.[1, 6] The mucosa is greyish-white, and small areas of superficial necrosis infrequently occur.[13] Necrosis is probably indicative of a transitional phase between PIA and NE. The mesenteric lymph nodes that drain affected portions of the intestine are usually enlarged.[1]

Necrotic enteritis is characterized by intestinal lesions which in essence are similar to those in PIA and occur in the same locations. In addition, however, the surface of the affected mucosa is covered by a necrotic or diphtheric pseudomembrane,[1, 2, 42, 44] which imparts a greyish-yellow to yellow colour to the affected surface.[2, 44] Oedema of the intestinal wall[44] and of the mesentery[2] may be observed in some instances. Pigs that have died from NE are invariably emaciated.[1, 2]

When RI is an incidental finding at slaughter, the carcass is usually well-fleshed,[8, 42] but in fatal cases the animal is often emaciated.[12] A marked thickening and rigidity ('hose-pipe gut') of the wall of the terminal ileum is the most consistent gross finding,[7, 8, 12, 30, 34, 44] the diameter of the intestine being up to three times that of normal pigs.[7] The increase in diameter is due to severe hypertrophy of the longitudinal and circular muscle layers of the tunica muscularis and, in most cases, concomitant thickening of the mucosa.[7, 8, 12, 30, 34, 44] The serosa of the terminal ileum and associated mesentery may be either thickened and oedematous[7, 12] or congested.[7, 34] In some cases there is a patchy, fibrinous, granulomatous or fibrous serositis.[7, 34] The mucosa may be whitish, greyish, yellowish or diffusely reddened,[7] and occasionally there are ulcers covered with necrotic debris and pseudomembranes.[7, 12, 34, 44] Peyer's patches and the ileocaecal lymph nodes may be hyperplastic,[7, 8, 12, 34] and ileocaecal lymphadenitis has also been described.[7] If perforation of the ileum occurs, it usually takes place at the attachment of the meso-ileum[7] and almost invariably results in a diffuse, fibrinous peritonitis.[7, 8, 30]

In pigs with PHE which are killed when clinical signs first appear, there is marked oedema of the ileomesenteric attachment[23, 33] and abundant clear ascitic fluid.[23, 25] At this time the intestinal content is blood-tinged and the mucosa diffusely reddened **(Figure 118.2)**. Twelve hours after the commencement of clinical signs, the mucosa is covered by a fibrinous pseudomembrane with discrete, fresh blood clots up to 10 mm in diameter trapped between the membrane and epithelium. Twenty-four hours after clinical signs have appeared, the lumen

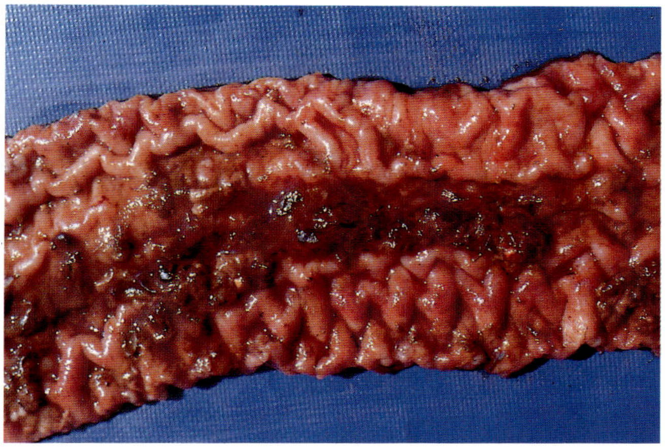

Figure 118.2 Haemorrhagic intestinal content of a pig suffering from porcine haemorrhagic enteropathy

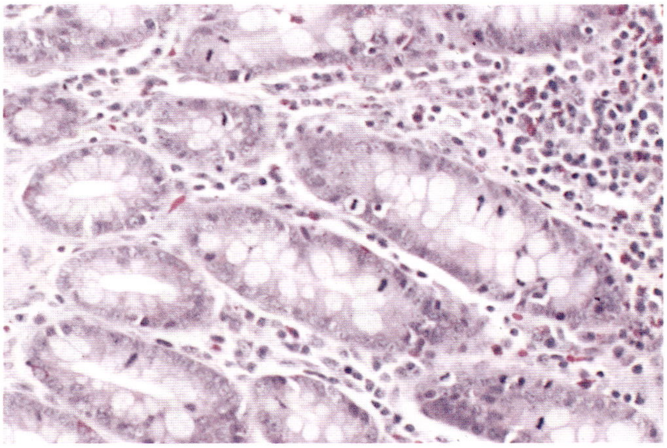

Figure 118.3 Section of a normal small intestinal tract

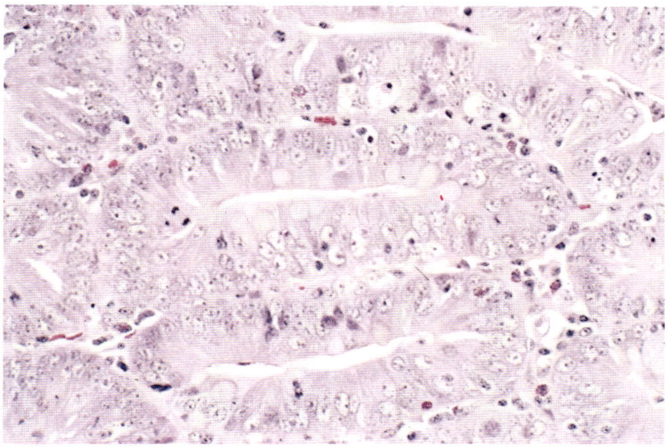

Figure 118.4 Immature, hypertrophied cells in hyperplastic mucosa of a pig suffering from porcine intestinal adenomatosis

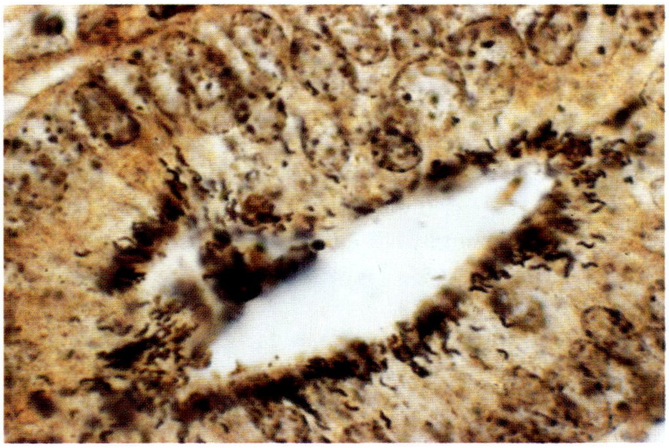

Figure 118.5 Histological section of the intestine demonstrating intracytoplasmic bacteria (Warthin-Starry silver impregnation)

is filled with blood, and a cast consisting of clotted blood covers the mucosal surface.[23, 25]

The carcass shows generalized pallor in pigs that have died of PHE.[31, 32, 33, 35, 49] Specific lesions in most cases are confined to the ileum, but the caecum may also be affected in some.[35] The serosa of the ileum has a characteristic reticulate appearance[23, 25, 35, 49] probably due to subserosal oedema.[49] The lumen of the ileum and colon contains a large amount of fluid or clotted blood. The ileal mucosa, as in PIA, is thickened and ridged[23, 25, 31, 32, 33, 35, 49] and pinkish-red to red. There may be mucosal petechiation.[33, 49]

Proliferation of immature mucosal epithelial cells, either as discrete islands within normal mucosa or as diffuse involvement of the entire mucosa, is the underlying, essential lesion common to PIA, NE, RI and PHE. This imparts the nodular or evenly thickened appearance to the intestine which can be observed macroscopically.[6, 7, 13, 49] There is a sharp demarcation between normal and abnormal (adenomatous) mucosa.[1, 6, 49] Villous atrophy causes a flattened mucosa,[6, 48, 49] while the glands themselves are often highly distorted and branched.[1, 7, 49]

The glandular epithelial cells are immature, being large, uniformly columnar, and often crowded onto the basal lamina to give an overlapping or pseudostratified appearance.[1, 6, 7, 49] The cytoplasm is deeply eosinophilic to slightly basophilic.[7] Most nuclei are either large and vesicular, containing one or two nucleoli, or elongated and densely stained.[7, 49] Numerous mitoses,[7, 49] but very few goblet cells,[1, 6, 7, 49] are evident in the adenomatous epithelium **(Figures 118.3 and 118.4)**. The marked immaturity of the proliferating epithelial cells is well demonstrated by positive pyroninophilia, poorly developed brush borders, and the slight cytoplasmic enzyme activity (alkaline phosphatase and adenosine triphosphatase). Taken as a whole, these staining reactions are typical of those of the undifferentiated epithelial cells at the base of mucosal glands.[48, 49] Warthin-Starry silver impregnation techniques stain numerous, irregularly curved bacteria with a morphology typical of *Campylobacter* spp. in the apical cytoplasm of the immature epithelial cells **(Figure 118.5)**.[13, 48]

Changes in the intestinal wall (apart from those in the epithelium) are absent or unremarkable in PIA. Increased numbers of lymphocytes and plasma cells and a few eosinophils may be found in the lamina propria.[6, 49]

In pigs killed immediately after the first appearance of clinical signs of PHE, histological evidence of an acute hypersensitivity reaction is found,[23] including extensive accumulation of proteinaceous fluid in the interstitium and lacteals of the lamina propria, severe congestion of the mucosal blood vessels and marked infiltration of eosinophils into the mucosa. Mast cells and thrombosed blood vessels have been noted in the affected intestine.[23]

In pigs which have died of PHE, cell debris and desquamated epithelium, either free in the lumen or attached to the mucosa, are invariably observed in addition to the adenomatous changes, blood and fibrin admixed with inflammatory cells.[35, 45, 49] Superficial epithelial desquamation[31, 49] and necrosis of single[45] or small groups[49] of epithelial cells occur. Many mucosal glands are dilated and contain inflammatory cells, cell debris and desquamated epithelial cells.[21, 31, 35, 45, 49] The lamina propria is usually moderately congested[49] and oedematous.[45] Haemorrhage is apparent in many areas in the lamina propria[45, 49] but this is not always seen.[35] Histological evidence of blood vessel wall lesions is not observed.[35, 45] A mild to moderate infiltration of inflammatory cells consisting of eosinophils, neutrophils, plasma cells and macrophages is usually present in the lamina propria.[32, 35, 45, 49] The submucosa is moderately to severely congested and oedematous,[35, 45, 49] and may contain small clusters of neutrophils[45, 49] and a few eosinophils.[49] Oedema of the intermuscular connective tissue in the tunica muscularis and of the subserosa has been described.[45, 49]

Necrotic enteritis is characterized by patchy[42, 44] to extensive[1, 6] coagulative necrosis and inflammation of the mucosa. In some cases there is granulation tissue proliferation in the mucosa,[44] while adenomatous epithelium may be found in non-necrotic areas of the mucosa.[1, 42, 44]

In RI the histological changes observed in the mucosa are variable. The mucosa may be adenomatous,[7, 12, 34, 44] chronically inflamed,[7, 8, 34, 42, 44] or essentially normal.[30] Typically there is subacute inflammation of varying degree with a mixed cell infiltration in the lamina propria, submucosa and serosa.[7, 12, 34, 44] This, together with marked hypertrophy of both layers of the tunica muscularis, is responsible for the thickening of the ileum observed macroscopically.[7, 12, 30, 34, 44]

Ultrastructurally, the epithelial cells in adenomatous areas of the mucosa resemble undifferentiated crypt cells.[43] They are elongated, have a narrow apex,[12, 43] and a basal nucleus[12, 48] which is round, oval, or irregular and deeply indented.[48] The cytoplasm contains numerous mitochondria of variable size,[48] and clusters of free ribosomes.[43, 48] The few microvilli that are present are of irregular shape.[12, 13, 43, 48] The lack of microvilli is more pronounced in cells which contain large numbers of intracytoplasmic bacteria.[23]

Intracellular bacteria are found in the immature cells in PIA,[47] PHE,[23] NE,[44] and RI.[11, 12] They are consistently found in the apical cytoplasm,[12, 13, 43, 45, 48] but in PHE they also occur free, in macrophages in the lamina propria and submucosa, and within capillaries and lymphatics.[21, 23]

Diagnosis

No reliable laboratory tests are currently available for confirmation of the PIA complex or the presence of either of the two organisms in a living animal.

Investigation into the serological response to infection has been confined to the use of the agglutination test. Most pigs suffering from PIA have agglutinating serum antibodies some time during the period that lesions are present,[17] but a positive agglutinating reaction is not indicative of clinical disease.[56] A large proportion of sera obtained from healthy adult pigs shows high antibody levels[5, 15, 56] against the antigens of both *C. hyointestinalis* and *C. mucosalis*. Agglutinating antibodies to *C. hyointestinalis* and *C. mucosalis* are transferred to neonatal pigs via colostrum,[5, 15, 56] but most have disappeared by the time the piglets are weaned. Seroconversion takes place at 9–13 weeks of age, when the disease might be expected, but clinical signs of the disease may not be apparent in all animals.[15]

Agglutination tests carried out on a collection of pig sera at the Veterinary Research Institute, Onderstepoort showed that most of the sera had low antibody levels against both *C. hyointestinalis* and *C. mucosalis* and/or against *C. mucosalis* only.[52]

There are a number of ways in which the causative bacteria can be demonstrated in affected tissues collected after death: silver-impregnated histology sections of the affected intestine, indirect immunofluorescence on tissue sections or smears, and culture of the organisms from affected tissue are the most suitable.

Since these organisms can only be demonstrated in macroscopically affected tissue and not in adjacent healthy tissue,[4, 16] material intended for examination for the presence of organisms should be taken only from such areas. Impression smears of intestinal mucosa at necropsy, stained with the modified Ziehl-Neelsen technique, are helpful in demonstrating the organisms in epithelial cells.

Immunofluorescent techniques are applied to cryostat sections or to smears of intestinal mucosal scrapings. Sections are treated with either *C. hyointestinalis* or *C. muco-salis* antisera.[4]

For bacterial isolation, short segments of macroscopically affected areas of the intestine are cut off without the intestine being opened, and the ends tied off with string. Specimens should be taken immediately after the death of the animal, as isolation of *Campylobacter* spp. from autolysed material is unsuccessful. The specimens should either be frozen immediately or transported on ice to the laboratory as soon as possible. The organism can easily be recovered in large numbers on ordinary media by a simple technique involving dilution of the homogenized mucosa from freshly killed cases of uncomplicated PIA.[17] Where there is damage to the mucosa, or when the animals are submitted dead for examination, selective media containing antimicrobials should be used.[17] Large numbers of organisms can be isolated from uncomplicated PIA and from cases of NE and RI, but isolation of organisms from PHE is difficult.[21] Organisms can be isolated in small numbers from the chyme or faeces of infected animals, as most organisms occur in the intestinal mucosa.[46] They may also be isolated from the gingival margins.[54] Colonies of either *C. hyointestinalis* or *C. mucosalis* appear after three to five days at 37 °C, and are then identified biochemically.

Differential diagnosis

Clinically the PIA complex may resemble many enteric, as well as some non-enteric, conditions. Porcine intestinal adenomatosis and NE may be confused with diseases causing diarrhoea or loose stools in post-weaners, such as colibacillosis, salmonellosis, swine dysentery and viral diarrhoea. Porcine haemorrhagic enteropathy may be clinically mistaken for diseases causing melaena and anaemia, such as gastric ulceration and intestinal haemorrhage syndrome (usually associated with whey feeding).

The lesions observed in the PIA complex at necropsy are fairly characteristic. Mucosal thickening in the ileum is usually obvious. In cases of NE, where the lesion may also involve the caecum and colon, the gross findings closely resemble chronic salmonellosis and swine dysentery. Mucosal thickening and severe enterorrhagia make the diagnosis of PHE relatively easy, as does the marked muscular hypertrophy of the ileum in RI. When at all possible, bacterial isolation and histopathological examination of the affected mucosa should be performed in order to confirm the diagnosis.

Control

Porcine intestinal adenomatosis complex is probably endemic in many piggeries, usually in covert form, only manifesting as sporadic outbreaks of PHE or as occasional cases of NE or RI. It is debatable whether control measures are economically justifiable for NE or RI. In a herd with an outbreak of PHE, the disease can be controlled by including antibiotics (chlortetracycline or tylosin at 100 g/ton) or furazolidone at 200 g/ton, in the ration.[24, 25, 35] Treatment of animals with clinical manifestations of PHE appears to be ineffective irrespective of the antibiotic used.[25, 35, 49, 50]

Porcine haemorrhagic enteropathy can be fairly effectively prevented in pigs introduced into an infected herd by placing them in a sty containing animals from the herd for three weeks and so exposing them to infection, and then feeding a medicated ration for several weeks.[24] The rationale is that these pigs become immune by means of controlled infection.

References

1 **BIESTER, H.E. & SCHWARTE, L.H., 1931.** Intestinal adenoma in swine. *American Journal of Pathology*, 7, 175–185.

2 **BIESTER, H.E., SCHWARTE, L.H. & EVELETH, D.F., 1939.** Studies on a rapidly developing intestinal adenoma in a pig. *American Journal of Pathology*, 15, 385–389.

3 **BOOSINGER, T.R., THACKER, H.L. & ARMSTRONG, C.H., 1985.** *Campylobacter sputorum* subsp. *mucosalis* and *C. hyointestinalis* infection in the intestine of gnotobiotic pigs. *American Journal of Veterinary Research*, 46, 2152–2156.

4 **CHANG, K., KURTZ, H.J., WARD, G.E. & GEBHART, C.J., 1984.** Immunofluorescent demonstration of *Campylobacter hyointestinalis* and *C. sputorum* subsp. *mucosalis* in swine intestines with lesions of proliferative enteritis. *American Journal of Veterinary Research*, 45, 703–710.

5 **CHANG, K., KURTZ, H.J., WARD, G.E. & GEBHART, C.J., 1984.** Campylobacter microagglutination test of swine with proliferative enteritis. *American Journal of Veterinary Research*, 45, 1373–1378.

6 **DODD, D.C., 1968.** Adenomatous intestinal hyperplasia (proliferative ileitis) of swine. *Pathologia Veterinaria*, 5, 333–341.

7 **EMSBO, P., 1951.** Terminal or regional ileitis in swine. *Nordisk Veterinaer Medicin*, 3, 1–28.

8 **FIELD, H.I., BUNTAIN, D. & JENNINGS, A.R., 1953.** Terminal or regional ileitis in pigs. *Journal of Comparative Pathology*, 63, 153–159.

9 **GEBHART, C.J., CHANG, K. & KURTZ, H.J., 1983.** *Campylobacter hyointestinalis* (new species) isolated from swine with lesions of proliferative ileitis. *American Journal of Veterinary Research*, 44, 361–367.

10 **GEBHART, C.J., EDMONDS, P., WARD, G.E., KURTZ, H.J. & BREWER, D.J., 1985.** *Campylobacter hyointestinalis* sp. nov. a new species of *Campylobacter* found in the intestines of pigs and other animals. *Journal of Clinical Microbiology*, 21, 715–720.

11 **GUNNARSSON, A., HURVELL, B., JONSSON, L., MARTINSSON, K. & REILAND, S., 1976.** Regional ileitis in pigs. Isolation of *Campylobacter* from affected ileal mucosa. *Acta Veterinaria Scandinavica*, 17, 267–269.

12 **JONSSON, L. & MARTINSSON, K., 1976.** Regional ileitis in pigs. Morphological and pathogenetical aspects. *Acta Veterinaria Scandinavica*, 17, 223–232.

13 **LANDSVERK, T. & NORDSTOGA, K., 1981.** Intestinal adenomatosis in pigs. A patho-morphological investigation. *Nordisk Veterinaer Medicin*, 36, 77–80.

14 **LAWSON, G.H.K., LEAVER, J.L., PETTIGREW, G.W. & ROWLAND, A.C., 1981.** Some features of *Campylobacter sputorum* subsp. *mucosalis* subsp. nov., nom. rev. and their taxonomic significance. *International Journal of Systematic Bacteriology*, 31, 385–391.

15 **LAWSON, G.H.K., ROBERTS, L., McCARTNEY, E., ROWLAND, A.C. & LUCKINS, A.G., 1982.** Presence of serum agglutinins to *Campylobacter sputorum* subsp. *mucosalis* in pigs. *Research in Veterinary Science*, 32, 89–94.

16 **LAWSON, G.H.K. & ROWLAND, A.C., 1974.** Intestinal adenomatosis in the pig; a bacteriological study. *Research in Veterinary Science*, 17, 331–336.

17 **LAWSON, G.H.K. & ROWLAND, A.C., 1984.** *Campylobacter sputorum* subsp. *mucosalis*. *In*: BUTZLER, J-P., (ed.) *Campylobacter Infection in Man and Animals*. Florida: CRC Press, Inc.

18 **LAWSON, G.H.K., ROWLAND, A.C. & ROBERTS, L., 1975.** Isolation of *Campylobacter sputorum* subsp. *mucosalis* from the oral cavity of pigs. *The Veterinary Record*, 97, 308.

19 **LAWSON, G.H.K., ROWLAND, A.C. & ROBERTS, L., 1976.** Studies on *Campylobacter sputorum* subsp. *mucosalis*. *Journal of Medical Microbiology*, 9, 163–171.

20 **LAWSON, G.H.K., ROWLAND, A.C. & ROBERTS, L., 1977.** The surface antigens of *Campylobacter sputorum* subsp. *mucosalis*. *Research in Veterinary Science*, 23, 378–382.

21 **LAWSON, G.H.K., ROWLAND, A.C., ROBERTS, L., FRASER, G. & McCARTNEY, E., 1979.** Proliferative haemorrhagic enteropathy. *Research in Veterinary Science*, 27, 46–51.

22 **LOMAX, L.G., GLOCK, R.D., HARRIS, D.L. & HOGAN, J.E., 1982.** Porcine proliferative enteritis: Experimentally induced disease in caesarean-derived colostrum-deprived pigs. *American Journal of Veterinary Research*, 43, 1622–1630.

23 **LOVE, D.N. & LOVE, R.J., 1979.** Pathology of proliferative haemorrhagic enteropathy in pigs. *Veterinary Pathology*, 16, 41–48.

24 **LOVE, R.J. & LOVE, D.N., 1977.** Control of proliferative haemorrhagic enteropathy in pigs. *The Veterinary Record*, 100, 473.

25 **LOVE, R.J., LOVE, D.N. & EDWARDS, M.J., 1977.** Proliferative haemorrhagic enteropathy of pigs. *The Veterinary Record*, 100, 65–68.

26 **MAPOTHER, M.E., JOENS, L.A. & GLOCK, R.D., 1987.** Investigations into the aetiology of porcine proliferative enteritis. *The Veterinary Record*, 121, 86.

27 **MAPOTHER, M.E., JOENS, L.A. & GLOCK, R.D., 1987.** Experimental reproduction of porcine proliferative enteritis. *The Veterinary Record*, 121, 533–536.

28 **MARTINSSON, K., EKMAN, L. & JONSSON, L., 1976.** Haematological and biochemical analysis of blood and serum in pigs with regional ileitis with special reference to the pathogenesis. *Acta Veterinaria Scandinavica*, 17, 233–243.

29 **McCARTNEY, E., LAWSON, G.H.K. & ROWLAND, A.C., 1984.** Behaviour of *Campylobacter sputorum* subsp. *mucosalis* in gnotobiotic pigs. *Research in Veterinary Science*, 36, 290–297.

30 **NIELSEN, S.W., 1955.** Muscular hypertrophy of the ileum in relation to 'terminal ileitis' in pigs – a preliminary report. *Journal of the American Veterinary Medical Association*, 127, 437–441.

31 **O'HARA, P.J., 1972.** Intestinal haemorrhage syndrome in the pig. *The Veterinary Record*, 91, 517–518.

32 **O'NEILL, P.A., 1970.** Observations on a haemorrhagic bowel syndrome involving pigs on three associated premises. *The Veterinary Record*, 87, 742–747.

33 **PILL, A.H., 1971.** A haemorrhagic bowel syndrome in pigs. *The Veterinary Record*, 87, 27–28.

34 **RAHKO, T. & SALONIEMI, H., 1972.** On the pathology of regional ileitis in the pig. *Nordisk Veterinaer Medicin*, 24, 132–138.

35 **REDMAN CHU, R.M. & HONG, C.B., 1973.** Haemorrhagic bowel syndrome in pigs in Taiwan. *The Veterinary Record*, 93, 562–563.

36 **ROBERTS, L., LAWSON, G.H.K. & ROWLAND, A.C., 1977.** Porcine intestinal adenomatosis associated with serologically distinct *Campylobacter sputorum* subsp. *mucosalis*. *Research in Veterinary Science*, 23, 257–258.

37 **ROBERTS, L., LAWSON, G.H.K. & ROWLAND, A.C., 1980.** The experimental infection of neonatal pigs with *Campylobacter sputorum* subsp. *mucosalis*. *Research in Veterinary Science*, 28, 145–147.

38 **ROBERTS, L., LAWSON, G.H.K. & ROWLAND, A.C., 1980.** The experimental infection of pigs with *Campylobacter sputorum* subsp. *mucosalis*. Weaned pigs, with special reference to pharmacologically mediated hypomotility. *Research in Veterinary Science*, 28, 148–150.

39 **ROBERTS, L., LAWSON, G.H.K. & ROWLAND, A.C., 1980.** Experimental infection of neonatal pigs with *Campylobacter sputorum* subsp. *mucosalis* with special reference to the oral cavity. *Veterinary Microbiology*, 5, 249–255.

40 **ROBERTS, L., LAWSON, G.H.K., ROWLAND, A.C. & LAING, A.H., 1979.** Porcine intestinal adenomatosis and its detection in a closed pig herd. *The Veterinary Record*, 104, 366–368.

41 **ROBERTS, L., ROWLAND, A.C. & LAWSON, G.H.K., 1977.** Experimental reproduction of porcine intestinal adenomatosis and necrotic enteritis. *The Veterinary Record*, 100, 12–13.

42 **ROWLAND, A.C. & HUTCHINGS, D.A., 1978.** Necrotic enteritis and regional ileitis in pigs at slaughter. *The Veterinary Record*, 103, 338–339.

43 **ROWLAND, A.C. & LAWSON, G.H.K., 1974.** Intestinal adenomatosis in the pig: Immunofluorescent and electron microscopic studies. *Research in Veterinary Science*, 17, 323–330.

44 **ROWLAND, A.C. & LAWSON, G.H.K., 1975.** Porcine intestinal adenomatosis: A possible relationship with necrotic enteritis, regional ileitis and proliferative haemorrhagic enteropathy. *The Veterinary Record*, 97, 178–180.

45 **ROWLAND, A.C. & LAWSON, G.H.K., 1975.** Intestinal adenomatosis in the pig: A possible relationship with a haemorrhagic enteropathy. *Research in Veterinary Science*, 18, 263–268.

46 **ROWLAND, A.C. & LAWSON, G.H.K., 1981.** Intestinal adenomatosis complex (porcine proliferative enteropathies). *In*: LEMAN, A.D., GLOCK, R.D. & MENGELING, W.L., (eds). *Diseases of Swine*. 5th edn. Ames, Iowa: Iowa State University Press.

47 **ROWLAND, A.C., LAWSON, G.H.K. & MAXWELL, A., 1973.** Intestinal adenomatosis in the pig: Occurrence of a bacterium in affected cells. *Nature*, 243, 417.

48 **ROWLAND, A.C., LAWSON, G.H.K. & ROBERTS, L., 1978.** Intestinal adenomatosis in the pig: Histochemical and electron microscopic studies of the mucosa. *Research in Veterinary Science*, 24, 191–199.

49 **ROWLAND, A.C. & ROWNTREE, P.G.M., 1972.** A haemorrhagic bowel syndrome associated with intestinal adenomatosis in the pig. *The Veterinary Record*, 91, 235–241.

50 **ROWNTREE, P.G.M., 1972.** A haemorrhagic bowel syndrome in the pig. *The Veterinary Record*, 91, 347–348.

51 **TAYLOR, D.J. & AL-MASHAT, R.R., 1984.** Enteric infections with catalase-positive campylobacters in cattle, sheep and pigs. *In*: BUTZLER, J-P., (ed.) *Campylobacter Infection in Man and Animals*.Boca Raton, Florida: CRC Press, Inc.

52 **VAN DER WALT, M.L., 1988.** Veterinary Research Institute, Onderstepoort, South Africa. Unpublished data.

53 **VAN DER WALT, M.L. & VAN DER LUGT, J.J., 1988.** The isolation of *Campylobacter hyointestinalis* from a pig in South Africa. *Onderstepoort Journal of Veterinary Research*, 55, 85–87.

54 **VAN DER WALT, M.L., SPENCER, B.T. & LOVEDAY, R.K., 1988.** The first isolation of *Campylobacter mucosalis* from pigs in South Africa. *Onderstepoort Journal of Veterinary Research*, 55, 165–168.

55 **WILLIAMS, M.C., 1978.** Faculty of Veterinary Science, University of Pretoria, Onderstepoort, South Africa. Unpublished data.

56 **WILSON, T.M., CHANG, K., GEBHART, C.J., KURTZ, H.J., BRAKE, T.R. & LINTNER, V., 1986.** Porcine proliferative enteritis. Serological, microbiological and pathological studies from three field epizootics. *Canadian Journal of Veterinary Research*, 50, 217–220.

57 **ZUMPT, I.F., 1979.** Regional Veterinary Laboratory, Stellenbosch, Cape Province, South Africa. Personal communication.

119

Campylobacter jejuni *infection*

M.L. van der Walt

Introduction

Campylobacter jejuni infection in cattle has been associated with enteric disease for over 50 years and was previously considered to be the cause of 'winter dysentery', a profuse watery diarrhoea of sudden onset and short duration in adult cattle.[32] It now seems that 'winter dysentery' is caused by a coronaviral infection.[44] *Campylobacter jejuni* has been isolated so frequently from the intestine of healthy animals that it is considered to be part of the normal intestinal flora. It is, however, possible that *C. jejuni*, either alone or in combination with other pathogens, may be involved in the development of a self-terminating enteritis in calves[51] and sheep,[49, 56] but its significance in such cases should be interpreted with care.

Campylobacter jejuni is also an occasional cause of mastitis[22, 23, 29, 36] and abortion[55] in cattle, of abortion in sheep,[12, 21, 57] and of abortion storms in goats[3] and blesbok (*Damaliscus dorcas*).[4]

Campylobacter jejuni is a primary enteric pathogen of humans and an important zoonosis which arises primarily from deficiencies in hygiene.

Statistics on the prevalence of *C. jejuni* infections in animals and humans in South Africa are not available, as it is not a notifiable disease. In contrast to other countries, where the organism and its effects are very prevalent in the more affluent sectors of society,[15, 45, 54] in South Africa it appears to be more prevalent in the lower socio-economic groups.

Aetiology and epidemiology

Campylobacter jejuni is micro-aerophilic and grows optimally in an atmospheric oxygen concentration of 6 per cent. The organisms are slender, spirally curved, Gram-negative rods of 0,2–0,8 µm in length. They vary in morphology and may have an increased number of spirals or may be gull-wing-shaped, while coccoid forms occur in older cultures. The bacteria are actively motile, the movement being characteristically darting or corkscrew-like. Motility is caused by polar flagella that may occur at one or both ends of the organism.[31, 48]

Strains are differentiated by serotyping, using heat-labile and heat-stable antigens,[54] phage-typing, outer membrane protein-typing[8] and restriction endonuclease digestion of DNA.[34, 39] Strains of different pathogenicity may be identified in outbreaks,[30] while serotypes also differ in pathogenicity and tropism.[21]

The organism can survive in a moist environment for several weeks at 4 °C, but it tends to die more rapidly at ambient temperatures. It survives in bovine faeces for at least 20 days at 25 °C and for eight weeks at 4 °C.[11] In cows' milk or water *C. jejuni* survives for two to five weeks when kept at 4 °C.[42, 59] The bacteria are sensitive to dehydration at room temperature,[15] while freezing drastically reduces the number of organisms on meat.[50] The organism is inactivated by iodine udder washes within eight minutes and is rapidly killed by hydrochloric acid at pH 2,3.[7] Campylobacters do not survive the temperatures of pasteurization. It requires 50 seconds at 92 °C and 40 seconds at 95,7 °C[11] for inactivation in skimmed milk and beef cubes respectively.

Campylobacter jejuni is shed in the faeces of both diarrhoeic and healthy cattle.[37, 41, 52] Faecal shedding by healthy animals is intermittent and only a few organisms are shed. There appears to be no difference in the carriage rates between healthy and diarrhoeic cattle, horses, pigs and dogs. Carriage rates do vary within a species and between animals from different sources.[40] Organisms are commonly present in the rumen of calves and less so in adult cattle. A similar situation is found on chilled carcasses, where organisms are more consistently cultured from those of calves. Isolation levels from fresh tissue are five times higher than those from frozen tissue,[50] and drastically reduced counts are seen after 40 hours of chilling. The carcasses of feedlot-fed cattle are also more likely to be contaminated than those of pasture-fed cattle.[14]

The organism is widely distributed and occurs particularly in avian species, experimental and domesticated animals including both farm animals and pets such as dogs and cats, and in humans. Food animals, especially poultry, are reservoirs of the infection, which follows consumption of untreated surface water, unpasteurized and incompletely cooked milk, and other contaminated food products such as meat.[46] Wild birds and poultry[15] constitute the main natural reservoir of infection for humans, and it appears that only about 5 per cent of the overall prevalence of this type of enteritis in humans is associated with the consumption of fresh milk.[20] Infection is contracted from milk and meat, particularly poultry carcasses[5, 38, 47] and minced meat.[13] No other dairy products act as a source of *C. jejuni*.[20]

Flies may be important in the transmission of the bacterium, particularly to humans. On poultry and pig farms, 50 and 43 per cent of *Musca domestica* contained *C. jejuni*, respectively.[43]

Pathogenesis

During a brief bacteraemia, which lasts no longer than 72 hours and develops soon after oral infection with inocula containing large numbers of *C. jejuni*, organisms are diseminated to the mesenteric lymph nodes, gastrointestinal tract, gall bladder and spleen. Disappearance of the bacteraemia coincides with the appearance of circulating antibodies.[53]

The initial colonization of the entire intestinal tract by *C. jejuni* after experimental infection changes in time, and after 96 hours bacteria persist only in the ileum, caecum and colon. Lesions in calves develop mostly in the large intestine, while in lambs they occur in the ileum.[53] This intestinal localization is associated with scouring four to five days after infection,[58] which also coincides with the development of a severe oedema and inflammatory reaction in the colon. The inflammatory reaction is characterized by a severe neutrophil infiltration, the development of microscopic ulcers, and focal goblet cell hyperplasia. The initial acute inflammatory reaction is followed by the infiltration of lymphocytes and macrophages.[9] In sheep, the onset of the gastroenteritis can be precipitated by the stress of transport and a change in diet.[49]

The enteritis appears not to be entirely due to the effect of an enterotoxin, but also to the results of invasion and cell damage and, possibly, the effect of a cytotoxin.[33, 51] The organisms colonize the mucosal surface, adhere to and invade the epithelial cells and mucosa.[27, 28] After colonization, the bacteria multiply and appear to produce toxins, including an enterotoxin which is immunologically related to cholera toxin,[24, 59] and other cytotoxic and cytolethal toxins.[17, 25] The intestinal lesions are also aggravated by bacteria which occur around small blood vessels in the lamina propria. The lesions caused in the blood vessels in the affected portions of the intestine by the bacteria include endothelial hypertrophy and an increase in the thickness of the basal lamina, and are probably also responsible for the development of oedema in the affected areas.[58]

Clinical signs

Cattle

Calves and older animals may suffer from the enteric syndrome.[2] After an incubation period of one to three days, there is a rise in temperature to 41 °C and passage of dark, mucoid or haemorrhagic faeces with a uniform consistency.[41, 52] The diarrhoea may last up to 18 days. Experimental infections are self-limiting[60] and the course of the disease is usually not longer than 20 days.[51]

Other syndromes associated with *C. jejuni* infections include abortion storms which occur during late gestation in cattle; the birth of live but weak calves,[55] and a purulent mastitis of varying degree in cattle.[29]

Sheep and goats

The morbidity in outbreaks of diarrhoea in fattening lambs may reach 30 per cent.[49] Abortions in experimentally infected ewes occur seven to 12 days after infection. In field outbreaks many ewes have a mild diarrhoea before the first abortions occur. In an outbreak up to 10 per cent or more of the ewes may abort, and weak lambs are also born.[12]

In goats, abortion may occur during late gestation. As in sheep, diarrhoea is seen in the does before or during the abortions.[3]

Pathology

Lesions in cattle suffering from the enteric syndrome occur primarily in the large intestine. Macroscopically the small intestine is flaccid and may contain a fluid ingesta, whereas the large intestine has a very fluid content containing strings of mucus and blood.[51] The mesenteric lymph nodes are consistently enlarged.[41, 52] In lambs, the ileum is more commonly affected.

Histologically *Campylobacter* is present in the mucosa at all levels of the gastrointestinal tract.[1] Bacteria occur close to the surface of the cells, sometimes in the lumen of crypts, and in the lamina propria surrounding the small blood vessels. In the ileum and the jejunum there is loss of superficial villar epithelium, stunting and fusion of villi, dilatation of crypts, thickening of the lamina propria, oedema and congestion and inflammatory cell infiltration of the mucosa,[41] and a prominent lymphoid hyperplasia.[52] Scattered crypt abscesses occur, as well as excessive mucus production.[53]

In cattle that have aborted there is a severe necrotizing placentitis and occasionally a bronchopneumonia in the foetus.[55]

Ewes that abort suffer from a severe purulent endometritis, an accompanying vasculitis, and a necropurulent placentitis. Bacterial colonies are present in the placenta.[21] Aborted foetuses have a severe purulent bronchopneumonia and multifocal hepatic necrosis.[21]

Diagnosis

A presumptive diagnosis can be based on the clinical signs but the diagnosis should be confirmed by the isolation and identification of the organism.

As *C. jejuni* is a labile organism and dies rapidly on exposure to air, heat and desiccation, and is also rapidly eliminated by putrefactive organisms, specimens should consist of fresh tissues which must be submitted in a transport medium such as Stuart's or Amies', be kept cool and moist, and reach the laboratories as soon as possible.

For successful culturing, prior filtering (pore size of 0,65 µm), the use of commercially available selective media such as Skirrow, Preston, Butzler, Blaser, Campy-BAP and others, and culturing the organisms in an atmosphere containing 6 per cent oxygen are required. Preferential growth is also obtained if the cultures are incubated at the upper range of the optimal incubation temperature of 37–42 °C.[48] After 48 hours of culturing, the colonies are typically small (2–4 mm in diameter) and low-convex with entire edges. Swarming colonies may extend along the line of incubation when moist media are used. Colonies are further identified by biotyping.[48]

The identity of organisms may also be confirmed in tissue sections by immunofluorescent or immunoperoxidase techniques,[21] and by commercial latex agglutination tests.[19] ELISA tests have also been applied successfully.[16]

When attempting the isolation of *C. jejuni* in live animals, it must be kept in mind that the bacteraemia and faecal shedding of organisms may occur sporadically[60] and that many animals are symptomless carriers. In fatal cases in cattle and sheep, organisms can be isolated from both normal and grossly inflamed intestinal mucosa.[1, 49, 52] Organisms may be isolated from the gall bladder in chronically affected animals.[51]

In abortion storms, organisms may be isolated in pure culture and in large numbers from the placenta, as well as from the organs and stomach content of aborted foetuses.[3, 4, 21, 55] Faecal cultures are of no help in the diagnosis of abortion, as in infected herds *C. jejuni* can be isolated with the same frequency from normal cows and those that have aborted, as well as from normal calves and those with diarrhoea.[55]

Milk from cows with a subclinical or mild mastitis due to infection with *C. jejuni* has an increased somatic cell count, and several strains of the bacterium, which have different drug sensitivities, may be isolated from the affected milk of different animals on the same farm.[36] Isolation of *C. jejuni* from milk is aided by the destruction of the lactoperoxidase system.[6] Different strains of the organism may be isolated from the milk and faeces of the same animal at the same time.[22] Variable numbers of organisms are excreted from affected quarters for as long as 73 days after infection.[30]

Differential diagnosis

Most cases of diarrhoea in cattle from which *C. jejuni* has been isolated in large numbers also yield other agents such as cryptosporidia, coccidia, rotavirus, coronavirus, enteropathogenic *Escherichia coli*, *Salmonella* serovars or nematodes. Clinical cases should in particular be differentiated from coccidiosis and paratyphoid.[51]

Control

No specific vaccines are available, but the ovine *C. fetus* bacterin has been used in goats and sheep with good effect.[3, 18] Multiple resistance to antibiotics is not uncommon[10, 26] but, in general, most strains appear to be susceptible to nitrofurans, gentamicin, and chloramphenicol.[19] In sheep, abortions can be controlled by daily injections of erythromycin at a dosage of 4 mg/kg followed by an intramuscular injection of long-acting oxytetracycline.[49] Orally administered chlortetracycline at a rate of 75 mg/kg per day for 14 days is also effective in controlling an outbreak of abortion.[3]

Permanent cure of intestinal infection appears to be difficult. In one report concerning the treatment of dogs with intestinal *C. jejuni* infection, both chloramphenicol and erythromycin failed to eliminate the infection, and the organism could be isolated again within nine days of discontinuing treatment.[35]

References

1 **AL-MASHAT, R.R. & TAYLOR, D.J., 1980.** Campylobacter spp. in enteric lesions in cattle. *The Veterinary Record*, 107, 31.

2 **AL-MASHAT, R.R. & TAYLOR, D.J., 1980.** Production of diarrhoea and dysentery in experimental calves by feeding pure cultures of *Campylobacter fetus* subsp. *jejuni*. *The Veterinary Record*, 107, 459.

3 **ANDERSON, K.L., HAMOUD, M.M., URBANCE, J.W., RHOADES, H.E. & BRYNER, J.H., 1983.** Isolation of *Campylobacter jejuni* from an aborted caprine fetus. *Journal of the American Veterinary Association*, 183, 90–92.

4 **ANON., 1984/1985.** Diagnostics of infertility and abortion. *Annual Report*, Veterinary Research Institute, Onderstepoort.

5 **BANFFER, J.R.J., 1985.** Biotypes and serotypes of *Campylobacter jejuni* and *Campylobacter coli* strains isolated from patients, pigs and chickens in the region of Rotterdam. *Journal of Infection*, 10, 277–281.

6 **BEUMER, R.R., CRUYSEN, J.J.M. & BIRTANTIE, I.R.K., 1988.** The occurrence of *Campylobacter jejuni* in raw cows' milk. *Journal of Applied Bacteriology*, 65, 93–96.

7 **BLASER, M.J., HARDESTY, B., POWERS, B. & WANG, W.L., 1980.** Survival of *Campylobacter fetus* subsp. *jejuni* in biological milieus. *Journal of Clinical Microbiology*, 11, 309–313.

8 **BLASER, M.J., HOPKINS, J.A., BERKA, R.M., VASIL, M.L. & WANG, W.L., 1983.** Identification and characterization of *Campylobacter jejuni* outer membrane proteins. *Infection and Immunity*, 42, 276–284.

9 **BOOSINGER, T.R. & POWE, T.A., 1988.** *Campylobacter jejuni* infections in gnotobiotic pigs. *American Journal of Veterinary Research*, 49, 456–458.

10 **BURRIDGE, R., WARREN, C. & PHILLIPS, I., 1986.** Macrolide, lincosamide and streptogramin resistance in *Campylobacter jejuni/coli*. *Journal of Antimicrobial Chemotherapy*, 17, 315–321.

11 **DEIBEL, K.E., 1985.** Study of *Campylobacter jejuni. Dissertation Abstracts International*, 46, 1812–1813.

12 **DIKER, K.S. & ISTANBULLUOGLU, E., 1986.** Ovine abortion associated with *Campylobacter jejuni. The Veterinary Record*, 118, 307.

13 **GARCIA, M.M., EAGLESOME, M.D., & RIGBY, C., 1983.** Campylobacters important in veterinary medicine. *Veterinary Bulletin*, 53, 793–818.

14 **GRAU, F.H. 1988.** *Campylobacter jejuni* and *Campylobacter hyointestinalis* in the intestinal tract and on the carcasses of calves and cattle. *Journal of Food Protection*, 51, 857–861.

15 **GRIFFITHS, P.L. & PARK, R.W.A., 1990.** Campylobacters associated with human diarrhoeal disease. *Journal of Applied Bacteriology*, 69, 281–301.

16 **GROHN, K. & GENIGEORGIS, C., 1985.** Adaption of ELISA for the detection of *Campylobacter* antibodies and its application in seroepidemiological studies in sheep and cattle herds. *Acta Veterinaria Scandinavica*, 26, 30–48.

17 **GUERRANT, R.L., WANKE, C.A., PENNIE, R.A., BARRETT, L.J. LIMA, A.A.M. & O'BRIEN, A.D., 1987.** Production of a unique cytotoxin by *Campylobacter jejuni. Infection and Immunity*, 55, 2526–2530.

18 **HANSEN, D.E., HEDSTROM, O.R., SONN, R.J., & SNYDER, S.P., 1990.** Efficacy of a vaccine to prevent *Chlamydia*- or *Campylobacter*-induced abortions in ewes. *Journal of the American Veterinary Medical Association*, 196, 731–734.

19 **HARIHARAN, H., WRIGHT, T. & LONG, J.R., 1990.** Isolation and antimicrobial susceptibility of *Campylobacter coli* and *Campylobacter jejuni* from slaughter hogs. *Microbiologica* (Italy), 13, 1–6.

20 **HARRIS, N.V., KIMBALL, T., WEISS, N.S. & NOLAN, C., 1986.** Dairy products, produce and other non-meat foods as possible sources of *Campylobacter jejuni* and *Campylobacter coli* enteritis. *Journal of Food Protection*, 49, 347–351.

21 **HEDSTROM, O.R., SONN, R.J., LASSEN, E.D., HULTGREN, B.D., CRISMAN, R.O., SMITH, B.B. & SNYDER, S.P., 1987.** Pathology of *Campylobacter jejuni* abortion in sheep. *Veterinary Pathology*, 24, 419–426.

22 **HUDSON, P.J., VOGT, R.L., BRONDUM, J., & PATTON, C.M., 1984.** Isolation of *Campylobacter jejuni* from milk during an outbreak of Campylobacteriosis. *Journal of Infectious Diseases*, 150, 789.

23 **HUTCHINSON, N.D., BOLTON, F.J., HINCHLIFFE, P.M., DAWKINS, H.C., HORSLEY, S.D., JESSOP, E.G., ROBERT SHAW, P.A. & COUNTER, D.E., 1985.** Evidence of udder excretion of *Campylobacter jejuni* as the cause of milk-borne *Campylobacter* outbreak. *Journal of Hygiene*, 94, 205–215.

24 **JOHNSON, W.M. & LIOR, H., 1986.** Cytotoxic and cytotonic factors produced by *Campylobacter jejuni, C. coli* and *C. laridis. Journal of Clinical Microbiology*, 24, 275–281.

25 **JOHNSON, W.M. & LIOR, H., 1988.** A new heat-labile cytolethal toxin (CLDT) of *Campylobacter* spp. *Microbial Pathogenesis*, 4, 115–126.

26 **KANEUCHI, C., ASHIHARA, M., SUGIYAMA, Y. & IMAIZUMI, T., 1988.** Antimicrobial susceptibility of *Campylobacter jejuni, Campylobacter coli*, and *Campylobacter laridis* from cats, dogs, pigs and seagulls. *Japanese Journal of Veterinary Science*, 50, 685–691.

27 **KONKEL, M.E., BABAKHANI, F. & JOENS, L.A., 1990.** Invasion-related antigens of *Campylobacter jejuni. Journal of Infectious Diseases*, 162, 888–895.

28 **KONKEL, M.E. & JOENS, L.A., 1989.** Adhesion to and invasion of HEp-2 cells by *Campylobacter* spp. *Infection and Immunity*, 57, 2984–2990.

29 **LANDER, K.P., 1984.** Studies on *Campylobacter jejuni* infection of the bovine udder. Phd. Thesis, London School of Hygiene and Tropical Medicine, University of London.

30 **LANDER, K.P. & BASKERVILLE, A., 1983.** *Campylobacter jejuni* mastitis in cows: Bacteriology and pathology. *Campylobacter. II. Proceedings of the Second International Workshop on Campylobacter Infections*, Brussels, 6–9 September, 1983.

31 **LANDER, K.P. & GILL, K.P.W., 1985.** Campylobacters. *In*: COLLINS, C.H. & GRANGE, J.M., (eds). *Isolation and Identification of Microorganisms of Medical and Veterinary Importance*. London: Academic Press.

32 **MACPHERSON, L.W., 1957.** Bovine virus enteritis (winter dysentery). *Canadian Journal of Comparative Medicine*, 21, 184–192.

33 **MANNINEN, K.I., PRESCOTT, J.F. & DOHOO, I.R., 1982.** Pathogenicity of *Campylobacter jejuni* isolates from animals and humans. *Infection and Immunity*, 38, 46–52.

34 **MEANGER, J.D. & MARSHALL, R.B., 1989.** Seasonal prevalence of thermophilic *Campylobacter* infections in dairy cattle and a study of infection of sheep. *New Zealand Veterinary Journal*, 37, 18–20.

35 **MONFORT, J.D., DONAHOE, J.P., STILLS, H.F. & BECH NIELSEN, S., 1990.** Efficacies of erythromycin and chloramphenicol in extinguishing fecal shedding of *Campylobacter jejuni* in dogs. *Journal of the American Veterinary Medical Association*, 196, 1069–1072.

36 **MORGAN, G., CHADWICK, P., LANDER, K.P. & GILL, K.P.W., 1985.** *Campylobacter jejuni* mastitis in a cow: A zoonosis-related incident. *The Veterinary Record*, 116, 111.

37 **MYERS, L.L., FIREHAMMER, B.D., BORDER, M.M. & SHOOP, D.S., 1984.** Prevalence of enteric pathogens in the faeces of healthy beef calves. *American Journal of Veterinary Research*, 45, 1544–1548.

38 **OOSTEROM, J., BANFFER, J.R.J., LAUWERS, S. & BUSSCHBACH, A.E., 1985.** Serotyping of, and hippurate hydrolysis by, *Campylobacter jejuni* isolates from human patients, poultry and pigs in the Netherlands. *Antonie van Leeuwenhoek*, 51, 65–70.

39 **OWEN, R.J., COSTAS, M. & DAWSON, C., 1989.** Application of different chromosomal DNA restriction digest fingerprints to specific and subspecific identification of *Campylobacter* isolates. *Journal of Clinical Microbiology*, 27, 2338–2343.

40 **PRESCOTT, J.F. & BRUIN-MOSCH, C.W., 1981.** Carriage of *Campylobacter jejuni* in healthy and diarrhoeic animals. *American Journal of Veterinary Research*, 42, 164–165.

41 **PRESCOTT, J.F. & MUNROE, D.L., 1982.** *Campylobacter jejuni* enteritis in man and domestic animals. *Journal of the American Veterinary Association*, 181, 1524–1530.

42 **REDWOOD, D.W., GILL, K.P.W. & LANDER, K.P., 1983.** The survival of *Campylobacter jejuni* in milk. *Campylobacter II. Proceedings of the Second International Workshop on Campylobacter Infections*, Brussels, 6–9 September 1983.

43 **ROSEF, O. & KAPPERUD, G., 1983.** House flies (*Musca domestica*) as possible vectors of *Campylobacter fetus* subsp. *jejuni. Applied and Environmental Microbiology*, 45, 381–383.

44 **SAIF, L.J., REDMAN, D.R., BROCK, K.V., KOHLER, E.M. & HECKERT, R.A., 1988.** Winter dysentery in adult dairy cattle: Detection of coronavirus in the faeces. *The Veterinary Record*, 123, 300–301.

45 **SALAMA, S.M. BOLTON, F.J. & HUTCHINSON, D.N., 1990.** Application of a new phagetyping scheme to campylobacters isolated during outbreaks. *Epidemiology and Infection*, 104, 405–411.

46 **SHANE, S.M. & MONTROSE, M.S., 1985.** The occurrence and significance of *Campylobacter jejuni* in man and animals. *Veterinary Research Communications*, 9, 167–198.

47 **SKIRROW, M.B., 1982.** *Campylobacter* enteritis — the first five years. *Journal of Hygiene*, 89, 175–184.

48 **SMIBERT, R.M., 1984.** *Campylobacter*. *In*: KRIEG, N.R. & HOLT, J.G., (eds). *Bergey's Manual of Systematic Bacteriology*. Vol. I. Baltimore and London: Williams & Wilkins.

49 **STANSFIELD, D.G., HUNT, B. & KEMBLE, P.R., 1986.** *Campylobacter* gastroenteritis in fattening lambs. *The Veterinary Record*, 118, 210–211.

50 **STERN, N.J., GREEN, S.S., THAKER, N., KRONT, D.J. & CHIU, J., 1984.** Recovery of *Campylobacter jejuni* from fresh and frozen meat and poultry collected at slaughter. *Journal of Food Protection*, 47, 372–374.

51 **TAYLOR, D.J., 1983.** *Campylobacter jejuni* infections in calves. *Veterinary Annual*, 23, 60–64.

52 **TAYLOR, D.J. & AL-MASHAT, R.R., 1984.** Enteric infections with catalase-positive campylobacters in cattle, sheep and pigs. *In*: BUTZLER, J-P., (ed.) *Campylobacter Infection in Man and Animals*. Florida: CRC Press.

53 **TERZOLO, H.R., LAWSON, G.H.K., ANGUS, K.W. & SNODGRASS, D.R., 1987.** Enteric *Campylobacter* infection in gnotobiotic calves and lambs. *Research in Veterinary Science*, 43, 72–77.

54 **TRESCHNAK, E., 1986.** Thermophilic *Campylobacter* species in veterinary medicine — a review. *Berliner und Münchener Tierärztliche Wochenschrift*, 99, 52–57.

55 **VAN DONKERSGOED, J., JANZEN, E., SCHUMANN, F., CLARK, E.G., ORR, J., COPELAND, S., CHIRINO-TREJO, M., BERRY, C. & SPINATO, M., 1989.** *Campylobacter jejuni* abortion in beef cattle. *Canadian Veterinary Journal*, 30, 680.

56 **VANDENBERGHE, J. & HOORENS, J., 1980.** *Campylobacter* species and regional enteritis in lambs. *Research in Veterinary Science*, 29, 390–391.

57 **VARGA, J., MEZES, B., FODOR, L. & HAJTOS, I., 1990.** Sero-groups of *Campylobacter fetus* and *Campylobacter jejuni* isolated in cases of ovine abortion. *Journal of Veterinary Medicine*, Series B, 1990, 37, 148–152.

58 **VITOVEC, J., KOUDELA, B., STERBA, J., TOMANCOVA, I., MATYAS, Z. & VLADIK, P., 1989.** The gnotobiotic piglet as a model for the pathogenesis of *Campylobacter jejuni* infection. *Zentralblatt für Bakteriologie, Mikrobiologie und Hygiene*, A., 271, 91–103.

59 **WALKER, R.I., CALDWELL, M.B., LEE, E.C., GUERRY, P., TRUST, T.J. & RUIZ-PALACIOS, G.M., 1986.** Pathophysiology of *Campylobacter* enteritis. *Microbiological Reviews*, 50, 81–94.

60 **WARNER, D.P. & BRYNER, J.H., 1984.** *Campylobacter jejuni* and *Campylobacter coli* inoculation of neonatal calves. *American Journal of Veterinary Research*, 45, 1822–1824.

GRAM-NEGATIVE AEROBIC RODS AND COCCI

Bacteria classified as Gram-negative aerobic rods and cocci are divided amongst eight families, most of which do not contain members that infect mammals. Only two of these families — Pseudomonadaceae and Neisseriaceae — contain genera that are significant in terms of diseases of livestock **(Table 1)**.

The family Pseudomonadaceae, one of the most complex groups of Gram-negative bacteria, contains bacteria that are straight or curved, and which are motile as a result of having polar flagella. The type genus is *Pseudomonas*. Differentiation between the genera in this family is difficult and requires specialized techniques which are often beyond the capabilities of most diagnostic laboratories. *Pseudomonas* is the only genus in the family that is of veterinary importance.[3] More information on the genus *Pseudomonas* is given in the ***Pseudomonas* spp. infections: Introduction**.

The family Neisseriaceae contains bacteria that are aerobic, non-motile and which may occur singly, in pairs, or in masses. They are coccal or rod-shaped, do not form endospores, and may be encapsulated. Although they are Gram-negative, they may be decolorized with difficulty, in which case they appear to be Gram-positive.[1] Three genera (*Moraxella*, *Brucella* and *Bordetella*) in this family are important to livestock; the diseases with which they are associated are listed in **Table 1**.

Bacteria of the genus *Moraxella*, many of which are avirulent or poorly pathogenic, occur on the mucous membranes of healthy humans and other warm-blooded animals. In cattle, *M. bovis* causes infectious bovine

Table 1 The most common diseases in livestock caused by bacteria belonging to the genera containing members that are classified as Gram-negative aerobic rods and cocci

BACTERIUM	DISEASE	SPECIES AFFECTED
Family: Pseudomonadaceae		
Pseumononas mallei	Glanders	Horses
Pseudomonas pseudomallei	Melioidosis	All domestic species
Pseudomonas aeruginosa	Fleece-rot and fleece discoloration	Sheep
	Mastitis	Cattle
	Endometritis	Horses
Family: Neisseriaceae		
Moraxella bovis	Infectious bovine keratoconjunctivitis	Cattle
Moraxella ovis	Infectious ophthalmia	Sheep
Moraxella equi	Keratoconjunctivitis	Horses
Moraxella osloensis	Pneumonia	Sheep and goats
	Abortions and mastitis	Cattle
Moraxella phenylpyruvica	Septicaemia	Cattle and sheep
Bordetella bronchiseptica	Atrophic rhinitis and bronchopneumonia	Pigs
Brucella abortus	Brucellosis (contagious abortion)	Cattle
Brucella ovis	Epididymitis/orchitis	Sheep
Brucella melitensis	Abortion and orchitis	Sheep and goats
Brucella suis	Abortion, stillbirth, sterility in sows, and orchitis	Pigs

keratoconjunctivitis which may occasionally be economically important. *Moraxella* infections in the other livestock species are sporadic, and in some, such as ovine infectious ophthalmia, the primary role of the bacteria as a cause of the diseases for which they are held responsible is in doubt.

Bacteria of the genus *Bordetella* are obligate parasites of humans and animals and commonly localize and multiply throughout the respiratory tract, between the cilia of the respiratory epithelial cells. Two species in this genus (particularly *B. pertussis*, the cause of whooping cough) are responsible for severe infections in humans. In livestock, *B. bronchiseptica* generally infects pigs, causing non-progressive atrophic rhinitis and progressive atrophic rhinitis, in which the infection occurs in combination with toxigenic strains of *Pasteurella multocida* types A and D. Pigs infected with *B. bronchiseptica* may remain carriers of the bacterium. *Bordetella bronchiseptica* is important in dogs as the cause of infectious tracheobronchitis (kennel cough) — either alone or in association with infection with any one of a number of epitheliotropic viruses (such as canine parainfluenza type 2, canine adenovirus 2 and canine distemper virus).[2]

Information on the genus *Brucella* is given in the ***Brucella* spp. infections: Introduction**.

References

1 **BOVRE, K., 1984.** Neisseriaceae. *In*: KRIEG, N.R. & HOLT, J.G., (eds). *Bergey's Manual of Systematic Bacteriology*. Vol. I. Baltimore, London: Williams & Wilkins.

2 **DUNGWORTH, D.L., 1993.** The respiratory system. *In*: JUBB, K.V.F., KENNEDY, P.C. & PALMER, N., (eds) *Pathology of Domestic Animals*. Vol II. 4th edn. San Diego: Academic Press, Inc.

3 **PALLERONI, N.J., 1984.** Pseudomonadaceae. *In*: KRIEG, N.R. & HOLT, J.G., (eds). *Bergey's Manual of Systematic Bacteriology*. Vol. I. Baltimore, London: Williams & Wilkins.

120

Moraxella *spp. infections*

A. van Halderen and M.M. Henton

Introduction

Of the known *Moraxella* spp., only *Moraxella bovis*, the cause of infectious bovine keratoconjunctivitis in cattle, is recognized as an important pathogen of livestock.[9] *Moraxella bovis* has also been isolated from sheep with keratoconjunctivitis on rare occasions, while *M. equi* (possibly a variant of *M. bovis*) has been isolated from horses with keratoconjunctivitis.[26] The role of *Moraxella (Branhamella, Neisseria) ovis* in infectious ophthalmia in sheep and goats is uncertain, as it has also been isolated from the conjunctiva of healthy animals.[9, 47] It has occasionally been associated with pneumonia and pleuritis in sheep and goats, and with pituitary abscesses in goats in South Africa.[24] *Moraxella osloensis* has been isolated from a lamb with pneumonia, aborted calves, and cattle with mastitis, while *M. phenylpyruvica* has been associated with septicaemia in a calf and a sheep.[9, 47]

MORAXELLA BOVIS *INFECTION*

Infectious bovine keratoconjunctivitis caused by *M. bovis* is characterized by lachrymation, conjunctivitis and keratitis.[5, 38] It has been described under a variety of names including New Forest disease, pink-eye, blight, and infectious keratitis.[38] This condition was first described as keratitis contagiosa by Billings in the USA in 1889 and has subsequently been reported throughout the world.[5, 23, 38]

Moraxella bovis is generally accepted as being the primary cause of infectious ophthalmia of cattle.[3, 6, 24, 32, 34, 38–40]

Aetiology

Moraxella bovis is a non-motile, non-sugar-fermenting, Gram-negative, short and plump diplobacillus.[43] Different strains of *M. bovis*, which vary in virulence, occur,[5, 27] but only haemolytic,[6, 33, 38–40] piliated or fimbriated[27, 38–40] strains are pathogenic. The production of certain enzymes, such as lipases and proteases,[27, 39, 40] and the presence of a dermonecrotic toxin[7, 39, 40] also play an important role in the virulence of *M. bovis*. The ability of *M. bovis* to change spontaneously from virulent to avirulent strains *in vivo* and *in vitro*[38, 43] may be the reason why many transmission experiments have been unsuccessful. Phase variation, which is a reversible genetic mechanism, controls pilus expression.[27, 32] Much confusion surrounds the description of colony morphology with regard to piliated or non-piliated strains — both kinds having been variously described as rough or smooth.[5, 27, 33, 34, 38, 43]

Epidemiology

Infectious bovine keratoconjunctivitis is highly contagious and usually occurs in epidemics; individual cases are rare.[5, 38] The prevalence in a herd may vary from 10–76 per cent[23] but although the morbidity rate is high, the mortality rate is negligible.[7] The disease is more common and usually more severe in young animals,[7, 29, 46, 48] although previously unexposed adult cattle may be affected.[48] There are definite breed differences in susceptibility — the Hereford and its crosses are most susceptible, while the *Bos indicus* breeds are least susceptible.[5, 38, 44, 48, 49] Animals with pigmented skin around the eye are more resistant to infection.

Clinically healthy carrier animals harbour the organism in the oculonasal tract,[32, 33, 37] and play an important role in maintaining the infection.[7, 29, 34, 37, 38] They may be responsible for introducing the disease into previously clean herds.[44] Transmission may be either direct, by means of droplet infection from oculonasal secretion,[31, 37] or indirect, by insect carriers such as the house fly (*Musca domestica*), face fly (*Musca autumnalis*) or stable fly (*Stomoxys calcitrans*)[5, 22, 31, 38] **(see Chapter 3: Vectors: Muscidae)**. *Moraxella bovis* has been transmitted experimentally by *Musca autumnalis*[4, 20] and by *Arcyophora longivalvis*, a moth that feeds on the ocular secretion of cattle. Other eye-frequenting Lepidoptera have also been implicated in southern Africa as possible transmitters of *M. bovis* and other microorganisms of the eyes.[12–14, 23]

Infectious ophthalmia is most prevalent during the summer months,[6, 37, 44, 48] as dust and other mechanical irritants, increased ultraviolet radiation, increased fly populations, and crowding of animals predispose to the infection,[5, 6, 10, 17, 31–33, 37, 44] while vitamin A deficiency has also been suggested as a possible predisposing factor.[5, 38] Stress such as transport may aggravate the disease,[37] as may concurrent or prior infection with other infectious agents such as *Chlamydia psittaci*, infectious bovine rhinotracheitis, parainfluenza-3, adenoviruses, and certain *Mycoplasma* spp.[1, 6, 38, 41, 42] The infection does not appear to be transmitted from cattle to sheep.[23]

Pathogenesis

Pathogenic strains of *M. bovis* have the ability to adhere to and penetrate the superficial epithelial cells of the cornea and conjunctiva. Adhesion appears to be mediated by the bacterial pili, although other 'adhesins' may also play a role.[39, 40] More bacteria adhere to the so-called 'dark' corneal epithelial cells (which contain fewer microplicae) than to the 'light' cells. Virulent *M. bovis* bacteria are cytotoxic to epithelial cells of the cornea, and invade these and the superficial stromal collagen even in the absence of prior mechanical injury.[38–40] After penetration, the bacteria are found inside the superficial epithelial cells of the cornea. This may be followed by oedema of the cornea and conjunctiva and the development of vesicles, erosions and ulcerations.[1, 29, 39, 40]

The earliest microscopic lesions develop in the bulbar conjunctiva and include oedema, hyperaemia and mononuclear cell infiltrates.[15, 29, 39, 40] In experimental cases bacteria are visible within swollen epithelial cells of the palpebral conjunctiva within one or two hours of inoculation, and may result in erosion and ulceration.[39, 40] The mechanism by which the erosions develop has not been elucidated; it has been suggested that *M. bovis* disrupts cell junctions without damaging the cells.[39, 40] The exact cytotoxic factor responsible for the damage has not been identified yet, but haemolysins, a dermonecrotic toxin, and lipase and protease enzymes have been incriminated.[7, 39, 40] No collagenase is produced.[39, 40] Pustules and erosions of varying extent develop on the nictitating membrane, palpebral conjunctiva and margins of the eyelids 10 – 72 hours after inoculation,[39, 40] and are accompanied by hyperaemia, oedema and neutrophil infiltration of the underlying lamina propria.[39, 40]

Corneal ulcers are usually smaller than 5 mm in diameter[27] and are centrally situated.[39, 40] The onset of corneal ulceration varies from one to four days after inoculation,[29, 39, 40] and in untreated cases a purulent keratitis develops.[27] When this happens, there is a neutrophil infiltration of the tissue surrounding the ulcer, the adjacent swollen epithelium and the underlying stroma.[1, 15, 39, 40]

After a week there is vascularization of the stroma extending from the limbus area.[29, 38] In uncomplicated cases the necrotic epithelium of the cornea sloughs off and healing occurs with gradual epithelialization.[29, 38]

Clinical signs and pathology

The incubation period of infectious bovine keratoconjunctivitis varies from two to three days to as long as three weeks in most natural and experimental cases.[1, 7, 16, 29] One or both eyes may be affected.[38] The first signs are lachrymation, blepharospasm and photophobia,[1, 5, 10, 15, 16, 35, 38] and conjunctivitis characterized by oedema, hyperaemia and swelling of the eyelids.[5, 35, 38] The ocular discharge is initially serous but later becomes purulent, causing the eyelids to be glued together.[5, 23, 38] The cornea is oedematous, and a whitish to yellowish-blue opaqueness, which spreads centrifugally, develops in its centre two to four days after the onset of clinical signs.[1, 5, 10, 15, 38] Corneal vascularization heralds the recovery phase,[10, 38] although in more severe cases the cornea may ulcerate.[1, 35] Complications include keratoconus, hypopyon, iridocyclitis or even lenticular enucleation.[5, 15, 38]

In most cases complete recovery of the eye (spontaneously or after treatment), with centrifugal disappearance of corneal opacity, occurs four to eight weeks after the initial clinical signs.[5, 7, 38] In severe cases permanent scarring of the cornea or even blindness may result.[5, 7, 23, 35, 38] Systemic signs are rarely encountered, although fever or decreased milk yield may accompany the infection.[7] Affected animals frequently fail to gain, or even lose, weight.[7]

Diagnosis

The provisional diagnosis of infectious ophthalmia in cattle usually presents few problems because of the explosive nature and characteristic signs of the disease. For isolation of the causative organism, ocular swabs must be taken from the cornea and conjunctiva (preferably from early, untreated cases) and appropriate methods used to culture the organism involved.[7, 15] Swabs should be submitted in a transport medium.

A diagnosis of infectious bovine keratoconjunctivitis can be confirmed by the fluorescent antibody technique, which is regarded as being more accurate and reliable than culture.[5, 33, 38] ELISA has been used to determine serum antibody titres after infection or vaccination and to distinguish between virulent or potentially virulent strains of *M. bovis*.[32, 34]

Differential diagnosis

Chemicals or foreign bodies (e.g., grass awns) sporadically cause keratoconjunctivitis in livestock. Other agents that have been incriminated as causes of infectious ophthalmia in cattle include *Chlamydia psittaci*, parainfluenza-3 and adenoviruses,[1, 5, 39, 40] *Mycoplasma bovoculi* and other *Mycoplasma* spp.,[1, 5, 6, 38–40] *Listeria monocytogenes*[5] and *Thelazia* spp. ('eyeworms').[5]

Keratoconjunctivitis also occurs in animals suffering from systemic infectious diseases such as infectious bovine rhinotracheitis, bovine virus diarrhoea and mucosal disease, bovine malignant catarrhal fever and rinderpest.

Control

When infectious ophthalmia appears in a herd it is important to separate affected animals from the rest of the herd and to keep them in a shady, dust-free area.[5, 7, 38] Although affected eyes may recover spontaneously, treatment should be initiated as soon as possible for a better therapeutic response and to reduce the risk of complications.[38, 44] Topical antibiotic therapy is the treatment of choice. Repeated treatment is usually necessary.[7, 36]

Subconjunctival administration of antibiotics is not recommended as it is very painful and irritating (especially with tetracyclines), and maintains therapeutic levels in the eye for short periods only, necessitating frequent administration.[11, 19, 38] Ointment formulations are better than aerosol or powder formulations as the latter result in increased lachrymation and are therefore washed out more rapidly.[36, 38] Many ophthalmic preparations contain benzathine cloxacillin, as therapeutic levels of this antibiotic are maintained for a long time in tear secretions.[11, 19] However, resistance of *M. bovis* to cloxacillin has been described,[3, 19, 38] as well as to streptomycin, tylosin, sulphonamides and lincomycin.[19, 38] Chloramphenicol formulations are regarded as the treatment of choice, but regulations regarding their use in food-producing animals restrict their usefulness.[38] Eye inserts and ring devices that result in the sustained release of antibiotics are under investigation.[5, 38] Bacterial culture from eye swabs and antibiograms may be necessary when selecting the most effective antibiotic.

Although the use of corticosteroids in conjunction with antibiotics[38] has been propagated, their use is generally not recommended, especially in cases with corneal ulceration. Local anaesthetics are not advised as their prolonged use may result in corneal ulceration,[38] and the administration of vitamins A, D and E is also of doubtful value.[5, 38] In complicated cases or where corneal lesions are advanced, the third eyelid may be sutured across the cornea.[5, 7]

Fly control by means of dipping, spraying animals with insecticides or the use of insecticide-impregnated ear-tags is important in the control of infectious ophthalmia.[4, 5, 20, 31]

Bacterial pili play an important role in the development of immunity to infectious bovine keratoconjunctivitis following both natural infection and vaccination with an inactivated, piliated bacterin.[5, 32] Vaccination with non-piliated bacterins does not confer immunity to challenge with *M. bovis*.[27, 32] Animals are usually immune to ocular challenge by homologous strains after natural infection or vaccination, but not to heterologous strains, although a degree of cross-immunity is reported between various strains.[5, 32, 34, 38] Serum antibodies to *M. bovis* can be detected by means of ELISA or the modified gel-diffusion precipitin test two to three weeks after infection or vaccination,[7, 27, 32] but it is still uncertain whether these are due to a general or a local immune response.[38]

An inactivated, piliated *M. bovis* bacterin vaccine is commercially available to control infectious bovine kertoconjunctivitis.[27, 32, 34] Annual revaccination is necessary.

Animals with pigmented skin around the eyes should be selected for breeding purposes.

MORAXELLA (BRANHAMELLA) OVIS *INFECTION*

In southern Africa, infectious ophthalmia, which may be caused in sheep and goats by a number of organisms, is widespread and responsible for economic losses.[2, 23] Ophthalmia is very common in these species, but the aetiology is largely unresolved.

Although *Moraxella (Branhamella) ovis* has been isolated from cases of infectious ophthalmia in sheep and goats,[10, 35] it is regarded by some authors as being of doubtful aetiological significance.[7] Recent isolates from various cases of infectious ophthalmia in sheep in South Africa yielded only *M. ovis* and *Mycoplasma* spp.[3] Attempts to reproduce the disease in lambs by using cultures of *M. ovis* obtained from these clinical cases were, however, unsuccessful.[3]

A number of other organisms have been incriminated in infectious ophthalmia in sheep and goats. *Rickettsia (Colesiota) conjunctivae* was first demonstrated in South Africa in conjunctival scrapings from sheep with infectious ophthalmia by Coles,[23] but the opinion has been expressed by some workers that it could have been *Chlamydia psittaci*.[8, 10] *Chlamydia psittaci* causes ophthalmia in various species including sheep[7, 8, 29] **(see Chapter 37: Chlamydiosis)**, and the organism can be demonstrated in conjunctival or corneal scrapings stained with Gimenez.[23] *Mycoplasma conjunctivae*, *M. arginini*, *M. agalactiae*, *M. mycoides mycoides*, and other *Mycoplasma* spp. have been incriminated as causes of infectious ophthalmia of sheep and goats. The condition has recently been experimentally reproduced in the United Kingdom and Europe, using cultures of *M. conjunctivae*.[7, 18, 25, 28, 29, 45, 46]

The general principles for the treatment and control of infectious ophthalmia in cattle also appear to apply to sheep and goats **(see *Moraxella bovis*, above)**. The intramuscular injection of long-acting oxytetracyclines has proved to be very effective in cases of infectious ophthalmia; a single injection is usually effective.[21, 30] No vaccine is available for use in sheep and goats.

References

1 **AIKMAN, J.G., ALLAN, E.M. & SELMAN, I.E., 1985.** Experimental production of infectious bovine keratoconjunctivitis. *The Veterinary Record*, 117, 234–239.

2 **ANON., 1979–86.** Annual Reports of the Directorate of Veterinary Services, South Africa.

3 **ANON., 1985.** Regional Veterinary Laboratory, Stellenbosch, South Africa. Unpublished data.

4 **ARENDS, J.J., WRIGHT, R.E., BARTO, P.B. & LUSBY, K.S., 1984.** Transmission of *Moraxella bovis* from blood agar cultures to Hereford cattle by face flies (Diptera: Muscidae). *Journal of Economic Entomology*, 77, 394–398.

5 **BAPTISTA, P.J.H.P., 1979.** Infectious bovine keratoconjunctivitis. A review. *British Veterinary Journal*, 135, 225–242.

6 **BARBER, D.M.L., JONES, G.E. & WOOD, A., 1986.** Microbial flora of the eyes of cattle. *The Veterinary Record*, 118, 204–206.

7 **BLOOD, D.C., RADOSTITS, O.M. & HENDERSON, J.A., 1983.** *Veterinary Medicine/Small Animal Clinician.* 6th edn. London: Baillière Tindall.

8 **BOGAARD, A.E.J.M. (Jr), 1984.** Inclusion keratoconjunctivitis ('pink-eye') in sheep. A proposal for a new name for chlamydial keratoconjunctivitis in sheep and comment on recent clinical trials. *The Veterinary Quarterly*, 6, 229–235.

9 **BOVRE, K., 1984.** Moraxella. *In*: KRIEG, N.R. & HOLT, J.G., (eds) *Bergey's Manual of Systematic Bacteriology.* Vol. I. Baltimore: Williams and Wilkins.

10 **BULGIN, M.S. & DUBOSE, D.A., 1982.** Pink-eye associated with *Branhamella ovis* infection in dairy goats. *Veterinary Medicine/Small Animal Clinician*, 77, 1791–1793.

11 **BUSWELL, J.F. & HEWETT, G.R., 1983.** Single topical treatment for bovine keratoconjunctivitis using benzathine cloxacillin. *The Veterinary Record*, 113, 621–622.

12 **BÜTTIKER, W., 1973.** Further records of eye-frequenting Noctuidae (Lepidoptera) from South Africa. *South African Journal of Science*, 69, 337–341.

13 **BÜTTIKER, W. & BEZUIDENHOUT, J.D., 1974.** First records of eye-frequenting Lepidoptera from South West Africa. *Journal of the Entomological Society of Southern Africa*, 37, 73–78.

14 **BÜTTIKER, W. & WHELLAN, J.A., 1966.** Records of eye-frequenting moths from Rhodesia. Bulletin 2306. Reprinted from March/April 1966 issue of the *Rhodesia Agricultural Journal*, Ministry of Agriculture, Government Printer, Salisbury, 1–4.

15 **CHANDLER, R.L., TURFREY, B.A. & SMITH, K., 1983.** Laboratory model for infectious bovine keratoconjunctivitis: The pathogenicity of different strains of *Moraxella bovis*, pathology and ultrastructure observations. *Research in Veterinary Science*, 35, 277–284.

16 **CHANDLER, R.L., TURFREY, B., SMITH, K. & GOURLAY, R.N., 1980.** Virulence of *Moraxella bovis* in gnotobiotic calves. *The Veterinary Record*, 106, 364–365.

17 **COX, P.J., LIDDELL, J.S. & MATTINSON, A.D., 1984.** Infectious bovine keratoconjunctivitis: Isolation of *Moraxella bovis* from two groups of young beef cattle in fly-control field trials during 1981. *The Veterinary Record*, 115, 29–32.

18 **EGWU, G.O., FAULL, W.B., BRADBURY, J.M. & CLARKSON, M.J., 1989.** Ovine infectious keratoconjunctivitis: A microbiological study of clinically unaffected and affected sheep's eyes with special reference to *Mycoplasma conjunctivae*. *The Veterinary Record*, 125, 253–256.

19 **GEORGE, L.W., WILSON, W.D., BAGGOT, J.D. & MIHALYI, J.E., 1984.** Antibiotic treatment of *Moraxella bovis* infection in cattle. *Journal of the American Veterinary Medical Association*, 185, 1206–1209.

20 **GLASS, H.W. (Jr), & GERHARDT, R.R., 1984.** Transmission of *Moraxella bovis* by regurgitation from the crop of the face fly (Diptera: Muscidae). *Journal of Economic Entomology*, 77, 399–401.

21 **GREIG, A., 1989.** Ovine keratoconjunctivitis. *In Practice*, 11, 110–113.

22 **HALL, R.D., 1984.** Relationship of the face fly (Diptera: Muscidae) to pink-eye in cattle: A review and synthesis of the relevant literature. *Journal of Medical Entomology*, 21, 361–365.

23 **HENNING, M.W., 1956.** *Animal Diseases in South Africa*, 3rd edn. Pretoria: Central News Agency.

24 **HENTON, M.M., 1988.** Veterinary Research Institute, Onderstepoort. Personal communication.

25 **HOSIE, B.D., 1988.** Keratoconjunctivitis in a hil1-sheep flock. *The Veterinary Record*, 122, 40–43.

26 **HUGHES, D.E. & PUGH, G.W. (Jr), 1970.** Isolation and description of a *Moraxella* from horses with conjunctivitis. *American Journal of Veterinary Research*, 31, 451–462.

27 **JAYAPPA, H.G. & LEHR, C., 1986.** Pathogenicity and immunogenicity of piliated and nonpiliated phases of *Moraxella bovis* in calves. *American Journal of Veterinary Research*, 47, 2217–2221.

28 **JONES, G.E., 1983.** Mycoplasmas of sheep and goats: A synopsis. *The Veterinary Record*, 113, 619–620.

29 **JUBB, K.V.F., KENNEDY, P.C. & PALMER, N., 1985.** *Pathology of Domestic Animals.* 3rd edn. Orlando: Academic Press.

30 **KÖNIG. C.D.W., 1983.** 'Pink-eye' or 'zere oogjes' or keratoconjunctivitis infectiosa ovis (KIO). Clinical efficacy of a number of antimicrobial therapies. *The Veterinary Quarterly*, 5, 122–127.

31 **KOPECKY, K.E., PUGH, G.W. (Jr) & McDONALD, T.J., 1986.** Infectious bovine keratoconjunctivitis — contact transmission. *American Journal of Veterinary Research*, 47, 622–624.

32 **LEHR, C., JAYAPPA, H.G., GOODNOW, R.A., 1985.** Controlling bovine keratoconjunctivitis with a piliated *Moraxella bovis* bacterin. *Veterinary Medicine/Small Animal Clinician*, 80, 96–100.

33 **LEPPER, A.W.D. & BARTON, I.J., 1987.** Infectious bovine keratoconjunctivitis — seasonal variation in cultural, biochemical and immunoreactive properties of *Moraxella bovis* isolated from the eyes of cattle. *Australian Veterinary Journal*, 64, 33–39.

34 **LEPPER, A.W.D. & HERMANS, L.R., 1986.** Characterisation and quantitation of pilus antigens of *Moraxella bovis* by ELISA. *Australian Veterinary Journal*, 63, 401–405.

35 **OSUAGWUH, A.I.A. & AKPOKODJE, J.W., 1979.** Infectious keratoconjunctivitis in sheep and goats in Nigeria. *The Veterinary Record*, 105, 125–126.

36 **PIERCY, B.W.T., 1985.** Factors influencing the penetration of therapeutic substances in the eye following topical application. *The Veterinary Record*, 116, 99–104.

37 **PUGH, G.W. (Jr), & McDONALD, T.J., 1986.** Identification of bovine carriers of *Moraxella bovis* by comparative cultural examinations of ocular and nasal secretions. *American Journal of Veterinary Research*, 47, 2343–2345.

38 **PUNCH, P.I. & SLATTER, D.H., 1984.** A review of infectious bovine keratoconjunctivitis. *Veterinary Bulletin*, 54, 193–207.

39 **ROGERS, D.G., CHEVILLE, N.F. & PUGH, G.W. (Jr), 1987.** Pathogenesis of corneal lesions caused by *Moraxella bovis* in gnotobiotic calves. *Veterinary Pathology*, 24, 287–295.

40 **ROGERS, D.G., CHEVILLE, N.F. & PUGH, G.W. (Jr), 1987.** Conjunctival lesions caused by *Moraxella bovis* in gnotobiotic calves. *Veterinary Pathology*, 24, 554–559.

41 **ROSENBUSCH, R.F., 1983.** Influence of *Mycoplasma* preinfection on the expression of *Moraxella bovis* pathogenicity. *American Journal of Veterinary Research*, 44, 1621–1624.

42 **ROSENBUSCH, R.F. & OSTLE, A.G., 1986.** *Mycoplasma bovoculi* infection increases ocular colonisation by *Moraxella bovis* in calves. *American Journal of Veterinary Research*, 47, 1214–1216.

43 **SCHURIG, G.G., LIGHTFOOT, D.R., TROUTT, H.F. & FINKLER, B.I., 1984.** Genotypic, phenotypic and biological characteristics of *Moraxella bovis*. *American Journal of Veterinary Research*, 45, 35–39.

44 **SINCLAIR, J.A., COOPER, B.S. & STEFFERT, I.J., 1986.** A survey of infectious bovine keratoconjunctivitis in the Gisborne and Hunterville regions of New Zealand. *New Zealand Veterinary Journal*, 34, 121–125.

45 **TER LAAK, E.A., SCHREUDER, B.E.C., KIMMAN, T.G. & HOUWERS, D.J., 1988.** Ovine keratoconjunctivitis experimentally induced by instillation of *Mycoplasma conjunctivae*. *The Veterinary Quarterly*, 10, 217–224.

46 **TER LAAK, E.A., SCHREUDER, B.E.C. & SMITH-BUYS, C.M.C., 1988.** The occurrence of *Mycoplasma conjunctivae* in the Netherlands and its associations with infectious keratoconjunctivitis in sheep and goats. *The Veterinary Quarterly*, 10, 73–83.

47 **VEDROS, N.S., 1984.** Neisseria. *In:* KRIEG, N.R. & HOLT, J.G., (eds) *Bergey's Manual of Systematic Bacteriology*. Vol. I. Baltimore: Williams and Wilkins.

48 **WEBBER, J.J. & SELBY, L.A., 1981.** Risk factors related to the prevalence of infectious bovine keratoconjunctivitis. *Journal of the American Veterinary Medical Association*, 179, 823–826.

49 **WILCOX, G.E., 1970.** Bacterial flora of the bovine eye with special reference to the *Moraxella* and *Neisseria*. *Australian Veterinary Journal*, 46, 253–257.

121

Bordetella bronchiseptica *infections (including atrophic rhinitis)*

Synonyms: Bordetellosis

P. Botha

Introduction

Infection with toxigenic strains of *Bordetella bronchiseptica* in pigs causes non-progressive atrophic rhinitis and, less commonly, bronchopneumonia in piglets three to four days old. Non-progressive atrophic rhinitis affects piglets aged up to about six weeks, and is characterized by distortion of the ventral scrolls of the ventral turbinates and nasal septum in particular, but without significant growth retardation of affected piglets. Lesions that develop during early life usually persist into adulthood.

Infection of the nasal cavity of piglets with toxigenic strains of *Pasteurella multocida* type A or D, either on their own or mixed with *B. bronchiseptica*, causes progressive atrophic rhinitis mainly in pigs 13–17 weeks of age, but younger and older pigs may also be affected. It is a more severe condition than non-progressive atrophic rhinitis, and is characterized by severe atrophy of the turbinate scrolls and by defects of the septum of the nasal cavity which may be accompanied by deformities of the snout and facial bones and growth retardation in affected animals.[1, 7, 9, 10, 13, 14, 38, 39]

From snout-cut examinations done at different abattoirs, and from bacterial isolations performed from nasal swabs collected in the Transvaal and Natal, it appears that non-progressive atrophic rhinitis is widespread in most intensive pig herds but that it is uncommon in extensively raised pigs in these provinces.[4, 29] This condition is probably also widespread in other parts of South Africa and in other countries in the subcontinent. It is a mild disease and does not seem to be of economic importance.

Progressive atrophic rhinitis occurs in most intensive pig-rearing countries of the world[10, 35] and is also widespread in South Africa. It has been confirmed in various herds in the Transvaal and Natal, while clinical findings indicate that it also occurs in the other provinces. It is of economic importance because it usually results in significant growth retardation in affected pigs.

Aetiology and epidemiology

Bordetella bronchiseptica is a small, motile, Gram-negative, bipolar-staining rod or coccobacillus belonging to the Enterobacteriaceae. It is an aerobic bacterium which grows rapidly on ordinary media such as blood or MacConkey agar and contains a heat-stable somatic O antigen and a common heat-labile agglutinogen. Toxigenic strains of *B. bronchiseptica* produce a heat-labile, dermonecrotic toxin.[43]

For information on the morphology, cultural characteristics and virulence factors of *P. multocida* consult the ***Pasteurella* spp. infections: Introduction**. Toxigenic strains of *P. multocida* types A and D produce an endotoxin which is heat-labile and necrotoxic when applied to the skin of guinea-pigs.[10, 33] This is referred to as the dermonecrotic toxin, and is cytotoxic to bovine embryo lung (EBL) cell cultures[40]—an effect which is used to identify toxigenic strains of *P. multocida*. It is lethal when administered parenterally at high dosage levels to piglets and mice.[7, 10] The dermonecrotic toxin causes progressive atrophic rhinitis when injected intraperitoneally or when administered intranasally to piglets.[7]

Bordetella bronchiseptica is widespread in pig populations throughout the world. It is an obligate parasite of the upper respiratory tract of pigs, dogs and rodents. Most isolates obtained from species other than pigs appear to be of low pathogenicity for pigs. *Pasteurella multocida* can be isolated from a wide range of animal species and is known to cause disease in most livestock species and poultry. *Pasteurella multocida* colonizes the tonsils, while both non-toxigenic and toxigenic type A strains can be isolated from the lungs of pigs with pneumonia. Toxigenic and non-toxigenic type D strains are more frequently isolated from the nose and less often from the lungs than type A strains.[15] Mixed infections of *P. multocida* and *B. bronchiseptica* can occur in the same pig.

The outcome of *B. bronchiseptica* infection in piglets is determined by the age and immunity of the animals and the number of organisms they are exposed to. Colostral immunity is important in protecting piglets against infection. Non-immune piglets aged between three and six weeks are the most susceptible to infection, as the bacteria adhere easily to the nasal epithelium at that age.[19] The most severe turbinate lesions occur when non-immune piglets become infected during the first week of life; piglets that are exposed to *B. bronchiseptica* after this age show mild or virtually no lesions.

Transmission of *B. bronchiseptica* and *P. multocida* between pigs is usually via aerosols following sneezing and snout contact.[24, 42, 43] Introduction of pigs that are carriers of *B. bronchiseptica* and *P. multocida* into a susceptible population is important in the spread of the infections.[43] Sows would seem to be the main source of infection for their piglets. Once they become infected, infection spreads horizontally between piglets in the same litter as well as between litters—particularly at weaning, when they are regrouped. Factors which promote the spread of *B. bronchiseptica* and *P. multocida* infections amongst piglets include high population density in pens, poor hygiene and ventilation, and mixing of piglets of different litters.[43] Infections may be subclinical. Piglets affected with progressive atrophic rhinitis may show clinical signs at four weeks of age, but evidence of the disease is most commonly seen in the young growing group of pigs when they are 13–17 weeks of age, and more rarely at 17–21 weeks.

Pathogenesis

After inhalation, *B. bronchiseptica* colonizes the ciliated respiratory epithelium of the nasal cavity and produces dermonecrotic toxin which is thought to play an important role in the production of the turbinate lesions of non-progressive atrophic rhinitis of pigs.[6, 11, 18, 30, 31]

If the toxigenic strains of *P. multocida* are to exert their pathogenic effects, they must colonize the nasal epithelium in large numbers and for prolonged periods.[9, 33] Infection of the nasal epithelium with *B. bronchiseptica* results in damage to the cilia of the epithelium cells, allowing toxigenic strains of *P. multocida* to colonize and multiply to high numbers.[9, 13, 33] Damage caused to the respiratory epithelium by agents such as ammonia and dust particles may also play a role in lowering the resistance of the nasal epithelium to invasion and colonization by *P. multocida*. Low concentrations of acetic acid have been used experimentally to enhance the growth of toxigenic *P. multocida* on the nasal epithelium and to induce progressive atrophic rhinitis.[10, 34]

In the nasal cavity, the dermonecrotic toxin of *P. multocida* not only stimulates the proliferation of osteoclasts that results in the resorption of bone in the nasal septum (and sometimes also of some of the facial bones), but it also gives rise to the uncontrolled proliferation of undifferentiated mesenchymal cells and inhibits the differentiation of these cells to osteoblasts, resulting in a reduction in the number and function of osteoblasts. These changes culminate in the defects in the turbinates, nasal septum and snout that are so characteristic of progressive atrophic rhinitis.[10, 32, 34, 37, 41]

Clinical signs and pathology

Sneezing and snuffling are the most common signs in young piglets during the early stages of infection with non-progressive atrophic rhinitis. Tear-staining of the hair and skin below the medial canthus of the eyes may also be evident in some of the affected piglets because of obstruction of the lachrymal ducts by exudate and/or defects in the ducts. Feed intake, growth rate and carcass quality are not noticeably affected, and externally visible snout deformities are not a feature of non-progressive atrophic rhinitis as only the scrolls of the turbinates and the nasal septum, and not the facial bones, are affected. Varying degrees of turbinate involvement may be present. The ventral scrolls of the ventral turbinates are most commonly affected in animals that are mildly to moderately affected.[24] In more severe cases there is also involvement of the dorsal scrolls of the ventral turbinates and the dorsal and ethmoid turbinates. The lesions during the early stages of infection comprise catarrhal rhinitis, severe congestion of the nasal mucosa and sloughing of parts of the epithelium. These lesions are followed by atrophy and bizarre distortion of the form and shape of the turbinates as a result of the changes in the bony tissue and attempts at regrowth. Large cavities develop particularly in the ventral scrolls. In some cases the nasal septum is thickened and deviated to one side. Secondary bacterial infections may exacerbate the lesions and result in a mucopurulent rhinitis.

The bronchopneumonic syndrome caused by *B. bronchiseptica* is uncommon and occurs mainly in piglets three to four days old. It is characterized by fever, anorexia, coughing, dyspnoea and reduced weight gain or weight loss. The morbidity and mortality rates in litters may be high. The lung lesions occur primarily in the cranial and middle lobes and are characteristic of those of an acute to chronic catarrhal to mucopurulent bronchopneumonia. Secondary infection by other bacteria, such as *P. multocida*, may exacerbate the pneumonic lesions. *Bordetella bronchiseptica* is often a secondary opportunist in pneumonic lesions in older pigs caused by other infectious agents **(see Chapter 188: Porcine respiratory disease)**.

Sneezing is a common sign in piglets suffering from progressive atrophic rhinitis and usually precedes the development of deformities of the snout. A catarrhal to mucopurulent nasal discharge is frequent in animals that are sneezing, and they may shake their heads in attempts to rid themselves of the discharge. Some show epistaxis which can be exacerbated by swabbing of the nasal cavity. Affected pigs may develop varying degrees of deviation of the snout: it is deviated to the side with the most severe turbinate lesions **(Figure 121.1)**. Shortening of the upper jaw (*brachygnathia superior*) as a result of growth depression of the nasal and maxillary bones gives the face a 'pushed-up' appearance which results in the development of skin folds over the dorsum of the shortened snout **(Figure 121.1)**. Snout deformities develop late

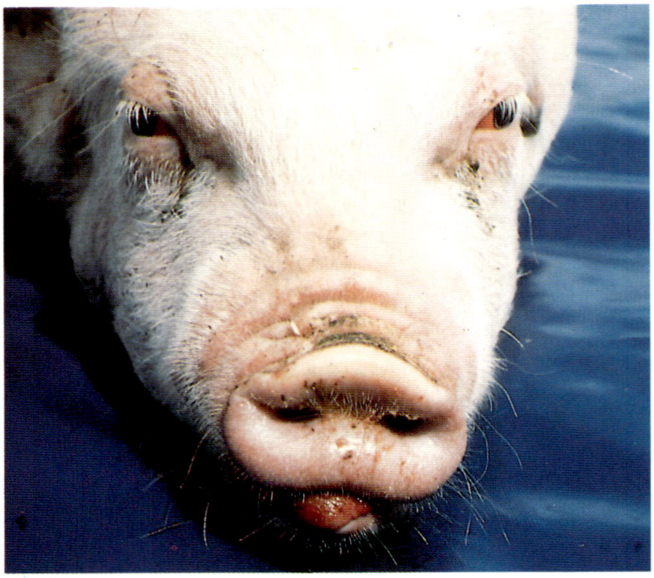

Figure 121.1 Progressive atrophic rhinitis. Note deviation of the snout, skin folds over dorsum of the snout and tear-staining below the medial canthus of the eye

in the course of the disease and may or may not be associated with growth retardation. Dirty streaks on the skin ventral to the medial canthi of the eyes are caused by dried tears and dust adhering to tears running down the skin of the face as a result of occlusion of the nasolachrymal ducts due to inflammatory exudate or deformities of the facial bones **(Figure 121.1)**. Pneumonia caused by *P. multocida* may occasionally occur in pigs suffering from progressive atrophic rhinitis, as a result of the lack of protection provided by healthy turbinates.[20] Although the morbidity rate may be 20–40 per cent in a herd, the mortality rate as a result of progressive atrophic rhinitis is negligible. Severely affected pigs show a reduction of up to 30 per cent in average daily weight gain and some may be stunted.

Pigs affected by progressive atrophic rhinitis have similar but more severe lesions of the turbinates and the nasal septum **(Figure 121.2)** than pigs suffering from non-progressive atrophic rhinitis. Some of the facial and snout bones, such as the nasal bones, maxillae and premaxillae, may also be deformed.[1] The lesions vary in extent. In mildly affected pigs, only the ventral scrolls of the ventral turbinates may be atrophic. In severe cases both scrolls of the ventral turbinates, as well as the dorsal and ethmoid turbinates, may show varying degrees of atrophy or may even be absent, and the nasal septum is deviated to one side or the other. The facial bones and those of the snout may also manifest some degree of atrophy. Histopathological changes include degeneration of osteoblasts, reduced numbers of osteoblasts, proliferation of osteoclasts, reduction of osseous tissue and cartilage, and disorderly proliferation of undifferentiated mesenchymal cells.[10, 19, 32, 34]

Diagnosis and differential diagnosis

A diagnosis of either non-progressive or progressive atrophic rhinitis is based on the clinical findings (particularly snuffling and sneezing and tear-staining ventral to the medial canthi of the eyes), bacterial culture of nasal and tonsillar swabs, and examination of the turbinates at abattoirs for the presence of lesions.[8, 17, 25, 43] The nasal cavity and turbinates are best exposed by transverse section of the snout at the level of the first to second upper premolar teeth. The lesions may be scored according to severity. To make a herd diagnosis, as many pigs as possible should be examined after slaughter for the presence

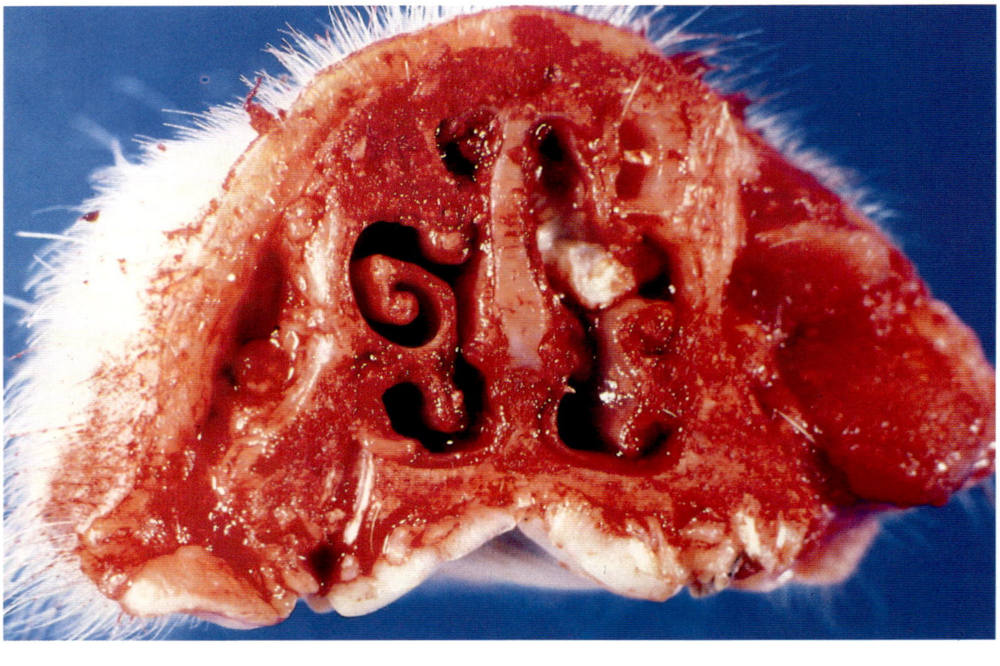

Figure 121.2 Progressive atrophic rhinitis. Note atrophy and distortion of the turbinates

of lesions, at intervals of about three to six months. The lesions of non-progressive atrophic rhinitis are very similar, but are usually milder than those present in pigs suffering from progressive atrophic rhinitis. The diagnosis may be further complicated as these two conditions often occur together in a herd. Differentiation between non-progressive and progressive atrophic rhinitis is problematic. Except for tear-staining and sneezing, non-progressive atrophic rhinitis is usually clinically inapparent in affected pigs because of the lack of snout deformities. On the other hand, progressive atrophic rhinitis can be diagnosed clinically in many affected animals as snout deformities and growth retardation are often prominent signs. On snout-cut examinations, non-progressive and progressive atrophic rhinitis are indistinguishable in pigs affected by low-scoring or mild lesions. If pigs in a herd are suffering from progressive atrophic rhinitis, some animals will exhibit higher-scoring or severe lesions.

An ELISA[21] can be applied for the detection of antibodies against the dermonecrotic toxin of *P. multocida* strains, especially in cases where isolation of the bacterium is unsuccessful.[7]

Other causes of sneezing, such as excessive dust in the environment and inclusion body rhinitis, should be considered as differential diagnoses. Clinically visible snout deformities of single pigs in a herd may be due to injury at a young age, infection of the tooth canal after clipping of teeth, and other infections of the snout, such as 'bull nose' which is caused by *Fusobacterium necrophorum*, or *Borrelia* spp.

Pigs of the Large White, Yorkshire and Duroc breeds seem to be more susceptible to progressive atrophic rhinitis than the Landrace breeds. Some Large White lines may show hereditary facial deformities which resemble progressive atrophic rhinitis. These pigs have deeply concave-shaped faces and shortened snouts, which give their faces a shrunken appearance. The snouts are not deviated laterally, as is often the case with progressive atrophic rhinitis, but some pigs may show a twist along the longitudinal axis.[4, 15]

The bronchopneumonic syndrome caused by *B. bronchiseptica* in pigs should not be confused with other causes of pneumonia, such as *P. multocida* and *Actinobacillus pleuropneumoniae* **(see Chapter 188: Porcine respiratory disease)**. Appropriate specimens of affected parts of the lungs should be cultured to establish a specific diagnosis.

Control

Measures to control progressive and non-progressive atrophic rhinitis in infected herds are aimed at reducing the prevalence of toxigenic strains of *B. bronchiseptica* and *P. multocida* types A and D by vaccination of the sows, and the provision of medicated feed and antimicrobial treatment of piglets. Pigs with an acute rhinitis should be treated to prevent growth impairment. Attention should be given to ensure good ventilation, hygiene and management and to prevent other predisposing factors, such as overcrowding and the mixing of pigs of different age groups.[15]

Bordetella bronchiseptica is susceptible to a wide range of antimicrobial drugs, including tetracyclines, cloxacillin, amoxycillin, streptomycin, erythromycin, sulphonamides and trimethoprim-potentiated sulphonamides.[43] Parenteral treatment by intramuscular injection is most effective for the treatment of individual animals suffering from non-progressive atrophic rhinitis or bronchopneumonia, but when large numbers of pigs are affected, feed or water medication at recommended therapeutic levels for three to six weeks is indicated.

The toxigenic strains of *P. multocida* types A and D that are involved in the aetiology of progressive atrophic rhinitis are highly sensitive to penicillin, ampicillin, amoxycillin, cephalexin, chloramphenicol, kanamycin, gentamicin and nitrofurans, but limited resistance to erythromycin, polymixin B, cotrimoxazole, neomycin and oxytetracyclines, and high resistance to lincomycin, streptomycin, oxacillin, spiramycin, sulphonamides and tylosin have been reported.[12]

Vaccines which contain bacterins of *B. bronchiseptica* and toxigenic strains of *P. multocida* as well as a formaldehyde-inactivated toxin (toxoid) of *P. multocida* are effective in the control of progressive and non-progressive atrophic rhinitis.[16, 23, 36, 44] The use of a genetically-engineered vaccine (Protech AR)[34] containing a single antigen of *P. multocida* (the so-called dO-protein) also gives good protection against progressive atrophic rhinitis.[3]

Two types of vaccines are available in South Africa:

- Nobivac-ART (Intervet), containing a *B. bronchiseptica* bacterin and a *P. multocida* toxoid; and
- Rhiniffa T (Rhône-Poulenc), containing bacterins of both *B. bronchiseptica* and *P. multocida* and a toxoid of *P. multocida*.

In order to protect piglets against progressive atrophic rhinitis it is recommended that pregnant sows be vaccinated with a *P. multocida* toxoid-containing vaccine six weeks and two weeks prior to farrowing in order to ensure the presence of high levels of antibodies in the colostrum.[2, 5, 36, 44] Only one vaccination is necessary two to four weeks before farrowing during subsequent pregnancies. Piglets born to vaccinated sows have a colostral immunity which protects them until the age of three to four weeks, but it does interfere with their response to vaccination. Vaccination of piglets born to unvaccinated sows affords good protection against clinical disease.[23]

A combined control regimen involving the vaccination and antimicrobial therapy of sows prior to farrowing and of post-weaning piglets has drastically reduced the prevalence of progressive atrophic rhinitis in herds in the Transvaal and Natal.[4] In addition to vaccination, antimicrobial treatment of sows after they have entered the farrowing crates protects piglets from being infected by their dams. This is generally achieved by the in-feed administration of an antimicrobial such as oxytetracycline for the last five days of pregnancy. This therapy, when extended to include in-feed medication of piglets for 28 days after weaning with a chlortetracycline-sulphonamide combination, is effective in reducing the clinical effects of the disease.[4]

A 'medicated-early-weaning' scheme, in which piglets are weaned at seven to ten days of age and various systemic or in-feed antimicrobial treatment regimes are used, is effective in controlling progressive atrophic rhinitis but it has the disadvantage that considerable economic losses are encountered because of the early weaning of piglets.[23]

It is essential that control programmes for progressive atrophic rhinitis be monitored by regularly assessing (at three- to six-monthly intervals) the prevalence of disease, clinical observation, using bacteriological examinations of nasal swabs for toxigenic *P. multocida* type A and D, and by 'snout scoring' at slaughter.[22, 26–28]

If new introductions must be made into commercial or breeding units, they should be quarantined for at least one month. During this time the new pigs should be given a full course of antimicrobial therapy in an attempt to eliminate any toxigenic *P. multocida* which they may be carrying.

References

1 **ANON., 1978.** Ministry of Agriculture, Fisheries and Food. Booklet LPD51, Pinner, UK. General indication of the composition of each grade.

2 **BAARS, J.C., PENNINGS, A. & STORM, P.K., 1986.** Challenge and field experiments with an experimental atrophic rhinitis vaccine containing *P. multocida* DNF-toxoid and *B. bronchiseptica*. *Proceedings of the Ninth Congress of the International Pig Veterinary Society.*

3 **BORDING, A, NYMARK, K., SMIDT, E. & HJALAGER, B., 1992.** Field studies with a new, genetically engineered vaccine against progressive atrophic rhinitis. *Proceedings of the Twelfth Congress of the International Pig Veterinary Society*, 179.

4 **BOTHA, P.D., 1993.** The Charles Street Veterinary Group, P.O. Box 95315, Waterkloof 0145, Pretoria. Unpublished data.

5 **BREUER, J. & SCHMIELPFENNIG, H., 1991.** Skin testing for *P. multocida* antitoxic antibodies in breeding herds. *Proceedings of the Eleventh Congress of the International Pig Veterinary Society*, 51.

6 **BYRD, D., ROOP, R.M., VEIT, H., HEWLETT, E., SCHRIG, G. & KORNEGAY, E., 1987.** Serum sensitivity of four strains of *Bordetella bronchiseptica* with defined virulence for neonate swine. *Abstracts of the Annual Meeting of the American Society for Microbiology*, 87, 39.

7 **CHANTER, N., 1990.** Advances in atrophic rhinitis and toxigenic *Pasteurella multocida* research. *Pig News and Information*, 11, 503–506.

8 **CHANTER, N., GOODWIN, R.F.W. & RUTTER, J.M., 1989.** Comparison of methods for the sampling and isolation of toxigenic *Pasteurella multocida* from the nasal cavity of pigs. *Research in Veterinary Science*, 47, 355–358.

9 **CHANTER, N., MAGYAR, T. & RUTTER, J.M., 1989.** Interactions between *Bordetella bronchiseptica* and toxigenic *Pasteurella multocida* in atrophic rhinitis of pigs. *Research in Veterinary Science*, 47, 48–53.

10 **CHANTER, N. & RUTTER, J.M., 1988.** *Pasteurella and Pasteurellosis*. San Diego, New York: Academic Press, Inc.

11 **CHUNG, W.B., COLLINS, M.T. & BÄCKSTROM, L.R., 1990.** Adherence of *Bordetella bronchiseptica* and *Pasteurella multocida* to swine nasal ciliated epithelial cells *in vitro*. *Acta Pathologica, Microbiologica et Immunologica Scandinavica*, 98, 453–461.

12 **CORBOZ, L., BUERGI, E., GRUBER, H. & GYSLING, P., 1992.** *Proceedings of the Twelfth Congress of the International Pig Veterinary Society*, 181.

13 **COWART, R.P., BÄCKSTRÖM, S. & BRIN, T.A., 1989.** *Pasteurella multocida* and *Bordetella bronchiseptica* in atrophic rhinitis and pneumonia in swine. *Canadian Journal of Veterinary Research*, 53, 295–300.

14 **DANIEL, G.M., FREESE, W., HENRY, S., STEVERMER, E., STRAW, B. & SWITZER, W.P., 1986.** An up-to-date review of atrophic rhinitis. *Veterinary Medicine*, 81, 735–744.

15 **DE JONG, M.F., 1992.** Progressive atrophic rhinitis. *In*: LEMAN, A.D., STRAW, B., MENGELING, W.L., D'ALLAIRE, S. & TAYLOR, D.J., (eds) *Diseases of Swine*. 7th edn. Ames, Iowa: Iowa State University Press.

16 **DE JONG, M.F., BOUWKAMP, F.T. & OOSTERWOUD, R.A., 1986.** The results of a field evaluation with the Nobivac AR vaccine after a period of three years. *Proceedings of the Ninth Congress of the International Pig Veterinary Society*, 243.

17 **DONE, J.T., UPCOTT, D.H., FREWIN, D.C. & HEBERT, C.N., 1984.** Atrophic rhinitis: Snout morphometry for quantitative assessment of conchal atrophy. *The Veterinary Record*, 114, 33–35.

18 **DUGAL, F., FIRARD, C. & JACQUES, M., 1990.** Adherence of *Bordetella bronchiseptica* 276 to porcine trachea maintained in organ culture. *Applied and Environmental Microbiology*, 56, 1523–1529.

19 **ELIAS, B., BOROS, G., ALBERT, M., TUBOLY, S., GERGELY, P., PAPP, L., BARNA VETRO, I., RAFAI, P. & MOLNER, E., 1990.** Clinical and pathological effects of the dermonecrotic toxin of *Bordetella bronchiseptica* and *Pasteurella multocida* in specific-pathogen-free piglets. *Japanese Journal of Veterinary Science*, 52, 677–688.

20 **ERLER, W. & SCHIMMEL, D., 1991.** On the importance of the dermonecrotic toxin of *Pasteurella multocida* for the pathogenesis of pneumonia in pigs. *Proceedings of the Twelfth Congress of the International Pig Veterinary Society*, 155.

21 **FOGED, N.T., NIELSEN, J.P. & BARFOD, K., 1991.** The use of ELISA—determination of *Pasteurella multocida* toxin antibodies in the control of progressive atrophic rhinitis. *Proceedings of the Eleventh Congress of the International Pig Veterinary Society*, 49.

22 **FOGED, N.T., NIELSEN, J.P. & JORSAL, S.E., 1989.** Protection against progressive atrophic rhinitis by vaccination with *Pasteurella multocida* toxin purified by monoclonal antibodies. *The Veterinary Record*, 125, 7–11.

23 **GEIGER, J.O., HARRIS, D.L., EDGERTON, S.L., JACKSON, W., KINYON, J.M., GLOCK, R.D., CONNOR, J.F. & HOUX, D.E., 1992.** Elimination of atrophic rhinitis utilizing Isowean^{SM} three-site production. *Proceedings of the Twelfth Congress of the International Pig Veterinary Society*, 166.

24 **GILES, G.J., 1986.** Bordetellosis. *In*: LEMAN, A.D., STRAW, B., GLOCK, R.O., MENGELING, W., PENNY, R.H.C. & SCHOLL, E., (eds) *Diseases of Swine*. 6th edn. Ames, Iowa: Iowa State University Press.

25 **GOODWIN, R.F.W., 1988.** Monitoring for atrophic rhinitis: The problem of higher snout scores. *The Veterinary Record*, 123, 566–568.

26 **GOODWIN, R.F.W., CHANTER, N. & RUTTER, J.M., 1990.** Detection and distribution of toxigenic *Pasteurella multocida* in pig herds with different degrees of atrophic rhinitis. *The Veterinary Record*, 126, 452–456.

27 **GOODWIN, R.F.W., CHANTER, N. & RUTTER, J.M., 1990.** Screening pig herds for toxigenic *Pasteurella multocida* and turbinate damage in a health scheme for atrophic rhinitis. *The Veterinary Record*, 127, 83–86.

28 **GOODWIN, R.F.W. & WHITTLESTONE, P., 1983.** Monitoring for atrophic rhinitis: Five years' experience with a pilot control scheme. *The Veterinary Record*, 113, 411–412.

29 **HENTON, M.M., 1991.** Veterinary Research Institute, Onderstepoort, South Africa. Personal communication.

30 **ISHIKAWA, H. & ISAYAMA, Y., 1987.** Evidence for sialyl gluco-conjugates as receptors for *Bordetella bronchiseptica* on swine nasal mucosa. *Infertility and Immunity*, 55, 1607–1609.

31 **ISHIKAWA, H. & ISAYAMA, Y., 1990.** Hydrophobic surface properties of *Bordetella bronchiseptica* X-mode cells and their possible role in adherence to porcine nasal mucosa. *Canadian Journal of Veterinary Research*, 54, 296–298.

32 **KAMP, E.M., KIMMAN, M.S. & KIMMAN, T.G., 1988.** Induction of nasal turbinate atrophy in germ-free pigs, using *Pasteurella multocida* as well as bacterium-free crude and purified dermonecrotic toxin of *P. multocida*. *American Journal of Veterinary Research*, 49, 1844–1849.

33 **NAKAI, T., KUME, K., YOSHIKAWA, H., OYAMADA, T. & YOSHIKAWA, T., 1988.** Adherence of *Pasteurella multocida* or *Bordetella bronchiseptica* to the swine nasal epithelial cell *in vitro*. *Information and Immunology*, 56, 234–240.

34 **PEDERSEN, K.B. & ELLING, F., 1984.** The pathogenesis of atrophic rhinitis in pigs induced by toxigenic *Pasteurella multocida*. *Journal of Comparative Pathology*, 94, 203–214.

35 **PEDERSEN, K.B., NIELSEN, J.P., FOGED, N.T., ELLING, F., NIELSEN, N.C. & WILLEBERG, P., 1988.** Atrophic rhinitis in pigs: Proposal for a revised definition. *The Veterinary Record*, 122, 190–191.

36 **PREVOST, P., REYNAUD, G., LACOSTE, F., CALMELS, F., PRATS, A. & STELLMANN, C., 1991.** Evaluation of the efficacy of a *B. bronchiseptica/P. multocida* type D bacterin toxoid vaccine against atrophic rhinitis. *Proceedings of the Eleventh Congress of the International Pig Veterinary Society*, 58.

37 **ROSENGURT, E., HIGGINS, T., CHANTER, N., LAX, A.J. & STRADDON, J.M., 1991.** *Pasteurella multocida* toxin is a novel potent mitogen for cultured fibroblasts. *Proceedings of the Eleventh Congress of the International Pig Veterinary Society*, 66.

38 **RUTTER, J.M., 1985.** The role of toxigenic *Pasteurella multocida* in atrophic rhinitis. *Proceedings of the International Pig Veterinary Society*, 16, 78–81.

39 **RUTTER, J.M., 1985.** Atrophic rhinitis in swine. *Advances in Veterinary Science Comparative Medicine*, 29, 239–279.

40 **RUTTER, J.M. & LUTHER, P.D., 1984.** Cell culture assay for toxigenic *Pasteurella multocida* from atrophic rhinitis in pigs. *The Veterinary Record*, 114, 393–396.

41 **RUTTER, J.M. & ROJAS, A.J., 1982.** Atrophic rhinitis in gnotobiotic piglets: Differences in the pathogenicity of *P. multocida* in combined infections with *B. bronchiseptica*. *The Veterinary Record*, 110, 531–535.

42 **STEHMANN, R., MEHLHORN, G. & NEUPARTH, V., 1989.** Nachweiss von *Bordetella bronchiseptica* in der Luft von Abferkel—und Absetzferkelställen. *Monatshefte für Veterinärmedizin*, 44, 307–311.

43 **TAYLOR, D.J., 1989.** *Pig Diseases*. 5th edn. Foxton, Cambridge: The Burlington Press.

44 **TRIGO, E., REESE, L. & SIMONSON, R., 1991.** Protection of piglets against atrophic rhinitis induced by the toxin of *P. multocida*. *Proceedings of the Twelfth Congress of the International Pig Veterinary Society*, 164.

Pseudomonas *spp. infections*

The genus *Pseudomonas* is a complex group of Gram-negative bacteria, which are aerobic, straight or slightly curved rods 0,5–1,0 x 1,5–5,0 µm in size, and motile. The cells contain one or several polar flagella. Some species produce lateral flagella and possess pili, which are important in the attachment of the bacteria to cell surfaces and affect phagocytosis.[2] Many of the *Pseudomonas* spp. produce pigments, the best-known being pyocyanin and the fluorescent pyoveridin, which are produced in profusion in media of low iron content. Members of this genus are characterized by their ability to grow in simple media of neutral reaction.

Glanders and melioidosis in animals are caused by *P. mallei* and *P. pseudomallei* respectively. They are also important zoonotic diseases. Glanders is a disease particularly of solipeds. It was a common and important disease at the time when equids were used extensively for draught and transport purposes, but it has since been eradicated from many countries, including South Africa. Currently, glanders still occurs in eastern Europe and Asia. Melioidosis, which is primarily a disease of rodents, is not an important disease of livestock. It has, however, been sporadically diagnosed in various livestock species in tropical countries, particularly in south-east Asia.

Pseudomonas spp. are frequently isolated from a variety of biological tissue and organ specimens obtained from diseased animals and humans.[2] They are often the cause of nosocomial infections, particularly in immunocompromised humans and animals. Infections by them (and particularly by *P. aeruginosa*) are opportunistic and of relatively little importance.[1] *Pseudomonas aeruginosa* is sporadically isolated from specimens collected from the lesions of bovine mastitis **(see Chapter 190: Mastitis)**, equine endometritis **(see Chapter 189: Infectious causes of equine reproductive failure)**, equine and bovine pyelonephritis and pyometra, bovine suppurative bronchopneumonia, and valvular endocarditis.[1]

Pseudomonas aeruginosa is also considered to be almost the sole causative agent of the disease known as fleece rot in woolled sheep, and it is responsible for the production of pigmented wool. Fleece rot, which is also known as wool rot, yolk rot or water rot, has been reviewed by Salisbury and Barrowman.[4] It is an acute superficial exudative dermatitis caused by prolonged wetting of the fleece and skin, and by marked proliferation of bacteria on the skin surface. The wet conditions provide a suitable environment for bacterial proliferation, which may occur within 24 hours of wetting. The pathogenicity of *P. aeruginosa* has been attributed mainly to its extracellular products, such as the pigments which may suppress the action of other microorganisms, proteases of localized activity, haemolytic toxins, enterotoxin, and the lethal toxin (exotoxin A), an acidic protein capable of inhibiting protein synthesis.[3] Sheep with well-grown fleeces are more prone to develop the disease, and in Merino sheep the lesion tends to develop particularly in the skin and fleece of the withers and backline. The skin in the affected area assumes a deep purple colour and the seropurulent exudate causes a band of matted fleece to develop. The wool appears saturated and has a leached and dingy appearance.[2] In severe cases the wool can be easily plucked from the lesion and the skin may tear when the fleece is parted.

Fleece rot is manifested by seropurulent exudation with resultant matting of the wool fibres and the formation of a band of matted fleece adjacent to the skin. Pigmentation of the fleece commonly accompanies the disease, in which case the affected fleece may assume shades of green, brown, orange, pink or blue. Bacterial discoloration of the fleece without skin exudation is not considered to be fleece rot.

The odours produced by bacterial decomposition in the lesion encourage blowfly strike, principally by *Lucilia cuprina*, which gives rise to the most economically significant feature of the disease. Fleece rot, together with the associated body blowfly strike, represents one of the major causes of production loss in the Australian sheep industry.

The two most important differential diagnoses of fleece rot are sheep scab due to *Psoroptes communis* var. *ovis* infestation and lumpy wool caused by *Dermatophilus congolensis* **(see Chapter 176: Dermatophilosis)**.

Pigmentation or discoloration of sheeps' wool in the

absence of fleece rot has been reviewed by van Tonder.[5] The condition is caused by the growth of a number of chromogenic bacteria in the fleece, including *P. aeruginosa, Chromobacterium violaceum, Serratia marcescens, Pseudomonas indigofera, Arthrobacter* sp. and others. The ensuing coloration may be green, brown, yellow, violet, blue, purple, pink or red, depending on the species of bacterium present. Bacterial wool pigmentation has been described in several countries, including Australia, New Zealand, the USA and South Africa, and is associated with very damp environmental conditions. In the case of *P. aeruginosa* infection the pigment pyocyanin that is elaborated by the organism is the responsible agent, and this produces a green discoloration of the wool. The soundness of the wool fibres is not affected, but the economic importance of the condition lies in the fact that the pigment cannot be removed by scouring, and this severely affects the usefulness of the fibres from the wool processors' point of view.

References

1 **JUBB, K.V.F., KENNEDY, P.C. & PALMER, N., 1993.** *Pathology of Domestic Animals.* Vols I-IV. 4th edn. San Diego: Academic Press, Inc.

2 **HAYMAN, R.H., 1953.** Studies in fleece-rot of sheep. *Australian Journal of Agricultural Research*, 4, 430–468.

3 **PALLERONI, N.J., 1984.** Pseudomonadaceae. *In*: KRIEG, N.R. & HOLT, J.G., (eds) *Bergey's Manual of Systematic Bacteriology*. Vol. I. Baltimore, London: Williams & Wilkins.

4 **SALISBURY, R.H. & BARROWMAN, P.R., 1984.** Fleece-rot: The epidemiology and significance of the disease in sheep. *Journal of the South African Veterinary Association*, 55, 147–151.

5 **VAN TONDER, E.M., KELLERMAN, G.E. & BOLTON, T.F.W., 1976.** Discoloration of wool: 1 Green discoloration. *Journal of the South African Veterinary Association*, 47, 223–226.

122

Glanders

Synonym: Droes

G.C. Bishop

Introduction

Glanders is a contagious disease of solipeds caused by the bacterium *Pseudomonas mallei*. It is characterized by nodules, ulcers and the formation of scars, particularly in the upper respiratory tract, lungs, skin, and less frequently in other organs. It may occur in an acute or chronic form, is usually fatal, and is of major importance in any infected equine population. Glanders once occurred extensively throughout the world, including South Africa. Presently it occurs only sporadically in eastern European countries, North Africa,[3] and Asia (including India,[11] Pakistan,[10] Turkey[1] and China[8]).

The disease was already recognized in 400 BC by Hippocrates, and a century later by Aristotle.[5, 6] The bacterium was first isolated by Loeffler and Schütz in 1882, but it was only four years later that Loeffler demonstrated beyond doubt that it was the cause of glanders. During 1891 and 1892 no less than seven European scientists died of the disease following accidental laboratory infection.[6]

Glanders was spread by animal movements through trade or war to most countries of the world.[6] Henning[5] expressed uncertainty about the way in which it was introduced into South Africa, but in his review of the disease, Hunting[6] mentions that during the Anglo-Boer War, in which 240 000 horses perished, South Africa was plagued by the spread of glanders throughout the entire country. According to Hunting, the disease was introduced into South Africa by remounts imported from Great Britain, America and Australia, and possibly also from Europe. Eventually, in 1929, glanders was restricted to the Cape Peninsula, from which it was eradicated soon afterwards by application of a slaughter-out policy **(Figures 122.1 and 122.2)**. This control measure and the use of the mallein test for diagnostic purposes were the major reasons for the successful eradication of the disease.

Glanders is unlikely to assume any great significance in southern Africa unless the pathogen is reintroduced under circumstances where large numbers of horses or other solipeds are kept under unsanitary conditions.

Aetiology

Glanders is caused by *Pseudomonas mallei* (Bergey) (syn. *Actinobacillus mallei, Malleomyces mallei* and *Pfeifferella mallei*), a Gram-negative, non-motile, non-encapsulated and non-spore-forming bacillus.[4] It is obligately aerobic except in media containing nitrate, is nutritionally versatile and does not require special growth factors. The best growth of *P. mallei* is obtained at 37 °C. Potato media are particularly suited for its cultivation.[5] *In vitro* DNA hybridization experiments suggest a close relationship to *P. pseudomallei*, the causative organism of false glanders (melioidosis).

The bacterium is not very resistant to external factors. It is destroyed by exposure to direct sunlight in 24 hours and is killed by most of the common disinfectants, e.g., phenol, potassium permanganate, copper sulphate, formalin and chlorine. In damp media the organism retains its vitality for three to five weeks and in decomposing material for 20–30 days. It may survive for about 20 days in clean water and for about six weeks in contaminated stables.[3, 5]

Epidemiology

Underfed animals and those kept in poor conditions are more susceptible than animals that are healthy and well-cared-for. Humans are also highly susceptible; the disease sometimes affects laboratory workers and individuals who are in intimate contact with affected horses or the organisms.

The natural disease occurs primarily in domestic equidae and only occasionally in carnivores, rodents, cattle, sheep, goats, pigs and humans.[3, 9] All domestic equidae are highly susceptible. Donkeys are apparently the most susceptible and frequently develop the acute form of the disease.[5] Horses are more resistant and commonly contract the chronic form. Mules occupy an intermediate position.

In acute glanders, the pathogen may be distributed throughout the body, whereas in chronic cases the organism appears to be confined to the affected organs and exudates from lesions. Although the urine, saliva, tears and faeces may be contaminated, nasal discharges and the pus from cutaneous ulcers are the most infective. The mode of infection is unclear, but it generally appears to result from contaminated food or water. Outbreaks of the disease are usually favoured where several animals are kept together and share feeding places and water troughs. The occurrence of glanders in lions in an Italian zoological park was traced back to contaminated meat originating from horses which were imported.[2, 5]

The frequency of lung involvement has led to the speculation that aerogenous infection is important, yet most attempts to produce chronic glanders via the respiratory tract have failed. Typical glanders has, however, been reproduced by intranasal and intratracheal injections and by feeding the animals infective material.

Cutaneous glanders, also referred to as farcy, occurs as a result of infection of the skin following injury, or from metastases of pulmonary origin.

The importance of asymptomatic carriers, and the transmission of the disease from them to healthy animals, should be emphasized. This form of transmission is considered to be more significant than that from clinical cases.[5] Once the disease has been introduced into a stable or a stud it spreads rapidly.

Pathogenesis

Infection taking place *per os* results in the acute form and is characterized by a septicaemia or bacteraemia.[3, 5] Localization in the lungs invariably occurs, and in some cases also in the skin and nasal mucosa. Nodules may also develop in organs such as the liver, spleen and testes.[5] In some animals nodular lesions appear to be the only sign of lung involvement, while in others there may be a bronchopneumonia.[3, 5]

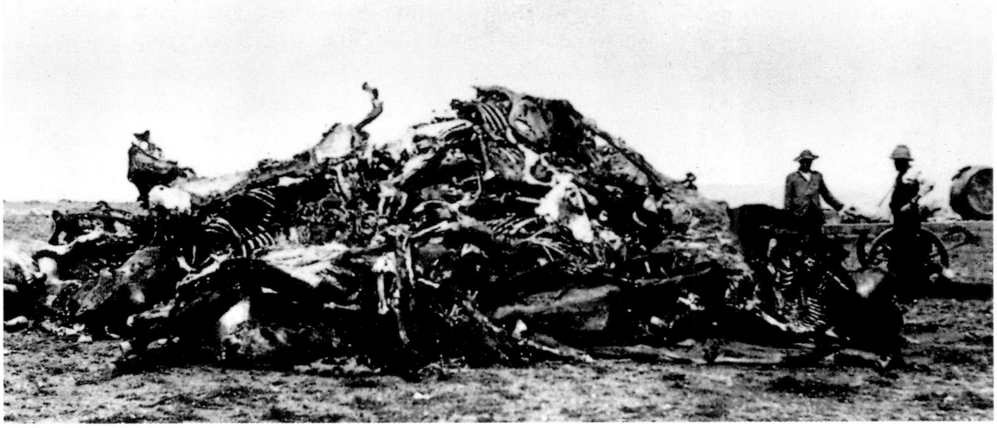

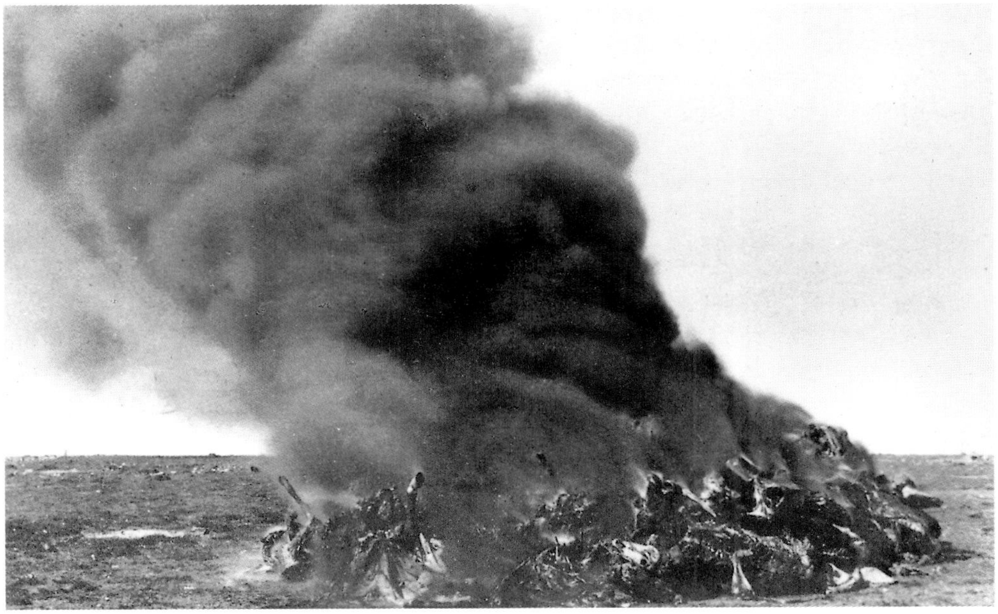

Figures 122.1 (above) and 122.2 (below)
Historic photographs depicting mass slaughter of horses and burning of carcasses during the glanders eradication campaign in the 1920s in South Africa

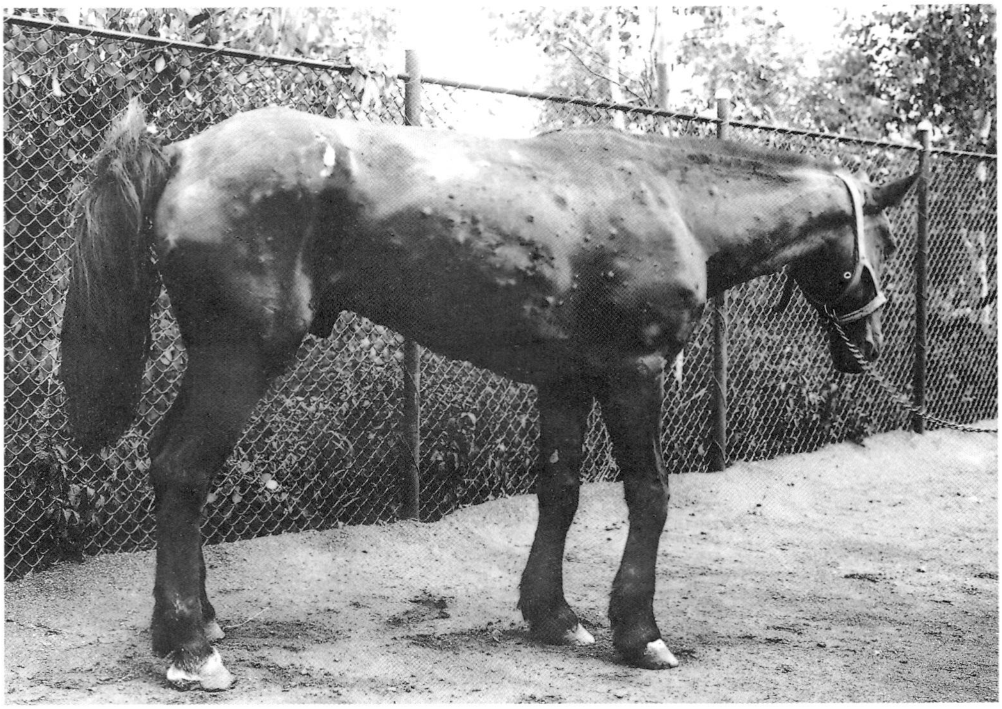

Figure 122.3 Farcy: skin form of glanders in a horse. Note the numerous cutaneous lesions on the side of the chest and the abdomen

Clinical signs

Following experimental infection, the incubation period varies according to the route and intensity of infection, and the natural resistance of the animal;[5] a fever appears after about three days and clinical signs after a week. Following natural infection, several weeks (on average two months) often elapse before the first signs are noticeable.[5]

In acute glanders there is a high fever, nasal discharge, coughing, and swelling of the submandibular lymph nodes.[3, 5] The nasal discharge, which is usually unilateral, may be yellowish-green or bloody and may partly accumulate around the nostrils. Nasal mucous membranes are swollen, may be covered by a diphtheritic exudate and contain several nodules which often eventually ulcerate. The ulcers may coalesce; their borders are raised and irregular and their bases are covered by yellowish granulation tissue. Peculiar rattling and roaring sounds may be heard during breathing. The superficial lymph nodes are swollen and sensitive, and may rupture to discharge a viscous, purulent exudate. Death due to septicaemia occurs within a week or two.

Chronic glanders is more common than the acute form in horses, particularly in countries where the disease is endemic.[3, 5, 9] This form may have a duration of years and can be so mild that it is easily overlooked. Intermittent and irregular exacerbations are associated with coughing and dyspnoea. Sometimes the submandibular lymph nodes adhere to the skin and the mandible, and they may be hard and knotty. The extremities, particularly the hind legs, are in some cases severely affected and thickened.

The pulmonary form of glanders may take several months to develop, and culminates in fits of coughing or a dry, persistent cough. Respiration becomes costosternal and laboured. Eventually, typical lesions also appear in the nasal mucous membranes and skin.

Nasal glanders usually starts with a unilateral nasal catarrh that becomes progressively worse, and is eventually characterized by a purulent and greenish-yellow nasal discharge sometimes containing streaks of blood or flakes of epithelium. Large quantities of exudate may be expelled during fits of coughing and snorting. Yellowish-grey nodules develop in the mucosa and when the covering epithelium sloughs, these give rise to ulcers with well-defined borders. Healed ulcers leave distinct, stellate scars. The submandibular lymph nodes are initially swollen and painful, but eventually they become firm and less painful and adhere to the mandible and surrounding skin.

The nodules which develop in the skin and subcutaneous tissue (cutaneous glanders or farcy), particularly of the limbs, sides of the chest and ventral abdomen, may be 10 mm in diameter **(Figure 122.3)**. On rupturing, these nodules become ulcers that may heal or spread to the surrounding tissue. Involvement of the lymphatic system is manifested by the presence of inflamed lymphatics which are thickened, nodular and cord-like. They often link nodules and ulcers to each other and the resultant lesions resemble strings of beads. Oedematous swelling of the legs can be so extensive that it interferes with movement.

Pathology

In the acute form, multiple petechiae are found throughout the body, while a severe catarrhal bronchopneumonia **(Figure 122.4)** and enlargement of the bronchial lymph nodes are typical.

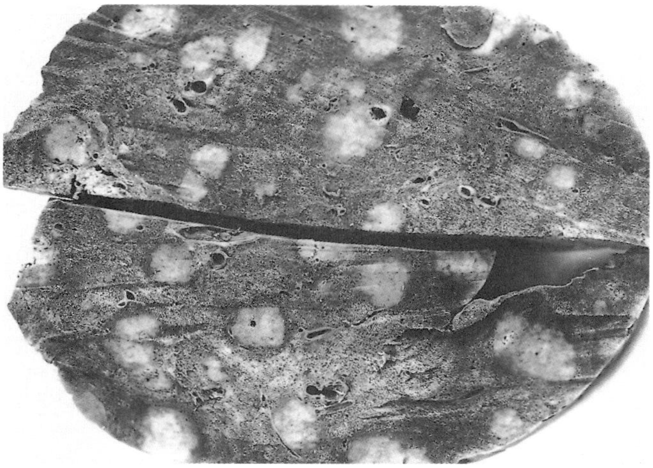

Figure 122.4 Partially encapsulated, focally disseminated, necrogranulomatous lesions characteristic of the chronic pulmonary form of glanders

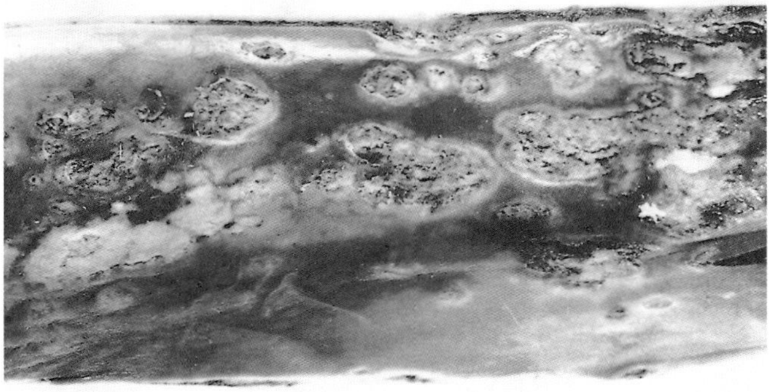

Figure 122.5 Ulcerative necrotic lesions in the nasal septum

In the more common chronic form, lesions are invariably present in the lungs and palpation reveals nodules resembling tubercles, or areas of bronchopneumonia. The nodules are firm, round, encapsulated and greyish.[3, 5, 9] Nodules and ulcers are frequently present in the upper respiratory tract, especially in the nasal septum **(Figure 122.5)**, larynx and trachea. Some of the ulcers may have healed to form bulging or flat, stellate scars **(Figure 122.6)**. Lymph nodes draining affected skin or deep-seated lesions are enlarged. Nodules similar to those in the lungs may also be seen in the liver, spleen and kidneys.

Lesions in the digestive system are rare. Occasionally lesions from the upper respiratory tract may extend into the pharyngeal mucous membrane.

Microscopically, the nodules are necrogranulomatous and are characterized by necrosis and liquefaction, and at a later stage by caseation and mineralization of their centres. These changes are surrounded by a mixture of inflammatory cells comprising many neutrophils, a few

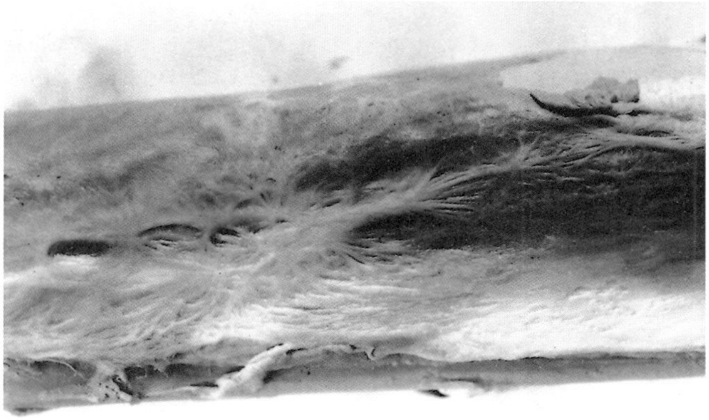

Figure 122.6 Stellate scars indicating healed lesions of glanders in the nasal septum

lymphocytes, macrophages, epithelioid cells, and a few giant cells. The nodules are well encapsulated. Vasculitis and thrombosis of the vessels immediately adjacent to the necrotic nodules are prominent features. Circumscribed, haemorrhagic foci are sometimes found in the lungs, and these may be infiltrated by many neutrophils and a few macrophages.[5, 6, 9]

The disease is accompanied by anaemia, a leukocytosis and neutrophilia.[3]

Diagnosis

The characteristic clinical signs of glanders appear late in the course of the disease and a definite diagnosis based on the clinical manifestation alone is seldom possible.[5] The mallein or complement fixation (CF) tests should be used to detect the occult or carrier cases, which are very important in the control of the disease.[3, 5, 6] The administration of mallein (a solution containing endo- and exotoxins of *P. mallei*), using the ophthalmic and subcutaneous routes,[5] has been largely replaced by the intradermal-palpebral test in which mallein is injected into the lower eyelid of the animal. In positive cases, a delayed hypersensitivity reaction, which is detectable after 48 hours, is responsible for the development of a mucopurulent ocular discharge and marked oedema of the eyelid. Certain strains of the bacterium may, however, cross-react with *Pseudomonas pseudomallei*.[3] Recently the sensitivity of the mallein test, the indirect haemagglutination test, the CF test and counter-immunoelectrophoresis (CIE) were compared by using serum samples obtained from 155 horses and 57 mules in India.[7] Although it was concluded that CIE is the most rapid, simple and economical test for dealing with large numbers of serum samples, the CF test is the most reliable serological test available.

Glanders may be confirmed by the bacteriological examination of swabs taken of pus from open lesions.[9]

The organism grows readily on blood agar, Loeffler's serum agar or glycerine–potato media incubated aerobically at 37 °C. Colonies are about 1 mm in diameter, white, semi-transparent and viscid.

The intraperitoneal injection of infective material into guinea-pigs results in death in 10–14 days.[9] The organism localizes in lymph nodes and on the tunica of the testes, producing a purulent exudate and causing swelling of the scrotum in two to three days.[5] This characteristic response is referred to as the Strauss reaction.

Differential diagnosis

Several conditions may be confused with glanders and laboratory examination is essential in differentiating the disease from strangles, botryomycosis, horsepox and such fungal conditions as sporotrichosis caused by *Sporothrix schenckii*, epizootic lymphangitis caused by *Histoplasma farciminosum* and ulcerative lymphangitis caused by *Actinomyces (Corynebacterium) pseudotuberculosis*.

Control

Treatment with sulphadiazine alone or in combination with formalized preparations of *P. mallei* has sometimes been successful. Most countries of the western world — including South Africa, in which it is a notifiable disease — provide for the slaughter of clinical cases and animals which show a reaction to the mallein test or to one of the serological tests.[5] Carcasses must be burnt or buried and thorough disinfection of the premises should be undertaken. Complete quarantine of affected and surrounding premises is necessary and equine traffic should be carefully monitored.

Horses may recover spontaneously from the disease, but their subsequent immunity is incomplete. It is not surprising, therefore, that immunization has never been considered successful in the control of the disease.

References

1 **ALIBASOGLU, M., YESILDERE, T., CALISLAR, T., INAL, T. & CALISKAN, U., 1986.** Outbreak of glanders in lions in the Istanbul zoological garden. *Berliner und Münchener Tierärtzliche Wochenschrift*, 99, 57–63.

2 **BATTELLI, C., CONTENTO, F., CORSALINI, T., GOFFREDO, G., LAZARI, P., PUCCINI, V. & SOBRERO, L., 1973.** Glanders in a group of lions in captivity. *Veterinaria Italiana*, 24, 87–112, 113–116.

3 **BLOOD, D.C., RADOSTITS, O.M. & HENDERSON, J.A., 1983.** *Veterinary Medicine*. 6th edn. London: Baillière, Tindall and Cox.

4 **BUCHANAN, R.E. & GIBBONS, N.E., 1974.** *Bergey's Manual of Determinative Bacteriology*. 8th edn. Baltimore: Williams & Wilkins.

5 **HENNING, M.W., 1956.** *Animal Diseases in South Africa*. 3rd edn. Pretoria: Central News Agency Ltd.

6 **HUNTING, W., 1913.** Glanders. In: HOARE, E.W., (ed.) *A System of Veterinary Medicine*. London: Ballière, Tindall and Cox.

7 **JANA, A.M., GUPTA, A.K., PANDYA, G., VERMA, R.D. & RAO, K.M., 1982.** Rapid diagnosis of glanders in equines by counter-immunoelectrophoresis. *Indian Veterinary Journal*, 59, 5–9.

8 **LIANG, S.Y., WEI, J.S., MEI, W.H., XIE, X., DUAN, X.W. & GONG, R.X., 1980.** Post-infection immunity after recovery from glanders. *Collected Papers of Veterinary Research*, 6, 77–82.

9 **MACAULAY, J.W., 1978.** Glanders. In: FRENCH, E.L. & GEERING, W.A., (eds). *Exotic Diseases of Animals: A Manual for Diagnosis*. 2nd edn. Canberra: Australian Government Publishing Service.

10 **VAID, M.Y., MUNEER, M.A. & NAEEM, M., 1981.** Studies on the incidence of glanders in Lahore. *Pakistan Veterinary Journal*, 1, 75.

11 **VERMA, R.D., 1981.** Glanders in India with special reference to incidence and epidemiology. *Indian Veterinary Journal*, 58, 177–183.

123

Melioidosis

Synonyms: Pseudoglanders, melioidose (Afrik.)

G.C. Bishop

Introduction

Melioidosis is a glanders-like disease of carnivores, rodents, cattle, sheep, goats, pigs, horses and occasionally humans. It is caused by *Pseudomonas pseudomallei,* and is characterized by suppurating or caseous lesions in the lymph nodes and other organs. It has not yet been described in animals in southern Africa, although Henning[3] quotes McDouell and Varney as reporting the disease in humans in South Africa in 1947. Melioidosis is of little or no importance to the livestock industry in southern Africa.

Aetiology and epidemiology

Melioidosis is caused by the bacterium *Pseudomonas pseudomallei* (synonyms: *Malleomyces pseudomallei, Loefflerella pseudomallei*), which can be readily isolated aerobically on ordinary culture media at 37 °C.[2] The organism is a Gram-negative, non-spore-forming rod and stains with the common bacterial stains. The bacillus is nutritionally versatile and can be isolated from the soil and water. Infection may therefore arise from the environment rather than by transmission from animal to animal. In humans and rodents the disease occurs almost exclusively in tropical areas. A fatal case of the disease in an ox in south-eastern Queensland in Australia is described,[4] where it was postulated that an unusually wet summer with prolonged flooding had favoured the saprophytic growth of the pathogen. In a survey conducted in northern Queensland, 75 strains of *P. pseudomallei* were isolated from 48 animals including birds, pigs, sheep, goats, horses and a kangaroo.[5]

Clinical signs, pathogenesis and pathology

In domestic animals, the disease is usually chronic and progressive with the clinical signs varying according to the location of the lesions.[3] Sheep usually show lameness and may become paralysed in the hind quarters. Suppuration of the nasal mucous membranes, polyarthritis and meningoencephalitis are often seen. Recumbency followed by death after a week is common. The characteristic lesion of the disease comprises small nodules and abscesses in the internal organs, muscles, bones, subcutis and sometimes the mucous membranes of the respiratory system. The progression and development of the disease is thought to be similar to glanders: an initial septicaemia and bacteraemia is followed by localization in various organs.[1]

Diagnosis, differential diagnosis and control

The typical nodules, multiple abscessation and debilitated condition of the animal may serve to differentiate melioidosis from caseous lymphadenitis in sheep.[1] Isolation of the bacterium provides a positive diagnosis and the organism is easily cultured from nasal exudates and suppurating abscesses. In horses, the disease must be differentiated from strangles and glanders. In melioidosis of equines there is no lymph node enlargement or involvement of the skin and nasal mucosa.

Although tetracycline has proved effective, treatment should not be undertaken because of the risk of human exposure. Control is based on the elimination of infected animals and the disinfection of premises. No effective vaccine is available.

References

1 **BLOOD, D.C., RADOSTITS, O.M. & HENDERSON, J.A., 1983.** *Veterinary Medicine.* 6th edn. London: Baillière Tindall.

2 **BUCHANAN, R.E. & GIBBONS, N.E., 1974.** *Bergey's Manual of Determinative Bacteriology.* 8th edn. Baltimore: Williams & Wilkins.

3 **HENNING, M.W., 1956.** *Animal Diseases in South Africa.* 3rd edn. Pretoria: Central News Agency Ltd.

4 **KETTERER, P.J., DONALD, B. & ROGERS, R.J., 1975.** Bovine melioidosis in south-eastern Queensland. *Australian Veterinary Journal,* 51, 395–398.

5 **THOMAS, A.D., 1981.** Prevalence of melioidosis in animals in northern Queensland. *Australian Veterinary Journal,* 57, 146–148.

Brucella *spp. infections*

Bacteria of the genus *Brucella* are Gram-negative cocci, coccobacilli or short rods. They are intracellular parasites transmissible to a wide range of animal species, in which they generally cause non-lethal infections. Early bacteraemia is followed by localization of the infection in the genital organs and cells of the monocyte-macrophage series.[1] The *Brucella* spp. and the diseases they cause are listed in **Table 1**. Of these diseases, those caused by *B. abortus* and *B. ovis* are of particular economic importance to cattle and sheep respectively in southern Africa.

The major clinical manifestations of infection with *B. abortus* in cattle are abortions, stillbirths and the birth of weak calves. In sheep, infection by *B. ovis* results in the development of epididymitis, occasionally accompanied by orchitis. The presence of this disease in sheep causes economic losses in the major sheep-farming regions of the world, primarily due to infertility in rams. Vaccines, when applied appropriately, limit the effects and spread of *B. abortus* and *B. ovis* infections.

Infections by *B. abortus* and *B. melitensis*, which are the causes of undulant and Malta fever respectively, are important zoonoses. Infection of humans with *B. melitensis* is, however, rare in southern African countries and the bacteria is not a practical problem from a human point of view. The natural hosts of *B. melitensis* are sheep and goats, and disease caused by it is particularly prevalent in countries that border the Mediterranean Sea, in the Near East and in South America.[2]

In pigs, *B. suis* produces a generalized infection which is followed by localization, particularly in the genital system. In boars, the testes, epididymides and seminal vesicles are most severely affected, while metritis, placentitis and abortions occur in pregnant females.[1]

Table 1
Most common diseases caused by *Brucella* spp. in livestock

BRUCELLA SPP.	DISEASE	LIVESTOCK SPECIES
B. abortus	Brucellosis (contagious abortion)	Cattle
B. ovis	Epididymitis/orchitis	Sheep
B. melitensis	Abortion and orchitis	Sheep and goats
B. suis	Abortion, stillbirth, sterility in sows, and orchitis	Pigs

References

1 **BOVRE, K., 1984.** Neisseriaceae. *In*: KRIEG, N.R. & HOLT, J.G., (eds) *Bergey's Manual of Systematic Bacteriology*. Vol. I. Baltimore, London: Williams & Wilkins.

2 **KENNEDY, P.D. & MILLER, R.B., 1993.** The female genital system. *In*: JUBB, K.V.F., KENNEDY, P.C. & PALMER, N., (eds) *Pathology of Domestic Animals*. Vol. III. 4th edn. San Diego: Academic Press, Inc.

124

Bovine brucellosis

Synonyms: Contagious abortion, besmetlike misgeboorte (Afrik.)

G.C. Bishop, P.P. Bosman and S. Herr

Introduction

Bovine brucellosis is a highly contagious disease caused by *Brucella abortus*, an intracellular bacterium. Apart from causing characteristic mid- to late-term abortion and infertility in cows, *B. abortus* also occasionally causes orchitis and inflammation of the accessory sex glands in bulls. Other livestock and wild animal species, though of varying susceptibility, are sometimes infected, and it is an important zoonosis.

It is suspected that bovine brucellosis was introduced into southern Africa with cattle imported from Europe,[55] but there is also a possibility that it was introduced into the subcontinent much earlier, during the migration of the black races and their cattle herds from other African countries.[76] The first reliable record of its existence in South Africa was that of Gray in 1906, when he reported a serious outbreak of abortion among cattle near Johannesburg.[55] Its presence was finally confirmed by Hall in 1913 when he isolated *B. abortus* from the stomach of an aborted bovine foetus.[55] Outbreaks of abortion thought to be bovine brucellosis were first observed in Zimbabwe in 1906, and the presence of brucellosis was confirmed in that country in 1914. According to an obituary notice in *The Veterinary Record* of 1957, Bevan, in Zimbabwe, was the first to show that *B. abortus*-infected cattle could transmit the pathogen to humans and that goats were not the source of the infection.[7]

The disease has a relatively high prevalence in southern Africa, especially in intensively farmed areas, and it is the most important bacterial cause of abortion on the subcontinent. It has an enormous economic impact on the beef and dairy cattle industries, especially as 14,7 per cent of the herds in South Africa are known to be infected and the losses to cattle farmers exceed R300 million per annum.[12]

Aetiology

Brucella abortus is a small, Gram-negative, non-sporulating, non-encapsulated coccus, coccobacillus or short rod, 0,6–1,5 µm in length and 0,5–0,7 µm in width.[5, 30] The organism is not acid-fast but does resist decolorization by weak acids and thus stains red with Stamp's modification of the Ziehl Neelsen stain.[101.]

Most wild strains are fastidious and slow-growing, and require CO_2 (5–10 per cent) supplementation for primary isolation at an optimal growth temperature of 36–38 °C. Strain 19, however, grows well in a normal atmosphere at 37 °C.[6] Complex media containing serum are required for growth and, although most strains grow on sheep-blood agar, the colonies may not be as distinctive as when grown on serum-dextrose agar. On primary isolation, growth is seldom clearly visible before 48 hours of incubation, at which stage the colonies are usually 0,5–1,0 mm in diameter. The use of selective media, such as Farrell's medium,[48] may substantially enhance the chances of isolation[5] by inhibiting the growth of contaminants. The growth rate of *B. abortus* may, however, be markedly retarded by selective media, and for this reason such cultures should be incubated for five days or longer.[6] Smooth colonies on a clear growth medium, such as serum-dextrose agar, are convex, entire-edged, have a smooth, shiny surface, and are pale yellowish-brown when viewed under transmitted light.[30] Considerable variation in colour and surface texture are found in the rough strains. Smooth forms are often markedly pathogenic, whereas the rough variants are usually less so.

There is no single test by which *B. abortus* may be identified with absolute certainty, but a combination of growth characteristics, colonial and cellular morphology, staining properties, agglutinating antisera and biochemical reactions will allow an accurate identification.[5, 6, 30, 31] Eight biovars (biotypes) are recognized (biovars 1, 2, 3, 4, 5, 6, 7 and 9) and these may be differentiated by phage typing, monospecific antisera, biochemical reactions and growth-inhibition tests.[5] There are no proven differences in the pathogenicity of field-strain biovars.[85] Biovar 7 is reported to be a mixed culture and, because no authentic isolate has been made for many years, it is expected to be deleted from the list.[5] Ninety per cent of isolates typed in South Africa are biovar 1 and 10 per cent biovar 2.[17, 56]

The abundance of erythritol in the pregnant uterus results in the massive multiplication of brucella organisms in this organ,[33] except that the growth of strain 19 is generally inhibited by the presence of erythritol. However, erythritol-tolerant isolates of strain 19, which arise by mutation, have been made from milk and aborted foetuses in South Africa and New Zealand.[14, 17] The mutation rate of strain 19 tolerance to erythritol is quite high and some strains may grow in the presence of this carbohydrate and yet resemble strain 19 in all other tests.[5] Interference with pregnancy has been associated with strain 19 vaccine; about 50 per cent of foetuses contained erythritol-utilizing organisms, probably due to colonization of the pregnant uterus by these variants.[14]

Epidemiology

No accurate figures are available on the prevalence of brucellosis in cattle in southern Africa, as most reports are based on non-representative laboratory results. The prevalence, which varies considerably within South Africa, is probably largely the consequence of regulatory measures that have been applied.

Since 1968, when compulsory calfhood vaccination was introduced, the control scheme in South Africa has made a considerable impact on the prevalence of the disease. The prevalence has decreased on a national scale from 10,5 per cent in 1976 to 6 per cent in 1979,[19] 1,9 per cent in 1984–5,[49] and 1,4 per cent in 1988–9.[10] The variation in prevalence is demonstrated by a survey of 90 per cent of the dairy and beef herds in the eastern Cape Province and Karoo between 1985 and 1989, which revealed a prevalence of less than 0,3 per cent.[67] The prevalence of brucellosis in about 5 000 adult beef cows slaughtered at a large Natal abattoir in 1981–2 was estimated to be less than 1,5 per cent.[15] Although these cows were drawn from all the provinces of South Africa they originated mostly from Natal.[9]

A prevalence of 4,5 per cent in dairy cattle[77] and an overall prevalence of 1,4 per cent in cattle herds tested in Zimbabwe have been reported,[76] even though generally intensive management systems employed in Zimbabwe seem to favour the spread of bovine brucellosis. Cattle in the communal areas of Manicaland province were free of brucellosis before 1985, while the prevalence was high in intensively managed herds in the Midlands and Mashonaland.[76] However, with the establishment of dairy cooperatives in resettlement areas in Zimbabwe in 1980, cattle of unknown disease status were mixed and often grazed together on communal pastures. As a result of this practice the prevalence of brucellosis in one settlement scheme in Manicaland province has risen from 0,7 per cent in 1986 to 3,3 per cent in 1988.[76] In Zimbabwe the prevalence of bovine brucellosis in the communal areas also varies from province to province. The prevalence is lowest in Mashonaland and highest in Manicaland and Matebeleland.[76] The patchy distribution of brucellosis in the provinces (some herds are free of the disease, while others have a high prevalence of brucellosis) may be explained by the fact that some communal herds have been kept closed whereas other cattle owners have purchased infected animals to upgrade their stock.[76]

The disease is reported to be widespread in Zambia[41] and Malawi,[111] but its prevalence in the two countries is unknown. The estimated prevalence of brucellosis in the commercial farming areas of Namibia is 0,5 per cent.[9]

There does not appear to be a specific breed-resistance to brucellosis in cattle,[82] but the smaller breeds such as the Jersey mature earlier in life and become susceptible to infection at an earlier age.[82] Sexually mature heifers (and especially pregnant cattle) are more susceptible to infection by *Brucella* than are sexually immature heifers, and they may remain infected for life. Calves may acquire infection *in utero* or they may become infected after the ingestion of infected colostrum or milk. Most will rid themselves of the infection within a few months.[85]

There appear to have been no controlled studies showing that bulls are more resistant to *B. abortus* than heifers and cows. Bulls may become infected *in utero* or during early calfhood by the oral route and retain the infection into adult life,[93] but spread of infection by these bulls during natural service is rare. It is possible that bulls are more resistant than sexually mature heifers but less resistant than sexually immature heifers.[85]

Both acquired and passive immunity affect the susceptibility of the host. Acquired immunity attained through natural infection and vaccination is referred to as 'relative immunity' as it does not impart complete protection.[83] Passive immunity acquired by the ingestion of colostrum has little long-term value, although it may reduce transmission of the infection via milk.[38]

Cattle usually become infected after ingesting contaminated feed or water or after licking an infected placenta, calf, foetus, or the genitalia of an infected cow soon after it has aborted or calved, when very large numbers of *B. abortus* are present, particularly in the placenta lochia.[1] Animals may also become infected by inhaling organisms or through the conjunctiva.[85] Congenital transmission may also occur after *in utero* infection, and these calves may retain the infection and spread the disease at their first and subsequent parturitions.[8, 38]

Although *B. abortus* has been isolated from ixodid ticks and their eggs in Brazil, ticks are probably not important in the transmission of the disease.[42] The transmission of brucellosis by ticks, fleas or mosquitoes from an infected herd to a non-infected herd has never been proved.[82]

Brucella abortus is sensitive to pasteurization temperatures and its survival outside the host is largely dependent on environmental conditions.[85] The pathogen may survive in an aborted foetus in the shade for up to eight months, for two to three months in wet soil, one to two months in dry soil, three to four months in faeces,[65] and for eight months in liquid-manure tanks.[92] Generally, removal of infected animals from contaminated premises for one month is sufficient to prevent infection, provided the facilities have been properly disinfected.[94] Large numbers of organisms are shed from the reproductive tract when infected cows abort. In cows which lactate following abortion, milk, including colostrum, is an important source of infection, and bacteria are excreted intermittently in milk throughout the lactation period. Urine and faeces of infected cattle are less important sources of the bacteria. The fluid in hygromas caused by *B. abortus* infection may contain large numbers of organisms,[8] but because of being restricted to the lesion they do not seem to be important in the spread of the disease. There is a rapid reduction in the numbers of organisms shed after calving and abortion, and cows are usually non-infective until the next pregnancy, when there is again a rapid increase of brucella organisms in the reproductive tract.[109] During subsequent pregnancies there is invasion of the gravid uterus and allantochorion,[38] but abortion rarely recurs. Ninety per cent of infected cows remain chronically infected, sometimes life-long, with the infection confined to the udder and lymph nodes.[38, 85]

A contaminated environment or equipment used for milking or artificial insemination are further sources of infection. Permanent calving camps and lush pastures, particularly if they are wet and muddy, may play a very important role in the spread of the disease.[85, 94]

Infected animals usually abort only once; subsequent calves are carried to full-term, although they may be infected.[8, 38, 85] Approximately 2,5 to 9 per cent of heifers born from seropositive cows may be latently infected but serologically negative until the middle of their first gestation or even later, when antibodies to *B. abortus* may be detectable for the first time.[8, 27, 44, 72, 73, 92, 114]

In bulls, the testes (one or both) and accessory sex glands may be affected. Infected bulls may shed brucellae in their semen, seminal fluid and urine, and therefore bulls in infected herds should always be viewed with suspicion,[91] particularly if artificial insemination using the semen of these bulls is contemplated.[78] The risk of introducing the disease into a herd through embryo transplantation is probably not significant.[25, 102]

Although *B. abortus* infection may occasionally cause sheep and goats to abort, the infection does not spread in these species and they are apparently not a real danger to cattle unless there is close association between the species.[82] Horses become infected particularly by ingestion of *B. abortus*-contaminated feed. In this species the organisms localize in bursae, tendons and joints, and they are thus an unlikely source of infection for cattle.[99]

Several species of wildlife [African buffalo (*Syncerus caffer*), hippopotamus (*Hippopotamus amphibius*), zebra (*Equus burchelli*), eland (*Taurotragus oryx*) and impala (*Aepyceros melampus*)] have tested serologically positive for brucellosis, but these species are probably not of great importance in the epidemiology of bovine brucellosis in southern Africa. This is possibly because of the relatively infrequent contact between cattle and wild-life.[28, 29, 43, 52, 70] There are few records of abortions in wildlife in southern Africa due to *Brucella*, although *B. abortus* biovar 1 has been isolated from the cotyledons of pregnant buffalo at slaughter.[52] Even though serological surveys have revealed up to 23 per cent[11, 59] positive reactors in buffalo from the Kruger National Park, these animals probably do not constitute a significant source of infection for cattle because of the strict control measures to prevent the spread of foot-and-mouth disease across the boundaries of the Park and from adjoining private nature reserves.

The typing of *B. abortus* isolates may yield important epidemiological information, as it allows sources of infection to be traced,[37] particularly in countries where a number of biovars are present.

Brucellosis or undulant fever in humans is chiefly an occupational disease, occurring most often in veterinarians, stock inspectors, abattoir workers, laboratory personnel and farmers who become infected by contamination of abraded or intact skin or mucous membranes, or by inhalation during contact with infected cattle, foetuses or foetal membranes, and calves. Humans may also become infected after ingesting unpasteurized dairy products containing field strains of *B. abortus* or after inadvertent self-inoculation with *B. abortus* strain 19 vaccine.[8, 40] After an incubation period of five to 30 days or longer, a mild, self-limiting or severe, prolonged disease may follow. Patients typically experience a fever which may be intermittent or irregular, and so is also known as undulant fever. Other common symptoms include chills, depression, weakness, headache, joint pain, generalized aches and sweating.[40]

Papular to pustular skin rashes which are sometimes evident on the arms of veterinarians following obstetric procedures have been attributed to allergy to *Brucella*, but sensitivity to other pathogens including *Salmonella dublin*, *Salmonella typhimurium* and *Listeria monocytogenes*, have also been incriminated.[8]

Pathogenesis

The establishment of infection is influenced by the size of the infective dose, virulence of the bacteria, and the resistance, age, sex and reproductive status of the animal.[109]

Brucella abortus readily penetrates mucous membranes such as those of the pharynx and alimentary tract, and survives and multiplies particularly in cells of the reticulo-endothelial system.[8, 99, 109] After penetration, the organisms are phagocytosed by neutrophils and macrophages which carry them to the regional lymph nodes, where they multiply and cause a lymphadenitis which may persist for months. Multiplication of the organism here may be followed by a bacteraemia which may last for several months, resolve itself, or be recurrent for at least two years in 5–10 per cent of animals. Recurrence occurs particularly at the time of parturition.

During the bacteraemia, organisms are carried intracellularly in neutrophils and macrophages or free in the plasma[20] and localize in various organs, especially the gravid uterus, udder, and supramammary lymph nodes.

Localization may also occur in other lymph nodes and the spleen, testes, and male accessory sex glands.[85] Occasionally bacterial localization occurs in synovial structures causing a purulent tendovaginitis, arthritis or bursitis.[50, 68]

Localization of the infection in the endometrium of the gravid uterus and in foetal membranes of cattle appears to be the result of the special affinity of the organism for erythritol,[38, 71, 99, 109, 115] elevated levels of which occur in the placenta and foetal fluids from about the fifth month of gestation. The chorionic epithelium becomes parasitized and infection extends to the placental stroma, blood vessels, and ultimately to the foetus.[109] There is considerable variation in the uterine and placental lesions in both natural and experimental *B. abortus* infections, and foetuses that become infected late in gestation may be aborted without any grossly recognizable placental lesions. Depending on the severity of the placentitis, abortion, premature birth or the birth of a viable or non-viable calf may result.[68] Because the non-pregnant uterus is not particularly susceptible to *B. abortus*, it is cleared of the organisms within a few weeks of abortion or parturition.

Tolerance to erythritol by some strain 19 variants may be the reason for occasional persistent infection with strain 19 and abortion,[14] but erythritol-sensitive strains do also occur.

Up to 35 per cent of cows may be resistant to *B. abortus* as a result of the greater bacteriostatic activity of their macrophages against *B. abortus* than is the case in susceptible cows.[53] Macrophage oxidative-burst activity and differences in macrophage bacteriostatic activity against *B. abortus* are significantly enhanced in cows that are resistant to infection. It is thought that the level of macrophage function, which is reduced in susceptible cows, plays a role in the establishment of chronic infections.[53]

In acute *Brucella* infections in cows an increase in the level of IgM in the serum is the first evidence of antibody response. IgG soon becomes the predominant antibody and usually persists for as long as the animal remains infected, while the IgM level wanes. Of the two subclasses of IgG in the serum, IgG_1 is the most abundant and predominant agglutinating and complement fixing antibody.[99]

The main antigenic stimulation is provided by antigens in the cell wall. Treatment with steroid hormones[82] and certain antibiotics (such as penicillin and oxytetracyclines) may induce the L-form due to interference with cell-wall synthesis.[8] This may result in the lack of a humoral antibody response.

Humoral antibodies do not provide the main protective immunity, whereas cell-mediated immunity against *Brucella* is the most important defence mechanism. Lymphocyte stimulation is greater in cattle infected by virulent strains of *B. abortus* than in animals vaccinated with strain 19.[69] In cattle infected with field strains of *B. abortus*, there is a direct correlation between cell-mediated immunity and humoral antibody response, whereas in those vaccinated with strain 19 there is no correlation as measured by lymphocyte stimulation and antibody titres. It is possible that *B. abortus* has developed multiple mechanisms to ensure its intracellular survival and it appears that these are more resistant to intracellular than extracellular defence mechanisms.[95]

Clinical signs

The length of the incubation period of bovine brucellosis varies tremendously and has been variously defined as the period between exposure and abortion,[22] the period between exposure and the first appearance of clinical disease, or the period before the first serological evidence of infection can be detected.[85] The latter definition is preferred in heifers and cows, as not all infected animals manifest clinical signs. In bulls this period is even more imprecise, as serological evidence of infection may be equivocal or lacking, and clinical signs may be absent. The length of the incubation period is also affected by the size of the infective dose, and the age, sex, stage of gestation, and immunity of the infected animal. In cows that eventually abort, the usual length of the incubation period varies according to the time at which infection occurred. Cows infected at service abort after an average interval of 225 days, whereas those infected at seven months gestation abort about 50 days later.[110] Congenitally infected calves may remain seronegative for at least 18 months, after which they manifest clinical signs. The longest recorded 'incubation period' in a cow is nine years.[73]

The abortion rate in infected herds is dependent on many factors and varies according to the susceptibility of the pregnant females, management practices, the severity of the challenge, the period for which the herd has been infected, and various environmental factors such as the quality of pastures (which may affect cattle density), the climate and the topography.[8, 38, 85] In fully susceptible herds, abortion rates vary from 30 to 70 per cent, but in South Africa it seldom exceeds 50 per cent. Increased public awareness, veterinary intervention, improved management practices and vaccination have all contributed to making the disease in these herds assume a more insidious, chronic form. In many closed herds very few or no abortions occur and the disease is almost impossible to recognize clinically.

Abortions typically occur at approximately five to seven months of gestation, although some occur earlier or later. Weak, full-term calves that often die shortly after birth are sometimes encountered. About 20 per cent of infected animals do not abort,[38] while 80 per cent of animals that abort as a result of *B. abortus* infection do so only once.[38] The placenta is not consistently retained after abortion but when it is retained, metritis is common. In an average outbreak, there is as much as a 20 per cent reduction in the milk production of the herd.[46] Early abortion results in a 40–50 per cent loss in the milk yield. Infection of the udder is clinically inapparent and the organ appears to be normal when palpated.[80, 81]

In bulls, an acute to chronic, uni- or bilateral orchitis, epididymitis, and seminal vesiculitis occasionally occur.[112] The scrotal circumference in these animals may be normal or severely increased.[18] Strain 19 vaccination may also cause orchitis.

Uni- or bilateral hygromas, especially of the carpal joints, may be evident in some animals in chronically infected herds,[49, 68, 116] or may occasionally follow inoculation of heifers with strain 19 vaccine.[32] A progressive, erosive, non-suppurative arthritis of the stifle joints has been reported in young cattle from brucellosis-free herds that were vaccinated with strain 19 vaccine.[116]

Pathology

Irrespective of the route of infection, the organism provokes a regional lymphadenitis which is characterized by reticuloendothelial cell and lymphoid hyperplasia, as well as the infiltration of large numbers of mononuclear cells and some neutrophils, and a few eosinophils and plasma cells.[68] Other lymph nodes in the body may be affected later in the course of the infection but to a lesser degree.[68, 88] Similar changes may be evident in the spleen.[88]

There is considerable variation in the severity of the uterine lesions at abortion.[68] As the disease progresses, lesions advance from an acute (mild to severe) to chronic endometritis. Microscopically, the endometrium is infiltrated by lymphocytes and plasma cells, and some neutrophils. Microgranulomas may be scattered in the endometrium.[68, 88]

The chorion is not uniformly affected and large parts may appear quite normal. The lesions in and at the periphery of the cotyledons, as well as those in the intercotyledonary area, vary in extent, appearing to be most severe adjacent to cotyledons. The affected cotyledons, or parts of them, are covered by a sticky, odourless, brownish exudate, and are yellowish-grey as a result of necrosis **(Figure 124.1)**. Parts of the intercotelydonary placenta are thickened, oedematous, yellowish-grey and may contain exudate on the surface. Microscopically, the stroma of the chorion is infiltrated by numerous mononuclear cells and some neutrophils. Some chorionic villi are necrotic, while a fibrinopurulent exudate and desquamated necrotic chorionic epithelial cells are accumulated between the villi. Many of the chorionic epithelial cells are packed with numerous intracytoplasmic bacteria **(Figure 124.2)**. Vasculitis, sometimes accompanied by thrombosis, may be evident in the chorion.

Some aborted foetuses have varying degrees of subcutaneous oedema and blood-tinged fluid in the thoracic and abdominal cavities, while the abomasal content is sometimes turbid, bright yellow and flaky. In some foetuses, greyish-white foci of pneumonia, 1 mm or larger in diameter, may be present, particularly in the apical lobes **(Figure 124.3)**. A fibrinous pleuritis sometimes accompanies the pneumonia. The liver is usually enlarged, discoloured orange-brown, and its surface may have a slightly uneven appearance. Many foetuses show no gross changes. Microscopically most aborted foetuses reveal a multifocal bronchopneumonia, bronchitis and bronchiolitis characterized by the accumulation of cellular debris, neutrophils and macrophages in the lumen of the bronchi and bronchioli, patchy desquamation of bronchial epithelial cells, and a mild to moderate infiltration of mononuclear cells and some neutrophils in the alveolar septa. Vasculitis of some of the pulmonary vessels may be seen. Isolated small foci of necrosis or microgranulomas are often found in the liver, but may also occur in the lymph nodes, spleen and kidneys. In most aborted foetuses it is not possible — or is very difficult — to demonstrate organisms in tissue sections, notwithstanding that they may have been specially stained for *Brucella*. However, it is easy to demonstrate the organisms in smears made from the abomasal content or wall and that have been stained with Stamp's modification of the Ziehl Neelsen stain.

The udder in infected cows does not show any gross lesions, although the supramammary lymph nodes may be somewhat enlarged.[80, 81] Microscopically, infection of the udder is characterized by a lymphoplasmacytic and histiocytic interstitial mastitis, while the regional lymph nodes show lymphoid hyperplasia, medullary plasmacytosis and sinus histiocytosis.[80, 81]

Acute orchitis is characterized by multifocal or diffuse necrosis of the testicular parenchyma, and a focal, necrotizing epididymitis may occur. Microscopically the seminal epithelial cells are necrotic and desquamate; large numbers of organisms are present in them, while numerous leukocytes, particularly neutrophils, and fibrin occur in the affected tubuli and interstitial tissues. In the chronic stage, spermatic granulomas develop in the testicular parenchyma and epididymis in response to dead sperm.[68, 113]

In horses, infection may localize in the bursa between the nuchal ligament, the atlas and axis causing poll evil. Fistulous withers caused by *B. abortus* is characterized by inflammation of the bursa between the nuchal ligament and the dorsal spines of the thoracic vertebrae.[99] Chronic draining sinuses are formed in both conditions.

Brucellae in cattle may localize in the carpal and other bursae, where hygromas containing large numbers of the pathogen may be found.[8] *Brucella abortus* strain 19 may cause gonitis in calves or arthropathy in cows.[32, 116]

Diagnosis

Because of the variable incubation period and the often subclinical nature of the disease in most animals, a definitive diagnosis should be based on the isolation and identification of *B. abortus* and on positive serological

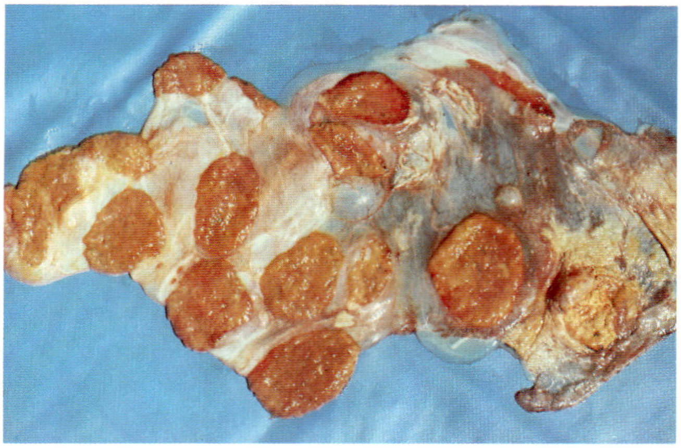

Figure 124.1 Note the mottled appearance of the cotyledons in the placenta of a cow infected with *Brucella abortus*

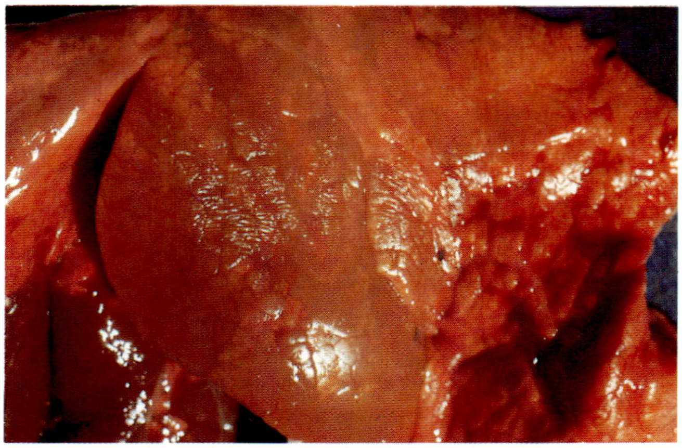

Figure 124.3 Bronchopneumonia in a *Brucella abortus*-infected foetus

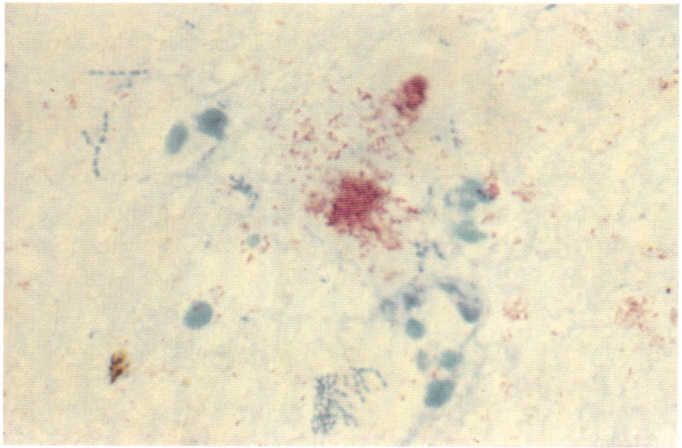

Figure 124.2 Large intracytoplasmic colony of *Brucella abortus* (Stamp's stain)

results based on the detection of antibodies in blood, milk, whey, vaginal mucus, or seminal plasma.

The isolation of *B. abortus* is mandatory when dealing with specific groups or herds of animals when there is doubt about their infection status. When a herd is known to be infected and where its environment is infected, serological reactors are viewed in a different light from those in a herd in which reactions might be due to the use of strain 19 vaccine. When assessing serological results it is difficult to prescribe strict cut-off points which will apply in all cases where a live vaccine has been used. It is preferable to interpret serological test results according to the known infection status of the herd. As stated by Brinley Morgan:[22]

> I have found in my experience over the past twenty-five years working with *Brucella* that you are invariably wearing at least two hats. One is where you are in a very clean environment where you can take an awful lot of chances and the other hat is where you are working in an infected environment where you cannot afford to take any chances at all.

Failure to isolate *B. abortus* in a herd may result in difficulty in interpreting serological results.

Diagnostic tests for bovine brucellosis are subdivided into three groups — tests for the demonstration of *B. abortus* organisms, those which detect immunoglobulins, and those dependent on allergic reactions to *B. abortus*.[47] The 'ideal' diagnostic test should detect infection early, during the long and variable incubation period; not be influenced by the presence of 'non-specific' antibodies; detect carriers; and differentiate between responses to vaccination and those due to field infection.[22] There is no single test available that completely satisfies all these requirements.

Tests for the demonstration of B. abortus

Culture

The specimens of choice include foetal membranes; the lungs, stomach-content, liver and spleen of aborted foetuses and full-term calves; and uterine discharge, milk or colostrum of infected cows.

The supramammary lymph node is the most suitable specimen from carcasses of adult animals, but the retropharyngeal, mandibular, iliac, or prescapular and parotid lymph nodes may also be collected. Other specimens which may be submitted include the uterus, milk and udder tissue, fluid aspirated from hygromas, and male accessory sex glands and testes.[34, 60, 112] Isolation may also be attempted from the semen or seminal plasma of infected bulls.

The supramammary lymph nodes are preferred for isolation of *B. abortus* from animals that have been slaughtered, and a 90 per cent recovery rate from infected animals may be achieved. Recovery of *B. abortus* on culture from infected adult cows may approach 100 per cent using the supramammary, parotid, mandibular and sub-iliac nodes. Isolation of the pathogen from infected heifers is best achieved through the culture of the mandibular lymph nodes, and this probably reflects the primary route of infection through the conjunctiva or the nasal or oral mucosa.[34] When specimens of larger groups of animals (five or more) must be cultured, collection of only the left and right supramammary lymph nodes will suffice.[16, 45]

Microscopic examination

Using Stamp's modification of the Ziehl Neelsen stain,[101] *B. abortus* stains red against a blue background in tissue sections and smears. However, this colour reaction is not specific for *Brucella*, as *Coxiella*, *Chlamydia* and *Nocardia* spp. are also weakly acid-fast, but *Nocardia* spp. can be differentiated from these organisms on morphological grounds, *Chlamydia* is much smaller than *Brucella* spp. while *Coxiella* is virtually indistinguishable from *Brucella* spp.

Tests for the detection of specific immunoglobulins

Serological diagnostic tests are suitable for use in large-scale campaigns and in the eradication of the disease from large herds.[5, 58] In South Africa, serum samples are screened with the Rose Bengal test (RBT), while the complement fixation test (CFT) is used as the definitive test. The slow (tube) agglutination test (SAT) is sometimes used as a supplementary test and has some value in detecting IgM, the persistent and often predominant immunoglobulin resulting from vaccination with strain 19 vaccine.[8, 22, 103] The milk-ring test (MRT) is also used to screen and monitor bulk milk samples.

The length of time between exposure and the consequent serological response is dependent on the stage of gestation. Following infection at four to six months gestation, the SAT and CFT become positive after about four weeks. If the animals are infected two months before or after insemination, these tests become positive about ten weeks later, but this pattern is not consistent in all animals, as some infected cows or heifers may remain serologically negative for up to 21 days or longer after calving or aborting.[92]

Colostral antibodies may cause calves to be serologically positive for about four months from birth.[18, 92]

Reliance on serological tests alone for the diagnosis of brucellosis in bulls can be misleading, because both false-negative and false-positive results may be obtained.[82, 91] All bulls from infected herds should be viewed with suspicion and the diagnosis should be based on clinical examination (including palpation of the seminal vesicles and ampullae), serological tests, and bacteriological and antibody examination of semen.[91]

Milk-ring test (MRT)

The milk-ring test is used to detect antibodies in milk, and the development of a positive reaction is dependent on two reactions: (a) the fat globules in the milk are aggregated by milk antibodies (fat-globule agglutinins); and (b) the added stained *Brucella* cells (antigen) are agglutinated by the *Brucella* antibody/fat-globule complexes which rise to form a coloured cream layer at the top.[21] This is a sensitive screening test used on bulk milk samples either to detect infected animals on a herd basis or to monitor clean herds. It should be carried out at least quarterly to ensure that all animals that come into lactation are screened. The sensitivity of the MRT is somewhat reduced when it is applied to large herds with few reactors (the probability of the MRT detecting one reactor in different-sized herds is indicated in **Table 124.1**[97]), but this loss in sensitivity in large herds of 150 or more animals can be counteracted to some extent by decreasing the ratio of antigen to milk in the test.[5] Despite its reduced sensitivity in these large herds, the MRT has been very successfully used to monitor the brucellosis-free status of dairy herds.[8, 46] When the MRT is applied to individual cows, a fairly high proportion of false-positive results may be obtained, but this can be countered by diluting the milk to be tested with known brucellosis-negative milk at a ratio of 1:10 and repeating the test, or by carrying out serial dilutions of the samples.[5] A titre of 1:16 or more can often be correlated with the presence of *B. abortus* in the milk.

Factors that may cause false-positive results include a high prevalence of mastitis; a high proportion of cows in early or late lactation; recent (within three to four months) vaccination with strain 19 vaccine; and souring of milk. Milk samples may be preserved for testing by adding a 0,5 ml formalin solution to a 10 ml milk sample (formalin solution is prepared by mixing 7,5 ml of 37 per cent formaldehyde with 1 litre of distilled water).[5] Milk samples have been successfully preserved with 0,2 ml 2-bromo-2 mitro-1,3 propane diol per ml of milk for simultaneous MRT and somatic cell counts.[16]

The duration and temperature at which samples are stored (in particular excessive heating, such as storing for longer than five minutes at 45 °C) may cause false negatives.[46] Pasteurized milk cannot be effectively tested by the MRT.[5]

Rose Bengal test (RBT)

The RBT is a modification of the plate-agglutination test. The antigen, which has been stained with Rose Bengal stain, is buffered at a pH of 3,65.[66] At this level of activity,

Table 124.1 The probability of the milk-ring test detecting one reactor cow in herds of different sizes[96]

Number of cows in production in the herd	Estimated probability of detecting one reactor cow
1	0,993
2	0,984
4	0,967
8	0,931
12	0,871
25	0,818
50	0,696
100	0,521
200	0,389
400	0,248

'non-specific' agglutinins are destroyed and IgG, normally the most abundant antibody in the serum of infected animals, agglutinates strongly.[22, 66] Equal volumes (25 µl) of test serum and antigen are mixed, shaken for four minutes and viewed over an x-ray viewer.[58] Any degree of agglutination is recorded as positive. Because of its very high sensitivity, this test is only used as a screening test in those herds where the prevalence of brucellosis is low and the percentage of vaccinated cattle high. In South Africa, all sera are first screened with the RBT and those that are negative are usually not tested further. All sera that test positive are subjected to the CFT. In order for a herd to qualify for accreditation in the official South African Bovine Brucellosis Scheme, all animals must be CFT-negative in the final two tests.

The test is inexpensive and easy to perform. False-negative results are rare and are usually obtained during the early stages of the incubation period of the disease. Despite improved specificity at an acid pH, a high percentage of false-positive reactions occur, usually due to the presence of IgM as a result of strain 19 vaccination.

Complement fixation test (CFT)

This test is very sensitive and specific and is regarded throughout the world as the definitive test of choice for the serological detection of infected animals. The CFT has been modified, standardized and adapted to a microtitre system.[58] In South Africa, warm fixation, as opposed to cold fixation which is used in certain countries, is preferred, mainly because it is quicker and more convenient. The test results are rarely complicated by non-specific reactions[22] and, unlike the SAT, the titres do not wane as the disease becomes chronic. Results are measured in International Units (IU/ml).[58, 62] In South Africa, 30 IU/ml or higher is considered positive in those animals that have been vaccinated during calfhood (four to eight months old), or in adult animals that have not been vaccinated, whereas 60 IU/ml or higher is regarded as positive in animals that have been vaccinated as adults.[58] These guidelines may be applied rigorously where strain 19 vaccine has not been used for several years, as is the case in most of the United Kingdom, but its strict application in countries enforcing compulsory vaccination (such as South Africa) is often problematic and sometimes leads to unacceptably large numbers of false positives. Considerable expertise and experience are needed to certify herds, or individual animals, free of brucellosis when they exceed these values, and a departure from these guidelines can be considered only if the following epidemiological criteria are taken into account:

- the herd is closed and has been closed for at least two years;
- the herd is closed except for introductions from certified-free herds;
- there is no evidence of spread within the herd (strain 19 infection does not spread);[54]
- all cows that aborted were tested negative for *B. abortus*;
- the lymph nodes of animals with high titres, and which have been slaughtered, are negative for wild strains of *B. abortus* and/or have yielded strain 19 on culture;
- the foetal membranes and uterine discharge of cows exhibiting high titres are negative on culture;
- milk samples from reactors yielded strain 19 or are negative for the wild strain of *B. abortus*;
- the possibility of infection having been introduced from a neighbouring infected herd is ruled out;
- vaccine titres, as a rule, tend to decline faster than those due to infection with wild strains.

Although the CFT is useful when differentiating calfhood vaccination titres from those due to wild-strain infection, there may be difficulty in distinguishing vaccine reactions from those caused by wild strains when animals have been repeatedly vaccinated or after they have become sexually mature.[14] Haphazard vaccination of heifers and vaccination of adult animals may result in much confusion in the interpretation of laboratory results, and it is therefore essential that accurate records of vaccination and birth dates be kept to allow correct interpretation of the results of the CFT. In Britain it has been estimated that persistent reactors in brucellosis-free herds occur in less than 0,5 per cent of vaccinated heifers,[22] but 16 per cent of cows in brucellosis-free herds in New Zealand have been shown to develop CFT titres of 1:8 or greater which persisted for at least 12 months after strain 19 vaccination.[14] Persistent titres are significantly fewer when sexually mature cows, which have been vaccinated as calves, are revaccinated. In South Africa the use of low-dose vaccination of sexually mature heifers causes a similar pattern.[16] Very high CFT titres are found in some adult animals that have not been vaccinated as calves and which have been inoculated immediately prior to, or after initial conception. Titres of *c.* 5 000 IU/ml may be found in up to 9 per cent of animals of some herds (mainly Jersey) that have been free of brucellosis for many years.

Slow (tube) agglutination test (SAT)

Notwithstanding its being less specific and less sensitive than the CFT, the SAT is still very useful as a supplementary test and may be used as an indicator of the levels of serum IgM, the predominant immunoglobulin after vaccination with strain 19 vaccine. When combined with the CFT, the SAT is used as an additional screening test for sera that are positive to the RBT. The probability of detecting false-negative CFT reactions due to the prozone phenomenon or human error can be improved, since there is no easy way to achieve a control on the CFT results.[22, 63, 64] Non-specific agglutination in sera is decreased by the addition of EDTA with no decrease in *B. abortus* agglutination titres of sera from infected cattle.[51, 75]

Indirect haemolysis test (IHLT)[89]

This test may be applied in the later stages of brucellosis eradication schemes and, when used as a supplementary test together with the CFT, detects a greater number of infected animals than the CFT used alone. Little advantage is gained by using the IHLT instead of the CFT as a definitive test, but used in conjunction with the CFT it can be a useful supplementary test.[89, 106, 107] The prozone phenomenon, which may be somewhat troublesome in the CFT, is not a factor with the IHLT. Strain 19 vaccination influences the interpretation of IHLT less than that of the CFT.[106]

The enzyme-linked immunosorbent assay (ELISA)

This test is considerably more sensitive when detecting antibodies to *Brucella* than are the RBT, SAT, CFT and IHLT,[26, 104, 105] but with the exception of the RBT, is less specific than any of these.[104] The ELISA assay may be used with telling effect in unvaccinated herds,[113] but great care must be exercised in animals vaccinated with strain 19 vaccine.[26, 104, 105] The use of monoclonal antibodies in the competitive ELISA has improved the specificity of the test.[98, 105]

The vaginal mucus agglutination test

This test may be an aid in detecting individual infected animals, but it appears to have no advantage over serological tests.[96]

Test to demonstrate the allergic reaction to B. abortus

There has been some disagreement over the value of this test, mainly because of problems with its sensitivity.[5] An intradermal brucellin test for the diagnosis of brucellosis has been used in extensively-managed herds in New Zealand,[74] and although the sensitivity of the test, compared to the CFT, varied between 52 and 62 per cent, its specificity exceeded 99 per cent. It is claimed that this test is a useful low-cost method of identifying infected herds rather than individual animals.[5] Calfhood vaccination using strain 19 does not appear to complicate interpretation of the brucellin test, whereas the use of an adjuvant vaccine, such as 45/20, causes prolonged sensitivity to *Brucella* allergens.

Differential diagnosis

Numerous infectious agents may cause foetal loss and abortion in cattle. A multidisciplinary approach involving pathology, microbiology and toxicology is of benefit when making a definitive diagnosis.[57] Microscopic examination of smears or histopathological sections, particularly of the placenta, stained with the modified Ziehl Neelsen method, may present difficulties in differentiating *B. abortus* morphologically from *Coxiella burnetii* or *Chlamydia psittaci*. *Brucella abortus* can be distinguished from *Coxiella* and *Chlamydia* spp. by fluorescent antibody techniques and serological tests.[30]

Brucella abortus may cross-react serologically, with *B. melitensis* in particular but also with *E. coli* serogroup 0:157, *Yersinia enterocolitica* serovar 0:9, *Salmonella* serovars of the Kaufmann-White group N, *Francisella tularensis, Pseudomonas maltophilia*, and *Vibrio cholerae*.[5] Such cross-reactions are probably not of great significance in eradication campaigns unless the prevalence of the disease has been reduced to a very low level.

Control

Treatment of bovine brucellosis is not normally undertaken. *Brucella abortus* may undergo L-transformation when exposed to certain antibiotics such as penicillin and oxytetracycline.[8] The effect that these cell-wall-deficient forms have in preventing serological detection and the resultant creation of carrier animals requires further investigation. The elimination of carrier cattle from infected herds by the use of oxytetracycline[92] likewise needs confirmation.

The planning and management of control or eradication programmes for brucellosis have been investigated in many countries, and recently by the World Health Organization.[8] Strategies based on the prevention of spread between animals, the monitoring of brucellosis-free herds and zones, the elimination of infected animals by test and slaughter, strict 'one-way' movement of infected and suspect cattle, mass immunization to reduce the infection rate, and supporting specific education and training programmes have all received attention.[8, 100]

In the Australian Brucellosis Control Plan, eradication areas were defined as being those with a prevalence of not more than 2 per cent.[46] In South Africa, herds with a prevalence of 10–20 per cent have been cleared of the disease while incurring losses that were still economically acceptable.[61]

In South Africa, bovine brucellosis is listed as a state-controlled disease, and its control and eradication are given high priority by the Directorate of Animal Health. The control and eradication of bovine brucellosis here is broadly based on a test-and-slaughter policy, the vaccination of heifer calves, and the prohibition of the sale and movement of infected cattle.

Good progress towards achieving eradication has been made in some regions in South Africa; in 1975 the prevalence in Natal was estimated at 9,0 per cent, and this had been reduced to 0,6 per cent by 1988.[10]

It is extremely difficult to be prescriptive when recommending a strategy for the control or eradication of brucellosis that will be applicable or practical in all circumstances. Broadly-based national strategies and policies will invariably differ according to the situation in each instance. The approaches to be adopted when attempting to eradicate the disease will vary markedly according to whether one is dealing with an infected herd or an uninfected (vaccine-reactions) herd. Application of control measures on individual farms is also frequently affected by a variety of other factors. These include the infection rate in the herd; duration of infection; the abortion rate; whether an extensive or intensive farming system is being practised; rainfall; whether it is a beef or dairy herd; vaccine cover; the availability of or necessity for replacement stock; the financial situation of the producer; the proximity to a veterinary laboratory; neighbourhood cooperation; milk and slaughter quotas; slaughter prices of dairy cows; the availability of camps and suitable calving facilities; availability of veterinary guidance; and handling facilities necessary to collect blood from large groups of cattle.[46, 100]

The following principles have been found to be crucial to the successful control or eradication of brucellosis:

- reliable diagnostic techniques;
- close cooperation and joint effort by the owner, laboratory and veterinarian;
- good records;
- education of the farming community and public awareness;
- established procedures for handling the disease;
- controlled movement of cattle; and
- permanent marking of infected animals.

Application of these principles has led to the successful eradication of bovine brucellosis in a number of countries throughout the world.[18]

Vaccination in conjunction with other measures can be used effectively in the control or eradication of brucellosis, and in general it is recommended that all heifer calves should be immunized where the prevalence of brucellosis in an area, region, province or country is high, and that cessation of immunization with strain 19 vaccine should be considered only when the prevalence of the infection is reduced to 0,2 per cent or less.[2, 8]

In 1906 Bang observed that cattle could be protected against brucellosis by vaccinating them with live cultures. Since then two avirulent strains of *B. abortus*, strain 19[24, 35] and strain 45/20,[79] that are used for the preparation of vaccine have been studied extensively. Strain 19 is stable, whereas strain 45/20 is inclined to lose its rough characteristics and revert to the smooth form when used as a live vaccine.[108] Strain 19 vaccines used in the USA prior to 1956 contained erythritol-tolerant variants, but those produced since then are erythritol-sensitive.[23]

Vaccination with strain 19 vaccine increases resistance to *B. abortus* but does not produce absolute immunity, and vaccination is not curative. This increase in resistance following vaccination has been termed 'relative immunity', since it is estimated to be only about 70 per cent effective against field challenge.[8, 83]

Strain 19 is the only brucellosis vaccine presently allowed in South Africa. It is of low virulence when used in cows, but it may cause orchitis in bulls and undulant fever in humans when they are accidentally injected. Systemic reactions are rare after the use of this vaccine, although they appear to be fairly frequent in the Jersey breed.[18] Temperature reactions varying from 40,5–42 °C, lasting for two to three days may occur in addition to swelling at the injection site. Abortion in less than 1 per cent of vaccinated cows in late pregnancy has also been reported.[84] The vaccine does not appear to interfere with the conception rate and there is no evidence of the spread of strain 19 to unvaccinated cattle.[83] It is thought that strain 19 vaccine raises immunity to field strains of *B. abortus* and, by preventing unrestricted multiplication in the uterus and mammary glands, excretion in the milk is less frequent than in non-vaccinated cattle.[83] Although it may be intermittently present in the milk of vaccinated cows, there is no evidence of infection in humans who have ingested milk containing strain 19 organisms.[84]

Strain 19 vaccine must be stored correctly and the cold chain maintained to retain its full potency. It is for this reason that lyophilization has proved so successful in the preservation of the vaccine.[8, 18] On reconstitution, the lyophilized vaccine should be used on the same day, preferably within three hours.

Traditionally the dose of strain 19 vaccine administered to heifer calves at four to eight months of age contains 5×10^{10} viable *Brucella* organisms.[8] The calfhood strain 19 vaccine produced at the Veterinary Research Institute, Onderstepoort, contains $4–12 \times 10^{10}$ viable organisms per dose, and a single dose of this vaccine inoculated at five months generally provides life-long relative immunity, although virtually all immunized female calves lose their serum-antibody titres by the age of 16 to 18 months. Because of interference by colostral antibodies, vaccination of heifers at five weeks is not as effective as at five months of age.[22, 38]

Vaccination of heifers practically eliminates the occurrence of abortions in a herd.[84] A gradual reduction in the prevalence of bovine brucellosis may be expected when 80 per cent of the female population has been vaccinated.[8] This vaccination pressure must be maintained for optimal results.

In the event of an outbreak, the vaccination of adult cattle with strain 19 vaccine may be advantageous — particularly in large dairy herds and in herds where a large proportion of the animals have not been previously vaccinated.[8] The rate of abortions may decrease a few months after vaccinating the adult cows.[84] The disadvantages of vaccinating adult animals include the development of vaccine reactions, a positive milk-ring test, and the stigma attached to vaccinated adult animals because of their association with positive herds.

In South Africa, adult vaccination is restricted by law to individual farms and may only be given when written permission by the state to do so has been given. However, since this practice complicates the interpretation of serological results for a considerable period, its use may be unacceptable in eradication campaigns.[14]

A strain 19 vaccine containing reduced numbers of organisms ($2 \times 10^8–3 \times 10^9$/dose) for use in adult animals has been extensively assessed,[3, 4, 13, 85, 87] and it was found that 15 per cent of cows which were vaccinated when three to five months pregnant developed CFT titres which persisted for 12 months or longer.[14] Similar results were obtained when sexually mature heifers were inoculated with a reduced-dose strain 19 vaccine.[16] The occurrence of these persistent titres was noticeably less in cows which had been subjected to calfhood vaccination. It has been suggested that adult vaccination of uninfected herds with reduced-dose strain 19 vaccine should not be undertaken because of its interference with serological and milk-ring tests.[14]

A policy of using a reduced-dose vaccine containing $3 \times 10^{8-9}$ organisms/dose in calves of four to 12 months of age has been introduced in the USA.[8]

Mature cows vaccinated with $3–10 \times 10^8$ organisms/dose are protected for at least 12 months,[8] but most (90–95 per cent) of the vaccinated animals lose their CFT titres within six months. Five to 10 per cent of animals, however, may remain serologically positive for eight to 12 months or longer and strain 19 organisms may be isolated from the milk of these animals.

Administration of strain 19 vaccine in the conjunctival sac (two doses of $5–10 \times 10^{10}$ at four and eight months of age, respectively) results in good protection and the almost complete elimination of serological reactions in heifers and adults.[86, 87]

Strain 45/20 has been used with considerable success in an inactivated vaccine incorporating an oil adjuvant,[38] but it is not as protective as strain 19 vaccine in animals less than nine months old. Two consecutive vaccinations with strain 45/20 vaccine are usually recommended six to 12 weeks apart. Large, unsightly granulomas may develop at the site of injection with some batches of strain 45/20.[38] Post-vaccinal agglutination and CFT titres as a result of vaccination with strain 45/20 vaccine are not as high as those caused by strain 19 vaccine.

A smooth strain of *B. suis*, Biovar 1 strain 2, has been in use as an oral vaccine to control brucellosis in cattle, sheep, goats and pigs in China since 1971.[8, 117] This vaccine protects cattle against *B. abortus*, is safe if administered orally, does not induce persistent antibody titres and can be administered without having to restrain the animal.[117] The *B. suis* vaccine can only be used orally as it causes abortion if injected intramuscularly or subcutaneously into pregnant sheep or goats. This vaccine has been used widely and with great success in China for nearly 20 years, but is unlikely to be allowed into South Africa as *B. suis* has not been diagnosed in this country or in the subcontinent.

Control by test-and-slaughter, management and hygiene

The reduction in numbers of infected animals and their rapid elimination are essential in the control or eradication of brucellosis. All calves in infected herds should be regarded as potential sources of infection.[8] The 'two-year breakdown syndrome' (previously infected herds which have been apparently clear for about two years and which break down after this period) has been ascribed to latently infected calves which remain serologically negative until at least mid-gestation or later during their first pregnancy.[38] However, brucellosis has been eradicated in several countries without slaughtering calves born to infected dams.

Cows should calve in an environment which can be thoroughly cleaned and disinfected with 2,5 per cent formalin. Wet and well-grassed calving camps should be avoided, and vehicles used for transporting infected animals should be disinfected after use. Isolation of cows prior to and after parturition contributes significantly to the control of brucellosis,[8] and in addition, cows that abort should be isolated immediately and tested serologically soon afterwards. If negative, they should be retested two to three weeks later. Positive animals should be culled. Foetuses, placentas and discharges must be disposed of, preferably by incineration. Chlorhexidine gluconate may be used to disinfect hands.

It is important to maintain regular blood-testing in infected herds.[36] Serological tests at intervals of two to three months and bacteriological examination of aborted foetuses, placentas, lochia and milk are often of great benefit. The judicious use of the MRT to monitor progress within a herd and to detect spread at an early stage can have telling effects. Milk from negative animals should be tested regularly at short intervals.

It is important to prevent, or in outbreaks at least limit, the spread of the disease. Depending on circumstances on a farm, the availability of spare camps can be advantageous, particularly where it is deemed necessary to split the herd into two or more groups. The two-herd system, based on the segregation of weaner heifers and adults, can be highly effective in extensive farming operations.[100] It is often not possible to cull all infected animals at the outset of the eradication campaign, but it is vitally important to separate them from the 'negative' herd. The creation of another 'suspect' group of animals, and the effective separation of cows from four months' gestation onwards may be beneficial. Replacement stock should be purchased from herds certified free of brucellosis.

Whatever strategy is to be adopted, the owner must be fully aware of the implications of the proposed control programme. The co-operation of neighbouring farmers may be of assistance in this respect.

Decisive action is important in dealing with an infected herd. The 'negative' herd must be maintained as such and any contact with infected animals avoided. All animals diagnosed as bacteriologically or serologically positive should be regarded as infected and must be identified permanently, preferably by branding. Undoubtedly an element of 'overkill' is built into a somewhat uncompromising and apparently ruthless approach in these programmes, but the long-term benefits far outweigh this short-term disadvantage. The economic implications of a test-and-slaughter eradication policy must also be taken into account.[39]

References

1 **ALEXANDER, B., SCHNURRENBERGER, P.R. & BROWN, R.R., 1981.** Numbers of *Brucella abortus* in the placenta, umbilicus and foetal fluid of two naturally infected cows. *The Veterinary Record*, 108, 500.

2 **ALTON, G.G., 1978.** Recent developments in vaccination against bovine brucellosis. *Australian Veterinary Journal*, 54, 551–557.

3 **ALTON, G.G. & CORNER, L.A., 1981.** Vaccination of heifers with a reduced dose of *Brucella abortus* strain 19 vaccine before first mating. *Australian Veterinary Journal*, 57, 548–550.

4 **ALTON, G.G., CORNER, L.A. & PLACKETT, P., 1980.** Vaccination of pregnant cows with doses of *Brucella abortus* strain 19 vaccine. *Australian Veterinary Journal*, 56, 369–372.

5 **ALTON, G.G., JONES, L.M., ANGUS, R.D. & VERGER, J.M., 1988.** *Techniques for the Brucellosis Laboratory*. 1st edn. Paris: Institut National de la Recherche Agronomique.

6 **ALTON, G.G., JONES, L.M. & PEITZ, D.E., 1975.** *Laboratory Techniques in Brucellosis*. 2nd edn. Monograph Series no. 55. Geneva: World Health Organization.

7 **ANON., 1957.** Obituary notice: L.E. Bevan. *The Veterinary Record*, 69, 421–422.

8 **ANON., 1986.** JOINT FAO/WHO Expert Committee on Brucellosis. *World Health Organization Technical Report Series*, 740, WHO, Geneva.

9 **ANON., 1987.** Directorate of Veterinary Services, Annual Report. South West Africa.

10 **ANON., 1988/89.** Annual Report, Director of Animal Health, Directorate of Veterinary Services, Private Bag X138, Pretoria, South Africa.

11 **ANON., 1989/90.** Annual Report, State Veterinarian, Skukuza, P.O. Box 12, Skukuza, South Africa.

12 **ANON., 1990.** Information pamphlet: *Brucellosis in Cattle (Contagious Abortion)*. Director of Animal Health, Directorate of Veterinary Services, Private Bag X138, Pretoria, South Africa.

13 **BARTON, C.E. & LOMME, J.R., 1980.** Reduced-dose whole-herd vaccination against brucellosis: A review of recent experience. *Journal of the American Veterinary Medical Association*, 177, 1218–1220.

14 **BECKETT, F.W. & MACDIARMID, S.C., 1985.** The effect of reduced-dose *Brucella abortus* strain 19 vaccination in accredited dairy herds. *British Veterinary Journal*, 141, 507–514.

15 **BISHOP, G.C., 1984.** A brucellosis serological survey of beef cattle slaughtered at Cato Ridge Abattoir. *Journal of the South African Veterinary Association*, 55, 185–186.

16 **BISHOP, G.C., 1990.** Allerton Veterinary Laboratory, Pietermaritzburg, South Africa. Unpublished data.

17 **BISHOP, G.C. & HAW, C.L., 1990.** Allerton Veterinary Laboratory, Pietermaritzburg, South Africa. Unpublished data.

18 **BLOOD, D.C., RADOSTITS, O.M. & HENDERSON, J.A., 1983.** *Veterinary Medicine*. 6th edn. London: Baillière Tindall.

19 **BOSMAN, P.P., 1980.** Scheme for the control and eradication of bovine brucellosis. *Journal of the South African Veterinary Association*, 51, 75–79.

20 **BRAUDE, A.I., 1951.** Studies in the pathogenesis of experimental brucellosis. II. The formation of the hepatic granuloma and its evolution. *Journal of Infectious Diseases*, 89, 87–94.

21 **BRINLEY MORGAN, W.J., 1967.** The serological diagnosis of bovine brucellosis. *The Veterinary Record*, 80, 612–621.

22 **BRINLEY MORGAN, W.J., 1977.** The diagnosis of *Brucella abortus* infection in Britain. *In*: CRAWFORD, R.P. & HIDALGO, R.J., (eds). *Bovine Brucellosis. An International Symposium*. College Station, London: Texas A&M University Press.

23 **BROWN, G.M., LOVE, E.L., PIETZ, D.E. & RANGER, C.R., 1972.** *Brucella abortus* strain 19. *American Journal of Veterinary Research*, 33, 759–764.

24 **BUCK, J.M., 1930.** Studies of vaccination during calfhood to prevent bovine infectious abortion. *Journal of Agricultural Research*, 41, 667–689.

25 **CAMPO, L.R., TAMAYO, R. & CAMPO, C.H., 1987.** Embryo transfer from brucellosis-positive donors: A field trial. *Theriogenology*, 27, 221.

26 **CARGILL, C., LEE, K. & CLARKE, I., 1985.** Use of an enzyme-linked immunoabsorbant assay in a bovine brucellosis eradication programme. *Australian Veterinary Journal*, 62, 49–52.

27 **CATLIN, J.E. & SHEEHAN, E.J., 1986.** Transmission of bovine brucellosis from dam to offspring. *Journal of the American Veterinary Medical Association*, 188, 867–869.

28 **CONDY, J.B. & VICKERS, D.B., 1972.** Brucellosis in Rhodesian wildlife. *Journal of the South African Veterinary Medical Association*, 43, 175–179.

29 **CONDY, J.B. & VICKERS, D.B., 1976.** Brucellosis in buffalo (*Syncerus caffer*) in Wankie National Park. *Rhodesian Veterinary Journal*, 7, 58–60.

30 **CORBEL, M.J. & BRINLEY MORGAN, W.J., 1984.** Genus *Brucella* Meyer and Shaw 1920. *In*: KRIEG, N.R. & HOLT, J.G., (eds). *Bergey's Manual of Systematic Bacteriology*. Baltimore, London: Williams & Wilkins.

31 **CORBEL, M.J., GILL, K.P.W. & THOMAS, E.L., revised by CORBEL, M.L. & HENDRY, D., 1983.** *Methods for the Identification of Brucella*. Weybridge, Surrey: Central Veterinary Laboratory.

32 **CORBEL, M.J., STUART, F.A., BREWER, R.A., JEFFREY, M. & BRADLEY, R., 1989.** Arthropathy associated with *Brucella abortus* strain 19 vaccination in cattle. I. Examination of field cases. *British Veterinary Journal*, 145, 337–346.

33 **CORNER, L.A. & ALTON, G.G., 1981.** Persistence of *Brucella abortus* strain 19 infection in adult cattle vaccinated with reduced doses. *Research in Veterinary Science*, 31, 342–344.

34 **CORNER, L.A., ALTON, G.G. & IYER, H., 1987.** Distribution of *Brucella abortus* in infected cattle. *Australian Veterinary Journal*, 64, 241–244.

35 **COTTON, W.E. & BUCK, J.M., 1934.** The status of vaccination against Bang's disease. *Journal of the American Veterinary Medical Association*, 84, 329–340.

36 **CRAWFORD, R.P., SANDERS, R.B. & ADAMS, L.G., 1988.** Early removal of cows with brucellosis and the effect in strain 19-vaccinated cattle herds. *Preventative Veterinary Medicine*, 5, 191–195.

37 **CRAWFORD, R.P., WILLIAMS, J.D., HUBER, J.D. & CHILDERS, A.B., 1979.** Biotypes of *Brucella abortus* and their value in epidemiologic studies of infected cattle herds. *Journal of the American Veterinary Medical Association*, 175, 1274–1277.

38 **CUNNINGHAM, B., 1977.** A difficult disease called brucellosis. *In*: CRAWFORD, R.P. & HIDALGO, R.J., (eds). *Bovine Brucellosis. An International Symposium*. College Station, London: Texas A&M University Press.

39 **CUNNINGHAM, B., 1977.** The National Brucellosis Programme of the Republic of Ireland. *In*: CRAWFORD, R.P. & HILDAGO, R.J., (eds). *Bovine Brucellosis. An International Symposium*. College Station, London: Texas A&M University Press.

40 **CURRIER, R.W., 1989.** Brucellosis. *Journal of the American Veterinary Medical Association*, 195, 595–597.

41 **D'CRUZ, S., 1987.** Zambia. Brucellosis in cattle and small ruminants: Diagnosis, control and vaccination. *Technical Series, Office International des Epizooties*, 6, 74–79.

42 **DE GODOY, A.M., PERES, J.N., BARG, L. & COSTA, J.O., 1985.** Ixodidae as a reservoir of animal brucellosis. *Arquivo Brasileiro de Medicina Veterinaria e Zootecnia*, 37, 369–375.

43 **DE VOS, V. & VAN NIEKERK, C.A., 1969.** Brucellosis in the Kruger National Park. *Journal of the South African Veterinary Medical Association*, 40, 331–334.

44 **DOLAN, L.A., 1980.** Latent carriers of brucellosis. *The Veterinary Record*, 106, 241–243.

45 **DUFFIELD, B.J., STREETEN, T.A. & SPINKS, G.A., 1984.** Isolation of *Brucella abortus* from supramammary lymph nodes of cattle from infected herds vaccinated with low-dose strain 19. *Australian Veterinary Journal*, 61, 411–412.

46 **ELLIOTT, R.E.W. & CHRISTIANSEN, K.J., 1977.** *Brucellosis: A Veterinarian's Guide to the Literature*. Ministry of Agriculture and Fisheries, Animal Health Division, Wellington, New Zealand.

47 **FARR, N.H., 1976.** The diagnosis of bovine brucellosis. *State Veterinary Journal*, 31, 144–160.

48 **FARRELL, I.D., 1974.** The development of a new selective medium for the isolation of *Brucella abortus* from contaminated sources. *Research in Veterinary Science*, 16, 280–286.

49 **FAUL, A. & BOSMAN, P.P., 1987.** South Africa. Bovine brucellosis and brucellosis of small ruminants. *Technical Series, Office International des Epizooties*, Paris, France, 6, 60–64.

50 **FENSTERBANK, R., 1978.** Congenital brucellosis in cattle associated with localization in a hygroma. *The Veterinary Record*, 103, 283–284.

51 **GARIN, B., TRAP, D. & GAUMONT, R., 1985.** Assessment of the EDTA seroagglutination test for the diagnosis of bovine brucellosis. *The Veterinary Record*, 117, 444–445.

52 **GRADWELL, D.V., SCHUTTE, A.P., VAN NIEKERK, C.A. & ROUX, D.J., 1977.** The isolation of *Brucella abortus* biotype I from African buffalo in the Kruger National Park. *Journal of the South African Veterinary Association*, 48, 41–43.

53 **HARMON, B.G., ADAMS, L.G., TEMPLETON, J.W. & SMITH, R., 1989.** Macrophage function in mammary glands of *Brucella abortus*-infected cows and cows that resisted infection after inoculation of *Brucella abortus*. *American Journal of Veterinary Research*, 50, 459–465.

54 **HENDRICKS, J.B., 1977.** *In*: CRAWFORD, R.P. & HIDALGO, R.J., (eds) *Bovine Brucellosis. An International Symposium*. College Station, London: Texas A&M University Press.

55 **HENNING, M.W., 1956.** *Animal Diseases in South Africa*. 3rd edn. Pretoria: Central News Agency, Ltd.

56 **HERR, S., 1989.** Veterinary Research Institute, Onderstepoort, South Africa. Unpublished data.

57 **HERR, S., 1989.** Causes of foetal death in cattle. *Zimbabwe Veterinary Journal*, 20, 167–168.

58 **HERR, S., BISHOP, G.C., BOLTON, T.F.W. & VAN DER MERWE, D., 1979.** *Onderstepoort Brucellosis Serology Manual*. Pretoria: Department of Agriculture and Fisheries.

59 **HERR, S. & MARSHALL, C., 1981.** Brucellosis in free-living African buffalo (*Syncerus caffer*): A serological survey. *Onderstepoort Journal of Veterinary Research*, 48, 133–134.

60 **HERR, S. & ROUX, D., 1981.** The efficacy of bacteriological procedures for the isolation of *Brucella abortus* from abattoir material. *Onderstepoort Journal of Veterinary Research*, 48, 7–12.

61 **HERR, S. & TE BRUGGE, L.A., 1984.** Experience with reduced-dose *Brucella abortus* strain 19 vaccination of adult cattle in infected herds in South Africa. *Proceedings of the Thirteenth World Congress on Diseases of Cattle*, 1, 359–365.

62 **HERR, S. & TE BRUGGE, L.A., 1985.** Profiles of serological reactions following adult cow inoculation with standard-dose *Brucella abortus* strain 19 vaccine. *Journal of the South African Veterinary Association*, 56, 93–96.

63 **HERR, S., TE BRUGGE, L.A. & GUINEY, M.C.M., 1982.** The value of the microtitre serum agglutination test as a second screening test in bovine brucellosis. *Onderstepoort Journal of Veterinary Research*, 49, 23–28.

64 **HERR, S., WILLIAMSON, C.C., PRIGGE, R.E. & VAN WYK, A., 1986.** The relationship between the microtitration serum-agglutination test and complement-fixation tests in bovine brucellosis serology. *Onderstepoort Journal of Veterinary Research*, 53, 199–200.

65 **HUDDLESON, I.F., 1943.** *Brucellosis in Man and Animals*. New York: The Commonwealth Fund.

66 **JONES, L.M., 1977.** *Brucella* antigens and serologic test results. *In*: CRAWFORD, R.P. & HILDALGO, R.J., (eds). *Bovine Brucellosis. An International Symposium*. College Station, London: Texas A&M University Press.

67 **JONKER, 1988.** Directorate of Animal Health, Eastern Cape Province and Karoo, Private Bag X12999, Centrahill. Personal communication.

68 **JUBB, K.V.F., KENNEDY, P.C. & PALMER, N., 1985.** *Pathology of Domestic Animals*. 3rd edn. London: Academic Press, Inc.

69 **KANEENE, J.M.B., JOHNSON, D.W., ANDERSON, R.K., ANGUS, R.D., PIETZ, D.E. & MUSCOPLAT, C.C., 1978.** Specific lymphocytic stimulation in cattle naturally infected with strains of *Brucella abortus* and cattle vaccinated with *Brucella abortus* S19. *American Journal of Veterinary Research*, 39, 585–589.

70 **KEEP, M.E. & BISHOP, G.C., 1985.** A brucellosis survey in Natal wildlife. *Lammergeyer*, 35, 47–48.

71 **KEPPIE, J., WILLIAMS, A.E., WITT, K. & SMITH, H., 1965.** The role of erythritol in the tissue localization of the brucellae. *British Journal of Experimental Pathology*, 46, 104–108.

72 **LA PRAIK, R.D. & MOFFAT, R., 1982.** Latent bovine brucellosis. *The Veterinary Record*, 111, 578–579.

73 **LA PRAIK, R.D., BROWN, D.D., MANN, H. & BRAND, T., 1975.** Brucellosis: A study of five calves from reactor dams. *The Veterinary Record*, 97, 52–54.

74 **MACDIARMID, S.C. & HELLSTROM, J.S., 1987.** An intradermal test for the diagnosis of brucellosis in extensively managed herds. *Preventative Veterinary Medicine*, 4, 361–369.

75 **MACMILLAN, A.P. & COCKREM, D.S., 1985.** Reduction of non-specific reactions to the *Brucella abortus* serum agglutination test by the addition of EDTA. *Research in Veterinary Science*, 38, 288–291.

76 **MADSEN, M., 1989.** The current state of brucellosis in Zimbabwe. *Zimbabwe Veterinary Journal*, 20, 133–148.

77 **MADZINA, W.M., 1987.** Zimbabwe. Bovine brucellosis and brucellosis of small ruminants: Diagnosis, control and vaccination. *Technical Series, Office International des Epizooties*, 75017 Paris, France, 6, 80–82.

78 **MANTHEI, C.A., DETRAY, D.E. & GOODE, E.R., 1950.** *Brucella* infection in bulls and the spread of brucellosis in cattle by artificial insemination. *Proceedings of the 87th Annual Meeting of the American Veterinary Medical Association*, 87, 177.

79 **McEWAN, A.D., 1937.** Experiments on contagious abortion. II. Field immunization experiments with a vaccine prepared from strain 45. *The Veterinary Record*, 49, 1585.

80 **MEADOR, V.P., DEYOE, B.L. & CHEVILLE, N.F., 1989.** Pathogenesis of *Brucella abortus* infection of the mammary gland and supramammary lymph node of the goat. *Veterinary Pathology*, 26, 357–368.

81 **MEADOR, V.P., DEYOE, B.L. & CHEVILLE, N.F., 1989.** Effect of nursing of *Brucella abortus* infection of mammary glands of goats. *Veterinary Pathology*, 26, 369–375.

82 **MEYER, M.E., 1977.** Serological odds and ends. *In*: CRAWFORD, R.P. & HIDALGO, R.J., (eds). *Bovine Brucellosis: An International Symposium*. College Station, London: Texas A&M University Press.

83 **NELSON, C.J., 1977.** Immunity to *Brucella abortus*. *In*: CRAWFORD, R.P. & HIDALGO, R.J., (eds). *Bovine Brucellosis: An International Symposium*. College Station, London: Texas A&M University Press.

84 **NICOLETTI, P., 1977.** Adult vaccination. *In*: CRAWFORD, R.P. & HIDALGO, R.J., (eds). *Bovine Brucellosis: An International Symposium*. College Station, London: Texas A&M University Press.

85 **NICOLETTI, P., 1980.** The epidemiology of bovine brucellosis. *Advances in Veterinary Science and Comparative Medicine*, 24, 69–98.

86 **NICOLETTI, P., 1984.** Vaccination of cattle with *Brucella abortus* strain 19 administered by different routes and doses. *Vaccine*, 2, 133–135.

87 **NICOLETTI, P., JONES, L.M. & BERMAN, D.T., 1978.** Comparison of the subcutaneous and conjunctival route of vaccination with *Brucella abortus* strain 19 vaccine in adult cattle. *Journal of the American Veterinary Medical Association*, 173, 1450–1456.

88 **PAYNE, J.M., 1959.** The pathogenesis of experimental brucellosis in the pregnant cow. *Journal of Pathology and Bacteriology*,

78, 447–463.

89 **PLACKETT, P., ALTON, C.G., CARTER, P.D. & CORNER, L.A., 1980.** The indirect haemolysis test (IHLT) for bovine brucellosis — comparisons with the complement-fixation test (CFT) in vaccinated and experimentally infected cattle. *Australian Veterinary Journal*, 56, 405–408.

90 **PLACKETT, P., COTTEW, G.S. & BEST, S.J., 1976.** An indirect haemolysis test (IHLT) for bovine brucellosis. *Australian Veterinary Journal*, 52, 136–140.

91 **PLANT, J.W., CLAXTON, P.D., JAKOVLJEVIC, M.B. & DE SARAM, W., 1976.** *Brucella abortus* infection in the bull. *Australian Veterinary Journal*, 52, 17–20.

92 **PLOMMET, M., 1977.** Studies on experimental brucellosis in cows in France. *In*: CRAWFORD, R.P. & HIDALGO, R.J., (eds). *Bovine Brucellosis: An International Symposium*, College Station, London: Texas A&M University Press.

93 **RANKIN, J.E.F., 1965.** *Brucella abortus* in bulls: A study of twelve naturally infected cases. *The Veterinary Record*, 77, 132–135.

94 **RAY, W.C., 1977.** The epidemiology of *Brucella abortus*. *In*: CRAWFORD, R.P. & HIDALGO, R.J., (eds). *Bovine Brucellosis: An International Symposium*. College Station, London: Texas A&M University Press.

95 **RILEY, L.K. & ROBERTSON, D.C., 1984.** Brucellacidal activity of human and bovine polymorphonuclear leukocyte granule extracts against smooth and rough strains of *Brucella abortus*. *Infection and Immunity*, 46, 231–236.

96 **ROBERTS, R.M., 1986.** The vaginal mucus agglutination test in the diagnosis of bovine brucellosis. *The Veterinary Record*, 118, 505–507.

97 **ROEPKE, M.H. & STILES, F.C., 1970.** Potential efficiency of the milk-ring test for detection of brucellosis. *American Journal of Veterinary Research*, 31, 2145–2149.

98 **RYLATT, D.B., WYATT, D.M. & BUNDESEN, P.G., 1985.** A competitive enzyme immunoassay for the detection of bovine antibodies to *Brucella abortus* using monoclonal antibodies. *Veterinary Immunology and Immunopathology*, 8, 261–271.

99 **SCANLAN, C.M., 1988.** *Introduction to Veterinary Bacteriology*, Ames, Iowa: Iowa State University Press.

100 **SLATTER, W., 1977.** Experiences with brucellosis under range conditions in northern Australia. *In*: CRAWFORD, R.P. & HIDALGO, R.J., (eds). *Bovine Brucellosis: An International Symposium*. College Station, London: Texas A&M University Press.

101 **STAMP, J.T., McEWAN, A.D., WATT, J.A.A. & NISBETT, D.I., 1950.** Enzootic abortion in ewes. *The Veterinary Record*, 62, 251–154.

102 **STRINGFELLOW, D.A., WOLFE, D.F., McGUIRE, J.A., LAUERMAN, L.A., GRAY, B.W. & SPARLING, P.H., 1986.** Effects of embryo-freezing and thawing techniques on the survivability of *Brucella abortus*. *Theriogenology*, 26, 553–560.

103 **SUTHERLAND, S.S., 1980.** Immunology of bovine brucellosis. *The Veterinary Bulletin*, 50, 359–368.

104 **SUTHERLAND, S.S., 1984.** Evaluation of the enzyme-linked immunosorbent assay in the detection of cattle infected with *Brucella abortus*. *Veterinary Microbiology*, 10, 23–32.

105 **SUTHERLAND, S., 1985.** An enzyme-linked immunosorbent assay for the detection of *Brucella abortus* in cattle using monoclonal antibodies. *Australian Veterinary Journal*, 62, 264–268.

106 **SUTHERLAND, S.S., LE CRAS, D.V. & EVANS, R.J., 1982.** Comparison of the complement-fixation test and the indirect haemolysis test for cattle vaccinated and infected with *Brucella abortus*. *Journal of Clinical Microbiology*, 16, 599–603.

107 **SUTHERLAND, S.S. & MACKENZIE, R.M., 1983.** Applied serology in the latter stages of the eradication of bovine brucellosis. *Australian Veterinary Journal*, 60, 240–242.

108 **TAYLOR, A.W. & MACDIARMID, A., 1949.** The stability of the avirulent characters of *Brucella abortus* strain 19 and 45/20 in lactating and pregnant cows. *The Veterinary Record*, 61, 317–318.

109 **THOEN, C.O. & ENRIGHT, F., 1986.** *Brucella*. *In*: GYLES, C.L. & THOEN, C.O., (eds). *Pathogenesis of Bacterial Infections in Animals*. 1st edn. Ames, Iowa: Iowa State University Press.

110 **THOMSON, A., 1950.** Experimental studies on the incubation period of infectious abortion in cattle. *British Veterinary Journal*, 106, 41–54.

111 **THYANGATHYANGA, G.A.A., 1987.** Malawi. Bovine brucellosis and brucellosis of small ruminants: Diagnosis, control and vaccination. *Technical Series, Office International des Epizooties*, 6, 50–55.

112 **TRICHARD, C.J.V., HERR, S., BASTIANELLO, S.S. & ROUX, D., 1982.** Unilateral orchitis in a bull caused by *Brucella abortus* Biotype 1. *Journal of the South African Veterinary Association*, 53, 60–62.

113 **VAN AERDT, A., BRIOEN, P., DE KEYSER, P., UYTTERHAEGAN, L., SIJENS, R.J. & BOEYE, A., 1984.** A comparative study of ELISA and other methods for the detection of *Brucella* antibodies in bovine sera. *Veterinary Microbiology* 10, 13–21.

114 **WILESMITH, J.W., 1978.** The persistence of *Brucella abortus* infection in calves: A retrospective study of heavily infected herds. *The Veterinary Record*, 103, 149–153.

115 **WILLIAMS, A.E., KEPPIE, J. & SMITH, H., 1962.** The chemical basis of the virulence of *Brucella abortus*. III. Foetal erythritol, a cause of the localization of *Brucella abortus* in pregnant cows. *British Journal of Experimental Pathology*, 43, 530–537.

116 **WYNN-JONES, G., BAKER, J.R. & JOHNSON, P.M., 1980.** A clinical and immunopathological study of *Brucella abortus* strain 19–induced arthritis in cattle. *The Veterinary Record*, 107, 5–9.

117 **XIE XIN, 1986.** Orally administrable brucellosis vaccine: *Brucella suis* strain 2 vaccine. *Vaccine*, 4, 212–216.

125

Brucella ovis *infection*

E.M. van Tonder, S. Herr, G.C. Bishop and P.P. Bosman

Introduction

Brucella ovis is one of the common causes of epididymitis in rams and a rare cause of abortion in ewes and neonatal mortality in lambs. Low reproductive rates, varying between 11 and 40 per cent, may occur in infected flocks.

Brucella-like organisms, which were first isolated from the lesions of rams with epididymitis and from ewes in Australia and New Zealand in 1953,[13, 76] were assigned to a new species, *Brucella ovis*, after comprehensive studies.[12]

In South Africa, rams with clinical or subclinical epididymitis and low fertility as a result of *B. ovis* infection were diagnosed for the first time in 1956.[84] Since then the disease has also been diagnosed in Namibia and Zimbabwe.[85]

Brucella ovis infections occur in many countries of the world. In Australia up to 80 per cent of young rams in certain studs or flocks are infected,[52, 68] and the infection is also widespread throughout South Africa.[28, 81, 82, 83] Results of a survey in 1984 revealed that 4,3 per cent of rams in the Orange Free State in South Africa were infected.[28]

Aetiology

Brucella ovis is a small, non-motile, non-sporulating, non-encapsulated bacillus or coccobacillus with rounded ends and a straight axis, ranging from 0,7–1,5 µm in length and 0,3–0,7 µm in width.[12, 13, 51] The organisms are Gram-negative and weakly acid-fast when stained with Stamp's modification of the Ziehl Neelsen staining method.[78] In smears the bacteria occur singly, in pairs, or more frequently in clumps.

Although *B. ovis* is generally similar to the other *Brucella* spp. in its morphology, staining properties and general cultural characteristics[12, 51, 62] **(see Chapter 124: Bovine brucellosis)**, it can be identified on the basis of biochemical reactions, its reactions with specific antisera, and phage susceptibility.[2, 23]

For primary culture the organism requires an atmosphere containing approximately 10 per cent CO_2[13, 51, 76] and enrichment of culture media with 5–10 per cent blood or serum.[13, 51, 54, 76] Optimum growth occurs at 37 °C, while no growth occurs at temperatures below 20 °C or above 40 °C.[13] On primary culture after 72 hours' incubation on media such as tryptose blood agar, the colonies are greyish-white, up to 0,5 mm in diameter, non-haemolytic, circular, convex, smooth, glistening, translucent and entire-edged.[12, 13, 51, 76]

Epidemiology

Only sheep are naturally infected by *B. ovis*, although billy goats[18, 35] and white-tailed deer (*Odocoileus virginianus*)[5] are susceptible to experimental infection.

The disease is spread primarily by infected rams. *Brucella ovis* may be excreted in the semen of infected rams even before the development of lesions.[16, 39, 53] Clinically or subclinically infected rams may excrete *B. ovis* in their semen for as long as four years.[12, 39]

Infection may spread from ram to ram as a result of homosexual activity or venereally during coitus when non-infected rams mate with ewes which passively harbour the bacteria.[4, 9, 18, 19, 39, 52, 65, 77, 88] Ewes generally only transfer organisms mechanically from infected to non-infected rams when they are mated in succession by different rams during the same heat period. Vasectomized and cryptorchid rams are equally vulnerable as a result of direct transmission through contact, homosexual activity and venereal spread through ewes.

Direct ram-to-ram and venereal transmission result in a higher prevalence of infection in flock rams than in stud rams.[4, 29, 30, 52, 66, 88, 92] This is probably due to the differences in mating and management practices between these two categories of rams, such as the regular examination of breeding rams and new introductions, individual versus mass-mating, and the more isolated rearing and housing of stud rams.

Ewes are relatively resistant to infection. Natural infection of ewes by *B. ovis* is sporadic, transient, and of a very low prevalence.[12, 20, 39, 52, 77] Ewe-to-ewe transmission of the infection during close contact has not been demonstrated.

Infected ewes rarely abort, but when this does occur, organisms may be present in large numbers in the uterine exudate, foetal membranes and in tissues such as the lungs, spleen, liver and abomasal content of the aborted foetuses.[13, 38, 39, 59] Organisms may also be recovered from the colostrum and milk of such ewes,[13, 92] and they usually persist for 10–14 days in uterine discharges of ewes that have aborted.[39, 43]

Pathogenesis

Rams become infected after penetration by *B. ovis* of the mucous membranes of the prepuce, penis, nasal cavity or conjunctiva.[7–9, 17, 69] This is followed by a bacteraemia and localization of the infection in lymph nodes and organs such as the epididymis, ampullae, seminal vesicles, bulbourethral glands, spleen, liver and kidneys. Organisms are first excreted in the semen from between 31 and 45 days following exposure.

Gross lesions develop only in the genitalia.[7] In rams the earliest lesions usually occur in the tail of the epididymis, but lesions in the head and/or body of the epididymis may develop later. Initially the bacteria cause degeneration and necrosis of the epididymal epithelium, resulting in leakage of semen into the interstitial tissues where it provokes a severe inflammatory reaction and the development of spermatic granulomas. Similar inflammatory changes may also occur in the vas deferens, ampullae, seminal vesicles, bulbourethral glands, and testes.

Bacterial products, inflammatory cells (particularly neutrophils) in the semen, and a decrease in the production and quality of sperm as a consequence of testicular degeneration all lead to lower fertility or infertility.[3, 53, 93] Infertility may also be caused by the total cessation of spermatogenesis or by obstruction of the epididymis by spermatic granulomas and the development of a spermatocoele. There is a direct relationship between the semen quality, extent of the epididymal lesions and the number of leukocytes present in the semen. The reduction in fertility is ascribed to both low spermatozoa counts and the high number of defective spermatozoa; defects of the spermatozoal head and neck being common.

Infection enters ewes mainly through the vaginal mucosa. In pregnant ewes, the ensuing bacteraemia rarely causes a placentitis that results in abortion or the birth of lambs with reduced birth weights.[49]

A detectable humoral immune response in rams initially appears two weeks after exposure, but uniformly positive titres are only obtained from the fourth week onwards. In rams, antibody titres increase rapidly and remain high until about the seventh month of infection, after which they steadily decline.[7]

Clinical signs

The interval between infection and the development of lesions in rams varies considerably, being anything from 50 to 250 days.[69, 84]

The most consistent clinical sign is enlargement, particularly of the tail of the epididymis, which may be barely perceptible or up to a four- or five-fold increase in size. The head, body or entire epididymis are less often affected.[7, 51, 68, 84, 93] The lesions often occur unilaterally, but bilateral involvement is relatively common.[47, 51, 60, 84]

Clinically detectable lesions may be acute to chronic. Although chronic lesions may follow a bout of acute epididymitis,[7, 60, 84] they more commonly develop insidiously without clinical evidence of the acute phase.

Most rams suffering from acute epididymitis are not systemically affected. The entire testis on the affected side may be hot, swollen and oedematous, but only a localized swelling of the epididymis is detectable in animals that are less severely affected.[47, 93] Lesions often commence as slight soft swellings of the tail of the epididymis. These localized early lesions may develop over one week into a severe, acute epididymitis, in which case the reaction may still be localized but hot and painful.

Chronic epididymitis is clinically characterized by enlargement and an increased consistency of the affected parts.[12, 47, 48, 60, 84] As a result of fibrous adhesions, the mobility of the affected testis in the scrotum is often reduced. The marked increase in scrotal circumference caused by the epididymal and testicular lesions can be seen from a distance.

The testis is seldom primarily affected. In some cases the testis on the affected side may be slightly atrophied and have a somewhat softer consistency than normal,[48] while in others with a severe, chronic epididymitis, the testis may be severely atrophied and firm.[48, 84]

Affected rams may be sterile, or have reduced fertility. The degree of impairment depends on whether the lesions are uni- or bilateral, and on the course and severity of the lesions.[20, 25, 52, 60, 63, 77] The libido of affected rams remains unaffected.

Ewes abort very rarely as a result of *B. ovis* infection.[56, 59, 61] In experimentally infected pregnant ewes, abortion occurred in about 30 per cent of the pregnant animals within a month of inoculation with *B. ovis*. In field cases as many as 50 per cent of the pregnant ewes may abort.[56] Accidental administration of the standard Rev. I vaccine to pregnant sheep and goats causes abortion.[40, 67]

Pathology

The typical lesions in the affected epididymis include solitary or multiple spermatocoeles and spermatic granulomas which contain a creamy fluid or inspissated, caseous material, thickening due to the presence of a low-grade, non-purulent inflammatory response, and fibrosis of the interductal connective tissue and the tunica albuginea. In most cases fibrous adhesions form between the tail of the epididymis, the parietal tunica vaginalis and the distal pole of the testis.[63]

Varying degrees of testicular atrophy, which is usually more severe in rams with widespread and severe adhesions, may accompany the epididymal lesions.[51, 63] In most cases, however, the changes in the testis are minimal

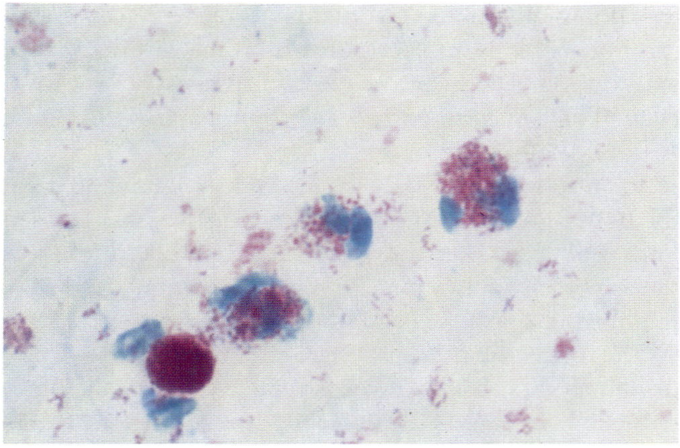

Figure 125.1
Semen smear stained by the modified Ziehl Neelsen method: note acid-fast *Brucella ovis* organisms

and non-specific.[7] Changes in the vas deferens and accessory sex glands may be similar to those in the epididymis.

The effect of clinical or subclinical infection on semen quality is determined by the extent and severity of the lesions in the epididymis, testes, and accessory glands.[3, 51–53, 77] Poor semen quality is characterized by reduced density of the ejaculate (due to decreased numbers of spermatozoa), reduced motility and longevity of spermatozoa, an increase in the proportion of abnormal spermatozoa such as those with detached sperm-heads, midpiece abnormalities, bent tails, coiled tails, and tails tightly coiled around the heads of spermatozoa,[29, 30, 87] and the presence, in many cases, of varying numbers of leukocytes, particularly neutrophils.[3, 53, 68, 86, 87]

The carcasses of aborted lambs are not autolyzed but are dehydrated, and they manifest fibrinous peritonitis. The accompanying placentitis is characterized by a yellowish fibrinous exudate which is present particularly in the intercotyledonary areas. Histologically the lesions in the placentas are characterized by a multifocal suppurative inflammation.[64] Foetal tissues manifest a suppurative bronchitis, bronchiolitis and bronchopneumonia.[56]

Diagnosis

Methods used to diagnose *B. ovis* infection in sheep include palpation of the external genitalia of rams, microscopic examination of stained semen smears, bacteriological culture of semen and exudate from lesions, and serology. A combination of two or more of these examinations should ensure a reliable diagnosis.[54, 91]

The presence of *B. ovis* and neutrophils in semen smears stained by the modified Ziehl Neelsen method **(Figure 125.1)**,[78] particularly in those rams which are subclinically affected, is essential for the diagnosis of ovine brucellosis.[16, 69, 79, 84, 93] Although there is usually a good correlation between the presence of neutrophils and *B. ovis* organisms in semen smears,[84, 93] the presence of neutrophils alone is not a reliable diagnostic criterion.[14]

As the excretion of *B. ovis* only occurs sporadically in the semen of infected rams, organisms may be absent at the time of sampling[11, 37] and repeated sampling may be required in order to confirm the diagnosis by bacteriological isolation of the organism.

In ewes which have aborted, *B. ovis* infection can be diagnosed by the demonstration of the organisms in smears made from uterine exudate and by the bacteriological culture of uterine exudate. In aborted foetuses bacteriological cultures of the abomasal content, spleen, lungs and liver should be made in order to isolate the organism.[38, 56]

A variety of serological and immunological tests, including the tube-agglutination, ELISA, Rose Bengal plate, complement fixation (CFT), gel-diffusion and FA tests may be used to detect *B. ovis* infections.[2] Of the available tests the CFT appears to be the most reliable. Although false-negatives[7] and false-positives occur in CFTs, no false-positives have been encountered in flocks known to be free of the disease,[44] but they do occur in infected flocks.[44, 73] A titre of 1:8 or higher in the microtitre CFT is considered positive.[18, 94] False-positive CFT results following the use of *B. melitensis* Rev. I vaccine apparently do not occur.[33, 86]

The results of gel-diffusion tests correspond well with those obtained with the CF test,[71, 94, 95] while ELISA has greater sensitivity than the CF test.[36, 55, 71, 94, 95] However, ELISA is not specific for *B. ovis* infections in areas where *B. melitensis* infection also occurs in sheep.[71]

The fluorescent antibody test[22] has been successfully adapted for the detection of *B. ovis* in semen and in cultures.[1, 24]

Differential diagnosis

Epididymitis in rams as a result of *B. ovis* should be differentiated from similar lesions caused by *Actinobacillus seminis*,[6] *Actinobacillus actinomycetemcomitans*,[27] other *Actinobacillus* spp.,[31] *Histophilus ovis*,[21] *Corynebacterium pseudotuberculosis*,[15] *Haemophilus somnus*,[15] *Haemophilus agni*,[96] and other *Haemophilus* spp.[10, 44–46] Nodular enlargement of the epididymis and testes detected clinically may also be caused by trauma,[70] paradidymal cysts, *Cysticercus tenuicollis* cysts, Sertoli-cell tumours and seminomas,[74, 75, 89, 90] and by spermatocoeles and spermatogranuloma resulting from non-infectious causes.[50] Nodular enlargement within the scrotum due to varicocoele should also be considered.

The possible involvement of *B. ovis* infection in abortion and perinatal lamb mortality should be considered.

Control

Control is based on the elimination of infected animals, vaccination, or a combination of the two approaches.[52, 65, 72, 77, 84]

Control programmes are aimed at preventing infection from taking place and reducing and eliminating infected rams. Management procedures such as the rearing and weaning of male replacement lambs in isolation from other rams, particularly breeding rams, timely weaning of ram lambs, early replacement of older rams, avoidance of the use of susceptible young rams in multiple-sire breeding systems, testing of rams before the mating season, and introduction of only tested and/or vaccinated rams are important in the control of the disease.

Vaccination with the Rev. I mutant strain of *B. melitensis*[41, 42] was introduced into South Africa by Van Drimmelen[80] and has proved highly effective in preventing *B. ovis* infection.[82, 83] In South Africa, ram lambs of between two and four months old should be vaccinated.[32, 34, 37, 41, 42, 80] The induced immunity against *B. ovis* infection lasts for up to four years.[37, 82, 83] A vaccine containing aluminium hydroxide-adsorbed *B. ovis* bacteria probably only protects rams from the clinical disease and does not prevent the establishment of a carrier state.[14] This vaccine is, however, not available in South Africa.

In areas where *B. melitensis* infection is known to exist, the use of Rev I vaccine via the conjunctival, as opposed to the subcutaneous, route may be advisable in rams, as the conjunctival inoculation results in immunity while minimizing a post-vaccinal serological response.[57]

The treatment of *B. ovis*-infected rams with long-acting oxytetracycline and dihydrostreptomycin results in a reduction in the shedding of the pathogen in the semen,[26, 58] but conclusive elimination of the infection from all rams has not been proved. Treatment with these antibiotics early in the course of the disease might enable a ram to be used for at least one more breeding season.

References

1 **AJAI, C.O., COOK, J.E. & DENNIS, S.M., 1980.** Diagnosing ovine epididymitis by immunofluorescence. *The Veterinary Record*, 107, 421–424.

2 **ALTON, G.G., JONES, L.H., ANGUS, R.D. & VERGER, J.M., 1988.** *Techniques for the Brucellosis Laboratory*. 1st edn. Paris: Institut National de la Recherche Agronomique.

3 **BAGLEY, C.V., BURRELL, W.C., ESPLIN, G.M. & WALTERS, J.L., 1984.** Effect of epididymitis on semen quality of rams. *Journal of the American Veterinary Medical Association*, 185, 876–877.

4 **BAGLEY, C.V., PASKETT, M.E., MATTHEWS, N.J. & STENQUIST, N.J., 1985.** Prevalence and causes of ram epididymitis in Utah. *Journal of the American Veterinary Medical Association*, 186, 798–801.

5 **BARRON, S.J., KOCAN, A.A., MORTON, R.J., THEDFORD, T.R. & McCAIN, C.S., 1985.** Susceptibility of male white-tailed deer (*Odocoileus virginianus*) to *Brucella ovis* infection. *American Journal of Veterinary Research*, 46, 1762–1764.

6 **BAYNES, I.D. & SIMMONS, G.C., 1960.** Ovine epididymitis caused by *Actinobacillus seminis* n. sp. *Australian Veterinary Journal*, 36, 454–459.

7 **BIBERSTEIN, E.L., McGOWAN, B., OLANDER, H. & KENNEDY, P.C., 1964.** Epididymitis in rams: Studies on pathogenesis. *Cornell Veterinarian*, 54, 27–41.

8 **BIBERSTEIN, E.L., McGOWAN, B., ROBINSON, E.A. & HARROLD, D.R., 1962.** Epididymitis in rams: Studies on immunity. *Cornell Veterinarian*, 52, 214–227.

9 **BROWN, G.M., PIETZ, D.E. & PRICE, D.A., 1973.** Studies on the transmission of *Brucella ovis* infection in rams. *Cornell Veterinarian*, 63, 29–40.

10 **BRUSS, M.L., BULGIN, M.S & ANDERSON, B.S., 1981.** Ram epididymitis caused by *Haemophilus*-like bacteria. *Proceedings: Second Annual Western Conference for Food Animal Veterinary Medicine*, Fort Collins, Colorado, 1981.

11 **BUDDLE, M.B., 1955.** Observations on the transmission of *Brucella* infection in sheep. *New Zealand Veterinary Journal*, 3, 10–19.

12 **BUDDLE, M.B., 1956.** Studies on *Brucella ovis* (n. sp.), a cause of genital disease of sheep in New Zealand and Australia. *The Journal of Hygiene*, 54, 351–364.

13 **BUDDLE, M.B. & BOYES, B.W., 1953.** A *Brucella* mutant causing genital disease of sheep in New Zealand. *Australian Veterinary Journal*, 29, 145–153.

14 **BULGIN, M.S., 1990.** *Brucella ovis* excretion in semen of seronegative, clinically normal breeding rams. *Journal of the American Veterinary Medical Association*, 196, 313–315.

15 **BULGIN, M.S. & ANDERSON, B.C., 1983.** Association of sexual experience with isolation of various bacteria in cases of ovine epididymitis. *Journal of the American Veterinary Medical Association*, 182, 372–374.

16 **BURGESS, G.W., McDONALD, J.W. & NORRIS, M.J., 1982.** Epidemiological studies on ovine brucellosis in selected ram flocks. *Australian Veterinary Journal*, 59, 45–47.

17 **BURGESS, G.W. & NORRIS, M.J., 1982.** Evaluation of the cold complement-fixation test for diagnosis of ovine brucellosis. *Australian Veterinary Journal*, 59, 23–25.

18 **BURGESS, G.W., SPENCER, T.L. & NORRIS, M.J., 1985.** Experimental infection of goats with *Brucella ovis*. *Australian Veterinary Journal*, 62, 262–264.

19 **CLAPP, K.H., KEOGH, J. & DOOLETTE, J.B., 1957.** Ovine brucellosis. 1. Epidemiology. Annual Report, Institute of Medical and Veterinary Science, South Australia, 61–65.

20 **CLAPP, K.H., KEOGH, J. & RICHARDS, R.D.A., 1962.** Epidemiology of ovine brucellosis in South Australia. *Australian Veterinary Journal*, 38, 482–486.

21 **CLAXTON, P.D. & EVERETT, R.E., 1966.** Recovery of an organism resembling *Haemophilus ovis* from a ram. *Australian Veterinary Journal*, 42, 457–458.

22 **COONS, A.H. & KAPLAN, M.H., 1950.** Localization of antigen in tissue cells. II. Improvements in a method for the detection of antigens by means of fluorescent antibody. *Journal of Experimental Medicine*, 91, 591–597.

23 **CORBELL, M.J., GILL, K.P.W. & THOMAS, E.L., revised by CORBELL, M.J. & HENDRY, D., 1983.** *Methods for the Identification of Brucella*. Central Veterinary Laboratory, Weybridge, Surrey, England.

24 **COX, J.C., GRORRIE, C.J.R., NAIRN, R.C. & WARD, H.A., 1977.** A comparison of methods for the serological diagnosis of *Brucella ovis* infection. *British Veterinary Journal*, 133, 442–445.

25 **CRENSHAW, G.L., SCHULTZ, G., BILLS, C.J., CAMERON, H.S. & TIMM, O., 1963.** Ram epididymitis in California. *California Veterinarian*, 17, 42–44.

26 **DARGATZ, D.A., SMITH, J.A., KNIGHT, A.P., FARIN, P.W. & KIMBERLING, C.V., 1990.** Antimicrobial therapy for rams with *Brucella ovis* infection of the urogenital tract. *Journal of the American Veterinary Medical Association*, 196, 605–610.

27 **DELONG, W.J., WALDHALM, D.G. & HALL, R.F., 1979.** Bacterial isolates associated with epididymitis in rams from Idaho and eastern Oregon flocks. *American Journal of Veterinary Research*, 40, 101–102.

28 **DE WET, J.A.L. & ERASMUS, J.A., 1984.** Epididymitis of rams in the central and southern districts of the Orange Free State. *Journal of the South African Veterinary Association*, 55, 173–179.

29 **EDGAR, D.G., 1959.** Examination of rams for fertility. *New Zealand Veterinary Journal*, 7, 61–63.

30 **EDGAR, D.G., 1959.** The detection of *Brucella ovis* infection in rams. *New Zealand Veterinary Journal*, 7, 64–66.

31 **EKDAHL, M.O., MONEY, D.F.L. & MARTIN, C.A., 1968.** Some aspects of epididymitis of rams in New Zealand. *New Zealand Veterinary Journal*, 16, 81–82.

32 **ELBERG, S.S. & MEYER, K.F., 1958.** Caprine immunization against brucellosis: A summary of experiments on the isolation, properties and behaviour of a vaccine strain. *Bulletin of the World Health Organization*, 19, 711–724.

33 **ERASMUS, J.A. & BERGH, E.C., 1985.** Ovine brucellosis: Repeated vaccination with Rev. I vaccine and the prevalence of the disease in the Winburg district. *Journal of the South African Veterinary Association*, 56, 205–208.

34 **FENSTERBANK, R., PARDON, P. & MARLY, J., 1982.** Efficacy of *Brucella melitensis* Rev. I vaccine against *Brucella ovis* infection in rams. *Annales Recherches Vétérinaires*, 13, 185–190.

35 **GARCIA-CARILLO, C., CASAS-OLASCOAGA, R., CUBA-CAPARO, A., LUCERO, N. & SZYFRES, B., 1977.** Infection experimental de caprinos machos con *Brucella ovis*. Estudio bacteriologica, serologico e histopatologico. *Revista de la Asociacion Argentina de Microbiologia*, 9, 101–108.

36 **GILL, T.J., 1970.** Methods for detecting antibody. *Immunochemistry*, 7, 997–1000.

37 **GRADWELL, D.V. & VAN ZYL, F.E., 1975.** Effectivity of Rev. I vaccine in rams against *Brucella ovis* infection. *Journal of the South African Veterinary Association*, 46, 349–351.

38 **HARTLEY, W.J., 1961.** The pathology of *Brucella ovis* infection in the pregnant ewe. *New Zealand Veterinary Journal*, 9, 115–120.

39 **HARTLEY, W.J., JEBSON, J.L. & MACFARLANE, D., 1955.** Some observations on natural transmission of ovine brucellosis. *New Zealand Veterinary Journal*, 3, 5–10.

40 **HERR, S., PIETERSON, M.P., GUMMOW, B., PEFANIS, S.M. & VENTER, C.G., 1987.** A *Brucella melitensis* similar to Rev. I. *Research in Reproduction*, 7.

41 **HERZBERG, M. & ELBERG, S.S., 1953.** Immunization against brucella infection. I. Isolation and characterization of a streptomycin-dependent mutant. *Journal of Bacteriology*, 66, 585–599.

42 **HERZBERG, M. & ELBERG, S.S., 1955.** Immunization against brucella infection. III. Response of mice and guinea-pigs to injection of viable and nonviable suspensions of a streptomycin-dependent mutant of *Brucella melitensis*. *Journal of Bacteriology*, 69, 432–435.

43 **HUGHES, K.L., 1972.** Experimental *Brucella ovis* infection in ewes. I. Breeding performance of infected ewes. *Australian Veterinary Journal*, 48, 12–17.

44 **HUGHES, K.L. & CLAXTON, P.D., 1968.** *Brucella ovis* infection. I. An evaluation of microbiological, serological and clinical methods of diagnosis in the ram. *Australian Veterinary Journal*, 44, 41–47.

45 **JANSEN, B.C., 1980.** The aetiology of ram epididymitis. *Onderstepoort Journal of Veterinary Research*, 47, 101–107.

46 **JANSEN, B.C., 1983.** The epidemiology of bacterial infection of the genitalia of rams. *Onderstepoort Journal of Veterinary Research*, 50, 275–282.

47 **JEBSON, J.L., HARTLEY, W.J., McCLURE, T.J. & McFARLANE, D., 1955.** Pathology of brucellosis in rams in New Zealand. *New Zealand Veterinary Journal*, 3, 100–104.

48 **JEBSON, J.L., HARTLEY, W.J. & McFARLANE, D., 1954.** The artificial infection of sheep with a *Brucella*-like organism. Part II. The artificial infection of rams. *New Zealand Veterinary Journal*, 2, 80–89.

49 **JOINT FAO/WHO EXPERT COMMITTEE ON BRUCELLOSIS, 1986.** *World Health Organization Technical Report Series 740*. Geneva: WHO.

50 **JUBB, K.V.F., KENNEDY, P.C. & PALMER, N., 1985.** *Pathology of Domestic Animals*. 3rd edn. Vol. III. New York, London: Academic Press.

51 **KENNEDY, P.C., FRAXIER, L.M. & McGOWAN, B., 1956.** Epididymitis in rams: Pathology and bacteriology. *Cornell Veterinarian*, 46, 303–309.

52 **KEOGH, J., DOOLETTE, J.B. & CLAPP, K.H., 1958.** The epidemiology of ovine brucellosis in South Australia. *Australian Veterinary Journal*, 34, 412–423.

53 **KIMBERLING, C.V., ARNOLD, S.K., SCHWEITZER, D.J., JONES, R.L., VON BYERN, H. & LUCAS, M., 1986.** Correlation of the presence of seminal white blood cells and the prevalence of separated spermatozoal heads with subclinical *Brucella ovis* infection in rams. *Journal of the American Veterinary Medical Association*, 189, 73–76.

54 **LAWRENCE, W.E., 1961.** Ovine brucellosis: A review of the disease in sheep manifested by epididymitis and abortion. *British Veterinary Journal*, 117, 435–447.

55 **LEE, K., CARGILL, C. & ATKINSON, H., 1985.** Evaluation of an enzyme-linked immunosorbent assay for the diagnosis of *Brucella ovis* infection in rams. *Australian Veterinary Journal*, 62, 91–93.

56 **LIBAL, M.C. & KIRKBRIDE, C.A., 1983.** *Brucella ovis*-induced abortion in ewes. *Journal of the American Veterinary Medical Association*, 183, 553–554.

57 **MARIN, C.M., BARBERAN, M., JIMENEZ DE BAGUES, M.P. & BLASCO, J.M., 1990.** Comparison of subcutaneous and conjunctival routes of Rev. I vaccination for the prophylaxis of *Brucella ovis* infection in rams. *Research in Veterinary Science*, 48, 209–215.

58 **MARIN, C.M., JIMENEZ DE BAGUES, M.P., BARBERAN, M. & BLASCO, J.M., 1989.** Efficacy of long-acting oxytetracycline alone or in combination with streptomycin for treatment of *Brucella ovis* infection of rams. *American Journal of Veterinary Research*, 50, 560–563.

59 **McFARLANE, D., SALISBURY, R.M., OSBORNE, H.G. & JEBSON, J.L., 1952.** Investigation into sheep abortion in New Zealand during the 1950 lambing season: Ram epididymitis, ewe abortion and lamb neonatal mortality. *Australian Veterinary Journal*, 28, 221–226.

60 **McGOWAN, B. & SCHULTZ, G., 1956.** Epididymitis of rams: Clinical description and field aspects. *Cornell Veterinarian*, 46, 277–281.

61 **MEINERSHAGEN, W.A., FRANK, F.W. & WALDHALM, D.G., 1974.** *Brucella ovis* as a cause of abortion in ewes. *American Journal of Veterinary Research*, 35, 723–724.

62 **MEYER, M.E., 1966.** Identification of *Brucella* organisms by immunofluorescence. *American Journal of Veterinary Research*, 27, 424–429.

63 **MILLER, S.J. & MOULE, G.R., 1954.** Clinical observations on the reproductive organs of Merino rams in pastoral Queensland. *Australian Veterinary Journal*, 30, 353–363.

64 **MOLLELO, J.A., JENSEN, R., FLINT, J.C. & COLLIER, J.R., 1963.** Placental pathology. I. Placental lesions of sheep experimentally infected with *Brucella ovis*. *American Journal of Veterinary Research*, 24, 897–903.

65 **MURRAY, R.M., 1969.** Scrotal abnormalities in rams in tropical Queensland with particular reference to ovine brucellosis and its control. *Australian Veterinary Journal*, 45, 63–67.

66 **OSBORNE, H.G., 1955.** Epididymitis of rams. *Australian Veterinary Journal*, 31, 11–16.

67 **PIETERSON, P.M., GUMMOW, B., PEFANIS, S., VENTER, C.G. & HERR, S., 1988.** The characteristics of a variant strain of *Brucella melitensis* Rev I. *Onderstepoort Journal of Veterinary Research*, 55, 15–17.

68 **PLANT, J.W., 1974.** Ovine brucellosis—still a cause of infertility. *Agricultural Gazette of New South Wales*, 85, 1–4.

69 **PLANT, J.W., EAMENS, G.J. & SEAMAN, J.T., 1986.** Serological, bacteriological and pathological changes in rams following different routes of exposure to *Brucella ovis*. *Australian Veterinary Journal*, 63, 409–412.

70 **PULSFORD, M.F., EASTICK, B.C., CLAPP, K.H. & ROBERTS, R., 1967.** Traumatic epididymitis of Dorset Horn and Poll Dorset rams. *Australian Veterinary Journal*, 43, 99–101.

71 **RIEZU-BOJ, J.I., MORIYON, I., BLASCO, J.M., MARIN, C.M. & DIAZ, R., 1986.** Comparison of lipopolysaccharide and outer membrane protein-lipopolysaccharide extracts in an enzyme-linked immunosorbent assay for the diagnosis of *Brucella ovis* infection. *Journal of Clinical Microbiology*, 23, 938–942.

72 **RYAN, F.B., 1964.** Eradication of ovine brucellosis. *Australian Veterinary Journal*, 40, 162–165.

73 **SEARSON, J.E., 1986.** Distribution of *Brucella ovis* in the tissues of rams reacting to the complement-fixation test for ovine brucellosis. *Australian Veterinary Journal*, 63, 30–31.

74 **SHORTRIDGE, E.H., 1962.** The lesions of the testicle and epididymis of rams. *New Zealand Veterinary Journal*, 10, 23–26.

75 **SHORTRIDGE, E.H. & CORDES, D.O., 1969.** Seminomas in sheep. *Journal of Comparative Pathology*, 79, 229–232.

76 **SIMMONS, G.C. & HALL, W.T.K., 1953.** Epididymitis of rams. Preliminary studies on the occurrence and pathogenicity of a *Brucella*-like organism. *Australian Veterinary Journal*, 29, 33–40.

77 **SNOWDON, W.A., 1958.** The epidemiology of ovine brucellosis in South Australia. Opening of discussion. *Australian Veterinary Journal*, 34, 417–423.

78 **STAMP, J.T., McEWEN, A.D., WATT, J.A.A. & NISBET, D.I., 1950.** Enzootic abortion in ewes. I. Transmission of the disease. *The Veterinary Record*, 62, 251–254.

79 **VAN DRIMMELEN, G.C., 1959.** Diagnosis of brucellosis in sheep and goats. *Journal of the South African Veterinary Medical Association*, 30, 259–269.

80 **VAN DRIMMELEN, G.C., 1960.** Control of brucellosis in sheep and goats by means of vaccination. *Journal of the South African Veterinary Medical Association*, 31, 129–138.

81 **VAN DRIMMELEN, G.C., 1974.** The distribution, incidence and control of brucellosis in the Republic of South Africa. *Bulletin de l'Office International des Épizooties*, 82, 97–105.

82 **VAN HEERDEN, K.M., 1964.** Results obtained by the use of Rev. I vaccine in sheep against infectious infertility suspected to be caused by ovine brucellosis. *Bulletin de l'Office International des Épizooties*, 62, 997–1002.

83 **VAN HEERDEN, K.M. & VAN RENSBURG, S.W.J., 1962.** The immunization of rams against ovine brucellosis. *Journal of the South African Veterinary Medical Association*, 33, 143–148.

84 **VAN RENSBURG, S.W.J., VAN HEERDEN, K.M., LE ROUX, D.J. & SNYDERS, A.J., 1958.** Infectious infertility in sheep. *Journal of the South African Veterinary Medical Association*, 39, 223–233.

85 **VAN TONDER, E.M., 1974–84.** Regional Veterinary Laboratory, Middelburg, Cape Province. Unpublished data.

86 **VAN TONDER, E.M., 1977.** Actinobacillus seminis *Infection in Sheep in South Africa*. D.V.Sc. Thesis, University of Pretoria.

87 **VAN TONDER, E.M., 1977.** Examination of rams for genital soundness. *Journal of the South African Veterinary Medical Association*, 48, 267–272.

88 **WALKER, R.L., LEAMASTER, B.R., STELLFLUG, J.N. & BIBERSTEIN, E.L., 1986.** Association of age of ram with distribution of epididymal lesions and etiologic agent. *Journal of the American Veterinary Medical Association*, 188, 393–396.

89 **WATT, D.A., 1971.** Congenital retention cysts of the epididymis in rams. *Australian Veterinary Journal*, 47, 287–288.

90 **WATT, D.A., 1971.** Seminoma in a sheep. *Australian Veterinary Journal*, 47, 405–406.

91 **WATT, D.A., 1972.** Testicular abnormalities and spermatogenesis of the ovine and other species. *Veterinary Bulletin, Weybridge*, 42, 181–190.

92 **WATTS, P.S., 1955.** Genital infections in sheep with particular reference to *Brucella*-like organisms. *Australian Veterinary Journal*, 31, 1–6.

93 **WEBB, R.F., QUINN, C.A., COCKRAM, F.A. & HUSBAND, A.J., 1980.** Evaluation of procedures for the diagnosis of *Brucella ovis* infection in rams. *Australian Veterinary Journal*, 56, 172–175.

94 **WORTHINGTON, R.W., STEVENSON, B.J. & DE LISLE, G.W., 1985.** Serology and semen culture for the diagnosis of *Brucella ovis* infection in chronically infected rams. *New Zealand Veterinary Journal*, 33, 84–86.

95 **WORTHINGTON, R.W., WEDDELL, W. & PENROSE, M.E., 1984.** A comparison of three serological tests for the diagnosis of *B. ovis* infection in rams. *New Zealand Veterinary Journal*, 32, 58–60.

96 **ZEKI, S., KUMAR, K.G.R. & KESHAVAMURTHY, B.S., 1981.** Isolation of *Haemophilus agni* from cases of purulent orchitis in rams. *Indian Journal of Comparative Microbiology*, 2, 30–31.

126

Brucella melitensis *infection*

S. Herr

Introduction

Infection with *Brucella melitensis* causes abortion, reduced milk yield and orchitis in goats and sheep, and undulant fever (also known as Malta fever or Mediterranean fever) in humans.

The organism responsible for undulant fever in humans was first discovered by Bruce on the island of Malta in 1887. Soon thereafter it was shown to be the cause of contagious abortion on the island, and also that humans contracted the infection by the consumption of fresh goats' milk.

Brucella melitensis has a high prevalence in Malta and the Mediterranean area, from whence came the original names for the disease in humans, Malta fever or Mediterranean fever, but it also occurs in many other parts of the world, such as Central America, the USA and Africa. Undulant fever in humans is also caused by *B. abortus* and *B. suis* infections; the resultant clinical diseases being indistinguishable from that caused by *B. melitensis*.

Confirmed cases of *Brucella melitensis* infection in goats and sheep in South Africa and Namibia are rare[11, 18, 19] — in recent years (1980 to 1988) only three isolates of *B. melitensis* biotype 1 from humans in northern Namibia have been recorded,[11] while in 1989 *B. melitensis* was isolated from two goats on a smallholding near Pretoria, but no spread from this property has been reported.[11] Until 1987 it was believed that *B. melitensis* did not occur in Zimbabwe, but since then two outbreaks in goats on commercial farms in the Gweru and Harare districts, and two in goats in communal areas in Matabeleland North and Mashonaland Central have been diagnosed.[16]

Aetiology and epidemiology

Brucella melitensis, which is the most pathogenic of the *Brucella* spp., is morphologically and tinctorially indistinguishable from *B. abortus*, but it can be identified serologically.[5, 8] For further information on the aetiology, **see Chapter 124: Bovine brucellosis.**

Outbreaks of *B. melitensis* infection in sheep and goats are sporadic in countries in southern Africa such as Zambia[15] and Zimbabwe.[16] Both sexes are equally susceptible to infection. In contrast to cattle, pregnant and non-pregnant goats and sheep do not differ in their susceptibility to the infection. All breeds of goats are equally susceptible to the infection, but resistance varies with breed in sheep; Maltese sheep are highly resistant, while certain fat-tailed breeds (such as Awassi) are highly susceptible.[1, 3, 6] Different breeds of sheep also differ in their serological response to the vaccine strain of the causative organism, *B. melitensis* Rev. I.[6]

Genital discharges of infected goats and sheep are usually copious and persist for up to three months following abortion, kidding or lambing. These often contain large numbers of the organism and are the prime sources of infection.[20] Although infection occurs by the ingestion of infected milk, inhalation is the most important route of infection in goats and sheep,[1] and the herding of goats and sheep into pens or kraals at night creates an ideal environment for the spread of the infection.[6]

Orchitis is a common sequel to infection in billy goats and rams, but even though organisms may be present in semen and urine, males do not play an important role in the dissemination of the disease.

Young animals usually recover spontaneously from the infection. However, adult animals seldom recover. Congenital, latent infection is suspected to occur, but has not been proven.[1]

Survival of *B. melitensis* in the environment is similar to that of *B. abortus*.[1]

Inoculation of the vaccine strain, *B. melitensis* Rev. I, into pregnant goats and sheep causes abortion, and results in the excretion of the vaccine strain in the milk in lactating nanny goats and ewes.

Cattle are readily infected with *B. melitensis* when in close contact with infected goats and sheep on communal grazing or at watering places, which leads to abortions in pregnant animals.[20] Humans are also highly susceptible to infection and are often the first reported cases of infection in an area where the disease has been newly introduced.[20] In addition to handling infective material, humans may become infected by the consumption of unpasteurized milk, and fresh cheese processed from infected milk, or by accidental inoculation with the *B. melitensis* Rev. I vaccine strain.[2, 4]

Pathogenesis and clinical signs

The pathogenesis of the disease is similar to that of *B. abortus* infection in cattle[6] **(see Chapter 124: Bovine brucellosis)**.

The first sign of the presence of the disease in a susceptible flock of goats or sheep is usually an abortion storm during which up to 60 per cent of the pregnant animals may abort, generally late in gestation. During subsequent breeding seasons the numbers of animals that abort declines progressively until abortions cease to occur. Such flocks do, however, remain infected for years. Milk yield following abortion is poor, and the general quality of the milk may be reduced. *Brucella melitensis* bacteria may persist in the udder for years. Orchitis is common in males (goats and sheep).[1, 6] Lambs from infected ewes may be born weak or may be asymptomatic but become persistent latent carriers of the infection.

In some flocks the prevalence of infection with *B. melitensis* may be high in the absence of obvious disease at any stage.

Pathology

The macroscopic lesions in ewes following infection with *B. melitensis* include oedema, greyish-white areas of necrosis of the placenta, and the presence of a brownish-red exudate between the allantochorion and the endometrium.[17]

Microscopically, foci of necrosis are evident in and around the placentomes. Intracytoplasmic bacteria are present in epithelial cells in the affected areas. Desquamated trophoblast cells and a few macrophages, neutrophils and plasma cells occur in the spaces between the chorionic villi and septa. The placental lesions are accompanied by an acute endometritis.[17]

Diagnosis

Smears made from the placenta, the content of the abomasum of the foetus, and vaginal discharges, stained with the Stamp's modification of the Ziehl Neelsen stain, should be examined for the presence of *B. melitensis*. Only a presumptive diagnosis can, however, be made by smear examination. This should be confirmed by isolation and typing of the organism. Attempts should be made to culture bacteria from the cotyledons, abomasal content and lungs of the foetus and, in slaughtered animals, from the mammary glands and supramammary lymph nodes in females, the seminal vesicles and testes in males, and the parotid, mandibular and retropharyngeal lymph nodes.[7] Selective and enriched media, such as Albimi *Brucella* medium or Farrell's medium, should be used. Isolates made from goats' milk and the supramammary lymph nodes are often in the rough phase and may be difficult to type.[1]

With some exceptions, the serological tests used for diagnosing *B. abortus* infection are also suitable for the diagnosis of *B. melitensis* infection.[13] *Brucella abortus* strain 99 is usually used as the antigen in serological tests for *B. melitensis*, but there may be an advantage to using a *B. melitensis* antigen where the disease is caused by biotype 1, as the reaction is then more specific.[10, 20] The milk-ring test does not give as clear-cut a reaction as it does in cattle infected with *B. abortus*, and it is thus not recommended as a flock test.[6] The serum-agglutination and Rose Bengal tests are less sensitive than the complement fixation test (CFT).[12] An allergic test, using brucellin, has also been recommended as a flock test.[3, 6, 13] Although it is not as sensitive or specific as it is in cattle infected with *B. abortus*, the CFT is considered the best for testing individual animals.[3, 6, 10] If lambs or kids between three and eight months of age are vaccinated with *B. melitensis* Rev. I, the CFT will be negative for 12 months after inoculation.[2, 3] The ELISA assay is more sensitive than the CFT and it can be automated,[10] but it has not been standardized and is not yet accepted for international trade purposes.

Differential diagnosis

Causes of abortion in sheep and goats must be established by laboratory examination. In stained smears prepared from infected material, *B. melitensis* may be confused with *Chlamydia* spp. and *Coxiella burnetii*, both of which are causes of abortion in sheep and goats in the subregion. Diseases such as Rift Valley fever and toxoplasmosis should also be considered.

The differentiation of the vaccine strain from wild *B. melitensis* is accomplished by additional laboratory tests such as sensitivity to penicillin and streptomycin, size of colony, and growth on dyes (thionin and basic fuchsin).[8] It is not possible to distinguish between *B. melitensis* and *B. abortus* by serological methods on serum because of the common antigens contained by the two bacteria.[10] This includes reaction to *B. abortus* strain 99 antigen, which is most commonly used in *B. melitensis* serology, and the reactions using strains 99 and Rev. I as antigens.[10, 11] However, no cross-reaction occurs with *B. ovis*.

Control

Vaccination with the *B. melitensis* Rev. I vaccine containing 10^9 viable organisms per dose is the most common method of control.[6] Lambs and kids between three and eight months of age should be vaccinated, as should adults at least two months prior to breeding. The attenuated bacteria do not persist in kids and lambs for longer than 14 weeks following inoculation, but immunity evoked by a single inoculation in lambs is protective for at least four years, and may be life-long.[2] Vaccination of pregnant goats and sheep causes abortion or excretion of the vaccine organisms in milk. Billy goats and rams vaccinated at one year of age react poorly immunologically.

Even though the duration of immunity following vaccination of adult females is unknown, it is recommended that they only be vaccinated once. Although eradication of the disease will not be achieved by vaccination alone, its prevalence can be dramatically reduced in goats and sheep.[3, 6, 9, 14]

Eradication of the disease can only be accomplished by a test-and-slaughter approach, but this can only be applied in small flocks where the prevalence of the disease is less than 2 per cent. Two negative CFT results (the test of choice) six months apart, on all the animals in a flock, is accepted as proof of eradication of the disease.[3, 6, 13, 14]

Incineration of infective material (such as foetuses, foetal membranes, contaminated bedding) and other general hygienic measures, including isolation of infected animals, should be applied to protect both animals and humans from infection.[13]

References

1 **ALTON, G.G., 1985.** The epidemiology of *Brucella melitensis* in sheep and goats. *In*: VERGER, J.M. & PLOMMET, M., (eds). *Brucella melitensis*. Dordrecht, Boston, Lancaster: Martinus Nijhoff Publishers.

2 **ALTON, G.G., 1985.** Rev. I and H38 *Brucella melitensis* vaccines. *In*: VERGER, J.M. & PLOMMET, M., (eds). *Brucella melitensis*. Dordrecht, Boston, Lancaster: Martinus Nijhoff Publishers.

3 **ALTON, G.G., 1987.** Control of *Brucella melitensis* infection in sheep and goats — A review. *Tropical Animal Health and Production*, 19, 65–74.

4 **ALTON, G.G. & ELBERG, S.S., 1967.** Rev. I *Brucella melitensis* vaccine. A review of ten years of study. *Veterinary Bulletin*, 37, 793–800.

5 **ALTON, G.G., JONES, L.M., ANGUS, R.D. & VERGER, J.M., 1988.** Techniques for the brucellosis laboratory. Paris: Institut National de la Recherche Agronomique (INRA).

6 **ANON., 1986.** JOINT FAO/WHO EXPERT COMMITTEE ON BRUCELLOSIS. *World Health Organization Technical Report Series 740*. Geneva: WHO.

7 **CORBEL, M.J., 1985.** Bacteriological procedures in the diagnosis of *Brucella melitensis* infection. *In*: VERGER, J.M. & PLOMMET, M., (eds). *Brucella melitensis*. Dordrecht, Boston, Lancaster: Martinus Nijhoff Publishers.

8 **CORBEL, M.J., GILL, K.P.W. & THOMAS, E.L. revised by CORBEL, M.J. & HENDRY, D., 1983.** *Methods for the Identification of Brucella*. Central Veterinary Laboratory, Weybridge, Surrey KT15 3NB, England.

9 **ELBERG, S.S., 1981.** Rev. I *Brucella melitensis* vaccine. Part II: 1968–80. *Veterinary Bulletin*, 51, 67–73.

10 **FARINA, R., 1985.** Current serological methods in *B. melitensis* diagnosis. *In*: VERGER, J.M. & PLOMMET, M., (eds). *Brucella melitensis*. Dordrecht, Boston, Lancaster: Martinus Nijhoff Publishers.

11 **HERR, S., 1990.** Veterinary Research Institute, Onderstepoort. Unpublished data.

12 **HOSIE, B.D., AL-BAKRI, O.M. & FUTTER, R.J., 1985.** Survey of brucellosis in goats and sheep in the Yemen Arab Republic: Comparison of the tests for *Brucella melitensis* infection in sheep. *Tropical Animal Health and Production*, 17, 93–99.

13 **KOLAR, J., 1984.** Diagnosis and control of brucellosis in small ruminants. *Preventive Veterinary Medicine*, 2, 215–225.

14 **LANTIER, F. & FENSTERBANK, R., 1985.** Kinetics of Rev I infection in sheep. *In*: VERGER, J.M. & PLOMMET, M., (eds). *Brucella melitensis*. Dordrecht, Boston, Lancaster: Martinus Nijhoff Publishers.

15 **LINYANGWE, P.G., 1991.** Central Veterinary Research Institute, P.O. Box 33980, Lusaka, Zambia. Unpublished data.

16 **MADSEN, M, 1989.** The current state of brucellosis in Zimbabwe. *Zimbabwe Veterinary Journal*, 20, 133–143.

17 **MOLELLO, J.A., FLINT, J.C., COLLIER, J.R. & JENSEN, R., 1963.** Placental pathology. II. Placental lesions of sheep experimentally infected with *Brucella melitensis*. *American Journal of Veterinary Research*, 24, 905–911.

18 **VAN DRIMMELEN, G.C., 1965.** The presence of *Brucella melitensis* infection in sheep in the Transvaal. *Bulletin de l'Office International des Épizooties*, 64, 745–756.

19 **VAN DRIMMELEN, G.C., 1966.** Brucellosis of sheep and swine. *Bulletin de l'Office International des Épizooties*, 66, 815–824.

20 **VERGER, J.M., 1985.** *Brucella melitensis* infection in cattle. *In*: VERGER, J.M. & PLOMMET, M., (eds). *Brucella melitensis*. Dordrecht, Boston, Lancaster: Martinus Nijhoff Publishers.

127

Brucella suis *infection*

G.C. Bishop and P.P. Bosman

Introduction

Brucella suis infection in pigs causes an acute or chronic disease that results in abortions, stillbirths, sterility of sows, orchitis in boars, and mortalities in piglets. Although the disease is widely distributed in the world,[2] it has not yet been diagnosed in southern Africa.

Aetiology and epidemiology

The morphological and cultural characteristics of *B. suis* are similar to those of the other members of the genus *Brucella*[4, 5] **(see Chapter 124: Bovine brucellosis)**. It does not, however, require an increased carbon dioxide tension for primary isolation, but needs blood- or serum-enriched media for optimal growth.[1] There are five recognized biovars (typed on the basis of biochemical tests, serological reactivity, and phage-susceptibility), which vary in their virulence for pigs, their host range, and the countries in which they occur. Biovars 1, 2 and 3 affect pigs, whereas the preferred hosts for biovars 4 and 5 are reindeer and wild rodents, respectively.[2]

Brucella suis biovars 1–3 are mainly pathogenic in pigs and humans, but other species such as horses, cattle, dogs, hares, reindeer and wild rodents are also susceptible. The susceptibility of pigs varies with age, the prevalence of infection usually being higher in older pigs.[3, 6] Both sexes are equally susceptible.

Infection is generally introduced into a herd by infected pigs. Boars are the main source of infection, and transmission occurs chiefly by coitus, but other routes, such as the ingestion of infected material, also play a role.[7] The course of the disease is usually acute in a herd of pigs.[2] Spread within a herd may be rapid and, although no durable immunity develops, there is a degree of herd resistance which causes the infection in some individuals to manifest in a chronic form.

Persistent granulomatous lesions occur in the uterus, urinary bladder, or in the testes and accessory male sex organs, from which bacteria can be shed in the semen for months or years.[9]

Pathogenesis, clinical signs and pathology

Bacteraemia follows multiplication of the organism at the portal of entry. *Brucella suis* has no predilection for specific tissues or organs; the infection may localize in the male and female genital organs, skeletal system, joints, mammary glands, lymph nodes, spleen, liver, kidneys and urinary bladder. Most lesions consist of progressively enlarging, caseating granulomas which may become calcified. In the uterus and Fallopian tube they are generally 2–5 mm in diameter and have a miliary distribution. In addition to the miliary granulomatous metritis, a mucoid endometritis may be present in which numerous *Brucella* organisms occur in the luminal exudate. Genital tract infections in sows result in irregular oestrus, small litters, abortion, stillbirths, and the birth of weak piglets. Abortion usually occurs between the second and third month of pregnancy. Sows usually do not abort more than once following infection, but may become infertile. Some piglets infected *in utero* may die within a few hours of birth, the mortality rate often being very high. However others survive and retain the infection into adulthood.[9] Orchitis and infection of the accessory sex glands are common in boars.[10] Mortality in older pigs is usually low. Chronic disease causes economic losses because of the forced culling of boars and sows as a result of infertility caused by lesions in the genital tract.

The inflammatory reaction in joints is fibrinopurulent. If the vertebrae (often the lumbar, in particular) are involved, an osteomyelitis develops which has a tendency to spread to and destroy adjacent intervertebral disks: such affected animals often clinically manifest posterior paresis.

No specific lesions occur in aborted foetuses.

Diagnosis and differential diagnosis

It is preferable to make the diagnosis on a herd basis, using the results of both bacteriological and serological tests (such as the complement fixation test and enzyme-linked immunosorbent assay).[2, 3, 8] As not all infected pigs react immunologically, all breeding pigs should be considered as being infected once a diagnosis has been made in a particular herd.

Abortion in sows as a result of *B. suis* infection should be differentiated from other causes of abortion, including infections with bacteria, such as *Leptospira* spp., *Erysipelothrix rhusiopathiae*, *Streptococcus* spp., *Staphylococcus* spp., *Corynebacterium* spp., and *Salmonella* serovars.

Control

Control on the basis of 'test and slaughter' has been widely used but, ultimately, because of the difficulties of detecting infection in all infected animals in a herd, complete disposal by slaughter of all the stock in infected herds is the best option. Restocking must then be based on the introduction of pigs free from *B. suis* infection.

The *B. suis* strain 2 vaccine has been successfully used in China as an oral vaccine.[11]

References

1 **ALTON, G.G., JONES, L.M., ANGUS, R.D. & VERGER, J.M., 1988.** *Techniques for the Brucellosis Laboratory*. 1st edn. Paris: Institut National de l'Université.

2 **ANON., 1986.** *Joint FAO/WHO Expert Committee on Brucellosis*, 1986. 6th report. Geneva: World Health Organization.

3 **BLOOD, D.C., HENDERSON, J.A. & RADOSTITS, O.M., 1983.** *Veterinary Medicine*. 6th edn. London: Baillière Tindall.

4 **CORBEL, M.J. & BRINLEY MORGAN, W.J., 1984.** *In*: KRIEG, N.R. & HOLT, J.G., (eds). *Bergey's Manual of Systematic Bacteriology*. Baltimore, London: Williams & Wilkins.

5 **CORBEL, M.J., GILL, K.P.W., THOMAS, E.L. & HENDRY, D., 1983.** *Methods for the Identification of Brucella*. Booklet No. 85. United Kingdom: MAFF Publications, Alnwick NE66 2PF.

6 **CRICHTON, R. & MEDVECZKY, N.E., 1987.** The identity, distribution and epizootiological significance of *Brucella* isolates in Australia, 1981 to 1985. *Australian Veterinary Journal*, 64, 48–52.

7 **JUBB, K.V.F., KENNEDY, P.C. & PALMER, N., 1985.** *Pathology of Domestic Animals*. 3rd edn. San Diego: Academic Press, Inc.

8 **ROGERS, R.J., COOK, D.R., KETTERER, P.J., BALOOCK, F.C., BLACKALL, P.J. & STEWART, R.W., 1989.** An evaluation of three serological tests for antibody to *Brucella suis* in pigs. *Australian Veterinary Journal*, 66, 77–80.

9 **TAYLOR, D.J., 1983.** *Pig Diseases*. Cambridge: The Burlington Press.

10 **THOEN, C.O. & ENRIGHT, F., 1986.** *In*: GYLES, C.L. & THOEN, C.O., (eds). *Pathogenesis of Bacterial Infections in Animals*. 1st edn. Ames, Iowa: Iowa State University Press.

11 **XIE XIN, 1986.** Orally administrable brucellosis vaccine: *Brucella suis* strain 2 vaccine. *Vaccine*, 4, 212–216.

FACULTATIVELY ANAEROBIC GRAM-NEGATIVE RODS

The genera of three families (Enterobacteriaceae, Pasteurellaceae, and Vibrionaceae) are classified as facultatively anaerobic, Gram-negative rods. As far as is currently known, only the genera within the families Enterobacteriaceae and Pasteurellaceae contain bacteria that are pathogenic to animals.[3]

FAMILY ENTEROBACTERIACEAE

Bacteria that belong to this family are Gram-negative straight rods, 0,3–1,0 x 1,0–6,0 µm in size, which are motile as a result of the presence of peritrichous flagella. They do not form endocysts, nor are they acid-fast. They are ubiquitous in nature, occurring in soil, water, fruit, vegetables, grains, flowering plants, trees, insects and mammals.

Of the eight genera (*Escherichia, Shigella, Salmonella, Klebsiella, Enterobacter, Serratia, Proteus* and *Yersinia*) belonging to the Enterobacteriaceae that contain members which infect humans and animals, only *Escherichia, Salmonella* and *Klebsiella* are important in terms of causing economically important diseases in livestock. Members of the other genera are associated with rare sporadic and often opportunistic infections in animals. *Shigella dysenteriae* often causes enterocolitis in a variety of captive, non-human primates.[2] *Enterobacter aerogenes* and *Serratia* spp. are occasionally reported as a cause of mastitis in cattle, while infection with *Proteus* spp., and particularly *Proteus mirabilis,* may cause severe enteritis following prolonged antibiotic treatment, and mastitis in goats. *Proteus* spp. are also commonly associated with the spoilage of meat.[1] Infection by the various *Yersinia* spp. is common, but these bacteria do not regularly infect livestock species. *Yersinia pestis,* the cause of bubonic plague in humans, has rarely been isolated from goats and donkeys. *Yersinia enterocolitica,* a cause of terminal ileitis in humans, has been occasionally identified as the cause of severe enteritis in sheep, goats and pigs.[1] *Yersinia pseudotuberculosis,* which is a common intestinal inhabitant of various animal species, is the cause of a septicaemic disease, sometimes accompanied by abscessation, in birds and rodents. Infection by it has been recorded as a very rare, sporadic cause of abortions in cattle and sheep, mastitis in goats, epididymitis and orchitis in rams, and abscessation, lymphadenitis and pneumonia in cattle.[2,4]

FAMILY PASTEURELLACEAE

This family contains three genera (*Pasteurella, Haemophilus,* and *Actinobacillus*). General information about the characteristics of each of the genera is contained in the introductions to the respective sections.

FAMILY VIBRIONACEAE

The two genera (*Vibrio and Aeromonas*) in this family do not contain any bacteria that are important in livestock species.

References

1 **BLOOD, D.C. & RADOSTITS, O.M., 1989.** *Veterinary Medicine.* 7th edn. London, Philadelphia, Sydney, Tokyo, Toronto: Baillière Tindall.

2 **HUNGERFORD, T.G., 1990.** *Diseases of Livestock.* 9th edn. Sydney: McGraw-Hill Book Company.

3 **KRIEG, N.R. & HOLT, J.G., 1984.** *Bergey's Manual of Systematic Bacteriology.* Vol. I. Baltimore, London: Williams & Wilkins.

4 **TIMONEY, J.S., GILLESPIE, J.H., SCOTT, F.W. & BARLOUGH, J.E., (eds), 1988.** *Hagan and Bruner's Microbiology and Infectious Disease of Domestic Animals.* 8th edn. Ithaca: Comstock Publishing Associates.

128

Klebsiella *spp. infections*

M.M. Henton

Introduction

Infections with *Klebsiella* spp. cause a variety of syndromes in livestock, the most important being endometritis, infertility and abortion in mares, mastitis in cows and sows, and neonatal septicaemia, particularly in foals. In southern Africa, the majority of infections are associated with the genital tract of Thoroughbred mares **(see Chapter 189: Infectious causes of equine reproductive failure)**. Antibiotic-resistant strains of *Klebsiella* commonly cause nosocomial infections in humans.[20]

Klebsiella was first described by Escherich in 1885 as *Bakterium lactis aerogenes*, but as this name was later also used for *Enterobacter*, it was changed to *Klebsiella*, after the German bacteriologist, Edwin Klebs.[20]

The pathogenic capsular types found in South Africa are similar to those in other parts of the world[3, 6, 8, 14, 21] **(Table 128.1)**.

Aetiology and epidemiology

The genus *Klebsiella* belongs to the family Enterobacteriaceae. *Klebsiella* spp. are facultative anaerobes and are large, non-motile, Gram-negative rods (0,3–1,0 µm wide and 0,6–6,0 µm long) usually containing a thick, mucoid capsule. In the laboratory they grow well on most growth media, forming large, moist and viscid colonies. *Klebsiella* spp. are inositol-positive, and most pathogenic strains are rapidly urease-positive. They are classified biochemically into *K. pneumoniae, K. oxytoca, K. terrigena,* and *K. planticola*.[20] *Klebsiella pneumoniae* is subdivided into three subspecies: *pneumoniae, ozaenae* and *rhinoscleromatis*. *Klebsiella pneumoniae* and *K. oxytoca* are isolated from various pathological processes in humans and animals, while *K. terrigena* and *K. planticola* are found mainly in soil and water.[20]

The biochemically defined species of *Klebsiella* are serotyped with one set of capsular typing antisera.[5] Presently, all strains of *Klebsiella* are serologically classified into 82 capsular types,[20] and numbered from 1 to 82. This classification gives a much clearer indication of pathogenicity than biochemical typing.[10, 18, 19]

Serotyping is done by means of the quelling (Neufeld) reaction;[5] live bacteria are mixed with capsular antisera, and the reaction indicated by refractile, precipitin patterns which are discernible microscopically on the surface of the bacterial capsule. The O-types of *Klebsiella* are usually not characterized, as they are few in number, and typing of the O-antigens is hampered by the large capsule.

Klebsiella spp. are ubiquitous and occur in soil and water, or are part of the normal flora in the gastrointestinal tract of animals, albeit often in low numbers. They are particularly common in contaminated wood shavings and soil containing shavings.[17] Wood shavings used as bedding are therefore an important source of infection, especially when severely contaminated with faeces.[19]

Klebsiella spp. are opportunistic pathogens. The pathogenicity of specific capsular types for livestock species other than horses is largely unknown. In South Africa, capsular types 2, 6, 21, 30 and 33 are most commonly isolated from non-equid livestock species. These types are usually associated with mastitis in cows and sows and septicaemia in neonatal calves, lambs and piglets.[7]

Identification of the capsular types of *Klebsiella* isolated from the genital tract of horses between 1972 and 1987 at the Veterinary Research Institute, Onderstepoort showed that certain types are more common than others **(Table 128.1)**. Stallions may be subclinical carriers of these types and may infect mares venereally.[4, 10, 11] It was found that capsular Types 1, 2 and 20 were responsible for endometritis in mares in about 50 per cent of all cases. Types such as 3, 31 and 64 occurred only as transient colonists of the uterus, whereas Types 6, 7, 20, 21 and 30, which commonly infect the immunocompromised uterus, were also regularly isolated from the cervix of healthy horses.

Endometritis in mares

Flaccid, gaping vulvar lips, a vulva which slants dorso-anteriorally, pneumovagina as a result of poor conformation in which the dorsal commissure of the vulva is displaced to a position dorsally of the ischeal arch, foaling injuries to the genitalia (e.g., recto-vaginal lacerations or fistulas), urovagina and/or urouterus, ageing of the mare, and poor condition may predispose to *Klebsiella* endometritis. Endometritis usually results from an ascending infection after faecal contamination of the vulval lips, vestibulum and clitoral fossa[22].

As *Klebsiella* is relatively resistant to most disinfectants, the injudicious use of disinfectants to wash the genitalia of mares and stallions may inhibit the normal genital flora and stimulate overgrowth of *Klebsiella*. Similarly, treatment of mares suffering from endometritis with antimicrobials not selected on the basis of an antibiogram may result in overgrowth of *Klebsiella*.

The strains of *K. pneumoniae* isolated from mares with endometritis are divided into:[21]

- *Venereal strains (capsular Types 1, 2 and 5):* These strains are mostly transmitted venereally, but may also be transmitted mechanically by stallions that are not carriers of the infection. Environmental spread through contamination of pastures or bedding is also possible.
- *Strains which infect the immunocompromised uterus (capsular Types 6, 7, 20, 21 and 30):* The term 'immunocompromised uterus', as defined by Ricketts,[21] embraces any malfunction of the uterus, be it structural or hormonal. Colonization of the external genitalia by these strains is common but transient in healthy animals.[21] Stallions may transmit these organisms mechanically.
- *Opportunists:* Any of the other 82 capsular types may cause opportunistic venereal infections in horses.

Klebsiella is transmitted venereally or mechanically to mares. Transmission of *Klebsiella* may also occur by using improperly disinfected specula in mares.[21] The bacteria may be isolated from the semen as well as from the sheath of stallions that are carriers.[9] The infection rate in mares served by a carrier stallion may be as low as 25 per cent, even with the most common pathogenic type (capsular Type 1).[7] Of those infected, more than 50 per cent recover spontaneously or after treatment.[1] Mares may, however, remain infected for prolonged periods and shed *Klebsiella* Type 1 from one to 17 months.[7] On rare occasions, mares may remain infected and barren for up to five years.[7]

As the breeding of Thoroughbreds is seasonal, more cases of *Klebsiella* infections are detected in the spring than at any other time of the year.

Pastures may be contaminated by vaginal discharges and faeces containing *Klebsiella*.[15] Horses grazing on these pastures may become infected and the bacteria may become part of their normal gastrointestinal tract flora[10].

Mastitis

Mastitis caused by *Klebsiella* in cows is most common in countries with a cold climate where cows are kept indoors, especially on wood shavings.[17] In South Africa, however, there is a marked preponderance of cases during the hot summer months of December to February.[7] This may be related to calving, as *Klebsiella* mastitis is more common during early lactation when the udder is oedematous and milk production is at its highest.[18, 19] Severe toxaemia, due to absorption of endotoxin, may occur in animals with peracute mastitis.[16] For more information consult **Chapter 190: Mastitis**.

Pathogenesis

In mares predisposed to endometritis, infection and colonization of *Klebsiella* usually result from contamination of the vulval, clitoral and/or vestibular areas. From these areas the infection ascends to involve the uterus. Depending on the strain of *Klebsiella* involved and the susceptibility of the mare, the genital tract may become infected for a variable period. Semen seems to promote *Klebsiella* infections; mares that are repeatedly served carry the infection longer than those that have sexual rest.[22]

For information on the pathogenesis of mastitis, consult **Chapter 190: Mastitis**.

Table 128.1 Number of common capsular types of *Klebsiella* spp. isolated from horses at the Veterinary Research Institute, Onderstepoort from 1972 to 1987

CAPSULAR TYPES	SUBCLINICAL Mares	SUBCLINICAL Stallions	DISEASED Mares	DISEASED Stallions	TOTAL NO.
1	4	8	20	–	32
2	1	1	16	–	18
3	1	15	4	–	20
6	7	2	12	1	22
7	21	11	11	–	43
20	1	–	10	–	11
21	11	9	10	–	30
22	1	1	5	–	7
27	4	2	3	–	9
30	7	1	7	–	15
31	8	–	–	–	8
33	3	3	6	–	12
64	6	0	1	–	7

Clinical signs

Endometritis in mares

Mares predisposed to endometritis may become infected and show clinical signs at any stage of the oestrous cycle or during pregnancy. Venereally infected mares usually develop a vaginal discharge within three to five days of being served by a shedder stallion and are usually temporarily barren.

Endometritis in mares is generally manifested clinically by the presence of a scant or profuse greyish, viscid vaginal discharge which may contain floccules of pus. In mares with a profuse vaginal discharge, the hair on the buttocks and tail may be matted by the exudate. The mucous membrane of the vagina and cervix is often dull and reddish-brown to purplish-red. In advanced cases, pyometra may result.[22] On rectal palpation, the uterus is enlarged and atonic. The oestrous cycle in affected mares may be irregular, especially if the infection is secondary to a hormonal imbalance. Generally, mares and stallions with genital infection do not show systemic illness.

If a foetus becomes infected, abortion may occur, a weak, septicaemic foal may be born, or the foal may be normal at birth and develop septicaemia soon afterwards.[24, 25] Septicaemic foals show anorexia, depression, high fever, and usually develop severe polyarthritis, pneumonia and/or meningoencephalitis. Such foals die within a few days of birth if left untreated.

Stallions rarely show any clinical signs but are commonly subclinically infected with *Klebsiella*. The prepuce is frequently colonized but *Klebsiella* may also infect the accessory sexual glands, kidneys or urinary bladder.[4, 10, 11]

Mastitis

The mastitis-metritis-agalactiae syndrome in sows is only rarely associated with *Klebsiella* infections in South Africa, and when it occurs, it usually does so during the immediate post-partum period.[2]

Klebsiella generally causes peracute mastitis in sows and cows, characterized by severe systemic signs which include fever, anorexia, and increased heart and respiratory rates. The milk is yellowish and watery and contains small floccules of pus. In animals with acute to chronic mastitis, systemic signs are mild or inapparent. The udder is usually not markedly swollen or painful in animals with peracute, acute or chronic mastitis.[2, 3] For more information **Chapter 190: Mastitis** should be consulted.

Other syndromes

Other syndromes caused by *Klebsiella*, such as septicaemia and pneumonia, occur sporadically. Young calves and piglets drinking milk from cows or sows with *Klebsiella* mastitis may die from septicaemia. Sporadic cases of septicaemia or pneumonia in livestock as a result of *Klebsiella* may occur.

Pathology

Endometritis in mares

The lesions in mares suffering from endometritis vary according to the stage of development of the lesions, stage of the oestrous cycle, type of *Klebsiella* involved and which predisposing factors **(see Aetiology and epidemiology)** are present. In mild cases, only the superficial layers of the endometrium are affected, but in severe cases the endometrium may be focally denuded and have a dull, red, granular appearance.[22] On histopathology, small abscesses may be present in the uterine glands and the luminal epithelium may be covered with small or copious amounts of pus, which is usually mucoid. As with other bacterial infections of the endometrium, a diffuse or focal neutrophilic infiltrate is present in one or more layers of the endometrium. In chronic infections, atrophy and fibrosis of the endometrium may be evident. Bacteria cannot always be found in histopathological sections of endometrial biopsies taken from *Klebsiella*-infected mares.

Endometrial or cervical cytology usually reveals a large number of neutrophils and increased numbers of epithelial cells, while bacteria may or may not be present but are generally more plentiful than in histopathological sections.

Mastitis

Apart from the usual inflammatory changes associated with mastitis, severe cases may also develop thrombosis and infarction of the parenchyma **(see Chapter 190: Mastitis)**.

Diagnosis and differential diagnosis

Endometritis in mares

Endometritis due to infection by *Klebsiella* spp. in mares is very similar clinically and pathologically to that caused by other bacteria, including *Streptococcus* spp., *Pseudomonas aeruginosa* and *Taylorella equigenitalis*.[12, 13] Endometrial bacterial culture and cytology are therefore necessary to confirm the diagnosis **(see Chapter 189: Infectious causes of equine reproductive failure)**. Swabs for bacterial isolation should be taken from the urethral fossa and sheath in stallions and from the endometrium of mares in oestrus. The bacteriological examination of swabs taken from the urethra, cervix and clitoral fossa of mares is a useful means of establishing persistent carriers.

Mastitis

Klebsiella mastitis may be confused with other causes of mastitis **(see Chapter 190: Mastitis)**, particularly *Escherichia coli* infection, and can be distinguished only on bacterial culture.

Other syndromes

Apart from *Klebsiella*, septicaemia in foals is frequently caused by infection of *Escherichia coli, Actinobacillus equuli, A. suis* or *Streptococcus* spp. acquired *in utero*, during parturition or during the early neonatal period.[25]

Control

Endometritis in mares

As *Klebsiella* is common in the intestinal tract of healthy animals and is also commonly found in the environment,[20] methods of controlling *Klebsiella* infections should be aimed at those strains residing in or infecting the genital tract.

To prevent spread of infection in a stud, it is important to take swabs from mares that are possibly infected before they are covered. Stallions should also be swabbed two or three times during the breeding season.

Structural defects of the genital tract which predispose to infection should be rectified surgically before any antimicrobial therapy is started. Mares and stallions carrying *Klebsiella* Types 1, 2 and 5 should preferably be given sexual rest for a year. Mares should be treated as soon as possible with intra-uterine antimicrobials, chosen with due regard to the antibiotic sensitivity of the isolate, to prevent endometrial fibrosis **(see Chapter 189: Infectious causes of equine reproductive failure)** and should only be bred again after they have been shown to have recovered completely from the infection. Carrier stallions may be treated with disinfectants such as chlorhexidine or antimicrobials instilled into the sheath, but as most stallions are transient carriers and self-cure will result, it is preferable not to treat them. The injudicious use of antimicrobials and disinfectants can diminish the resident flora of the sheath and actually promote the multiplication of *Klebsiella*. If such stallions are to be used for breeding, artificial insemination with semen incubated in a diluent containing an appropriate antibiotic is effective in preventing the transmission of the infection to mares. Where artificial insemination is not allowed or practically impossible to perform, the semen diluent can be instilled into the mare's uterus immediately prior to natural service. Such mares should then be treated with an appropriate antibiotic for at least three days after service.

Mares and stallions should be swabbed at least three times at seven- to 14-day intervals with at least one swab taken during oestrus, after treatment or sexual rest to ensure that they are free of infection. During this time infected mares should be kept in isolation and the swabbing repeated if necessary until all three swabs are found to be free of *Klebsiella*.

Strict hygiene should be applied at service and during any veterinary examination. Recovered mares should preferably only be mated once (as close as possible to ovulation), and antibiotic therapy as indicated by an antibiogram is usually necessary.[23]

Faeces should be removed from the stables at least once a day to minimize faecal contamination, and straw should be used instead of wood shavings. Efforts should be made to keep the bedding as dry as possible. All tail bandages and reproductive instruments should be disposable or sterilized after each use.

Mastitis

General mastitis therapy, as well as supportive therapy using corticosteroids and intravenous fluids, is necessary in *Klebsiella* mastitis **(see Chapter 190: Mastitis)**.

References

1 **BAKER, B., 1982.** P.O. Box 787, Hillcrest, 3650, South Africa. Personal communication.

2 **BERTSCHINGER, H.U., POHLENZ, J. & ROSS, R.F., 1986.** Coliform mastitis. *In:* LEMAN, A.D., STRAW, B., GLOCK, R.D., MENGELING, W.L., PENNY, R.H.C. & SCHOLL, E., (eds). *Diseases of Swine.* 6th edn. Ames, Iowa: Iowa State University Press.

3 **BRAMAN, S.K., EBERHART, R.J., ASBURY, M.A. & HERMANN, G.J., 1973.** Capsular types of *Klebsiella pneumoniae* associated with bovine mastitis. *Journal of the American Veterinary Medical Association,* 162, 109–111.

4 **CROUCH, J.R.F., ATHERTON, J.C. & PLATT, H., 1972.** Venereal transmission of *Klebsiella aerogenes* in a thoroughbred stud from a persistently infected stallion. *The Veterinary Record,* 90, 21–28.

5 **EWING, W.H., 1986.** *Edwards and Ewing's Identification of Enterobacteriaceae.* 4th edn. New York: Elsevier Science Publishing Company.

6 **FLOER, W., 1974.** *Klebsiella* organisms in the genital organs and foetuses of thoroughbred horses. *Deutsche Tierärztliche Wochenschrift,* 81, 20–22.

7 **HENTON, M.M., 1992.** Onderstepoort Veterinary Institute, South Africa. Unpublished data.

8 **KENNEY, R.M., 1990.** Hofmann Fertility Clinic, School of Veterinary Medicine, University of Pennsylvania, Kennett Square, Pennsylvania 19348, USA.

9 **KENNEY, R.M., BERGMAN, R.V., COOPER, W.L. & MORSE, G.W., 1975.** Minimal contamination techniques for breeding mares: Technique and preliminary findings. *Proceedings of the American Association of Equine Practitioners,* S8–S15.

10 **KIKUCHI, N., IGUCHI, I.. & HIRAMUNE, T., 1987.** Capsule types of *Klebsiella pneumoniae* isolated from the genital tract of mares with metritis, extragenital sites of healthy mares and the genital tract of stallions. *Veterinary Microbiology,* 15, 219–228.

11 **KIKUCHI, N., TAKAYANAGI, N., KOSAKA, T., HIRAMUNE, T. & YANAGAWA, R., 1988.** Presence of less heavily encapsulated *Klebsiella pneumoniae* capsular Type 1 in semen of healthy stallions and cervical swabs of mares suffering from metritis and comparison of virulence between heavily and less heavily encapsulated strains. *Japanese Journal of Veterinary Science,* 50, 313–323.

12 **LE BLANC, M.M., 1989.** Treatment protocols and preventive practices for mares with endometritis. *Veterinary Medicine,* 84, 906–911.

13 **LIU, I.K.M., 1989.** Uterine infections in the mare. *Equine Practice,* 11, 26–32.

14 **MERKT, H., KLUG, E. BÖHM, K.H. & WEISS, R., 1974.** *Klebsiella* organisms as agents of genital infection in horses. *Berliner und Münchener Tierartztliche Wochenschrift,* 87, 405–409.

15 **MERKT, H., KLUG, E., BÖHM, K.H. & WEISS, R., 1975.** Recent observations concerning *Klebsiella* infections in stallions. *Journal of Reproduction and Fertility,* suppl. 23, 143–145.

16 **NEUMANN, P. & WENDT, K., 1985.** Aetiopathogenesis of bovine mastitis due to *Klebsiella pneumoniae. Monatschrifte für Veterinärmedizin,* 40, 120–123.

17 **NEWMAN, L.E. & KOWALSKI, J., 1973.** Fresh sawdust bedding as a potential source of *Klebsiella* organisms. *American Journal of Veterinary Research,* 34, 979–980.

18 **NOMURA, T., SUGIURA, H., MORIYA, H., KIKUCHI, N., HIRAMUNE, T. & YANAGAWA, R., 1989.** Species and capsular types of *Klebsiella* isolated from cows and their environment. *Journal of Rakuno Gakuen University, Natural Science,* 14, 57–61.

19 **NONNECKE, B.J. & NEWBOULD, F.H., 1984.** Biochemical and serologic characterization of *Klebsiella* strains from bovine mastitis and the environment of the dairy cow. *American Journal of Veterinary Research,* 45, 2451–2454.

20 **ORSKOV, I., 1984.** Genus V. *Klebsiella. In:* KRIEG, N.R. &

HOLT, J.G., (eds). *Bergey's Manual of Systematic Bacteriology*. Baltimore, London: Williams Wilkins.

21 **RICKETTS, S.W., 1981.** Bacteriological examinations of the mare's cervix: Techniques and interpretation of results. *The Veterinary Record*, 108, 46–51.

22 **ROBERTS, S.J., 1971.** *Veterinary Obstetrics and Genital Diseases*. Ithaca, New York: Edwards Brothers.

23 **VOLKMANN, D.H., 1992.** Minimal contamination breeding techniques. *Proceedings of Equine Practitioners Group Congress*, 24–27 February 1992, Badplaas: 117–119.

24 **WHITWELL, K.E., 1988.** Infective placentitis in the mare. *Equine Infectious Diseases, Proceedings of the Fifth International Conference*. University of Kentucky, USA.

25 **WILSON, W.D. & MADIGAN, J.E., 1989.** Comparison of bacterologic culture of blood and necropsy specimens for determining the cause of foal septicaemia: 47 cases (1978–87). *Journal of the American Veterinary Medical Association*, 195, 1759–1763.

129

Escherichia coli *infections*

Synonym: Colibacillosis

M.M. Henton and P. Hunter

Introduction

Escherichia coli is the predominant bacterium of the facultatively anaerobic flora of the intestine of many animal species. While most E. *coli* strains are non-pathogenic, certain of them may cause disease. The main syndromes produced by *E. coli* are enteritis (white scours, enteric colibacillosis) and septicaemia (colisepticaemia) in young calves, lambs, kids, piglets and foals, and oedema disease in pigs. *Escherichia coli* occasionally also causes pyogenic infections in a variety of tissues and is responsible for some forms of mastitis **(see Chapter 190: Mastitis)**, uterine infection and abortion in certain livestock species. Enteric colibacillosis occurs most commonly in new-born animals in intensive farming systems, but only rarely in animals raised under extensive conditions.

Escherichia coli infections occur worldwide,[19, 35, 85, 98] and can be of major economic significance. In southern Africa, enteric colibacillosis occurs most commonly in piglets, and less frequently in calves, lambs and kids.[33, 49]

Aetiology

Escherichia coli is a straight, Gram-negative, usually motile rod, 1,1–1,5 µm wide and 2–6 µm long, that belongs to the Enterobacteriaceae. It is facultatively anaerobic, having both respiratory and fermentative types of metabolism, and some strains possess peritrichous flagella. Most colonies on nutrient agar are either smooth or rough, but intermediate forms and mucoid colonies do occur. Smooth forms are low-convex and shiny, possess an entire, regular circumference, and are easily dispersible in saline, while rough colonies are dry, have a dull appearance, are usually flattish, have an irregular outline, and are difficult to disperse in saline. As a result of mutation, rough forms have lost the polysaccharide side chains of the lipopolysaccharide of the outer membrane of the cell wall. They autoagglutinate in saline and are therefore impossible to serotype by conventional means.

Escherichia coli is distinguishable from *Citrobacter* in that citrate cannot be used as its sole carbon source. Lactose is fermented by most strains of *E. coli*, and the colonies are therefore pink on McConkey agar. *Escherichia coli* is usually a strong indole producer, which distinguishes it from *Enterobacter*. Unlike *Klebsiella*, *E. coli* does not ferment inositol or adonitol.[70]

Different strains of *E. coli* are typeable according to the characteristics of capsular (K), somatic (O) and flagellar (H) antigens. Many strains, especially those isolated from extra-intestinal sites, possess polysaccharide capsules that are used for typing K antigens. The cell wall of the bacterium is used for O-antigen typing and is partially composed of lipopolysaccharide, of which the lipid-A portion is responsible for the endotoxic activities. Flagellar (H) antigens can also be used to serotype strains that are motile as a result of the flagella they possess.[70] If a strain possesses neither a capsule nor flagella, it is characterized by the O antigen alone.

The classification of *E. coli* is based both on biochemical tests and serotyping of the O, K and H antigens, which is one of the most useful ways of identifying pathogenic types. At present more than 170 O antigens, 80 K antigens, and 50 H antigens are recognized. The number of possible serovars or serotypes is great, as there is considerable variation in the combinations of the three antigens. There is, however, a group of *E. coli* with O and K antigens in which the K antigen is considered to be merely a different expression of the basic O antigen. As many O and K antigens were described before this was known, many authors still use the older nomenclature, for example *E. coli* O149:K91. Where K91 is the capsular equivalent of O149, it is not necessary to add K91, as it is implied.

A plasmid, of which there may be more than one in a bacterial cell, may code for only one virulence factor, or it may have a multifactorial function. Virulence factors coded for by plasmids are toxin production, possession of pili (fimbriae), and antibiotic resistance. The virulence of enteropathogenic *E. coli* is mainly attributed to the presence of pili and the production of toxins **(see Pathogenesis)**.[62] Certain serotypes are usually associated with specific virulence factors. Although most of the virulence factors are coded for by transmissible plasmids, and while in theory any serotype could harbour them, in practice there is usually no environmental pressure for most of them to be transmitted. The only exception is for the plasmids coding for antibiotic resistance, which is usually complex and involves multiple antibiotic resistance.[86, 89, 98]

In addition to flagella, many strains possess antigenic proteinaceous pili (also referred to as fimbriae), some of which function as adherence factors and are therefore responsible for the attachment of *E. coli* to mucosal epithelial cells of the intestinal tract.[79, 84] When these pili antigens were first described, their chemical nature was unknown. The first two discovered were thought to be capsular antigens and were named K88 and K99.[70] These are now known, respectively, as F4 and F5 (F for fimbrial antigen). Similarly, the F6 pilus was first isolated from a porcine strain 987P. Both the 'K' and 'F' appellations are used in the designation of pili antigens in this text. The important pili in strains of *E. coli* in animals are K99 (F5) in ruminants, K88 (F4) and 987P (F6) in pigs, and F41 in both ruminants and pigs. Three antigenic types of K88 are recognized (K88 a,b; K88 a,c and K88 a,d). Pili K88 and K99 are relatively easy to detect by agglutination, and the presence of the other two important pili, 987P and F41, is determined by ELISA. Adherence factors are produced in the greatest quantity in the small intestine but are only elaborated under certain circumstances in culture. The factors K88 and K99 are produced in culture media incubated at 37 °C but not at 20 °C, while the factors 987P and F41 develop poorly in laboratory culture media.

Table 129.1 Most important factors that play a role in the epidemiology of *Escherichia coli* infections

HOST	
Species	
Age	
Adhesion sites (receptors) in intestines	
Antibody levels (colostrum intake, lacteal antibodies)	
Stress (hygiene, weaning, crowding, transportation, castration)	
Concomitant infections	
Decreased gastric acidity	
Lack of competition from other gut flora	
ENVIRONMENT	BACTERIAL
Quantity of pathogenic strains (hygiene)	Serotype involved
Introduction of new strains	Ability to colonize the intestine
Loss of maternal contact	Presence of adherence factors
Changes in pens or penmates, crowding	Ability to produce toxins
Transport, shipping	Antibiotic resistance
Rapid temperature changes	
Changes in diet	
Hypersensitivity to antigens in diet	

Epidemiology

General comments

Whether or not disease is caused after an animal is infected with *E. coli* depends on a complex interaction between the susceptibility of the host, pathogenicity of the specific strain of the organism **(see Aetiology and Pathogenesis)**, and environmental predisposing factors **(Table 129.1)**.

A number of host factors are important in the establishment of infection or disease. The pili allow *E. coli* to attach to specific receptor sites on the intestinal mucosa. Once attached, the organisms are protected from being washed down the intestinal tract by normal peristaltic movements, and they can multiply rapidly. The role of attachment is well demonstrated by the situation in pigs, in which a recessive hereditary factor codes for the lack of K88 receptor sites. Pigs possessing the factor in its homozygous form are not susceptible to organisms possessing K88 pili, since they lack the specific receptors and are disease-resistant, while heterozygous pigs are fully susceptible.[8] Selection of pigs resistant to K88 pilar attachment is therefore desirable, although at present it is not a feasible method of control as there is no test available to determine the presence or absence of the factor in live animals.

Certain serotypes are species-specific, while others are pathogenic for several species. For example, *E. coli* O149:K91 is considered to be pathogenic only for pigs, O119:K69 serotype causes problems in ruminants, and other serotypes, such as O78:K80, are regarded as universal pathogens, as they are pathogenic to a variety of animal species including poultry and humans. As a rule, however, a particular pathogenic *E. coli* strain is limited to only one animal species on a farm. Nevertheless, colibacillosis may occur in calves after the consumption of chicken litter containing a strain such as *E. coli* O78:K80 which is considered to be pathogenic for both cattle and poultry.[86]

New-born and young animals are most susceptible to enteric colibacillosis. Enteric colibacillosis generally occurs in calves under ten days of age, and in lambs and kids under two weeks of age.[76] In pigs it occurs in two distinct age groups: neonates, and those in the immediate post-weaning period.

Colostrum-derived antibodies are very important in the protection of new-born animals against *E. coli* infections.[50] These antibodies against specific serotypes occur in the colostrum of dams which have been exposed to natural infection with them or inoculated with vaccines containing them. The offspring of dams that are young or have recently arrived on a farm, and which have not been exposed to the pathogenic strains that are prevalent on the farm, are particularly prone to developing disease.[4, 90] Colostrum should be ingested as soon after birth as possible, preferably within a few hours, in order to provide effective protection, as the enterocytes of neonates lose their ability to absorb antibodies in the colostrum as the animal gets older. The longer the interval between birth and the first ingestion of colostrum, the fewer antibodies are absorbed. This leads to inadequate protection.

The antibody classes in colostrum that are of particular importance in protection against *E. coli* infections are IgM and IgG in the case of colisepticaemia,[81] and IgA in enteric colibacillosis.[74, 89]

Infection with other infectious agents, such as rota- and coronaviruses, and *Eimeria* and *Cryptosporidium* spp., may predispose young animals to enteric colibacillosis.[1, 91]

As animals suffering from colibacillosis may excrete very large numbers of the pathogenic strain concerned in almost pure culture, poor sanitary hygiene may result in massive faecal contamination of the environment and the build-up of very large numbers of pathogenic *E. coli*. In addition, dampness of the environment plays an important role in the survival of *E. coli* and consequent spread of the infection.[1]

Pathogenic strains of *E. coli* which animals on a farm have not previously been exposed to may be introduced into a herd or flock by newly arrived animals or, conversely, newly arrived animals may become infected with strains with which they have not previously been in contact. These factors play a particularly significant role in calf-rearing units where the calves are purchased from many different sources. Stresses such as transportation and overcrowding also play major predisposing roles.[9, 85]

Pigs

Colibacillosis in pigs occurs in two distinct age groups: neonates, and those in the immediate post-weaning period. The percentage of pathogenic strains of *E. coli* relative to non-pathogenic strains that is carried by the sow increases markedly at farrowing. This facilitates their transmission to piglets early in life.[2, 55] Whether or not neonatal colibacillosis develops in piglets which are exposed to pathogenic strains of *E. coli* depends to a large extent on the presence or absence of colostral and lacteal antibodies; other factors play a lesser role. On the other hand, stress plays an important predisposing role in the development of the disease in weaned piglets. Piglets are exposed to many stress factors at weaning, including loss of maternal contact, movement to new pens, new penmates, overcrowding, and erratic environmental temperature caused in part by lack of maternal warmth. In addition, declining levels of lacteal IgA may play a role. Weaning stress also results in a temporary increased gastric pH, which results in decreased gastric bactericidal activity.[77] Previously, changes in dietary composition at weaning or after transport to a different farm were believed to predispose to colibacillosis in piglets. It is now believed that if piglets are fed a creep-feed while still suckling their dams, hypersensitivity to dietary antigens may develop. This could predispose to enteric colibacillosis after weaning if they are fed a weaning diet containing the ingredients to which they developed sensitivity in the creep-feed.[53] The addition of antibiotics to feed enables antibiotic-resistant organisms in the intestine to multiply at the expense of the non-resistant ones. In the case of *E. coli*, pathogenic strains are often antibiotic-resistant.[35]

On analysis of the results of bacterial isolation from specimens of cases of colibacillosis in pigs submitted to the Veterinary Research Institute, Onderstepoort over a 20-year period (1971–91), it was found that serotypes O149:K91 and O141:K85 comprised 70 per cent of isolates. Strain O149:K91 was the predominant pathogenic serotype in pigs, accounting for 55 per cent of all pathogenic strains of *E. coli* that were isolated. Infection with this serotype is particularly common in the immediate post-weaning period (**Table 129.2**).[33] Nearly 90 per cent of these isolates possessed the pilar attachment factor K88. *Escherichia coli* O141:K85 was the next most common isolate, of which about 40 per cent possessed the K88 antigen. This isolate accounted for about 15 per cent of the cases of colibacillosis in pigs. It is found in a wider age range of piglets, and was also isolated from aborted pig foetuses. All other pathogenic serotypes individually accounted for 5 per cent or less of the total number of isolates. The most common of these were *E. coli* O20, O139:K82, O9:K30, O9:K28 and O78:K80.

The two main syndromes seen in pigs are enteric colibacillosis (about 60 per cent of cases) and colisepticaemia (about 40 per cent). There has been a marked decrease in the prevalence of both syndromes in suckling piglets in South Africa since 1981. This may be a reflection of the greater number of sows that are vaccinated (with consequent transfer of colostral antibodies to piglets), increased hybrid vigour due to the more frequent use of first-cross sows because they possess a greater non-specific disease resistance, and the improvement in farrowing housing.[33]

Table 129.2 The number of serotypes of *Escherichia coli* associated with disease in piglets of different age groups in South Africa for the period 1977–87[33]

AGE OF PIGS	0149:K91(88)	0141:K85(88)	OTHER	TOTAL (%)
Foetus		1	2	3 (1,0)
1–3 days	6	1	15	22 (7,6)
Under 1 week	10	2	9	21 (7,3)
1 week – weaning	25	5	16	46 (16,0)
Post-weaning	105	25	28	158 (55,0)
2–4 months	12	4	10	26 (9,0)
Adults	3	2	6	11 (3,8)
Total	161	40	86	287 (99,7)

Table 129.3 Common *Escherichia coli* serotypes isolated from calves over a 10–year period (1977–87) in South Africa[33]

SEROTYPES OF *E. COLI*	NO. OF SEROTYPES ISOLATED				NO. OF SEROTYPES WITH K99 (%)	TOTAL
	Enteritis	Septicaemia	Abortion	Other		
09:K28	24	27		3	18 (33,3)	54
078:K80	15	17	2	3	2 (5,4)	37
0141:K85	10	7	2	1	6 (30,0)	20
0119:K69	10	8		1	0 (0)	19
09:K30	4	11		3	6 (33,3)	18
026:K60	11	2		3	0 (0)	16

The prevalence of oedema disease in South Africa is relatively low. *Escherichia coli* serotypes O139:K82, O138:K81 and O141:K85 are the most common causes of the syndrome on a worldwide basis. In South Africa serotypes O139:K82 and O138:K81 are usually associated with it. Other serotypes which may be associated with oedema disease are O149 and O8, which do occur in South Africa, and O147 and O45, which as yet have not been isolated from pigs in this country.[33, 68]

Calves

Colibacillosis in calves is much more common in those fed milk surrogates than in ranched calves. It occurs mostly in spring. Insufficient ingestion of colostrum soon after birth appears to be the most important predisposing factor **(Table 129.1)**.

In South Africa the most common pathogenic *E. coli* serotypes isolated from specimens from new-born calves submitted to the Veterinary Research Institute, Onderstepoort, were O9:K28, O78:K80, O141:K85, O119:K69, O9:K30 and O26:K60, comprising 70 per cent of all serotypes isolated **(Table 129.3)**.

Escherichia coli O9:K28 and O9:K30 usually occur in calves under one week of age, with the majority being less than three days old. *Escherichia coli* serotypes O78:K80, O26:K60 and O141:K85 occur in a much wider age range of calves than O9:K28. Three serotypes (O78:K80, O26:K60 and O141:K85) are pathogenic not only for neonatal animals, but also for calves up to one month old, and have also been found to be responsible for abortions in cattle.[34] In calves more than two weeks old, *E. coli* infections often occur in association with other diseases, such as paratyphoid, chlamydiosis or pasteurellosis. Poor housing conditions and nutrition enhance their pathogenicity.

Table 129.4 Common *Escherichia coli* serotypes isolated from sheep and goats over a 10–year period (1977–87) in South Africa[33]

SEROTYPE	SHEEP	GOATS	TOTAL
078:K80	16	9	25
026:K60	7	1	8
09:K28	6	1	7
09:K30	3	1	4
055:K59	3	1	4

Lambs and kids

Escherichia coli infections (colisepticaemia being much more common than enteric colibacillosis) in lambs and kids occur in many parts of the world, including South Africa, mainly in intensively raised animals.[29, 85] More cases in sheep occur in autumn than in spring. *Escherichia coli* O78:K80 and O26:K60 serotypes were most commonly isolated from specimens of affected lambs and kids in South Africa over a 10-year period **(Table 129.4)**. The adhesive factor K99 rarely occurs in serotypes of *E. coli* of small stock in South Africa, and was only present in a limited number of strains of the O9:K30 and O141:K85 serotypes. This is probably the main reason for the rare occurrence of enteric colibacillosis in this country.[33]

Foals

Escherichia coli is a rare cause of endometritis and abortion in mares and of colisepticaemia in foals.[29, 37, 85] Worldwide, including southern Africa, enterotoxigenic *E. coli* infection is implicated only occasionally as a cause of disease in foals.[33, 37, 94] *Escherichia coli* serotypes O9:K28 and O9:K30 have been isolated from diseased foals in South Africa, but in general *E. coli* infection tends to complicate diseases caused by infection with *Salmonella*, *Pasteurella* or *Actinobacillus* spp.[33] The enterotoxigenic *E. coli* serotypes isolated from horses carry F41, K88 (F4), K99 (F5) and 987P (F6), inconsistently.[37, 94]

Pathogenesis

Escherichia coli, particularly non-pathogenic strains, is part of the normal intestinal flora of warm-blooded animals. Pathogenic strains form only a small part of the total *E. coli* population of adult animals.[85] It is usually transmitted by the faecal–oral route, and is one of the first organisms to establish itself in the large intestine soon after birth,[85] with the small intestine being colonized subsequently. Once established, and irrespective of age, few *E. coli* are present in the cranial part of the small intestine, relatively large numbers are present in the caudal part, while the largest numbers occur in the large intestine.[29, 85]

A number of factors determine the success of the establishment in the intestinal tract and the age of susceptibility of very young animals to infection with pathogenic *E. coli*. Ingestion of very large numbers of pathogenic *E. coli* increases their chances of survival in the intestinal tract, where they are able to multiply and cause disease. The localization within the intestinal tract, and specific age-association with different strains appear to be chiefly related to the presence or absence of receptors for specific pili (such as K88, K99, K41, 987P) on the small intestinal epithelial cells and mucus in the lumen. There is an age-related decrease in the number of small intestinal receptors for K99 pili, which is directly related to the decrease in susceptibility of calves, lambs and pigs older than five days to the effects of strains of *E. coli* bearing K99 pili.[59, 60] On the other hand, the persistence of K88 and 987P receptors in older animals is reflected in the equal susceptibility of both neonatal and recently-weaned piglets to strains of the bacterium bearing the respective pili. It appears that receptors on mucus may be more important in the age-associated susceptibility than receptors on the epithelial cells.[18, 20] Localization of the bacteria within a specific section of the intestinal tract similarly appears to be a function of the presence or the absence of these receptors.[30]

Pathogenic strains of *E. coli* produce several toxins categorized either as enterotoxins or cytotoxins. The enterotoxigenic strains produce two main toxins, designated heat-labile toxin, which is chemically closely related to cholera toxin, and heat-stable toxin. Each toxin may be produced alone or they may be produced in combination. The toxins are usually associated with specific serotypes, and toxin production is coded for by specific plasmids. The heat-labile toxin is antigenic, while the heat-stable toxin is not. Only human and porcine *E. coli* strains, particularly those of the K88 serotypes, have been shown to produce heat-labile toxin.[30] The heat-labile toxins produced by different animal-derived strains of *E. coli* are antigenically similar. In southern Africa, heat-labile toxin is mainly associated with *E. coli* O149:K91. Both toxins induce biochemical changes in the epithelial cells of the mucosa (the cells of the mucosa remain intact and show no morphological changes) that result in the hypersecretion of fluids and electrolytes into the intestinal lumen.[48]

The heat-labile enterotoxin consists of two polypeptide subunits designated A and B, each toxin molecule consisting of five B subunits and one A subunit. The B subunits have a receptor function and bind to ganglioside GM_1 on enterocytes of the small intestine. After entry into the cell, the A subunit activates adenylate cyclase by nicotinamide adenine dinucleotide (NAD)-dependent adenosine diphosphate (ADP)-ribosylation of its regulatory subunit,[26] thereby increasing the concentration of cyclic-adenosine monophosphate (cAMP) in the cells. In enterocytes on the small intestinal villi, cAMP inhibits the absorption of Na^+, and hence of Cl^- and water, while in epithelial cells in the crypts cAMP exerts a direct secretory effect by increasing Na^+ secretion and causing a simultaneous loss of Cl^- and water.[25] The net effect is the accumulation of large volumes of fluid and electrolytes in the small intestinal lumen, and the consequent development of diarrhoea.

The heat-stable toxin (ST) is divided into STa, which is produced by *E. coli* strains from humans as well as by those that cause neonatal diarrhoea in piglets and calves, and STb, which is only produced by *E. coli* strains that cause diarrhoea in weanling pigs. STa can be further divided into STaH, which is only obtained from human sources, and STaP, which is obtainable from human, bovine and porcine sources.[52] STaH and STaP toxins differ genotypically; the differences can be demonstrated by DNA sequence analysis. The STa and STb toxins are often produced by the same enterotoxigenic *E. coli* strains isolated from pigs, with STb being more common.[61] They are, however, two totally distinct toxins, and have different molecular sizes. STa is an 18 or 19 amino-acid peptide that binds to a unique receptor located in the membrane of the brush border of intestinal epithelial cells, where it activates particulate guanylate cyclase (GMP). Increased levels of cyclic GMP inactivate the ionic pump in affected epithelial cells, resulting in an efflux of Na^+ and water into the lumen, and a reduced absorption of Cl^- ions.[89] Relatively little is known about the effects of STb. It is a 48 amino-acid, lysine-rich peptide, which induces fluid secretion into the intestinal lumen by an unknown mechanism.[93] In South Africa, STa has been found to be associated with *E. coli* O20, O154, O9:K30 and O9:K35.[33]

Enteropathogenic *E. coli* produce Vero cytotoxins (VT),[10, 71] also known as Shiga-like toxins (SLT), which are similar to the toxins of *Shigella dysenteriae* type 1. These toxins are cytotoxic for HeLa and Vero cells, enterotoxic in ligated rabbit ileal segments, and lethal for mice.[69] Three types of toxin are known: VT1, which can be neutralized by anti-Shiga toxin; VT2; and VTe, the latter being a variant which was previously known as 'Edema Disease Principle (EDP)' or 'oedema disease toxin'. VT1 is bacterial cell-associated and is usually present in large amounts, while VT2 is found outside the bacterial cell, usually in moderate amounts. As the production of VT1 and VT2 is largely determined by bacteriophages, the amount and type of toxin produced depend on the specific phage as well as on other unknown factors. The VTe toxin responsible for the development of oedema disease is probably chromosomally determined.[42] The various VT toxins bind to receptors in the glycolipid outer membrane of epithelial cells of the intestine and to endothelial cells. The toxins enter the cells by receptor-mediated endocytosis, act on the ribosomes (where they inhibit protein synthesis), and cause cellular damage which results in the lesions that occur in the intestinal tract and vascular endothelium. The toxin causes vasculitis which eventually leads to necrosis and haemorrhage.[13]

Escherichia coli also produces a number of less well-known toxins. These include a cytotoxic necrotizing factor (CNF) associated with infant enteritis in humans,[15] piglet enteritis[27] and calf enteritis,[21] and a protein Vir toxin, which is lethal for mice, chickens and calves.[51, 83]

The CNF and Vir toxins may be found together, but are distinguished by their effects on HeLa and Vero cell cultures. There is a slight cross-neutralization between the two toxins.[21]

Endotoxin (or lipopolysaccharide (LPS)) which mimics the effects of septicaemic *E. coli* infections is present in the cell wall of all Gram-negative bacteria, and is comprised of lipid-A, polysaccharide and a protein (core) portion. Though the antigenicity of LPS is determined by its polysaccharide component, lipid-A is considered to be responsible for the endotoxic effects. In healthy animals, LPS is prevented from entering the circulation by being bound by bile acids in the intestinal tract, by the integrity of the intestinal barrier, and by small amounts of LPS being removed by the liver from the portal circulation. High concentrations of LPS occur in the systemic circulation, where endotoxin exert its effects, following breakdown of the intestinal barrier and in invasive Gram-negative infections such as occur in colisepticaemia. The effects of endotoxin, which develop as a consequence of the activation of inflammatory mediators and direct cellular injury, are species-specific. In livestock the lungs are the main target organ. Following exposure to LPS, a transient and mild pulmonary hypertension and bronchoconstriction develop, followed within hours by severe pulmonary oedema and increasing pulmonary hypertension. Endotoxin also causes a leukopenia, followed by leukocytosis in animals that survive for longer than 24 hours, thrombocytopenia, lactic acidosis, hypoxaemia, transient hyperglycaemia followed by hypoglycaemia, haemoconcentration and intravascular coagulation. Neutrophils, vascular endothelium and macrophages, each being an important source of mediators of toxic substances, are specifically targeted and destroyed by endotoxin. Damage to these cells is followed by the release of primary mediators such as cytokines—primarily tumour necrosis factor and interleukin-1—and lipid mediators such as thromboxane, prostacyclin, leukotrienes, and platelet-activating factor. Numerous secondary mediators are activated as a consequence of the activation of these primary mediators. The subsequent cytotoxicity occurs as a consequence of the direct effects of endotoxin, the affects of the various mediators, the generation of oxygen radicals, and the effects of the release of lysosomal enzymes as a consequence of cell death.[31]

The pathogenesis of disease caused by *E. coli* is determined by many factors (**Table 129.1**). Five separate mechanisms (enterotoxigenic, enteropathogenic, enterohaemorrhagic, enteroinvasive, enteroadherent) are involved in the pathogenesis of enteric colibacillosis or diarrhoeagenic *E. coli* disease. Each mechanism is dependent upon a variety of factors, including distinct virulence properties of the *E. coli* serotype involved, different interactions between the *E. coli* strain and the intestinal mucosa, distinct O:H serotypes, and production of certain toxins. Based on these factors, and the effects on the animals, enterotoxigenic, enteropathogenic, enterohaemorrhagic, enteroinvasive and enteroadherent infections can be identified.

Enterotoxigenic E. coli *(ETEC) infections*

Most cases of enteric colibacillosis in calves and piglets are in this category. Diarrhoea caused by ETEC in calves occurs most commonly in animals less than one week old.[1] Although piglets are susceptible to ETEC enteritis until they are three months of age, most cases occur during the first week of life or during the first two weeks after weaning. In southern Africa, ETEC infections are most commonly caused by *E. coli* serotypes O8, O9, O15, O20, O101, O141 and O149.[33]

The ETEC strains adhere loosely to the brush border of the enterocytes of the small intestines by means of their pili. Following adherence, the local biochemical effects of LT, STa and STb toxins result in the accumulation of increased amounts of fluid in the intestinal tract, leading to an acute, profuse, watery diarrhoea, culminating in dehydration, metabolic acidosis, and death in severe cases.[29] The degree of intestinal colonization varies among strains of ETEC and is affected by serotype as well as host factors. The number of *E. coli* present in the mid-jejunum in healthy animals is in the order of 10^4 per gram of intestinal content, but in animals with enteric colibacillosis it is about 10^9 per gram.[29] The largest number of bacteria usually occurs with strains that are both pilated and capsulated.

Enteropathogenic E. coli *(EPEC) infections*

Although strains of *E. coli* with enteropathogenic effects were identified in human infants as long ago as 1945,[12] their pathogenic mechanisms were only recently resolved. Some of the strains induce a characteristic lesion described as 'attaching and effacing', which has been reported in humans,[48] calves,[16, 97] pigs, lambs, dogs,[41] and rabbits.[14] Strains of 'attaching and effacing' *E. coli* (AEEC) in lesions of the small and large intestine are closely adherent to the plasmalemma of enterocytes, with the membrane often cupping or partially enveloping the bacteria.[48] The plasmid of Class I EPEC strains codes for a protein-localized adherence factor, named EPEC adherence factor (EAF), while Class II EPEC strains are EAF-negative.[67] Enteropathogenic *E. coli* strains produce VT which damages enterocytes and vascular endothelial cells by blocking protein synthesis by ribosomes. Diarrhoea is thought to be due to a diminution of absorption caused by villous damage. Enterocytes to which bacteria are attached are usually shorter than adjacent unaffected ones, and clumps of rounded-up, bacteria-covered cells slough into the intestinal lumen.[41] The microvilli are stunted, thickened and occasionally fused,[97] and the mucosa is irregularly eroded and has a scalloped appearance as a result of the cellular damage.

Calves of up to four months old (the average age being two weeks) are affected by EPEC strains. Some animals contain traces or moderate amounts of blood in their faeces as a result of a haemorrhagic colitis. Although the entire intestinal tract may be affected, the colon is the site most commonly colonized.[41] Similar lesions occur in pigs, lambs and dogs.[40] Animals which have suffered from a severe EPEC infection sometimes do not recover completely, and often remain 'poor doers'.

The most common EPEC serotypes in animals are O5, O111 and O26, but O4, O8, O119, O149 and O168 have also been implicated.[40, 41, 48]

Enterohaemorrhagic E. coli *(EHEC) infections*

Enterohaemorrhagic *E. coli* strains produce large amounts of VT, in contrast to EPEC strains, which produce variable amounts of VT. *Escherichia coli* O157:H7 strains are all potent producers of VT1 and VT2 and are associated with haemorrhagic colitis and the haemolytic-uraemic syndrome in humans.[95] Cattle have been found to be a reservoir of these strains.[10, 71] *Escherichia coli* O157 strains have long been recognized as enterohaemorrhagic in animals, although they rarely possess the flagellar antigen H7 and do not appear to belong to the same clonal type as the human *E. coli* O157:H7 strain.[95] In South Africa, *E. coli* O157 has been isolated on ten occasions from pigs; nine isolates being from pigs suffering from haemorrhagic enteritis, and one from the uterus of a sow with metritis.[33] Enterohaemorrhagic *E. coli* strains that cause haemorrhagic enteritis in animals have not been well studied other than in pigs.

The EHEC strains adhere intimately to intestinal epithelial cells. Some EHEC strains may also produce AEEC lesions in the same way as EPEC.[92]

The lesions caused by EHEC and EPEC differ from each other only in respect of severity and in terms of distribution in the intestinal tract. The lesions in EPEC infections involve the entire intestine, whereas only the caecum and colon are affected in EHEC infections. The lesions caused by EPEC infections are generally less severe than the profuse haemorrhagic colitis and typhlitis caused by EHEC infections. There is some infiltration of neutrophils in EPEC infections, but not in EHEC infections.[48]

Enteroinvasive E. coli *(EIEC) infections*

Enteroinvasive strains of *E. coli* have not been found in farm animals as yet. They are biochemically and serologically similar to *Shigella* spp. (which are pathogens of humans and primates), and also cause a haemorrhagic erosive colitis such as that caused by *Shigella*. The EIEC strains possess a large 140-megadalton plasmid, similar to that of *Shigella flexneri*, which codes for invasion of the epithelial cells of the mucosa of the colon.[32] The toxin of EIEC has not yet been fully characterized, but is thought to be a Shiga-like cytotoxin with enterotoxic properties, which probably also causes vascular damage.[48]

Enteroadherent E. coli *(EAEC) infections*

Enteroadherent *E. coli* strains have been isolated only from human infants suffering from chronic diarrhoea.[48]

Colisepticaemia

Colisepticaemia may develop terminally in animals suffering from enteric colibacillosis or it may occur without any evidence of enteric involvement. Infection may be contracted *per os* (tissue invasion taking place in the nasopharynx or intestinal tract) or via the umbilicus.[9] Very young animals, and particularly those that are hypogammaglobulinaemic due to insufficient absorption of colostral antibodies, are prone to contracting colisepticaemia.[43] Increased intestinal permeability to macromolecules in the new-born may also predispose to the invasion of tissues by septicaemia-inducing *E. coli* strains.[63]

Strains that cause colisepticaemia are usually invasive and have special properties (including resistance to the bactericidal activity of normal serum and the ability to extract iron from serum and transport it into their own cell bodies) enabling them to resist the defence mechanisms of the host, and to multiply and cause damage to its tissues.[29] Iron is essential for the growth of *E. coli*, and any strain that possesses the colicin V plasmid, which codes for colicin V synthesis and for iron-chelating hydroxamates, therefore has a competitive advantage.[89]

The exact pathogenesis of colisepticaemia has not been extensively studied, but endotoxin is known to play an important role in causing shock **(see Pathogenesis)**. Animals which survive the septicaemic disease may develop fibrinopurulent meningitis or arthritis.

Oedema disease

There are a number of important steps in the pathogenesis of oedema disease. The susceptibility of weaned pigs to the effect of the toxin causing oedema disease is variable and may be hereditary. After initial infection of the pigs with a toxigenic, oedema disease-producing strain of *E. coli*, the bacteria multiply in the digestive tract and colonize the small intestine. Colonization and adherence by virtue of the presence of pili occur particularly at the tips of the villi in the mid-jejunum and the ileum. Following its production, VTe toxin is absorbed into the systemic circulation. In circulation, the B subunit of the toxin, which determines its cytotoxic specificity, binds preferentially to globotetraosylceramide and galactosylgloboside which occur, amongst others, on the epithelial cells in the small intestine of piglets, as well as on certain endothelial cells in the blood-vascular system. The cytotoxic effects on the vascular endothelium, which develop in the intestine, subcutaneous tissue and the brain, are caused by the toxin's RNA-N-glycosidase activity, which causes inactivation of cellular protein synthesis. This leads to endothelial damage and the development of oedema and the nervous signs that are characteristic of oedema disease.[38]

Clinical signs

Pathogenic strains of *E. coli* are most commonly associated with enteric colibacillosis and colisepticaemia in the

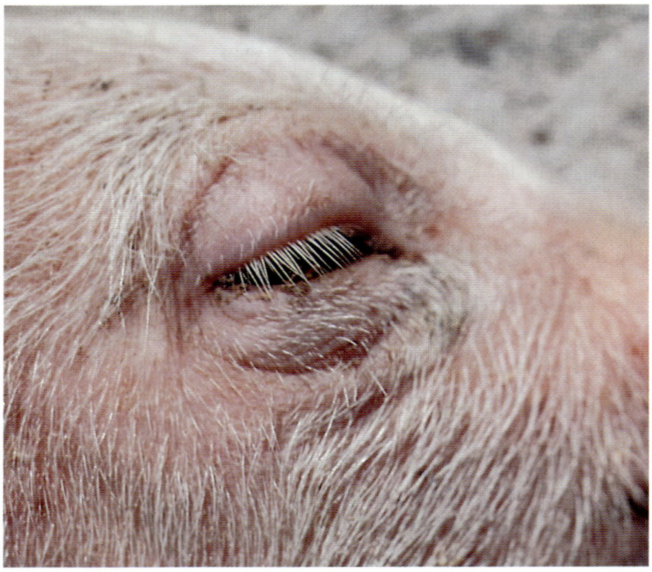

Figure 129.1
Oedema disease. Note oedematous swelling of the eyelids

first few weeks of life of livestock species, but they may also cause other syndromes such as cystitis, mastitis, metritis and abortion in older animals.

Pigs

Enteric colibacillosis is the most common syndrome caused by *E. coli* in new-born and post-weaning pigs. The incubation period in new-born piglets may be as short as two to three hours.[96] Only a few piglets in a litter may be affected, or the entire litter. The mortality rate may approach 100 per cent, particularly in very young piglets. In the peracute to acute disease, affected neonatal piglets may be found dead without clinical signs having been noticed, or they may be moribund with or without evidence of diarrhoea. If diarrhoea is present, the faeces are watery and are usually whitish to yellowish.[96] In the longer-standing disease piglets may show weakness, anaemia due to reduced absorption of nutrients (especially iron), dehydration, loss of condition, nervous signs, dyspnoea and cyanosis.[85, 96]

In pigs that develop post-weaning enteric colibacillosis, clinical signs usually occur within about a week of weaning. In a litter, piglets which are in the best condition are generally the ones affected first. Affected pigs commonly show fever and diarrhoea, but some animals may be found dead without having shown any signs of illness. The faeces are usually watery and greyish or brownish, and may be haemorrhagic, especially if *E. coli* O149:K91 is involved. The diarrhoea in most animals usually resolves within a few days, but it may persist and result either in death from dehydration or in chronic enteritis and stunting.[87] The morbidity rates may be as high as 50 per cent and the mortality rate is usually about 10 per cent.[87]

Animals affected by colisepticaemia (whether primary, or secondary following enteric colibacillosis) are initially febrile and listless but soon become recumbent and unconscious, or may show paddling limb movements before death.[87] Terminally, the body temperature is usually subnormal.

Oedema disease is not as commonly reported in southern Africa as it is in certain other parts of the world, such as the United Kingdom, some parts of Europe and the USA, where it is recognized as an economically important disease.[6, 45] It occurs sporadically, is stress-associated, and most commonly affects recently weaned piglets in good condition. The duration of an outbreak of oedema disease in a group of piglets is generally short, with no new cases occurring four to five days after its first appearance.[88] One or more piglets in a group may be found dead without clinical signs having been noticed, while some of the others show nervous signs such as opisthotonus, incoordination, dullness, apparent blindness and head-pressing.[87, 88] Paddling movements are seen once pigs are recumbent. The subcutaneous tissues of the head, especially the eyelids **(Figure 129.1)**, nose and ears are oedematous, and affected animals often have a hoarse, squeaky voice attributable to laryngeal oedema.[82] Fever may be present in the early stages of the disease, and the neurological signs may be preceded by diarrhoea if the *E. coli* strain associated with the disease produces enterotoxin.[6, 45] Death usually occurs within four to 36 hours of the onset of clinical signs.[87] The morbidity rate in a herd affected with the disease is usually low (about 15 per cent),[68] but the mortality rate of affected animals is about 50 per cent.[6, 45]

Apart from enteric colibacillosis, colisepticaemia and oedema disease, *E. coli* may also occasionally cause abortion, metritis, mastitis and agalactia in sows.[7]

Cattle

Enteric colibacillosis caused by enterotoxigenic strains in calves occurs in the first two to three days of life. In the peracute disease, calves usually die before enteritis is clinically evident. Acutely affected animals are listless, dull, disinclined to drink, and usually show a profuse, watery diarrhoea which is whitish-yellow or greyish, giving rise to the common name 'white scours'. Blood is present only rarely in the stool. Depending on the severity of diarrhoea, calves show variable degrees of dehydration. The umbilicus in some cases may be swollen and inflamed, and the inflammatory process may extend into the abdominal cavity.[1] Calves are rarely febrile, and generally have a lowered body temperature due to dehydration and collapse.[36] The morbidity and mortality rates may be high.

Colisepticaemia may be primary or develop as a sequel to enteric colibacillosis, and is more commonly seen in agammaglobulinaemic calves.[50] Many of the clinical signs correspond to those of shock due to the endotoxin produced by *E. coli*.[29] The course of disease is usually acute, ranging from one to three days. Calves are initially depressed and feverish, but the temperature drops rapidly as they become moribund. Affected calves show incoordination, opisthotonus, recumbency and leg-paddling movements. *Escherichia coli* may localize in the joints, causing polyarthritis in calves that survive the acute illness.[9]

Strains of 'attaching and effacing' enteropathogenic *E. coli* (AEEC) may cause disease in calves of up to four months of age, but calves less three weeks old are usually affected. Diarrhoea, which is often haemorrhagic or contains mucus, is the predominant clinical sign, but affected calves usually also show a fever and dehydration and refuse to drink.[40] The disease may be mild or severe and life-threatening.[40]

Abortion due to *E. coli* in cattle is rare and usually occurs at a late stage of gestation. *Escherichia coli* may be isolated in pure culture from all organs of such aborted foetuses. In South Africa, *E. coli* O78:K80 is the strain which is most commonly associated with abortion.[33]

Escherichia coli is the cause of sporadic cases of acute mastitis in cows in early lactation **(see Chapter 190: Mastitis)**. Affected animals show a severe systemic reaction. The serotypes involved are very diverse as they are generally of faecal origin.[89]

Sheep and goats

Clinical signs of enteric colibacillosis and colisepticaemia in lambs and kids are generally similar to those in calves. However, acute colisepticaemia occurs more commonly in these species than in calves.[9, 36, 40, 85]

Horses

The clinical signs in foals affected by enteric colibacillosis or colisepticaemia are similar to those in the other animal species. Endometritis and abortion in mares have also been reported, but are rare.

Pathology

In both enteric colibacillosis and colisepticaemia lesions are non-specific.

Animals that are affected by enteric colibacillosis are usually dehydrated and their hind quarters are soiled with faeces as a result of diarrhoea. At necropsy there is usually congestion of the small intestine, the contents of which are fluid and greyish to yellowish, and the mesenteric lymph nodes are oedematous and congested. For more information on the lesions associated with enteric colibacillosis, consult the section on **Pathogenesis** in this chapter.

Gross lesions in the acute septicaemic disease include generalized congestion and the presence of petechiae and ecchymoses in serosal surfaces (especially the epi- and endocardium and capsule of the adrenals), severe congestion and various degrees of oedema of the meninges, congestion of the gastric or abomasal mucosa, congestion and oedema of the lungs, and there may or may not be evidence of diarrhoea and congestion of the small intestinal mucosa.[44] In less acute cases, there may be evidence of organ or tissue localization of the bacterium, with lesions such as fibrinopurulent pleuritis, pericarditis, peritonitis, polyarthritis, pneumonia and meningitis being manifested. Calves may also show a meningoventriculitis.[78] In some animals, fibrinopurulent omphalophlebitis may be evident. In addition, in calves surviving the septicaemic disease, 'white-spotted kidneys' due to focal disseminated interstitial nephritis have been attributed to *E. coli* infection.

Pigs that have died from oedema disease are generally in good condition. The severity and distribution of the lesions vary considerably from case to case; in some they are quite obvious, while in others they must be actively sought during a necropsy, in which case making a diagnosis may be difficult. In some animals there may be reddish or purple patches of discoloration of the skin over the abdomen and on the inside of the fore and hind legs.[88] The conjunctivae are sometimes swollen and congested. The degree of oedema present varies from case to case, and the oedematous fluid is generally clear and somewhat jelly-like, but it may be slightly blood-stained. There may be obvious subcutaneous oedema of the eyelids and ears, and over the nasal bones, and the subcutaneous tissues of the jowl region and ventral abdomen may be moist.[88] Some or all of the superficial lymph nodes may be normal or oedematous and congested.[88] There is generally an increased amount of peritoneal fluid, varying from slight to very marked in quantity. A few or numerous strands of fibrin in the peritoneal cavity and between the abdominal viscera are present in almost all cases.[88] The mesocolon and the wall of the greater curvature of the stomach, particularly the submucosa of the cardiac area, generally show some degree of oedema.[88] The gastric mucosa may be normal in appearance or show areas of congestion. In cases in which there is pronounced oedema of the mesocolon, the submucosa of the spiral colon is thickened due to oedema. The colonic lymph nodes are often oedematous and may be congested. Some degree of hydrothorax and hydropericardium is generally encountered, and the pericardial fluid may contain a fibrin clot.[88] Epi- and endocardial haemorrhages and submucosal laryngeal and oesophageal oedema may be present.

Histopathologically, apart from the oedema, the most significant lesion of oedema disease is that of a degenerative angiopathy affecting the small arteries and arterioles in many organs and tissues.[6, 17, 46] The initial change in affected blood vessels is perivascular oedema, followed by necrosis of smooth muscle cells of the *tunica media*, which then undergoes fibrinoid necrosis.[46] This is followed by proliferation of cells in the *tunica adventitia*. Swelling of endothelial cells has also been observed, but thrombosis is not a prominent feature.[46] These vascular changes may be difficult to discern in acute cases. In animals which survive for several days, foci of encephalomalacia are often present in the brain stem, frequently with a bilaterally symmetrical distribution, as well as cerebral vascular lesions. The encephalomalacia is probably the result of ischaemia following the vascular damage.[46]

Diagnosis

The clinical characteristics of enteric colibacillosis, namely a short incubation period, depression, anorexia, diarrhoea and dehydration, are similar to those manifested in infections caused by the majority of enteropathogens, such as rotavirus, coronavirus, *Salmonella* serovars, and *Eimeria* and *Isospora* spp. The age of the affected animal and the colour of the faeces are sometimes of value in the making of a presumptive diagnosis, but to a large extent the diagnosis of disease caused by *E. coli* is made only after the results of bacteriological examinations are taken into account.

Specimens for bacteriological examination should consist of short sections of affected intestinal tract, several mesenteric lymph nodes, and appropriate-sized tissue blocks from organs such as the liver, spleen, kidneys and brain, preferably from animals that have not been treated with antimicrobial drugs. Specimens from the brain are useful in order to determine whether or not septicaemic spread has occurred. Tissue specimens must be collected using aseptic techniques, as soon after the death of the animal as possible, and must be placed in individual, sterile containers. In an outbreak of the disease, specimens from more than one animal should be taken. As *E. coli* forms part of the normal intestinal flora, post-mortal spread in carcasses is extremely rapid. It is therefore imperative to note in a report the interim time between death and the necropsy, as well as the amount of decomposition that has taken place.

Rectal swabs are less satisfactory as specimens for bacteriological examination, as the faecal flora in the rectum may bear little relation to the situation in the small intestine. If there is reluctance on the part of the owner to sacrifice one or more of the affected animals so that specimens of a good quality for bacteriological examination can be collected, rectal swabs from at least ten untreated animals suffering from enteritis should be taken if possible.[1, 11, 35, 85]

The samples should be cultured on a medium suitable for differentiating *E. coli* from other bacteria, such as McConkey agar. A general medium such as blood agar should also be routinely inoculated in order to detect other possible bacterial causes of the disease in question. Most Enterobacteriaceae form colonies with a similar appearance on blood agar. The majority of porcine pathogenic strains of *E. coli* are haemolytic on blood agar, but those of other animal species are not.[85]

Smooth and rough colonies of *E. coli* are best distinguished after several days' growth on McConkey agar. A crude test to determine roughness is to emulsify a colony in a 1:500 dilution of acriflavine in normal saline. If the emulsified bacteria autoagglutinate, the isolate is considered to be rough and is then untypable.

It is essential to select several (3–5) smooth colonies per culture for serotyping, as non-pathogenic intestinal strains may be present together with pathogenic strains, particularly if some post-mortal decomposition has occurred. Mixed growths may, however, also be obtained from the intestine of fresh carcasses. In such cases, bacteriological examination of the mesenteric lymph nodes is very useful, as it usually yields a pure culture of the pathogen.

Serotyping is usually carried out by slide agglutination using antisera developed against capsules and flagella in live cultures and antisera developed against O antigens in heated cultures. Serotyping may be confirmed by tube agglutination. Two of the adhesive pili types (K88 and K99) are detected in the same way.

Once the bacterial colonies under review (isolated from specimens taken from several animals showing signs of disease) have been typed, they should be assessed and the relative proportions noted of each serotype isolated. The pathogenic serotype is usually clearly predominant. If enteric colibacillosis is not the cause of the disease, a mixed growth of various serotypes in more-or-less equal numbers is found. In order to arrive at a final conclusion, all the factors concerned—including the epidemiology, clinical signs, and necropsy and laboratory results—must be taken into consideration.

Tests for virulence factors should also be performed. Pili (K88 and K99) can be detected by slide agglutination, fluorescent antibody, electron micrographs, haemagglutination tests and ELISA.[89] Heat-labile enterotoxin can be assayed by a number of methods: vascular permeability assay in ligated intestinal loops, its effect on Chinese hamster ovary and Vero cells, haemagglutination, solid-phase radioimmunoassay, ELISA, and its ability to bind to polystyrene-absorbed GM_1 ganglioside.[48, 75] Heat-stable enterotoxin can be assayed in ligated intestinal loops, and STa is also assayed in infant mice. These tests can only be carried out in specialized laboratories.

The diagnosis of oedema disease is based on the epidemiology, clinical signs, gross pathology, the presence of microscopic angiopathy in various organs and tissues, and the isolation of haemolytic *E. coli* from the small intestine. It must be borne in mind, however, that the number of *E. coli* may decrease as the disease progresses. Oedema disease toxin can be detected in Vero cell culture or by the use of a mouse test, as it causes posterior paralysis in mice.[22]

Although uncomplicated enteric colibacillosis is usually confined to specific age groups, strains of pathogenic *E. coli* are often isolated together with other pathogens, such as *Pasteurella*, *Salmonella* and *Chlamydia* spp.

Differential diagnosis

As the epidemiology, clinical signs and pathology of many enteropathic diseases are very similar, a specific diagnosis is generally based on laboratory results.

The most commonly encountered diseases which may be confused with enteric colibacillosis are nutritional scours, caused by ingestion of too much milk by neonatal animals, and, depending on the animal species involved, infections caused by agents such as rotavirus, coronavirus, *Campylobacter jejuni, Salmonella* serovars, *Clostridium perfringens* types A, B and C, *Treponema hyodysenteriae*, and *Cryptosporidium, Eimeria* and *Isospora* spp.

Peracute or acute oedema disease in pigs should be differentiated from mulberry heart disease (Vitamin E selenium deficiency) and the subacute or chronic disease manifested by neurological signs from conditions such as bacterial meningoencephalitis caused by *Haemophilus parasuis* or *Streptococcus suis*, haemagglutinating encephalomyelitis virus, and water deprivation (salt poisoning).[6]

Control

The factors mentioned under epidemiology **(Table 129.1)** should be examined and those pertaining to the outbreak concerned corrected. The most common predisposing factors include the quality and quantity of colostrum taken in, climatic changes, mixing of young animals from different origins, and general hygiene. Cold can exacerbate or precipitate scours in piglets.[3] An environmental temperature of 28–30 °C should be maintained for newly weaned piglets.[96]

Control of neonatal colibacillosis in animals can be achieved by vaccination of pregnant females in order to ensure that their colostrum will contain an adequate quantity of specific antibodies which, after absorption, will provide passive protective immunity to their offspring. The non-specific factors in colostrum, namely lactoferrin and transferrin, and the immunoglobulin fraction do afford some protection against colisepticaemia and enteric colibacillosis.[1]

Ingestion of specific colostral antibodies by the offspring, induced by vaccination of the pregnant female, is essential if diarrhoea caused by enterotoxigenic *E. coli* infections is to be prevented.[1] The intake of colostrum should equal at least 10 per cent of a young animal's body weight by 24 hours after birth,[99] and the initial ingestion of colostrum should occur within the first few hours of life to maximize the absorption of antibodies.[47, 80] The factors which promote successful colostral intake have been reviewed by Petrie.[72] Mismothering, teat defects and agalactia must be identified by the stockman, who must administer colostrum by bottle when the need arises. Colostrum banks, frozen or freeze-dried, should be kept for such emergencies. It is worth noting that some cows produce colostrum which has a low globulin content and their calves subsequently remain hypogammaglobulinaemic despite ingestion of the correct amount of colostrum.[72] In order to induce the presence of high concentrations of colostral antibodies, two vaccinations should be given to pregnant animals at a monthly interval, the second one preferably a month before the birth of piglets, lambs or calves. In subsequent pregnancies, previously vaccinated pregnant animals need be given only a single vaccination about one month before parturition.

Specific antibodies to the K antigens of pathogenic *E. coli* serotypes have been shown to be protective[24, 59] and vaccines containing whole bacterial cells or purified K antigens of specific serotypes have been formulated. The wide variety of K antigens and lack of cross-protection between the different antigens have, however, limited the usefulness of this type of bacterin, as the inclusion of all the antigens into one vaccine is not feasible.

The two vaccines prepared by the Veterinary Research Institute at Onderstepoort, one for cattle and sheep and the other for pigs, contain formalinized whole-cell bacterins from smooth strains which are emulsified in oil. The strains included are reviewed from time to time, so that common southern African pathogenic strains of *E. coli* are always represented. The vaccine for cattle and sheep always contains K99 pili, and the one for pigs, K88 pili. Septicaemia-causing strains such as *E. coli* O78:K80 are included in the cattle and sheep vaccines, while the two most common South African serotypes occurring in pigs, *E. coli* O149:K91 and O141:K85, are always incorporated into the porcine vaccine.

The discovery of pili as virulence factors of enterotoxigenic *E. coli* and the fact that they are immunogenic proteins and occur in a wide range of serotypes have led to their selection as ideal immunizing antigens for enterotoxigenic *E. coli* infections. Anti-pilus antibody has an anti-adhesive effect which successfully prevents the attachment and toxin production of enterotoxigenic *E. coli* in cattle, sheep and pigs.[28, 39, 64, 66] Neonatal scours can therefore be prevented if the vaccine used to immunize pregnant animals contains pilus antigen homologous to that of the infecting strain. Bovine vaccines should contain K99 pilus antigen, ovine vaccines F41 and K99, and porcine vaccines K99, K88 and 987P. Specific monoclonal antibody to K99 is available commercially and is administered to ensure that calves receive sufficient specific K99 antibody. It should not, however, be used as a replacement for colostrum-derived antibodies.

Live, pilus-bearing enterotoxigenic *E. coli* fed orally to sows also induce the formation of colostral antibodies which will protect piglets.[56, 58] However, this method is ineffective for immunizing cows.[57]

There is, as yet, no consensus on the methods that should be used to control post-weaning diarrhoea and oedema disease in piglets, probably because the pathogenesis of both is poorly understood. Weaner piglets are capable of mounting an immune response but their active response to enterotoxigenic *E. coli* may be suppressed by antibody which they receive from their dams.[65] Stimulating active immunity by feeding inactivated enterotoxigenic *E. coli* during the suckling period is claimed to be effective against post-weaning infections,[73] but it is not widely practised.

Some researchers have attributed post-weaning scours in piglets to an association between *E. coli* and microscopic lesions caused by dietary hypersensitivity. Post-weaning diarrhoea can be controlled by using hypoallergenic rations[53] and by the abrupt weaning of piglets which have not received creep feed.[54] The restriction of piglets' feed intake at weaning[5] or the increase of the total amount of fibre in their diet[23] have been advocated as methods to prevent post-weaning scours.

Animals with diarrhoea should be treated to restore the fluid balance, as death usually results from dehydration. Oral or parenteral electrolytes may be administered, depending on the severity of the disease. Acidosis develops in severe cases, therefore bicarbonate may need to be given. Oral antibiotic therapy is sometimes advocated to suppress the growth of enterotoxigenic *E. coli*, but antibiotic resistance due to the addition of antibiotics to feed is a major problem.

An antibiogram should be performed on the isolate causing an outbreak. Ideally, minimal inhibitory concentration determinations should be performed on the antibiotic of choice as indicated by the results of the antibiogram.

The use of antimicrobials in animals suffering from enteric colibacillosis is controversial. The absorption of antimicrobials from the affected intestine is unpredictable, especially if kaolin, aluminium gel or other protectants are used. Many *E. coli* isolates demonstrate multiple resistance to antimicrobials, and antimicrobial sensitivity should be carried out if possible before therapy is applied. Various preparations containing combinations of antimicrobials, electrolytes and intestinal protectants such as kaolin are available as general treatments. These should be selected with due regard to the sensitivity of the isolate. Antimicrobials in feed or water should be administered for four to five consecutive days, bearing in mind that the appetite of affected animals may be depressed. Colistin can be used in feed or drinking water at a rate of 1–2 g/10 kg body weight. Furazolidone may be mixed into the feed of piglets at 1–3 kg/ton of feed, or a trimethoprim/sulphonamide combination at a rate of 20 g/50 kg body weight.

Colisepticaemia should be treated with injectable antimicrobials such as trimethoprim/sulphonamide (at 15–25 mg/kg), colistin (at 50 000 iu/kg) or kanamycin (at 20 mg/kg).

As an alternative to the administration of antimicrobials, the therapeutic use of lactic-acid bacteria to treat scours has been claimed to be successful, but their usage has not yet gained momentum.

As with post-weaning scours, no single recommendation can be made for the control of oedema disease. Restricting feed intake, controlling the ambient temperature, and antibiotic therapy to reduce levels of enterotoxigenic *E. coli* may reduce the prevalence of the disease.

References

1 **ACRES, S.D., 1985.** Enterotoxigenic *Escherichia coli* infections in newborn calves: A review. *Journal of Dairy Science*, 68, 229–256.

2 **ARBUCKLE, J.B.R., 1968.** The occurrence of *Escherichia coli* somatic antibody in pig serum, colostrum and milk and an investigation of its possible significance in immunity. *British Veterinary Journal*, 124, 273–281.

3 **ARMSTRONG, W.D. & CLINE, T.R., 1977.** Effects of various nutrient levels and environmental temperatures on the incidence of colibacillary diarrhoea in pigs: Intestinal fistulation and titration studies. *Journal of Animal Science*, 45, 1042–1050.

4 **BANKS, K.L. & McGUIRE, T.C., 1989.** Neonatal immunology. *In*: HALLIWELL, R.E.W. & GORMAN, N.T., (eds). *Veterinary Clinical Immunology*. Philadelphia, London, Toronto, Montreal, Sydney, Tokyo: W.B. Saunders Company.

5 **BERTSCHINGER, H.U., EGGENBERGER, E., JUCKER, H. & PFIRTER, H.P., 1979.** Evaluation of low-nutrient, high-fibre diets for the prevention of porcine *Escherichia coli* enterotoxaemia. *Veterinary Microbiology*, 3, 281–290.

6 **BERTSCHINGER, H.U. & NIELSEN, N.O., 1992.** Edema disease. *In*: LEMAN, A.D., STRAW, B., MEGELING, W.L., D'ALLAIRE, S. & TAYLOR, D.J., (eds). *Diseases of Swine*. 7th edn. Ames, Iowa: Iowa State University Press.

7 **BERTSCHINGER, H.U., POHLENZ, J. & ROSS, R.F., 1986.** Coliform mastitis. *In*: LEMAN, A.D., STRAW, B., GLOCK, R.D., MENGELING, W.L., PENNY, R.H.C. & SCHOLL, E., (eds). *Diseases of Swine*. 6th edn. Ames, Iowa: Iowa State University Press.

8 **BIJLSMA, I.G.W., DE NIJS, A., VAN DER MEER, C. & FRIK, J.F., 1982.** Different pig phenotypes affect adherence of *Escherichia coli* to jejunal brush borders by K88ab, K88ac or K88ad antigen. *Infection and Immunity*, 37, 891–894.

9 **BLOOD, D.C. & RADOSTITS, O.M., 1989.** *Veterinary Medicine*. 7th edn. London, Philadelphia, Sydney, Tokyo, Toronto: Baillière Tindall.

10 **BORCZYK, A.A., KARMALI, M.A., LIOR, H. & DUNCAN, L.M.C., 1987.** Bovine reservoir for verotoxin-producing *Escherichia coli* O157:H7. *Lancet*, 1, 98.

11 **BOYD, J.W., 1974.** Neonatal diarrhoea in calves. *The Veterinary Record*, 95, 310–313.

12 **BRAY, J., 1945.** Isolation of antigenically homogeneous strains of *Bacterium coli neapolitanum* from summer diarrhoea of infants. *Journal of Pathology*, 57, 239–247.

13 **BROWN, J.E., ECHEVERRIA, P, & LINDBERG, A.A., 1991.** Digalactosyl-containing glycolipids as cell-surface receptors for Shiga toxin of *Shigella dysenteriae* 1 and related cytotoxins of *Escherichia coli*. *Reviews of Infectious Diseases*, 13 (Suppl. 4), S298–303.

14 **CANTEY, J.R. & BLAKE, R.K., 1977.** Diarrhoea due to *Escherichia coli* in the rabbit: A novel mechanism. *Journal of Infectious Diseases*, 135, 454–462.

15 **CAPRIOLI, A., FALBO, V., RODA, L.G., RUGGERI, F.M. & ZONA, C., 1983.** Partial purification and characterization of an *Escherichia coli* toxic factor that induces morphological cell alterations. *Infection and Immunity*, 39, 1300–1306.

16 **CHANTER, N., MORGAN, J.H., BRIDGER, J.C., HALL,**

G.A. & REYNOLDS, D.J., 1984. Dysentery in gnotobiotic calves caused by atypical *Escherichia coli*. *The Veterinary Record*, 114, 71.

17 **CLUGSTON, R.E., NIELSEN, N.O. & SMITH, D.L.T., 1974.** Experimental edema disease of swine (*E. coli* enterotoxaemia). III. Pathology and pathogenesis. *Canadian Journal of Comparative Medicine*, 38, 34–43.

18 **CONWAY, P.L., WELIN, A. & COHEN, P.S., 1990.** Presence of K88-specific receptors in porcine ileal mucus is age-dependent. *Infection and Immunity*, 58, 3178–3182.

19 **COOKE, E.M., 1985.** *Escherichia coli* — an overview. *Journal of Hygiene, Cambridge*, 95, 523–530.

20 **DEAN, E.A., 1990.** Comparison of receptors for 987P pili of enterotoxigenic *Escherichia coli* in the small intestine of neonatal and older pigs. *Infection and Immunity*, 58, 4030–4035.

21 **DE RYCKE, J., GUILLOT, J.F. & BOIVIN, R., 1987.** Cytotoxins in non-enterotoxigenic strains of *Escherichia coli* isolated from faeces of diarrhoeic calves. *Veterinary Microbiology*, 15, 137–150.

22 **DOBRESCU, L., 1983.** New biological effect of edema disease principle (*Escherichia coli* neurotoxin) and its use as an *in vitro* assay for this toxin. *American Journal of Veterinary Research*, 44, 31–34.

23 **DUNNE, H.W., 1975.** Colibacillosis and edema disease. *In*: DUNNE, H.W. & LEMAN, A.D, (eds). *Diseases of Swine*. 4th edn. Ames, Iowa: Iowa State University Press.

24 **GAY, C.C., McKAY, K.A. & BARNUM, D.A., 1964.** Studies on colibacillosis of calves. I. The antibody acquired by calves as the result of vaccination of the dam. *Canadian Veterinary Journal*, 5, 248–261.

25 **GILL, D.M., CLEMENTS, J.D., ROBERTSON, D.C. & FINKELSTEIN, R.A., 1981.** Subunit number and arrangement in *Escherichia coli* heat-labile enterotoxin. *Infection and Immunity*, 33, 677–682.

26 **GILL, D.M. & RICHARDSON, S.H., 1980.** Adenosine diphosphate-ribosylation of adenylate cyclase catalyzed by heat-labile enterotoxin *Escherichia coli*: Comparison with cholera toxin. *Journal of Infectious Diseases*, 141, 64–70.

27 **GONZALES, E.A. & BLANCO, J., 1985.** Production of cytotoxin VT in enteropathogenic and non-enteropathogenic *Escherichia coli* strains of porcine origin. *FEMS Microbiological Letters*, 26, 127–130.

28 **GREGORY, D.W., CARDELLA, M.A. & MYERS, L.L., 1983.** Lamb model in the study of immunity to enteropathogenic *Escherichia coli* infections. *American Journal of Veterinary Research*, 44, 2073–2077.

29 **GYLES, C.L., 1986.** *Escherichia coli*. *In*: GYLES, C.L. & THOEN, O., (eds). *Pathogenesis of Bacterial Infections in Animals*. Ames, Iowa: Iowa State University Press.

30 **GYLES, C.L. & THOEN, C.O., 1986.** *Pathogenesis of Bacterial Infections in Animals*. Ames, Iowa: Iowa State University Press.

31 **HARDIE, E.M. & KRUSE-ELLIOT, K., 1990.** Endotoxic shock. Part 1: A review. *Journal of Veterinary Internal Medicine*, 4, 258–266.

32 **HARRIS, J.R., WACHSMUTH, I.K., DAVIS, B.R. & COHEN, M.L., 1982.** High molecular-weight plasmid correlates with *Escherichia coli* enteroinvasiveness. *Infection and Immunity*, 37, 1295–1298.

33 **HENTON, M.M., 1993.** Section of Bacteriology, Veterinary Research Institute, Onderstepoort. Unpublished data.

34 **HERR, S., 1993.** Section of Bacteriology, Veterinary Research Institute, Onderstepoort. Unpublished data.

35 **HINTON, M., 1985.** The sub-specific differentiation of *Escherichia coli* with particular reference to ecological studies in young animals including man. *Journal of Hygiene, Cambridge*, 95, 595–609.

36 **HUNT, E., 1993.** Diarrhoeal diseases of neonatal ruminants. *In*: HOWARD, J.L., (ed.). *Current Veterinary Therapy 3: Food Animal Practice*. Philadelphia: W.B. Saunders Company.

37 **IKE, K., KAMADA, M., ANZAI, T., IMAGAWA, H., KUMANOMIDO, T., NAKAZAWA, M., KASHIWAZAKI, M. & KUME, T., 1987.** Some properties of *Escherichia coli* isolated from foals with diarrhoea and mares with metritis. *Bulletin of the Equine Research Institute*, 24, 33–41.

38 **IMBERECHTS, H., DE GREVE, H. & LINTERMANS, P., 1992.** The pathogenesis of edema disease in pigs. A review. *Veterinary Microbiology*, 31, 221–233.

39 **ISAACSON, R.E., DEAN, E.A., MORGAN, R.L. & MOON, H.W., 1980.** Immunization of suckling pigs against enterotoxigenic *Escherichia coli*-induced diarrhoeal disease by vaccinating dams with purified K99 or 987P pili: Antibody production in response to vaccination. *Infection and Immunity*, 29, 824–826.

40 **JANKE, B.H., FRANCIS, D.H., COLLINS, J.E., LIBAL, M.C., ZEMAN, D.H. & JOHNSON, D.D., 1989.** Attaching and effacing *Escherichia coli* infections in calves, pigs, lambs, and dogs. *Journal of Veterinary Diagnostic Investigation*, 1, 6–11.

41 **JANKE, B.H., FRANCIS, D.H., COLLINS, J.E., LIBAL, M.C., ZEMAN, D.H., JOHNSON, D.D. & NEIGER, R.D., 1990.** Attaching and effacing *Escherichia coli* infection as a cause of diarrhoea in young calves. *Journal of the American Veterinary Medical Association*, 196, 897–901.

42 **JOHNSON, W.M., POLLARD, D.R., LIOR, H., TYLER, S.D. & ROZEE, K.R., 1990.** Differentiation of genes coding for *Escherichia coli* verotoxin 2 and the verotoxin associated with porcine edema disease (VTe) by the polymerase chain reaction. *Journal of Clinical Microbiology*, 28, 2351–2353.

43 **JOHNSTON, N.E., ESTRELLA, R.A. & OXENDER, W.D., 1977.** Resistance of neonatal calves given colostrum diet to oral challenge with a septicaemia-producing *Escherichia coli*. *American Journal of Veterinary Research*, 38, 1323–1326.

44 **JUBB, K.V.F., KENNEDY, P.C. & PALMER, N., 1985.** *Pathology of Domestic Animals*. 3rd edn. New York: Academic Press, Inc.

45 **KAUSCHE, F.M., DEAN, E.A., ARP, L.H., SAMUEL, J.E. & MOON, H.W., 1992.** An experimental model for subclinical edema disease (*Escherichia coli* enterotoxaemia) manifest as vascular necrosis in pigs. *American Journal of Veterinary Research*, 53, 281–287.

46 **KURTZ, H.J., BERGELAND, M.E. & BARNES, D.M., 1969.** Pathologic changes in edema disease of swine. *American Journal of Veterinary Research*, 30, 791–806.

47 **LECCE, J.G. & MORGAN, D.O., 1962.** Effect of dietary regimen on cessation of intestinal absorption of large molecules (closure) in the neonatal pig and lamb. *Journal of Nutrition*, 78, 263–268.

48 **LEVINE, M.M., 1987.** *Escherichia coli* that cause diarrhoea: Enterotoxigenic, enteropathogenic, enteroinvasive, enterohaemorrhagic and enteroadherent. *Journal of Infectious Diseases*, 155, 377–389.

49 **LLOYD, J.C. & HENTON, M.M., 1993.** Veterinary Research Institute, Onderstepoort. Unpublished data.

50 **LOGAN, E.F., 1974.** Colostral immunity to colibacillosis in the neonatal calf. *British Veterinary Journal*, 130, 405–412.

51 **LOPEZ-ALVAREZ, J. & GYLES, C.L., 1980.** Occurrence of the Vir plasmid among animal and human strains of invasive *Escherichia coli*. *American Journal of Veterinary Research*, 41, 769–774.

52 **MAINIL, J.G., MOSELEY, S.L., SCHNEIDER, R.S., SUTCH, K., CASEY, T.A. & MOON, H.W., 1986.** Hybridization of bovine *Escherichia coli* isolates with gene probes for four enterotoxins (StaP, STaH, STb, LT) and one adhesion factor (K99). *American Journal of Veterinary Research*, 47, 1145–1148.

53 **MILLER, B.G., NEWBY, T.J., STOKES, C.R. & BOURNE, F.J., 1984.** Creep feeding and post-weaning diarrhoea in piglets. *The Veterinary Record*, 114, 296–297.

54 **MILLER, B.G., NEWBY, T.J., STOKES, C.R., HAMPSON, D.J. & BOURNE, F.J., 1983.** The role of dietary antigen in the aetiology of post-weaning diarrhoea. *Annales de Recherches Vétérinaires*, 14, 487–492.

55 **MOON, H.W., 1969.** Enteric colibacillosis in the newborn pig:

Problems of diagnosis and control. *Journal of the American Veterinary Medical Association*, 155, 1853–1859.

56 **MOON, H.W., 1981.** Protection against enteric colibacillosis in pigs suckling orally vaccinated dams: Evidence for pili as protective antigens. *American Journal of Veterinary Research*, 42, 173–177.

57 **MOON, H.W. & McDONALD, J.S., 1983.** Antibody response of cows to *Escherichia coli* pilus antigen K99 after oral vaccination with live or dead bacteria. *American Journal of Veterinary Research*, 44, 493–496.

58 **MOON, H.W., ROGERS, D.G. & ROSE, R., 1988.** Effects of an orally administered live *Escherichia coli* pilus vaccine on duration of lacteal immunity to enterotoxigenic *Escherichia coli* in swine. *American Journal of Veterinary Research*, 49, 2068–2071.

59 **MOON, H.W. & RUNNELS, P.L., 1983.** Trials with somatic (O) and capsular (K) polysaccharide antigens of enterotoxigenic *Escherichia coli* as protective antigens in vaccines for swine. *Proceedings of the Fourth International Symposium on Neonatal Diarrhoea*, University of Saskatchewan, 558–569.

60 **MOON, H.W. & RUNNELS, P.L., 1984.** The K99 adherence system in cattle. *In*: BOEDEKER, E.C., (ed.). *Attachment of Organisms to the Gut Mucosa*. Vol. I. Boca Raton, Florida: CRC Press.

61 **MOON, H.W., SCHNEIDER, R.A. & MOSELEY, S.L., 1986.** Comparative prevalence of four enterotoxin genes among *Escherichia coli* isolated from swine. *American Journal of Veterinary Research*, 47, 210–212.

62 **MORRIS, J.A., THORNS, C.J., WELLS, G.A.H., SCHOTT, A.C. & SOJKA, W.J., 1983.** The production of F41 fimbriae by piglet strains of enterotoxigenic *Escherichia coli* that lack K88, K99 and 987P fimbriae. *Journal of General Microbiology*, 129, 2753–2759.

63 **MURATA, H., YAGUCHI, H. & NAMIOKA, S., 1979.** Relationship between the intestinal permeability to macromolecules and invasion of septicaemia-inducing *Escherichia coli* in neonatal piglets. *Infection and Immunity*, 26, 339–347.

64 **MYERS, L.L., 1976.** Vaccination of cows with an *Escherichia coli* bacterin for the prevention of naturally occurring diarrhoeal disease in their calves. *American Journal of Veterinary Research*, 37, 831–834.

65 **MYERS, L.L. 1986.** Vaccine development against enterotoxigenic *Escherichia coli*. *Progress in Veterinary Microbiology and Immunology*, 2, 145–157.

66 **NAGY, B., 1980.** Vaccination of cows with a K99 extract to protect new-born calves against experimental enterotoxic colibacillosis. *Infection and Immunity*, 27, 21–24.

67 **NATARO, J.P., SCALETSKY, I.C.A., KAPER, J.B., LEVINE, M.M. & TRABULSI, L.R., 1985.** Plasmid-mediated factors conferring diffuse and localized adherence of enteropathogenic *Escherichia coli*. *Infection and Immunity*, 48, 378–383.

68 **NIELSEN, N.O., 1986.** Edema disease. *In*: LEMAN, A.D., STRAW, B., GLOCK, R.D., MENGELING, W.L., PENNY, R.H.C. & SCHOLL, E., (eds). *Diseases of Swine*. 6th edn. Ames, Iowa: Iowa State University Press.

69 **O'BRIEN, A.D. & HOLMES, R.K., 1987.** Shiga and Shiga-like toxins. *Microbiological Reviews*, 51, 206–220.

70 **ORSKOV, F., 1984.** Genus 1. *Escherichia*. *In*: KRIEG, N.R. & HOLT, J.G., (eds). *Bergey's Manual of Systematic Bacteriology*. Baltimore, London: Williams & Wilkins.

71 **ORSKOV, F., ORSKOV, I. & VILLAR, J.A., 1987.** Cattle as a reservoir of verotoxin-producing *Escherichia coli* O157:H7. *Lancet*, i, 276.

72 **PETRIE, L., 1984.** Maximizing the absorption of colostral immunoglobulins in the new-born calf. *The Veterinary Record*, 114, 157–163.

73 **PORTER, P., 1972.** Immunoglobulins in bovine mammary secretions. Quantitative changes in early lactation and absorption by the neonatal calf. *Immunology*, 23, 225–238.

74 **PORTER, P., NOAKES, D.E. & ALLEN, W.D., 1970.** Secretory IgA and antibodies to *Escherichia coli* in porcine colostrum and milk and their significance in the alimentary tract of the young pig. *Immunology*, 18, 245–257.

75 **RASKOWA, H. & RASKA, K., 1980.** Enterotoxins from Gram-negative bacteria relevant for *Veterinary Medicine*. *Veterinary Research Communications*, 41, 195–224.

76 **SCANLAN, C.M., 1988.** *Introduction to Veterinary Bacteriology*. Ames, Iowa: Iowa State University Press.

77 **SCHULMAN, A., 1973.** Effects of weaning on the pH changes of the contents of the piglet stomach and duodenum. *Nordisk Veterinaermedicin*, 25, 220–225.

78 **SEIMIYA, Y., OHSHIMA, K., ITOH, H., OGASAWARA, N., OKUTOMO, M. & TANAKA, S., 1992.** Central nervous system lesions due to *Escherichia coli* infection in neonatal calves. *Journal of Veterinary Medical Science*, 54, 767–768.

79 **SELLWOOD, R., 1984.** The K88 adherence system in swine. *In*: BOEDEKER, E.C., (ed.). *Attachment of Organisms to the Gut Mucosa*. Vol. I. Boca Raton, Florida: CRC Press.

80 **SELMAN, I.E., DE LA FUENTE, G.H., FISHER, E.W. & McEWAN, A.D., 1971.** The serum immune globulin concentrations of new-born dairy heifer calves: A farm survey. *The Veterinary Record*, 88, 460–464.

81 **SETO, A., OKABE, T., SASAKI, N. & ITO, Y., 1976.** Opsonic activity and O-agglutinins against *Escherichia coli* in bovine colostrum. *American Journal of Veterinary Research*, 37, 635–638.

82 **SHANKS, P.L., 1938.** An unusual condition affecting the digestive organs of the pig. *The Veterinary Record*, 12, 356–358.

83 **SMITH, H.W., 1974.** A search for transmissible pathogenic characters in invasive strains of *Escherichia coli*: The discovery of a plasmid-controlled toxin and a plasmid-controlled lethal character closely associated or identical with colicin V. *Journal of General Microbiology*, 83, 95–111.

84 **SMITH, H.W. & HUGGINS, M.B., 1978.** The influence of plasmid-determined and other characteristics of enteropathogenic *Escherichia coli* on their ability to proliferate in the alimentary tracts of piglets, calves and lambs. *Journal of Medical Microbiology*, 11, 471–492.

85 **SOJKA, W.J., 1965.** *Escherichia coli* in domestic animals and poultry. Review Series No. 7 of the Commonwealth Bureau of Animal Health, Weybridge.

86 **SOJKA, W.J., 1973.** Enteropathogenic *Escherichia coli* in man and farm animals. *Canadian Institute of Food Science and Technology Journal*, 6, 52–63.

87 **TAYLOR, D.J., 1983.** *Pig Diseases*. 3rd edn. Cambridge: The Burlington Press (Cambridge) Ltd.

88 **TIMONEY, J.F., 1950.** Oedema disease of swine. *The Veterinary Record*, 49, 748–755.

89 **TIMONEY, J.F., GILLESPIE, J.H., SCOTT, F.W. & BARLOUGH, J.E., 1988.** *Hagan and Bruner's Microbiology and Infectious Diseases of Domestic Animals*. 8th edn. Ithaca, London: Comstock Publishing Associates.

90 **TIZARD, I., 1987.** Immunity in the foetus and newborn. *In*: TIZARD, I., (ed.). *Veterinary Immunology. An Introduction*. 3rd edn. Philadelphia, London, Toronto, Sydney, Tokyo, Hong Kong: W.B. Saunders Company.

91 **TZIPORI, S., 1981.** The aetiology and diagnosis of calf diarrhoea. *The Veterinary Record*, 108, 510–514.

92 **TZIPORI, S., KARCH, H., WACHSMUTH, K.I., ROBINS-BROWNE, R.M., O'BRIEN, A.D., LIOR, H., COHEN, M.L., SMITHERS, J. & LEVINE, M.M., 1987.** Role of a 60-megadalton plasmid and Shiga-like toxins in the pathogenesis of infection caused by enterohaemorrhagic *Escherichia coli* O157:H7 in gnotobiotic piglets. *Infectioi and Immunity*, 55, 3117–3125.

93 **URBAN, R.G., PIPPER, E.M., DREYFUS, L.A. & WHIPP, S.C., 1990.** High-level production of *Escherichia coli* STb heat-stable enterotoxin and quantification by a direct enzyme-linked immunosorbent assay. *Journal of Clinical Microbiology*, 28, 2383–2388.

94 **WARD, A.C.S., SRIRANGANATHAN, N., EVERMANN, J.F. & TRAUB-DARGATZ, J.L., 1986.** Isolation of pilated

Escherichia coli from diarrhoeic foals. *Veterinary Microbiology*, 12, 221–228.

95 **WHITTAM, T.S. & WILSON, R.A., 1988.** Genetic relationships among pathogenic *Escherichia coli* of serogroup O157. *Infection and Immunity*, 56, 2467–2473.

96 **WILSON, M.R., 1986.** Enteric colibacillosis. *In*: LEMAN, A.D., STRAW, B., GLOCK, R.D., MENGELING, W.L., PENNY, R.H.C. & SCHOLL, E., (eds). *Diseases of Swine*. 6th edn. Ames, Iowa: Iowa State University Press.

97 **WRAY, C., McLAREN, I. & PEARSON, G.R., 1989.** Occurrence of 'attaching and effacing' lesions in the small intestine of calves experimentally infected with bovine isolates of verocytoxic *E. coli*. *The Veterinary Record*, 125, 365–368.

98 **WRAY, C. & MORRIS, J.A., 1985.** Aspects of colibacillosis in farm animals. *Journal of Hygiene, Cambridge*, 95, 577–593.

99 **WOODS, P.R. & ROUSSEL, A.J., 1993.** Colostrum and passive immunity. *In*: HOWARD, J.L., (ed.). *Current Veterinary Therapy 3: Food Animal Practice*. Philadelphia: W.B. Saunders Company.

Salmonella *sp. infections*

Introduction

Salmonellosis in livestock is caused by infection with both host-specific and non-host-specific *Salmonella* serovars, and results in enteritis, septicaemia or abortion. It is an economically important disease of cattle in many parts of the world, including southern Africa, but may also be responsible for serious sporadic outbreaks of disease in sheep, horses and pigs. Carrier animals and contaminated environments are important sources of infection. The most common serovars associated with disease in livestock are listed in **Table 1**.

The genus *Salmonella* is classified in the family Enterobacteriaceae, whose members are Gram-negative coccobacilli.[3] With the exception of *S. gallinarumpullorum*, all salmonellas are motile, as they have peritrichous flagella.

The genus *Salmonella* consists of a single species, *S. enterica*, which comprises seven subspecies (*enterica, salamae, arizonae, diarizonae, houtenae, bongori, indica*), the distinction between subspecies being based on biochemical reactions.[8, 15–18, 22] *Salmonella enterica* subsp. *enterica* contains all the serovars found in warm-blooded animals — those formerly assigned to subgenus I.

The members of the genus *Salmonella* are typed into serovars which are differentiated from each other by the combinations of their somatic (O) and flagellar (H) antigens and, to a lesser extent, by their biochemical reactions. The serovars, of which over 1 700 have been identified, do not have a species status allocated to them in the current classification of the genus, and the names of the serovars (such as Typhimurium or Dublin) should be used without italicization or underlining, e.g. *S. enterica* subsp. *enterica* ser. Typhimurium. As it is tedious and impractical to adopt this long, formal nomenclature for everyday use, it is common to refer to serovars as, for example, *Salmonella* Typhimurium, or as serovar Typhimurium. In this book, however, the 'older' (e.g. *Salmonella dublin*) form of nomenclature is used.[8, 16]

Antigenic composition

The O antigen is part of the lipopolysaccharide component of the cell wall that also contains lipid A and a core portion. The O antigen, or O-specific side chain consists of repetitive oligosaccharide units of which the type, order, and repetition of sugar moieties differ between serovars. These differences and those in the flagella antigens are used to type *Salmonella* into serovars. Sixty-seven different O antigens are currently known and they are identified by arabic numerals 1 to 67. Some of these occur singly (e.g. 11), while others occur in combination (e.g. 1, 4, 5, 12; and 6, 7) **(Table 2).**[15, 22]

Table 1 Most common serovars of *Salmonella* that infect livestock and the syndromes they induce

SPECIES AFFECTED	SEROVARS	COMMON SYNDROMES
Cattle	*S. dublin* and *S. typhimurium*	Septicaemia, acute and chronic enteritis and abortion
Sheep	*S. typhimurium*	Septicaemia, typhlocolitis and abortion
Pigs	*S. choleraesuis*, *S. typhimurium* and *S. typhisuis*	Septicaemia and enterotyphlocolitis
Horses	*S. typhimurium*	Septicaemia, acute colitis and abortion

Table 2 Antigenic composition of common *Salmonella* serovars

SEROVARS	O-ANTIGENS	H-ANTIGENS	
		Phase 1	Phase 2
S. abortus ovis	4,12	c	1,6
S. derby	1,4,5,12	f,g	1,2
S. typhimurium	1,4,5,12	i	1,2
S. abortus equi	4,12		e, n, x
S. choleraesuis	6,7	c	1,5
S. typhisuis	6,7	c	1,5
S. thompson	6,7	k	1,5
S. bovismorbificans	6,8	r	1,5
S. typhi	9,12	d	
S. enteritidis	1,9,12	g,m	1,7
S. dublin	1,9,12	g,p	
S. gallinarumpullorum	1,9,12		

Some *Salmonella* mutants have defects in the synthesis of the oligosaccharide O-specific side chain, with the result that the oligosaccharide is not fully synthesized when cultured. The colonies of such mutant strains have a ground-glass appearance and are therefore referred to as 'rough' strains. Colonies of strains which possess the complete oligosaccharide O-specific side chain are smooth and the strains are therefore referred to as 'smooth'. Rough strains are untypable as they do not agglutinate with O typing antisera.[22]

The complete O antigen is not only the major immunogen of bacteria in this genus, but it also possesses virulence properties **(see Virulence factors)**. It elicits both humoral and cellular immune responses to infections by salmonellas. Strains with incomplete O antigens (rough strains) are therefore used for the production of live attenuated vaccines, such as the calf paratyphoid (*Salmonella dublin*) vaccine.

The H antigens are heat-labile and are an integral part of the flagella in those serovars which possess them. The antigens are designated by a combination of letters of the alphabet and numerals (e.g. a to z, z1 to z32 and 1 to 7).[8] Two antigenic forms (also referred to as 'phases') of the flagella may occur in culture. A culture may therefore contain cells in which the flagella are all in the same phase, or cells which possess flagella of both phases. Most of the serovars contain flagella of two phases, but in some (e.g. *S. dublin*) the flagella occur in only one phase **(Table 2)**.

In order to establish the complete antigenic composition of any *Salmonella* serovar, antigens of both flagellar phases must be known, as well as the O antigens.[15] This is done by testing suspensions of the bacteria against antisera produced in rabbits against individual O and H antigens by means of a series of slide agglutination tests.[8] For identification purposes the results from these agglutination tests are then compared with known antigenic formulae contained in the Kauffmann-White diagnostic scheme. In this scheme the antigenic formula has three parts: the O antigens, the phase-1 H antigens, and finally the phase-2 H antigens. As new serovars of *Salmonella* are constantly emerging, the Kauffmann-White scheme is updated annually.[8, 16]. The antigenic composition of some of the more common *Salmonella* serovars is given in **Table 2**.

Virulence factors

The biological effects of the virulence factors of salmonellas are interrelated and are responsible for enteric and systemic clinical signs and lesions of salmonellosis.

- Lipopolysaccharide (LPS): Apart from the fact that the O-specific side chain of the LPS is immunogenic and is recognized by the host's immune system, it has also been associated with invasiveness of salmonellas and enterotoxin production.[21] For example, *Salmonella* strains with incomplete O-specific side chains (rough mutants) are not as invasive as those strains with a complete O-specific side chain, and are also less successful in avoiding phagocytosis and lysis by phagolysosomes after invasion.

  Endotoxin-mediated effects **(see Chapter 129: *Escherichia coli* infections)** in clinically affected animals are attributed to the lipid A portion of the LPS. Vasculitis and thrombosis which may be present in the intestine, liver, spleen and other tissues of affected animals are thought to be the result of absorption of large amounts of endotoxin through the damaged intestinal mucosa, or of endotoxin that is released locally in infected tissues. The cytotoxin may also be involved in the pathogenesis of the vascular lesions.[1, 5, 6, 10, 12, 14, 19, 21, 24–29]
- Enterotoxin: Several serovars of *Salmonella* produce an enterotoxin similar to the heat-labile toxin of *Escherichia coli* and the cholera toxin produced by *Vibrio cholerae*[5, 21] **(see Chapter 129: *Escherichia coli* infections)**. The enterotoxin binds to intestinal epithelial cells and stimulates increased intracellular cyclic adenosine monophosphate, which lead to the net secretion of Cl^-, HCO_3^-, Na^+ and water into the intestinal lumen, resulting in diarrhoea.
- Cytotoxin: Some serovars of *Salmonella* produce a cytotoxin[5, 21] that causes increased permeability of intestinal epithelial cell membranes. The cytotoxin appears to chelate cations such as Ca^{++} and Mg^{++}, which appears to cause structural changes in the cell membrane, resulting in rounding of cells and selective leakage of molecules.[21]
- Adhesion pili (fimbriae): Salmonellas possess type 1 pili which facilitate the adhesion of bacteria to epithelial cells.[10, 21]
- Plasmids: The virulence of the most common serovars (e.g. *S. dublin, S. typhimurium* and *S. choleraesuis*) that cause disease in livestock is enhanced by serovar-specific plasmids, which provide these serovars with the ability to survive in macrophages.[9, 11, 14] Salmonellas may carry R-plasmids that provide resistance to some antimicrobial drugs.[13]

Isolation and identification

Salmonellas have simple nutrient requirements and growth *in vitro* is therefore possible in simple salt-glucose media,[4] occurring over a temperature range of 10–49 °C.[2] At temperatures between 0 and 5 °C the organisms remain viable even though there is no growth.[2]

Selective procedures are used for the isolation of salmonellas from specimens such as faeces that contains a mixed bacterial flora. Enrichment media, such as a liquid-nutrient broth that contains agents which selectively inhibit the growth of other bacteria, are used for this purpose. The three enrichment media commonly used are tetrathionate medium, Kauffmann-Muller tetrathionate medium, and a selenite broth.[7] Small pieces of tissue from the spleen, liver, mesenteric lymph nodes or the

Table 3 Biochemical differentiation of non-lactose-fermenting enterobacteria. (Adapted from Brenner[3])

GENUS	BIOCHEMICAL REACTION				
	Lactose fermentation	H_2S production	Urease production	Indole production	Lysine production
Salmonella	–	+	–	–	+
Proteus	–	+	+	+/–	–
Enterobacter	+/–	–	+/–	–	+/–
Citrobacter	+/–	+/–	+/–	+/–	–

\+ Positive
– Negative
+/– Positive or negative

small and large intestines, or small amounts of faeces are each inoculated into the enrichment medium and, after incubation at 37 °C for 48 hours, a loopful of the medium is plated onto a discriminating agar medium such as MacConkey agar, deoxycholate agar or *Salmonella-Shigella* agar.[7] These media differentiate the genera of the family Enterobacteriaceae according to differences in lactose fermentation and other biochemical reactions.[3] Serovars of the genus *Salmonella* are non-lactose fermenting, as are members of the genus *Proteus*, and some strains of *Citrobacter* and *Enterobacter* **(Table 3)**. As all these bacteria are morphologically indistinguishable from each other, they are further characterized by the biochemical reactions that they induce in suitably prepared media.[15]

Salmonellas are facultatively anaerobic and, with a few exceptions, all produce gas from fermentable sugars.[15] In culture, nitrates are reduced to nitrites, and hydrogen sulphide (but not indole and urease) is produced. Glucose and maltose are fermented, dulcitol and inositol are variably used, and sucrose is not fermented. The other non-lactose-fermenting genera of the family Enterobacteriaceae which also produce hydrogen sulphide are *Proteus* and some strains of *Citrobacter*.[3] The biochemical differentiation of these enterobacteria is given in **Table 3**.[3]

Factors affecting growth and survival

Salmonellas are killed when exposed to temperatures of 55 °C for one hour or 60 °C for 15–20 minutes, and by pasteurization at 71 °C for 15 seconds or 63 °C for 30 minutes.[2] The cooking of food will destroy salmonellas if the internal temperature of the food reaches 74–77 °C.[2, 4] Salmonellas in animal feeds and feed ingredients are killed by a process where the feed is heated to boiling point in steam-jacketed agitating cookers (110 °C for 2,5–3,5 hours).[4, 20, 23] There is a marked reduction in the number of salmonellas during freezing and long-term frozen storage, but not all are destroyed.[4]

Salmonellas are able to grow in media with a pH range of 4,5–9,0 (optimum 6,5–7,5);[4, 23] lower or higher pH values cause the bacteria to die.

References

1 **ABOU-SHLEIB, H., ELKHOULY, A.E. & ROANTREE, R.J., 1986**. Effect of selected plasmids on the serum sensitivity of *Salmonella typhimurium* strains with defined lipopolysaccharide core defects. *FEMS Microbiology Letters*, 36, 27–30.

2 **BOWMER, E.J., 1965**. Salmonellae in food—A review. *Journal of Food Protection*, 28, 74–86.

3 **BRENNER, D.J., 1984.** Facultatively anaerobic Gram-negative rods. *In*: KRIEG, N.R. & HOLT, J.G., (eds). *Bergey's Manual of Systematic Bacteriology*. Vol. I. Baltimore, London: Williams & Wilkins.

4 **BRYAN, F.L., FANELLI, M.J. & RIEMANN, H., 1979**. *Salmonella* infections. *In*: RIEMANN, H. & BRYAN, F.L., (eds). *Food-borne Infections and Intoxications*. New York, San Francisco, London: Academic Press, Inc.

5 **CLARKE, R.E. & GYLES, C.L., 1986.** *In*: GYLES, C.L. & THOEN, C.O., (eds). *Pathogenesis of Bacterial Infections in Animals*. Ames, Iowa: Iowa State University Press.

6 **COLLINS, L.V., ATTRIDGE, S. & HACKETT, J., 1991.** Mutations at rfc or pmi attenuated *Salmonella typhimurium* virulence for mice. *Infection and Immunity*, 59, 1079–1085.

7 **CRUICKSHANK, R., DUGUID, J.P., MARMION, B.P. & SWAIN, R.H.A., 1975.** *Medical Microbiology*. Vol. II. 12th edn. Edinburgh, London, New York: Churchill Livingstone.

8 **EWING, W.H., 1986.** *Edwards and Ewing's Identification of Enterobacteriaceae*. 4th edn. New York: Elsevier Science Publishing Co., Inc.

9 **FIERER, J., KRAUSE, M., TAUXE, R. & GUINEY, D., 1992.** *Salmonella typhimurium* bacteremia: Association with the virulence plasmid. *Journal of Infectious Diseases*, 166, 639–642.

10 **FINLAY, B.B. & FALKOW, S., 1988.** Virulence factors associated with *Salmonella* species. *Microbiological Sciences*, 5, 324–328.

11 **GULIG, P.A., 1990**. Virulence plasmids of *Salmonella typhimurium* and other Salmonellae. *Microbial Pathogenesis*, 8, 3–11.

12 **JOINER, K.A., HAMMER, C.H., BROWN, E.J. & FRANK, M.M., 1982**. Studies on the mechanism of bacterial resistance to complement-mediated killing. II. C8 and C9 release C5b76 from the surface of *Salmonella minnesota* S218 because the terminal complex does not insert into the bacterial outer membrane. *Journal of Experimental Medicine*, 155, 809–819.

13 **JONES, C. & STANLEY, J., 1992**. *Salmonella* plasmids of the pre-antibiotic era. *Journal of General Microbiology*, 138, 189–197.

14 **JUBB, K.V.F., KENNEDY, P.C. & PALMER, N., 1993**. *Pathology of Domestic Animals*. 4th edn. Vol. II. San Diego: Academic Press, Inc.

15 **LE MINOR, L., 1984**. *Salmonella*. *In*: KRIEG, N.R. & HOLT, J.G., (eds). *Bergey's Manual of Systematic Bacteriology*. Vol. I. Baltimore, London: Williams & Wilkins.

16 **LE MINOR, L. & POPOFF, M.Y., 1987.** Designation of *Salmonella enterica* sp. nov., nom. rev., as the type and only species of the genus *Salmonella*. *International Journal of Systematic Bacteriology*, 37, 465–468.

17 **LE MINOR, L., POPOFF, M.Y., LAURENT, B. & HERMANT, D., 1986**. Description of a seventh *Salmonella* subspecies: *S. choleraesuis* subsp. *indica* subsp. nov. *Annales Institut Pasteur/Microbiologie*, 137B, 211–217.

18 **LE MINOR, L., VERON, M. & POPOFF, M.Y., 1982**. A proposal for *Salmonella* nomenclature. *Annales Institut Pasteur/ Microbiologie*, 133B, 245–254.

19 **LINDBERG, A.A., 1980.** Bacterial virulence factors—with particular reference to *Salmonella* bacteria. *Scandinavian Journal of Infectious Diseases*, Suppl. 24, 86–92.

20 **MEARA, P.J., 1973.** Salmonellosis in slaughter animals as a source of human food poisoning. *Journal of the South African Veterinary Association*, 44, 215–233.

21 **MURRAY, M.J., 1986.** *Salmonella*: Virulence factors and enteric salmonellosis. *Journal of the American Veterinary Medical Association*, 189, 145–147.

22 **PARKER, M.T., 1983.** *Salmonella*. *In*: WILSON, G.S., MILES, A.A. & PARKER, M.T., (eds). *Topley and Wilson's Principles of Bacteriology, Virology and Immunity*. 7th edn. Vol. II. London: Edward Arnold.

23 **PROST, E. & RIEMANN, H., 1967**. Food-borne salmonellosis. *Annual Review of Microbiology*, 21, 495–528.

24 **ROWLEY, D., 1968.** Sensitivity of rough Gram-negative bacteria to the bactericidal action of serum. *Journal of Bacteriology*, 95, 1647–1650.

25 **STINAVAGE, P.S., MARTIN, L.E. & SPITZNAGEL, J.K., 1989**. O antigen and lipid A phosphoryl groups in resistance of *Salmonella typhimurium* LT-2 nonoxydative killing in human polymorphonuclear neutrophils. *Infection and Immunity*, 57, 3894–3900.

26 **STINAVAGE, P.S., MARTIN, L.E. & SPITZNAGEL, J.K., 1990**. A 59-kilodalton outer membrane protein of *Salmonella typhimurium* protects against oxidative intraleukocytic killing due to human neutrophils. *Molecular Microbiology*, 4, 283–293.

27 **TAGESSEN, C. & STENDAHL, O., 1973**. Influence of the cell surface lipopolysaccharide structure of *Salmonella typhimurium* on resistance to intracellular bactericidal systems. *Acta Pathologica Microbiologica Scandinavica*, Section B, 81, 473–480.

28 **TAKASAKI, C.L., SAXEN, H., MAKELA, P.H. & LEIVE, L., 1983**. Complement activation by polysaccharide of lipopolysaccharide: An important virulence determinant of *Salmonella*. *Infection and Immunity*, 41, 563–569.

29 **VALTONEN, V.V., 1970**. Mouse virulence of *Salmonella* strains: The effect of different smooth-type O side chains. *Journal of General Microbiology*, 64, 255–268.

130

Bovine salmonellosis

Synonyms: Paratyphoid, paratifus (Afrik.)

B.J. Venter, J.G. Myburgh and M.L. van der Walt

Introduction

Bovine salmonellosis usually manifests clinically as a syndrome of septicaemia, acute or chronic enteritis, or abortion. One or more of these syndromes may occur simultaneously in the same animal or herd. Calves less than three months of age are most commonly affected, while animals exposed to stressful situations are particularly prone to contracting the disease. Although salmonellosis in cattle is caused by a number of different serovars, *Salmonella dublin* and *S. typhimurium* are by far the most common. The source of infection is usually an environment contaminated by the faeces of either clinically affected or carrier animals. Salmonellosis is a zoonosis.

A disease of calves that was subsequently considered to be paratyphoid was first diagnosed in South Africa by Hutcheon in 1893.[31] It was similar to the condition described by O. Henning in 1894 as 'lewerziekte' (liver disease) or 'yellow liver'.[31] *Salmonella dublin* as a cause of abortion in cattle in South Africa was first reported in 1943.[6]

Salmonellosis in both calves and adult cattle occurs in most countries of the world and has been shown to be economically important in Europe and North America.[7, 39, 90] In South Africa the disease is frequently diagnosed in calves, but is only rarely encountered as a clinical problem in adult cattle.[32, 76] Although an accurate estimate of the occurrence of salmonellosis in southern Africa is not available, its importance (especially in calves) is likely to be similar to that in many other parts of the world.[37]

Aetiology

Serovars of the genus *Salmonella* are identified on the basis of specific combinations of somatic and flagellar antigens and, to a lesser extent, by their biochemical reactions **(see *Salmonella* sp. infections: Introduction)**.

Salmonella dublin and *S. typhimurium* are the serovars most frequently associated with bovine salmonellosis;[7, 32, 50] other serovars are incriminated only rarely.[4] Henning in 1939[30] and 1953 reported that more than 95 per cent of cases of calf paratyphoid in South Africa were due to *S. dublin*, while Botes in 1965[8] recorded that *S. typhimurium* infection was responsible for up to 19,1 per cent of cases of calf paratyphoid.

For information on the general characteristics of the salmonellas consult the ***Salmonella* sp. infections: Introduction.**

Epidemiology

The diseases in cattle caused by *S. dublin* and *S. typhimurium* are clinically indistinguishable, but they differ epidemiologically **(Table 130.1)**.[1, 71, 91] The host preferences[88] and the ability of the two serovars to establish carriers in animals following initial infection also differ.[1, 10, 13, 29, 66, 88, 91, 92]

Salmonella dublin is regarded as a serovar specific to cattle and only rarely infects other species of animals and humans.[10, 73, 85] On the other hand, most other serovars, including *S. typhimurium*, are not host-specific,[92] and direct or indirect transmission between cattle as well as between cattle and other domestic or wild animals may occur.[10, 92]

Calves aged between three and 12 weeks of age are the most frequent victims of salmonellosis, but mature cattle may also suffer from clinical disease.[1, 2, 8, 32, 66, 88] The

Table 130.1 Important epidemiological differences between *Salmonella dublin* and *Salmonella typhimurium* infections in cattle

SALMONELLA DUBLIN	*SALMONELLA TYPHIMURIUM*
Bovine-specific[88]	Not host-specific[92]
Usually endemic herd problem[91]	Usually sporadic disease outbreaks: calf rearing units[38, 76, 91]
Bovine carriers important as source of infection[10, 66]	Various animal species and their products are important sources of infection[48, 66, 94]
Carriers excrete organisms for long periods (sometimes life-long)[88]	Carriers excrete organisms for short periods (usually 3–4 months)[66, 88]
Septicaemia common[1]	Septicaemia uncommon: enteritis more common[1]
Abortions relatively common[39, 91]	Abortions uncommon[88, 91]

disease is much more common in dairy than in beef calves, mainly because of the differences in management practices.[10] In contrast to the general husbandry practices applied to beef calves, dairy calves are usually removed from their mothers at a very early age and many of them are then subjected to the stresses of transportation, starvation, changes in environment and feed, and the mixing of calves from different farms. These factors all predispose them to salmonellosis.[3, 29, 95] In calves infected with *S. dublin*, salmonellosis usually occurs at between six and 12 weeks of age, whereas disease caused by *S. typhimurium* is most common in the first three weeks of life.[8, 94] The probable explanation for this difference is that *S. dublin* infection is more prevalent in adult cattle than *S. typhimurium*,[92] and the presence of colostral immunity to *S. dublin* is therefore more common in calves than immunity to *S. typhimurium*.[94]

Managemental, physiological and nutritional factors, as well as intercurrent infections,[88, 92] not only predispose animals to salmonellosis, but they may also precipitate clinical disease in infected cattle and the excretion of the bacteria by carrier animals.[49, 66, 88] Predisposing factors include unhygienic conditions,[95] overcrowding, transportation,[29, 49] insufficient intake of colostrum, inadequate availability of water and food,[14] inclement weather, hospitalization, surgery and parturition.[36, 76] Intercurrent infections which may play a role include bovine virus diarrhoea and mucosal disease, infectious bovine rhinotracheitis viruses and *Escherichia coli*, or infestation with parasites such as *Fasciola hepatica*.[88, 91] The effects of these 'stress factors' are probably related to the suppression of cell-mediated immunity.[5]

The most important sources of *Salmonella* organisms are clinically affected and carrier animals, and faecally contaminated environments, water and feedstuffs (e.g. bone, fish and soya-bean meals).[26, 92] Clinically affected animals excrete large numbers of bacteria, particularly in their faeces. Adult cattle are important in the dissemination of salmonellas as they act as carriers, particularly of *S. dublin*.[66, 89, 91] Carrier animals harbour organisms in their mesenteric lymph nodes, gut-associated lymphoid tissue, macrophages in the lamina propria of the intestine, and the gall bladder.[5, 71, 72] Stressed animals shed the organisms more readily and in higher numbers than non-stressed carriers.[19, 49]

Animals that graze with active carriers (animals that are faecal excretors of the organism) may ingest and shed salmonellas in their faeces, presumably by voiding the ingested bacteria.[10, 66] These animals are referred to as 'passive carriers', as they stop excreting the bacteria when they are removed from the source of infection.[66] Carriers that do not excrete salmonellas in their faeces are referred to as 'latent carriers'.

Cattle carrying *S. dublin* may eventually lose the infection or remain life-long carriers,[66, 90] shedding organisms intermittently or continuously in large numbers in their faeces.[66, 71, 74, 88] In contrast, cattle carrying *S. typhimurium* shed the bacteria for a limited period only, in most instances no longer than three or four months.[66, 88] In addition to cattle, a wide range of other domestic and wild animals, particularly rodents and birds, may also be carriers of *S. typhimurium* and shed the organism into the environment.[28, 31, 52]

Seven per cent of cattle in Botswana have been reported to be carriers of *Salmonella* infections, but the overall situation in southern Africa is unknown.[50] Prevalence rates of carriers from a number of non-southern African countries have ranged from 5 to 15 per cent in dairy cattle, and a rate of 4 per cent has been recorded in beef cattle.[7] However, these estimates are likely to be low because cattle may excrete organisms intermittently, and stress could precipitate excretion by latent carriers.[88]

Apart from faecal excretion of salmonellas, organisms may also be excreted in the urine[10] and the saliva (originating from the tonsils or salivary glands) of diseased calves[2, 67, 88] as well as in the milk of cows in which salmonellas have colonized the udder.[55, 85, 88] *Salmonella dublin* may be excreted in the milk, faeces and urine of cows for up to four weeks after parturition or abortion.[10, 36]

Apart from carrier or diseased animals, other sources of salmonellas include animal feedstuffs whose constituents may be infected prior to formulation or become contaminated thereafter,[3, 9, 66] poultry manure and litter (which are commonly used as a feed supplement for cattle in southern Africa because of their high nitrogen content),[88] and water contaminated by sewage.[17, 88] The practice of using farm wastes to irrigate pastures may disseminate the infection widely and expose large numbers of cattle to salmonellosis.[40, 88] Rivers, particularly in the vicinity of informal settlements with unsatisfactory sewage-disposal facilities, may become contaminated with salmonellas and can also widely disseminate the bacteria.[17, 88]

Salmonella organisms may survive in the environment for variable periods when suitable conditions of moisture and organic material are present.[69, 92] For example, *S. dublin* has been found to survive in the environment for over a year under a wide range of climatic conditions,[48, 65] and *S. typhimurium* has been reported to persist in contaminated pastures and soil for between four months and two years.[48, 88]

Most *Salmonella* infections occur by the oro-faecal route.[28, 56, 58, 92] Aerosol transmission has been reported but is rare.[28, 63, 84] Calves may occasionally become infected transplacentally.[20, 66] Intensive farming units with close contact between calves favour the transmission of salmonellas.[2, 3, 88]

The minimal oral dose of various serovars required to induce clinical disease varies from 10^4 to 10^{11} organisms;[5, 53, 92, 93] the oral route requiring about 25 per cent more bacteria than respiratory infection.[63] Clearly, therefore, the larger the number of organisms in the environment, the more likely it is that a susceptible animal will contract clinical salmonellosis.[74]

Salmonellosis is a zoonosis, *S. typhimurium* being more commonly involved than *S. dublin*.[10, 29] The organisms can readily be transmitted from animals to humans by ingestion or inhalation.[3, 13, 21, 29, 92] Animal-derived food, especially raw milk, meat and eggs, is the most important source.[3] The organisms are protected from the acidic environment of the stomach by the high fat content of milk and are able to pass through it unscathed.[10] The transmission of infection by direct contact between humans is rare, except under special circumstances such as those that may prevail in hospitals.[3] People working with animals are at risk of contracting the disease during the treatment of animals suffering from salmonellosis.[13] Likewise, humans who are excretors of *Salmonella* organisms can provide a source of infection for animals.[3, 52, 88] For example, calves may become infected when they are taught to drink milk from a bucket by attendants who are themselves infected.[88]

Pathogenesis

The outcome of infection with salmonellas depends essentially on three factors: the infective dose, predisposing factors influencing the host, and the level of immunity.[5, 69, 88]

In bovine salmonellosis only the intestinal tract may be involved or, if the organisms manage to spread beyond the intestinal mucosa and mesenteric lymph nodes, septicaemia or bacteraemia may develop and result in dissemination to many organs, including the lungs, joints, brain and placenta.[5, 69, 86]

The pathogenesis of the enteric lesions has two stages; colonization and invasion of the intestine by the bacteria, followed by increased secretion of fluid and electrolytes.[5, 54]

Colonization and invasion of the intestine

Salmonellas must be ingested in sufficient numbers (generally a minimal infective dose of 10^4 – 10^{11} organisms is required) for colonization of the distal small intestine and colon to occur.[5, 53, 92, 93] Factors which interfere with and disrupt the normal intestinal flora, such as antimicrobial therapy and food and water deprivation, result in reduced peristalsis and enhance colonization and temporary overgrowth by salmonellas, especially in the small intestine.[16, 33, 80] Colonization tends to occur more readily in stressed animals.[5, 80]

The ability of the bacteria to attach to and invade enterocytes is essential to the development of enteric salmonellosis.[5] The possession of adhesion pili enables the bacteria to become attached to the surface of enterocytes, which facilitates their entrance into the cells through the brush border. The bacteria may also enter the mucosa through intercellular junctional complexes.[5] Most salmonellas remain intact within membrane-bound vacuoles in the cytoplasm of enterocytes, where they multiply and produce enterotoxin.[5] Although many bacteria may be present in a single enterocyte during the early stages of infection, cellular damage is mild.[5, 92] After 24 hours of infection most of the bacteria are located in membrane-bound vacuoles within macrophages and neutrophils in the lamina propria,[5, 16] from whence they may spread to the regional lymph nodes, in which further multiplication takes place.

Stimulation of secretion of increased amounts of fluids and electrolytes

Enterotoxin and the inflammatory response that follows invasion of the intestinal mucosa[54, 77, 80] by salmonellas cause the release of prostaglandins that activate mucosal adenyl-cyclase, resulting in a net secretion of water, Na^+, HCO_3^-, and Cl^- into the lumen of the intestine.[54, 69, 81] Malabsorption and maldigestion develop as a result of cellular infiltration in the affected intestine and damage to the villi, which restricts lymph and blood flow and diminishes the absorptive surface.[69]

Septicaemia may develop after intestinal infection, resulting in localization of the bacteria in other organs and tissues (e.g., liver, spleen, lungs, joints, brain). Pregnant animals may abort. The role of the virulence factors, including that of the lipid A portion (endotoxin) of the lipopolysaccharide of the cell wall, that are associated with septicaemic salmonellosis is discussed in the ***Salmonella* sp. infections: Introduction.**[5, 54] For more information on the composition and pathophysiological effects of endotoxin, consult the section on pathogenesis in **Chapter 129**: ***Escherichia coli* infections**.

The relative roles of cell-mediated and humoral immunity in protection against, and recovery from, salmonellosis are not well understood,[15] but both are probably involved.[11, 18, 41, 42]

Clinical signs

In cattle the enteric and septicaemic syndromes of salmonellosis are more common[1, 66, 88] than the abortion syndrome.[35] One or more of the syndromes may occur simultaneously in an outbreak of salmonellosis in a herd, or even in a single affected animal.[92] *Salmonella dublin* is more often the cause of septicaemia than *S. typhimurium*,[1, 59] and adult animals are less likely than calves to suffer septicaemic infections.[5]

Calves

Calves may develop peracute, acute or chronic salmonellosis.[69]

The peracute disease is usually a septicaemic condition. It is often fatal, and calves may die suddenly without being seen to be ill.[69] Some, however, develop enteritis and diarrhoea in addition to septicaemia.[1, 88] When the course of the septicaemia is protracted, signs of hepatitis, pneumonia, meningoencephalitis, polyarthritis and osteomyelitis may develop.[1, 10, 59, 62, 66]

Acute enteric salmonellosis is the most common syndrome of salmonellosis encountered in calves.[1, 4, 69, 92]

Following an incubation period which may vary from one to five days, calves develop a high fever,[93] inappetence, lethargy, diarrhoea, polypnoea, and frequently a serous nasal discharge followed by a slight cough.[59, 71] Scouring may only occur terminally.[67] The faeces of affected calves are foul-smelling, have a putty-like consistency, and contain large amounts of mucus, sloughed mucosa and flecks of blood.[1] These animals show signs of colic, become gradually weaker, are unthrifty and may collapse into sternal recumbency. At this time the body temperature may be normal or subnormal.[93] The mortality rate is generally much higher among purchased than home-bred calves; it may reach 75 per cent, but mortality rates are generally between 5 and 10 per cent.

Chronic salmonellosis in calves is characterized by unthriftiness, long and scruffy hair coats, and stunting.[69, 92] Diarrhoea is not always present and signs of chronic pneumonia with persistent coughing may occur.[39, 69]

Calves that survive either peracute, acute or chronic disease may develop pneumonia, meningoencephalitis, purulent polyarthritis (particularly of the carpal and tarsal joints), and osteomyelitis of the vertebrae and bones of the distal parts of the limbs, resulting in lameness, paresis or even almost complete paraplegia.[25, 62, 69, 82] Dry gangrene of the skin of the lower limbs (often between the carpus/tarsus and the coronary band)[45] and the tips of the ears and tail, resembling ergotism, is rarely encountered.[66] The affected parts are cold and sharply demarcated from the normal tissues.

Adult cattle

Adult cattle generally contract either acute or subacute enteric salmonellosis, and pregnant animals may abort.[88, 91, 92]

During the early stages of the acute enteric disease, severely affected animals show fever, depression, inappetence, and a drop in milk yield. These signs are followed by diarrhoea which is foul-smelling, the faeces being mucoid and usually containing clots of blood and shreds of necrotic intestinal mucosa.[66, 76] Signs of colic, congested mucous membranes and dehydration may be evident. The acute disease lasts for about a week. The case fatality rate in adult animals with dysentery is usually about 50 per cent, but may be higher.[65, 68] Complete recovery may take up to two months.[38, 88]

Similar but less severe signs are present in animals suffering from subacute enteric salmonellosis,[76, 88] and most affected animals recover without treatment.[88]

Salmonella dublin in particular, but also other serovars, may cause abortion in cows at any stage of pregnancy.[27, 35, 36] Abortions may either precede the onset of dysentery or follow it within two to four weeks. Alternatively, abortion may occur in cows that show no signs of ill health,[36] septicaemia and/or placentitis being the cause of death of the foetus.[35] Retention of the placenta occurs in approximately 70 per cent of cows that abort, but subsequent fertility is not usually affected.[27]

In humans a number of disease syndromes are caused by infection with salmonellas. These include food poisoning characterized by diarrhoea and vomition, septicaemia, arthritis, meningitis, and pustular dermatitis on the arms and hands of animal handlers and veterinarians who perform obstetric manipulations on infected cows.[3, 10, 35, 46]

Pathology

Calves suffering from peracute septicaemic salmonellosis show marked leukopenia with a left shift. Metabolic acidosis may be present, even in the absence of diarrhoea or dehydration.[69]

In calves with enteritis, leukopenia is present during the early stage, but those that survive for three or four days develop a leukocytosis and elevated plasma fibrinogen levels. During the initial stage of enteric disease dehydration results in elevated packed cell volume and plasma protein levels, but plasma protein levels drop after some time due to loss into the gastrointestinal tract.[69] Diarrhoeic calves have decreased serum sodium and chloride levels, and serum potassium values may be either elevated or depressed, despite the body's tendency towards a metabolic acidosis.[69]

Calves that have died from peracute septicaemic salmonellosis usually have widespread subcutaneous, mucosal and serosal petechial haemorrhages, generalized congestion, oedema and congestion of the lungs, splenomegaly and hepatomegaly.[5, 69]

The carcasses of calves that have died from the acute enteric disease reveal varying degrees of dehydration and in some cases mild icterus.[88, 93] There is moderate hepatomegaly, and the liver is bronze or orange-brown with a few to numerous greyish-white foci of necrosis, 0,5–1,0 mm in diameter, and a few petechiae disseminated throughout the parenchyma.[32] In order to see the necrotic foci with the naked eye, it is often necessary to examine several cut surfaces of the liver very carefully in good light, sunlight being preferable. The gall bladder wall is oedematous and there may be focal necrosis of its mucosa. The spleen is moderately enlarged and on cut section may reveal inconspicuous necrotic foci in the red pulp, similar to those in the liver.[5] Small areas of acute bronchopneumonia (sometimes accompanied by haemorrhages in the lung parenchyma) and swelling of the kidneys with whitish-grey foci of necrosis (0,5–1,0 mm in diameter) in the renal cortex may be evident in some animals.[5, 88] The lesions in the gastrointestinal tract vary in severity and location, but in most calves the jejunum and ileum are affected. Depending on the severity of the disease, catarrhal, necrotizing or diphtheritic jejunitis and ileitis may be present.[5, 92] In some animals the caecum and colon show similar lesions to those in the small intestine. The contents of the intestine, particularly the affected parts, are watery, foul-smelling, and usually contain copious amounts of an admixture of fibrin, mucus, desquamated mucosa and digested blood.[92] The mesenteric lymph nodes are invariably enlarged and oedematous, and may reveal petechiae on cut surface.

The carcasses of calves that have died from the chronic disease manifest many of the lesions present in the acute disease but, in addition, have signs of localization of the infection in a variety of organs and tissues.[69] These include fibrinopurulent synovitis of the larger joints (particularly of the limbs), bronchopneumonia and abscessation in the lungs, and occasionally meningoencephalitis, osteomyelitis of one or more of the vertebrae and bones of the limbs, and ischaemic necrosis of the skin of the tips of the ears and the distal parts of the tail and limbs.[62, 69, 88]

The histopathological lesions in the liver comprise small foci of coagulative necrosis which are infiltrated by a few macrophages and mononuclear cells.[5] These foci are present in most livers and are referred to as 'typhoid nodules'. They are randomly scattered in lobules throughout the liver, some of which are associated with thrombosis of central veins or blood vessels in portal triads. Other lesions include mild to moderate infiltration of mononuclear cells into most portal triads, vasculitis sometimes accompanied by thrombosis of some of the larger blood vessels in the triads, moderate Kupffer cell proliferation and bile stasis. Vascular lesions and necrotic foci similar to those in the liver are usually present in the spleen and sometimes also in the lungs, lymph nodes (particularly the mesenteric lymph nodes), kidneys, and bone marrow.[5] The lesions in the affected parts of the intestines are characterized by necrosis and ulceration of the mucosa, presence of moderate numbers of mononuclear cells and neutrophils in the lamina propria and submucosa, and vasculitis and thrombosis of some of the blood vessels in the submucosa. Copious amounts of cellular debris, mucus and fibrin adhere to the necrotic mucosa or are present in the lumen of the affected parts of the intestines. *Salmonella* organisms may be observed microscopically as individual bacteria or colonies of organisms, associated with the areas of inflammation and necrosis.

The macro- and microscopic lesions of salmonellosis in adult cattle are similar to those in calves except that the enteritis is generally more haemorrhagic and fibrinous.[5, 76]

The hepatic lesions in aborted foetuses are similar to those described for calves.

Diagnosis

The diagnosis of salmonellosis is based on the isolation of the causative organism, supported by the history, clinical signs, and lesions at necropsy.[1, 76]

In live animals with diarrhoea, faecal specimens (2–20 g) or rectal swabs should be submitted for bacterial isolation.[61, 88, 92] In animals suffering from severe diarrhoea the large volume of fluid may dilute the number of organisms in the faeces to such an extent that rectal swabs contain insufficient organisms to enable successful isolation.[69, 74] *Salmonella* organisms may be isolated from the blood of septicaemic animals.[76, 88, 92]

Apart from the examination of faecal specimens and rectal swabs, rectal mucosal biopsies provide an easy and safe method that increases the chance of isolating *Salmonella* organisms,[61] the reason being the adherent and invasive nature of salmonellas which results in their concentration on the mucosa.[61]

From dead animals, specimens comprising tissue blocks of the liver and spleen, one or more mesenteric lymph nodes, and a section of the affected part of the intestine should be submitted at 4 °C for bacterial isolation. In addition, specimens from the liver, spleen, kidneys, brain, lungs and intestine should be collected and placed in a 10 per cent buffered formalin solution for histopathological examination. The presence of the typical necrotic foci and thrombosis, particularly in the liver and spleen, are highly suggestive of salmonellosis.

The identification of carrier animals is not always easy, as such animals may shed bacteria intermittently and it may be necessary to examine specimens taken from them on a number of occasions before a positive culture is obtained.[92]

Salmonellas can be isolated from the organs (liver, spleen, lungs) and stomach content of aborted foetuses.[35] The placenta and vaginal mucus of cows that abort should also be submitted for bacterial isolation.[65, 88]

Specimens submitted to a laboratory for *Salmonella* isolation are incubated in enrichment broth to enhance the chances of isolating the organisms **(see *Salmonella* sp. infections: Introduction)**.

Serological tests, such as ELISA, serum agglutination and complement fixation,[12, 92] can be used for the retrospective diagnosis of salmonellosis or the detection of carriers. These tests are, however, rarely used for diagnostic purposes and are only reliable when applied on a herd or flock basis, or when both acute and convalescent phase sera are tested.[7, 80] Antibody responses are much more consistent in animals that have suffered systemic infections, i.e. bacteraemia or septicaemia.[36, 80] Many infected animals may not have positive titres, either because the serum was collected too early during the course of infection (less than 14 days) or because the infection was not severe enough to stimulate a detectable humoral immune response.[7, 80, 90] Some latently infected cattle remain serologically negative.

Differential diagnosis

The clinical signs of enteric salmonellosis in calves are non-specific and are very similar to those caused by many other infectious and non-infectious agents that affect the gastrointestinal tract. The most important of these include viruses (e.g. rota-, corona-, Breda- and bovine virus diarrhoea and mucosal disease viruses), bacteria (e.g. *Escherichia coli, Clostridium perfringens* types A,

B or C), *Chlamydia psittaci*, protozoa (e.g. *Eimeria* spp., *Cryptosporidium* sp.) and nutritional causes (over-feeding, incorrect feeding and the feeding of milk-replacers containing heat-denatured whey proteins).[7, 32, 69] The clinical signs and lesions of salmonellosis in calves may be very similar to those of Rift Valley fever **(see Chapter 71: Rift Valley fever)**.

The diarrhoea, which may be bloody or dysenteric, associated with enteric salmonellosis in adult cattle should be differentiated from those caused by bovine virus diarrhoea-mucosal disease virus, helminths (e.g. *Geigeria pachyscelis*, *Bunostomum phlebotomum*, and *Paramphistomum microbothrium*), toxic plants (e.g. *Ornithogalum* spp., *Ornithoglossum* spp., *Homeria* and *Moraea* spp. and *Quercus* spp.) and ingestion of pollen beetles (*Astylus atromaculatus*).[43]

Abortion caused by *Salmonella* serovars should be differentiated from that induced by other agents, the most important of these in southern Africa being *Brucella abortus*, *Leptospira* spp., Rift Valley fever virus and Palyam serogroup viruses.

Control

Different approaches to the therapy of salmonellosis, particularly the enteric disease, have been reported.[44, 69] The use of antimicrobial drugs in the treatment of enteric salmonellosis, although controversial, may have beneficial effects, especially if applied during the early stages of the disease.[2, 38, 44, 69] Parenteral antimicrobial therapy has been shown to be more beneficial than oral treatment.[69] Those antimicrobial drugs that have been shown to be effective in preventing the development of bacteraemia or septicaemia in animals suffering from enteric disease.[57] They also prevent localization of *Salmonella* organisms in extraintestinal organs and the subsequent development of lesions.[5, 69]

Antimicrobial drugs generally recommended for parenteral use are ampicillin, amoxycillin, gentamicin, trimethoprim-sulphonamide combinations and fluoroquinolones.[7, 22, 57, 69, 87] Bacterial resistance has been demonstrated towards several antimicrobials e.g. neomycin, tetracyclines and sulphonamides.[44] An antibiogram could be of help to the practitioner, because antimicrobial sensitivity of *Salmonella* organisms may vary geographically.[44]

The oral administration of antimicrobial drugs in cattle is a satisfactory method of treatment,[7] but it must be used with caution.[51] Some antimicrobial drugs e.g. neomycin, chloramphenicol, tetracycline and ampicillin may cause diarrhoea due to malabsorption after three days of treatment.[51] Disturbance of the gastrointestinal flora by the use of antimicrobial drugs in the presence of resistant *Salmonella* may involve the intestinal flora responsible for restricting the multiplication of *Salmonella*, resulting in overgrowth and conversion of an enteric infection into a septicaemic form. Antimicrobial drugs administered orally may also increase the colonization of the gut by other Gram-negative bacteria and the development of multiple drug resistance, and prolong the carrier state.[23, 24, 70, 75, 78]

Antimicrobial therapy does not usually eliminate the carrier state in cattle.[7, 44] The number of animals that shed the organism and the duration and amount of shedding may be increased if the *Salmonella* strain involved is resistant to the drug used.[7] Chloramphenicol facilitates the persistence of salmonellas, particularly the antimicrobial-resistant serovars.[47, 60, 79]

It is generally agreed that supportive therapy and good nursing are important. These include oral or parenteral rehydration, correction of electrolyte imbalances and stabilization of the acid-base equilibrium. Symptomatic treatment with opioids, alpha-2-agonists, parasympatholytics and anti-inflammatory drugs may have a beneficial effect.[83] Non-steroidal anti-inflammatory drugs, such as flunixin meglumine, may be of benefit in cases with endotoxic shock and to block intestinal prostaglandin production.[44] Most anti-inflammatory drugs are, however, potentially dangerous, especially in dehydrated animals.[83] There is no consensus on the value of intestinal adsorbents and protectants, such as activated charcoal and kaolin, in animals affected by enteric disease.[44]

In programmes designed to control salmonellosis the following should be applied:

Measures directed towards protecting cattle

Improving the resistance of animals in high-risk groups by immunization is important, as is correct feeding to maintain the intestinal flora in a balanced state. Separation of age groups and the prevention of contact with other infected carrier animals lessen the risk of exposure; while the isolation of diseased animals and the elimination of potential sources of infection prevent the spread of the infection and contamination of the environment.

Measures aimed at the agent

Treatment, isolation or elimination of animals suffering from salmonellosis, as well as disinfection of sheds and stables, should be implemented to prevent the build-up of environmental contamination. *Salmonella* organisms are destroyed by most disinfectants that are effective against vegetative bacteria. Some specific disinfectants e.g., diethylpyrocarbonate + hydrogen peroxide, are recommended for use in feedstuffs[64] but are generally too expensive to use as disinfectants for the external environment or fomites. Salmonella-contaminated areas, such as stables, concrete areas, equipment and transport vehicles should be cleaned and then disinfected with phenolic, or chlorine or iodine based disinfectants.[34, 44, 74] Yards with earthen flooring can be decontaminated with several successive sprayings of 5 per cent formalin.[50]

Measures aimed at the environment

These include the institution and maintenance of hygiene and good animal husbandry practices, such as the regular removal of faeces; keeping food stores rodent-free; the use of separate milk pails for each calf, which are then thoroughly washed and disinfected after use; provision of suitable housing; and the prevention of overcrowding.

Vaccination

The use of vaccines is important in the control of salmonellosis in cattle, but immunization on its own is often insufficiently effective to be relied upon entirely, and other means of limiting the spread of infection (such as those described above) also need to be implemented.

Generally, both live attenuated vaccines produced from rough strains and bacterins precipitated on aluminium hydroxide are available commercially. The Veterinary Research Institute, Onderstepoort produces two vaccines against bovine salmonellosis:

- a trivalent, formalin-inactivated bacterin prepared from isolates of *S. dublin*, *S. typhimurium* and *S. bovismorbificans*, and
- a live, attenuated vaccine containing an avirulent rough mutant of *S. dublin*.

Live attenuated vaccines should be administered as a single inoculation to calves at two to four weeks of age.[7]

Bacterins, to be effective, require to be administered twice at an interval of two weeks, but are usually ineffective in calves under six weeks of age.[7] For this reason, the administration of bacterins to pregnant cows is sometimes recommended in order to provide their calves with colostral immunity which persists at protective levels for approximately six weeks.[7] On farms on which calf paratyphoid is a particular problem, calves whose dams were immunized with a bacterin during pregnancy should be immunized at six weeks of age with a live attenuated vaccine against *S. dublin*. In this way it is usually possible to ensure that these calves have an adequate level of immunity during the danger period for calf paratyphoid, viz. three to 12 weeks of age.

Antimicrobial drugs should not be administered to calves during the week prior to and for two weeks after immunization with live attenuated *Salmonella* vaccines, as immunity is dependent upon the multiplication of the bacteria contained in the vaccine.

References

1 **ANDERSON, M. & BLANCHARD, P., 1989.** The clinical syndromes caused by *Salmonella* infection. *Veterinary Medicine*, 84, 816–819.

2 **ANDREWS, A.H., 1983.** Calf management and disease notes. Hertfordshire: Nynwood Arts Ltd.

3 **ANON., 1981.** Salmonellosis in animals and man. *The Veterinary Record*, 109, 438–440.

4 **ANON., 1988.** Onderstepoort Vaccines. Veterinary Research Institute, Onderstepoort. Directorate of Agricultural Information, Private Bag X144, Pretoria 0001.

5 **BARKER, I.K. & VAN DREUMEL, A.A., 1991.** The alimentary system. *In*: JUBB, K.V.F., KENNEDY, P.C. & PALMER, N., (eds). *Pathology of Domestic Animals*. 4th edn. San Diego: Academic Press, Inc..

6 **BISHOP, G., SCHATZ, W., & CANHAM, A.S., 1943.** *Salmonella enteriditis* var. *dublin* infection in adult cattle. *Journal of the South African Veterinary Medical Association*, 14, 67–72.

7 **BLOOD, D.C. & RADOSTITS, O.M., 1989.** *Veterinary Medicine*. 7th edn. London: Baillière Tindall.

8 **BOTES, H.J.W., 1965.** Live vaccines in the control of salmonellosis. *Journal of the South African Veterinary Medical Association*, 36, 461–474.

9 **BRANDER, G.C. & ELLIS, P.R., 1977.** *Animal and Human Disease, the Control of Disease*. London: Baillière Tindall.

10 **BULGIN, M.S., 1983.** *Salmonella dublin*: What veterinarians should know. *Journal of the American Veterinary Medical Association*, 182, 116–118.

11 **CAMERON, C.M. & FULS, W.J.P., 1976.** Immunization of mice and calves against *Salmonella dublin* with attenuated live and inactivated vaccines. *Onderstepoort Journal of Veterinary Research*, 43, 31–37.

12 **CARLSSON, H.E., LINDBERG, A.A. & HAMMARSTRÖM, S., 1973.** Titration of antibodies to *Salmonella* O-antigens by enzyme-linked immunosorbent assay. *Infection and Immunity*, 6, 703–708.

13 **CARTER, A.P., 1991.** Transmission of salmonellae to veterinarians. *The Veterinary Record*, 11, 415.

14 **CHAMBERS, P.G. & LYSONS, R.J., 1979.** The inhibitory effect of bovine rumen fluid on *Salmonella typhimurium*. *Research in Veterinary Science*, 26, 273–276.

15 **CHATURVEDI, G.C. & SHARMA, V.K., 1981.** Cell-mediated immunoprotection in calves immunized with rough *Salmonella dublin*. *The British Veterinary Journal*, 137, 421–430.

16 **CLARKE, R.C., GYLES, C.L. & VAN DREUMEL, A.A., 1986.** Pathogenesis of acute experimental salmonellosis in calves. *Fourth International Symposium of Veterinary Laboratory Diagnosticians*, 2–6 June 1986, Amsterdam.

17 **CLEGG, F.G., CHIEJINA, S.N., DUNCAN, A.L., KAY, R.N. & WRAY, C., 1983.** Outbreaks of *Salmonella newport* infection in dairy herds and their relationship to management and contamination of the environment. *The Veterinary Record*, 112, 580–584.

18 **COLLINS, F.M. & CHAMPBELL, S.G., 1981.** Immunity to intracellular bacteria. *In*: KIRSTENSEN, F. & ANTCZAK, D.F., (eds). *Advances in Veterinary Immunology. Developments in Animal and Veterinary Science*, 9, 5–66.

19 **CORRIER, D.E., PURDY, C.W. & DELOACH, J.R., 1990.** Effects of marketing stress on fecal excretion of *Salmonella* spp. in feeder calves. *American Journal of Veterinary Research*, 51, 866–869.

20 **COUNTER, D.E. & GIBSON, E.A., 1980.** *Salmonella dublin* infection in self-contained dairy herds in East Anglia: Excretion at calving. *The Veterinary Record*, 107, 191–193.

21 **DE VOS, A. & DE VRIESE, L., 1975.** Epidemiologie en bestrijding van *Salmonella* infecties. *Vlaams Diergeneeskundig Tijdscrift*, 44, 309–323.

22 **EL BAHRI, L. & BLOUIN, A., 1991.** Fluoroquinolones: A new family of antimicrobials. *The Compendium of Continuing Education for the Practising Veterinarian*, 13, 1429–1434.

23 **FRETER, R., 1955.** The fatal enteric cholera infection in the guinea-pig, achieved by inhibition of normal enteric flora. *Journal of Infectious Diseases*, 97, 57–65.

24 **FRETER, R., 1956.** Experimental enteric *Shigella* and *Vibrio* infections in mice and guinea-pigs. *Journal of Experimental*

Medicine, 104, 411–418.

25 **GITTER, M., WRAY, C., RICHARDSON, C. & PEPPER, R.T., 1978.** Chronic *Salmonella dublin* infection in calves. *The British Veterinary Journal*, 134, 113–121.

26 **GLICKMAN, L.T., McDONOUGH, P.L., SHIN, S.J., FAIRBROTHER, J.M., LADUE, R.L. & KING, S.E., 1981.** Bovine salmonellosis attributed to *Salmonella anatum*-contaminated haylage and dietary stress. *Journal of the American Veterinary Medical Association*, 178, 1268–1272.

27 **HALL, G.A. & JONES, P.W., 1979.** Experimental oral infections of pregnant heifers with *Salmonella dublin*. *The British Veterinary Journal*, 135, 75–82.

28 **HARDMAN, P.M., WATHES, C.M. & WRAY, C., 1991.** Transmission of salmonellae among calves penned individually. *The Veterinary Record*, 129, 327–329.

29 **HENDERSON, J.M., 1989.** Salmonellosis in dairy calves and humans. *Canadian Veterinary Journal*, 30, 903.

30 **HENNING, M.W., 1939.** The antigenic structure of salmonellas obtained from domestic animals and birds in South Africa. *Onderstepoort Journal of Veterinary Research*, 13, 79–189.

31 **HENNING, M.W., 1953.** Calf Paratyphoid. I. A general discussion of the disease in relation to animal and man. *Onderstepoort Journal of Veterinary Research*, 26, 3–23.

32 **HENNING, M.W., 1958.** *Die Kalf, sy Versorging, Voeding en Siektes*. Johannesburg: Voortrekkerpers beperk.

33 **HENTGES, D.J. & MAIER, B.R., 1970.** Inhibition of *Shigella flexineri* by the normal intestinal flora. III. Interactions with *Bacteroides fragilis* strains *in vitro*. *Infections and Immunology*, 2, 364–370.

34 **HESS, G.W., MOULTROP, J.I. & NORTON, H.R., 1970.** New decontamination efforts and techniques for elimination of *Salmonella* from animal protein-rendering plants. *Journal of the American Veterinary Medical Association*, 157, 1975–1980.

35 **HINTON, M., 1971.** *Salmonella* abortion in cattle. *The Veterinary Bulletin*, 41, 973–980.

36 **HINTON, M., 1974.** *Salmonella dublin* abortion in cattle. Studies on the clinical aspects of the condition. *The British Veterinary Journal*, 130, 556–562.

37 **HOBBS, B.C., 1974.** Microbiological hazards of meat production. *Food Manufacture*, 49, 29–31.

38 **HUGHES, L.E., GIBSON, E.A., ROBERTS, H.E., DAVIES, E.T., DAVIES, G. & SOJKA, W.J., 1971.** Bovine salmonellosis in England and Wales. *The British Veterinary Journal*, 127, 225–238.

39 **HUNGERFORD, T.G., 1990.** *Diseases of Livestock*. 9th edn. Sydney: McGraw-Hill Book Company.

40 **JACK, E.J. & HEPPER, P.T., 1969.** An outbreak of *Salmonella typhimurium* infection in cattle associated with the spreading of slurry. *The Veterinary Record*, 84, 196–199.

41 **JOHNSON, E.M., HIETALA, S. & SMITH, B.P., 1985.** Chemiluminescence of bovine alveolar macrophages as an indicator of developing immunity in calves vaccinated with aromatic-dependent *Salmonella*. *Veterinary Microbiology*, 10, 451–464.

42 **JÖRBECK, H.J.A., SVENSON, S.B. & LINDBERG, A.A., 1981.** Artificial *Salmonella* vaccines: *Salmonella typhimurium* O-antigen-specific oligosaccharide-protein conjugates elicit opsonizing antibodies that enhance phagocytosis. *Infection and Immunity*, 32, 497–502.

43 **KELLERMAN, T.S., COETZER, J.A.W. & NAUDÉ, T.W., 1988.** *Plant Poisonings and Mycotoxicoses of Livestock in Southern Africa*. Cape Town: Oxford University Press Southern Africa.

44 **KENNEDY, G.A. & HIBBS, C.M., 1993.** Salmonellosis. *In*: HOWARD, J.L., (ed.). *Current Veterinary Therapy. Food Animal Practice*. 3rd edn. Philadelphia: W.B. Saunders Co.

45 **KERSJES, A.W., FRIK, J.F. & VAN DER WATERING, C.C., 1966.** Bacteriële ostitis bij runderen. *Tijdschrift voor Diergeneeskunde*, 91, 1537–1546.

46 **LUND, L.J., ATKINSON, W.I. & HOLT, G.J., 1991.** Transmission of salmonellae to veterinarians. *The Veterinary Record*, 11, 415.

47 **MARTIN, S.W., MEEK, A.H. & CURTIS, R.A., 1983.** Antimicrobial use in feedlot calves: Its association with culture rates and antimicrobial susceptibility. *Canadian Journal of Comparative Medicine*, 47, 6–10.

48 **McLAREN, I.M. & WRAY, C., 1991.** Epidemiology of *Salmonella typhimurium* infection in calves: Persistence of salmonellae on calf units. *The Veterinary Record*, 129, 461–462.

49 **McORIST, S. & MILLER, G.T., 1981.** Salmonellosis in transported feral goats. *Australian Veterinary Journal*, 57, 389–390.

50 **MEARA, P.J., 1973.** Salmonellosis in slaughter animals as a source of human food poisoning. *Journal of the South African Veterinary Association*, 44, 215–233.

51 **MERO, K.N., ROLLIN, R.E. & PHILLIPS, R.W., 1985.** Malabsorption due to selected oral antibiotics. *Veterinary Clinics of North America: Food Animal Practice*, 1, 581–588.

52 **MINGA, U.M., LICHT, H.H. & SHLUNDT, J., 1985.** Four outbreaks of salmonellosis due to *Salmonella typhimurium* among cattle in one district in Denmark: Case reports. *The British Veterinary Journal*, 141, 490–497.

53 **MORSE, E.V. & DUNCAN, M.A., 1974.** Salmonellosis—An environmental health problem. *Journal of the American Veterinary Medical Association*, 165, 1015–1019.

54 **MURRAY, M.J., 1986.** Salmonella: Virulence factors and enteric salmonellosis. *Journal of the American Veterinary Medical Association*, 189, 145–147.

55 **OGILVIE, T.H., 1986.** The persistent isolation of *Salmonella typhimurium* from the mammary gland of a dairy cow. *The Canadian Veterinary Journal*, 27, 329–331.

56 **OSBORNE, A.D., 1978.** Some aspects of salmonellosis in calves. *Proceedings of the Second International Symposium on Neonatal Diarrhoea*, 3–5 October 1978, University of Saskatchewan.

57 **OSBORNE, A.D., NAZER, A.H.K. & SHIMELD, C., 1978.** Treatment of experimental calf salmonellosis with amoxycillin. *The Veterinary Record*, 103, 233–237.

58 **OSBORNE, A.D., PEARSON, H., LINTON, A.H. & SHIMELD, C., 1977.** Epidemiology of *Salmonella* infection in calves: The source of calfhood infection by *Salmonella dublin*. *The Veterinary Record*, 101, 513–516.

59 **OVERGOOR, G.H.A., KÖNIG, C.D.W., MICHIELSEN, W.H. & ROSEBOOM, M., 1978.** Enkele gegevens over een *Salmonella dublin* epizoötie bij vleeskalveren in Gelderland. *Tijdschrift voor Diergeneeskunde*, 103, 532–537.

60 **PACER, R.E., SPIKA, J.S., THURMOND, M.C., HARGRETT-BEAN, N. & POTTER, M.E., 1989.** Prevalence of *Salmonella* and multiple antimicrobial-resistant *Salmonella* in California dairies. *Journal of the American Veterinary Medical Association*, 195, 59–63.

61 **PALMER, J.E., WHITLOCK, R.H., BENSON, C.E., BECHT, J.L., MORRIS, D.D. & ACLAND, H.M., 1985.** Comparison of rectal mucosal cultures and fecal cultures in detecting *Salmonella* infection in horses and cattle. *American Journal of Veterinary Research*, 46, 697–698.

62 **POWER, E.P. & O'KEEFFE, F., 1991.** Osteomyelitis of the cervical vertebrae of a calf due to *Salmonella dublin*. *Irish Veterinary News*, 13, 31, 33.

63 **PRITULIN, P.L., 1959.** Paratyphoid in sheep and cattle resulting from airborne infection. *Veterinariya*, 36, 26–27.

64 **PROST, E. & RIEMANN, H., 1967.** Food-borne salmonellosis. *Annual Review of Microbiology*, 21, 495–528.

65 **RICHARDSON, A., 1974.** *Salmonella dublin* infections in cattle. *Australian Veterinary Journal*, 50, 463–465.

66 **RICHARDSON, A., 1975.** Salmonellosis in cattle. *The Veterinary Record*, 96, 329–331.

67 **RICHARDSON, A. & FAWCETT, A.R., 1973.** *Salmonella dublin* infection in calves: The value of rectal swabs in diagnosis and epidemiological studies. *The British Veterinary Journal*, 129, 151–155.

68 **RICHARDSON, A. & WATSON, W.A., 1971.** A contribution to the epidemiology of *Salmonella dublin* infection in cattle.

The British Veterinary Journal, 127, 173–183.

69 **RINGS, D.M., 1985.** Salmonellosis in calves. *Veterinary Clinics of North America: Food Animal Practice*, 1, 529–539.

70 **ROWE, B., THRELFALL, E.J., WARD, L.R. & ASHLEY, A.S., 1979.** International spread of multiresistant strains of *Salmonella typhimurium* phage types 204 and 193 from Britain to Europe. *The Veterinary Record*, 105, 468–469.

71 **ROY, J.H.B., 1990.** *The Calf. Management of Health.* Vol. I. 5th edn. London: Butterworths.

72 **SAMUEL, J.L., O'BOYLE, D.A., MATHERS, W.J. & FROST, A.J., 1979.** Isolation of *Salmonella* from mesenteric lymph nodes of healthy cattle at slaughter. *Research in Veterinary Science*, 28, 238–241.

73 **SMALL, R.G. & SHARP, J.C.M., 1979.** A milk-borne outbreak due to *Salmonella dublin*. *Journal of Hygiene*, 82, 95–100.

74 **SOJKA, W.J., THOMSON, P.D. & HUDSON, E.B., 1974.** Excretion of *Salmonella dublin* by adult bovine carriers. *The British Veterinary Journal*, 130, 482–488.

75 **SPIKA, J.S., WATERMAN, S.H., SOO HOO, G.W., ST. LOUIS, M.E., PACER, R.E., JAMES, S.M., BISSETT, M.L., MAYER, L.W., CHIU, J.Y., HALL, B., GREENE, K., POTTER, M.E., COHEN, M.L. & BLAKE, P.A., 1987.** Chloramphenicol-resistant *Salmonella newport* traced through hamburgers to dairy farms: A major persisting source of human salmonellosis in California. *The New England Journal of Medicine*, 316, 565–570.

76 **STADLER, P. & NESBIT, J.W., 1990.** Salmonellosis in an adult dairy cow. *Journal of the South African Veterinary Association*, 61, 65–67.

77 **TAKEUCHI, A., 1967.** Electron microscope studies of experimental *Salmonella* infection. I. Penetration into the intestinal epithelium by *Salmonella typhimurium*. *American Journal of Pathology*, 50, 109–136.

78 **THRELFALL, E.J., ROWE, B., FERGUSON, J.L. & WARD, L.R., 1985.** Increasing incidence of resistance to gentamicin and related aminoglycosides in *Salmonella typhimurium* phage type 204c in England, Wales and Scotland. *The Veterinary Record*, 117, 355–357.

79 **TIMONEY, J.F., 1978.** The epidemiology and genetics of antibiotic resistance of *Salmonella typhimurium* isolated from diseased animals in New York. *Journal of Infectious Diseases*, 137, 67–73.

80 **TIMONEY, J.F., GILLESPIE, J.H., SCOTT, F.W. & BARLOUGH, J.E., 1988.** *Hagan and Bruner's Microbiology and Infectious Diseases of Domestic Animals.* 8th edn. Ithaca: Comstock Publishing Associates.

81 **TURNBULL, P.C.B., 1979.** Food poisoning with special reference to *Salmonella*—Its epidemiology, pathogenesis and control. *Clinics in Gastroenterology*, 8, 663–714.

82 **VAN DEN HEEVER, L.W., 1955.** Vertebral osteitis in a calf due to *Salmonella dublin*. *Journal of the South African Veterinary Medical Association*, 26, 299–300.

83 **VAN MIERT, A.S., BOGAERT, M.G. & DEBACKESE, M., 1985.** *Comparative Veterinary Pharmacology and Therapy*, Proceedings of the Third Congress of the European Association for Veterinary Pharmacology and Toxicology, 25–29 August 1985, Ghent, Belgium.

84 **WATHES, C.M., ZAIDAN, W.A.R., PEARSON, G.R., HINTON, M. & TODD, N., 1988.** Aerosol infection of calves and mice with *Salmonella typhimurium*. *The Veterinary Record*, 123, 590–594.

85 **WERNER, S.B., HUMPHREY, G.L. & KAMEI, I., 1979.** Association between raw milk and human *Salmonella dublin* infection. *The British Medical Journal*, 2, 238–241.

86 **WHITE, G., PIERCY, D.W.T., CLAMPITT, R.B., MORGAN, R.J.I. & WEST, B., 1981.** Appraisal of the suitability of a disease model of acute salmonellosis in calves for chemotherapeutic studies. *Research in Veterinary Science*, 31, 19–26.

87 **WHITE, G., PIERCY, D.W.T. & GIBBS, H.A., 1981.** Use of a calf salmonellosis model to evaluate the therapeutic properties of trimethoprim and sulphadiazine and their mutual potentiation *in vivo*. *Research in Veterinary Science*, 31, 27–31.

88 **WILLIAMS, B.M., 1980.** Bovine salmonellosis. *The Bovine Practitioner*, 15, 122–128.

89 **WILLIAMS, D.R., BELLHOUSE, R. & DAVIDSON, C.L., 1978.** The prevalence of *Salmonella* in healthy cattle at slaughter. *The Veterinary Record*, 103, 359–360.

90 **WRAY, C., 1985.** Is salmonellosis still a serious problem in veterinary practice? *The Veterinary Record*, 116, 485–489.

91 **WRAY, C., 1991.** Salmonellosis in cattle. *In Practice*, 13, 13–15.

92 **WRAY, C. & SOJKA, W.J., 1977.** Reviews of the progress of dairy science: Bovine salmonellosis. *Journal of Dairy Research*, 44, 383–425.

93 **WRAY, C. & SOJKA, W.J., 1978.** Experimental *Salmonella typhimurium* infection in calves. *Research in Veterinary Science*, 25, 139–143.

94 **WRAY, C., TODD, J.N. & HINTON, M., 1987.** Epidemiology of *Salmonella typhimurium* infection in calves: Excretion of *S. typhimurium* in the faeces of calves in different management systems. *The Veterinary Record*, 121, 293–296.

95 **WRAY, C., TODD, N., McLAREN, I., BEEDELL, Y. & ROWE, B., 1990.** The epidemiology of *Salmonella* infection of calves: The role of dealers. *Epidemiology and Infection*, 105, 295–305.

131

Ovine and caprine salmonellosis

J.A. Neser

Introduction

Salmonella infections in sheep and goats are manifested by the development of two distinct syndromes: an acute to subacute septicaemic disease with an associated diarrhoea, and abortion. The septicaemic syndrome is precipitated by stress and is characterized by the development of a watery-green to blood-tinged diarrhoea, the consequence of a severe necrohaemorrhagic ileitis, typhlitis and colitis.

Although the septicaemic disease in sheep is less prevalent than bovine salmonellosis, its occurrence and economic importance appear to be increasing in South Africa with the development of the sheep feedlot industry.

In the United Kingdom and Australia, *Salmonella abortus ovis*,[23, 50] *Salmonella dublin*,[3, 49] and *Salmonella typhimurium*[9, 22] infections have been incriminated as causes of abortion in sheep. Abortions due to infections by *Salmonella* serovars have not been documented in South Africa.

Aetiology

Salmonella typhimurium is most frequently isolated from sheep in South Africa while *S. dublin*, *S. enteritidis* and others are only rarely encountered.[1] For information on the characteristics of the salmonellas, consult ***Salmonella* sp. infections: Introduction**.

Epidemiology

Salmonellosis in sheep and goats occurs under both intensive and extensive farming conditions. Sheep of all age groups are susceptible, but two- to four-toothed sheep are most commonly affected when they are marketed from pasture and consigned to abattoirs or feedlots.[47] Since 1936, when *S. typhimurium* and *S. onderstepoort* infections of sheep were first reported in South Africa,[19] salmonellosis has often been associated with mortality in sheep which have been railed over long distances to the Veterinary Research Institute, Onderstepoort.[1] With few exceptions, there is therefore a history of preceding transport lasting several hours.[1]

Most outbreaks of the disease in South Africa occur within two to four weeks of the introduction of sheep from pastoral grazing into feedlots where diets comprising high proportions of grain and insufficient amounts of roughage are fed. Other nutritional practices, such as a too-rapid change to finishing rations with a high (12,5 per cent) non-protein nitrogen content which favours the proliferation of salmonellas in the digestive tract,[42] are considered to be a major predisposing factor to the development of the disease in feedlots in the USA. Stressful situations, such as those resulting from starvation during transportation, dietary disturbances and overcrowding, are further important predisposing factors.[7, 13, 21] The disease also occurs under pastoral grazing conditions after sheep have been crowded during dipping and shearing.[22, 47]

Although the source of infection in outbreaks is often obscure, it can sometimes be traced back to animals that have been exposed to poor hygienic conditions along the course of transit. Heavy contamination of holding pens, road or railway vehicles, water troughs, abattoir or feedlot yards, dams and streams by *Salmonella*-infected faeces of carrier animals and birds has been reported.[9, 18, 21, 22, 47] *Salmonella typhimurium* has been shown to survive for at least 251 days in soil and for 168 days on pastures.[22, 25]

Under field conditions, infection by the oral route is the most important mode, but sheep may also become infected by the nasal route.[23, 46, 47] Although *S. abortus ovis* has been isolated from the male genital tract on several occasions, venereal transmission has not been demonstrated, and the role of *S. abortus ovis* in the causation of abortion awaits confirmation.[23] Stress-inducing factors, such as mobbing, starvation, and a high saline content of drinking water have been associated with abortions due to *S. dublin* and *S. typhimurium*.[3, 9, 48]

Sheep, and possibly goats, which have recovered from clinical disease may become subclinical carriers of *Salmonella* serovars and excrete organisms in their faeces intermittently. Vaginal discharges or products of abortion may also contaminate the environment.[7, 15, 23, 31, 45, 53] Infected cattle, which excrete salmonellas in their faeces for up to 12 months[22] or even indefinitely,[20] and

Salmonella-contaminated animal products such as blood, carcass and bone meal[17, 39, 55, 56] serve as additional sources of infection for sheep.

Pathogenesis

The pathogenesis of systemic infections of *S. typhimurium* in sheep[6, 40] and goats[31] is very similar to that of experimental *S. typhimurium* infections in rabbits,[14] pigs[43] and calves,[51, 63] and to *S. dublin*[52] and *S. enteritidis* infections in calves[41] **(see Chapter 130: Bovine salmonellosis)**.

The pathogenesis of salmonellosis and the determinants of virulence of the bacteria have been reviewed.[33] There appears to be a correlation between the dosage level of *S. typhimurium* and the severity of the disease; severe disease develops in 50–100 per cent of lambs that receive 2×10^{11}–2×10^{13} *S. typhimurium* organisms *per os*.[6] However, fasting renders animals more susceptible to the disease; lambs fed *ad lib* withstand at least six times the oral dose of organisms lethal for those which are fasted for 48 hours prior to infection.[38]

The virulence of certain *S. typhimurium*, *S. dublin* and *S. enteritidis* strains in mice appears to be plasmid-mediated.[27, 34, 54] Salmonellas also possess flagella which prolong their survival in macrophages.[62]

The lipopolysaccharide component of the endotoxin contained in the outer cell wall of the bacteria contributes to many aspects of the pathogenesis of salmonellosis. Invasiveness, and survival time of *S. typhimurium* in the animal, amongst other factors, have been related to the structure of the O-side chain of the lipopolysaccharide.[30] It also triggers the release of mediators of acute inflammation, such as interleukin-1 and prostaglandins, and the clotting cascade.[33] Endotoxic shock, characterized by pulmonary hypertension, prolonged systemic hypotension and decreased perfusion of vital organs, appear to be mediated by prostaglandins.[8, 11, 44]

Acute enteritis, initially affecting the duodenum, develops within 24 hours of infection.[6] By three to eight days after infection, a severe acute typhlitis and colitis occur, with the presence of blood-stained mucus and fluid in the intestinal lumen, and lymphadenitis of the mesenteric lymph nodes. Most lambs manifest a multifocal, necrotic hepatitis and nephrosis by the sixth day. Many lambs also exhibit a mild, interstitial pneumonia[40] which bears some resemblance to the endotoxin-mediated lung lesions evoked by the experimental intravenous infusion of endotoxin.[32] Penetration of the intestinal mucosa by bacteria, and the consequent inflammatory process, promotes the development of diarrhoea. Entrance of the salmonellas into the circulation may lead to septicaemia, coagulopathy and circulatory shock accompanied by lactacidosis. The effects of diarrhoea and dehydration aggravate these haemodynamic disturbances, thereby causing organ failure and death. Virulence factors contained by the bacteria, which promote diarrhoea, include adhesion pili, and cyto- and enterotoxins which cause increased permeability and increased secretion by mucosal epithelial cells, respectively.[26, 27, 29, 33]

Clinical signs

The incubation period varies from one to seven days in experimentally induced cases,[6, 47] but the natural disease usually manifests from six to 30 days after the animals have been exposed to any one or more of the predisposing stress factors.[47]

Under field conditions, morbidity and mortality rates of 2 to 50 per cent have been reported.[9, 21, 37, 38] Affected sheep usually have a fever of 40 °C or higher, and show loss of appetite, listlessness, weakness, disinclination to move, a watery-green to blood-tinged diarrhoea, and soiling of the perineum. Severely affected animals become recumbent and usually die within seven days. Sheep which survive for more than seven days are often severely dehydrated, lose weight, and stand with arched backs and tucked-up bellies. Affected animals may recover and regain their normal body weight within three to four weeks.[21, 35, 37, 61]

Clinical signs associated with the abortion syndrome vary to some extent according to the serovar of *Salmonella* involved and the stage of pregnancy. About 10 per cent (range 1–60 per cent) of ewes which become infected with *S. abortus ovis*, *S. dublin* or *S. typhimurium*, may abort or give birth to stillborn or diseased lambs.[3, 9, 23, 49, 60] Ewes that abort as a result of *S. dublin* and *S. typhimurium* infection usually become more severely affected and may die. The remaining animals usually show lethargy, inappetence, a purulent vaginal discharge, retained placenta, a break in the wool, and diarrhoea. Aborted foetuses due to infection with *S. dublin* are often in an advanced state of decomposition when expelled.[9, 15, 23, 49, 60] Ewes which abort due to *S. abortus ovis* infection rarely show signs of illness, except for a small percentage which succumb to metritis as a result of secondary infections.[23]

Pathology

Depending on the course of the disease, the condition of affected sheep or goats varies from poor to good.[13, 31] Acutely affected animals usually show generalized congestion, variable degrees of pulmonary oedema, hepatomegaly, splenomegaly, focal necrosis in the mucosa of the gall bladder, atrophy of the rumen, sparse and poorly mixed rumen content or the rumen may contain large amounts of water, severe congestion of the mucosa of the abomasum and the small intestine, a fibrinous to necrohaemorrhagic ileitis, typhlitis and colitis **(Figure 131.1.)**, and enlargement, congestion and oedema of the mesenteric lymph nodes.[6, 13, 35] The contents particularly of the distal parts of the small intestine and the entire large intestine are very watery and foul-smelling.[6, 7, 13, 21, 31, 35, 37, 38]

Microscopically, the most severe lesions occur in the caecum and colon, while milder changes are usually present in the small intestine. These lesions include congestion, oedema, haemorrhage, degeneration and necrosis of the mucosa, and infiltration mainly of neutrophils but also of lymphocytes, plasma cells and macrophages into the lamina propria and submucosa. Fibrin thrombi may be present in submucosal blood vessels. In acute cases, foci of necrosis and infiltration of neutrophils occur in the mesenteric lymph nodes, while in more protracted cases, the lymph nodes manifest only lymphoid and reticuloendothelial hyperplasia.

In the liver, disseminated foci of parenchymal necrosis, Kupffer cell proliferation, the presence of a few thrombi and leukostasis in the sinusoids, and a mild to moderate neutrophilic and mononuclear leukocyte infiltration in portal tracts are consistent findings in experimentally infected lambs.[40] Focal areas of hepatocellular necrosis are not invariably present in the livers in naturally infected cases.[31, 35]

Ewes that abort may show a necropurulent metritis, blood-tinged pleural and peritoneal transudates, haemorrhagic enterocolitis and swollen, oedematous mesenteric lymph nodes. Foetal membranes may be necrotic.[3, 9]

Infected lambs which die shortly after birth may reveal pneumonia, gastroenteritis, enlarged mesenteric lymph nodes, a clear to haemorrhagic ventral, subcutaneous oedema, fibrinous peritonitis, arthritis and foci of necrosis in the liver.[3, 23]

Diagnosis

Salmonellosis should be suspected in sheep or goats which develop fever, severe diarrhoea, and a necrohaemorrhagic ileitis, typhlitis and colitis of sudden onset following transportation or recent introduction into feedlots.[6, 13, 31, 35, 40]

In live animals, a diagnosis of salmonellosis is confirmed by the isolation of the bacteria from the faeces or from blood collected during the febrile phase of the disease.[46] In animals that have died of the acute disease, salmonellas can be isolated from the liver, spleen, lungs and mesenteric lymph nodes regional to the affected parts of the intestinal tract.[6]

The detection of subclinical infections in individual sheep may constitute a problem as shedding of the bacteria in the faeces may be intermittent.[6, 16, 46] The isolation of *Salmonella* serovars on a flock basis is, therefore, generally more successful. For the recovery of the bacteria from carriers after they have been slaughtered, cultures should be made of the gastrointestinal tract and its regional lymph nodes.

The methodology, laboratory isolation, and cultural procedures have been described in the ***Salmonella* sp. infections: Introduction.** It must be remembered that exposure to heat, freezing or disinfectants reduces the viability of *Salmonella* serovars. It is important to use non-inhibitory enrichment media, or to add a factor, such as yeast extract, when frozen specimens are examined.

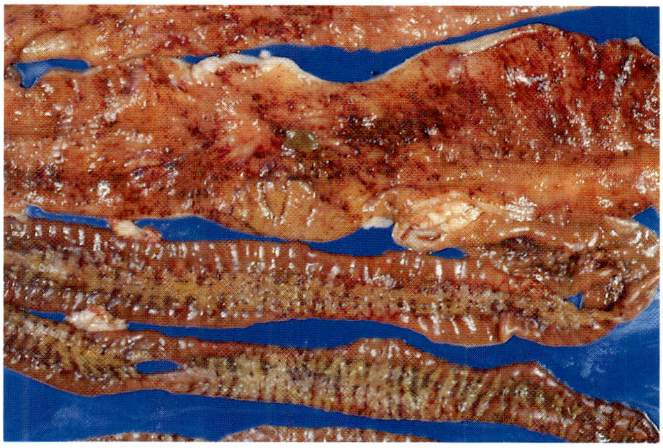

Figure 131.1
Ovine salmonellosis: severe necrohaemorrhagic typhlocolitis

Prolonged incubation is recommended for blood and bone marrow cultures.[46]

Serology is of limited value in the detection of previous infections.[6, 46]

Differential diagnosis

Infectious and non-infectious diseases which cause enteritis and diarrhoea should be distinguished from ovine and caprine salmonellosis. In new-born and pre-weaned lambs, the most important conditions include colibacillosis due to enterotoxigenic strains of *Escherichia coli*, lamb dysentery caused by *Clostridium perfringens* type B, rota- and coronavirus infections, coccidiosis and verminosis. The diagnosis in each case should be confirmed by the isolation or identification of the causative agent from faeces and/or tissue specimens.[4] Plant poisonings caused by *Ornithogalum* spp. (chinkerinchee), *Ornithoglossum* spp. (slangkop) and *Gnidia polycephala* (Januariebos), and intoxication by the trichothecene mycotoxins may also be confused clinically with salmonellosis.[28]

A number of diseases, such as Q-fever, chlamydiosis, toxoplasmosis, Rift Valley fever, Wesselsbron disease, campylobacteriosis and listeriosis cause abortion and neonatal death and should be considered in the differential diagnosis of ovine abortion caused by *Salmonella* serovars.

Control

Therapy with combinations of trimethoprim and sulphadiazine, or with members of the aminoglycoside group, such as gentamicin and neomycin, may be of value in reducing mortalities during an outbreak of salmonellosis in sheep. Oral treatment can effect clinical cure but may cause rumen dysfunction.[4] It is, however, doubtful whether antimicrobial therapy can eliminate salmonellas from the digestive tract of recovered animals in order to stop their excretion in the faeces.[57]

The performance of an antibiogram on isolates of salmonellas is imperative in order to formulate a strategy for the most effective form of antimicrobial treatment because drug-resistant strains of salmonellas have become an obstacle in the effective chemotherapy of the disease.[46] These strains may infect humans via food. Such resistance can also be transferred to other Enterobacteriaceae in both *in vitro* and *in vivo* situations.[10, 46, 59]

Antimicrobial therapy is not always beneficial in the treatment of salmonellosis and other Gram-negative bacterial infections since destruction of these bacteria may result in the liberation of highly toxic lipopolysaccharides which are then responsible for the endotoxin-mediated effects associated with them. Early treatment with cyclooxygenase inhibitors, such as indomethacin, aspirin and flunixin meglumine, counteract the detrimental effects of endotoxin.[5, 11, 12] Immunotherapy with polyvalent anti-lipopolysaccharide hyperimmune serum is a highly effective adjunct in the treatment of endotoxin-mediated diseases. Appropriate electrolyte and acid-base solutions should be administered. Digestive disturbances should be corrected with rumenotorics and other appropriate measures. The crutch and tail should be washed with an insecticidal solution to prevent blowfly strike due to faecal soiling of these areas.

A most important aspect in the control of salmonellosis in sheep and goats is the elimination or minimization of the predisposing stress factors. Where possible, sheep should be well fed on a good quality roughage, such as lucerne hay, in holding pens before they are subjected to a long journey. After the introduction of animals to a feedlot their dietary programme should provide roughage of good quality while the amount of concentrates fed should be gradually increased over a period. Scrupulous hygiene measures should be applied in transport vehicles, abattoir lairages, feedlots or wherever the congregation or temporary starvation of sheep is expected to occur.[46] An all-in-all-out policy with sufficient time for cleaning and disinfection between different batches of sheep may be of great advantage in feedlots.

The isolation of scouring or moribund animals is imperative and the carcasses of dead sheep should either be incinerated or deeply buried to prevent contamination of the environment. Feedstuffs of animal origin and organic fertilizers should be carefully screened in order to determine that they have not been contaminated with salmonellas as a result of ineffective processing or following recontamination during storage.

In New Zealand, the use of a killed vaccine consisting of a combination of *S. typhimurium* and *S. bovismorbificans* administered twice at an interval of 21 days has been found to reduce mortalities due to salmonellosis in sheep on pastures.[46, 58] Favourable results have also been obtained in South Africa after vaccination of lambs twice at an interval of 14 days with the Onderstepoort Inactivated Polyvalent Calf Paratyphoid Vaccine containing *S. typhimurium*, *S. dublin* and *S. bovismorbificans*.[36] Less promising results have been obtained following the use in sheep of the live gal-e mutant vaccine from Australia[24] and the Onderstepoort Live Calf Paratyphoid Vaccine in South Africa.[2, 36] Although live vaccines are more immunogenic, there is the potential risk of dissemination of the attenuated bacteria following their excretion in faeces or by contamination of meat and other foods.[46]

References

1 **ANON, 1978–88.** *Annual Reports*, Veterinary Research Institute, Onderstepoort.

2 **ANON, 1988.** *Onderstepoort Vaccines*, Veterinary Research Institute, Onderstepoort. Reprinted 1990.

3 **BAKER, J.R., FAULL, W.B. & RANKIN, J.E.F., 1971.** An outbreak of salmonellosis in sheep. *The Veterinary Record*, 88, 270–277.

4 **BLOOD, D.C., RADOSTITS, O.M. & HENDERSON, J.A., 1983.** *Veterinary Medicine*. 6th edn. London: Baillière Tindall.

5 **BOTTOMS, G.D., TEMPLETON, C.B., FESSLER, J.F., JOHNSON, M.A. & ROESEL, O.F., 1982.** Thromboxane, prostaglandin I_2 epoprostenol and the hemodynamic changes in equine endotoxin shock. *American Journal of Veterinary Research*, 43, 999–1002.

6 **BROWN, D.D., ROSS, J.G. & SMITH, A.F., 1976.** Experimental infections of sheep with *Salmonella typhimurium*. *Research in Veterinary Science*, 21, 335–340.

7 **BULGIN, M.S. & ANDERSON, B.C., 1981.** Salmonellosis in goats. *Journal of the American Veterinary Medical Association*, 178, 720–723.

8 **DEMLING, R.H., SMITH, M., GUNTHER, R., FLYNN, J.T. & GEE, M.H., 1981.** Pulmonary injury and prostaglandin production during endotoxaemia in conscious sheep. *American Journal of Physiology*, 240, 348–353.

9 **DENNIS, S.M. & ARMSTRONG, J.M., 1965.** Ovine abortion due to *Salmonella typhimurium* in Western Australia. *Australian Veterinary Journal*, 41, 178–181.

10 **DURAND, A.M., BARNARD, M.L., SWANEPOEL, M.L. & ENGELBRECHT, M.M., 1987.** Resistance to various antibiotics of *Salmonella* and *Escherichia coli* isolates from registrable farm feeds. *Onderstepoort Journal of Veterinary Research*, 45, 21–26.

11 **EMAU, P., GIRI, S.N. & BRUSS, M.L., 1984.** Role of prostaglandins, histamine and serotonin in the pathophysiology induced by *Pasteurella haemolytica* endotoxin in sheep. *Circulatory Shock*, 12, 47–59.

12 **FLETCHER, J.R. & RAMWELL, P.W., 1977.** Modification by aspirin and indomethacin of the hemodynamic and prostaglandins-releasing effects of *E. coli* endotoxin. *British Journal of Pharmacology*, 61, 175–181.

13 **GARDINER, M.R. & CRAIG, J., 1970.** Factors affecting survival in the transportation of sheep by sea in the tropics and subtropics. *Australian Veterinary Journal*, 46, 65–69.

14 **GIANELLA, R.A., FORMAL, S.B., DAMMIN, G.J. & COLLINS, H., 1973.** Pathogenesis of salmonellosis. *The Journal of Clinical Investigation*, 52, 441–453.

15 **GITTER, M. & SOJKA, W.J., 1970.** *Salmonella dublin* abortion in sheep. *The Veterinary Record*, 87, 775–778.

16 **GRAU, F.H., BROWNLIE, L.E. & SMITH, M.G., 1969.** Effects of food intake on numbers of *Salmonellae* and *Escherichia coli* in rumen and faeces of sheep. *Journal of Applied Bacteriology*, 32, 112–117.

17 **GRAY, D.F., LEWIS, P.F. & GORRIE, C.J.R., 1958.** Bone meal as a source of bovine salmonellosis. *The Australian Veterinary Journal*, 62, 345–351.

18 **HEMMINGSEN, P., MONTGOMERY, R.A., WARD, C.G. & HENDERSON, T.G., 1982.** A fatal disease outbreak in sheep associated with *Salmonella enteritidis* ser. Havana. *New Zealand Veterinary Journal*, 30, 98.

19 **HENNING, M.W., 1936.** *Salmonella onderstepoort*: A new type of *Salmonella* from a sheep. *Journal of Hygiene*, 36, 525–531.

20 **HENNING, M.W., 1956.** *Animal Diseases in South Africa*. Pretoria: Central News Agency.

21 **HINDMARSH, W.L., 1940.** Dysentery in sheep due to *Salmonella* infection. *The Australian Veterinary Journal*, 16, 112–117.

22 **HUNTER, A.G., CORRIGALL, W., MATHIESON, A.O. & SCOTT, J.A., 1976.** An outbreak of *S. typhimurium* and its consequences. *The Veterinary Record*, 98, 126.

23 **JACK, E.J., 1971.** *Salmonella* abortion in sheep. *Veterinary Annual*, 12, 57–63.

24 **JELINEK, P.D., ROBERTSON, G.M. & MILLAR, C., 1982.** Vaccination of sheep with a live gal-e mutant of *Salmonella typhimurium*. *Australian Veterinary Journal*, 59, 31–32.

25 **JOSLAND, S.W., 1951.** Survival of *Salmonella typhimurium* on various substances under natural circumstances. *Australian Veterinary Journal*, 1, 264–266.

26 **JONES, G.W., RABERT, D.K., SVINARICH, D.M. & WHITFIELD, H.J., 1982.** Association of adhesive, invasive and virulent phenomous 60–megadalton plasmids. *Infection and Immunity*, 38, 476–481.

27 **JONES, G.W. & RICHARDSON, L.A., 1981.** The attachment to and invasion of HeLa cells by *Salmonella typhimurium*. The contribution of mannose-sensitive and mannose-resistant hemagglutination activities. *Journal of General Microbiology*, 127, 361–370.

28 **KELLERMAN, T.S., COETZER, J.A.W. & NAUDÉ, T.W., 1988.** *Plant Poisonings and Mycotoxicoses of Livestock in Southern Africa*. Cape Town: Oxford University Press Southern Africa.

29 **KOO, F.C.W., PETERSON, J.W., HOUSTON, C.W., 1984.** Pathogenesis of experimental salmonellosis. Inhibition of protein synthesis by cytotoxin. *Infection and Immunity*, 43, 93–100.

30 **MAKELA, P., VALTONEN, V.V. & VALTONEN, M., 1973.** Role of O-antigen (lipopolysaccharide) factors in the virulence of *Salmonella*. *Journal of Infectious Diseases*, 128, S81–S85.

31 **McORIST, S. & MILLER, G.T., 1981.** Salmonellosis in transported feral goats. *The Australian Veterinary Journal*, 57, 389–390.

32 **MEYRICK, B. & BRIGHAM, K.L., 1983.** Acute effects of *Escherichia coli* endotoxin on the pulmonary microcirculation of anesthetized sheep. *Laboratory Investigation*, 48, 458–470.

33 **MURRAY, M.J., 1986.** *Salmonella*: Virulence factors and enteric salmonellosis. *Journal of the American Veterinary Medical Association*, 189, 145–147.

34 **NAKAMURA, M., SATO, S., OHYA, T., SUZUKI, S. & IKEDA, S., 1985.** Possible relationship of a 36–megadalton *Salmonella enteritidis* plasmid to virulence in mice. *Infection and Immunity*, 47, 831–833.

35 **NESER, J.A., 1988.** Veterinary Research Institute, Onderstepoort. Unpublished data.

36 **NESER, J.A., CAMERON, C.M. & HENTON, M.M., 1984.** Veterinary Research Institute, Onderstepoort. Unpublished data.

37 **NEWSOM, I.E. & CROSS, F., 1924.** An outbreak of paratyphoid dysentery in lambs. *Journal of the American Veterinary Medical Association*, 66, 289–300.

38 **NEWSOM, I.E. & CROSS, F., 1935.** Third outbreak of paratyphoid dysentery in lambs. *Journal of the American Veterinary Medical Association*, 86, 534–536.

39 **OGONOWSKI, K., BARNARD, M.L. & GIESECKE, W.H., 1984.** Bacteriological findings regarding the hygienic safety of poultry litter intended as an ingredient of feeds for ruminants. *Onderstepoort Journal of Veterinary Research*, 51, 249–252.

40 **ORR, M.B., HUNTER, A.R., BROWN, D.D. & SMITH, A.F., 1977.** The histopathology of experimental infections of sheep with *Salmonella typhimurium*. *Veterinary Science Communications*, 1, 191–195.

41 **PETRIE, L., SELMAN, I.E., GRINDLAY, M. & THOMPSON, H., 1977.** Salmonellosis in young calves due to *Salmonella enteritidis*. *The Veterinary Record*, 101, 398–402.

42 **PIERSON, R.E., PODUSKA, P.J., CHOLAS, G. & BROWN, G., 1972.** Relationship of management and nutrition to salmonellosis in feedlot lambs. *Journal of the American Veterinary Medical Association*, 161, 1217–1220.

43 **REED, W.M., OLANDER, H.J. & THACKER, H.L., 1986.** Studies on the pathogenesis of *Salmonella typhimurium* and *Salmonella choleraesuis* var. kunzendorf infection in weanling pigs. *American Journal of Veterinary Research*, 47, 75–83.

44 **RIETSCHEL, E.T., SCHADE, U., JENSEN, M., WOLLENWEBER, H.W., LUDERITZ, O. & GREISMAN, S.G., 1982.** Bacterial endotoxins: Chemical structure, biological activity and role in septicaemia. *Scandinavian Journal of Infectious Diseases* (Supplement), 31, 8–21.

45 **ROBINSON, R.A., 1966.** *Salmonella* excretion by sheep following yarding. *New Zealand Veterinary Journal*, 125, 24–25.

46 **ROBINSON, R.A., 1970.** *Salmonella* infection: Diagnosis and control (Review Article). *New Zealand Veterinary Journal*, 18, 259–277.

47 **ROBINSON, R.A. & ROYAL, W.A., 1971.** Field epizootiology of *Salmonella* infection in sheep. *New Zealand Journal of Agricultural Research*, 14, 442–456.

48 **SALISBURY, R.M., 1958.** *Salmonella* infections in animals and birds in New Zealand. *The New Zealand Veterinary Journal*, 6, 76–86.

49 **SHEARER, G.C., 1957.** An outbreak of abortion in ewes due to *Salmonella dublin*. *The Veterinary Record*, 69, 693–695.

50 **SOJKA, W.J., WRAY, C., SHREEVE, J.E. & BELL, J.C., 1983.** The incidence of *Salmonella* infection in sheep in England and Wales, 1975 to 1981. *British Veterinary Journal*, 139, 386–392.

51 **SMITH, B.P., HABASHA, F., REINA-GUERRA, M. & HARDY, B.S., 1979.** Bovine salmonellosis: Experimental production and characterization of the disease in calves, using oral challenge with *Salmonella typhimurium*. *American Journal of Veterinary Research*, 40, 1510–1513.

52 **SMITH, H.W. & JONES, J.E., 1967.** Observations on experimental oral infection with *Salmonella dublin* in calves and *Salmonella choleraesuis* in pigs. *Journal of Pathology and Bacteriology*, 93, 141–156.

53 **TANNOCK, G.W. & SMITH, J.M., 1971.** A *Salmonella* carrier state of sheep following intranasal inoculation. *Research in Veterinary Science*, 12, 371–373.

54 **TERAKADO, N., SEKIZAKI, T., HASHIMOTO, K. & NAITOH, S., 1983.** Correlation between the presence of a fifty-megadalton plasmid in *Salmonella dublin* and virulence for mice. *Infection and Immunity*, 41, 443–444.

55 **VAN DEN HEEVER, L.W. & VAN DER MADE, H.N., 1977.** The effect of sample size and culture method on the recovery of *Salmonella* spp. from naturally contaminated carcass meal. *Journal of the South African Veterinary Association*, 48, 51–52.

56 **VAN DER MADE, H.N., VAN STADEN, J.J., DU TOIT, J. DE V., JORDAAN, E., BARRETT, E.L. & COETZEE, J.D., 1980.** Determination of the physiochemical and microbiological quality of carcass, bone and blood meal. *Onderstepoort Journal of Veterinary Research*, 47, 197–201.

57 **VAN DER WALT, K., JENKINS, W.L. & BOTES, H.J., 1967.** The therapeutic control of calf paratyphoid (*S. dublin*) infection. *Journal of the South African Veterinary Medical Association*, 38, 425–430.

58 **WALLACE, G.V. & MURCH, O., 1967.** Field trials to assess the value of a bivalent killed *Salmonella* vaccine in the control of ovine salmonellosis. *New Zealand Veterinary Journal*, 15, 62–65.

59 **WALTON, J.R., 1968.** Infectious drug resistance. *The Veterinary Record*, 82, 448–454.

60 **WATSON, W.A., 1960.** *Salmonella dublin* infection in a lambing flock. *The Veterinary Record*, 72, 62–65.

61 **WATTS, P.S. & WALL, M., 1952.** The 1951 *Salmonella typhimurium* epidemic in sheep in South Australia. *The Australian Veterinary Journal*, 28, 165–168.

62 **WEINSTEIN, D.L., CARSIOTIS, M., LISSNER, C.R. & O'BRIAN, A., 1984.** Flagella help *Salmonella typhimurium* survive within murine macrophages. *Infection and Immunity*, 46, 819–825.

63 **WRAY, C. & SOJKA, W.J., 1978.** Experimental *Salmonella typhimurium* infection in calves. *Research in Veterinary Science*, 25, 139–143.

132

Porcine salmonellosis

Synonym: Salmonellose van varke (Afrik.)

J.A. Neser

Introduction

Porcine salmonellosis, depending on the specific serovar involved, manifests either as septicaemia, which may include signs of diarrhoea, or as a primary, acute, subacute or chronic enterocolitis. The septicaemic form is often characterized by pneumonia and generalized lymphadenitis. The disease mainly affects post-weaner pigs.[23, 26, 40, 54] Apart from its importance as an animal disease, porcine *Salmonella* infection also constitutes a public health hazard.[1, 58]

The first isolation of *Salmonella* was in 1886 by Salmon and Smith from pigs in the USA suffering from hog cholera. The bacterium isolated from these cases was named *Salmonella choleraesuis* in honour of Salmon.[5] *Salmonella choleraesuis* was first isolated in South Africa from pigs affected by a septicaemic disease resembling African swine fever.[7] Since then, *S. choleraesuis, S. typhimurium, S. thompson* and *S. enteritidis* have been isolated sporadically from tissues of pigs submitted to the Veterinary Research Institute, Onderstepoort for diagnostic purposes.[2] However, salmonellosis in pigs is an uncommon disease in the subcontinent. Although it occurs throughout the world, there are few reports on its prevalence in any particular country. The prevalence of the disease should not be equated with reported figures of the occurrence of the bacteria isolated from necropsy material or from animals surveyed at abattoirs.

Aetiology

For general information on the morphology, physicochemical and other properties of salmonellas, the ***Salmonella* sp. infections: Introduction** should be consulted.

Only a few of the large number of *Salmonella* serovars which have been isolated from carcasses and products of pigs are associated with clinical disease. Disease results most commonly from infection with *S. choleraesuis, S. typhimurium* or *S. typhisuis*, but under conditions of stress or as a result of intercurrent infections other serovars such as *S. dublin* and *S. enteritidis* may also cause frank disease.[3, 7, 13, 15, 21, 26, 31, 32, 53] Recent surveys in the USA,[4] England, Wales[24, 64] and South Africa[2] indicate that *S. typhimurium* is surpassing *S. choleraesuis* in importance as the cause of porcine salmonellosis.[27, 34]

Epidemiology

Salmonella choleraesuis is a host-adapted pathogen of pigs and its spread is related more specifically to the movement of pigs. The host range of *S. typhimurium* is wider, however, and other animal species such as birds, rodents, and other mammals may become infected and contaminate the environment, water and feed.[17, 28, 36, 39, 49]

Porcine salmonellosis occurs most commonly in pigs that are 12 to 13 weeks of age, but pigs from one week of age to adulthood may also be affected.[26, 32, 45] In general, the scarcity of the disease prior to weaning is attributed to the presence of colostral immunity. However, infection and faecal excretion of *Salmonella* in the absence of clinical disease have been demonstrated in animals of this age group.[16, 52]

Pigs that are carriers constitute the most important source of infection in piggeries, as they excrete the bacteria in their faeces and are probably the cause of recurrent incidents of clinical disease in the same herd.[27] The ratio between the number of infected pigs and those excreting salmonellas varies considerably according to the nutritional state of the pigs and their exposure to stress, such as that caused by transportation and intercurrent disease.[18, 39, 60]

The duration of the carrier state in pigs has not been determined. Following experimental infection of weanling pigs, *S. typhimurium* persisted in the liver for only one to two weeks, but the bacteria may be found in the digestive tract and mesenteric lymph nodes at least until marketing age.[57, 63] Pigs ingesting contaminated feed and drinking water may retain small numbers of salmonellas in their mesenteric lymph nodes without developing clinical disease, lesions or permanent faecal excretion of the organisms.

On infected farms, attendants wearing faecally contaminated clothing and footwear may carry salmonellas from pen to pen. Water supplies contaminated with human or porcine sewage and feeds containing ingredients from *Salmonella*-infected animals may also be sources of salmonellas in piggeries.[9, 19, 20, 38, 39, 51, 59, 61]

Natural infection with serovars of *Salmonella* in pigs occurs via the oral route following the ingestion of infected faeces, drinking water or feed.[39]

Because of the occurrence of asymptomatic carriers, faecal soiling of carcasses at slaughter constitutes a health hazard to humans.[22, 24, 35, 39, 43, 47] Faecal contamination of carcasses occurs particularly in dehairing machines, scalding tanks, and during the processing of the end-products of the slaughtering process.[6, 39, 43, 47, 53]

The most important mode of spread of salmonellas from animals to humans is via contaminated food of animal origin such as meat, milk or eggs. Surveys conducted on slaughter pigs and pig products, both in South Africa and abroad, have revealed significant rates of contamination of these products.[10, 22, 33, 43] When contaminated products are left at room temperature or are incompletely refrigerated in too large a quantity, organisms may multiply to infective doses of several million within a few hours.[58, 62]

The most common syndrome caused by *Salmonella* infection in humans is gastroenteritis, usually manifested by anorexia, headache, fever, vomition, abdominal cramps and diarrhoea which may last from about seven to ten days. Disturbances of the normal intestinal flora by antibiotic therapy, gastrointestinal surgery or severe gastroenteritis greatly increases the susceptibility of the host to the septicaemic form, which may be fatal. Chronic disease and neoplastic conditions may also predispose to septicaemic salmonellosis, especially among old people. *Salmonella typhimurium*, *S. enteritidis*, *S. heidelberg* and *S. oranienburg* have been the most prevalent serotypes to be isolated from human cases of salmonellosis. Septicaemic infections may be fatal or may give rise to localized purulent infections in the lungs, heart, kidneys, brain and joints, especially in infants.[58]

Salmonella typhimurium and *S. choleraesuis* may stay alive on contaminated pasture for 451 days, while *S. typhimurium* remains viable for more than 291 days at 22–25 °C in dried pig faeces. In water contaminated with organic material, *S. typhimurium* may remain viable for 98 days.[50]

Pathogenesis

The course and nature of the disease and the severity of the lesions in pigs are determined by the size of the infective dose and the virulence of the specific serovar, as well as by the presence or absence of acquired immunity and the degree of natural resistance of the host.[25, 44, 54] Virulence factors, such as adhesion pili, flagella, cytotoxin, enterotoxin and the lipopolysaccharides of the outer cell wall, contribute to mucosal invasion and the development of diarrhoea and septicaemia[37] **(see *Salmonella* sp. infections: Introduction).**

The pathogenesis of salmonellosis can be divided into four phases, namely:[44]

- proliferation of the organisms in the intestinal lumen;
- bacterial invasion of the mucosal epithelium and lamina propria;
- stimulation of excessive fluid secretion into the lumen; and
- spread to the mesenteric lymph nodes and internal organs, at which stage various bacterial toxins are also elaborated into the circulation.

Invasion of the mucosa of the intestine by salmonellas is a prerequisite for the development of both the intestinal and the septicaemic forms of the disease.[14] After penetration of the intestinal mucosa, the bacteria locate in the mesenteric lymph nodes as soon as eight hours after infection, and bacteraemia is present 48 hours after infection. In general, oral administration of *S. typhimurium* mainly causes enterocolitis and diarrhoea, while infection with *S. choleraesuis* results in septicaemia followed by enterocolitis in some of the affected pigs.[44]

Bacterial multiplication in the mucosa of the intestine gives rise to an acute inflammatory reaction, initially characterized by a predominantly neutrophil infiltration, followed by the presence of mononuclear leukocytes and macrophages. The most pronounced mucosal destruction is found in areas where gut-associated lymphoid aggregates are present. Subsequent thrombosis and infarction in the lamina propria result in ulceration. Intestinal lesions are accompanied by impaired fluid resorption from the intestinal lumen.[44] Excessive intestinal fluid secretion and diarrhoea are the result of the combined action of the inflammatory response, bacterial enterotoxin and the endotoxin-mediated effects attributable to the lipid A portion of the lipopolysaccharides in the bacterial cell wall. The enterotoxin specifically binds to epithelial cells and induces increased intracellular cyclic AMP synthesis which stimulates the secretion of water and electrolytes into the intestinal lumen. In systemic infections, the reaction between endotoxin and macrophages produces interleukin-1, which stimulates B and T lymphocyte activity, and various chemical mediators, thus activating prostaglandin synthesis, intravascular coagulation and thrombosis.[37] Endotoxic shock **(see Chapter 129: *Escherichia coli* infections)** frequently complicates the hypovolaemia caused by the fluid loss as a consequence of diarrhoea.[8, 12, 37, 46]

Clinical signs

The clinical signs of salmonellosis in pigs are, in general, determined by the serovar involved: the disease usually manifests as an acute septicaemia in pigs infected with *S. choleraesuis* or as an enterocolitis in *S. typhimurium* infections.[44, 54]

In the septicaemic form, the incubation period after oral infection is usually 24–48 hours. It occurs most commonly in pigs of 12–13 weeks of age and is characterized by fever, lethargy, inappetence, huddling, erythema, and blue discoloration of the ears. Although the morbidity and the mortality rates may vary greatly, the morbidity is usually low (less than 10 per cent), while the mortality rate is higher than 90 per cent. Diarrhoea is not a constant sign, but a yellowish watery diarrhoea may develop in about 40 per cent of cases after animals have been ill for three or four days.[26, 53]

Enterocolitis caused by *S. typhimurium* also occurs most frequently in pigs that are 12–13 weeks old, and manifests as an intermittent, sometimes haemorrhagic diarrhoea which persists for several weeks. Although the disease may spread rapidly and involve most of the piglets in the piggery, the mortality rate is usually low. Deaths occur in animals that have been ill for several days, usually as a result of dehydration. Piglets that survive may become carriers and excrete salmonellas in their faeces for several months.[53]

Sporadic cases of septicaemic salmonellosis caused by *S. dublin*, *S. enteritidis* and *S. choleraesuis* in piglets of one to ten weeks old manifest nervous signs, including incoordination and circling, in the absence of scouring.[32, 45, 56]

Pathology

The nature of the lesions depends on the form of the disease.

The carcasses of animals that have died of the septicaemic form show severe congestion of the skin (particularly of the legs, abdomen, head and ears) and internal organs. The congested skin may also reveal focal necrosis because of thrombosis of vessels in the dermis.[23, 26, 40, 54] Petechiae occur widely throughout the carcass, but are particularly prevalent in lymph nodes (especially the pharyngeal and mesenteric), on serosal surfaces and in organs such as the lungs, heart, kidneys, urinary bladder and ureters.[23, 26, 54] Lesions in the lungs occur frequently and are characterized by an acute fibrinous pneumonia and numerous fibrin thrombi in blood vessels. Splenomegaly is frequently present, and scattered small foci of necrosis 0,1–0,4 mm in diameter may be present in the liver. Most affected animals show isolated foci of necrosis of the renal cortex, but complete bilateral renal cortical necrosis may be present in very severely affected pigs.[25, 26, 41] The mucosa of the stomach, particularly that of weaned pigs infected with *S. choleraesuis*, may be dark red to black due to thrombosis, infarction and congestion. There may be a catarrhal enteritis which is usually more pronounced in the ileum, fibrinopurulent colitis and typhilitis.[23, 25, 26, 42]

The lesions of pigs that have died of salmonellosis caused by *S. typhimurium* are usually characterized by a diffuse catarrhal to fibrinonecrotic enterocolitis. In chronic cases, the lesions may progress to an ulcerative colitis and chronic proctitis which eventually may result in rectal stricture.[23, 54, 55] The intestinal lesions caused by *S. typhisuis* are characterized by well-circumscribed 'button' ulcers in the ileum, caecum and colon.[3, 23] Microscopically, the ulcers consist of necrosis of the mucosa and submucosa, and a mixed inflammatory cell reaction (predominantly of lymphocytes an macrophages) and hyaline to granular thrombi are present in some blood vessels in the submucosa, particularly those at the base of large ulcers. In some cases, phlebitis or periphlebitis, with or without thrombosis, may be evident in the submucosa and subserosa.[23, 26, 42, 44, 54]

Other lesions that have been described include a caseous necrotic tonsillitis and regional lymphadenitis as a result of *S. typhisuis* infection,[3] and a serofibrinous to fibrinopurulent lobular pneumonia and fibrinohaemorrhagic pericarditis in pigs suffering from the septicaemic form of the disease caused by *S. typhimurium*.[23, 26, 54]

Histologically, thrombosis commonly occurs in organs such as lymph nodes, lungs, spleen and liver. Congestion, leukocytosis, varying numbers of disseminated necrotic foci and haemorrhages are consistent changes in the liver of animals that have died of the septicaemic form of the disease. The necrotic foci vary from small (comprising only a few hepatocytes) to larger areas (which include entire lobules). Necrotic foci in the liver contain infiltrated histiocytes and are referred to as microgranulomas or typhoid nodules.[23, 54] Bacteria are absent from the lesions in the liver. The spleen shows congestion and severe reticuloendothelial cell proliferation. In the kidneys, an acute, diffuse glomerulitis, exudative vasculitis and thrombosis may be seen, the latter being associated with the development of isolated necrotic foci or bilateral renal cortical necrosis.[23, 26, 40, 41]

Diagnosis

The clinical signs and lesions in the septicaemic and enterocolitic forms of the disease may permit a presumptive diagnosis.[39] However, isolation of the bacteria from intestinal and tissue samples, including mesenteric lymph nodes, spleen and liver is necessary to confirm the diagnosis.

Detection of asymptomatic carriers is difficult as faecal excretion of salmonellas by infected pigs occurs intermittently. The sampling of the faeces of pigs on a group basis for bacteriological examination provides satisfactory results: the collection of pooled samples of approximately 10 g of freshly voided faeces from each pen yields accurate results since the majority of pigs in a particular pen probably share the same infection.[19, 29, 39, 53] A more accurate method of establishing infection rates in pigs would be to culture multiple specimens of the wall of the ileum, as well as specimens of the internal organs, such as the mesenteric lymph nodes, the liver and the spleen, collected at abattoirs.[39, 53]

The isolation of salmonellas from materials such as sewage, polluted drinking water, feeds, organs or faeces of carrier animals in which only small numbers of organisms are usually present, requires special enrichment and pre-enrichment of culture media.[48, 53] Material from clinical cases and carcasses, such as faeces or organ specimens, can be directly plated onto culture media. The use of simple standardized enrichment procedures as set out by the International Committee on the study of Salmonellosis facilitates the bacteriological diagnosis and generally ensures a satisfactory result.[11, 29, 53]

Differential diagnosis

Septicaemic salmonellosis should be differentiated from the septicaemic forms of erysipelas, *Haemophilus parasuis* and *Streptococcus* spp. infections, and acute viral diseases such as hog cholera and African swine fever.[23, 30] In all cases, the isolation of the specific pathogen from the lymphoid tissues and organs such as the liver and lungs should confirm the diagnosis.

The diarrhoea caused by the enterocolitic form of salmonellosis must be differentiated from other post-weaning bacterial infections, such as colibacillosis, swine dysentery and the intestinal adenomatosis complex. Virus diseases, such as rota- and coronavirus infections and coccidiosis, should also be borne in mind.[23, 53]

Control

The inclusion of various antimicrobial drugs in the feed or water is recommended for the treatment and control of salmonellosis in pigs.

Feeding of medicated feed for prolonged periods will substantially reduce the frequency and severity of cases in a piggery, but few beneficial effects have been reported with this type of medication when it is commenced after the onset of disease. In addition, only pigs given the medication uninterruptedly will show any beneficial effects. Pigs may excrete salmonellas for periods of up to 209 days despite prolonged antibiotic treatment, and the bacteria can still be isolated from the intestinal tract (ileum and caecum) and mesenteric lymph nodes.[57]

The effect of control measures on salmonellosis in pigs appears to differ according to the serovar. *Salmonella choleraesuis* infection, which is restricted to pigs, may be eliminated from a herd by stringent sanitation measures, culling of known carriers and restriction of the introduction of pigs into the herd. In non-host-adapted serovars, the above measures are futile and will at best reduce the level of contamination of the environment and the number of clinical cases.

The application of control measures will achieve some degree of success only if the herd is a closed one, the source of infection is controlled, and the faeces from infected animals are not allowed to come into contact with healthy stock.[20] Features aimed specifically at the prevention of the distribution of infections such as salmonellosis in a piggery should be incorporated into the design of pig units.

No effective vaccine is available.

References

1 **ACHA, P.N. & SZYFRES, B., 1987.** Salmonellosis in swine. *In: Zoonoses and Communicable Diseases Common to Man and Animals.* 2nd edn. Scientific Publications No. 503, World Health Organization.

2 **ANON., 1970–93.** Annual reports of the section of bacteriology, Veterinary Research Institute, Onderstepoort, Republic of South Africa.

3 **BARNES, D.M. & BERGELAND, M.E., 1968.** *Salmonella typhisuis* infection in Minnesota swine. *Journal of the American Veterinary Medical Association*, 152, 1766–1770.

4 **BLACKBURN, B.O., SUTCH, K. & HARRINGTON, R., 1982.** *Salmonella* and Arizona serotypes from animals and related sources reported during fiscal year 1981. *Proceedings of the United States Animal Health Association*, 86, 454–471.

5 **BLOOMFIELD, S.A., 1986.** Daniel Salmon. *PHLS Microbiology Digest*, 3, 18.

6 **CHAMBERS, P.G., 1977.** *Salmonella* in Rhodesia: Sources and serotypes of some isolates from abattoirs, domestic animals, birds and man. *Journal of the South African Veterinary Association*, 48, 241–244.

7 **DE KOCK, G., ROBINSON, E.M. & KEPPEL, J.J.G., 1940.** Swine fever in South Africa. *Onderstepoort Journal of Veterinary Science and Animal Industry*, 14, 31–89.

8 **DEMLING, R.H., SMITH, M., GUNTHER, R., FLYNN, J.T. & GEE, M.H., 1981.** Pulmonary injury and prostaglandin production during endotoxaemia in conscious sheep. *American Journal of Physiology*, 240, H348–H353.

9 **DURAND, A.M., GIESECKE, W.H., BARNARD, M.L., VAN DER WALT, M.L. & STEYN, H.C., 1990.** Salmonellae isolated from feeds and feed ingredients during the period 1982–1988: Animal and public health implications. *Onderstepoort Journal of Veterinary Research*, 57, 175–181.

10 **EDEL, W., GUINEE, P.A.M., VAN SCOTHORST, M. & KAMPELMACHER, E.K., 1973.** *Salmonella* cycles in foods with special reference to the effects of environmental factors, including feeds. *Journal of the Canadian Institute of Food Science Technology*, 6, 64–67.

11 **EDEL, W. & KAMPELMACHER, E.H., 1969.** *Salmonella* isolation in nine European laboratories using a standardized technique. *Bulletin of the World Health Organization*, 41, 297–306.

12 **EMAU, P., GIRI, S.M. & BRUSS, M.L., 1984.** Role of prostaglandins, histamins and serotonin in the pathophysiology induced by *Pasteurella haemolytica* endotoxin in sheep. *Circulatory Shock*, 12, 47–59.

13 **GANGULY, S., PRAMANIK, A.K., CHAKRABORTY, D. & BISWAS, C.R., 1980.** Pneumonia in pigs due to *Salmonella typhisuis* infection. *Indian Journal of Animal Health*, 19, 63–65.

14 **GIANNELLA, R.A., FORMAL, S.B., DAMMIN, G.J. & COLLINS, H., 1973.** Pathogenesis of salmonellosis: Studies of fluid secretion, mucosal invasion and morphologic reaction in the rabbit ileum. *Journal of Clinical Investigation*, 52, 441–453.

15 **GLASSER, K., 1909.** Zum heutigen Stande der Schweinepestfrage und zu den weiteren Untersuchungen von Uhlenhuth, Hubener, Xylander und Bohtz über das Wesen und die Bekämpfung der Schweinepest und über die bakteriologie der hog cholera (Paratyphosus B)—Gruppe. *Deutsche Tierärztliche Wochenschrift*, 17, 513–516, 529–534.

16 **GOOCH, J.M. & HADDOCK, R.L., 1969.** Swine salmonellosis in a Hawaiian piggery. *Journal of the American Veterinary Medical Association*, 154, 1051–1054.

17 **GOODCHILD, W.M. & TUCKER, J.F., 1968.** Salmonellae in British wild birds and their transfer to domestic fowl. *British Veterinary Journal*, 124, 95–96.

18 **GUINEE, P.A.M., KAMPELMACHER, E.H., HOFSTRA, K. & VAN KEULEN, A., 1965.** Salmonellae in young piglets in the Netherlands. *Zentralblatt für Veterinärmedizin*, 12, 250–257.

19 **HEARD, T.M. & LINTON, A.H., 1966.** An epidemiological survey in a closed pig herd. *Journal of Hygiene, Cambridge*, 64, 411–417.

20 **HEARD, T.M., JENNETT, N.A. & LINTON, A.H., 1968.** The control and eradication of salmonellosis in a closed pig herd. *The Veterinary Record*, 82, 92–99.

21 **HENNING, M.W., 1939.** The antigenic structure of salmonellas obtained from domestic animals and birds in South Africa. *Onderstepoort Journal of Veterinary Science and Animal Industry*, 13, 79–120.

22 **HORTON, B. & VENTER, A., 1981.** Results of a survey to determine the number of *Salmonella* spp. isolations from pig carcasses and offal at the Estcourt and Heidelberg abattoirs between 1973 and 1981. State Veterinarian, Post Office Box 4, Olifantsfontein, 1666.

23 **JUBB, K.V.F., KENNEDY, P.C. & PALMER, N., 1985.** Salmonellosis in swine. *In: Pathology of Domestic Animals*, Vol. II. New York: Academic Press, Inc.

24 **KIRBY, F.D., 1985.** Epidemiological notes. Surveillance of animal salmonella infection 1976–84. *The Veterinary Record*, 117, 456 –457.

25 **LAWSON, G.H.K. & DOW, C., 1965.** The pathogenesis of oral *Salmonella choleraesuis* infection in pigs. *Journal of Comparative Pathology*, 75, 75–81.

26 **LAWSON, G.H.K. & DOW, C., 1966.** Porcine salmonellosis. *Journal of Comparative Pathology*, 76, 363–371.

27 **LEMAN, A.D., 1991.** *Salmonella choleraesuis. Proceedings of the Annual Congress of the Pig Veterinary Society of the South African Veterinary Association*, Mont-aux-Sources, South Africa.

28 **LI, H. & DAVIS, D.E., 1952.** The prevalence of carriers of *Leptospira* and *Salmonella* in Norway rats of Baltimore. *American Journal of Hygiene*, 56, 90–100.

29 **LINTON, A.H., 1981.** Salmonellosis in pigs. *Pig News and Information*, (CAB) 25–28.

30 **MAURER, F.D., GRIESEMER, R.A. & JONES, T.C., 1958.** The pathology of African swine fever, a comparison with hog cholera. *American Journal of Veterinary Research*, 19, 517–539.

31 **McCAUGHEY, W.J., McCLELAND, T.G. & RODDY, R.M., 1973.** *Salmonella* isolations in pigs. *The Veterinary Record*, 92, 191–194.

32 **McERLEAN, B.A., 1968.** *Salmonella dublin* meningitis in piglets. *The Veterinary Record*, 82, 257–258.

33 **MEARA, P.J., 1973.** Salmonellosis in slaughter animals as a source of human food poisoning. *Journal of the South African Veterinary Association*, 44, 215–233.

34 **MILLS, K.W. & KELLY, B.L., 1986.** Antibiotic susceptibilities of swine *Salmonella* isolates from 1979 to 1983. *American Journal of Veterinary Research*, 47, 2349–2350.

35 **MORGAN, I.R., KRAUTIL, F.L. & CRAVEN, J.A., 1987.** Effect of time in lairage on caecal and carcass *Salmonella* contamination of slaughter pigs. *Epidemiology and Infection*, 98, 323–330.

36 **MULLER, G., 1965.** *Salmonella* in bird faeces. *Nature*, 5003, 1315.

37 **MURRAY, M.J., 1986.** *Salmonella*: Virulence factors and enteric salmonellosis. *Journal of the American Veterinary Medical Association*, 189, 145–147.

38 **NEWELL, K.W., MACCLAREN, R., MURDOCK, C.R., MACDONALD, W.N. & HUTCHINSON, H.L., 1959.** Salmonellosis in Northern Ireland, with special reference to pigs and *Salmonella*-contaminated pig meal. *Journal of Hygiene*, 57, 92–105.

39 **NEWELL, K.W. & WILLIAMS, L.P., 1971.** The control of salmonellae affecting swine and man. *Journal of the American Veterinary Medical Association*, 158, 89–98.

40 **NORDSTOGA, K., 1970.** Porcine salmonellosis. I. Gross and microscopic changes in experimentally infected animals. *Acta Veterinaria Scandinavica*, 11, 361–369.

41 **NORDSTOGA, K. & FJOLSTAD, M., 1970.** Porcine salmonellosis. II. Production of the generalized Schwartzman reaction by intravenous injections of disintegrated cells of *Salmonella choleraesuis. Acta Veterinaria Scandinavica*, 11, 370 –379.

42 **NORDSTOGA, K. & FJOLSTAD, M., 1970.** Porcine salmonellosis. III. Production of fibrinous colitis by intravenous injections of a mixture of viable cells of *Salmonella choleraesuis* and disintegrated cells of the same agent, or haemolytic *Echerichia coli. Acta Veterinaria Scandinavica*, 11, 380–389.

43 **PRIOR, B.A. & BADENHORST, L., 1974.** Incidence of salmonellae in some meat products. *South African Medical Journal*, 48, 2532–2533.

44 **REED, W.M., OLANDER, H.J. & THACKER, H.L., 1986.** Studies on the pathogenesis of *Salmonella typhimurium* and *Salmonella choleraesuis* var *kunzendorf* infection in weanling pigs. *American Journal of Veterinary Research*, 46, 2300–2310.

45 **REYNOLDS, I.M., MINER, P.W. & SMITH, R.E., 1967.** *Salmonella enteritis* from porcine meningitis. A case report. *Cornell Veterinarian*, 58, 180–185.

46 **RIETSCHEL, E.T., SCHADE, U., JENSEN, M., WOLLENWEBER, H.W., LUDERITZ, O. & GREISMAN, S.G., 1982.** Bacterial endotoxins: Chemical structure, biological activity and role in septicaemia. *Scandinavian Journal of Infectious Disease*, Supplement. 31, 8–21.

47 **ROBERTS, T.A., 1980.** Contamination of meat: The effects of slaughtering practices on the bacteriology of the red meat carcass. *Royal Society of Health Journal*, 100, 3–10.

48 **ROBINSON, R.A., 1970.** *Salmonella* infection: Diagnosis and control (review article). *New Zealand Veterinary Journal*, 18, 259–277.

49 **SNOEYENBOS, G.H., MOREN, E.W. & WETHERBEE, D.K., 1967.** Naturally occurring *Salmonella* in blackbirds and gulls. *Avian Diseases*, 11, 642– 646.

50 **TANNOCK, G.W. & SMITH, J.M., 1971.** Studies on the survival of *Salmonella typhimurium* and *Salmonella bovis morbificans* on pasture and in water. *Australian Veterinary Journal*, 47, 557–559.

51 **VAN DEN HEEVER, L.W. & VAN DER MADE, H.N., 1977.** The effect of sample size and culture method on the recovery of *Salmonella* spp. from naturally contaminated carcass meal. *Journal of the South African Veterinary Association*, 48, 51–52.

52 **WILCOCK, B.P., 1979.** Experimental *Klebsiella* and *Salmonella* infection in neonatal swine. *Canadian Journal of Comparative Medicine*, 43, 200–206.

53 **WILCOCK, B.P., 1986.** Salmonellosis: *In*: LEMAN, A.D., STRAW, B., GLOCK, R.D., MENGELING, W.L., PENNY, R.H. & SCHOLL, E., (eds). *Diseases of Swine*. 6th edn. Ames, Iowa: Iowa State University Press.

54 **WILCOCK, B.P., ARMSTRONG, C.H. & OLANDER, H.J., 1976.** The significance of the serotype in the clinical pathological features of naturally occurring porcine salmonellosis. *Canadian Journal of Comparative Medicine*, 40, 80–88.

55 **WILCOCK, B.P. & OLANDER, H.J., 1977.** The pathogenesis of porcine rectal stricture. II. Experimental salmonellosis and ischaemic proctitis. *Veterinary Pathology*, 14, 43–55.

56 **WILCOCK, B.P. & OLANDER, H.J., 1977.** Neurologic disease in naturally occurring *Salmonella choleraesuis* infection in pigs. *Veterinary Pathology*, 14, 113–120.

57 **WILCOCK, B.P. & OLANDER, H.J., 1978.** Influence of oral antibiotic feeding on the duration and severity of clinical disease, growth performance and pattern of shedding in swine inoculated with *Salmonella typhimurium. Journal of the American Veterinary Medical Association*, 172, 472– 477.

58 **WILLIAMS, L.P., 1982.** Salmonellosis. *In*: STEELE, J.H., (ed.). *Handbook Series in Zoonoses. Section A, Bacterial Diseases.* Vols I, II & III. Boca Raton, Florida: CRC Press.

59 **WILLIAMS, L.P. & NEWELL, K.W., 1968.** Sources of salmonellas in market swine. *Journal of Hygiene,* Cambridge, 66, 281–293.

60 **WILLIAMS, L.P. & NEWELL, K.W., 1970.** *Salmonella* excretion in joy-riding pigs. *American Journal of Public Health,* 60, 926–929.

61 **WILLIAMS SMITH, H., 1960.** The effect of feeding pigs on food naturally contaminated with salmonellae. *Journal of Hygiene,* Cambridge, 58, 381–389.

62 **WILLIAMS SMITH, H., 1969.** *Salmonella* food poisoning in human beings. The part played by domestic animals. *Royal Society of Health Journal,* London, 6, 271–275.

63 **WOOD, R.L., POPISCHIL, A. & ROSE, R., 1989.** Distribution of persistent *Salmonella typhimurium* infection in internal organs of swine. *American Journal of Veterinary Research,* 50, 1015–1021.

64 **WRAY, C., 1985.** Is salmonellosis still a serious problem in veterinary practice? *The Veterinary Record,* 116, 485–489.

133

Equine salmonellosis

Synonym: Salmonellose by perde (Afrik.)

C.A. Wilkens

Introduction

Equine salmonellosis is a peracute, acute, chronic or inapparent disease of horses of all ages, but foals and aged, debilitated or stressed horses are particularly susceptible. It manifests as several different clinical syndromes — acute colitis accompanied by profuse diarrhoea, and septicaemia with or without diarrhoea are the most common. Other syndromes are chronic diarrhoea and colic, and more rarely polyarthritis, fistulous withers, orchitis and abortion.[8, 39] Salmonellosis occurs either sporadically or, at times, in extensive outbreak form in groups of horses that are at risk. Nosocomial *Salmonella* infections are common and may create serious problems in large equine clinics or hospitals, as horses may die from salmonellosis after surgical operations or therapy for unrelated conditions.[7, 20] Severe outbreaks in such institutions may force their temporary closure in order to control the disease.[3] Outbreaks in foals on stud farms have been reported in several countries.[2, 17, 39]

Equine disease caused by the non-host-specific salmonellas (most commonly *Salmonella typhimurium*) occurs in many countries and is diagnosed sporadically in South Africa. Although infection with the host-specific *Salmonella abortus equi* is often quoted as a cause of abortion in mares,[13] this only seems to be a problem in India,[31] where other *Salmonella* serovars are also implicated in the syndrome.[16] It has only been documented twice as being a cause of outbreaks of abortion in mares in the USA,[20] and has not been reported there as a cause of abortion since the late 1960s.[21] *Salmonella abortus equi* may also cause arthritis in foals and orchitis in stallions.[31] Although Henning (1956) reported *S. abortus equi* as the cause of purulent tendovaginitis, bursitis and pneumonia in horses in South Africa, it has not been isolated in the country since 1970.[10]

Aetiology

For the general morphological and physicochemical properties of the salmonellas, consult ***Salmonella* sp. infections: Introduction.**

At least 40 of the known serovars of *Salmonella* have been isolated from horses. Several serovars may occur in contaminated environments at the same time, and the simultaneous infection of an animal with two or even more serovars is not uncommon. When this does occur, it is usually reason for a poor prognosis.[21] Apart from *S. typhimurium*, other serovars isolated from cases of equine salmonellosis include *S. enteritidis*, *S. anatum*, *S. newport*, *S. heidelberg*, *S. typhimurium* var. *copenhagen*, *S. kottbus*, and *S. saint-paul*.[3, 20] Infections with *S. typhimurium* and *S. typhimurium* var. *copenhagen* appear to be the most pathogenic when compared with the effects of infections caused by the other serovars.[3] Numerous phage types of *S. typhimurium* have been shown to be involved in different infections. The variety is such, however, that no clear conclusion can be reached regarding the origin of the various types, even of known phage types that originate from wild birds, such as finches and sparrows. It appears that the reaction in horses, when exposed to sufficient numbers of salmonellas — irrespective of sero- or phage type — is similar to that in other animal species.[8]

Epidemiology

Salmonellosis in horses on stud farms may have a prevalence varying from 0,36–27 per cent; it has been estimated that up to 10 per cent of horses in the USA may be infected with the organism at some time or another.[20]

Horses most frequently become infected via the oral route, although infection may also take place through the mucous membranes of the eyes and the nose via aerosol droplets.[34] There are many environmental sources of infection, but particular problems are posed by contamination of water by effluent, contaminated feed (meat or bone meal and milk products) and dietary additives, and carrier birds, rodents, horses and other farm animal species that excrete the bacteria.[8] Asymptomatic carrier horses may be active shedders of the bacteria for at least 14 months, or non-shedders.[21, 33] A frequent site for the harbouring of bacteria by carrier animals is the mesenteric lymph nodes.[21]

Shedders of salmonellas appear to play a major role in the dissemination of the organisms.[21] It seems that stress can activate the infection in carrier animals, and not only enhance the faecal excretion of *Salmonella* organisms but also sometimes precipitate overt clinical disease. Faecal excretion of the bacteria is intermittent, and while the numbers of organisms excreted are usually low, the quantities are sufficient to contaminate the environment to a threatening extent, particularly in areas of close confinement such as veterinary hospitals.[1] Horses requiring treatment for conditions unrelated to salmonellosis may be hospitalized as carriers either shedding or not shedding the bacteria. Alternatively they may be admitted to hospital suffering from diarrhoea and excreting the bacteria.[35] The close confinement of large numbers of horses with a variety of medical and surgical problems in hospitals or clinics creates an ideal situation for the development of outbreaks of salmonellosis.[12]

Various serovars of *Salmonella* may be isolated from carriers but, in keeping with the prevalence of specific serovars, *S. typhimurium* is the one which is isolated from most carriers or diseased animals.[1, 3, 20] Two or even three serovars may, however, be isolated from an animal at any specific time.[21]

The pathogenesis of equine enteric or septicaemic salmonellosis is multifaceted and the appearance of overt disease is generally regarded as being a sequel to one or more predisposing causes.[8] Although horses of all ages may be affected, it is most often associated with foals or aged animals. Other factors which play a prominent role are debility, stress (such as that induced by transport, a new stable environment, new stable-mates, hot humid weather, changed feeding regimes, unfamiliar handlers, surgical operations, overwork and intercurrent disease) and anthelmintic or tetracycline medication.[8, 21] It appears that the changes in gut flora that occur during stress or antimicrobial therapy allow salmonellas to multiply.[33] Colic and the oral administration of antibiotics appear to be the two most important risk factors for the induction of *Salmonella* infections;[11] the chances of isolating salmonellas from horses are about 10 times greater in those that are receiving antibiotic therapy than in those that are not. In addition, combined oral and parenteral antibiotic treatment increases 40-fold the chance of contracting salmonellosis.[11] The probability of salmonellas being isolated from horses suffering from colic is two to five times higher than it is from those presenting with other medical complaints.[11, 12, 28]

The epidemiology of the diseases caused by *S. abortus equi* is poorly understood. The bacterium occurs exclusively in horses, in which it causes genital infections, orchitis and arthritis.[31] It does not occur in the intestinal tract and has not been isolated from faeces. The role played by stallions in the dissemination of the organisms is unknown, but transmission during coitus does appear to be a distinct possibility.[31] *Salmonella abortus equi* is disseminated on stud farms by direct or indirect contact with abortion products which contain large numbers of organisms. A high prevalence of abortion generally only occurs in the first foaling season after the infection has been introduced. Thereafter abortion is restricted to new arrivals. Foals may contract the infection before or after birth, and may be born suffering from the disease.[13] The organism may also be the cause of abortion in donkey mares.[37]

Pathogenesis

The pathogenesis of salmonellosis in horses has been poorly studied but it is probably similar to that in other domestic species **(see Chapter 130: Bovine salmonellosis and Chapter 131: Ovine and caprine salmonellosis).**

The stress and other factors mentioned above play significant roles in the initiation, course and outcome of the disease.[21] Pathogenic salmonellas invade the mucosa of the intestinal tract. Bacterial virulence factors and the inflammatory response by the host against the infection appear to contribute to the development of the disease.[24]

Clinical signs

The clinical signs of enteric or septicaemic salmonellosis in horses are similar to those occurring in the comparable disease in other species.

Animals may manifest clinical signs within 24–48 hours of being exposed orally to the bacteria[35] or subjected to stress[9] or other predisposing factors. In studies on experimentally induced disease in ponies, it was found that there is an elevated body temperature during the first five days, which is accompanied by a severe neutropenia, also lasting for five days, after which a neutrophilia sets in.[26] Plasma fibrinogen levels may be slightly elevated.[32, 39] Animals suffering from diarrhoea may exhibit a decrease in plasma proteins and marked electrolyte and acid-base abnormalities.[33]

In general, three overlapping clinical forms of salmonellosis occur. The most severe is a peracute, fatal septicaemic disease, often affecting foals one to six months of age, in which the animals show fever, weakness, depression and reduced appetite. Signs of enteritis may be absent or there may be a severe, foetid diarrhoea. Affected animals usually die within 24–72 hours. The acute disease, which may extend over a period of three weeks, is characterized initially by pyrexia, loss of appetite, a severe enteritis (typified by green or brown watery faeces containing mucus, blood and shreds of intestinal mucosa) and dehydration. The fever and diarrhoea become intermittent as the disease progresses. These animals usually recover despite rapid loss of weight and accompanying dehydration, but in some, septicaemia may give rise to tissue or organ localization of the infection and result in such lesions as acute, fatal, purulent meningitis,[36] particularly in foals, and septic arthritis in one or more joints.[33] The chronic form, which has a duration of three weeks to several months, is characterized by loose faeces, intermittent fever, poor appetite, weight loss and dehydration. Animals suffering from the chronic form of the disease but with a shorter course often recover, while those that remain ill for more extended periods usually die after a spell of recumbency due to severe weakness.[21]

Other manifestations of the infection in horses have been reported. Adult horses may only manifest fever, anorexia and severe depression in the absence of any other clinical signs,[32] and usually recover spontaneously without being treated with antimicrobial drugs. Mild infections may manifest only as colic.[27] Pregnant mares infected with *S. abortus equi* usually abort during the latter half of gestation.[31]

Pathology

Lesions in animals that have died of the disease vary according to the syndrome from which they suffered.

Petechial and ecchymotic haemorrhages are present in the peracute or acute septicaemic disease, especially in serosal membranes (particularly the pericardium and peritoneum), and there is splenomegaly.[14] The gastric mucosa is intensely hyperaemic, with some scattered haemorrhages and oedema. There may be congestion of the small intestine, and the visceral lymph nodes are enlarged, oedematous, and may be haemorrhagic. In animals that have died from the acute enteritis syndrome, lesions are usually present in the mucosa of the entire caecum and proximal large colon, and occasionally in the distal ileum, and are those of a severe acute fibrinonecrotic inflammatory process, often with small ulcers and occasionally with multiple small abscesses in the gut wall.[2, 33] Affected parts of the gut wall may be oedematous. The contents of the large intestine are watery and foul-smelling. The associated regional lymph nodes are usually enlarged and oedematous.[39] There may be macroscopic or microscopic evidence of localization of the infection in other sites, with the development of lesions such as suppurative meningitis and arthritis, and cerebral abscessation.[29, 39] Lesions in chronic salmonellosis are not nearly as marked as they are in the acute disease;[14] a patchy fibrinous or ulcerative colitis or typhlitis may be present.

Diagnosis

Because of the non-specific clinical signs of the disease, the diagnosis should be confirmed by isolation of salmonellas from affected horses. Serological tests are of limited value in the establishment of a diagnosis, as most horses contain antibodies to salmonellas and because a rise in titre is not always marked.[26] A reliable diagnosis, determination of the origin of the causative bacteria, and control require a detailed investigation which includes the serotyping, biotyping and phage-typing of the organism, application of biochemical and antibiotic sensitivity tests, and perusal of hospital case-records.[1]

In order to diagnose the condition in live animals it is essential that serial faecal cultures be made over a period of time, as the isolation of *Salmonella* from infected animals, even during the course of clinical disease, is inconsistent.[32] Culture of the organism from affected animals is more successful when specimens of the faeces and rectal mucosa are cultured concurrently. When rectal specimens alone are used for culturing purposes, the results obtained are superior to those when faecal specimens alone are used. In the latter instance, a success rate of only about 32 per cent can be expected, whereas when the two are used in combination the success rate may rise to 60 per cent.[28] *Salmonella* serovars are readily cultured from specimens of the intestinal tract and the internal organs collected at necropsy from animals that have died of the septicaemic form of the disease.[39] In general, it can be expected that 50 per cent more *Salmonella*-infected animals will be identified at necropsy than when they are alive.[3] In many cases in which the results of the culturing of faeces from the rectum have proved negative, salmonellas can be isolated from specimens of the contents of the ileum and the colon.[3] Necropsy specimens for bacteriological examination should always include mesenteric and ileocolonic lymph nodes and sections of the wall of the caecum and proximal large colon, liver and spleen in separate containers.[33]

Specimens of faeces should consist of 5–10 g of faeces submitted in a selective medium such as tetrathionate or selenite broth and in brilliant green or Salmonella-Shigella agar.[22]

In cases of abortion due to *S. abortus equi* infection, the organism can be isolated from tissues of the aborted foetus, such as heart blood, internal organs, stomach and intestinal contents, and from the foetal membranes and swabs of the vaginal exudate of the mare.[31]

Differential diagnosis

Depending on the syndrome, several diseases may be confused with salmonellosis.

In young foals suffering from the septicaemic form, a number of other bacterial diseases (particularly those caused by *Actinobacillus equuli*, *Klebsiella* spp., *Escherichia coli* and beta-haemolytic streptococci) should be considered.[29] In the enteric syndrome with diarrhoea in foals, conditions such as nutritional diarrhoea, rotavirus infection, cryptosporidiosis, enteric infection with *Clostridium perfringens* type A, B or C, and *Rhodococcus equi*, and helminth-related diarrhoeas should be considered as differential diagnoses.[15, 30]

In older animals suffering from acute clinical salmonellosis with diarrhoea, colitis X, *C. perfringens* type A infection, acute peritonitis, and typhlocolitis due to *Rhodococcus equi* and *Ehrlichia risticii* (Potomac horse fever) infections should be considered as differential diagnoses. Lesions of colitis X are very similar to those of enteric salmonellosis, and the distinction between the two conditions is dependent on culturing the organism from the content or the wall of the intestinal tract.[25] The administration of excessive dosages of non-steroidal anti-inflammatory drugs has been associated with diarrhoea in horses.[23] Chronic salmonellosis should be differentiated from strongyle larval migrans, granulomatous enteritis, alimentary lymphosarcoma, chronic peritonitis, chronic *R. equi* infection, coccidiosis, sand enteropathy and chronic liver disease.[18, 19]

Apart from salmonellas, common causes of infectious synovitis in young foals—often with evidence of systemic illness—are *E. coli*, *Klebsiella* spp., beta-haemolytic streptococci, *A. equuli* and *R. equi*.[38]

The diseases responsible for equine abortions, and their differentiating features, are discussed in **Chapter 189: Infectious causes of equine reproductive failure**.

Control

Antimicrobial therapy with drugs such as the nitrofurans, neomycin, polymyxin B, and chloramphenicol for the treatment of intestinal salmonellosis is of questionable value and does not necessarily result in the elimination of salmonellas from the intestinal tract; they may still be isolated from the faeces and tissues during and after the completion of the course of treatment.[20] Horses may still succumb to the disease in spite of intensive antimicrobial treatment.[1, 21] Trimethroprim alone, or in combination with sulphadiazine, appears to give the best results.[8, 34] Particularly in peracute cases, up to 66 per cent of affected animals may die in spite of intensive treatment. Animals may survive the chronic disease but fail to ever reach their previous level of performance.[20] Antimicrobial therapy is more effective when initiated prior to the development of diarrhoea, or when it is used to control systemic or septicaemic *Salmonella* infections.[8] It should be kept in mind that once diarrhoea has developed, oral antibiotic treatment, particularly with oxytetracycline, may aggravate the severity of the diarrhoea,[8] and the use of this drug is contraindicated when diarrhoea has already developed. Antimicrobial therapy, preferably after determining drug sensitivity, is indicated in the case of foals suffering from the septicaemic syndrome or in horses with indwelling intravenous catheters.

In the treatment of salmonellosis, symptomatic and supportive treatment with the emphasis on fluid replacement, correction of electrolyte deficiencies and acid-base status, and good nursing are important.[5] Successful treatment of the disease in animals in which diarrhoea has developed is dependent on the rapid replacement of lost fluid. Oral fluid replacement is considered to increase the severity of the diarrhoea. The administration of plasma containing antibodies to Gram-negative core antigens is also beneficial.[34] Antidiarrhoeal drugs such as bismuth subsalicylate or activated charcoal may be used, but these should be discontinued after three days if they have not produced a beneficial effect. Non-steroidal anti-inflammatory drugs, such as low doses of flunixin meglumine, may be used for their anti-endotoxic effects. Plasma transfusions may help to alleviate the hypoproteinaemia which develops as a consequence of the enteropathy.[5]

During an outbreak, affected animals should be isolated and their faeces and bedding burnt. Attendants should be acquainted with the dangers of carrying infection and instructed in proper hygienic procedures. Other precautions for containing the infection should include the prevention of the contamination of the feed and water of all the horses in the establishment, and the control of flies and rodents.[8] An animal which has been infected with salmonellas should not be returned to its farm of origin until five consecutive specimens of its faeces have proved to be negative for salmonellas. It has been suggested that daily faecal cultures for three to four weeks may be necessary to be reasonably certain that an animal is not shedding the bacteria.[34]

To reduce the possibility of salmonellosis developing in horses admitted to a veterinary hospital, every effort must be made to minimize stress. Horses with normal haemograms should be operated on within the first 48 hours of administration, or, if the haemogram is not within normal limits, the operation should be delayed for at least a week. Animals should be sent home as soon as possible after the operation.[7]

The extensive use of a killed whole-cell vaccine has been reported in a number of countries, but controlled studies have not been undertaken to determine its efficacy.[1] When a vaccine is used, it is imperative that the serovars prevailing in the outbreak in question be monitored against those present in the vaccine in order to determine whether or not its use is warranted. In order that colostral-derived passive immunity can be provided in foals, pregnant mares should be vaccinated 30 days prior to foaling, while foals should be vaccinated at two to three months of age to effect control of the condition.[6] It appears that no equine salmonellosis vaccine is currently available commercially. Preliminary studies on the development of an *S. abortus equi* vaccine for the control of outbreaks of abortion have shown that experimentally a beta-propriolactone-inactivated chrome alum vaccine provides better protection in mice than a formalin-inactivated vaccine.[37] When required, autogenous vaccines are prepared for use in specific outbreaks.[34]

Management practices should lessen exposure of horses to possible sources of infection and also minimize the stressful situations that may precipitate the disease.[5]

References

1 **BEGG, A.P., JOHNSTONE, K.G., HUTCHINS, D.R. & EDWARDS, D.J., 1988.** Some aspects of the epidemiology of equine salmonellosis. *Australian Veterinary Journal*, 65, 221–223.

2 **BRYANS, J.T., FALLON, E.H. & SHEPHARD, B.P., 1961.** Equine salmonellosis. *Cornell Veterinarian*, 51, 467–477.

3 **CARTER, J.D., HIRD, D.W., FARVER, T.B. & HJERPE, C.A., 1986.** Salmonellosis in hospitalized horses: Seasonality and case fatality rates. *Journal of the American Veterinary Medical Association*, 188, 163–167.

4 **CARTER, J.D., WHITLOCK, R.H., BENSON, C.E., BECHT, J.L., MORRIS, D.D. & ACLAND, H.M., 1985.** Comparison of rectal cultures and fecal cultures in detecting *Salmonella* infection in horses and cattle. *American Journal of Veterinary Research*, 46, 697–698.

5 **COLAHAN, P.T., MAYHEW, I.G., MERRITT, A.M. & MOORE, J.N., 1991.** *Equine Medicine and Surgery*. Goleta: American Veterinary Publications.

6 **CONBOY, H.S., 1982.** Preventive medicine on the broodmare farm. *In*: MANSMANN, R.A., McALLISTER, E.S. & PRATT, P.W., (eds). *Equine Medicine and Surgery*. 3rd edn. Santa Barbara, California: American Veterinary Publications.

7 **DORN, C.D, COFFMAN, J.R., SCHMIDT, D.A., GARNER, H.E., ADDISON, J.B. & McCUNE, E.L., 1975.** Neutropenia and salmonellosis in hospitalized horses. *Journal of the American Veterinary Medical Association*, 166, 65–67.

8 **GIBBONS, D.F., 1980.** Equine salmonellosis: A review. *The Veterinary Record*, 106, 356–359.

9 **GRAHAM, R., REYNOLDS, H.K. & HILL, J.F., 1920.** Bacteriological studies of a peracute disease of horses and mules. *Journal of the American Veterinary Medical Association*, 56, 378–393.

10 **HENTON, M.M., 1992.** Onderstepoort Veterinary Institute. Personal communication.

11 **HIRD, D.W., CASEBOLT, D.B., CARTER, J.D., PAPPAIOANOU, M. & HJERPE, C.A., 1986.** Risk factors for salmonellosis in hospitalised horses. *Journal of the American Veterinary Medical Association*, 188, 173–177.

12 **HIRD, D.W., PAPPAIOANOU, M. & SMITH, B.P., 1984.** Case-control study of risk factors associated with isolation of *Salmonella saint-paul* in hospitalized horses. *American Journal of Epidemiology*, 120, 852–864.

13 **HORSCH, F., 1984.** Infectious diseases of the digestive system. *In*: DIETZ, O. & WIESNER, E., (eds). *Diseases of the Horse. A Handbook for Science and Practice*. Berlin: S. Karger.

14 **JUBB, K.V.F., KENNEDY, P.C. & PALMER, N., 1985.** *Pathology of Domestic Animals*, 3rd edn. New York: Academic Press.

15 **KOTERBA, A.M., DRUMMOND, W.H. & KOSCH, P.C., 1990.** *Equine Clinical Neonatology*. Philadelphia: Lea & Febiger.

16 **KUMAR, S. & GUPTA, B.K., 1972.** *Salmonella anatum* from an aborted foal. *British Veterinary Journal*, 128, lxiv.

17 **MAHAFFEY, L.W., 1952.** *Salmonella typhimurium* in foals in Western Australia. *Australian Veterinary Journal*, 28, 8.

18 **MERRITT, A.M., 1982.** Chronic diarrhoea. *In*: MANSMANN, R.A., McALLISTER, E.S. & PRATT, P.W., (eds). *Equine Medicine and Surgery*. 3rd edn. Santa Barbara, California: American Veterinary Publications.

19 **MERRITT, A.M., BOLTON, J.R. & CIMPRICH, R., 1975.** Differential diagnosis of diarrhoea in horses over six months of age. *Journal of the South African Veterinary Association*, 46, 73–76.

20 **MORSE, E.V. & DUNCAN, M.A., 1976.** The treatment of salmonellosis in equidae. *Modern Veterinary Practice*, 57, 47–57.

21 **MORSE, E.V., DUNCAN, M.A., PAGE, E.A. & FESSLER, J.F., 1976.** Salmonellosis in equidae: A study of 23 cases. *Cornell Veterinarian*, 66, 198–213.

22 **MURRAY, M.J., 1989.** Diarrhea. *In*: BROWN, C.M., (ed.). *Problems in Equine Medicine*. Philadelphia: Lea & Febiger.

23 **MURRAY, M.J., 1992.** Acute colitis. *In*: ROBINSON, N.E., (ed.). *Current Therapy in Equine Medicine*. Philadelphia: W.B. Saunders Company.

24 **MURRAY, M.J., DORAN, R.E., PFEIFFER, C.J., TYLER, D.E., MOORE, J.N. & SRIRANGANATHAN, T., 1989.** Comparative effects of cholera toxin, *Salmonella typhimurium* culture lysate, and viable *Salmonella typhimurium* in isolated colon segments in ponies. *American Journal of Veterinary Research*, 50, 22–28.

25 **OWEN, R.R., 1975.** Post-stress diarrhoea in the horse. *The Veterinary Record*, 96, 267–270.

26 **OWEN, R.R., FULLERTON, J.N., TIZARD, I.R., LUMSDEN, J.H. & BARNUM, D.A., 1979.** Studies on experimental enteric salmonellosis in ponies. *Canadian Journal of Comparative Medicine*, 43, 247–254.

27 **PALMER, J.E., BENSON, C.E. & WHITLOCK, R.H., 1982.** Subclinical salmonellosis in horses with colic. *Proceedings of the Equine Colic Research Symposium*, Athens, Georgia: University of Georgia Press.

28 **PALMER, J.E., BENSON, C.E. & WHITLOCK, R.H., 1985.** *Salmonella* shed by horses with colic. *Journal of the American Veterinary Medical Association*, 187, 256–257.

29 **PLATT, H., 1973.** Septicaemia in the foal. A review of 61 cases. *British Veterinary Journal*, 129, 221–229.

30 **SENRAD, S.D. & SHAFTOE, S., 1992.** Gastrointestinal diseases of the neonatal foal. *In*: ROBINSON, N.E., (ed.). *Current Therapy in Equine Medicine*. Philadelphia: W.B. Saunders Company.

31 **SINGH, I.P., SHARMA, V.K. & KAURA, Y.K., 1971.** Some aspects of the epidemiology of *Salmonella abortus-equi* infection in equines. *British Veterinary Journal*, 127, 378–383.

32 **SMITH, B.P., 1979.** Atypical salmonellosis in horses: Fever and depression without diarrhoea. *Journal of the American Veterinary Medical Association*, 175, 69–71.

33 **SMITH, B.P., 1985.** Salmonella infections in horses. The Compendium Collection. Fifth Anniversary Series. *Equine Medicine and Surgery in Practice*, 16–25.

34 **SMITH, B.P., 1990.** Salmonellosis: Paranoia or reason to worry? *Compendium on Continuing Education for the Practising Veterinarian*, 10, 1459–1461.

35 **SMITH, B.P., RIENA-GUERRA, M. & HARDY, A.J., 1978.** Prevalence and epizootiology of equine salmonellosis. *Journal of the American Veterinary Medical Association*, 172, 353–356.

36 **STUART, B.P., MARTIN, B.R., WILLIAMS, L.P. & VON BYERN, H., 1973.** *Salmonella*-induced meningoencephalitis in a foal. *Journal of the American Veterinary Medical Association*, 162, 211–213.

37 **UPPAL, P.K. & KATARIA, J.M., 1987.** Epidemic of *Salmonella abortus equi* abortion in horses and some studies on the development of a vaccine. *Journal of Reproduction and Fertility*, 35, 669–670.

38 **WAGNER, P.C., WATROUS, B.J. & DARIEN, B.J., 1992.** Septic arthritis and osteomyelitis. *In*: ROBINSON, N.E. (ed.). *Current Therapy in Equine Medicine*. Philadelphia: W.B. Saunders Company.

39 **WENKOFF, M.S., 1973.** *Salmonella typhimurium* septicaemia in foals. *Canadian Veterinary Journal*, 14, 284–287.

Haemophilus *spp. infections*

The members of the genus *Haemophilus* are classified in the family Pasteurellaceae. The bacteria in this genus are pleomorphic and vary in morphology from minute to medium-sized coccobacilli or rods (usually less than 1 µm wide and of variable length) to filaments. *Haemophilus* spp. may have capsules, and, as is the case with other Gram-negative bacteria, they have cell walls with endotoxic activity—attributes that may be important in the pathogenesis of the diseases that they cause.[3]

Haemophilus spp. are Gram-negative, aerobic or facultatively anaerobic, and require preformed growth factors such as factor X (protoporphyrin IX) and/or factor V (nicotinamide adenine dinucleotide [NAD] or NAD phosphate [NADP]) in culture media. Both these factors are present in blood, and this dependence on blood for their growth gave rise to the name of the genus. Factor V is also present in yeast extract and is elaborated by staphylococci, the latter giving rise to the phenomenon known as satellitism which occurs when a mixed culture of *Haemophilus* organisms and staphylococci are grown on a solid medium. *Haemophilus* spp. grow more luxuriantly when adjacent to colonies of staphylococci because of the diffusion of factor V from them into the surrounding medium.[1]

Haemophilus spp. are part of the resident bacterial flora of the mucous membranes of the upper respiratory tract and oral cavity of a variety of animal species including humans, but they may also be isolated from the vagina and the intestinal tract. With the exception of *H. parainfluenza*, the individual species of *Haemophilus* are host-specific.[3]

Of the *Haemophilus* spp., only *H. parasuis* is of veterinary importance, while the other two which cause disease in livestock, *H. somnus* and *H. agni,* do not qualify for inclusion in the genus. It has been suggested that *H. somnus, H. agni,* and *Histophilus ovis* may belong to a single taxon.[3] For practical purposes, and until such time as they are finally reclassified, the two species will be retained under this heading.

Haemophilus parasuis is the cause of Glässer's disease, a peracute to acute disease of young pigs that is characterized by a serofibrinous polyserositis, polyarthritis and meningitis. *Haemophilus somnus* infections are responsible for a variety of syndromes in cattle, including septicaemia, thrombotic meningoencephalitis, pneumonia, myocarditis, arthritis, mastitis, and infections of the reproductive tract of cows and bulls. *Haemophilus agni* very rarely causes septicaemia in sheep. The disease in lambs is fulminating and is associated with sudden death, whereas in adult sheep it is less severe. At necropsy, the disease is a typical haemorrhagic septicaemia, which is also characterized by the presence of scattered haemorrhages throughout the carcass, and multifocal small areas of hepatic necrosis.[2]

Both *H. parasuis* and *H. somnus* are ubiquitous, but *H. agni* is rarely encountered.[2]

References

1 **BUXTON, A. & FRASER, G., 1977.** *Animal Microbiology.* Vol. I. Oxford: Blackwell Scientific Publications.

2 **KENNEDY, P.C., FRAZIER, L.M., THEILER, G.H. & BIBERSTEIN, E.L., 1958.** A septicaemic disease of lambs caused by *Haemophilus agni* (new species). *American Journal of Veterinary Research*, 19, 645–654.

3 **MANNHEIM, W., 1984.** Pasteurellaceae. *In*: KRIEG, N.R. & HOLT, J.G., (eds). *Bergey's Manual of Systematic Bacteriology.* Vol. I. Baltimore, London: Williams & Wilkins.

134

Haemophilus parasuis infection

Synonyms: Glässer's disease, porcine polyserositis and arthritis

M.M. Henton

Introduction

Glässer's disease, caused by *Haemophilus parasuis*, is a peracute to acute disease of young pigs characterized by a serofibrinous polyserositis, polyarthritis and meningitis. It generally occurs sporadically, involving single or several animals, but may occur in outbreak form, and is frequently associated with some form of managemental or environmental stress, particularly that relating to transport, weaning, adverse environmental conditions, or changes in housing or diet. Glässer's disease rarely occurs in South Africa.

A disease syndrome manifested by fibrinous pleuritis, pericarditis and peritonitis, and often accompanied by arthritis, was described by Glässer in 1910.[4] He was able to demonstrate Gram-negative bacilli in the exudate but could not cultivate them. Some decades later it was observed that meningitis was often an associated lesion in animals suffering from the syndrome.[8] In 1939, a bacterium thought to be *Haemophilus suis*, which had first been described in 1931 in association with lesions caused by swine influenza,[27] was isolated from the joints of pigs suffering from arthritis.[26] This was followed some years later by the isolation of the same bacterium from typical cases of Glässer's disease and by the experimental production of the disease in pigs by inoculation of *H. suis*.[8]

In 1969, a new species of *Haemophilus* (*H. parasuis*) from pigs was proposed.[1] This organism required factor V or nicotinamide adenine dinucleotide (NAD) for growth, but did not require factor X (protoporphyrin IX or protohaeme). During recent years this has been the most frequent bacterium isolated from cases of Glässer's disease.[24] Most strains in culture collections identified as *H. suis* are only V-factor-requiring and belong to *H. parasuis*.[12] *Haemophilus suis* requires both factors X and V and it seems, therefore, that this organism, as described in the earlier literature, may be invalid as the cause of Glässer's disease. For this reason, only *H. parasuis* is considered here.

Aetiology

Bacteria of the genus *Haemophilus* (meaning blood-loving) belong to the family Pasteurellaceae. *Haemophilus parasuis* (the prefix, *para*, meaning alongside or resembling — *parasuis* therefore meaning *suis*-like) is a small, thin, pleomorphic, Gram-negative rod generally less than 1 μm in width and variable in length.[12] The bacterium is factor V-dependent and therefore requires the addition of this factor to the culture medium. Growth on chocolate agar is very feeble after 48–72 hours; in the absence of the factor V, the colonies are smooth, greyish and translucent, and reach a diameter of about 0,5 mm. There is, however, a marked enhancement of growth on blood agar if the medium is streaked with a *Staphylococcus* feeder culture (as staphylococci, as well as certain other bacteria, produce the critical growth factor in excess), with colonies attaining a diameter of 1–2 mm around the streak.[12] This is known as satellite growth or satellitism. Chocolate agar and Levinthal media (agar and broth) are satisfactory media for propagation of the bacterium.[12] Growth is also improved if the carbon dioxide level is raised to about 5 per cent.

Haemophilus parasuis is not haemolytic, ferments glucose, sucrose, maltose, galactose, mannose, fructose, ribose and insulin, and is urease- and Camp-negative.[12] Identification of *H. parasuis* is based on morphological and colonial characteristics, factor V dependency and biochemical testing. For this purpose reference should be made to *Bergey's Manual of Systematic Bacteriology*.[14]

As reported by Smart *et al.*,[29] Bakos, Nilsson and Thal in 1952 proposed a serological classification of *H. parasuis* based on a tube agglutination test of whole-cell preparations. Isolates of groups A, B or C are serologically related organisms; all other strains are placed in an ill-defined group D. In an attempt to provide a more comprehensive system, Morozumi and Nicolet in 1986, as cited by Smart *et al.*,[30] proposed an alternative typing system based on an immunodiffusion test that used antigens extracted from either the capsule or, in the case of unencapsulated strains, from the outer membrane. They described seven serovars. Serovars 2 and 5 correspond to the serovars A and B, respectively, of Bakos *et al.* Using either serotyping system, 20–40 per cent of strains cannot be typed.[30] Subsequently Smart *et al.*[30] used restriction endonuclease fingerprinting (REF) analysis to group isolates of *H. parasuis* to be classified. Of the 69 isolates that they examined, 24 were unique, while the remaining 45 isolates could be placed into one of 13 REF profile groups.

In a given herd, many strains of *H. parasuis* can be isolated, but in most cases one or two strains predominate.[30]

Epidemiology

Glässer's disease is widely distributed throughout the world[7, 19] but is of sporadic occurrence. The disease generally occurs in pigs between the ages of two and 16 weeks,[7] but older animals of all ages are also susceptible.[21, 24] Pigs seem to be particularly susceptible soon after they are weaned. In South Africa, where the disease occurs rarely, it has been diagnosed more frequently in young piglets two to six weeks of age.[5]

Haemophilus spp. occur as obligate parasites on the mucous membranes of humans and a variety of animal species.[12] *Haemophilus parasuis* is a common member of the flora of the upper respiratory tract and pharynx of healthy pigs,[7, 17, 25, 28] and piglets acquire the organism soon after birth,[24, 28] but natural immunity to Glässer's disease has usually developed by the age of seven to eight weeks and the disease thus occurs only sporadically.[24, 28] It appears that under certain conditions, particularly those associated with stress such as transport, weaning, changes in diet or weather (especially chilling), movement to new quarters, and mixing of animals from different sources,[19, 21] animals become predisposed to the disease. The disease is more common in winter than in summer.

Glässer's disease often affects all the piglets in a single litter in a piggery, presumably because they all have a similar immune status and are all subject to the same amount and type of stress.[5]

Experimentally, an acute disease with a short incubation period of less than 24 hours can readily be produced following intratracheal inoculations of *H. parasuis* in pigs.[16, 18] In addition, the condition can be reproduced by inoculation of the organism by other routes, such as the intraperitoneal, intravenous and subdural.[7, 25]

Pathogenesis

The pathogenesis of *H. parasuis* infection is poorly understood.[19] Piglets become infected with *H. parasuis* soon after birth but usually do not develop clinical disease because of the presence of maternal immunity. Under conditions of stress, *H. parasuis* invades the mucosa of the upper respiratory tract or pharynx and enters the surrounding tissues, from which it is disseminated haematogenously throughout the body. The bacterium has a predilection for serosal surfaces, such as those lining the large body cavities, joints and meninges, where it localizes[24] to produce its pathological effects. The immunological status of the host probably plays a paramount role in the establishment of the disease,[19] as is exemplified not only by the age predilection for the disease, which is generally at the stage when piglets' maternally acquired antibodies are probably waning, but also by the fact that specific pathogen-free animals are more susceptible even in the absence of any apparent predisposing factors.[21] Even in non-specific, pathogen-free herds, precipitating stress factors cannot always be identified.[30]

Clinical signs

The duration of the incubation period of the disease under field conditions is not known, but it is likely to be short, as clinical signs can become evident within two to three days of animals being stressed.[6]

The manifestations of the clinical disease depend upon the localization and severity of the lesions. In some animals, clinical signs may not be noticed — the animals simply expire suddenly.[29] In those in which signs are apparent, the disease is generally of sudden onset with a peracute to acute course of one to two days, and is characterized by fever in which the rectal temperature may be as high as 42 °C. The affected animals also manifest anorexia, listlessness, respiratory distress (respiration is shallow and rapid, and may be accompanied by extension of the neck and opening of the mouth with breathing), increased heart rate, lameness and nervous signs.[2, 7, 9, 23, 29, 31] Coughing may be present, and auscultation of the thoracic cavity may reveal the presence of pleural and pericardial frictional rubbing sounds. The skin may show cyanosis before death supervenes.

Most animals show some degree of lameness and develop a shuffling gait as the result of pain due to polyarthritis. One or several of the joints of the limbs, particularly the larger ones, are swollen, hot and tender.

Involvement of the nervous system is manifested in many animals by depression, muscular tremors, ataxia, paresis or paralysis, and convulsions.

In piggeries where the disease occurs, the morbidity rate is variable[19] but the mortality rate in untreated cases may be very high.[7] Survivors may reveal evidence of persistent disease in the form of chronic arthritis, meningitis or intestinal obstruction due to the presence of peritoneal adhesions.[2, 31]

Pathology

In typical cases of Glässer's disease, the macroscopical pathology is characterized by the presence of a serofibrinous meningitis of the brain and spinal cord, pleuritis, pericarditis, peritonitis and polyarthritis,[7] but in individuals not all these lesions are equally evident or even present; in some they may be difficult to detect, particularly in those that have died of the peracute disease.[25, 29]

In the central nervous system, the meninges of the brain are generally more severely affected than those of the spinal cord. The cerebrospinal fluid is frequently cloudy.[7]

In animals suffering from polyarthritis, the atlanto-occipital joint and the larger joints of the limbs are particularly involved.[7] In these joints the inflammatory reaction is characterized by an excessive amount of synovial fluid, which is turbid, and the presence of yellowish-grey flecks or deposits of fibrinous exudate which are adherent to the synovial membranes or joint surfaces.

The pleural, pericardial and peritoneal cavities contain increased amounts (which may be slight) of serous fluid in which yellowish floccules of fibrin may be floating. The serosal surfaces may contain flecks and strands of fibrin, which in some cases may be very delicate and difficult to detect unless the observer is aware of the possibility of their existence.[7, 32] Mucosal congestion of the gastrointestinal tract, particularly in the fundus of the stomach, and multiple petechial haemorrhages in the renal cortices may be present.[25] A few animals exhibit bronchopneumonia with or without the presence of the other typical lesions of Glässer's disease.[11]

The histological changes reflect those of the gross pathology with, in addition, thrombosis of some vessels in the meninges, renal glomeruli and dermal papillae.[9, 22, 25]

Diagnosis and differential diagnosis

In a typical case of Glässer's disease, the presence of serofibrinous polyserositis, polyarthritis and meningitis is sufficient to make a provisional diagnosis, which is often reinforced if the history includes the existence of a predisposing stress factor and the clinical signs are characteristic.

Affected tissues or swabs of the exudate should be submitted for bacterial isolation to confirm the diagnosis. The meningeal exudate and the cerebrospinal fluid seem to be the most suitable for this purpose.[7]

In most cases, the organism can be isolated from the lungs, but very seldom from other organs, such as the liver, kidneys and spleen.[7] Swabs should be placed in a transport medium (such as Amies or Stuarts) for submission to a diagnostic laboratory, as *H. parasuis* grows poorly and is susceptible to drying out.

Generally, the isolation of *H. parasuis* presents no difficulties[7] unless the material from which cultures are made is grossly contaminated, and provided that a suitable selective medium, such as modified Levinthal agar containing 1,6 units of bacitracin per ml, chocolate agar containing 1 in 25 000 dilution of crystal violet and 1,6 units of bacitracin,[15] or broth with factor V added[19] is used.

As most herds are subclinically infected, most animals will show low complement fixation titres, whereas in fully susceptible animals high titres are present soon after exposure.[20]

In the differential diagnosis of Glässer's disease several diseases should be considered. Mycoplasmal infections, such as that caused by *Mycoplasma hyorhinis*, may show similar clinical signs and lesions but are usually milder and more chronic than Glässer's disease.[7, 9] Erysipelas may present a similar picture, but the range of the ages of affected animals is usually wider. *Streptococcus suis* type II infections cause a similar disease picture to *H. parasuis* infection but the exudate is of a more purulent nature, while *Actinobacillus pleuropneumoniae* infections may occasionally mimic Glässer's disease. Teschen and Aujeszky's disease should also be considered in countries where these diseases occur.[31]

Control

Most cases or outbreaks of the disease are sporadic in nature and not anticipated. Factors which may lead to stress should be reduced or avoided as far as possible.

Several agents may be used for the treatment or prophylaxis of Glässer's disease, including penicillin, tetracycline, chloramphenicol, and sulphanomides potentiated with trimethoprim.[3] Treatment should be by parenteral administration of the agent, and it is imperative that it be commenced as early as possible in the course of the disease. In addition, all the animals in the group in which the disease has occurred should be treated, whether or not clinical signs are apparent.[19, 31] It has been suggested that, in practice, penicillin should be the treatment of choice, followed by tetracyclines, with chloramphenicol being held in reserve.[10] For chemoprophylaxis, the addition of one of the agents to feed or water can also be considered. It should be borne in mind, however, that strains with reduced sensitivity or with resistance to penicillin, tetracyclines and other chemotherapeutics have been encountered, so the sensitivity of the organism should be continuously monitored in all herds which experience disease as a result of *H. parasuis* infection.[10, 11]

Although vaccines are not generally available, they have been used to good effect.[28] In one outbreak in a specific pathogen-free herd in Denmark which was associated with a very high morbidity rate, prophylactic use of a formalized autovaccine prepared from cultures of *H. parasuis* and containing aluminium hydroxide as adjuvant provided significant protection.[21] A commercial vaccine (Glassinord R, Northern Drugs and Chemicals Ltd, Copenhagen) was subsequently developed and has been successfully used to control the disease in Denmark and Switzerland.[24] Despite these good results following immunization, the presence of poor cross-immunization between serotypes, and the absence of homologous immunity to the SV5 serotype in specific pathogen-free pigs, immunoprophylaxis may not always be successful.[13]

References

1 **BIBERSTEIN, E.L. & WHITE, D.C., 1969.** A proposal for the establishment of two new *Haemophilus* species. *Journal of Medical Microbiology*, 2, 75–78.

2 **BLOOD, D.C. & HENDERSON, J.A., 1963.** *Veterinary Medicine*. 2nd edn. Baltimore: Williams & Wilkins.

3 **EAVES, L.E., BLACKWELL, P.G. & FEGAN, M., 1989.** Characterization and antimicrobial sensitivity of haemophili isolated from pigs. *Australian Veterinary Journal*, 66, 1–4.

4 **GLÄSSER, K., 1910.** Untersuchungen über die Schweineseuche mit besonderer Berücksichtigung ihrer Atiologie und Patologie. *Deutsche Tierärztliche Wochenschrift*, 18, 729–733.

5 **HENTON, M.M., 1992.** Veterinary Research Institute, Onderstepoort. Unpublished data.

6 **HIRASAWA, H., SATHO, Y., MOROZUMI, K., MOROZUMI, T., NAKAGAWA, Y., OTA, T., TANAKA, K., OSADA, N. & TAKADA, T., 1987.** Outbreak of *Haemophilus parasuis* infection in swine associated with purulent fibrinous meningitis. *Journal of the Japan Veterinary Medical Association*, 40, 519–522.

7 **HJARRE, A., 1958.** Enzootic virus pneumonia and Glässer's disease of swine. *Advances in Veterinary Science*, 4, 235–263. New York & London: Academic Press.

8 **HJARRE, A. & WARMBY, G., 1942.** cited by Nielsen, R. & Damielsen, V.

9 **JUBB, K.V.F., KENNEDY, P.C. & PALMER, N., 1985.** *Pathology of Domestic Animals*. 3rd edn. Orlando: Academic Press, Inc.

10 **KIELSTEIN, P., 1985.** Zur Glässerschen Krankheiten und Chemotherapeutika-Empfindlicheit ihres Erregers. *Monatshefte für Veterinärmedizin*, 40, 806 – 809.

11 **KIELSTEIN, P. & LEUER, R., 1990.** Zur Glässerschen Krankheit des Schweines — Atiologisch-epizootiologische Untersuchungen zum Erregspektrum. *Monatshefte für Veterinärmedizin*, 45, 577–582.

12 **KILIAN, M. & BIBERSTEIN, E.L., 1984.** Genus II. *Haemophilus*. In: KRIEG, N.R. & HOLT, J.G., (eds). *Bergey's Manual of Systematic Bacteriology*. Vol. 1. Baltimore: Williams & Wilkins.

13 **KLEINSTEIN, P. & RASSBACH, A., 1991.** Serologische Typisierung und Nachweiss immunoger Kreuzreaktionen von *Haemophilus parasuis* (Glässersche Krankheit). *Monatshefte für Veterinärmedizin*, 46, 586–589.

14 **KRIEG, N.R. & HOLT, J.G., 1984.** *Bergey's Manual of Systematic Bacteriology*. Vol. 1. Baltimore: Williams & Wilkins.

15 **LITTLE, T.W.A., 1970.** *Haemophilus* infection in pigs. *The Veterinary Record*, 87, 399–402.

16 **LITTLE, T.W.A. & HARDIUNG, J.D.J., 1971.** The comparative pathogenicity of two porcine *Haemophilus* species. *The Veterinary Record*, 88, 540–545.

17 **MOLLER, K. & KILLIAN, H., 1990.** V factor-dependent members of the family Pasteurellaceae in the porcine upper respiratory tract. *Journal of Clinical Microbiology*, 28, 2711–2716.

18 **NEIL, D.H., McKAY, K.A., L'ECUYER, C.L. & CORNER, A.H., 1969.** Glässer's disease of swine produced by intratracheal inoculation of *Haemophilus suis*. *Canadian Journal of Comparative Medicine*, 33, 187–193.

19 **NICOLET, J., 1986.** *Haemophilus* infections. In: LEMAN, A.D., STRAW, B., GLOCK, R.D., MENGELING, W.L., PENNY, R.H.C. & SCHOL, E., (eds). *Diseases of Swine*. 6th edn. Ames, Iowa: Iowa State University Press.

20 **NIELSEN, R., 1981.** *Haemophilus* infections in Danish swine herds. In: KILIAN, M., FREDERIKSEN, W. & BIBERSTEIN, E.L., (eds). *Haemophilus, Pasteurella and Actinobacillus*. London, New York, Toronto, Sydney, San Francisco: Academic Press, Inc.

21 **NIELSEN, R. & DANIELSEN, V., 1975.** An outbreak of Glässer's disease. Studies on the etiology, serology and the effect of vaccination. *Nordisk Veterinaer Medicin*, 27, 20 –25.

22 **PEET, R.L., FRY, J., LLOYD, J., HENDERSON, J., CURRAN, J. & MOIR, D., 1983.** *Haemophilus parasuis* septicaemia in pigs. *Australian Veterinary Journal*, 60, 187.

23 **RADOSTITS, O.M., RUHNKE, H.L. & LOSOS, G.J., 1963.** An outbreak of meningitis in swine caused by *Haemophilus* species or organism. *Canadian Veterinary Journal*, 4, 265–270.

24 **RIISING, H.J., 1981.** Prevention of Glässers disease through immunity to *Haemophilus parasuis*. *Zentralblatt für Veterinärmedizin*, Reihe B, 28, 630–638.

25 **RILEY, M.G.I., 1977.** *Haemophilus parasuis* infection in swine. *Journal of the American Veterinary Medical Association*, 171, 649–651.

26 **SHANKS, P.L., 1939.** Acute arthritis in pigs. *The Veterinary Record*, 51, 783–784.

27 **SHOPE, R.E., 1931.** Swine influenza. I. Experimental transmission and etiology. *Journal of Experimental Medicine*, 54, 349–385.

28 **SMART, N.L. & MINIATS, O.P., 1989.** Preliminary assessment of a *Haemophilus parasuis* bacterin for use in specific pathogen-free swine. *Canadian Journal of Veterinary Research*, 53, 390–393.

29 **SMART, N.L., MINIATS, O.P. & FRIENDSHIP, R.M., 1989.** Glasser's disease and prevalence of subclinical infection with *Haemophilus parasuis* in swine in southern Ontario. *Canadian Veterinary Journal*, 53, 339–343.

30 **SMART, N.L., MINIATS, O.P. & MACINNES, J.I., 1988.** Analysis of *Haemophilus parasuis* isolates from southern Ontario swine by restriction endonuclease fingerprinting. *Canadian Journal of Veterinary Research*, 52, 319–324.

31 **TAYLOR, D.J., 1983.** *Pig Diseases*. 3rd edn. Cambridge: The Burlington Press (Cambridge) Ltd.

32 **TUSTIN, R.C., 1992.** Faculty of Veterinary Science, University of Pretoria. Personal communication.

135

The Haemophilus somnus *disease complex in cattle*

Synonym: Haemophilosis

J.P. Kitching and G.C. Bishop

Introduction

Haemophilus somnus is the cause of a variety of clinical syndromes in cattle, including those associated with septicaemia, thrombotic meningoencephalitis, pneumonia, myocarditis, arthritis, mastitis, and disease of the reproductive tract in cows and bulls. Disease caused by *H. somnus* occurs in many countries, but it is rare in southern Africa and has only been reported from South Africa[42] and Zimbabwe.[61]

Disease due to *H. somnus* was first described in 1956 in feedlots in the USA.[4, 21, 40] This disease manifested in the form of an infectious meningoencephalitis, and has been variously termed the 'sleeper syndrome', thromboembolic meningoencephalitis (TEME), infectious thromboembolic meningoencephalitis (ITEME) and, more recently, thrombotic meningoencephalitis (TME). The last name for this syndrome is preferred because it has been established that embolism does not play a role in the pathogenesis of the lesions.[25] Although TME was thought to be the major disease problem, fewer cases of it are being encountered, while some of the other syndromes are becoming more common and new manifestations of infection are being identified.[25]

When disease due to *H. somnus* first breaks out in a region, it is predominantly seen as TME, but as the infection becomes endemic, there is a gradual change in its manifestation, and the respiratory form attains a high profile.[50]

Haemophilus somnus has been isolated from cattle in many parts of South Africa, but clinical disease as a consequence of the infection has only been diagnosed on a few occasions.[29, 43]

There are several excellent reviews on *H. somnus* and the disease syndromes that it produces.[6, 25, 35, 46, 73]

Aetiology

Bacteria of the genus *Haemophilus* (meaning blood-loving) belong to the family Pasteurellaceae and occur as obligate parasites on the mucous membranes of humans and a variety of animal species.[41] *Haemophilus somnus* is a facultatively anaerobic, micro-aerophilic, small, pleomorphic, non-motile, Gram-negative and non-acid-fast coccobacillus.[35, 41]

The taxonomic status of *H. somnus* is still unresolved.[41] It has been suggested that *H. somnus*, *H. agni* and *Histophilus ovis* may belong to a single taxon.[71] Further investigation into the relationship between them and *Actinobacillus seminis* is required.

Although all isolates of *H. somnus* are probably potentially pathogenic, they differ in virulence.[23, 35, 77]

An atmosphere containing 5–20 per cent CO_2 is required for primary isolation of *H. somnus*. The organism grows well at 37° C on media supplemented with 10 per cent blood of cattle or sheep, although brain-heart infusion agar supplemented with 0,5 per cent yeast extract may also be used.[17, 19] *Haemophilus somnus* is easily overgrown by most contaminants, and a selective medium incorporating vancomycin, neomycin, sodium azide, nystatin and cyclohexamide in 5 per cent horse-blood agar is more successful for primary isolation.[70]

Haemophilus somnus is both factor X (protoporphyrin, or protohaeme) and factor V (nicotinamide adenosine dinucleotide or NAD) independent, whereas most other *Haemophilus* spp. require the heat-stable factor X and/or the heat-labile factor V for *in vitro* growth.[68] The colonies are about 1–2mm in diameter after two to three days' growth and are non-haemolytic, convex, circular and have a pale yellow colour. This colour of the colonies is more conspicuous when the colonies are raised on a bacteriological loop.[82] Identification of *H. somnus* is based on morphological and colonial characteristics, the fact that it is not dependent on either factors X or V, and biochemical testing (for these purposes reference should be made to *Bergey's Manual of Systematic Bacteriology*[45] and to a review of the organism[35]), as well as gel-diffusion tests with reference antisera,[71] disc electrophoresis of acid-phenol-soluble proteins[12] and an API ZYM system (API System S.A., La Balme les Grottes, France) which is a commercially available technique that measures bacterial enzyme activity.[12]

Epidemiology

Thrombotic meningoencephalitis has been recorded in North and South America, Europe, Russia, Japan, New

Zealand, South Africa and Zimbabwe.[21, 26, 35, 42, 50, 61, 78] The organism has been isolated from the respiratory and reproductive tracts of cattle in North America, Europe and South Africa.[7, 35] Abortions in cattle as a result of *H. somnus* infection have been reported in several countries,[25, 75] but have not yet been diagnosed in South Africa.

Cattle between one and three years of age which have been in a feedlot for four weeks or longer are more likely to develop TME.[5, 42, 67] However, the disease has also been diagnosed in calves less than four months of age, in adult dairy animals[67] and in cattle on pasture.[62, 78] It is most prevalent during the winter months,[42, 51,] and may be associated with recent transportation,[51, 62] while the mixing of cattle from different sources may also enhance the possibility of outbreaks.[67]

Potentially, *H. somnus* can be an important cause of mortality in feedlots.[35] A survey of feedlot cattle in Ontario, Canada in 1983 indicated that the population mortality rate due to TME was about 0,1 per cent of all feedlot animals, while 12 per cent of overall cattle mortality was due to this condition.[35]

In another survey in a large feedlot in Saskatchewan, haemophilosis was determined to be the most significant cause of mortality in calves.[79] Common manifestations of fatal *H. somnus* infection were myocarditis and pleuritis, occasionally TME, peracute septicaemia, and pneumonia, while circumstantial evidence suggested that *H. somnus* may have been a pathogen in polyarthritis. Deaths from pneumonia occurred mainly during the first five weeks in the feedlot, while those from myocarditis, pleuritis, TME, septicaemia, and euthanasia because of polyarthritis occurred mainly after the third week in the feedlot.

The respiratory syndrome is most common in calves under four months of age, but also occurs in feedlot cattle and adults.[10, 67] Calves are most susceptible when passive immunity wanes.[9] Respiratory disease is most prevalent in spring and summer.[67] It has been suggested that *H. somnus* infection may be part of the 'shipping fever' or bovine respiratory disease complex of feedlot cattle.[25, 35, 67, 69]

Several studies have indicated that subclinical carriers of *H. somnus* probably play an important role in the epidemiology of the disease syndromes attributed to the organism, as they act as potential reservoirs of infection. That *H. somnus* is maintained in the reproductive and respiratory tracts is suggested by the fact that it is isolated from these sites in healthy cattle with relative frequency.[7, 10, 33, 34, 66] It seems that the organism is harboured in the reproductive tract more frequently than it is in the upper respiratory tract of healthy animals,[10] while it can be isolated from the prepuce of a much higher percentage of bulls than it can from the vagina of cows.[10, 33–35, 50] In one study of healthy cattle, cultures made from the prepuce, vagina and nasal cavity showed that 61 per cent, 15 per cent and 1,2 per cent respectively were positive for *H. somnus*.[10] Similar results were obtained in an abattoir survey of the urogenital tract of normal bulls while, in addition, *H. somnus* was recovered from the bladder, accessory sex glands and ampullae of about 20 per cent of the animals.[50]

In an endemic region it has been shown that as many as 40–60 per cent of cows in an asymptomatic herd may carry the genital infection and that calves pick up the infection soon after birth so that by the time they are seven months of age, they are also carriers of *H. somnus* in their genital tracts.[50] In addition, up to 50 per cent or more of healthy animals may be seropositive.[14, 15, 25, 31, 50, 65]

Little seems to be known about the possible role that fomites play in the spread of infection. *Haemophilus somnus* can survive for more than 70 days in secretions and discharges at freezing temperatures. At summer temperatures in Canada it may survive for more than 70 days when mixed with blood and nasal mucus, but it survives for less than 15 minutes in urine.[14, 50] Despite this latter short survival period, it is thought that it is not sufficient to impede transmission by inhalation of urinary aerosols in cattle kept in close contact with each other.[50] The respiratory system seems to be the most likely route of infection in natural cases of the disease,[13, 25] with animals becoming infected by inhaling aerosols containing the organism. In addition to inhalation, other possible means of transmission from the urogenital tracts of infected animals are by ingestion (licking) and venereally.[35]

Pathogenesis

The exact pathogenetic mechanisms involved in naturally occurring *H. somnus*-induced disease syndromes have not been established; nor have the reasons why so few animals which do become infected manifest clinical signs or lesions. There does not appear to be any correlation between animals' susceptibility to the experimentally induced disease and serum antibody levels.[23, 72] While differences in virulence of various *H. somnus* isolates have been shown to exist in *in vivo* and *in vitro* experiments,[23, 50] no differences between strains based on morphological, cultural, biochemical, electrophoretic and serological criteria have been reported.[25, 54] The possibility that virulence is lost in subcultured organisms has been considered.[50, 73] Isolates from the prepuce may be apathogenic or produce mild lesions, while those from the brain may experimentally cause severe nervous lesions but little evidence of pneumonia, and similarly those from the lung may cause severe pneumonia but few lesions in the brain.[23, 50]

Intranasal inoculation or aerosol exposure may result in transient fever and bacteraemia in the absence of clinical signs. *Haemophilus somnus* may possess specific adhesions for respiratory tract epithelium, and adherence to such epithelium may be an initial event in the pathogenesis of the disease.[35, 60] It seems probable that invasion of the surrounding tissues occurs after colonization of the respiratory mucosa, followed by bacteraemia or septicaemia, and eventual localization in distant organs and tissues.[25] The nature and severity of clinical signs will depend on the site(s) and extent of such localization. A possible alternative route for organisms invading the central nervous system from the reproductive tract via Batson's veins (*plexi venosi vertebralis*) has been suggested.[54, 55] Direct retrograde spread of infection from the orbital or nasal cavities and sinuses to intracranial veins should also be considered as a posible pathogenetic mechanism in TME.

Experimentally, although syndromes resembling those of the natural disease may be produced by inoculation of the bacterium by several different routes, the results obtained are not always predictable.[50] Thrombotic meningoencephalitis may be experimentally reproduced following the intravenous, intracarotid and intracisternal administration of the organisms.[35, 50, 62] It has been shown that while there does seem to be a predilection for the central nervous system following intravenous administration, this is not an inevitable site of localization. Other preferential sites of localization are the cerebrospinal fluid, kidneys and urine, with smaller numbers being present in other organs.[35, 73] Thrombotic meningoencephalitis has not been reproduced by the administration of the bacterium by other routes, such as intratracheal, intraperitoneal or intramuscular, which supports the hypothesis that a bacteraemia or septicaemia is an essential feature in the pathogenesis of the nervous syndrome and probably also of many of the other syndromes.

The pneumonic syndrome has been more successfully reproduced following intratracheal or intrabronchial installation of virulent strains of *H. somnus* than it has following nasal installation, aerosol exposure or intravenous inoculation.[10, 23]

Abortion has been caused after the inoculation of *H. somnus* into the middle uterine artery and into the amnion[54, 55] of pregnant cows as well as by the jugular intravenous route.[81] A severe metritis and abortion may result after intracervical inoculation.[35] Introduction of *H. somnus* into the uterus or cervix of non-pregnant cows may cause transient endometritis, cervicitis, vaginitis or vulvitis with persistence of the organism, particularly in the major vestibular glands.[46]

The primary lesion in the pathological process is considered to be damage to the endothelial cells of small vessels, which predisposes to vasculitis, thrombosis, ischaemic necrosis (infarction) and haemorrhage.[5, 77] Bacteria are often observed in the thrombi, and there is an intense neutrophilic response around the affected blood vessels and in the necrotic tissue of the infarcts. The probable pathogenetic role that the initial endothelial cell damage plays has been confirmed in *in vitro* organ cultures of segments of arteries infected with *H. somnus*.[77] It has been shown that many bacteria become adherent to the endothelial cells and that widespread contraction and desquamation of these cells occur, which exposes large areas of subendothelial collagen.[77] It is suggested that the exposed collagen initiates the clotting cascade through activation of factor XII, the Hageman factor, and allows the organism direct access to the underlying tissue.[50, 77] Disseminated intravascular coagulation has been demonstrated in natural cases of *H. somnus* infection and it has been suggested that it might play a role in the pathogenesis of the disease.[56]

It has been established that bovine neutrophils are able to phagocytose opsonized *H. somnus* in an *in vitro* system but fail to kill them.[13] Soluble bacterial fractions from *H. somnus* inhibit neutrophil ingestion of opsonized *Staphylococcus aureus* and iodination of protein.[32] In addition, monocytes and alveolar macrophages phagocytose opsonized organisms; but not only do they fail to kill them, the organisms can actually multiply and persist in these cells,[49] which suggests that these cell types may play a role in the pathogenesis of the disease.

Clinical signs

The most common clinical syndromes associated with *H. somnus* involve the central nervous, respiratory and reproductive systems, and joints.[35, 46] In addition, the organism may also occasionally cause mastitis,[27, 30] conjunctivitis,[47, 58] otitis[58] and myocarditis.[24]

Thrombotic meningoencephalitis

The thrombotic meningoencephalitic syndrome is considered to be the outcome of the peracute or acute septicaemic form of the disease. In some animals, however, evidence of respiratory disease may precede or accompany the nervous signs.[35, 51, 62, 67]

The occurrence of sudden deaths or animals being found moribund may herald an outbreak of TME.[5, 21, 35] In the very early stage animals show a high fever (up to 42° C) and often profound depression,[25] the latter being the most important clinical finding. Other early signs are reluctance to move, stiffness of the legs and knuckling of the fetlocks.[25, 35, 42] Evidence of involvement of the nervous system soon widens to include such signs as muscle tremors, blindness, excitement, irritability, circling, ataxia, paresis, paralysis and paddling movements.[35] Affected animals generally become comatose in the terminal stages.[35, 42, 51]

During the course of the disease, the preservation and pupillary light reflexes of the eyes may be absent,[80] and ophthalmoscopic examination may reveal the presence of scattered focal retinal haemorrhages with ill-defined borders which, when present, provide a reliable presumptive diagnosis. Hyphaema and hypopyon may also be present.[16, 35]

Animals suffering from the advanced neurological syndrome invariably die,[40] but those treated in the very early stage of clinical disease may recover, although in some recovered cases mild neurological signs may persist.[43]

Other clinical signs indicative of localization of *H. somnus* in tissues or organs other than the central

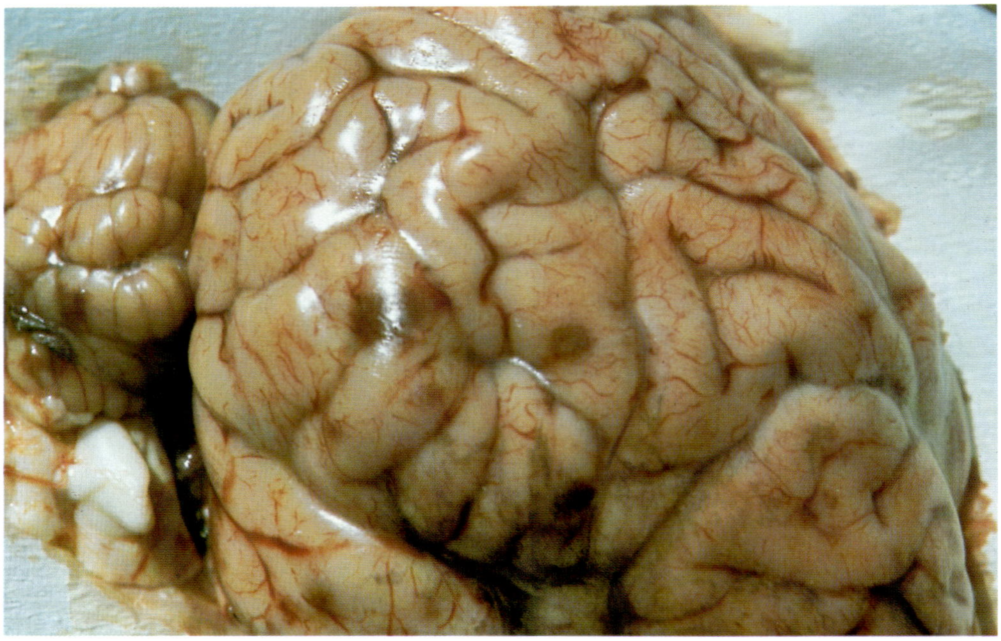

Figure 135.1 Multifocal infarction in the brain of an ox that died of TME due to *Haemophilus somnus* infection

nervous system may be present,[25, 35] both in the acute and the more protracted or subacute disease. These are represented, for example, by the presence of one or more swollen joints due to arthritis resulting in lameness and stiffness, or by myocardial involvement, or sudden death as a result of acute heart failure.[25]

Respiratory disease syndrome

Apart from the respiratory signs present in some cases of TME, a syndrome characterized by acute fibrinous pneumonia with or without an accompanying pleuritis is associated with *H. somnus* infections, particularly in calves but also sometimes in older cattle.[2, 64, 67] Other bacteria, particularly *Actinomyces pyogenes*, *Pasteurella haemolytica* and *Pasteurella multocida* increase the severity of the pneumonia as secondary invaders.[68] In addition to the pneumonic syndrome, *H. somnus* can cause laryngitis[25] as well as tracheitis, which results in chronic coughing.[35]

Reproductive disease syndromes

Haemophilus somnus has been isolated from the genital tract of cows with metritis, endometritis, vaginitis and infertility,[7, 74, 80] as well as from aborted foetuses and their placentas.[67, 75, 80] Spontaneous abortion due to *H. somnus* is generally sporadic rather than occurring as an 'abortion storm', and usually occurs between the seventh and ninth months of gestation. It is associated with retention of the placenta and a severe placentitis.[46] The abortion rate may vary from 3 to 12 per cent.[80]

Although *H. somnus* can frequently be isolated from the semen, prepuce and elsewhere in the urogenital system of bulls without any indication of disease,[7, 34] the organism has been associated with a purulent ejaculate.[11] Suppurative orchitis associated with *H. somnus* has been encountered in two calves.[44, 53]

Other disease syndromes

Spontaneously developing cases of acute mastitis have been reported in cows with persistent clinical signs due to resistance of *H. somnus* to antibiotic therapy.[3, 30] Acute gangrenous mastitis and chronic mastitis have been produced by inoculation of the organism into the udder.[28] In the case of the chronic form of the disease, affected cows shed the bacterium in their milk for up to a year. In contrast to this, *H. somnus* has been isolated from the milk of a cow suffering from mastitis which responded well to antibiotic therapy.[20]

Outbreaks of otitis externa have been described in feedlot cattle in Canada,[52, 58] and *H. somnus* has been isolated in pure culture and in large numbers from two of the affected animals. Morbidity is generally low, but can reach 10 per cent in some feedlots. The otitis is generally unilateral, but may be bilateral. The affected ear is held lower than normal and there is a copious serous discharge to the externum. There may or may not be concurrent respiratory disease, but in many outbreaks there is not, and TME has not occurred at the same time in affected herds. Sudden death due to a unilateral suppurative otitis media and interna and meningitis has been noted in a heifer.[48]

A case has been described of pyelonephritis in a cow from which *H. somnus* was cultured.[48]

Pathology

Haematological examination of both the naturally occurring and experimentally induced TME reveals that there is an initial neutropenia followed by a neutrophilia.[35, 59]

Macroscopically, in animals that have died from TME, the characteristic lesions are multiple infarcts which present as reddish-brown foci of haemorrhagic necrosis, varying in diameter from pin-point to 40 mm, in the central nervous system **(Figure 135.1)**.[42, 62, 73] The extent and distribution of these infarcts in the brain and spinal cord are variable, but they occur in both the grey and white matter. In some animals most of the foci are very small (sometimes microscopic) and occur mainly in the spinal cord, while in others only a few very large lesions are present. Lesions may be more prevalent in the thalamus, subthalamic nuclei and cerebrum, frequently near the junction of the grey and white matter.[62]

Accompanying focal fibrinopurulent meningitis may be associated with infarcts, or meningitis may be more diffuse.[62] Fibrinopurulent meningitis in the absence of encephalitic lesions may also occur.[36] The cerebrospinal fluid is usually cloudy, yellowish-tinged and contains flocculent debris, and it may coagulate within minutes on exposure to air.[62] Analysis of the cerebrospinal fluid may disclose a pleocytosis, with neutrophils predominating, increased globulin content, and a total protein content greater than 200 mg/100 ml, while the glucose content may be very depressed.[51]

The pathology and other aspects of disease produced by *H. somnus* have been reviewed by Humphrey and Stephens.[35] In cases of TME, gross lesions are frequently present in tissues and organ systems other than those of the central nervous system. These include, *inter alia*, fibrinopurulent polyarthritis and synovitis; rhinitis; sinusitis; necrotizing or ulcerative laryngitis; fibrinonecrotic tracheitis; exudative or interstitial pneumonia;[1] serofibrinous pleuritis, pericarditis and peritonitis; enteritis; infarcts in the myocardium[24, 38] and kidneys; and regional or generalized lymphadenitis as evidenced by enlargement, congestion, oedema and haemorrhage of the affected lymph nodes.[62]

Microscopically, the lesions in TME are typified by severe vasculitis, thrombosis with or without infarction, and a cellular exudate composed almost entirely of neutrophils.[62] Such lesions are seen consistently in the brain and cerebral meninges but may be present in many other tissues, such as the myocardium, kidneys, skeletal musculature, liver, thymus, urinary bladder, and optic tract and retina.[35, 38, 51, 62] Large numbers of Gram-negative coccobacilli are often present in some of the smaller thrombosed blood vessels.[35, 42, 51]

Several forms of pneumonia have been described in calves which have suffered from the respiratory disease syndrome caused by *H. somnus* and that are unassociated with TME.[35] The experience of Humphrey and Stephens[35] is that the pneumonia frequently presents as a severe, acute fibrinohaemorrhagic bronchopneumonia and fibrinous pleuritis resembling those seen in *Pasteurella haemolytica* infections. Histologically in acute cases there is extensive alveolar and interstitial fibrin deposition, haemorrhage, vascular thrombosis, pulmonary necrosis, and an intense alveolar and interstitial leukocyte infiltration. A necrotizing bronchiolitis may also be present.[1] Lung lesions resembling those of the natural disease have been reproduced experimentally by introducing *H. somnus* into the bronchi or trachea of calves.[18, 37, 63]

There are few studies relating to the lesions produced by *H. somnus* in the reproductive tract of cattle and in aborted foetuses and their membranes.[35, 46, 54, 55] Gross lesions that have been observed are oedema and necrosis of cotyledons in the placenta, and pronounced, diffuse oedema of the foetal extremities. Microscopically, fibrinoid necrosis of arteries of the placenta may be present and the foetus may show vascular necrosis, thrombosis and leukocytosis of the vessels in the brain, lungs, myocardium and renal glomeruli, infiltration of neutrophils into the alveoli of the lungs and bronchioli, interstitial pneumonia and myocarditis.

The vaginitis, cervicitis and endometritis in both the naturally occurring and experimentally induced disease seem to be mainly of a purulent nature.

Diagnosis and differential diagnosis

Since infection by *H. somnus* can present as a variety of non-specific syndromes, clinical differentiation of these syndromes from others of different aetiology may be difficult.[25] Thrombotic meningoencephalitis may be confused clinically with conditions such as viral encephalitides (e.g. rabies, and meningoencephalitis caused by bovine herpesvirus-1), heartwater, cerebral redwater, cerebral theileriosis, listeriosis, sporadic bovine encephalomyelitis caused by *Chlamydia psittaci*, bacterial meningitis caused, for example, by *Pasteurella haemolytica* or *P. multocida*, pituitary or cerebral abscessation, polioencephalomalacia (or cerebrocortical necrosis) caused by a deficiency of thiamine, and certain intoxications, for example, lead poisoning, botulism (lamsiekte), diplodiosis, *Aspergillus clavatus* mycotoxicosis, and pesticide poisoning.

Two important clinical findings which may help to differentiate some of these diseases are the very profound depression[25] or somnolence (hence the coining of the term 'sleeper syndrome') which commences in the early stages of TME, and the focal retinal haemorrhages visible on ophthalmoscopic examination which, when present, provide a reliable presumptive diagnosis.[16, 35] Depression of such severity that affected animals are described as 'drowsy' or having the appearance of being drugged has been noted in *Ornithogalum* spp. (chinkerinchee) and *Matricaria nigellifolia* poisonings.[39] The blindness that occurs in cattle poisoned by chinkerinchee is, however, an amaurosis. Amaurosis in cattle may also occur in cerebrocortical necrosis and lead poisoning.

From a pathological viewpoint the haemorrhagic infarcts in the central nervous system in TME are considered to be characteristic and are macroscopically visible in the majority of cases. Thrombosis and infarcts are also present in the central nervous system of animals suffering from cerebral theileriosis; differentiation between the two diseases is accomplished by the microscopical detection, in the case of cerebral theileriosis, of Koch's bodies in smears made from the contents of thrombosed blood vessels, or by histopathology.

The 'sudden death' syndrome in haemophilosis that results in death from acute heart failure following focal myocardial infarction should be differentiated from other possible causes of this syndrome in feedlot cattle, such as acute pneumonic pasteurellosis, blackquarter, ruminal acidosis and tympany, and poisonings (e.g. urea and salinomycin poisonings).

The respiratory disease syndrome caused by *H. somnus* should primarily be differentiated from the 'shipping fever' complex, but as this cannot readily be achieved on clinical or pathological grounds, a definitive diagnosis rests on the results of bacteriological examination of pneumonic lesions. It should be borne in mind that *H. somnus*, when cultured, is a relatively slow grower and may be outgrown by other bacteria such as *Pasteurella* spp. when mixed infections are present in pneumonic lesions, as is frequently the case. Use of a selective medium is therefore advocated, such as the one incorporating vancomycin (5 µg/ml), neomycin (5 µg/ml), sodium azide (50 µg/ml), nystatin (100 iu/ml) and cyclohexamide (100 µg/ml) into 5 per cent horse-blood agar.[70]

While the clinical signs and history may be helpful in making a tentative diagnosis of TME, confirmation of it depends on histopathological and bacteriological examination of the affected tissues. Bacteriological examination of the blood and cerebrospinal fluid in clinical cases yields *H. somnus* inconsistently.[25, 73] The organism does not survive for a prolonged period in commonly used transport media.[8, 25] Swabs for bacterial culture should be kept moist and if possible refrigerated, and they should be transported rapidly to the laboratory.[25]

The use of serological tests for the diagnosis of clinical cases of haemophilosis is equivocal. It is not known whether *H. somnus* carrier animals have antibody titres or if they are immune to TME.[72] In herds in which TME has been diagnosed, more than 50 per cent of normal cattle may be seropositive, indicating that while TME is generally sporadic, most animals that become infected do not show evidence of the disease. Even rising antibody titres in successive examinations do not necessarily provide meaningful evidence, as this phenomenon has also been detected in asymptomatic cattle.[25, 35]

Another problem in the interpretation of serological data is lack of specificity, as *H. somnus* cross-reacts with other bacteria, such as other *Haemophilus* spp., *Actinobacillus lignieresii*, *Listeria monocytogenes*, *Bordetella bronchiseptica*, and others.[35, 73]

Serological tests used are the microagglutination test, tube agglutination tests, complement fixation test and ELISA.[25, 35] A technique for the identification of *H. somnus* antigen by the use of monoclonal antibodies has been described.[76]

Control

In vitro tests indicate that *H. somnus* is susceptible to most commonly used antimicrobials.[35] In animals suffering from TME, treatment must commence as early in the course of the disease as possible, as once neurological signs are well established, treatment is generally not successful. Oxytetracycline injected intravenously early in the course of TME is successful in preventing mortality.[25, 42]

In North America, where the disease is most prevalent, it is a standard recommendation in the event of an outbreak to increase surveillance and to institute immediate treatment with an antimicrobial. Mass medication with antibiotics in the feed, or the treatment of every animal in the group which contains affected animals with a long-acting antibiotic, has yielded variable results.[25]

A commercially produced vaccine (Somnugen, Boehringer Ingelheim, Burlington, Ontario) consisting of a bacterin containing killed whole bacteria in aluminium hydroxide adjuvant is available in North America and its use has yielded beneficial results.[22, 35, 57, 66, 72, 82] Good antibody responses have occurred when cationic and anionic components of the outer membranes of *H. somnus* were used as antigens in cattle. The latter provided complete protection against experimental challenge, while the cationic component did not,[35] which indicates that protection can not necessarily be equated with serum antibody levels.

References

1 **ANDREWS, J.J., ANDERSON, T.D., SLIFE, L.N. & STEVENSON, G.W., 1985.** Microscopic lesions associated with the isolation of *Haemophilus somnus* from pneumonic bovine lungs. *Veterinary Pathology*, 22, 131–136.

2 **ANDREWS, J.J., SLIFE, L.N. & STEVENSON, G.W., 1983.** Naturally occurring *Haemophilus somnus* pneumonia in cattle. *Proceedings of the Third International Meeting of Veterinary Laboratory Diagnosticians*, 377–384.

3 **ARMSTRONG, K.R., OSBORNE, A.D. & JANZEN, E.D., 1986.** *Haemophilus somnus* mastitis in a dairy cow. *Canadian Veterinary Journal*, 27, 211–212.

4 **BAILIE, W.E., 1969.** Characterization of *Haemophilus somnus* (new species), a microorganism isolated from infectious thromboembolic meningoencephalitis of cattle. *Dissertation Abstracts*, 30B: 2482.

5 **BAILIE, W.E., ANTHONY, H.D. & WEIDE, K.D., 1966.** Infectious thromboembolic meningoencephalitis (sleeper syndrome) in feedlot cattle. *Journal of the American Veterinary Medical Association*, 148, 162–166.

6 **BEEMAN, K.B., 1985.** *Haemophilus somnus* of cattle: An overview. *The Compendium on Continuing Education for the Practising Veterinarian*, 7, S259–S263.

7 **BISHOP, G.C. & KITCHING, J.P., 1992.** Allerton Regional Veterinary Laboratory, Pietermaritzburg. Unpublished data.

8 **BREWER, R.A., CORBEL, M.J. & STUART, F.A., 1985.** Development of improved methods for the transport and

isolation of *Haemophilus somnus*. *Research in Veterinary Science*, 39, 299–306.

9 **CORBEIL, L.B., WATT, B., CORBEIL, R., BENZEN, T.G., BROWNSON, R.K. & MORRIL, J.L., 1984.** Immunoglobulin concentrations in serum and nasal secretions of calves at the onset of pneumonia. *American Journal of Veterinary Research*, 45, 773–778.

10 **CORBEIL, L.B., WIDDERS, P.R., GOGLEWSKI, R., INZANA, I. & WARD, A.C.S., 1986.** *Haemophilus somnus*: Bovine reproductive and respiratory disease. *Canadian Veterinary Journal*, 27, 90–93.

11 **CORBOZ, L. & WILD, P., 1981.** Epidemiologie der *Haemophilus somnus*-Infektion beim Rind: Vergleich von Stämmen in der Polyacrylamidgel-Elektrophorese (PAGE). *Schweizer Archiv für Tierheilkunde*, 123, 79–88.

12 **COUSINS, D.V. & LLOYD, J.M., 1988.** Rapid identification of *Haemophilus somnus, Histophilus ovis* and *Actinobacillus seminis* using the API ZYM system. *Veterinary Microbiology*, 17, 75–81.

13 **CZUPRYNSKI, C.J. & HAMILTON, H.L., 1985.** Bovine neutrophils ingest but do not kill *Haemophilus somnus in vitro*. *Infection and Immunity*, 50, 431–436.

14 **DEWEY, K.J. & LITTLE, P.B., 1984.** Environmental survival of *H. somnus* and influence of secretions and excretions. *Canadian Journal of Comparative Medicine*, 48, 23–26.

15 **DIERKS, R.E., HANNA, S.A. & DILLMAN, R.C., 1973.** Epizootiology and pathogenesis of *Haemophilus somnus* infection. *Journal of the American Veterinary Medical Association*, 163, 866–869.

16 **DUKES, T.W., 1971.** The ocular lesions in thromboembolic meningoencephalitis (TEME) of cattle. *Canadian Veterinary Journal*, 12, 180–182.

17 **GARCIA-DELGADO, G.A., LITTLE, P.B. & BARNUM, D.A., 1977.** A comparison of various *Haemophilus somnus* strains. *Canadian Journal of Comparative Medicine*, 41, 380–388.

18 **GOGOLEWSKI, R.P., LEATHERS, C.W., LIGGITT, H.D. & CORBEIL, L.B., 1987.** Experimental *Haemophilus somnus* pneumonia in calves and immunoperoxidase localization of bacteria. *Veterinary Pathology*, 24, 250–256.

19 **GOSSLING, J., 1966.** The bacteria isolated from lesions of embolic meningoencephalitis of cattle. *Illinois Veterinarian*, 9, 14–18.

20 **GREER, D., McCONNELL, W. & BALL, H., 1989.** Isolation of *Haemophilus somnus* from bovine milk. *The Veterinary Record*, 125, 381–382.

21 **GRINER, L.A., JENSEN, R. & BROWN, W.W., 1956.** Infectious embolic meningo-encephalitis in cattle. *Journal of the American Veterinary Medical Association*, 129, 417–421.

22 **GROOM, S.C. & LITTLE, P.B., 1988.** Effects of vaccination of calves against induced *Haemophilus somnus* pneumonia. *American Journal of Veterinary Research*, 49, 793–800.

23 **GROOM, S.C., LITTLE, P.B. & ROSENDAL, S., 1988.** Virulence differences among three strains of *Haemophilus somnus* following intratracheal inoculation of calves. *Canadian Journal of Veterinary Research*, 52, 349–354.

24 **GUICHON, P.T., PRITCHARD, J. & JIM, G.K., 1988.** *Haemophilus somnus* myocarditis in a feedlot steer. *Canadian Veterinary Journal*, 29, 1012–1013.

25 **HARRIS, F.W. & JANZEN, E.D., 1989.** The *Haemophilus somnus* complex (Haemophilosis): A review. *Canadian Veterinary Journal*, 30, 816–822.

26 **HASE, M., 1984.** Outbreaks of *Haemophilus somnus* infection in cattle in Kagoshima Prefecture. *Journal of the Japan Veterinary Medical Association*, 37, 431–435.

27 **HAZLETT, M.J., LITTLE, P.B. & BARNUM, D.A., 1983.** Experimental production of mastitis with *Haemophilus somnus* in the lactating bovine mammary gland. *Canadian Veterinary Journal*, 24, 135.

28 **HAZLETT, M.J., LITTLE, P.B., BARNUM, D.A., MAXIE, M.G., LESLIE, K.E. & MILLER, R.B., 1985.** *Haemophilus somnus*: Investigations of its potential role in bovine mastitis. *American Journal of Veterinary Research*, 46, 2229–2234.

29 **HENTON, M.M., 1989.** Veterinary Research Institute, Onderstepoort. Unpublished data.

30 **HIGGINS, R., MARTIN, J.R., LAROUCHE, Y. & GOYETTE, G., 1987.** Mastitis caused by *Haemophilus somnus* in a dairy cow. *Canadian Veterinary Journal*, 28, 117–118.

31 **HOERLEIN, A.B., GOTO, K. & YOUNG, S., 1973.** *Haemophilus somnus* agglutinins in cattle. *Journal of the American Veterinary Medical Association*, 163, 1375–1377.

32 **HUBBARD, R.D., KAEBERLE, M.L., ROTH, J.A. & CHIANG, Y.W., 1986.** *Haemophilus somnus*-induced interference with bovine neutrophil functions. *Veterinary Microbiology*, 12, 77–85.

33 **HUMPHREY, J.D., LITTLE, P.B., BARNUM, D.A. DOIG, P.A., STEPHENS, L.R. & THORSEN, J., 1982.** Occurrence of *Haemophilus somnus* in bovine semen and in the prepuce of bulls and steers. *Canadian Journal of Comparative Medicine*, 46, 215–217.

34 **HUMPHREY, J.D., LITTLE, P.B., STEPHENS, L.R., BARNUM, D.A., DOIG, P.A. & THORSEN, J., 1982.** Prevalence and distribution of *Haemophilus somnus* in the bovine reproductive tract. *American Journal of Veterinary Research*, 43, 791–795.

35 **HUMPHREY, J.D. & STEPHENS, L.R., 1983.** *Haemophilus somnus*: A review. *The Veterinary Bulletin*, 53, 987–1004.

36 **ISHIKAWA, Y., TSUKUDA, S. NAKAJIMA, Y. & OHSHIMA, K., 1984.** Atypical nervous lesion in *Haemophilus somnus* infection of cattle. *Cornell Veterinarian*, 74, 349–353.

37 **JACKSON, J.A., ANDREWS, J.J. & HARRIS, J.W., 1987.** Experimental *Haemophilus somnus* pneumonia in calves. *Veterinary Pathology*, 24, 129–134.

38 **JANZEN, E.D., 1987.** Myocardial lesions caused by *H. somnus* in cattle. *Canadian Veterinary Journal*, 28, 208.

39 **KELLERMAN, T.S., COETZER, J.A.W. & NAUDÉ, T.W., 1988.** *Plant Poisonings and Mycotoxicoses of Livestock in Southern Africa*. Cape Town: Oxford University Press.

40 **KENNEDY, P.C., BIBERSTEIN, E.L., HOWARTH, J.A., FRAZIER, L.M. & DUNGWORTH, D.L., 1960.** Infectious meningoencephalitis in cattle, caused by a *Haemophilus*-like organism. *American Journal of Veterinary Research*, 21, 403–409.

41 **KILIAN, M. & BIBERSTEIN, E.L., 1984.** Genus *Haemophilus*. *In*: KRIEG, N.R. & HOLT, J.G., (eds). *Bergey's Manual of Systematic Bacteriology*. Baltimore, London: Williams & Wilkins.

42 **KITCHING, J.P., BISHOP, G.C. & MAPHAM, P.H., 1985.** Thromboembolic meningoencephalitis diagnosed in Natal. *Journal of the South African Veterinary Association*, 56, 97–98.

43 **KITCHING, J.P., BISHOP, G.C. & MAPHAM, P.H., 1992.** Allerton Regional Veterinary Laboratory, Pietermaritzburg. Unpublished data.

44 **KREPLIN, C., 1991.** Suppurative orchitis associated with *Haemophilus somnus* in a calf. *Canadian Veterinary Journal*, 32, 567.

45 **KRIEG, N.R. & HOLT, J.G., 1984.** *Bergey's Manual of Systematic Bacteriology*. Baltimore, London: Williams & Wilkins.

46 **KWIECIEN, J.M. & LITTLE, P.B., 1991.** *Haemophilus somnus* and reproductive disease in the cow: A review. *Canadian Veterinary Journal*, 32, 595–601.

47 **LAMONT, H.H. & HUNT, B.W., 1982.** *Haemophilus somnus* and conjunctivitis. *The Veterinary Record*, 117, 21.

48 **LANE, M.V. & LEDER, R.L., 1988.** Unilateral nephrectomy for chronic *Haemophilus somnus*-associated nephritis in a cow. *Compendium on Continuing Education for the Practising Veterinarian*, 10, 522–525.

49 **LEDERER, J.A., BROWN, J.F. & CZUPRYNSKI, C.J., 1987.** *Haemophilus somnus*, a facultative intracellular pathogen of bovine mononuclear phagocytes. *Infection and Immunity*, 55, 381–387.

50 **LITTLE, P.B., 1986.** *Haemophilus somnus* complex: Pathogenesis of the septicaemic thrombotic meningoencephalitis.

Canadian Veterinary Journal, 27, 94–96.

51 **LITTLE, P.B. & SORENSEN, D.K., 1969.** Bovine polioencephalomalacia, infectious embolic meningoencephalitis, and acute lead poisoning in feedlot cattle. *Journal of the American Veterinary Medical Association*, 155, 1892–1903.

52 **McEWEN, S.A. & HULLAND, T.J., 1985.** *Haemophilus somnus*-induced otitis and meningitis in a heifer. *Canadian Veterinary Journal*, 26, 7–8.

53 **METZ, A.L., HAGGARD, D.L. & MAKOMAKI, M.R., 1984.** Chronic suppurative orchiepididymitis associated with *Haemophilus somnus* in a calf. *Journal of the American Veterinary Medical Association*, 184, 1507–1508.

54 **MILLER, R.B., LEIN, D.H., McENTEE, K.E., HALL, C.E. & SHIN, S., 1983.** *Haemophilus somnus* infection of the reproductive tract of cattle: A review. *Journal of the American Veterinary Medical Association*, 182, 1390–1392.

55 **MILLER, R.B., VAN CAMP, S.D. & BARNUM, D.A., 1983.** The effects of intra-amniotic inoculation of *Haemophilus somnus* on the bovine fetus and dam. *Veterinary Pathology*, 20, 574–583.

56 **MOMOTANI, E., YABUKI, Y., MIHO, H., ISHIKAWA, Y. & YOSHINO, T., 1985.** Histopathologic evaluation of disseminated intravascular coagulation in *Haemophilus somnus* infection in cattle. *Journal of Comparative Pathology*, 95, 15–23.

57 **MORTER, R.L. & AMSTUTZ, H.E., 1983.** Evaluating the efficacy of a *Haemophilus somnus* bacterin in a controlled field trial. *The Bovine Practitioner*, 18, 82–83.

58 **NATION, P.N., FRELIER, P.F., GIFFORD, G.A. & CARNAT, B.D., 1983.** Otitis in feedlot cattle. *Canadian Veterinary Journal*, 24, 238.

59 **NAYER, P.S.G., WARD, G.E., SAUNDERS, J.R. & MACWILLIAMS, P., 1977.** Diagnostic procedures in experimental *Haemophilus somnus* infection in cattle. *Canadian Veterinary Journal*, 18, 159–163.

60 **NIVARD, J.L., WARD, G.E., STEPHENS, J.B. & MAHESWARAN, S.K., 1982.** Model infection of the chicken embryo with *Haemophilus somnus*. *American Journal of Veterinary Research*, 43, 1790–1792.

61 **ODIAWO, G.O., OBIVOLO, J.M. & NDIKUWERA, J., 1990.** A case of bovine thromboembolic meningoencephalitis on two farms near Harare. *Bulletin of Animal Health and Production in Africa*, 38, 33–38.

62 **PANCIERA, R.J., DAHLGREN, R.R. & RINKER, H.B., 1968.** Observations on septicaemia of cattle caused by a *Haemophilus*-like organism. *Pathologia Veterinaria*, 5, 212–226.

63 **POTGIETER, L.N.D., HELMAN, R.G., GREENE, W., BREIDER, M.A., THURBER, E.T. & PEETZ, R.H., 1988.** Experimental bovine respiratory tract disease with *Haemophilus somnus*. *Veterinary Pathology*, 25, 124–130.

64 **PRITCHARD, D.G., SHREEVE, J. & BRADLEY, R., 1979.** The experimental infection of calves with a British strain of *Haemophilus somnus*. *Research in Veterinary Science*, 26, 7–11.

65 **SANFACON, D. & HIGGINS, R., 1983.** Epidemiology of *Haemophilus somnus* infection in dairy cattle in Quebec. *Canadian Journal of Comparative Medicine*, 47, 456–459.

66 **SAUNDERS, J.R. & JANZEN, E.D., 1980.** *Haemophilus somnus* infections. II. A Canadian field trial of a commercial bacterin: Clinical and serological results. *Canadian Veterinary Journal*, 21, 219–224.

67 **SAUNDERS, J.R., THIESSEN, W.A. & JANZEN, E.D., 1980.** *Haemophilus somnus* infections. I. A ten-year (1969–78) retrospective study of losses in cattle herds in western Canada. *Canadian Veterinary Journal*, 21, 119–123.

68 **SCANLAN, C.M., 1988.** *Introduction to Veterinary Bacteriology*, Ames, Iowa: Iowa State University Press.

69 **SCHIEFER, B., WARD, G.E. & MOFFAT, R.E., 1978.** Correlation of microbial and histological findings in bovine fibrinous pneumonia. *Veterinary Pathology*, 15, 313–321.

70 **SLEE, K.J. & STEPHENS, L.R., 1985.** Selective medium for isolation of *Haemophilus somnus* from cattle and sheep. *The Veterinary Record*, 116, 215–217.

71 **STEPHENS, L.R., HUMPHREY, J.D., LITTLE, P.B. & BARNUM, D.A., 1983.** Morphological, biochemical, antigenic, and cytochemical relationships among *Haemophilus somnus, Haemophilus agni, Haemophilus haemoglobinophilus, Histophilus ovis* and *Actinobacillus seminis*. *Journal of Clinical Microbiology*, 17, 728–737.

72 **STEPHENS, L.R., LITTLE, P.B., WILKIE, B.N. & BARNUM, D.A., 1981.** Humoral immunity in experimental thromboembolic meningoencephalitis in cattle caused by *Haemophilus somnus*. *American Journal of Veterinary Research*, 42, 468–475.

73 **STEPHENS, L.R., LITTLE, P.B., WILKIE, B.N. & BARNUM, D.A., 1981.** Infectious thromboembolic meningoencephalitis in cattle: A review. *Journal of the American Veterinary Medical Association*, 178, 378–384.

74 **STEPHENS, L.R., SLEE, K.J., POULTON, P., LARCOMBE, M. & KOSIOR, E., 1986.** Investigation of purulent vaginal discharge in cows, with particular reference to *Haemophilus somnus*. *Australian Veterinary Journal*, 63, 182–185.

75 **STUART, F.A., CORBEL, M.J., RICHARDSON, C., BREWER, R.A., BRADLEY, R. & BRIDGES, A.W., 1990.** Experimental *Haemophilus somnus* infection in pregnant cattle. *British Veterinary Journal*, 146, 57–67.

76 **THOMSON, M.S., LAUERMANN, L.H. & WILT, G.R., 1990.** Monoclonal antibody in the identification of *Haemophilus somnus*. *Journal of Veterinary Diagnostic Investigation*, 2, 116–119.

77 **THOMPSON, K.G. & LITTLE, P.B., 1981.** Effect of *Haemophilus somnus* on bovine endothelial cells in organ culture. *American Journal of Veterinary Research*, 42, 748–754.

78 **THOMPSON, K.G., VICKERS, M.C., STEVENSON, B.J. & DAVIDSON, G.W., 1987.** Thromboembolic meningoencephalitis caused by *Haemophilus somnus* in a bull calf — a new disease in New Zealand. *New Zealand Veterinary Journal*, 35, 5–7.

79 **VAN DONKERSGOED, J., JANZEN, E.D. & HARLAND, R.J., 1990.** Epidemiological features of calf mortality due to haemophilosis in a large feedlot. *Canadian Veterinary Journal*, 31, 821–825.

80 **VAN DREUMEL, A.A. & KIERSTEAD, M., 1975.** Abortion associated with *Haemophilus somnus* infection in a bovine fetus. *Canadian Veterinary Journal*, 16, 367–370.

81 **WIDDERS, P.R., PAISLY, I.G., GOGOLEWSKI, R.P., EVERMANN, J.F., SMITH, J.W. & CORBEIL, I.B., 1986.** Experimental abortion and the systemic immune response to *Haemophilus somnus* in cattle. *Infection and Immunity*, 54, 555–560.

82 **WILLIAMS, J.M., SMITH, G.L. & MURDOCK, F.M., 1978.** Immunogenicity of a *Haemophilus somnus* bacterin in cattle. *American Journal of Veterinary Research*, 39, 1756–1762.

Actinobacillus *spp. infections*

M.M. Henton

Actinobacillus spp. cause a variety of diseases in livestock **(Table 1)**, although most are relatively uncommon in southern Africa. Of these diseases, epididymitis and orchitis in rams (caused by *A. seminis*), sleepy foal disease (caused by *A. equuli*), porcine pleuropneumonia (caused by *A. pleuropneumoniae*) and pyogranulomatous lesions of the soft tissues of the head—in particular the oral cavity — or the forestomachs of cattle, sheep and goats (caused by *A. lignieresii*) occur most commonly.[1]

Actinobacillus spp. are closely related to bacteria of two other genera, *Pasteurella* and *Haemophilus*. These three genera are grouped together in the family Pasteurellaceae, the members of which are obligate parasites of vertebrates.[5, 7] They particularly favour the mucous membranes of the respiratory tract, but some species also infect the genital and alimentary tracts. Pathogenic strains of these bacteria are part of the normal microbial flora on the mucous membranes of healthy animals, albeit in low numbers.[6] Bacteria that belong to the Pasteurellaceae grow slowly and are easily overgrown by the other bacteria in the normal flora that populate the mucous membranes. Selective media are therefore required for their isolation.

Actinobacillus spp. are labile in the environment, and are particularly susceptible to dessication.[2]

Actinobacillus spp. are Gram-negative, non-motile, pleomorphic rods interspersed with coccal forms, giving a 'Morse code' appearance. They ferment sugars,

Table 1 Diseases caused by *Actinobacillus* spp. in livestock

ACTINOBACILLUS SPP.	ANIMAL SPECIES AFFECTED	MOST COMMON DISEASES
A. lignieresii	Cattle, sheep, goats	Pyogranulomatous lesions of particularly the soft tissues of the head, oral cavity, and forestomachs
	Pigs	Pyogranulomatous lesions of the teats and udder, septicaemia (piglets)
A. equuli	Horses	Neonatal septicaemia (sleepy foal disease), abortion (rare), other purulent infections (rare)
	Pigs	Neonatal septicaemia, metritis, abortion, abscesses
A. suis	Pigs	Neonatal septicaemia
	Horses	Neonatal septicaemia
A. seminis	Sheep (rarely goats and cattle)	Epididymitis, orchitis, vaginitis
A. actinomycetemcomitans	Sheep	Epididymitis, orchitis
Actinobacillus sp. 'Ross'	Pigs	Normal in vagina (pathogenic potential unclear)

Table 2 Biochemical characteristics of *Actinobacillus* spp.

	A. EQUULI	*A. LIGNIERESII*	*A. PLEUROPNEUMONIAE*	*A. SUIS*	*A. A COMITANS A. SEMINIS*	*A.* SP. 'ROSS'
Beta-haemolysis	−	−	+	+	−	+
Staphylococcus-dependent	−	−	+	−	−	−
Growth on McConkey	+	+	−	+	−	d
Catalase	d	d	d	+	+(−)	+
Urease	+	+	+	+	−	+
Trehalose	+	−	−	+	−	−
Mannitol	+	+	+	−	+(−)	+
Aesculin hydrolysis	−	−	−	+	−	−

d 11–89 per cent of species are positive
+(−) most strains positive, a few are negative

producing acid but no gas, and they reduce nitrates to nitrites.[9] They are indole-negative.

Actinobacillus equuli, A. lignieresii and *A. suis* grow readily on ordinary bacterial growth media.[9] Growth in primary cultures made from lesions is often sparse, and adding blood or serum to the media, and incubation in an atmosphere consisting of 5–10 per cent CO_2 in air aids isolation.[9] However, *A. pleuropneumoniae* requires a *Staphylococcus* feeder culture or a nicotinamide adenine dinucleotide (NAD) supplement in media intended for its growth.[4]

Actinobacillus colonies are small, greyish and usually 'sticky' on primary isolation. If touched with a wire loop, a mucoid string is formed between the loop and the colony. This characteristic is most marked in *A. equuli*,[9] but it may be lost on repeated subculture. When a broth culture of *A. equuli* is swirled, the growth at the bottom of the tube twists in a mucoid, ropy spiral.[3, 9]

Distinguishing biochemical characteristics of the *Actinobacillus* spp. are rather variable **(Table 2)**, and many isolates are not easily identifiable.[7–9] As the antigens of *Actinobacillus* spp. are complex, the results of serotyping by different methods may produce conflicting results. For this reason the results of serotyping should be interpreted with care.[9]

References

1 **BIBERSTEIN, E.L., 1981.** *Haemophilus–Pasteurella–Actinobacillus*: Their significance in veterinary medicine. *In*: KILIAN, M., FREDERIKSEN, W. & BIBERSTEIN, E.L. (eds). *Haemophilus, Pasteurella and Actinobacillus*. London, New York, Toronto, Sydney, San Francisco: Academic Press, Inc.

2 **BIBERSTEIN, E.L., 1990.** Our understanding of the Pasteurellaceae. *Canadian Journal of Veterinary Research*, 54 (suppl.), S78–S82.

3 **COTTEW, G.S. & RILEY, J.W., 1952.** *Shigella equirulis* infection in a foal. *Australian Veterinary Journal*. 28, 302–306.

4 **KILIAN, M., 1976.** A taxonomic study of the genus *Haemophilus*, with the proposal of a new species. *Journal of General Microbiology*. 93, 9–62.

5 **KILIAN, M. & BIBERSTEIN, E.L., 1984.** *Haemophilus*. *In*: KRIEG, N.R. & HOLT, J.G., (eds). *Bergey's Manual of Systematic Bacteriology*. Vol. I. Baltimore, London: Williams & Wilkins.

6 **KILIAN, M. & FREDERIKSEN, W., 1981.** Ecology of *Haemophilus, Pasteurella* and *Actinobacillus*. *In*: KILIAN, M., FREDERIKSEN, W. & BIBERSTEIN, E.L., (eds). *Haemophilus, Pasteurella and Actinobacillus*. London, New York, Toronto, Sydney, San Francisco: Academic Press, Inc.

7 **MANNHEIM, W., 1984.** *Pasteurellaceae*. *In*: KRIEG, N.R. & HOLT, J.G., (eds). *Bergey's Manual of Systematic Bacteriology*, Vol. I. Baltimore, London: Williams & Wilkins.

8 **MUTTERS, R., MANNHEIM, W. & BISGAARD, M., 1989.** Taxonomy of the group. *In*: ADLAM, C. & RUTTER, J.M., (eds). *Pasteurella and Pasteurellosis*. London, San Diego, New York, Berkeley, Boston, Sydney, Tokyo, Toronto: Academic Press, Inc.

9 **PHILLIPS, J.E., 1984.** *Actinobacillus*. *In*: KRIEG, N.R. & HOLT, J.G., (eds). *Bergey's Manual of Systematic Bacteriology*. Vol. I. Baltimore, London: Williams & Wilkins.

136

Actinobaccillus lignieresii infections

Synonyms: Actinobacillosis, wooden tongue, houttong (Afrik.)

M.M. Henton

Introduction and aetiology

Actinobacillosis caused by *Actinobacillus lignieresii* is a ubiquitous, but usually sporadic, disease of cattle, sheep and goats. The disease is generally chronic and is characterized by pyogranulomatous inflammation, particularly of the skin and other soft tissues of the head and mouth, and of the regional lymph nodes. Infection in the tongue of cattle, a common site in this species, induces a marked fibroplastic response that gives the disease its common name, 'wooden tongue'. The bacterium occasionally causes abscesses or granulomas in the teats and udders of sows.[8]

The cultural, morphological and other characteristics of *A. lignieresii* are outlined in the ***Actinobacillus* spp. infections: Introduction**.

Epidemiology, pathogenesis, clinical signs and pathology

Actinobacillus lignieresii occurs as a commensal of the oral mucosae of ruminants in particular. Disease may follow injury to the mucous membranes in cattle, sheep and goats. Such injuries might be caused by coarse feeds, grass awns, or teeth abrasions or eruptions. Injuries to the skin, such as those inflicted by thorns and tick bites, may also lead to disease. In cattle the disease tends to occur sporadically, with only single cases being encountered, but in sheep it may occur as outbreaks involving several or many animals in a flock. Because of the differences in prehension of feed between cattle and sheep (cattle use their tongues, while sheep use their lips and generally feed with their heads closer to the ground), the lesions in cattle occur most frequently in the tissues of the tongue. The site of entry of the organisms is often the lingual groove because of injuries to the tongue epithelium that have followed the entrapment there of sharp objects, such as the awns of grasses. Lesions in sheep, on the other hand, tend to occur initially in the cutaneous and subcutaneous tissues of the lips and cheeks, with multiple cases occurring in sheep as a result of the nature of the feed.[11] In one outbreak, sheep that had been fed the leaves of prickly pears (*Opuntia* sp.) developed lesions in the mouth, pharynx, and forestomachs.[10]

In cattle, sheep and goats, pyogranulomas caused by *A. lignieresii* occur most commonly in the soft tissues of the head and oral cavity and less commonly in other sites such as the forestomachs, lungs and skin. Lesions spread by extension, as well as via the lymphatic system to regional lymph nodes which are frequently affected and become enlarged and firm. The lesions are initially hard, circumscribed nodules, varying in size from a few to several millimetres in diameter. Some eventually become soft and fluctuate, discharging their contents through the skin or mucous membrane, leaving deep ulcers or fistulae **(Figures 136.1 and 136.2)**. These lesions may expand and extend into surrounding tissues. When the tongue is involved, part of the organ becomes indurated, enlarged and immobile. This interferes with mastication and deglutition, and results in salivation and loss of weight. In some, the surface of the tongue becomes unevenly elevated. In severe cases the enlarged tongue may protrude from the mouth. Similarly, when the skin and subcutaneous tissues of the lips, cheeks and submandibular region of the head of sheep are affected, the thickened indurated lesions interfere progressively with prehension and mastication of feed, and animals gradually starve to death.

Abscesses and granulomas may occur in the teats and udders of sows as a result of small wounds inflicted by the sharp teeth of sucking pigs.

Other bacteria such as *Actinomyces (Corynebacterium) pyogenes*, *Streptococcus* spp. and *Pseudomonas aeruginosa* are commonly found together with *A. lignieresii* in lesions, and it is likely that they all gain entry to tissues in the same way.

The lesions are pyogranulomatous and contain barely visible colonies of the organism. In some lesions, or parts of lesions, the granulation tissue is hard and firm and somewhat resembles a fibroma,[4] the colonies standing out as yellowish-white specks which are referred to as 'sulphur granules'; in others the affected tissue has a nodular appearance and has more numerous granules dispersed in the fibromatous connective tissue. Lesions may coalesce to form large nodules which may be of a softer consistency and which show evidence, on cut surface, of suppuration and consequently abscessation.

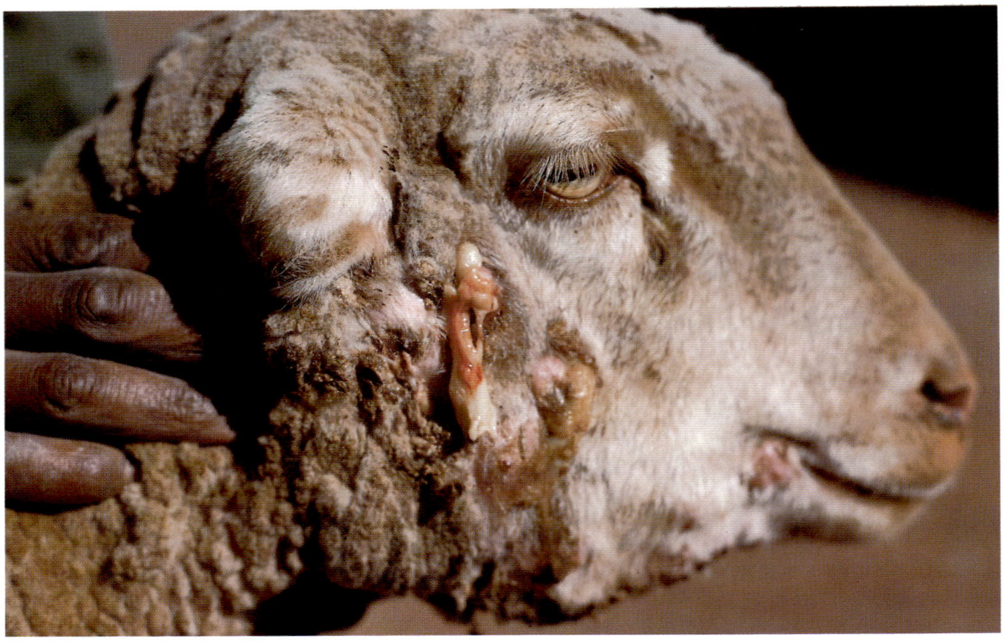

Figure 136.1 Multiple abscesses in the skin of the face and oral commissure of a sheep. Note the yellowish-green, blood-stained, tenacious pus

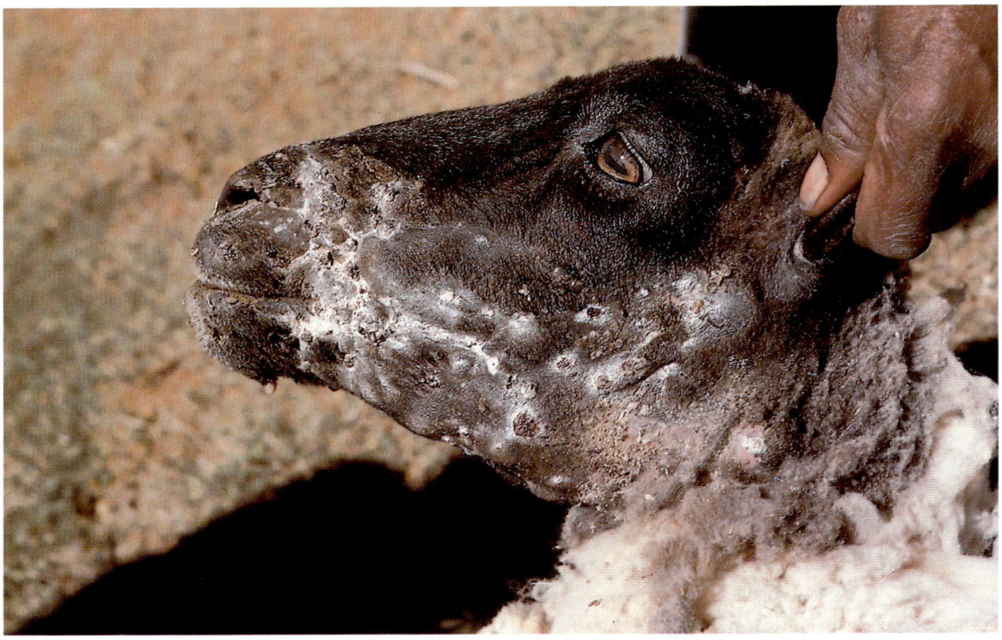

Figure 136.2 Extensive scarring of the skin of the face of a sheep following healing of lesions caused by *Actinobacillus lignieresii*

The pus is thick, mucoid, greenish-yellow and odourless, and contains numerous granules which have the appearance of grains of sand. Ulcers and discharging fistulae and sinuses are sometimes formed when lesions break out into the lumen of hollow organs or to the externum. Frank abscessation does not often occur in tongue lesions.[4] Affected lymph nodes may contain only a few nodules or they may be considerably enlarged and oedematous. In long-standing cases the nodes are fibrous and nodular, the nodules containing greenish-yellow pus and characteristic granules.[4] Affected nodes, if superficially located, may adhere to the skin and some may form sinuses and discharge pus. Histologically, the sulphur granules consist of masses of coccobacilli which are embedded in a homogeneous eosinophilic material that has a palisaded outer circumference consisting of radiating finger-like or club-shaped structures. The coccobacilli stain negatively by Gram's method. Around the granules is a zone containing mainly neutrophils but also macrophages and a few giant cells. Lymphocytes and plasma cells occur peripherally in the encompassing fibrous connective tissue, which may be very dense in parts, and replace normal tissue structures in the vicinity.

Diagnosis and differential diagnosis

Actinobacillus lignieresii may be difficult to culture from pus, and only a few colonies may grow in primary cultures prepared from fresh lesions.[7] If sulphur granules are present, the pus should be vigorously shaken in sterile physiological saline in a test tube in order to liquify it. This enables the granules to sink to the bottom of the tube, where they may be collected and utilized either for the preparation of smears or for culturing.

For smears, granules are placed on a glass slide, crushed by firm application of a cover-slip and examined microscopically, either directly or after staining. The peripheral club-shaped structures, which are thought to consist of immune complexes, may be seen in both unstained and stained preparations. Gram's staining reveals the presence of the negatively staining coccobacilli in the centres of the granules, which are surrounded by radiating red-staining clubs.[3, 9] Granules used for the preparation of bacteriological cultures should also be crushed prior to the inoculation of media.

Actinomycosis, caused by *Actinomyces bovis*, botryomycosis, caused by *Staphylococcus aureus*, and tuberculosis are the most important differential diagnoses to be considered. Granules resembling those of actinobacillosis may be encountered in the pus of both actinomycotic and botryomycotic lesions. *Actinomyces bovis* infection in cattle frequently causes a chronic purulent and proliferative inflammation of bony structures (particularly the mandible), the resultant disease being known as 'lumpy jaw'. In addition, in contrast to actinobacillosis, the regional lymph nodes tend not to be affected in actinomycosis. The granules in actinomycosis are larger than those of actinobacillosis, in which they are generally less than 1 mm in diameter. They also tend to be harder in the former disease, centres consisting of Gram-positive filamentous organisms. Botryomycosis is a chronic disease characterized by the formation of granulomas that contain suppurative foci.[4] The essential feature is the presence in the pus of the so-called botryomycotic granules, which in histological sections are seen to consist of closely-packed Gram-positive cocci embedded in a homogeneous matrix, although the latter may not be discernible in younger granules. Numerous cocci are present when granules are placed on a glass slide, crushed with a cover-slip and then stained and examined.

The macroscopic lesions caused by *A. lignieresii* may also be confused with those caused by other pyogenic bacteria such as *Actinomyces pyogenes*, *Corynebacterium pseudotuberculosis*, *Staphylococcus* spp. and *Streptococcus* spp.

Control

Disease caused by *A. lignieresii* occurs sporadically and may be controlled to some extent by the application of sound managemental procedures, such as the timely and appropriate treatment of wounds and the minimization of injuries to the lips and oral mucosa.[2, 5, 12] Cases or even outbreaks can be anticipated and early preventative measures and treatment adopted when animals are, for example, fed prickly pear (the thorns of which should be burned off with a blowlamp before feeding) or other material (such as barley) likely to injure soft tissues in and around the mouth.

Iodine is a satisfactory disinfectant. Treatment is more successful when applied during the initial stages of infection than in the chronic stage.[1]

Lesions that are well circumscribed and accessible can be surgically excised under local anaesthesia and the wound cavity packed with gauze tampons soaked in tincture of iodine. If surgical excision cannot be carried out, fistulae, if present, should be curetted and packed with gauze saturated with tincture of iodine. In some cases it may be advisable to make an incision into a lesion which is then irrigated with iodine. Lugol's iodine can be injected directly into lesions.[6]

Prior to the advent of modern antimicrobial drugs, the oral administration of iodine preparations was widely recommended, whether surgical procedures had been performed or not.[6] Potassium iodide, at a dosage level of 6–10 g/day, should be administered orally or in the drinking water for two to four weeks. During or shortly after this form of therapy an animal may develop signs of catarrh of the nose and eyes, dandruff, loss of hair, cutaneous eruptions and loss of appetite. These are indicative of iodism—the maximum systemic level of iodine that can be tolerated has been reached. The administration of iodine should then be suspended for about a week and then resumed if the full course of iodine has not been given.[1] Potassium iodide should never be administered parenterally.

Actinobacillus lignieresii is usually sensitive to the sulphanomides or trimethoprim-sulphanomide combinations, ampicillin, streptomycin, tetracyclines and chloramphenicol. Antibiotic treatment should be chosen with due regard to the sensitivity of the isolate. As abscesses and purulent foci are generally enclosed in a thick, fibrous tissue capsule, antimicrobial preparations may not be able to penetrate them to reach the causative organisms, and prolonged (longer than five days) therapy may be necessary to achieve this.[13]

References

1 **BLOOD, D.C., HENDERSON, J.A. & RADOSTITS, O.M., 1979.** *Veterinary Medicine*. 5th edn. London: Baillière Tindall.

2 **CAMPBELL, S.G., WHITLOCK, R.H., TOMONEY, J.F. & UNDERWOOD, A.M., 1975.** An unusual epizootic of actinobacillosis in dairy heifers. *Journal of the American Veterinary Medical Association*, 166, 604–606.

3 **CARTER, G.R., 1984.** *Diagnostic Procedures in Veterinary Bacteriology and Mycology*. 4th edn. Springfield: Charles C. Thomas. 122–125.

4 **DAVIES, G.O., 1947.** *Gaiger and Davies' Veterinary Pathology and Bacteriology*. 3rd edn. London: Baillière Tindall.

5 **HEBELER, H.F., LINTON, A.H. & OSBORNE, A.D., 1961.**

Atypical actinobacillus in a dairy herd. *The Veterinary Record*, 73, 517–521.

6 **HENNING, M.W., 1956.** *Animal Diseases in South Africa*. 3rd edn. South Africa: Central News Agency Ltd.

7 **PHILLIPS, J.E., 1984.** *Actinobacillus*. *In*: KRIEG, N.R. & HOLT, J.G., (eds). *Bergey's Manual of Systematic Bacteriology*. Vol. I. Baltimore, London: Williams & Wilkins.

8 **SANDERS, D.A. & RISTIC, M., 1956.** *Actinobacillus* of cattle. *Journal of the American Veterinary Medical Association*, 129, 478–481.

9 **SMITH, H.A. & JONES, T.C., 1966.** *Veterinary Pathology*, Philadelphia: Lea & Febiger.

10 **THOMAS, A.D., 1931.** Actinobacillosis and other complications in sheep which may arise from the feeding of prickly pear (*Opuntia* sp.). *Seventeenth Report of the Director of Veterinary Services and Animal Industry of the Union of South Africa*, 215–229.

11 **TUSTIN, R.C., 1993.** 293 Julius Jeppe Street, Waterkloof, Pretoria. Personal observations.

12 **WALKER, R.D., 1993.** Actinobacillosis and actinomycosis. *In*: HOWARD, J.L., (ed.). *Current Veterinary Therapy 3: Food Animal Practice*. Philadelphia: W.B. Saunders Co.

13 **WILLSON, P.J., 1990.** *Haemophilus, Actinobacillus, Pasteurella*: Mechanisms of resistance and antibiotic therapy. *Canadian Journal of Veterinary Research*, 54, S73–S77.

137

Actinobacillus equuli infections

Synonym: Sleepy foal disease

M.M. Henton

Introduction and aetiology

Actinobacillus equuli is the cause of a peracute to chronic septicaemic condition of new-born foals, referred to as sleepy foal disease. Localization of the bacteria may occur in many tissues or organ systems, including the joints, lungs, heart and kidneys. This results in lesions such as purulent polyarthritis, bronchopneumonia, valvular endocarditis, myocarditis and embolic suppurative nephritis. It may also occasionally be the cause of abortions in mares and of septicaemia and arthritis in new-born piglets.

Diseases caused by *A. equuli* probably occur in most countries, but they are sporadic. Only 33 cases of disease caused by *A. equuli* in horses and 21 cases in pigs were diagnosed bacteriologically at the Veterinary Research Institute, Onderstepoort between 1977 and 1987.[5]

Actinobacillus equuli was first described by Meyer in 1910 in South Africa, after the bacterium had been isolated from kidney abscesses in foals. Meyer originally named it *Shigella nephritidis equi*.[4] In the older literature a variety of other names have been used for the organism, including *Bacterium viscosum equi* and *Shigella equirulis*.[1]

The cultural, morphological and other characteristics of *A. equuli* are outlined in the ***Actinobacillus* spp. infections: Introduction**.

Epidemiology

Actinobacillus equuli infection and resultant disease occur in horses and occasionally in pigs. Healthy mares and sows may be carriers of the bacterium in their genital tracts (cervix and vagina), and less often in their upper respiratory tracts, particularly the tonsils.[11]

Foals most commonly become infected during or soon after parturition, by direct contact with the infected genital tracts of carrier mares, but transplacental infections and infection via the umbilicus may also occur. Foals less than two weeks old are usually affected, and particularly those which have a deficient colostral immunity.[1, 2, 6, 11]

Although piglets are rarely affected by *A. equuli*, septicaemia complicated by arthritis and meningoencephalitis occurs most commonly in piglets during the first week of life and immediately after weaning.[12] *Actinobacillus equuli* may also rarely cause metritis and abortion in sows.[9, 10]

Clinical signs

Signs of septicaemia are usually evident in foals suffering from peracute or acute sleepy foal disease, while those affected by the subacute or chronic disease generally have suppurative lesions in various tissues.

Foals afflicted by peracute disease are born weak, refuse to suck, or do so sluggishly, and are feverish, dull, listless and lethargic. They stand with their heads hanging and their ears drooping, before eventually becoming recumbent and dying. They seldom live for more than 24 hours.[7, 11]

The clinical signs of the acute disease in foals are characterized by listlessness, lethargy, inappetence and fever one to three days after birth. Affected foals either abstain from sucking or may suck for a short while before apparently 'falling asleep' with the teat in their mouth (from whence the name 'sleepy foal disease'). Some foals may show swelling and inflammation of the umbilicus, evidence of abdominal pain, shallow and laboured respiration, diarrhoea and frequent micturition before death supervenes—usually within a week.[1, 7, 11]

Foals affected with the subacute or chronic disease reveal signs of purulent arthritis and/or bronchopneumonia, which usually develop two or three weeks after birth, but these signs may appear sooner or be delayed for several weeks. The first sign of illness is usually lameness, associated with a variable amount of swelling of one or more joints. The lameness soon increases in severity. Foals often lie down, rise with difficulty, and progressively become weak and emaciated. In some cases a suppurative omphalophlebitis is present. Many affected foals also show signs of purulent bronchopneumonia, such as an increased respiratory rate, painful cough and purulent nasal discharge. The organisms are frequently localized in other organs or tissues (particularly the kidneys and myocardium), and evidence of this may be manifested clinically.[1, 7, 11] The course of the subacute or chronic disease is protracted, and the mortality rate is

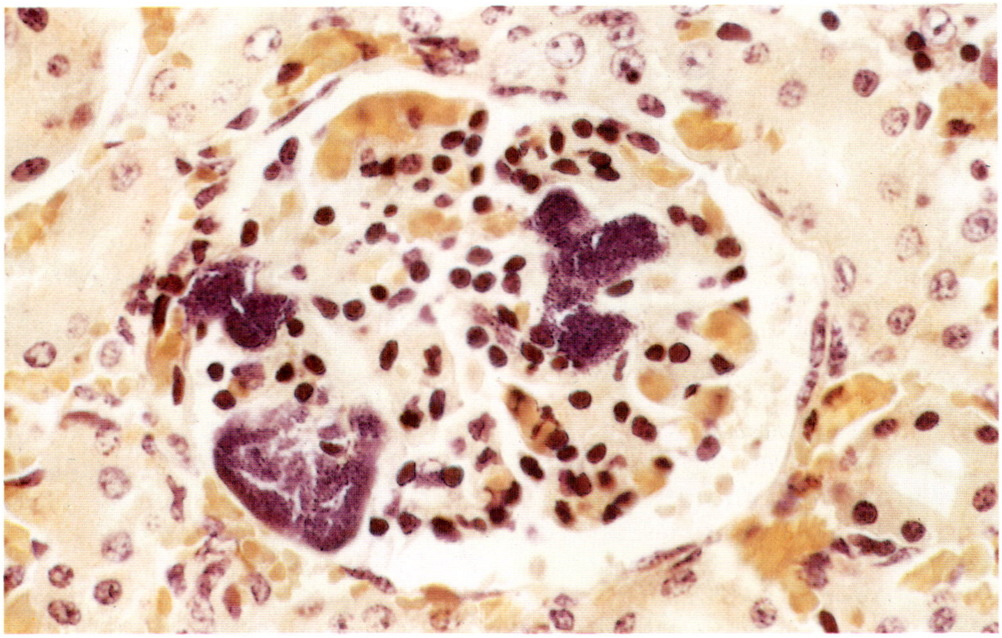

Figure 137.1 Histological section of a kidney manifesting colonies of *Actinobacillus equuli* in a renal glomerulus (Gram's stain)

usually not as high as in the peracute and acute disease. The older the foal when clinical signs appear, the greater its chances of recovery. In foals which survive, convalescence is slow and the animals may be emaciated for a protracted period before improvement becomes apparent.[4]

Actinobacillus equuli is a rare cause of abortion in mares at any stage of gestation. The organism either reaches the genital tract haematogenously or, more frequently, as an ascending infection. Other manifestations of infection are purulent rhinitis, pneumonia, polyarthritis and tendovaginitis in older foals. Wound infections, abscessations and peritonitis may occur in adult horses.[3, 8]

Clinical signs of the septicaemic disease in piglets are similar to those in foals;[12] the bacterium may localize in the joints, brain and kidneys. Some piglets may only show clinical signs of nervous involvement.

Pathology

Foals that die of peracute or acute disease show lesions of septicaemia, including petechiae in serosal surfaces and mucous membranes, generalized congestion, splenomegaly, and oedema and congestion of lymph nodes. There may be a slight increase in the volume of serous fluids in the pericardial and pleural cavities, and bronchopneumonia may be evident in some foals that die of the acute disease.

In the subacute or chronic disease, *A. equuli* localizes in many organs and tissues after a bacteraemic phase. The outstanding lesions are purulent polyarthritis (particularly of the hock and knee joints), tendovaginitis and bronchopneumonia. Miliary abscessation is present in the cortex of the kidneys and in the myocardium in some animals, the abscesses varying in size from microscopic to a maximum diameter of 3 mm. Suppurative omphalophlebitis may be present. The microscopic lesions in the kidneys are those of a purulent embolic nephritis. Colonies of bacteria are usually evident in glomerular and other cortical capillaries **(Figure 137.1)**.

Lesions similar to those in foals may be evident in piglets infected with *A. equuli*.

Diagnosis and differential diagnosis

Because the clinical signs of sleepy foal disease may be confused with those of other infections, the diagnosis should be confirmed by the isolation of *A. equuli* from the blood and kidneys of septicaemic foals, or from other affected tissues (pneumonic lesions, kidney abscesses) or exudates from foals in which the course of the disease is more prolonged. There is usually no difficulty in culturing *A. equuli* on blood-agar medium, and growth is characteristically profuse.[5] In new-born foals that die of the disease, microscopic lesions compatible with purulent embolic glomerular and interstitial nephritis are highly suggestive of sleepy foal disease.

In foals, neonatal septicaemia caused by *A. equuli* may be confused with septicaemia caused by *Escherichia coli*, *Streptococcus* spp. or *Klebsiella* spp.

Control

Apart from maintaining a high level of general hygiene and disinfecting the umbilicus at birth, very little can be done to prevent infection of new-born foals. *Actinobacillus equuli* is sensitive to streptomycin, tetracycline, chloramphenicol, ampicillin and trimethoprim-sulphonamide combinations. Affected animals should be treated parenterally with these antimicrobial drugs at the recommended dosages for three to five days.[3]

References

1 **COTTEW, G.S. & RYLEY, J.W., 1952.** *Shigella equirulis* infection in a foal. *Australian Veterinary Journal*, 28, 302–306.

2 **DIMOCK, W.W., EDWARDS, P.R. & BRUNER, D.W., 1947.** Infections of fetuses and foal. *Kentucky Agricultural Experimental Station Bulletin*, 509.

3 **GAY, C.C. & LORDING, P.M., 1980.** Peritonitis in horses associated with *Actinobacillus equuli*. *Australian Veterinary Journal*, 56, 296–300.

4 **HENNING, M.W., 1956.** *Animal Diseases in South Africa*. 3rd edn. South Africa: Central News Agency Ltd.

5 **HENTON, M.M., 1993.** Veterinary Research Institute, Onderstepoort. Unpublished observations.

6 **KAMADA, M., KUMANOMIDO, T., KANEMARU, T., YOSHIHARA, T., TOMIOKA, Y., KANEKO, M., SENBA, H. & OHISHI, H., 1985.** Isolation of *Actinobacillus equuli* from neonatal foals with death in colostrum-deficiency or failure of maternal immunity transfer. *Bulletin of Equine Research Institute*, 22, 38–42.

7 **LITTLEJOHN, A., 1959.** Sleepy foal disease in Natal. *Journal of the South African Veterinary Medical Association*, 30, 143–147.

8 **MAGUIRE, L.C., 1958.** The role of *Bacterium viscosum equi* in the causation of equine disease. *The Veterinary Record*, 70, 989–991.

9 **PEDERSEN, K.B., 1977.** *Actinobacillus* infections in swine. *Nordisk Veterinaer Medizin*, 29, 137–140.

10 **PHILLIPS, J.E., 1984.** *Actinobacillus*. *In*: KRIEG, N.R. & HOLT, J.G., (eds). *Bergey's Manual of Systematic Bacteriology*. Vol. I. Baltimore, London: Williams & Wilkins.

11 **PLATT, H., 1973.** Septicaemia in the foal: A review of 61 cases. *British Veterinary Journal*, 129, 221–229.

12 **WINDSOR, R.S., 1973.** *Actinobacillus equuli* infection in a litter of pigs and a review of previous reports on similar infections. *The Veterinary Record*, 92, 178–180.

138

Actinobacillus seminis *infections*

E.M. Van Tonder and J.A. Erasmus*
* Deceased

Introduction

Actinobacillus seminis is the cause of epididymitis, particularly in young rams, but it is also rarely associated with purulent vaginitis and cervicitis in ewes, and purulent arthritis in lambs. Epididymitis may occasionally occur in ennobled Boer and Angora goats, and in cattle.

Actinobacillus seminis, the first Gram-negative, pleomorphic bacterium isolated from rams suffering from clinical epididymitis, was isolated in Australia in 1960.[5] Subsequently, epididymitis as a result of this bacterium has been reported in the USA[31, 34, 43] and South Africa.[35, 36, 39, 41, 49] There is no record of *A. seminis* infection in other countries in southern Africa.

Aetiology

There is much confusion in the literature regarding the nomenclature, identification and characterization of the different species or variants of aerobic bacteria which are isolated from the lesions of young rams suffering from epididymitis, or from other sites of the genitalia of sheep. These organisms are collectively referred to as Gram-negative pleomorphs, and include members of the *Haemophilus-Pasteurella-Actinobacillus* group of bacteria, such as *A. seminis, Histophilus ovis, A. actinomycetemcomitans, P. haemolytica, P. multocida* and *Haemophilus somnus*.[10] *Actinobacillus seminis* and *H. ovis* share many characteristics[29, 47] but nevertheless seem to be distinct from each other.[25, 27] Although the bacteria listed above may cause epididymitis in rams, they are opportunistic and may be part of the normal flora of the genital tract.[17]

Actinobacillus seminis is non-capsulated, Gram-negative, non-sporulating and non-motile, and varies in shape from that of a coccobacillus to rod-shaped. Most *A. seminis* strains are non-haemolytic, but some may show a degree of alpha haemolysis.[33]

Although *A. seminis* grows under aerobic conditions, its growth is more luxuriant in a micro-aerophilic or carboxophilic atmosphere in which 10–20 per cent of air is replaced by carbon dioxide. Bacterial growth is poor on ordinary nutrient media but is greatly enhanced on a variety of media enriched by the addition of 5 per cent horse blood or inactivated horse serum.[5, 33, 36, 40, 49]

Epidemiology

Epididymitis caused by *A. seminis* is mainly a problem of virgin rams up to one year of age which are maintained in intensive or semi-intensive systems on a high plane of nutrition.[4, 10, 31, 34, 36, 42, 43] It has also occasionally been reported in ennobled Boer and Angora goats[35] and in cattle.[14, 20, 41] *Actinobacillus seminis* has also been isolated from the vaginas of six-month-old lambs and from the prepuces of 12- to 20-week-old ram lambs.[42] Epididymitis caused by Gram-negative pleomorphs is seldom encountered in older rams used for stud or flock mating purposes.[4, 7, 9, 10, 15, 18–21, 23, 30, 31, 35, 36, 42, 43]

Rams that are clinically or subclinically infected are important in the venereal transmission of *A. seminis* to ewes for long periods—sometimes even life-long.[9, 16, 36] Ewes served by these rams may become subclinical carriers—rarely do they show evidence of overt disease—and then act as a source of infection to other ewes through mechanical transmission by rams from one ewe to another during mating. It would seem, however, that infected ewes, as well as the ewe lambs born to them, may indefinitely transmit the infection transplacentally to their offspring.[36]

Pathogenesis

The nutritional[10, 18, 21, 31, 36, 43] and hormonal status of young ram lambs,[18, 21, 42, 43] as well as stressful situations brought about by conditions such as transportation,[4, 9, 23, 34] may predispose to the disease.

Young ram lambs receiving a high plane of nutrition manifest early, probably hormone-induced, sexual development, which apparently creates a favourable environment for the rapid growth and multiplication of *A. seminis* and other organisms harboured in the genital tract.[8, 22, 28, 44, 48] There is a difference of opinion as to how infection of young virgin ram lambs occurs. Some consider that transmission occurs largely transplacentally from infected ewes to their offspring, followed by localization in the genitalia (including the prepuce) as a result of a descending infection, while others are of the opinion that primary colonization of the preputial cavity occurs as a result of contact with a contaminated environment, such as stable floors and bedding, and that infection of the epididymis and possibly other parts of the genital tract follows ascending infection.[1, 18, 21, 25, 26]

Clinical signs and pathology

Actinobacillus seminis infection in young ram lambs may manifest clinically as peracute, acute, subacute or chronic epididymitis or epididymo-orchitis. In older rams the disease tends to be more subacute to chronic. However, subclinical epididymitis in all age groups is also common.[5–7, 12, 13, 16, 23, 30, 31, 35, 36, 38, 41, 43, 49]

Peracute disease is characterized by severe, rapidly developing uni- or bilateral swelling and pain of the scrotum, high fever, listlessness, loss of appetite and body weight, and a stiff and straddled gait.[5, 7, 12, 18, 30, 31, 34, 35, 43] On incision, the cavity of the *tunica vaginalis* contains copious amounts of a fibrinous to fibrino-purulent exudate **(Figure 138.1)**. The swelling usually subsides after four days to a week and the enlarged epididymis (usually the tail) can then be palpated.[7, 12, 23, 30, 35, 43] In some animals scrotal fistulae develop, which discharge a slimy, greyish-white to greenish-yellow exudate to the externum.[18, 19, 31, 35, 43]

Acute epididymitis is characterized by rapid enlargement of the tail of the epididymis without apparent concomitant swelling and pain of the scrotum, although if the cavity of the *tunica vaginalis* is exposed by incision,[7, 30, 35, 36, 41, 43, 49] variable amounts of fibrinous exudate are usually found adhering to the surface of the thickened *tunica albuginea* and *tunica vaginalis*.[1, 18, 31] Microscopically, lesions in the affected part of the epididymis are characterized by necrosis, desquamation of the epithelium and cystic changes of the tubules, infiltration of numerous neutrophils and some macrophages and lymphocytes, and degeneration and necrosis of neutrophils and spermatozoa.[7, 18, 19]

A subacute to chronic epididymitis is characterized by a slow, progressive enlargement and induration of the epididymis which is seldom detected clinically unless the part concerned is palpated. The tail of the epididymis of one or both testes is most commonly enlarged, sometimes by as much as five times, but the head and body of the epididymis may also be affected **(Figure 138.2)**. The affected epididymis is freely moveable and is not attached, as there are generally no adhesions between the visceral and parietal layers of the *tunica vaginalis*.[5, 7, 9, 12, 13, 18, 19, 30, 35, 36, 43] On incision of the affected part, the *tunica albuginea* is found to be thickened, the epididymal tissue is fibrotic and enlarged, and a greyish-white, purulent exudate or a granular, cheesy or calcified material is liberated **(Figure 138.3)**. Microscopic lesions are

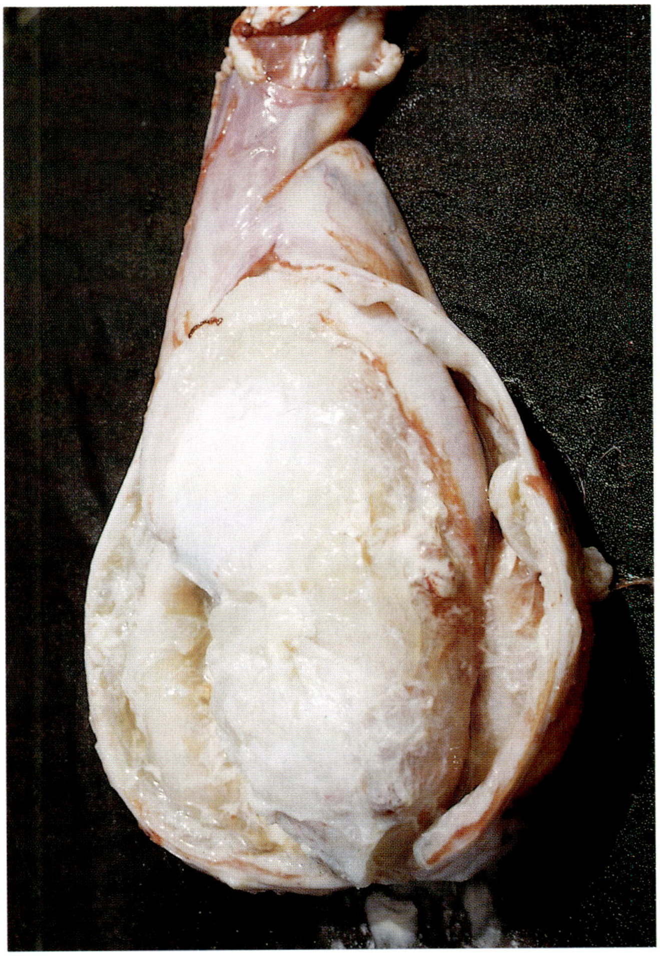

Figure 138.1 Peracute *Actinobacillus seminis* infection. Note the severe fibrinous periorchitis

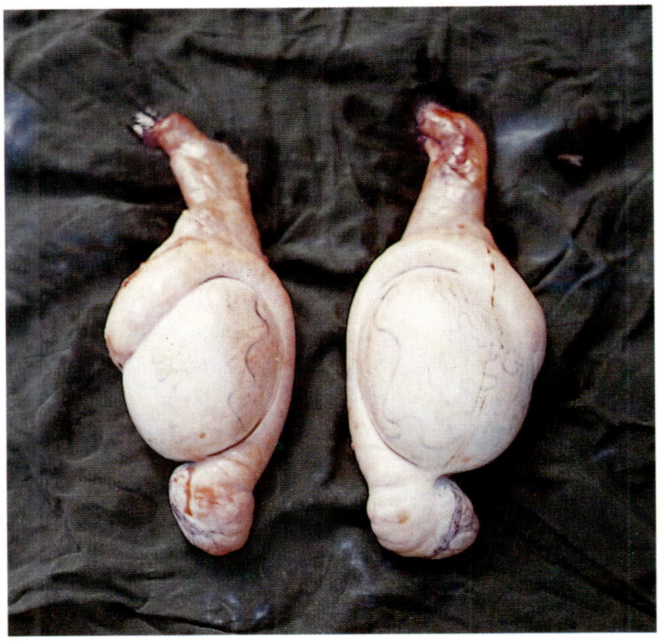

Figure 138.2 Subacute to chronic *Actinobacillus seminis* infection. Note the bilateral lesions in the tail of the epididymis, mild involvement of the head of the epididymis and unilateral testicular atrophy

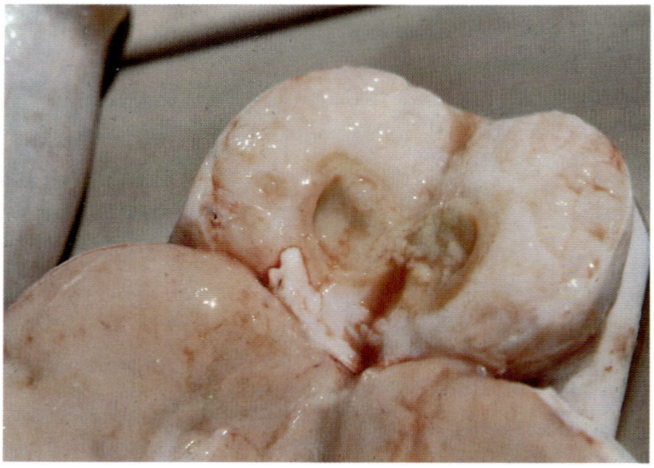

Figure 138.3 Cut surface of the tail of an epididymis showing extensive fibrosis, and lysis and cavitation of the content of a spermatic granuloma

characterized by fibrosis and infiltration of lymphocytes and plasma cells into the interstitium. The ductular epithelium may be hyperplastic and focally infiltrated by neutrophils. Spermatic granulomas, often present in the affected part of the epididymis, are characterized by central masses of sperm cells surrounded by foreign-body giant cells, neutrophils, macrophages, lymphocytes, plasma cells, fibroblasts and fibrous connective tissue.[7, 18, 19] Testicular atrophy may occur in rams with chronic epididymitis. Increased fibrous connective tissue, infiltration of lymphocytes and plasma cells in the interstitium, and amorphous mineralized material in some of the seminiferous tubules may also be evident in the testis.[18, 19] The epididymitis may be accompanied by orchitis, ampullitis, seminal vesiculitis, prostatitis, bulbo-urethritis, urethritis, balanoposthitis, chronic pyelonephritis and hydronephrosis.[1, 7, 18, 46]

Microscopic examination of stained semen smears of a clinically or subclinically affected ram generally shows varying numbers of bacteria, neutrophils, and desquamated epithelial cells.[18, 19, 35–37]

Apart from lesions in the urogenital system of rams, *A. seminis* has also been associated with epididymitis in ennobled Boer and Angora goats[35] and cattle,[14, 20, 41] acute purulent anterior vaginitis and cervicitis in ewes within two days of mating with infected rams,[36] and acute purulent polyarthritis in young lambs. Experimentally, an acute gangrenous mastitis has been produced in ewes by infection of the mammary gland.[2, 3, 46]

Diagnosis

The diagnosis of epididymitis as a result of *A. seminis* and other Gram-negative pleomorphs is based on epidemiological data, clinical signs and pathology, examination of stained semen smears, and bacteriological examinations.[36, 37]

Semen smears stained with Giemsa or the modified Ziehl Neelsen technique (to exclude *Brucella ovis* as a cause of epididymitis)[32, 45] should be examined for the presence of neutrophils, epithelial cells and bacteria, the latter usually being found in close proximity to neutrophils. The examination of smears is useful in the diagnosis of both the clinical and subclinical disease, provided the epididymal ducts are patent.

The isolation of Gram-negative pleomorphs from infected semen samples presents no difficulties. However, the Gram-negative pleomorphic bacteria isolated from the genital tract of rams may be opportunistic pathogens and part of the normal flora,[17] and the presence of such bacteria, with or without neutrophils, in semen samples does not signify that they are, in fact, the actual cause of the lesions.

At present there are no reliable serological tests that can be used to confirm a diagnosis of disease or infection caused by Gram-negative pleomorphs.

Differential diagnosis

Epididymitis in rams caused by *A. seminis* should be distinguished from epididymitis caused by other Gram-negative pleomorphs and *Brucella ovis*. The latter generally affects older rams and those used for flock breeding purposes, whereas epididymitis caused by Gram-negative pleomorphs occurs more frequently in virgin rams on a high plane of nutrition.[10, 11, 24] *Brucella ovis* can be distinguished from the Gram-negative pleomorphs in semen smears by the fact that it stains positively with the modified Ziehl Neelsen technique. It also has specific growth requirements and other bacteriological characteristics; and serological tests, such as the complement fixation test, can be used to identify *B. ovis*-infected rams.

In addition to *A. seminis*,[13, 16, 23, 24, 31, 41–43, 49] other Gram-negative pleomorphs such as *A. actinomycetemcomitans*,[10, 11] *Actinobacillus* spp.,[24] *Actinobacillus*-like organisms,[36, 38] *Histophilus ovis*,[36, 38, 43] *Haemophilus* spp., *Moraxella* spp.,[10] *Pasteurella* spp.,[18] and pyogenic bacteria such as *A. (Corynebacterium) pyogenes* and *Corynebacterium pseudotuberculosis* may be involved in epididymitis. Differentiation of these organisms can only be done by specific laboratory methods.

Control

The treatment of rams suffering from clinical or subclinical epididymitis is of limited value.[10, 12] As the majority of latently infected young rams seem to clear themselves of infection between weaning and the late two-tooth stage, they should not be culled from the flock at too early an age.[37] Final judgement as to the status of infection should preferably be made only when the rams are older than 15 months and after at least three examinations at monthly intervals have been conducted.[36, 37] It is suggested that rams subclinically or latently infected at this age should undergo a course of parenterally administered tetracycline therapy.

It is well known that young rams may excrete

neutrophils in their semen for some time, and that the semen may clear spontaneously without any form of treatment having been applied. For this reason, in a treated animal, it is often difficult to decide whether such a positive response is the result of therapy or self-cure.

It is advised that the breeding rams be tested for infection before the onset of the mating season. Similarly, rams should be tested before they are purchased or introduced to the flock for the first time.

The maintenance after weaning of young ram lambs in open-range systems with minimal supplementary feeding has proved effective in the control of epididymitis caused by Gram-negative pleomorphs, but in the highly competitive field of ram production this method is not very attractive.

At present there is no vaccine available against *A. seminis* infection.

References

1 **AL-KATIB, W,A-K,H., 1981.** Experimental *Actinobacillus seminis* infection of rams. Dissertation Abstracts International, 41, No. 07, 2415–B. Ph.D. thesis, Kansas State University, Manhattan, USA, (1980). *Veterinary Bulletin Abstracts*, 50, 944.

2 **ALSENOY, A.M., 1984.** Comparative light and electron microscopic study of experimental *Actinobacillus seminis* mastitis in ewes. *Veterinary Bulletin Abstracts*, 54, 914.

3 **ALSENOY, A.M. & DENNIS, S.M., 1985.** Pathology of acute experimental *Actinobacillus seminis* mastitis in ewes. *Australian Veterinary Journal*, 62, 234–237.

4 **BAGLEY, C.V., PASKETT, M.E., MATTHEWS, N.J. & STENQUIST, N.J., 1985.** Prevalence and causes of ram epididymitis in Utah. *Journal of the American Veterinary Medical Association*, 186, 798–801.

5 **BAYNES, I.D. & SIMMONS, G.C., 1960.** Ovine epididymitis caused by *Actinobacillus seminis* sp. *Australian Veterinary Journal*, 36, 454–459.

6 **BAYNES, I.D. & SIMMONS, G.C., 1966.** *Actinobacillus seminis* in sheep. *Australian Veterinary Journal*, 42, 225.

7 **BAYNES, I.D. & SIMMONS, G.C., 1968.** Clinical and pathological studies of Border Leicester rams naturally infected with *Actinobacillus seminis*. *Australian Veterinary Journal*, 44, 339–343.

8 **BELONJE, P.C., 1965.** Observations on the post-natal development of the penis in Merino ram lambs and wethers: The possible relationship to the passage of urinary calculi. *Journal of the South African Veterinary Medical Association*, 36, 381–383.

9 **BRUERE, A.N., WEST, D.M., MACLACHLAN, N.J., EDWARDS, J.D. & CHAPMAN, H.M., 1977.** Genital infection of ram hoggets associated with a Gram-negative pleomorphic organism. *New Zealand Veterinary Journal*, 25, 191–193.

10 **BULGIN, M.S. & ANDERSON, B.C., 1983.** Association of sexual experience with isolation of various bacteria in cases of ovine epididymitis. *Journal of the American Veterinary Medical Association*, 372–374.

11 **DE LONG, W.J., WALDHALM, D.G. & HALL, R.F., 1979.** Bacteria isolates associated with epididymitis in rams from Idaho and Eastern Oregon flocks. *American Journal of Veterinary Research*, 40, 101–102.

12 **DE WET, J.A.L., 1985.** Siektes by kleinvee. 6. Bybalontsteking (2). *Landbouweekblad*, 12 April 1985, 38–41.

13 **DE WET, J.A.L. & ERASMUS, J.A., 1984.** Epididymitis of rams in the central and southern districts of the Orange Free State. *Journal of the South African Veterinary Association*, 55, 173–179.

14 **DIXON, R.J., STEVENSON, B.J. & SIMS, K.R., 1983.** *Actinobacillus seminis* isolated from cattle. *New Zealand Veterinary Journal*, 31, 122–123.

15 **EKDAHL, M.O., MONEY, D.F.L. & MARTIN, C.A., 1968.** Some aspects of epididymitis of rams in New Zealand. *New Zealand Veterinary Journal*, 16, 81–82.

16 **ERASMUS, J.A., DE WET, J.A.L. & PROZESKY, L., 1982.** *Actinobacillus seminis* infection in a Walrich ram. *Journal of the South African Veterinary Association*, 53, 129.

17 **HEALY, M.C., HWANG, H.H., KLEINSCHUSTER, S.J., JOHNSON, A.V. & SYMONS, K.S., 1988.** Comparison and partial characterization of the protein profiles and other membrane antigens of *Actinobacillus* species isolated from ram lambs with epididymitis. *American Journal of Veterinary Research*, 49, 1824–1832.

18 **JANSEN, B.C., 1980.** The aetiology of ram epididymitis. *Onderstepoort Journal of Veterinary Research*, 47, 101–107.

19 **JANSEN, B.C., 1980.** A surgical technique for the experimental reproduction of epididymitis in rams. *Onderstepoort Journal of Veterinary Research*, 47, 281–283.

20 **JANSEN, B.C., 1981.** The pathogenicity of *Actinobacillus seminis* in cattle. *In: Landbounavorsing (Agricultural Research)*. Pretoria, South Africa; Department of Agriculture.

21 **JANSEN, B.C., 1983.** The epidemiology of bacterial infection of the genitalia in rams. *Onderstepoort Journal of Veterinary Research*, 50, 275–282.

22 **JOHNSTONE, I.L., 1948.** The growth and development of the penis in sheep: Their possible relationship to posthitis. *Australian Veterinary Journal*, 24, 86–88.

23 **LIVINGSTON, C.W. & HARDY, W.J., 1964.** Isolation of *Actinobacillus seminis* from ovine epididymitis. *American Journal of Veterinary Research*, 25, 660–663.

24 **LOZANO, E.A., 1986.** Etiological significance of bacterial isolates from rams with palpable epididymitis. *American Journal of Veterinary Research*, 47, 1153–1156.

25 **McGILLIVERY, D.J., WEBBER, J.J. & DEAN, H.F., 1986.** Characterisation of *Histophilus ovis* and related organisms by restriction endonuclease analysis. *Australian Veterinary Journal*, 63, 389–393.

26 **OSTER, G., 1978.** Research review: The blood testis barrier in rats and monkeys. *Research in Reproduction*, 10, 4.

27 **PIECHULA, K., MUTTERS, R., BURBACH, S., KLUSSMEIER, R., POHL, S. & MANNHEIM, W., 1986.** Deoxyribonucleic acid relationships of *'Histophilus ovis/ Haemophilus somnus'*, *Haemophilus haemoglobinophilus* and *Actinobacillus seminis*. *International Journal of Systematic Bacteriology*, 1–7.

28 **PRETORIUS, P.S. & MARINCOWITZ, G., 1968.** Post-natal penis development, testes descent and puberty in Merino lambs on different planes of nutrition. *South African Journal of Agricultural Science*, 11, 319–334.

29 **RAHALEY, R.S., 1978.** Serological comparison between *Histophilus ovis*, *Actinobacillus seminis* and *Brucella ovis*. *Australian Veterinary Journal*, 54, 423–425.

30 **SIMMONS, G.C., BAYNES, I.D. & LUDFORD, C.G., 1966.** Epidemiology of *Actinobacillus seminis* in a flock of Border Leicester sheep. *Australian Veterinary Journal*, 42, 183–187.

31 **SPONENBERG, D.P., CARTER, M.E., CARTER, G.R., CORDES, D.O., STEVENS, S.E. & VEIT, H.P., 1983.** Suppurative epididymitis in a ram infected with *Actinobacillus*

seminis. *Journal of the American Veterinary Medical Association*, 182, 990–991.

32 **STAMP, J.T., McEWEN, A.D., WATT, J.A.A. & NISBET, D.I., 1950.** Enzootic abortion in ewes. 1. Transmission of the disease. *The Veterinary Record*, 62, 251–254.

33 **SWANEPOEL, M.L., 1984.** A study for the differentiation of *Actinobacillus seminis*, *A. actinomycetemcomitans*, *Histophilus ovis* and *Pasteurella haemolytica*. *Onderstepoort Journal of Veterinary Research*, 51, 41–46.

34 **SWIFT, B.L., CRADDOCK, F., HANCOCK, R.J., THOMAS, G.M., TRUEBLOOD, M.S. & WEIBEL, J., 1982.** Ram epididymitis: A clinical report. *Theriogenology*, 17, 344–347.

35 **VAN TONDER, E.M., 1973.** Infection of rams with *Actinobacillus seminis*. *Journal of the South African Veterinary Association*, 44, 235–240.

36 **VAN TONDER, E.M., 1977.** *Actinobacillus seminis* infection in sheep in South Africa. DVSc thesis, University of Pretoria, Pretoria.

37 **VAN TONDER, E.M., 1977.** Examination of rams for genital soundness. *Journal of the South African Veterinary Association*, 48, 267–272.

38 **VAN TONDER, E.M., 1979.** *Actinobacillus seminis* infection in sheep in the Republic of South Africa. I. Identification of the problem. *Onderstepoort Journal of Veterinary Research*, 46, 129–133.

39 **VAN TONDER, E.M., 1979.** *Actinobacillus seminis* infection in sheep in the Republic of South Africa. II. Incidence and geographical distribution. *Onderstepoort Journal of Veterinary Research*, 46, 135–140.

40 **VAN TONDER, E.M., 1979.** *Actinobacillus seminis* infection in sheep in the Republic of South Africa. III. Growth and cultural characteristics of *A. seminis*. *Onderstepoort Journal of Veterinary Research*, 46, 141–148.

41 **VAN TONDER, E.M. & BOLTON, T.F.W., 1970.** The isolation of *Actinobacillus seminis* from bovine semen: A preliminary report. *Journal of the South African Veterinary Medical Association*, 41, 287–288.

42 **WALKER, R.L. & LEAMASTER, B.R., 1986.** Prevalence of *Histophilus ovis* and *Actinobacillus seminis* in the genital tract of sheep. *American Journal of Veterinary Research*, 47, 1928–1980.

43 **WALKER, R.L., LEAMASTER, B.R., STELLFLUG, J.N. & BIBERSTEIN, E.L., 1986.** Association of age of ram with distribution of epididymal lesions and etiologic agent. *Journal of the American Veterinary Medical Association*, 188, 393–396.

44 **WATSON, R.H., SAPSFORD, C.S. & McCANE, I., 1956.** The development of the testis, epididymis and penis in the young Merino ram. *Australian Journal of Agricultural Research*, 7, 574–590.

45 **WATT, D.A., 1970.** Investigations of ovine brucellosis in Merino rams of Western Australia. *Australian Veterinary Journal*, 46, 506–508.

46 **WATT, D.A., BAMFORD, V. & NAIRN, M.E., 1970.** *Actinobacillus seminis* as a cause of polyarthritis and posthitis in sheep. *Australian Veterinary Journal*, 46, 516.

47 **WEBB, R.F., 1983.** Bacteriological characteristics of *Histophilus ovis* and its relationship to similar bacteria. *Research in Veterinary Science*, 35, 25–29.

48 **WIGGINS, E.L. & TERRILL, C.E., 1953.** Variation in penis development in ram lambs. *Journal of Animal Science*, 12, 524–535.

49 **WORTHINGTON, R.W. & BOSMAN, P.P., 1968.** Isolation of *Actinobacillus seminis* in South Africa. *Journal of the South African Veterinary Medical Association*, 39, 81–85.

139

Porcine pleuropneumonia

Synonym: *Actinobacillus (Haemophilus) pleuropneumoniae* infection

M.M. Henton and C.M. Veary

Introduction

Porcine pleuropneumonia, caused by *Actinobacillus (Haemophilus) pleuropneumoniae*, is a highly contagious and often fatal disease which particularly affects pigs aged between 12 and 15 weeks, although animals of all ages are susceptible.[10, 46, 52, 53] It may manifest clinically as a peracute, acute, subacute or chronic disease, the more acute forms being characterized by the presence of a fibrinous to fibrinonecrotic bronchopneumonia, and the chronic by the development of pulmonary sequestra and reduced weight gain. Apparently recovered animals, as well as healthy ones may be carriers of the infection.

A *Haemophilus*-like organism was first described from cases of porcine pleuropneumonia in England in 1957.[39] Since the late 1960s, porcine pleuropneumonia has been of major economic importance in European countries, particularly Scandinavia,[46] and has also become increasingly important to the pig industry in many countries throughout the world. In South Africa the organism was isolated for the first time in 1985. In contrast to most countries, where it initially caused explosive outbreaks of disease with high mortality, the first cases diagnosed in South Africa were characterized by the development of an insidious form of chronic pneumonia which was complicated by simultaneous infections with either *Pasteurella multocida, Streptococcus equisimilis, Streptococcus suis* or *Actinomyces (Corynebacterium) pyogenes*. Subsequently the more typical peracute, acute, subacute and chronic forms of the disease have occurred in South Africa. Most outbreaks have been reported in the Transvaal and have almost exclusively involved pigs aged between two and six months.

Outbreaks of porcine pleuropneumonia are the cause of severe economic losses as a result of the high mortality rate, high cost of chemotherapy and, in the chronic form of the disease, reduced herd performance.[19, 53]

Aetiology

The genus *Actinobacillus* belongs to the family Pasteurellaceae, which comprises short, Gram-negative, non-motile, non-spore-forming, pleomorphic rods (with a tendency to occur mainly in coccobacillary forms). The other two members of the family are *Haemophilus* and *Pasteurella*. The genus *Haemophilus* is defined by its need for specific growth factors for optimal growth, the growth-factor requirements also having been used as a criterion for speciation within the genus.[19] These factors may be plasmid controlled[8] and are Factor X (protoporphyrin IX or protohaeme) and Factor V (nicotinamide adenine dinucleotide or NAD).

As most strains of *A. pleuropneumoniae* require Factor V, or Factor V-related compounds, it was initially placed in the genus *Haemophilus*. However, on the basis of DNA:DNA hybridization data it is now classified as an *Actinobacillus*[41] and is divided into two biovars: biovar 1, which requires Factor V and occurs worldwide, and biovar 2, which is Factor V-independent (although it still appears to require Factor V-related compounds) and has only been isolated in Switzerland.[28]

Actinobacillus pleuropneumoniae is Factor V-dependent (excepting biovar 2) but Factor X-independent, urease-positive, CAMP-positive, ferments mannitol and is beta-haemolytic on 5 per cent calf- or sheep-blood agar[19] **(Table 139.1)**. It forms small, whitish, opaque colonies (1–2 mm in diameter) within 48 hours of incubation on chocolate blood agar. Two types of colonies have been described:[19] a rough, round, hard, waxy type which adheres to wire inoculating loops, and a flatter, soft and more readily serotypable, glistening colony. Most virulent strains are heavily capsulated and produce iridescent colonies on Levinthal agar.[18]

The antigenic properties of *A. pleuropneumoniae* have been extensively researched.[27, 31, 35] There are antigenic, serotype-specific, membrane lipopolysaccharides and capsular polysaccharides.[20] Non-encapsulated mutants are generally avirulent and rapidly cleared by host defences.[14] The serospecific polysaccharide capsules inhibit the bactericidal and opsonic activity of normal serum. Based on differences in the capsular polysaccharides, *A. pleuropneumoniae* biovar 1 is divided into 12 serovars. Common antigens (lipopolysaccharide and outer membrane proteins)[14, 24, 33] exist which complicate serodiagnostic and sero-epidemiological studies.[37] Cross-reactions are common between serovars 1, 9 and 11,

Table 139.1 Simplified bacteriological differentiation criteria of *Actinobacillus* spp. that may be isolated from pigs[31]

CHARACTERISTIC	*A. PLEUROPNEUMONIAE* Biovar 1	*A. PLEUROPNEUMONIAE* Biovar 2	*A. SUIS*	*A. EQUULI*	*A. LIGNIERESII*
NAD-requirement	+	–	–	–	–
Haemolysis	+	+	+	+	–
Urease	+	+	+	+	+
Aesculin	–	–	+	–	–
CAMP	+	+	+	–	–
Trehalose	–	–	+	+	–
Mannitol	+	+	–	+	+
Raffinose	V	V	–	+	+

v = variable

between 4 and 7, and between 3, 6 and 8,[20, 24, 33] but cross-reactivity between virtually all serovars can occur, depending on the antigen and test method used.[9]

Whilst coagglutination and slide agglutination are the tests of choice for routine typing, serovars can only conclusively be identified by the agar gel diffusion and indirect haemagglutination tests.[33] In spite of low sensitivity, the slide agglutination test would seem to be the best for serotyping isolates.[40] The coagglutination test has the advantage that antigen can be detected directly from lung samples of pigs with acute or chronic respiratory problems, and from those of apparently healthy carriers.[26]

Epidemiology

Actinobacillus pleuropneumoniae is a primary pathogen of the respiratory tract of pigs. It rarely affects other animals, having only been isolated from a case of arthritis in a lamb and a brain abscess in a steer.[16] Porcine pleuropneumonia occurs particularly in pigs of about 12–15 weeks of age,[53] but other age groups may also be affected, particularly when the infection is first introduced into a herd. With the disappearance of colostral immunity at six weeks, pigs become susceptible to the disease.[34]

The occurrence of different serovars may be restricted to certain regions or countries. In South Africa serovars 7 and 12 (which are related to serovars 3 and 6) are the most common, but serovars 1, 2, 3, 5, 6, 8, 9 and 10 have also been found.[11] Although *A. pleuropneumoniae* occurs in all four provinces of South Africa, most cases have been reported from the Transvaal. *Actinobacillus pleuropneumoniae* has not been reported from any other southern African country.

Pigs suffering from the acute disease shed large numbers of organisms in nasal discharges and in aerosols.[44] Transmission occurs mainly through the respiratory route, by the inhalation of such aerosols, in pigs which are maintained in close contact with each other.[19] Environmental and managemental factors often contribute to the development of the disease[47, 50] **(see Chapter 188: Porcine respiratory disease)**. Conditions conducive to aerosol formation, humidity changes, close confinement and overcrowding—including the crowding which often occurs in cold weather—facilitate spread of the disease among pigs. Aerosols containing small droplets are formed under conditions of low temperatures and low-to-medium humidity levels, and these may penetrate the respiratory system as far as the alveoli.[44, 51]

Pigs which have recovered from clinical disease may serve as inapparent carriers for many months or even years. In these animals the organisms are located mainly in sequestra in the lungs and/or the tonsillar crypts, and infrequently in the nasal cavity.[19, 53] In addition, in infected herds a variable number of apparently healthy pigs which have never manifested clinical signs may carry the bacterium in their tonsillar crypts and nasal cavities; in one herd as many as 53 per cent of the animals were recorded as being healthy carriers.[17] Such animals are important reservoirs of the bacterium and introduction of them into susceptible herds may result in spread of the infection.[19] The appearance of overt disease is usually triggered by environmental or managemental stress. Transportation of pigs is a common stressor; because of the short incubation period, susceptible animals in contact with carriers during transportation to abattoirs can develop acute pleuropneumonia and die before slaughter. An abrupt change of climate, such as a sudden increase or decrease in the prevailing environmental temperature, can also precipitate clinical disease. The prevalence of the disease in infected herds may gradually increase from a low rate in summer to a peak in winter or spring.[19] In South Africa, the number of cases of pleuropneumonia peaks in the early summer.[11]

Because of the susceptibility of the organism to common disinfectants such as 2 per cent chlorine dioxide fogging,[44] and to dessication and sunlight, it is unlikely to survive for longer than a day in the environment,[29] and it is therefore probably not disseminated mechanically by vectors. It can, however, survive for a few days in, and be transmitted by, nasal discharges and mucus,[31] and because of the massive nasal excretion of exudate during the acute phase of the disease, indirect transmission by fomites and farm personnel cannot be excluded.[31]

Pathogenesis

The exact pathogenesis of porcine pleuropneumonia is unknown, although the determinants of virulence of

A. pleuropneumoniae have been extensively studied.[1, 15] *Actinobacillus pleuropneumoniae* organisms initially reach the alveoli of the lungs either from primary sites of infection in the tonsillar crypts or nasal cavity during stressful situations or as a result of the direct inhalation of infected aerosols. Virulence factors (their presence or absence being variable) of the organism, including the capsule, endotoxin, exotoxins (haemolysins and cytotoxins) and others, are important in the pathogenesis of the disease. *Actinobacillus pleuropneumoniae* has an antiphagocytic capsule and produces leukotoxins which impair the function of, and eventually kill, leukocytes.[5] The capsule also inhibits the bactericidal effect of serum, thus further protecting the bacterium from the host defences.[15] The ability of *A. pleuropneumoniae* to resist the lethal effects of complement *in vitro* may also reflect a virulence mechanism that *in vivo* renders pulmonary defences inactive and promotes bacterial invasion of the lungs.[43] Pathogenic *A. pleuropneumoniae* strains also release an IgA protease that cleaves mucosal IgA, whereas non-pathogenic strains, as well as non-pathogenic *Haemophilus* strains that merely colonize the upper airways, lack this enzyme.[1] The endotoxin (lipopolysaccharide), which is similar to that of other Gram-negative bacteria **(see Chapter 129: *Escherichia coli* infections)**, acts synergistically with other toxins of this bacterium and, among other effects, inactivates the phagocytic function of pulmonary alveolar macrophages.[7] *Actinobacillus pleuropneumoniae* activates intravascular coagulation (probably by way of endotoxin) which, in association with prostaglandin, plays an important role in the development of the lesions in the lungs.[1]

Several other toxins, including haemolysins that are cytotoxic, lethal for pigs or antiphagocytic, are also produced by *A. pleuropneumoniae*. They play an important role in the pathogenesis of the disease and can act synergistically with *Staphylococcus aureus* beta toxin. When injected parenterally into pigs, they induce some of the characteristic lesions which occur in natural *A. pleuropneumoniae* infections.[1]

The immune response against *A. pleuropneumoniae* is not fully understood. Following natural infection, circulating antibodies develop within two weeks. Colostral immunity is conferred upon piglets by immune sows.

Clinical signs

The incubation period may vary from six to 12 hours[34] to a few days, depending on the size of the infective dose and the susceptibility of the host.

The disease may present in a peracute, acute, subacute or chronic form. In susceptible herds with no natural immunity, and especially if predisposing factors are present, its onset is generally sudden and the spread rapid, with fatalities occurring in all age groups. The mortality rate can be as high as 40 per cent in these herds.[44]

The first signs in peracutely affected pigs are usually a sudden loss of appetite and a high rectal temperature (up to 40,5 °C), but some individuals die without clinical signs having been observed. Other signs in the peracute disease include cyanosis of the skin and mucous membranes, a roughened hair coat, dyspnoea, respiratory distress, a moist, suppressed cough, vomition, epistaxis and a copious, foamy, blood-tinged discharge from the mouth and nostrils.[35] Death usually occurs within 24 hours of the onset of the disease. In neonatal pigs, in which the mortality rate is usually 100 per cent, signs of nervous involvement, such as incoordination, may be a feature.

Acute cases begin with high fever, lethargy, anorexia and, as the disease progresses, show signs of respiratory distress and dyspnoea when forced to move. A short, suppressed cough may be heard. The disease may lead to death in one or two days, or may proceed to the subacute and chronic stage.[34, 49]

Chronically affected animals show no characteristic clinical signs, but their food intake is reduced, growth rate retarded, and they may suffer from a chronic cough and elevated body temperature. Chronically infected herds may contain many subclinical cases of the disease, in which the presence of the lung lesions may exacerbate the clinical signs caused by other concurrent respiratory infections.

Sequelae after septicaemic spread of the organism include arthritis, endocarditis and abscess formation in the lungs;[32] such dissemination of *A. pleuropneumoniae* occurs more commonly after infection with serovar 3 than with the other serovars.[32] Pregnant sows may abort as a sequel to the acute disease.[32]

Pathology

The gross and microscopic pathology varies according to the nature and course of the disease, but the most prominent lesions are usually found in the thoracic cavity.[30, 38] In the peracute form, blood-tinged, frothy exudate may ooze from the nares and fill the upper respiratory passage. The mucosa of the nasal cavity, trachea and bronchi is congested, and may contain haemorrhages. The lungs show blood-tinged alveolar and interstitial oedema, congestion, petechiation and uni- or bilateral multilobular red patches of pneumonia, particularly at the dorsal and hilar regions, and well-circumscribed, necrotic and haemorrhagic areas **(Figures 139.1 and 2)**. Serosanguineous hydrothorax and hydropericardium, and fibrinous pericarditis are frequently present. The intrathoracic lymph nodes are enlarged but not haemorrhagic.[1, 30, 38] Evidence of septicaemia is present in some cases. Microscopically in peracutely affected animals there is congestion, haemorrhage, oedema and serofibrinous exudate in the alveoli and interstitial tissues of the lungs **(Figure 139.3)**. The bronchial lymph nodes show accumulation of some neutrophils in their sinuses.

In the acute form, the lung lesions are characterized by a fibrinous, fibrinohaemorrhagic or fibrinonecrotic bronchopneumonia, giving the organ a mottled appearance.[21] These lesions are similar in distribution to the

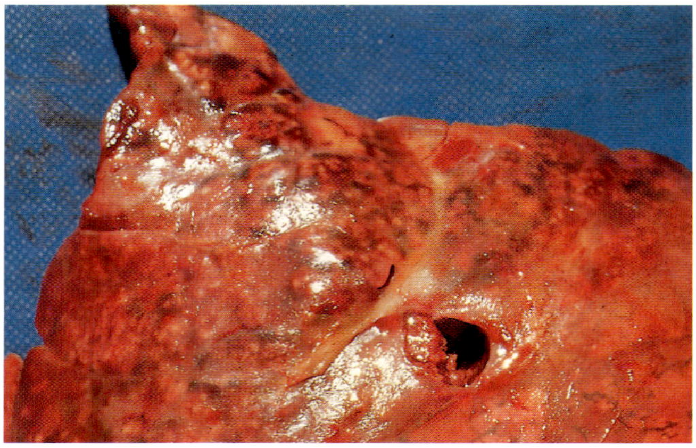

Figure 139.1 Porcine pleuropneumonia. Mottled appearance of the pleural surface imparted by congestion, haemorrhage and multifocal areas of acute pneumonia

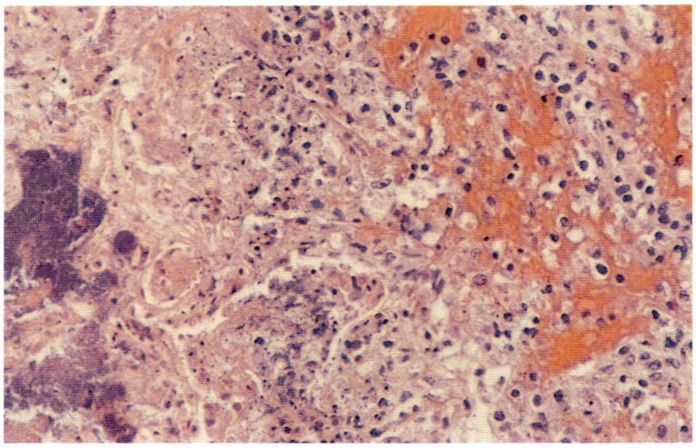

Figure 139.3 Photomicrograph of lung showing focal haemorrhage, a scant cellular infiltrate and a serofibrinous exudate in addition to locally extensive necrosis

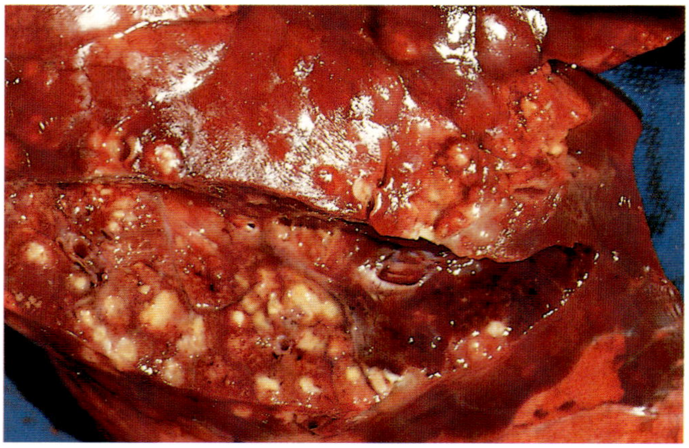

Figure 139.2 Cut surface of the lung manifesting multiple, sometimes confluent areas of necrosis

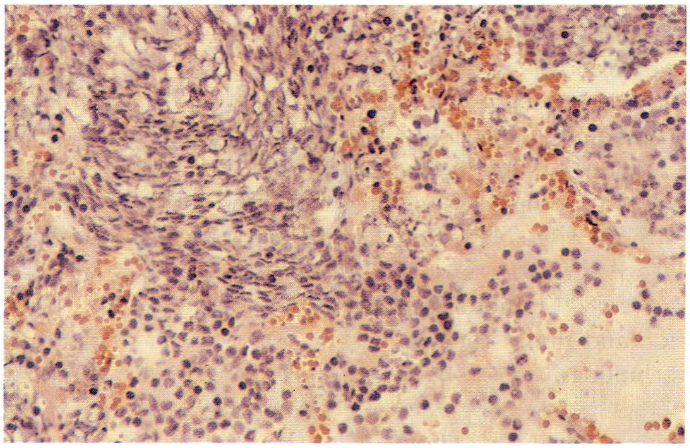

Figure 139.4 Acute porcine pleuropneumonia. Note the prominent mononuclear infiltrate and elongated streaming macrophages arranged in a swirling pattern

haemorrhagic lesions seen in the peracute form of the disease. The interlobular septa of the lungs are widened by hyperaemia and oedema and a fibrinous pleuritis is usually present on the pleural surfaces over pneumonic areas, causing the lungs to adhere to the thoracic wall.[38] A fibrinous polyarthritis and fibrinopurulent meningo-encephalitis may be present in some cases. Histologically, neutrophils are absent from the pneumonic lesions, but there are abundant mononuclear leukocytes.[19] These cells also infiltrate the interlobular septa. The presence of numerous elongated macrophages orientated in a swirling pattern is characteristic of the lesion **(Figure 139.4)**.[19]

Pigs that survive more than four or five days show necrotic foci up to 100 mm in diameter situated particularly in the dorsal or hilar regions of the lungs. In the sub-acute to chronic forms, the extent of the lesions usually correlates with the severity of clinical disease. However, extensive lung lesions and chronic pleuritis have been found at slaughter in apparently healthy pigs. The lesions in the lungs may resolve completely in pigs that recover from the disease, but often small, encapsulated pulmonary sequestra remain, in which the causative organisms persist, accounting largely for the carrier state of the disease. If the sequestra become secondarily invaded, for example by *A. pyogenes*, *P. multocida* or streptococci, they may be transformed into abscesses. Occasionally severe pyothorax and an extensive fibrinous or chronic adhesive pleuritis are evident. A pericarditis is sometimes associated with the lung lesions.

Diagnosis

A presumptive diagnosis of porcine pleuropneumonia can be made on the clinical signs and on the necropsy and histopathological findings, but isolation of *A. pleuropneumoniae* and serology are necessary to confirm it.

Specimens for bacteriological examination from fatal cases of the more acute disease should comprise tissue samples of lung lesions, and bronchial and mediastinal lymph nodes. Specimens from the lungs should preferably be taken from the caudal lobes, if lesions are present in them, as they tend to contain fewer contaminants than the cranial lobes. Recovery of the organism from other tissues and organs in the septicaemic disease tends to be erratic.

It is generally easier to recover *A. pleuropneumoniae* from the affected tissues of more acute cases. It is often difficult to isolate the organism from pulmonary lesions and sequestra in subacutely and chronically affected pigs because it may have been overgrown or even killed by other species of bacteria,[12, 53] such as *P. multocida*, alpha- and beta-haemolytic streptococci, and *A. pyogenes*. In such cases, a definitive diagnosis is not always possible.

The organism may also be isolated from swabs of nasal discharges in live animals, from the joint fluid of joints affected by arthritis,[12] and from the tonsillar crypts. In the latter case, the material for bacteriological culture should originate preferably from the tissue side rather than from the pharyngeal side, in order to minimize contamination.

Actinobacillus pleuropneumoniae usually survives for at least four days under various storage conditions at temperatures lower than 20°C. Apart from possible co-infection of the lesions with other species of bacteria, its isolation may be hampered by post-mortem decomposition of affected tissues, or if the animal has been treated with an antibiotic prior to collection of the specimens.[12] In order to overcome some of these problems, selective media,[17, 51] rapid detection methods such as coagglutination and fluorescent antibody techniques,[26] and dilution techniques have been used. One technique which incorporates the use of selective media and dilution requires the lung sample to be homogenized, and eight subsequent ten-fold dilutions made in serum broth. Each dilution is then streaked at right angles onto blood agar inoculated with a *Staphylococcus epidermidis* feeder culture. A more simple dilution technique is one in which the affected tissue contained in an inoculating wire loop is streaked onto four consecutive blood agar plates without flaming the loop between plates.[36] This technique has been found to be adequate in diluting out *P. multocida* and other concomitant bacteria whilst retaining *A. pleuropneumoniae*, and is much less time-consuming than serial dilution. Once isolated, the strain may be serotyped. Several colonies should be chosen, as more than one strain may be present.

Immunoperoxidase techniques are of diagnostic value in formalin-fixed tissues.[13]

In order to determine whether or not a herd is infected, serological and bacteriological examinations of more than one animal should be conducted. A number of pigs should be bled in order to determine antibody levels. This is more conveniently done at the abattoir than on the farm. When analysing the results of serological examinations, it should be borne in mind that cross-reactivity with serovar groupings, for example 3, 6 and 8, is associated with IgG antibodies, and that a combination of tests is essential in order to eliminate overlapping type-specific determinants.[25] The indirect fluorescent antibody test is most sensitive for multiple serovars, but the coagglutination test is less time-consuming, easier to read and preferred when many serum samples have to be tested.[3] However, both are of limited value for the detection of serovars 2, 7 and 9. The enzyme-linked immunosorbent assay (ELISA) is approximately 90 per cent sensitive and is specific on a herd basis.[54] The sensitivity of the ELISA is higher, but its specificity is lower, than those of the complement fixation test (CFT). The CFT is reasonably serovar-specific and a direct relationship has been found between positive CF titres and the presence of *A. pleuropneumoniae* in the lungs.[12] The CFT is the test of choice if a single test is preferred in diagnostic laboratories and, when interpreted on a herd basis, the results accurately reflect whether the organism is present or not. This is particularly true when clinical signs are mild or absent, as is often the case in chronically infected herds. For the detection of infection a herd should be tested twice at an interval of three weeks for all the serovars prevalent in the country.

The physical examination of the lungs of pigs at an abattoir is another important way of diagnosing chronic pneumonia on a herd basis, and is also a good method of monitoring the effectiveness of control programmes.

It is essential that the results of serological tests be interpreted by an experienced serologist or bacteriologist so that the correct decisions are made about the purchase of replacement stock, sale of animals, and culling and vaccination programmes.[12]

Differential diagnosis

Porcine pleuropneumonia should be differentiated from pneumonia caused by a variety of microorganisms **(see Chapter 188: Porcine respiratory disease)**, including *Haemophilus parasuis*, *Mycoplasma hyopneumoniae* and *Pasteurella* spp.

Control

Control of the disease is based on its early diagnosis and therapy, effective environmental control measures, reduction of stress, serological testing in an attempt to maintain a disease-free herd in an all-in/all-out system, and vaccination.[19, 22, 23, 35, 44, 45]

It is important to ensure that pigs are maintained under high standards of environmental hygiene in well-ventilated, uncrowded pens which are separated from each other by solid partitions. As *A. pleuropneumoniae* outbreaks are closely related to stress, this should be minimized.

A closed herd should be maintained as far as possible, but if pigs do have to be introduced, they should originate only from uninfected piggeries that are serologically negative to the disease. This will help to avoid introducing subclinical carriers. As not all affected pigs reveal clinical evidence of disease, regular and thorough inspection of the lungs at abattoirs is advocated in order to confirm that *A. pleuropneumoniae* infection is absent from the herd.

If newly introduced pigs do originate from unknown sources, some authors recommended that they be quarantined for at least 30 days and receive treatment consisting either of the parenteral administration of a long-acting oxytetracycline at a dosage rate of 22,5 mg/kg once a day for three to five days, or of oxytetracycline in the feed for two weeks at the rate of 400 g/ton of feed. The feeding of the medicated ration should commence at the start of the quarantine period.[4, 51] The administration of antimicrobials does not eliminate infection in all carriers.

Actinobacillus pleuropneumoniae is susceptible to many antimicrobials but it is advisable to do an antibiogram to select the most effective drug before therapy is instituted. In South Africa the organism is generally susceptible to ampicillin, cephalosporins and oxytetracycline.[11] In outbreaks of acute disease, these antimicrobials should be administered parenterally at recommended dosages, as the affected pigs usually do not eat or drink. Antimicrobial therapy of acute cases does reduce the mortality from porcine pleuropneumonia, and subsequently improves daily weight gains. In chronically infected herds, the appetite of infected pigs is not affected, and antimicrobial medication may therefore be administered in the feed or water, according to the manufacturer's recommendations. Animals suffering from the chronic disease do not generally respond well to antimicrobial therapy. Treated animals may continue to harbour the organisms in pulmonary sequestra, and prolonged treatment with high levels of antimicrobials is necessary to eliminate them, although this is not usually successful.[19]

The long-term administration of antimicrobials in feed may induce the development of resistance of *A. pleuropneumoniae* to the drug used. In the Netherlands, tiamulin, lincomycin, tylosin and spiramycin have been found to be inactive against the organism.

Capsular antigens are important protective antigens following natural exposure or immunization.[42]

It seems that vaccination does prevent acute deaths but not the development of subclinical and chronic infections.[23, 42] Because there are different serovars of *A. pleuropneumoniae*, the serotyping of the isolate or isolates responsible for an outbreak of the disease is an extremely important procedure, which enables the correct vaccine to be selected in order to control the particular outbreak.[40] Natural infection results in a high level of cross-protection between serovars,[35] but, as far as the selection of a vaccine is concerned, monovalent vaccines give the best results.[6] However, variable results have been reported following the use of vaccines.[6, 32] Oil-adjuvanted vaccines prepared from young cultures are highly immunogenic, but the oil may induce the development of unacceptably large granulomas at the injection site.[48] A formalinized polyvalent vaccine (serovars 1, 2, 3, 4, 6 and 8) has been successfully used to reduce mortalities.[2, 6, 32] Vaccines should only be administered to animals older than five to six weeks, to avoid the suppression of the development of active immunity in piglets protected by colostrum-acquired passive immunity.

References

1 **BERTRAM, T.A., 1990.** *Actinobacillus pleuropneumoniae*: Molecular aspects of virulence and pulmonary injury. *Canadian Journal of Veterinary Research*, 54, S53–56.

2 **BLOXHAM, P.A., 1987.** Preliminary results on the efficacy of a *Haemophilus pleuropneumoniae* vaccine in pigs. *Irish Veterinary News*, 9, 37–38.

3 **BUNKA, S., 1987.** Direct demonstration of *Haemophilus (Actinobacillus) pleuropneumoniae* in lungs of swine. Inaugural Dissertation, Tierärztliche Hochschule, Hannover, Federal Republic of Germany, 1–68.

4 **BURCH, D.G.S., JONES, G.T., HEARD, T.W. & TUCK, R.E., 1986.** The synergistic activity of tiamulin and chlortetracycline: In-feed treatment of bacterially complicated enzootic pneumonia in fattening pigs. *The Veterinary Record*, 119, 108–112.

5 **CZUPRYNSKI, C.J. & SAMPLE, A.K., 1990.** Interactions of *Haemophilus-Actinobacillus-Pasteurella* bacteria with phagocytic cells. *Canadian Journal of Veterinary Research*, 54, 536–540.

6 **EWALD, C., APPEL, G. & VON MICKWITX, G., 1989.** Experiences with vaccination against *Haemophilus pleuropneumoniae* in pigs. *Berliner und Münchener Tierärztliche Wochenschrift*, 102, 6–11.

7 **FENWICK, B.W., OSBURN, B.I. & OLANDER, H.J., 1986.** Isolation and biological characterisation of two lipopolysaccharides and a capsular-enriched polysaccharide preparation from *Haemophilus pleuropneumoniae*. *American Journal of Veterinary Research*, 47, 1433–1441.

8 **GROMKOVA, R. & KOORNHOF, H., 1990.** Naturally occurring NAD-independent *Haemophilus parainfluenzae*. *Journal of General Microbiology*, 136, 1031–1035.

9 **GUTIERREZ, C.B., TASCON, R.I., VAZQUEZ, J.A. & RODRIGUEZ FERRI, E.F., 1991.** Cross-reactivity between *Actinobacillus pleuropneumoniae* serotypes comparing different antigens and serological tests. *Research in Veterinary Science*, 50, 308–310.

10 **HENRY, S.C., 1986.** Evaluating the alternative therapies for swine respiratory disease. *Food Animal Practice/Veterinary Medicine*, 81, 763–771.

11 **HENTON, M.M., 1993.** Veterinary Research Institute, Onderstepoort. Unpublished data.

12 **HOFFMAN, L.J., 1989.** *Actinobacillus (Haemophilus) pleuropneumoniae*: Use of coagulation and complement fixation to determine the relationship between presence of organism and antibody titre in slaughterhouse pigs. *Journal of Veterinary Diagnostic Investigation*, 1, 12–15.

13 **IBARGOYEN, G.S., PERFUMO, C.J., MASSONE, A.R., MARTIN, A.A. & GRIMENO, E.J., 1989.** The use of immunoperoxidase techniques for the identification of *Actinobacillus pleuropneumoniae* in tissue sections. *Israel Journal of Veterinary Medicine*, 45, 18–20.

14 **INZANA, T.J., 1990.** Capsules and virulence in the HAP group of bacteria. *Canadian Journal of Veterinary Research*, 54, 522–529.

15 **INZANA, T.J., 1991.** Virulence properties of *Actinobacillus pleuropneumoniae. Microbial Pathogenesis*, 11, 305–316.

16 **KILIAN, M. & BIBERSTEIN, E.L., 1984.** Genus II. *Haemophilus. In*: KRIEG, N.R. & HOLT, J.G., (eds). *Bergey's Manual of Systematic Bacteriology*. Vol. I. Baltimore, London: Williams & Wilkins.

17 **KUME, K., NAGANO, I. & NAKAI, T., 1986.** Bacteriological, serological and pathological examinations of *Haemophilus pleuropneumoniae* infection in 200 slaughtered pigs. *Japanese Journal of Veterinary Science*, 48, 965–970.

18 **LEVINSHAL, W., 1918.** Bakteriologische und serologische influenzastudien. *Zeitschrift für Hygiene und Infektionskrankheiten*, 86, 1.

19 **LEWIS, D.H. & SCHWARTZ, W.L., 1987.** *Haemophilus pleuropneumoniae* in swine. *Compendium Food Animal*, 9, 7–12.

20 **LIDA, J., SMITH, I.M. & NICOLET, J., 1990.** Use of monoclonal antibodies for classifying *Actinobacillus (Haemophilus) pleuropneumoniae. Research in Veterinary Science*, 49, 8–13.

21 **LIGGETT, A.D. & HARRISON, L.R., 1987.** Sequential study of lesion development in experimental *Haemophilus pleuropneumoniae. Research in Veterinary Science*, 42, 204–221.

22 **MACINNES, J.L. & ROSENDAL, S., 1988.** Prevention and control of *Actinobacillus (Haemophilus) pleuropneumoniae* infection in swine: A review. *Canadian Veterinary Journal*, 29, 572–574.

23 **MARTINEAU, G.P., HIGGINS, R., LARIVIRE, S., MITTAL, K.R., VAILLANCOURT, J. & DESROSIERS, R., 1985.** Elimination and control measures for swine pleuropneumonia in Quebec. *Compendium on Swine Haemophilus Pleuropneumonia*, 39–42.

24 **MITTAL, K.R., 1990.** Cross-reactions between *Actinobacillus (Haemophilus) pleuropneumoniae* strains of serotypes 1 and 9. *Journal of Clinical Microbiology*, 28, 535–539.

25 **MITTAL, K.R., HIGGINS, R. & LARIVIRE, S., 1988.** Serologic studies of *Actinobacillus (Haemophilus) pleuropneumoniae* strains of serotype 3 and their antigenic relationship with other *Actinobacillus pleuropneumoniae* serotypes in swine. *American Journal of Veterinary Research*, 49, 152–155.

26 **MITTAL, K.R., HIGGINS, R., LARIVIRE, S. & MARTINEAU, G., 1985.** Use of coagglutination test for direct detection and serotyping of *Haemophilus pleuropneumoniae. Compendium on Swine Haemophilus Pleuropneumonia*, 28–33.

27 **MITTAL, K.R., HIGGINS, R., LARIVIRE, S. & MARTINEAU, G.P., 1987.** Effect of heat treatment on the surface antigens of *Haemophilus pleuropneumoniae. The Veterinary Record*, 120, 62–65.

28 **MOLLER, K. & KILIAN, M., 1990.** V factor-dependent members of the family *Pasteurellaceae* in the porcine upper respiratory tract. *Journal of Clinical Microbiology*, 28, 2711–2716.

29 **MOROZUMI, T. & HIRAMUNE, T., 1982.** Effect of temperature on the survival of *Haemophilus parasuis* in physiological saline. *National Institute of Animal Health (Tokyo)*, 22, 90–91.

30 **MYLREA, P.J., FRASER, G., MACQUEEN, P. & LAMBOURNE, D.A., 1974.** Pleuropneumonia in pigs caused by *Haemophilus parahaemolyticus. Australian Veterinary Journal*, 50, 255–259.

31 **NICOLET, J., 1985.** *Haemophilus pleuropneumoniae*—Bacteriology and epidemiology. *Compendium on Swine Haemophilus Pleuropneumonia*, 7–11.

32 **NICOLET, J., 1986.** *Haemophilus* infections. *In*: LEMAN, A.D., STRAW, B., GLOCK, R.D., MENGELING, W.L., PENNY, R.H.C. & SCHOLL, E., (eds). *Diseases of Swine*. 6th edn. Ames, Iowa: Iowa State University Press.

33 **NICOLET, J., 1988.** Taxonomy and serology identification of *Actinobacillus pleuropneumoniae. Canadian Veterinary Journal*, 29, 578–579.

34 **NIELSEN, R., 1982.** *Haemophilus pleuropneumoniae* infection in pigs. Thesis, Veterinaer-og Landbohojskoles, Copenhagen, Denmark.

35 **NIELSEN, R., 1985.** *Haemophilus pleuropneumoniae* diagnosis, immunity and control. *Compendium on Swine Haemophilus Pleuropneumonia*, 18–22.

36 **NIELSEN, R., 1986.** State Veterinary Serum Laboratory, Bärowsvey 27, Copenhagen, Denmark. Personal communication.

37 **NIELSEN, R., 1988.** Seroepidemiology of *Actinobacillus pleuropneumoniae. Canadian Veterinary Journal*, 29, 580–582.

38 **OLANDER, H.J., 1985.** The pathology of *Haemophilus pleuropneumoniae* infection of swine. *Compendium on Swine Haemophilus Pleuropneumonia*, 12–17.

39 **PATTISON, I.H., HOWELL, D.C. & ELLIOTT, J., 1957.** A *Haemophilus*-like organism isolated from pig lung and the associated pneumonic lesion. *Journal of Comparative Pathology*, 67, 320–329.

40 **PIJOAN, C., 1985.** Serology and immunology of *Haemophilus pleuropneumoniae. Compendium on Swine Haemophilus Pleuropneumonia*, 23–27.

41 **POHL, S., BERSTSCHINGER, H.U., FREDERIKSEN, W. & MANNHEIM, W., 1983.** Transfer of *Haemophilus pleuropneumoniae* and the *Pasteurella haemolytica*-like organism causing porcine necrotic pleuropneumonia to the genus *Actinobacillus (Actinobacillus pleuropneumoniae* comb. nov.) on the basis of phenotypic and deoxyribonucleic acid relatedness. *International Journal of Systematic Bacteriology*, 33, 510–514.

42 **RAPP, V.J. & ROSS, R.F., 1988.** Immunogenicity of outer membrane components of *Haemophilus (Actinobacillus) pleuropneumoniae. Canadian Veterinary Journal*, 29, 585–587.

43 **RYCROFT, A.N. & CULLEN, J.M., 1990.** Complement resistance in *Actinobacillus (Haemophilus) pleuropneumoniae* infection of swine. *American Journal of Veterinary Research*, 51, 1449–1453.

44 **SCHULTZ, R.A., 1985.** *Haemophilus pleuropneumoniae* of swine: Prevalence, treatment, control and prevention. *Compendium on Swine Haemophilus Pleuropneumonia*, 34–38.

45 **SCHULTZ, R.A., 1985.** *Haemophilus*: Overview of diagnostic tests and potential treatment. *Agri-Practice*, 6, 25–28.

46 **SEBUNYA, T.N.K. & SAUNDERS, J.R., 1983.** *Haemophilus pleuropneumoniae* infection in swine: A review. *Journal of the American Veterinary Medical Association*, 182, 1331–1337.

47 **STRAW, B., 1986.** A look at the factors that contribute to the development of swine pneumonia. *Food Animal Practice/Veterinary Medicine*, 81, 747–756.

48 **STRAW, B., SHIN, S., CALLIHAN, D. & PETERSEN, M., 1990.** Antibody production and tissue irritation in swine vaccinated with *Actinobacillus* bacterins containing various adjuvants. *Journal of the American Veterinary Medical Association*, 196, 600–604.

49 **TARASIUK, K., PEJSAK, Z., PALKA, E. & BLASZCZYK, B., 1991.** Acute form of pleuropneumonia in pigs caused by *Actinobacillus pleuropneumoniae* serotype 9. *Medycyna Weterynaryjna*, 47, 348–350.

50 **THOMAS, P., 1984.** The influence of housing design and some management systems on the health of the growing pig, particularly in relation to pneumonia. Commonwealth Agricultural Bureaux: *Pig News and Information*, 5, 343–349.

51 **TUBBS, R.C., 1988.** Managing the swine herd that has been infected with *Haemophilus pleuropneumoniae. Food Animal Practice/Veterinary Medicine*, 83, 220–229.

52 **UDEZE, F.A., LATIMER, K.S. & KADIS, S., 1987.** Role of *Haemophilus pleuropneumoniae* lipopolysaccharide endotoxin in the pathogenesis of porcine *Haemophilus pleuropneumoniae. American Journal of Veterinary Research*, 48, 768–773.

53 **WILSON, P.J., FALK, G. & KLASHINSKY, S., 1987.** Detection of *Actinobacillus pleuropneumoniae* infection in pigs. *Canadian Veterinary Journal*, 28, 111–116.

54 **WILSON, P.J., SCHIPPER, C. & MORGAN, E.D., 1988.** The use of an enzyme-linked immunosorbent assay for diagnosis of *Actinobacillus pleuropneumoniae* infection in pigs. *Canadian Veterinary Journal*, 29, 583–585.

140

Actinobacillus suis *infections*

M.M. Henton

Actinobacillus suis is a rare cause of a rapidly fatal septicaemia particularly of piglets younger than two months of age. Adult sows, especially those in minimal-disease herds, may also succumb to septicaemic disease, and may show signs very similar to those of acute erysipelas.[3] Pathogenic *Escherichia coli* infections may occur together with *A. suis* in piglets. The clinical signs and lesions in affected animals are similar to those which occur in foals suffering from *A. equuli* septicaemia **(see Chapter 137: *Actinobacillus equuli* infections)**.

Horses may carry *A. suis* in the upper respiratory and genital tracts, but the role of the organism in the production of disease — if indeed there is a role — is unclear.[2]

Actinobacillus equuli and *A. suis* have similar biochemical properties; earlier publications have not always differentiated clearly between the two species.[5, 6]

Only nine cases of *A. suis* infection were diagnosed in pigs at the Veterinary Research Institute, Onderstepoort in the period from 1979 to 1991.[1]

Actinobacillus suis is susceptible to ampicillin, chloramphenicol, trimethoprim-sulphonamide combinations, tetracyclines and streptomycin, and treatment at recommended dosages with any of these is usually effective.[3, 4]

References

1 **HENTON, M.M., 1993.** Veterinary Research Institute, Onderstepoort. Unpublished observations.

2 **KIM, B.H., PHILLIPS, J.G. & ATHERTON, J.G., 1976.** *Actinobacillus suis* in the horse. *The Veterinary Record*, 98, 239.

3 **MINIATS, O.P., SPINATO, M.T. & SANDFORD, S.E., 1989.** *Actinobacillus suis* septicaemia in mature swine. Two outbreaks resembling erysipelas. *Canadian Veterinary Journal*, 30, 943–947.

4 **TAYLOR, D.J., 1986.** Miscellaneous bacterial infections. *In:* LEMAN, A.D., STRAW, B., GLOCK, R.D., MENGELING, W.L., PENNY, R.H.C. & SCHOLL, E., (eds). *Diseases of Swine*. 6th edn. 634–636.

5 **VAN DORSSEN, C.A. & JAARSVELD, F.H.J., 1962.** *Actinobacillus suis* (novo species). A bacterium occurring in swine. *Tijdschrift Diergeneeskunde*, 87, 450–458.

6 **WINDSOR, R.S., 1973.** *Actinobacillus equuli* infection in a litter of pigs and a review of previous reports on similar infections. *The Veterinary Record*, 92, 178–180.

Pasteurella *spp. infections*

J.W. Nesbit

Pasteurellosis signifies disease produced by infection of animals (domestic and wild mammals, birds and reptiles) and humans by species of the ubiquitous bacterial genus, *Pasteurella*.[5]

The family Pasteurellaceae includes a large group of bacteria with phenotypic and genomic similarities and currently includes the genera *Pasteurella, Actinobacillus* and *Haemophilus* amongst other, less well-defined, groups.[23] The Pasteurellae and allied bacteria are Gram-negative, chemo-organotrophic, facultatively anaerobic, fermentative bacteria linked by DNA affiliation. Despite these similarities, it is a heterogeneous group.[23, 26] DNA hybridization studies, in particular, have emphasized the heterogeneity of the species within the group.[23] Consequently, the taxonomic position of many of the species within the family Pasteurellaceae is the topic of debate; a debate that has prompted proposals for nomenclatural changes and reclassification of some species.[23, 26] Notwithstanding this sometimes confusing state of affairs, the nomenclature adopted in this chapter is a reflection of the familiarity of common usage in the literature up to the present time.

The genus *Pasteurella* comprises a number of species, of which *Pasteurella multocida* and *P. haemolytica* are of significance in disease processes in domestic livestock.[5] Although *P. multocida* was only finally accepted as the type species as recently as 1985, its nomenclatural origin goes back to before the turn of the century.[16, 23] The causative agent of a disease in poultry (subsequently referred to as fowl cholera), first described by Rivolta in 1877 and then by Revolee in 1879, was named *Micrococcus gallicidus* by Burrill in 1883. The microorganism underwent several name changes until 1887, when an Italian, Count Trevisan, named the genus *Pasteurella* in honour of Louis Pasteur for his efforts in elucidating the aetiology of fowl cholera in turkeys.[23] In spite of this signal occurrence, the nomenclatural inconsistency prevailed. Kitt is credited with the introduction of the species epithet when the microorganism was designated *Bacterium (bipolare) multocidum* in his Bacterienkunde II Auflage, 1893.[16] In 1900, the name *Bacterium (bipolare) multocidum* was used synonymously with *Bacterium bovisepticum* by Migula[16] and *Bacillus boviseptica* by Lignieres[22] in their texts on bacterial systematics. The latter two names referred to the causative agent of haemorrhagic septicaemia in cattle.[22] The genus name of *Pasteurella* was apparently accepted thereafter, but isolates of the microorganism were named according to their origin: *P. bovicida* or *P. boviseptica* from cattle, for example.[26] The name *P. septica*, mooted by Topley and Wilson in 1929, was used until 1939, after which the combination *Pasteurella multocida*, proposed by Rosenbusch and Merchant, gained wide acceptance.[16, 23, 26] Species with phenotypic similarities were either separated from the type species (*Pasteurella haemolytica* in 1932) or added to the genus (*Pasteurella pneumotropica* in 1950, *Pasteurella gallinarum* in 1955, *Pasteurella ureae* in 1962 and *Pasteurella aerogenes* in 1974, amongst others).[23] The different species may be distinguished by their biochemical characteristics.[6]

Pasteurella multocida is a species that exhibits heterogeneity in several respects.[26] The microorganism measures 0,6–2,5 x 0,2–0,4 μm and is a non-motile, non-sporogenous, Gram-negative, encapsulated, facultatively anaerobic coccobacillus or short rod. Bipolar staining is evident in Giemsa- or Wright-stained preparations of young cultures. While not the only factor involved, the polysaccharide constituent of the capsule plays a role in adherence, colonization, invasiveness and virulence, and is therefore an important determinant of pathogenicity. Other chemical determinants of pathogenicity identified to date include:

- the lipopolysaccharide (LPS) of the outer cell membrane, which has endotoxic activity—an activity indistinguishable from that of LPS derived from other Gram-negative bacteria **(see below)**, and
- the protein (dermonecrotic) toxin elaborated by certain serotypes, serotype D in particular, that plays an integral role in the pathogenesis of progressive atrophic rhinitis in pigs.

The remaining (chemical) determinants of pathogenicity await elucidation. Plasmids that encode for antibiotic resistance have been identified in this species. Based on the passive haemagglutination test, five serotypes: A, B, D, E and F, of *P. multocida* are recognized. In addition, untypable isolates are also encountered.

Pasteurella multocida has a wide geographic distribution and an almost unlimited host range amongst mammals and birds in both terrestrial and aquatic environments.[5, 26] The biological behaviour of the microorganism varies, however. It may exist as a commensal in the upper respiratory tract (nasopharynx) or it may act as a primary or secondary pathogen in different animals. Most strains of the microorganism are, however, singularly pathogenic for laboratory mice.[5] An association between the different serotypes and the different disease syndromes in domestic livestock is apparent.[5, 12] Thus, serotypes B and E are the causative agents of haemorrhagic septicaemia (epidemic pasteurellosis) of cattle and water buffaloes, serotype A is occasionally associated with pneumonic pasteurellosis in cattle and pigs, while serotype D is most frequently implicated in the aetiology of progressive atrophic rhinitis in pigs and occasionally with pneumonic pasteurellosis in pigs, sheep and goats.

Although structurally similar, *Pasteurella haemolytica* differs from the other *Pasteurella* spp. in its biochemical reactivity; most significantly in the production of a narrow zone of haemolysis when grown on blood-enriched agar.[1] Two biotypes and 16 serotypes, as well as numerous untypable strains, are acknowledged in the intraspecies classification of the microorganism.[1, 6] The biotypes are distinguished on the basis of differences in sugar fermentation: biotype A referring to arabinose fermentation and biotype T to trehalose fermentation. Twelve of the serotypes (1, 2, 5–9, 11–14 and 16) are incorporated with biotype A, and four serotypes (3, 4, 10 and 15) with biotype T. Because of its pivotal role in pneumonic pasteurellosis in cattle, the determinants of pathogenicity of *P. haemolytica* biotype A serotype 1 (A1) have been subjected to the most intensive investigation.[1, 9, 15, 37] *In vitro* cultivation of the microorganism is characterized by an initial period of exponential proliferation (the logarithmic phase or log-phase of bacterial growth) that is succeeded by a stationary growth phase during which replication is minimal.[36] During the log-phase of growth, factors which determine bacterial virulence are produced in large quantities.[2, 8, 10, 13, 14, 18, 25, 27, 36] It is not as yet known whether all the virulence factors identified in *P. haemolytica* A1 are shared with the other biotype or serotypes of the species.[1] The pathogenicity of *P. haemolytica* A1 rests with certain cellular components (virulence factors)[9, 19] that include:

- fimbriae (cell-surface pili),
- proteolytic enzymes, neuramidase in particular,
- capsular polysaccharides,
- leukotoxin (cytotoxin), and
- lipopolysaccharide (LPS) of the outer cell membrane.

Each factor fulfils a specific function or set of functions that subserve initiation and amplification of the infectious and inflammatory process in the bovine respiratory tract. The fimbriae may act as specific adhesins facilitating bacterial attachment to, and colonization of, the upper and lower respiratory tract; the former an essential prelude to production of pneumonic pasteurellosis.[1, 13, 14, 21] The purported action of the proteolytic enzymes is twofold.[1, 2, 10] Firstly, enzymatic breakdown of mucus in the airways with a consequent loss of viscosity and adhesiveness may interfere with the mucociliary clearance function. Secondly, enzymatic removal of fibronectin from the surface of the epithelial cells lining the airways may facilitate bacterial attachment and colonization. Production of capsular polysaccharides and leukotoxin is maximal during the logarithmic growth phase of *P. haemolytica* A1.[11, 29] Capsular polysaccharides and leukotoxin are released into the inflammatory exudate but remain localized within the alveolar lumen.[37] The putative pathogenic functions of the capsular polysaccharides[9, 10] include:

- facilitation of bacterial adherence to bronchiolar and alveolar epithelium,
- chemotaxis of neutrophils,
- inhibition of phagocytic and microbicidal mechanisms of neutrophils and macrophages, and
- inhibition of complement-mediated microbicidal mechanisms.

These functions are largely owed to the net negative surface charge and hydrophilic properties of the capsular polysaccharides.[10] Leukotoxin is an exotoxin that is heat-labile, antigenic and specifically toxic for alveolar macrophages and circulating blood lymphocytes, neutrophils and platelets of ruminants.[8, 17, 20, 28] In low concentrations it may induce inappropriate activation of alveolar macrophages and neutrophils, resulting in pro-inflammatory effects while inhibiting phagocytosis of the microorganisms.[1, 9, 37] In high concentrations it causes cytolysis of the target cells. Release of lysosomal enzymes from alveolar macrophages and neutrophils lysed by leukotoxin may augment local tissue injury,[15, 35, 37] while fibrinogenesis may ensue after the release of procoagulant mediators from escaped blood platelets which are then subsequently damaged by leukotoxin.[9] The pathogenic effects of leukotoxin are, therefore indirect.[9, 15, 35, 37] The pathogenic effects of LPS are attributable to its endotoxic activity[1, 9] and it is estimated that between 12 and 25 per cent of the dry weight of *P. haemolytica* consists of LPS.[19] The route of administration is the major determinant of the response to LPS,[33, 34] of which both systemic and local effects are recognized.[9] The onset of the effects of LPS is rapid (within 15 minutes) upon intravenous administration but is considerably longer (up to 6 hours) when administered by other routes.[3, 33, 35] Systemic effects are characterized by biphasic pyrexia, activation of complement, alterations in clotting homeostasis with resultant disseminated intravascular coagulopathy (DIC), progressive leukopenia (granulocytopenia in particular), progressive thrombocytopenia and alterations in systemic and pulmonary haemodynamics and function.[3, 32–34] The haemodynamic and functional deficits in the lungs that follow intratracheal instillation of LPS are biphasic: phase I consists of eicosanoid-dependent hypertension (and either ventilation-perfusion mismatching or diffusion impairment leading to hypoxaemia), and phase II is characterized by neutrophil-dependent pulmonary oedema.[33, 35] The progressive nature of the leukopenia and thrombocytopenia with *P. haemolytica* is attributable to the combined effects of LPS and leukotoxin.[3] An immunohistochemical study found that LPS is released into the inflammatory exudate and is present on epithelial surfaces and in the cytoplasm of alveolar macrophages and neutrophils in experimental pneumonic pasteurellosis in cattle and, in contrast to capsular polysaccharides and leukotoxin, may cross the alveolar wall and be present within the cytoplasm of endothelial cells, monocytes and neutrophils in vascular sites of the interstitium.[37] The pathogenic effects of LPS at the alveolar level[4, 9, 24, 37] include:

- direct damage to endothelial cells, with induction of increased vascular permeability and oedema,
- activation of the clotting mechanism, resulting in fibrinogenesis,
- activation of complement, resulting in activation of alveolar macrophages as well as chemotaxis and activation of neutrophils, and
- complex formation with surfactant leading to increased surface tension and predisposing to atelectasis, oedema and haemorrhage.

However, the discrepancies noted between the pathogenic effects of purified LPS and live *P. haemolytica* A1 in experimental models emphasize that LPS, albeit an important component, is but one of several potential virulence factors.[33] In addition, plasmids that encode for resistance to certain antibiotics have been identified in this species.[1]

Pasteurella haemolytica has a global distribution, but a fairly restricted mammalian host range that includes cattle, sheep, goats, pigs and humans.[5] Its occurrence in species other than ruminants has been questioned.[23]

Bovine pasteurellosis refers to infection in cattle by either *P. multocida* or *P. haemolytica*.[5, 12] Although there is overlapping in certain respects, infections by these two species of *Pasteurella* give rise to different manifestations of disease in cattle. Thus, besides haemorrhagic septicaemia, *P. multocida* is also implicated in the aetiology of pneumonia, meningoencephalitis, polyarthritis and mastitis, while *P. haemolytica*, the predominant causal agent of pneumonic pasteurellosis, may also have an aetiological association with septicaemic conditions, localized infections (pericarditis, pleuritis, peritonitis), mastitis and abortion in cattle.[5, 12, 15] The reaction in the localized infections is invariably acute and associated with fibrinous or fibrinopurulent, occasionally haemorrhagic, exudation.[12] Localized infections may be significant on an individual basis but tend to occur sporadically. Hence, the subsequent account relates exclusively to the two cardinal pasteurelloses of cattle: haemorrhagic septicaemia and pneumonic pasteurellosis.

The first report of haemorrhagic septicaemia, called 'wild und rinderseuche' because of the involvement of deer as well as cattle, emanated from Germany in 1878.[7] The disease was reproduced in cattle. In 1892, Nocard reproduced acute fibrinous pneumonia in a juvenile bovine, utilizing bacteria isolated from cattle that had died acutely with similar lesions following transshipment to France from North America.[30, 31] Nocard appreciated the distinction between this disease and haemorrhagic septicaemia.[30] Nevertheless, around this period, the similarities between the aetiological agents responsible for haemorrhagic septicaemia and acute fibrinous pneumonia in cattle (bipolar staining amongst other features), led to the hypothesis that the latter disease was merely the pectoral (pneumonic) form of haemorrhagic septicaemia.[22, 31] Although cultural differences between the microorganisms associated with haemorrhagic septicaemia and its so-called pectoral variant were recognized in 1921, it was only in the 1930s that separation of haemorrhagic septicaemia and pneumonic pasteurellosis into distinct disease entities was finally accepted.[22, 30, 31] This coincided with reclassification of *Bacillus (Pasteurella) boviseptica*: *P. haemolytica* materialized in 1932, while the remaining bacteria were grouped into *P. multocida* in 1939.[23]

References

1 **ADLAM, C., 1989.** The structure, function and properties of cellular and extracellular components of *Pasteurella haemolytica*. *In*: ADLAM, C. & RUTTER, J.M., (eds). *Pasteurella and Pasteurellosis*. London: Academic Press, Inc.

2 **BABIUK, L.A. & ACRES, S.D., 1984.** Models for bovine respiratory disease. *In:* LOAN, R.W., (ed.). *Bovine Respiratory Disease*. Proceedings of the North American Symposium on Bovine Respiratory Disease. College Station: Texas A & M University Press.

3 **BOWERSOCK, T.L., WALKER, R.D., MADDUX, J.M., FENNER, D. & MOORE, R.N., 1990.** Haematological changes in calves exposed to a mixture of lipopolysaccharide and crude leukotoxin of *Pasteurella haemolytica*. *Canadian Journal of Veterinary Research*, 54, 415–421.

4 **BROGDEN, K.A., ADLAM, C., LEHMKUHL, H.D., CUTLIP, R.C., KNIGHTS, J.M. & ENGEN, R.L., 1989.** Effect of *Pasteurella haemolytica* (A1) capsular polysaccharide on sheep lung *in vivo* and on pulmonary surfactant *in vitro*. *American Journal of Veterinary Research*, 50, 555–559.

5 **CARTER, G.R., 1967.** Pasteurellosis: *Pasteurella multocida* and *Pasteurella haemolytica*. *Advances in Veterinary Science*, 11, 321–379.

6 **CARTER, G.R., 1984.** *In:* KRIEG, N.R. & HOLT, J.G., (eds). *Bergey's Manual of Systematic Bacteriology*. Vol. I. Baltimore, London: Williams & Wilkins.

7 **CARTER, L.R. & DE ALWIS, M.C.L., 1989.** Haemorrhagic septicaemia. *In:* ADLAM, C. & RUTTER, J.M., (eds). *Pasteurella and Pasteurellosis*. London: Academic Press, Inc.

8 **CHANG, Y.F., RENSHAW, H.W. & YOUNG, R., 1987.** Pneumonic pasteurellosis: Examination of typable and untypable *Pasteurella haemolytica* strains for leukotoxin production, plasmid content, and antimicrobial susceptibility. *American Journal of Veterinary Research*, 48, 378–384.

9 **CONFER, A.W., PANCIERA, R.J., CLINKENBEARD, K.D. & MOSIER, D.A., 1990.** Molecular aspects of virulence of *Pasteurella haemolytica*. *Canadian Journal of Veterinary Research*, 54, S48–S52.

10 **CORBEIL, L.B. & GOGOLEWSKY, R.P., 1985.** Mechanisms of bacterial injury. *Veterinary Clinics of North America: Food Animal Practice*, 1, 367–375.

11 **CORSTVET, R.E., GENTRY, M.J., NEWMAN, P.R., RUMMAGE, J.A. & CONFER, A.W., 1982.** The demonstration of age-dependent capsular material on *Pasteurella haemolytica* serotype 1. *Journal of Clinical Microbiology*, 16, 1123–1126.

12 **DUNGWORTH, D.L., 1985.** The respiratory system. *In:* JUBB, K.V.F., KENNEDY, P.C. & PALMER, N., (eds). *Pathology of Domestic Animals*. Vol. 2. 3rd edn. Orlando: Academic Press, Inc.

13 **FRANK, G.H., 1984.** Bacteria as etiological agents in bovine respiratory disease. *In:* LOAN, R.W., (ed.). *Bovine Respiratory Disease*. Proceedings of the North American Symposium on Bovine Respiratory Disease. College Station: Texas A & M University Press.

14 **FRANK, G.H., 1986.** The role of *Pasteurella haemolytica* in the bovine respiratory disease complex. *Veterinary Medicine*, 81, 838–846.

15 **FRANK, G.H., 1989.** Pasteurellosis of cattle. *In:* ADLAM, C. & RUTTER, J.M., (eds). *Pasteurella and Pasteurellosis*. London: Academic Press, Inc.

16 **FREDERICKSEN, W., 1989.** A note on the name *Pasteurella multocida*. *In:* ADLAM, C. & RUTTER, J.M., (eds). *Pasteurella and Pasteurellosis*. London: Academic Press, Inc.

17 **HIMMEL, M.E., YATES, M.D., LAUERMAN, L.M. & SQUIRE, P.G., 1982.** Purification and partial characterization of a macrophage cytotoxin from *Pasteurella haemolytica*. *American Journal of Veterinary Research*, 43, 764–767.

18 **JONES, C.D.R., 1987.** Proliferation of *Pasteurella haemolytica* in the calf respiratory tract after an abrupt change in climate. *Research in Veterinary Science*, 47, 179–186.

19 **KEISS, R.E., WILL, D.H. & COLLIER, J.R., 1964.** Skin toxicity and hemodynamic properties of endotoxin derived from *Pasteurella haemolytica*. *American Journal of Veterinary Research*, 25, 935–941.

20 **MARKHAM, R.J.F., RAMNARIANE, M.L.R. & MUSCOPLAT, C.C., 1982.** Cytotoxic effect of *Pasteurella haemolytica* on bovine polymorphonuclear leucocytes and impaired production of chemotactic factors by *Pasteurella haemolytica*-infected alveolar macrophages. *American Journal of Veterinary Research*, 43, 417–422.

21 **MORCK, D.W., OLSON, M.E., ACRES, S.D., DAOUST, P-Y. & COSTERTON, J.W., 1989.** Presence of bacterial glycocalyx and fimbriae on *Pasteurella haemolytica* in feedlot cattle with pneumonic pasteurellosis. *Canadian Journal of Veterinary Research*, 53, 161–171.

22 **MOSIER, D.A., CONFER, A.W. & PANCIERA, R.J., 1989.** The evolution of vaccines for bovine pneumonia pasteurellosis. *Research in Veterinary Science*, 47, 1–10.

23 **MUTTERS, R., MANNHEIM, W. & BISGAARD, M., 1989.** Taxonomy of the group. *In:* ADLAM, C. & RUTTER, J.M., (eds). *Pasteurella and Pasteurellosis*. London: Academic Press, Inc.

24 **PAULSEN, D.B., MOSIER, D.A., CLINKENBEARD, K.D. & CONFER, A.W., 1989.** Direct effects of *Pasteurella haemolytica* lipopolysaccharide on bovine pulmonary endothelial cells *in vitro*. *American Journal of Veterinary Research*, 50, 1633–1637.

25 **RENSHAW, H.W., 1984.** A molecular approach to bacteria. *In:* LOAN, R.W., (ed.). *Bovine Respiratory Disease*. Proceedings of the North American Symposium on Bovine Respiratory Disease. College Station: Texas A & M University Press.

26 **RIMLER, R.B. & RHOADES, K.R., 1989.** *Pasteurella multocida*. *In:* ADLAM, C. & RUTTER, J.M., (eds). *Pasteurella and Pasteurellosis*. London: Academic Press, Inc.

27 **ROTH, J.A., 1984.** Immunosuppression and immunodulation in bovine respiratory diseases. *In:* LOAN, R.W., (ed.). *Bovine Respiratory Disease*. Proceedings of the North American Symposium on Bovine Respiratory Disease. College Station: Texas A & M University Press.

28 **SHEWEN, P.E., 1983.** The role of the *Pasteurella haemolytica* cytotoxin in bovine pneumonic pasteurellosis. *Dissertation Abstracts International* B, 43, 2471.

29 **SHEWEN, P.E. & WILKIE, B.N., 1985.** Evidence for *Pasteurella haemolytica* cytotoxin as a product of actively growing bacteria. *American Journal of Veterinary Research*, 46, 1212–1214.

30 **SHOO, M.K., 1989.** Experimental pneumonic pasteurellosis. A review. *The Veterinary Record*, 124, 141–144.

31 **SINHA, S.K. & ABINANTI, F.R., 1962.** Shipping fever of cattle. *Advances in Veterinary Science*, 7, 225–271.

32 **SLOCOMBE, R.F., DERKSEN, F.J. & ROBINSON, N.E., 1984.** Interactions of cold stress and *Pasteurella haemolytica* in the pathogenesis of pneumonic pasteurellosis in calves: Pathologic changes in pulmonary function. *American Journal of Veterinary Research*, 45, 1764–1770.

33 **SLOCOMBE, R.F., DERKSEN, F.J. & ROBINSON, N.E., 1989.** Comparison of pathophysiologic changes in the lungs of calves exposed to *Escherichia coli*-derived endotoxin and *Pasteurella haemolytica*, alone or in combination. *American Journal of Veterinary Research*, 50, 701–707.

34 **SLOCOMBE, R.F., MULKS, M., KILLINGWORTH, C.R., DERKSEN, F.J. & ROBINSON, N.E., 1990.** Effect of *Pasteurella haemolytica*-derived endotoxin on pulmonary structure and function in calves. *American Journal of Veterinary Research*, 51, 433–438.

35 **THOMAS, L.H., GOURLAY, R.N., WYLD, S.G., PARSONS, K.R. & CHANTER, N., 1989.** Evidence that blood-borne infection is involved in the pathogenesis of bovine pneumonic pasteurellosis. *Veterinary Pathology*, 26, 253–259.

36 **WALKER, R.D., SCHULTZ, T.W., HOPKINS, F.M. & BRYANT, J.J., 1984.** Growth phase-dependent phagocytosis of *Pasteurella haemolytica* by bovine pulmonary macrophages. *American Journal of Veterinary Research*, 45, 1230–1234.

37 **WHITELEY, L.O., MAHESWARAN, S.K., WEISS, D.J. & AMES, T.R., 1990.** Immunohistochemical localization of *Pasteurella haemolytica* A1–derived endotoxin, leukotoxin and capsular polysaccharide in experimental bovine pasteurella pneumonia. *Veterinary Pathology*, 27, 150–161.

141

Pneumonic pasteurellosis in cattle

J.W. Nesbit and S.R. van Amstel

Introduction

Bovine pneumonic pasteurellosis refers to respiratory disease of cattle in which the clinical and pathological features are referable to acute fibrinous pneumonia caused by *Pasteurella*, predominantly *P. haemolytica*, infection.[10, 18, 24, 72, 74, 94]

Pneumonic pasteurellosis is of considerable economic significance, particularly in feedlot cattle in North America[94] and elsewhere (including South Africa), and in single suckled calves in the United Kingdom.[27] Initially referred to as the pectoral form of haemorrhagic septicaemia, its association with feedlots and trans-shipment led to it being named 'stockyards pneumonia' and 'shipping fever' in North America, and 'transit fever' in the United Kingdom.[74] Bacteriological examination of the lungs of fatal cases of 'shipping fever' consistently yielded a pure culture of *P. haemolytica*.[10, 74] Experimental reproduction of the disease with isolates of *P. haemolytica*, however, proved extremely difficult.[94] Subsequently, a multiplicity of infectious agents including a variety of viruses,[57] mycoplasmas, chlamydiae[63] and bacteria,[35, 85, 90] either alone or in concert, have been incriminated in the aetiology of pneumonic pasteurellosis.[24, 94] The interaction of viruses and bacteria in the bovine lung has provided evidence of the multifactorial nature of the disease and has reinforced the putative secondary role of the pasteurellae.

Inhibition of bacterial clearance in the lungs of cattle exposed to a prior parainfluenza-3 (PI-3) virus infection was demonstrated in 1976,[53] while two years later fibrinous pneumonia, similar to natural cases of 'shipping fever', was reproduced in cattle superinfected with *P. haemolytica* four days after a priming infection with bovine herpesvirus 1 (BHV-I).[42] Continuing investigation of the problem led to an increased awareness of the role played by stress in the pathogenesis of the disease.[94] Environmental, physical, physiological and psychological factors were identified, in addition to transport stress, and their role in 'shipping fever' partially characterized. In an attempt to define the specific components of the disease, the term 'shipping fever' gave way to a new term: bovine respiratory disease (BRD).[94] The conventional wisdom of the period between 1950 and 1980 was that 'shipping fever' or BRD is a disease complex rather than a single disease entity.[24, 94] Nevertheless, not all investigators subscribed to this view. While conceding the potential significance of stress and other infectious agents, some research workers, in deference to the undoubted central role of *P. haemolytica* in the pathogenesis of the disease, opted for the term 'pneumonic pasteurellosis'.[18, 27, 64, 72]

Between 50 and 60 per cent of mortality in feedlot cattle in the USA is attributable to pneumonic pasteurellosis.[39] A similar profile pertains to the situation in South Africa.[62] The economic cost is, however, difficult to quantify. Besides the direct losses associated with mortality, the final account should take cognizance of the indirect losses, such as those related to condemnation of carcasses at slaughter and investigative effort, as well as morbidity.[94] Nevertheless, the losses in the USA are estimated at $800 million per annum or just over $30 per head.[24] Extrapolation to the situation in South Africa indicates a potential loss of R30 million (about US$10 million) per annum.

Aetiology

Both *P. haemolytica* and *P. multocida* are implicated in the aetiology of pneumonic pasteurellosis of cattle.[10, 18, 24, 94]

Reports emanating from North America and the United Kingdom suggest a prevalence of *P. haemolytica* biotype A serotype 1 (designated *P. haemolytica* A1) in more than 75 per cent[22, 94] and frequently more than 90 per cent[93] of cases from natural outbreaks of the disease. Although a recent South African study yielded the relatively low 45 per cent isolation rate of *P. haemolytica* from clinical material,[85] the ratio of isolates from pneumonic pasteurellosis in cattle during the six years preceding 1989 was in the order of 70 per cent for *P. haemolytica* and 30 per cent for *P. multocida* in South Africa.[34] In concert with the international experience, *P. haemolytica* A1 accounted for 80 per cent of these isolations, followed by 12 per cent for serotype 6 and 2 per cent each for serotypes 4, 9, 12 and 13, while serotype A was predominant for *P. multocida*.[34] Although occasionally isolated together with other infectious agents, *P. haemolytica*, and in particular[94] *P. haemolytica* A1, is frequently isolated in pure culture.[26, 93, 94]

The role of *P. haemolytica* as a primary pathogen has been questioned[94] because of the equivocal results obtained in attempts to reproduce the disease using the bacteria alone, the recovery of the bacteria from healthy animals, the occurrence of the disease in association with stress, and the limited therapeutic efficacy of specific bacterins and immune serum to control the infection. *Pasteurella multocida* is readily isolated from the nasopharynx of healthy cattle, whereas *P. haemolytica* (dominated by A2) is only rarely detected from that locality in the same animals.[22] However, in cattle subjected to stress or suffering from a viral infection, *P. haemolytica* A1 is isolated with much greater frequency, indicating an increase in colonization as well as proliferation by this microorganism in these animals.[24] In earlier investigations, successful experimental transmission of the infection could only be accomplished with considerable manipulation of the host. Animals received either a priming infection with chlamydiae, mycoplasmas, PI-3 virus or BHV-I, or were subjected to prolonged transportation, forced exercise or extreme fluctuations in ambient temperature in order to induce stress prior to bacterial challenge.[22, 94] Alternatively, the defence mechanisms of the upper respiratory tract were either obviated through direct bacterial instillation into the lungs or artificially overcome through administration of solutions of acetic acid into the trachea before bacterial inoculation.[22] Since 1977 it has become evident that *P. haemolytica* A1 may fulfil the role of primary pathogen in experimental reproduction of the disease provided the following conditions are met:

- use of non-immune (susceptible) animals, and
- tracheal or pulmonic administration of *P. haemolytica* A1 in the logarithmic growth phase in numbers greater than 5×10^9 colony-forming units.[72]

The biotype and serotype of the bacterial species, the growth phase and the dose are the critical factors; stress and viral infection are not essential prerequisites.

Pasteurella multocida serotype A is most frequently associated with naturally-occurring pneumonia in cattle.[94] However, it is mostly incriminated in secondary infections.[22, 23, 36, 68, 83, 94] Houghton and Gourlay[36] concluded that although *P. multocida* is occasionally the cause of acute fatal septicaemia, it is not a primary pathogen of the bovine lung. Based on a correlation of microbiological and histological criteria, it was pointed out that *P. multocida* was the dominant isolate only when evidence of a concurrent viral infection was present.[68]

Epidemiology

Although recognized in other cattle enterprises, pneumonic pasteurellosis is essentially a problem when cattle are kept in feedlots.[24, 94] The nature of the feedlot industry generally involves the congregation of cattle of diverse origins in large groups[45, 50] and entails the transfer of cattle from their farm of origin, either by road or rail, often over vast distances and frequently at a time of year when the climate is least favourable. During transit, in the feedlots and at auction saleyards, the animals are subjected to a variety of predisposing factors **(Table 141.1)**. Exposure to other stressed or sick cattle results in the dissemination of potential respiratory pathogens which are essential for the development of the disease.[24, 94]

Table 141.1 Predisposing factors of importance in pneumonic pasteurellosis

Infectious agents
Chlamydiae
Mycoplasmas
Respiratory viruses
Other bacteria
Noxious gases
Ammonia
Carbon monoxide
Diesel fumes
Dust
Vaccination
Viruses of the respiratory tract
Bacterins
High daily ambient temperature fluctuation
Nutrition
Diet high in carbohydrate
Stressors
Weaning
Transportation
Surgical procedures
Exhaustion
Starvation
Overcrowding
Co-mingling
Heat and cold
Rearrangement of the social hierarchy

The contributory role of other infectious agents, notably chlamydiae, mycoplasmas and viruses, has been the subject of considerable investigation.[24, 94] Evidence for synergistic interaction between *P. haemolytica* and other infectious agents has only been adequately demonstrated in experimental models using *Chlamydia psittaci*,[63] *Mycoplasma bovis*,[31, 36] PI-3 virus[53] or BHV-1.[42]

Most investigations have centred on the role of the viruses that affect the respiratory tract and their potential for interaction with bacteria.[66, 94] Bovine herpesvirus-1 (BHV-1), bovine herpesvirus-3 (BHV-3), respiratory syncytial virus (RSV), bovine viral diarrhoea (BVD) virus, and possibly bovine herpesvirus-4 (BHV-4) and PI-3 virus possess the capacity to inflict severe lesions in the bovine lung.[48, 57] In the context of bovine pneumonia, the viruses considered most important in the USA are BHV-1, adenovirus (serotypes 3, 4 and 7 in particular), PI-3 virus, RSV, and, although controversial, BVD virus.[66] Based on a reduction in the prevalence of disease following vaccination, Morter and Amstutz[58] considered RSV to be a significant contributory cause of BRD in North America, while circumstantial evidence supports the contention that prior RSV infection predisposes to pneumonic pasteurellosis in calves in the United Kingdom[8] and the Netherlands. The evidence for the role of BVD virus is equivocal, as some authors[15] claim success and others[51] failure in experimental attempts to reproduce acute fibrinous pneumonia in cattle when this virus was employed in the priming infections. Serological studies indicate that BHV-1, PI-3 virus, BVD virus, adenovirus (serotype 3), rhinovirus (serotype undetermined)[5] and RSV[86] are potentially significant in bovine pneumonia in feedlot cattle in South Africa.

Experimental infection with any of the viruses is not always associated with detectable clinical illness.[57, 66] Their significance in the aetiology of pneumonic pasteurellosis, as with *C. psittaci* and the mycoplasmas, lies in their capacity to predispose to secondary bacterial infection.[4, 37, 49, 67, 83, 91, 94] Virus infection may result in reduced mucociliary clearance, lowered fibronectin levels in the surface epithelium of the airways, decreased production of alveolar lining material, and dysfunction of the neutrophils, lymphocytes and alveolar macrophages, all of which facilitate enhanced susceptibility to bacterial attachment and colonization. Loss of adequate function of the alveolar macrophage would appear to be the most important determinant,[37, 49] and is due to disturbances in chemotaxis, immunological bacterial adherence and ingestion, phagolysosome formation, intracellular killing and bacterial degradation by these cells, and to the mounting of an immune-mediated cytolytic reaction directed against virus-infected cells. Paradoxically, this occurs at a time when the antiviral immune response is maximal. Much of the evidence in support of this hypothesis has been derived by extrapolation from the murine viral/bacterial model of experimental pneumonia.[37] In this model, bacterial pulmonary clearance mechanisms remain intact during the acute phase of the viral infection but become refractory seven to eight days after challenge. Moreover, the degree of refractoriness is proportional to the quantum of virus used in the priming infection. Similar data have been acquired from the study of PI-3 virus- and BHV-1-dependent models of *P. haemolytica* pneumonia in cattle.[42, 53, 95] Impairment of bacterial pulmonary clearance is maximal between seven and 11 days after PI-3 virus infection, whereas an interval of four days is required for demonstrable synergism between BHV-1 and *P. haemolytica*. In the latter model, furthermore, at least 10^6 plaque-forming units of BHV-1 are required to induce sufficient impairment of pulmonary clearance for significant bacterial impact.[4] The purported viral effect on the defence mechanisms of the bovine respiratory tract may underpin the contention that vaccination against the respiratory viruses is not necessarily beneficial and may, indeed, predispose to development of pneumonic pasteurellosis.[49, 55]

Other risk factors that have been identified as potentially significant in pneumonic pasteurellosis of feedlot cattle may exert their effects directly or indirectly.

Noxious gases such as ammonia, carbon monoxide and diesel fumes,[87] and chilling as a result of transportation or inclement weather[65, 87] may predispose to the development of bovine pneumonia by interfering with both mucociliary clearance and alveolar macrophage function. Dust particles of 2–3,3 µm in diameter are capable of reaching the alveoli and are associated with a higher prevalence of the disease.[54] The interval between exposure to dust and pneumonia development is approximately 10 days, and is possibly related to satiety of the phagocytic capabilities of the alveolar macrophages. Thermoregulation in the bovine has a ventilatory component, so overheating may result in an increase in minute ventilation and a greater pulmonary exposure to potential respiratory pathogens.[35, 87] Although heat and cold are important, there is also a positive correlation between the prevalence of pneumonic pasteurellosis and the daily range of the prevailing ambient temperature.[54] The higher prevalence of the disease in autumn and winter may be due to the fact that the difference between diurnal and nocturnal temperatures is often extreme during these seasons of the year. The potentially deleterious effect of vaccination against viruses of the respiratory tract on admission to the feedlot has already been referred to.

The mixing of cattle originating from different sources predisposes to the development of pneumonia as a result of both the increased risk of exposure to potential respiratory pathogens[56] and the stress associated with rearrangement of the social hierarchy.[35, 90] In one investigation in which farm-derived cattle adapted to a 10 per cent grain ration were compared with those assembled at auction salesyards and subsequently confronted with high levels of grain in their diet, it was found that animals from the latter group were 4,9 times more likely to be treated for and 6,7 times more likely to die of respiratory disease than the former group. Inclusion of high carbohydrate levels in the ration prior to ruminal adaptation may induce rumen and systemic acidosis. The resultant suppression of alveolar macrophage function may interfere with bacterial pulmonary clearance.[35, 56, 90]

Stress resulting in the release of high levels of glucocorticoids and their induction of purportive alveolar macrophage dysfunction and suppression of specific immunological responsiveness has received much emphasis as a predisposing factor.[7, 21, 35, 39, 67, 81, 96] High cortisol levels cause decreased production of interleukin-2 by helper T-lymphocytes, with consequent reduction in antigen-dependent blastogenesis of effector T- and B-lymphocytes as well as inhibition in the activity of natural killer cells.[7, 96] High cortisol levels could also reactivate latent, particularly viral, infections and increase the potential for their dissemination.[21, 81] Many stress factors in cattle have been identified **(Table 141.1)**. Transit time, particularly when longer than 24 hours, is apparently the most potent of all the stress factors and is the cause of excessive dehydration, electrolyte disturbances and rumen dysfunction.

In feedlots in South Africa, outbreaks of pneumonic pasteurellosis occur throughout the year but are more frequent in autumn and winter, especially following cold and windy spells.[62] This period coincides with major cattle sales and movements. Furthermore, whereas at other times of the year 60 per cent of the cattle which are placed in feedlots are farm-derived and 40 per cent originate in auction salesyards, this trend is frequently reversed in autumn. With the exception of brindled Brahman/Sussex crosses, which rarely develop the disease in South Africa, cattle of any breed, age or sex are equally susceptible.[62] Cattle may succumb at any stage of the feeding process, but the majority of cases occur during the first 45 days following their admission to a feedlot; the first cases are generally observed on the fourth day and the highest number on the 21st day. Only isolated cases occur after the initial 45-day period.[62] The morbidity rate is about 10–12 per cent[84] but may reach 33–50 per cent in exceptional circumstances.[62] The prevalence is higher in weaners which have been purchased at an auction saleyard than in either yearlings (regardless of origin) or weaners derived directly from a single cow-calf farming operation.[35, 56, 90] The higher prevalence of pneumonic pasteurellosis in calves is probably related to a decline of maternally-conferred immunity to potential respiratory pathogens.[8] In South Africa, although the mortality rate rarely exceeds 1 per cent (except in autumn, when a mortality rate approaching 4 per cent is not unusual), it may occasionally reach 20 per cent.[62, 84]

Various managerial procedures prior or subsequent to admission to a feedlot affect the prevalence of the disease in the USA and Canada.[35, 56, 90] Preweaning and preconditioning programmes instituted at the farm of origin result in a reduction in morbidity rates. Preweaning entails the training of calves to take water and feed from troughs during the weaning process at least three weeks before sale. Preconditioning involves eartagging, dehorning, castration, treatment for parasites, and vaccination against blackquarter, malignant oedema, and infections of PI-3 virus, BHV-1, *Pasteurella* spp. and, occasionally, BVD virus and *Haemophilus somnus*, before admission of animals to the feedlot. However, the benefits associated with the latter programme cannot be justified when measured against the cost. Although preconditioning is not practised in South Africa, the results of a pilot trial indicated that, all other parameters being equal, vaccination against PI-3 virus, BHV-1 and *Pasteurella* spp. four weeks prior to admission accrued minimal benefit with respect to the prevalence of pneumonic pasteurellosis when compared to that following vaccination of the animals on their arrival at the feedlot.[61] The morbidity rate in the group of calves vaccinated earlier was higher than in the group vaccinated on arrival. Nevertheless, there was a reduction in the duration of illness in those animals that did contract the disease and an increase in the average weight gain in the vaccinated animals.

Pathogenesis

The lungs are not sterile; the lower respiratory tract is subjected to continual exposure to aerolized particles, including potential respiratory pathogens, derived from environmental air, ruminal gases, and nasopharyngeal infections.[44, 50] The number of pathogens in the upper respiratory tract determines the quantum delivered to the lungs.[44] Thus, the first step in the pathogenesis of pneumonic pasteurellosis is colonization of the nasopharynx by specific bacterial pathogens.[4, 14, 23, 24, 33, 40, 43, 83] The introduction of stress, whether environmental, physical, physiological or psychological, predisposes to the establishment of bacteria—*P. haemolytica* A1 in particular—in the upper respiratory tract.[22, 24] Whether this is dependent on the high cortisol levels associated with stress is uncertain. It has been found that high cortisol levels associated with transportation and handling render cattle more susceptible to BHV-1 but not to *P. haemolytica* A1 infection.[21] Although the other predisposing factors **(Table 141.1)** may also facilitate the process, bacterial virulence factors contribute to the subsequent proliferation in the nasopharynx.[4, 14, 22, 23] This is followed by pulmonary colonization; access to the lungs is achieved primarily by inhalation of infective material derived by aerosol formation in the nasopharynx, and secondarily by progressive colonization down the trachea.[4, 14, 22, 23, 33, 40, 43, 83] The relative shortness of the airways and gravitational influences result in greater particulate impaction in the cranioventral regions of the lungs.[50, 87] Increased rate or depth of respiration associated with heat or cold stress, respectively, may enhance the process.[76] Although the aerogenous route is the most probable route of infection, the haematogenous route may be important in the pathogenesis for two reasons:

- *P. haemolytica* may be isolated from the blood of cattle with natural disease, and
- not only does *P. haemolytica* exhibit specific tropism for the bovine lung following intravenous administration, but the pneumonic lesion is essentially similar to that produced by intratracheal infection in experimental disease.[82]

Regardless of the route of infection, the critical factors in consequence of bacterial deposition in the lungs are the efficiency of the pulmonary defence system and the virulence factors of the invading microorganism.[4, 14] Ninety per cent of the bacteria delivered by the aerogenous route may be cleared within four hours in healthy animals.[43, 83] Impairment of the pulmonary clearance mechanisms as a consequence of high dust-loads, preceding viral, chlamydial, mycoplasmal or bacterial infection and/or stress-associated factors may allow the bacteria to gain a foothold in the lungs.[33, 94] Alternatively, proliferation of *P. haemolytica* A1 in the nasopharynx would increase the quantum of bacteria in the log-phase of growth aspirated into the lungs.[4, 43] The virulence factors produced in large quantities by proliferating *P. haemolytica* A1 organisms impede phagocytic clearance by alveolar macrophages and neutrophils.[11, 89] Thus, a cycle of bacterial replication, impairment of pulmonary clearance mechanisms, extension of the infectious process and bacterial replication is initiated.

The ensuing tissue damage in the lungs is attributed to extrinsic and intrinsic factors. A functional study of experimental pneumonic pasteurellosis[76] showed that ventilation–perfusion mismatching precedes an increase in airways resistance predicating initiation of injury in the parenchyma rather than the bronchioles. This correlates with the confluent nature and parenchymal predominance of the lesion.[41] The subsequent impairment of gas exchange with resultant hypoxaemia is ascribed to oedema due to neutrophil influx and activation, pulmonary hypertension and an increase in vascular permeability.[77, 82] Both effects are a sequel to the presence of bacterial virulence factors, particularly lipopolysaccharide.[12] Other contributory effects include activation of the complement and coagulation pathways.[14, 75] Whilst a major effect of complement activation is chemotaxis of leukocytes, particularly neutrophils, split products of complement contribute to initiation and maintenance of other aspects of the inflammatory reaction.[52, 75] Activation of the coagulation pathway results in both intravascular and extravascular fibrinogenesis.[75] The relatively high fibrinogen content in the blood, together with the paucity of pulmonary fibrinolytic mechanisms in the bovine, predisposes to the prominence of fibrin in acute pulmonary injury in this species.[18, 75, 87] Capillary thrombosis, together with bacterial endotoxin and cytotoxin, is assigned a causal role in the associated focal coagulative necrosis.[18, 41] Another factor is complete compartmentalization due to the lack of collateral ventilation in the lungs, which predisposes to atelectasis and hypoxia in regions distal to airways occluded by transudate or exudate.[87] This results in further inhibition of alveolar macrophage function.[65, 87] Although these factors are significant, possibly the most important contributory factor in the pneumonic process is the action of neutrophils.[4, 24, 49, 52, 75, 78, 79] Neutrophil depletion prior to bacterial exposure in experimental systems results in the total lack of development of the clinical and pathological features of pneumonic pasteurellosis.[79] Influx of neutrophils is rapid and substantial; they become the dominant cell type in the alveolar lumens within four hours of exposure to bacterial aerosols.[52] Neutrophils are more effective microbicidal agents than alveolar macrophages in the pneumonic lung because of their greater functional and secretory capability and their greater content of reactive products.[49, 75] Moreover, neutrophils are capable of functioning in a hypoxic environment. However, uncontrolled accumulation, activation and, ultimately, disintegration, of these cells may induce injury to the lungs that is of greater consequence than the insult which elicited the reaction. The injurious consequences are attributed to the effects of exported free-oxygen radicals and lysosomal enzymes.[24] Although a contentious issue,[80] leukotoxin may be the virulence factor responsible for the release of the tissue-damaging products from neutrophils.[11, 24]

Death of cattle suffering from pneumonic pasteurellosis is ascribed to hypoxaemia, anoxia, toxaemia, endotoxaemia, shock and right-heart failure, either individually or collectively.[39, 94] In survivors, the nature and extent of the preceding lung injury, in conjunction with complete compartmentalization and lack of collateral ventilation characteristic of the bovine lung, inevitably result in the development of complications, notably extensive scarring, chronic suppurative pneumonia, bronchiectasis and pulmonary abscessation.[18] Extension of the infection may occur, resulting in pleuritis, pericarditis, peritonitis and, less frequently, meningitis and polyarthritis.[18]

Clinical signs

The course of pneumonic pasteurellosis may vary from acute to chronic.[94] However, a small proportion of cases may die suddenly without having shown any premonitory signs.[65, 83] Although some affected animals reveal no evidence of disease, detectable clinical signs usually occur within two days of the onset of pneumonia.[3]

The clinical signs in the early stages of disease include fever, staring coat, inappetence, nasal discharge and tachypnoea,[26, 27, 35, 90, 94] which may develop over a period of three to seven days.[89] A serous nasal discharge is invariably present and may be associated with lachrymation and photophobia, resulting in partial closure of the eyes due to swelling of the eyelids. Adventitious sounds are occasionally audible on auscultation of the cranioventral lung-fields.

In the advanced stages of the disease there is marked depression and inappetence together with prominent signs resulting from respiratory involvement.[26, 35, 90, 94] The nasal discharge becomes profuse and mucopurulent, resulting in extensive crusting of the external nares. Affected animals show tachypnoea (with respiratory rates up to 100 per minute) and hyperpnoea, and a cough is frequently present but is usually soft and protective rather than productive and can be elicited upon laryngeal palpation.[26, 94] Auscultation reveals a decrease in vesicular sounds and an accentuation of bronchial tones and/or expiratory sounds which progress to coarse râles, initially moist and then dry, of the cranioventral areas of the lungs.[90, 94] Pleuritic friction rubs are occasionally detected. In particularly severe cases, dyspnoea is an outstanding clinical feature, manifested by extension of the

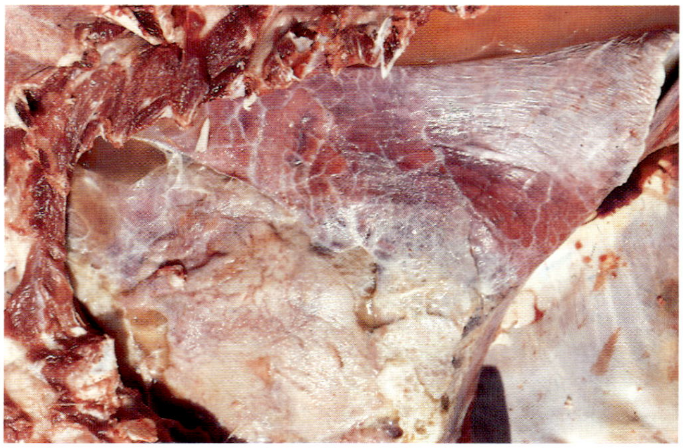

Figure 141.1 Severe, acute fibrinous pleuropneumonia in a calf with a *Pasteurella haemolytica* infection

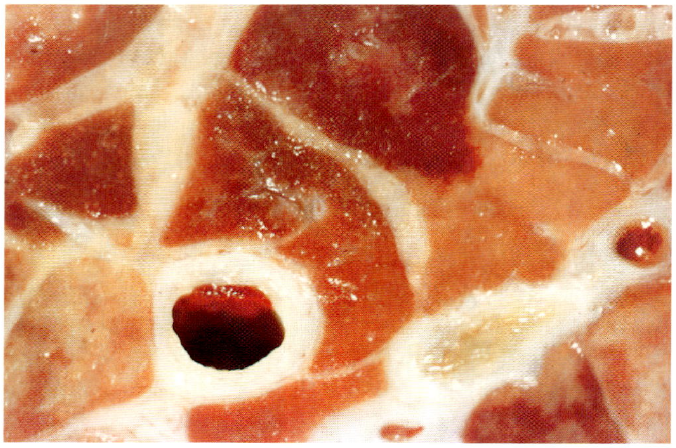

Figure 141.2 Close-up view of red and grey hepatization in pneumonic pasteurellosis

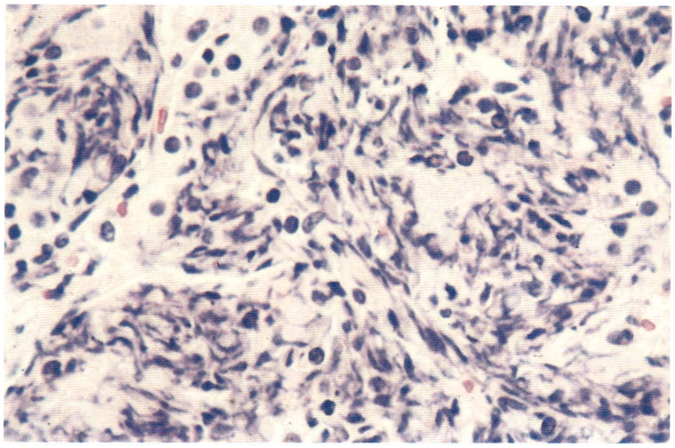

Figure 141.3 'Streaming macrophages' in a lung of an ox affected by pneumonic pasteurellosis

head and neck, abduction of the elbows, and open-mouth breathing which is accompanied by an expiratory grunt.[35, 94] Diarrhoea is an inconstant sign in some affected animals at this stage. Weight loss is profound.

Death may supervene at any time during the course of the disease. Although exceptions occur, spontaneous recovery in the absence of treatment is inevitably prolonged and attended by relapses. These animals never do well and are referred to as 'poor doers'[84, 94] or 'pulmonary cripples'.[47] The duration of illness seldom exceeds seven days in treated individuals.[90] Provided treatment is efficacious, recovery may be complete and the finishing process only temporarily interrupted.[35]

The clinical findings in experimental pneumonic pasteurellosis attest to the short incubation period and rapid course of the disease.[27, 79, 94] Following the nasal or tracheal administration of *P. haemolytica*, depression develops within six hours, tachypnoea within 24 hours, fever within 30 hours and exaggerated respiratory sounds within 48 hours.[27] Coughing is not a prominent clinical feature and only commences after four days. In other respects the experimental and natural disease are similar.

Pathology

Although centred on the respiratory system and regional lymph nodes, lesions are also found in other organ systems.[3, 18] The carcass reflects a fevered, deep red or occasionally cyanotic appearance which is frequently accompanied by congestion of individual organs. Fibrinous pericarditis, epi- and endocardial petechiae and ecchymoses, and, occasionally, fibrinous peritonitis, polyarthritis and/or meningitis may be present. Degenerative changes in parenchymal organs and renal infarction may also be evident.[35]

The upper respiratory tract is usually only mildly affected.[3] An initial serous rhinitis and tracheitis may be followed by congestion, oedema, petechiation, erosions and ulcerations of the mucosa and a thick, voluminous mucopurulent exudate. In cases in which BHV-1 infection may have initiated the illness, rhinotracheitis may be particularly severe and extensive, with pseudomembranous inflammation predominating.[3, 18, 83, 94] An acute, fulminating, fibrinous lobar pneumonia **(Figure 141.1)**,[18, 64, 68] distributed bilaterally but asymmetrically,[93] and fibrinous pleuritis are noted.[3, 18, 35, 40, 64, 68, 94] Up to 90 per cent of the lungs below a horizontal line drawn through the dorsal third of the thoracic inlet may be affected.[40, 68] The fibrinous exudate on the pleura may result in adhesion of contiguous lobes and attachment of the affected lung tissue to the thoracic wall.

In the affected portions of the lungs, the interlobular septa are distinct and distended with gelatinous material, and the lung tissue is variously discoloured and consolidated. Discrete, tan-coloured foci of coagulative necrosis of irregular size and shape are frequently present.[16] The necrotic foci may be outlined by distinct yellowish-white borders. Small white foci of necrosis may impart a faintly mottled appearance to the cut surface, which may exhibit large white areas following confluence of the foci. The lesions have a lobular distribution and are made up of oedema, haemorrhage, red and grey hepatization and/or necrosis of the parenchyma **(Figure 141.2)**. A distinct, fibrous connective tissue capsule encloses the necrotic areas in the later stages.[3] Mucopurulent material may be expressed from incised bronchioles. The dorsal, relatively unaffected portions of the lungs may reveal slight congestion, oedema, petechial or ecchymotic haemorrhages on the pleural surface, and emphysema. Besides an associated tonsillitis, the bronchial and mediastinal lymph nodes are enlarged and congested.[3]

The microscopic features of the pulmonic lesion include hyperaemia and oedema, inundation of the alveolar ducts and alveoli with serofibrinous exudate, haemorrhage, accumulation of alveolar macrophages and neutrophils, thrombosis of blood and lymphatic vessels, and multifocal coagulative necrosis.[3, 16–18, 64, 68, 94] An overlying acute fibrinous pleuritis may be a prominent finding. A conspicuous and characteristic feature of the leukocytic reaction within the alveoli is a swirling aggregation of fusiform cells with elongated, hyperchromatic, pyknotic nuclei **(Figure 141.3)**. These cells are referred to as 'oat cells' or 'streaming macrophages',[18, 94] and apparently owe their origin to the effect of *P. haemolytica* A1 leukotoxin upon alveolar macrophages and/or neutrophils, although the precise cellular derivation has yet to be determined.[3] Gram-negative bacteria are present in profusion, particularly at the periphery of the necrotic foci, but also in the alveoli and interstitium during the acute stage. The presence of fibrinous thrombi within the associated lymphatics is a prominent feature. In contrast, although vasculitis may be detected in the severely inflamed regions, thrombi are difficult to demonstrate. The bronchi and bronchioles contain the products of the inflammatory reaction in the distal regions of the lungs.[94] Occasionally, specific lesions may be encountered in these and related structures, particularly in the relatively unaffected portions of the lungs. The lesions may signify prior or concurrent viral, chlamydial, mycoplasmal or bacterial infection.[18, 48, 83]

The microscopical features of the lesions may be utilized to stage the pneumonic process: appearance of necrosis at three days, fibroblasts at four to five days, collagen fibres at seven days and birefringence of collagen fibres under polarized light at 21 days.[16] However, in experimental pneumonic pasteurellosis,[3, 25, 27, 29, 41, 52, 76, 79] lesions are discernible four hours after aerosol challenge and reach a maximum two or three days later with the development of an acute fibrinous pneumonia. Resolution and organization commence thereafter and by the ninth day there is fibrous encapsulation of the necrotic foci, and, in addition to the other inflammatory cells, the affected tissue is infiltrated with lymphocytes and plasma cells. Vascular thrombosis is of greater consequence and extent during the later stages of the infection.[3, 27]

Diagnosis and differential diagnosis

The epidemiological, clinical and pathological considerations may be sufficient to make a presumptive diagnosis of pneumonic pasteurellosis. However, a substantive diagnosis is dependent upon the isolation of the causative organism.[10, 24] Nasal swabs from the live animal and specimens of pneumonic areas removed aseptically during performance of a necropsy may be utilized for this purpose.[24] Isolation from specimens of affected lung are preferable, as the responsible bacteria are usually present in large numbers and in pure culture, whereas cultures made from nasal swabs frequently yield mixed bacterial populations.[24] Furthermore, greater success in bacterial isolation attempts is achieved when material from untreated cases is cultured.[34] Besides contributing to the epidemiological and diagnostic aspects of the disease, an important adjunct of bacterial isolation and identification rests upon the subsequent determination of the antibiotic sensitivity of the organism, which allows the development of specific therapeutic strategies.[24]

Pneumonic pasteurellosis is an important component of the bovine respiratory disease complex in feedlot cattle and should be differentiated from the other disease entities in the complex such as infectious bovine rhinotracheitis, intrapleural or intrapulmonary rupture of a lung abscess, pulmonary embolic aneurysm and interstitial pneumonia.[39, 84] Other conditions that should be considered in the differential diagnosis, and particularly in the clinical context, include foreign-body or aspiration pneumonia, necrobacillosis of the upper respiratory tract, salmonellosis, contagious bovine pleuropneumonia and pneumonia caused by *Haemophilus somnus*. With the exception of contagious bovine pleuropneumonia, which may require additional diagnostic procedures for confirmation, the conditions listed above are generally readily distinguished by the findings at necropsy.[18]

Control

Control of the immediate problem is attained through the institution of a therapeutic regimen. Efficacy of treatment is dependent upon a number of measures including the early detection of illness, selection of appropriate antibacterial agent, route and duration of drug administration, supportive therapy, and provision of adequate hospital facilities and nutrition.[35, 59] Any delay in the initiation of therapy is accompanied by a commensurate prolongation of the course of the disease and an exponential increase in the mortality and relapse rates.[35]

The criteria that determine antibacterial drug selection include the spectrum and duration of its effect, its quantum and persistence in tissue residues, and its cost.[35, 92] *Pasteurella haemolytica* and *P. multocida* are sensitive to most antibacterial agents, such as sulphonamides (including potentiated sulphonamides), penicillin G, ampicillin, amoxycillin, tetracyclines (including long-acting tetracyclines), chloramphenicol, spectinomycin, neomycin, kanamycin, gentamicin, polymixin B, cephalosporins, tylosin and erythromycin. More recently, tilmicosin (a tylosin derivative), ceftiofur (a cephalosporin) and

Table 141.2 Antimicrobial drugs that are commonly used to treat cattle suffering from pneumonic pasteurellosis

DRUG	DOSAGE RATE AND ROUTE OF ADMINISTRATION
Procaine penicillin G	45 000 IU/kg, im or sc once a day
Oxytetracycline	10 mg/kg, im once a day
Long-acting oxytetracycline	20 mg/kg, im once every three days
Trimethoprim-sulfadoxine	1 ml/15 kg, im once a day
Tylosin	2–10 mg/kg, im once a day
Amoxycillin	2–7 mg/kg, im or sc once a day
Ceftiofur sodium	1 mg/kg, im once a day
Tilmicosin	10 mg/kg, sc once every three days
Danofloxacin	1,25 mg/kg, im once a day

im Intramuscularly
sc Subcutaneously

danofloxacin (a fluoroquinolone) have been released, with the bovine respiratory disease complex as one of their main indications. The dosage rates and routes of administration of the antimicrobial drugs commonly used to treat pneumonic pasteurellosis are given in **Table 141.2**.[6, 20, 28, 73, 85] The prolonged withdrawal period following use of the long-acting oxytetracycline drugs, tilmicosin and ceftiofur must be considered when these drugs are used. Despite its undoubted efficacy, the use of chloramphenicol in food-producing animals is restricted by statute which was first brought into effect in South Africa in 1991. Consequently, the drug of first choice in most countries on a worldwide basis has been oxytetracycline, followed as second choice by procaine penicillin G, and as third choice by sulphadiazine combined with trimethoprim.[73, 92] The efficacy and prolonged therapeutic levels in pulmonary tissue following a single injection of low volume confers distinct advantages upon tilmicosin, a recently introduced semi-synthetic macrolide.[30, 321] Regardless of the antibiotic selected, it should be administered at the correct dose, for the recommended period, and by the correct route.[35] Although alternative routes are feasible, the most practical is by intramuscular injection as, besides ease of administration, therapeutic levels are readily attained and maintained. Lack of a positive response within two days of commencement of treatment justifies selection of an alternative antibiotic or other therapeutic agent.[6, 59] Treatment should continue for at least two days after abatement of the clinical signs, as premature termination of the therapeutic schedule may increase the relapse rate and predispose towards the development of microbial resistance.[35, 73]

Although there is an inherent resistance to dihydrostreptomycin and tylosin in most species of *Pasteurella*, antibiotic resistance to penicillin G, ampicillin, oxytetracycline and sulphadiazine is increasing in this genus.[73, 92] Most of this resistance is mediated by genetic encodation in plasmids and/or transposons[1, 92] and, while it is transferable, it tends to fluctuate in bacterial populations. Certain *Pasteurella* spp. isolates contain plasmids encoded for production of beta-lactamase, which inactivates the penicillins, including ampicillin.[28, 92] However, ampicillin combined with sulbactam, an inhibitor of beta-lactamase, remains effective against strains of *P. haemolytica* resistant to ampicillin alone.[28]

Supportive therapy is a controversial issue.[19, 35, 59] The value of mucolytic, spasmolytic and anti-inflammatory agents has been questioned, as their use merely induces relief of clinical signs and is unlikely to influence the end result.[35] Indeed, an associated disadvantage is the unwarranted cessation of antibiotic therapy. At the recommended dosages, corticosteroids may exert a beneficial effect,[19] but their immunosuppressive actions may result in enhanced predisposition to and/or reactivation of infections, particularly those of a viral aetiology.[21, 67]

Sick cattle should be sheltered from inclement weather, penned with animals of similar size, and provided with clean water and hay of good quality together with starting ration.[35]

In addition to the putative infectious agents which are ubiquitous in bovine populations, environmental and stress-associated factors **(see Aetiology)** are important determinants in the occurrence of the disease in the feedlot situation and should be eliminated or at least limited as far as possible.[45, 90] Animals should be acquired directly from the farm of origin rather than from an auction saleyard,[35] and mixing of cattle from different sources should be avoided in order to minimize stress and reduce the potential for cross-infection. Animals of similar size, type and gender should be penned together, and the pen population should be held at below 200 head. Adaptation to the environment and the diet must be encouraged. Handling of recent arrivals, except for initial processing, should be curtailed for at least 21 days. The starting ration should be palatable, balanced, and introduced incrementally while good-quality grass hay is freely available. Dust may present a considerable problem.[54, 88] Feed dust may be controlled by adjusting the water, molasses and fat content of the ration. The latter, when included at 4 per cent of the ration, also contributes to reduction of manure dust. Water sprinkling systems and regular removal schedules are the predominant means of dust control during periods of high environmental loads.

Preweaning and preconditioning programmes offer a theoretical basis for the control of pneumonic pasteurellosis. Evaluation of the available data suggests that either programme is equally effective, which places a question mark against the validity of vaccination, the essential difference between the two programmes.[38] Attempts to establish effective immunity against *P. haemolytica* and/or *P. multocida* in cattle have met with variable success.[60] Largely because of its predilective involvement and because immunity is serotype-specific, most research has centred upon immunity to *P. haemolytica* A1.[60, 72]

Although not entirely understood, immunity to the microorganism is comprised of both humoral and cell-mediated mechanisms directed against bacterial cell components including capsular polysaccharides, other cell-surface antigens, leukotoxin and, to a minor extent, lipopolysaccharide.[60, 71] The lack of leukotoxin in inactivated vaccines offers an explanation for the frequent failures associated with the use of bacterins in the past.[71] Although specific opsonizing antibody against bacterial cell-surface antigens enhances the phagocytic process, this facilitates destruction of the alveolar macrophages and augmentation of the infectious process in the absence of antileukotoxin antibody.[69]

An improved vaccine is the subject of intensive research, particularly in North America, and future prospects utilizing subunit, synthetic polypeptide, adjuvanted, recombinant and live attenuated vaccines are promising.[60, 96] The current options that use vaccines containing leukotoxin and live vaccines have yielded excellent results in most experimental studies.[9, 33, 46, 60, 70]

References

1 **ADLAM, C., 1989.** The structure, function and properties of cellular and extracellular components of *Pasteurella haemolytica*. *In*: ADLAM, C. & RUTTER, J.M., (eds). *Pasteurella and Pasteurellosis*. London: Academic Press, Inc.

2 **ALLAN, E.M., GIBBS, H.A., WISEMAN, A. & SELMAN, I.E., 1982.** *Pasteurella haemolytica* pneumonia in weaned, housed, single suckled calves. *The Veterinary Record*, 112, 327.

3 **ALLAN, E.M., GIBBS, H.A., WISEMAN, A. & SELMAN, I.E., 1985.** Sequential lesions of experimental bovine pneumonic pasteurellosis. *The Veterinary Record*, 117, 438–442.

4 **BABIUK, L.A. & ACRES, S.D., 1984.** Models for *Bovine Respiratory Disease*. *In*: LOAN, R.W., (ed.). *Bovine Respiratory Disease*. Proceedings of the North American Symposium on *Bovine Respiratory Disease*. College Station: Texas A & M University Press.

5 **BARNARD, B.J.H., 1977.** Virus diseases in feedlot cattle in South Africa. *Bulletin de l'Office International des Épizooties*, 153–160.

6 **BATEMAN, K.G., MARTIN, S.W., SHEWEN, P.E. & MENZIES, P.I., 1990.** An evaluation of antimicrobial therapy for undifferentiated bovine respiratory disease. *Canadian Veterinary Journal*, 31, 689–697.

7 **BLECHA, F., BOYLES, S.L. & RILEY, J.G., 1984.** Shipping suppresses lymphocyte blastogenic responses in Angus and Brahman X Angus feeder calves. *Journal of Animal Science*, 59, 576–583.

8 **BRYSON, D.G., 1985.** Calf pneumonia. *Veterinary Clinics of North America: Food Animal Practice*, 1, 237–257.

9 **CARDELLA, M.A., ADVIENTO, M.A. & NERVIG, R.M., 1987.** Vaccination studies against experimental bovine *Pasteurella* pneumonia. *Canadian Journal of Veterinary Research*, 51, 204–211.

10 **CARTER, G.R., 1967.** Pasteurellosis: *Pasteurella multocida* and *Pasteurella haemolytica*. *Advances in Veterinary Science*, 11, 321–379.

11 **CHANG, Y.F., RENSHAW, H.W. & YOUNG, R., 1987.** Pneumonic pasteurellosis: Examination of typable and untypable *Pasteurella haemolytica* strains for leukotoxin production, plasmid content, and antimicrobial susceptibility. *American Journal of Veterinary Research*, 48, 378–384.

12 **CLARK, C.R., BURROWS, G.E. & AMES, T.R., 1991.** Therapy of bovine bacterial pneumonia. *Veterinary Clinics of North America: Food Animal Practice*, 7, 669–694.

13 **CONFER, A.W., PANCIERA, R.J., CLINKENBEARD, K.D. & MOSIER, D.A., 1990.** Molecular aspects of virulence of *Pasteurella haemolytica*. *Canadian Journal of Veterinary Research*, 54, S48–S52.

14 **CORBEIL, L.B. & GOGOLEWSKY, R.P., 1985.** Mechanisms of bacterial injury. *Veterinary Clinics of North America: Food Animal Practice*, 1, 367–375.

15 **CORSTVET, R.E. & PANCIERA, R.J., 1982.** Effect of infectious bovine rhinotracheitis virus and bovine virus diarrhoea virus on *Pasteurella haemolytica* infection in the bovine lung. *American Association of Veterinary Laboratory Diagnosticians*, 25th Annual Proceedings, 363–368.

16 **DAOUST, P-Y., 1989.** Morphological study of bacterial pneumonia of feedlot cattle: Determination of age of lesions. *Canadian Veterinary Journal*, 30, 155–160.

17 **DUNGWORTH, D.L., 1982.** Interstitial pulmonary disease. *Advances in Veterinary Science and Comparative Medicine*, 26, 172–200.

18 **DUNGWORTH, D.L., 1985.** The respiratory system. *In*: JUBB, K.V.F., KENNEDY, P.C. & PALMER, N., (eds). *Pathology of Domestic Animals*. Vol. 2. 3rd edn. Orlando: Academic Press, Inc.

19 **ESPINASSE, J., ALLAIRE, R., RAYNAUD, J.P., VAN GOOL, F. & TIXIER, G., 1986.** Combined corticosteroid and antibiotic therapy in bovine respiratory disease (BRD) of young cattle: Clinical results. *Bovine Practitioner*, 21, 59–61.

20 **FALES, W.H., SELBY, L.A., WEBBER, J.J., SMITH, D.R., KINTNER, L.D., NELSON, S.L., MILLER, R.B., THORNE, J.G. & McGINITY, J.T., 1981.** Antibiotic-resistant *Pasteurella* recovered from Missouri cattle with bovine respiratory disease complex. *American Association of Veterinary Laboratory Diagnosticians*, 24th Annual Proceedings, 43–50.

21 **FILION, L.G., WILLSON, P.J., BIELEFELDT-OHMANN, H., BABIUK, L.A. & THOMSON, R.G., 1984.** The possible role of stress in the induction of pneumonic pasteurellosis. *Canadian Journal of Comparative Medicine*, 48, 268–274.

22 **FRANK, G.H., 1984.** Bacteria as etiological agents in *Bovine Respiratory Disease*. *In*: LOAN, R.W., (ed.). *Bovine Respiratory Disease*. Proceedings of the North American Symposium on Bovine Respiratory Disease. College Station: Texas A & M University Press.

23 **FRANK, G.H., 1986.** The role of *Pasteurella haemolytica* in the bovine respiratory disease complex. *Veterinary Medicine*, 81, 838–846.

24 **FRANK, G.H., 1989.** Pasteurellosis of cattle. *In*: ADLAM, C. & RUTTER, J.M., (eds). *Pasteurella and Pasteurellosis*. London: Academic Press, Inc.

25 **FRIEND, S.C.E., THOMSON, R.G. & WILKIE, B.N., 1977.** Pulmonary lesions induced by *Pasteurella haemolytica* in cattle. *Canadian Journal of Comparative Medicine*, 41, 212–223.

26 **GIBBS, H.A., ALLAN, E.M., WISEMAN, A. & SELMAN, I.E., 1983.** Pneumonic pasteurellosis in housed, weaned, single suckled calves. *The Veterinary Record*, 112, 87.

27 **GIBBS, H.A., ALLAN, E.M., WISEMAN, A. & SELMAN, I.E., 1984.** Experimental production of bovine pneumonic pasteurellosis. *Research in Veterinary Science*, 37, 154–166.

28 **GIFFORD, G.A., POTTER, A.A. & BABIUK, L.A., 1988.** Clinical and pathological evaluation of sulbactam/ampicillin for treatment of experimental bovine pneumonic pasteurellosis. *Canadian Veterinary Journal*, 29, 142–148.

29 **GILKA, F., THOMSON, R.G. & SAVAN, M., 1974.** Microscopic findings in the lungs of calves aerosolysed with *Pasteurella haemolytica* and treated to alter pulmonary clearance. *Zentralblatt für Veterinärmedizin*, 21B, 774–786.

30 **GORHAM, P.E., CARROLL, L.H., McASKILL, J.W., WATKINS, L.E., OSE, E.E., TONKINSON, L.V. & MERRILL, J.K., 1990.** Tilmicosin as a single injection treatment for respiratory disease of feedlot cattle. *Canadian Veterinary Journal*, 31, 826–829.

31 **GOURLAY, R.N. & HOUGHTON, S.B., 1985.** Experimental pneumonia in conventionally reared and gnotobiotic calves by dual infection with *Mycoplasma bovis* and *Pasteurella haemolytica*. *Research in Veterinary Science*, 38, 377–382.

32 **GOURLAY, R.N., THOMAS, L.H., WYLD, S.L. & SMITH, C.J., 1989.** Effect of a new macrolide antibiotic (tilmicosin) on pneumonia experimentally induced in calves by *Mycoplasma bovis* and *Pasteurella haemolytica*. *Research in Veterinary Science*, 47, 84–89.

33 **HENRY, C.W., 1984.** Shipping fever pneumonia: A new look at an old enemy. *Veterinary Medicine*, 79, 1200–1206.

34 **HENTON, M.M., 1985.** Veterinary Research Institute, Onderstepoort, South Africa. Unpublished data.

35 **HJERPE, C.A., 1983.** Clinical management of respiratory disease in feedlot cattle. *Veterinary Clinics of North America: Large Animal Practice*, 5, 119–142.

36 **HOUGHTON, S.B. & GOURLAY, R.N., 1984.** Bacteria associated with calf pneumonia and their effect on gnotobiotic calves. *Research in Veterinary Science*, 37, 194–198.

37 **JAKAB, G.J., 1982.** Viral–bacterial interactions in pulmonary infection. *Advances in Veterinary Science and Comparative Medicine*, 26, 155–171.

38 **JANZEN, E.D., 1991.** Clinical management of bovine respiratory disease. *Canadian Veterinary Journal*, 32, 215–218.

39 **JENSEN, R. & MACKEY, D.R., 1979.** *Diseases of Feedlot Cattle.* 3rd edn. Philadelphia: Lea & Febiger.

40 **JENSEN, R., PEIRSON, R.E., BRADDY, P.M., SAARI, D.A., LAUERMAN, L.H., ENGLAND, J.J., KEYVANFAR, H., COLLIER, J.R., HORTON, D.P., McCHESNEY, A.E., BENITZ, A. & CHRISTIE, R.M., 1976.** Shipping fever pneumonia in yearling feedlot cattle. *Journal of the American Veterinary Medical Association*, 169, 500–506.

41 **JERICHO, K.W.F., 1983.** Histological changes in the respiratory tract of calves exposed to aerosols of bovine herpesvirus 1 and *Pasteurella haemolytica*. *Journal of Comparative Pathology*, 93, 73–82.

42 **JERICHO, K.W.F. & LANGFORD, E.V., 1978.** Pneumonia in calves produced with aerosols of bovine herpesvirus 1 and *Pasteurella haemolytica*. *Canadian Journal of Comparative Medicine*, 42, 269–277.

43 **JONES, C.D.R., 1987.** Proliferation of *Pasteurella haemolytica* in the calf respiratory tract after an abrupt change in climate. *Research in Veterinary Science*, 47, 179–186.

44 **JONES, C.D.R. & WEBSTER, A.J.F., 1984.** Relationships between counts of nasopharyngeal bacteria, temperature, humidity and lung lesions in veal calves. *Research in Veterinary Science*, 37, 132–137.

45 **KAHRS, R.F., 1984.** Perspectives into the future of bovine respiratory disease research. *In*: LOAN, R.W., (ed.). *Bovine Respiratory Disease.* Proceedings of the North American Symposium on Bovine Respiratory Disease. College Station: Texas A & M University Press.

46 **KEE, J., GUICHON, T. & SHAW, G., 1988.** Protecting feedlot calves from pneumonic pasteurellosis. *Veterinary Medicine*, 83, 1084–1087.

47 **KENNEDY, P.C., 1968.** Comments on gross and histological aspects of field cases of bovine respiratory disease. *Journal of the American Veterinary Medical Association*, 152, 756–757.

48 **KERSCHEN, R.P., BENNETT, B.W., FLACK, D.E., JENSEN, R. & COLLINS, J.K., 1987.** Bovine respiratory syncytial virus infection in yearling feedlot cattle. *Agri-Practice*, 8, 23–26.

49 **LIGGITT, H.D., 1985.** Defence mechanisms in the bovine lung. *Veterinary Clinics of North America: Food Animal Practice*, 1, 347–366.

50 **LILLIE, L.E., 1974.** The bovine respiratory disease complex. *Canadian Veterinary Journal*, 15, 233–242.

51 **LOPEZ, A., MAXIE, M.G., RUHNKE, L., SAVAN, M. & THOMSON, R.G., 1982.** The pulmonary clearance of *Pasteurella haemolytica* in calves infected with bovine virus diarrhea or *Mycoplasma bovis*. *Canadian Journal of Comparative Medicine*, 46, 302–306.

52 **LOPEZ, A., MAXIE, M.G., RUHNKE, L., SAVAN, M. & THOMSON, R.G., 1986.** Cellular inflammatory response in the lungs of calves exposed to bovine viral diarrhea virus, *Mycoplasma bovis* and *Pasteurella haemolytica*. *American Journal of Veterinary Research*, 47, 1283–1286.

53 **LOPEZ, A., THOMSON, R.G. & SAVAN, M., 1976.** The pulmonary clearance of *Pasteurella haemolytica* in calves infected with bovine parainfluenza-3 virus. *Canadian Journal of Comparative Medicine*, 40, 385–391.

54 **MACVEAN, D.W., FRANZEN, D.K., KEEFE, T.J. & BENNETT, B.W., 1986.** Airborne particle concentration and meteorologic conditions associated with pneumonia incidence in feedlot cattle. *American Journal of Veterinary Research*, 47, 2676–2682.

55 **MARTIN, S.W., 1983.** Vaccination: Is it effective in preventing respiratory disease or influencing weight gains of feeder calves? *Canadian Veterinary Journal*, 24, 10–19.

56 **MARTIN, S.W., MEEK, A.H., DAVIS, D.L., THOMSON, R.G., JOHNSON, J.A., LOPEZ, A., STEPHENS, L., CURTIS, R.A., PRESCOTT, J.F., ROSENDAL, S., SAVAN, M., ZUBAIDY, A.J. & BOLTON, M.R., 1982.** Factors associated with mortality and treatment costs in feedlot calves: The Bruce county beef project, years 1978, 1979, 1980. *Canadian Journal of Comparative Medicine*, 46, 341–349.

57 **MOHANTY, S.B., 1978.** Bovine respiratory viruses. *Advances in Veterinary Science and Comparative Medicine*, 22, 83–109.

58 **MORTER, R.L. & AMSTUTZ, H.E., 1986.** Effectiveness of vaccination of feedlot cattle with bovine respiratory syncytial virus (BRSV). *Bovine Practitioner*, 21, 65–69.

59 **MORTER, R.L., BOYCE, J.R. & AMSTUTZ, H.E., 1986.** Treatment of bovine respiratory disease with erythromycin and amoxicillin. *Bovine Practitioner*, 21, 62–64.

60 **MOSIER, D.A., CONFER, A.W. & PANCIERA, R.J., 1989.** The evolution of vaccines for bovine pneumonia pasteurellosis. *Research in Veterinary Science*, 47, 1–10.

61 **NESBIT, J.W., ORSMUND, L.M., BARNARD, B.J.H. & VAN AMSTEL, S.R., 1987.** Faculty of Veterinary Science, University of Pretoria. Unpublished data.

62 **ORSMOND, L.M., 1987.** P.O. Box 356, Middelburg, Transvaal. Unpublished data.

63 **PALOTAY, J.L. & CHRISTENSEN, N.R., 1959.** Bovine respiratory infections: Lymphogranuloma venereum group of viruses as etiologic agents. *Journal of the American Veterinary Medical Association*, 134, 222–230.

64 **REHMTULLA, A.J. & THOMSON, R.G., 1981.** A review of the lesions in shipping fever of cattle. *Canadian Veterinary Journal*, 22, 1–8.

65 **ROBINSON, N.E., SLOCOMBE, R.F. & DERKSEN, F.J., 1984.** Physiology of the bovine lung. *In*: LOAN, R.W., (ed.) *Bovine Respiratory Disease.* Proceedings of the North American Symposium on Bovine Respiratory Disease. College Station: Texas A & M University Press.

66 **ROSENQUIST, B.D., 1984.** Viruses as etiologic agents of bovine respiratory disease. *In*: LOAN, R.W., (ed.). *Bovine Respiratory Disease.* Proceedings of the North American Symposium on Bovine Respiratory Disease. College Station: Texas A & M University Press.

67 **ROTH, J.A., 1984.** Immunosuppression and immunodulation in bovine respiratory diseases. *In*: LOAN, R.W., (ed.). *Bovine Respiratory Disease.* Proceedings of the North American Symposium on Bovine Respiratory Disease. College Station: Texas A & M University Press.

68 **SCHIEFER, B., WARD, G.E. & MOFFATT, R.E., 1978.** Correlation of microbiological and histological findings in bovine fibrinous pneumonia. *Veterinary Pathology*, 15, 313–321.

69 **SHEWEN, P.E., 1983.** The role of the *Pasteurella haemolytica* cytotoxin in bovine pneumonic pasteurellosis. *Dissertation Abstracts International* B, 43, 2471.

70 **SHEWEN, P.E., SHARP, A. & WILKIE, B.N., 1988.** Efficacy testing a *Pasteurella haemolytica* extract vaccine. *Veterinary Medicine*, 83, 1078–1083.

71 **SHEWEN, P.E. & WILKIE, B.N., 1984.** Immunity to *Pasteurella haemolytica* serotype 1. *In*: LOAN, R.W., (ed.). *Bovine Respiratory Disease*. Proceedings of the North American Symposium on Bovine Respiratory Disease. College Station: Texas A & M University Press.

72 **SHOO, M.K., 1989.** Experimental pneumonic pasteurellosis. A review. *The Veterinary Record*, 124, 141–144.

73 **SHOO, M.K., 1990.** The treatment and prevention of bovine pneumonic pasteurellosis using antimicrobial drugs. *Veterinary Research Communications*, 14, 341–345.

74 **SINHA, S.K. & ABINANTI, F.R., 1962.** Shipping fever of cattle. *Advances in Veterinary Science*, 7, 225–271.

75 **SLAUSON, D.O., 1982.** The mediation of pulmonary inflammatory injury. *Advances in Veterinary Science and Comparative Medicine*, 26, 99–153.

76 **SLOCOMBE, R.F., DERKSEN, F.J. & ROBINSON, N.E., 1984.** Interactions of cold stress and *Pasteurella haemolytica* in the pathogenesis of pneumonic pasteurellosis in calves: Pathologic changes in pulmonary function. *American Journal of Veterinary Research*, 45, 1764–1770.

77 **SLOCOMBE, R.F., DERKSEN, F.J. & ROBINSON, N.E., 1989.** Comparison of pathophysiologic changes in the lungs of calves challenge-exposed with *Escherichia coli*-derived endotoxin and *Pasteurella haemolytica*, alone or in combination. *American Journal of Veterinary Research*, 50, 701–707.

78 **SLOCOMBE, R.F., DERKSEN, F.J., ROBINSON, N.E., TRAPP, A., GUPTA, A. & NEUMAN, J.P., 1984.** Interactions of cold stress and *Pasteurella haemolytica* in the pathogenesis of pneumonic pasteurellosis in calves: Method of induction and hematologic and pathologic changes. *American Journal of Veterinary Research*, 45, 1757–1763.

79 **SLOCOMBE, R.F., MALARK, J., INGERSOLL, R., DERKSEN, F.J. & ROBINSON, N.E., 1985.** Importance of neutrophils in the pathogenesis of acute pneumonic pasteurellosis in calves. *American Journal of Veterinary Research*, 46, 2253–2258.

80 **STYRT, B., WALKER, R.D., WHITE, J.C., DAHL, L.D. & BAKER, J.C., 1990.** Granulocyte plasma membrane damage by leukotoxic supernatant from *Pasteurella haemolytica* A1 and protection by immune serum. *Canadian Journal of Veterinary Research*, 54, 146–150.

81 **THIRY, E., SALIKI, J., BUBLOT, M. & PASTORET, P.-P., 1987.** Reactivation of infectious bovine rhinotracheitis virus by transport. *Comparative Immunology, Microbiology and Infectious Diseases*, 10, 59–63.

82 **THOMAS, L.H., GOURLAY, R.N., WYLD, S.G., PARSONS, K.R. & CHANTER, N., 1989.** Evidence that blood-borne infection is involved in the pathogenesis of bovine pneumonic pasteurellosis. *Veterinary Pathology*, 26, 253–259.

83 **THOMSON, R.G., 1984.** Pathogenesis of pneumonia in feedlot cattle. *In*: LOAN, R.W., (ed.). *Bovine Respiratory Disease*. Proceedings of the North American Symposium on Bovine Respiratory Disease. College Station: Texas A & M University Press.

84 **VAN AMSTEL, S.R., 1987.** Faculty of Veterinary Science, University of Pretoria. Unpublished data.

85 **VAN AMSTEL, S.R., HENTON, M., WITCOMB, M.A., FABIAN, B. & VERVOORT, P., 1987.** Antibiotic sensitivity of *Pasteurella haemolytica* isolated by means of a fibreoptic endoscope from cases of pneumonic pasteurellosis in cattle. *Onderstepoort Journal of Veterinary Research*, 54, 551–552.

86 **VAN VUUREN, M., 1990.** Serological studies of bovine respiratory syncytial virus in feedlot cattle in South Africa. *Journal of the South African Veterinary Association*, 61, 168–169.

87 **VEIT, H.P. & FARRELL, R.L., 1978.** The anatomy and physiology of the bovine respiratory system relating to pulmonary disease. *Cornell Veterinarian*. 68, 555–581.

88 **VESTWEBER, J.G., 1981.** Pneumonia. *In*: HOWARD, J.L., (ed.). *Current Veterinary Therapy: Food Animals Practice*. Philadelphia: W.B. Saunders Company.

89 **WALKER, R.D., SCHULTZ, T.W., HOPKINS, F.M. & BRYANT, J.J., 1984.** Growth phase-dependent phagocytosis of *Pasteurella haemolytica* by bovine pulmonary macrophages. *American Journal of Veterinary Research*, 45, 1230–1234.

90 **WIKSE, S.E., 1985.** Feedlot cattle pneumonias. *Veterinary Clinics of North America: Food Animal Practice*, 1, 289–310.

91 **WILKIE, B.N., 1984.** Humoral and cell-mediated resistance mechanisms of cattle. *In*: LOAN, R.W., (ed.). *Bovine Respiratory Disease*. Proceedings of the North American Symposium on Bovine Respiratory Disease. College Station: Texas A & M University Press.

92 **WILLSON, P.J., 1990.** *Haemophilus, Actinobacillus, Pasteurella*: Mechanisms of resistance and antibiotic therapy. *Canadian Journal of Veterinary Research*, 54, 573–577.

93 **WISEMAN, A., ALLAN, E.M., GIBBS, H.A. & SELMAN, I.E., 1985.** Production of transit fever with isolates of *Pasteurella haemolytica* A1. *Bovine Practitioner*, 20, 141–143.

94 **YATES, W.D.G., 1982.** A review of infectious bovine rhinotracheitis, shipping fever pneumonia and viral–bacterial synergism in respiratory diseases of cattle. *Canadian Journal of Comparative Medicine*, 46, 225–263.

95 **YATES, W.D.G., JERICHO, K.W.F. & DOIGE, C.E., 1983.** Effect of bacterial dose on pneumonia induced by aerosol exposure of calves to bovine herpesvirus-1 and *Pasteurella haemolytica*. *American Journal of Veterinary Research*, 44, 238–243.

96 **YILMA, T. & BREEZE, R., 1985.** New technology for prevention and control of infectious bovine respiratory diseases. *Veterinary Clinics of North America: Food Animal Practice*, 1, 419–439.

142

Haemorrhagic septicaemia

S.S. Bastianello and J.W. Nesbit

Introduction and aetiology

Haemorrhagic septicaemia is a peracute to acute, often fatal disease, principally of cattle and water buffaloes (*Bubalus bubalis*), caused by *Pasteurella multocida* serotype B or E. It occurs almost exclusively in Asia and Africa.[9] The Asian form is caused by serotype B and the African form (East African haemorrhagic fever) primarily by serotype E.

For information on the characteristics of *Pasteurella* spp. consult ***Pasteurella* spp. infections: Introduction**.

Epidemiology

The disease occurs commonly in several countries in Africa, including Senegal, Mali, Ivory Coast, Nigeria, Cameroon, Egypt, Sudan, Congo, Zaïre, Zambia, and Namibia,[2, 5, 16, 23, 24] and in Asia, particularly southern and south-east Asia.[9, 21] It has also been recorded in the USA and Canada, where in both cases bison (*Bison bison*) were principally affected,[19, 22] and in cattle in Argentina, southern Europe, Russia[4, 26] and South Africa.[6] In all countries in Africa except Egypt and Sudan, serotype E is the causative serotype.[6, 16, 24] In Egypt and Sudan both serotypes B and E have been isolated,[23, 24] probably because these are the two African countries closest to Asia, in which only serotype B has been implicated as the cause of haemorrhagic septicaemia.

The African form of haemorrhagic fever occurs sporadically. Outbreaks are usually of limited extent and tend to be associated with stress conditions. It is recorded predominantly in countries which have a tropical or subtropical climate and a high seasonal rainfall.[16, 25] In Namibia, the disease occurs more commonly in the wetter northern and central parts of the country, such as the Caprivi and Ovamboland, and the Otjiwarongo, Okahandja, Gobabis and Grootfontein districts, but it has also been reported from drier parts such as the Keetmanshoop and Windhoek districts.[5, 7] There is only one record of the disease in South Africa — in calves in the north-western Transvaal.[6]

The Asian form of haemorrhagic septicaemia occurs in countries with a high seasonal rainfall. It is frequently endemic in marshy zones or along river deltas.[25]

In the endemic regions of Africa and Asia, haemorrhagic septicaemia occurs throughout the year but its prevalence increases at the onset of, or during, the rainy season.[2, 3, 14, 16–18, 25] It has been reported following a sudden increase in rainfall and humidity with a concomitant severe drop in temperature.[2]

Under natural conditions, haemorrhagic septicaemia occurs mainly in cattle and water buffaloes but it has also been reported in pigs, sheep, goats, horses, donkeys, camels, fallow deer (*Dama dama*), bison and Indian elephants (*Elephas sengalensis*).[1, 5, 9] Water buffaloes are more susceptible than cattle.[9] In endemic regions, it usually affects young animals (cattle or water buffaloes between six months and two years of age) and it is seldom reported in cattle older than four years.[11, 13] In non-endemic regions, all age groups of animals, including calves, may be affected.[14, 19]

Carrier animals probably play an important role in the epidemiology of the disease.[4] Animals which are subclinically infected or which have recovered from the disease and are carriers are important sources of infection.[9, 23] Up to 40 per cent of an animal population may be carriers; the bacteria being harboured in the nasopharynx and tonsils. The nasopharyngeal infection is apparently short-lived (four to six weeks) and the latent carrier state is fulfilled by tonsillar infection.[9] Recent evidence indicates that it is the animals which develop high antibody levels following infection which undergo so-called 'arrested infection' and become persistent or latent carriers of the infection. These animals are important in the spread of the disease. An outbreak is believed to arise when a latent carrier animal becomes an active shedder of bacteria and infects in-contact susceptible animals.[12]

Various stress factors, including intercurrent protozoal and bacterial infections, transport over long distances, administration of intramuscular injections, and starvation, may trigger carrier animals to shed virulent organisms.[2, 6, 19]

Transmission of the infection is via aerosol or by direct or indirect contact between affected and susceptible animals. The excretion of the bacteria in the saliva, urine, faeces and milk results in contamination of the environment and infection of in-contact animals.[1, 9, 20] Experimentally, animals have been infected via the subcutaneous or intramuscular routes.

The magnitude of an outbreak of haemorrhagic septicaemia is dependent upon the level of immunity in the animal population.[9] An explosive outbreak with high morbidity and mortality rates is likely when an animal that is shedding the bacteria is introduced into a herd with minimal immunity. On the other hand, in endemic areas where large proportions of adult animals are immune, disease tends to be restricted to young animals with declining passive immunity or recently introduced animals from non-endemic areas. Mortality rates can vary from 1 to 10 per cent in endemic regions and 20 to 98 per cent in non-endemic regions.[9, 14]

Pathogenesis

In natural cases the organisms probably enter via the nasal and oral routes and multiply initially in the tonsils. Fever, salivation and dullness occur a few hours after infection. Bacteraemia has been detected within 12 hours of experimental infection; at this stage the organisms are usually present in the saliva.

The effects of the infection are dependent upon the virulence and dose of the organism and the susceptibility of the host.[9] Virulence of the organism is associated with the presence of capsules; virulent organisms produce smooth, iridescent colonies on culture.[9, 20] Overwhelming of the host's defence mechanisms results in overt disease.[9] There is mounting evidence that lipopolysaccharide (endotoxin) of the bacterial cell wall is responsible for the lethal effects of the infection.[9, 26]

As the disease progresses, affected animals may show respiratory distress, a reluctance to move and may become recumbent. At this stage the venous blood pressure falls and the bacteria appear in the faeces, urine and milk.

Clinical signs

The incubation period of the natural disease is two to three days but may be as short as 30 hours in experimentally induced infections.[9] The disease may run a peracute, acute or subacute course. The peracute disease is characterized by sudden death in cattle, generally with no premonitory signs being noticed, but some animals may manifest dyspnoea, grunting and prostration for a few hours to 24 hours prior to death.[6, 19, 20] Acutely and subacutely affected animals may be pyretic and show anorexia, depression, profuse salivation and nasal discharge, and rapid respiratory and pulse rates before death.[9, 16]

Subacute disease is characterized by the development of a firm, subcutaneous swelling of the submandibular region which may extend to the neck, brisket and fore legs.[1, 5, 6, 9, 18] Some animals may show circling movements and incoordination.[5] Clinical signs are usually present for periods ranging from eight to ten days.[5, 6, 19] The disease is generally fatal if animals are not treated.[18, 19]

Pathology

The peracute and acute septicaemic disease is usually characterized by severe generalized congestion and widespread petechiae and ecchymoses of the serosal surfaces and subcutis, the presence of suggillations in the abomasum, mild to moderate ascites, hydrothorax and hydropericardium, focal oedema at the thoracic inlet, and congestion, oedema and petechiation of lymph nodes.[6, 9, 19, 26] Some animals may show severe oedema of the lungs or a focal fibrinopurulent pneumonia, oedema and haemorrhages of the tracheal mucosa and adventitia, and peritracheal connective tissue, and localized serofibrinous myositis of one or more muscles.[6, 26] Microscopically, the acute disease is characterized by hyperaemia and leukostasis throughout the body, the presence of bacteria in lymph vessels in the lungs and occasionally in blood vessels in other organs and tissues, and myositis marked by necrosis of the muscle fibres, interstitial oedema, haemorrhage and serofibrinous exudation.[6, 19]

Subacute disease is characterized by severe localized cellulitis, fasciitis and myositis with micro-abscessation and fibroplasia of the submandibular region, neck, brisket and/or fore legs, and lymphadenitis of the draining lymph nodes.[2, 5, 6] Other lesions may include generalized congestion, widespread serosal haemorrhages, pulmonary oedema, serofibrinous or blood-stained fluid in the thoracic cavity, focal fibrinous pleuritis and pericarditis, serofibrinous polyarthritis and periarthritis, myocarditis and myocardial and/or renal infarcts, pseudomembranous erosive or ulcerative rhinitis, and serofibrinous meningitis.[5, 6] Fibrin thrombi and bacteria are frequently encountered in lymphatics and venules in the affected areas.

Diagnosis

A presumptive diagnosis of haemorrhagic septicaemia can be made on the epidemiology, clinical signs and pathology, and the demonstration of *Pasteurella* organisms in blood or tissue smears or organ sections stained with Giemsa or by the Gram method.[9] A definitive diagnosis rests on the isolation of the causative organisms. Blood from live animals is seldom useful for this purpose, as septicaemia often only develops terminally just before death.[12] Specimens of blood from dead animals, or in the case of those that have been dead for some time, specimens of bone marrow, should be submitted for diagnostic purposes.[12]

Specific identification of the organism as to species and serotype (*P. multocida* B or E) can be done by using an ELISA.[10] With this assay, serotypes responsible for causing haemorrhagic septicaemia are readily distinguished from those *P. multocida* that do not.

Differential diagnosis

Acute haemorrhagic septicaemia should be differentiated from other causes of acute mortality, such as anthrax, blackquarter (blackleg), rinderpest, and acute toxic conditions such as arsenic poisoning. The subacute form may be confused with conditions that cause submandibular, peripharyngeal and brisket oedema, such as calf diphtheria, snake bite or congestive heart failure.[9]

Control

The acute nature of most cases of the disease limits the efficacy of antimicrobial therapy of sick animals.[9, 16] However, an outbreak may be effectively controlled by administering a sulphonamide (sulphadimidine or sulphamethazine) or an antibiotic (oxytetracycline, penicillin, ampicillin or chloramphenicol) to purportedly healthy animals that show a febrile reaction.[9]

Immunity may be actively acquired through natural exposure or vaccination, or, in the new-born animal, passively following ingestion of colostrum from immune dams.[11] A solid, long-lasting immunity is conferred on animals that recover from the natural disease.[9] Vaccination programmes in countries in Asia decrease the prevalence of the disease.[1, 14, 17] Considerable success has been obtained in Asia by the immunization of buffaloes with alum-precipitated or oil-adjuvant vaccines.[9] The immunity is, however, only of six to nine months' duration following primary vaccination, and 12 months after a second administration of the vaccine.[9] It is recommended, therefore, that animals at risk receive the first vaccination at four to six months of age. This should be followed with a booster three months later and thereafter with annual administration of the vaccine. Since mice can be effectively immunized with inactivated vaccines prepared from serotype E strains,[8] it is probable that cattle could be equally effectively immunized against the African form of haemorrhagic septicaemia.

Large-scale vaccination of cattle against haemorrhagic septicaemia is not practised in Africa. An outbreak of the disease in Zambia was eventually controlled by using a formalinized vaccine obtained from the Sudan.[16] In South Africa, a combined bacterin/alum-precipitated vaccine containing *P. multocida* serotypes A, D and E and *P. haemolytica* is available for use in cattle.[15]

References

1 **ANON., THE INDONESIAN DELEGATION, 1977.** Haemorrhagic septicaemia and eradication program in Indonesia. *Bulletin de l'Office International des Épizooties*, 87, 609–612.

2 **ANOSA, V.O. & ISOUN, T.T., 1975.** An outbreak of haemorrhagic septicaemia in Holstein cattle in Nigeria: Possible role of associated factors. *Bulletin of Animal Health and Production in Africa*, 23, 337–340.

3 **BAHARSEFAT, M. & FIROUZI, Sh., 1977.** Progress in control of haemorrhagic septicaemia (pasteurellosis) in cattle in Iran. *Bulletin de l'Office International des Épizooties*, 67, 621–625.

4 **BAIN, R.V.S., 1963.** Haemorrhagic septicaemia. *In*: *FAO Agricultural Studies*, 62, 1–78. Rome: Food and Agricultural Organization of the United Nations.

5 **BASSON, P.A., 1987.** Haemorrhagic septicaemia (septicaemic pasteurellosis) in South West Africa. Paper presented at Annual Meeting of State Veterinarians in South West Africa, Grootfontein.

6 **BASTIANELLO, S.S. & JONKER, M.R., 1981.** A report on the occurrence of septicaemia caused by *Pasteurella multocida* type E from southern Africa. *Journal of the South African Veterinary Association*, 52, 99–104.

7 **BIGGS, H., 1989.** National Parks Board, Private Bag X402, Skukuza. Personal communication.

8 **CAMERON, C.M. & BESTER, F.J., 1986.** Respondence of sheep and cattle to combined polyvalent *Pasteurella haemolytica* vaccines. *Onderstepoort Journal of Veterinary Research*, 53, 1–7.

9 **CARTER, L.R. & DE ALWIS, M.C.L., 1989.** Haemorrhagic septicaemia. *In*: ADLAM, C. & RUTTER, J.M., (eds). *Pasteurella and Pasteurellosis*. London: Academic Press, Inc.

10 **DAWKINS, H.J.S., JOHNSON, R.B., SPENCER, T.L. & PATTEN, B.E., 1990.** Rapid identification of *Pasteurella multocida* organisms responsible for haemorrhagic septicaemia using an enzyme-linked immunosorbent assay. *Research in Veterinary Science*, 49, 261–267.

11 **DE ALWIS, M.C.L., 1981.** Mortality among cattle and buffaloes in Sri Lanka due to haemorrhagic septicaemia. *Tropical Animal Health and Production*, 13, 195–202.

12 **DE ALWIS, M.C.L., 1992.** Haemorrhagic septicaemia — A general review. *British Veterinary Journal*, 148, 99–112.

13 **DE ALWIS, M.C.L. & KODITUWAKKU, A.O., 1976.** Haemorrhagic septicaemia — an analysis of two outbreaks of disease among buffaloes. *Ceylon Veterinary Journal*, 14, 18–21.

14 **DE ALWIS, M.C.L. & VIPULASIRI, A.A., 1980.** An epizootiological study of haemorrhagic septicaemia in buffaloes and cattle in Sri Lanka. *Ceylon Veterinary Journal*, 28, 24–35.

15 **ERASMUS, B.J., CAMERON, C.M., HUNTER, P., CILLIERS, J.A., OBEREM, P.T., STOLTSZ, W.H. & DE WAAL, D.T., 1988.** *Onderstepoort Vaccines*. Directorate of Agricultural Information, Private Bag X144, Pretoria 0001, Republic of South Africa.

16 **FRANCIS, B.K.T., SCHELS, H.F. & CARTER, G.R., 1980.** Type E *Pasteurella multocida* associated with haemorrhagic septicaemia in Zambia. *The Veterinary Record*, 107, 135.

17 **GAJAPATHI, V.S. & D'SOUZA, B.A., 1968.** Epidemiological studies on haemorrhagic septicaemia, blackquarter and foot-and-mouth disease in Madras state for the period 1957–64. *Indian Veterinary Journal*, 45, 175–186.

18 **KHERA, S.S., 1979.** The incidence and distribution of epizootic diseases in India. *Bulletin de l'Office International des Épizooties*, 91, 331–347.

19 **KRADEL, D.C., HEDDLESTON, K.L., RISSER, J.V. & MANSPEAKER, J.E., 1969.** Septicemic pasteurellosis (hemorrhagic septicemia) in young dairy cattle. *Veterinary Medicine and Small Animal Clinician*, 64, 145–147.

20 **LOSOS, G.J., 1986.** Haemorrhagic septicaemia. *In*: LOSOS, G.J., (ed.). *Infectious Tropical Diseases of Domestic Animals*. New York: Longman Scientific and Technical.

21 **LUK'YANCHENKO. A.V., 1977.** Pasteurellosis and methods of its control. *Bulletin de l'Office International des Épizooties*, 87, 613–619.

22 **MARSHALL, C.J., 1922.** Haemorrhagic septicaemia. *Journal of the American Veterinary Medical Association*, 14, 238–242.

23 **MUSTAFA, A.A., GHALIB, H.W. & SHIGIDI, M.T., 1978.** Carrier rate of *Pasteurella multocida* in a cattle herd associated with an outbreak of haemorrhagic septicaemia in the Sudan. *British Veterinary Journal*, 134, 275–378.

24 **PERREAU, P., 1961.** Contribution à l'étude immunologique de *Pasteurella multocida*. Existence et importance d'un nouveau type, agent de la septicémie hémorragique des bovidés africains. *Revue d'Élevage et de Médecine Vétérinaire des Pays Tropicaux*, 14, 245–256.

25 **PERREAU, P., PETIT, J.-P. & THORNE, M., 1964.** Epizootologie de la pasteurellose bovine en République du Tchad. Importance de l'immunité naturelle acquise. *Revue d'Élevage et de Médecine Vétérinaire des Pays Tropicaux*, 17, 587–597.

26 **RHOADES, K.R., HEDDLESTON, K.L. & REBERS, P.A., 1967.** Experimental hemorrhagic septicemia: Gross and microscopic lesions resulting from acute infections and from endotoxin administration. *Canadian Journal of Comparative Medicine and Veterinary Science*, 31, 226–233.

143

Ovine and caprine pasteurellosis

J.W. Nesbit, S.S. Bastianello and G. Bath

Introduction and aetiology

Pasteurellosis in sheep and goats may manifest in a variety of forms, the most common being pneumonia.[18, 20, 21, 24, 35, 50] Although implicated in an outbreak of pneumonia in sheep in southern Africa for the first time in 1936,[28] the importance of pasteurellosis as a cause of economic losses in sheep and goats in South Africa has only been appreciated since 1960,[3] and then more in sheep than in goats.[50]

Pasteurella haemolytica is divided into biotypes according to cultural characteristic — biotype A (= arabinose fermenters) and biotype T (= trehalose fermenters) — as well as 16 serotypes. For more information on the characteristics of the *Pasteurella* spp. consult ***Pasteurella* spp. infections: Introduction**.

In sheep, *P. haemolytica* infection is associated with four specific syndromes.[18, 20, 21, 24, 35] Disease due to infection with *P. haemolytica* biotype A causes septicaemia in lambs, pneumonia in sheep of all ages, and mastitis ('blou-uier') in postparturient ewes, whereas *P. haemolytica* biotype T is the cause of systemic (embolic) pasteurellosis (occasionally also referred to as septicaemic pasteurellosis) in subadult, predominantly feedlot, sheep.[16, 45] The distinction in the nomenclature between septicaemic pasteurellosis due to infection with *P. haemolytica* biotype A and systemic (embolic) pasteurellosis due to infection with *P. haemolytica* biotype T is preferred because it affords an accurate reflection of the different pathogenetic pathways of the two syndromes.[17, 24] Infection with *P. multocida* serotypes B and E may result in haemorrhagic septicaemia **(see Chapter 142: Haemorrhagic septicaemia)** in sheep, goats and other animal species.[13] In addition, *P. multocida* types A and D infection is a cause of pneumonia in sheep of all ages. Apart from acute fibrinous bronchopneumonia, infection by *P. haemolytica* or *P. multocida*, individually or together, may occasionally be responsible for fibrinous or fibrinopurulent meningitis, encephalitis, pericarditis, pleuritis, peritonitis, polyarthritis and/or epididymitis,[16, 18, 20, 21, 32, 35] and has been implicated in the aetiology of a hepatogenous bacterial icterus in sheep.[48]

The situation in goats is less clear. Pneumonia in goats has been attributed to infection by both *P. haemolytica*[39] and *P. multocida*,[8, 42, 52] whilst *P. haemolytica* has been incriminated as a cause of mastitis.[4]

In sheep and goats in South Africa, disease due to *P. haemolytica* is more prevalent than that caused by *P. multocida*. Based on 893 isolations of *Pasteurella* spp. from specimens submitted to the Veterinary Research Institute, Onderstepoort, *P. haemolytica* accounts for 87,2 per cent of the isolates, compared with 12,8 per cent for *P. multocida*.[29] Fifteen serotypes of *P. haemolytica* have been isolated in South Africa. The prevalence of the serotypes in tissue samples from sheep and goats examined at the Institute between 1983 and 1989 are reflected in **Table 143.1**. The dominant serotypes from sheep and goats with pneumonia were 6, 2 and 1 (in that order), whilst serotypes 7, 2 and 6 were the most frequent isolates from cases with mastitis. Over 36 per cent of the isolates were untypable. Serotype A and, to a lesser extent, serotype E were identified more frequently than other serotypes of *P. multocida*.

Table 143.1 Prevalence of serotypes of 589 *Pasteurella haemolytica* isolates from sheep and goats between 1983 and 1989[29]

SEROTYPE	PREVALENCE RATE %*
1	5,4
2	12,2
3	1,9
4	3,6
5	3,9
6	10,6
7	6,3
8	2,2
9	5,3
10	3,1
11	3,7
12	1,7
13	0,5
14	0,9
15	2,2
Untypable	36,7

* Percentages rounded off to the nearest 0,1 per cent

Because disease due to *P. haemolytica* predominates, the four syndromes associated with it in sheep [pneumonic pasteurellosis, mastitic pasteurellosis, systemic (embolic) pasteurellosis and septicaemic pasteurellosis] are considered here.

PNEUMONIC PASTEURELLOSIS IN SHEEP

Synonym: Bont-long (Afrik.)

Introduction

Ovine pneumonic pasteurellosis refers to respiratory disease of sheep characterized by acute, fibrinopurulent pneumonia due predominantly to *P. haemolytica* infection.[24] It is the most common syndrome of pasteurellosis in sheep, and affects particularly animals that are sub-optimally nourished, although it also occurs occasionally in well-nourished animals.[18, 20]

Epidemiology

Infection of the nasopharynx and tonsils serves as the carrier state for *P. haemolytica* in healthy sheep.[24] Transmission of *Pasteurella* spp. from ewe to lamb, resulting in tonsillar colonization, occurs shortly after birth and is dominated by biotype A.[2] After nine weeks of age, biotype T becomes increasingly dominant in the tonsils, to the virtual exclusion of biotype A by six months of age. However, biotype A may still be recovered from the nasopharynx of these animals.[24] Up to 95 per cent of animals may be carriers of *P. haemolytica*; a high percentage may become carriers during outbreaks of disease.[24] In the United Kingdom, the percentage of animals that become carriers of biotype A peaks during outbreaks of pneumonic pasteurellosis, while biotype T predominates during outbreaks of systemic (embolic) pasteurellosis.[24]

The prevalence of pneumonic pasteurellosis is highest in autumn and spring,[18, 20, 24] and is often predisposed by sudden changes in weather, especially to cold, wet weather.[7, 21, 35] Other factors which may be important predisposing factors include:

- gathering, handling and mixing of animals from different sources and of different age groups, such as the situation generally prevailing in feedlots;[7, 21, 35]
- the age of sheep: lambs are more susceptible to the disease than adult animals;[24]
- transportation, overcrowding, dehydration, starvation, dipping, trauma (castration and taildocking), shearing, verminosis, and exposure to dusty atmospheres; and
- prior or concomitant bacterial, chlamydial, mycoplasmal, protozoal or viral infection.[7, 18, 20, 21, 24, 35]

A number of infectious agents have been associated with *P. haemolytica* infections, including *P. multocida*, *Actinomyces (Corynebacterium) pyogenes*, *Corynebacterium pseudotuberculosis (C. ovis)*,[15, 16, 29] *Trypanosoma congolense*,[36] *Chlamydia psittaci*,[18, 20] *Cytoecetes phagocytophila*,[9, 23] *Mycoplasma ovipneumoniae*,[12, 15, 20, 21, 37] adenovirus,[6] parainfluenza virus type 3,[15, 21, 37, 43, 44] respiratory syncytial virus,[1, 46] jaagsiekte retrovirus,[40, 51] and lentivirus.[40] The role played by these infectious agents in the pathogenesis of pneumonic pasteurellosis in sheep is uncertain. *Pasteurella multocida* may be a primary, concomitant or secondary invader. *Actinomyces pyogenes* and *C. pseudotuberculosis* are probably opportunists.[29] Although *C. psittaci* and *M. ovipneumoniae* may often be isolated together with *P. haemolytica* from natural cases of pneumonia in sheep, their role in the production of pneumonic pasteurellosis has been questioned.[12, 16] However, *M. ovipneumoniae* and *P. haemolytica* biotype A are implicated in the aetiology of atypical pneumonia, a predominantly subclinical proliferative exudative pneumonia of the cranioventral aspects of the lungs in sheep reared under intensive systems.[24] The role of prior trypanosomal, rickettsial (*C. phagocytophila*) and viral infections as significant predisposing factors is a little more substantive.[1, 9, 15, 21, 23, 36, 37, 40, 43, 46]

Pathogenesis

Certain viral infections of the respiratory system, such as those caused by adenovirus, parainfluenza virus type 3, respiratory syncytial virus, jaagsiekte retrovirus and lentivirus, result in impairment of the pulmonary clearance mechanism (including the phagocytic mechanisms) and cause local immunosuppression, which facilitates subsequent bacterial infection[15, 40] in which *P. haemolytica* biotype A predominates.[15] Although not as extensively investigated as in cattle, prior viral infection is not an essential requirement in experimental ovine pneumonic pasteurellosis; the condition is readily induced by *P. haemolytica* alone.[12] Other diseases, such as ovine trypanosomiasis and tick-borne fever caused by *C. phagocytophila*, cause diminution of the humoral and cellular immune responses to bacterial infection.[9, 23, 36] In addition, there is impaired neutrophil function in tick-borne fever.[9]

Although certain serotypes are isolated more frequently than others from field cases of pneumonic pasteurellosis in sheep,[29] the individual serotypes of *P. haemolytica* are apparently not as significant an aetiological factor as in cattle. The clinical and pathological features of experimental disease in sheep induced by serotypes 1, 2, 7 and 9 are indistinguishable.[25] In other respects the pathogenesis is assumed to be similar to that pertaining to cattle **(see Chapter 141: Pneumonic pasteurellosis in cattle)**, where bacteria, having first proliferated in the upper respiratory tract, are transferred to the lower respiratory tract where they result in pneumonia.[18]

Infection may be facilitated by a number of components (virulence factors) contained by the bacteria, including the surface glycocalyx and fimbriae, proteolytic enzymes, capsular polysaccharide, leukotoxin (cytotoxin) and lipopolysaccharide.[10] The subsequent inflammatory reaction is initiated by the lipopolysaccharide, which is largely responsible for the vascular events and the associated influx of neutrophils.[11] Accelerated destruction of neutrophils (induced by leukotoxin) may trigger neutrophil-dependent tissue necrosis as well as augmentation of the inflammatory reaction.[10, 11] The severity of the reaction is dependent on the quantum of bacteria that gains access to the lungs.[15, 18, 35] For more information on the different virulence factors and their effects consult ***Pasteurella* spp. infections: Introduction** and **Chapter 141: Pneumonic pasteurellosis in cattle: Pathogenesis.**

Clinical signs

The disease occurs commonly as outbreaks,[21] particularly in feedlots,[35] but sporadic cases involving individual animals may be found in a flock. The morbidity rate may vary from 10–50 per cent and the mortality rate seldom exceeds 10 per cent. Clinical disease usually follows exposure to predisposing factors within a few days, but the interval may be as long as several weeks.[15, 18]

The disease may have an acute, subacute or chronic course.[21, 35] In acutely affected animals, particularly lambs, death may occur without premonitory signs,[21, 35] but most animals show fever, depression, anorexia, weight loss, serous to mucopurulent nasal discharge, lachrymation, coughing, tachypnoea and dyspnoea induced by exercise.[24, 35] Frothing at the mouth and harsh pulmonary sounds are indicative of severe, advanced pulmonary involvement.[21]

The clinical signs in subacutely and chronically affected animals are generally non-specific, and are dominated by unthriftiness in survivors.[24, 35]

Pathology

Depending on the course, pneumonic pasteurellosis is characterized by acute, fibrinopurulent bronchopneumonia **(Figure 143.1)** predominantly affecting the cranioventral portions of the lungs.[1, 16, 18, 20, 30] In the early stages of the acute disease the affected areas are consolidated, deep red to reddish-purple, and tend to merge with the relatively unaffected lung tissue; the subpleural and interlobular interstitium in the affected parts are distended with serosanguineous exudate, and discrete foci of necrosis of varying size may be present in the lungs. In the later stages of the acute disease, affected and unaffected areas are well demarcated from each other and affected areas show haemorrhage, a fibrinous exudate in the distended interlobular septa and various stages of red or grey hepatization on a lobular basis which has given rise to the Afrikaans name of 'bont-long' (literally meaning 'mottled- or pied-lung') for the disease. On cut surface of the affected parts of the lungs a serofibrinous to fibrinopurulent exudate may be expressed from the bronchioles. The pneumonic lesion is almost invariably accompanied by an acute fibrinous pleuritis and pericarditis **(Figure 143.2)**.[18, 20] The subacute and chronic pneumonic lesions are usually characterized by abscessation of the lungs and, occasionally, the regional lymph nodes, and extensive pulmonary scarring and focal fibrous adhesions between the parietal and visceral pleura and the pericardium.[16]

The histological features of acutely affected lungs include hyperaemia and oedema, serofibrinous exudate admixed with variable numbers of macrophages and neutrophils in alveoli, bronchioles, bronchi and interstitium of the lungs, haemorrhages, thrombosis of blood and lymphatic vessels, and multiple foci of coagulative necrosis.[1, 16, 20, 30] The necrotic areas are frequently confluent, extend across interlobular septa, and are surrounded by parenchyma in which 'oat cells' or 'streaming macrophages' are abundant. Gram-negative bacteria are particularly prevalent at the periphery of the necrotic foci. Inflammatory changes which indicate a prior viral, chlamydial or mycoplasmal infection, such as the presence of a necrotizing, lymphocytic, or proliferative bronchiolitis, may also be present.[16] In subacutely and chronically affected lungs there is evidence of organization of the affected areas, fibroplasia, abscessation and fibrous pleuritis and pericarditis.

Diagnosis and differential diagnosis

A provisional diagnosis can be made on the clinical and pathological findings, but confirmation of the diagnosis is dependent upon the isolation of the causative organism in sufficient numbers from specimens of affected parts of the lungs, lesions, pleural exudate, blood and spleen collected aseptically at necropsy.[24] As *P. haemolytica* may be present in the lungs of sheep without causing disease, a high infection load of approximately 10^6 colony-forming units per gram of lung in acute cases and 10^3–10^5 colony-forming units per gram of lung in subacutely and chronically affected animals should be present in order to substantiate the diagnosis.[24] However, isolation of the causative organism may be difficult from chronic pneumonic lesions or from animals that have been treated with antibiotics.

Similar lesions may be encountered in pneumonia caused by other bacteria, notably *P. multocida* and, rarely, *Escherichia coli*.[5] Aspiration pneumonia may be distinguished from *P. haemolytica* pneumonia on the basis of the distribution of the lesions (predilective involvement of the right cranial lobe) and the type of reaction (often gangrenous).[16] Chronic pneumonia due to *P. haemolytica* should be differentiated clinically and pathologically from jaagsiekte,[51] pneumonic corynebacteriosis (caused by *Corynebacterium pseudotuberculosis* or *Actinomyces pyogenes*), lungworm infestation and maedi or ovine progressive pneumonia.[18] Histological examination is useful to differentiate between these conditions. Secondary

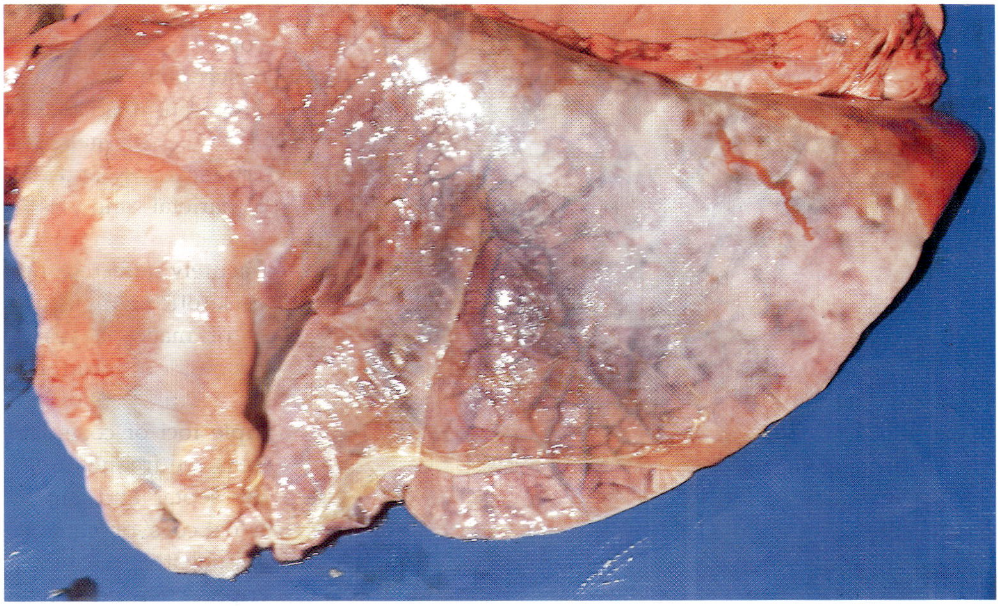

Figure 143.1 Acute, fibrinous pleuropneumonia in a sheep. Note the cranioventral distribution of the lesions

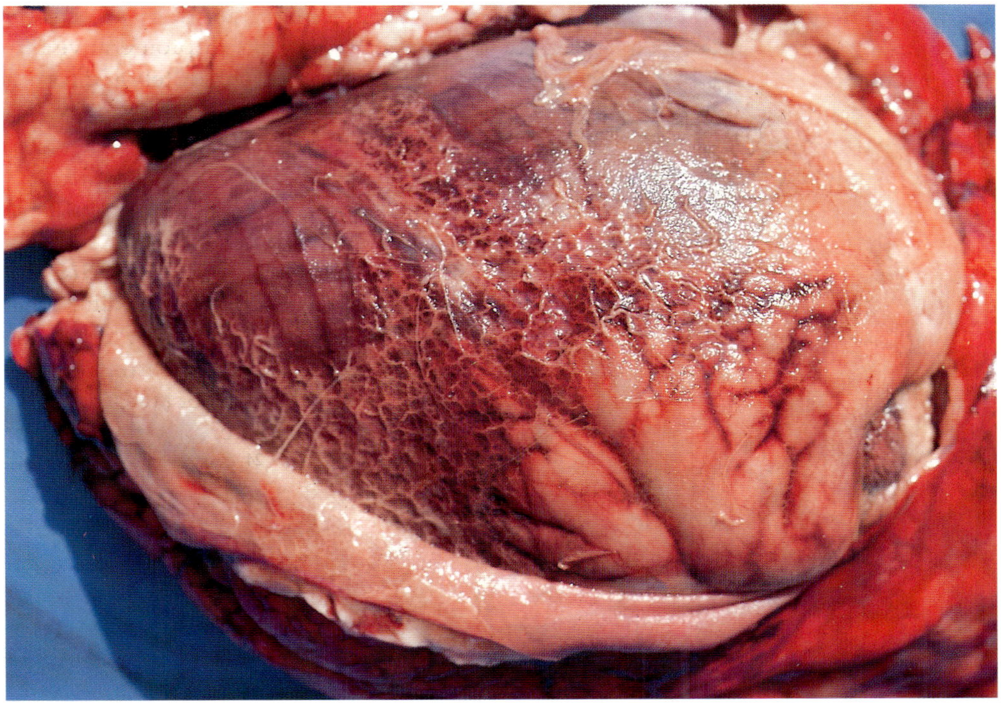

Figure 143.2 Acute, fibrinous pericarditis in a sheep suffering from acute pasteurellosis

bacterial infections of the lungs occur commonly in animals that are affected by lungworm infestation, jaagsiekte and maedi or ovine progressive pneumonia.

Control

Treatment may be successful provided that the disease is not too severe or chronic.[18] Sulphonamides (trimethoprim-sulphonamide combinations) or antibiotics, such as penicillin, ampicillin, or preferably oxytetracycline (all serotypes of *P. haemolytica* are sensitive to it) may be used,[21, 24, 26, 35] and should be accompanied by supportive therapy and proper nursing.[18] In experimentally induced pneumonic pasteurellosis in lambs, the clinical signs have been controlled within 24 hours by the administration of long-acting oxytetracycline at 20 mg/kg body weight. The beneficial effect was maintained for six days, whereafter reactivation of the infection occurred,[26] suggesting that a follow-up treatment of oxytetracycline four to six days later would be advisable. This experimental finding of recrudescence of the disease following treatment is borne out by field experience involving the treatment of affected sheep with tetracyclines and other antibiotics, such as penicillin and ampicillin.[5]

Protection of sheep against pneumonic pasteurellosis may be afforded through vaccination and appropriate management. The Onderstepoort *Pasteurella* Vaccine for Sheep and Goats (Reg. No. G 479 Act 36/1947) produced by the Veterinary Research Institute, Onderstepoort, is suitable for vaccination of sheep at risk.[19] The vaccine is a bacterin that consists of a combination of *P. multocida* types A and D, and *P. haemolytica* serotypes 1, 2 and 6. The recommended procedure of immunization entails administration of two injections at an interval of four weeks, followed by a booster injection which should be administered six to eight weeks before anticipated exposure to stressful situations. Vaccination should commence as early as one month of age. While good immunity is obtained against infection with homologous serotypes of *P. multocida*, the vaccine produces poor immunity against infection by others. In such cases, an autogenous vaccine may be prepared from isolates of the causative organism.[29] In many instances, good management will largely obviate the necessity for vaccination.[5] Adequate nutrition, protection from inclement weather and environmental and feed dust, reduction of crowding and mixing of disparate groups, control of other infectious diseases and of parasitic infestations, and limiting of stress may help to reduce the prevalence of disease. Supplementation of the feed ration with a sulphonamide or tetracycline preparation has also been used to reduce the risk of pneumonic pasteurellosis in sheep and goats in feedlots.[35]

MASTITIC PASTEURELLOSIS IN POSTPARTURIENT EWES

Synonyms: Blue-udder, blou-uier (Afrik.)

Introduction, aetiology and epidemiology

Ovine mastitic pasteurellosis in sheep is caused predominantly by infection with *P. haemolytica*.[24] The disease occurs in postparturient ewes at or near the end of lactation and it is therefore associated with the lambing seasons.[38, 47] Environmental contamination is an important source of infection. Trauma induced by the vigorous bumping and suckling of distended udders predisposes to infection. Lambs of mastitic ewes often attempt to obtain milk from other ewes, and in this way may transmit the infection to uninfected animals.[5] Infection is believed to be galactogenic.[33, 34]

Clinical signs and pathology

Outbreaks of the disease are sporadic; the morbidity rate seldom exceeds 5 per cent, but the mortality rate may reach 50 per cent of affected sheep.[47] The initial clinical signs include fever, anorexia, tachypnoea and signs of acute mastitis (lameness of the hind leg on the side corresponding to that of the affected half of the udder, and refusal by the ewe to let the lamb suckle).[47] The udder is usually unilaterally affected.[38, 47] The acutely affected gland is swollen, firm, reddish to bluish-red, and painful on palpation. A watery, flocculent exudate may be expressed from the teat.[33, 34] Death may follow in two or three days [47] or the acute reaction may subside within a few days but may be followed by abscessation of the udder. The abscesses may rupture and form fistules, and necrotic parts of the udder may eventually slough. Because ewes refuse to allow their lambs to suckle, the lambs may die of starvation.[5]

At necropsy, the affected part is enlarged, firm, congested and cyanotic, and contains a watery flocculent exudate.[33, 34] Foci of necrosis of varying size are disseminated throughout the affected tissue. Microscopical examination of affected udder tissue reveals the presence of fibrinopurulent exudate in the acini and interstitial tissues, hyperaemia, oedema, haemorrhages, thrombosis of blood vessels, and multiple foci of coagulative necrosis and the presence of numerous Gram-negative bacteria.[33, 34] The leukocytic reaction is characterized by an accumulation of 'oat cells' or 'streaming macrophages' within the lumens of the acini of the affected parts of the gland.[41]

Diagnosis and differential diagnosis

Confirmation of the diagnosis is dependent upon isolation of the causative organism from milk expressed from the affected half of the udder,[38, 47] or from specimens of the affected gland collected at necropsy. The differential diagnoses should include mastitis caused by other bacteria, particularly *Staphylococcus aureus*, but others, such as *Actinomyces pyogenes*, *Streptococcus* spp. and *Escherichia coli*, should also be considered.[33, 34]

Control

Treatment may be life-saving, but unless instituted within the first 24 hours of the disease will not save the affected part of the udder from severe damage and loss of function.[47] Untreated survivors are frequently culled for this reason. Antibiotics (oxytetracycline in particular) may be administered either parenterally or via the intramammary route to counter the infection, while supportive therapy should include frequent stripping of both the affected and unaffected glands, and, in severe cases, the use of oxytocin to stimulate milk let-down and corticosteroids to counter shock.[5] Mastectomy may be indicated to save the lives of animals suffering from gangrenous mastitis.[5]

Vaccination may assist in the control of the disease in ewes at risk.[19] The Onderstepoort Blue-udder Vaccine for Sheep (Reg. No. G 710 Act 36/1947) produced by the Veterinary Research Institute, Onderstepoort is a combination of the bacterin(s) of *P. haemolytica* serotypes 7 and 9 and a toxoid prepared from two strains of *Staphylococcus aureus*. Ewes should initially be inoculated twice: the first injection is given six weeks and the second two weeks before the onset of lambing. A single booster injection should be given two weeks before subsequent lambing seasons. Other precautionary measures which may reduce the prevalence of the disease include substantially reducing the feed intake of ewes for three days prior to weaning of their lambs, in order to limit milk production and avoid the subsequent distension of the udder, and the prophylactic administration of a specific intramammary antibiotic preparation (a combination of cephalexin and neomycin in a slow-release base) when the udder becomes distended after lambs have been weaned.[5, 31]

During an outbreak, mastitic ewes and their lambs should immediately be separated from the rest of the flock in order to prevent transmission of the infection to healthy animals, while chronically ill animals should be culled for the same reason.

SYSTEMIC (EMBOLIC) PASTEURELLOSIS

Introduction and aetiology

Systemic (embolic) pasteurellosis due to infection with *P. haemolytica* biotype T is an acute, often fatal disease of sheep of all ages.[18, 20] It is well documented in the veterinary literature of the United Kingdom and North America,[18, 21, 35] but only unconfirmed cases of the disease are on record in South Africa.[49]

Epidemiology

Although sheep of any age are susceptible,[20, 21] animals five to 12 months old are at greatest risk.[17, 18] A study of colonization of the tonsils of lambs by *P. haemolytica* showed that the early establishment of biotype A serotypes (derived from the dam) is succeeded in time by increasing dominance of biotype T serotypes.[2] By the time lambs are six months old, tonsillar colonization by T serotypes is almost exclusive.

The prevalence of disease is highest in autumn,[45] although outbreaks may occur at other times of the year.[20, 21] Its prevalence increases in cold, wet weather conditions.[17] Stress associated with weaning, transportation, vaccination and shearing, as well as a change in diet, particularly from a low-quality ration to succulent pastures or feed high in carbohydrate, are important predisposing factors.[45] The disease may therefore be a significant problem in feedlots.

Pathogenesis

Stress is presumed to result not only in corticosteroid-dependent bacterial proliferation in the tonsillar region, with consequent tonsillitis and pharyngitis,[17] but also in corticosteroid-dependent injury to the alimentary tract, the abomasum and duodenum in particular, with consequent ulceration.[45] The lesions may be exacerbated by an acidosis associated with a change in diet.[45] The injured pharyngeal, abomasal and duodenal mucosa serve as portals of entry for *P. haemolytica* biotype T derived from the tonsils.[2, 17, 45] From these sites bacteria gain access to the blood as emboli, most of which impact in the capillary bed of the lungs,[17] whilst bacterial invasion of the lower alimentary tract results in primary embolization of the hepatic sinusoids.[45] Rapid multiplication of bacteria in these sites results in embolic dissemination to other organs and tissues.[17, 45] Death is attributed to endotoxaemia.[17, 45]

Clinical signs

Clinical disease usually follows within several days of exposure to the predisposing factors, and an outbreak is heralded by unexpected deaths, almost invariably in the absence of premonitory clinical signs.[18, 20, 21, 35] Very rarely, affected animals show a fever, reluctance to move, dyspnoea, blood-stained frothy discharge from the nose and mouth, and recumbency followed by death.[20, 21] The mortality rate seldom exceeds 5 per cent of the sheep at risk, but occasionally may be as high as 20 per cent.[21]

Pathology

Systemic (embolic) pasteurellosis is characterized by involvement of multiple organs.[18] The carcass is in good condition and petechiae and ecchymoses are frequently present in the subcutis (particularly of the neck and thorax), pleura and peritoneum.[16, 18, 20, 22] The cranial, cervical and mesenteric lymph nodes are oedematous and haemorrhagic. Necrosis, sometimes accompanied by linear ulcers in the tonsils and the proximal oesophagus, is a characteristic feature[17] and may be accompanied by erosions and ulcers in the mucosa of the pyloric region of the abomasum and proximal duodenum.[16, 18] Copious amounts of clear or blood-stained froth in the trachea and bronchi, as well as from the cut surface of the lungs, attest to the severity of pulmonary congestion and oedema.[16, 18, 20, 22] In addition, multiple, acute infarcts may be present, predominantly subpleurally, in the lungs,[22] while the liver shows fatty changes and focal disseminated necrosis; the necrotic areas are yellowish-white to grey and measure 0,5–5 mm in diameter.[18, 20] Other findings such as hydropericardium, haemorrhages in the epicardium, endocardium and atrioventricular valves, acute fibrinous pleuritis, pneumonia, pericarditis, meningitis, choroiditis and polyarthritis, and focal malacia of the brain, are inconsistent and more often associated with the experimentally induced disease.[17, 22]

Microscopic examination of tissues reveals the presence of bacterial emboli in many organs and tissues[16, 17, 22] which give rise to multifocal infarcts. Infarcts may be found in the spleen, adrenals and, to a lesser extent, in the kidneys and lungs. Apart from the presence of Gram-negative bacteria in these tissues, bacteria are also discernible in necrotic lesions in the tonsils, oesophagus, lower alimentary tract and liver.

Diagnosis and differential diagnosis

The epidemiological and pathological findings may be of diagnostic significance, but isolation of the specific causative organism in large numbers (more than 10^6 colony-forming units per gram of tissue) from specimens, preferably of the lungs, liver and spleen collected aseptically during performance of a necropsy, is necessary to substantiate the diagnosis.[18, 24]

Systemic (embolic) pasteurellosis needs to be differentiated from enterotoxaemia and acute pneumonic pasteurellosis.[18]

Control

The acute course of systemic (embolic) pasteurellosis precludes chemotherapy.[18] No suitable vaccine is available[18] and the control of the disease is therefore non-specific and aimed at limiting exposure to stress and allowing adequate time for dietary adaptation.

SEPTICAEMIC PASTEURELLOSIS IN LAMBS

Although animals up to three months of age are susceptible, lambs less than two months old are at greatest risk of contracting septicaemic pasteurellosis caused by *P. haemolytica* biotype A.[18, 20, 27]

Five per cent of the lambs in a flock may be affected. An outbreak of pneumonic pasteurellosis in older animals,[20] manifested by dyspnoea and occasionally diarrhoea, may occur at the same time in the flock.[20, 27]

The lesions are non-specific and include petechiation of the serosal surfaces, congestion and oedema of the lungs, fatty changes of the liver, and oedema and haemorrhages in the lymph nodes.[18, 20] Acute fibrinous pleuritis and pericarditis may be present,[18] particularly in older lambs. Occasionally ecchymoses in the lungs and acute catarrhal to haemorrhagic enteritis of segmental distribution may be the predominant lesions.[27]

Confirmation of the diagnosis is dependent upon isolation, preferably in pure culture, of the causative organism from specimens of blood, brain, lungs, liver, spleen and lymph nodes collected aseptically at necropsy.

Septicaemic pasteurellosis should be differentiated from viral and bacterial infections that cause acute mortality in lambs, such as colibacillosis,[18] Rift Valley fever,[14] pulpy kidney disease, lamb dysentery ('bloedpens'), and *Clostridium perfringens* type C infection.

The acute course of the syndrome precludes treatment of the condition and prevention is the most effective control measure. Lambs at risk may be inoculated at two weeks of age and again four weeks later with the Onderstepoort *Pasteurella* Vaccine for Sheep and Goats (Reg. No. G 479 Act 36/1947) produced by the Veterinary Research Institute, Onderstepoort.[19]

References

1 **AL-DARRAJI, A.M., CUTLIP, R.C., LEMKUHL, H.D. & GRAHAM, D.L., 1982.** Experimental infections of lambs with bovine respiratory syncytial virus and *Pasteurella haemolytica*: Pathologic studies. *American Journal of Veterinary Research*, 43, 224–229.

2 **AL-SULTAN, I.I. & AITKEN, I.D., 1985.** The tonsillar carriage of *Pasteurella haemolytica* in lambs. *Journal of Comparative Pathology*, 95, 193–201.

3 **ANON., 1960–89.** Annual Reports, Director of Veterinary Services, South Africa.

4 **BAGADI, H.O. & RAZIG, S.E., 1976.** Caprine mastitis caused by *Pasteurella mastitidis* (*P. haemolytica*). *The Veterinary Record*, 99, 13.

5 **BATH, G., 1989.** Faculty of Veterinary Science, University of Pretoria. Unpublished data.

6 **BELAK, S., PALFI, V. & PALYA, P., 1976.** Adenovirus infection in lambs. I. Epizootiology of the disease. *Zentralblatt für Veterinärmedizin*, 23, 320–330.

7 **BEVERIDGE, W.I.B., 1983.** Bacterial diseases of cattle, sheep and goats. *In*: *Animal Health in Australia*, Vol. IV. Canberra: Australian Government Publishing Service.

8 **BORGMAN, R.F. & WILSON, C.E., 1955.** Pasteurellosis and enzootic pneumonia in goats. *Journal of the American Veterinary Medical Association*, 126, 198–204.

9 **BRODIE, T.A., HOLMES, P.H. & URQUHART, G.M., 1986.** Some aspects of tick-borne diseases of British sheep. *The Veterinary Record*, 118, 415–418.

10 **BROGDEN, K.A., ADLAM, L.C., LEHMKUHL, H.D., CUTLIP, R.C., KNIGHTS, J.M. & ENGEN, R.L., 1989.** Effect of *Pasteurella haemolytica* (A1) capsular polysaccharide on sheep lung *in vivo* and on pulmonary surfactant *in vitro*. *American Journal of Veterinary Research*, 50, 555–559.

11 **BROGDEN, K.A., CUTLIP, R.C. & LEHMKUHL, H.D., 1984.** Response of sheep after localized deposition of lipopolysaccharide in the lung. *Experimental Lung Research*, 7, 123–132.

12 **BUDDLE, B.M., HERCEG, M. & DAVIES, D.H., 1984.** Experimental infection of sheep with *Mycoplasma ovipneumoniae* and *Pasteurella haemolytica*. *Veterinary Microbiology*, 9, 543–548.

13 **CARTER, G.R., 1967.** Pasteurellosis: *Pasteurella multocida* and *Pasteurella haemolytica*. *Advances in Veterinary Science and Comparative Medicine*, 11, 321–379.

14 **COETZER, J.A.W., 1989.** Faculty of Veterinary Science, University of Pretoria. Personal communication.

15 **DAVIES, D.H., 1985.** Aetiology of pneumonias in young sheep. *In*: PANDEY, R., (ed.). *Infection and Immunity in Farm Animals*. Basel: S. Karger.

16 **DUNGWORTH, D.L., 1985.** The respiratory system. *In*: JUBB, K.V.F., KENNEDY, P.C. & PALMER, N., (eds). *Pathology of*

Domestic Animals. Vol. II. 3rd edn. Orlando, Florida: Academic Press, Inc.

17 **DYSON, D.A., GILMOUR, N.J.L. & ANGUS, F.W., 1981.** Ovine systemic pasteurellosis caused by *Pasteurella haemolytica* biotype T. *Journal of Medical Microbiology*, 14, 89–95.

18 **ELLIS, J.A., 1984.** *Pasteurella haemolytica* infections in sheep. *The Compendium of Continuing Education*, 6, 5360–5366.

19 **ERASMUS, B.J., CAMERON, C.M., HUNTER, P., CILLIERS, J.A., OBEREM, P.T., STOLTSZ, W.H. & DE WAAL, D.T., 1988.** *In*: *Onderstepoort Vaccines*. Pretoria: Department of Agriculture and Water Affairs.

20 **GILMOUR, N.J.L., 1978.** Pasteurellosis in sheep. *The Veterinary Record*, 102, 100–102.

21 **GILMOUR, N.J.L. & ANGUS, K.W., 1983.** Pasteurellosis. *In*: MARTIN, W.B., (ed.). *Diseases of Sheep*. London: Blackwell Scientific Publications.

22 **GILMOUR, N.J.L., ANGUS, K.W. & SHARP, J.M., 1980.** Experimental pulmonary infections of sheep caused by *Pasteurella haemolytica* biotype T. *The Veterinary Record*, 106, 507–508.

23 **GILMOUR, N.J.L., BRODIE, T.A. & HOLMES, P.H., 1982.** Tick-borne fever and pasteurellosis in sheep. *The Veterinary Record*, 111, 512.

24 **GILMOUR, N.J.L. & GILMOUR, J.S., 1989.** Pasteurellosis of sheep. *In*: ADLAM, C. & RUTTER, J.M., (eds). *Pasteurella and Pasteurellosis*. London: Academic Press.

25 **GILMOUR, J.S., JONES, G.E., RAE, A.G. & QUIRIE, M., 1986.** Comparison of single strains of four serotypes of *Pasteurella haemolytica* biotype A in experimental pneumonia in sheep. *Research in Veterinary Science*, 40, 136–137.

26 **GILMOUR, N.J.L., SHARP, J.M. & GILMOUR, J.S., 1982.** Effect of oxytetracycline therapy in experimentally induced pneumonic pasteurellosis in lambs. *The Veterinary Record*, 111, 97–99.

27 **HARRIS, G., 1974.** An outbreak of pasteurellosis in lambs. *The Veterinary Record*, 94, 84–85.

28 **HENNING, M.W. & BROWN, M.H.V., 1936.** Pasteurellosis: An outbreak amongst sheep. *Onderstepoort Journal of Veterinary Research*, 7, 113–130.

29 **HENTON, M.M., 1989.** Veterinary Research Institute, Onderstepoort 0110. Unpublished data.

30 **HERCEG, M., THURLEY, D.C. & DAVIES, D.H., 1982.** Oat cells in the pathology of ovine pneumonia-pleurisy. *New Zealand Veterinary Journal*, 30, 170–173.

31 **IMMELMAN, A., 1989.** Roodeplaat Research Laboratories, Roodeplaat, Pretoria, South Africa. Unpublished data.

32 **JANSEN, B.C., 1980.** The aetiology of ram epididymitis. *Onderstepoort Journal of Veterinary Research*, 47, 101–107.

33 **JONES, T.C. & HUNT, R.D., 1983.** *Veterinary Pathology*. 5th edn. Philadelphia: Lea & Febiger.

34 **JUBB, K.V.F., KENNEDY, P.C. & PALMER, N., 1985.** *Pathology of Domestic Animals*. Vol. III. 3rd edn. Orlando: Academic Press, Inc.

35 **KIMBERLING, C.V., 1988.** *Jensen and Swift's Diseases of Sheep*. 3rd edn. Philadelphia: Lea & Febiger.

36 **MACKENZIE, P.K.I., BOYT, W.P., ENSLIE, V.W., LANDER, K.P. & SWANEPOEL, R., 1975.** Immunosuppression in ovine trypanosomiasis. *The Veterinary Record*, 97, 452–453.

37 **MALONE, F.E., McCULLOUGH, S.J., McCLOUGHLIN, M.F., BALL, H.J. & O'HAGAN, J., 1988.** Infectious agents of respiratory disease of housed, fattening lambs in Northern Ireland. *The Veterinary Record*, 122, 203–207.

38 **MARSH, H., 1932.** Mastitis in ewes caused by a *Pasteurella*. *Journal of the American Veterinary Medical Association*, 81, 376–382.

39 **MIDWINTER, A.C., CLARKE, J.K. & ALLEY, M.R., 1986.** *Pasteurella haemolytica* serotypes from pneumonic goat lungs. *New Zealand Veterinary Journal*, 34, 35–36.

40 **MYER, M.S., HUCHZERMEYER, H.F.A.K., YORK, D.F., HUNTER, P., VERWOERD, D.W. & GARNETT, H.M., 1988.** The possible involvement of immunosuppression caused by a lentivirus in the aetiology of jaagsiekte and pasteurellosis in sheep. *Onderstepoort Journal of Veterinary Research*, 55, 127–133.

41 **NESBIT, J.W., 1989.** Faculty of Veterinary Science, University of Pretoria. Unpublished data.

42 **OJO, M.H., 1977.** Caprine pneumonia. *Veterinary Bulletin*, 47, 73–578.

43 **SHARP. J.M., GILMOUR, N.J.L., THOMPSON, D.A. & RUSHTON, B., 1978.** Experimental infection of specific pathogen-free lambs with parainfluenza virus type 3 and *Pasteurella haemolytica*. *Journal of Comparative Pathology*, 88, 237–243.

44 **ST. GEORGE, T.D., 1972.** Investigations of respiratory disease of sheep in Australia. *Australian Veterinary Journal*, 48, 318–322.

45 **SUAREZ-GÜEMES, F., COLLINS, M.T. & WHITEMAN, C.E., 1985.** Experimental reproduction of septicemic pasteurellosis in feedlot lambs: Bacteriologic and pathologic examinations. *American Journal of Veterinary Research*, 46, 193–201.

46 **TRIGO, F.J., BREEZE, R.G., LIGGITT, H.D., EVERMANN, J.F. & TRIGO, E., 1984.** Interaction of bovine respiratory syncytical virus and *Pasteurella haemolytica* in the ovine lung. *American Journal of Veterinary Research*, 45, 1671–1676.

47 **TUNNICLIFF, E.A., 1949.** *Pasteurella* mastitis in ewes. *Veterinary Medicine*, 44, 498–502.

48 **TUSTIN, R.C., ADELAAR, T.F. & CAMERON, C., 1960.** An outbreak of bacterial icterus in sheep. *Journal of the South African Veterinary Medical Association*, 31, 275–283.

49 **VAN RENSBURG, I.B.J. & TUSTIN, R.C., 1987.** Faculty of Veterinary Science, University of Pretoria. Unpublished data.

50 **VAN TONDER, E.M., 1975.** Notes on some disease problems in Angora goats in South Africa. *Veterinary Medical Review*, 1, 109–138.

51 **VERWOERD, D.W., TUSTIN, R.C. & PAYNE, A.-L., 1985.** Jaagsiekte: An infectious pulmonary adenomatosis of sheep. *In*: OLSEN, R.G., KRAKOWKA, S. & BLAKESLEE, J.R., (eds). *Comparative Pathobiology of Viral Diseases*. Vol. II. Boca Raton, Florida: CRC Press.

52 **YOUNG, J.D. & GRIFFITH, J.W., 1985.** Spontaneous *Pasteurella* pneumonia in adult laboratory goats complicated by superinfection with *Corynebacterium pseudotuberculosis* and *Meullerius capillaris*. *Laboratory Animal Science*, 35, 409–411.

144

Porcine pasteurellosis

S.S. Bastianello and J.W. Nesbit

Introduction

Porcine pasteurellosis may manifest as septicaemic or pneumonic forms.[5–7, 11, 12] Septicaemic pasteurellosis occurs in both neonatal and juvenile pigs, while pneumonic pasteurellosis is predominantly a disease of juvenile animals. The infection, in conjunction with other infectious agents, *Bordetella bronchiseptica* in particular, is also implicated in the aetiology of atrophic rhinitis, a syndrome peculiar to pigs.[2, 3, 5, 8, 13] **(see Chapter 121: *Bordetella bronchiseptica* infections including atrophic rhinitis)**.

Aetiology

In pigs, infection by *Pasteurella multocida* is more prevalent than that by *P. haemolytica*. Of the isolations made from the specimens submitted to the Veterinary Research Institute, Onderstepoort, about 92 per cent were *P. multocida*, 6 per cent *P. haemolytica* and 2 per cent comprised *P. pneumotropica* or untypable species of *Pasteurella*.[9] *Pasteurella multocida* serotypes A and D predominate in isolates from specimens obtained from pigs that have suffered from septicaemia or pneumonia in South Africa.[9] Haemorrhagic septicaemia caused by *P. multocida* serotype B has not been recorded in pigs in the region. It has, however, been implicated in an outbreak of the disease in India.[11] Whilst of rare occurrence in pigs, *P. haemolytica* (biotype and serotype undetermined) has been isolated from aborted foetuses and neonatal piglets suffering from septicaemia[5, 6] and from pneumonic lesions in juvenile pigs.[8, 15]

Toxigenic strains of *P. multocida* serotype D are also associated with progressive atrophic rhinitis in pigs.[2–5, 8, 13]

SEPTICAEMIC PASTEURELLOSIS IN PIGLETS

Septicaemic pasteurellosis caused by *P. multocida* has been reported in juvenile and adult pigs.[5, 11] Although specific pathogen-free animals are apparently at greatest risk,[5] the prevalence of this form of the malady, irrespective of whether it is caused by *P. multocida* or *P. haemolytica*, is higher in neonatal pigs.[5–7, 15] The mode of transmission is unknown, although infection via the umbilicus and/or the respiratory tract have been mooted.[7, 10]

The course of the disease is peracute: death supervenes after a period of illness that lasts no more than 12 hours in most cases, but rarely 24–48 hours.[5, 6, 11] Clinical signs usually include bluish-red discoloration of the skin of the snout, ears, and ventral regions of the neck, flanks and abdomen, lowered habitus, fever, dyspnoea and reluctance to move.[6, 11] Generalized congestion, cutaneous lividity, subcutaneous oedema and petechiation, serosanguineous effusions in the body cavities, and extensive ecchymotic haemorrhages in the lungs and epicardium are often present at necropsy.[5, 6, 11] Acute catarrhal to fibrinous pharyngitis may be encountered,[5] accompanied by peripharyngeal oedema, severe congestion of the cranial cervical lymph nodes,[11] and occasionally also acute fibrinous meningitis, particularly in neonatal pigs.

The diagnosis is confirmed on the basis of isolation of the bacterium in pure culture from specimens of blood, brain, or other suitable tissues (spleen, lymph nodes and liver). The differential diagnosis should include other diseases associated with sudden death, such as African swine fever, colibacillosis, salmonellosis, erysipelas, *Haemophilus* septicaemia, streptococcal septicaemia, porcine pleuropneumonia and leptospirosis.

Specific antibacterial therapy is hampered by the sporadic nature and acute course of the disease. Control may be best achieved by separating diseased animals from healthy susceptible pigs and improving the standards of housing, nutrition and hygiene.

PNEUMONIC PASTEURELLOSIS IN PIGS

Epidemiology

Pneumonic pasteurellosis is the most prevalent form of *Pasteurella* spp. infection in pigs.[2, 5, 7, 12, 15] Fattening pigs in overcrowded conditions are at greatest risk.[7, 15]

As in other species, the causative organism is a normal constituent of the flora of the upper respiratory tract, and stress factors (such as overcrowding, transportation, commingling, handling, exposure to excessive amounts of environmental or feed dust, and poor hygienic conditions), sometimes in association with concomitant pulmonic infection, probably trigger dissemination of *P. multocida* to the lung parenchyma. Intercurrent viral and bacterial infections, such as hog cholera, Aujeszky's disease and swine influenza, and infections with *Bordetella bronchiseptica, Actinobacillus pleuropneumoniae* and *Salmonella choleraesuis* have been implicated as predisposing factors in pig-producing countries elsewhere in the world.[2, 5, 7] However, enzootic mycoplasmal pneumonia is the most important predisposing infectious condition on a worldwide basis, including South Africa.[5, 7, 12, 15] In South Africa pneumonic pasteurellosis occurs only very rarely, except as a complication of mycoplasmal pneumonia.[14]

Pathogenesis

The available information on the pathogenesis of pneumonic pasteurellosis in pigs is incomplete and refers mostly to the infection as a complication of mycoplasmal pneumonia.[5, 7] The infection is acquired through aerosol transmission.[7, 15] Injury to the lungs that has been induced by prior infection by *Mycoplasma hyopneumoniae* presumably provides not only a portal of entry for *P. multocida* but also the environment for local proliferation of the bacteria. Adherence to ciliated epithelial cells and evasion of phagocytosis by alveolar macrophages in the porcine respiratory tract are presumed to be functions of the capsule of *P. multocida*.[2] The extent of the inflammatory reaction in the lungs is dependent upon the severity of the preceding injury and the quantum of bacteria that colonizes the lungs.[7, 12]

Clinical signs

Clinical signs vary in intensity according to the severity and extent of the pneumonic process.[7] Infections may be inapparent or associated with a dry, non-productive cough that may persist for weeks or months in mildly affected animals. Most of the more severely affected cases initially show a non-productive cough which becomes productive, depression, inappetence, fever, dyspnoea, and mucopurulent discharge from the nostrils. Auscultation reveals harsh pulmonary sounds. After a period of five to ten days pigs that suffer from severe disease almost inevitably die in the absence of effective antibacterial therapy. Recovery may be incomplete and characterized by persistent coughing that lasts for up to five weeks, emaciation and eventual death.[2] Relapses may occur in fully recovered animals.

Pathology

Acute, fibrinous pleuropneumonia succeeded by chronic, suppurative pneumonia is the usual course of events.[5, 7, 12] The cranioventral areas of the lungs are most commonly affected, although the caudal lobes may also be involved. In acute disease, the affected lungs are consolidated, reddish-purple in colour and frequently attached to the pleura and pericardium by fibrinous adhesions. The subpleural and interlobular tissues are distended by inflammatory oedema, and the regional lymph nodes are enlarged. The histological features include all the hallmarks of acute fibrinous bronchopneumonia, multifocal necrosis, and the presence of 'oat cells' or 'streaming macrophages'.[1] Gram-negative bacteria are present throughout the affected lungs.[5, 7] This reaction is frequently superimposed upon broncho-interstitial or 'cuffing' pneumonia indicative of a preceding mycoplasmal infection.[5] Extrathoracic lesions may include generalized congestion, some degree of icterus, fibrinous or ulcerative pharyngitis and pronounced peripharyngeal oedema, fibrinous pericarditis and polyarthritis.[5, 7]

Emaciation, chronic suppurative pneumonia, bronchiectasis and extensive fibrosis are common sequelae of the acute disease[5, 7, 12] and may be complicated by chronic adhesive pleuritis and pericarditis, and chronic polyarthritis.[5]

Diagnosis and differential diagnosis

A definitive diagnosis of pneumonic pasteurellosis is based on isolation of the causative organism from mucous nasal secretions and blood of clinically affected animals, or pneumonic tissues, blood, and pleural and pericardial exudates collected at necropsy.

Porcine pleuropneumonia caused by *Actinobacillus pleuropneumoniae* should be considered as a possible differential diagnosis.

Control

Parenteral administration of antimicrobial agents (sulphonamides or antibiotics) to affected pigs may be beneficial.[7, 15] This procedure should be supplemented by the provision of medicated feed or water for the entire group of pigs for three to five days. Certain strains of *P. multocida* are, however, resistant to some of the antibacterial agents in common usage and it is preferable to treat according to the results obtained from an antibiogram.

Although there is no specific vaccine available against pneumonic pasteurellosis in pigs in South Africa, autogenous bacterins or live attenuated vaccines have been utilized with some success in other parts of the world.[7] In addition, protection against the disease may be afforded by correcting husbandry procedures that are likely to predispose to the infection. This may include providing adequate housing, nutrition and hygiene, the reduction of commingling, handling and exposure to dusty conditions,[7, 15] and the prevention of the primary infections which predispose to secondary *P. multocida* infection of the porcine lung.[2]

References

1 **BASTIANELLO, S.S., 1989.** Veterinary Research Institute, Onderstepoort, 0110. Personal communication.

2 **CHANTER, N. & RUTTER, R.M., 1989.** Pasteurellosis in pigs. *In*: ADLAM, C. & RUTTER, R.M., (eds). *Pasteurella and Pasteurellosis*. London: Academic Press, Inc.

3 **DOMINICK, M.A. & RIMLER, R.B., 1986.** Turbinate atrophy in gnotobiotic pigs intranasally inoculated with protein toxin isolated from Type D *Pasteurella multocida*. *American Journal of Veterinary Research*, 47, 1532–1536.

4 **DOMINICK, M.A. & RIMLER, R.B., 1988.** Turbinate osteoporosis in pigs following intranasal inoculation of purified *Pasteurella* toxin: Histomorphometric and ultrastructural studies. *Veterinary Pathology*, 25, 17–27.

5 **DUNGWORTH, D.L., 1985.** The respiratory system. *In*: JUBB, K.V.F., KENNEDY, P.C. & PALMER, N., (eds). *Pathology of Domestic Animals*. 3rd edn. New York: Academic Press, Inc.

6 **EDWARDS, B.L., 1959.** A note on haemorrhagic septicaemia in neonatal pigs. *The Veterinary Record*, 71, 208.

7 **FARRINGTON, D.O., 1986.** Pneumonic pasteurellosis. *In*: LEMAN, A.D., STRAW, B., GLOCK, R.D., MENGELING, W.L., PENNY, R.H.C. & SCHOLL, E., (eds). *Diseases of Swine*. 6th edn. Ames, Iowa: Iowa State University Press.

8 **GILES, C.J., 1986.** Atrophic rhinitis. *In*: LEMAN, A.D., STRAW, B., GLOCK, R.D., MENGELING, W.L., PENNY, R.H.C. & SCHOLL, E., (eds). *Diseases of Swine*. 6th edn. Ames, Iowa: Iowa State University Press.

9 **HENTON, M.M., 1989.** Veterinary Research Institute, Onderstepoort, 0110. Personal communication.

10 **JUBB, K.V.F. & KENNEDY, P.C., 1970.** *Pathology of Domestic Animals*. 2nd edn. New York: Academic Press, Inc.

11 **MURTY, D.K. & KAUSHIK, R.K., 1965.** Studies on an outbreak of acute swine pasteurellosis due to *Pasteurella multocida* type B (Carter, 1955). *The Veterinary Record*, 77, 411–416.

12 **PIJOAN, C. & FUENTES, M., 1987.** Severe pleuritis associated with certain strains of *Pasteurella multocida* in swine. *Journal of the American Veterinary Medical Association*, 191, 823–826.

13 **RUTTER, J.M. & ROJAS, X., 1982.** Atrophic rhinitis in gnotobiotic piglets: Differences in the pathogenicity of *Pasteurella multocida* in combined infections with *Bordetella bronchiseptica*. *The Veterinary Record*, 110, 531–535.

14 **SPENCER, B.T., 1989.** National Pig Health Scheme, Meat Board, 556 Vermeulen St., Arcadia, Pretoria, 0083. Personal communication.

15 **TAYLOR, D.J., 1986.** *Pig Diseases*. 4th edn. Cambridge: Burlington Press.

ANAEROBIC, GRAM-NEGATIVE, IRREGULAR RODS

Within this group of bacteria, the family Bacteroidaceae contains 13 genera of which only two—*Fusobacterium* and *Bacteroides*—are relatively commonly associated with specific **(Table 1)** or non-specific (abscesses in a variety of organs and tissues, dental and oral lesions, chronic pleuropneumonia, and chronic sinusitis) diseases in livestock and humans. *Fusobacterium necrophorum* is the most important pathogenic species in this group and, apart from the diseases with which it is primarily associated, it may secondarily infect and complicate lesions of infectious diseases in which the mucous membranes of the gastrointestinal tract are involved, such as foot-and-mouth disease, rinderpest and orf.

Members of the family Bacteroidaceae are obligately anaerobic, Gram-negative, non-spore-forming bacteria that commonly occur on mucous membranes of the mouth, the upper respiratory tract and the gastrointestinal and urogenital systems of healthy animals and humans. They often occur in lesions in association with aerobic or other facultatively anaerobic bacteria e.g. *Actinomyces (Corynebacterium) pyogenes*. *Fusobacterium necrophorum* and *Bacteroides* spp. appear, in many instances, to depend on these bacteria to reduce the redox potential in the affected tissues to a level that allows their growth and subsequent tissue invasion.[8, 25, 26, 30, 35, 36]

In 1968 Biberstein and his colleagues wrote that, apart from *F. necrophorum* and the organisms implicated in ovine foot rot, the Gram-negative, non-sporulating anaerobes are a relatively neglected group of organisms in veterinary microbiology.[7] The same situation probably still applies 25 years later. The presumed reason that they gave for this state of affairs involves two characteristics of these bacteria: they are fastidious in their nutritive and atmospheric requirements, and they are usually found in association with other microorganisms such as *A. pyogenes, Pasteurella multocida, Escherichia coli*, streptococci and others, and are therefore possibly overlooked. In these mixed infections it does, however, seem likely that anaerobic species such as *Bacteroides* act synergistically with the other bacteria in order to produce suppurative and necrotizing lesions.[7] This emphasizes how important it is that bacteriological examinations of exudates should include both aerobic and strict anaerobic culturing techniques.

One of the hallmarks of infection by anaerobic bacteria, including *Bacteroides*, is an exudate with a putrid odour, although the absence of such an odour does not preclude an anaerobic infection.[7, 46] The odour is primarily the result of metabolic end products such as volatile amines, short chain fatty acids, and organic acids.[46]

There is considerable doubt about the validity of conclusions concerning the involvement of *F. necrophorum* in diseases appearing in publications prior to 1970, because it was referred to by a variety of names (e.g. *Fusiformis, Bacteroides, Sphaerophorus*).[28] In 1970 a subcommittee of the International Committee on Nomenclature of Bacteria published a report recommending that members of the genera *Sphaerophorus* and *Fusobacterium* be incorporated into a single genus *Fusobacterium*, and that the genus *Bacteroides* should be retained because of the inability of its species to produce butyric acid—a feature which distinguishes them from the *Fusobacterium* spp.[1]

Of all the species in the *Fusobacterium* and *Bacteroides* genera, *F. necrophorum, Prevotella melaninogenica (Bacteroides melaninogenicus)* and *Dichelobacter (Bacteroides) nodosus* are of the greatest veterinary importance **(Table 1)**.

Fusobacterium necrophorum

Fusobacterium necrophorum is an obligately anaerobic, Gram-negative, non-spore-forming, non-motile and pleomorphic bacterium which varies in shape from small cocci (0,5–1,75 µm in diameter) to filaments. The bacteria have irregular swellings along their length, and blunt or tapering ends.[31]

On blood agar, colonies of *F. necrophorum* are convex, translucent to opaque, 1–2 mm in diameter, and have a circular outline with scalloped to eroded edges. The colonies are often ridged or uneven.

Fusobacterium necrophorum produces haemolysin and indole, but does not reduce nitrate. Most strains cause either alpha or beta haemolysis on rabbit blood agar. Generally, beta-haemolytic strains are lipase-positive, and alpha-haemolytic and non-haemolytic strains are

Table 1 Most common specific diseases in livestock in which *Fusobacterium necrophorum, Dichelobacter nodosus* or *Prevotella melaninoginica (Bacteroides melaninogenicus)* are the primary causative agent. Bacteria that may play a secondary role are indicated in brackets

DISEASE	ANIMAL SPECIES AFFECTED	INFECTIOUS AGENT
Bovine foot rot	Cattle	*F. necrophorum* *(Actinomyces pyogenes, P. melaninogenica, D. nodosus)*
Ovine foot rot	Sheep and goats	*D. nodosus* (*F. necrophorum, A. pyogenes*)
Interdigital dermatitis	Cattle	*D. nodosus*: benign strains
	Sheep and goats	*F. necrophorum, A. pyogenes*
Digital dermatitis	Cattle	*F. necrophorum*?
Heel erosion	Cattle	*P. melaninogenica*?
Foot abscess	Sheep and goats	*F. necrophorum, A. pyogenes*
Toe abscess	Sheep	*F. necrophorum, A. pyogenes*
Hepatic necrobacillosis	Cattle, sheep and goats	*F. necrophorum* (*A. pyogenes* and other bacteria)
Rumenitis	Cattle	*F. necrophorum*
Necrotic and ulcerative stomatitis and laryngitis	Calves, lambs and kids	*F. necrophorum*
Necrotic rhinitis (bull nose)	Pigs	*F. necrophorum* (spirochaetes and other bacteria)
Porcine foot rot	Pigs	*F. necrophorum* (*A. pyogenes*, spirochaetes and other bacteria)
Cara inchada	Cattle	*P. melaninogenica*? (*A. pyogenes, Bacteroides bivius, F. nucleatum, Actinomyces israelii*)

lipase-negative. No lecithinase is produced.[28]

Strains of *F. necrophorum* are grouped into biovars (phases) A, AB, B and C.[3, 12, 20, 37, 40] The pathogenic strains of biovars A, B and AB are haemolytic and produce a leukocidin; strains of biovar B are, however, less pathogenic than those of biovars A and AB. The strains of biovar C are neither haemolytic nor pathogenic and are now known as *F. pseudonecrophorum*. Strains of biovars A are commonly found in cattle, while those of biovars B and C are more often isolated from humans than from animals.[32]

The cell wall of *F. necrophorum* contains a lipopolysaccharide with endotoxic activities similar to those of the Enterobacteriaceae **(see Chapter 129: *Escherichia coli* infections)**.[5, 27, 34] Pili (fimbriae) have been observed in a few isolates of *F. necrophorum* but their role in the pathogenesis of disease is not clear.[19, 33]

Dichelobacter (Bacteroides) nodosus

Dichelobacter nodosus was formerly known as *Bacteroides nodosus*.[16] The designation '*nodosus*', meaning 'knobbed', refers to the terminal (sometimes central) enlarged areas of the cells of *D. nodosus*. Terminal enlargements are more pronounced in bacteria that are present in lesions than in those grown in cultures. These bacteria are fairly large (1–1,7 x 3,0–6,0 µm), non-motile, straight or slightly curved rods. Varying numbers of pili are found on the surface of different strains of *D. nodosus*. Reports differ as to whether or not *D. nodosus* possesses a capsule.[28]

Surface colonies of the type strain of *D. nodosus* are 0,5–2,0 mm in diameter, smooth, convex, and translucent or semi-opaque. Colonies often etch into the surface of the medium immediately beneath them, producing a sunken appearance. Three basic colony types, namely papillate or beaded (B) type, mucoid (M) type, and circular (C) type, have been described.[4, 41]

Nine major serogroups, designated A to I, have been defined according to the antigenicity of their pili which is determined by employing a slide agglutination technique.[9–11, 24, 43] Cross-reactions between strains of specific serogroups have been reported.[10] At least 18 different serovars of *D. nodosus* are recognized among the nine serogroups, and their distribution varies around the world. Serovars belonging to serogroups A, B, C and G have been found in South Africa.[2]

Agglutinating antibodies against pili of *D. nodosus* are the most important in protective immunity induced by killed whole-cell vaccines.[21, 24, 43, 45, 48]

Various factors appear to influence the pathogenicity

of *D. nodosus*. Earlier studies suggested that increased virulence is correlated with the increased production and activity of protease (of which there are two forms, thermostable and thermolabile), the presence of large numbers of pili, increased degree of motility of the bacteria, and specific types of colony morphology on culture. Variation in colony morphology has also been linked to the degree of piliation of *D. nodosus*.[13–15, 18, 23, 41, 44, 47] Recent studies, however, indicate that the virulence of *D. nodosus* strains appears to be coupled with the combined effect of the thermostable protease and the degree of motility of *D. nodosus*, and that it is not strongly correlated to the total protease activity, colony morphology (other than size) or the degree of piliation.[4, 15, 48] Based on these studies, it has been suggested that strains of *D. nodosus* may be grouped into two major categories:

- benign strains which have thermolabile, extracellular protease and a low degree of motility. These strains cause benign foot rot of sheep and interdigital dermatitis in cattle and goats; and
- intermediate and virulent strains which produce thermostable protease. These cause intermediate and virulent foot rot in sheep, which varies in severity according to the degree of motility of the strain.

The gene regions associated with virulence have recently been mapped.[29]

The isolation of *D. nodosus* is often unsuccessful, notwithstanding the application of correct procedures in the collection and transportation of tissue specimens and the use of recommended culturing media and methods. To ensure optimal results when attempting to isolate *D. nodosus*, specimens should be collected by detaching pieces of affected skin or hoof from active and untreated lesions. These are placed in a suitable transport medium such as Thorley's medium. Stringent anaerobic conditions should be maintained during transportation of the specimens to the laboratory. The best results are obtained when hoof agar plates are inoculated in the field and then placed in an anaerobic jar with an attached anaerobic gas-generating kit, in which the agar plates are transported to the laboratory.[4] *Dichelobacter nodosus* has fastidious growth requirements. Variable success has been achieved when media such as Thorley's, Stuart's, and modified Stuart's containing L-cystine are used to isolate *D. nodosus*.[4, 17] It grows well in solidified trypicase-arginine-serine (TAS) medium at 37 °C under anaerobic conditions.[48]

Dichelobacter nodosus is an obligate parasite of the skin of the feet of sheep, goats, cattle and deer, and cannot survive in the environment for more than 14 days.[42]

Other Bacteroides *spp. and related genera* (Porphyromonas *and* Prevotella)

Because many previous studies of organisms called *Bacteroides melaninogenicus* included strains that might have been members of any of nine presently recognized species, earlier literature is difficult to correlate with present designations.[28]

Pigmented species of *Bacteroides* have been reclassified into the genera *Porphyromonas* and *Prevotella*.[38, 39] For example, *Bacteroides melaninogenicus* is now known as *Prevotella melaninogenica*.[22, 39]

Members of *Bacteroides, Porphyromonas* and *Prevotella* are all Gram-negative pleomorphic rods which produce as fermentation products succinate, acetate, lactate, formate or propionate and only rarely small amounts of butyrate. This distinguishes them from *Fusobacterium* spp, in which butyrate is a major product.[28]

Historically, the predominant differentiating characteristic of *P. melaninogenica (B. melaninogenicus)* was its production of darkly pigmented colonies on a blood-containing medium. This pigmentation is the result of the production of a dark brown to black pigment, protohemin, and not of melanin as was originally thought. Surface colonies of *P. melaninogenica* on blood agar are 0,5–2,0 mm in diameter, circular, entire, convex and shiny. They are usually darker in the centre of the colony, with the edges being grey to light brown. The colonies become darker as they age and the pigmentation usually develops more rapidly when laked blood, rather than blood containing intact red blood cells, is used. All strains produce pigment when cultured on agar containing rabbit blood, while only certain strains produce pigment when cultured on agar containing horse blood. A few strains are beta-haemolytic on rabbit blood agar.[28]

Bacteroides, Porphyromonas and *Prevotella* spp. cause a variety of purulent conditions of soft tissues, including liver abscesses and bite wounds. These infections are generally polymicrobial (i.e. more than one species of bacterium are involved): *Actinomyces pyogenes*, which requires oxygen for its multiplication, is often present in lesions.

References

1 **ANON., 1970.** Report of the International Committee on Nomenclature of Bacteria. Taxonomic subcommittee for Gram-negative anaerobic rods. *International Journal of Systematic Bacteriology*, 20, 297–300.

2 **ANON., 1985.** Annual Report, Allerton Regional Veterinary Laboratory, Private Bag X2, Cascades 3202, South Africa.

3 **BEERENS, H., FIEVAZ, L., WATTRE, P., 1971.** Observations concernant souches appartenant aux espèces *Sphaerophorus necrophorus, Sphaerophorus funduliformis, Sphaerophorus pseudonecrophorus. Annales Institut Pasteur (Paris)*, 121, 37–41.

4 **BELFIELD, A.J.M., 1986.** Evaluation of laboratory tests for distinguishing between field strains of *Bacteroides nodosus. In*: STEWART, D.J., PETERSON, J.E., McKERN, N.M. & EMERY, D.L., (eds). Proceedings of a workshop, Melbourne 1985, CSIRO Division of Animal Health, Australian Wool Corporation, Australia.

5 **BERG, J.N. & SCANLAN, C.M., 1982.** Studies of *Fusobacterium necrophorum* from bovine hepatic abscesses: Biotypes, quantitation, virulence, and antibiotic susceptibility. *American Journal of Veterinary Research* 43, 1580–1586.

6 **BERKHOFF, G.A., 1977.** Recovery and identification of anaerobes in veterinary medicine: A two-year experience. *Veterinary Microbiology*, 2, 237–252.

7 **BIBERSTEIN, E.L., KNIGHT, H.D. & ENGLAND, K., 1968.** *Bacteroides melaninogenicus* in diseases of domestic animals. *Journal of the American Veterinary Medical Association*, 153, 1045–1049.

8 **BROOK, I. & WALKER, R.I., 1986.** The relationship between *Fusobacterium* species and other flora in mixed infection. *Journal of Medical Microbiology*, 21, 93–100.

9 **CLAXTON, P.D., 1981.** Serogrouping of *Bacteroides nodosus* in relation to protection by vaccination. *In*: BEVERIDGE, W.I.B. & EGERTON, J.R., (eds). *Ovine footrot.* A report of a workshop at the University of Sydney, 3–6 May 1981. Revesby, N.S.W.: Craig Copying Co.

10 **CLAXTON, P.D., 1986.** Serogrouping of *Bacteroides nodosus* isolates. *In*: STERWART, D.J., PETERSON, J.E., McKERN, N.M. & EMERY, D.L., (eds). Proceedings of a workshop, Melbourne 1985, CSIRO Division of Animal Health, Australian Wool Corporation, Australia.

11 **CLAXTON, P.D., RIBEIRO, L.A. & EGERTON, J.R., 1983.** Classification of *Bacteroides nodosus* by agglutination tests. *Australian Veterinary Journal*, 60, 331–334.

12 **COYLE-DENNIS, J.E., LAUERMAN, L.H., 1978.** Biological and biochemical characteristics of *Fusobacterium necrophorum* leukocidin. *American Journal of Veterinary Research*, 39, 1790–1793.

13 **DEPIAZZI, L.J. & RICHARDS, R.B., 1979.** A degrading proteinase test to distinguish benign and virulent ovine isolates of *Bacteroides nodosus. Australian Veterinary Journal*, 55, 25–28.

14 **DEPIAZZI, L.J. & RICHARDS, R.B., 1985.** Motility in relation to virulence of *Bacteroides nodosus. Veterinary Microbiology*, 10, 107–116.

15 **DEPIAZZI, L.J., RICHARDS, R.B., McQUADE, N.C. & ROOD, J.I., 1986.** Virulence, protease, pilus and motility characteristics of *Bacteroides nodosus. In*: STERWART, D.J., PETERSON, J.E., McKERN, N.M. & EMERY, D.L., (eds). Proceedings of a workshop, Melbourne 1985, CSIRO Division of Animal Health, Australian Wool Corporation, Australia.

16 **DEWHIRST, F.E., PASTER, B.J., LA FONTAINE, S. & ROOD, J.I., 1990.** Transfer of *Kingella indologenes* (Snell & La Page, 1976) to the genus *Suttonella* gen. nov. as *Suttonella indologenes* comb. nov., transfer of *Bacteroides nodosus* (Beveridge, 1941) to the genus *Dichelobacter* gen. nov. as *Dichelobacter nodosus* comb. nov. and assignment of the genera *Cardiobacterium, Dichelobacter* and *Suttonella* to *Cardiobacteriaceae* fam. nov. in the gamma division of *Proteobacteria* based on 16 S ribosomal ribonucleic acid sequence comparisons. *International Journal of Systematic Bacteriology*, 40, 426–433.

17 **DUNCAN, S.P., VALERA, R.C., MANZANO, J.V. & MACHOTA, S.V., 1990.** Isolation and identification of anaerobic bacteria from ovine foot rot in Spain. *Research in Veterinary Science*, 49, 245–247.

18 **EGERTON, J.R. & PARSONSON, I.M., 1969.** Benign footrot—a specific interdigital dermatitis of sheep associated with infection by less proteolytic strains of *Bacteroides nodosus. Australian Veterinary Journal*, 45, 345–349.

19 **EMERY, D.L., 1987.** Immunity against anaerobic bacterial infections. *Veterinary Immunology and Immunopathology*, 15, 1–57.

20 **EMERY, D.L., DUFTY, J.H. & CLARK, B.L., 1984.** Biochemical and functional properties of a leucocidin produced by several strains of *Fusobacterium necrophorum. Australian Veterinary Journal*, 61, 382–387.

21 **EMERY, D.L., STEWART, D.J., CLARK, B.L. & ELLEMAN, T.C., 1986.** Protective parts of pili from *Bacteroides nodosus. In*: STEWART, D.J., PETERSON, J.E., McKERN, N.M. & EMERY, D.L., (eds). Proceedings of a workshop, Melbourne 1985, CSIRO Division of Animal Health, Australian Wool Corporation, Australia.

22 **ENGELKIRK, P.G., DUBEN-ENGELKIRK, J. & DOWELL, V.R., 1992.** Principles and practice of clinical anaerobic bacteriology. Belmont, California: Star.

23 **EVERY, D., 1982.** Proteinase isoenzyme patterns of *Bacteroides nodosus*: Distinction between ovine virulent isolates, ovine benign isolates and bovine isolates. *Journal of General Microbiology*, 128, 809–812.

24 **EVERY, D. & SKERMAN, T.M., 1982.** Protection of sheep against experimental footrot by vaccination with pili purified from *Bacteroides nodosus. New Zealand Veterinary Journal*, 30, 156–158.

25 **GYLES, L.C. & THOEN, C.O., 1986.** *Pathogenesis of Bacterial Infections in Animals.* Ames, Iowa: Iowa State University Press.

26 **HITE, K.E., LOCKE, M. & HESSELTINE, H.C., 1949.** Synergism in experimental infections with nonsporulating anaerobic bacteria. *Journal of Infectious Diseases*, 84, 1–9.

27 **HOFSTAD, T., 1982.** Immunochemical studies of partially hydrolysed lipopolysaccharide from *Fusobacterium nucleatum* ATCC 10953. *Acta Pathologica, Microbiologica et Immunologica Scandinavica*, B90, 289–293.

28 **HOLDEMAN, L.V., KELLY, R.W. & MOORE, W.E.C., 1984.** Family 1 Bacteroidaceae. *In*: KRIEG, N.R. & HOLT, J.G., (eds). *Bergey's Manual of Systematic Bacteriology.* Vol. I. Baltimore, London: Williams & Wilkins.

29 **KATZ, M.E., HOWARTH, P.M., YONK, W.K., RIFFKIN, G.G., DEPIAZZI, L.J. & ROOD, J.I., 1991.** Identification of three gene regions associated with virulence in *Dichelobacter nodosus*, the causative agent of ovine footrot. *Journal of General Microbiology*, 137, 2117–2124.

30 **KELLY, M.J., 1978.** The quantitative and histological demonstration of pathogenic synergy between *Escherichia coli* and *Bacteroides fragilis* in guinea-pig wounds. *Journal of Medical Microbiology*, 11, 513–523.

31 **LANGWORTH, B.F., 1977.** *Fusobacterium necrophorum*: Its characteristics and role as an animal pathogen. *Bacteriological Reviews*, 41, 373–390.

32 **MOORE, W.E.C., HOLDEMAN, L.V. & KELLY, R.W., 1984.** Genus II *Fusobacterium. In*: KRIEG, N.R. & HOLT, J.G., (eds). *Bergey's Manual of Systematic Bacteriology.* Vol. I. Baltimore, London: Williams & Wilkins.

33 **NAGAI, S., KANOE, M. & TODA, M., 1984.** Purification and partial characterization of *Fusobacterium necrophorum* haemagglutinin. *Zentralblatt für Bakteriologie, Microbiologie und Hygiene*, Series A, 258, 232–241.

34 **OKAHASHI, N., KOGA, Y., NISHIHARA, T., FUJIWARA, T. & HAMADA, S., 1988.** Immunobiological properties of lipopolysaccharides isolated from *Fusobacterium nucleatum* and *F. necrophorum. Journal of General Microbiology*, 134, 1707–1715.

35 **ROBERTS, D.S., 1967.** The pathogenic synergy of *Fusiformis necrophorus* and *Corynebacterium pyogenes*. I. Influence of the leucocidal exotoxin of *F. necrophorus. British Journal of Experimental Pathology*, 48, 665–673.

36 **ROBERTS, D.S., 1967.** The pathogenic synergy of *Fusiformis necrophorus* and *Corynebacterium pyogenes*. II. The response of *F. necrophorus* to a filterable product of *C. pyogenes. British Journal of Experimental Pathology*, 48, 674–679.

37 **ROBERTS, D.S., 1970.** Toxic, allergenic and immunogenic factors of *Fusiformis necrophorus. Journal of Comparative Pathology*, 80, 247–257.

38 **SHAH, H.N. & COLLINS, M.D., 1988.** Proposal for reclassification of *Bacteroides asaccharolyticus, Bacteroides gingivalis* and *Bacteroides endodontalis* in a new genus, *Porphyromonas. International Journal of Systematic Bacteriology*, 38, 128–131.

39 **SHAH, H.N. & COLLINS, M.D., 1990.** *Prevotella*, a new genus to include *Bacteroides melaninogenicus* and related species formerly classified in the genus *Bacteroides. International Journal of Systematic Bacteriology*, 40, 205–208.

40 **SHINJO, T., HIRAIWA, K. & MIYAZATO, S., 1990.** Recognition of biovar C of *Fusobacterium necrophorum* (Flugge) Moore and Holdeman as *Fusobacterium pseudonecrophorum* sp. nov., nom. rev. (ex Prevot 1940). *International Journal of*

Systematic Bacteriology, 40, 71–73.

41 **SKERMAN, T.M., ERASMUSON, S.K. & EVERY, D., 1981.** Differentiation of *Bacteroides nodosus* biotypes and colony variants in relation to their virulence and immunoprotective properties in sheep. *Infection and Immunity*, 32, 788–795.

42 **SMITH, L.D.S., 1975.** *The Pathogenic Anaerobic Bacteria.* 2nd edn. Illinois: Charles C. Thomas.

43 **STEWART, D.J., 1978.** The role of various antigenic fractions of *Bacteroides nodosus* in eliciting protection against footrot in vaccinated sheep. *Research in Veterinary Science*, 24, 14–19.

44 **STEWART, D.J., 1979.** The role of elastase in the differentiation of *Bacteroides nodosus* infections in sheep and cattle. *Research in Veterinary Science*, 27, 99–105.

45 **STEWART, D.J., CLARK, B.L., PETERSON, J.E., GRIFFITHS, D.A. & SMITH, E.F., 1982.** Importance of pilus-associated antigen in *Bacteroides nodosus* vaccines. *Research in Veterinary Science*, 32, 140–147.

46 **SWEENEY, C.R., DIVERS, T.J. & BENSON, C.E., 1985.** Anaerobic bacteria in 21 horses with pleuropneumonia. *Journal of the American Veterinary Medical Association*, 187, 721–724.

47 **THORLEY, C.M., 1976.** A simplified method for the isolation of *Bacteroides nodosus* from ovine footrot and studies on its colony morphology and serology. *Journal of Applied Bacteriology*, 40, 301–309.

48 **YONG, W.K., MOSES, E.K. & RIFFKIN, G.G., 1986.** Characterisation of virulence-associated antigens for differentiating virulent and benign strains of *Bacteroides nodosus. In*: STEWART, D.J., PETERSON, J.E., McKERN, N.M. & EMERY, D.L., (eds). Proceedings of a workshop, Melbourne 1985, CSIRO Division of Animal Health, Australian Wool Corporation, Australia.

145

Fusobacterium necrophorum, Dichelobacter (Bacteroides) nodosus *and* Bacteroides *spp. infections*

B.J. Venter and S.R. van Amstel

INFECTIOUS DISEASES OF THE FEET OF CATTLE

Introduction

The lack of a standardized terminology is a serious limitation when studying the various infectious and non-infectious diseases of the feet of cattle.[148] Different terms are often used to describe the same condition. In an effort to clarify the situation it has been decided that the name given to a particular disease should be based on the anatomical structures and the part of the feet involved **(Figure 145.1)** rather than on the aetiology, which is often of a multifactorial nature or uncertain.[148]

Lameness in cattle is most commonly caused by conditions affecting the interdigital skin or horn and corium of the claws, whereas that which results from conditions affecting parts of the leg proximal to the feet (non-digital conditions) is relatively rare.[43, 101, 109] The hind feet are affected by a greater variety of diseases and are also far more commonly involved than the front feet;[4, 5] 85 per cent of lesions involve the abaxial (or lateral) digits of the hind feet. In contrast, the prevalence of disease conditions in the axial and the abaxial digits of the front feet is more or less the same.

Infectious conditions (foot rot, interdigital dermatitis, digital dermatitis and heel erosion) of the feet, of which foot rot is the most important economically, account for approximately 70 per cent of cases of lameness.[4, 5, 31, 109] Foot rot and interdigital dermatitis are common diseases worldwide which occur particularly in dairy and beef cattle kept under intensive conditions, but they may also have a similar prevalence in cattle farmed under extensive conditions in areas with high rainfall and where muddy conditions prevail for prolonged periods.[25, 84] Although foot rot usually occurs as sporadic cases, 20 per cent or more of the animals in a herd may be affected over a period of several months.[25] During wet conditions, between 40 and 60 per cent of cattle are likely to be affected by interdigital dermatitis, but because it is a mild disease it is usually not diagnosed clinically and is of little or no consequence.[25]

Collectively, the different conditions that affect the feet

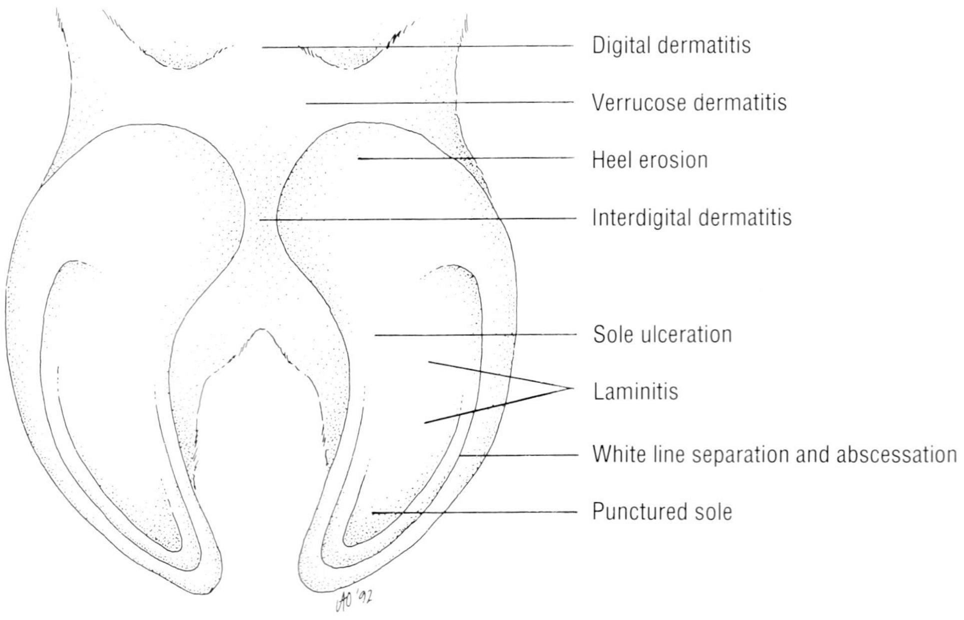

Figure 145.1 A sketch indicating the location of the different diseases of the feet of cattle

of cattle may cause significant economic losses. Studies have been done to determine the prevalence rates of some of them in affected herds in a number of countries.[4, 5] There is, however, very little information available on the prevalence of the various conditions in southern Africa.

In this chapter the conditions of the feet of cattle (namely, foot rot, interdigital dermatitis, digital dermatitis and heel erosion) which are caused, or thought to be caused, primarily by *Fusobacterium necrophorum*, *Dichelobacter (Bacteroides) nodosus* or *Prevotella melaninogenica (Bacteroides melaninogenicus)*, are discussed, while the other conditions that affect the feet are only described briefly, and particularly with a view to distinguishing them from some of the infectious conditions.

Aetiology

The aetiologies of infectious conditions of the feet of cattle are multifactorial because of the interrelationships which exist between the infectious agents on the one hand, and the host and environmental factors on the other (**see Epidemiology and Pathogenesis**).

Several infectious agents, including *F. necrophorum*, *D. nodosus*, *P. melaninogenica*, and *Actinomyces (Corynebacterium) pyogenes*, as well as other facultative, spirochaetal and diphtheroid bacteria, have been isolated from cases of foot rot and other diseases of the feet of cattle.[14, 25] Of these bacteria, *F. necrophorum* is considered to be of primary importance in the aetiology of foot rot, while the others, particularly *P. melaninogenica*, *D. nodosus* and *A. pyogenes*, may in some instances play a contributory role.[14] Interdigital dermatitis is caused by benign strains of *D. nodosus* and is considered to predispose to foot rot.[25, 34, 49, 73, 132, 136, 146, 148] The cause of digital dermatitis is largely unknown, but benign strains of *D. nodosus*, *F. necrophorum*, zinc deficiency and unhygienic housing conditions are all believed to play a role.[11] Although the aetiology of heel erosion is not well defined, *P. melaninogenica* and subclinical laminitis have been implicated in its aetiology. It has also been suggested that there is a linkage between interdigital dermatitis and heel erosion.[49, 136]

Fusobacterium necrophorum is a frequent inhabitant of the gastrointestinal tract of healthy herbivores and pigs and is therefore commonly found in faecally contaminated environments. The pathogenic isolates of *F. necrophorum* that cause foot rot belong to either biovars A or AB and produce a soluble leukocidin and a haemolysin, while isolates that belong to biovar B produce little, if any, leukocidin or haemolysin, and are less pathogenic.[40]

Most sheep, goats, cattle and farmed deer are carriers of benign strains of *D. nodosus* on the interdigital skin. In contrast to *F. necrophorum*, which can survive for several months in faecally contaminated, muddy conditions, *D. nodosus* cannot survive in the external environment for more than two weeks under ideal conditions.[122, 124, 143]

For information on the general characteristics of *F. necrophorum*, *D. nodosus* and *P. melaninogenica* consult **Anaerobic, Gram-negative irregular rods: Introduction**.

Epidemiology

One or more of several factors may play a role in the development of infectious diseases of the feet of cattle in a problem herd. These factors include the following:

- Certain anatomical features of the feet contribute to their susceptibility to infection. The relatively unprotected epidermis of the interdigital skin is frequently exposed not only to unhygienic muddy conditions, which are the most important predisposing factor to foot rot and interdigital dermatitis, but also to trauma caused by a variety of objects such as stones, cinders of walkways, stubble of harvested grain fields, plant awns and thorns, and tick bites. A favourable environment for the growth of bacteria and a portal for their entry into the underlying tissues are provided by changes in the integrity of the surface of the interdigital skin, if these are of a sufficient degree.[63] Infections of the interdigital skin that extend into the deeper tissues may cause infection of the distal interphalangeal joint because of the superficial position of the dorsal pouch of the joint capsule.[144]
- Infectious interdigital skin diseases, including foot rot in cattle, often have a seasonal occurrence because wet environmental conditions predispose to them.[63]
- *Bos indicus* cattle breeds are generally more resistant to foot rot than *Bos taurus* breeds.[45, 84] A genetic predisposition to certain other conditions, such as interdigital hyperplasia, corkscrew claw, sole ulceration and laminitis appears to be present in some lines of dairy cattle and this renders them more susceptible to these diseases.[9, 146]
- Zinc deficiency may predispose to interdigital dermatitis because of the production of a poorer quality of hoof horn and interdigital skin. High concentrations of zinc are present in colostrum, with the result that a marginal zinc deficiency may occur in cows during early lactation. This deficiency can be exacerbated in cows that are fed a diet high in calcium during late pregnancy and early lactation. Even when the levels of zinc are adequate, excessive levels of calcium diminish effective absorption and metabolism of zinc.

Other less important factors which predispose to foot rot and other conditions of the feet in individual animals include conformational anomalies, which often only develop late in an animal's life and result in increased mechanical stress on the claws,[47, 135, 144] and metabolic stresses associated with pregnancy, parturition and lactation that result in softer, poorer-quality hoof horn.[6, 32, 114] Changes in management and nutrition that many cows are subjected to before or after calving may also play an important role in the occurrence of foot lesions.[52] For example, the behavioural changes associated with the re-introduction of particular animals to the milking herd and the resumption of oestrus, together with possible changes in housing conditions, may all increase the risk of injury to the feet.[114]

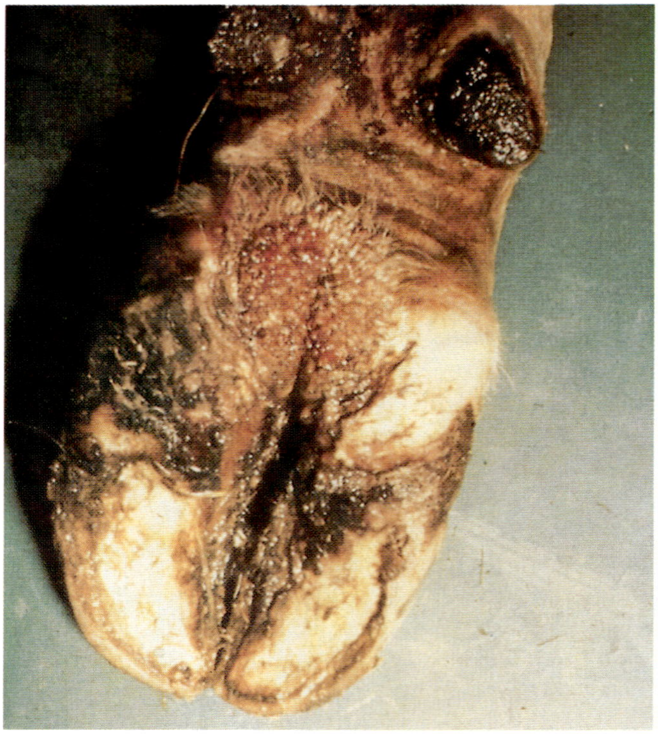

Figure 145.2 Chronic foot rot. (By courtesy of Prof. S.S. van den Berg, Department of Surgery, Faculty of Veterinary Science, Onderstepoort)

Pathogenesis

Fusobacterium necrophorum, D. nodosus, P. melaninogenica and *A. pyogenes* are not able to invade intact skin. They can only penetrate when there is prior damage which, in the interdigital region, is usually in the form of maceration or mechanical trauma of the skin.[71]

In infected tissues, *A. pyogenes* produces a diffusible factor which stimulates *F. necrophorum* to multiply. It also consumes oxygen, resulting in a lowered redox potential in the tissues, thus enabling *F. necrophorum, D. nodosus* and *P. melaninogenica* to grow.[14, 25] *Fusobacterium necrophorum* produces a leukocidin that is cytotoxic to phagocytic cells, thus protecting itself and *A. pyogenes* from phagocytosis. It also elaborates a dermonecrotic toxin and a vitamin K-like substance that is a growth factor required by *P. melaninogenica*. A collagenase that breaks down proteins to peptides and amino acids is produced by *P. melaninogenica*. The latter products contribute to tissue damage and are utilized by *F. necrophorum* during multiplication, but they in turn have a negative effect on collagenase production by *P. melaninogenica*.

Clinical signs and pathology

Bovine foot rot [foul-in-the-foot, interdigital phlegmon, infectious pododermatitis, interdigital necrobacillosis, foot abscess, phlegmona interdigitalis, *vrotpootjie (Afrik.)]*

Foot rot **(Figure 145.2)** usually affects only one foot, most commonly that of a hind leg. Mild to severe lameness and fever are common signs. Foot rot is characterized by interdigital dermatitis and cellulitis that cause symmetrical swelling of the tissues between the digits and around the heels, which in severe cases may extend to include the fetlock area. As a result of the necrosis which occurs in the affected tissues, discharging sinus tracts which open to the externum in the skin of the interdigital region and coronary band are sometimes present. If the distal interphalangeal joint, whose capsule is in close proximity to the interdigital skin, becomes infected by extension of the lesion, septic arthritis may result, with consequent severe and prolonged lameness, rapid loss of weight and a marked drop in milk production. Septic tendovaginitis of the flexor tendons, culminating in their rupture, abscessation of the interdigital tissues and osteomyelitis of the digital bones may be complications of foot rot.[25, 48, 100, 102, 144, 146]

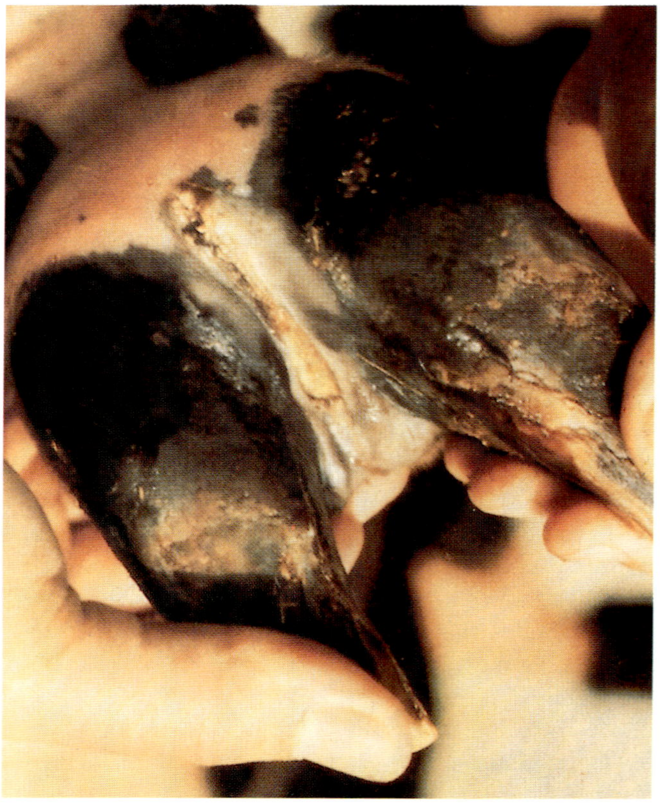

Figure 145.3 Acute bovine interdigital dermatitis. Note erosion of interdigital skin. (By courtesy of Prof. S.S. van den Berg, Department of Surgery, Faculty of Veterinary Science, Onderstepoort)

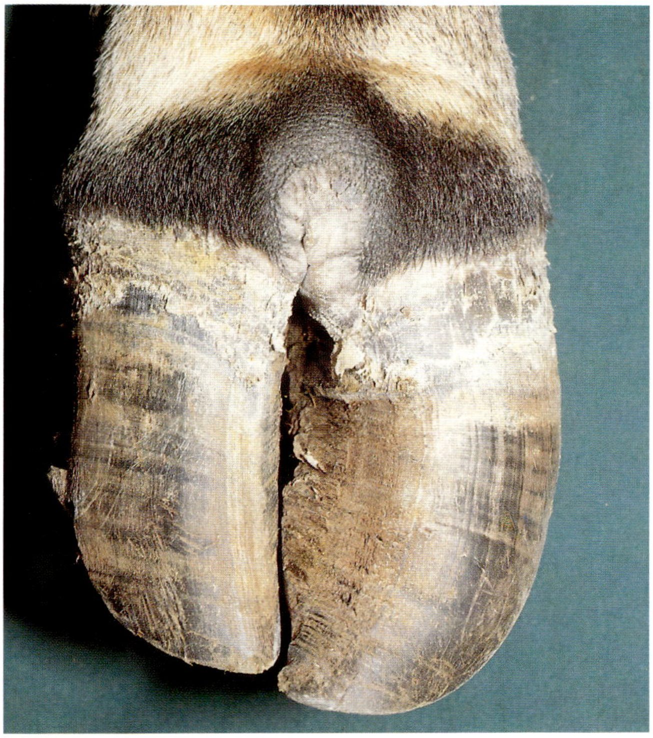

Figure 145.4 Chronic bovine interdigital dermatitis. Note the thickening of dorsal commissure of interdigital skin. (By courtesy of Prof. S.S. van den Berg, Department of Surgery, Faculty of Veterinary Science, Onderstepoort)

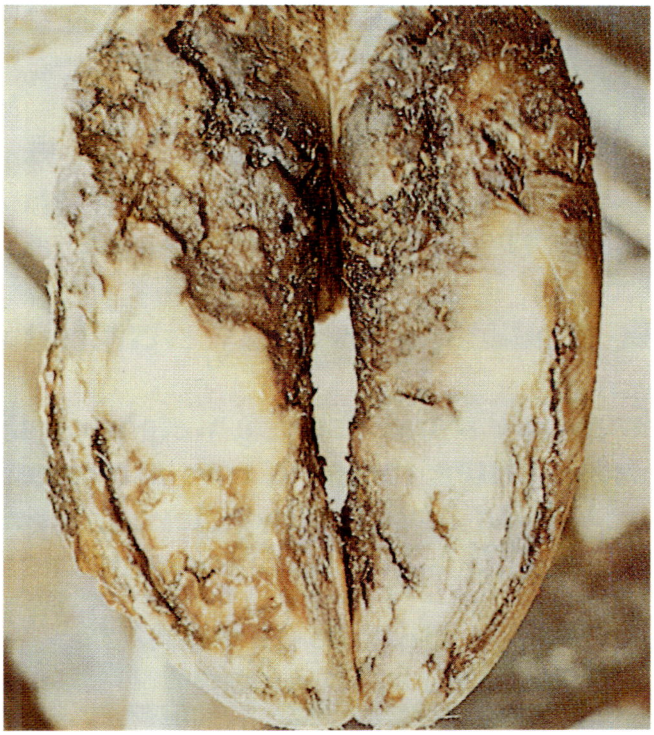

Figure 145.6 Heel erosion (severe case). Claw also shows signs of white line disease. (By courtesy of Prof. S.S. van den Berg, Department of Surgery, Faculty of Veterinary Science, Onderstepoort)

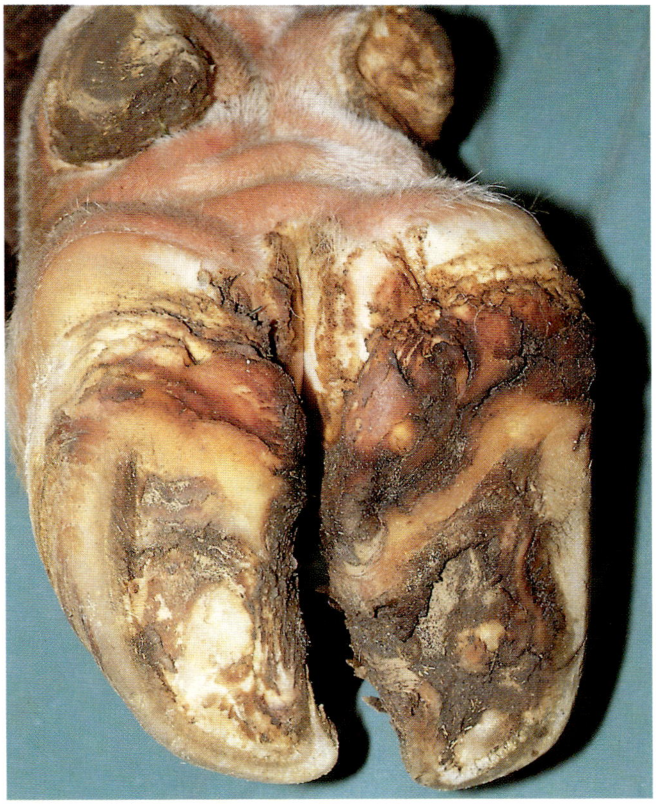

Figure 145.5 Heel erosion (mild case). (By courtesy of Prof. S.S. van den Berg, Department of Surgery, Faculty of Veterinary Science, Onderstepoort)

Interdigital dermatitis (stable foot rot, scalb, dermatitis interdigitalis*)*

Interdigital dermatitis is characterized by erosion and hyperkeratosis of the interdigital skin **(Figures 145.3 and 145.4)**, usually without fissure formation or extension of the inflammatory process into the deeper tissues of the feet.[25, 49, 100] A foul odour may be present. The lesions are usually most obvious at the heels and result in mild swelling of the adjacent soft tissues. This may be followed by separation of the horn on the inner aspects of the heels, which facilitates the entry of foreign material between the horn and the underlying corium, resulting in a proliferative inflammatory reaction. In most uncomplicated cases there is no evidence of lameness, although some animals may be mildly lame.

*Heel erosion (*erosio ungulae*)*

Heel erosion is characterized by the development of lines of erosions that appear as black marks, circular craters or deep terraces on the plantar/palmar convexity of the heels[49] **(Figures 145.5 and 145.6)**. As the condition progresses, the lines of erosions form V-shaped clefts with the apex of the 'V' pointing dorsally.[49] Heel erosion is relatively unimportant as a direct cause of lameness but, because of the gradual loss of heel horn which leads to a reduced shock-absorption capacity of the digital cushions and a consequent reduction in their ability to transfer concussion to the sole, it predisposes to other claw conditions (interdigital dermatitis, laminitis, insufficient wear of the wall of the hoof, sole ulcer).[49]

Digital dermatitis (dermatitis digitalis)

Digital dermatitis is an uncommon condition characterized by dermatitis followed by erosion and superficial ulceration of the skin bordering the perioplic band above the heels. The lesion has a white border and a surrounding area of proliferative dermatitis.[146] It causes no (or only mild) lameness.

Table 145.1 Classification of some diseases of the interdigital skin, or the horn and corium of the claws of cattle. (Adapted from Weaver[147])

SKIN	HORN AND CORIUM
Foot rot	Sole ulceration
Interdigital dermatitis	Punctured sole
Interdigital hyperplasia	White line separation
Verrucose dermatitis	Laminitis
Digital dermatitis	Heel erosion

Diagnosis and differential diagnosis

As lameness in cattle is most commonly caused by disease of the feet, their careful and thorough examination, after they have been cleaned and trimmed, is of the utmost importance in order to establish an accurate diagnosis.

Conditions responsible for lameness in cattle may for convenience be divided into

- those that involve the interdigital skin,
- those that affect the horn and corium of the claws, and
- those that affect the tissues of the limbs proximal to the feet.

Conditions that affect the interdigital skin or the horn and corium of the claws **(Table 145.1)** may be collectively termed digital diseases.[5] For information on the conditions that affect the tissues proximal to the feet, other sources should be consulted.[58]

The locations of some of the common conditions that affect the feet are illustrated in **Figure 145.1** and listed in **Table 145.1**. Of these, sole ulceration, punctured sole, white line disease, laminitis and heel erosion are inextricably intermingled—the production of poor-quality horn being the common factor **(Figure 145.7)**.[147]

Although any condition that results in lameness could probably be confused with foot rot, retroarticular abscess, interdigital foreign body, septic pedal arthritis, septic sandcrack, white line disease and interdigital dermatitis are most commonly confused clinically with it.[49] The swelling that is associated with retroarticular abscess is symmetrical and restricted to the heel of only one digit, in contrast to foot rot, in which there is symmetrical swelling of the affected region of both digits. Septic pedal arthritis can be distinguished from foot rot in that the oedematous swelling is proximal to the coronary band, and that it

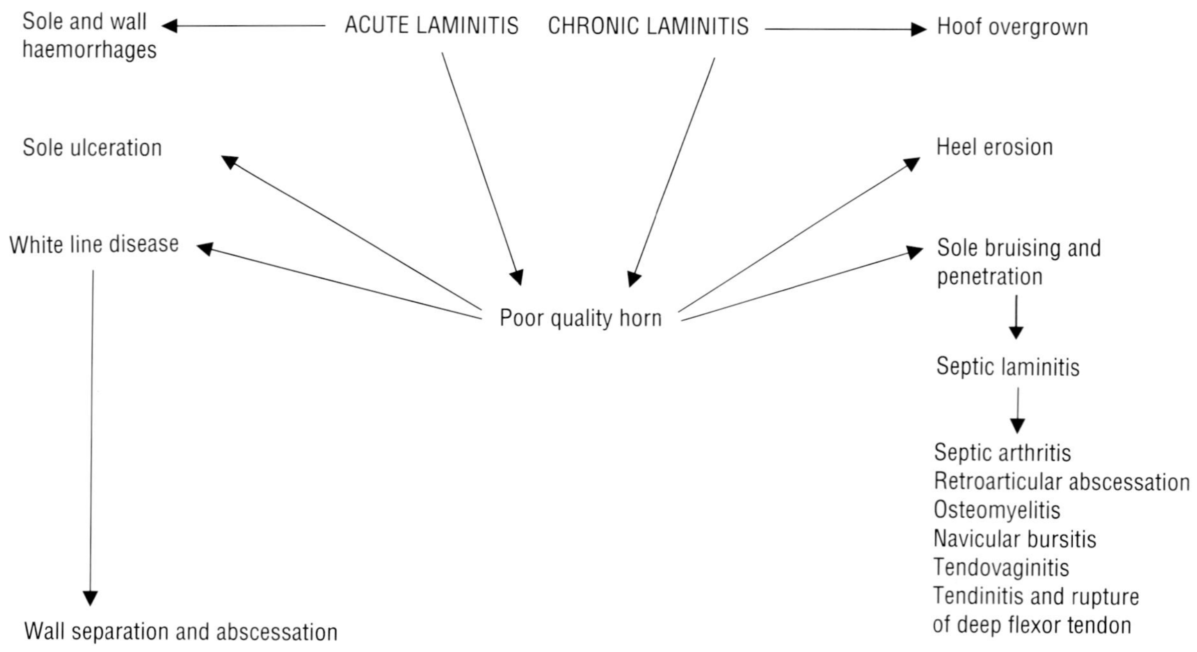

Figure 145.7 Conditions of the bovine claw that are associated with acute and chronic laminitis. (Adapted from Weaver[147])

affects only one digit and is first noticed on the dorsal surface of the digit. A distinguishing characteristic of a septic sandcrack is that the inflammatory oedema proximal to the coronary band is localized to the dorso-abaxial quarter of the digit. In white line disease the oedema is proximal to the coronary band and is confined to the area just dorsal to the heel. Interdigital dermatitis is sometimes confused with foot rot, but it produces only mild swelling of the feet, no systemic signs, and usually no (or only mild) lameness, all of which are usually pronounced features of severe foot rot.

The following conditions may also affect the claws and cause lameness.

Verrucose dermatitis (heel warts, dermatitis verrucosa*)*

Verrucose dermatitis is a chronic, moist, proliferative, wart-like inflammation of the plantar or palmar skin above the heels of the hind claws that is characterized by a mass of filiform fronds. Affected animals show slight lameness as a result of the mass of abnormal tissue.[100, 146] Generally the occurrence of verrucose dermatitis is sporadic, but occasionally a number of cases may be present simultaneously in a herd. While the precise aetiology remains undetermined, factors that cause chronic irritation could play a causative role.[100, 146]

Interdigital hyperplasia or interdigital fibroma (interdigital warts, corns, keloids, hyperplasia interdigitalis*)*

This is a chronic, symmetrical hyperplastic inflammation of the interdigital skin that commonly affects both hind feet **(Figure 145.8)**. Lameness may be evident if the mass of hyperplastic tissues is abraded as a result of necrosis caused by pressure against the axial side of the horny walls of the claw, or if it becomes infected. The degree of lameness usually depends on the severity of hyperplasia and superimposed bacterial infections.[100, 144, 146]

If interdigital hyperplasia occurs symmetrically in animals less than two years old it is probably precipitated by an inherited anatomical defect such as an abnormally wide interdigital space and abaxial angulation of the middle and distal phalanges.[146] Chronic mechanical irritation and infectious agents may also play a role in inducing or exacerbating the condition.

Laminitis (founder, pododermatitis aseptica diffusa *or* coreitis aseptica diffusa*)*

Laminitis is an acute, subacute, or chronic aseptic inflammation of the corium or sensitive laminae of the hoofs.[9, 48] Acute laminitis is characterized by sole and wall haemorrhages **(Figure 145.9)**, warm and painful claws, severe lameness, stiffness, elevated body temperature, increased heart and respiratory rates, and loss of appetite.[93] All four feet are involved.

In the chronic disease there are no generalized systemic signs, but lameness and stiffness are present. The shape of the claws may be altered, the dorsal wall becoming concave and showing irregular transverse grooves and ridges which diverge towards the bulb **(Figure 145.10)**. There is often a yellow or red discoloration of the horn of the sole. A widening of the white line is seen **(Figure 145.11)**, often combined with deviation of the distal phalanx. There is a widening and flattening of the hoofs, and differences in height between the lateral and medial claws as a result of sole overgrowth. Because it causes poorer horn quality, laminitis is a major predisposing factor for many of the other conditions of the claws **(Figure 145.7)**.[24, 52, 53, 94, 147]

The aetiology of laminitis is not clearly defined. Factors which have been incriminated include damage to the vascular bed of the corium by endotoxin following

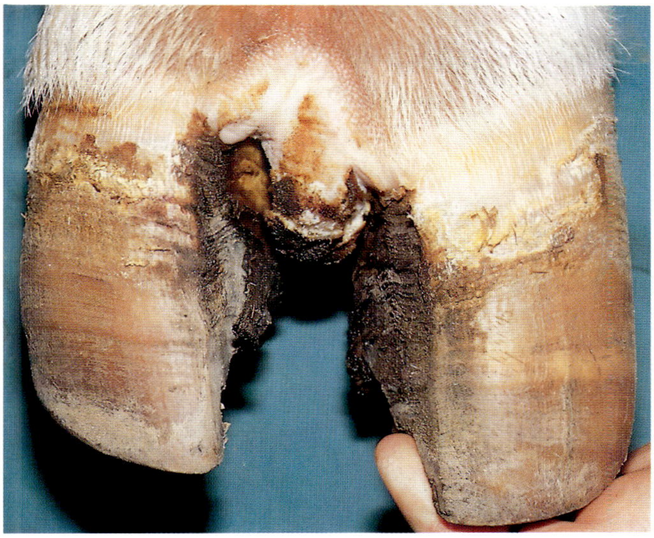

Figure 145.8 Interdigital hyperplasia. (By courtesy of Prof. S.S. van den Berg, Department of Surgery, Faculty of Veterinary Science, Onderstepoort)

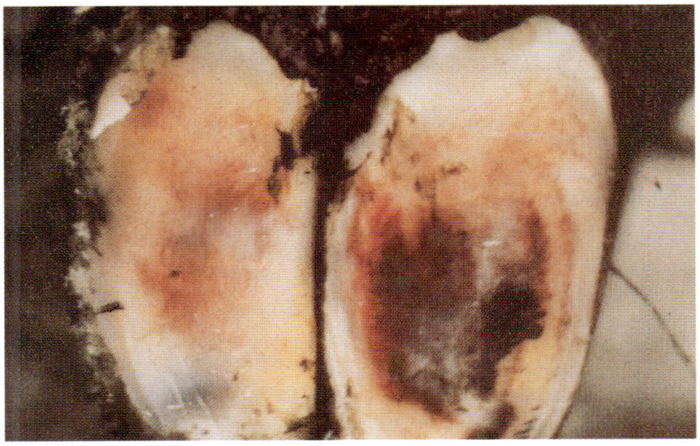

Figure 145.9 Acute laminitis. Note severe haemorrhages in the sole. (By courtesy of Prof. S.S. van den Berg, Department of Surgery, Faculty of Veterinary Science, Onderstepoort)

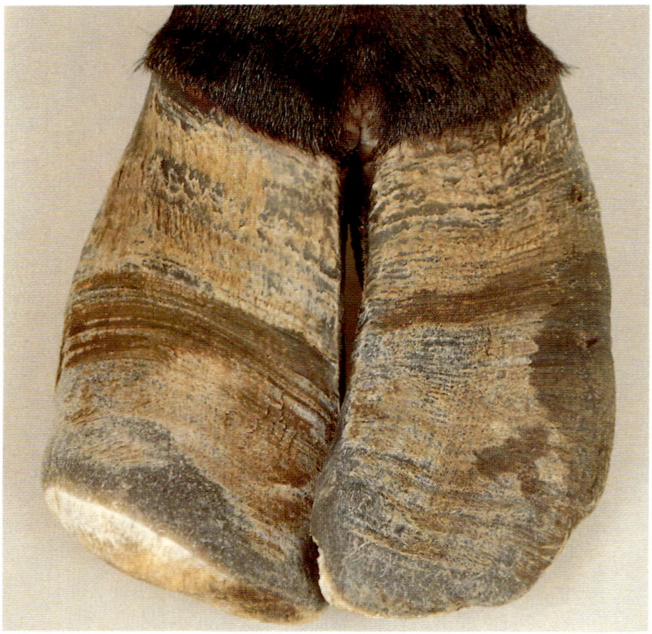

Figure 145.10 Chronic laminitis. Note concave dorsal wall of the hoof and transverse ridges in the horn. (By courtesy of Prof. S.S. van den Berg, Department of Surgery, Faculty of Veterinary Science, Onderstepoort)

ruminal acidosis, metritis and mastitis, and trauma of the claws as a result of obesity or rough ground surfaces. A genetic predisposition to it may also be a factor.[48] Lesions of subclinical or chronic laminitis can also occur as a result of overburdening of the claws during trekking, which is a common practice in Africa.[85]

Sole ulceration (sole ulcer, solear ulceration, Rusterholz ulcer, pododermatitis circumscripta*)*

Sole ulceration is a circumscribed ulcer of the horny sole which exposes the corium and is specifically located at the sole-heel junction, slightly towards the axial border **(Figure 145.12)**. Bilateral involvement of the lateral digit of the hind feet is common but the lesion is often more advanced in one of the claws. Lameness is usually not severe unless granulation tissue is formed which extends from the corium and prolapses through the defect in the sole.[100] Sepsis may complicate sole ulceration and result in septic laminitis, osteomyelitis, digital arthritis and abscessation.

Sole ulceration occurs almost exclusively in cattle kept intensively on hard surfaces which cause pressure on the sole. Laminitis as a result of ruminal acidosis may also predispose to the condition **(Figure 145.7)**.[100, 147]

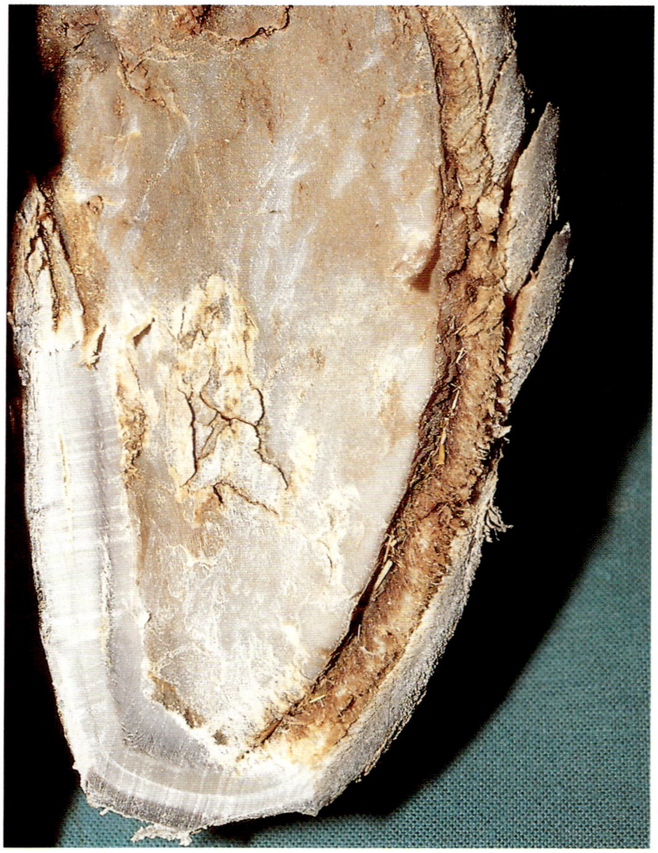

Figure 145.11 White line disease. Note widening of white line and accumulation of debris in the space where the wall has separated. (By courtesy of Prof. S.S. van den Berg, Department of Surgery, Faculty of Veterinary Science, Onderstepoort)

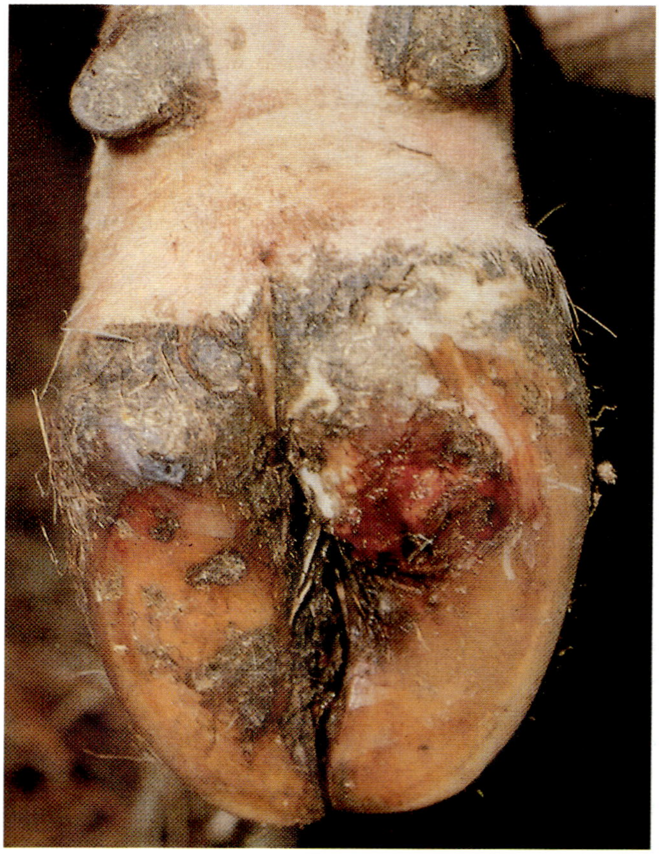

Figure 145.12 Sole ulceration. (By courtesy of Prof. S.S. van den Berg, Department of Surgery, Faculty of Veterinary Science, Onderstepoort)

Punctured sole (sole abscess, white line disease, septic traumatic pododermatitis, pododermatitis septica *or* coreitis septica*)*

This is a diffuse or localized septic inflammation of the pododerm. The condition often has a traumatic origin involving nails, sharp stones or excessive abrasion. The horny capsule is penetrated and infection leads to a septic pododermatitis.[102] It is a common condition of the claws.

Sandcrack or vertical fissure

Sandcracks occur on the dorsal and dorso-abaxial side of the horn of the hoof, particularly that of the fore limbs **(Figure 145.13)**. The length of sandcracks varies, but those that do not extend to the coronary band do not result in lameness, while those that involve the coronary band and become secondarily infected are serious and may result in infection of the joint capsule. A sandcrack develops when hoof horn becomes dehydrated and splits, such as when the periople, which restricts evaporation of water from the wall, is damaged by windy and sandy conditions, or following subclinical laminitis.[51, 100]

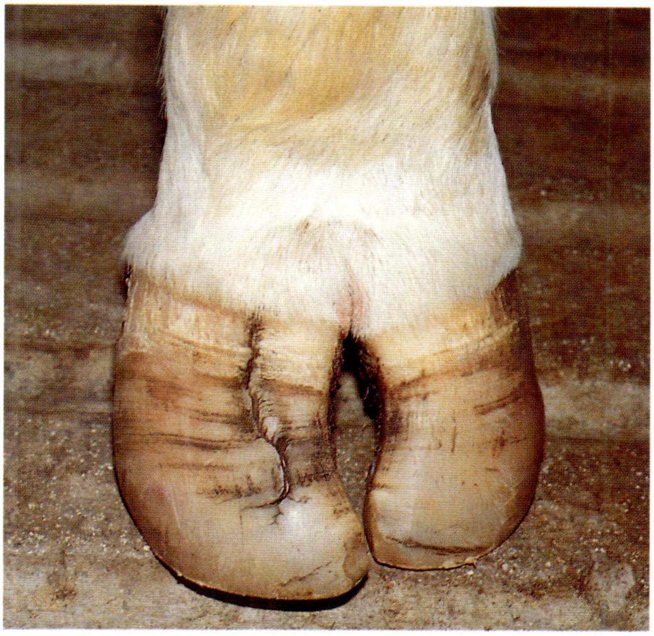

Figure 145.13 Sandcrack or vertical fissure. (By courtesy of Prof. S.S. van den Berg, Department of Surgery, Faculty of Veterinary Science, Onderstepoort)

Thimble or horizontal fissure

A thimble is a deep crack or fault in the hoof wall that runs parallel with the rugae (ridges) **(Figure 145.14)**.[51, 100] It develops secondarily to any disturbance in horn production that may follow dystocia, post-partum complications, acute febrile diseases and drastic nutritional changes.[51, 100] The disturbance in horn growth varies in severity; if severe, the integrity of the hoof wall is lost and the hoof wall sloughs partially as it grows out.

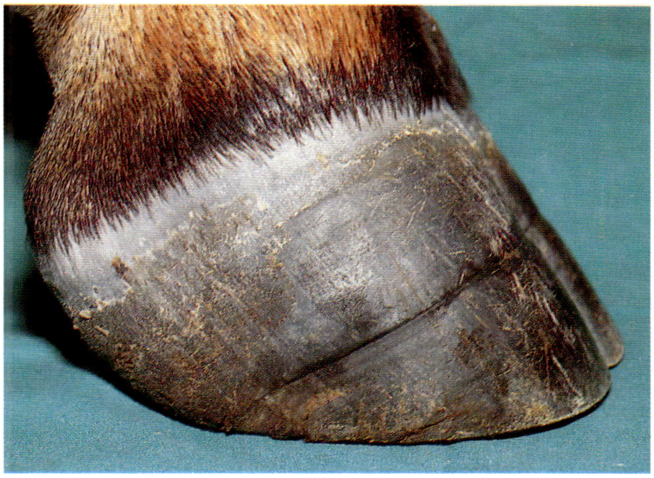

Figure 145.14 Thimble or horizontal fissure. (By courtesy of Prof. S.S. van den Berg, Department of Surgery, Faculty of Veterinary Science, Onderstepoort)

Control

The main methods used in the control of foot rot are the elimination or reduction of the exposure of the feet of cattle to the major risk factors (wet, muddy conditions and trauma), the use of prophylactic foot-bathing, and the prompt application of chemotherapy (parenteral or topical). Vaccination to prevent foot rot has been applied, but with variable success.

Adequate restraint of an affected animal is necessary in order to allow proper examination of the claws and to apply effective local treatment. This can be achieved by the use of mechanical leg lifters or tilt tables, casting the animal on the ground, or lifting the affected leg by means of a rope using one of several well-tried methods.[100, 102] Chemical restraint can also be used to quieten an animal, particularly during examinations of the hind legs; in most cattle a small dose of xylazine (10–20 mg) given intravenously will make it possible to lift a hind leg without the use of ropes. However, this form of restraint is not usually suitable for examining a front foot, as the animal tends to lie down when a front foot is lifted.

In animals suffering from a very painful digit, regional anaesthesia by interdigital nerve block or regional intravenous anaesthesia may have to be resorted to in order to carry out an adequate examination and application of local treatment. Both techniques are quick and simple. An interdigital nerve block anaesthetizes mainly the medial aspects of the digit. It is performed by injecting 20 ml of a suitable local anaesthetic between the digits distal to the fetlock while the animal is in a standing position and lightly sedated, at the same time restraining it by lifting its tail and pushing the latter forward. Either the lateral or medial digital vein can be used when applying regional intravenous anaesthesia. A tourniquet is placed around the limb just below the carpal or tarsal region and the vein palpated immediately proximal to the fetlock joint. The area over the vein is disinfected and 20 ml of a 2 per cent plain lignocaine solution (without adrenaline) is injected intravenously using a 20 gauge needle. Anaesthesia commences at once and is complete within five minutes. After releasing the tourniquet, sensation returns to normal in about five minutes.

Once restraint of the animal has been achieved, the affected foot is cleaned thoroughly. The affected interdigital skin, heel horn and surrounding soft tissue, including the coronets, are carefully examined to assess the depth of penetration of the infection, and the presence of cellulitis, heel horn erosion and discharging sinuses which usually occur in neglected or advanced cases of foot rot and indicate that the infection has spread to the deeper structures of the digit. Swelling at the coronary band or in the interdigital area may indicate a build-up of pus under the sole. Hoof testers may be used to assist in the location of painful areas in the sole, but if xylazine was used as a means of restraint or if regional anaesthesia was applied, the response of the animal to hoof testers will be affected to some degree. Sloughed and necrotic interdigital tissue and heel and sole horn should be removed using a pair of sharp scissors or a hoof knife. During this procedure attention should be given to the axial region to ensure that the interdigital space is sufficiently exposed to prevent dirt and dung from being trapped.

After removal of necrotic and under-run horn, all cracks should be trimmed and cleaned out and excessive granulation tissue removed. If the heel is overgrown, the excess heel horn should be pared away. The toe should be shortened so that the vertical weight-bearing axis is moved forward.

The type of local chemotherapy to be applied will depend on the nature and severity of the infectious condition. In cases of interdigital dermatitis, topical dressing with a 1:1 mixture of anhydrous copper sulphate and sulphamethazine usually results in rapid healing.[49] Formalin (2–10 per cent) footbaths may be used to control the condition. Good results will be obtained if it is used as a 5 per cent solution on alternate days for two weeks.

Various therapeutic agents used in the local treatment of foot rot and other infectious diseases of the feet are listed in **Table 145.2**.

Bandaging of the affected foot can be considered if the housing conditions are unhygienic or if the lesions are extensive. Medicated gauze, cotton wool padding and adhesive bandage are used. The interdigital area should be bandaged loosely to assist drainage. The bandage should be removed after five to seven days and replaced if necessary.

Systemic antimicrobials should be administered in cases of infectious digital disease where there are signs of deep penetration of the infection, as is often the case in foot rot. A list of the common antimicrobial agents used in the therapy of infectious disease of the feet is given in **Table 145.3**.

Table 145.2 Some common therapeutic agents used for the topical treatment of foot rot and other digital diseases in cattle

AGENT	METHOD OF USE
Metacresolsulphonic acid	Daily topical application of concentrate
Hydrogen peroxide	Daily topical application of concentrate
Acriflavine:glycerine mixture	Commonly used under a bandage (as a 1:100 concentration)
Glycerine ichthamol BPC	Commonly used under a bandage
Povidone iodine	Apply as an ointment or a spray
Antibiotic and antimicrobial mixtures. Commonly contain sulphanilamide, sulphadiazine, oxytetracycline, chloramphenicol, nitrofuran	Apply as an ointment, a powder or an aerosol
Gentian violet	Apply as a spray in combination with antimicrobial mixtures

Table 145.3 Antibiotic and antimicrobial drugs commonly used for the systematic treatment of infectious digital diseases in cattle

ANTIBIOTIC/ANTIMICROBIAL	DOSAGE AND ROUTE
Procain penicillin G	20 000–30 000 IU/kg body weight im twice a day
Ampicillin trihydrate	5–10 mg/kg sc or im once a day for three days
Oxytetracycline	10 mg/kg body weight im or iv once a day
Sulphamethazine 33$^{1}/_{3}$% solution	0,2 gm/kg initial dose followed by 0,1 gm/kg iv once a day
Sulphadimethoxine	1 ml/10 kg im daily
Sulphonamide-trimethoprim combination	15–24 mg/kg im or iv daily
Tylosine	10 mg/kg im once a day

im intramuscularly
iv intravenously
sc subcutaneously

Non-steroidal anti-inflammatory drugs should be administered to animals in severe pain. One such drug is phenylbutazone, which only needs to be administered at a dosage rate of 8 mg/kg every second day for 10–14 days because of its half-life of 32 to 60 hours.[147]

When complications such as septic joint disease, sole ulceration or suppurative tendosynovitis occur, a support block may be attached to the normal claw in order to lift the affected claw off the ground. The wooden block should be shaped to resemble that of the normal claw and fixed to it with an adhesive compound. Care must be taken that the normal weight-bearing mechanism of the claw is not disturbed after the block has been fixed in position. Other procedures such as the provision of adequate drainage, induction of ankylosis of an infected joint, or even claw amputation may also be considered.

The best way to control infectious digital disease is by eliminating or restricting exposure to predisposing factors such as faecally contaminated muddy conditions. Poor claw care increases the exposure of the interdigital skin to trauma and wet conditions. Where practical, claws should be trimmed twice a year.[3]

Foot-bathing can be used to prevent infectious conditions of the feet. It not only cleans the claws and interdigital skin, but also inhibits the growth of bacteria and hardens the interdigital skin. Two footbaths should be used, one containing only water to wash the claws and interdigital skin and the other a 5–10 per cent solution of copper sulphate or formalin. Copper sulphate and formalin may cause irritation, and for this reason cattle should not be exposed to them more frequently than twice a week.[3] A convenient and practical prophylactic programme for dairy cows may be to expose them to a footbath before or after four successive milkings every five days, the footbath being drained and refilled with water between each course of treatment.[147] Zinc sulphate as a 10 per cent solution may also be used in a footbath. As it is non-toxic and non-irritating, cattle should be exposed to it daily for the best results.[3] Footbaths should be properly constructed to ensure that the feet are exposed to the solution and that the floors are not slippery.[147]

Although some studies indicate that the addition of ethylenediamine dihydriodide (0,156 per cent) to the diet may reduce the severity and prevalence of foot rot in experimental animals,[76] others[3] determined no such beneficial effects and reported that herds treated with oral iodides for prolonged periods develop a chronic upper respiratory irritation and cough.

Zinc supplementation should be considered under circumstances where a zinc deficiency plays a role in the prevalence of foot rot or other interdigital skin diseases.[28]

Immunization of cattle against foot rot with an autogenous *D. nodosus* vaccine has been used.[25] Although vaccination appears to decrease the severity of foot rot, it has only a minor effect on the prevalence of the condition.[25]

Information on the diagnosis, therapy and control of the conditions of the bovine claw that are discussed in the differential diagnosis may be obtained from the relevant publications.[4, 5, 48, 51, 100, 102, 146, 147]

OVINE INTERDIGITAL DERMATITIS

Synonyms: Scald, brandpoot (Afrik.)

Introduction

Ovine interdigital dermatitis (OID) is an acute inflammatory condition, mainly of the interdigital skin of the feet of sheep, caused by *F. necrophorum* in association with *A. pyogenes*, although other non-specific bacteria may also be involved.[96, 153] It is usually accompanied by maceration and erosion of the affected parts. Pitting of the soft horn is occasionally present in severely affected animals. An identical disease occurs in goats, cattle and farmed deer, and is caused by benign strains of *D. nodosus*. Lameness usually occurs in only a small proportion of affected sheep, although it is generally this clinical sign which draws attention to the fact that the disease is present in a flock. In some outbreaks, however, a large number of animals in the flock may become lame. Excessive moisture and heavy faecal contamination of the environment are two of the most important predisposing factors.[36, 96] *Fusobacterium necrophorum* may survive for several months in faecally contaminated muddy conditions and occurs in the gastrointestinal tract as part of the microbial flora of different animal species.

Aetiology and epidemiology

Ovine interdigital dermatitis (OID), foot abscess, toe abscess and foot rot are distinct infectious conditions of the feet, particularly of sheep and occasionally of goats, which are caused by infections with *Fusobacterium necrophorum* and/or *Dichelobacter (Bacteroides) nodosus* in association with other infectious agents such as *Actinomyces (Corynebacterium) pyogenes*. Of these conditions, ovine interdigital dermatitis is the mildest, but it may predispose to foot rot and foot abscess, which are much more severe conditions.[35, 106]

Although foot abscess and toe abscess are often confused with each other and described as though they were the same entity, they are two distinct suppurative conditions with different pathogeneses. Foot abscess is the more common of the two conditions.

The seasonal occurrence of OID in Australia[96] and New Zealand,[151] and its association with wet conditions following prolonged rainfall are well known. In South Africa the prevalence of OID is dependent on suitable climatological conditions. It occurs in the coastal area of Natal and those parts of the eastern, southern and western Cape Province which have a high annual rainfall, but favourable conditions for its occurrence may also develop in other parts of the country during periods of prolonged rainfall. It may also occur on farms where wet underfoot conditions prevail, such as in the vicinity of leaking drinking troughs, or in poorly-drained camps, pens or irrigated pastures.

A number of other factors may also adversely affect the integrity of the interdigital skin and lead to outbreaks of OID. Inadequate dietary levels of zinc, or its unavailability due to mineral antagonism, may result in the formation of a poor quality interdigital skin and horn which enhances the probability of invasion by *F. necrophorum*.[112] Overgrowth of the horn of the feet, particularly of the walls and heel, which prevents the claws from opening and drying out, tends to trap mud and faeces and keeps *F. necrophorum* in continuous contact with the feet.[10, 86]

Differences in breed susceptibility are recognized, with Merinos being most susceptible under conditions of moderate challenge.[86] Individuals within breeds may be more than usually susceptible and are prone to successive attacks of OID.

Although all age groups of sheep are susceptible, young rams about eight months of age are the most commonly affected. Because of the behavioural patterns of young rams, the pastures on which they are kept are often trampled and the soil becomes and remains muddy. They frequently mount each other, which increases the risk of physical damage to the interdigital skin.[153]

Apart from the abovementioned conditions, other diseases may also cause lameness in sheep and goats **(see Ovine foot rot: Differential diagnosis)**.

Pathogenesis

Trauma or maceration of the interdigital skin permits invasion of *F. necrophorum*.[96] Once invasion of the interdigital skin by *F. necrophorum* has been accomplished, the dermonecrotic properties of the bacterium establish the infection. *Fusobacterium necrophorum* produces a leukocidin that is effective in protecting both itself and *A. pyogenes* against phagocytosis. Conversely, *A. pyogenes* produces a diffusible growth factor for *F. necrophorum*, so these bacteria grow synergistically.[96]

Clinical signs and pathology

Clinical signs of OID are usually absent or mild.[87, 96] Usually only a small proportion of affected sheep are lame: the signs are particularly evident when underfoot conditions are moist and muddy. If the feet of supposedly unaffected animals in the flock are examined, it will be observed that many of them are also affected. In mildly affected animals, the lesions are characterized by erythema, swelling, and in some cases erosion of the interdigital skin of one or more of the feet. Severely affected animals, which usually manifest marked lameness, have macerated, eroded, suppurating interdigital tissues, and only rarely erosion and pitting of the soft horn.[87, 96, 151] Histologically, the epidermis shows superficial necrosis and sloughing, infiltration with numerous neutrophils and invasion with *F. necrophorum* and other bacteria.[96]

Diagnosis and differential diagnosis

The feet of as many sheep as possible in an affected flock should be examined after they have been washed and scrubbed clean with a soft brush.[153]

It is usually not difficult to differentiate OID from foot abscess, as the former is almost invariably a mild infection limited mainly to the interdigital skin,[151] while in foot abscess the deeper tissues are also involved and the affected digit is generally very painful and swollen, especially in the area above the coronet of its abaxial aspect. Pus may drain through sinus tracts in the skin of the coronet and interdigital area. On the other hand, the clinical differentiation of OID from benign foot rot or early cases of intermediate or virulent foot rot is not always possible.

Lameness in small stock is also associated with other conditions **(see Ovine foot rot: Differential diagnosis)**.

Control

Mildly affected animals usually recover spontaneously if they are transferred from wet or muddy pastures to dry areas. Walk-through foot-bathing at two- to four-week intervals using 10 per cent zinc sulphate or 5 per cent formalin markedly reduces the prevalence of OID. Treated sheep should be allowed to stand on a dry surface in order to enable the disinfectant to dry on the feet before they are returned to pasture. Severely affected sheep should be treated as potential cases of foot abscess; the parenteral administration of penicillin may prevent spread of the infection to the distal interphalangeal joints.[153]

FOOT ABSCESS

Synonyms: Infective bulbar necrosis, heel abscess, sweerklou (Afrik.)

Introduction and aetiology

Foot abscess **(Figure 145.15)** is an acute to chronic, purulent, infectious but non-contagious disease of sheep and goats that usually involves a single digit of one of the feet. It usually follows ovine interdigital dermatitis or trauma of the interdigital skin and is caused by a mixed infection with *F. necrophorum* and *A. pyogenes*[104, 106, 151] that extends into the distal interphalangeal joint of the affected digit. Foot abscess is the most common infectious condition affecting the feet of sheep in South Africa. It also occurs commonly in goats.

The prevalence of foot abscess is usually less than 5 per cent in a flock of sheep, but it is nevertheless an important disease because of the severity of the lesion and because it generally affects the more valuable animals, such as rams and heavily pregnant ewes. Losses in production may occur as a result of the breeding programme being interrupted and of the development of pregnancy toxaemia as a consequence of the severe lameness which is associated with the disease.[153]

The general bacteriological characteristics of *F. necrophorum* and *A. pyogenes* are given in the **Anaerobic, Gram-negative, irregular rods: Introduction** and **Chapter 170**: ***Actinomyces pyogenes* infections** respectively.

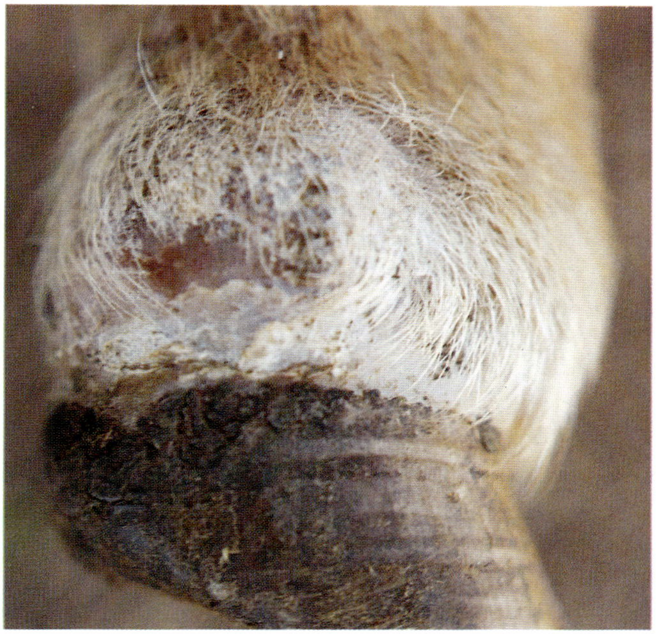

Figure 145.15 Foot abscess in a sheep. Note severe swelling above coronary band

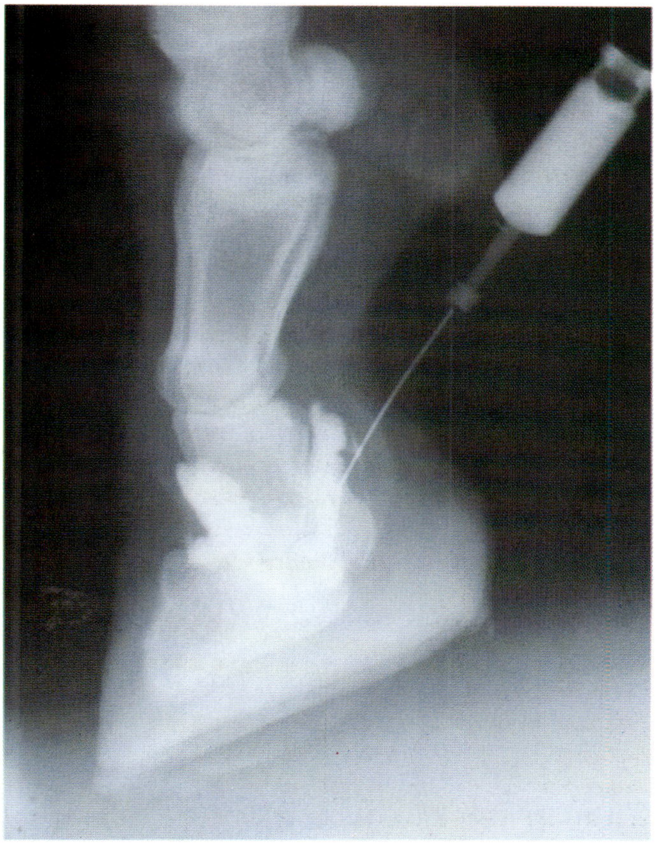

Figure 145.16 A radio-opaque substrate is injected into the distal interphalangeal joint to demonstrate the dorsal and volar pouches of the joint capsule. (By courtesy of Dr D.M. West, New Zealand)

Epidemiology

Any damage to the interdigital skin, such as that caused by excessive moisture, sharp stones, stubble, ticks, the too frequent use of formalin-containing footbaths or the use of too high a concentration of formalin in a footbath may predispose to foot abscess.

Prolonged and continuous wet or moist and muddy conditions in yards or pastures accompanied by stocking densities which give rise to high levels of faecal contamination of the environment are commonly associated with ovine interdigital dermatitis, which may subsequently lead to the development of foot abscess.[104, 106, 151] However, in one study in South Africa no significant correlation could be established between rainfall and the number of abscessed feet of Angora and Boer goats, but there was a statistically significant correlation between the prevalence of foot abscesses and the seasonal abundance of the smooth brown tick (*Rhipicephalus glabroscutatum*) and the bont tick (*Amblyomma hebraeum*).[77] The trauma of the skin between the claws that is associated with the common attachment site of both these ticks or that of *Hyalomma* spp. provides an excellent portal of entry for microorganisms such as *F. necrophorum* and *A. pyogenes*.

In southern Africa there are three *Rhipicephalus* spp. that have a strong predilection for the feet, and sometimes the legs, of sheep and goats, and to a lesser extent of other animals. *Rhipicephalus glabroscutatum*, a two-host tick, is probably the best known of these species. It occurs most commonly in a fairly restricted area of the south-eastern Cape Province, and its habit of attaching to the feet between the claws often leads to extremely painful lameness in sheep and goats.[131] *Rhipicephalus lounsburyi*,[142] previously described as *R. follis*,[130] is a three-host tick. Sheep are the only domestic animals on which its adults have been detected. They attach to the skin of the heels and feet between the claws. *Rhipicephalus lounsburyi* was first detected in the Dordrecht district but has since also been identified in the Maclear, Aliwal North, and Queenstown districts of the eastern Cape Province, as well as in other parts of the Cape Province, such as the Mountain Zebra National Park near Cradock, the Bontebok National Park near Swellendam, and the Calvinia district, and in the Impendle district of Natal. The adult ticks are most active from May to September. They occur mainly, but not exclusively, in mountainous and hilly areas covered with vegetation that ranges from succulent Karoo, Cape shrubland (fynbos) and coastal renosterbosveld to various types of grassland.[142] The third species, *Rhipicephalus neumanni*, also has a three-host life cycle.[142] Sheep are the most common hosts of the adult ticks, but they have also been found on Boer goats. *Rhipicephalus neumanni* is present in southern Namibia, where it has been found in the Bethanien, Luderitz and Keetmanshoop districts. It also occurs in scattered localities in the Karoo of the Cape Province: in the Prieska, Williston, Fraserburg and Victoria West districts, but is probably widely distributed in the rest of the Karoo.[142]

Pathogenesis

Foot abscess usually develops as a complication of ovine interdigital dermatitis or trauma of the interdigital skin. The inflammatory process extends from the skin into the subcutis and ultimately into one of the distal interphalangeal joints (coffin joints) **(Figure 145.16)**. These joints are vulnerable to infection, particularly those on the axial side (interdigital area) of the digit, in which the joint capsules protrude above the coronary borders as the dorsal and volar pouches **(Figure 145.16)**.[153] These pouches are protected only by skin and a small amount of subcutaneous tissue. During the early stages of the development of foot abscess, the nature of the inflammatory process is necrotic rather than suppurative because *F. necrophorum* is not a pyogenic bacterium; hence the term 'infective bulbar necrosis' is more appropriate than foot abscess.[106] At a later stage in the inflammatory process *A. pyogenes* becomes dominant and suppuration is evident. The infection in the joints may spread to surrounding tissues, resulting in rupture of the axial collateral and interdigital ligaments and subsequent deformity of the affected digit. Resolution may take many weeks, with eventual fibrosis and synarthrosis.

Clinical signs and pathology

An outbreak of foot abscess may start insidiously in a flock and present as sporadic cases of severe lameness, or it may be characterized by the sudden occurrence of a number of lame sheep. Usually, but not invariably, only one digit of one foot is affected.

On examination of the affected foot there is heat, pain and severe swelling in the interdigital area and above the coronary band **(Figure 145.15)**. As a result of the swelling, the affected digit becomes displaced abaxially (laterally). Blood, necrotic material and pus, which is often creamy-white, are discharged from sinus tracts which usually break out in the interdigital area, although occasionally they may open in the skin at one or more points above the coronet. In about 50 per cent of cases infection of the joint results in rupture of the axial collateral ligaments and the interdigital ligament giving rise to exaggerated movement of the affected digit, displacement of the digit during locomotion, and permanent deformity. Healing is slow and takes about two to four months. The development of excessive granulation tissue frequently occurs in the skin and subcutis, especially at sites where the sinuses discharge into the interdigital space. In severely affected animals neighbouring joints may also be affected, and the inflammatory process may extend along the tendons to the fetlock region or even higher.[54, 149]

Diagnosis and differential diagnosis

The initial lesions of foot abscess are clinically indistinguishable from OID and the earliest lesions of the different forms of foot rot. In general, foot abscess differs from foot rot in that the lesions in the latter disease only involve the interdigital skin and the matrix of the hoof, while in the former, the distal interphalangeal joint and, in some, the associated ligaments and tendons are affected. Foot abscess is almost invariably restricted to one digit of one foot, while foot rot usually affects more than one foot. In foot abscess the characteristic odour associated with *D. nodosus* infection is not present, and the prevalence rarely exceeds 5 per cent. Radiology is useful in establishing the involvement of the distal interphalangeal joint in cases of foot abscess.[153] Other distinguishing features are given in **Table 145.4**.

Control

Treatment of foot abscess should include cleansing of the lesions with disinfectants, drainage of the infected area, and parenteral administration of antimicrobial drugs. Penicillin alone or in combination with streptomycin is effective against *F. necrophorum* and *A. pyogenes*. Early cases, before or very soon after the infection reaches the joint, may benefit from aggressive and prolonged antimicrobial therapy. Nevertheless, eventual recovery cannot always be ascribed to the treatment used, as resolution of infection occurs in most animals after three to four months, although the affected digit may be deformed.[149] The prognosis is therefore usually good if animals can be given supportive treatment in the form of rest, shelter and hand-feeding until the disease has run its course.

Control is based on minimizing the factors which predispose to OID. Footbaths containing 5 per cent formalin or 10 per cent zinc sulphate used at weekly intervals may lower the prevalence of OID. The use of too high a concentration of formalin, however, may have the opposite effect and actually increase the prevalence of foot abscess, as it causes drying and cracking of the interdigital skin.[152] Where the bites of ticks are incriminated as the predisposing factor, tick control using acaricides which are applied either in the form of a footbath or spot treatment of the feet, should be instituted.

TOE ABSCESS

Synonyms: Lamellar suppuration, toonsweer (Afrik.)

In toe abscess it is presumed in most cases that infection gains entry through minute fissures in, or trauma to, the horn of the hoof, especially at the sole-wall junction (white line).[153] The toe of one digit of a fore foot is usually involved. Sheep with misshapen or overgrown hoofs, or those whose hoofs have been subjected to injudicious paring, are particularly prone to toe abscess. However, toe abscess is an uncommon condition. In contrast to the association between foot abscess, foot rot and ovine interdigital dermatitis, the latter is not involved in the pathogenesis of toe abscess.

Table 145.4
Comparison of the most important clinical aspects of foot rot, foot abscess and toe abscess in sheep. (Adapted from Walker[143])

	FOOT ROT	FOOT ABSCESS	TOE ABSCESS
Primary infectious agents involved	*D. nodosus* and *F. necrophorum*	*F. necrophorum* and *A. pyogenes*	*F. necrophorum* and *A. pyogenes*
Swelling	None	Usually above coronary band	None
Exudate	No pus; greyish-black slimy substance may be present	Discharge of creamy-white pus	Blackish pus and gas bubbles may be evident when exposed
Odour	Putrid odour. Lesions may be fly-blown	Slight odour. Lesions are rarely fly-blown	Odour distinct from that of foot rot. Lesions may be fly-blown
Sheep affected	All ages under conditions favourable to its development	Usually confined to heavy animals, e.g. rams and pregnant ewes	All classes of sheep
Location of lesion	No break in the skin of the coronet but separation of the inner sensitive horn from the outer hard horn	Sinus tracts usually break out at the coronet or the interdigital skin	Usually under horn of toe. May open in a line above coronary band but usually needs to be exposed by paring
Hoof	Often markedly misshapen	Usually normal	Slight distortion over the lesions

Toe abscess is caused by a mixed infection of bacteria, in which *F. necrophorum* predominates. *Actinomyces pyogenes* is also commonly implicated as one of the pathogens. Although it has been suggested by Van Tonder[138] that most cases of toe abscess in South Africa are probably caused by *A. pyogenes* and other pyogenic bacteria, his hypothesis is not generally accepted, mainly because *F. necrophorum* may be difficult or impossible to isolate during the later stages of the disease, giving the impression that *A. pyogenes* is the only (or principal) pathogen.[149]

The earliest sign of toe abscess in a flock of sheep is the appearance of acute lameness affecting one limb of one or more sheep. These animals tend to 'carry' the affected leg as a result of the severe pain. In the early stage of the disease clinical examination may fail to reveal any obvious lesion, although one claw is generally found to be hot and painful on palpation. Careful paring away of the horn at the toe will, however, reveal the presence of greyish pus of fairly thick consistency in the affected part. In more advanced cases the suppurative process may be found to have spread posteriorly under the sole, or to have 'broken out' to the externum through sinus tracts above the coronet. Because it primarily affects the lamellae of the hoof, it is also known as 'lamellar suppuration'.

Toe abscess must be distinguished from foot abscess and foot rot **(Table 145.4)**. It should also be differentiated from the condition known as shelly toe [also referred to as shelly hoof, white line disease or dopklou (Afrik.)], a non-infectious disease characterized by separation of the hoof horn from the sensitive laminae. The cavity that forms as a result of the separation is often packed with debris. The condition seldom causes lameness.

The therapy for toe abscess consists of exposing the lesion and treating it as an open wound. Parenteral antimicrobial therapy is indicated.

OVINE FOOT ROT

Synonym: vrotpootjie (Afrik.)

Introduction and aetiology

Foot rot is a highly contagious, painful and debilitating bacterial disease, particularly of sheep, usually affecting more than one foot. It is caused primarily by synergistic infection with *Dichelobacter (Bacteroides) nodosus* and *Fusobacterium necrophorum*. Other organisms such as *Actinomyces pyogenes* and *Spirochaeta penortha* are often isolated from affected feet, but they do not play a primary role. Environmental factors such as wet, muddy conditions are important predisposing factors to foot rot, but other factors may also be involved.[36, 86, 105] An outbreak in a flock is usually heralded by the presence of a few limping sheep as a result of the disease, which rapidly spreads to affect a large proportion of sheep. Based on the severity of the lesions, three forms of foot rot are recognized—benign (non-progressive, mild), intermediate, and virulent (progressive). The severity of the disease is dependent upon the virulence of the infecting strain of *D. nodosus*.[2] A high proportion of cattle are carriers of benign strains of *D. nodosus*. These strains cause interdigital dermatitis in cattle if suitable conditions prevail.

Foot rot is an ubiquitous disease of sheep.[143] It is economically important in Australia, New Zealand, the USA, and the United Kingdom and other countries in Europe.

Probably the first publication pertaining to an infectious disease affecting the feet of sheep in South Africa was by Theiler in 1911.[129] During the years following Theiler's publication there was confusion and controversy over the nature of diseases of the feet of sheep, because most farmers and many veterinarians used the term foot rot to describe a variety of infectious lamenesses, whatever the apparent cause. The first isolation of *D. nodosus* in South Africa was made only in 1984,[12] from foot rot lesions of sheep in Natal, but clinical cases of what was probably foot rot in sheep and goats have been recognized for many years in South Africa.[133, 137] Subsequently its presence has been confirmed in cases of foot rot in sheep in the south-western region of the Cape Province and in goats in Natal, as well as in cases of interdigital dermatitis in cattle from both these provinces. The disease has also been diagnosed clinically in sheep in the eastern Cape Province and eastern Orange Free State.

Foot rot is an important disease because it causes losses in production as a result of reduced body and fleece weights, decreased length and tensile strength of wool fibres, and reduced fertility. The lesions are prone to blowfly strike, which aggravates the effects of the disease.[10, 123, 124, 143] The labour and costs involved in control and eradication programmes contribute further to its economic importance.

Consult **Anaerobic, Gram-negative, irregular rods: Introduction** for information on the general characteristics of *D. nodosus* and *F. necrophorum*.

Epidemiology

Dichelobacter nodosus is an obligate parasite of the skin of the feet of sheep, goats, cattle and deer.[122] It cannot survive in the environment for more than 14 days, and infected animals, particularly sheep, are the main reservoir of infection. A proportion of sheep are carriers of *D. nodosus*, which persists in small pockets in the sole or wall of the hoof. These asymptomatic carriers may remain infected for two to three years or longer, and may develop lesions if conditions become favourable for the development of foot rot. They therefore complicate eradication programmes.[18, 143] Cattle may also be a source of infection, as they are frequently infected with strains of *D. nodosus* that cause benign foot rot in sheep. Benign strains have also been isolated from farmed deer in Australia and New Zealand.[143] For this reason, benign foot rot may occur on properties from which virulent foot rot has been eradicated or after the introduction of apparently healthy sheep, goats or cattle infected with *D. nodosus* strains of low virulence.[124, 143]

Fusobacterium necrophorum is part of the normal microflora of the intestinal tract of ruminants and may therefore occur in the environment through faecal contamination. It may survive for several months in faecally contaminated, muddy conditions.[66, 74, 107, 117]

Prolonged wet and muddy conditions with ambient temperatures above 10 °C are the most important factors predisposing the interdigital skin to infection. Other predisposing factors include traumatic injury to the skin, such as that caused by the penetration of *Strongyloides papillosus* larvae,[18] grasses, such as kikuyu (*Pennisetum clandestinum*), and thorns, as well as hoof cracks and over-grown hoofs, which increase the susceptibility of the feet to bacterial invasion.[112]

Merinos are more susceptible to virulent foot rot than the British breeds, but there is individual variation in susceptibility within breeds;[39] horn quality and the degree to which the claws can open seem to be the major determining factors. All ages and both sexes of sheep are susceptible.

Pathogenesis

Foot rot starts as an infection of the interdigital skin which, depending on the form of disease (benign, intermediate or virulent), then progressively spreads down the inside of the inner (medial) wall of the hoof and across the sole, causing under-running and separation of the horn **(Table 145.5)**. In very severely affected animals the infection also extends from the sole and up the outer (lateral) wall of the hoof. The severity of the disease is mainly determined by the virulence of the strain of *D. nodosus* involved, but environmental factors (e.g. temperature, moisture) and breed of sheep also play a role.[143]

In foot rot, *F. necrophorum* is critical for initial tissue destruction. *Dichelobacter nodosus* enhances the infection by producing a growth factor which enables *F. necrophorum* to multiply in the deeper parts of the lesion. In these areas *D. nodosus* grows slowly but persistently and prevents healing during periods when *F. necrophorum* is quiescent. The pili of *D. nodosus* allow the bacterium to adhere to the epidermal matrix of the horn while the protease it produces digests the horn, thus promoting its separation and facilitating invasion by other species of bacteria. The latter aggravate the lesion and help to provide the anaerobic conditions which enable *D. nodosus* and *F. necrophorum* to grow.

Table 145.5 Scoring of lesions of sheep suffering from foot rot. (Adapted from Walker[143])

SCORE	LESIONS
0	Normal, dry interdigital skin
1	Mild, localized interdigital dermatitis; slight to moderate inflammation which includes erosion of the epidermis
2	Moderate interdigital dermatitis and necrotizing inflammation of part or all the soft horn of the medial wall of the digit
3	Severe interdigital dermatitis and under-running of the horn of the heel and sole; the necrotizing inflammation does not extend to the outer edge of the sole
4	Under-running extending to the outer edge of the sole of the hoof
5	Necrotizing inflammation of the deeper layers of the hoof resulting in separation of the hoof

Clinical signs and pathology

The severity of lesions of foot rot in sheep may be scored **(Table 145.5)** in order to differentiate the three forms of foot rot and also as an aid to decide which control programme should be implemented.

In benign foot rot, sometimes also referred to as 'scald', the interdigital skin lesions are characterized by hyperaemia, moistening and, in some, granulation tissue formation. The lesions rarely progress to an under-running of the horn (score 3 or 4). There is often ridging of the horn on the medial posterior wall. More than one foot is usually affected. Lameness is usually only apparent in heavy sheep such as rams or ewes in late pregnancy. Many animals in a flock may be affected under conditions that are favourable to the spread of foot rot. Most cases of benign foot rot resolve without treatment if the animals are moved to dry pastures, and the lesions usually do not become chronic. It has a minimal effect on production of meat and wool.[124, 143]

Next in order of severity of lesions is intermediate foot rot. These lesions usually develop more slowly than those of benign foot rot **(Table 145.6)**. The severity of lameness is commensurate with the severity of lesions. A variable proportion of the flock may be affected. Up to 10 per cent of sheep may have lesions with a score of 4. Self-cure of affected animals may occur if environmental conditions become drier.

Table 145.6 Time-scale of development of lesions of foot rot in sheep. (Adapted from Walker[143])

LESIONS	TIME SCALE		
	BENIGN	INTERMEDIATE	VIRULENT
Interdigital dermatitis	3–4 days	3–4 days	3–4 days
Separation of the skin/horn junction at heel (score 3)		30 days	7–14 days
Separation of entire sole to outside wall (score 4)			21 days
Chronic infection			Months

Virulent foot rot spreads rapidly in a flock; under ideal environmental conditions for the development of foot rot, up to 90 per cent of a flock may become infected within six weeks. Affected sheep are severely lame and lose weight. The disease commences as an interdigital dermatitis but the subsequent lesions develop rapidly, and in one to two weeks **(Table 145.6)** there is severe under-running of the hoof **(Figure 145.17)**. More than 10 per cent of sheep may have lesions with a score of 4. Only in a small proportion of cases with virulent foot rot do the lesions resolve spontaneously as environmental conditions become drier. Sheep suffering from chronic virulent foot rot often have overgrown and misshapen hoofs, while the soft tissue beneath the horn is destroyed and may have a greyish-black, tarry appearance **(Figure 145.18)**. Myiasis of the lesions may occur, and this compounds the severity of the disease.

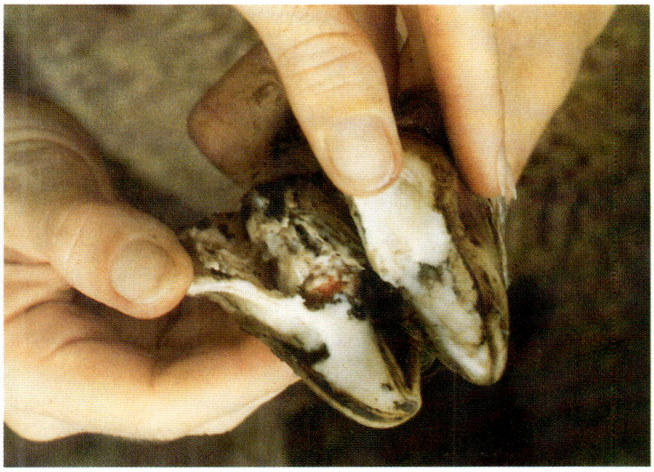

Figure 145.17 Virulent ovine foot rot. Note separation of the sole

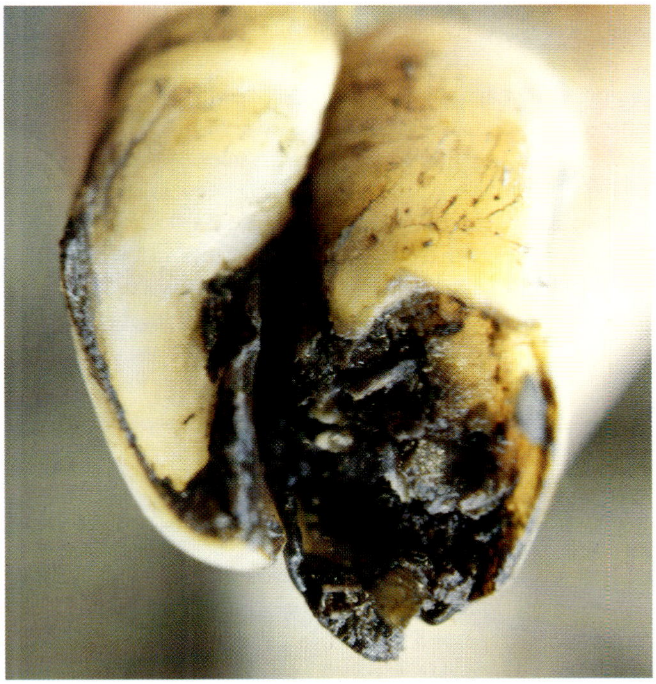

Figure 145.18 Virulent ovine foot rot. Note greyish-black material where the sole has separated

Both virulent and benign strains of *D. nodosus* have been isolated from goats with foot rot.[143] The predominant lesion in goats is severe interdigital dermatitis characterized by hyperkeratosis, erosions and necrosis, with only occasional under-running of the sole. Some granulation tissue formation may accompany the interdigital dermatitis. Severely affected goats may exhibit marked lameness and weight loss.[124, 143]

Diagnosis and differential diagnosis

Visual and manual inspection of all the feet of as many sheep as possible is the most practical way of diagnosing foot rot.[33] No reliable serological or other *in vitro* tests for detecting infected sheep have so far been developed. The lesions should be graded and scored 0–5 to determine which form of foot rot is prevalent in the flock **(Table 145.5)**. Severe under-running of the hoofs in a large proportion of sheep will indicate virulent foot rot. Benign foot rot is characterized generally by interdigital lesions with little under-running, even under the worst environmental conditions. The severity of the lesions of intermediate foot rot is between those of virulent and benign foot rot.

If foot rot is suspected and environmental conditions are not favourable for its development, the 'progressive test' is a useful diagnostic aid. In this test, 10–20 sheep with score 2–3 lesions are identified and placed on wet rubber mats, wet straw or irrigated pastures at ambient temperatures above 10 °C for seven days.[143] After one to three weeks the lesions are re-assessed, and if they have progressed rapidly a diagnosis of virulent foot rot is justified.

Microscopic examination of smears prepared from material obtained from interdigital skin lesions or other active lesions, such as the margin of the most recent under-run part of a hoof or an active lesion that has been exposed by paring, may be used to determine the presence of *D. nodosus*. The smears should be stained with the Gram's staining method or a fluorescent antibody staining technique. The rod-shaped bacteria have characteristic terminal enlargements. False negative results by both these methods are sometimes obtained when recently treated sheep are examined or at times of the year when conditions unfavourable for the multiplication of the bacteria prevail.[143]

Ideally, an attempt should also be made to culture *D. nodosus* from active lesions to confirm the diagnosis. Best results are obtained if material from the lesions is inoculated onto plates containing a specialized medium known as hoof agar. The plates are placed immediately in an anaerobic jar and sent to a laboratory familiar with culturing *D. nodosus*.[143] Alternatively, special transport media should be used. Once *D. nodosus* is isolated, its virulence and the serogroup to which it belongs should be determined. For information on the morphological characteristics and cultural requirements of *D. nodosus*, as well as its identification, consult **Anaerobic, Gram-negative, irregular rods: Introduction**.

Foot rot is most commonly confused with foot abscess. Some characteristics which will help to differentiate foot rot, foot abscess and toe abscess from each other are summarized in **Table 145.4**. Other causes of lameness in sheep include injury or trauma to the feet (such as those caused by thorns of *Tribulus terrestris* or 'dubbeltjies' and bites of ticks) or joints of the legs, orf lesions around the coronet, heels and in the interdigital skin, coronitis caused by bluetongue, strawberry foot rot caused by *Dermatophilus congolensis*, post-dipping lameness caused by *Erysipelothrix rhusiopathiae*, polyarthritis due to a variety of infectious agents, laminitis due to the feeding of excessive amounts of carbohydrates, and white muscle disease (nutritional myopathy).

Control

The economic benefits of control (reducing the prevalence of ovine foot rot to acceptable levels) versus eradication strategies should be discussed with the flock owner, and the expected extent of his or her co-operation assessed, before any programme is implemented.[2, 33]

In the case of virulent foot rot in sheep, implementation of an eradication strategy is usually indicated, but control may be the best option where the prospects for eradication are poor. If control is the objective, vaccination or foot-bathing will reduce the prevalence of virulent foot rot in a flock.[33, 103] Once the prevalence has been reduced to a low level, its eradication may become feasible. Where benign foot rot is the problem, control should be attempted during the wet seasons, as its eradication has proved difficult. In the case of intermediate foot rot, an eradication strategy of the disease in young sheep may be undertaken initially, and if successful could be expanded to include the other age groups.[2]

Various methods may be applied to control foot rot. These include the removal of affected flocks from wet pastures to dry areas, parenteral or topical antimicrobial therapy, foot-bathing and vaccination.[143] Paring of affected hoofs to expose pockets of infection may be useful prior to topical or parenteral antimicrobial therapy or foot-bathing, but it is very time-consuming and thus expensive. Depending on the situation on the farm, one or more of these methods could be combined. Preventive measures (foot-bathing and vaccination) are applied before or during wet conditions which favour transmission, while therapeutic measures (antimicrobial therapy and paring) are most effective during dry conditions (the non-transmission phase).[33]

Walk-through foot-bathing should be instituted prior to and during the wet season in order to reduce the prevalence of overt disease in any carriers.[143] Before this programme is instituted, however, all sheep on the property should be inspected and, where appropriate, the hoofs pared in order to expose pockets of infection.[33] At the same time the sheep should be segregated into 'clean', 'salvage' and 'cull' categories; those in the latter group should be disposed of as soon as possible. Only the clean and salvage groups should be foot-bathed and re-inspected three weeks after treatment.[143]

The preparations used in footbaths are usually 10 per cent zinc sulphate, 5 per cent formalin, or commercial products [e.g. Footrite; Hardman Chemical (Pty) Ltd] which contain zinc sulphate and sodium lauryl sulphate, the latter substantially enhancing the penetration of zinc sulphate into the hoof.[7, 22, 57] Portable or permanent troughs may be used as footbaths; the former can be placed, for example, in gateways. Fresh solutions should be made up regularly. The disadvantages of walk-through foot-bathing programmes are that they lead to a low cure rate in comparison to parenteral antimicrobial treatment and are labour-intensive. Generally, control of benign foot rot and most cases of intermediate foot rot is satisfactorily effected if the animals walk through, or preferably stand in, the footbath for up to five minutes every two to four weeks, to ensure that all four feet are treated. Sheep should stand on dry areas for 10–20 minutes following foot-bathing to allow the solution to dry on the feet if the chemical it contains is to have a lasting effect. The principle of a walk-through foot-bathing programme is that the chemical used makes contact with the interdigital skin and the area of under-running so that *D. nodosus* is killed. Foot-bathing (particularly with formalin) will also harden the hoof and interdigital skin, rendering them less susceptible to infection.

Vaccination or more intensive foot-bathing (weekly 'walk-through', or 'stand-in' every two to three weeks) prior to or during the wet season will be required to control virulent foot rot.[2] With Footrite, which contains both zinc sulphate and sodium lauryl sulphate, the interval could be up to 21 days between treatments.[143] A high cure rate is usually obtained with Footrite without prior paring.[22]

Paring and topical antimicrobial treatment can be applied to control foot rot.[33] However, parenteral antimicrobial therapy offers a good alternative to conventional paring and topical antimicrobial treatment or foot-bathing.[2, 33] Parenteral chemotherapy has the advantage of not requiring the extensive paring which is a prerequisite for effective topical treatment.[140] Once-only parenteral treatment of infected sheep during the dry season with combinations of procaine penicillin and dihydro-streptomycin at 50 000–70 000 IU/kg body weight and 50–70 mg/kg respectively, or a mixed solution containing 50 mg lincomycin and 100 mg spectinomycin/ml given at a dose rate of 1 ml/10 kg body weight will result in the cure of more than 90 per cent of affected sheep.[140, 143] Treated animals should be identified and thereafter kept under dry conditions for 24 hours. Some chronically affected sheep do not respond to antimicrobial treatment and should be culled.[143]

Various inactivated adjuvanted (mostly oil) vaccines containing different strains of *D. nodosus* serogroups are commercially available in Europe, Australia and New Zealand. The use of vaccines gives a farmer an alternative method for the control of foot rot in wet conditions other than simply foot-bathing.[33] Vaccination is used to reduce the prevalence of foot rot in flocks to manageable levels and it has the advantage that it is less labour-intensive than foot-bathing. Vaccination not only induces immunity which prevents the infection from becoming established in 80 per cent of sheep, but it also has a curative effect; the lesions resolve in at least 60 per cent of affected sheep that are vaccinated.[33, 143] Once the prevalence of foot rot in a flock has been reduced through vaccination, eradication could be attempted either by disposal or by chemotherapy of affected sheep.[33]

Depending on the make of the vaccine, the interval between the administration of the first and second dose of vaccine varies, but it is generally two weeks.[103, 143] An effective immunity develops only after the second dose of vaccine, and maximum protection lasts for only 10–12 weeks after administration of the second dose. The administration of a single booster dose of vaccine prior to the wet season in the subsequent year will provide good protection.[23, 103, 143] The vaccination programme should be planned so that maximum protection occurs during the period when the prevalence of foot rot is most likely to be increasing.[103, 143] Vaccinated ewes confer colostral immunity to their lambs, and maternal antibodies may interfere with the response to vaccination in lambs less than eight weeks of age.[103]

Dietary zinc improves the quality of the horn of the hoof and interdigital skin and therefore decreases the susceptibility of animals to infection.[112] Oral administration of zinc sulphate to adult sheep at the rate of 0,5 g daily for 21 days has been found to be useful, both therapeutically and prophylactically, especially when the sheep receive inadequate levels of dietary zinc.[112]

Several strategies can be applied to eradicate virulent foot rot.[33, 143] Methods that can be applied to achieve eradication of foot rot fall into three categories:[33]

- disposal of the entire flock and restocking with sheep free of foot rot,
- identification and disposal of affected sheep in a flock, and
- elimination of infection by chemotherapy.

If the first of these strategies, i.e. disposal and restocking, is not instituted it usually takes two to three years to achieve eradication. The best results are generally obtained if eradication is attempted during the dry summer months by applying chemotherapy. Sheep free of foot rot should be identified and isolated from infected sheep, while the infected ones are either treated or culled. Any eradication strategy must incorporate regular surveillance of the flock after affected sheep have been removed.[33]

BOVINE HEPATIC NECROBACILLOSIS

Synonym: Rumenitis/liver abscess complex

Introduction

There is a close association between rumenitis in cattle and the development of hepatic necrobacillosis. In many cases *Fusobacterium necrophorum*, particularly biovar A, may be isolated in pure culture from these lesions, but more often the infection is mixed, with *Actinomyces (Corynebacterium) pyogenes* being the most common bacterium to accompany *F. necrophorum*. The lesion in the liver produced by uncomplicated *F. necrophorum* is frequently described as an abscess, but this is not so if the strict definition of the term is applied. *Fusobacterium necrophorum* causes localized areas of hepatic necrosis which are initially coagulative in nature. The necrotic tissue may later undergo liquefaction, become invaded by pyogenic organisms, and then resemble pus, and the lesion as a whole resemble an abscess **(see Clinical signs and pathology)**. Nevertheless, in order to conform with general practice the word abscess is used in this section.

Hepatic necrobacillosis or the rumenitis/liver abscess complex in cattle, which occurs most frequently in feedlot animals,[60, 61, 79, 83, 92, 113] may cause considerable economic loss, primarily because of the condemnation of affected livers at slaughter. In some animals the liver lesions result in acute or chronic systemic disease. Surveys conducted in the USA between 1967 and 1969 indicated that approximately 10 per cent of cattle slaughtered had abscesses in their livers. However, abscesses only occurred rarely in other organs. In South Africa the situation is less clear because of a paucity of relevant data. Average yearly liver condemnations due to abscesses at four abattoirs in South Africa varied from 4,3 to 12,7 per cent over four years.

Aetiology

Fusobacterium necrophorum can be isolated in pure culture from 81 to 97 per cent of small or newly-formed hepatic abscesses in cattle.[67, 79, 92, 117] As the abscesses increase in size and age, they usually become secondarily infected by one or more of a variety of anaerobic or facultatively anaerobic bacteria.

Biovars A, B and AB of *F. necrophorum* are usually associated with hepatic abscesses.[1, 15, 67, 69] Strains of biovar A are usually isolated in pure culture from liver abscesses[15, 67, 117] and may be isolated from as many as 50 per cent of all cases.[75] They have a greater potential to cause liver abscess, which is attributed to virulence factors in their cell walls and the production of more leukocidin than the other two biovars.[42] Strains of biovar B are most often isolated from lesions in the rumen.[69] Biovar B strains are less virulent than biovar A and they invariably occur in association with other microorganisms, particularly *A. pyogenes*, on which they depend in order to exert their pathogenic effects.[15, 75] Biovar AB strains are rarely isolated and their pathogenicity is intermediate between those of biovars A and B[75] **(see Epidemiology and pathogenesis)**.

Consult **Anaerobic, Gram-negative, irregular rods: Introduction** for further information on the general characteristics of *F. necrophorum*.

Epidemiology and pathogenesis

Fusobacterium necrophorum is a frequent inhabitant of the alimentary tract, especially the rumen, of healthy cattle.[46, 66, 107, 117] It does not penetrate normal intact epithelium; devitalization of the tissue is essential if this is to happen.[38]

The prevalence of liver abscesses is highest in cattle that pass through feedlot systems. In order to appreciate the reason for this phenomenon, it is necessary to understand the processes involved in the adaptation of these animals to the nutrition they receive while in the feedlot. The intense economic pressure to move these animals through the system as quickly as possible is opposed by several biological constraints. Most cattle entering a feedlot have come from open grazing systems, where most, if not all, of the animals' feed intake consisted of high-fibre veld or pasture grasses. Since few cattle in southern Africa are grazed on mixed pasture, some of which may contain the more digestible clovers, most of these animals are adapted to a diet containing a large proportion of fibre and little soluble carbohydrate. As a result, the physiology and ecology of their digestive tracts are adapted to optimize the fermentation and digestion of the cellulose and hemicellulose fractions of the diet. In other words, rate of passage of digesta through the tract will be slow, retention of particles in the rumen will be long, saliva volume will be copious but it will not contain much bicarbonate, and the cellulolytic and hemicellulolytic microorganisms will be well represented in the ruminal ecology, while lactilytic groups will be present in small numbers.

In principle, it is possible to adapt cattle from the more natural high-fibre diet to one containing very little fibre (as little as 10–20 per cent) and large quantities of highly digestible carbohydrates such as starch. This adaptation results in an increase in the rate of passage of digesta through the digestive tract, which includes a considerable shortening of the retention time of digesta in the rumen, and the production of more bicarbonate in the saliva. In addition, extensive population changes must occur in the ruminal ecology if an animal is to cope with this change in substrate. There are always groups of microorganisms, containing bacteria such as *Selenomonas ruminantium* and *Streptococcus bovis*, which can rapidly ferment soluble carbohydrate, thereby producing small amounts of lactate as end-product.[110] This lactate is then rapidly transformed to propionate by the lactilytic group of microorganisms, which include *Veillonella parvula (V. alcalescens), Megasphaera elsdenii* and *Selenomonas ruminantium*.[78] However, when the influx of soluble carbohydrate increases suddenly, as often happens when cattle are first introduced to a feedlot diet, several factors combine to exacerbate the situation. Firstly, reduced tactile stimulation of the rumen wall by grass fibres leads to a reduction in saliva production and hence in its buffer capacity. Secondly, the amount of lactate produced in the rumen from the soluble carbohydrate is more than the lactilytic bacteria can metabolize, and this hydroxy acid then accumulates in the rumen. The Gram-positive *S. bovis* and other lactobacilli normally produce acetate, propionate and ethanol as end-products at low growth rates, but switch to lactate production at high growth rates.[110] As a result, the pH in the rumen declines rapidly from the normal range of 6,5–7,2 to 4,5–6,5 as lactate (pK_a = 3,73) is a stronger acid than the volatile fatty acids (pK_a = 4,76 to 4,82). This decline in pH suppresses several important groups of microorganisms in the rumen, including those that ferment the fibre component of the diet, as well as those responsible for removing the excess lactate. However, low pH does not have an effect on *F. necrophorum*. Rumen acidosis, if it is not fatal in itself, may persist in a subclinical form and result in superficial necrosis of the ruminal epithelium or even in a low-grade rumenitis.[60]

The areas of the rumen affected are usually located in the cranial ventral sac,[60] and if they are invaded by *F. necrophorum* the destructive effect of leukocidin produced by the organism on the plasma membrane of ruminal epithelial cells increases the severity of the lesions.[68]

Once *F. necrophorum* has penetrated into the rumen wall it may metastasize via branches of the portal vein to the liver.[61]

Infection by *F. necrophorum* alone may result in liver abscessation, but it does appear that the chances of establishing the infection in the liver are enhanced by a number of factors. Endotoxin produced in the rumen during acidosis by various Gram-negative bacteria may contribute to the development of hepatic abscessation[29, 89, 134] by impairing the phagocytic ability of cells in the liver, initiating disseminated intravascular coagulation, and causing focal hepatic necrosis.[72] Based on experimental data, it appears that most of these effects are mediated through the Schwartzman reaction.[90, 91] In addition to the effects of endotoxin in the liver, platelet aggregation mediated by haemolysin and a toxic metabolite of *F. necrophorum*[70] also predisposes to the development of hepatic necrosis.[65, 90] Once the bacteria have lodged in the liver, the synergistic effect of toxic substances produced by the bacterium causes enlargement of the areas of necrosis.[90]

It has been shown experimentally that the development of liver abscesses caused by *F. necrophorum* is enhanced by the presence in the lesion of sublethal numbers of *A. pyogenes*.[127] Thus the minimal intravenous infective dose of *Fusobacterium* required for the causation of liver abscesses may be reduced from more than one million organisms to less than ten. Other bacteria that are able to fulfil the role of helper agent include *Staphylococcus aureus*, *Bacillus cereus* and *Klebsiella oxytoca*. The ability of *Bacillus subtilus*, *Pasteurella haemolytica*, *Proteus mirabilis*,[120, 121] *Citrobacter freundi*, alpha-haemolytic streptococci and *Bacillus fragilis* to help in the formation of these lesions is less developed.[119]

In addition to ruminal acidosis, foreign objects, such as pieces of wire, nails and other metal fragments that are inadvertently ingested with the feed, may also cause injury to the rumen wall and provide portals of entry for *F. necrophorum*[44, 62] or other bacteria. Umbilical infections of new-born animals with *F. necrophorum* may also result in disseminated liver abscesses.

The infectivity of *F. necrophorum* appears to be enhanced by faecal contamination of wounds. It has been shown experimentally that the addition of *F. necrophorum* to a suspension of faeces reduces the minimal infective dose of the organism when the suspension is injected subcutaneously. A similar outcome may be obtained when *F. necrophorum* is inoculated into a subcutaneous site in which faecal material has previously been injected. *Fusobacterium necrophorum* may metastasize from the liver to the lungs, where similar lesions develop.[62]

Clinical signs and pathology

Hepatic abscesses are rarely diagnosed clinically and are usually only detected at slaughter or necropsy. Occasionally, however, systemic disease or even fatality results when the number of abscesses in the liver is large enough to cause hepatic insufficiency or toxaemia, or when an abscess ruptures and is followed by peritonitis.[62]

When large numbers of abscesses develop simultaneously, affected cattle manifest fever, depression and abdominal pain, while some may be icteric.[62] The presence of abscesses in the liver may induce a marked neutrophilia in some animals, and liver function tests may indicate hepatic involvement. An increased sialic acid content of serum appears to be a reliable indicator of the development of hepatic abscesses.[59]

Single or multiple abscesses of varying size may be present in the liver. They may be located deep in the parenchyma or close to the capsule; in the latter case the inflammatory reaction may involve the capsule of the liver and cause a localized perihepatitis. The lesions from which pure cultures of *F. necrophorum* are isolated characteristically consist of round, raised or sunken areas of dry coagulative necrosis **(Figure 145.19)** which may be surrounded by a zone of hyperaemia. Histologically, the peripheral rim of the necrotic lesion contains scattered basophilic debris of nuclear material amongst which numerous filamentous, non-branching, granular, Gram-negative *F. necrophorum* organisms are visible. The inflammatory reaction is principally mononuclear. Older lesions, particularly those containing mixed bacterial populations, may resemble typical abscesses and become encapsulated. The lesions may be accompanied by a severe focal or diffuse fibrinous peritonitis, or in more chronic cases by fibrous adhesions to neighbouring structures.

Liver abscesses often occur concurrently with rumenitis (51 per cent of cases), and less often with hyperkeratosis of the forestomachs (14 per cent), abomasal ulcer (10 per cent), and traumatic reticulitis (4 per cent).[55]

In the rumen, lesions caused by *F. necrophorum* are generally superficial and consist of focal or diffuse areas of thickened and fused ruminal papillae, some of which may show necrosis or ulceration. Acute lesions **(Figure**

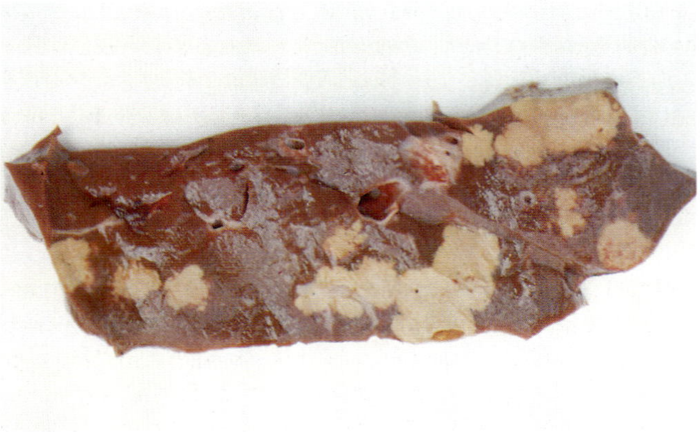

Figure 145.19 Bovine hepatic necrobacillosis. Note yellowish-grey areas of coagulative necrosis

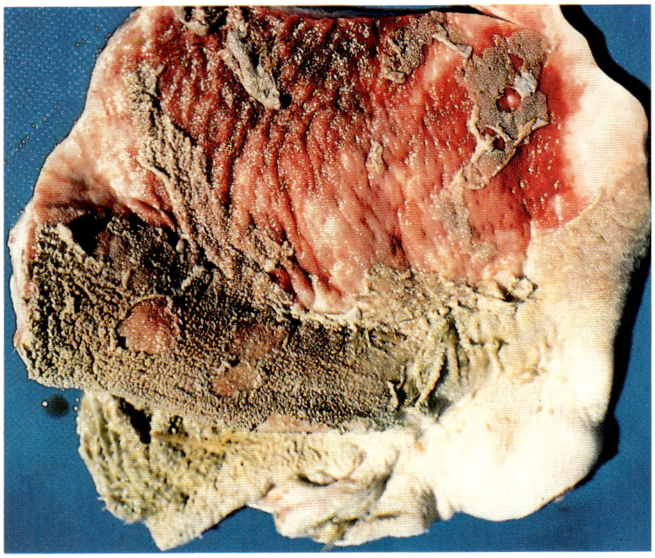

Figure 145.20 Rumenitis caused by *Fusobacterium necrophorum*. Note sloughing of the mucosa and hyperaemia of the exposed areas

145.20), characterized additionally by the presence of oedema, hyperaemia and haemorrhage, may progress to a chronic stage which is characterized by loss of papillae, depigmentation and the presence of star-shaped ulcers that heal by granulation and scar tissue formation.

Thrombophlebitis of the caudal vena cava is a possible sequel to hepatic abscessation and arises when a lesion extends into a hepatic vein. Caval thrombophlebitis **(see Pulmonary thrombo-embolism in cattle)** is accompanied in a large proportion of cases by pulmonary embolism, pneumonia, pulmonary abscessation or endocarditis.

Diagnosis and differential diagnosis

Liver abscesses are infrequently diagnosed in live animals. Acute clinical cases may be confused with acute peritonitis or traumatic reticuloperitonitis, while chronic cases may be confused with a number of conditions associated with chronic debility and emaciation. Pathologically, rumenitis caused by *F. necrophorum* must be differentiated from that caused by fungi, usually by members of the genera *Mucor*, *Rhizopus* and *Absidia* **(see Chapter 185: Mycoses)**. Mycotic rumenitis is a more severe, deeper (often involving the entire thickness of the rumen wall due to infarction) and extensive lesion, and is often fatal.[64] A definitive diagnosis of hepatic necrobacillosis rests upon histopathological confirmation or the isolation of *F. necrophorum* which may be difficult in cases in which the abscesses are of long duration,[41] and the use of selective media may have to be resorted to.

Control

The prevalence of rumenitis and the subsequent development of hepatic abscesses may be reduced by adapting cattle to high-concentrate–low-roughage rations gradually over a period of two to three weeks. Care should be taken that the feed does not contain foreign objects, such as nails, pieces of wire or glass. The inclusion of up to 1,2 per cent calcium carbonate in the diet of cattle in feedlots to counteract low pH levels reduces the occurrence of ruminal lesions to negligible levels. Though the addition of antimicrobial drugs to the diet may detrimentally affect rumen functions, the occurrence of liver abscesses can be reduced by continuous feeding, throughout the fattening process, of tylosine at a rate of 100 mg per animal per day or chlortetracycline or oxytetracycline at subtherapeutic dosage levels. The latter has the advantage of having a lesser effect on the rumen bacteria.

In individual animals, parenteral administration of antimicrobial drugs such as broad spectrum penicillin and ceftiofur may have a beneficial effect.[8] However, relapses are common after antimicrobial treatment, as most drugs are unable to penetrate the liver lesions.

OVINE AND CAPRINE HEPATIC NECROBACILLOSIS

Necrobacillosis occurs sporadically in sheep and goats but the predisposing factors and portals of entry have not been defined as clearly as in cattle. Necrobacillosis may occur in adults or in lambs and kids; in the latter it may be a consequence of umbilical infection. Lambs and kids kept in wet, intensive conditions are most commonly affected.

In sheep, *F. necrophorum* may be isolated as the only bacterium involved in up to 45 per cent of cases, or it may be isolated in association with other aerobic and anaerobic bacteria such as *A. pyogenes*, *Staphylococcus aureus*, *Pseudomonas aeruginosa*, *Bacteroides fragilis*, *Peptostreptococcus anaerobius*, *Escherichia coli* and *Clostridium perfringens*.[155] Abscesses caused by *F. necrophorum* in sheep livers are similar in appearance and nature to those in cattle, but contrary to the situation in cattle, biovar B is isolated more commonly than biovar A, and often in pure culture.[111] Lambs and kids that die of hepatic necrobacillosis are usually in good condition.

Goats affected by hepatic abscesses may develop septicaemia, which in pregnant does may result in abortion.

NECROTIC AND ULCERATIVE STOMATITIS AND LARYNGITIS

Synonyms: Calf diphtheria, oral necrobacillosis, kalwerdifterie (Afrik.)

Introduction, aetiology, epidemiology and pathogenesis

Calf diphtheria is a rare but frequently fatal, acute or chronic, non-contagious, infectious disease, characterized by localized, necrotic inflammation of the mucous membranes of the oral cavity, pharynx and/or larynx. Ulcers may develop in the later stages. It is usually a disease of young calves, but may be encountered in older cattle. A similar disease also occurs in sheep, goats and pigs.

When first described in calves in 1876 it was considered to be closely related to human diphtheria,[26] which is caused by *Corynebacterium diphtheriae*. However, Loeffler in 1884 proved that it was a distinct disease, and demonstrated that *Fusobacterium necrophorum*, found invariably along the borders of the lesions, is the cause. Jensen subsequently reported in 1903 that although the primary lesions usually appear in the mouth, metastatic lesions frequently develop in the lungs and result in bronchopneumonia and, in some animals, serofibrinous or purulent pleuritis.

The condition is widely distributed in the world and is most commonly found in malnourished, bucket-fed calves and those that are housed or closely confined.[56] Its prevalence is highest in young calves from a few weeks to a few months of age. Predisposing factors are poor hygiene, improper housing, neglect, improper and insufficient feeding, debilitating diseases, close confinement in dark, dirty, damp quarters,[56] and abrasions to the pharyngeal mucosa. It may also affect Boergoat kids grazing on vegetation consisting largely of thorny shrubs and species of grass containing large awns, which cause small injuries to the buccal and pharyngeal mucosa.[139]

Fusobacterium necrophorum is common in feedlot manure and soil, and in the mouth, forestomachs and intestines of healthy and diseased ruminants. The organism is unable to penetrate healthy, intact mucous membrane or skin, but it readily invades injured tissues to cause extensive necrosis. In calf diphtheria the marked inflammatory reaction in the mucosa, submucosa and deeper tissues of the pharynx and larynx often causes partial obstruction of the respiratory tract. Other sites at which lesions may arise are the tongue, gums, cheeks, palate, and dorsal angles of the larynx, and in the mucous membrane that covers the vocal processes of the arytenoid cartilages. In some animals lesions may be present in the trachea, nasal passages, oesophagus and forestomachs.

Consult **Anaerobic, Gram-negative, irregular rods: Introduction** for the general characteristics of *F. necrophorum*.

Clinical signs and pathology

The clinical signs of calf diphtheria depend on the location, extent and severity of the lesions. Initial signs include loss of appetite, listlessness, salivation, frequent sucking or swallowing movements and, in some affected animals, swelling of the cheek or throat regions. A purulent exudate may be discharged from the nostrils.[56] Depending on the extent of the necrosis and tissue involvement, the body temperature may rise to 41 °C, and loss of weight, due at least partially to profound anorexia, may be rapid. Animals suffering from laryngeal involvement breathe with difficulty and develop a cough. Respiration, especially during inspiration, is often noisy. More severely affected calves may be dyspnoeic. They extend their heads and necks in an effort to breathe, which they do through the mouth. Digital compression of the larynx or trachea usually evokes coughing and exaggerates the dyspnoea. Death may result from asphyxia. If lesions are present in the tongue or elsewhere in the oral cavity they may seriously interfere with feeding. In some cases the tongue may be swollen and protrude from the mouth.[56] The lesions impart an offensive odour to the breath. Exudate from lesions in the upper respiratory tract may be inhaled into the lungs, resulting in abscess formation and bronchopneumonia.[62]

The course of the disease varies from case to case. Some calves may recover spontaneously, but therapy is usually necessary in order to effect recovery. Death in untreated calves may occur in four or five days in the more acute disease, or the animal may live for another two to three weeks, eventually dying from toxaemia or pneumonia.[27] In chronic cases, although the appetite may improve to some extent during the course of the disease, body weight is gained only slowly.[62]

In the outbreaks of necrotic stomatitis in Boergoat kids that have been recorded in South Africa, the clinical signs and lesions were similar to those in calves.[139]

The initial lesions of calf diphtheria consist of one or more irregular, sharply circumscribed, whitish-grey areas of coagulative necrosis up to about 50 mm in diameter, which may be surrounded by a zone of hyperaemia. The necrotic material is raised slightly above the surrounding normal tissue and is firmly adherent to the underlying tissue, but as the disease progresses, some or all of it may slough, leaving deep ulcers which heal by granulation.[27]

Microscopically, the lesions consist of coagulation necrosis of the mucosa and submucosa of affected areas. Colonies of *F. necrophorum*, as well as other bacteria, are discernible particularly at the periphery of the lesions.

Highly pleomorphic *F. necrophorum* organisms, which are filamentous and non-branching, are present in acute, active lesions, while in chronic lesions they are coccoid and rod-shaped.

Diagnosis and differential diagnosis

The condition may be diagnosed on the basis of the clinical signs and characteristic appearance of the lesions in the oral cavity, pharynx or upper respiratory tract. The diagnosis can be confirmed by isolation of *F. necrophorum* from swabs of the lesions taken from live animals, or from specimens taken aseptically from the affected tissues at necropsy.

Similar clinical signs may be induced by abscesses caused by *A. pyogenes* or *Corynebacterium pseudotuberculosis* and acute or chronic pharyngitis caused by trauma that may be induced by dosing procedures, sharp objects in the feed, and, in piglets, erupting teeth or the removal of teeth as a managemental procedure.

Control

Calves may recover spontaneously, but debridement of the necrotic tissue is advisable, if possible, followed by local treatment with povidone iodine oral solution and parenteral antimicrobial treatment with oxytetracycline at 10 mg/kg or trimethoprim/sulphonamide combination at 1 ml/10 kg. It is advisable to continue therapy for three weeks.

In the control of calf diphtheria, strict attention should be given to the general principles of hygiene. The provision of coarse feed that may injure the oral mucous membrane should be avoided.

OTHER CONDITIONS CAUSED BY FUSOBACTERIUM NECROPHORUM, BACTEROIDES *SPP. AND MEMBERS OF RELATED GENERA*

Pulmonary thromboembolism in cattle

Pulmonary thromboembolism in cattle is one of the possible complications associated with hepatic abscessation caused by *Fusobacterium necrophorum* and other species of bacteria **(see Bovine hepatic necrobacillosis)**. It is a sporadic condition and is the sequel to the development of septic thrombophlebitis of the caudal vena cava or one of the larger branches of a hepatic vein, with subsequent involvement of the caudal vena cava. The thrombophlebitis arises most commonly by direct extension of the inflammatory process of a hepatic abscess located in close proximity to the blood vessel concerned, but it may similarly arise as a result of an abscess lying outside the liver, but adjacent to the caudal vena cava, such as one situated between the liver and the diaphragm.[115] Selman and his colleagues reviewed the clinical and pathological aspects of 12 cases of thromboembolism in cattle.[115] The thrombi which develop in the caudal vena cava may extend from the liver to the right atrium of the heart and may totally or partially occlude the vessel and result in chronic venous congestion of the liver. Septic thrombi dislodged from the thrombus metastasize to the lungs, where the principal lesions to develop are multiple pulmonary abscesses, suppurative pneumonia, and erosion of pulmonary arterial walls with intrapulmonary haemorrhage. In some cases the latter may be massive and prove to be fatal. An endocarditis may be present in a small percentage of animals.[141]

The history of the disease in affected animals varies from that of a 'sudden death' syndrome to one associated with a respiratory disease that has a course that varies in length from a few to more than 100 days. One or several of the following clinical signs may be manifested:[115] loss of weight, fever (not constant), tachypnoea, hyperpnoea, dyspnoea, widespread rhonci on auscultation, coughing, thoracic pain, tachycardia, evidence of cardiac failure, hepatomegaly, anaemic mucous membranes (as a result of pneumorrhagia), haemoptysis, and melaena (the result of swallowing blood from the lungs). The three most constant presenting signs of diagnostic value appear to be anaemia, haemoptysis and widespread rhonci, while thoracic pain and hepatomegaly are commonly encountered.[115] Death frequently takes place soon after pulmonary haemorrhage has occurred, but is usually preceded by respiratory signs of at least several days' duration.[115]

Necrotic rhinitis of pigs

Synonym: Bull nose

Necrotic rhinitis or bull nose is a disease of young, growing pigs characterized by severe, irregular, asymmetrical swelling and deformity of the snout and face as a result of localized necrosis, suppuration and connective tissue proliferation following infection of the soft and bony tissues of the region by *Fusobacterium necrophorum*, in some cases together with spirochaetes **(see Chapter 115: *Borrelia suilla* infection)** and other bacteria. The skin is usually intact.

Bacteria gain entry through injuries, which are often inconspicuous, to the oral and nasal mucosa or face. Bite wounds may play a role. A common portal of entry of organisms in piglets is the injury to the gums that may arise if the needle teeth are clipped too short,[116] spread to bony tissue with resultant osteitis occurring via gingival lymphatics.[64] The condition is also associated with unhygienic environmental conditions.

The prevalence of necrotic rhinitis in herds is generally low, with only one or two pigs being affected.[116] The disease is often accompanied by partial obstruction of the upper respiratory tract, which is accompanied by snuffling, sneezing, a foul-smelling nasal discharge and occasional epistaxis.[116] Loss of appetite, interference in mastication, loss of weight and death may occur. Some animals may show a purulent ocular discharge.[116]

The localized swelling is usually hard, and when incised reveals a mass of greyish, foul-smelling, necrotic tissue with massive connective tissue proliferation.[108, 116] Soft tissues, facial bones and sinuses are usually involved in the inflammatory process.

The treatment of early cases is by surgical intervention and the topical application of sulphonamides or tincture of iodine.[116] The oral administration of sulphadimidine has proved successful;[37] probably therapy with other antimicrobial drugs to which *F. necrophorum* is susceptible would have a similar result in controlling the infection if applied in the early stage of the disease. It is doubtful whether treatment of advanced cases is advisable.[116] Prevention lies in the general hygiene of piggeries. Great care should be taken in the clipping of needle teeth in herds where the disease occurs repeatedly.[116]

Necrotic rhinitis should be differentiated from progressive atrophic rhinitis **[see Chapter 121: *Bordetella bronchiseptica* infections (including atrophic rhinitis)]**. Pigs suffering from progressive atrophic rhinitis often show deviation of the snout but no swelling of the region.[116]

Foot rot in pigs

Foot rot in pigs is a term used to describe the disease which results when a lesion in the claw of a pig of any age becomes invaded by infectious agents.[128] The commonest claw lesions involved are a sandcrack (including false sandcrack) in the wall of a hoof; heel, toe and sole erosions; and a lesion of the white line.[98] Bruising of the heel-sole junction may precede the development of erosive lesions.[154] Common invading organisms are *Fusobacterium necrophorum, Actinomyces (Corynebacterium) pyogenes* and spirochaetes. Once the infection has gained entrance in a claw it may spread to the deeper tissues of the claw and neighbouring structures such as tendons, joints, ligaments and bone. Although all claws may be affected, lesions appears to be most common in the abaxial (lateral) claws of the hind feet.[98]

Factors which predispose to foot lesions are the abrasive effect of rough concrete floors, the chemical effects of newly laid concrete floors, poor bedding and damp, unhygienic conditions.[98, 128, 154]

Foot rot may spread rapidly and become a herd problem. The infection may be introduced into a piggery by infected pigs.

The affected claw is usually swollen, warm and painful. The degree of lameness depends on the extent of the lesions. Severe lameness is manifested when sinus tracts and abscesses break out at the coronet, and swelling due to cellulitis extends higher up the limb to reach the carpus or hock.[128] Pain and lameness may lead to production losses, while lameness in sows may cause clumsiness and bad mothering, and in boars lead to *impotentia coeundi*.[95, 98]

To control foot rot, possible predisposing causes should be prevented. Treatment of individual cases includes cleaning and surgical paring of hoof lesions, and topical and/or systemic administration of antimicrobial drugs. Exposing pigs to a footbath containing a 5–10 per cent solution of formalin or copper sulphate two or three times a week may reduce the prevalence of foot rot.[154] In addition, it should be ensured that the herd is not suffering from a biotin deficiency, as biotin supplementation to gilts in one trial resulted in fewer and less severe foot lesions.[97]

Cara inchada

Cara inchada (Portuguese for 'bulging face' or 'swollen face') is a progressive periodontal disease of young cattle aged mainly between two and 14 months. It occurs in central and northern Brazil, where in some regions it constitutes a serious economic problem.[20] In some herds the prevalence rate exceeds 50 per cent. Clinically it is characterized by a unilateral or bilateral bulging of the part of the face which is over the lesion in the maxilla or mandible. The lesion is a progressive periodontitis of one or more of the premolar or molar teeth, which leads to localized bone resorption with cavitation, proliferation of bone, and loosening and eventual loss of the tooth or teeth involved. Loss of teeth leads to malnutrition and occasionally to death.

The precise pathogenesis of cara inchada has not been elucidated. Several species of bacteria have been associated with the lesions, however. *Prevotella melaninogenica (Bacteroides melaninogenicus)*, in association with *Actinomyces (Corynebacterium) pyogenes, Bacteroides bivius, Fusobacterium nucleatum* and *Actinomyces israelii*, is consistently isolated from the lesions.[21] It has been suggested that enzymes and endotoxin produced by the bacteria are actively involved in the pathogenesis of the lesions. *Prevotella melaninogenica* produces deoxyribonuclease, collagenase, chondroitin sulfatase, fibrinolysin, gelatinase, hyaluronidase, lipase and protease.[30]

Removal of diseased cows and calves from a herd reduces the prevalence of the condition.[21] The bacterial species which have been isolated from the lesions are susceptible *in vivo* to penicillin, tetracycline and erythromycin.[20]

Other Bacteroides *spp. infections*

Bacteroides spp. are associated with different non-specific disease conditions in livestock.[16, 17, 19, 88, 125] For example, *Prevotella melaninogenica (Bacteroides melaninogenicus)* has been isolated from cattle suffering from phlegmon, traumatic pericarditis and peritonitis, suppurative arthritis or fibrinous pneumonia; from sheep with fibrinous pneumonia, polyarthritis, purulent rhinitis, septicaemic pasteurellosis or suppurative meningitis; from horses affected by pleuropneumonia and deep, draining wounds; and from pigs with preputial ulceration, pneumonia and enteritis. *Bacteroides fragilis* has been isolated from calves, lambs and foals with diarrhoea; from horses with pleuropneumonia and deep, draining wounds; and from pigs with preputial ulceration.

Species other than *P. melaninogenica* and *B. fragilis* that have been associated with equine pleuropneumonia are *B. oralis, B. asaccharolyticus, B. splanchnicus, B. uniformis, B. thetaiotaomicron, B. ruminicola* and an unnamed species.[125] Unnamed species have also been isolated from septic arthritis in horses[81] and a cerebral abscess in a heifer.[82]

The relatively high prevalence of *Bacteroides* spp. infections in pleuropneumonic lesions in horses indicates that specimens for both anaerobic and aerobic culture should be submitted from every horse with pleural effusion, irrespective of whether or not the specimen has a putrid odour.[125] The breath of such animals may also have a similar unpleasant odour.

Antimicrobial therapy of *Bacteroides* spp. infections should always be based on the result of an antibiogram[17] as well as on the nature and sensitivity of the other species of bacteria with which the organism is usually associated in the lesions. The results of aerobic cultures may dictate that a combination of drugs is necessary. In human medicine, metronidazole, chloramphenicol and clindamycin are routinely used against *B. fragilis* infections,[17] but penicillin is the drug of choice if the anaerobe is not *B. fragilis*.[17]

Prevotella melaninogenica, Fusobacterium necrophorum, Actinomyces pyogenes, Peptostreptococcus indolicus, and *Streptococcus dysgalactiae* are among the factors that have been implicated in the complex aetiology of summer mastitis in cattle.[80] For more information on summer mastitis, **Chapter 190: Mastitis** should be consulted.

References

1 **AALBAK, B., 1971.** *Sphaerophorus necrophorus.* A study of 23 strains. *Acta Veterinaria Scandinavica,* 12, 344–364.

2 **ALLWORTH, B., 1990.** Footrot—control and eradication. *In: Sheep Medicine,* Proceedings of the Sandy and Georgina Reid Memorial Refresher Course for Veterinarians, 16–20 July 1990, University of Sydney, Australia.

3 **AMSTUTZ, H.E., 1985.** Prevention and control of lameness in dairy cattle. *Veterinary Clinics of North America,* 1, 25–37.

4 **ARKINS, S., 1981.** Lameness in dairy cows. *Irish Veterinary Journal,* 35, 163–170.

5 **ARKINS, S., 1981.** Lameness in dairy cows. *Irish Veterinary Journal,* 35, 135–140.

6 **ARKINS, S., 1982.** Lameness: An often neglected factor in dairy cow health. *Farm and Food Research,* 13, 90.

7 **ATKINS, J.W., 1986.** The use of a zinc sulphate formulation for the eradication of footrot during a period favouring spread of the disease. *In:* STEWART, D.J., PETERSON, J.E., McKERN, N.M. & EMERY, D.L., (eds). *Footrot in Ruminants,* Proceedings of a workshop, Melbourne 1985, CSIRO Division of Animal Health, Australian Wool Corporation, Australia.

8 **BABA, E., FUKATA, T., ARAKAWA, A., IKAWA, H. & TAKEDA, M., 1989.** Antibiotic susceptibility of *Fusobacterium necrophorum* from bovine hepatic abscesses. *British Veterinary Journal,* 145, 195–197.

9 **BAGGOTT, E., 1982.** Hoof lameness in dairy cattle. *In Practice* (a supplement to *The Veterinary Record*), September, 133–141.

10 **BARBER, D.M.L., 1979.** Foot rot in sheep. *The Veterinary Record,* 104, 194–195.

11 **BASSET, H.F., MONAGHAN, M.L., LENHAN, P., DOHERTY, M.L. & CARTER, M.E., 1990.** Bovine digital dermatitis. *The Veterinary Record,* 126, 164–165.

12 **BATH, G. & BISHOP, G., 1984.** Allerton Regional Veterinary Laboratory, Private Bag X2, Cascades 3202, South Africa. Unpublished data.

13 **BAZELEY, K. & PINSETT, P.J.N., 1984.** Preliminary observations on a series of outbreaks of acute laminitis in dairy cattle. *The Veterinary Record,* 115, 619–622.

14 **BERG, J.N. & LOAN, R.W., 1975.** *Fusobacterium necrophorum* and *Bacteroides melaninogenicus* as etiologic agents of foot rot in cattle. *American Journal of Veterinary Research* 36, 1115–1122.

15 **BERG, J.N. & SCANLAN, C.M., 1982.** Studies of *Fusobacterium necrophorum* from bovine hepatic abscesses: Biotypes, quantitation, virulence, and antibiotic susceptibility. *American Journal of Veterinary Research* 43, 1580–1586.

16 **BERKHOFF, G.A., 1977.** Recovery and identification of anaerobes in veterinary medicine: A two-year experience. *Veterinary Microbiology,* 2, 237–252.

17 **BERNARD-STROTHER, S. & MANSMANN, R.A., 1985.** Diagnosis and treatment of anaerobic bacterial pleuropneumonia in six horses. *The Compendium on Continuing Education for the Practising Veterinarian,* 7, S341–S349.

18 **BEVERIDGE, W.I.B., 1941.** Foot rot in sheep: A transmissible disease due to infection with *Fusiformis nodosus* (n. sp.). Studies on its cause, epidemiology and control. *Bulletin of the Council for Scientific and Industrial Research of Australia,* 140, 1–53.

19 **BIBERSTEIN, E.L., KNIGHT, H.D. & ENGLAND, K., 1968.** *Bacteroides melaninogenicus* in diseases of domestic animals. *Journal of the American Veterinary Medical Association,* 153, 1045–1049.

20 **BLOBEL, H., DÖBEREINER, J., LIMA, F.G.F. & ROSA, I.V., 1984.** Bacterial isolations from 'cara inchada'-like lesions of cattle. *Pesquisa Veterinária Brasileira,* 4, 73–77.

21 **BLOBEL, H., DÖBEREINER, G., ROSA, I.V., LIMA, F.G.F. & DOS SANTOS DURA, I., 1987.** Bacterial investigations of a periodontal disease—cara inchada—in Brazilian cattle. *Tierärztliche Umschau,* 42, 152–157.

22 **CASEY, R.H. & MARTIN, P.A.J., 1988.** Effect of foot paring of sheep affected with footrot in response to zinc sulphate/sodium lauryl sulphate foot bathing treatment. *Australian Veterinary Journal,* 65, 258–259.

23 **CHETWIN, D.H., LAIRDET, D.M., KINGSLEY, D.F. & HINDMARSH, F.H., 1986.** The serological response in sheep to immunisation at varying intervals with a multistrain footrot vaccine. *In:* STEWART, D.J., PETERSON, J.E., McKERN, N.M. & EMERY, D.L., (eds). *Footrot in Ruminants,* Proceedings of a workshop, Melbourne, 1985. CSIRO Division of Animal Health, Australian Wool Corporation, Australia.

24 **CHOQUETTE-LEVY, L., BARIL, J., LEVY, M. & ST-PIERRE, H., 1985.** A study of foot disease of dairy cattle in Quebec. *Canadian Veterinary Journal,* 26, 278–281.

25 **CLARK, B.L., EMERY, D.L. & STEWART, D.J., 1986.** *In*: STEWART, D.J., PETERSON, J.E., McKERN, N.M. & EMERY, D.L., (eds). The aetiology and prevention of interdigital necrobacillosis (foot abscess) in cattle. Proceedings of a workshop, Melbourne, 1985. CSIRO Division of Animal Health, Australia, Wool Corporation, Australia.

26 **DAMMANN, C. 1876.** Die Diphtherie der Kalber eine neue, auf den Menschen übertraglare Zoonose. *Deutsch Zeitschrift für Tiermedizin und Vergleichende Pathologie*, 3, 1–27.

27 **DAVIES, G.O., 1947.** *Gaiger and Davies' Veterinary Pathology and Bacteriology*. 3rd edn. London: Baillière, Tindall & Cox.

28 **DEMERTZIS, P.N. & MILLS, C.F., 1973.** Oral zinc therapy in the control of infectious pododermatitis in young bulls. *The Veterinary Record*, 93, 219–222.

29 **DOHERTY, R.M., RILEY, J.L., BAETZ, A.L., *et al.*, 1975.** Physiologic studies of experimentally grain-engorged cattle and sheep. *American Journal of Veterinary Research*, 36, 833–835.

30 **DOS SANTOS DURA, I., KANOE, M. & BLOBEL, H., 1986.** Enzymatic and endotoxic activities of bacteria isolated from periodontal lesions of calves with 'cara inchada'. *Pesquisa Veterinária Brazileira*, 6, 59–63.

31 **EDWARDS, B., 1980.** Foot lameness in cattle. *In Practice*, 2, 25–31.

32 **EDWARDS, G.B., 1972.** Foot lameness in cattle. *Veterinary Annual*, 7–14.

33 **EGERTON, J.R., 1986.** Control and eradication of ovine footrot. *In*: STEWART, D.J., PETERSON, J.E., McKERN, N.M. & EMERY, D.L., (eds). *Footrot in Ruminants*. Proceedings of a workshop, Melbourne, 1985. CSIRO Division of Animal Health, Australian Wool Corporation, Australia.

34 **EGERTON, J.R. & PARSONSON, I.M., 1966.** Isolation of *F. nodosus* from cattle. *Australian Veterinary Journal*, 42, 425–429.

35 **EGERTON, J.R., ROBERTS, D.S., GRAHAM, N.P.H. & PARSONSON, I.M., 1966.** Ovine interdigital dermatitis and its relationship to foot-rot and foot abscess. *Australian Veterinary Journal*, 42, 440.

36 **EGERTON, J.R., ROBERTS, D.S. & PARSONSON, I.M., 1969.** The aetiology and pathogenesis of ovine foot-rot. I. A histological study of the bacterial invasion. *Journal of Comparative Pathology*, 79, 207–216.

37 **EIELAND, E. & FAANES, T., 1950.** *Actinomyces necrophorum* infection in suckling pigs and experiment on treatment with sulphamethazine. *Nordisk Veterinaermedicin*, 2, 204–208.

38 **EMERY, D.L., 1987.** Immunity against anaerobic bacterial infections. *Veterinary Immunology and Immunopathology*, 15, 1–57.

39 **EMERY, D.L., STEWART, D.J. & CLARK, B.L., 1984.** The comparative susceptibility of five breeds of sheep to foot-rot. *Australian Veterinary Journal*, 61, 85–88.

40 **EMERY, D.L., VAUGHAN, J.A., CLARK, B.L., DUFFY, J.H. & STEWART, D.J., 1985.** Cultural characteristics and virulence of strains of *Fusobacterium necrophorum* isolated from the feet of cattle and sheep. *Australian Veterinary Journal*, 62, 43–46.

41 **FALES, W.H. & TERESA, G.W., 1972.** A selective medium for the isolation of *Sphaerophorus necrophorus*. *American Journal of Veterinary Research*, 33, 2317–2321.

42 **FALES, W.H., WARNER, J.F. & TERESA, G.W. 1977.** Effects of *Fusobacterium necrophorum* leukotoxin on rabbit peritoneal macrophages *in vitro*. *American Journal of Veterinary Research*, 38, 491–495.

43 **FAYE, B. & LESCOURRET, F., 1989.** Environmental factors associated with lameness in dairy cattle. *Preventive Veterinary Medicine*, 7, 267–287.

44 **FREDERICK, L.D., 1943.** The economic and nutritional importance of bovine hepatic disturbances. *Journal of the American Veterinary Medical Association*, 102, 338–345.

45 **FRISCH, J.E., 1976.** The comparative incidence of foot rot in *Bos taurus* and *Bos indicus* cattle. *Australian Veterinary Journal*, 52, 228–229.

46 **GARCIA, M.M., NEIL, D.H. & McKAY, K.A., 1971.** Application of immunofluorescence to studies on the ecology of *Sphaerophorus necrophorus*. *Applied Microbiology*, 21, 809–814.

47 **GREENOUGH, P.R., 1980.** The conformation of cattle. *Bovine Practice*, 1, 20–34.

48 **GREENOUGH, P.R., 1987.** An illustrated compendium of bovine lameness. Part 1. *Modern Veterinary Practice*, January, 6–9.

49 **GREENOUGH, P.R., 1987.** An illustrated compendium of bovine lameness. Part 2. *Modern Veterinary Practice*, February, 94–97.

50 **GREENOUGH, P.R., 1987.** An illustrated compendium of bovine lameness. Part 3. *Modern Veterinary Practice*, March, 148–152.

51 **GREENOUGH, P.R., 1987.** An illustrated compendium of bovine lameness. Part 4. *Modern Veterinary Practice*, April, 216–220.

52 **GREENOUGH, P.R., 1990.** Observations on bovine laminitis. *In Practice*, July, 169–173.

53 **GREENOUGH, P.R. & VERMUNT, J.J., 1991.** Evaluation of subclinical laminitis in a dairy herd and observations on associated nutritional and management factors. *The Veterinary Record*, 128, 11–17.

54 **GREGORY, T.S., 1939.** Foot-rot in sheep. *Australian Veterinary Journal*, 15, 160–167.

55 **HAN, I.K., SEO, B.K., CHANG, K.J. & YOON, H.J., 1985.** Abattoir survey of liver abscesses in cattle in Korea. *Korean Journal of Veterinary Public Health*, 9, 17–24.

56 **HENNING, M.W., 1962.** *The Calf in Health and Disease*. Johannesburg: Central News Agency, Ltd.

57 **HINTON, D.G., 1991.** Eradication of actively spreading ovine footrot. *Australian Veterinary Journal*, 68, 118–119.

58 **HULL, B.L., 1993.** Diseases of the musculoskeletal system. *In*: HOWARD, J.L., (ed.). *Current Veterinary Therapy 3: Food Animal Practice*. Philadelphia: W.B. Saunders Company.

59 **ITABISASHI, T., YAMIYA, K., YAMAMOTIO, R. & SATOH, M., 1987.** Serum sialic acid levels in cattle inoculated with *Fusobacterium necrophorum*. *Japanese Journal of Veterinary Science*, 49, 673–680.

60 **JENSEN, R., CONNEL, W.E. & DEEM, A.W., 1954.** Rumenitis and its relation to rate of change of ration and the proportion of concentrate in the ration of cattle. *American Journal of Veterinary Research*, 15, 425–428.

61 **JENSEN, R., DEANE, H.M., COOPER, L.J., MILLER, V.A. & GRAHAM, W.R., 1954.** The rumenitis-liver abscess complex in beef cattle. *American Journal of Veterinary Research*, 15, 202–216.

62 **JENSEN, R. & MACKEY, D.R., 1971.** *Diseases of Feedlot Cattle*. Philadelphia: Lea & Febiger.

63 **JOHNSON, D.W., DOMMER, A.R. & KIGER, D.G., 1969.** Clinical investigations of infectious foot rot of cattle. *Journal of the American Veterinary Medical Association*, 155, 1886–1891.

64 **JUBB, K.V.F., KENNEDY, P.C. & PALMER, N., 1985.** *Pathology of Domestic Animals*. 3rd edn. San Diego: Academic Press, Inc.

65 **KANOE, M., 1990.** *Fusobacterium necrophorum* haemolysin in bovine hepatic abscess. *Journal of Veterinary Medicine*, 37, 770–773.

66 **KANOE, M., IMAGAWA, H. & TODA, M., 1975.** Distribution of *Fusobacterium necrophorum* in bovine alimentary tracts. *Bulletin of the Faculty of Agriculture, Yamaguti University*, 26, 161–172.

67 **KANOE, M., IMAGAWA, H., TODA, M. & SATO INOUE, M., 1976.** Bacteriology of bovine hepatic abscesses. *Japanese Journal of Veterinary Science*, 38, 263–268.

68 **KANOE, M., ISHII, T. & KAI, K., 1987.** Effects of *Fusobacterium necrophorum* leukocidin on bovine ruminal cell *in vitro*. *Microbios Letters*, 35, 119–123.

69 **KANOE, M., IZICHI, Y. & TODA, M., 1979.** Isolation of *Fusobacterium necrophorum* from bovine ruminal lesions. *Japanese Journal of Veterinary Science*, 40, 275–281.

70 **KANOE, M. & YAMANAKA, M., 1989.** Bovine platelet aggregation by *Fusobacterium necrophorum*. *Journal of Medical Microbiology*, 29, 13–17.

71 **KASARI, T.R., MARQUIS, H. & SCANLAN, C.M., 1987.** Septic arthritis and osteomyelitis in a bovine digit: A mixed infection of *Actinomyces pyogenes* and *Fusobacterium necrophorum*. *Cornell Veterinarian*, 78, 215–219.

72 **KOLB, V.E., 1979.** Ernährungsbiochemische und pathobiochemische Aspekte der Bildung und Resorption von Endotoxinen in den Vormägen, unter besonderer Berücksichtigung der Verhältnisse bei der Parakeratose, bei der Azidose und bei der Ausbildung von Leberabszessen. *Monatsschriftung für Veterinärmedizin*, 34, 914–918.

73 **LAING, E.A., EGERTON, J.R., 1978.** The occurrence, prevalence and transmission of *Bacteroides nodosus* infection in cattle. *Research in Veterinary Science*, 24, 300–304.

74 **LANGWORTH, B.F., 1977.** *Fusobacterium necrophorum*: Its characteristics and role as an animal pathogen. *Bacteriological Reviews*, 41, 373–390.

75 **LECHTENBERG, K.F., NAGARAJA, T.G., LEIPOLD, H.W. & CHENGAPPA, M.M., 1988.** Bacteriologic and histologic studies of hepatic abscesses in cattle. *American Journal of Veterinary Research*, 49, 58–62.

76 **MAAS, J., DAVIS, L.E., HEMSTEAD, C., BERG, J.N. & HOFFMAN, K.A., 1984.** Efficacy of ethylenediamine dihydriodide in the prevention of naturally occurring foot rot in cattle. *American Journal of Veterinary Research*, 45, 2347–2350.

77 **MACIVOR, K.M. de F. & HORAK, I.G., 1987.** Foot abscess in goats in relation to the seasonal abundance of adult *Amblyomma hebraeum* and adult *Rhipicephalus glabroscutatum* (Acari: Ixodidae). *Journal of the South African Veterinary Association*, 58, 113–118.

78 **MACKIE, R.I., GILCHRIST, F.M.C. & HEATH, S., 1984.** An *in vitro* study of ruminal microorganisms influencing lactate turnover and its contribution to volatile fatty acid production. *Journal of Agricultural Science, (Cambridge)*, 103, 37–51.

79 **MADIN, S.H., 1949.** A bacteriologic study of bovine liver abscesses. *Veterinary Medicine*, 44, 248–251.

80 **MADSEN, M., SORENSEN, G.H., AALBAEK, B., HANSEN, J.W. & BJORN, H., 1992.** Summer mastitis in heifers: Studies on the seasonal occurrence of *Actinomyces pyogenes*, *Peptostreptococcus indolicus* and Bacteroidaceae in clinical healthy cattle in Denmark. *Veterinary Microbiology*, 30, 243–255.

81 **MARTENS, R.G., AUER, J.A. & CARTER, K.C., 1986.** Equine pediatrics: Septic arthritis and osteomyelitis. *Journal of the American Veterinary Medical Association*, 188, 582–585.

82 **McCORMACK, J.E., 1973.** Papilledema related to left cerebral hemisphere abscess in a heifer. *Veterinary Medicine: Small Animal Clinician*, 68, 1249–1252.

83 **McFADYEAN, M.J., 1891.** Disseminated necrosis of the liver of the ox and sheep. *Journal of Comparative Pathology and Therapeutics*, 4, 346–353.

84 **MGASA, M.N., 1987.** Footrot in cattle in Morogoro, Tanzania. *Bulletin of Animal Health and Production in Africa*, 35, 332–335.

85 **MGASA, M.N., AMAYA-POSADA, G. & HESSELBOLT, M., 1984.** Pododermatitis aseptica diffusa (laminitis) in free range beef cattle in tropical Africa. *The Veterinary Record*, 115, 413–414.

86 **MORGAN, K., 1987.** Footrot. *In Practice*, July, 124–129.

87 **MURNANE, D., 1933.** Footrot in sheep. *Journal of the Council for Scientific and Industrial Research of Australia*, 6, 252–259.

88 **MYERS, L.L., SHOOP, D.S. & BYARS, T.D., 1987.** Diarrhea associated with enterotoxic *Bacteroides fragilis* in foals. *American Journal of Veterinary Research*, 48, 1565–1567.

89 **NAGARAJA, T.G., BARTLEY, E.E. & FINA, L.R., 1978.** Evidence of endotoxins in the rumen bacteria of cattle fed hay or grain. *Journal of Animal Science*, 47, 226–234.

90 **NAKAJIMA, Y., UEDA, H. & TAKEUCHI, S., 1988.** Synergistic effects of *Fusobacterium necrophorum* lipopolysaccharide, cytoplasmic and cultural supernatant fractions on induction of acute necrosis in rabbits. *American Journal of Veterinary Research*, 49, 125–129.

91 **NAKAJIMA, Y., UEDA, H., TAKEUCHI, S. & FUJIMOTO, Y., 1987.** The effects of *Escherichia coli* endotoxin as a trigger for hepatic infection in rabbits with *Fusobacterium necrophorum*. *Journal of Comparative pathology*, 97, 207–215.

92 **NEWSOM, L.E., 1938.** A bacteriologic study of liver abscesses in cattle. *Journal of Infectious Diseases*, 63, 232–233.

93 **NILSSON, S.A., 1963.** Clinical, morphological and experimental studies of laminitis in cattle. *Acta Veterinaria Scandinavica*, (supplement), 4, 124–139.

94 **NILSSON, S.A., 1966.** Recent opinions about causes of ulceration of the hoof in cattle. *Nordisk Veterinaermedicin*, 18, 241.

95 **OSBORNE, H.G., 1950.** Foot-rot in pigs. *Australian Veterinary Journal*, 26, 316–317.

96 **PARSONSON, I.M., EGERTON, J.R. & ROBERTS, D.S., 1967.** Ovine interdigital dermatitis. *Journal of Comparative Pathology*, 77, 309–313.

97 **PENNY, R.H.C., CAMERON, R.D.A., JOHNSON, S., KENYON, P.J., SMITH, H.A., BELL, A.W.P., COLE, J.P.L. & TAYLOR, J., 1980.** Foot rot of pigs: The influence of biotin supplementation on foot lesions in sows. *The Veterinary Record*, 107, 350–351.

98 **PENNY, R.H.C., OSBORNE, A.D. & WRIGHT, A.I., 1963.** The causes and incidence of lameness in store and adult pigs. *The Veterinary Record*, 75, 1225–1240.

99 **PETERSE, D.J., 1979.** Nutrition as a possible factor in the pathogenesis of ulcers of the sole in cattle. *Tijdschrift voor Diergeneeskunde*, 104, 966–970.

100 **PETERSEN, G.C. & NELSON, D.R., 1984.** Foot diseases in cattle: Part II. Diagnosis and treatment. *The Compendium of Continuing Education*, 5565–5573.

101 **RAUTENBACH, G.H., 1985.** The incidence of clinical cases in a peri-urban farm animal practice. *Journal of the South African Veterinary Association*, 56, 85–88.

102 **REBHUN, W.C. & PEARSON, E.G., 1982.** Clinical management of the bovine foot problems. *Journal of the American Veterinary Medical Association*, 181, 572–577.

103 **ROBERTS, D.S. & EGERTON, J.R., 1969.** The aetiology and pathogenesis of ovine foot-rot. II. The pathogenic association of *Fusiformis nodosus* and *F. necrophorum*. *Journal of Comparative Pathology*, 79, 217–227.

104 **REED, G.A., 1986.** The role of footrot vaccines in Australia. *In*: STEWART, D.J., PETERSON, J.E., McKERN, N.M. & EMERY, D.L., (eds). *Footrot in Ruminants*. Proceedings of a workshop, Melbourne, 1985. CSIRO Division of Animal Health, Australian Wool Corporation, Australia.

105 **ROBERTS, D.S., 1967**. The pathogenic synergy of *Fusiformis necrophorus and* Corynebacterium pyogenes. II. The response of *F. necrophorus* to a filterable product of *C. pyogenes*. *British Journal of Experimental Pathology*, 48, 674–679.

106 **ROBERTS, D.S., GRAHAM, N.P.H., EGERTON, J.R. & PARSONSON, I.M., 1968.** Infective bulbar necrosis (heel-abscess) of sheep, a mixed infection with *Fusiformis necrophorus* and *Corynebacterium pyogenes*. *Journal of Comparative Pathology*, 78, 1–8.

107 **ROBINSON, T.J., JASPER, D.E. & GUILBERT, H.R., 1951.** The isolation of *Spherophorus necrophorus* from the rumen together with some feedlot data on abscess and telangiectasis. *Journal of Animal Science*, 10, 733–741.

108 **RUNNELS, R.A., MONLUX, W.S. & MONLUX, A.W., 1960.** *Principles of Veterinary Pathology*. Ames, Iowa: Iowa State University Press.

109 **RUSSEL, A.M., ROWLANDS, G.J., SHAW, S.R. & WEAVER, A.D., 1982.** Survey of lameness in British dairy cattle. *The Veterinary Record*, 111, 155–160.

110 **RUSSELL, J.B. & HINO, T., 1985.** Regulation of lactate production in *Streptococcus bovis*: A spiralling effect that

contributes to rumen acidosis. *Journal of Dairy Science*, 68, 1712–1721.

111 **SCANLAN, C.M. & EDWARDS, J.F., 1990.** Bacteriological and pathologic studies of hepatic lesions in sheep. *American Journal of Veterinary Research*, 51, 363–366.

112 **SCANLAN, C.M., GARRET, P.D. & CAMPBELL, E.F., 1985.** Ovine contagious foot rot. *The Compendium on Continuing Education*, 7, S15–S18.

113 **SCANLAN, C.M. & HATHCOCK, T.L., 1983.** Bovine rumenitis-liver abscess complex: A bacteriological review. *Cornell Veterinarian*, 73, 288–297.

114 **SCOTT, G.B., 1988.** Lameness and pregnancy in Friesian dairy cows. *British Veterinary Journal*, 144, 273–281.

115 **SELMAN, I.E., WISEMAN, A., PETRIE, L. & PIRIE, H.M., 1974.** A respiratory syndrome in cattle resulting from thrombosis of the posterior vena cava. *The Veterinary Record*, 94, 459–466.

116 **SIEGMUND, O.H., 1979.** *The Merck Veterinary Manual*. 5th edn. Rahway, New Jersey: Merck Publishing Co.

117 **SIMON, P.C. & STOVELL, P.L., 1969.** Diseases of animals associated with *Sphaerophorus necrophorus*: Characteristics of the organism. *The Veterinary Bulletin*, 39, 311–315.

118 **SIMON, P.C. & STOVELL, P.L., 1971.** Isolation of *Sphaerophorus necrophorus* from bovine hepatic abscesses in British Columbia. *Canadian Journal of Comparative Medicine*, 35, 103–106.

119 **SMITH, G.R., BARTON, S.A. & WALLACE, L.M., 1987.** Further observations on the enhancement of the infectivity of *Fusobacterium necrophorum* by other bacteria. *Epidemiology and Infection*, 100, 305–310.

120 **SMITH, G.R., TILL, D., WALLACE, L.M. & NOAKES, D.E., 1989.** Enhancement of the infectivity of *Fusobacterium necrophorum* by other bacteria. *Epidemiology and Infection*, 102, 447–458.

121 **SMITH, G.R., WALLACE, L.M. & NOAKES, D.E., 1990.** Experimental observations on the pathogenesis of necrobacillosis. *Epidemiology and Infection*, 104, 73–78.

122 **SMITH, L.D.S., 1975.** *The Pathogenic Anaerobic Bacteria*. 2nd edn. Illinois: Charles C. Thomas.

123 **STEWART, D.J., CLARK, B.L. & JARRETT, R.G., 1984.** Differences between strains of *Bacteroides nodosus* in their effects on the severity of footrot, bodyweight and woolgrowth in Merino sheep. *Australian Veterinary Journal*, 61, 348–352.

124 **STEWART, D.J., PETERSON, J.E., VAUGHAN, J.A., CLARK, B.L., EMERY, D.L., CALDWELL, J.B. & KORTT, A.A., 1986.** Clinical and laboratory diagnosis of benign, intermediate and virulent strains of *Bacteroides nodosus*. *In*: STEWART, D.J., PETERSON, J.E., McKERN, N.M. & EMERY, D.L., (eds). *Footrot in Ruminants*. Proceedings of a workshop, Melbourne, 1985. CSIRO Division of Animal Health, Australian Wool Corporation, Australia.

125 **SWEENEY, C.R., DIVERS, T.J. & BENSON, C.E., 1985.** Anaerobic bacteria in 21 horses with pleuropneumonia. *Journal of the American Veterinary Medical Association*, 187, 721–724.

126 **SYMONS, L.E.A., 1978.** Experimental foot rot, wool growth, and body mass. *Australian Veterinary Journal*, 54, 362–363.

127 **TAKEUCHI, S., NAKAJIMA, Y. & HASHIMOTO, K., 1983.** Pathogenic synergism of *Fusobacterium necrophorum* and other bacteria in formation of liver abscess in BALB/c mice. *Japanese Journal of Veterinary Science*, 45, 775–781.

128 **TAYLOR, D.J., 1989.** *Pig Diseases*. Cambridge: The Burlington Press (Cambridge) Ltd.

129 **THEILER, A., 1911.** An infectious foot disease in sheep. *Veterinary Journal*, March, 659–663.

130 **THEILER, A. & ROBINSON, B.N., 1953.** Ticks in the South African Zoological Survey Collection. Part VIII. Six lesser-known African rhipicephalids. *Onderstepoort Journal of Veterinary Research*, 26, 93–136.

131 **THEILER, G., 1962.** The Ixodoidea parasites of vertebrates in Africa south of the Sahara (Ethiopian Region). Project S 9958. *Report to the Director of Veterinary Services, Onderstepoort*.

132 **THORLEY, C.M., CALDER, H.A. McL. & HARRISON, W.J., 1977.** Recognition in Great Britain of *Bacteroides nodosus* in foot lesions in cattle. *The Veterinary Record*, 100, 387.

133 **THOROLD, P.W., 1964.** Some common bacterial infections of sheep in South Africa. *Journal of the South African Veterinary Medical Association*, 35, 549–565.

134 **TODD, G.C. & KROOK, L., 1966.** Nutritional hepatic necrosis in beef cattle. Sawdust liver. *Pathologica Veterinaria*, 3, 379–400.

135 **TOUSSAINT-RAVEN, E., 1973.** Lameness in cattle and foot care. *Netherlands Journal of Veterinary Science*, 5, 2.

136 **TOUSSAINT-RAVEN, E. & CORNELISSE, J.L., 1971.** Specific contagious inflammation of the interdigital skin in cattle. *Veterinary Medical Review*, 2/3, 223–247.

137 **VAN TONDER, E.M., 1975.** Notes on some disease problems in Angora goats in South Africa. *Veterinary Medical Review*, 1/2, 109–138.

138 **VAN TONDER, E.M., 1983.** Foot infections and other conditions of small stock. *Ugqira*, 16, 19.

139 **VAN TONDER, E.M., KELLERMAN, G.E. & BOLTON, T.F.W., 1976.** An outbreak of diphtheria in boergoat kids. *Journal of the South African Veterinary Association*, 47, 123–124.

140 **VENNING, C.M., CURTIS, M.A. & EGERTON, J.R., 1990.** Treatment of virulent footrot with lincomyin and spectinomycin. *Australian Veterinary Journal*, 67, 258–260.

141 **WAGENAAR, G., 1963.** Trombose van de vena cava posterior bij het rund. *Tijdschrift voor Diergeneeskunde*, 88, 30–33.

142 **WALKER, J.B., 1990.** Two new species of tick from southern Africa whose adults parasitize the feet of ungulates: *Rhipicephalus lounsburyi* n. sp. and *Rhipicephalus neumanni* n. sp. (Ixodoidea, Ixodidae). *Onderstepoort Journal of Veterinary Research*, 57, 57–75.

143 **WALKER, R., 1990.** *Footrot Technical Information Manual*. 2nd edn. New South Wales Department of Agriculture and Fisheries, Australia.

144 **WEAVER, A.D., 1974.** Lameness in cattle: The interdigital space. *The Veterinary Record*, 95, 115–120.

145 **WEAVER, A.D., 1985.** Lameness in cattle—Investigational and diagnostic check lists. *British Veterinary Journal*, 141, 27–33.

146 **WEAVER, A.D., 1988**. Cattle foot problems. Part 1: Introduction and interdigital skin disease. *Agri-Practice*, 9, 34–38.

147 **WEAVER, A.D., 1988.** Cattle foot problems. Part 2: Diseases of the horn and corium. *Agri-Practice*, 9, 35–40.

148 **WEAVER, A.D., ANDERSON, L., DE LAISTRE BANTING, L., DEMERZIS, P.N., KNEZEVIC, P.F., PETERSE, D.J. & SANKOVIC, F., 1981.** Review of disorders of the ruminant digit with proposals for anatomical and pathological terminology and recording. *The Veterinary Record*, 108, 117–120.

149 **WEST, D.M. 1981.** A study of foot abscess in sheep. PhD thesis, Massey University, New Zealand.

150 **WEST, D.M., 1983.** Anatomical consideration of the distal interphalangeal joint of sheep. *New Zealand Veterinary Journal*, 31, 58–60.

151 **WEST, D.M., 1983.** Observations on an outbreak of foot abscess in sheep. *New Zealand Veterinary Journal*, 31, 71–74.

152 **WEST, D.M., 1989.** Foot abscess in sheep. *In*: EGERTON, J.R., YOUNG, W.K. & RUFFKIN, G.G., (eds). *Footrot and Foot Abscess of Ruminants*. CRC Press.

153 **WEST, D.M., 1990.** Foot abscess and other lameness problems of sheep. *In: Sheep Medicine*. Proceedings of the Sandy and Georgina Reid Memorial Refresher Course for Veterinarians, 16–20 July 1990, University of Sydney, Australia.

154 **WRIGHT, A.I., OSBORNE, A.D., PENNY, R.H.C. & GRAY, E., 1972.** Foot-rot in pigs: Experimental production of the disease. *The Veterinary Record*, 90, 93–99.

155 **ZIENAB EL-SAYED, M., EL-SEEDY, F.R., EL-BARDISY M., & KAMEL, M., 1991.** A bacteriological study of sheep liver abscesses. *Veterinary Medical Journal, Giza*, 39, 91–103.

GRAM-POSITIVE COCCI

The fifteen genera in this group of bacteria are diverse: all are Gram-positive, but they have few other characteristics in common. They vary in their oxygen requirements, with some being aerobic, while others are facultatively anaerobic or anaerobic. Other variable features include their reaction to the catalase test, whether or not they contain cytochromes, differences in their major fermentation products, and the nature of their peptidoglycan and cell wall components. According to these criteria, the Gram-positive cocci have been classified into two families, the Micrococcaceae (which contains the genus *Staphylococcus*) and the Deinococcaceae, as well as a host of genera, including the genus *Streptococcus,* that are not currently included in any specific family.[1] Only the genera *Staphylococcus* and *Streptococcus,* which are facultatively anaerobic, are of veterinary importance. Their taxonomic status, growth characteristics and the diseases they cause are contained in the introductory sections to the relevant chapters.

Reference

1 **SCHLIEFER, K.H., 1986.** Gram-positive cocci. *In:* SNEATH, P.H.A., MAIR, N.S., SHARPE, M.E. & HOLT, J.G., (eds). *Bergey's Manual of Systematic Bacteriology.* Vol. II Baltimore: Williams & Wilkens.

Staphylococcus *spp. infections*

M.M. Henton

Staphylococcus spp., which are classified in the family Micrococcaceae, are Gram-positive bacteria, some of which cause suppurative disease processes in animals and humans. Of the 19 species recognized at present **(Table 1)**,[9] only four (*Staphylococcus aureus, S. epidermidis, S. intermedius* and *S. hyicus* subsp. *hyicus*) are significant in livestock. These cause various suppurative infections, especially abscesses, mastitis and pyoderma **(Table 2)**. They occur as part of the normal microbial flora on the skin and mucous membranes of healthy humans and animals, and, to a lesser extent, in the environment.

The causation of lesions in the skin and mucous membranes by *Staphylococcus* depends on a number of factors, such as trauma, the immune status of the animal, disturbance of the normal microflora and whether or not the particular *Staphylococcus* strain produces certain toxins and enzymes.

Table 1 Currently recognized *Staphylococcus* spp.

Coagulase-positive (or variable) pathogens	
S. aureus	
S. intermedius	
S. hyicus subsp. *hyicus*	
Coagulase-negative opportunists or non-pathogens	
S. epidermidis group	*S. epidermidis*
	S. capitis
	S. warneri
	S. haemolyticus
	S. hominis
	S. saccharolyticus
S. saprophyticus group	*S. saprophyticus*
	S. cohnii
	S. xylosus
S. simulans group	*S. simulans*
	S. carnosus
S. sciuri group	*S. sciuri*
	(*S. lentus*)
Other unrelated species	*S. auricularis*
	S. caseolyticus
	S. gallinarum
	S. caprae

The family Micrococcaceae consists of four distantly related genera, namely *Micrococcus, Staphylococcus, Stomatococcus,* and *Planococcus*.[15] *Micrococcus* spp. are common in the environment and on skin but they are not regarded as pathogenic and are distinguished from *Staphylococcus* spp. only in that they are strict aerobes. *Stomatococcus mucilaginosus*, the only species in the genus, is a facultative anaerobe, as are *Staphylococcus* spp., but it differs from the latter by forming mucoid, adherent colonies on commonly used media such as blood tryptose agar. *Stomatococcus mucilaginosus* occurs on the mucous membranes of the oral cavity and upper respiratory tract of humans, and is an opportunistic pathogen. *Planococcus* spp. are found only in marine habitats, and in clams, shrimps and prawns.[10]

Staphylococcus spp. are Gram-positive cocci (0,8–1,0 μm in diameter), non-motile, facultatively anaerobic, and catalase-positive, and in pus they form clusters like bunches of grapes. They grow well on conventional culture media such as blood tryptose agar or nutrient agar, forming white to yellowish-orange, butyrous colonies, the colour being due to the production of a carotenoid pigment. The colonies of some species, especially *S. aureus*, may be surrounded by a zone of haemolysis, due to the effect of haemolysins, such as alpha and delta haemolysins, produced by them. The individual species of *Staphylococcus* are biochemically distinct **(Table 3)** and ferment sugars with the formation of acid but not gas.

Staphylococcus organisms are among the most resistant of the non-sporing bacteria to dehydration, are relatively heat-resistant (they are destroyed by a temperature of 60 °C maintained for 30 minutes), tolerate common disinfectants better than most other bacteria, and are generally resistant to many of the commonly used antimicrobial drugs.[12]

Staphylococcus, depending on the species, may be ubiquitous or may occupy very specific ecological niches. An example is *S. epidermidis*, which inhabits the skin of mammals, especially humans and domestic animals. Its preferred site is the skin close to natural openings, where it is well placed to opportunistically infect adjacent organs such as the udder **(see Chapter 190: Mastitis)** or

Table 2 Most common diseases caused by *Staphylococcus* spp. in livestock

STAPHYLOCOCCUS SPP.	DISEASE	ANIMAL SPECIES AFFECTED
Staphylococcus aureus	Mastitis	Cattle, sheep, goats
	Botryomycosis	Horses, cattle, pigs
	Suppurative wound infections	All livestock species
	Abscesses	All livestock species
	Tick pyaemia	Lambs
S. hyicus subsp. *hyicus*	Exudative epidermitis (greasy pig disease)	Pigs
	Polyarthritis	Pigs
S. epidermidis	Causes no specific disease entity: occurs on normal skin (opportunistic pathogen)	Wide variety of animal species and humans

to cause wound infections. In contrast, *S. saccharolyticus* is only found on the skin of the human forehead and *S. auricularis* in the external auditory meatus of humans, while *S. gallinarum* occurs on the skin of poultry, and *S. lentus* on the skin of goats and sheep.[9]

Phage-typing and biochemical differences are used to differentiate between biotypes of *S. aureus*,[3, 8, 13, 18] of which four are now recognized. These are *S. aureus* biovar A (human), biovar B (porcine), biovar C (bovine and ovine) and biovar D (hares). The biovars previously referred to as E and F are not species-specific (dogs, pigeons, mink and horses), and are now considered to be *S. intermedius*.[7, 8] Reference to coagulase-positive *S. aureus* strains in the older literature may include *S. intermedius*.

The cell wall of *Staphylococcus* spp. contains peptidoglycan, in which L-lysine is the diamino acid, and teichoic acid.[9] *Staphylococcus aureus* also contains a small basic protein, protein A, in its cell wall, that reacts with the Fc fragment of the IgG molecules, and is antiphagocytic and fixes complement.[16]

Various toxins and enzymes are produced by *S. aureus* but, with the exception of the exfoliative toxin produced by *S. hyicus* subsp. *hyicus*, few, if any, toxins or enzymes are produced by the other *Staphylococcus* spp. Toxins produced by *S. aureus* include haemolysins (alpha, beta, gamma and delta), leukocidin and enterotoxin. The alpha haemolysin is dermonecrotic and leukocidal, and produces complete haemolysis of erythrocytes of rabbits, sheep and cattle, but it has no effect on those of humans and horses.[1] This haemolysin is thought to play a major role in the pathogenesis of blue udder or gangrenous mastitis in sheep, not only because of its haemolytic and leukocidal effects, but also because it destroys blood platelets and causes vasoconstriction.[2] The beta haemolysin is unique to animal biotypes of *S. aureus*. It is a sphingomyelinase C and produces incomplete haemolysis of sheep and bovine erythrocytes, but it does not affect those of horses when incubated at 37 °C. Complete haemolysis does, however, occur when cultures containing horse red blood cells are stored at 4–15 °C after being incubated.[17] The gamma haemolysin only produces weak haemolysis, while the delta haemolysin is a phospholipase with effects similar to those of alpha haemolysin in that it causes haemolysis of erythrocytes of humans, sheep, rabbits, guinea-pigs and horses, and is also leukocidal and dermonecrotic.

Many strains of *S. aureus* produce heat-stable enterotoxins, which, when ingested by humans in food, cause food poisoning manifested by gastroenteritis. Six (A–F) serologically distinct enterotoxin types are recognized. The enterotoxin types produced do not correspond to *S. aureus* biotypes, which are also alphabetically named. About 40 per cent of human strains produce enterotoxin.[5] Enterotoxin-producing strains of *S. aureus* may produce

Table 3 Characteristics that differentiate the pathogenic *Staphylococcus* spp.[9]

CHARACTERISTIC	*S. AUREUS*	*S. EPIDERMIDIS*	*S. INTERMEDIUS*	*S. HYICUS* SUBSP. *HYICUS*
Pigment	+w	–	–	–
Haemolysis	+	–w	d	–
Maltose	+	+	w	–
Mannitol	+	–	d	–
Coagulase	+	–	+	d
Clumping factor	+	–	d	–
Deoxyribonuclease	+	–w	+	+

\+ 90 per cent or more strains positive
– 90 per cent or more strains negative
d 11–89 per cent of strains positive
w weak reaction

more than one type of enterotoxin. Strains of *S. aureus* that produce enterotoxin A, or both enterotoxins A and B are responsible for about 70 per cent of outbreaks of food poisoning.[6] Enterotoxins are relatively heat-resistant proteins, and the usual boiling of food inactivates them slowly, e.g. enterotoxins A and B are both slowly inactivated at 100 °C, requiring between 10 and nearly 40 minutes depending on the concentration of the toxin and the substrate,[5] but temperatures used in canning food usually destroy any enterotoxin present. Enterotoxins can withstand the action of proteases such as trypsin and chymotrypsin.[5] Strains implicated in food poisoning should be examined for enterotoxin production.[9]

Enterotoxin is optimally produced in foods which can support satisfactory growth of the contaminating *S. aureus* strain at a temperature of 35–40 °C; lesser amounts are produced at lower temperatures.[6] Milk of mastitic cows infected with *S. aureus* may contain enterotoxins and may therefore cause food poisoning in humans who consume it **(see Chapter 190: Mastitis)**.

Certain strains of *S. aureus* may also produce a number of other enzymes, including coagulase, deoxyribonuclease, hyaluronidase, fibrinolysin, lipase and protease. The presence of coagulase and deoxyribonuclease correlates positively with virulence of the bacterium and is used for identification purposes.[9] Hyaluronidase,[4] fibrinolysin (staphylokinase) which causes the lysis of thrombi by activating plasminogen, and protease enhance the spread of *Staphylococcus* in tissues, while the lipase degrades bacterial fatty acids on the skin.[12]

Coagulase has the ability to clot plasma prepared from blood which has been treated with an anticoagulant such as heparin, EDTA or oxalate. Two forms of coagulase are produced: bound coagulase or clumping factor, which is produced by *S. aureus* and most strains of *S. intermedius*, and free coagulase, which is produced by *S. aureus*, *S. intermedius* and some strains of *S. hyicus* subsp. *hyicus*.[9, 14] Bound coagulase is detected by a slide test, while free coagulase is detected by a tube test. The slide test is usually used as a screening test as it is rapidly performed, and the tube coagulase test is regarded as the definitive test. Rabbit or human plasma is used and must always be tested with known coagulase-positive and -negative strains before being put into general use, as the plasma from certain individuals may not react correctly in the test.[11] The coagulase test should be carried out under carefully standardized conditions to ensure optimal results.[9, 11]

References

1 **ARBUTHNOTT, J.P., 1970.** Staphylococcal alpha-toxin. *In*: MONTIE, T.C., KADIS, S. & AJL, S.J., (eds). *Microbial Toxins*. Vol. III. New York, London: Academic Press, Inc.

2 **BROWN, R.W. & SHERER, R.K., 1958.** A study of the necrotising action of staphylococci alpha toxin. *American Journal of Veterinary Research*, 19, 354–362.

3 **DAVIDSON, I., 1961.** A set of bacteriophages for typing bovine staphylococci. *Research in Veterinary Science*, 2, 396 – 407.

4 **DURAN-REYNALS, F., 1942.** Tissue permeability and the spreading factors in infection. *Bacteriological Reviews*, 6, 197–252.

5 **EASMON, C.S.F. & GOODFELLOW, M., 1990.** *Staphylococcus* and *Micrococcus*. *In*: PARKER, M.T. & COLLIER, L.H., (eds). *Topley and Wilson's Principles of Bacteriology, Virology and Immunity*. 8th edn. London: Edward Arnold.

6 **GILBERT, R.J., ROBERTS, D. & SMITH, G., 1984.** Food-borne diseases and botulism. *In*: WILSON, G.S., MILES, A.A. & PARKER, M.T., (eds). *Topley and Wilson's Principles of Bacteriology, Virology and Immunity*. 7th edn. Bacterial Diseases. London: Edward Arnold.

7 **HÁJEK, V., 1976.** *Staphylococcus intermedius*, a new species isolated from animals. *International Journal of Systematic Bacteriology*, 26, 401–408.

8 **HÁJEK, V. & MARSÁLEK, E., 1971.** The differentiation of pathogenic staphylococci and a suggestion for their taxonomic classification. *Zentralblatt für Bakteriologie, Parasitenkunde, Infectionskrankheiten und Hygiene*, Abteilung 1 Original A 217, 176–182.

9 **KLOOS, W.E. & SCHLEIFER, K.H., 1986.** Genus IV. *Staphylococcus*. *In*: SNEATH, P.H.A., MAIR, N,S., SHARPE, M.E. & HOLT, J.G., (eds). *Bergey's Manual of Systematic Bacteriology*. Vol. II. Baltimore: Williams & Wilkins.

10 **KOCUR, M., 1986.** Genus III. *Planococcus*. *In*: SNEATH, P.H.A., MAIR, N.S., SHARPE, M.E. & HOLT, J.G., (eds). *Bergey's Manual of Systematic Bacteriology*. Vol. II. Baltimore: Williams and Wilkins.

11 **MACFADDIN, J.F., 1980.** *Biochemical Tests for Identification of Medical Bacteria*. 2nd edn. Baltimore: Williams & Wilkins.

12 **PARKER, M.T., 1983.** *Staphylococcus* and *Micrococcus*; the anaerobic Gram-positive cocci. *In*: PARKER, M.T., (ed.). *Topley and Wilson's Principles of Bacteriology, Virology and Immunity*. 7th edn. London: Edward Arnold.

13 **PARKER, M.T., 1983.** The significance of phage-typing patterns in *Staphylococcus aureus*. *In*: EASMON, C.S.F. & ADLAM, C., (eds). *Staphylococci and Staphylococcal Infections*, London: Academic Press, Inc.

14 **PHILLIPS, W.E. & KLOOS, W.E., 1981.** Identification of coagulase-positive *Staphylococcus intermedius* and *Staphylococcus hyicus* subsp. *hyicus* isolates from veterinary clinical specimens. *Journal of Clinical Microbiology*, 14, 671–673.

15 **SCHLEIFER, K.H., 1986.** Gram-positive cocci. *In*: SNEATH, P.H.A., MAIR, N.S., SHARPE, M.E. & HOLT, J.G., (eds). *Bergey's Manual of Systematic Bacteriology*. Vol. II. Baltimore: Williams & Wilkins.

16 **SJOQUIST, J., MOVITZ, J., JOHANSSON, I-B. & HJELM, H., 1972.** Localization of Protein A in the bacteria. *European Journal of Biochemistry*, 30, 190 –194.

17 **TIMONEY, J.F., GILLESPIE, J.H., SCOTT, F.W. & BARLOUGH, J.E., 1989.** *Hagan and Bruner's Microbiology and Infectious Diseases of Domestic Animals*. 8th edn. Ithaca, London: Comstock Publishing Associates.

18 **WANG, C.T., 1978.** Bacteriophage typing of canine staphylococci. I. Typing by use of the international phage sets for human and bovine staphylococci. *Japanese Journal of Veterinary Science*, 40, 401–405.

146

Staphylococcus aureus *infections*

M.M. Henton

Introduction

Staphylococcus aureus is a commensal bacterium of animals and humans that most commonly occurs on the skin and in the nasopharynx, but may also be present in the alimentary and genital tracts.[18] It is a potential pathogen and may cause a range of pyogenic conditions, the major one in livestock being mastitis in cattle, sheep and goats. Other conditions for which it is periodically responsible include tick pyaemia of lambs;[11] chronic pyogranulomatous inflammation known as 'botryomycosis' which may occur in horses, cattle and pigs; folliculitis and furunculosis in horses, goats and sheep;[12] pyoderma in goats, piglets and cattle;[9] staphylococcal dermatitis in sheep (also known as facial or periorbital eczema[10]); polyarthritis in young animals; impetigo or subcorneal pustular dermatitis of piglets; and dermatitis of the udder in goats.[17] Wounds may become infected with *S. aureus*, and it may play a primary or secondary role in a great variety of infections. These include purulent bronchopneumonia and pyothorax, osteomyelitis, salpingitis and abscess formation. In addition, many strains of *S. aureus* are an important cause of food poisoning in humans.[18]

Staphylococcus aureus of cattle, pigs, horses, poultry and humans can be distinguished from each other, and may be regarded as representing different ecovars (or biovars).[18]

Some of the conditions mentioned above, and of which *S. aureus* is the cause, are discussed below. Mastitis caused by *S. aureus* (except for botryomycotic mastitis) is dealt with in **Chapter 190: Mastitis**.

TICK PYAEMIA OF LAMBS

Synonym: Cripples

Tick pyaemia of lambs is a pyogenic staphylococcal infection of two- to ten-week-old animals reported in the United Kingdom and Ireland, resulting from infestation with the tick, *Ixodes ricinus*. Affected animals often suffer concurrent tick-borne fever caused by *Cytoecetes phagocytophila* **(see Chapter 36: Lesser-known rickettsias infecting livestock)**.[2, 23] The syndrome has not been reported in southern Africa.

Staphylococcus aureus appears to be transmitted by *I. ricinus*, although the process would seem to be purely mechanical: the bacteria enter the skin of lambs via the wounds produced by the mouth parts of infected ticks. From these primary sites of infection the bacteria spread haematogenously to localize in many organs and tissues of the body, particularly the joints, where they produce a suppurative inflammatory reaction.

As only young lambs between two and ten weeks of age are affected, it seems probable that an acquired immunity to *S. aureus* develops in older animals.[11] It appears that tick-borne fever, though it is usually a mild disease, may predispose to the development of tick pyaemia by the suppression of the humoral and cell-mediated immune responses which occur during the course of the disease.[1] Additionally, the parasites also infect neutrophils, thus further impairing the defence against infection with *S. aureus*.[11]

The disease occurs most often on hill farms in Scotland, Wales, north-east England and Ireland, and can result in serious economic losses. Prevalence rates as high as 29 per cent have been reported on some farms, although they are generally less than this; a figure of about 5 per cent is usual on farms on which the disease occurs.[11]

The most commonly recognized forms of tick pyaemia are characterized by the development of suppurative polyarthritis that results in lameness (crippling) and multiple abscesses in other organs and tissues, or of vertebral abscessation with pressure on the spinal cord and consequent paresis or paralysis. Abscesses may, however, develop in virtually any organ or tissue, resulting in lambs which are thin, dull and unthrifty, or even in sudden death if one of the vital organs is involved.[11]

Conditions such as joint ill (both suppurative and non-suppurative polyarthritides), lameness caused by foot rot, foot abscess or toe abscess **[see Chapter 145: *Fusobacterium necrophorum, Dichelobacter* (*Bacteroides*) *nodosus* and *Bacteroides* spp. infections]**, nutritional muscular dystrophy (white muscle disease), ill-thrift, and tick paralysis should be considered in the differential diagnosis of tick pyaemia.

The treatment of lambs suffering from tick pyaemia is often disappointing, as by the time the disease is noticed, lesions are well advanced and irreparable damage has occurred.[11] The control of the disease is primarily dependent upon the control of the vector tick. Alternatively, holding ewes and their lambs in a fenced, tick-free—or relatively tick-free—pasture until the lambs are about six weeks old is effective. In addition, suppression of either the *S. aureus* or *C. phagocytophila* infections by the administration of long-acting antibiotics to which the organisms are susceptible may reduce the prevalence of tick pyaemia.[2, 11] Long-acting benzathine penicillin given to lambs at three weeks of age produced a marked decrease in the prevalence of tick pyaemia, while long-acting tetracycline protected them against experimental tick-borne fever for about three weeks.[2]

STAPHYLOCOCCAL DERMATITIS IN SHEEP

Synonyms: Facial or periorbital eczema, facial dermatitis, necrotic or ulcerative dermatitis

An apparently contagious purulent dermatitis, frequently termed facial or periorbital eczema, which affects mainly the face of sheep and which is associated with infection by some strains of *S. aureus,* has been described in the United Kingdom, particularly Scotland.[15] The disease has been reviewed by Martin.[10]

The term 'facial eczema' used for this disease is a misnomer and should not be used, as this name is more generally reserved for the form of photosensitization of unpigmented skin that is caused by the hepatotoxic mycotoxin sporidesmin, which is elaborated by the fungus *Pithomyces chartarum*.[15] The term 'periorbital eczema' is also inappropriate, as the condition is not eczematous according to the strict definition of the word.[15]

A form of staphylococcal folliculitis and furunculosis has been encountered in sheep and goats in South Africa in association with the bites of *Simulium* flies (black flies).[19] Lesions occur on the parts of the body that are not covered by wool—chiefly the face and pinnae, but also the perineum. Papules develop which may give rise to pustules, ulceration and scab formation. Healing lesions may be confused with ringworm.

While staphylococci are commensal bacteria on the skin and in the nose, mouth and vagina of sheep,[10, 22] it is not known whether dermatopathogenic strains are frequent or regular inhabitants of the skin.[10] Numerous organisms are present in the exudate of the lesion in staphylococcal dermatitis, and it appears that strains of the staphylococci isolated from cases of the disease are more pathogenic for the skin than those that cause other conditions in sheep.[10] Such dermatopathogenic strains are coagulase-positive, produce alpha and beta haemolysins, and most also elaborate delta haemolysin. However, no other characteristics which could specifically identify them have been established. Although it appears that the staphylococci are the primary pathogens, mixed infections with a variety of other bacteria are quite common.[10]

The pathogenesis of the condition is not known, but it is thought that the bacteria gain entrance to the skin through minor injuries; the skin of the head may be subjected to more infection because it is not protected by wool. Close contact during feeding seems to facilitate the spread of infection between sheep.[15] The history is frequently that of sheep being fed from troughs, and it is possible that head-to-head contact during feeding, particularly in overcrowded conditions, could cause skin abrasions which then become invaded by the staphylococci.

The disease is more prevalent in adult sheep, although younger animals may occasionally be affected. As many as 50 per cent of the animals in affected flocks may develop the disease over a period of several months.[10] The lesions are generally confined to the woolless parts of the head, particularly the skin over bony prominences. Common sites are around the eyes and ears, the pinnae of the ears, over the nasal and maxillary bones, and at the base of the horns, where irregularly shaped, deep, suppurative ulcers, 10–60 mm in diameter, form at one or more of these sites. They are covered with blackish scabs and surrounded by inflamed zones of alopecic and thickened skin. These lesions exude pus and bleed easily, the blood and exudate adhering to the surrounding skin. Some sheep have red, thickened areas of skin which exude a serous fluid. Severely affected sheep are said to present an 'alarming and distressing' appearance, but the disease does not appear to cause systemic disturbances.[16] Infections that spread to involve an eye may result in blindness. On rare occasions, ulcerative dermatitis in sheep can involve only the legs (particularly the skin adjacent to the coronary bands)[20] or teats.[5] Healing of the skin lesions is by scar tissue formation and in individual animals takes place slowly over a period of five to six weeks. It commences at the periphery and in the depth of the ulcers. Recovered sheep do not seem to develop immunity against reinfection,[4] and the disease may reappear in affected flocks in consecutive years.[10]

Staphylococcal skin lesions of lesser severity may manifest only as folliculitis in early post-natal lambs.[13] The lesions in these animals are confined to one or more of the hairless sites of the body, which include the lips, especially the anterior aspect of the upper lips, around the nostrils, the ventral aspect of the tail, perineum, and near the teats.

In the differential diagnosis of staphylococcal dermatitis, orf **(see Chapter 54: Orf)** and dermatophilosis **(see Chapter 176: Dermatophilosis)** should be considered. In the case of staphylococcal dermatitis, removal of a scab reveals a deep ulcer, whereas in orf the scabs cover areas of granulation tissue.[16] Dermatophilosis can be distinguished from staphylococcal dermatitis by making a smear of the exudate below the crusts and by demonstrating *Dermatophilus congolensis* after the smear has been stained with Giemsa or other suitable strains.

In order to control the disease, affected sheep should be isolated and treated and, if trough feeding is practised, provision of adequate trough-space for each individual must be ensured so that head bumping is minimized.[10] Isolates of the causative organism are sensitive to most antibiotics, and affected sheep can be treated either by topical application of an antibiotic together with other accepted forms of wound therapy or, in serious cases, by topical therapy combined with parenteral antibiotic administration.[10]

BOTRYOMYCOSIS

Botryomycosis is a chronic, localized, pyogranulomatous condition of horses, cattle, pigs, dogs, cats and humans that is caused by several species of bacteria, most commonly staphylococci. The term botryomycosis is technically erroneous.[14] Etymologically it is derived from the Greek word *botrys*, meaning a bunch of grapes, and 'mycosis' because it was originally thought to be caused by a fungus. The use of the term has persisted because of the close clinical and histopathological resemblance of the disease to fungal granulomas.[3]

Most reported cases of botryomycosis are caused by *S. aureus*, but *Escherichia coli*, *Pseudomonas aeruginosa*, *Actinobacillus lignieresii*, species of *Bacteroides*, *Streptococcus* and *Proteus*, and *Actinobacillus equuli*[3, 14] have also been implicated. The lesion caused by *A. lignieresii* in the bovine tongue ('wooden tongue') **(see Chapter 136: *Actinobacillus lignieresii* infections)** is actually a form of botryomycosis, as is the chronic granulomatous mastitis caused by *S. aureus* in cows, sows and mares.[3, 9]

Well-known botryomycotic conditions are 'scirrhous cord' (from scirrhus = hard, indurated growth with predominance of fibrous tissue) which is a chronic, persistent funiculitis resulting from the bacterial contamination of the incised end of the spermatic cord following castration, particularly of horses **(Figure 146.1)** and pigs; 'breast boil' in horses; and chronic staphylococcal mastitis in cows and sows.

Lesions of botryomycosis generally involve the skin and adjacent tissues, but also the viscera. Grossly botryomycotic lesions consist of single or multiple firm nodules or tumorous growths which contain pockets of pus of varying sizes, and suppurative tracts. They frequently ulcerate and exude pus in which small granules, such as those found in certain mycoses, may be just visible to the naked eye as whitish or yellowish grains.[9, 14] Some lesions, such as those of scirrhous cord in geldings, may become very large. Histologically the granules consist of masses of bacteria surrounded by eosinophilic material, known as Splendore-Hoeppli material, from which

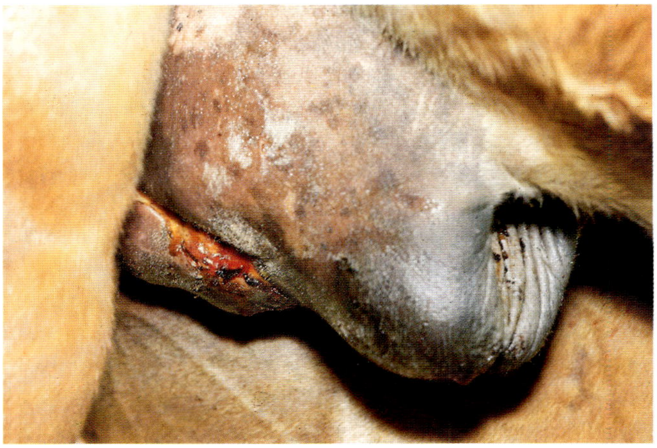

Figure 146.1 Scirrhous cord in a horse caused by *Staphylococcus aureus* infection following castration. Note swelling of the prepuce and protrusion of granulation tissue through the incision. (By courtesy of Prof. R.D. Gottschalk, Department of Surgery, Faculty of Veterinary Science, University of Pretoria, Onderstepoort)

club-like bodies sometimes radiate at the periphery. This material probably represents glycoprotein antigen-antibody complexes and stains positively with the periodic-acid Schiff stain.[9] The cell reaction generally consists of varying proportions of neutrophils, epithelioid cells, macrophages, lymphocytes, plasma cells and, in some, giant cells. There is often exuberant fibroplasia.

Predisposing causes of scirrhous cord in horses subsequent to castration are the spermatic cord being cut too close to the testicle, resulting in the protrusion of the cord through the scrotal wound after the operation; undue tension on the cord during the procedure; and adherence of the edge of the scrotal wound to the incised end of the cord.[6, 7] The lesion, which consists of a firm, irregular, cauliflower- or mushroom-like (hence its French name of champignon) mass of connective tissue permeated by small abscesses and purulent sinus tracts, continues to expand slowly in size over many months or even years. In horses, it may attain the size of a human head. The lesion may extend into the inguinal canal, assuming the shape of a cone, and even into the abdominal cavity, or it may hang down from the scrotum, sometimes reaching the hocks. Alternatively it may fill the scrotal sac, giving the impression that the animal still possesses a testicle. Pus discharges intermittently from the mass. Extensive adhesions develop between the growth and normal surrounding tissues and hamper surgical intervention, which is usually accompanied by severe haemorrhage. Well-developed lesions are associated with pain, fever and loss of condition.[6, 7]

The condition in horses known as 'breast boil' is encountered particularly in draught animals and is essentially a botryomycotic myositis of the neck and pectoral regions.[9] The organisms gain entrance to the muscles through skin lesions caused by ill-fitting harnesses. This results in typical botryomycotic lesions, with swelling of the affected part which slowly enlarges until it interferes with the horse's work. The skin over the lesion becomes tense and eventually ruptures, with pus being discharged. The swelling may then subside to some extent and the skin wound heals. The swelling recurs and the whole process is periodically repeated, with the muscle lesion progressively increasing in size.[8]

The definitive diagnosis of botryomycosis rests on the results of bacteriological and histopathological examination of the lesions. In the latter case, the application of special staining techniques may be required **(Figure 146.2)**. Botryomycotic granulomas have an identical macroscopic appearance to those of eumycotic mycetomas **(see Chapter 185: Mycoses)** caused by true fungi, and granulomas caused by *Actinomyces* and *Nocardia* spp.[3]

The location of the lesions in botryomycosis often presents difficulties in its treatment, because simple surgical drainage of the lesions and the systemic administration of antimicrobial drugs are usually ineffective.[14] The Splendore-Hoeppli material that surrounds the bacterial colonies and the granulomatous reaction with its large component of fibrous connective tissue apparently impede the penetration of drugs and protect the organism. The best therapeutic results are obtained by complete surgical excision of the lesion, if this is possible, or by radical surgical debulking followed by prolonged systemic antibiotic therapy, with the selection of the drug based on an antibiogram of the organism.[14] Prevention lies in attention to aseptic surgical techniques and postoperative hygiene, or, in the case of botryomycosis developing secondarily to mechanical injury of the skin (such as that caused by the harness or plant thorns or bristles), in removal of the cause if at all possible. Most cases of botryomycosis in horses involve wound infections of the skin, with or without the presence of a foreign body.[12, 14]

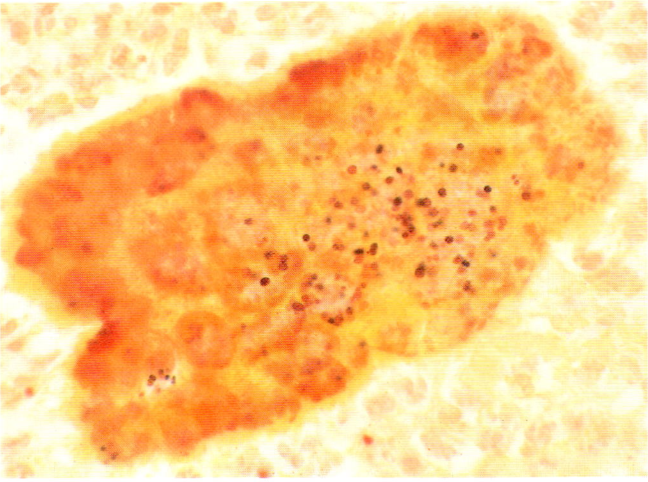

Figure 146.2 Microscopic appearance of a granule in a botryomycotic granuloma depicting Gram-positive cocci of *Staphylococcus aureus* (Gram's staining)

FOLLICULITIS AND FURUNCULOSIS

Folliculitis and furunculosis due to staphylococcal infection are more common in horses, goats and sheep than in other livestock species. Most are caused by cutaneous trauma, and physiological stress is the predisposing factor.[14]

In horses there are three common forms, namely pastern folliculitis, truncal folliculitis and tail pyoderma. These conditions have been reviewed by Mullowney and Fadok.[12] In pastern folliculitis, which occurs infrequently, lesions develop on the posterior aspect of the pastern and fetlock regions of one or more limbs. Initial lesions consist of papules and pustules which, if left untreated, coalesce to produce large, painful areas of ulceration and suppuration. Treatment consists of clipping the hairs from the affected area, washing the lesion, and the regular application of an antimicrobial ointment. The systemic administration of antibiotics is not usually necessary. The condition should be differentiated from greasy heel (pastern dermatitis).[14]

Most lesions in truncal folliculitis and furunculosis, which is also known by a variety of other names including saddle boil, saddle scab, acne, and summer rash, occur in the areas of the skin that are covered by saddles or harness. In temperate climates, it is encountered mainly in the spring and early summer. The condition is associated with sweating and friction, and is less common in well-groomed horses. The lesions may persist for two or more weeks, and may be so painful that the animal is rendered unfit for work. Treatment consisting of the daily washing of the affected area with a povidone-iodine scrub and the intramuscular administration of penicillin for seven days is usually successful. However, the condition may recur.

Tail pyoderma of horses usually occurs as a result of skin trauma produced by tail-rubbing, which is provoked by insect bites, mange, lice or pinworm (*Oxyuris equi*) infestations, or as a vice. Small pustules form on the dorsal surface of the tail. The affected skin is pruritic, which compounds the self-mutilation. The disease progresses to a chronic pyoderma which responds poorly to treatment. Therapy includes the removal of predisposing causes, prevention of tail-rubbing, protection of the tail by bandaging, and topical and systemic application of antimicrobials.

Caprine staphylococcal folliculitis and furunculosis have been reviewed by Scott *et al.*[17] Moist and filthy environments, trauma, and the stress of parturition predispose to the condition, which is manifested by the development in the skin of superficial to deep papules, pustules, erosions and ulcers which are covered by scabs. They may be painful and result in systemic disturbances. Lesions commonly start on the udder and may spread to the ventral abdomen, medial thighs, distal limbs, perineum, face, and pinnae. Therapy consists of topical and systemic application of antimicrobial drugs to which the organism is susceptible, while the administration of an autogenous bacterin may be helpful. Infections by *Corynebacterium pseudotuberculosis, Actinomyces (Corynebacterium) pyogenes* and *Pseudomonas aeruginosa* may produce a similar disease but are much rarer than the staphylococcal condition.

References

1 **BATUNGBACAL, M.R. & SCOTT, G.R., 1982**. Suppression of the immune response to clostridial vaccine by tick-borne fever. *Journal of Comparative Pathology*, 92, 409–413.

2 **BRODIE, T.A., HOLMES, P.H. & URQUHART, G.M., 1986**. Some aspects of tick-borne disease of British sheep. *The Veterinary Record*, 118, 415–418.

3 **DONOVAN, G.A. & GROSS, T.L., 1984**. Cutaneous botryomycosis (bacterial granulomas) in dairy cows caused by *Pseudomonas aeruginosa*. *Journal of the American Veterinary Medical Association*, 184, 197–198.

4 **FRASER, J., SCOTT, F.M.M., ANGUS, K.W. & MARTIN, W.B., 1982**. Experimental re-infection of the skin of sheep with *Staphylococcus aureus*. *The Veterinary Record*, 111, 485–486.

5 **GUNNING, R.F. & BOSWORTH, P.A., 1989**. Staphylococcal dermatitis involving the teats of lactating ewes. *The Veterinary Record*, 124, 146–147.

6 **HAYES, M.H., 1952**. *Veterinary Notes for Horse Owners. A Manual of Horse Medicine and Surgery*. London: Hurst & Blackett Ltd.

7 **HOBDAY, F.T.G., 1913**. *Manual of the Practice of Veterinary Medicine*. London: Baillière, Tindall & Cox.

8 **HUNGEFORD, T.G., 1990**. *Diseases of Livestock*. 9th edn. Sydney: McGraw-Hill Book Company.

9 **JUBB, K.V.F., KENNEDY, P.C. & PALMER, N., 1985**. *Pathology of Domestic Animals*. 3rd edn. New York: Academic Press, Inc.

10 **MARTIN, W.B., 1983**. Staphylococcal dermatitis in sheep. *The Veterinary Annual*, 23, 104–108.

11 **MITCHELL, G.B.B., BRODIE, T.A. & WEBSTER, K.A., 1988**. Tick pyaemia (enzootic staphylococcal infection): Recent developments. *The Veterinary Annual*, 28, 69–73. London: Butterworth & Co.

12 **MULLOWNEY, P.C. & FADOK, V.A., 1984**. Dermatologic diseases of horses. Part II. Bacterial and viral skin diseases. *The Compendium on Continuing Education for the Practising Veterinarian*, 6, S16–S22.

13 **PARKER, B.N.J., BONSON, M.D. & CARROL, P.J., 1983**. Staphylococcal dermatitis in unweaned lambs. *The Veterinary Record*, 113, 570–571.

14 **SCOTT, D.W., 1988**. *Large Animal Dermatology*. Philadelphia: W.B. Saunders Company.

15 **SCOTT, F.M.M., FRASER, J. & MARTIN, W.B., 1980**. Staphylococcal dermatitis in sheep. *The Veterinary Record*, 107, 572–574.

16 **SCOTT, F.M.M., FRASER, J. & SCOTT, G.R., 1991**. Pyoderma. *In*: MARTIN, W.B. & AITKEN, I.D., (eds). *Diseases of Sheep*. 2nd edn. London: Blackwell Scientific Publications.

17 **SCOTT, D.W., SMITH, M.C. & MANNING, T.O., 1984**. Caprine dermatology. Part I. Normal skin and bacterial and fungal disorders. *The Compendium on Continuing Education for the Practising Veterinarian*, 6, S190 – S221.

18 **SCHLEIFER, K.H., 1986**. Family 1. Micrococcaceae Prevot 1961. *In*: SNEATH, P.H.A., MAIR, N.S., SHARPE, M.E. & HOLT, J.G., (eds). *Bergey's Manual of Systematic Bacteriology*. Baltimore: Williams & Wilkins.

19 **SCHNEIDER, D.J., 1993**. Veterinary Diagnostic Laboratory, Stellenbosch. Personal communication.

20 **SYNGE, B.A., SCOTT, F.M.M. & MACDOUGALL, D.C., 1985**. Dermatitis of the legs of sheep associated with *Staphylococcus aureus*. *The Veterinary Record*, 116, 459–460.

21 **WATSON, W.A., 1964**. Studies on the distribution of the sheep tick (*Ixodes ricinus* L.) and the occurrence of enzootic staphylococcal infection of lambs in North-West Yorkshire and North-East Lancashire. *The Veterinary Record*, 76, 743–747.

22 **WATSON, W.A., 1965**. The carriage of pathogenic staphylococci by sheep. *The Veterinary Record*, 77, 477–478.

23 **WEBSTER, K.A. & MITCHELL, G.B.B., 1986**. Experimental production of tick pyaemia. *The Veterinary Record*, 119, 186–187.

147

Exudative epidermitis of pigs

Synonym: Greasy pig disease

M.M. Henton

Introduction

Exudative epidermitis of pigs is an often fatal, peracute to subacute, contagious, generalized, superficial dermatitis of sudden onset, caused by *Staphylococcus hyicus* subsp. *hyicus*. The disease usually affects piglets between five days and ten weeks of age, but it may occur in older piglets and even in adult pigs. Although the bacterium is predominantly associated with skin lesions, it occasionally causes septicaemia, arthritis and abortions in pigs.

The disease characteristically has a sudden onset and a short course, during which the piglets become severely dehydrated but do not manifest pruritis. The morbidity and mortality rates vary from farm to farm.[14] Piglets suffering from the peracute or acute forms of the disease usually die.

Spinola in 1842 was the first to publish the results of research on exudative epidermitis,[11] but it was more fully described by Hjärre in 1948.[9] The causative bacterium, *Staphylococcus hyicus* subsp. *hyicus*, was first isolated by Sompolinsky in 1953,[23] when he referred to it as *Micrococcus hyicus*.

The disease is not seasonal,[11] and is of sporadic occurrence. It may be so mild or insignificant that its presence in a pig herd is of no consequence, or it may reach such proportions and persist for such a time that it forces the closure of the operation and removal of all pigs from the farm.[14] Economic losses due to death or ill-thrift as a consequence of the infection may be considerable, as the mortality rate may be close to 100 per cent in piglets on farms where the disease is newly introduced.

Aetiology

Staphylococcus hyicus subsp. *hyicus*, previously known as *Micrococcus hyicus* or as *Staphylococcus epidermidis* biotype 2, is a coagulase-positive bacterium (when pig—but not guinea-pig, dog or sheep—serum is used as substrate) that contains substances in the cell wall with protein A-like IgG Fc-receptors, a characteristic that is restricted to isolates from pigs. In addition, the glycosyl-glycerol teichoic acid contained in the cell wall of the bacterium is specific for *S. hyicus* subsp. *hyicus* and may be used, in association with other tests, in its differentiation from other staphylococcal species. The teichoic acid may also be used for the production of *S. hyicus*-specific antibodies for use in serological surveys. It produces specific enzymes with a bacteriolytic effect, and on blood agar plates it causes a characteristic dark brown discoloration of the medium in addition to the haemolysis which is induced in media containing rabbit blood, but not in those containing sheep or chicken blood.[13] A heat-labile exfoliative toxin has been isolated from *S. hyicus* subsp. *hyicus*.[21]

For further information on the bacterium and its differentiation from other pathogenic *Staphylococcus* spp. refer to ***Staphylococcus* spp. infections: Introduction: Table 3.**

Epidemiology

The disease has been reported in Europe, Australia, Canada, the USA, Japan[21] and South Africa. Only pigs are affected by *S. hyicus* subsp. *hyicus*, although the bacterium has also been isolated from the skin of cattle, horses, donkeys, goats, dogs and chickens.[13] The disease is usually restricted to suckling piglets less than 35 days old, but older piglets and adults are more rarely affected.[11] The severity and frequency of occurrence decrease with increasing age of piglets—the younger the animal, the shorter the course and the higher the morbidity and mortality rates.[11] The morbidity and mortality rates are highly variable, however, and susceptibility may vary from litter to litter and from farm to farm.[15] Entire litters or only some piglets may be affected. During outbreaks a proportion of piglets on one farm may contract the acute disease, while others are only mildly affected.

Infection is introduced into a susceptible population by healthy carriers or animals suffering from clinical disease—usually the mild, subacute form. Alternatively, when susceptible piglets or non-immune sows are introduced onto a contaminated property they may contract the disease.[14] Healthy pigs may carry the organism on their skin[1] or as part of the normal bacterial flora in the tonsils (from which it may be isolated in more than 90 per cent of animals), nares, nasal cavity, conjunctiva, ears and vagina.[7, 8, 22] The bacterium may persist for some weeks on fittings in animals' housing.[26]

Exudative epidermitis of pigs is highly contagious and easily spreads by direct contact between infected and susceptible pigs. Infection often occurs through skin wounds, usually bite wounds inflicted during fighting.[24] Spread may be hastened by ectoparasites and poor hygiene of pens. Abrasions on the skin, such as those caused by coarse straw or sawdust bedding or rough concrete flooring, also appear to predispose to the spread of the disease.[14, 25] Inadequate ventilation and high humidity in the animals' housing may increase the prevalence of the disease.[26]

Poor management, nutritional deficiencies or imbalances, mange and secondary infections appear to increase the severity of the disease and the mortality rate.

Pathogenesis

Experimentally, exudative epidermitis may be induced by applying cultures of *S. hyicus* subsp. *hyicus* to the skin of susceptible pigs.[16, 27] Irrespective of the route of infection, even when it is intravenous, the organism proliferates profusely in the skin and the resultant lesions are, for reasons unknown, essentially restricted to the epidermis.[16]

Macroscopic skin lesions only develop when more than 10^5 colony-forming units of the bacterium occur per square centimetre of skin.[1] Other less well-known factors, such as the observation that colonization of the skin by *S. hyicus* subsp. *hyicus* is inhibited by avirulent *S. hyicus* subsp. *hyicus* strains which are often present on the skin of normal pigs, determine the initial stages of the infection and whether or not the disease will develop.[1, 10]

It is probable that the local effect of the exfoliative toxin is responsible for the development of the skin lesions in exudative epidermitis. The toxic effect is similar to that caused by the exfoliative toxins (serine proteases) produced by certain strains of *Staphylococcus aureus*.[5] The exfoliative toxin produced by toxigenic strains of *S. hyicus*, when applied intradermally or subcutaneously to the skin, causes cleavage between the epidermal cells at the level of the junction between the *stratum corneum* and *stratum granulosum*, the primary lesion being in the latter.[21] The lesions commence as swelling and vacuolization of the cells of the *stratum intermedium* and those in the outer layer of the *stratum spinosum*. Subsequently the desmosomes and tonofibrils of these cells are reduced in size and number, there is total disappearance of keratohyaline granules from the *stratum granulosum*, and the intercellular spaces become enlarged and are filled with an opaque material.[19] Consequent lack of thickening of the plasma membrane of the cells in the *stratum corneum* and absence of intercellular discs cause poor adhesion between these cells and allow the loss of large amounts of tissue fluid. In addition to these changes, the extensive purulent inflammation which occurs in the skin further contributes to the fluid loss and the development of the marked dehydration which appears to be the major cause of death.[14]

In many pigs that have died from exudative epidermitis there are changes in the urinary system, which consist of purulent ureteritis with some distension of the ureters, pyelonephritis with dilation of the renal pelves, and desquamation of epithelial cells of collecting tubules in the kidneys.[11, 12, 17] The pathogenesis of these lesions, however, is unclear. They may be caused by the local effect of the bacteria which can be isolated from, or detected histologically in, the epithelium of the renal pelves and ureters of affected animals.[1, 17]

Clinical signs and pathology

The incubation period of the disease is not well defined, but piglets usually manifest clinical signs within one or two weeks of being introduced onto infected premises. Macroscopic skin lesions are observed four days after animals are infected experimentally.[1]

Irrespective of the severity of the disease, the first indication of its presence is the appearance of a scant, flaky, brown exudate at the base of hairs over the openings of sweat glands in focal areas of the skin. Rarely, small vesicles that may coalesce can be seen where the initial lesions develop,[11] but they soon rupture. Progression of the lesions is characterized by the development of papules which expand, the centres of the areas becoming covered by a reddish-brown, greasy exudate. These lesions are accompanied by hyperaemia and thickening of the skin on the ears, flanks or the lateral aspects of the thorax and abdomen, after which the animals either recover fully, or the lesions progress to involve the entire surface of the skin.

Microscopically, lesions of an acute exudative epidermitis are present—including hyperkeratosis, parakeratosis, pronounced acanthosis, oedema and hydropic degeneration of the upper layer of the *stratum spinosum* and the *stratum granulosum*, and subcorneal vesiculation and pustule formation. Afterwards there is exocytosis of neutrophils; the reaction extends to the hair follicles, causing severe purulent folliculitis. Ultimately the inflammatory process expands to involve the entire thickness of the epidermis and may be followed by ulceration, particularly around the hair follicles. Numerous colonies of coccoid bacteria occur in the superficial layers of the epidermis and in the exudate surrounding the hair shafts. The dermis is severely congested and infiltrated by neutrophils and eosinophils. In severe cases the epidermis may be six to seven times its normal thickness due to the accumulation of exudate, acanthosis, and para- and hyperkeratosis.[16, 17]

Generalization of the skin lesions is dependent on the expansion of the localized lesions, as well as on the development of new foci elsewhere on the skin. Affected piglets are not pruritic. The regional lymph nodes are markedly hyperplastic and purulent lymphadenitis is evident in them in severely affected piglets.[17]

Vesicles, erosions and ulcers occur on the lips and the tongue of about a third of piglets suffering from the disease. The severity and location of these oral lesions differ markedly, the most consistent manifestation being that of marked focal erosions and ulcers on the dorsum of the tongue. Multiple erosions may also rarely occur on the hard palate.[3]

On the basis of the extent and severity of the lesions, the disease can be subdivided into peracute, acute or subacute forms.

In the peracute disease the lesions spread to involve the entire skin within a matter of 24–48 hours. By this time the exudate becomes malodorous, thick, brownish and greasy, and has the appearance of dried serum. The exudate is usually most abundant on the ears and the face, and the eyelids are encrusted with it. Masses of the exudate may accumulate at the mucocutaneous junctions of the eyes, nose and oral cavity.[11, 17] Ocular lesions may be seen as mild purulent conjunctivitis, but may progress to a severe purulent inflammation in which the eyelids are glued together by the exudate. The coronary bands are severely inflamed, resulting in detachment of the hoof, particularly in the interdigital area. The cornified area of the bulb detaches regularly and may slough. Affected piglets have an increased body temperature and are severely depressed, anorexic, dehydrated, and reluctant to move. They become recumbent, severely emaciated and die within three to five days of the onset of clinical signs. During the course of the disease the piglets usually become constipated, although some may have diarrhoea.[11] These animals develop leukopenia within four or five days of the commencement of clinical signs, and marked neutrophilia as the disease progresses.[17] The mortality rate may be close to 100 per cent.[11]

At necropsy the only consistent lesions elsewhere in the carcass may be found in the ureters, renal pelves and kidneys. During the initial stages of the disease there may be slight uni- or bilateral dilatation of the ureters. This is the result of obstruction caused by a local acute inflammatory reaction that is characterized by the infiltration of neutrophils and mucoid degeneration of the epithelium as well as the desquamation of necrotic ureteral epithelium. During the later stages of the disease there is also mild hydronephrosis and peripelvic oedema.[17] Similar changes to those in the ureters may be present in the transitional epithelium of the renal pelves, with dilation of the latter as well as hydropic degeneration and desquamation of epithelial cells of dilated collecting tubules of the kidneys. The latter phenomenon may be macroscopically visible as white linear deposits. The urine in distended ureters and renal pelves has a mucoid consistency and contains cellular casts and debris.[11, 12, 17, 27] Small numbers of coccoid bacteria are present on the surface of the affected ureteral and pelvic epithelium.

The lesions of the acute disease are very similar to those of the peracute disease, although they develop over a longer period of time. In animals suffering from the acute disease the exudate tends to dry out, assuming the appearance of rough, brown fish scales. Raw areas are left when the scales are removed, or raw fissures are formed when dried-out scabs crack.[11, 14] Affected animals become severely dehydrated and most eventually die. The majority of deaths, which occur after five to eight days, appear to be the consequence of secondary bacterial infections causing purulent pneumonia, pleuritis or peritonitis. Some animals may linger on for about three weeks before they die.[11] Survivors recover slowly, remain stunted and often have residual skin lesions such as subcutaneous abscesses.

The subacute disease is characterized by focal lesions on the head, ears, neck and the sides of the body. Affected pigs do not lose their appetite, nor do they show a reduction in growth rate. The focal lesions vary from 10–40 mm in diameter, their surfaces becoming dry and changing in colour from brownish to dark brown or black. The skin lesions heal within 15 days without the formation of scars.

Staphylococcus hyicus subsp. *hyicus* occasionally causes acute fibrinous polyarthritis[20] and abortion in pigs.[6]

Diagnosis

A presumptive diagnosis of exudative epidermitis can be based on the characteristic macroscopic and histologic lesions, and the age group of animals affected. The diagnosis should, however, be confirmed by the isolation of the causative bacterium from superficial scrapings of the skin. *Staphylococcus hyicus* subsp. *hyicus* may also occasionally be isolated from the lungs, liver and kidneys of such animals.[1] *Staphylococcus hyicus* subsp. *hyicus* can be readily isolated on most common bacteriological media **(see *Staphylococcus* spp. infections: Introduction: Table 3)**. Smears made from the skin lesions reveal the presence of Gram-positive cocci.

Differential diagnosis

Exudative epidermitis has distinctive clinical signs, but it may be confused with parakeratosis caused by zinc deficiency. In parakeratosis, which occurs in weaners, the lesions are usually bilaterally symmetrical and dry. Other conditions that may superficially resemble exudative epidermitis include mange, ringworm, rare conditions such as *pityriasis rosea* and *dermatosis vegetans*, and dermatitis and abscessation following the infection of skin wounds.[17, 26]

Control

Prompt antimicrobial treatment of entire litters during the early stages of the development of the lesions is essential if it is to be successful. Affected animals respond differently to the addition of antimicrobials to their feed: in some instances it may have a curative effect, whereas in others the disease will run its course uninterruptedly in spite of the addition of chlortetracycline, sulphamethazine or penicillin.[14, 18] Antimicrobial therapy should be based on the results of antibiograms. Supportive treatment of piglets, including intravenous fluids, can be given if economically justifiable.

Local treatment, such as cleansing of the skin with preparations containing iodine or other disinfectants, is also helpful.[4] If ectoparasites are present they should be controlled.

Management practices should be directed to limiting the possibility of introducing the disease into susceptible herds, and limiting the spread on farms by restrictions on the intermingling of pigs from different sources. Attention should be given to general hygiene and reducing the causes of skin trauma (such as coarse bedding, rough floors and walls), prevention of fighting and clipping of teeth. Farrowing pens and other enclosures should be disinfected regularly.

Exudative epidermitis can be controlled by the use of formalinized bacterins or a vaccine containing the exfoliative toxin of *S. hyicus*.[2] Where the disease is a problem, the preparation and use of autogenous bacterins in pregnant sows (to induce colostral immunity in their piglets after birth), or in piglets when the disease occurs at weaning is advised.[25] These have been shown to reduce the duration of outbreaks.[25] Such vaccines are not currently available in South Africa.

References

1 **ALLAKER, R.P., LLOYD, D.H. & SMITH, I.M., 1988.** Prevention of exudative epidermitis in gnotobiotic piglets by bacterial interference. *The Veterinary Record*, 123, 597–598.

2 **AMTSBERG, G., 1978.** Infection experiments with *Staphylococcus hyicus* in actively and passively immunized pigs. *Berliner und Münchener Tierärtzliche Wochenschrift*, 91, 201–206.

3 **ANDREWS, J.J., 1979.** Ulcerative glossitis and stomatitis associated with exudative epidermitis in suckling pigs. *Veterinary Pathology*, 16, 432–437.

4 **BENNETT, P.C., 1970.** Necrotic rhinitis and exudative epidermitis. *In*: DUNNE, H.W., (ed.). *Diseases of Swine*. 3rd edn. Ames, Iowa: Iowa State University Press.

5 **DANCER, S.J., GARRATT, R., SALDANHA, J., JHOTI, H. & EVANS, R., 1990.** The epidermolytic toxins are serine proteases. *FEBS Letters*, 268, 129–132.

6 **DUNCAN, M. & SMITH, D., 1992.** Isolation of *Staphylococcus hyicus* from aborted piglets. *Canadian Veterinary Journal*, 33, 75–76.

7 **ELLIOT, G., 1986.** Porcine bacterial flora. *The Veterinary Record*, 118, 251.

8 **HAJSIG, D., BABIC, T. & MADIC, J., 1985.** Exudative epidermitis in piglets. II. Distribution of *Staphylococcus hyicus* subsp. *hyicus*. Findings in healthy piglets. *Veterinarski Archiv*, 55, 45–51.

9 **HJÄRRE, A., 1948.** Kontagios pyodermi hos svin (Impetigo contagiosa). *Skandinavish Veterinärtidskrift*, 38, 662–682.

10 **HUNTER, D., TODD, J.N. & LARKIN, M., 1970.** Exudative epidermitis of pigs. *The British Veterinary Journal*, 126, 225–229.

11 **JONES, L.D., 1956.** Exudative epidermitis of pigs. *American Journal of Veterinary Research*, 17, 179–193.

12 **JUBB, K.V.F., KENNEDY, P.C. & PALMER, N., 1985.** *Pathology of Domestic Animals*. 3rd edn. San Diego: Academic Press, Inc.

13 **LÄMMLER, C.H., 1990.** *Staphylococcus hyicus*, der Erreger der exsudativen Epidermitis der Schweines. *Berliner und Münchener Tierärztliche Wochenschrift*, 103, 60–63.

14 **L'ECUYER, C., 1966.** Exudative epidermitis in pigs. Clinical studies and preliminary transmission trials. *Canadian Journal of Comparative Medicine and Veterinary Science*, 30, 9–16.

15 **L'ECUYER, C. & ALEXANDER, D.C., 1969.** Exudative epidermitis in pigs. Treatment trials. *Canadian Veterinary Journal*, 10, 227–234.

16 **L'ECUYER, C. & JERICHO, K., 1966.** Exudative epidermitis in pigs: Etiological studies and pathology. *Canadian Journal of Comparative Medicine and Veterinary Science*, 30, 94–101.

17 **MEBUS, C.A., UNDERDAHL, N.R. & TWEIHAUS, M.J., 1968.** Exudative epidermitis. Pathogenesis and pathology. *Pathologia Veterinaria*, 5, 146–163.

18 **NOBLE, W.C. & ALLAKER, R.P., 1992.** Staphylococci on the skin of pigs: Isolates from two farms with different antibiotic policies. *The Veterinary Record*, 130, 466–468.

19 **OBEL, A-L. & NICANDER, L., 1970.** Epithelial changes in porcine exudative epidermitis. *Pathologia Veterinaria*, 7, 329–345.

20 **PHILLIPS, W.E., KING, R.E. & KLOOS, W.E., 1980.** Isolation of *Staphylococcus hyicus* subsp. *hyicus* from a pig with septic polyarthritis. *American Journal of Veterinary Research*, 41, 274–276.

21 **SATO, H., TANABE, T., KURAMOTO M., TANAKA, K., HASHIMOTO, T. & SAITO, H., 1991.** Isolation of exfoliative toxin from *Staphylococcus hyicus* subsp. *hyicus* and its exfoliative activity in the piglet. *Veterinary Microbiology*, 27, 263–275.

22 **SHIMIZU, A., KAWANO, J., TERANISHI, H., HAZUE, S., FUJINAMI, T., KIMURA, S. & SUGIHARA, K., 1987.** Isolation of *Staphylococcus* species from the tonsils of healthy pigs and phage patterns of isolates. *Japanese Journal of Veterinary Science*, 49, 703–709.

23 **SOMPOLINSKI, D., 1953.** De l'impetgo contagiosa suis et du *Micrococcus hyicus* n. sp. *Schweitzer Archiv für Tierheilkunde*, 95, 302–309.

24 **STUKER, G., 1976.** Contribution to the epizootiology of exudative epidermitis: Spread of *Staphylococcus hyicus* by animal contact. *Schweitzer Archiv für Tierheilkunde*, 118, 335–340.

25 **TAYLOR, D.J., 1989.** *Pig Diseases*. 5th edn. Cambridge: The Burlington Press (Cambridge) Ltd.

26 **TAYLOR, D.J., 1992.** Exudative epidermitis. *In*: LEMAN, A.D., STRAW, B.E., MENGELING, W.L., D'ALLAIRE, S. & TAYLOR, D.J., (eds). *Diseases of Swine*. 7th edn. Wolfe Publishing Ltd.

27 **UNDERDAHL, N.R., GRACE, O.D. & YOUNG, G.A., 1963.** Experimental transmission of exudative epidermitis of pigs. *Journal of the American Veterinary Medical Association*, 142, 754–762.

148

Other Staphylococcus *spp. infections*

M.M. Henton

Apart from *Staphylococcus intermedius*, *S. aureus*, *S. epidermidis* and *S. hyicus* var. *hyicus*, other *Staphylococcus* spp. are only associated with disease as opportunists.

Staphylococcus intermedius is generally found on the skin and nasal mucous membranes of carnivores and is most commonly associated with canine pyoderma. It also occurs on the skin of horses and pigeons, but rarely of humans unless they have a close association with carnivores. *Staphylococcus intermedius* has also been associated with otitis externa in dogs, wound infection in various animal species, and mastitis in cattle **(see Chapter 190: Mastitis)**.[1]

Staphylococcus epidermidis as an occasional opportunistic pathogen causes mastitis in cows **(see Chapter 190: Mastitis)**.[2]

References

1 **PHILLIPS, W.E. & KLOOS, W.E., 1981.** Identification of coagulase-positive *Staphylococcus intermedius* and *Staphylococcus hyicus* subsp. *hyicus* isolates from veterinary clinical specimens. *Journal of Clinical Microbiology*, 14, 671–673.

2 **SCHLEIFER, K.H., 1986.** Gram-positive cocci. *In*: SNEATH, P.H.A., MAIR, N.S., SHARPE, M.E. & HOLT, J.G., (eds). *Bergey's Manual of Systematic Bacteriology*. Vol. II. Baltimore: Williams & Wilkins.

Streptococcus *spp. infections*

M.M. Henton

Introduction

Infections by *Streptococcus* spp. in livestock cause a great variety of primary or secondary suppurative conditions **(Table 1)**, including strangles, mastitis, genital tract infections, cervical lymphadenitis, septicaemia, endocarditis, meningoencephalitis and arthritis.

The name 'Streptococcus' was first coined by Billroth and Ehrlich in 1877[2] for the chain-forming coccus found in infected wounds. Since then the *Streptococcus* spp. have been extensively studied and a large number of species have been identified. Their taxonomy is currently in a state of flux following new findings that resulted from hybridization studies.[8, 19] The species in this chapter, however, are referred to by their established names.

In South Africa, *S. equisimilis* and *S. zooepidemicus* affect livestock species most commonly **(Tables 2 to 4)**, while *S. agalactiae* is the most important cause of bovine mastitis **(see Chapter 190: Mastitis)**. The isolation of *S. dysgalactiae* in cattle, and *S. suis* and *S. porcinus* in pigs, is also regularly reported **(Tables 2 to 4)**. *Streptococcus equi*, the cause of strangles in equidae, and to a lesser extent *S. suis*, are the only streptococci which infect animals and which are relatively host-specific.

Streptococcus spp. are facultatively anaerobic, Gram-positive, spherical or ovoid cocci that usually occur in chains, but may also be single or in pairs. They are catalase-negative and ferment sugars without the production of gas.[8]

Streptococci grow best on media enriched by blood or tissue extracts at 37°C, suggesting that they are adapted to a parasitic rather than a saprophytic existence. Surface colonies are small and transparent to semi-opaque, and a wide zone of complete (beta) haemolysis is evident around the colonies of most pyogenic streptococci. The pathogens in serological groups B and D are often either non-haemolytic or cause alpha haemolysis.[18] Alpha-haemolytic strains, which cause greening of blood agar, were previously placed in the 'Viridans Group' of Sherman, but this is now not considered to be a reliable taxonomic feature.[8] In most veterinary diagnostic laboratories Group C streptococci are identified on the basis of their fermentation reactions.[5]

Streptococcus spp. are traditionally divided into serologic groups (Lancefield groups) based on their dominant carbohydrate cell wall antigens. These group-specific antigens (or C-substances) are either polysaccharides associated with the cell wall (e.g. Groups A, B, C, E, F and G) or teichoic acids (e.g. Groups D and N) situated in the region between the cell membrane and the inner surface of the cell wall.[8] There are 20 Lancefield groups, designated A to H and K to V. The use of this system of classification is being abolished, as its main value was to distinguish between pathogenic beta-haemolytic streptococci. It could not be used, however, to classify all streptococcal species, such as the alpha-haemolytic viridans streptococci and the non-haemolytic streptococci.[11, 15] To a large extent these latter groups comprise strains found normally in the oral cavity and upper respiratory tract, and seldom cause disease.[8]

Depending on the *Streptococcus* spp. involved, the virulence of the bacterium is determined by a number of factors including cell wall-associated components such as the capsule, fimbriae, M-protein, lipoteichoic acids, and peptidoglycan, and other extracellular products such as nucleases, proteinase, neuraminidase, nicotinamide adenine dinucleotidase (NADase), streptolysins O and S, hyaluronidase, and streptokinase (fibrinolysin).[1, 8, 14] Abscesses or purulent infections are produced as a result of the response of neutrophils to the products of the bacteria. While antibodies directed against the protein antigens are protective, those formed in response to carbohydrate antigens are not.[18]

Only a few of the streptococcal species form a capsule, and when they do, for example in the case of *S. pyogenes*, the capsule is composed of hyaluronic acid[14] and is formed during the early stages of growth.[8] The capsule is not important in terms of pathogenesis except in the case of *S. pneumoniae* (which rarely causes disease in animals), where the capsular polysaccharide is the virulence factor and enables *S. pneumoniae* to evade phagocytosis in the absence of type-specific antibody.[14]

Peptidoglycan, the main component of the cell wall, has similar systemic effects to those produced by the endotoxins of Gram-negative bacteria[8] **(see Chapter 129: *Escherichia coli* infections)**.

Table 1 Most common diseases caused by *Streptococcus* spp. in livestock and humans. (Adapted from Carter & Thoen,[5] and Schleifer *et al.*[19])

STREPTOCOCCUS SPP.	ANIMAL SPP.	DISEASE
PYOGENIC STREPTOCOCCI		
Group A streptococci		
S. pyogenes	Humans	Septic sore throat, scarlet fever, pyoderma, lymphadenitis and erysipelas
	Cattle	Mastitis
Group B streptococci		
S. agalactiae	Cattle, sheep and goats	Mastitis
Group C streptococci		
S. equi	Horses	Strangles
S. zooepidemicus	Horses	Endometritis, cervicitis, placentitis, embryonal loss, abortion, secondary respiratory infections, pneumonia, abscesses, omphalophlebitis, neonatal septicaemia and polyarthritis
	Cattle	Mastitis, abscesses, neonatal septicaemia and pneumonia
	Goats	Mastitis and abscesses
	Sheep	Abscesses, neonatal septicaemia and pneumonia
	Pigs	Cervical lymphadenitis, neonatal septicaemia and arthritis, abortion and abscesses
S. equisimilis	Pigs	Neonatal purulent arthritis, lymphadenitis (cervical nodes), genital infections, mastitis-metritis-agalactiae syndrome, abortion, stillbirths and weak piglets at birth
	Horses	Suppurative conditions, abscesses, neonatal septicaemia, polyarthritis and enteritis, secondary infection to viral infection of the respiratory tract and endometritis
S. dysgalactiae	Cattle	Mastitis and neonatal septicaemia
	Pigs	Metritis, pneumonia, neonatal septicaemia, polyarthritis and genital infections
	Sheep	Mastitis, abscesses, neonatal septicaemia and polyarthritis
Group D enterococci		
Enterococcus faecium *E. faecalis* *E. avium* *E. gallinarum* *E. casseliflavus* *E. durans* *E. hirae* *E. malodoratus* *E. mundtii*	All livestock species	Meningoencephalitis, sporadic cases of valvular endocarditis and urinary tract infections
OTHER STREPTOCOCCI		
S. uberis	Cows	Mastitis
S. porcinus (Groups E, P, U and V)	Pigs	Cervical lymphadenitis (jowl abscesses), neonatal septicaemia, pneumonia, infertility, arthritis, pleuritis and peritonitis
	Cows	Mastitis
S. suis	Pigs	Septicaemia, meningitis, arthritis, pharyngitis, endocarditis, abscesses, lymphadenitis (cervical nodes), genital tract infections (vaginitis, endometritis), abortion and stillbirths
ANAEROBIC STREPTOCOCCI		
S. mobillorum	All species	Abscesses

Streptolysin O is produced by all Group A and some Group B, C, F and G streptococci. It causes beta haemolysis as well as the destruction of leukocytes, macrophages and platelets in certain animal species.[8, 18] The effects of streptolysin S are similar to, but less pronounced than, those of streptolysin O.

Hyaluronidase is produced by *S. suis* and streptococci in Groups A, B and C. It causes lysis of the ground substance of connective tissue and may play a role in the local spread of infection. Streptokinase (fibrinolysin) produced by Group A and some members of Groups C and G, is a fibrinolytic protease and interferes with the formation of a fibrin barrier around lesions, thereby promoting the spread of streptococcal infections.[18] Streptodornase, which degrades DNA, is the collective term for the four distinct deoxyribonucleases (A, B, C and D) of which type B is most common.[1, 18]

Table 2 Common *Streptococcus* spp. isolated from pigs from 1977 to 1987 at the general diagnostic laboratory, Veterinary Research Institute, Onderstepoort

	S. EQUISIMILIS	*S. SUIS*	*S. PORCINUS*	*S. ZOOEPIDEMICUS*	*S. DYSGALACTIAE*	TOTAL NUMBER OF CASES
Mastitis-metritis-agalactia syndrome	49	5	3	3	2	62
Septicaemia	27	10	9	2	–	48
Pneumonia	12	8	2	1	2	25
Abscessation	6	3	1	1	1	12
Polyserositis	3	5	3	–	1	12
Abortion	8	1	1	1	–	11
Arthritis	6	1	1	–	2	10
Lymphadenitis	5	1	1	1	1	9
Pyoderma	3	1	2	–	–	6
Meningitis	1	1	–	–	–	2
Cystitis	–	–	–	2	–	2
Myositis	–	–	1	–	–	1

Table 3 Percentage of isolations of *Streptococcus* spp. made from livestock species from 1977 to 1987 at the general diagnostic laboratory, Veterinary Research Institute, Onderstepoort

STREPTOCOCCUS SPP.	HORSES	PIGS	CATTLE	SHEEP	GOATS
S. zooepidemicus	89,9	5,4	7,1	39,1	33,31
S. equisimilis	8,7	56,9	12,5	13,0	66,62
S. dysgalactiae	0,4	4,9	62,5	39,1	–
S. suis	–	20,1	1,8	2,2	–
S. porcinus	–	10,3	1,8	–	–
S. agalactiae	–	1,3	10,7	–	–
S. uberis	–	0,4	3,6	2,2	–
Streptococcus G	–	0,4	–	4,3	–
S. equi	0,9	–	–	–	–

Table 4 Isolates of *Streptococcus* spp. made from a variety of conditions in livestock from 1977 to 1980 at the general diagnostic laboratory, Veterinary Research Institute, Onderstepoort

CONDITION	HORSES	PIGS	CATTLE	SHEEP	GOATS	TOTAL NUMBER OF CASES
Metritis	164	66	7	2	–	239
Septicaemia	8	50	10	9	2	79
Pneumonia	11	26	–	11	1	49
Abscessation	5	13	5	6	–	29
Abortion	8	12	3	3	–	26
Arthritis	2	10	1	2	–	15
Nasal discharge	13	–	–	–	–	13
Polyserositis	–	12	–	–	–	12
Lymphadenitis	–	9	1	–	–	10
Skin infections	4	6	–	–	–	10
Meningitis	–	2	–	2	–	4
Cellulitis	2	–	1	–	–	3
Cystitis	–	2	–	–	–	2
Myositis	–	1	–	–	–	1
Otitis	1	–	–	–	–	1

Nucleases, proteinase and neuraminidase are produced by Group A streptococci. M-protein (in *S. pyogenes*), which is also antiphagocytic, is a determinant of virulence.

Epidemiology

Streptococcus spp. inhabit the mucous membranes of the upper respiratory, alimentary and lower urogenital tracts of healthy animals as commensals. They may also be found in feed, faecally contaminated water, and the environment contaminated by purulent exudates which develop as a consequence of streptococcal infections. They are destroyed by the usual strengths of disinfectant but may survive for months in dust in buildings.[21] Some species, such as *S. faecium* var. *casseliflavus*, thrive as epiphytes on plants.[13]

Bacteria gain entrance to the tissues of the body through the mucous membranes of the respiratory, genital and gastrointestinal tracts, wounds in the skin, and the umbilicus. Infections may spread *per continuitatum*, ascend or descend in the duct systems or lumens of hollow organs or tissues that contain them, or lymphogenously or haematogenously to distant organs or tissues.[6]

Infection with many of the *Streptococcus* spp. may occur in animals of either sex and of all age groups. Exceptions to this occur when infection is dependent on the existence of certain predisposing circumstances, such as metritis that occurs particularly in the post-partum period, mastitis in the lactating udder, and omphalophlebitis in neonates, while in some infections, such as equine strangles, an age-dependent immunity seems to play a role, since the condition is infrequently encountered in the older age group.[3, 22] As many of the streptococcal infections in livestock in South Africa occur in neonates and in the genital tract of adult animals, there is an increased incidence of these infections in spring.[9]

Pathogenic streptococci selectively colonize specific anatomical sites. The infections result either in the development of subclinical carrier states (for example, the tonsils in the case of *S. pyogenes* in humans, *S. equi* in horses, and *S. suis* in pigs) or in clinical disease. In mares and sows, *S. zooepidemicus* and *S. equisimilis* occur commonly in the vagina, and occasionally in the cervix and uterus (especially immediately post-partum). *Streptococcus zooepidemicus* may be part of the normal flora of the vagina and clitoral fossa in mares, and occasionally also of the skin and upper respiratory tract. In boars and stallions respectively, *S. equisimilis* and *S. zooepidemicus* may be part of the normal flora of the preputial mucosa, but their prevalence in this locality is much lower than in the female genital tract of sows and mares.[10] *Streptococcus agalactiae* is an obligate intramammary parasite of the mucosa of the lactiferous ducts of cattle, sheep and goats.[7] It may also be found, however, in the mouth and vagina, and on the skin of the udder of domestic ruminants.[8] *Streptococcus uberis* may be isolated from many sites of the body, including the skin, tonsils, vagina, rectum, teats and udder, and in the faeces of cattle.[4, 7] Faecal streptococci (= enterococci) such as *S. faecalis, S. faecium*, and *S. mobillorum* occur normally in the intestinal tract of all animals. They are opportunistic pathogens usually associated with abscesses in various internal organs and tissues following the occurrence of trauma, omphalophlebitis, or septicaemia.[10, 11, 17, 18, 20]

Mixed infections of streptococci with one or more other organisms, such as *Salmonella* serovars., *Klebsiella* spp., pathogenic strains of *Escherichia coli, Pasteurella* spp., *Actinobacillus* spp., *Corynebacterium* spp. and *Chlamydia psittaci*, are sometimes encountered.[9, 16]

Most streptococci (with the exception of enterococci) are sensitive to penicillin, which is the therapeutic drug of choice.[1, 12]

References

1 **BARNUM, D.A., 1986.** *Streptococcus. In:* GYLES, C.L. & THOEN, C.O., (eds). *Pathogenesis of Bacterial Infections in Animals.* Ames, Iowa: Iowa State University Press.

2 **BILLROTH, T. & EHRLICH, F., 1877.** *Archive für klinische Chirurgie*, 20, 403.

3 **BLOOD, D.C., HENDERSON, J.A. & RADOSTITS, O.M., 1979.** *Veterinary Medicine.* 5th edn. London: Baillière Tindall.

4 **BRAMLEY, A.J., 1982.** Sources of *Streptococcus uberis* in a dairy herd. *Journal of Dairy Research*, 46, 369–373.

5 **CARTER, G.R. & THOEN, C.O., 1984.** *Diagnostic Procedures in Veterinary Bacteriology and Mycology.* 4th edn. Springfield, Illinois: C.C. Tokoma.

6 **ERICKSON, E.D., 1993.** Streptococcal disease. *In:* HOWARD, J.L., (ed.). *Current Veterinary Therapy: Food Animal Practice 3.* Philadelphia, London, Toronto, Montreal, Sydney, Tokyo: W.B. Saunders.

7 **GILLESPIE, J.H. & TIMONEY, J.F., 1981.** *Hagan and Bruner's Infectious Diseases of Domestic Animals.* 7th edn. Ithaca: Cornell University Press.

8 **HARDIE, J.M., 1986.** Genus *Streptococcus* Rosenbach 1884. *In:* SNEATH, P.H.A., MAIR, N.S., SHARPE, M.E. & HOLT, J.G., (eds). *Bergey's Manual of Systematic Bacteriology.* 9th edn. Baltimore: Williams & Wilkins.

9 **HENTON, M.M., 1993.** Veterinary Research Institute, Onderstepoort 0110, South Africa. Unpublished observations.

10 **JONES, J.E.T., 1976.** The carriage of beta-haemolytic streptococci by healthy pigs. *British Veterinary Journal*, 132, 276–283.

11 **KRANTZ, G.E. & DUNNE, H.W., 1965.** An attempt to classify streptococcic isolates from domestic animals. *American Journal of Veterinary Research*, 26, 951–959.

12 **LE BLANC, M.M., 1989.** Treatment protocols and preventive practices for mares with endometritis. *Veterinary Medicine/Small Animal Clinician*, 84, 906–911.

13 **MUNDT, J.O. & GRAHAM, W.F., 1968.** *Streptococcus faecium* var. *casseliflavus*, nov. var. *Journal of Bacteriology*, 95, 2005–2009.

14 **PARKER, M.T., 1983.** Streptococcus and Lactobacillus. *In:* WILSON, G.S., MILES, A.A. & PARKER, M.T., (eds). *Topley and Wilson's Principles of Bacteriology, Virology and Immunity.* 7th edn. Vol. II. *Systematic Bacteriology.* London: Edward Arnold.

15 **RIISING, H.-J., NIELSEN, N.C., BILLE, N. & SVENDSEN, J., 1976.** Streptococcal infections in sucking pigs. *Nordisk Veterinaermedicin*, 28, 65–79.

16 **ROBERTS, S.J., 1971.** *Veterinary Obstetrics and Genital Diseases.* 2nd edn. Ann Arbor: Edwards Brothers.

17 **ROBERTSON, I.D. & BLACKMORE, D.K., 1989.** Prevalence of *Streptococcus suis* type 1 and 2 in domestic pigs in Australia and New Zealand. *The Veterinary Record*, 124, 391–394.

18 **SCANLAN, C.M., 1988.** *Introduction to Veterinary Bacteriology.* Ames, Iowa: Iowa State University Press.

19 **SCHLEIFER, K.H. & KILPPER-BALZ, R., 1987.** Molecular and chemotaxonomic approaches to the classification of streptococci, enterococci and lactococci: A review. *Systematic and Applied Microbiology,* 10, 1–19.

20 **SWANN, A.I. & KJAR, H.A., 1980.** Streptococcal infection as a cause of reproductive tract problems of swine. *Veterinary Microbiology,* 5, 135–142.

21 **WILSON, G.S. & MILES, A., 1975.** *Topley and Wilson's Principles of Bacteriology, Virology and Immunity.* Vol. I. London: Edward Arnold.

22 **WINDSOR, R.S., 1978.** Streptococcal infections in young pigs. *Veterinary Annual,* 18, 134–143.

149

Strangles

Synonyms: *Streptococcus equi* infection, nuwesiekte (Afrik.)

C.A. Wilkens

Introduction

Strangles is an acute contagious disease of horses, mules and donkeys caused by *Streptococcus equi*. It is characterized, in the typical disease, by fever, acute mucopurulent inflammation of the upper respiratory tract and purulent lymphadenitis and abscessation of particularly the submandibular and retropharyngeal lymph nodes. A serious and often fatal, but uncommon, complication is known as 'bastard strangles', in which metastasis of *S. equi* occurs, with resultant abscess formation in other organs and tissues, such as the lungs, liver, spleen, kidneys, brain and, most frequently, mesenteric and mediastinal lymph nodes. Purulent tendosynovitis and arthritis may also be a sequel. It has been suggested that the occurrence of this form of strangles is largely determined by the animal having an inadequate immune response.[5]

The disease was recognized as long ago as 1251 AD, and the causative *Streptococcus* was first described by Ravolta in 1873.[14] The disease was reproduced experimentally in 1888 by three independent researchers using pure cultures of this *Streptococcus*.[14]

Strangles still occurs throughout the world; sporadic outbreaks occur in mainland Europe, Australia, New Zealand, Japan, North America, Ireland and the United Kingdom.[1–3, 15, 40] At the annual meeting of the International Breeders' Secretariat in 1991 it was established from information derived from reports submitted by 20 countries to the International Collating Centre of the Animal Health Trust, Newmarket, England that during the previous four years three diseases were of major importance: abortion attributable to equid herpesvirus I, equine influenza, and strangles.[3]

The disease is uncommon in southern Africa, but can be expected to occur in any situation where horses, particularly the younger age group, originating from different sources are crowded together. As far as can be ascertained, the last major series of outbreaks occurred in Thoroughbred mares and foals during the period November 1977 to February 1978, after the mares had visited the Western Cape for service during the 1977 breeding season. Many contracted the disease during the visit before returning to their home stud farms in the Eastern Cape, Karoo and Natal.[19] Quite high mortality rates were associated with these outbreaks. Theiler[33] reported on the occurrence in South Africa of sporadic cases and epidemics in the earlier part of this century and considered that aged horses were to a very great extent immune to it as they had 'passed through the disease at an earlier age — very few horses escaping it altogether whilst young.' This was before the major decline in equine populations took place throughout the world. During World War II thousands of horses and mules were shipped from South Africa to India to be used as pack animals in the Burma Campaign. Many of these animals were congregated at a military base camp in Pinetown before shipment from Durban harbour. Periodic outbreaks of strangles occurred in this camp.[39]

Aetiology

Streptococcus equi is a catalase-negative, facultatively anaerobic coccus. Individual cells are ovoid or spherical, 0,6–1,0 µm in diameter; sometimes in pus the long axis of the cells is transverse to the long axis of the chain, but at other times it is parallel.[25] Bacillary forms may occur. It grows in pairs and in short or long chains.[25] A hyaluronic capsule is demonstrable in some strains when young cultures are examined or when serum is added to the growth medium.[25] Growth in common laboratory media is poor unless serum is added.[25] The organism is Gram-positive when cultures are young, but the bacteria obtained from old cultures may stain negatively. Based on the group-specific antigen (Component C), it is placed in Lancefield's Group C. It is strongly ß-haemolytic and produces mucoid (smooth) or matt (wrinkled) colonies on primary isolation.[26] Both matt-colony and mucoid-colony strains of the organism may be isolated from infected horses in one outbreak, and although matt-colony strains have been associated with a less severe form of the disease,[17] there does not appear to be any difference in virulence between the two strains.[36] *Streptococcus equi* contains lipoteichoic acid, which is antigenically similar to antigens of *S. pyogenes*, as well as to a species-specific, trypsin-labile antigen, the 'M-protein'.[4]

Epidemiology

Strangles affects only domestic equidae and is more severe in horses than in either donkeys or mules.[14] It occurs in animals of all ages, but is more common in those less than two years old.[31, 32] Immune mares will confer passive immunity to their foals which will protect the foals until the age of three months.[12] Adult animals which have grown up in relative isolation are fully susceptible and may become severely ill following exposure to *S. equi*.[22] While the majority of animals which recover from an initial attack of strangles are subsequently immune, some may contract the disease a second or even a third time.[38]

Transmission of *S. equi* occurs through both the oral and nasal routes, the former being the more common. It occurs by direct contact with a diseased animal or indirectly through stable attendants and infected fomites. Contaminated feed, water, bedding, stables and stable utensils, including tack or harnesses, are most important in the spread of the infection.[14, 31] Flies may also play a role in its spread. Infection may be transmitted by diseased foals to their dams during suckling, with the subsequent development of purulent mastitis, and by stallions to mares while 'nosing' prior to coitus, with resultant metritis.[14] Contamination of surgical and other wounds may also occur, but in these cases typical strangles does not occur — the infection remains localized at the site and its regional lymph node.[10]

Streptococcus equi is very resistant. In pus and purulent discharges it remains viable for several weeks or months, particularly in a moist environment. It is generally believed that an infected stable, unless very carefully cleaned and disinfected, may remain infective for several months.[14]

The streptococci are shed in nasal discharges and in exudates which may discharge from abscesses for four weeks or more. A carrier state may develop in convalescent and apparently recovered animals, and some 20 per cent of these animals shed *S. equi* in their nasal secretions for up to one month.[31] *Streptococcus equi* has been isolated from the nasal mucosa and pharynx for as long as ten months after initial infection.[14, 31]

On farms and in stables which have a high population density of horses and a rapid turnover of animals, there is an increased risk of infection. In a survey of 179 stud farms in Australia during the period 1985 to 1988 it was found that the risk of strangles increased progressively and dramatically with the total horse population. Stud farms with a population of more than 100 horses had 26,2 times more risk than those with less than 15 horses. Stress, particularly transportation, overcrowding, and concurrent viral infections and parasitism, increases the susceptibility of animals and may precipitate strangles in animals with latent infections. From these the disease then spreads rapidly to other susceptible horses in a stable.[14]

Pathogenesis

Bacteria enter via the oral and respiratory routes, after which they adhere to the epithelium of the nasal cavity and oropharynx. Adherence appears to be a function of the M-protein[24, 28] and is independent of the group-specific carbohydrate, lipoteichoic acid, and the bacterial capsule.[29] Tissue invasion, however, is enhanced by the ability of both the M-protein and the capsule of the organism to inhibit phagocytosis.[4] After penetration of the mucosa it is assumed that bacteria reach the regional lymph nodes of the area via the lymphatic vessels, where they initiate abscessation.

Clinical signs and pathology

In outbreaks the morbidity varies from 10–100 per cent,[31] but the mortality rate is low and ranges from about 1–5 per cent.[11, 14, 32]

The course of strangles in mild and uncomplicated cases is seldom longer than two to four weeks and generally terminates in complete recovery, but it may sometimes be protracted and then lasts for several months. A chronic form of the disease develops in animals with an inadequate immune response.[38]

After an incubation period which usually lasts for between three and eight days, clinical signs are heralded by a sudden sharp rise in temperature to 41 °C. This is often accompanied by anorexia and depression and is soon followed by the development of a serous nasal discharge which, during the course of two to three days, becomes mucopurulent, then purulent and finally thick and yellow. The discharge is generally bilateral but may be more profuse from one nostril than the other. It can be very abundant. A soft, moist cough may be present and can usually be elicited by compression of the pharynx or larynx. Large quantities of exudate are expelled from the nostrils during bouts of coughing, snorting or blowing. The pharyngeal area is painful and the animal stands with its head lowered and extended. The act of swallowing may be impeded. These clinical signs are the result of an acute purulent rhinitis, pharyngitis and, in some cases, laryngitis with hyperaemia and swelling of the mucosa and accumulation of pus in the nasal cavities. Small abscesses may develop in the lymphoid follicles of the soft palate.[11, 35] A catarrhal or purulent conjunctivitis with ocular discharge may be present.

In typical cases of strangles it soon becomes apparent that there is concurrent involvement of the regional lymph nodes draining the nasopharynx, particularly the submandibular and retropharyngeal areas, and, in some animals, other areas in the region, such as the submaxillary and parotid **(Figure 149.1)** may be involved. Affected nodes are hot, swollen and painful, and are initially firm on palpation for about four to six days but with the development of abscessation and suppuration within them, they become softer and considerably larger. The skin over them is extended and becomes very thin

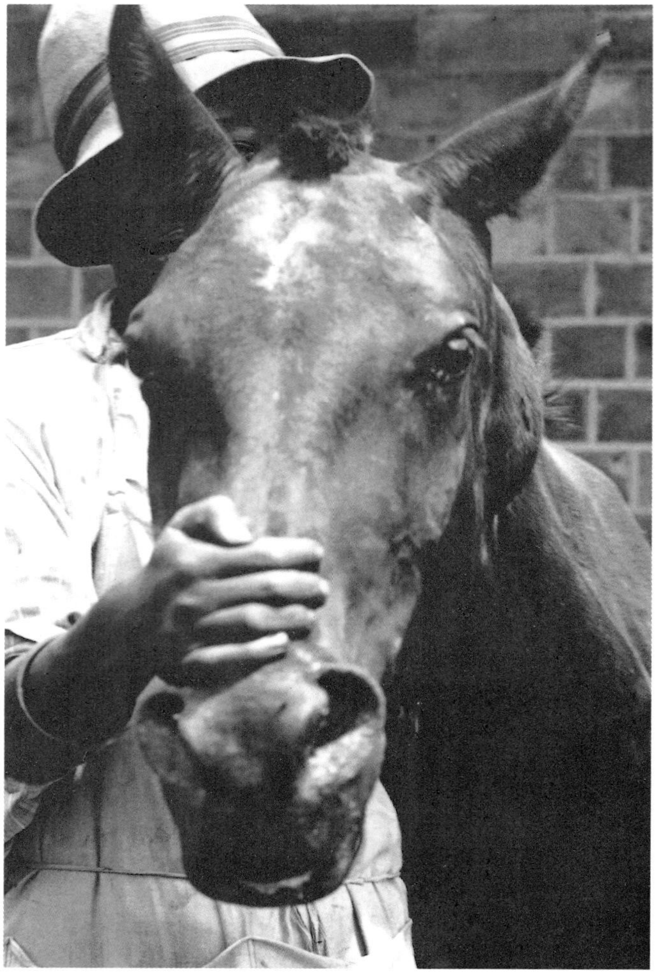

Figure 149.1 Horse with strangles. Note the marked swelling of the parotid region due to lymphadenitis

and may exude a serum-like fluid. The severe lymph node enlargement, together with mucosal changes, may impede mastication, swallowing and respiration and may be so severe as to result in asphyxiation. Finally, after about ten days the abscess or abscesses rupture, discharging large quantities of thick, yellow, creamy pus. Abscesses in the retropharyngeal lymph nodes may rupture externally or internally, i.e. discharge their contents into the pharynx. Rupture is commonly followed by a rapid decline in the fever and an improvement in the habitus of the animal.[8, 14] Occasionally small vesicles, ulcers and scabs form in the skin of various parts of the body, particularly on the cheeks, nose, mouth, sides of the neck, and chest.[14] Haematological examination will reveal the presence of a severe neutrophilia.

The clinical signs in affected animals may range from mild to severe.[11, 14] In the mild form, which occurs most commonly in older horses, manifestations of the disease remain confined to a catarrhal inflammation of the upper respiratory tract, generally without regional lymphadenopathy; if the latter does occur, abscesses in the nodes either do not develop or, if they do, often become encapsulated without rupturing.

The complications of strangles may take on one or more of several forms, some of which may result in a fatal outcome. They include: spread of infection to the guttural pouches via the Eustachian tubes to cause empyema of them, or to the sinuses with resultant purulent sinusitis; periorbital abscessation; paravertebral abscessation; roaring following recurrent nerve involvement in the inflammatory process; purulent pneumonia as the result of aspiration of pus into the lungs following the internal rupture of an abscess in a retropharyngeal lymph node; agalactia in lactating mares;[14, 32] asphyxiation following upper respiratory tract obstruction; myocarditis which may cause significant electrocardiographic abnormalities that persist for several months;[20] endocarditis; pyaemia; and purpura haemorrhagica.[14, 32]

Pyaemia may result in the form of strangles known as 'bastard strangles', in which *S. equi* has metastasized to lymph nodes other than those regional to the upper respiratory tract, and to organs, such as the liver, kidneys, lungs, and brain, with resultant abscess formation, as well as to synovial structures of the limbs with purulent arthritis and tendosynovitis. Of the internal organs, the mesenteric and mediastinal lymph nodes are most commonly affected. Although abscesses in them may become very large, they rarely rupture, but the infection may spread *per continuitatum* from them to reach nearby serosal surfaces with the development of purulent peritonitis or pleuritis. Enlarged mesenteric lymph nodes may result in digestive disturbances and emaciation.[14] A chronic debilitating disease in donkeys has been reported as a result of abscessation of abdominal lymph nodes in the absence of prior upper respiratory tract disease.[42]

Purpura haemorrhagica in horses is a disease of uncertain aetiology and occurs most often two to four weeks after an episode of upper respiratory tract disease, such as strangles, in which it can be a serious, if not fatal, complication.[23] It is thought to be an immune complex-mediated condition in which soluble immune complexes form in the circulation, activate the complement system and cause endothelial cell injury. The resultant increase in capillary permeability leads to the development of widespread oedema and petechiation, but the pathophysiology of the disease is not simple and direct.[18] Thrombocytopenia or other coagulation defects are not features of this condition.[6] Despite its name, oedema is its most outstanding feature in horses. In fatal cases, death is generally due to pulmonary oedema, but there is also widespread oedema of the subcutis (particularly of the head, ventral abdomen and upper parts of the limbs), intermuscular fasciae, larynx, trachea, gastrointestinal tract and body cavities. Scattered petechiae may be found in the skin and in serosal and mucosal membranes, as well as in the kidneys and liver capsule. Foci of degeneration and necrosis may be present in some skeletal muscles. It is generally not possible to make a definitive diagnosis of this condition, but it should always be borne in mind that severe cases of this form of purpura haemorrhagica very closely resemble African horsesickness, both clinically and on necropsy.

Agalactia (in the absence of detectable physical abnormalities in the mammary glands) may be secondary to the high fever, anorexia and depression associated with the disease.[32] Though this complication is not life-threatening, it may become a serious management problem, as alternative sources of milk have to be found for the foals of mares suffering from the condition.

Signs of septicaemia and polyarthritis are commonly seen in foals infected with *S. equi* in the first few weeks of life. Central nervous system involvement commonly follows the septicaemia and causes hyperaesthesia, neck rigidity and terminal paralysis. Because of the generally poor response to treatment, foals with polyarthritis frequently develop chronic arthritis and permanent joint damage.[7]

Diagnosis and differential diagnosis

A provisional diagnosis is based on the clinical signs and demonstration of bacteria in Gram-stained smears made from nasal exudates or obtained from abscesses. Laryngoscopic examination of the upper respiratory tract[41] and radiological demonstration of enlarged lymph nodes and infection of the guttural pouches would add further supportive evidence. The diagnosis is confirmed by the culturing of *S. equi* from the exudate of affected tissues or organs.

The early stages of strangles may be confused with respiratory signs associated with equine viral rhinopneumonitis, equine viral arteritis, equine influenza and acute bronchitis, but in all of these conditions any enlargement of the regional lymph nodes is only slight.[7] Advanced cases of strangles may be confused with other pyogenic infections of the upper respiratory tract, particularly that caused by *Streptococcus zooepidemicus*.

Control

There is controversy surrounding the treatment of strangles with antibiotics. One school of thought claims that antibiotics should not be used because they interfere with the development of immunity and may cause cold abscesses which do not mature. The other advocates rigorous antibiotic therapy, especially with penicillins, throughout the course of the disease. In cases where there is a fever or where life-threatening situations such as pneumonia develop, antibiotic treatment should immediately be instituted and maintained for at least seven days after the abscesses have drained and the temperature has returned to normal. Early antibiotic therapy may in fact be successful in preventing the formation of abscesses. If abscesses have developed to the stage where they are detectable, antibiotics should be withheld until they rupture. Nursing should accompany antibiotic therapy.[8] In some cases, heat treatment of the abscesses until they are soft and fluctuating, followed by lancing, is advised. After lancing, abscesses must be thoroughly drained and then flushed daily with an iodine solution.[16] In some cases, tracheotomy may have to be resorted to.

Particularly when outbreaks occur in fully susceptible horses, all possible precautions must be taken to prevent the spread of the disease. The strict isolation of affected animals should be enforced for at least four to five weeks,[31] and should include the attending grooms, as well as utensils, tack and harnesses used on affected horses. Stables should be thoroughly cleaned and disinfected, and bedding burned. All animals in the stable should be monitored routinely and antibiotic therapy instituted immediately if a rise in body temperature is noticed. The prophylactic use of antibiotics may be considered where large numbers of valuable foals are at risk. Most strains of *S. equi* are sensitive to penicillins, sulphonamide, kefalothin and chloramphenicol, but are resistant to streptomycin, tetracycline, kanamycin and gentamycin.[40]

Following recovery, animals generally have a solid immunity which lasts for more than a year, although some may lose it within six months and become reinfected.[7, 13, 21, 27] Passive transfer of antibodies to *S. equi* in foals occurs via colostrum.[12] The importance of foal management cannot be overemphasized, and foals must be given adequate amounts of colostrum within two days of birth.

The protection afforded by vaccines against *S. equi* infection has been disappointing.[9] Vaccines developed with an acid extraction of the M-protein appear to give the best results.[30, 31, 37] Intra-nasal application of recently developed avirulent strains of *S. equi* gives promise for the development of a successful vaccine.[34]

The treatment of horses suffering from purpura haemorrhagica includes good nursing care and the administration of penicillin (the preferred drug for streptococcal infection), corticosteroids such as prednisone and dexamethasone, and diuretics such as furosemide.[18] The prognosis is guarded, pending response to therapy, and relapses may occur. Steroid therapy might be needed for several weeks.[18]

References

1 **ANON., 1984.** Disease incidence among horses in France, Ireland and the United Kingdom during 1983. *The Veterinary Record*, 114, 56.

2 **ANON., 1985.** Infectious disease incidence among horses in France, Ireland and the United Kingdom during 1984. *The Veterinary Record*, 116, 145.

3 **ANON., 1991.** *International Breeders' Meeting Secretariat Report*. Newmarket, England.

4 **BARNUM, D.A., 1986.** *Streptococcus*. *In*: GYLES, C.L. & THOEN, C.O., (eds). *Pathogenesis of Bacterial Infections*. Ames, Iowa: Iowa State University Press.

5 **BEECH, J., 1991.** *Equine Respiratory Diseases*. Philadelphia: Lea & Febiger.

6 **BIGGERS, J.D., INGRAM, P.L. & MURRAY, C.B., 1949.** Studies on equine purpura haemorrhagica. Haematology. *The British Veterinary Journal*, 105, 191–199.

7 **BLOOD, D.C., RADOSTITS, O.M. & HENDERSON, J.A., 1983.** *Veterinary Medicine*. 6th edn. London: Baillière Tindall.

8 **BLUE, M.G., 1985.** Strangles in horses — the clinical syndrome and a modern immunological approach to its prevention by local vaccination. *Immunology in Clinical Practice, Faculty of Veterinary Science, Massey University*, 11–15 February, 279–282.

9 **BRYANT, S., BROWN, K.K., LEWIS, S., STEWART, R.C. & PARIZEH, R., 1985.** Protection against strangles with enzymatic *Streptococcus equi* extract. *Veterinary Medicine*, 80, 58–70.

10 **DAVIES, G.O., 1947.** *Gaiger and Davies' Veterinary Pathology and Bacteriology*. 3rd edn. London: Baillière, Tindall & Cox.

11 **FALLON, E.H., 1969.** The clinical aspects of streptococcal infections of horses. *Journal of the American Veterinary Medical Association*, 155, 413–414.

12 **GALAN, J.E., TIMONEY, J.F. & LENGEMAN, F.W., 1986.** Passive transfer of mucosal antibodies to *Streptococcus equi* in the foal. *Infection and Immunity*, 54, 202–206.

13 **GEORGE, J.L., REIF, J.S., SHIDELER, R.K., SMALL, C.J., ELLIS, P.P., SNYDER, S.P. & McCHESNEY, A.E., 1983.** Identification of carriers of *Streptococcus equi* in a naturally infected herd. *Journal of the American Veterinary Medical Association*, 183, 80–84.

14 **HENNING, M.W., 1956.** *Animal Diseases in South Africa*. 3rd edn. Pretoria: Central News Agency.

15 **JORM, L.R., 1990.** Strangles in horse studs: Incidence, risk factors and effect of vaccination. *Australian Veterinary Journal*, 67, 436–439.

16 **KNIGHT, A.P., VOX, J.L., McCHESNEY, A.E. & BIGBEE, H.G., 1975.** Experimentally induced *Streptococcus equi* infections in horses with resultant guttural pouch empyema. *Veterinary Medicine/Small Animal Clinician*, 70, 1194–1199.

17 **MAHAFFEY, L.W., 1962.** Respiratory conditions in horses. *The Veterinary Record*, 74, 1295–1313.

18 **MANNING, T. & SWEENEY, C., 1986.** Immune-mediated equine skin diseases. *Compendium on Continuing Education for the Practising Veterinarian*, 8, 979–987.

19 **MARLOW, C.H.B., 1992.** PO Box 138, Cradock 5880, South Africa. Personal communication.

20 **McALLISTER, E.S., 1983.** Bacterial respiratory infections. *In*: MANSMANN, R.A., McALLISTER, E.S. & PRATT, P.W., (eds). *Equine Medicine and Surgery*. 3rd edn. Vol. II. Santa Barbara, California: American Veterinary Publications.

21 **NARA, P.L., KRAHOWHA, S., POWERS, T.E. & GRAG, R.C., 1983.** Experimental *Streptococcus equi* infection in the horse: Correlation with *in vivo* and *in vitro* immune responses. *American Journal of Veterinary Research*, 44, 529–534.

22 **PICHE, C.A., 1984.** Clinical observations on an outbreak of strangles. *Canadian Veterinary Journal*, 25, 7–11.

23 **SCHALM, O.W. & CARLSON, G.P., 1982.** The blood and blood-forming organs. *In*: MANSMANN, R.A., McALLISTER, E.S. & PRATT, P.W., (eds). *Equine Medicine and Surgery*. 3rd edn. Vol. I. Santa Barbara, California: American Veterinary Publications.

24 **SMALL, C. & ELLIS, R., 1982.** Purification and characterization of an M-like protein from *Streptococcus equi*. *Abstracts of papers presented at the 63rd Annual Meeting of the Conference of Research Workers in Animal Disease*. American Congress Hotel, 520 South Michigan, Chicago, Illinois, 8–9 November 1982.

25 **SNEATH, P.H.A., MAIR, N.S., SHARPE, M.E. & HOLT, J.G., 1986.** *Bergey's Manual of Bacteriology*. Vol. 2. Baltimore: Williams & Wilkins.

26 **SPANIER J. & TIMONEY, J.F., 1977.** Bacteriophages from *Streptococcus equi*. *Journal of General Virology*, 35, 369–372.

27 **SRIVASTAVA, S.K. & BARNUM, D.A., 1981.** The serological response of foals to vaccination against strangles. *Canadian Journal of Comparative Medicine*, 45, 20–25.

28 **SRIVASTAVA, S.K. & BARNUM, D.A., 1983.** The role of lipoteichoic acids on the adherence of *Streptococcus equi* to epithelial cells. *Veterinary Microbiology*, 8, 485–492.

29 **SRIVASTAVA, S.K. & BARNUM, D.A., 1983.** Adherence of *Streptococcus equi* on tongue, cheek and nasal epithelial cells of ponies. *Veterinary Microbiology*, 8, 493–504.

30 **SRIVASTAVA, S.K. & BARNUM, D.A., 1985.** Studies on the immunogenicity of *Streptococcus equi* vaccine in foals. *Canadian Journal of Comparative Medicine*, 49, 351–356.

31 **SWEENEY, C.R., BENSON, C.E., WHITLOCK, R.H., MEIRS, D.A., BARRINGHAM, S.O., WHITEHEAD, S.C. & COHEN, D., 1989.** Description of an epizootic and persistence of *Streptococcus equi* infections in horses. *Journal of the American Veterinary Medical Association*, 194, 1281–1286.

32 **SWEENEY, C.R., WHITLOCK, R.H., MEIRS, D.A., WHITEHEAD, S.C. & BARRINGHAM, S.O., 1987.** Complications associated with *Streptococcus equi* infection on a horse farm. *Journal of the American Veterinary Medical Association*, 191, 1446–1448.

33 **THEILER, A., 1918.** Observations on an epizootic contagious catarrh of the respiratory organs of equines and its relation to purpura haemorrhagica. *Seventh and Eighth Reports of the Director of Veterinary Services, Department of Agriculture, Union of South Africa*, 361–393.

34 **TIMONEY, J.F. & GALAN, J.E., 1985.** The protective response of the horse to an avirulent strain of *Streptococcus equi*. *In*: KIMURA, Y., KOTAMI, S. & SHIOKOWA, Y., (eds). *Proceedings of the IXth Lancefield International Symposium on Streptococci and Streptococcal Diseases*.

35 **TIMONEY, J.F., GILLESPIE, J.H., SCOTT, F.W. & BARLOUGH, J.E., 1988.** *Hagan and Bruner's Microbiology and Infectious Diseases of Domestic Animals*. 8th edn. Ithaca: Comstock Publishing Associates.

36 **TIMONEY, J.F., TIMONEY, P.J. & STRICKLAND, K.L., 1984.** Lysogeny and the immunologically reactive proteins of *Streptococcus equi*. *The Veterinary Record*, 115, 148–149.

37 **TIMONEY, J.F. & TRACHMAN, J., 1985.** Immunologically reactive proteins of *Streptococcus equi*. *Infection and Immunity*, 48, 29–34.

38 **TODD, A.G., 1910.** Strangles. *Journal of Comparative Pathology and Therapeutics*, 23, 212–219.

39 **TUSTIN, R.C., 1992.** Pretoria. Personal communication.

40 **VAISSAIRE, J., PLATEAU, E., LAROCHE, M. & MIRIAL, G., 1986.** The strangles situation in France. *Douzième Journal de la Recherche Chevaline*, 129–137.

41 **VON KELLER, H. & JAESCHKE, G., 1984.** Klinische und labordiagnostik bakterieller Infectionen der Atmungsorgane des Pferdes. *Praktische Tierärtztkunde*, 7, 565–570.

42 **WISECUP, W.G., SCHRODER, C. & PAGE, N.P., 1967.** Isolation of *Streptococcus equi* from burros. *Journal of the American Veterinary Medical Association*, 150, 303–306.

150

Streptococcus suis *infections*

M.M. Henton

Introduction and aetiology

Streptococcus suis is an important pathogen of pigs. Although infection with it usually results in bacteraemia and meningitis in pigs, it may also be associated with porcine respiratory disease **(see Chapter 188: Porcine respiratory disease)**, often together with other pathogens, valvular endocarditis, and genital infections. It occasionally causes purulent infections such as abscesses, pneumonia and arthritis in ruminants and horses,[4, 13] and abortions in pigs and cattle.[10]

Isolates of *S. suis* are serologically grouped into Lancefield groups R, S, RS and T, although certain isolates are ungroupable.[14, 16] At one time *S. suis* was considered to resemble Lancefield group D streptococci, and, although this belief has been perpetuated by some authors,[6] it is no longer regarded as valid.[8, 14] *Streptococcus suis* can also be subdivided into serotypes 1 to 8.[17, 24] *Streptococcus suis* type 2 is regarded as being identical to Lancefield group R, whereas *S. suis* type 1 is identical to Lancefield group S.[22]

Humans are also susceptible to *S. suis* type 2 infection and, as the organism may circulate in the blood of both diseased and apparently healthy pigs, infection is a potential occupational health hazard for abattoir workers, pig farmers, meat handlers and veterinarians who work with pigs or handle their products.[1, 18] Disease due to this infection in humans is rare, but it may cause conditions such as meningitis, purulent arthritis, purulent pharyngitis, endophthalmitis, diarrhoea, lymphadenopathy, and disseminated intravascular coagulation.[1] Permanent vestibular and auditory dysfunctions may occur in patients who have recovered from streptococcal meningitis.

Although all strains of *S. suis* are pathogenic, *S. suis* type 2 (Group R) is most commonly the cause of disease in pigs which is similar to but more severe than that caused by *S. suis* type 1.

Infection with *S. suis* type 1 is generally encountered in sucking piglets two to four weeks of age, whereas *S. suis* type 2 infections usually occur in older piglets.[16] Although the syndrome resulting from *S. suis* type 1 infection is similar to that produced by type 2, the mortality rate is not as high.[18]

Infection with *S. suis* type 2 principally causes a syndrome characterized by septicaemia, meningitis, and arthritis in growing pigs.[7, 18] The organism is also the cause of pneumonia among fatteners,[7] valvular endocarditis, neonatal deaths in piglets, and genital infections.[20] It may be a secondary invader of the lungs of pigs suffering from enzootic pneumonia[18] or bronchopneumonia caused by *Pasteurella multocida, Escherichia coli,* or *Actinobacillus pleuropneumoniae.*

Disease due to *S. suis* type 2 has been recorded in the Netherlands, Denmark, Germany, France, Ireland, Czechoslovakia, Brazil, the USA, Canada, New Zealand, Australia[1, 18, 20] and South Africa.[9]

Epidemiology

The syndrome characterized by septicaemia, meningitis, and arthritis is most prevalent in intensive pig-farming systems in which there is a high stocking density. Poor ventilation and heating, sudden changes in weather, overcrowding, and the stress associated with weaning or mixing of pigs predispose to outbreaks of disease.[1] Less than 5 per cent of the weaned animals are usually affected in outbreaks, but higher morbidity rates have been reported.[1]

Carrier pigs are the most important source of infection. The organisms are predominantly harboured in the palatine tonsils and occasionally in the nose, but may rarely be isolated from other organs and tissues of healthy carriers, such as the supramammary and submandibular lymph nodes, joints, blood, vagina and uterus.[1, 18] Infections harboured in the genital tracts of sows also serve as a source of infection for piglets. Piglets born from apparently normal carrier sows with vaginal infections may be infected orally during, or shortly after, the birth process.[3, 18]

Carriers occur in all age groups in herds in which no clinical evidence of infection has been encountered, as well as in herds in which disease has occurred.[1] The carrier rate in different pig herds may vary from 0–100 per cent, although most herds have a prevalence of less than 20 per cent.[3]

Pigs may also become infected after being exposed to environments contaminated with the bacterium, such as the floors and feed troughs of piggeries. *Streptococcus suis* type 2 can survive in dust and faeces at 0°C for between 54 and 104 days.[2, 19] It is killed under experimental conditions by cleaners and disinfectants commonly used in piggeries at concentrations more dilute than those recommended by the manufacturers, and also by dilute soap and water solutions.[1]

The house fly (*Musca domestica*) can carry *S. suis* type 2 for at least four days, and may therefore play a role in the dissemination of the disease in piggeries.[5]

Clinical signs and pathology

The syndrome manifested by septicaemia, meningitis, and arthritis in growing pigs affects animals aged between two and 22 weeks, the majority of cases occurring in the three- to 12-week-old group.[12] Clinical signs are seen within 10–14 days of the occurrence of predisposing factors, or within five days of being in contact with carrier pigs.[1] During outbreaks pigs may suffer from peracute disease and may be found dead without any premonitory signs being noticed. In the acute disease, evidence of septicaemia, loss of appetite, depression, and reddening of the skin may be present initially. The disease rapidly progresses and manifestations of meningitis, characterized by the adoption of unusual postures, swaying gait, circling, incoordination and convulsions, become apparent. These signs are followed by paddling movements of the legs, opisthotonus and tetanic spasms and paralysis.[1, 22] Affected pigs may be deaf and have staring eyes and nystagmus, or become blind.[1, 22] Some animals, particularly the younger ones, may show evidence of arthritis. The course of the disease syndrome is often very short and pigs may die within a matter of hours.

On necropsy, the nature and extent of the lesions depend on the length of the clinical disease. In a typical case, there is marked congestion of the carcass,[1, 22] the lymph nodes are enlarged and congested, and there is congestion of the parenchymatous organs. A fibrinous peritonitis is often present. Gross evidence of meningitis may or may not be visible. When lesions do occur, the meninges are congested, discoloured, yellowish and thickened due to the presence of exudate. The cerebrospinal fluid may be turbid and excessive. Histopathologically, the lesions in untreated pigs are those of an acute purulent leptomeningitis and choroiditis, but the cellular reaction is predominantly lymphocytic in animals which have received antibiotic treatment and where the course of the disease is prolonged.[22] In some pigs an acute purulent polyarthritis is present.

Little information is available about the disease in ruminants, as *S. suis* infection is so sporadic.[11, 13]

Diagnosis

A preliminary diagnosis is based on the history (frequently involving recent weaning or mixing of animals), age group involved, clinical signs, and macroscopic and microscopic pathology which includes the demonstration of the organism. For confirmation of the diagnosis, isolation and identification of *S. suis* are required. The specimens that are necessary for bacteriological examination comprise brain, cerebrospinal fluid, blood, peritoneal and pleural fluids, internal organs, and synovial membrane and joint fluids.[1] Identification of *S. suis* is performed by demonstrating the type-specific polysaccharide capsule using hyperimmune rabbit antiserum, or by direct or indirect fluorescent antibody tests of the organism in smears.[1, 18] The methods used for the identification of *S. suis* have been reviewed.[10]

Control

Pigs affected by *S. suis* type 2 respond well to antimicrobial treatment. Penicillin is the drug of choice in the parenteral treatment of individual cases,[21, 23] but *S. suis* is also susceptible to other antimicrobials such as amoxyllin, ampicillin, and lincomycin.[21] In an outbreak it is recommended that all pigs in the group containing affected animals be treated either by individual parenteral administration of a suitable antimicrobial drug or by the feeding of a medicated ration. Treatment of an affected individual should commence as early as possible in the course of the disease, and good nursing — particularly ensuring an adequate fluid intake and removal to a quiet environment — is essential.[23]

In the control of the disease, predisposing factors should be eliminated or minimized. Strategic medication through the feed or water during periods of heightened risk will reduce the prevalence of the disease. Blanket medication of the feed in order to eliminate the disease from herds has been attempted without success, although it does temporarily decrease the number of cases.[1, 15] Feed may be medicated with procaine penicillin G or a mixture of chlortetracycline hydrochloride, sulphadimidine and procaine penicillin G.[15] When penicillin is used in medicated feeds, only freshly mixed rations should be used.

Apart from depopulation and restocking with clean stock, eradication of the disease can also be achieved by application of medicated early weaning techniques. The use of autogenous bacterins and commercial antisera and vaccines that are now available in the USA have yielded encouraging results.[19] These products are not available in South Africa.

References

1 **CLIFTON-HADLEY, F.A., 1983.** *Streptococcus suis* type 2 infections. *British Veterinary Journal,* 139, 1–5.

2 **CLIFTON-HADLEY, F.A., ALEXANDER, T.J.L. & ENRIGHT, M.R., 1986.** The epidemiology, diagnosis, treatment and control of *Streptococcus suis* type 2 infection. *Proceedings of the American Association of Swine Practitioners.*

3 **CLIFTON-HADLEY, F.A., ALEXANDER, T.J.L., UPTON, I. & DUFFUS, W.P.H., 1984.** Further studies on the subclinical carrier state of *Streptococcus suis* type 2 in pigs. *The Veterinary Record,* 114, 513–518.

4 **DEVRIESE, L.A., CEYSSENS, K., HOMMEZ, J., KILPPER-BÄLZ, R. & SCHLEIFER, K.H., 1991.** Characteristics of different *Streptococcus suis* ecovars and description of a simplified identification method. *Veterinary Microbiology,* 26, 141–150.

5 **ENRIGHT, M.R., ALEXANDER, T.J.L. & CLIFTON-HADLEY, F.A., 1987.** Role of house flies (*Musca domestica*) in the epidemiology of *Streptococcus suis* type 2. *The Veterinary Record,* 121, 132–133.

6 **ERICKSON, E.D., 1993.** Streptococcal disease. In: HOWARD, J.L., (ed.). *Current Veterinary Therapy: Food Animal Practice 3.* Philadelphia: W.B. Saunders Co.

7 **GUISE, H.J., PENNY, R.H.C. & PETHERICK, D.J., 1986.** Streptococcal meningitis in pigs: Field trails to study the prophylactic effect of trimethoprim/sulphadiazine medication in feed. *The Veterinary Record,* 119, 395–400.

8 **HARDIE, J.M., 1986.** Genus *Streptococcus* Rosenbach 1884. *In:* SNEATH, P.H.A., MAIR, N.S., SHARPE, M.E. & HOLT, J.G., (eds). *Bergey's Manual of Systematic Bacteriology.* 9th edn. Baltimore: Williams & Wilkins.

9 **HENTON, M.M., 1993.** Veterinary Research Institute, Onderstepoort 0110, South Africa. Unpublished data.

10 **HIGGINS, R. & GOTTSCHALK, M., 1990.** An update on *Streptococcus suis* identification. *Journal of Veterinary Diagnostic Investigation,* 2, 249–252.

11 **HIGGINS, R., GOTTSCHALK, M., FECTEAN, G., SANVAGEEN, R., DE GUISE, S. & DU TREMBLAY, D., 1990.** Isolation of *Streptococcus suis* from cattle. *Canadian Veterinary Journal,* 31, 259.

12 **HOFFMAN, L.J. & HENDERSON, L.M., 1985.** The significance of *Streptococcus suis* in swine disease: Clinical, pathologic and bacteriologic data from a two-year study. *American Association of Veterinary Laboratory Diagnosticians,* 28th Annual Proceedings, Milwaukee, Wisconsin, Oct. 27–29.

13 **HOMMEZ, J., WULLEPIT, J., CASSIMON, P., CASTRYCK, F., CEYSSENS, K. & DEVRIESE, L.A., 1988.** *Streptococcus suis* and other streptococcal species as a cause of extramammary infection in ruminants. *The Veterinary Record,* 123, 626–627.

14 **KILPPER-BÄLZ, R. & SCHLEIFER, K.H., 1987.** *Streptococcus suis* sp. nov., nom. rev. *International Journal of Systematic Bacteriology,* 37, 160–162.

15 **McKELLAR, Q. H., BAXTER, P., TAYLOR, D. & BOGAN, J.A., 1987.** Penicillin therapy of spontaneous streptococcal meningitis in pigs. *The Veterinary Record,* 121, 347–350.

16 **PEDERSEN, K.B., KJEMS, E., PERCH, B. & SLOT, P., 1981.** Infection with RS streptococci in pigs. *Acta Pathologica et Microbiologica Scandanavia,* Section B, 89, 161–165.

17 **PERCH, B., PEDERSEN, K.B. & HENRICHSEN, J., 1983.** Serology of capsulated streptococci pathogenic for pigs: Six new serotypes of *Streptococcus suis. Journal of Clinical Microbiology,* 17, 993–996.

18 **ROBERTSON, I.D. & BLACKMORE, D.K., 1989.** Prevalence of *Streptococcus suis* type 1 and 2 in domestic pigs in Australia and New Zealand. *The Veterinary Record,* 124, 391–394.

19 **SANFORD, S.E. & HIGGINS, R., 1992.** Streptococcal diseases. *In:* LEMAN, A.D., STRAW, B.E., MENGELING, W.L., D'ALLAIRE, S. & TAYLOR, D.J., (eds). *Diseases of Swine,* 7th edn. Ames, Iowa: Iowa State University Press.

20 **SANFORD, S.E. & TILKER, A.M.E., 1982.** *Streptococcus suis* type 2-associated disease in swine: Observations of a one-year study. *Journal of the American Veterinary Medical Association,* 181, 673–676.

21 **TAYLOR, D.J., 1983.** *Pig Diseases.* 3rd edn. Cambridge: The Burlington Pess (Cambridge) Ltd.

22 **WINDSOR, R.S., 1977.** Meningitis in pigs caused by *Streptococcus suis* type 2. *The Veterinary Record,* 101, 378–379.

23 **WINDSOR, R.S., 1978.** Streptococcal infections in young pigs. *In:* GRUNSELL, C.S. & HILL, F.W.G., (eds). *The Veterinary Annual.* 18th issue. Bristol: Scientechnica.

24 **WINDSOR, R.S. & ELLIOTT, S.D., 1975.** Streptococcal infection in young pigs. IV. An outbreak of streptococcal meningitis in weaned pigs. *Journal of Hygiene,* 75, 69–78.

151

Streptococcus porcinus *infections*

Synonyms: Cervical lymphadenitis, jowl abscess

M.M. Henton

Introduction and aetiology

Streptococcus porcinus (Lancefield groups E, P, U or V) is commonly involved in purulent infections in pigs.[8] Streptococcal cervical lymphadenitis of pigs is by far the most important of these infections. It is a contagious, usually non-fatal disease caused principally by *S. porcinus* group E, and is characterized clinically by the development of abscesses in the lymph nodes of the cephalic and cervical regions.[3, 6, 13, 15] It may be responsible for severe economic losses as a result of the condemnation of the heads of affected pigs when slaughtered at abattoirs.[4, 14] *Streptococcus porcinus* groups P, U and V have also been associated with cervical lymph node abcessation, but may be isolated from pigs suffering from pneumonia or septicaemia and from certain forms of mastitis in cows **(see Chapter 190: Mastitis)**.[8]

Epidemiology

Asymptomatic carrier animals harbour the organisms in their palatine tonsils for up to 21 months after their initial exposure,[6, 17] and are responsible for the spread of infection to other animals via nasal droplets or by contaminating drinking water, feed and soil.[6, 13] Infection in susceptible animals occurs in their palatine tonsils and nasal cavity, from whence the organism spreads lymphogenously to regional lymph nodes.[6, 22]

Pigs younger than eight weeks of age and older than two-and-a-half years are less susceptible than animals of other ages;[1, 14, 17] it appears that animals between the ages of nine and 14 weeks are the most susceptible.[1, 16] The reason for the differences in resistance to the infection is not understood. Streptococcal lymphadenitis may occur endemically in some pig herds, with the disease occurring yearly in young pigs.[5] When healthy adult animals from streptococcal lymphadenitis-free herds are introduced into infected herds, the disease may develop in them within a few weeks.

Pathogenesis

In the experimentally induced disease, abscesses develop most commonly in the mandibular lymph nodes but are also frequently found in the retropharyngeal and parotid lymph nodes.[3] Microscopically, streptococci and neutrophils may be present in affected lymph nodes as soon as two hours after oral infection.[11] Scattered miliary, encapsulated abscesses about 1 mm in diameter may be macroscopically visible in lymph nodes seven days after experimental infection.[3, 11] By the 15th day, the abscesses may have enlarged to 5–10 mm in diameter, and by the 21st day to 70 mm in diameter.[3] When fully developed the abscesses have a dense, fibrous tissue capsule and contain greenish, viscous or semi-fluid pus which does not have an offensive odour.[4]

Clinical signs and pathology

Following experimental transmission of *S. porcinus* to susceptible pigs, an acute febrile reaction develops between eight and 15 days after exposure, and persists for five to eight days.[6] An inversion of the neutrophil to lymphocyte ratio in the blood occurs simultaneously with the fever and is followed some days later by a leukocytosis. During the febrile stage, pigs have a reduced feed intake and may be constipated and depressed. Abscesses may be detected about 14 days after the onset of the fever, by deep palpation of the tissues medial to the rami of the mandibles. The first visible evidence of the progressively enlarging abscesses in the lymph nodes may be a bulging of the skin in the region 21 days after the onset of the acute febrile stage. Skin necrosis over abscesses may occur in the fifth week after infection, with spontaneous rupture of the abscesses and drainage of the exudate in the seventh or eighth week, after which healing occurs. Healing may be complete by the tenth week.[4]

The natural disease resembles that produced experimentally. The abscesses may be multiple and up to 100 mm in diameter. In many pigs, however, they are not noticed until the animals are slaughtered, when they are observed during meat inspection.[4] In the USA, the condemnation of heads as a result of the abscesses in slaughtered pigs may be as high as 94 per cent for some herds.[14, 17] Abscesses caused by *S. porcinus* group E are occasionally encountered in atypical sites, such as the popliteal lymph nodes.[17]

Diagnosis

The diagnosis of streptococcal lymphadenitis is based on the clinical signs and pathology, and the bacteriological isolation of *S. porcinus* from the exudate. A direct fluorescent antibody test has been developed and is used not only to identify the organism in smears of cultures and exudates, but also to detect the organism in the tonsils of carriers.[20] Serological tests, including haemagglutination, tube and plate agglutination, microtitration agglutination, and precipitation, have been applied in attempts to detect infected pigs, but none has proved satisfactory as a reliable diagnostic tool, as cross-reactions with antibodies to other groups of streptococci and other complicating factors do occur.[2, 13, 21]

Differential diagnosis

Other bacteria such as *Streptococcus equisimilis, Actinomyces (Corynebacterium) pyogenes, Pasteurella multocida, Escherichia coli and Mycobacterium* spp. may also cause cervical lymphadenitis,[3, 4] which should be distinguished by bacteriological means from that caused by *S. porcinus*.

Control

Individual animals suffering from large abscesses should be treated surgically if possible, as therapy with antimicrobial drugs is ineffective.[16]

There are three basic approaches to the control of streptococcal lymphadenitis on a herd basis: the adoption of and rigid adherence to a specific pathogen-free system of management; the prophylactic and therapeutic treatment of pigs either by the addition of antimicrobial drugs to their diet or by parenteral administration; and vaccination. The addition of chlortetracycline (125 g/ton for six weeks after weaning) to the diet of pigs will significantly reduce the prevalence of the disease, if the isolate is not resistant to the antibiotic.[10] Simultaneous treatment of all the breeding stock with chlortetracycline at 400 g/ton of feed, and of all the pigs to be marketed with 200 g chlortetracycline per ton for one month, also results in fewer abscesses in all groups.[18, 19] Managemental procedures, such as the isolation of groups of pigs after weaning, the maintenance of smaller numbers of pigs per pen, and keeping the same pigs together throughout the finishing period, should also be instituted to control the disease.[14]

Streptococcus porcinus group E-infected pigs are immune to the organism after recovery from clinical disease.[4] A less virulent immunogenic strain of the bacterium is used for the production of a commercial vaccine (Jowl Vac, Fort Dodge Laboratories, Fort Dodge, Iowa) which is administered orally.[7, 9] The protection rate following vaccination with this vaccine varies between 88 and 100 per cent.[9, 12] No such vaccine is available in South Africa.

References

1 **ARMSTRONG, C.H., BOEHM, P.N. & ELLIS, R.P., 1970.** Experimental transmission of streptococci lymphadenitis (jowl abscess) of swine. *American Journal of Veterinary Research*, 31, 823–829.

2 **ARMSTRONG, C.H., WOOD, R.C. & WESSMAN, G.E., 1982.** A microtitration agglutination test for detecting group E *Streptococcus* infection in swine. *Canadian Journal of Comparative Medicine*, 46, 201–205.

3 **COLLIER, J.R., 1956.** Streptococcic lymphadenitis of the pharyngeal region of swine. *Journal of the American Veterinary Medical Association*, 129, 543–548.

4 **COLLIER, J.R., 1965.** Abscesses of swine. *Journal of the American Veterinary Medical Association*, 146, 344–347.

5 **COLLIER, J.R. & NOEL, J., 1971.** Streptococcic lymphadenitis of swine: A contagious disease. *American Journal of Veterinary Research*, 32, 1501–1505.

6 **COLLIER, J.R. & NOEL, J., 1974.** Streptococcal lymphadenitis of swine: Prolonged carrier state and bacterial dynamics in the introduction of disease. *American Journal of Veterinary Research*, 35, 799–801.

7 **COLLIER, J.R., SHAFFER, H.D. & SCHULTZ, M., 1976.** Evaluation of a vaccine for control of streptococcic lymphadenitis of swine. *Journal of the American Veterinary Medical Association*, 169, 697–699.

8 **COLLINS, M.D., FARROW, J.A.E., KATIC, V. & KANDLER, O., 1984.** Taxonomic studies on streptococci of serological groups E, P, U and V: Description of *Streptococcus porcinus* sp. nov. *Systematic and Applied Microbioloby*, 5, 402–413.

9 **ENGELBRECHT, H. & DOLAN, M., 1968.** Vaccination of swine for jowl abscesses. *Veterinary Medicine/Small Animal Clinician*, 63, 872–875.

10 **ERICKSON, E.D., 1993.** Streptococcal disease. In: HOWARD, J.L., (ed.). *Current Veterinary Therapy: Food Animal Practice 3*. Philadelphia: W.B. Saunders Co.

11 **GOSSER, H.S. & OLSON, L.D., 1973.** Chronologic development of streptococcic lymphadenitis in swine. *American Journal of Veterinary Research*, 34, 77–82.

12 **ISAKI, L.S., BAINEY, M.H. & VAN PATTEN, L.K., 1973.** Response of vaccinated swine to group E *Streptococcus* exposure. *Cornell Veterinarian*, 63, 578–588.

13 **MILLER, R.B. & OLSON, L.D., 1983.** Distribution of abscesses and shedder state of swine inoculated with group E streptococci via routes other than oral. *American Journal of Veterinary Research*, 44, 937–944.

14 **MILLER, R.B. & OLSON, L.D., 1983.** Frequency of jowl abscesses in feeder and market swine exposed to group E streptococci as nursing pigs. *American Journal of Veterinary Research*, 44, 945–948.

15 **SANFORD, S.E. & HIGGINS, R., 1992.** Streptococcal diseases. *In:* LEMAN, A.D., STRAW, B.E., MENGELING, W.L., D'ALLAIRE, S. & TAYLOR, D.J., (eds). *Diseases of Swine*. 7th edn. Ames, Iowa: Iowa State University Press.

16 **SCHMITZ, J.A. & OLSON, L.D., 1972.** Susceptibility of swine of various ages to streptococcic lymphadenitis. *American Journal of Veterinary Research*, 33, 1995–2001.

17 **SCHMITZ, J.A. & OLSON, L.D., 1973.** Transmission of streptococcic lymphadenitis by carrier swine. *American*

Journal of Veterinary Research, 34, 189–190.

18 **SCHMITZ, J.A. & OLSON, L.D., 1973.** Prevention of streptococcic lymphadenitis in swine: Effectiveness of medication with chlortetracycline and isolation from other swine in an infected herd. *Journal of the American Veterinary Medical Association*, 162, 55–57.

19 **SCHMITZ, J.A. & OLSON, L.D., 1973.** Prevention of streptococcic lymphadenitis in swine: Effectiveness of selected antibiotics and a modified live-GES vaccine. *Journal of the American Veterinary Medical Association*, 162, 58–60.

20 **SCHUELER, R.L., MOREHOUSE, L.G. & OLSON, L.D., 1973.** A direct fluorescent antibody test for identification of group E streptococci. *Canadian Journal of Comparative Medicine*, 37, 327–329.

21 **WESSMAN, G.E., SHUMAN, R.D., WOOD, R.L. & NORD, N., 1971.** Swine abscesses caused by Lancefield's group E streptococci. IX. Comparison of the precipitin, haemagglutination and agglutination tests for their detection. *Cornell Veterinarian*, 61, 400–415.

22 **WOOD, R.L. & WESSMAN, G.E., 1984.** Immune response of swine vaccinated with a group E *Streptococcus* whole-culture bacterin. *American Journal of Veterinary Research*, 45, 1933–1936.

152

Other Streptococcus *spp. infections*

M.M. Henton

Introduction

Many varied primary and secondary purulent infections are caused by *Streptococcus* spp. **(see *Streptococcus* spp. infections: Introduction: Table 1)**. Miscellaneous streptococcal infections, particularly those associated with genital tract disease and neonatal septicaemia and its consequences, are dealt with in this chapter. The introductory section should be consulted for information on the microbiologic and epidemiological characteristics of the various *Streptococcus* spp. *Streptococcus agalactiae, S. dysgalactiae* and *S. uberis* as causes of mastitis are discussed in **Chapter 190: Mastitis**.

Genital tract infections and neonatal disease

Streptococcus zooepidemicus is a common cause of genital tract disease in mares.[7] Mares suffering from genital tract disease show a slight to copious purulent vulval discharge which varies in nature from a cloudy, thin fluid to a thick, yellowish exudate which may be frothy; it is more prominent at oestrus than during dioestrus. The vulva of affected mares may gape and the vaginal mucous membrane is congested and inflamed. In severe cases the cervix and uterus are enlarged on rectal palpation. Streptococcal infections in mares usually cause reduced conception rates as a result of early embryonic death (usually before 35 days of gestation), but abortions or the birth of infected foals may also occur.[9] Stallions usually act only as carriers; they harbour *S. zooepidemicus* as a commensal in the prepuce. For broad guidelines on the diagnosis and control of endometritis in mares, **see Chapter 189: Infectious causes of equine reproductive failure**.

Streptococcus equisimilis is the most common bacterium associated with vaginal discharges, lowered conception rates, metritis and abortion in sows in South Africa.[5] Infection with beta-haemolytic streptococci of several serotypes is also associated with infertility and abortion in sows.[11] The effects of, and clinical signs caused by, *S. equisimilis* infections in sows are similar to those of *S. zooepidemicus* infection in mares. Dual infection by *S. equisimilis* and parvovirus in sows may cause abortions at any stage of pregnancy,[3, 11] a high percentage of stillbirths, and the birth of weak piglets.[10] *Streptococcus* spp. are not known to cause disease in the reproductive tract of boars.

On rare occasions, streptococcal infections are associated with abortions and genital infections in sheep, goats and cattle. In the *Streptococcus* spp. infections of the genital tract in ruminants, *S. dysgalactiae* is the most common of the streptococci causing infertility, and may be isolated from normal semen and the sheath (where it rarely causes inflammation) of bulls and rams. These bacteria may be isolated together with *Mycoplasma* serovars from cases of ulcerative balanoposthitis and vulvovaginitis in sheep and goats **(see Chapter 192: Ulcerative balanoposthitis and vulvovaginitis of sheep and goats)**.

In neonates of all livestock species, septicaemia, arthritis and meningitis or meningoencephalitis may be caused by *Streptococcus* spp. (in addition to a variety of other bacteria, such as *Escherichia coli, Salmonella* serovars, *Klebsiella* spp. and *Actinobacillus equuli*). Streptococcal septicaemia is, however, encountered particularly in foals and piglets.

Neonatal streptococcal septicaemia is often a sequel to purulent omphalophlebitis, but it may also follow infection via the oral or cutaneous routes. In South Africa, streptococcal septicaemia in foals is rare, but when it does occur it is usually caused by *S. zooepidemicus,* and only infrequently by *S. equisimilis.* Neonatal septicaemia in South African piglets is predominantly caused by *S. equisimilis* infection, although such infections by *S. suis* and *S. porcinus* are reasonably common.[5]

The initial clinical signs in neonates suffering from septicaemia are subtle, and include fever, listlessness, increased respiratory and heart rates and a disinclination to suckle. These are often followed by signs which indicate localization of infection in one or more tissues or organs, such as the meninges, joints, lungs and endocardium. If the route of entry to the body was via the umbilical cord, the umbilicus may show signs of slight or marked omphalophlebitis. When the infection is severe, the umbilicus is markedly swollen and may discharge pus.[10] Omphalophlebitis and subsequent septicaemia are also caused by infection with bacteria belonging to the Enterobacteriaceae (such as *Escherichia coli* and *Salmonella* serovars) or *Actinobacillus* spp., but these are usually more acute and rapidly fatal than those caused by *Streptococcus* spp. *Erysipelothrix rhusiopathiae* infection in pigs may be difficult to distinguish clinically from streptococcal infections, as it also causes septicaemia, arthritis and valvular endocarditis.[6]

Streptococcal arthritis occurs in the young of all livestock species.[2] *Streptococcus equisimilis* is the most common cause of a suppurative, proliferative arthritis of piglets from birth to six weeks of age, following infection in the birth canal or of skin wounds, tonsils or the umbilicus, but it also occurs in older animals.[1, 4, 8] Affected animals are disinclined to move and their joints are swollen and painful. The larger joints (hock, stifle and knee) are generally more severely affected, and in these cases the infection may extend to involve tendon sheaths in the vicinity of affected joints. The arthritis may become chronic, in which case joints may eventually become ankylosed. Arthritis and synovitis in pigs are also caused by a wide variety of microorganisms, including *Erysipelothrix rhusiopathiae, Actinomyces (Corynebacterium) pyogenes, Staphylococcus aureus, Haemophilus parasuis, Eschericia coli, Salmonella* serovars, and *Mycoplasma hyorhinis* and *M. hyosynoviae*.[12–14]

Streptococcal meningitis or meningoencephalitis is often encountered in piglets **(see Chapter 150: *Streptococcus suis* infections)** but may also occur in neonates of other livestock species. Affected animals (several in a litter may be affected) show nervous signs such as incoordination, swaying, circling, paddling movements and convulsions.[1, 4]

Other purulent infections

Abscesses and other purulent inflammations affecting a variety of tissues or organs may occur as a result of streptococcal infection **(see *Streptococcus* spp. infections: Introduction: Tables 2-4)**. The clinical signs vary according to the site and severity of the infection.

Streptococcal abscessation caused by *S. equisimilis, S. suis, S. zooepidemicus, S. dysgalactiae* and *S. porcinus* in lymph nodes, especially in the cervical nodes in pigs, may macroscopically resemble tubercular granulomas. They should also be differentiated from abscesses caused by *A. pyogenes*.

In horses, *S. zooepidemicus* in particular, but also *S. equisimilis*, are responsible for abscessation, 'poll evil' and 'fistulous withers'.[5] *Streptococcus zooepidemicus* is also the cause of wound infections or pneumonia (either alone or together with *Rhodococcus equi*) in horses, or it may complicate viral infections of the respiratory tract.[2]

Control

Application of the general principles of hygiene is important in the control of streptococcal infections. Attention should be given to the removal and destruction of purulent exudates from the environment, and to proper disinfection of the umbilicus in new-born animals.

Most streptococci are sensitive to penicillin, which remains the drug of choice.[1, 7]

References

1 **BARNUM, D.A., 1986.** *Streptococcus. In:* GYLES, C.L. & THOEN, C.O., (eds). *Pathogenesis of Bacterial Infections in Animals.* Ames, Iowa: Iowa State University Press.

2 **BLOOD, D.C., HENDERSON, J.A. & RADOSTITS, O.M., 1979.** *Veterinary Medicine.* 5th edn. London, Sydney, Auckland, Toronto, Johannesburg: Baillière Tindall.

3 **DOTY, M.K. & VORHIES, M.W., 1971.** The role of *Streptococcus equisimilis* in swine infertility, fetal death, and abortion. *Iowa State University Veterinarian,* 33, 89–91.

4 **GILLESPIE, J.H. & TIMONEY, J.F., 1981.** *Hagan and Bruner's Infectious Diseases of Domestic Animals.* 7th edn. Ithaca: Cornell University Press.

5 **HENTON, M.M., 1993.** Veterinary Research Institute, Onderstepoort 0110. Unpublished data.

6 **KUNESH, J.P., 1993.** Swine erysipelas. *In:* HOWARD, J.L., (ed.). *Current Veterinary Therapy: Food Animal Practice 3.* Philadelphia: W.B. Saunders Co.

7 **LE BLANC, M.M., 1989.** Treatment protocols and preventive practices for mares with endometritis. *Veterinary Medicine/ Small Animal Clinician,* 84, 906–911.

8 **RIISING, H.-J., NIELSEN, N.C., BILLE, N. & SVENDSEN, J., 1976.** Streptococcal infections in sucking pigs. *Nordisk Veterinaermedicin,* 28, 65–79.

9 **ROBERTS, S.J., 1971.** *Veterinary Obstetrics and Genital Diseases.* 2nd edn. Ann Arbor: Edwards Brothers.

10 **SANFORD, S.E. & ROSS, R.F., 1986.** Streptococcal diseases. *In:* LEMAN, A.D., STRAW, B., GLOCK, R.D., MENGELING, W.L., PENNY, R.H.C. & SCHOLL, E., (eds). *Diseases of Swine.* 6th edn. Ames, Iowa: Iowa State University Press.

11 **SWANN, A.I. & KJAR, H.A., 1980.** Streptococcal infection as a cause of reproductive tract problems of swine. *Veterinary Microbiology,* 5, 135–142.

12 **TURNER, G.V.S., 1977.** The aetiology, nature and public health significance of arthritis in slaughter pigs at a South African abattoir. Thesis, M. Med. Vet. (Hyg.), University of Pretoria, South Africa.

13 **TURNER, G.V.S., 1982.** A microbiological study of polyarthritis in slaughter pigs. *Journal of the South African Veterinary Association,* 53, 99–101.

14 **TITTIGER, F. & ALEXANDER, D.C., 1971.** Studies on the bacterial flora of condemned portions from arthritic hogs. *Canadian Journal of Comparative Medicine,* 35, 244–248.

ENDOSPORE-FORMING GRAM-POSITIVE RODS AND COCCI

The genera included in this group have diverse characteristics and are only grouped together for convenience because of their ability to form endospores.[1] Of the six genera contained within the group, only species in the genera *Bacillus* and *Clostridium* are of veterinary importance. The characteristics of these two genera and the species contained within them are dealt with in the introductory sections preceding or within the relevant chapters that deal with them.

The endospores that are characteristic for the members of this group are round or oval and form within the bacterial cells. These spores are highly resistant to the lethal effects of heat, desiccation and disinfectants, and this allows them to survive in nature for prolonged periods, sometimes for decades—a factor that is important in the persistence of the bacteria in the environment and in the epidemiology of the diseases caused by them. In general, the taxonomic relationship between the genera in this group is uncertain, but it does appear that the *Bacillus* and *Clostridium* genera belong to a major group of bacteria that includes genera such as *Staphylococcus* and *Streptococcus*. It is likely that both *Clostridium* and *Bacillus* may in future be subdivided into a number of different genera.[1]

Species of bacteria within the two relevant genera in this group cause some of the oldest and most destructive diseases known. *Bacillus anthracis*, which causes anthrax, a highly fatal and contagious disease of humans and animals, is the only species of the genus that is an important pathogen, although some of the others, such as *Bacillus cereus* may be opportunistic pathogens. Numerous clostridial species, on the other hand, are causes of disease; their pathogenicity is largely dependent on their ability to produce a range of toxins that have diverse effects, including histotoxicity, haemolysis and neurotoxicity. These toxins are elaborated in and absorbed from either the lumen of the intestinal tract of an animal, resulting in an enterotoxaemia (e.g. pulpy kidney disease), or foci of necrotic tissue (e.g. tetanus and gas gangrene), or they are produced in feed or decomposing matter of animal or vegetable origin (e.g. botulism, which is a form of food poisoning).

Reference

1 **SNEATH, P.H.A., 1986.** Endospore-forming Gram-positive rods and cocci. *In*: SNEATH, P.H.A., MAIR, N.S., SHARPE, M.E. & HOLT, J.G., (eds). *Bergey's Manual of Systematic Bacteriology*. Baltimore: Williams & Wilkins.

153

Anthrax

Synonym: Miltsiekte (Afrik.)

V. de Vos

Introduction

Anthrax is a peracute, acute or subacute, highly contagious disease of domestic and wild animals and humans caused by the bacterium *Bacillus anthracis*. In most species of animals it is characterized terminally by the development of a rapidly fatal septicaemia that results in sudden death, and by the presence of the organism in blood and body fluids at death. The principal lesions are those of widespread oedema, haemorrhage and necrosis.

The first record of anthrax is considered to be that in the Bible (Exodus, Chapters 7–9) which refers to the fifth and sixth plagues of Egypt — believed to be systemic and cutaneous anthrax, respectively — which occurred in about 1491 BC.[57, 109, 117, 201, 258] Virgil (70–19 BC) not only described major periodic outbreaks of anthrax in animals and humans in ancient Rome, but also associated the occurrence of anthrax in humans with the consumption of meat or contact with hair or hides of animals that had died of the disease.[54] Reference is also made to anthrax in the 'Hippokratika', a collection of veterinary documents dating from the 10th century.[109]

Anthrax is thought to have originated in early Mesopotamia and northern Africa,[109, 117, 118, 201] from whence its spread was associated with the process of domestication of wild ungulates which were subsequently disseminated into areas such as Eurasia,[118] the USA[86, 208, 258] and Australia.[187]

The more recent history of anthrax is intimately associated with the history of bacteriology and infectious diseases.[109, 124, 201, 231, 238, 259] Anthrax appears to be the first disease of humans and animals that was shown to be caused by a microorganism. Barthelémy in 1823 demonstrated that it was transmissible by inoculation, and Rayer and Davaine in 1850 observed filiform bodies in the blood of animals that had died of the disease. This organism, referred to as *Bacterium* by Davaine in 1864, was named *Bacillus anthracis* by Cohn in 1875.[259] Final proof of its causative role was furnished in 1876 by Koch, who, in a classic masterpiece subsequently referred to as 'Koch's postulates', described not only the organism, its ability to form resistant spores and its cultivation *in vitro*, but also the reproduction of the disease by injection of pure cultures, and the recovery of the organism at necropsy from animals that had died as a result of experimental infection.[115] Anthrax was also the first disease against which avirulent strains of the causative organism were used as immunizing agents in vaccines. In spite of the fact that Pasteur's 1881 vaccine against anthrax[169] has long been credited with being history's first bacterial vaccine, it has since been pointed out that Greenfield prepared an effective vaccine against anthrax and described his results some months before Pasteur's experiments were conducted.[227]

The pathogenesis of anthrax was extensively studied during the first half of the twentieth century,[231] but interest in it has fluctuated since then. The development of Sterne's effective livestock vaccine in 1937,[216] and the successful application of penicillin therapy[112, 160] lessened concern about the disease, but the threat of *Bacillus anthracis* being used as an agent in biological warfare during and after World War II reawakened interest in it.[38, 41, 143, 215] After the signing of the 1972 Biological Weapons Convention, interest in *B. anthracis* waned to the extent that the subsequent period, albeit short, has been referred to as a 'dark age' for research into anthrax.[231] However, the Sverdlovsk incident in April 1979, when an epidemic of anthrax in humans occurred near a facility suspected of being utilized for the production of materials for use in biological warfare, rekindled interest in the disease.[12, 182, 237, 244] Continuing threats to use *B. anthracis* as an agent for biological warfare have been made as recently as 1990 during the Gulf war.

The histories of anthrax and domestic animals in Africa probably have a common origin on the continent; the Nile Valley is where the disease was first recorded. Although Egypt is considered to be the main gateway through which precursors of the present African domestic breeds of cattle entered the continent,[58, 177] and it is conceivable that the dispersion of domestic cattle could have been an important route for the invasion of Africa by anthrax, the actual situation remains unknown. It is also possible that the tribes and their domesticated animals, during their migration through Africa, encountered anthrax along the way, where it already existed endemically amongst free-living wild animals. If the latter is true, anthrax must be considered indigenous to all parts of Africa.

There is no doubt that anthrax occurred much earlier in southern Africa than is documented in the records of early historians, explorers and travellers in which the disease is mentioned. Livingstone[139] has often been wrongly credited with the first report of anthrax in southern Africa. As early as 1838 Alexander[5] described a condition which occurred at Henkrees, close to the Orange River in the Cape Province, which in the light of present-day knowledge of the disease was undoubtedly anthrax. The relevant passage from his book is as follows:

> A respectable old Bastaard lived at Henkrees, Balli by name; he was the owner of a thousand head of cattle, of many horses and sheep. Unlike the generality of the people of the land, he and his sons were very lusty. The united families formed a small community of about thirty persons, in mat huts. Balli was suffering under the disease called blood sickness. Sheep occasionally get this, which is a corrupted state of the blood; the natives then kill them, and strange to say, eat them. The disease is very often communicated to those partaking of the impure flesh; and it appears in angry sores on the arms and on other parts of the body. It is very difficult to cure.

It would also appear that in 1842 the missionary Robert Moffat was the first to chronicle the disease in a human of European descent in southern Africa. He also described the disease as being particularly prevalent in humans and livestock of the indigenous tribes in the north-eastern Cape Province in an area near the Kuruman Missionary Station. From a veterinary-medical point of view, his account is so interesting that the following relevant passage from his book is quoted:

> On the 30th of March 1825, we were deeply affected to hear of the death of Peclu, the young prince. He died of what is called kuatsi, a disease which appears to be endemial, which assumes the form of a carbuncle, and carries off many cattle, and as the natives will on no account abstain from eating the dead meat, they are often attacked by it. If it happens to be near a vital part, as in the case of Peclu, it is very frequently fatal; if internal and not suppurating outwardly it is always so. The meat of the goat which has died of this disease is particularly noxious, and I have known persons after having eaten it, cut off in five days. It is always accompanied by considerable swelling attended with great stupor, though with comparatively little pain. I write from experience, having had one on my right eyebrow, which gave my constitution a severe shock, and from its position my recovery was considered very doubtful.

In what can probably be considered the first record of anthrax in wild animal species in southern Africa, Livingstone[139] reported a very virulent disease in the Marico district, which he called 'horsesickness', but which, from the following descriptions from his book, can now without doubt be identified as anthrax:

> Cattle, too, are subject to it, but only at intervals of few, sometimes many, years; but it never makes a clean sweep of the whole cattle of a village, as it would do of a troop of fifty horses. When the flesh of animals that have died of this disease is eaten, it causes a malignant carbuncle; which, when it appears over any important organ, proves rapidly fatal. It is more especially dangerous over the pit of the stomach. The effects of the poison have been experienced by missionaries who had eaten improperly cooked food, the flesh of sheep really but not visibly affected by the disease. The virus in the flesh of the animal is destroyed neither by boiling nor roasting. This disease attacks wild animals too. During our residence at Chonuane great numbers of tolos, or koodoos, were attracted to the gardens of the Bakwains, abandoned at the usual period of harvest because there was no prospect of the corn (*Holcus sorghum*) bearing that year. The koodoo is remarkably fond of the green stalks of this kind of millet. Free feeding produced that state of fatness favourable for the development of the disease, and no fewer than twenty-five died on the hill opposite our house. Great numbers of gnus and zebras perished from the same cause, but the mortality produced no sensible dimunition in the numbers of game, any more than the deaths of many of the Bakwains who persisted, in spite of any remonstrance, in eating the dead meat, caused any sensible decrease in the strength of the tribe.

Commenting on diseases of wild animals in general, Livingstone also wrote:

> Reference has already been made to peripneumonia which cuts off horses, tolos or koodoos. Great numbers also of zebras are found dead with masses of foam at the nostrils, exactly as occurs in the common 'horse-sickness'. The production of the malignant carbuncle called kuatsi, or selonda, by the flesh when eaten, is another proof of the disease of the tame and wild being identical.

Livingstone made the observations on which the foregoing accounts are based whilst residing at a place called Chonuane during the period 1845 to 1849. There is, however, some uncertainty as to the exact location of this station. Viljoen, Curson and Fourie in 1928[242] mention that the Government Secretary for the then Bechuanaland Protectorate, C.L. O'Brien Dutton Esq., had been informed that Chonuane 'was situated on a farm managed by Mr Ruben, 14 miles east of Ramoutsa, Bechuanaland Protectorate, and that it is now called Sechele's Old Stat'. If this is indeed the case, then the village was actually situated in the Marico district of Transvaal, Republic of South Africa, and not in the Republic of Botswana.

As can be inferred from the accounts by Moffat in 1842[158] and Livingstone in 1857,[139] the use of the term 'kuatsi' for a condition which was undoubtedly anthrax, was apparently in general use in the north-eastern Cape Province and adjacent parts of western Transvaal and Botswana at the time. Mr. A.C. Campbell, Curator of the National Museum and Art Gallery, Gaborone, Botswana, has given the modern version of this term in a letter dated 21 March 1975, from which the following passage is quoted:

> 'The disease is well known in Botswana. In the modern orthography it is spelt 'kwatsi'. It refers to anthrax in both animals and humans.'

A salient feature of these initial observations on anthrax in southern Africa, made during the approximate period 1838 to 1857, is that they all indicate that the disease occurred in a region that incorporates the north-eastern part of the Cape Province (Griqualand West) and the adjoining parts of western Transvaal and Botswana . The accounts of Alexander in 1838,[5] Moffat in 1842[158] and Livingstone in 1857[139] also suggest a high degree of familiarity with the disease on the part of the indigenous populations, which could only have been acquired after prolonged experience of it. It can therefore be assumed that the existence of anthrax in this region preceded the first Europeans travelling or living in this part of southern Africa. This assumption is corroborated by the fact that virulent *B. anthracis* was isolated from bones collected at the archaeological diggings of an early African settlement in the far northern regions of the Kruger National Park in the

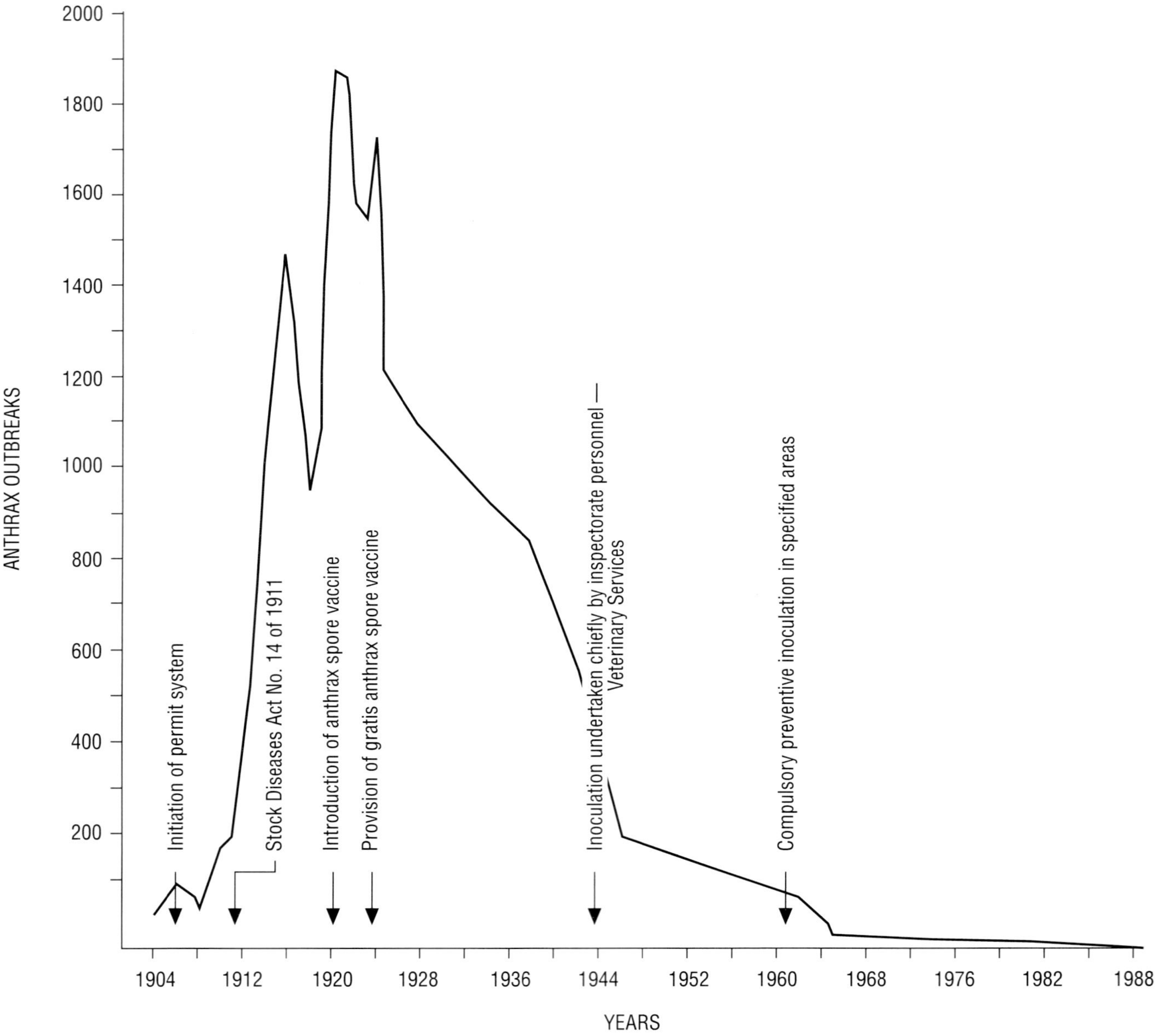

Figure 153.1 Distribution and spread of anthrax in southern Africa demonstrating peak periods of the disease

Transvaal.[50] These bones were subsequently radiocarbon-dated as being 200 ± 50 years old (i.e. AD 1770 ± 50), and can be considered as providing the first confirmed date of the occurrence of anthrax in southern Africa.

While the first scientific report indicating the existence of anthrax in South Africa was made by Branford in 1876,[23] the first reliable record of its occurrence in the country was that of Hutcheon in 1880.[94] Anthrax was placed on the list of scheduled diseases in the Orange Free State in 1891, and governmental control measures were instituted in the Transvaal in 1903.

Prior to 1904, anthrax spread slowly from its apparent original locus, and there was a tendency to confuse anthrax and horsesickness in horses.[94, 102, 125] In spite of the fact that by 1905 anthrax had extended beyond the borders of this locus to include larger areas of Griqualand West, the western Transvaal and parts of the Orange Free State, it was still regarded as being 'a very insignificant item in the catalogue of South African diseases'.[222] Thereafter, however, outbreaks escalated exponentially **(Figure 153.1)**. Around the time of Union in 1910, Gray[81] repeatedly referred to the increasing prevalence of the scourge, while Dixon warned that unless more stringent measures were taken to control the disease, it was likely to become much more serious. Dixon's prediction was realized, and by 1923–24 the disease had not only spread into new districts, but had also become markedly more prevalent **(Figure 153.1)**. In 1923, the year in which its prevalence peaked in South Africa, it was estimated that 30 000 to 60 000 animals died of anthrax.[218]

The development of an effective vaccine, the so-called 'spore-vaccine', turned the tide against anthrax in 1920. The decision by the government to issue vaccine free of charge to all stock owners in South Africa in 1923 was followed by an immediate and drastic reduction in the number of outbreaks of anthrax. From 1945, when compulsory inoculation of cattle became a legal requirement, a further decline in reported outbreaks resulted, which, if expressed in five-year periods, is reflected in the following dramatic results (year period: number of anthrax outbreaks): 1960–65: 311; 1966–70: 70; 1971–75: 30; 1976–80: 20; 1981–85: 14. During the last 25 years, the annual number of outbreaks of anthrax has declined from about 100 to less than three. Information provided by the South African Department of Health reflects a similar decline in the prevalence of anthrax in humans in South Africa, thus demonstrating the existence of a relationship between the occurrence of anthrax in humans and in animals.

A similar decline in the occurrence of anthrax has been experienced in many countries throughout the world, with the disease approaching near-eradication in a number of countries.[92] This decline has been ascribed to the availability of reliable vaccines, the liberal use of antibiotics, and the implementation of quarantine regulations.[256] There are, however, still a large number of countries such as India, Indonesia, Greece, and the countries of tropical Africa, where the situation has remained unchanged.[218] History has shown that anthrax remains a potential danger in many regions of the world should anything happen to upset recognized practices of hygiene and control.[218, 231] This was vividly illustrated in Zimbabwe when the programme of livestock vaccination was interrupted during the war years of the late 1970s. A massive outbreak of anthrax started in 1978, and resulted in more than 10 000 cases in humans and untold numbers in cattle.[46, 47, 236]

Because of practical difficulties encountered in vaccinating free-living wild animals, anthrax remains a major threat to them.[35, 53] Major epidemics have been, and periodically still are, recorded in wildlife conservation areas such as the Ruwenzori National Park in Uganda, the Selous Nature Reserve in Tanzania, the Etosha National Park in Namibia, and the Kalahari Gemsbok, Vaalbos and Kruger National Parks in South Africa.[35, 50, 52, 53, 56, 57, 68, 174, 231]

Aetiology

Bacillus anthracis[39] is a bacterium belonging to the family Bacillaceae. The genus *Bacillus* includes many species which have a great diversity of properties, but which are all aerobic and spore-bearing.

Before 1950, the taxonomy of the aerobic spore-bearing bacteria was in a state of confusion. However, Smith *et al.*[199, 200] brought some order into the taxonomy of the genus *Bacillus*, to which noteworthy contributions had been made by Wolf and Barker,[261] Gordon *et al.*,[78] Gordon,[76, 77] Gibson and Gordon,[69] the Subcommittee on the Taxonomy of the genus *Bacillus*,[6] and Berkeley and Goodfellow.[11] The work of Parry *et al.*[168] provides an excellent review of the taxonomic interrelationships of those members of the genus *Bacillus* which have some clinical significance. The taxonomic status of *B. anthracis* as a distinct and homogeneous species distinct from *B. cereus*, *B. mycoides* and *B. thuringiensis* was confirmed by DNA hybridization and G+C content determinations.[16]

The following description of *B. anthracis* is based on the above-mentioned taxonomically oriented works and the descriptions of Sterne,[217] and Wilson and Miles.[259]

Actively growing (vegetative) *B. anthracis* organisms are typically rod-shaped, measure 1,0–1,5 by 3,0–10,0 µm, and in stained smears of blood or tissue fluid obtained from infected animals, the organisms appear truncated, commonly occur singly or in short chains, and are surrounded by a well-developed capsule **(Figures 153.2 and 153.3)**. Capsules are not formed in culture unless special conditions for their development are provided. In unstained preparations, the organisms are robust, non-motile, transparent rods and, in contrast to those in animal tissues, have rounded ends. *In vitro*, *B. anthracis* grows in long, undulant chains composed of many individuals which resemble the segments of a bamboo pole.

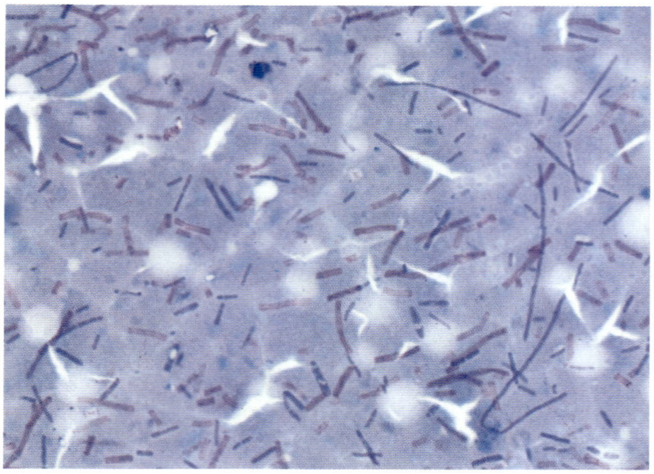

Figure 153.2 Giemsa-stained blood smear from a decomposed carcass of a waterbuck that died of anthrax. Note numerous clostridial bacteria

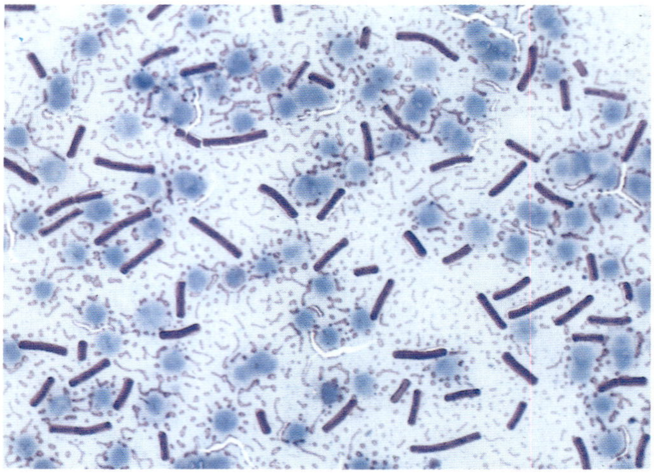

Figure 153.3 Giemsa-stained blood smear from a fresh carcass of a kudu that died of anthrax

The spores, which are never found in the animal body during life, are ellipsoidal or oval, and are formed equatorially without causing a swelling of the sporangium. Spores develop under suitable environmental conditions and are liberated by lysis of the bacilli. They germinate by polar rupture. Sporulation, in cultures on the surface of solid media, commences at about the end of logarithmic growth, is far advanced by 24 hours, and is usually complete by 48 hours.

The shape, wall thickness and size of the spores relative to the sporangium are important criteria in the taxonomy of the genus *Bacillus* and are of considerable assistance in distinguishing *B. anthracis* from other members of the genus. The aerobic spore-bearers have been classified into three distinct morphological groups on the basis of these criteria.[78, 168, 199, 200] *Bacillus anthracis* is placed in Morphological Group I (absence of sporangial swelling, and ellipsoidal spores). Other *Bacillus* spp., such as *B. megatherium, B. cereus, B. cereus* var. *mycoides, B. thuringiensis, B. licheniformis, B. subtilus,* and several others, however, also possess these characteristics; consequently other methods must be used to differentiate between them **(Table 153.1).**

Bacillus anthracis is generally Gram-positive, but this attribute is often lost with age.[69] Gram's staining of smears of the organism grown in culture should therefore be carried out as soon as possible, usually within 24 hours of the commencement of growth. The capsule, although also Gram-positive, is more easily decolourized than the body of the young bacilli, with the result that individual Gram-positive bacilli may be enveloped by a Gram-negative capsule. Several *Bacillus* spp., including *B. anthracis, B. subtilis, B. licheniformis* and *B. megatherium* under appropriate growth conditions, produce carbohydrate capsules containing varying amounts of the polypeptide poly-D-glutamic acid. The organisms are readily stained by the usual stains.[168] In contrast to the other polysaccharide capsule-producing bacilli, the capsule of *B. anthracis* consists predominantly of poly-D-glutamate **(see below)** and only shows up well with Wright's and Giemsa stains, polychrome methylene blue (M'Fadyean reaction stain), and 0,1 per cent toluidine blue in a 1 per cent aqueous solution of alcohol, or by the application of immunofluorescence techniques. Of the techniques described, the Giemsa and M'Fadyean staining techniques are preferred by most laboratories **(Figure 153.3)**.[168] Demonstration of the capsule by staining blood smears helps in the confirmation of the diagnosis of anthrax. Other *Bacillus* spp., such as *B. subtilus, B. licheniformis* and *B. megatherium,* also have capsules that contain polypeptides which impart similar staining characteristics. These species are, however, unlikely to be encountered in specimens of blood or tissues from animals or humans suspected of having anthrax.

Although the spores of *B. anthracis* can be stained by the usual spore stains, Schaeffer and Fulton's malachite green technique is recommended.[168] Relief methods which leave the spores uncoloured are sometimes useful. The use of phase-contrast microscopy is also helpful in the examination of spores.

Wild, virulent types of *B. anthracis* are aerobic, but do grow in partial anaerobic atmospheres. The optimum temperature for growth is between 35 and 37 °C; growth is slower at lower temperatures. *Bacillus anthracis* utilizes simple sources of nitrogen and carbon for energy and growth, and grows on most of the ordinary culture media, but the provision of suitable concentrations of thiamine and metallic ions, particularly potassium, magnesium, calcium, iron and manganese, is important.[25, 34, 110, 178] After 24 hours' growth on nutrient agar, the colonies are 3–5 mm in diameter and have a grey, frosted appearance, especially when viewed with transmitted, oblique light from above **(Figures 153.4 to 153.6)**. The margins of colonies are very irregular because of highly tangled outgrowths of bacterial filaments from the edges of the colonies which impart the so-called 'Medusa head' appearance. Typically these outgrowths taper and recurve in the same direction so that the colony as a whole almost appears to be spinning. This feature is best demonstrated by placing a cover slip on top of a young colony growing on an agar surface and examining the colony edges under a microscope using a x10 objective lens. This appearance is also seen in colonies of many strains of *B. cereus*, *B. thuringiensis*, *B. cereus* var. *mycoides*[168] and *B. megatherium*,[31] although the recurvature of the outgrowths of *B. cereus* colonies is less noticeable than that which can be seen in the other *Bacillus* spp.[217]

Tenacity is another characteristic feature of cultures of *B. anthracis*.[168] Typical colonies are very viscid and have a marked tenacity. The effect produced by drawing a bacteriological loop across them has been described as 'strings' or 'tacky, resembling drying glue'.[168] Such 'strings' can be made to stand up perpendicular to the agar surface without support.[63] This form of growth is probably responsible for 'spiking' or 'tailing' along the inoculation line[168] which, in turn, is associated with virulence; avirulent strains tend to lack these outgrowths.[168]

After 24 hours, growth is less characteristic and colonies become whitish-opaque and contain scattered, darker lacunae. Colonies are then also typically butyrous, lack the tenacity of young growth, and are easily emulsifiable.

Bacillus anthracis does not produce a capsule when grown on or in ordinary culture media; capsules develop after inoculation of the bacteria into suitable animal hosts. Capsule formation can, however, be induced *in vitro* by special conditions such as a high partial pressure of CO_2 and media containing serum,[216] bicarbonate,[73, 226] activated charcoal with or without serum,[150] or milk.[249] Capsule formation in bicarbonate agar is an effective way of differentiating between *B. cereus* and *B. anthracis*.[168] Capsulated *B. anthracis* cultures on solid media are thick, smooth and very slimy and have no resemblance to the usual dry, flat, tough 'Medusa head' type of growth.

Nutrient broth, when inoculated with *B. anthracis*, becomes turbid, and as the floccules which develop become more dense they sediment to the bottom. Freshly isolated strains usually form a deposit in broth.

In gelatin stab cultures, delicate, lateral projections grow out from the needle tract, with the longest projections at the upper part of the culture and the others decreasing in length progressively downwards, giving the growths an inverted fir tree-effect. Liquefaction is slow and crateriform. This has some diagnostic application as *B. cereus* has a more pronounced arborescent, filamentous growth and causes saccate liquefaction.

Biochemically, *B. anthracis* is much less active than other morphologically similar but nonpathogenic *Bacillus* spp.[55, 71, 76, 168, 203, 217, 259] These biochemical characteristics are not specific enough to differentiate it from other *Bacillus* spp.

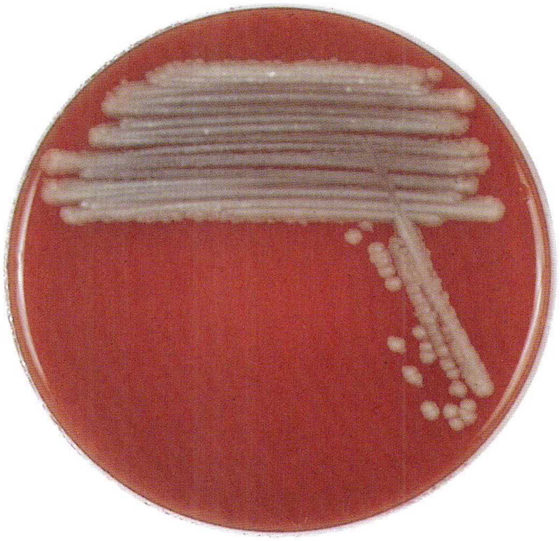

Figure 153.4
Typical *Bacillus anthracis* colonies on culture (24 hours' growth)

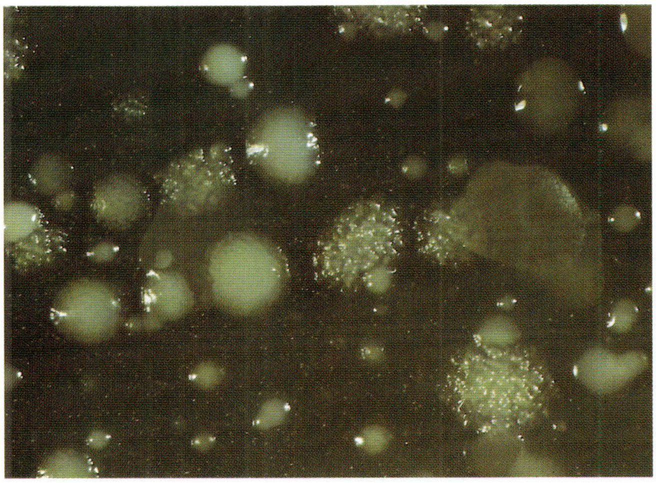

Figure 153.5 BTA medium with *Bacillus anthracis* colonies

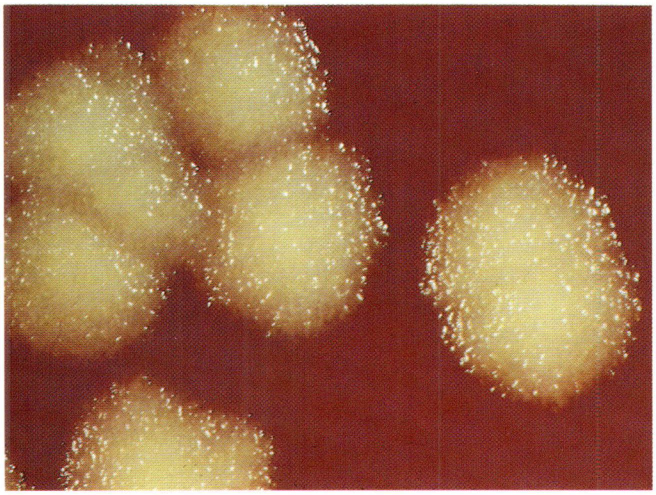

Figure 153.6 PLET medium with *Bacillus anthracis* colonies

Table 153.1 Proposed tests to differentiate *Bacillus anthracis* from other members of the *Bacillus cereus* group. (Adapted from Parry *et al.*[168])*

	B. ANTHRACIS	*B. CEREUS*
Motility	–	+ (sometimes slight)
'Cotton wool' growth in broth culture	+/–	–
Haemolysis on 5% blood agar	–	+
L V reaction	–/+	+
Sensitivity to penicillin (10 units)	+	–
Susceptible to gamma phage	+	–
'Inverted pine tree' growth in gelatin stab	–/+	–/+
Capsule formation – fresh animal isolates	+	–
Capsule formation on bicarbonate medium	+	–
Reduction of methylene blue (48 hours)	–	–/+
Pathogenicity (0,2 ml 18 hours' broth culture subcutaneously):		
Mice	–	–/+
Guinea-pigs	+	–/+
Rabbits	–	–
Lethal toxin (0,5 ml cell-free culture filtrate intravenously in mice)	–	+
Requiring thiamine	+	–
Growth at 45 °C	–	+
Tyrosine decomposition	–	+

* Considered by Parry *et al.*,[168] together with colony, tenacity and Gram stain appearance, to constitute the basic and most practical tests to differentiate *B. anthracis* from other members of the *B. cereus* group.

Bacillus anthracis produces a tripartite extracellular toxin consisting of three distinct, relatively unstable protein components known as oedema factor (EF) or Factor I, protective antigen (PA) or Factor II, and lethal factor (LF) or Factor III.[10, 65, 87, 103, 128, 129, 131, 194, 196–198, 207] Various combinations of these factors cause oedema or are lethal.[207] Thus oedema factor is not toxic when given alone, but when mixed with purified PA and applied to the skin of rabbits it causes oedema, and is lethal to mice. Lethal factor is nonlethal to mice when injected alone or mixed with EF and only lethal when mixed with PA. A mixture of all three components is the most lethal combination **(see Pathogenesis)**.

Oedema factor is an adenylate cyclase which is considered to be 'the archetype of a novel category of bacterial toxins'.[128] Its activation requires the synergistic presence of PA, whereas LF blocks its action. Conversely, EF also blocks the action of LF.[61] It is hypothesized that PA binds to receptors on eukaryotic cells to create a receptor recognized by EF and LF.[129]

Plasmids appear to be involved in the production by *B. anthracis* of the three distinct protein components of the toxin.[151] Strains of *B. anthracis* cured of the plasmid PX01 lose their toxigenicity and their virulence.[62, 152, 153, 183, 243] In addition, cured strains exhibit an altered colonial morphology, a marked increase in the rate and frequency of sporulation, altered growth characteristics in synthetic media, and increased sensitivity to *B. cereus* phages.

Virulent and some avirulent strains of *B. anthracis* also harbour a smaller plasmid (PX02), which is involved in the synthesis of the capsule.[82] Without PX02, capsule formation is impossible, which explains why the avirulent Sterne vaccine strain which carries PX01 but not PX02 has remained stable. In the past, bacilli which resemble *B. anthracis* but which failed to produce the capsule or to induce anthrax in test animals have been dismissed in clinical and veterinary laboratories as *B. cereus* or simply as unidentified *Bacillus* spp., and thereupon discarded as inconsequential.[234] However, the application of a newly available DNA probe, polymerase chain reaction and specific toxin antigen detection technology has revealed that a proportion of such strains are actually *B. anthracis* which lack the plasmid carrying the capsule gene (PX02).[234]

Mutants, or Pasteur strains, either arise spontaneously or can be induced in culture and may differ considerably from the wild type of *B. anthracis*. Pasteur in 1881[169] showed that *B. anthracis* loses much of its virulence permanently and irreversibly when cultivated at 42 °C for two or more weeks, and that these colonies are smoother and more glistening than those of the virulent type. Observations of this changed appearance of the colony, which apparently correlated with a loss of virulence, initiated and perpetuated the almost universally held view that *B. anthracis* is virulent in its rough colony form and attenuated when smooth.[217] However, variants of *B. anthracis* similar to those described by Pasteur have since been obtained by a variety of procedures, usually involving growth under unfavourable conditions. Such variants also tend to develop spontaneously in old laboratory strains.[217] In 1937,[216] however, Sterne showed that wild, virulent strains are always smooth, mucoid and fully capsulated on serum agar under a moderately high partial pressure of CO_2, and that the mucoid outgrowth upon further incubation consistently gives rise to rough, noncapsulated, avirulent mutants which retain, to a high degree, the ability to elicit immunity to anthrax. Such a noncapsulated, spore-forming, immunogenic variant of *B. anthracis* forms the basis for the Sterne vaccine, which is the safest, most effective vaccine currently available for the prevention of anthrax in livestock.

The vegetative cells of *B. anthracis* are not particularly resistant to adverse environmental conditions, whilst spores, which form rapidly under suitable conditions, are very resistant and can withstand the action of physical and chemical agents for considerable periods.[15]

Epidemiology

Anthrax occurs virtually worldwide. It is, however, uncommon in most of western Europe, Canada, the USA and Australia. It is common in southern and eastern

Europe, the countries of the former USSR, southern and central America, Africa and Asia.

The initiation of an outbreak or an epidemic of anthrax depends on interrelated factors which include specific properties of the bacterium, environmental factors, factors affecting dissemination of the organism, and certain human activities **(Figure 153.7)**. In anthrax, the abilities of the bacterium to survive outside its host, to enter and successfully infect its host, and to multiply *in vivo* are of particular importance.

The characteristic terminal septicaemia which is a constant feature of the fatal disease in most animal species ensures persistence of the disease. Sporulation and subsequent dissemination of the spores are dependent on the carcass being opened, as the bacteria are rapidly killed by putrefaction. A high partial pressure of CO_2, as occurs in intact carcasses, inhibits sporulation and explains why, in nature, sporulation occurs only after the tissues of an infected carcass have been exposed to the surrounding air when they have been opened. Sporulation is slow at temperatures below 20 °C, and even in opened carcasses the organisms are rapidly killed by putrefactive organisms at low environmental temperatures.[154, 209, 217, 229]

With few exceptions, anthrax bacilli do not remain alive in most of the tissues of an unopened carcass for

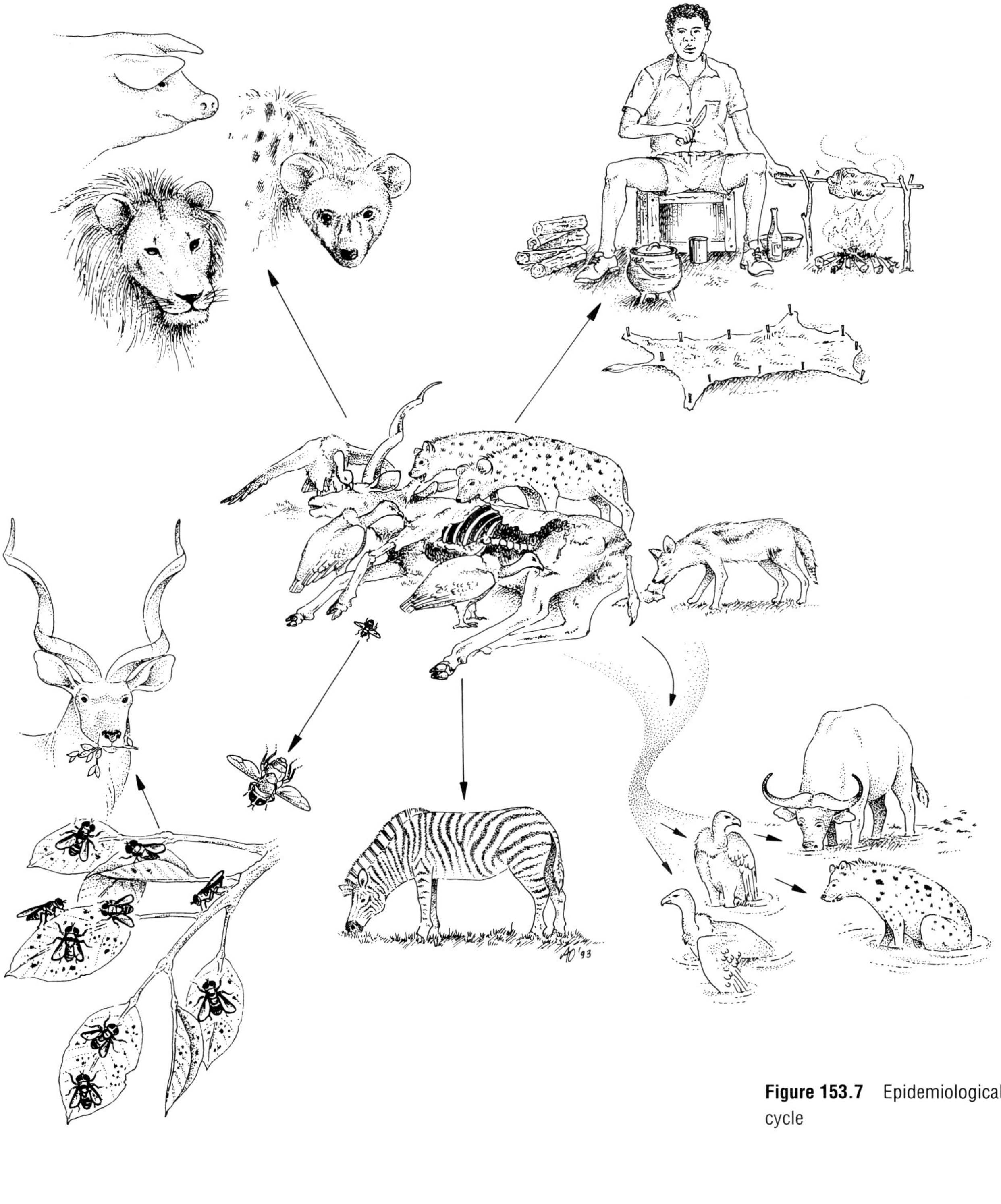

Figure 153.7 Epidemiological cycle

longer than three days at temperatures of 25–30 °C or higher.[209] They do, however, survive in bone marrow for a week, and in skin for two weeks.[154] At temperatures of 5–10 °C the rate of decomposition of a carcass is reduced, and *B. anthracis* can still be recovered from it for up to four weeks after death.[255]

The clotting ability of the blood of an animal suffering from septicaemic anthrax is impaired. This often results in the formation of pools of blood and tissue fluid in and around the carcass of such an animal after it has been opened. In these pools, sufficiently aerobic conditions are present which, when favourable temperatures also prevail, allow *B. anthracis* to multiply and sporulate at the end of the growth phase.[51]

When the carcasses of animals that have died of anthrax are opened by predators, scavengers, carrion-eating birds or humans, the spores produced are liberated into the environment. Many of them remain at the site of the dead animal, but some are dispersed mechanically by run-off water, scavengers (mammals, birds and insects) and humans.

Because dormant bacterial spores can remain in a cryobiotic state for more than 500 million years (as has been demonstrated by the isolation of the related *Bacillus circulans* from palaoezoic slate plugs[224]), it appears that under ideal conditions anthrax spores are able to survive almost indefinitely. Viable and fully pathogenic spores have been isolated from bones carbon-dated as being 200±50 years old.[50] In the dry state under laboratory conditions, they retain their viability and pathogenicity for at least 40 years.[148, 193, 260]

In nature, the survival of anthrax spores in the soil is dependent on a variety of factors, such as their initial numbers, the climate, topography of the terrain, and the presence of soil saprophytes,[35, 217, 259] certain chemicals, plant material and anthrax bacteriophages. Thus, in soils of high biological activity that contain a great diversity of microbial life, the survival period of spores is probably limited to not more than three or four years.[255] Anthrax spores may, however, remain viable in soil for 50 years,[143] and even for up to 250 years [50] if the soil is dry and has either a very low[142, 143] or very high[50] pH which adversely affects the biological activity of other microbial organisms.

The interdependency between length of the survival period of *B. anthracis* and the environment in which it is present gave rise to the hypothesis that *B. anthracis* behaves as a saprophyte during its abiotic phase, and that it multiplies in 'incubator areas' outside the animal body.[116, 240] The basis of this 'incubator area' or 'soil capability' concept of Van Ness[240] is that *B. anthracis* survives in soil in a dynamic state in which it undergoes cycles of germination and sporulation dependent on fluctuating conditions in the micro-environment.

The 'persistent spore' concept has greater credibility than the 'incubator area' theory, since *B. anthracis* does not appear to behave as a saprophyte in nature and is unable to multiply in competition with the microbes that synthesize antibiotic substances.[50, 156, 241, 263] This theory is supported by the fact that under suitable conditions of moisture and temperature *B. anthracis* can be grown artificially in the laboratory in sterilized, but not in unsterilized, soil.[156] In addition, anthrax bacilli disappear from soils in the presence of certain plants, probably because of the bactericidal/bacteriostatic properties of substances produced by the root systems.[263]

Data collected during a long-term survey of soil samples from an endemic anthrax area in the Kruger National Park for the presence of *B. anthracis* spores, indicate that the disease is maintained by a biotic-abiotic cycle.[50] During the biotic phase, animals die from anthrax, the carcasses are opened by scavengers, and the anthrax spores which form contaminate the environment. During the abiotic phase, spores are washed down drainage channels (particularly during seasons of above-average rainfall) to low-lying, poorly drained areas (such as flood plains) where they accumulate almost exclusively in the upper few centimetres of the soil . The spores become suspended in drinking water, or become concentrated in the water, particularly during droughts, when water levels are low and stagnant pools dry up. Animals are then infected when they use water holes.

In countries with a warm climate which favours the growth and sporulation of *B. anthracis* in body fluids in the carcass and in pools of blood or serum in the immediate surroundings of an opened carcass (resulting in contamination of the soil and vegetation), the occurrence of anthrax is closely integrated with a soil phase. In countries with a cold climate, the temperature is unfavourable for sporulation for much of the year, and anthrax tends to be self-limiting.[218] Its occurrence in cold countries is, to a great extent, independent of the soil phase, and the peak of anthrax outbreaks occurs in winter,[155] since most of the outbreaks of anthrax in animals are caused by the consumption during winter of imported fodder and feed supplements originating from endemic anthrax areas.[24, 98]

Germination of *B. anthracis* spores occurs at temperatures between 20 and 40 °C at a relative humidity greater than 80 per cent.[45, 228]

The susceptibility of different animal species to anthrax varies considerably, and most warm-blooded vertebrate species have been infected either naturally or artificially at one time or another.[217] In South Africa deaths have been recorded in at least 36 species in anthrax outbreaks **(Table 153.2)**.[56, 162, 174] Both wild and domesticated herbivorous animals are the most susceptible, and the disease occurs most commonly in cattle, sheep, goats, horses, donkeys and wild herbivores. Pigs, dogs, commercial mink and ostriches are less susceptible, although outbreaks in these species do occur. Cold-blooded animals may have to be warmed, while birds may have to be cooled, to render them susceptible to the disease.[204]

The susceptibility of animals to natural infection does not correlate with their susceptibility to experimental infection.[217] Experimentally, cattle, horses and donkeys appear to possess a far greater degree of natural resistance than sheep and goats, but under field conditions, the former species are affected much more commonly than small stock.[90] Thus, sheep, in which the disease can be induced by the parenteral inoculation of one to ten virulent spores, may remain unaffected even when cattle are dying of anthrax on the same property.[217] Goats are even more susceptible to anthrax than sheep, but the 'dwarf pig' is very resistant, if not fully refractive, to *B. anthracis* infection.[245] Discrepancies between susceptibility and prevalence of disease can probably also be explained in terms of differences in behaviour, such as feeding habits, and in routes of infection. In the Kruger National Park the browsers have a higher vulnerability to anthrax than the grazers.[50] In phosphorous-deficient areas in South Africa, osteophagia may increase the likelihood of cattle contracting anthrax; sheep do not usually suffer osteophagia under the same circumstances.[37]

In contrast to herbivores, pigs and carnivores are highly resistant to anthrax, and the ingestion of large numbers of *B. anthracis* in infected meat is generally required to induce infection in them. The feeding behaviour of these animals exposes them to much higher levels of infection than is the case with herbivores. Carnivores in the Kruger National Park, in zoological gardens, and on fur farms (most often when fed meat from animals subjected to emergency slaughter without having first been adequately inspected) have contracted the disease in this manner,[1, 51, 96, 141, 174] but recovery, even without treatment, is not uncommon in these species.[24, 64, 245]

Although the mortality rate is high and few animals which contract the disease recover spontaneously, evidence does exist that a carrier state can develop in individual animals and some animal species. For example, dormant spores of *B. anthracis* may circulate in the blood of 'black rats' for 30 days,[245] and viable, virulent *B. anthracis* has been isolated not only from the lymph nodes of several apparently normal, fully susceptible impalas (*Aepyceros melampus*) slaughtered four weeks after experimental infection with the organism,[50] but also from the 'abdominal' lymph nodes of apparently healthy cattle from an endemic anthrax area in Tchad.[179] In addition, it has been reported that a carrier state may develop in cattle that are inadequately immunized and subsequently infected, in immune animals challenged with an 'overwhelming' infective dose,[50, 179] and in pigs that have recovered from the disease.[64] It has been postulated that such carrier animals in an endemic anthrax area, being subjected to low-grade infection over a period of time, could develop a mild form of anthrax which, when they are exposed to severe environmental stress, could conceivably convert into the peracute disease.[68] At present it is unknown whether a carrier state plays a role in the epidemiology of the disease.

Age also affects the susceptibility of animals to anthrax — adults being generally more vulnerable than the young or subadults.[27, 50] Different behavioural patterns and feeding habits may predispose to this phenomenon, although there may also be a specific, but as yet not understood, physiological basis.

Apart from the role that scavengers and predators, such as spotted hyenas (*Crocuta crocuta*), jackals, lions and vultures, play in the dissemination of anthrax organisms by opening up and dismembering infected carcasses and dragging around portions of them, they also ingest spores together with the tissues of the carcasses, which are then widely disseminated in their faeces. After gorging themselves on carcasses, vultures usually visit watering places,[50, 91, 174] where they contaminate the water by bathing and defecating in the water or around its edge, and on occasion by regurgitating ingested, spore-infected material into it. Spores of *B. anthracis* occur in the faeces of white-backed vultures (*Gyps africana*) for up to two weeks after they have fed on contaminated carcasses in which bacteria have sporulated. Vegetative forms do not constitute a source of infection.[50]

Although *B. anthracis* has been isolated from the crops of house sparrows (*Passer domesticus*) and it has been shown that other bird species may carry the organism accidentally, they are unimportant in the epidemiology of anthrax.[190]

Bacillus anthracis may be transmitted mechanically by insect vectors, such as house flies (*Musca domestica*) and other arthropods including biting flies, mosquitoes and ticks.[83, 84, 157] Horse flies (members of the Tabanidae family) have been incriminated in the transmission of *B. anthracis* to horses.[90, 102] Although it has been suggested that biting insects smaller than the tabanids generally pick up too few organisms from a sick animal consistently to transmit the disease,[83, 84] transmission by stable flies (*Stomoxys calcitrans*) and mosquitoes (*Aedes aegypti* and *Aedes taeniorrhynchus*) has been reported.[113, 123, 230] The cumulative effects of a large number of bites and numerous interrupted feedings by one or many of these insects probably favour transmission.

Tabanids appear to transmit *B. anthracis* more consistently.[48, 119, 120, 122, 159, 163, 188] In the former USSR and Java, this method of transmission appears to be important, astabanids have been held responsible for transmitting the infection in 80 per cent of cases in horses and cattle.[119, 167] However, in South Africa and the USA biting flies are not considered to be of great significance in the transmission of anthrax.[51, 240]

Non-biting flies can act as carriers and transmitters of *B. anthracis* spores[80, 137, 188] but, except under certain circumstances, they generally do not play an important role in the epidemiology of the disease. However, in the Kruger National Park, blowflies (mainly *Chrysomyia albiceps* and *C. marginalis*) play an important role in the transmission chain of anthrax, particularly to browsing animals such as kudu (*Tragelaphus strepsiceros*), because

Table 153.2 Anthrax host list and patterns of occurrence in individual populations from southern Africa

HOST			PATTERNS OF DISEASE OCCURRENCE	REFERENCE
Classification	Scientific name	Vernacular name		
PERISSODACTYLA				
Rhinocerotidae	*Ceratotherium simum*	Square-lipped rhinoceros	Rare	51
Rhinocerotidae	*Diceros bicornis*	Hook-lipped rhinoceros	Rare	
Equidae	*Equus burchelli*	Burchell's zebra	Epidemic in KNP Sporadic in Etosha	50, 56, 174
Equidae	*Equus zebra hartmannae*	Hartmann's mountain zebra	Rare	
Equidae	*Equus caballus*	Horse	Rare to sporadic*	242
Equidae	*Equus asinus*	Donkey	Rare	242
Equidae	*Equus caballus* x *Equus asinus*	Mule	Rare	242
Proboscidea	*Loxodonta africana*	African elephant	Rare to sporadic in KNP Sporadic to epidemic in Etosha	51, 56, 174
ARTIODACTYLA				
Suidae	*Potamochoerus porcus*	Bushpig	Exceptional	174
Suidae	*Phacochoerus aethiopicus*	Warthog	Exeptional	51, 174
Suidae	*Sus scrofa*	Domestic pig	Rare to sporadic*	90, 242
Hippopotamidae	*Hippopotamus amphibius*	Hippopotamus	Sporadic to epidemic	50, 174
Giraffidae	*Giraffa camelopardalis*	Giraffe	Rare to sporadic	51, 56
Bovidae	*Connochaetes taurinus*	Blue wildebeest	Sporadic in KNP Epidemic in Etosha	51, 56
Bovidae	*Damaliscus dorcas phillipsi,*	Blesbok	Experimental	162
Bovidae	*Damaliscus lunatus*	Tsessebe	Rare	51
Bovidae	*Sylvicapra grimmia*	Common duiker	Rare	50, 174
Bovidae	*Antidorcas marsupialis*	Springbok	Sporadic	56
Bovidae	*Oreotragus oreotragus*	Klipspringer	Rare	50
Bovidae	*Raphicerus campestris*	Steenbok	Rare	50, 174
Bovidae	*Raphicerus sharpei*	Sharpe's grysbok	Rare	50, 174
Bovidae	*Aepyceros melampus*	Impala	Endemic to sporadic in KNP	50, 174
Bovidae	*Hippotragus equinus*	Roan antelope	Sporadic	50, 174
Bovidae	*Hippotragus niger*	Sable antelope	Rare	51
Bovidae	*Oryx gazella*	Gemsbok	Sporadic	56
Bovidae	*Syncerus caffer*	African buffalo	Sporadic to epidemic	50, 51, 174
Bovidae	*Tragelaphus strepsiceros*	Kudu	Endemic to epidemic in KNP Sporadic in Etosha	50, 56, 174
Bovidae	*Tragelaphus angasii*	Nyala	Rare to sporadic	50, 174
Bovidae	*Tragelaphus scriptus*	Bushbuck	Rare to sporadic	174
Bovidae	*Taurotragus oryx*	Eland	Rare to sporadic	50, 56
Bovidae	*Redunca arundinum*	Reedbuck	Rare to sporadic	50, 174

Table 153.2 *(continued)*

HOST			PATTERNS OF DISEASE OCCURRENCE	REFERENCE
Classification	Scientific name	Vernacular name		
Bovidae	*Kobus ellipsiprymnus*	Waterbuck	Rare to sporadic	51, 174
Bovidae	*Bos taurus*	Ox	Rare to sporadic*	90, 242
Bovidae	*Capra hircus*	Goat	Rare*	90, 242
Bovidae	*Ovies aries*	Sheep	Rare*	90, 242
CARNIVORA				
Hyaenidac	*Crocuta crocuta*	Spotted hyena	Exceptional	51
Felidae	*Acinonyx jubatus*	Cheetah	Exceptional	174
Felidae	*Panthera pardus*	Leopard	Exceptional	174
Felidae	*Panthera leo*	Lion	Rare to sporadic	51, 174
Canidae	*Lycaon pictus*	Wild dog	Exceptional	51
Canidae	*Canis mesomelas*	Black-backed jackal	Exceptional	51
Mustelidae	*Mellivora capensis*	Honey badger	Exceptional	174
Viverridae	*Civettictis civetta*	African civet	Exceptional	51, 174
Viverridae	*Genetta* spp.	Genet	Exceptional	174
LAGOMORPHA				
Leporidae	*Oryctolagus cuniculus*	Rabbit	Experimental	216
RODENTIA				
Eavidae	*Cavia porcellus*	Guinea-pig	Experimental	216
Muvidae	*Mus musculus*	Albino mouse	Experimental	216
PRIMATES				
Cercopithecidae	*Papio ursinus*	Chacma baboon	Exceptional	51
Cercopithecidae	*Cercopithecus aethiops*	Vervet monkey	Exceptional	51
Hominidae	*Homo sapiens*	Humans	Rare to sporadic	5, 126, 158
STRUTHIONIFORMES				
Struthionidae	*Struthio camelus*	Ostrich	Exceptional	56, 90
FALCONIFORMES				
Accipitridae	*Gyps africanus*	White-backed vulture	Exceptional	51, 174

The abbreviation 'KNP' refers to Kruger National Park, South Africa, and 'Etosha' to Etosha National Park, Namibia

Endemic — Predictable regularity of anthrax in a population unit within a specific area. The prevalence rate is usually low, but can progress into a sporadic or epidemic outbreak. Over a prolonged time (years) the incidence rate will show a clustering in time with a typical bell-shaped incidence curve developing. These species are considered primary or main hosts and are important in maintaining the disease in a specific area

Epidemic — A major flare-up of anthrax over a given time with relatively widespread occurrence. These species act as primary or main hosts and are co-responsible for maintaining the specific outbreak. Prevalence rating is high at the height of the outbreak, with a bell-shaped incidence curve to be expected

Sporadic — A flare-up of disease events with a relatively limited occurrence. These species usually act as secondary or incidental hosts and are not responsible for maintaining the disease or outbreak. Prevalence rating is never high and a point or spike frequency distribution of anthrax deaths can be expected during an outbreak

Rare — Deaths due to anthrax are rare and only a few can be expected during an outbreak. The prevalence and incidence rates are therefore very low, with a rather flat frequency distribution of anthrax deaths to be expected

Exceptional — Deaths due to anthrax are exceptional and also occur incidentally during an outbreak in the main hosts

* — Although epidemic or sporadic outbreaks have occurred in domestic species in earlier years, effective immunization procedures have made it a rare occurrence at present. It can, however, revert where the social order and disease control are disrupted

Unexpected patterns may develop under unnatural conditions of intensification, such as zoological gardens by their feeding and post-feeding habits they provide a link between a carcass and its environment. They feed on the body fluids from opened and unopened carcasses before flying to rest on the bushes, trees and grass in the immediate vicinity of the carcass, on which they deposit discard droplets and sometimes vomit droplets which teem with bacilli **(Figure 153.8 and 153.9)**. The extent of the contamination of the vegetation in the vicinity of a carcass is in direct proportion to its distance from the carcass; the contamination level reduces with increasing distance from the carcass. Blowflies may disperse as far as 63,5 km from a carcass at a dispersal rate of up to 2,35 km per day.[19] Droplets are usually deposited on nearby twigs, at a level of one to three metres above the ground, which coincides with the preferred feeding height of kudus,[18] and thus accounts for the high vulnerability rating of this species. After a contaminated-blood meal, blowflies may be life-long carriers of *B. anthracis* spores, but vegetative cells disappear from their digestive tract within about two weeks.[51]

Ticks from terminally ill animals have been found to contain *B. anthracis*,[3, 29, 51, 221] but they do not seem to play a role in the transmission of the disease as interhost transference of adult ticks is rare.

Most tropical and subtropical countries have a peak of infection during dry summer seasons and a low point six months after the peak.[155, 239, 240] This also applies to South Africa, judging by the monthly figures for anthrax outbreaks during the mid-1920s, when anthrax was at its peak in South Africa.

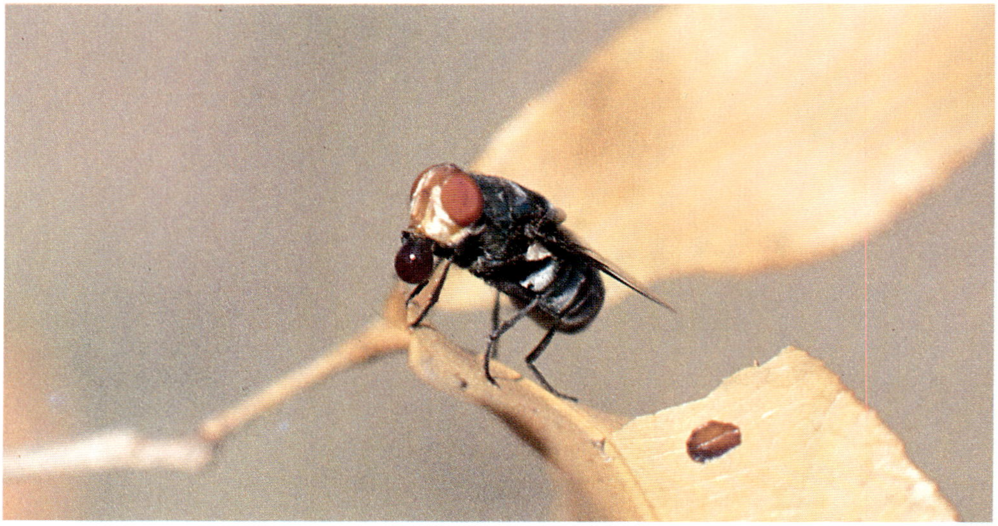

Figure 153.8 Engorged blowfly in the process of disgorging a droplet of ingested carcass material

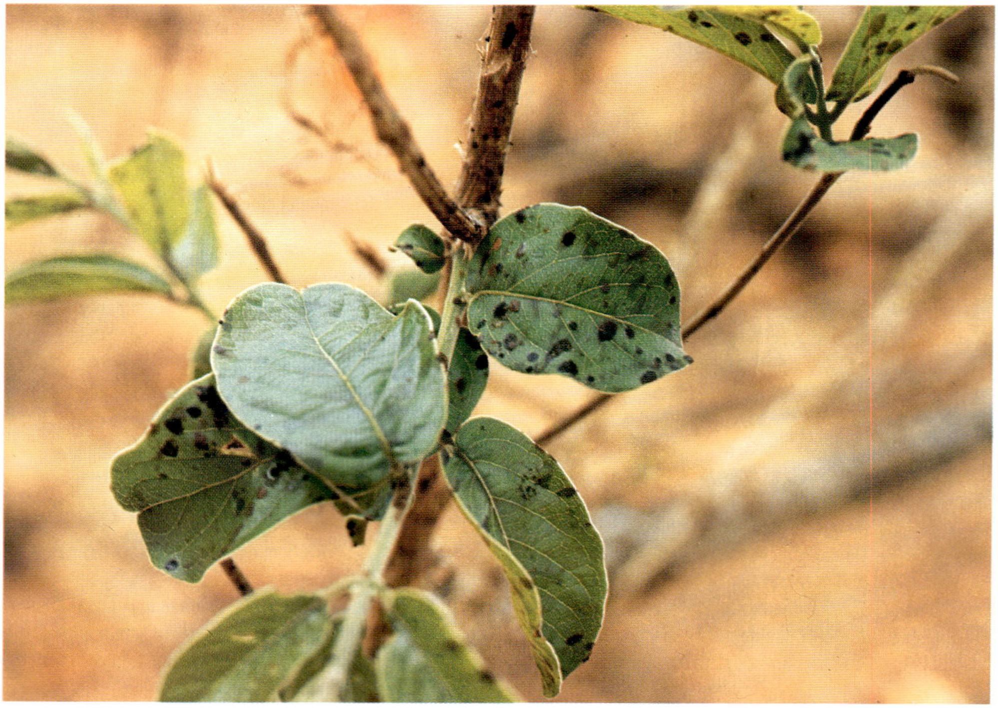

Figure 153.9 Faecal and vomit droplets deposited on leaves by blowflies which have fed on a carcass

Outbreaks of anthrax in wildlife in the Etosha National Park, Kalahari Gemsbok National Park and Kruger National Park in southern Africa are associated with the concentration of game, over-utilization of vegetation (local overabundance), animals suffering from nutritional stress, dwindling of water in watering points, and concentration of game around water resources, but outbreaks occur at different times of the year. In the Etosha[56] and Kalahari Gemsbok National Parks,[51] anthrax outbreaks peak in summer after the major rains, following the availability of water in man-made gravel pits which attracts and causes the concentration of large numbers of game in certain areas. On the other hand, in the Kruger National Park, outbreaks of anthrax typically occur towards the end of winter and during early summer, before the first major rains, when water is scarce and animals are concentrated around the remaining watering points.[50] Cyclic patterns of outbreaks, as in the Kruger National Park, where it occurs approximately every ten years, are also related to the concentration of susceptible hosts in an area.[50]

Outbreaks of anthrax in domestic stock are usually of short duration and rarely progress beyond the primary cases which contracted the disease from a common source. Control measures, which are usually effective, result in abrupt termination of the outbreaks, giving rise to typical 'point epidemics'. However, if an outbreak does progress beyond the primary cases, major epidemics may ensue, such as those which occur in game parks in Africa.[50, 56, 67, 68]

There has been a significant human influence on the epidemiology of anthrax. The introduction of animals into endemic areas, the overpopulation of livestock in intensive farming ventures within such areas, the dissemination of infective material over long distances, and the placing of undue pressure on rivers all tend to increase the prevalence of the disease. In addition, poor socio-economic conditions seem to be one of the principle determinants of the occurrence of anthrax in domestic stock and humans.[46, 47, 126, 149]

Human infection generally occurs after direct contact with tissues of diseased animals or their products. In South Africa, cases of anthrax have been traced to the use of riems (thongs of raw leather) made from infected hides, and shaving brushes, blankets and cardigan jackets made from infected hair or wool. In Europe many outbreaks of anthrax have been traced to infected, imported, raw animal products. Hides from carcasses infected with *B. anthracis* should be regarded as being permanently infected and may contaminate articles with which they come into contact; even final products made after the tanning or curing of raw hides are not free from spores.[90]

Farm labourers, butchers, workers in tanneries, and handlers of wool, hides and hair are most commonly affected. Infection is usually percutaneous (cutaneous anthrax). During the 1979–80 human epidemic of anthrax in Zimbabwe, in which more than 10 000 cases (with about 100 deaths) occurred, the vast majority were of the cutaneous form, the intestinal and pneumonic forms being extremely rare. It is thought that transmission of the disease by contact with infected meat and by biting flies, particularly horse-flies (tabanids), played equally important roles in the epidemic in humans.[236] Pulmonary anthrax, or woolsorter's disease, occurs in humans who work in factories where wool and hair are handled, and results from the inhalation of dust containing spores of *B. anthracis*. Although food is rarely a source of infection in humans, several cases of the disease in which lesions develop in the gastrointestinal tract (intestinal anthrax) have been recorded following ingestion of contaminated products, especially in areas where socio-economic conditions are poor.[2, 238, 256]

Pathogenesis

Natural infection of animals is usually acquired by the ingestion of spores which germinate and gain entrance to the animal's tissues, either in the pharynx or lower down the gastrointestinal tract, but infection also occurs through the abraded skin or cutaneous lesions caused by insect bites. Infection via the respiratory tract by inhalation of spores is rare.[50, 135, 262]

Experimentally, animals species vary in their susceptibility to infection by different routes of administration of the organism. Infection is established most readily through the intramuscular route. The oral route is the least successful way of inducing the disease,[205] and generally requires a large dose of organisms to produce a fatal infection.[50, 72] Cattle, however, are easily infected *per os*, but appear to be relatively resistant to subcutaneous challenge.[99, 186] The oral administration of 15 million spores is required to produce disease and death in 50 per cent of impalas infected via this route, whilst 100 spores via the intramuscular route will consistently kill all impalas in the experimental group.

The outcome of infection is influenced both by the host and the strain of *B. anthracis*.[61, 97, 105, 136, 138, 232, 235, 248, 251] As animal species differ greatly not only in their resistance to lethal infection, but also in their susceptibility to the effects of lethal toxin, the resistance to infection and intoxication appears to be based on separate mechanisms. Innate resistance appears to be dependent on the inhibition of the initial germination and/or multiplication of the bacteria.[60, 105, 136, 251] On this basis it has been suggested that host species can be grouped into two categories:[136]

- species resistant to infection [e.g. immune guinea-pigs, rats (NIH black and Fischer strains), dogs and pigs] but which once infected are highly susceptible to the effects of the toxin. These species develop a low terminal bacteraemia (i.e. septicaemia);
- species that are easily infected but resistant to the effects of the toxin (e.g. chimpanzees, guinea-pigs,

rabbits, mice, rhesus monkeys, goats, sheep, horses, and cattle). Most species show a high terminal bacteraemia (i.e. septicaemia).

Mice and guinea-pigs are the most susceptible of the laboratory animals. Rabbits are far more refractory than guinea-pigs, whilst rats are very, but not totally, resistant. In many large animal species, *B. anthracis* bacilli are, terminally, usually plentiful in the blood,[223] although pigs and horses may die before the organisms have proliferated sufficiently to be detected microscopically in blood smears. The greater kudu (*Tragelaphus strepsiceros*), nyala (*Tragelaphus angasii*), waterbuck (*Kobus ellipsiprymnus*) and roan antelope (*Hippotragus equinus*) show a high terminal septicaemia, whilst in African buffalo (*Syncerus caffer*) few or no bacilli are found in blood smears.[51, 147] These observations correlate well with vulnerability ratings of wild animals for anthrax during outbreaks in the Kruger National Park.[50] In humans, invasion of the blood stream may occur, but the number of organisms is seldom as great as in some of the larger animal species.[59]

The pathogenesis of anthrax has been studied in laboratory animals.[65, 74, 101, 104, 134, 184, 192, 251–254, 256] Following subcutaneous injection, the spores soon germinate to form actively dividing, encapsulated, vegetative cells which produce toxin. Within about two hours of inoculation, oedema, which extends progressively as further bacterial multiplication takes place, begins to develop at the site. The bacteria are usually confined to the initial site of infection and are not present in the extensive oedema fluid surrounding the primary lesion.[42] The bacilli are transported from the primary site via lymphatics to regional lymph nodes, where further multiplication takes place and whence vegetative bacilli continuously enter the blood stream. Initially bacteria are filtered out by the reticuloendothelial system, particularly in the spleen,[101, 104] until this system is overwhelmed. During the final 10–14 hours of the host's life, the bacteraemia increases progressively (at a doubling rate of 50 minutes in mice, guinea-pigs and rhesus monkeys, 95 minutes in sheep, 125 minutes in rats and 150 minutes in chimpanzees) to reach a fairly constant terminal level (respectively 10^4 in Fischer rats, 10^6 in NIH black rats, 10^7 in mice, and 10^8 bacteria/ml in sheep).[101, 103, 106, 134, 136, 232, 248, 251]

The variation in the severity and extent of lesions that develop is dependent on the virulence of the organisms, the susceptibility of the animal, the infective dose, and the route and site of infection.[90, 95, 217] At the site of the invading organism, highly susceptible hosts show a mild inflammatory response followed by generalized necrosis and haemorrhage involving many tissues and organs, whilst resistant hosts reveal only a severe localized inflammatory response.[74]

Infection with organisms possessing a high virulence, or with a large number of organisms, results in disease with a short course, thereby limiting the time available for the body to respond to infection.

Anthrax bacilli possess two primary virulence factors: the poly-D-glutamate capsule and the tripartite protein toxin.[9, 10, 61, 65, 129, 131, 133, 207] The summative effect of the individual components of the toxin and of the capsule is to inhibit phagocytosis, increase capillary endothelial permeability and delay blood clotting. Protective antigen, an adenylate cyclase, which is activated by calmodulin from the eukaryotic host cell,[128, 129] binds to specific receptors on cells producing an uptake system competitively recognized by both EF and LF.[129, 130] That the pathogenicity of *B. anthracis* is dependent on the amount of toxin and not the organism itself has been demonstrated by the fact that once the number of bacteria in the blood stream passes a certain threshold, death will occur, even if all bacilli are destroyed by antibiotic therapy. *Bacillus anthracis* evades the host's immune system by inhibiting immune-cell function. Both EF and LF, and the capsule of virulent anthrax bacilli, which physically inhibits phagocytosis and appears to interfere with opsonization through the negatively charged poly-D-glutamate contained in the capsule,[103] are associated with this protective mechanism.

The exact mechanism of action of the toxin produced by *B. anthracis* has not been substantiated, but extreme hypoxia, hypoglycaemia and alkalosis seem to contribute to most of the clinical signs observed.

Loss of body fluids into the tissues (oedema) and body cavities, such as the lungs, mediastinum, and peritoneal, pleural and pericardial cavities, causes haemoconcentration in diseased animals.[60, 198] Respiratory distress and severe hypoxia in animals *in extremis*, have been attributed to pulmonary oedema,[198] utilization of available oxygen by the massive numbers of circulating bacilli[60] and/or depression of the central nervous system.[17, 107, 135, 247] Hypoglycaemia,[14, 247] decreased levels of serum calcium, and increased levels of serum potassium and chlorine occur during the terminal phases of the disease.[247] In some host species, leukocyte counts and the haematocrit increase concurrently with the changes in calcium, with myocardial involvement occurring just before respiration ceases.[247] The neuromuscular irritability and convulsions exhibited by some animals in the terminal stages of anthrax are probably the consequence of the decreased serum calcium and increased serum potassium. Extreme hypoxia and hypoglycaemia prevent the development of convulsions.[247]

Clinical signs

The incubation period of anthrax under natural conditions is not known, but probably ranges from one to 14 days.[13, 211] Under experimental conditions it varies considerably, and is influenced by the virulence of the organisms, the resistance of the animal, the route of infection and the number of infecting organisms.

Most animals suffering from anthrax develop a fever, but its severity is extremely variable,[4, 75, 161, 164, 195, 217, 246] appears to be characteristic for a species, and may depend on the number of infecting organisms.[246] After an animal has been infected subcutaneously, pyrexia is usually observed within one to two days.[90] Small numbers of infecting bacteria may increase this period four- or five-fold. The fever usually declines before death.[135]

Three different manifestations of anthrax are recognized: peracute or apoplectic, acute, and subacute to chronic forms. Cattle, sheep, goats and some wild ruminants such as kudus, roan antelopes and impalas mainly manifest the peracute and acute forms. Horses, donkeys and zebras suffer from the acute form, and omnivores (e.g. pigs), carnivores and immune animals (i.e. animals challenged with high doses of infective material, or animals with low-grade immunity) from the subacute to chronic form.

In peracute anthrax, the course of the disease is always short, usually less than two hours. The majority of animals are found dead without having shown signs of illness. In those in which clinical signs occur, pyrexia (depending on the species), restlessness or anxiety, muscle tremors, dyspnoea, congestion of mucous membranes, ruminal stasis, collapse, and terminal convulsions may be observed. Blood-stained fluid sometimes exudes from the nostrils, mouth and anus. Experimentally, impalas and most wild ruminant species under natural conditions rarely show clinical signs until immediately before death. At death they are afebrile and manifest pronounced dyspnoea due to lung oedema, convulsions, and paddling movements with the legs. Terminally, the front legs are usually extended rigidly and they show opisthotonus. Similar clinical signs are regularly seen in wild ruminants dying of the disease **(Figures 153.10 and 153.11)**.[51, 147]

The course of acute anthrax is usually less than 72 hours. A rise in body temperature is an inconsistent feature. At first, affected animals remain standing, with head hanging and eyes staring; they are depressed, lag behind the others, walk about listlessly, and lie down frequently. Respiration is laboured and fast, and scattered small haemorrhages occur in the visible mucous membranes. The appetite is lost, rumination is suppressed and acute digestive disturbances may set in. Some animals may develop diarrhoea, which is usually haemorrhagic. In lactating cows, milk production decreases and the small amount of milk still secreted is either blood-stained or yellow. Pregnant animals usually abort. Oedema of the tongue and subcutaneous oedematous swellings in the region of the throat and ventral parts of the thorax, abdomen and perineum may occur. Horses may develop oedematous foci or more generalized subcutaneous swelling of the ventral parts of the body and perineum, usually at the sites where the infection due to the bites of stable or horse flies took place. Horses that become infected orally develop enteritis, colic, a high fever, and depression. They generally die within two to four days of infection or appearance of the first clinical signs, but some animals may survive longer.

In the subacute to chronic form of the disease, the course usually extends for more than three days before recovery or death occurs. The most frequent sign is an oedematous swelling of the throat and neck following primary infection of the pharynx, peripharyngeal tissues and regional lymph nodes. The swelling in the pharyngeal region may become so extensive that it interferes with respiration (and may result in asphyxia) and the ingestion of food and water. The infection may remain localized or it may progress to a septicaemia, which is often fatal. In those animals in which primary invasion has occurred lower down in the gastrointestinal tract, with the development of localized lesions there, clinical signs are not always obvious, although digestive disturbance such as loss of appetite, vomiting, and haemorrhagic diarrhoea and depression may be evident.

Carnivores and pigs have some degree of natural resistance to anthrax and so may recover.[24, 64, 245] Pigs that recover from the disease may remain carriers of *B. anthracis*.[64]

Anthrax takes one of three clinical forms in humans (cutaneous, pulmonary or intestinal), and meningitis and septicaemia may develop during the course of any one of these.[20, 46, 47, 114, 202, 238] The cutaneous form accounts for more than 95 per cent of reported cases of anthrax.[20, 114, 180, 202] There is no evidence that *B. anthracis* can penetrate the intact skin, and the infection usually enters the body through abraded skin or by means of an insect bite. The most prevalent sites of cutaneous anthrax are the exposed areas of the body, such as the head, face, neck, arms, hands and legs. The incubation period varies from one to 12 days.[20] Cutaneous lesions are characterized by the development of a malignant carbuncle or pustule surrounded by a zone of hyperaemia and oedema of adjoining tissues.[180] Central necrosis of the lesion occurs with the formation of an eschar, and is followed by ulceration. The cutaneous lesion is generally not painful, and, despite the designation 'malignant pustule', there is an absence of pus and suppuration at all stages.[236] The subsequent course depends greatly on the virulence of the bacilli and the site of the lesion. In approximately 90 per cent of cases cutaneous lesions regress and spontaneous recovery occurs, but in about 10 per cent of cases the infection spreads to the regional lymph nodes and develops into a fatal septicaemia.

Pulmonary anthrax (woolsorter's disease or mediastinal anthrax) occurs when dust particles laden with anthrax spores are inhaled and deposited in the alveoli, where they are phagocytosed and transported to the mediastinal lymph nodes, in which the bacilli multiply. From here, bacteria may enter the blood and initiate a rapidly fatal septicaemia.[184] This form usually manifests as an acute atypical pneumonia or influenza followed by signs of cardiac failure.[4, 21, 22, 184, 262] Virtually all untreated cases are fatal.

Intestinal anthrax is caused by eating uncooked or underdone *B. anthracis*-infected meat. Although this route of infection is considered most unlikely in developed countries,[21, 238] it is relatively common in people residing in developing countries with poor social services.[46, 47, 114, 180] Organisms penetrate the mucosa and form lesions similar to the cutaneous carbuncle, most commonly in the wall of the terminal ileum or caecum — but the oropharynx, stomach and other parts of the intestines are occasionally affected. The nature of the clinical signs depends on where the lesion is located. Involvement of the oropharynx results in fever, necrotic pseudomembranous mucosal lesions and cervical lymphadenopathy and oedema, whereas involvement of the intestines causes nausea, vomition, anorexia, fever, abdominal pain and a haemorrhagic enteritis.[46, 47, 191, 238]

Pathology

The principal lesions in septicaemic anthrax in animals comprise oedema, haemorrhage and necrosis.[74] Depending on the route of infection, host susceptibility and virulence of the bacteria, lesions vary at necropsy. Thus in some carcasses only lesions consistent with septicaemia are evident, while in others localized necrotizing lesions are also found. Rarely, only an enlarged lymph node,[210] the so-called 'carbon bacteridian cryptique',[179] may be found at meat inspection in pigs[24, 64] and in impalas infected experimentally.[50]

In ruminants, in which the course of the disease is usually peracute or acute, the most consistent changes at necropsy include evidence of rapid post-mortem decomposition of the carcass (resulting in marked bloating soon after death); incomplete development of rigor mortis; oozing of blood or blood-stained fluid from the natural body openings such as the nose, mouth and anus; dark red, poorly clotted blood; petechiae and ecchymoses throughout the carcass **(Figures 153.12 and 153.13)**; degenerative changes in parenchymatous organs; extensive pulmonary oedema; excessive amounts of blood-tinged serous fluids in the peritoneal, pleural and pericardial cavities; oedema and haemorrhage in individual lymph nodes; and an enlarged pulpy spleen, the red pulp being blackish-red, soft and sometimes semi-fluid. As indicated by the names 'splenic disease' and 'miltsiekte', severe splenomegaly **(Figure 153.14)** is considered by many to be the most characteristic change at necropsy. However, certain species such as sheep,[74] horses, pigs and impalas[51] rarely develop splenomegaly.

Other less frequent macroscopic lesions include localized inflammation and haemorrhages in the mucosa of the gastrointestinal tract **(Figure 153.15)**, particularly in or in close proximity to lymphoid follicles and Peyer's patches, and free blood in the colon; drops of blood exuding through the skin; localized oedema in the subcutaneous tissue, gastrointestinal tract and around lymph nodes; haematuria;[256] and congestion of subcutaneous blood vessels imparting a 'fiery' appearance to the carcass.[51] Microscopically, large numbers of *B. anthracis* vegetative cells are present in the peripheral blood of some animal species during the terminal phase of the disease, but their numbers vary significantly in other species.

Pigs may suffer from septicaemic, pharyngeal or intestinal forms of the disease. In those which have died from the subacute to chronic disease resulting from primary invasion of *B. anthracis* through the mucous membrane of the pharynx, the cause of death may be the result of asphyxia[90] following severe oedematous swellings of the mucosa and submucosa of the pharynx and glottis, and of the peripharyngeal and subcutaneous connective tissues of the throat and neck regions. There is often evidence of a diphtheric to necrotic pharyngitis and tonsilitis,[44, 90] or of carbuncle development at the site of entry of the organisms, while the regional lymph nodes are enlarged to several times their normal size and are bright to dark red[64] due to severe lymphadenopathy resulting from oedema, hyperaemia, haemorrhage and necrosis. In more chronic cases, lesions resembling tuberculous granulomas may occur in affected lymph nodes.[24, 185] Evidence of septicaemia is often absent from such cases. In those animals in which primary infection has occurred lower down the gastrointestinal tract, localized lesions may be present at the site of entry of the organism. These consist of focal or multifocal regions of intense, acute, haemorrhagic inflammation with oedematous swelling of the wall of the intestine and associated mesentery, and regional lymphadenopathy. Mucosal ulceration may occur.[90]

Pigs, horses, donkeys and zebras may also suffer from septicaemic anthrax,[64, 217] but more often the primary lesion in pigs is swelling of the pharyngeal region and lower part of the neck.[64] Horses also manifest localized swellings, but on the lower parts of the thorax and abdomen, shoulders, legs, perineum and around the external genitalia.[90, 214, 217]

Severe inflammation of the soft tissues of the head, tongue and throat, stomach and intestines are characteristic features of anthrax in carnivores.[35, 51, 256] Peripheral blood smears in these animals reveal few to numerous *B. anthracis* organisms at death.

Wild ruminants that die of anthrax manifest a vasogenic brain oedema and the presence in blood vessels of poorly formed and disintegrating thrombi containing numerous encapsulated bacteria.[121]

Diagnosis

In animals it is generally very difficult to demonstrate the presence of *B. anthracis* in the blood during the early stages of the disease, but later on the organisms may be cultured from specimens of blood. The organisms are seldom present in sufficient numbers in the blood to be demonstrable in blood smears of live animals, unless these are made when the disease is terminal, but they may be found — sometimes with difficulty — in smears made from local swellings if these are present.[90]

In order to prevent or minimize the contamination of

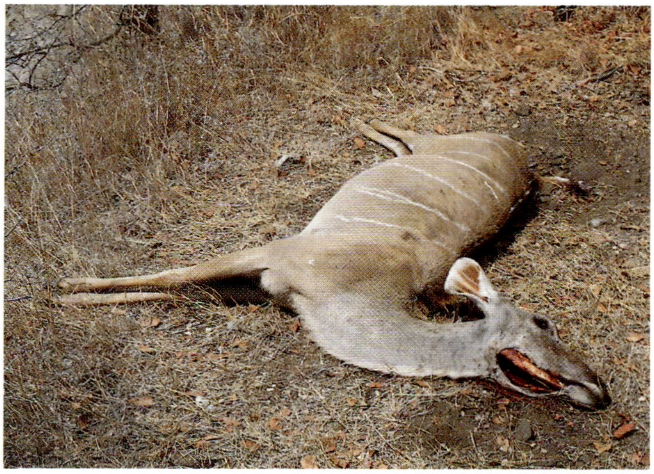

Figure 153.10 Typical appearance of the carcass of a kudu that died of anthrax

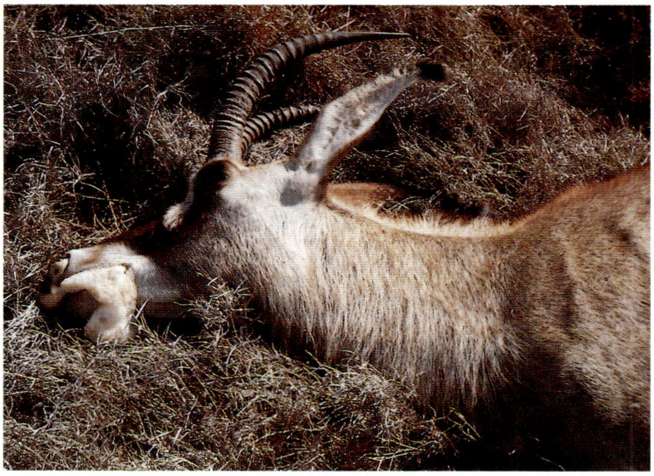

Figure 153.11 Carcass of an antelope that died of anthrax with froth at the nostrils and mouth due to lung oedema

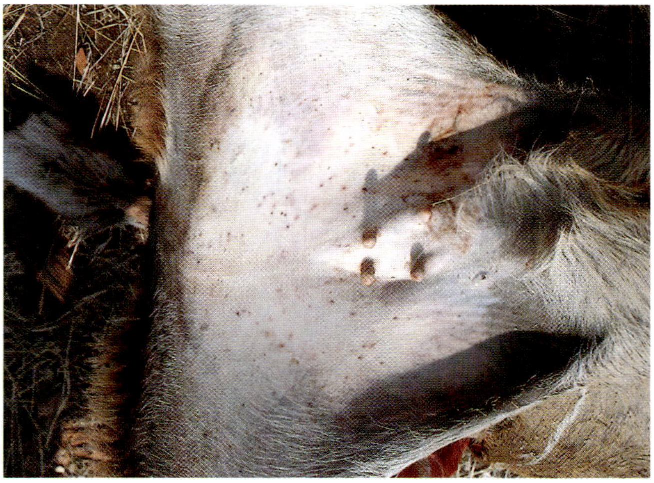

Figure 153.12 Multiple haemorrhages in the skin of a kudu that died of anthrax

the immediate surroundings of the carcass with *B. anthracis* spores, and also to avoid possible infection of the prosector, a necropsy should not be performed if the history and clinical signs indicate anthrax. An

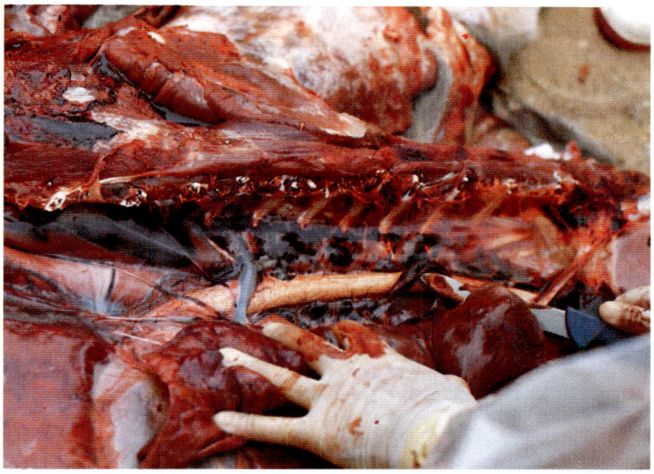

Figure 153.13 Multiple serosal haemorrhages in a kudu that died of anthrax

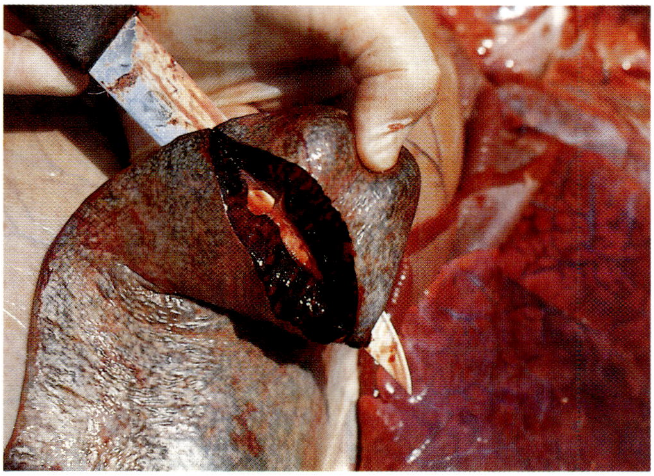

Figure 153.14 Marked splenomegaly in a kudu that died of anthrax

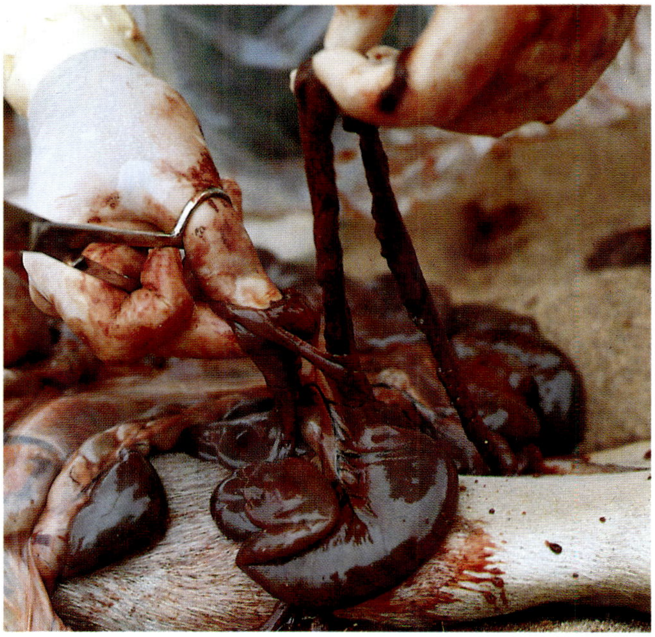

Figure 153.15 Severe, acute, diffuse fibrinohaemorrhagic enteritis in a kudu that died of anthrax

appropriately stained blood smear using blood obtained from a small wound made by puncturing the skin of the lip, ear or hoof coronet with a sharp instrument should be examined microscopically (refer to aetiology for staining procedures). It must be borne in mind that as soon as an animal dies, the anthrax bacillus in the unopened carcass undergoes changes in its morphology. The capsule starts to disintegrate and the protoplasm to degenerate, as is shown by it taking the stain more and more faintly until only ghost-like bacilli are seen **(Figure 153.2)**. The capsular material is the last to disappear.[44] At death only a few, if any, *B. anthracis* are usually present in the peripheral blood of horses, pigs, carnivores, and some wild animal species. A diagnosis may be made by preparing smears from the oedematous fluid that surrounds localized lesions, such as that which occurs in the region of the throat and neck of many pigs which die from the disease.[30]

If, after the examination of a blood smear, anthrax is still suspected but unconfirmed, suitable samples should be collected and submitted to a laboratory for bacteriological examination. The isolation and identification of *B. anthracis* from specimens originating from a relatively fresh carcass are not particularly difficult, but attempts to carry out these procedures using material obtained from severely decomposed carcasses are often unsuccessful.[256] Usually by 48 hours after death, organisms can only be isolated with difficulty,[209] but in cool environments it may be possible to isolate them for as long as four weeks after death.[209, 256] The preferred specimens for diagnostic purposes depend on the length of time that has elapsed between the animal's death and the collection of the specimens, and the state of the carcass.

In fresh, unopened carcasses, blood collected from peripheral blood vessels or the jugular vein and kept at 4 °C should be submitted for bacteriological examination. In carcasses in which decomposition is well advanced, blood should be obtained from the extremities furthest away from the gastrointestinal tract.[51] Specimens obtained from the coronets of the hooves offer the best chance of detecting the organism in smears or by isolation. In carcasses in which only bones are left, *B. anthracis* can be isolated most regularly from chips taken from the surface of bones in areas such as the eye sockets, lower jaw and ischium. Soil from below the carcass may also be submitted for culturing.

If a suitable blood sample is unobtainable, the tip of the tongue or a superficial lymph node, such as the prescapular, is the specimen of choice. If the carcass has been opened for necropsy, a specimen taken from the spleen or consisting of several lymph nodes is preferred. When carcasses are dehydrated and putrefaction is advanced, samples should be collected from areas which might have been contaminated with blood at an earlier stage where sporulation of *B. anthracis* could have taken place, such as at natural body openings or parts of the body mutilated by scavengers. Even when bones are all that remains of a carcass, bacteria may be more readily isolated from specimens of the bones forming the eye sockets, mandible and ischium than from those taken randomly.

Bacillus anthracis grows readily on artificial culture, and when isolation is attempted from uncontaminated fresh specimens, nutrient agar can be used for this purpose, but best results are generally obtained on media containing serum or blood. Severely contaminated material, such as samples of soil or bone meal, should be cultured on selective media, of which there are several available. The PLET medium of Knisely,[111] is the one most frequently used.[32, 43, 51, 143, 168] It consists of Difco Heart Infusion Agar as basal medium with 30 IU/ml polymixin, 40 µg/ml lysozyme, 300 µg/ml disodium ethylenediamine tetra-acetate, and 40 µg/ml thallous acetate. Refined lysozyme, however, inhibits the growth of *B. anthracis*, and its concentration can be decreased or it can be omitted from the formula without substantially affecting its selectivity. PLET medium is suitable for the purpose of isolating *B. anthracis* spores in soil, even when they are present in concentrations as low as three spores per gram.[143]

Seeded plates should be incubated for 12 to 24 hours at 37 °C and thereafter examined under a stereomicroscope with transmitted light from the side and above. Colonies suspected on the grounds of colonial morphology and tenacity of being *B. anthracis* are lifted with a bacteriological needle and seeded onto a 5 per cent blood agar plate. If no haemolysis occurs within 24 hours at 37 °C and the organisms conform to Morphological Group I bacilli, further tests[168] are required to differentiate *B. anthracis* from the other members of this group **(Table 153.1)**.

Additional tests in laboratory animals are considered essential if *B. anthracis* is to be conclusively identified.[168] In this respect, no universal standardized procedures have been formulated, and several variations of the methods that can be used are described in the literature, concerning the infection rate, route and site of inoculation of the organisms, and the species of laboratory animals to be used. It is generally recommended that 0,2 ml of a broth suspension should be inoculated subcutaneously into mice or guinea-pigs, intramuscularly into guinea-pigs, or intraperitoneally into mice. The intraperitoneal injection in mice of 1×10^5 to 5×10^5 *B. anthracis* spores is favoured.[234]

An API *Bacillus* system (API Laboratory Products, Ltd) has been developed to aid in the identification of *Bacillus* spp. and to facilitate the identification of both typical and atypical strains of *B. anthracis*.[168] Separation of slightly virulent and avirulent strains of *B. anthracis* from closely related *Bacillus* spp. is based on API and phage-sensitivity tests.[140]

Lysis by bacteriophage (gamma, W and Y) is a highly specific differential test for *B. anthracis*[26, 140, 145, 146, 168] and is becoming increasingly popular as a diagnostic aid in laboratories dealing with anthrax.

When *B. anthracis* is grown in the presence of low concentrations of penicillin, the bacilli swell and filaments of them appear as chains of spores or of round cellular forms referred to as 'strings of pearls'. This phenomenon, which was first described by Jensen and Kleemeyer,[100] is specific for *B. anthracis*, although exceptions do occur as some strains of *B. anthracis* do not grow under these circumstances.[28] Because of the specificity and relative ease with which it can be performed, this is a useful diagnostic test for the identification of *B. anthracis*.[33]

Generally, serological and immunofluorescent diagnostic methods are unreliable for the diagnosis of anthrax.[66, 231] Direct and indirect immunofluorescence assays, immunoradiometric assay and the enzyme-linked immunosorbent assay may be developed in future for determining the serological relatedness of *B. anthracis* and other *Bacillus* spp.[171–173] An enzyme immunoassay[8] and the production of monoclonal antibodies against the protective antigen of *B. anthracis*[108] have also been considered for diagnostic purposes.

An intracutaneous test using the Russian allergen 'Anthraxin' is highly specific and sensitive for the recognition of an actual infection and for retrospective diagnosis,[170] and it is also suitable for gauging post-vaccination immunity.[189]

The Ascoli test[7] is used for the detection of *B. anthracis* antigen in dried-out tissues of animals that have been dead for a long time, but is not approved in South Africa as a diagnostic test because of possible cross-reactions with antigens from other *Bacillus* spp.

A highly sensitive and specific enzyme-linked lectin-sorbent assay can be used to differentiate *B. anthracis* from its close relatives.[40, 79]

For practical purposes a battery of tests may be required to confirm a diagnosis of anthrax.[168, 217]

Differential diagnosis

In general, all causes of sudden death and of haemorrhagic septicaemia in animals may be confused with the peracute or acute form of anthrax. Causes of localized oedematous lesions should be considered in those species where the infection remains localized.

Control

Several efficient measures, used singly or in combination, may be employed to control anthrax.

The first effective vaccine, which consisted of capsulated non-toxogenic strains of *B. anthracis*[169] — the Pasteur duplex vaccine — was developed in 1879 by Pasteur, who had discovered that cultivation of the organism at 43 °C reduced its virulence. Vaccines based on this method of preparation remained in use until about 1935. Though effective and valuable, these heat-attenuated vaccines varied in virulence and were superseded by a live, avirulent, spore vaccine which was developed in South Africa by Sterne.[216, 219] This Sterne vaccine remains to this day, essentially as originally formulated, the major agent for the control of anthrax throughout the world.[231] It has been used primarily in animals and has been of great economic value to the livestock industry and to wildlife conservation.[218, 220]

The Sterne vaccine is, for all practical purposes, non-pathogenic in domestic[219] and many wild animal species.[53] A single inoculation provides effective immunity for about nine months, but annual revaccination is generally considered to be adequate to ensure permanent protection in most situations.[219] Effective immunity generally develops within a week of vaccination, although in horses it may take a month or more.[217] Outbreaks of anthrax in livestock are usually brought under control within a week to ten days of vaccination of affected herds. As the induction of anthrax in animals is dependent on the number of infecting organisms, high infection rates may cause disease even in immunized animals.[50, 135]

Despite the success of vaccines such as those of Pasteur and Sterne in the control of anthrax in livestock, there is general concern about the use of live, attenuated vaccines in humans.[85] Several vaccines consisting essentially of cell-free filtrates of Sterne-strain cultures, alum-precipitated or adsorbed on aluminium hydroxide gel, are available for use in humans.[85, 97, 181, 225, 231, 233, 235]

In South Africa, the recent changes in the regulations with regard to the government's responsibility for immunization of cattle against anthrax have shifted this responsibility to the farmer, and this has led to a dramatic decline in the number of animals vaccinated annually. The past success which has been achieved in the control of anthrax in livestock appears to have caused a complacent attitude in farmers, which may well be reflected in the recurrence of outbreaks of anthrax in South Africa. In this respect, the large anthrax outbreak which occurred in Zimbabwe during the late 1970s serves as a vivid reminder of what can happen if vaccination of livestock is interrupted.[46–48, 114, 180, 236]

To prevent sporulation of *B. anthracis*, carcasses should not be opened but should be incinerated intact or, if this is not possible, buried at a depth of two metres after being covered liberally with a mixture of one part chloride of lime, containing at least 25 per cent active chlorine, to three parts soil, before the grave is filled in. All excreta, blood, or other material that might be contaminated, such as bedding, must be similarly disposed of. In-contact articles must also be properly disinfected. The practical procedures for sterilizing materials contaminated with anthrax spores have recently been reviewed.[15]

Dry heat is less effective than moist heat in killing both the vegetative forms and the spores of *B. anthracis*. Vegetative forms are killed by a temperature of 60 °C for 30 minutes.[30] By contrast, the spores are highly resistant and are inactivated by dry heat at 140 °C for up to three hours, whilst under conditions of moist heat up to

14,2 minutes are necessary at temperatures of 100–115 °C.[15]

Viable spores of *B. anthracis* escape with the steam when open cultures are heated in an open vessel or glass tube,[213] and they can also escape from the tip of a bacteriological needle when this is singed in a flame. The common method of heat fixation of smears of anthrax organisms onto glass slides by passing them through the flame of a Bunsen burner for five to six seconds may not be lethal to spores, as smears prepared in this way and stored for several years have been shown to contain viable infective spores.[206]

The spores of *B. anthracis* are generally quite resistant to exposure to alcohols, phenols, quaternary ammonium compounds, ionic or non-ionic surfactants, acids or alkalis.[15, 127, 148, 212] High concentrations of chemicals such as formaldehyde, glutaraldehyde, hydrogen peroxide or peracetic acid are required to inactivate spores,[15, 93] with the result that the disinfection of livestock sheds and laboratories is difficult.[15]

The World Health Organization (WHO) has laid down guidelines for the disinfection of *B. anthracis*-infected material.[257] The following are the most relevant.

Premises

It is essential that preliminary disinfection precedes any cleaning process. The following disinfectant solutions can be used for this purpose: 10 per cent hot caustic soda solution, 4 per cent formaldehyde solution, chlorine-containing disinfectants (e.g. calcium hypochlorite containing 5 per cent active chlorine), 7 per cent hydrogen peroxide or 2 per cent glutaraldehyde. Disinfection with these solutions is conducted twice, with an interval of two hours between each application and at a rate of 1 l/m^2 for animal premises. After the final application of disinfectant the premises should be closed for three hours and then ventilated.

Transport vehicles

These can be disinfected by hot solutions of 3 per cent cresylic disinfectant or 1 per cent o-phenylphenate.

Clothing and small implements

These should be decontaminated by placing them in a 1 per cent activated chloramine solution, or 4 per cent formaldehyde solution for four hours, or by subjecting them to boiling in 2 per cent calcined ash for not less than 90 minutes.

Articles which are likely to be damaged by liquid disinfectants

These should be subjected to formaldehyde gas fumigation involving the use of 250 ml of a 38–40 per cent formaldehyde solution/m^3 of the chamber volume, at 58–59 °C for three hours.

Milk should be disposed of after decontamination by adding chloride of lime containing not less than 25 per cent active chlorine at a rate of 1 kg/20 l of milk. Milk can be considered decontaminated after being treated for 6 hours.

Animal by-products

Formaldehyde is recommended for wool, and a solution containing a mixture of hydrochloric acid and salt (2,5 per cent and 15 per cent respectively) for the disinfection of hides. Hair can be disinfected by boiling or autoclaving (120 °C for 20 minutes). It can also be disinfected by dry heat at 95 °C for 24 hours or by steaming for six hours.

Bone meal

After it was determined in South Africa in 1938/39 that anthrax-contaminated bone meal was still infective after it had been steam-treated for 15 minutes at 115 °C or treated with dry heat for three hours at 140 °C, De Kock *et al.*[49] prescribed a choice of one of several methods for the sterilization of bone-meal or broken bones:

- steam sterilization at 2,7 bar for two hours in a digester of not more than four-ton capacity;
- treatment of broken bones with benzene vapour at 95–115 °C for not less than four hours, followed by two hours of treatment with live steam at 5,4 bar;
- treatment of broken bones for eight hours with benzene vapour at 95–115 °C.

Heat sterilization for at least three hours has been found to be an efficient method for the sterilization of bone-meal,[255] which, nevertheless, should be monitored by the subsequent examination of random samples of the material.

Soil

A 4 per cent formaldehyde solution at 5 l/m^2, or a 10 per cent caustic soda solution, 5 per cent clarified lime solution, 10 per cent neutral calcium hypochlorite solution, or 15 per cent basic calcium hypochlorite or sodium dichlorisocyanurate solution, all of which are applied at a rate of 10 l/m^2, may be used. Exposure time in all instances should be at least 24 hours.

The effect of treating large areas of soil with sporicidal chemicals, such as potassium permanganate, formaldehyde, glutaraldehyde, dodecylamine and peracetic acid, has been investigated and it was found that only dodecylamine fails to kill the *B. anthracis* spores in the soil.[142–144] Formaldehyde (5 per cent) is suitable for large-scale application because it is effective and relatively cheap.[144] Formaldehyde was used for the decontamination of Gruinard Island, a site which was used during World War II for the first scientific trial of *B. anthracis* as a potential biological warfare agent. Since then *B. anthracis* spores have persisted in the soil of Gruinard Island. In 1986 the contaminated part of the island was successfully treated with a 5 per cent formaldehyde solution to a depth of 15 cm.[144]

Prophylactic methods to minimize the spread of *B. anthracis* in many countries are regulated by law. In

South Africa these are covered by the Animal Diseases Act No. 35 of 1984. This Act is administered by government veterinary officials and aims at the establishment of an immune population through the compulsory annual vaccination, by their owners, of all cattle in South Africa. During an outbreak, all livestock and domesticated game that have been exposed to possible infection should be vaccinated as soon as possible. They should be removed from the infected premises and kept in isolation under the observation and supervision of a government veterinary officer or other authorized person for two weeks after vaccination. Infected animals should be isolated, destroyed and disposed of under the supervision of a government veterinary officer or other authorized person. In South Africa these methods have been so successful that anthrax has been virtually eradicated from domestic animals.[218]

Anthrax is, however, still a major threat to wildlife populations throughout the world.[35] Earlier investigations were in agreement that parenteral treatment and vaccination of large populations of free-ranging wildlife are largely impractical and in some instances almost impossible.[35, 88, 176] Nevertheless, herd animals such as Burchell's zebra (*Equus burchelli*), blue wildebeest (*Connochaetes taurinus*), African buffalo (*Syncerus caffer*) and American bison (*Bison bison*) which can be corralled or captured can be vaccinated.[36] Long-stemmed, hand-held automatic vaccinating syringes are used from the sides of a crush[166, 175] but, needless to say, the strength and the wild and unruly nature of these animals makes this method very hazardous and difficult.

In 1973 De Vos *et al.*[53] achieved a breakthrough in the field of nature conservation by the use of an aerial method of immunizing free-ranging roan antelope in the Kruger National Park against anthrax. This method involves the incorporation of one dose of the vaccine in a disposable dart-like projectile syringe fitted with a hypodermic needle and a device which will effectively mark the animal which receives the vaccine with a dye for subsequent identification. The syringe is fired from a gun specifically constructed for the purpose. A helicopter is used to bring the operator within effective firing range of the animal to be darted. This method was improved by the use of a ballistic implantation method instead of the disposable darts.[51] It consists of a gun-like device capable of accurately delivering, over short distances, lightweight biodegradable implant projectiles (bio-bullets) containing the vaccine.

Apart from immunization, the control of anthrax in wildlife populations depends upon the elimination of sources of infection and its prevention through management practices,[35] such as the fencing-off of known 'anthrax areas'; the institution of continuous surveillance and an 'early warning' system in order to give early warning of outbreaks; location and incineration or burial of carcasses as soon as possible so as to prevent their dismemberment by scavengers and, thereby, the dissemination of spores (a helicopter or fixed-wing aircraft is virtually essential to locate such carcasses in an extensive area); the replacement of natural waterholes by concrete drinking troughs in which the water can be disinfected; the fencing-off of open waters in ground dams that have been infected by vultures; and the prevention of infection of drinking water by vultures by the erection of a branch barrier around the edges of the water in dams.

In many herbivorous animal species the course of anthrax is generally so rapid that death usually occurs before a diagnosis can be made while the animal is still alive. Treatment is therefore not always possible. In humans and 'resistant' animals, such as pigs, carnivores and horses, treatment is possible and advisable. In special situations, such as an outbreak in dairy cows, prophylactic antibiotic therapy on a herd basis might also be indicated.[70]

The successful treatment of anthrax is dependent upon the elimination of *B. anthracis* organisms from the system as soon as possible so as to prevent further production of toxins, as well as the speedy neutralization of the toxins already present.[135] Immune serum can be used as an effective prophylactic and therapeutic agent in experimental infection.[135] A commercial antiserum is not available in South Africa.

All strains of *B. anthracis* appear to be susceptible to tetracycline, erythromycin and chloramphenicol, whilst most are sensitive to gentamycin, streptomycin, and penicillin.[132, 165]

In advanced cases, antibiotics delay, but do not prevent, death.[89] In order to prevent the organisms from producing further toxins, antibiotics should be selected on the basis of their bactericidal effects.[135] Penicillin and dihydrostreptomycin are therefore recommended in preference to the bacteriostatic antibiotics (oxytetracycline, chlortetracycline and chloramphenicol) for the treatment of diseased animals.

Combined penicillin and streptomycin therapy repeated at 12-hour intervals for three successive treatments, and thereafter administered at 24-hour intervals for five days, is recommended.[135] For particularly valuable animals the use of benzathine penicillin for 21 days is recommended. Supportive therapy could be beneficial.[135]

Concurrent antibiotic treatment and vaccination with a live spore vaccine is not recommended.[250]

References

1 **ABDULLA, P.K., JAMES, P.C., SULOCHANA, S., JAYAPRAKASAN, V. & PILLAI, R.M., 1982.** Anthrax in a jaguar (*Panthera onca*). *Journal of Zoo Animal Medicine*, 13, 151.

2 **ACHA, P.N. & SZYFRES, B., 1987.** *Zoonoses and Communicable Diseases Common to Man and Animals.* Scientific Publication No. 503. Washington D.C., USA: Pan American Health Organization, Regional Offices of the World Health Organization.

3 **AKHMEROV, D.S., KUSOV, V.N. & CHERNOVA, A.A., 1982.** Survival of *Bacillus anthracis* in the tick *Dermacentor marginatus*. *Sbornik Nauchmykh Trudov, Kazanskii Veterinaryi Institut*, 101–103.

4 **ALBRINK, W.S., BROOKS, S.M., BIRON, R.E. & KOPEL, M., 1960.** Human inhalation of anthrax. *American Journal of Pathology*, 36, 457–471.

5 **ALEXANDER, J.E., 1838.** *An Expedition of Discovery into the Interior of Africa*, Vol. I. London: Henry Colburn.

6 **ANON., 1980.** Approved list of bacterial names. *International Journal of Systematic Bacteriology*, 30, 256.

7 **ASCOLI, A., 1911.** Die Präzipitendiagnose bei Milzbrand. *Zentralblatt für Bakteriologie, Parasitenkunde, Infektionskrankheiten und Hygiene*. 58, 63–70.

8 **BÄRBEL, N. & BÖHM, R., 1990.** Enzyme immunoassay for rapid detection of *Bacillus anthracis*. *Salisbury Medical Bulletin*, 68 (special suppl.), 24–25.

9 **BEAL, F.A. & DALDORF, F.G., 1966.** The pathogenesis of the lethal effect of anthrax toxin in the rat. *Journal of Infectious Diseases*, 116, 377–389.

10 **BEAL, F.A., TAYLOR, M.J. & THORNE, C.B., 1962.** Rapid lethal effect in rats of a third component found upon fractioning the toxin of *Bacillus anthracis*. *Journal of Bacteriology*, 83, 1274–1280.

11 **BERKELY, R.C.W. & GOODFELLOW. M., 1981.** *The Aerobic Endospore-forming Bacteria: Classification and Identification*. Special publication of the Society for General Microbiology. London: Academic Press, Inc.

12 **BEZDENEZHRYKH, O.S. & NIKIFOROV, V.N., 1980.** Epidemiological analysis of anthrax in Sverdlovsk. *Zhurnal Mikrobiologii, Epidemilogii, Immunobiologii*, 5, 111–113.

13 **BLOOD, D.C., HENDERSON, J.A. & RADOSTITS, O.M., 1983.** Diseases caused by *Bacillus* spp. *In: Veterinary Medicine*. 6th edn. London, Philadelphia, Toronto, Mexico City, Rio de Janeiro, Sydney, Tokyo, Hong Kong: Baillière Tindall.

14 **BLOOM, W.L., McGHEE, W.J., CROMARTJE, W.J. & WATSON, D.W., 1947.** Studies on infections with *B. anthracis*. VI. Physiological changes in experimental animals during the course of infection with *B. anthracis*. *Journal of Infectious Diseases*, 80, 137–144.

15 **BÖHM, R., 1990.** Resistance, survival, sterilization and disinfection of spores of *Bacillus anthracis*. *Salisbury Medical Bulletin*, 68 (special suppl.), 99–101.

16 **BÖHM, R. & SPÄTH, G., 1990.** The taxonomy of *Bacillus anthracis* according to DNA-DNA hybridization and G+C content. *Salisbury Medical Bulletin*, 68 (special suppl.), 29–31.

17 **BONVENTRE, P.F., SUEOKA, W., TRUE, C.W., KLEIN, F. & LINCOLN, R.L., 1967.** Attempts to implicate the central nervous system as a primary site of action of *Bacillus anthracis* lethal toxin. *Federation Proceedings*, 26, 1549–1553.

18 **BRAACK, L.E.O. & DE VOS, V., 1990.** Feeding habits and flight range of blowflies (*Chrysomyia* spp.) in relation to anthrax transmission in the Kruger National Park, South Africa. *Onderstepoort Journal of Veterinary Research*, 57, 141–142.

19 **BRAACK, L.E.O. & RETIEF, P.F., 1986.** Dispersal, density and habitat preference of the blowflies *Chrysomyia marginalis* Diptera Calliphoridae. *Onderstepoort Journal of Veterinary Research*, 53, 13–18.

20 **BRACHMAN, P.S., 1966.** Human anthrax in the United States. *Antimicrobial Agents and Chemotherapy*. USA: American Society for Microbiology.

21 **BRACHMAN, P.S., 1981.** Inhalation anthrax. *Annals of the New York Academy of Sciences*, 353, 83–93.

22 **BRACHMAN, P.S. & FEKETY, F.R., 1958.** Industrial anthrax. *Annals of the New York Academy of Sciences*, 70, 574–584.

23 **BRANFORD, W.C., 1876.** Meltziekte or splenic apoplexy. *Annual Report of the College of Veterinary Surgeons, Cape of Good Hope*, 19–20.

24 **BRENNAN, A.D.J., 1953.** Anthrax, with special reference to the recent outbreak in pigs. *The Veterinary Record*, 65, 255–258.

25 **BREWER, C.R., McCULLOUGH, W.G., MILLS, R.C., ROESSLER, W.G., HERBST, E.J., HOWE, A.F., 1946.** Studies on the nutritional requirements of *Bacillus anthracis*. *Archives of Biochemistry and Biophysics*, 19, 65–75.

26 **BROWN, E.R., CHERRY, W.B., MOODY, M.D. & GORDON, M.A., 1955.** The introduction of motility in *Bacillus anthracis* by means of bacteriophage lysates. *Journal of Bacteriology*, 69, 590–602.

27 **BRUNSDON, J.R., 1968.** Unusual features in anthrax outbreaks. *The Veterinary Record*, 82, 747–748.

28 **BUĆK, C.A., ANACKER, R.L., NEWMAN, F.S. & EISENSTARK, A., 1963.** Phage isolated from lysogenic *Bacillus anthracis*. *Journal of Bacteriology*, 85, 1423–1430.

29 **BURIRO, S.N., 1980.** Experimental inoculation of bacterial isolates obtained from *Argas (persicargas) persicus* in poultry. *Zeitschrift für Angewandte Entomologie*, 89, 324–330.

30 **BUXTON, A. & FRASER, G., 1977.** *Bacillus*. *In*: BUXTON, A. & FRASER, G., (eds). *Animal Microbiology*. Oxford, London, Edinburgh, Melbourne: Blackwell Scientific Publications.

31 **CANDELI, A., DE BARTOLOMEO, A., MASTRANDEA, V. & TROTTA, F., 1979.** Contribution to the characterization of *Bacillus megatherium*. *International Journal of Systematic Bacteriology*, 29, 25.

32 **CARMAN, J.A., HAMBLETON, P. & MELLING, J., 1985.** *Bacillus anthracis*. Isolation and identification of microorganisms of medical and veterinary importance. *In*: COLLINS, C.H. & GRANGE, J.M., (eds). *Society for Applied Bacteriology*, Technical Series No. 21.

33 **CHARLTON, R., 1980.** Anthrax and the string of pearls. *Zimbabwe Medical Technology Journal*, 9, 71.

34 **CHARNEY, J., FISHER, W.P. & HEGARTY, C.P., 1951.** Manganese as an essential element for sporulation in the genus *Bacillus*. *Journal of Bacteriology*, 62, 145–148.

35 **CHOQUETTE, L.P.E. & BROUGHTON, E., 1981.** Anthrax. *In*: DAVIS, J.W., KARSTAD, L.H. & TRAINER, D.O., (eds). *Infectious Diseases of Wild Mammals*. 2nd edn. Ames, Iowa: Iowa State University Press.

36 **CHOQUETTE, L.P.E., BROUGHTON, E., CURRIER, A.A., COUSINEAU, J.G. & NOVAKOWSKI, N.S., 1972.** Parasites and diseases of bison in Canada. III. Anthrax outbreaks in the last decade in northern Canada and control measures. *Canadian Field Naturalist*, 86, 127–132.

37 **CLARK, R., 1938.** Speculations on the incidence of anthrax in bovines. *Journal of the South African Veterinary Medical Association*, 9, 5–12.

38 **COGGINS, C.H., 1963.** Weapons of mass destruction. *Military Review*, 42, 43–50.

39 **COHN, F., 1875.** Untersuchungen über Bacterien. IV. Beitrage zur Biologie der Bacillen. *Beiträge zur Biologie der Pflanzen*, 2, 249–277.

40 **COLE, H.B., EZZELL, J.W. JR., KELLER, K.F. & DOYLE, R.J., 1984.** Differentiation of *Bacillus anthracis* and other *Bacillus* species by lectins. *Journal of Clinical Microbiology*, 19, 48–53.

41 **CONSTABLE, A., 1991.** Chemical and biological weapons. *Time*, 4 February, 29.

42 **CROMARTIE, W.J., BLOOM, W.L. & WATSON, D.W., 1947.** Studies on infection with *Bacillus anthracis*. I. A histopathological study of skin lesions produced by *B. anthracis* in susceptible and resistant animal species. *Journal of Infectious Diseases*, 80, 1–13.

43 **CRUICKSHANK, R., DUGUID, J.P., MARMION, B.P. & SWAIN, R.H.A., 1975.** *Medical Microbiology*. 12th edn. Vol. II. Edinburgh: Churchill, Livingstone.

44 **DAVIES, G.O., 1947.** *Gaiger and Davies' Veterinary Pathology and Bacteriology*. 3rd edn. London: Baillière, Tindall and Cox.

45 **DAVIES, D.G., 1960.** The influence of temperature and humidity on spore formation and germination in *Bacillus anthracis*. *Journal of Hygiene*, 58, 177–186.

46 **DAVIES, J.C.A., 1982.** A major epidemic of anthrax in Zimbabwe. Part I. *Central African Journal of Medicine*, 28,

291–298.
47 **DAVIES, J.C.A., 1983.** A major epidemic of anthrax in Zimbabwe. Part II. Distribution of cutaneous lesions. *Central African Journal of Medicine*, 29, 8–12.
48 **DAVIES, J.C.A., 1983.** Anthrax and flies. *Zimbabwe Science News*, 17, 11–12.
49 **DE KOCK, G.v.d.W., STERNE, M. & ROBINSON, E.M., 1940.** Sterilization of bone meal. *Journal of the South African Veterinary Medical Association*, 11, 138–141.
50 **DE VOS, V., 1990.** The ecology of anthrax in the Kruger National Park, South Africa. *Salisbury Medical Bulletin*, 68 (special suppl.), 19–23.
51 **DE VOS, V., 1991.** Private Bag X402, Skukuza, South Africa. Unpublished data.
52 **DE VOS, V. & LAMBRECHTS, M.C., 1971.** Emerging aspects of wildlife diseases in Southern Africa. *Proceedings of the SARCCUS Symposium on Nature Conservation as a Form of Land Use.* 13–17 September. Gorongosa National Park, Mozambique.
53 **DE VOS, V., VAN ROOYEN, G.L., KLOPPERS, J.J., 1973.** Anthrax immunization of free-ranging roan antelope *Hippotragus equinus* in the Kruger National Park. *Koedoe*, 16, 11–25.
54 **DIRCKX, J.M., 1981.** Virgil on anthrax. *American Journal of Dermatopathology*, 3, 191–195.
55 **DOYLE, R.J., KELLER, K. & EZZEL, J.W., 1985.** Bacillus. *In*: LENETTE, E.H., BALOWS, A., HAUSLER, W.J. & SHADOMY, H.J., (eds). *ASM Manual for Clinical Microbiology.* Washington, D.C.: American Society of Microbiology.
56 **EBEDES, H., 1977.** Anthrax epizootics in Etosha National Park. *Madoqua*, 10, 99–118.
57 **EBEDES, H., 1981.** A new look at anthrax. *In*: FOWLER, M.W., (ed.). *Proceedings of the Fourth International Conference of the Wildlife Disease Association.* Sydney, Australia.
58 **EPSTEIN, H., 1971.** *The Origin of the Domestic Animals of Africa.* Vols I & II. New York, London, Münich: Africana Publishing Corporation.
59 **EURICH, F.W., 1933.** Some notes on industrial anthrax. *British Medical Journal*, 2, 50–53.
60 **EZZEL, J.W., Jr., 1986.** *Bacillus anthracis. In*: GYLES, C.L. & THOEN, C.O., (eds). *Pathogenesis of Bacterial Infections in Animals.* Ames, Iowa: Iowa State University Press.
61 **EZZELL, J.W., IVINS, B.E. & LEPPLA, S.H., 1984.** Immunoelectrophoretic analysis, toxicity, and kinetics of *in vitro* production of the protective antigen and lethal factor components of *Bacillus anthracis* toxin. *Infection and Immunity*, 45, 761–767.
62 **EZZELL, J.W., MIKESELL, P., IVINS, B.E. & LEPPLA, S.H., 1985.** The genetic basis of Pasteur's attenuation of *Bacillus anthracis* cultures. *In*: KAPROWSKI, H.P., (ed.). *World's Debt to Pasteur.* The Wistar Symposium Series, Vol. III. New York: Allan R. Liss, Inc.
63 **FEELEY, J.C. & PATTON, C.M., 1980.** Bacillus. *In*: LENNETTE, E.H., BALOWS, A., HAUSLER, W.J. & TRUANT, J.P., (eds). *Manual of Clinical Microbiology.* 3rd edn. Washington D.C.: American Society for Microbiology.
64 **FERGUSON, L.C., 1981.** Anthrax. *In*: LEMAN, A.D., GLOCK, R.D., MENGELING, W.L., PENNY, R.H.C., SCHOLL, E. & STRAW, B., (eds). *Diseases of Swine.* 5th edn. Ames, Iowa: Iowa State University Press.
65 **FISH, D.C. & LINCOLN, R.E., 1968.** *In vivo*-produced anthrax toxin. *Journal of Bacteriology*, 95, 919–924.
66 **FLUCK, R., BOHM, R. & STRAUCH, D., 1977.** Fluoreszenzserologische Untersuchungen von Kreuzreaktion zwischen Sporen von *Bacillus anthracis* und Sporen anderer aerober Sporenbildner. *Zentralblatt für Veterinärmedizin*, 24, 497–507.
67 **GAINER, R., 1972.** Preliminary report of investigations into the dying of animals at the Katavie Game Reserve. Unpublished report. Miombo Research Centre, Dar-es-Salaam. Ministry of Natural Resources and Tourism.
68 **GAINER, R.S., 1987.** Epizootiology of anthrax and Nyasa wildebeest in the Selous Game Reserve, Tanzania. *Journal of Wildlife Diseases*, 23, 175–178.
69 **GIBSON, T. & GORDON, R.E., 1974.** Genus *Bacillus. In*: BUCHANAN, R.E. & GIBBONS, N.E., (eds). *Bergey's Manual of Determinative Bacteriology.* 8th edn. Baltimore: Williams & Wilkins.
70 **GILL, I.J., 1982.** Antibiotic therapy in the control of an outbreak of anthrax in dairy cows. *Australian Veterinary Journal*, 58, 214–215.
71 **GILLESPIE, J.H. & TIMONEY, J.F., 1981.** The genus *Bacillus. Hagan and Bruner's Infectious Diseases of Domestic Animals.* 7th edn. Ithaca, London: Comstock Publishing Associates, Division of Cornell University Press.
72 **GIOVANARDI, A., 1931.** Untersuchungen über die pathogenese des darmmilzbrandes. *Krankheitsforschung*, 9, 13–33.
73 **GLADSTONE, G.P., 1946.** Immunity to anthrax. Protective antigen present in cell-free culture filtrates. *British Journal of Experimental Pathology*, 27, 394–418.
74 **GLEISER, C.A., 1967.** Pathology of anthrax infection in animal hosts. *Federation Proceedings*, 26, 1518–1521.
75 **GOLD, H., 1967.** Treatment of anthrax. *Federation Proceedings*, 26, 1563–1568.
76 **GORDON, R.E., 1973.** The genus *Bacillus. In*: LASKIN, A.I. & LECHEVALIER, H.A., (eds). *Handbook of Microbiology.* Vol. I. Cleveland, Ohio: CRC Press, Inc.
77 **GORDON, R.E., 1981.** One hundred and seven years of the genus *Bacillus. In*: BERKELY, R.C.W. & GOODFELLOW, M., (eds). *The Aerobic Endosporeforming Bacteria: Classification and Identification.* London: Academic Press, Inc.
78 **GORDON, R.E., HAYNES, W.C. & PANG, C.H-N., 1973.** The genus *Bacillus. United States Department of Agriculture, Agricultural Research Service, Agriculture Handbook No. 427.* Washington, D.C.
79 **GRAHAM, K., KELLER, K., EZZELL, J. & DOYLE, R., 1984.** Enzyme-linked lectinsorbent assay (ELA) for detecting *Bacillus anthracis. European Journal of Clinical Microbiology*, 3, 210–212.
80 **GRAHAM-SMITH, G.S., 1913.** Flies in relation to disease on blood-sucking flies. Cambridge: Cambridge University Press.
81 **GRAY, C.E., 1906, 1907, 1910, 1914, 1918.** *Annual Reports, Principal Veterinary Surgeon*, Transvaal, Union of South Africa.
82 **GREEN, B.D., BATTISTI, L., KOEHLER, T.M., THORNE, C.B., IVINS, B.E., 1985.** Demonstration of a capsule plasmid in *Bacillus anthracis. Infection and Immunity*, 49, 291–297.
83 **GREENBERG, B., 1971.** *Flies and Disease.* Vol. I. Princeton, New Jersey: Princeton University Press.
84 **GREENBERG, B., 1973.** *Flies and Disease.* Vol. II. Princeton, New Jersey: Princeton University Press.
85 **HAMBLETON, P., CARMAN, J.A. & MELLING, J., 1984.** Anthrax: The disease in relation to vaccines. *Vaccine*, 2, 125–132.
86 **HANSON, R.P., 1959.** The earliest account of anthrax in man and animals in North America. *Journal of the American Veterinary Medical Association*, 135, 463–465.
87 **HARRIS-SMITH, P.W., SMITH, H. & KEPPIE, J., 1958.** Production *in vitro* of the toxin of *Bacillus anthracis* previously recognized *in vivo. Journal of General Microbiology*, 19, 91–103.
88 **HARTHOORN, A.M. & LOCK, J.A., 1960.** A note on the prophylactic vaccination of wild animals. *The British Veterinary Journal*, 116, 252–254.
89 **HENDERSON, D.W., PEACOCK, S. & BELTON, F.C., 1956.** Observations on the prophylaxis of experimental pulmonary anthrax in the monkey. *Journal of Hygiene*, 54, 28–36.
90 **HENNING, M.W., 1956.** Anthrax. *In: Animal Diseases in South Africa.* 3rd edn. South Africa: Central News Agency Ltd.
91 **HOUSTON, D.C. & COOPER, J.E., 1975.** The digestive tract of the whiteback griffon vulture and its role in disease transmission among wild ungulates. *Journal of Wildlife Diseases*, 11, 306–313.
92 **HUGH-JONES, M.E., 1990.** Global trends in the incidence of anthrax in livestock. *Salisbury Medical Bulletin*, 68, 2–4.

93 **HUSSAINI, S.N. & RUBY, K.R., 1976.** Sporicidal activity of peracetic acid against *B. anthracis* spores. *The Veterinary Record*, 98, 257–259.

94 **HUTCHEON, D., 1880, 1881, 1882, 1883, 1884, 1896, 1898, 1903.** *Annual Reports of the College of Veterinary Surgeons*, Cape of Good Hope.

95 **HUTYRA, F., MAREK, J. & MANNINGER, R., 1938.** *Special Pathology and Therapeutics of the Diseases of Domestic Animals*. 4th edn. London: Baillière, Tindall and Cox.

96 **IKEDE, B.O., FALADE, S. & GOLDING, R.R., 1976.** Anthrax in captive carnivores in Ibadan, Nigeria. *Journal of Wildlife Diseases*, 12, 130–132.

97 **IVINS, B.E. & WELKOS, S.L., 1988.** Recent advances in the development of an improved, human anthrax vaccine. *European Journal of Epidemiology*, 4, 12.

98 **JACKSON, SIR R., 1930.** The introduction into Great Britain of anthrax infection by means of products of animal origin. *Journal of Comparative Pathology and Therapeutics*, 43, 95–98.

99 **JACKSON, F.C., WRIGHT, G.C. & ARMSTRONG, J., 1957.** Immunization of cattle against experimental anthrax with alum-precipitated protective antigen or spore vaccine. *American Journal of Veterinary Research*, 18, 771–777.

100 **JENSEN, J. & KLEEMEYER, H., 1953.** Die bakterielle differentialdiagnose des anthrax mittels eines neuen spezifischen testes ('parlschnurtest'). *Zentralblatt für Bakteriologie, Parasietenkunde, Infektionskrankheiten und Hygiene*, 56, 349–350.

101 **JONES, W.I. & KLEIN, F., 1967.** *In vivo* growth and distribution of anthrax bacilli in resistant, susceptible and immunized hosts. *Journal of Bacteriology*, 94, 600–608.

102 **KEHOE, D., 1917.** Anthrax in South Africa. *Fifth and Sixth Reports of the Director of Veterinary Education and Research, Union of South Africa*.

103 **KEPPIE, J., HARRIS-SMITH, P.W. & SMITH, H., 1963.** The chemical basis of the virulence of *Bacillus anthracis*. IX: Its aggressions, and their mode of action. *British Journal of Experimental Pathology*, 44, 446–453.

104 **KEPPIE, J., SMITH, H. & HARRIS-SMITH, P.W., 1955.** The chemical basis of the virulence of *Bacillus anthracis*. III: The role of the terminal bacteraemia in death of guinea-pigs from anthrax. *British Journal of Experimental Pathology*, 36, 315–322.

105 **KLEIN, F., HAINES, B.W., MAHLANDT, B.G., DEARMON, I.A. & LINCOLN, R.E., 1963.** Dual nature of resistance mechanisms as revealed by studies of anthrax septicemia. *Journal of Bacteriology*, 85, 1032–1033.

106 **KLEIN, F., MAHLANDT, B.G., LINCOLN, R.E., DEARMON, I.A. & FERNELIUS, A.L., 1961.** Immunization as a factor affecting the course of septicaemic anthrax. *Science*, 133, 1021–1022.

107 **KLEIN, F., WALKER, J.S., FITZPATRICK, D.F., LINCOLN, R.E., MAHLANDT, B.G., JONES, W.I. JR., DOBBS, J.P. & HENDRIX, K.J., 1966.** Pathophysiology of anthrax. *Journal of Infectious Diseases*, 116, 123–138.

108 **KLEINE-ALBERS, C. & BÖHM, R., 1990.** Possible applications of monoclonal antibodies against the protective antigen of *Bacillus anthracis* for diagnostic purposes. *Salisbury Medical Bulletin*, 68 (special suppl.), 73–74.

109 **KLEMM, D.M. & KLEMM, W.R., 1959.** A history of anthrax. *Journal of the American Veterinary Medical Association*, 135, 458–462.

110 **KNIGHT, B.C.J.G. & PROOM, H., 1950.** A comparative survey of the nutrition and physiology of mesophilic species in the genus *Bacillus*. *Journal of General Microbiology*, 4, 508–538.

111 **KNISELY, R.F., 1966.** Selective medium for *Bacillus anthracis*. *Journal of Bacteriology*, 92, 784–786.

112 **KNUDSON, G.B., 1986.** Treatment of anthrax in man: History and current concepts. *Military Medicine*, 151, 71–77.

113 **KNUDSON, G.B. & TURRELL, M.J., 1987.** Mechanical transmission of *Bacillus anthracis* by the stable fly *Stomoxys calcitrans*. *Abstract of the Annual Meeting of the American Society of Microbiology*, 87, 355.

114 **KOBUCH, W.E., DAVIS, J., FLETSCHER, K., ISAACSON, M. & TURNBULL, P.C.B., 1990.** A clinical and epidemiological study of 621 patients with anthrax in western Zimbabwe. *Salibury Medical Bulletin*, 68, 34–38.

115 **KOCH, R., 1876.** The aetiology of anthrax based on the ontogeny of the anthrax bacillus. *Medical Classics (1938)*, 2, 745–820. Originally published in *Beiträge zür Biologie der Pflanzen*, 1876, 277–310.

116 **KOLONIN, G.V., 1969.** Nosogeography of anthrax in the USSR in association with its landscape epizootiology (English translation). *Zhurnal Mikrobiologii Epidemiologii i Immunobiologii*, 46, 91–97.

117 **KOLONIN, G.V., 1970.** Evolution of anthrax. Report I. Peculiarities of circulation of the causative agent and the origin of the disease. *Zhurnal Mikrobiologii Epidemiologii i Epidemiologii*, 47, 98–102.

118 **KOLONIN, G.V., 1971.** Evolution of anthrax. Report II. History of spread of the disease. *Zhurnal Mikrobiologii Epidemiologii i Immunobiologii*, 48, 118–122.

119 **KRANEVELD, F.C. & DJAENOEDIN, R., 1940.** Experiments on the transmission of anthrax by *Tabanus rubidus* to horses and buffaloes. *Veeartsenykundig Mededelingen*, 83, 42.

120 **KRANEVELD, F.C. & MANSJOER, M., 1939.** De miltvuurbacil in het digestie-apparaat van den *Tabanus rubidus* wied. *Nederlands-Indische Bladen Voor Diergeneeskunde*, 51, 62–75.

121 **KRIEK, N.P.J. & DE VOS, V., 1991.** Department of Pathology, Faculty of Veterinary Science, University of Pretoria, South Africa. Unpublished data.

122 **KRISHNA, R.N.S. & MOHIYUDEEN, S., 1958.** *Tabanus* flies as transmitters of anthrax — a field experience. *The Indian Veterinary Journal*, 35, 348–353.

123 **KUSOV, V.N., AKHMEROV, D.S. & CHERNOVA, A.A., 1983.** Role of blood-sucking mosquitoes in the transmission of anthrax. *Sbornik Nauchnykh Trudov, Kazanskii Veterinarnyi Institut*, 120–126.

124 **LAMANNA, C., 1967.** The anthrax question. *Federation Proceedings*, 26, 1491–1492.

125 **LAMBERT, J., 1882.** Horse-sickness or anthrax in South Africa. *Veterinary Journal*, 14, 118–128.

126 **LAWRENCE, J.A., FOGGIN, C.M. & NORVAL, R.A.I., 1980.** The effects of war on the control of diseases of livestock in Rhodesia (Zimbabwe). *The Veterinary Record*, 107, 82–85.

127 **LENSING, H.H. & OEI, H.L., 1984.** Een onderzoek naar de werkzaamheid van ontsmettingsmiddelen ten opzichte van miltvuursporen. (A study on the efficacy of disinfectants against anthrax spores). *Tijdschrift Diergeneeskunde*, 109, 557–563.

128 **LEPPLA, S.H., 1982.** Anthrax toxin edema factor: A bacterial adenylate cyclase that increases cyclic AMP concentrations in eukaryotic cells. *Biochemistry*, 79, 3162–3166.

129 **LEPPLA, S.H., 1984.** *Bacillus anthracis* calmodulin-dependent adenylate cyclase: Chemical and enzymatic properties and interactions with eukaryotic cells. *Advances in Cyclic Neucleotide and Protein Phosphorylation Research*, 17, 189–198.

130 **LEPPLA, S.H., FRIEDLANDER, A.M., SINGH, Y., CORA, E.M. & BHATNAGAR, R., 1990.** A model for anthrax toxic action at the cellular level. *Salisbury Medical Bulletin*, 68 (special suppl.), 41–43.

131 **LEPPLA, S.H., IVINS, B.E. & EZZELL, J.W. JR., 1985.** Anthrax toxin. *In*: LEIVE, L. (ed.). *Microbiology*. Washington, D.C.: American Society for Microbiology.

132 **LIGHTFOOT, N.F., SCOTT, R.J.D. & TURNBULL, P.C.B., 1990.** Antimicrobial susceptibility of *Bacillus anthracis*. *Salibury Medical Bulletin*, 68 (special suppl.), 95–98.

133 **LINCOLN, R.E. & FISH, D.C., 1970.** Anthrax toxin. *In*: MONTIE, T.C., KADIS SAND AJL, S.J., (eds). *Microbial Toxins*. New York, London: Academic Press, Inc.

134 **LINCOLN, R.E. & RHIAN, M.A., 1950.** Pathogenesis as related to physiological state of anthrax spore and cell. *In*: HALVORSON, H., (ed.). *Spores II*. Minneapolis: Burgess Publishing Company.

135 **LINCOLN, R.E., WALKER, J.S., KLEIN, F. & HAINES, B.W., 1964.** Anthrax. *In*: BRANDLEY, C.A. & JUNGHERR, E.L., (eds). *Advances in Veterinary Science*. Vol. IX. New York, London: Academic Press, Inc.

136 **LINCOLN, R.E., WALKER, J.S., KLEIN, F., ROSENWALD, A.J. & JONES, W.I. JR., 1967.** Value of field data for extrapolation in anthrax. *Federation Proceedings*, 26, 1558–1562.

137 **LINDSAY, D.R. & SCUDDER, H.I., 1956.** Nonbiting flies and disease. *Annual Review of Entomology*, 1, 323–346.

138 **LITTLE, S.F. & KNUDSON, G.B., 1986.** Comparative efficacy of *Bacillus anthracis* live spore vaccine and protective antigen against anthrax in the guinea-pig. *Infection and Immunity*, 52, 509–512.

139 **LIVINGSTONE, D., 1857.** *Missionary Travels and Researches in South Africa*. London: John Murray.

140 **LOGAN, N.A., CARMAN, J.A., MELLING, J. & BERKELEY, R.C.W., 1985.** Identification of *Bacillus anthracis* by API tests. *Journal of Medical Microbiology*, 20, 75–85.

141 **LYON, D.G., 1973.** An outbreak of anthrax at the Chester Zoological Gardens. *The Veterinary Record*, 92, 334–337.

142 **MANCHEE, R.J., BROSTER, M.G., ANDERSON, I.S., HENSTRIDGE, R.M. & MELLING, J., 1983.** Decontamination of *Bacillus anthracis* on Gruinard Island. *Nature*, 303, 239–240.

143 **MANCHEE, R.J., BROSTER, M.G., MELLING, J., HENSTRIDGE, R.M. & STAGG, A.J., 1981.** *Bacillus anthracis* on Gruinard Island. *Nature*, 294, 254–255.

144 **MANCHEE, R.J., BROSTER, M.G., STAGG, A.J., HIBBS, S.E. & PATIENCE, B., 1990.** Out of Gruinard Island. *Salisbury Medical Bulletin*, 68 (special suppl.), 17–18.

145 **McCLOY, E.W., 1951.** Studies on a lysogenic bacillus strain. I. A bacteriophage specific for *Bacillus anthracis*. *Journal of Hygiene*, 49, 114–125.

146 **McCLOY, E,W., 1958.** Lysogenicity and immunity to *Bacillus* phage W. *Journal of General Microbiology*, 18, 198–220.

147 **McCONNELL, E.E., TUSTIN, R.C. & DE VOS, V., 1972.** Anthrax in an African buffalo (*Syncerus caffer*) in the Kruger National Park. *Journal of the South African Veterinary Medical Association*, 43, 181–187.

148 **McCULLOUGH, E.C., 1936.** *Disinfection and Sterilization. Effect of Temperature upon Microbial Life*. Philadelphia: Lea & Febiger.

149 **McKENDRICK, A.G., 1940.** The dynamics of crowd infections. *Edinburgh Medical Journal*, New Series, 47, 117–136.

150 **MEYNELL, E. & MEYNELL, G.G., 1964.** The roles of serum and carbon dioxide in capsule formation by *Bacillus anthracis*. *Journal of General Microbiology*, 34, 153–164.

151 **MIKESELL, P., DREIER, T., RISTROPH, J.D. & KNUDSON, G.B., 1982.** Plasmid isolation in virulent and avirulent strains of *Bacillus anthracis*. *Abstracts of the Annual Meeting of the American Society of Microbiology*, 82, 118.

152 **MIKESELL, P., IVINS, B.E., RISTROPH, J.D. & DREIER, T.M., 1983.** Evidence for plasmid-mediated toxin production in *Bacillus anthracis*. *Infection and Immunity*, 39, 371–376.

153 **MIKESELL, P. & VODKIN, M., 1985.** Plasmids of *Bacillus anthracis*. *In*: LEIVE, L., (ed.). *Microbiology*. Washington, D.C.: American Society for Microbiology.

154 **MINETT, F.C., 1950.** Sporulation and viability of *B. anthracis* in relation to environmental temperature and humidity. *Journal of Comparative Pathology*, 60, 161–176.

155 **MINETT, F.C., 1952.** The annual and seasonal incidence of anthrax in various countries. Climatic effects and sources of infection. *Bulletin de l'Office International des Épizooties*, 37, 238–300.

156 **MINETT, F.C. & DHANDA, M.R., 1941.** Multiplication of *B. anthracis* and *B. chauvoei* in soil and water. *The Indian Journal of Veterinary Science and Animal Husbandry*, 11, 308–321.

157 **MITZMAIN, M.B., 1914.** Insect transmission of anthrax. *Journal of Tropical Medicine and Hygiene*, 17, 61–62.

158 **MOFFAT, R., 1842.** *Missionary Labours and Scenes in Southern Africa*. London: John Snow.

159 **MORRIS, H., 1920.** Some carriers of anthrax infection. *Journal of the American Veterinary Medical Association*, 56, 606–608.

160 **MURPHY, T.D., LA BOCCETTA, A.C. & LOCKWOOD, J.S., 1944.** Treatment of human anthrax with penicillin: Report of three cases. *Journal of the American Medical Association*, 126, 948–950.

161 **NARASIMHAM, C.V., 1954.** An interesting outbreak of anthrax. *Indian Veterinary Journal*, 30, 512–514.

162 **NEITZ, W.O., 1965.** A check-list and host-list of the zoonoses occurring in mammals and birds in South and South West Africa. *Onderstepoort Journal of Veterinary Research*, 32, 189–374.

163 **NIESCHULZ, O., 1928.** Enkele miltvuuroverbrengingsproeven met tabaniden, musciden, en muskieten. *Nederlands-Indische Bladin voor Diergeneeskunde*, 40, 355–377.

164 **NORDBERG, B.K., SCHMITERLOW, G.G. & HANSEN, N.J., 1961.** Pathological investigations into the terminal course of experimental anthrax in the rabbit. *Acta Pathologica et Microbiologica Scandanavica*, 53, 295–318.

165 **ODENDAAL, M.W., PIETERSON, P.M. & DE VOS, V., 1991.** The antibiotic sensitivity patterns of *Bacillus anthracis* isolated from the Kruger National Park. *Onderstepoort Journal of Veterinary Research*, 58, 17–19.

166 **OELOFSEN, J., 1969.** Cited by: PIENAAR, U. DE V., 1973. The capture and restraint of wild herbivores by mechanical methods. *In*: YOUNG, E., (ed.). *The Capture and Care of Wild Animals*. Cape Town and Pretoria: Human & Rousseau.

167 **OLSUFEV, N.G. & LELER, P.P., 1935.** On the importance of tabanids in the spread of anthrax. Abstr. in *Reviews of Applied Entomology* (1936), 24, 177–179.

168 **PARRY, J.M., TURNBULL, P.C.B., GIBSON, R.J., 1983.** *A Colour Atlas of Bacillus Species*. London: Wolfe Medical Publications Ltd.

169 **PASTEUR, L., 1881.** De l'attenuation des virus et de leur retour à la virulence (Attenuation of viruses and their return to virulence). *Comptes Rendus de l'Académie des Sciences*, 92, 429–435.

170 **PFISTERER, R.M., 1990.** Retrospective verification of the diagnosis of anthrax by means of intracutaneous skin test with the Russian allergen 'anthraxin' in a recent epidemic in Switzerland. *Salisbury Medical Bulletin*, 68 (special suppl.), 80.

171 **PHILLIPS, A.P. & MARTIN, K.L., 1983.** Assessment of immuno-fluorescence measurements of individual bacteria in direct and indirect assays for *Bacillus anthracis* and *Bacillus cereus* spores. *Journal of Applied Bacteriology*, 53, 223–232.

172 **PHILLIPS, A.P., MARTIN, K.L. & BROSTER, M.G., 1983.** Differentiation between spores of *Bacillus anthracis* and *Bacillus cereus* by a quantitative immunofluorescence technique. *Journal of Clinical Microbiology*, 17, 41–47.

173 **PHILLIPS, A.P., MARTIN, K.L., CROSS, N.L., & DRAKE, R.G., 1984.** Evaluation of immunoradiometric and ELISA versions of a microtitre plate assay for *Bacillus anthracis* spores. *Journal of Immunological Methods*, 70, 75–82.

174 **PIENAAR, U. DE V., 1967.** Epidemiology of anthrax in wild animals and the control of anthrax epizootics in the KNP, South Africa. *Federation Proceedings*, 26, 1496–1501.

175 **PIENAAR, U. DE V., 1973.** The capture and restraint of wild herbivores by mechanised methods. *In*: YOUNG, E., (ed.). *The Capture and Care of Wild Animals*. Cape Town, Pretoria: Human & Rousseau.

176 **PLOWRIGHT, W., 1982.** The effects of rinderpest and rinderpest control on wildlife in Africa. *In*: EDWARDS, M.A. & McDONNEL, U., (eds). *Animal Diseases in Relation to Animal Conservation: Symposium of the Zoological Society of London*, No. 50, 1–58. London: Academic Press, Inc.

177 **POSNANSKY, M., 1966.** *Prelude to East African History — a Collection of Papers given at the First East African Vacation School in Pre-European African History and Archaeology in December*

1962. London: Oxford University Press.

178 **PROOM, H. & KNIGHT, B.C.J.G., 1955.** The minimal nutritional requirements of some species in the genus *Bacillus*. *Journal of General Microbiology*, 13, 474–480.

179 **PROVOST, A. & TROUETTE, M., 1957.** Reflexions sur quelques cas de charbon bacteridien (cryptique) chez des bovins. *Revue d'Élevage et de Médecine Vétérinaire des Pays Tropicaux*, 10, 25–26.

180 **PUGH, A.O. & DAVIES, J.C.A., 1990.** Human anthrax in Zimbabwe. *Salisbury Medical Bulletin*, 68 (special suppl.), 32–33.

181 **PUZISS, M. & WRIGHT, G.G., 1963.** Studies on immunity in anthrax. X. Gel-adsorbed protective antigen for immunization in man. *Journal of Bacteriology*, 85, 230–236.

182 **RICH, V., 1980.** Incident at military village no 19. *Nature*, 284, 294.

183 **ROBILLARD, N.K., KOEHLER, T.M., MURRAY, R. & THORNE, C.B., 1983.** Effects of plasmid loss on the physiology of *Bacillus anthracis*. *Abstracts of the Annual Meeting of the American Society of Microbiology*, 83, 115.

184 **ROSS, J.M., 1957.** The pathogenesis of anthrax following the administration of spores by the respiratory route. *Journal of Pathology and Bacteriology*, 73, 485–494.

185 **SAUNDERS, J.E., 1939.** Cited by Stableforth, A.W. & Galloway, I.A., 1959. *Infectious Diseases of Animals. Diseases Due to Bacteria*. Vol. I. London: Butterworths Scientific Publications.

186 **SCHLINGMAN, A.S., DEVLIN, H.B., WRIGHT, G.G., MAINE, R.J. & MANNING, M., 1956.** Immunizing activity of alum-precipitated protective antigen of *Bacillus anthracis* in cattle, sheep and swine. *American Journal of Veterinary Research*, 17, 256–261.

187 **SEDDON, H.R., 1965.** Diseases of domestic animals in Australia. Part V. (2nd edn). *Bacterial Diseases*. Vol I. Commonwealth of Australia, Department of Health.

188 **SEN, S.K., MINETT, F.C., 1944.** Experiments on the transmission of anthrax through flies. *Indian Journal of Veterinary Science and Animal Husbandry*, 14, 149–158.

189 **SHLYAKHOV, E.N., 1971.** Correlation of anthraxin test indices with specific protection of guinea-pigs. *Journal of Hygiene and Epidemiological Microbial Immunology*, 15, 207–211.

190 **SHREWSBURY, J.F.D. & BARSON, G.F.A., 1952.** A bacteriological study of the house sparrow, *Passer domesticus domesticus*. *Journal of Pathology and Bacteriology*, 64, 605–618.

191 **SIRISANTHANA, T., NAVACHAREON, N., THARAVICHITKUL, P., SIRISANTHANA, V. & BROWN, A.E., 1984.** Outbreak of oral-oropharyngeal anthrax: An unusual manifestation of human infection with *Bacillus anthracis* from beef. *American Journal of Tropical Medicine and Hygiene*, 33, 144–150.

192 **SMITH, H., 1990.** Anthrax, clinical manifestations and pathogenesis: Much unknown and much just forgotten. *Salisbury Medical Bulletin*, 68 (special suppl.), 31.

193 **SMITH, G. & FURTHER, G.S., 1941.** Observations on the longevity of dry spores of *B. anthracis*. *Journal of Hygiene*, 41, 5–6.

194 **SMITH, H. & KEPPIE, J., 1954.** Observations on experimental anthrax: Demonstration of a specific lethal factor produced *in vivo* by *Bacillus anthracis*. *Nature*, 173, 869–870.

195 **SMITH, H. & KEPPIE, J., 1962.** The terminal phase of anthrax. *British Journal of Experimental Pathology*, 43, 684–686.

196 **SMITH, H., KEPPIE, J. & STANLEY, J.L., 1955.** The chemical basis of the virulence of *Bacillus anthracis*. V. The specific toxin produced by *B. anthracis in vivo*. *British Journal of Experimental Pathology*, 36, 460–472.

197 **SMITH, H. & STANLEY, J.L., 1962.** Purification of the third factor of anthrax toxin. *The Journal of General Microbiology*, 29, 517–521.

198 **SMITH, H. & STONER, H.B., 1956.** Anthrax toxic complex. *Federation Proceedings*, 26, 1554–1557.

199 **SMITH, N.R., GORDON, R.E. & CLARK, F.E., 1946.** Aerobic mesophilic spore-forming bacteria. *United States Department of Agriculture, Miscellaneous Publication 559*.

200 **SMITH, N.R., GORDON, R.E. & CLARK, F.E., 1952.** Aerobic spore-forming bacteria. *United States Department of Agriculture, Agriculture Monograph, No. 16*.

201 **SMITHCORS, J.F., 1957.** *Evolution of the Veterinary Art*. Kansas City, Missouri: Veterinary Medicine Publishing Co.

202 **SMYTH, H.F. & HIGGINS, W.D., 1945.** Anthrax in the United States 1939–43. Report of the Committee on Industrial Anthrax. *American Journal of Public Health*, 35, 850.

203 **SNEATH, P.H.A., 1986.** Endospore-forming Gram-positive rods and cocci. *In*: SNEATH, P.H.A., MAIR, N.S., SHARPE, M.E. & HOLT, J.G., (eds). *Bergey's Manual of Systematic Bacteriology*. Vol. II. Baltimore, London, Los Angeles, Sydney: Williams & Wilkins.

204 **SOBERNHEIM, G., 1931.** *Handbuch der Pathogen Mikroorganismen*. Jena, Berlin, Viena: Gustav Fischer Urban und Schwarzenberg.

205 **SOBERNHEIM, G. & MURATA, H., 1924.** Vergleichende Untersuchungen ü ber die Bedeutung des Infektionsmodus bei der experimentellen Milzbrandinfektion. *Zeitschrift für Hygiene und Infektionskrankheiten*, 103, 691–698.

206 **SOLTYS, M.A., 1948.** Anthrax in laboratory workers with observations on possible source of infection. *Journal of Pathology and Bacteriology*, 60, 253–257.

207 **STANLEY, J.L. & SMITH, H., 1961.** Purification of Factor I and recognition of a third factor of the anthrax toxin. *Journal of General Bacteriology*, 26, 49–63.

208 **STEIN, C.D., 1945.** The history and distribution of anthrax in livestock in the USA. *Veterinary Medicine and Small Animal Clinician*, 40, 340–349.

209 **STEIN, C.D., 1947.** Some observations on the tenacity of *Bacillus anthracis*. *Veterinary Medicine*, 42, 13–22.

210 **STEIN, C.D., 1948.** Incidence of anthrax in livestock during 1945, 1946 and 1947 with special reference to control measures in the various states. *Veterinary Medicine*, 43, 463–469.

211 **STEIN, C.D., 1955.** Anthrax. *Farmers' Bulletin*, 1736, 1–14.

212 **STEIN, C.D. & ROGERS, H., 1945.** Observations on the resistance of anthrax spores to heat. *Veterinary Medicine*, 40, 406–410.

213 **STEIN, C.D. & ROGERS, H., 1946.** Recovery of viable anthrax spores from vapors of heated anthrax spore suspensions and from the distillate from anthrax spore suspensions. *American Journal of Veterinary Research*, 7, 481–485.

214 **STEIN, C.D. & VAN NESS, G.B., 1955.** A ten-year survey of anthrax in livestock with special reference to outbreaks in 1954. *Veterinary Medicine*, 50, 579.

215 **STEPHEN, J., 1981.** Anthrax toxin. *International Encyclopedia of Pharmacology and Therapeutics*, 119, 381–395.

216 **STERNE, M., 1937.** The effects of different carbon dioxide concentrations on the growth of virulent anthrax strains. Pathogenicity and immunity tests on guinea-pigs and sheep with anthrax variants derived from virulent strains. *Onderstepoort Journal of Veterinary Science and Animal Industry*, 9, 49–67.

217 **STERNE, M., 1959.** Anthrax. *In*: STABLEFORTH, A.W. & GALLOWAY, I.A., (eds). *Infectious Diseases of Animals. Diseases due to Bacteria*. Vol. I. London: Butterworths Scientific Publications.

218 **STERNE, M., 1967.** Distribution and economic importance of anthrax. *Federation Proceedings*, 26, 1493–1495.

219 **STERNE, M., NICOL, J. & LAMBRECHTS, M.C., 1942.** The effect of large-scale active immunization against anthrax. *Journal of the South African Veterinary Medical Association*, 13, 53–63.

220 **STERNE, M., NICOL, J. & LAMBRECHTS, M.C., 1945.** Field results with avirulent anthrax vaccine. *Journal of South African Veterinary Medical Association*, 16, 12–13.

221 **STILES, G.W., 1944.** Isolation of the *Bacillus anthracis* from

spinose ear ticks *Ornithodorus megnini*. *American Journal of Veterinary Research*, 5, 318–319.

222 **STOCKMAN, S., 1905.** Anthrax. *Annual Report of the Department of Agriculture, Transvaal.*

223 **STOCKMAN, S., 1911.** The epizootiology of anthrax. *Journal of Comparative Pathology and Therapeutics*, 24, 97–108.

224 **SUSSMAN, A.S. & HALVORSON, H.O., 1966.** *Spores, their dormancy and germination.* New York: Harper & Row.

225 **THORNE, C.B. & BELTON, F.C., 1957.** An agar-diffusion method for titrating *Bacillus anthracis* immunizing antigen and its application to a study of antigen production. *Journal of General Microbiology*, 17, 505–516.

226 **THORNE, C.B., GOMEZ, C.G. & HOUSEWRIGHT, R.D., 1952.** Synthesis of glutamic acid and glutamyl polypeptide by *Bacillus anthracis*. *Journal of Bacteriology*, 63, 363.

227 **TIGERTT, W.D., 1980.** Anthrax. William Smith Greenfield, Professor Superintendent, The Brown Animal Sanitary Institution, London, England, 1878–81. The priority due to him for the production of the first vaccine against anthrax. *Journal of Hygiene*, 85, 415–420.

228 **TITBALL, R.W. & MANCHEE, R.J., 1987.** Factors affecting the germination of spores of *Bacillus anthracis*. *Journal of Applied Bacteriology*, 62, 269–274.

229 **TOSCHKOFF, A. & VELJANOV, D., 1970.** Sporulation und Virulenz von *Bacillus anthracis* in geöffneten und nicht geöffneten Tierleichen. *Archiv für Experimentelle Veterinärmedizin*, 24, 1153–1160.

230 **TURELL, M.J. & KNUDSON, G.B., 1987.** Mechanical transmission of *Bacillus anthracis* by stable flies (*Stomoxys calcitrans*) and mosquitoes (*Aedes aegypti* and *Aedes taeniorhynchus*). *Infection and Immunity*, 55, 1859–1861.

231 **TURNBULL, P.C.B., 1986.** Thoroughly modern anthrax. Bureau of Hygiene and Tropical Disease. *Abstracts on Hygiene and Tropical Diseases*, 61, 1–13.

232 **TURNBULL, P.C.B., 1990.** Terminal bacterial and toxin levels in blood of guinea-pigs dying of anthrax. *Salisbury Medical Journal*, 68 (special suppl.), 53–55.

233 **TURNBULL, P.C.B. & BROSTER, M.G., 1986.** Development of antibodies to protective antigen and lethal factor components of anthrax toxin in humans and guinea-pigs and their relevance to protective immunity. *Medical Microbiology and Immunology*, 177, 293.

234 **TURNBULL, P.C.B., HUDSON, R.A., WARD, M.J., JONES, M.N., QUINN, C.P., FINNIE, N.J., DUGGLEBY, C.J., KRAMER, J.M. & MELLING, J., 1992.** *Bacillus anthracis* but not always anthrax. *Journal of Applied Bacteriology*, 72, 21–28.

235 **TURNBULL, P.C.B., QUINN, C.P., HEWSON, M.C., STOCKBRIDGE, M.C. & MELLING, J., 1990.** Protection conferred by microbially supplemented UK and purified PA vaccine. *Salisbury Medical Journal*, 68 (special suppl.), 89–91.

236 **TURNER, M., 1980.** Anthrax in humans in Zimbabwe. *Central African Journal of Medicine*, 26, 160–161.

237 **TWINING, D.T., 1981.** Biological warfare opens Pandora's box in Sverdlovsk anthrax outbreak. *Air Force (US) Magazine*, 64, 124–128.

238 **VAN DER HOEDEN, J., 1964.** Anthrax. *In*: VAN DER HOEDEN, J., (ed.). *Zoonoses*. Amsterdam, London, New York: Elsevier Publishing Company.

239 **VAN NESS, G.B., 1959.** Soil relationship in the Oklahoma-Kansas anthrax outbreak of 1957. *Journal of Soil and Water Conservation*, 14, 70–71.

240 **VAN NESS, G.B., 1971.** Ecology of anthrax. *Science*, 172, 1303–1307.

241 **VASILEVA, V.M., 1958/59.** A study of soil bacteria as antagonists of anthrax bacilli. *Sbornik Nanchmykh Trudov Lvovskii Zooveterinarnyi Institut*, 9, 149–153.

242 **VILJOEN, P.R., CURSON, H.H. & FOURIE, P.J.J., 1928.** Anthrax in South Africa. *Thirteenth and Fourteenth Reports of the Director of Veterinary Education and Research*, 431–528.

243 **VODKIN, M.H. & LEPPLA, S.H., 1983.** Cloning of the protective antigen gene of *Bacillus anthracis*. *Cell*, 34, 693–697.

244 **WADE, N., 1980.** Death at Sverdlovski: A critical diagnosis. An anthrax outbreak. *Science*, 209, 1501–1502.

245 **WALKER, J.S., KLEIN, F., LINCOLN, R.E. & FERNELIUS, A.L., 1967.** A unique defence mechanism against anthrax demonstrated in dwarf swine. *Journal of Bacteriology*, 93, 2031–2032.

246 **WALKER, J.S., KLEIN, F., LINCOLN, R.E. & FERNELIUS, A.L., 1967.** Temperature response in animals infected with *Bacillus anthracis*. *Journal of Bacteriology*, 93, 552–556.

247 **WALKER, J.S., LINCOLN, R.E. & KLEIN, F., 1967.** Pathophysiological and biochemical changes in anthrax. *Federation Proceedings*, 26, 1539–1544.

248 **WARD, M.K., McGANN, V.G., HOGGE, A.L., HUFF, M.L., KANODE, R.G. & ROBERTS, E.O., 1965.** Studies on anthrax infections in immunized guinea-pigs. *Journal of Infectious Diseases*, 115, 59–67.

249 **WEAVER, R.E., BRACHMAN, P.S. & FEELEY, J.C., 1970.** Anthrax. *In*: BODILY, H.L., UPDIKE, E.L. & MASON, J.O., (eds). *Diagnostic Procedures for Bacterial, Mycotic and Parasitic Infections*. 5th edn. New York: The American Public Health Association Inc.

250 **WEBSTER, A., 1973.** Inhibiting effect of antibiotics on anthrax vaccination. *Australian Veterinary Journal*, 49, 545.

251 **WELKOS, S.L., BECKER, D., FRIEDLANDER, A. & TROTTER, R., 1990.** Pathogenesis and host resistance to *Bacillus anthracis*: A mouse model. *Salisbury Medical Bulletin*, 68, 49–52.

252 **WELKOS, S.L. & FRIEDLANDER, A.M., 1988.** Pathogenesis and genetic control of resistance to the Sterne strain of *Bacillus anthracis*. *Microbial Pathogenesis*, 4, 53–69.

253 **WELKOS, S.L., KENNET, T.J. & GIBBS, P.H., 1986.** Differences in susceptibility of inbred mice to *Bacillus anthracis*. *Infection and Immunity*, 51, 795–800.

254 **WELKOS, S.L., TROTTER, R.W., BECKER, D.M. & NELSON, G.O., 1989.** Resistance to the Sterne strain of *B. anthracis*: Phagocytic cell responses of resistant and susceptible mice. *Microbial Pathogenesis*, 7, 15–35.

255 **WHITFORD, H.W., 1978.** Factors affecting the laboratory diagnosis of anthrax. *Journal of the American Veterinary Medical Association*, 173, 1467–1469.

256 **WHITFORD, H.W., 1979.** Anthrax. *In*: STEELE, J.H., (ed.). *CRC Handbook Series in Zoonoses, Section A: Bacterial, Rickettsial and Mycotic Diseases*. Vol. I. Boca Raton, Florida: CRC Press, Inc.

257 **WHITFORD, H.W., 1987.** *A Guide to the Diagnosis, Treatment and Prevention of Anthrax*. World Health Organization.

258 **WILLIAMS, N., 1932.** Anthrax. *Journal of the American Veterinary Medical Association*, 81, 9–25.

259 **WILSON, G.S. & MILES, A.S., 1966.** Anthrax. *In: Topley and Wilson's Principles of Bacteriology and Immunity*. Vol. I. 5th edn. London: Edward Arnold (Publishers) Ltd.

260 **WILSON, J.B. & RUSSELL, K.E., 1964.** Isolation of *Bacillus anthracis* from soil stored for 60 years. *Journal of Bacteriology*, 87, 237–238.

261 **WOLF, J. & BARKER, A.N., 1968.** The genus *Bacillus*: Aids to the identification of the species. *In*: BERKELEY, R.C.W. & GOODFELLOW, M., (eds). *The Aerobic Endospore-forming Bacteria: Classification and Identification*. London: Academic Press, Inc.

262 **YOUNG, G.A. JR., ZELLE, M.R. & LINCOLN, R.E., 1946.** Respiratory pathogenicity of *Bacillus anthracis* spores. *Journal of Infectious Diseases*, 79, 233–271.

263 **ZARUBKINSKY, V.S., 1958/59.** Self-purification of soil and water of *Bacillus anthracis* spores. *Sbornik Nanchnykh Trudov, Lvovskii Zoovererinarnyi Institut*, 9, 51–58.

Clostridium perfringens *group*

Synonym: *Clostridium welchii*

M.W. Odendaal

General introduction

Clostridium perfringens, previously referred to as *C. welchii,* was first described in 1891 by Achalme as the *Bacillus of Acute Articular Rheumatism.*[72] In the historical literature it was also known by names such as *Bacillus phlegmonis emphysematosae, Bacillus emphysematis vaginae, Bacillus cadaveris butyricus, Bacillus aerogenes capsulatus, Granulobacillus saccharobutyricus liquefaciens immobilis,* and *Bacillus perfringens.*[72, 75]

Clostridium perfringens is a typical representative of the genus *Clostridium,* which requires anaerobic growth conditions. It is widely distributed in nature and occurs in soil, sewage and water, as well as in the intestinal tract of humans and warm-blooded animals. *Clostridium perfringens* is absent from the stomach, but present in small numbers (vegetative bacteria and spores) in the small and large intestine of most animal species. Vegetative organisms may multiply in soil,[74] and counts as high as 5×10^4 *C. perfringens* organisms per gram of soil have been recorded.[74, 91] Normal human intestinal contents can contain as many as 10^9 organisms per gram,[1] the number being dependent on the diet of the host.[2, 88] In pigs fed on a high-protein diet, the number of *C. perfringens* is significantly higher than in pigs fed on a standard protein diet.[40] Higher faecal counts of *C. perfringens* are found in calves aged between one and ten days than in older animals.[4]

Clostridium perfringens types produce four major lethal toxins (alpha, beta, epsilon and iota toxins) which are used to type them into toxin types A, B, C, D and E **(Table 1)**.[54, 75] Each one of these types also produces a number of minor, less lethal toxins, each of which has also been designated a letter of the Greek alphabet. Under certain *in vivo* and *in vitro* conditions the major and minor toxins, also referred to as virulence factors, are produced alone or in combination, depending on the specific type, and are responsible for the virulence of the bacterium.[72, 75, 82] These toxins, alone or in combination, are responsible for the various syndromes associated with this group of organisms. They cause disease as a consequence of their local effects on the intestinal tract, which may vary from insignificant to outspoken, or as a consequence of the systemic effect of absorbed toxins — a situation referred to as enterotoxaemia. Traditionally in South Africa, however, the designation 'enterotoxaemia' refers to pulpy kidney disease. The effects of these toxins are divided into three groups, namely,[73]

- the alpha and kappa toxins, which are phospholipase C (lecithinase) and collagenase enzymes, respectively, hydrolyze substances essential to the integrity of cellular membranes or other body structures;
- a group which includes the beta, epsilon and iota toxins, that acts primarily on the vascular endothelium, causing increased vascular permeability; and
- a group which includes the haemolytic toxins such as the theta and delta toxins.

Clostridium perfringens is associated with a wide variety of diseases **(Table 2)** that affect most domestic animal species and humans, and include enterotoxaemia, haemorrhagic and necrotic enteritis, traumatic wound infection, cellulitis and myonecrosis, post-abortion septicaemia, intravascular haemolysis, and puerpural infections.[48, 75, 82, 87] It is one of the most widespread and potentially pathogenic organisms in nature. Although small numbers of *C. perfringens* are present in a wide range of meats or products prepared from meat, it does not often play a role in spoilage. It is, however, one of the causes of food poisoning in humans.[71, 89]

Clostridium perfringens grows well on rabbit, human, ovine, bovine and equine blood agar at 35–37 °C in an anaerobic atmosphere. After 18–24 hours' incubation, the colonies are 2–5 mm in diameter, white or grey and translucent with a glossy appearance, low convex, and

Table 1 The major lethal toxins of the different types of *C. perfringens.* (Adapted from Smith & Williams[75])

C. PERFRINGENS TYPE	TOXIN TYPE			
	ALPHA	BETA	EPSILON	IOTA
A	+	–	–	–
B	+	+	+	–
C	+	+	–	–
D	+	–	+	–
E	+	–	–	+

Table 2
Diseases associated with *C. perfringens* in humans and animals

C. PERFRINGENS TYPE	DESCRIPTION OF DISEASE	ANIMAL AFFECTED
	WOUND INFECTION	
A	Gas gangrene, myonecrosis	Humans and animals
A	False blackleg	Cattle
A	Gangrenous mastitis	Cattle
A	Post-abortion septicaemia	Humans
	ENTEROTOXAEMIA	
A	Haemorrhagic/necrotic enteritis	Lambs, sheep
A	Yellow lamb disease	Lambs
A	Enterotoxaemia	Lambs, calves, piglets, water buffalo, deer, elk
A	Sudden death	Cattle
A	Equine intestinal clostridiosis	Horses
A	Equine grass sickness	Horses
A	Enterotoxin food poisoning	Humans and animals
B	Lamb dysentery	Lambs
B	Haemorrhagic entero-toxaemia	Sheep, goats
B	Haemorrhagic enteritis, dysentery	Foals, calves
C	Struck	Sheep
C	Haemorrhagic necrotic enteritis	Lambs, calves, piglets, foals
C	Necrotic enteritis	Humans
D	Pulpy kidney disease (enterotoxaemia, overeating disease)	Sheep, goats
D	Enterotoxaemia	Cattle

round with edges that may vary from irregular/serrated in certain isolates to entire in most isolates. Pure cultures of *C. perfringens* frequently contain two or more colony forms, with aberrant forms sometimes occurring alongside the typical colony forms. On ovine, bovine, rabbit, and human blood agar, colonies are surrounded by a narrow zone of complete haemolysis caused by the theta toxin, around which is a wider zone of partial haemolysis caused by the alpha toxin. On horse blood agar, only the theta toxin is responsible for haemolysis. The alpha toxin has relatively little effect on horse and goat red blood cells.[56, 72] *Clostridium perfringens* tolerates a wide temperature range when incubated and, although optimal range is 35–37 °C, temperatures of 43–45 °C favour its growth when it occurs in mixed cultures. Growth takes place over a pH range varying from 5,5–8,0. When grown under optimal conditions the generation time (i.e. the time it takes an organism to double itself) of *C. perfringens* may be as short as eight minutes, which makes it probably the most rapidly growing organism known.[75].

Different media have been composed for the selective isolation of *C. perfringens* in the presence of other organisms. The addition of antibiotics, such as neomycin, to the tryptone-sulphite-neomycin medium of Marshall, Steenbergen & McClung,[41] allows selective growth of the *C. perfringens* organism whilst suppressing the growth of contaminants. The OPSP medium of Handford & Cavett[25] and Handford[24] contains oleandomycin-polymyxin-sulphadiazine which suppresses the growth of *Clostridium bifermentans,* a common contaminant, more effectively than the tryptose-sulphite-cycloserine medium of Harmon, Kautter & Peeler.[27] More recently, another selective medium containing lactose and metabisulphite has been found to be more effective than tryptose-sulphite-cycloserine agar.[51] The addition of 0,1 per cent sodium metabisulphite to an agar medium containing *C. perfringens* results in the formation of black colonies due to the presence of ferrous sulphide which is formed by the reduction of sulphite to sulphide by *C. perfringens* in the medium.[70] This facilitates the selection of *C. perfringens* for the preparation of pure subcultures on the same or other media.

Clostridium perfringens grows in a variety of liquid media. Of these, Robertson's cooked-meat medium is probably the best known, since it has been extensively and successfully used for culturing the clostridia for the last 60–70 years.[17, 39, 79, 82, 90] The compilation of a fluid medium for the production of one of the exotoxins of *C. perfringens* is common practice, and one that is frequently used is made up of a peptone base, such as proteose peptone, to which salts and carbohydrates are added.[34, 44, 50] A synthetic medium, which facilitates the purification of toxin produced in it, consists of purified amino acids, vitamins, purine and pyrimidine bases, salts, carbohydrates and reducing agents.[46, 47] Synthetic media require more time to prepare and are usually much more expensive to produce. They are used more for research than for routine diagnostic purposes.

For routine diagnostic purposes, fluid media (such as thioglycolate broth, cooked-meat broth and brain-heart infusion broth) are commonly used. These are commercially available, easy to prepare, and relatively inexpensive and are used for the primary inoculation of different carbohydrate media to determine their fermentation reactions and the toxin-producing ability of each strain.

Clostridium perfringens is a Gram-positive, short, squat, thick, straight-sided, non-motile bacillus, measuring 0,6–0,8 x 1,2–4 µm. Very short forms occur in conditions that facilitate rapid growth of the organism. The bacteria usually occur singly or in pairs, and rarely in chains.[6, 87]

In animal tissues, but only in certain media, the organisms form a capsule which is demonstrated by negative staining with Indian ink. The capsule is composed of complex polysaccharides combined with peptides of acidic amino acids.[75]

Although the members of the genus *Clostridium* are characterized as being a spore-forming group of organisms, spores of *C. perfringens* are rarely seen on standard artificial media or in animal tissues. Media have been compiled which encourage the organisms to produce spores under artificial laboratory conditions; yields of up to 10^{6-7} spores per millilitre have been recorded.[58] It appears that there is considerable variation from one strain to another in the conditions required for sporulation.[45] Spores are oval and located subterminally. Sporulation is usually associated with the formation of an enterotoxin[30] which in humans causes a form of food poisoning characterized by abdominal pain, diarrhoea and nausea.[89] The spores are heat resistant, but here also there is considerable variation between different strains, some surviving exposure to 100 °C for one to five hours, while others do not.[86] The majority of spores from heat resistant strains require heat activation (75–100 °C for 10 minutes or more) in order to germinate.[75]

A variety of carbohydrates and other substances metabolized by *C. perfringens* is used in the identification and classification of isolates of the organism. For all practical purposes the biochemical reactions should be the same for all *C. perfringens* types A, B, C, D and E. Ninety per cent of *C. perfringens* strains ferment fructose, galactose, glucose, inositol, lactose, maltose, mannose, starch, and sucrose; liquefy gelatine; produce toxin; and are pathogenic for laboratory animals. Eleven to 89 per cent of strains ferment cellobiose, glycerol, glycogen, inulin, raffinose, ribose, salicin, and trehalose; hydrolyse casein; and reduce nitrates and acetylmethyl carbinol, while only about 1 per cent produce urease. Ninety per cent of *C. perfringens* strains do not ferment adonitol, amygdalin, arabinose, cellulose, dulcitol, erythritol, esculin, mannitol, melezitose, melibiose, rhamnose, sorbitol, sorbose, trehalose, or xylose.[79] The fermentation products formed include acetic and butyric acids, with or without butanol. These reactions play an important confirmatory role in the identification of *C. perfringens* but have no bearing on the toxin type. Once biochemically characterized, toxin-neutralization tests are performed in mice or guinea-pigs so that the toxin type can be established.[82, 83]

Major and minor toxins produced by the perfringens *group of clostridia, and their effects*

Alpha toxin

From a historic viewpoint, the alpha toxin (phospholipase C) was the first bacterial toxin ever to have its biochemical mode of action elucidated. It is a protein, enzymic in action, slightly heat-stable and antigenic, and can be toxoided. The alpha toxin is a phospholipase C enzyme specifically defined as phosphatidylcholine cholinephosphohydrolase (EC 3.1.4.3.), and has marked preference for phospholipids including sphingomyelin, phosphatidylcholine (lecithin), phosphatidylethanolamine, phosphatidylserine and glycerophosphatides. It catalyzes the hydrolysis of the phosphodiester bond in position three of the lecithin molecule to produce phosphorylcholine and water-insoluble 1,2-diacylglyceride.

The alpha toxin has a molecular weight ranging between 49 000 and 53 000 daltons and an isoelectric point of 5,4.[43, 77] The alpha toxin is produced by *C. perfringens* type A in both continuous and batch cultures containing pre-reduced media, with optimal production occurring at a pH of 7,0 and at 37 °C.[53] Phospholipase C is a comparatively thermo-stable enzyme which can retain 45 per cent of its activity when heated for 10–15 minutes at 100 °C. As zinc stabilizes the phospholipase C in the presence of proteases, it is believed that this enzyme is a zinc metalloenzyme.[69] Zinc ions confer a certain resistance to the haemolysis of sheep erythrocytes by the phospholipase C, probably by stabilizing their membranes. The enzyme activity is dependent on the presence of calcium, which acts on the substrate rather than on the enzyme itself. Divalent cations and positively-charged detergents activate the phospholipase C by inducing a positive charge on the substrate which optimizes the attachment of the negatively-charged enzyme. Under normal *in vitro* conditions, the phospholipase C is inhibited by phosphate, citrate, fluoride and substances that bind calcium.[69]

The main biological features of the alpha toxin include its ability to cause localized necrosis of skin when sublethal doses are injected intradermally in guinea-pigs or rabbits, its lethality to laboratory animals, such as mice, guinea-pigs and rabbits when administered parenterally, and its *in vitro* ability to cause haemolysis of erythrocytes of certain animals.[11, 19] These three activities of the alpha toxin were regarded as inseparable, but each may be expressed separately by chemically modifying the highly purified toxin.[60]

The alpha toxin exhibits its phospholipase C action by producing an opalescent reaction, the outcome of which is visible as a white precipitate in agar media containing lecithin, egg yolk or human serum. This enzyme reaction was initially and individually observed in 1939 by Nagler and Seifert, and is referred to as the Nagler reaction.[49] This reaction is used to assay the alpha toxin activity in culture supernatant fluid and during purification procedures of the toxin.[43, 57] The hydrolysis of p-nitrophenylphoshorylcholine also facilitates the detection of alpha toxin enzyme activity.[38]

Erythrocytes of cattle and mice are the most susceptible to the haemolytic activity of alpha toxin, those of rabbits, sheep and humans are moderately so, while horse erythrocytes are relatively insensitive.[32] Erythrocytes of some animal species, such as sheep, exhibit a 'hot-cold' lysis phenomenon; the erythrocytes do not lyse when exposed to the toxin at 37 °C but do when they are cooled down to 4 °C.[75] Apart from its effect on erythrocytes, the alpha toxin also lyses blood platelets and leukocytes, stimulates the *in vivo* and *in vitro* release of histamine from mast cells, and damages the cell membranes of fibroblasts and muscle cells. In one study it was found that purified alpha toxin alone does not alter the viability, chemotactic responsiveness or morphology of human polymorphonuclear leukocytes. It does evoke leukocytolytic activity, but only in the presence of theta toxin.[84] The formation of thrombi in venules, capillaries and arterioles is an important early event in the pathogenesis of necrosis caused by the alpha toxin.[42] The intravenous administration of alpha toxin results in the aggregation and lysis of platelets, a preliminary reduction followed by an increase in the blood clotting time, the formation of abnormally soft and friable clots, massive intravascular haemolysis, and damage to capillary endothelial cells with a resultant increase in their permeability.[73, 75] Alpha toxin is a vigorous inhibitor of the calcium pump of cardiac sarcoplasmic reticulum (Ca-Mg ATP-ase) which may lead to the depletion of releasable Ca^{++} in myocytes,[55] which in turn causes a reduction of systolic myocardial function and a decrease in contractility. If this decrease in myocardial function is significant, a substantial decrease in cardiac output may be responsible for the induction of shock which occurs in *C. perfringens* infections. These *in vivo* lethal and shock effects of alpha toxin and the direct myocardial-depressant effect seen *in vitro*, are well documented.[85] Experimentally, following a single intravenous injection, alpha toxin disappears from the blood stream within 10–20 minutes,[12] the liver being responsible for 72 per cent of its uptake from the blood.

Beta toxin

The beta toxin produced by *C. perfringens* types B and C is a single chain protein with a molecular mass of 28 000 daltons and isoelectric point of 5,4–5,5.[35,92] It is heat-labile; it loses 75 per cent of its biological activity after five minutes at 50 °C, and is destroyed by trypsin after 30 minutes at 37 °C.[59]

Purified beta toxin has a minimum lethal dose of 4 mg in mice, while 2 mg elicits a dermonecrotic effect after intradermal injection.[16] Following administration in ligated intestinal loops *in vivo* in guinea-pigs, it causes haemorrhage and necrosis of the intestinal mucosa,[35] and in rabbits, paralysis of the jejunum and ileum.[42] The *in vitro* addition of beta toxin to guinea-pig monocytes produces changes in their cytoplasm and nuclei which are followed by cell lysis.[28]

Epsilon toxin

Epsilon prototoxin has a molecular mass in the region of 23 200 to 25 000 daltons and a toxicity of 3,0–4,2 x 10^6 MLD/mg protein[22, 23, 95]. The prototoxin is produced during the logarithmic phase of growth, apparently within the cell, from which it diffuses into the surrounding medium. This prototoxin has been demonstrated in the vegetative cell and spores of type D isolates. It is believed that some spontaneous activation of the prototoxin takes place in the culture by proteolytic enzymes, such as the kappa and lambda toxins, which are also produced by the isolate in the same culture.[72] The isoelectric point for the major peak of prototoxin is 8,02, while the activated epsilon toxin has two major peaks with values of 5,36 and 5,74 respectively.[94] This significant change in the isoelectric point and the small change in molecular mass which occurs after the activation of the prototoxin has led to the suggestion that activation results in removal of a small and highly basic peptide from the molecule. The activation also results in some conformational change. It would seem that there is a tendency of the cleavage product to bind to the remaining active toxin molecule, which gives the toxin a conformational and serological identity similar to that of the prototoxin. Under certain conditions, however, this rebinding of the cleavage product can be prevented. It is not clear whether or not the conformation change that results from activation is a necessary prerequisite for toxicity.[5] The epsilon toxin has been purified by a number of researchers.[28]

The epsilon toxin is not haemolytic, but it is locally necrotizing when injected intradermally into guinea-pigs and rabbits and highly lethal when administered parenterally to laboratory animals, such as mice, rabbits, guinea-pigs and lambs.[19, 82] Following its intradermal administration, a circular white area of necrosis is produced, which in some cases is speckled with pinpoint haemorrhages.[82]

Numerous descriptions of the biological effects of the epsilon toxin have been reported. It causes an increased vascular permeability, which is independent of the release of histamine,[8] in the intestine and central nervous system,[7, 8, 13–15, 20, 21, 93] and in the skin of guinea-pigs. In rats, epsilon toxin has an effect on the blood pressure, which is increased without there being changes in electrocardiographic recordings or heart rate. This is accompanied by a decrease in cutaneous blood flow, suggesting that the toxin possesses a vasoconstrictor effect.[67]

Contraction of the rat ileum is induced by the epsilon toxin due to the activation of Na^{+} channels, releasing acetylcholine from cholinergic nerve endings, which in turn promotes the availability of Ca^{++}, causing contraction of the smooth muscle.[68] Loss of its lethal activity can be achieved by the addition of ethoxyformic anhydride to solutions containing the toxin. This has led to the suggestion that a single histidine residue on the surface of the toxin is responsible for its lethal activity.[64] It has also been reported that one tryptophan residue,[61, 62] one tyrosine residue,[65] several lysine residues[63] and several carboxyl groups are necessary to maintain the lethal activity of the epsilon toxin.[66]

Guinea-pig peritoneal macrophages are readily killed *in vitro* by epsilon toxin, but guinea-pig lymphocytes and pulmonary alveolar macrophages remain viable after similar treatment.[9] Rabbit peritoneal macrophages, although also susceptible to the action of the epsilon toxin, are less so than the guinea-pig cells. Rabbit lymphocytes and pulmonary alveolar macrophages possess the same measure of resistance to the toxin[9] as those of guinea-pigs. No demonstrable *in vitro* effect has been noted in other cell types from guinea-pigs, rabbits, mice and sheep.

Iota toxin

The iota toxin is produced as a prototoxin only by type E strains. It is similar to the epsilon toxin in that it has to be activated by proteolytic enzymes, such as trypsin or proteinase, to its toxic form. Not much is known about iota toxin, which has a molecular mass of 45 000 daltons and is heat-labile (it is inactivated after 15 minutes at 53–60 °C). When injected intradermally in guinea-pigs it is dermonecrotic, and after intravenous injection it is lethal. *Clostridium perfringens* type E has been isolated only very rarely from diseased animal species, and will not be discussed further.[42]

Delta toxin

The delta toxin has a molecular mass of 42 000 daltons and an isoelectric point of 9,1. The delta toxin is immunogenic in rabbits and lethal to mice, is not necrotizing on intradermal injection, and haemolyses red blood cells of sheep, cattle, goats and pigs, but not of other species, such as humans, rabbits and horses.[3, 42] The delta toxin, although produced by *C. perfringens* type C, does not seem to play a role in the pathogenesis of the enterotoxaemia caused by this organism.

Theta toxin

The theta toxin, which is also referred to as perfringolysin O, is produced by *C. perfringens* types A–E. It is an oxygen-labile haemolysin as it is reversibly inactivated on exposure to air and is reactivated by thiol-reducing agents, such as cysteine, 2-mercaptoethanol, dithiothreitol and sodium thioglycolate.[78] This toxin is better known as a thiol- or SH-activated cytolysin, and has a cytolytic activity on many cell types, including erythrocytes. It contains SH-groups which are essential for its haemolytic activity. The theta toxin has a molecular mass of 59 000–74 000 daltons, and an isoelectric point of 6,5.[76] It is thermo-labile, being destroyed by heating to 60 °C for 30 minutes. Its activity is temperature-dependent: activity rises sharply with increasing temperatures to 37 °C, but drops off sharply at temperatures above 37 °C. The haemolytic reaction occurs optimally at pH 6,7–6,8.[42]

One of the main characteristics of the theta toxin is its irreversible loss of biological activity if cholesterol is added to solutions containing it. It is lethal, necrotizing and cardiotoxic, and it lyses erythrocytes of a number of animal species, though mouse erythrocytes are characteristically resistant to its effect.[78] The most intense haemolysis is found on horse blood agar.[33] A number of other clostridia species, including *Clostridium tetani*, *C. septicum*, and *C. histolyticum*, produce toxins with a similar haemolytic action which are cross-neutralized by hyperimmune sera from these organisms.[81] The theta toxin also causes the release of histamine from platelets and an increase in vascular permeability.

The actual role of the theta toxin in the pathogenesis of disease is not clear. Experimental studies have revealed its potent leukocytolytic activity for human polymorphonuclear leukocytes[84] and an indirect cardiodepressant effect induced by the release of endogenous myocardial depressant mediators, such as platelet-activating factor in rabbits.[85] The theta toxin is formed under the same physical growth conditions as the alpha toxin in both pre-reduced batch and continuous cultures.[53] It is responsible for the zone of clear haemolysis that surrounds colonies of *C. perfringens* on blood agar plates.

Enterotoxin

The enterotoxin is a heat-labile protein produced primarily by *C. perfringens* type A strains and is responsible for natural outbreaks of food poisoning in humans, and an experimentally induced disease in lambs[29, 31] and several other animal species.[42] It has a molecular mass of 34 000–36 000 daltons and an isoelectric point of 4,3. In contrast to the alpha toxin, it is not produced during active, vegetative growth of the organism, but is synthesized during sporulation.[30] It is regarded as a sporulation-specific gene product, and in a culture medium it is dependent upon pH, temperature and the availability of carbohydrates for its production. Recently, however, enterotoxin production has been detected in cultures of a mutant, non-sporulating strain of *C. perfringens* growing in a chemically defined medium.[18] The enterotoxin is mainly produced by type A strains, but may also be produced by certain *C. perfringens* type C and D strains. It is heat-labile, as its biological properties are destroyed when it is heated at 60 °C for five minutes; some of its serological properties are, however, retained after such treatment. Some of the biological assays used to evaluate the presence of the enterotoxin include the rabbit ligated ileal loop test, the intradermal erythemal test, the mouse lethality test, and the plating efficiency inhibition activity test on Vero cells.[42, 80] Serological assays with excellent sensitivities have been developed which allow the detection of enterotoxin, ranging in amount from 0,5 mg/ml to 1 mg/ml. These assays include the Ouchterlony double-immunodiffusion method, which is not as sensitive as the electro-immunodiffusion, counter-immunoelectrophoresis, single gel diffusion tube, and reverse passive haemagglutinin techniques.[42]

The role of the enterotoxin in the pathogenesis of intestinal disease is not clear. It causes fluid accumulation in the intestinal loops of rabbits and lambs.[10, 11, 29] Parasympathomimetic effects develop after intravenous administration to rabbits, lambs and guinea-pigs. These include increased capillary permeability and vasodilation of intestinal blood vessels and increased intestinal motility. Other systemic effects include diarrhoea, lachrymation, salivation, lassitude, nasal discharge, dyspnoea, and congestion of the liver, lungs, spleen and kidneys.[52]

In the rat ileum, enterotoxin induces a reversal of fluid transfer — from absorption to secretion. In rabbits, *C. perfringens* enterotoxin is most active in the ileum, mildly active in the jejunum and almost inactive in the duodenum. The action of the *C. perfringens* enterotoxin is different from that of the other enterotoxins. In the intestine it inhibits the uptake of glucose, energy production and macromolecular synthesis, and it causes breakdown of the membrane structure and function by an apparently direct interaction with the outer cell membrane. The primary site where the enterotoxin appears to be active is the membrane of the brush border of epithelial cells of the tips of intestinal villi, eventually resulting in necrosis and desquamation of the affected cells.[42]

Kappa toxin

The kappa toxin, with a molecular mass of approximately 80 000 daltons, is a protein free of carbohydrate, heat-labile (enzyme activity is destroyed by heating to 60 °C for 10 minutes) and sensitive to low pH (the activity is destroyed at pH 4,5 or below). It has been purified by gel filtration and ion-exchange chromatography.[36, 42, 72, 75] It has collagenase and gelatinase activities, catalysing the non-polar region of the collagen molecule. This enzyme is primarily produced by *C. perfringens* types A, D and E, and possibly also by types B and C.

The kappa toxin is lethal when injected intravenously into mice and causes necrosis when injected intracutaneously into rabbits. Parenteral administration of the toxin to guinea-pigs results in extensive destruction of connective tissue and severe pulmonary haemorrhage. It has been suggested that it plays a role in the development of gas gangrene (myonecrosis) by softening the infected muscle tissue, thus facilitating the spread of the alpha toxin[42, 72, 75] and promoting the invasiveness of the causative pathogen.[81]

Mu toxin

The mu toxin is a hyaluronidase produced by most strains of types A and B, some strains of type D and a few strains of type C.[72, 75] It acts by releasing glucosamine from hyaluronic acid and, like most other proteins, it is heat-labile, being destroyed by temperatures above 50 °C, and remains active at pH levels varying from 3,9–8,5.[42] The toxin has haemolytic, necrotic and lethal activities and causes an increase in skin permeability.[72]

The role played by the mu toxin in the pathogenesis of disease is unknown, as there is no definite proof of the existence of a relationship between the production of the toxin and the virulence of the organism. It has, however, been suggested that while it does not seem to be essential for the development of gas gangrene, it may well contribute to the severity or rapidity of development and expansion of the lesions.[42]

Nu toxin

The nu toxin is a deoxyribonuclease that is produced by all strains of *C. perfringens* except certain type C strains isolated from humans. It is secreted into the culture medium in which it is growing during the logarithmic growth phase of the organism, is very thermolabile, and is inhibited by the divalent metal ions of copper and zinc, as well as by citrate.[33] It is assumed that the nu toxin exhibits lethal and haemolytic activities, and it has been demonstrated that it has definite cytotoxic activities in that it destroys the nuclei of polymorphonuclear leukocytes and muscle cells in gas gangrene — the absence of leukocytes in clinical gas gangrene lesions bears testimony to this.[42, 75]

Specimens that should be collected for the diagnosis of the C. perfringens *group of diseases*

To confirm a diagnosis of disease caused by *C. perfringens* it is necessary to isolate and identify the organism and type the toxins produced by it. Such specimens should be collected as soon after the death of the animal as possible. The specimens collected and investigation performed will vary according to the specific disease but in general will comprise the following:

- Several smears of affected tissues or of the affected intestinal mucosa (from which the contents have first been removed) and intestinal contents of the affected part prepared on glass slides for microscopical examination after Gram-staining.
- In the event of an enterotoxaemia, a specimen comprising about 30 ml (or, in the case of small animals, as much as possible) of the contents of the affected part of the intestine (in pulpy kidney disease of sheep the ileal contents are preferred) is required for bacteriological and toxicological investigation. The best way to obtain this specimen is to 'milk' the contents of the unopened section of the intestine into an empty sterile glass jar, working as aseptically as possible. In addition, several swabs of the intestinal mucosa should also be taken for bacteriological investigation. These specimens should immediately be refrigerated and kept at 4 °C until dispatched on ice to the investigating laboratory.
- Tissue specimens for bacteriological examination. In the case of a condition such as gas gangrene, specimens should comprise several blocks of affected tissue (about 50 mm x 50 mm x 25 mm in size) each being taken from a different part of the lesion. These are placed in sterile, wide-mouthed, screw-capped bottles. In enterotoxaemias, specimens are collected in a similar manner from the liver, spleen and kidneys.

Specimens should be collected as aseptically as possible and each tissue specimen should be placed in a separate container. Specimens should be refrigerated immediately and kept at 4 °C until they are dispatched on ice to the laboratory.

- Toxicological investigation of intestinal contents. The intestinal contents (5–10 ml) are centrifuged in order to remove as much particulate matter as possible. The resulting supernatant fluid is filter-sterilized, and the filtrate used for toxin-neutralization tests in mice or the intradermal test in guinea-pigs, utilizing *C. perfringens* type A, B, C, D and E antisera.[82]
- Bacteriological investigations of gut contents and tissue specimens include the anaerobic culturing of organisms on blood agar plates or other selective agar media. Organisms resembling *C. perfringens* are subjected to further investigation, which includes microscopical appearance, Gram-staining reactions, haemolytic properties, lecithinase reaction, and assessment of biochemical and carbohydrate fermentation properties.[6, 56, 72, 75]
- In some instances it is deemed necessary to determine the immune status of a herd or flock of animals. For this purpose, 10 ml of serum is required for antitoxin determination from each of 10 or more animals. The animals are bled, and the blood of each animal collected individually and separately in a sterile, rubber-stoppered tube (without anticoagulants) in which it is allowed to clot, first at room temperature for two hours, then overnight in a refrigerator. The serum from each tube is then decanted into another similar container, refrigerated, and submitted to the laboratory packed on ice.
- Specimens of food for human consumption suspected of having caused food poisoning should be collected in sterile containers using aseptic techniques and refrigerated until received by the investigating laboratory. These are subjected to cultural and enumeration methods for identification of the organisms and enterotoxin.[26]

Drug sensitivity of the perfringens *group of clostridia*

Most strains of *C. perfringens* are susceptible to metronidazole, penicillin G, erythromycin, chloramphenicol and amoxycillin with clavulanic acid. Antibiotics such as tetracycline and clindamycin are not always effective against these anaerobes. *Clostridium perfringens* is completely resistant to the aminoglycosides, which include neomycin, streptomycin, gentamycin and kanamycin, and most of the cephalosporins.[56] Strains isolated from pig faeces are resistant to tetracycline, erythromycin, lincomycin and clindamycin, a situation possibly associated with the extensive use of these antibiotics in animal feeds. *Clostridium perfringens* isolated from the intestinal contents of calves is susceptible to chloramphenicol, chlortetracycline, erythromycin, penicillin G, ampicillin, nitrofurantoin, furazolidone and trimethoprim, and resistant to neomycin, streptomycin, kanamycin, gentamycin and polymyxin.[4] In strains isolated from poultry, ampicillin, penicillin G, rifampicin, salinomycin and tylosin appear to be the most effective antibiotics.[37] Antimicrobial agents, such as the aminoglycosides, bacitracin, monensin, nalidixic acid and the tetracyclines, are much less effective.

References

1 **AKAMA, K. & OTANI, S., 1970.** *Clostridium perfringens* as the flora in the intestine of healthy persons. *Japanese Journal of Medical Science and Biology*, 23, 161–175.

2 **ALLISON, M.J., ROBINSON, I.M., DOUGHERTY, R.W. & BUCKLIN, J.A., 1975.** Grain overload in cattle and sheep: Changes in microbial populations in the cecum and rumen. *American Journal of Veterinary Research*, 36, 181–185.

3 **ALOUF, J.E. & JOLIVET-REYNAUD, C., 1981.** Purification and characterization of *Clostridium perfringens* delta toxin. *Infection and Immunity*, 31, 536–546.

4 **AMTSBERG, G., BISPING, W., KRABISCH, P. & MATTHIESEN, I., 1977.** Zum vorkommen und zur pathogenen Bedeutung von *Clostridium perfringens* beim Kalb. I. Mitteilung: Quantitative bakteriologische Untersuchungen zum *Clostridium perfringens*-Keimgehalt im Kot und Darminhalt von gesunden und erkrankten Kälbern. *Zentralblatt für Veterinärmedizin Reihe B*, 24, 104–113.

5 **BHOWN, A.S. & HABEEB, A.F., 1977.** Structural studies on epsilon prototoxin of *Clostridium perfringens* type D localization of the site of tryptic scission necessary for activation to epsilon toxin. *Biochemical and Biophysical Research Communications*, 78, 889–896.

6 **BISPING, W. & AMTSBERG, G., 1988.** *Colour Atlas for the Diagnosis of Bacterial Pathogens in Animals*. Berlin & Hamburg: Paul Parey Scientific Publishers.

7 **BULLEN, J.J. & BATTY, I., 1957.** Experimental enterotoxaemia of sheep: The effect on the permeability of the intestine and the stimulation of antitoxin production in immune animals. *Journal of Pathology and Bacteriology*, 73, 511–518.

8 **BUXTON, D., 1978.** Further studies on the mode of action of *Clostridium welchii* type D epsilon toxin. *Journal of Medical Microbiology*, 11, 293–298.

9 **BUXTON, D., 1978.** *In vitro* effects of *Clostridium welchii* type D epsilon toxin on guinea-pig, mouse, rabbit and sheep cells. *Journal of Medical Microbiology*, 11, 299–302.

10 **DUNCAN, C.L. & STRONG, D.H., 1969.** Ileal loop fluid accumulation and production of diarrhoea in rabbits by cell-free products of *Clostridium perfringens*. *Journal of Bacteriology*, 100, 86–94.

11 **DUNCAN, C.L. & STRONG, D.H., 1969.** Experimental production of diarrhoea in rabbits with *Clostridium perfringens*. *Canadian Journal of Microbiology*, 15, 765–770.

12 **ELLNER, P.D., 1961.** Fate of partially purified C^{14} labelled toxin of *Clostridium perfringens*. *Journal of Bacteriology*, 82, 275–283.

13 **GARDNER, D.E., 1973.** Pathology of *Clostridium welchii* type

D enterotoxaemia. I. Biochemical and haematological alterations in lambs. *Journal of Comparative Pathology*, 83, 499–507.

14 **GARDNER, D.E., 1973.** Pathology of *Clostridium welchii* type D enterotoxaemia. II. Structural and ultrastructural alterations in the tissues of lambs and mice. *Journal of Comparative Pathology*, 83, 509–524.

15 **GARDNER, D.E., 1973.** Pathology of *Clostridium welchii* type D enterotoxaemia. III. Basis of the hyperglycaemic response. *Journal of Comparative Pathology*, 83, 525–529.

16 **GILL, M., 1987.** Bacterial toxins: Description. *In:* LASKIN, A.I. & LECHEVALIER, H.A., (eds). *CRC Handbook of Microbiology*. Vol. VIII. 2nd edn. Toxin and Enzymes. Florida: CRC Press, Inc.

17 **GLENNY, A.T., BARR, M., LLEWELLYN-JONES, M., DALLING, T. & ROSS, H.E., 1933.** Multiple toxins produced by some organisms of the *Clostridium welchii* group. *Journal of Pathology*, 37, 53–74.

18 **GOLDNER, S.B., SOLBERG, M., JONES, S. & POST, L.S., 1986.** Enterotoxin synthesis by nonsporulating cultures of *Clostridium perfringens*. *Applied and Environmental Microbiology*, 52, 407–412.

19 **GORDON, W.S., STEWART, J., HOLMAN, H.H. & WILSON-TAYLOR, A., 1940.** Blood changes and post-mortem findings following intravenous inoculation of sheep with culture filtrates of *C. welchii* types A, C and D. *Journal of Pathology and Bacteriology*, L, 251–269.

20 **GRINER, L.A., 1961.** Enterotoxaemia of sheep. I. Effects of *Clostridium perfringens* type D on the brains of sheep and mice. *American Journal of Veterinary Research*, 22, 429–442.

21 **GRINER, L.A. & CARLSON, W.D., 1961.** Enterotoxaemia of sheep. II. Distribution of I^{131} radioiodinated serum albumin in brains of *Clostridium perfringens* type D-intoxicated lambs. *American Journal of Veterinary Research*, 22, 443–446.

22 **HABEEB, A.F., 1964.** Studies on the E prototoxin of *Clostridium perfringens* type D. *Canadian Journal of Biochemistry*, 42, 545–554.

23 **HABEEB, A.F., 1969.** Studies on E prototoxin of *Clostridium perfringens* type D. I. Purification methods: Evidence for multiple forms of E prototoxin. *Archives in Biochemistry and Biophysics*, 130, 430–440.

24 **HANDFORD, P.M., 1974.** A new medium for the detection and enumeration of *Clostridium perfringens* in foods. *Journal of Applied Bacteriology*, 37, 559–570.

25 **HANDFORD, P.M. & CAVETT, J.J., 1973.** A medium for the detection and enumeration of *Clostridium perfringens (welchii)* in foods. *Journal of the Science of Food and Agriculture*, 24, 487.

26 **HARMON, S.M., 1984.** *Clostridium perfringens:* Enumeration and identification. *In: Bacteriological Analytical Manual of the Division of Microbiology, Centre for Food Safety and Applied Nutrition, US Food and Drug Administration.* 6th edn. Virginia: Association of Official Analytical Chemists.

27 **HARMON, S.M., KAUTTER, D.A. & PEELER, J.T., 1971.** Improved medium for the enumeration of *Clostridium perfringens*. *Applied Microbiology*, 22, 688–692.

28 **HAUSCHILD, A.H.W., 1971.** *Clostridium perfringens* toxins types B, C, D and E. *In:* KADIS, S., MONTIE, T.C. & AJL, S.J., (eds). *Microbial Toxins*. Vol. IIA. New York, London: Academic Press, Inc.

29 **HAUSCHILD, A.H.W., NIILO, L. & DORWARD, W.J., 1970.** Response of ligated intestinal loops in lambs to an enteropathogenic factor of *Clostridium perfringens*, type A. *Canadian Journal of Microbiology*, 16, 339–343.

30 **HAUSCHILD, A.H.W., NIILO, L. & DORWARD, W.J., 1970.** Enteropathogenic factors of food poisoning: *Clostridium perfringens* type A. *Canadian Journal of Microbiology*, 16, 331–338.

31 **HAUSCHILD, A.H.W., NIILO, L. & DORWARD, W.J., 1971.** The role of enterotoxin in *Clostridium perfringens* type A enteritis. *Canadian Journal of Microbiology*, 17, 987–991.

32 **IKEZAWA, H. & MURATA, R., 1964.** Comparative kinetics of hemolysis of mammalian erythrocytes by *Clostridium perfringens* alpha toxin (phospholipase C). *Journal of Biochemistry*, 55, 217–224.

33 **ISPOLATOVSKAYA, M.V., 1971.** Type A *Clostridium perfringens* toxin. *In:* KADIS, S., MONTIE, T.C. & AJL, S.J., (eds). *Microbial Toxins*. Vol. IIA. New York, London: Academic Press, Inc.

34 **JAYKO L.G. & LICHSTEIN, H.C., 1959.** Nutritional factors concerned with growth and lecithinase production by *C. perfringens*. *Journal of Infectious Diseases*, 104, 142–151.

35 **JOLIVET-REYNAUD, C., POPOFF, M.R., VINIT, M.A., RAVISSE, P., MOREAU, H. & ALOUF, J.E., 1985.** Enteropathogenicity of *Clostridium perfringens* beta toxin and other clostridial toxins. *Zentralblatt für Bakteriologie, Mikrobiologie und Hygiene*, suppl. 15, 145–151.

36 **KAMEYAMA, S. & AKAMA, K., 1971.** Purification and some properties of kappa toxin of *Clostridium perfringens*. *Japanese Journal of Medical Science and Biology*, 24, 9–23.

37 **KONDO, F., 1988.** *In vitro* lecithinase activity and sensitivity to 22 antimicrobial agents of *Clostridium perfringens* isolated from necrotic enteritis of broiler chickens. *Research in Veterinary Science*, 45, 337–340.

38 **KURIOKA, S. & MATSUDA, M., 1976.** Phospholipase C assay using p-nitrophenylphosphorylcholine together with sorbitol and its application to studying the metal and detergent requirement of the enzyme. *Analytical Biochemistry*, 75, 281–289.

39 **MACFARLANE, M.G. & KNIGHT, B.C.J.G., 1941.** The biochemistry of bacterial toxins. The lecithinase activity of *Clostridium welchii*. *Biochemical Journal*, 35, 884–901.

40 **MANSSON, I., NORBERG, R., OLHAGEN, B. & BJORKLUND, N.E., 1971.** Arthritis in pigs induced by dietary factors. Microbiologic, clinical and histologic studies. *Clinical and Experimental Immunology*, 9, 677–693.

41 **MARSHALL, R.S., STEENBERGEN, J.F. & McCLUNG, L.S., 1965.** Rapid technique for the enumeration of *Clostridium perfringens*. *Applied Microbiology*, 13, 559–563.

42 **McDONEL, J.L., 1986.** *Clostridium perfringens* toxins (type A, B, C, D, E). *Pharmacology and Therapy*, 10, 617–655.

43 **MITSUI, K., MISUI, N. & HASE, J., 1973.** *Clostridium perfringens* exotoxins. I. Purification and properties of alpha toxin. *Japanese Journal of Experimental Medicine*, 43, 65–80.

44 **MÖLLBY, R., HOLME, T., NORD, C.E., SMYTH, C.J. & WADSTRÖM, T., 1976.** Production of phospholipase C (alpha toxin), haemolysins and lethal toxins by *C. perfringens* types A to D. *Journal of General Microbiology*, 96, 137–144.

45 **MUHAMMED, S.E., MORRISON, S.M. & BOYD, W.L., 1975.** Nutritional requirements for growth and sporulation of *Clostridium perfringens*. *Journal of Applied Bacteriology*, 38, 245–253.

46 **MURATA, R. & YAMAMOTO, A., 1964.** A synthetic medium for production of alpha toxin by *C. perfringens*. *Japanese Journal of Medical Science and Biology*, 17, 211–213.

47 **MURATA, R. & YAMAMOTO, A., SODA, S. & ITO, A., 1965.** Nutritional requirements of *C. perfringens* PB6K for alpha toxin production. *Japanese Journal of Medical Science and Biology*, 18, 189–202.

48 **MYRVIK, Q.N. & WEISER, R.S., 1988.** *Fundamentals of Medical Bacteriology and Mycology*. Philadelphia: Lea & Febiger.

49 **NAGLER, F.P.O., 1940.** Observations on a reaction between lethal toxins of *Cl. welchii* (Type A) and human serum. *British Journal of Experimental Pathology*, 20, 473–485.

50 **NAKAMURA, M., COOK, J.A. & CROSS, W.R., 1968.** Lecithinase production by *Clostridium perfringens* in chemically defined media. *Applied Microbiology*, 16, 1420–1421.

51 **NEUT, C., PATHAK, J., ROMOND, C. & BEERENS, H., 1985.** Rapid detection of *Clostridium perfringens:* Comparison of lactose sulfite broth with tryptose-sulfite-cycloserine agar. *Journal of the Association of Official Analytical Chemists*, 68, 881–883.

52 **NIILO, L., 1971.** Mechanism of action of the enteropathogenic factor of *Clostridium perfringens* type A. *Infection and Immunity*, 3, 100–106.

53 **NORD, C.E., MÖLLBY, R., SMYTH, C. & WADSTRÖM, T., 1974.** Formation of phospholipase C and theta-haemolysin in pre-reduced media in batch and continuous culture of *Clostridium perfringens* type A. *Journal of General Microbiology*, 84, 117–127.

54 **OAKLEY, C.L. & WARRACK, G.H., 1953.** Routine typing of *Clostridium welchii*. *Journal of Hygiene*, 51, 102–107.

55 **PHILIPSON, K.D., FRANK, J.S. & NISHIMOTO, A.Y., 1983.** Effects of phospholipase C on the Na^{+}– Ca^{2+} exchange and Ca^{2+} permeability of cardiac sarcolemmal vesicles. *Journal of Biological Chemistry*, 258, 5905–5910.

56 **PHILLIPS, K.D., BRAZIER, J.S., LEVETT, P.N. & WILLIS, A.T., 1985.** Clostridia. *In:* COLLINS, C.H. & GRANGE, J.M., (eds). *Isolation and Identification of Micro-organisms of Medical and Veterinary Importance.* London: Academic Press, Inc.

57 **RIGBY, G.J., 1981.** An egg-yolk agar diffusion assay for monitoring phospholipase C in cultures of *Clostridium welchii*. *Journal of Applied Bacteriology*, 50, 11–19.

58 **SACKS, L.E. & THOMPSON, P.A., 1978.** Clear defined medium for the sporulation of *C. perfringens*. *Applied and Environmental Microbiology*, 35, 405–410.

59 **SAKURAI, J. & DUNCAN, D.L., 1977.** Purification of beta toxin from *Clostridium perfringens* type C. *Infection and Immunity*, 18, 741–745.

60 **SAKURAI, J., FUJII, Y., TORII, K. & KOBAYASHI, K., 1989.** Dissociation of various biological activities of *Clostridium perfringens* alpha toxin by chemical modification. *Toxicon*, 27, 317–323.

61 **SAKURAI, J. & NAGAHAMA, M., 1985.** Tryptophan content of *Clostridium perfringens* epsilon toxin. *Infection and Immunity*, 47, 260–263.

62 **SAKURAI, J. & NAGAHAMA, M., 1985.** Role of one tryptophan residue in the lethal activity of *Clostridium perfringens* epsilon toxin. *Biochemical and Biophysical Research Communications*, 28, 760–766.

63 **SAKURAI, J. & NAGAHAMA, M., 1986.** Amino groups in *Clostridium perfringens* epsilon prototoxin and toxin. *Microbial Pathogenesis*, 1, 417–423.

64 **SAKURAI, J. & NAGAHAMA, M., 1987.** Histidine residues in *Clostridium perfringens* epsilon toxin. *FEMS Microbiology Letters*, 41, 317–319.

65 **SAKURAI, J. & NAGAHAMA, M., 1987.** The inactivation of *Clostridium perfringens* epsilon toxin by treatment with tetranitromethane and N-acetylimidazole. *Toxicon*, 25, 279–284.

66 **SAKURAI, J. & NAGAHAMA, M., 1987.** Carboxyl groups in *Clostridium perfringens* epsilon toxin. *Microbial Pathogenesis*, 3, 469–474.

67 **SAKURAI, J., NAGAHAMA, M. & FUJII, Y., 1983.** Effect of *Clostridium perfringens* epsilon toxin on the cardiovascular system of rats. *Infection and Immunity*, 42, 1183–1186.

68 **SAKURAI, J., NAGAHAMA, M. & TAKAHASHI, T., 1989.** Contraction induced by *Clostridium perfringens* epsilon toxin in the isolated rat ileum. *FEMS Microbiology Letters*, 58, 269–272.

69 **SATO, H., YAMAKAWA, Y., ITO, A. & MURATA, R., 1978.** Effect of zinc and calcium ions on the production of alpha toxin and proteases by *Clostridium perfringens*. *Infection and Immunity*, 20, 325–333.

70 **SHAHIDI, S.A. & FERGUSON, A.R., 1971.** New quantitative, qualitative and confirmatory media for rapid analysis of food for *Clostridium perfringens*. *Applied Microbiology*, 21, 500–506.

71 **SMART, J.L., ROBERTS, T.A., STRINGER, M.F. & SHAH, N., 1979.** The incidence and serotypes of *Clostridium perfringens* on beef, pork and lamb carcasses. *Journal of Applied Bacteriology*, 46, 377–383.

72 **SMITH, L.D.S, 1975.** *The Pathogenic Anaerobic Bacteria.* 2nd edn. Springfield, Illinois: Charles C. Thomas.

73 **SMITH, L.D.S., 1979.** Virulence factors of *Clostridium perfringens*. *Reviews of Infectious Diseases*, 1, 254–262.

74 **SMITH, L.D.S. & GARDNER, V.M., 1949.** Vegetative cells of *Clostridium perfringens* in soil. *Journal of Bacteriology*, 58, 407–408.

75 **SMITH, L.D.S. & WILLIAMS, B.L., 1984.** *The Pathogenic Anaerobic Bacteria.* 3rd edn. Springfield, Illinois: Charles C. Thomas.

76 **SMYTH, C.J., 1975.** The identification and purification of multiple forms of theta-haemolysin (theta toxin) of *Clostridium perfringens* type A. *Journal of General Microbiology*, 87, 219–238.

77 **SMYTH, C.J. & ARBUTHNOTT, J.P., 1974.** Properties of *Clostridium perfringens (welchii) type* A alpha toxin (phospholipase C) purified by electrofocusing. *Journal of Medical Microbiology*, 7, 41–66.

78 **SMYTH, C.J. & DUNCAN, C.L., 1978.** *In:* JELJASZEWICZ, J. & WADSTRÖM, T., (eds). *Bacterial Toxins and Cell Membranes.* New York: Academic Press, Inc.

79 **SNEATH, P.H.A., MAIR, N.S., SHARPE, M.E. & HOLT, J.G., 1986.** *Bergey's Manual of Systematic Bacteriology.* Vol. 2. Baltimore, London: Williams & Wilkins.

80 **STARK, R.L. & DUNCAN, C.L., 1971.** Biological characteristics of *Clostridium perfringens* type A enterotoxin. *Infection and Immunity*, 4, 89–96.

81 **STEPHEN, J. & PIETROWSKI, R.A., 1986.** *Bacterial Toxins.* 2nd edn. England: Van Nostrand Reinhold.

82 **STERNE, M. & BATTY, I., 1975.** *Pathogenic Clostridia.* London, Boston: Butterworths.

83 **STERNE, M. & WARRACK, H.G., 1964.** The types of *C. perfringens*. *Journal of Pathology and Bacteriology*, 88, 279–283.

84 **STEVENS, D.L., MITTEN, J. & HENRY, C., 1987.** Effects of alpha and theta toxins from *Clostridium perfringens* on human polymorphonuclear leukocytes. *Journal of Infectious Diseases*, 156, 324–333.

85 **STEVENS, D.L., TROYER, B.E., MERRICK, D.T., MITTEN, J. & OLSON, R.D., 1988.** Lethal effects and cardiovascular effects of purified alpha and theta toxins from *Clostridium perfringens*. *Journal of Infectious Diseases*, 157, 272–279.

86 **SUNAGAWA, H., TSUZUKI, T., TAKESHI, K., ANDO, Y. & OKA, S., 1987.** Enterotoxigenicity of heat-resistant and heat-sensitive strains of *Clostridium perfringens*. *Japanese Journal of Veterinary Science*, 49, 853–858.

87 **TIMONEY, J.F., GILLESPIE, J.H., SCOTT, F.W. & BARLOUGH, J.E., 1988.** *Hagan and Bruner's Microbiology and Infectious Diseases of Domestic Animals.* Ithaca & London: Comstock Publishing Associates (a division of Cornell University Press).

88 **VANCE, H.N., 1967.** A survey of the alimentary tract of cattle for *Clostridium perfringens*. *Canadian Journal of Comparative Medicine in Veterinary Science*, 31, 260–267.

89 **VARNAM, A.H. & EVANS, M.G., 1991.** *Food-borne Pathogens. An Illustrated Text.* London: Wolfe Publishing Ltd.

90 **WILLIS, A.T., 1977.** *Anaerobic Bacteriology: Clinical and Laboratory Practice.* London, Boston: Butterworths.

91 **WILSON-TAYLOR, A. & GORDON, W.S., 1940.** A survey of the types of *C. welchii* present in soil and in the intestinal contents of animals and man. *Journal of Pathology and Bacteriology*, 50, 271–277.

92 **WORTHINGTON, R.W. & MÜLDERS, M.S.G., 1975.** The partial purification of *Clostridium perfringens* beta toxin. *Onderstepoort Journal of Veterinary Research*, 42, 91–98.

93 **WORTHINGTON, R.W. & MÜLDERS, M.S.G., 1975.** The effect of *Clostridium perfringens* epsilon toxin on the blood-brain barrier of mice. *Onderstepoort Journal of Veterinary Research*, 42, 25–28.

94 **WORTHINGTON, R.W. & MÜLDERS, M.S.G., 1979.** Physical changes in the epsilon prototoxin molecule of *Clostridium perfringens* during enzymatic activation. *Infection and Immunity*, 18, 549–551.

95 **WORTHINTON, R.W., MÜLDERS, M.S.G. & VAN RENSBURG, J.J., 1973.** Enzymatic activation of *Clostridium perfringens* epsilon prototoxin and some biological properties of activated toxin. *Onderstepoort Journal of Veterinary Research*, 40, 153–156.

154

Clostridium perfringens *type A infections*

Synonyms: Sudden death, haemorrhagic enteritis, enterotoxaemia, necrotic enteritis, equine intestinal clostridiosis, yellow lamb disease

M.W. Odendaal, N.P.J. Kriek and P. Hunter

Introduction

Although there is uncertainty about the pathogenicity of *C. perfringens* type A for animals, a number of diseases have been associated with it in domestic and wild animals, poultry and wild birds. Despite its frequent isolation from diseased animals and necropsy specimens, it is usually disregarded as the aetiological agent because of its apparently innocuous ubiquity. Currently, *C. perfringens* type A is considered to be one of the causes of gas gangrene or malignant oedema arising from trauma associated with penetrating wounds in cattle,[73, 75] horses[26, 39, 57] and humans.[34, 68] It is also a rare cause of gangrenous mastitis in cattle[19, 31, 62] and acute mastitis in sheep.[37] The enterotoxaemia caused by *C. perfringens* is characterized in several domestic and wild animal species by a number of distinct syndromes that are usually associated with, and therefore referred to as, 'sudden death'.[4, 49]

Clostridium perfringens type A has been associated with lambs that succumb to an enterotoxaemic condition known as yellow lamb disease in California and Oregon,[38] and with enterotoxaemic jaundice in cattle and sheep in Australia in the 1930s.[60] In addition, enterotoxaemia in sheep and lambs considered to have been caused by *C. perfringens* type D has, on occasion, revealed only *C. perfringens* type A.[55]

In South Africa, a form of haemorrhagic enteritis occurs sporadically in sheep in the winter rainfall area of the south-western Cape Province. This is a peracute to acute, fatal disease associated with the isolation of *C. perfringens* type A in pure culture from the intestines of affected sheep.[79] In the United Kingdom a similar disease of unknown cause in lambs has been described as an intestinal haemorrhagic syndrome.[54, 64]

In cattle, *C. perfringens* type A is associated with, or is considered to cause, several disease syndromes. It has been isolated from calves suffering from an acute abdominal syndrome caused by abomasitis and abomasal ulceration.[59] Enterotoxaemia caused by *C. perfringens* type A has been described in calves,[5, 41, 47] wild deer[2] and water buffaloes (*Bubalus bubalis*).[77] It has also been associated with fatal gastroenteritis or sudden death of cattle in Canada[61] and the United Kingdom,[65, 72] and with other enteric lesions in cattle.[3]

Clostridium perfringens type A in horses is associated with intestinal clostridiosis.[76] Serological evidence also suggests that the enterotoxin of *C. perfringens* type A may be involved in equine grass sickness, either as an aetiological agent or as a complicating factor,[50] but this has not been confirmed.[20]

Clostridium perfringens type A has been reported as a cause of enterotoxaemia and death in pigs,[51, 52] and of diarrhoea and emaciation in piglets one to three weeks old.[4, 42] It has, however, been suggested that no special importance should be attached to the presence of *C. perfringens* type A in pigs suffering from enteritis.[4]

Clostridium perfringens type A is recognized as the cause of necrotic enteritis in conventionally reared broiler chickens,[33] as well as in germ-free chickens,[18] while fatal cases of enterotoxaemia in birds of prey have been directly attributed to the feeding of meat contaminated with *C. perfringens* type A.[32]

Certain strains of *C. perfringens* type A produce an enterotoxin **(see *Clostridium perfringens* group: Introduction)** which causes enteritis in humans and, experimentally, in lambs, calves, monkeys and rabbits.[14, 15, 24, 25, 36, 44, 45, 48] This enterotoxin is not regarded as playing an integral role in the pathogenesis of the classical enterotoxaemia syndrome in animals, although it has been detected in pigs, sheep, goats and cattle.[71] The enterotoxin exerts a local effect on the intestines, inducing a mild and non-fatal disease.

In South Africa, *C. perfringens* type A is considered to be a minor cause of deaths in sheep, although it can become a problem on individual farms.[8]

Aetiology

The cultural, morphological and biochemical characteristics of *C. perfringens* type A are dealt with in ***Clostridium perfringens* group: Introduction**. Although all five toxin types of *C. perfringens* are produced, the alpha toxin (a phospholipase C) is the main lethal toxin produced by type A. The term lecithinase, used in the older literature, is a synonym for phospholipase C.

Epidemiology

The epidemiology of the various syndromes associated, or thought to be associated, with *C. perfringens* type A infection is poorly defined, primarily because of uncertainty about the aetiological role of the organism. There is no doubt, however, about its ubiquitous occurrence in the environment. *Clostridium perfringens* type A is regarded as being a facultative pathogen, in contrast to *C. perfringens* types B, C, D and E, which are regarded as obligate parasites and, while widespread, are not as ubiquitous as type A. *Clostridium perfringens* type A is considered to be the most common of the five types of *C. perfringens* and occurs as a vegetative organism in the intestinal tract of almost all warm-blooded animal species and humans, and in soil.[28, 66–70]

As far as gas gangrene is concerned, it would appear that the microbial composition of the soil in the area in which the infection has occurred plays an important role in its development and severity. Poor and arid soils contain fewer organisms than fertile and cultivated soil. Direct and indirect faecal contamination of the skin play an additional important role in wound infections, but the advent of antibiotics and vaccines has minimized the importance of these infections and the development of gas gangrene in humans and animals.[69, 70] Humans suffering from malignant neoplasia are prone to the development of *C. perfringens*-associated infections, such as fatal sepsis and massive haemolysis,[9] and necrotizing pneumonia and empyema.[7, 53]

In South Africa, young sheep which graze on lush pastures, or which are fed quality carbohydrate and protein rich diets, are particularly susceptible to haemorrhagic enteritis, but it can occur sporadically under conditions of stress such as deworming, weaning and transport.[8]

In calves, type A enterotoxaemia occurs in pail-fed animals in intensive systems under good management.[41] Several instances have been reported in which water buffalo, stag and elk subjected to transport stress and a sudden change in diet suffered rumen and intestinal stasis and death from *C. perfringens* type A enterotoxaemia.[2, 77]

Animal feeds may be a source of *C. perfringens* type A and may contribute to its distribution. Feeds play a role in the occurrence of disease produced by *C. perfringens* type A in a variety of animal species, from livestock to laboratory animals.[21, 56]

Pathogenesis

Clostridium perfringens type A, either alone or in combination with other clostridia, is one of a group of anaerobes involved in clostridial wound infection. The spores of these organisms, which are present in soil and faeces, are carried into the wound at the time of injury, where, under conditions which are not well understood, they germinate, proliferate, synthesize toxin and invade surrounding tissues.[46, 63, 68, 69]

The bacteriology of wound contamination and gas gangrene is extremely complex.[34] Only rarely does the infection of wounds by clostridia alone result in gas gangrene. In the majority of clostridial wound infections, the organisms grow slowly and die within 10 days of the commencement of the infection. The conditions in clean and fresh wounds are barely suitable for clostridial infection to establish itself, but the presence of a watery, seropurulent exudate provides the initial nutriments for some proteolytic organisms (including the clostridia) to proliferate. Even then, only a slow growth of *C. perfringens* without toxin production may occur.[70]

Three types of wound infection involving clostridia occur: simple wound contamination, anaerobic cellulitis (also regarded as a form of malignant oedema), and gas gangrene or clostridial myonecrosis.[68] Simple wound contamination is the most frequently encountered but the least serious of the three types of infection. Invasion of the surrounding tissues rarely occurs and it normally terminates in uneventful recovery. Anaerobic cellulitis (malignant oedema) is limited to necrotic tissue initially caused by ischaemia or trauma, which supports active growth of *C. perfringens* accompanied by toxin production. It is initially limited to ischaemic and necrotic tissue, but then becomes self-perpetuating as a result of the synthesis of its own toxins which enhance the formation of the necrotic tissue required for multiplication of the organism. The alpha toxin causes destruction of erythrocytes, necrosis of tissue cells and increased permeability of the capillary endothelial cells. The production of some minor lethal toxins, which are proteolytic enzymes, contributes significantly to the infection by *C. perfringens* type A and its spread along fascial planes and loose connective tissues.[23, 30, 46] As the infection spreads, inflammatory oedema (mostly a serosanguineous exudate) and gas are produced.

Gas gangrene (clostridial or anaerobic myonecrosis) is an invasive, anaerobic infection of traumatized or ischaemic muscle and is characterized by destruction of tissue, extensive local oedema, the production of gas, and profound toxaemia. It is the consequence of the effect of alpha toxin, which has a direct toxic effect on muscle.[1] Impairment of the blood supply to the traumatized areas facilitates the growth and toxin production of the organism. These conditions enhance reduction of the oxidation-reduction potential in the muscle, which is conducive to the growth of anaerobic pathogenic organisms. The anaerobic conditions and reduction in pH increase activation of lysosomal enzymes and the breakdown of muscle protein. The toxins produced by the bacteria cause death of the living tissue in their immediate surroundings, which allows the organisms to spread slowly through the muscle.[68] The massive local destruction of tissue and production of toxins result in toxaemia and shock.[13]

In clostridial mastitis, the organism gains access to the udder, probably through the teat canal or wounds on the teats, during the pre- and post-partum periods. Growth of the organism is accompanied by an acute gangrenous mastitis and the presence of gas in the affected glandular tissue, milk, and subcutaneous tissues of the udder.

The role of *C. perfringens* type A in the pathogenesis of enterotoxaemia is based on the isolation of the organism and the demonstration of its toxin in the contents of the affected areas of the small intestine. This has been well documented in sheep, cattle, water buffaloes, wild raptors, horses, pigs, dogs, reindeer and goats. Small numbers of *C. perfringens* type A are normally present in the intestinal tract of most animals, but their number varies with the diet of the animal — an abundance of fodder rich in carbohydrate and proteins and low in fibre and cellulose leads to a greater number. Overeating on such diets results in overloading of the rumen and excessive amounts of carbohydrates and proteins reaching the small intestine. This in turn establishes the appropriate conditions for the growth of *C. perfringens* and the production of its toxin. Under these circumstances *C. perfringens* is an exceptionally active and fast-growing organism. It has a generation time of eight to ten minutes, which is one of the fastest known for bacteria and which probably allows it to outgrow most other organisms in the intestinal tract. It has also been established *in vitro* that it produces toxins and other metabolically active substances during exponential growth, the quantities produced depending greatly on the available nutrients and carbohydrate sources.

The administration of tetracyclines to horses has been reported to be responsible for an increase in the intestinal and faecal counts of *C. perfringens*. The alpha toxin appears to be responsible for the locally occurring extensive hyperaemia, haemorrhage, and oedema, and the poor coagulability of blood which is characteristic of the disease in horses.[76] The degenerative changes in the liver and kidneys, which also occur, are caused by mitochondrial damage inflicted by the alpha toxin.[10–12, 16] In addition, the nu toxin (deoxyribonuclease) appears to be responsible for leukopenia or leukocytosis, the theta toxin (thiol-activated haemolysin) for the myocardial changes, and the kappa toxin (collagenase), with its lethal and necrotizing properties, and the mu toxin (hyaluronidase) for the spread of infection in tissues.[76]

For more information on the properties of the *perfringens* group and the effects of their toxins, ***Clostridium perfringens* group : Introduction** should be consulted.

Clinical signs and pathology

The length of the incubation period of gas gangrene depends on the number of *C. perfringens* in the wound, the presence and amount of necrotic tissue, and the location of the wound — it may be as short as four to six hours or as long as 72 hours. Inflammatory changes such as swelling, pain, erythema and a local temperature increase develop around the wound or infected area. The intensity of the swelling and tenderness of the lesion increase progressively. Anaerobic cellulitis remains localized, whereas in gas gangrene, muscular tissue is extensively involved. The inflammatory oedema may remain localized, gravitate to lower areas, or spread to adjacent areas along fascial planes. The affected tissue may crepitate due to the presence of gas. Systemic involvement due to toxaemia causes animals to become inappetent, have an increased rectal temperature of up to 41–43 °C, walk with a stiff gait, have decreased mental alertness and eventually become prostrate. If a limb is affected, the animal will be lame and, with progression of the lesion, will eventually refuse to move. A serosanguineous, gaseous and malodorous fluid may exude from the wound. Focal areas of skin may become necrotic and slough.[23, 26, 29, 30, 57] Clostridial myonecrosis is complicated by shock and often terminates in death.

Ewes suffering from *C. perfringens* type A mastitis are depressed, pyrexic, and have an increased heart rate. The affected mammary gland is hot, swollen, emphysematous and painful, and a brown, flocculent secretion may be expressed from the teat. Other signs include haemoglobinuria, anaemia and icterus.[37]

Dairy cattle which develop a gangrenous mastitis present with a rapidly developing acute mastitis in one or more quarters. They are depressed, anorexic, pyrexic and have congested mucous membranes. The affected quarter or quarters are hot, swollen, hyperaemic, and oedematous, and the subcutaneous tissue over the affected parts may be emphysematous. The supramammary lymph nodes are palpable and the milk from affected quarters has a brownish to reddish colour, contains bubbles of gas and has a foul odour. Necrosis of the skin may subsequently develop on the ventral aspect of the udder at the base of the teats, and this will result in sloughing. Animals may die within 48 hours from the initial appearance of clinical signs.[19, 43, 58, 62]

The acute abdominal syndrome in neonatal calves (two to 21 days old) is characterized by ruminal and abomasal tympany, depression and colic, and in some instances by sudden death.[59] Some develop diarrhoea. In calves that have suffered from the acute abdominal syndrome with tympany, various degrees of abomasitis, which may be erosive or ulcerative in nature, are present; lesions being found particularly in the fundus. Ulcers, when present, are circular or linear, accompanied by submucosal oedema and haemorrhages, and may perforate.[59] Milk cows that have died from the 'sudden death' syndrome show marked abomasitis and severe haemorrhagic enteritis.[65]

Clinical signs in calves aged two weeks to four months that are affected by *C. perfringens* type A enterotoxaemia are generally evident only six to 24 hours before death,[60] but in some cases only five to 20 minutes before death. Affected animals are haemoglobinuric, inappetent and depressed, and have increased pulse and respiration rates. They soon become prostrate and die. The mortality rate is high. The morbidity rate on a farm may also be high.[61] Lesions in the enterotoxaemic disease of calves are said to resemble those of pulpy kidney disease in lambs, and include congested, nephrotic kidneys, splenomegaly, cloudy swelling of the liver, mild congestion and oedema of the lungs, epicardial haemorrhages, abomasitis, and severe congestion of the duodenal and jejunal mucosa.[61]

Adult sheep[60] and young nursing lambs[38] suffer from peracute to chronic *C. perfringens* type A enterotoxaemia. In the peracute and acute forms, animals are sick for only a few hours, become separated from the flock, show signs of depression and lassitude, increased pulse and respiratory rates and body temperature, and haemoglobinuria. The animals become icteric, recumbent and usually die.

The carcasses of both sheep and calves that die from enterotoxaemic jaundice undergo a very rapid onset and progression of putrefaction. In fresh carcasses, icterus and other evidence of intravascular haemolysis are outspoken, the liver is degenerated, and haemoglobinuria is consistently present.[38, 60]

In the case of the haemorrhagic enteritis syndrome, animals may be found dead without any evidence of illness having been noticed, but in those that are seen alive, signs of colic may be evident. Rapid decomposition occurs in the carcasses of sheep dying from haemorrhagic enteritis. Blood-stained fluid may ooze from the nostrils and anus. The characteristic lesions are segments of intense congestion and haemorrhage of the small intestine and a haemorrhagic intestinal content. A scant, blood-stained hydrothorax and ascites are present.

Equine intestinal clostridiosis has an acute onset and is associated with apathy, inappetence, a foul-smelling diarrhoea, discoloured mucous membranes, and an elevated pulse rate and body temperature. The severity of the diarrhoea is variable; the consistency of the faeces, which are often dark-coloured and malodorous, varies from watery to almost normal. Signs of mild colic are generally present. The conjunctival mucosae may be hyperaemic. Severely affected horses move with great difficulty and reluctance, and are eventually unable to stand. The body temperature in most animals is raised to 39–40 °C, although in some animals it is normal. The heart rate is greatly increased in cases of severe illness, accompanied by slight elevation of the respiratory rate. Other signs that may be observed include dehydration, sweating and laminitis. Horses manifesting acute severe clinical signs may die within 24–48 hours.[76] Mortality rates of about 40 per cent have been recorded.[76]

The predominant lesion in equine intestinal clostridiosis is a severe, acute typhlocolitis in which the exudate varies from catarrhal to haemorrhagic or necrotic. Degenerative changes occur in the heart, liver and kidneys.[76]

Diagnosis and differential diagnosis

The disease syndromes caused by *C. perfringens* type A are not specific and the diagnosis should be confirmed by isolation of the organism and detection of the toxin **(see *Clostridium perfringens* group: Introduction)**. *Clostridium perfringens* type A is always present in the intestines of animals and humans and invades the skeletal musculature and parenchymatous organs shortly after death. Thus, to be significant as a cause of death, *C. perfringens* type A must be present in large numbers and isolated in virtually pure culture from specimens of animals suspected as having died of the infection. Depending on the syndrome, appropriate specimens should be collected to confirm the diagnoses **(see *Clostridium perfringens* group: Introduction)**.

The morphology of the organisms observed in the smears, the outcome of the toxin-typing tests of the intestinal contents, and the isolation and toxin typing of the strains isolated from the specimens should be correlated with the clinical signs and lesions at necropsy before a final diagnosis is made. The presence of alpha toxin in the intestinal contents, and the absence of beta and epsilon toxins, may contribute to the decision to make a final diagnosis of *C. perfringens* type A enterotoxaemia.

Any disease which has a rapid course, or that causes sudden death in any of the susceptible species, should be considered as a possible differential diagnosis. Depending on the specific syndrome, copper and plant poisonings should be considered, along with other diseases in sheep and calves in which icterus occurs,[40] milk fever in cows[65] and vitamin E/selenium deficiency in calves[61] and sheep. Enterotoxaemia caused by one of the other *C. perfringens* toxin types should also be borne in mind. Haemorrhagic enteritis of sheep should not be confused with red gut of sheep (torsion of the intestinal tract[22]). The differential diagnosis of gas gangrene is discussed in **Chapter 158: *Clostridium chauvoei* infections,** and the various causes of mastitis in **Chapter 190: Mastitis**.

Control

The passive immunization of susceptible animals against the various syndromes caused by *C. perfringens* type A following the administration of hyperimmune serum affords immediate protection which persists for up to three weeks, and this should be considered during an outbreak.[13, 60] Specific hyperimmune serum is not currently commercially available in South Africa.

Since the late 1930s formalin toxoids have been used for immunoprophylaxis against gas gangrene and other diseases produced by *C. perfringens* and its toxins.[6, 27, 35, 78] A combined bacterin/toxoid of *C. perfringens* type A is available for use in cattle in India[74] and in South Africa.[17]

In South Africa, the Onderstepoort lamb dysentery vaccine provides partial protection against *C. perfringens* type A in sheep.[8]

References

1 **AIKAT, B.K. & DIBLE, J.H., 1956.** The pathology of *Clostridium welchii* infection. I. Experimental observations *in vivo*. *Journal of Pathology and Bacteriology*, 71, 461–476.

2 **AL-KHATIB, G., KÖHLER, B. & ILCHMAN, G., 1968.** Enterotoxämie durch *Clostridium perfringens* typ A bei Hirschen und einem Elch in einem Quarantänegehege. *Monatshefte für Veterinärmedizin*, 10, 381–384.

3 **AL-MASHAT, R.R. & TAYLOR, D.J., 1983.** Bacteria in enteric lesions of cattle. *The Veterinary Record*, 112, 5–10.

4 **AMTSBERG, G., BISPING, W., EL SUKHON, S.N., MATTHIESEN, I. & KRABISCH, P., 1976.** Untersuchungen zum Vorkommen und zur pathogenen Bedeitung von *Clostridium perfringens* Typ A beim Schwein. *Berliner und Münchener Tierärztliche Wochenschrift*, 89, 409–414.

5 **AMTSBERG, G., BISPING, W., KRABISCH, P. & MATTHIESEN, I., 1977.** Zum vorkommen und zur pathogenen Bedeutung von *Clostridium perfringens* beim kalb. I. Mitteilung: Quantitative bakteriologische Untersuchungen zum *Clostridium perfringens*-Keimgehalt im Kot und Darminhalt von gesunden und erkrankten Kälbern. *Zentralblatt für Veterinärmedizin* Reihe B, 24, 104–113.

6 **ARDEHALI, M. & DOWRAN, H., 1973.** Preparation of standard clostridial antitoxins in sheep. *Archives of the Institute Razi*, 25, 17–21.

7 **BASHIR, Y. & BENSON, M.K., 1990.** Necrotizing pneumonia and empyema due to *Clostridium perfringens* complicating pulmonary embolus. *Thorax*, 45, 72–73.

8 **BATH, G., 1992.** Faculty of Veterinary Science, University of Pretoria, Private Bag X04, Onderstepoort 0110, South Africa. Personal communication.

9 **BECKER, R.C., GUILIANI, M., SAVAGE, R.A. & WEICK, J.K., 1987.** Massive hemolysis in *C. perfringens* infections. *Journal of Surgical Oncology*, 35, 13–18.

10 **BERG, M. & LEVINSON, S.A., 1957.** Hyperglycemia induced in dogs by *Clostridium perfringens* toxin. *Archives of Pathology*, 64, 633–642.

11 **BERG, M. & LEVINSON, S.A., 1959.** Hyperglycemia and histochemical changes induced in dogs by *Clostridium perfringens* toxin. *Archives of Pathology*, 68, 83–93.

12 **BERG, M., LEVINSON, S.A. & WANG, K.J., 1951.** Effect of experimental shock induced by *Clostridium perfringens* toxin on the kidneys of dogs. *Archives of Pathology*, 51, 137–153.

13 **BULLEN, J.J., 1970.** Role of toxins in host–parasite relationships. *In*: KADIS, S., MONTIE, T.C. & AJL, S.J., (eds). *Microbial Toxins*, Vol. IIA. New York, London: Academic Press, Inc.

14 **DUNCAN, C.L. & STRONG, D.H., 1969.** Ileal loop fluid accumulation and production of diarrhoea in rabbits by cell-free products of *Clostridium perfringens*. *Journal of Bacteriology*, 100, 86–94.

15 **DUNCAN, C.L. & STRONG, D.H., 1969.** Experimental production of diarrhoea in rabbits with *Clostridium perfringens*. *Canadian Journal of Microbiology*, 15, 765–770.

16 **ELLNER, P.D., 1961.** Fate of partially purified C14 labeled toxin of *Clostridium perfringens*. *Journal of Bacteriology*, 82, 275–283.

17 **ERASMUS, B.J., CAMERON, C.M., HUNTER, P., CILLIERS, J.A., OBEREM, P.T., STOLTZ, W.H. & DE WAAL, D.T., 1990.** *Onderstepoort Vaccines*. Booklet issued by the Department of Agricultural Development and obtained from the Directorate of Agricultural Information, Private Bag X144, Pretoria 0001.

18 **FUKATA, T., HADATE, Y., BABA, E., UEMURA, T. & ARAKAWA, A., 1988.** Influence of *Clostridium perfringens* and its toxin in germ-free chickens. *Research in Veterinary Science*, 44, 68–70.

19 **GIESECKE, W.H., TUSTIN, R.H., MALAN, F.S. & DE WAAL, G.H., 1969.** Bovine mastitis due to *Clostridium perfringens* type A and *Bacillus cereus*. *Journal of the South African Veterinary Association*, 40, 342.

20 **GILMOUR, J.S., BROWN, R. & JOHNSON, P., 1981.** A negative serological relationship between cases of grass sickness in Scotland and *Clostridium perfringens* type A. *Equine Veterinary Journal*, 13, 56–58.

21 **GREENHAM, L.W., HARBER, C., LEWIS, E. & SCULLION, F.T., 1987.** *Clostridium perfringens* in pelleted feed. *The Veterinary Record*, 120, 557.

22 **GUMBRILL, R.C., 1973.** Red gut syndrome in lambs grazing lucerne. *New Zealand Veterinary Journal*, 21, 178–179.

23 **GYLES, C.L., 1986.** Histotoxic clostridia. *In*: GYLES, C.L. & THOEN, C.O., (eds). *Pathogenesis of Bacterial Infections in Animals*. Ames, Iowa: Iowa State University Press.

24 **HAUSCHILD, A.H.W., NIILO, L. & DORWARD, W.J., 1971.** The role of enterotoxin in *Clostridium perfringens* type A enteritis. *Canadian Journal of Microbiology*, 17, 987–991.

25 **HAUSCHILD, A.H.W., WALCROFT, M.J. & CAMPBELL, W., 1971.** Emesis and diarrhoea induced by enterotoxin of *Clostridium perfringens*. *Canadian Journal of Microbiology*, 17, 1141–1143.

26 **HORNER, R.F., 1982.** Malignant oedema caused by *Clostridium perfringens* type A in a horse. *Journal of the South African Veterinary Association*, 53, 122–123.

27 **ITO, A., 1970.** Alpha toxoid of *Clostridium perfringens*. II. Immunogenicity of the toxoid. *Japanese Journal of Medical Science and Biology*, 23, 21–30.

28 **ITODO, A.E., ADESIYUN, A.A., ADEKEYE, J.O. & UMOH, J.U., 1986.** Toxin types of *Clostridium perfringens* strains isolated from sheep, cattle and paddock soils in Nigeria. *Veterinary Microbiology*, 12, 93–96.

29 **JENSEN, R. & MACKEY, D.R., 1971.** *Diseases of Feedlot Cattle*. 2nd edn. Philadelphia: Lea & Febiger.

30 **JENSEN, R. & SWIFT, B.L., 1982.** *Diseases of Sheep*. 2nd edn. Philadelphia: Lea & Febiger.

31 **JOHNSTON, A.M., 1986.** A successfully treated case of mastitis in bovine associated with *Clostridium perfringens* type A. *The Veterinary Record*, 118, 728–729.

32 **KÖHLER, B. & BAUMGART, W., 1970.** Toxi-Infektionen durch *Clostridium perfringens* Typ A bei Greivögeln. *Monatshefte für Veterinärmedizin*, 9, 348–352.

33 **KONDO, F., 1988.** *In vitro* lecithinase activity and sensitivity to 22 antimicrobial agents of *Clostridium perfringens* isolated from necrotic enteritis of broiler chickens. *Research in Veterinary Science*, 45, 337–340.

34 **MACLENNAN, J.D., 1962.** The histotoxic clostridial infections of man. *Bacteriological Reviews*, 26, 177–276.

35 **MASON, J.H. & ROBINSON, M., 1963.** Immunization against the toxin of *Clostridium welchii type A*, with dissolved toxoid-antitoxin floccules. *South African Journal of Medical Science*, 28, 93–101.

36 **McDONEL, J.L. & DEMERS, G.W., 1982.** *In vivo* effects of enterotoxin from *Clostridium perfringens* type A in the rabbit colon: Binding vs. biologic activity. *The Journal of Infectious Disease*, 145, 490–493.

37 **McDONNEL, A.M. & HOLMES, L.A., 1990.** Haemoglobinuria due to *Clostridium perfringens* type A mastitis in a ewe. *British Veterinary Journal*, 146, 380–381.

38 **McGOWAN, B., MOULTON, J.E. & ROOD, S.E., 1958.** Lamb losses associated with *Clostridium perfringens* type A. *Journal of the American Veterinary Medical Association*, 133, 219–221.

39 **McKAY, R.J., CARLSON, G.P. & HIRSH, D.C., 1979.** *Clostridium perfringens* associated with a focal abscess in a horse. *Journal of the American Veterinary Medical Association*, 175, 71–72.

40 **MONTGOMERIE, R.F., 1961.** *Clostridium perfringens* (*Cl. welchii*) enterotoxaemia in the ruminant. *Canadian Veterinary Journal*, 2, 439–450.

41 **MUMFORD, D.H., 1961.** Enterotoxaemia in cattle. *The Australian Veterinary Journal*, 37, 122–126.

42 **NABUURS, M.J.A., HAAGSMA, J., VAN DER MOLEN, E.J. & VAN DER HEIJDEN, P. J., 1983.** Diarrhea in one- to three-week-old piglets associated with *Clostridium perfringens* type A. *Annales de Recherches Vétérinaires,* 14, 408–411.

43 **NESBAKKEN, T. & VARDEN, S.A., 1975.** Acute bovine mastitis caused by *Clostridium perfringens* type A. *Nordisk Veterinaer Medicin,* 27, 150–152.

44 **NIILO, L., 1971.** Mechanism of action of the enteropathogenic factor of *Clostridium perfringens* type A. *Infection and Immunity,* 3, 100–106.

45 **NIILO, L., 1978.** Enterotoxigenic *Clostridium perfringens* type A isolated from intestinal contents of cattle, sheep and chickens. *Canadian Journal of Comparative Medicine,* 42, 357–363.

46 **NIILO, L., 1980.** *Clostridium perfringens* in animal disease: A review of current knowledge. *The Canadian Veterinary Journal,* 21, 141–148.

47 **NIILO, L. & AVERY, R.J., 1963.** Bovine enterotoxaemia. I. *Clostridium perfringens* types isolated from animal sources in Alberta and Saskatchewan. *Canadian Veterinary Journal,* 4, 31–36.

48 **NIILO, L. & DORWARD, W.J., 1971.** The effect of enterotoxigenic *Clostridium welchii (perfringens)* type A on the bovine intestine. *Research in Veterinary Science,* 12, 376–378.

49 **NIILO, L., MOFFAT, R.E. & AVERY, R.J., 1963.** Bovine enterotoxaemia. II. Experimental reproduction of the disease. *Canadian Veterinary Journal,* 4, 288–298.

50 **OCHOA, R. & DE VELANDIA, S., 1978.** Equine grass sickness: Serologic evidence of association with *Clostridium perfringens* type A enterotoxin. *The American Journal of Veterinary Research,* 39, 1049–1051.

51 **OKEWOLE, P.A., ITODA, A.E., OYETUNDE, I.L., CHIMA, J.C., IROKANULO, E.A. & OCHOLI, R.A., 1991.** *Clostridium perfringens* type A enterotoxaemia in pigs: A report of five cases. *British Veterinary Journal,* 147, 484–4.

52 **OLUBUNMI, P.A. & TAYLOR, D.J., 1985.** *Clostridium perfringens* type A in enteric diseases of pigs. *Tropical Veterinarian,* 3, 28–33.

53 **PATEL, S.B. & MAHLER, R., 1990.** Clostridial pleuropulmonary infections: Case report and review of the literature. *Journal of Infection,* 21, 81–85.

54 **PENNING, P.D., TREACHER, T.T. & WOODS, A.J., 1971.** Intestinal haemorrhage syndrome in artificially reared lambs. *The Veterinary Record,* 88, 613–615.

55 **POPOFF, M.R., 1984.** Bacteriological examination in enterotoxaemia of sheep and lamb. *The Veterinary Record,* 114, 324.

56 **PRINCEWELL, T.J.T., AGBA, M.I. & JEMITOLA, S.O., 1985.** Animal feeds as likely vehicles of clostridial infections in livestock. *Microbios,* 42, 155–162.

57 **REEF, V.B., 1983.** *Clostridium perfringens* cellulitis and immune-mediated hemolytic anemia in a horse. *Journal of the American Veterinary Medical Association,* 182, 251–254.

58 **ROBINSON, A. & MANSER, P.A., 1977.** Mastitis in a heifer caused by *Clostridium welchii* type A. *The Veterinary Record,* 101, 37.

59 **ROEDER, B.L., CHENGAPPA, M.M., NAGARAJA, T.T., AVERY, T.B. & KENNEDY, G.A., 1987.** Isolation of *Clostridium perfringens* from neonatal calves with ruminal and abomasal tympany, abomastitis and abomasal ulceration. *Journal of the American Veterinary Medical Association,* 190, 1550–1555.

60 **ROSE, A.L. & EDGAR, G., 1936.** Enterotoxaemic jaundice of sheep and cattle. A preliminary report on the aetiology of the disease. *The Australian Veterinary Journal,* 12, 212–220.

61 **SCHOFIELD, F.W., 1955.** Enterotoxaemia (sudden death) in calves due to *Clostridium welchii. Journal of the Veterinary Medical Association,* 126, 192–194.

62 **SCHOONDERWOERD, M., LEWIS, L.M. & SCHOLTEN, J.A., 1990.** Acute gangrenous mastitis due to *Clostridium perfringens* type A and *Escherichia coli* in a cow. *Canadian Veterinary Journal,* 31, 523–524.

63 **SEIFERT, H.S.H., BÖHNEL, H. & RANAIVOSON, A., 1983.** Prophylaxis of anaerobic infections of ruminants in Madagascar by the intradermal application of ultrafiltered toxoids from local strains of clostridia. *Deutsche Tierärztliche Wochenschrift,* 7, 274–279.

64 **SHAW, W.B., 1971.** Intestinal haemorrhage syndrome in artificially reared lambs. *The Veterinary Record,* 88, 700.

65 **SHIRLEY, G.N., 1958.** Clostridial enteritis in cattle. *The Veterinary Record,* 70, 478–480.

66 **SINHA, M., 1972.** Vorkommen und Eigenschaften von *C. perfringens* isoliert aus der Darmflora von Pferden, Rindern, Schweinen, Hunden, Katzen und Hühnern. *Wiener Tierärztliche Monatschrift,* 59, 191–193.

67 **SINHA, M., WILLINGER, H. & TRCKA, J., 1977.** Untersuchungen über das Auftreten von *Clostridium perfringens* bei Haustieren (Pferde, Rinder, Schweine, Hunde, Katzen und Hühner). *Wiener Tierärztliche Monatschrift,* 62, 163–169.

68 **SMITH, L.D.S., 1975.** *The Pathogenic Anaerobic Bacteria.* 2nd edn. Springfield, Illinois: Charles C. Thomas.

69 **SMITH, L.D.S., 1979.** Virulence factors of *Clostridium perfringens. Reviews of Infectious Diseases,* 1, 254–262.

70 **SMITH, L.D.S. & WILLIAMS, B.L., 1984.** *The Pathogenic Anaerobic Bacteria.* 3rd edn. Springfield, Illinois: Charles C. Thomas.

71 **VAN BAELEN, D. & DEVRIESE, L.A., 1987.** Presence of *Clostridium perfringens* enterotoxin in intestinal samples from farm animals with diarrhoea of unknown origin. *Journal of Veterinary Medicine* B, 34, 713–716.

72 **VANCE, H.N., 1967.** *Clostridium perfringens* as a pathogen of cattle: A literature review. *Canadian Journal of Comparative Medicine and Veterinary Science,* 31, 248–250.

73 **VERMA, N.D., 1984.** Isolation and characterization of *Clostridium perfringens* type A causing blackquarter-like disease of cattle in Manipur. *Indian Journal of Animal Sciences,* 54, 1078–1108.

74 **VERMA, N.D., 1986.** Comparative efficacy of formalized, alum-precipitated and aluminium hydroxide gel-adsorbed bacterin toxoid of *Clostridium perfringens* type A. *Indian Veterinary Journal,* 63, 704–710.

75 **VERMA, N.D., 1988.** Antibiotic susceptibility of *Clostridium perfringens* type A isolated from 'false blackleg' of cattle. *Indian Veterinary Journal,* 65, 263–264.

76 **WIERUP, M., 1977.** Equine intestinal clostridiosis. *Acta Veterinaria Scandinavica* Supplementum, 62, 1–182.

77 **WORRALL, E.E., NATALIA, L., RONOHARDJO, P., PARTOUTOMO, S. & TARDMUDSI, 1987.** Enterotoxaemia in water buffaloes caused by *Clostridium perfringens* type A. *The Veterinary Record,* 121, 278–279.

78 **YAMAMOTO, A., ITO, A., MURATA, R., UEMATSU, N., NAGAI, K. & MINOMO, K., 1970.** Hyperimmunization of horses with alpha toxoid of *Clostridium perfringens. Japanese Journal of Medical Science and Biology,* 23, 111–115.

79 **ZUMPT, I.F., 1980.** P.O. Box 3080, Stellenbosch 7602, South Africa. Personal communication.

155

Clostridium perfringens *type B enterotoxaemia*

Synonyms: Lamb dysentery, bloedpens (Afrik.)

N.P.J. Kriek, M.W. Odendaal and P. Hunter

Introduction

Lamb dysentery, or 'bloedpens', is a peracute to chronic enterotoxaemia caused primarily by the action of the beta toxin and, to a lesser extent, the epsilon toxin, produced by *Clostridium perfringens* type B in the intestines. It usually affects lambs less than 14 days old. It is characterized clinically by an acute haemorrhagic to mucohaemorrhagic enteritis, resulting in death after a few hours or one or two days in the peracute and acute cases, and after four or more days in chronic cases. This type of enterotoxaemia has also been described in foals and calves.[4, 10, 15, 17, 18, 26]

The disease in lambs has been well known in the United Kingdom, western Europe and in the USA for many years. It is probable that the condition described in 1811 as 'Milk-ill' was lamb dysentery. In Europe it was described in 1871,[2] while in 1927 Jungherr and Welch first described a disease that resembles lamb dysentery in the USA.[9]

Lamb dysentery was prevalent and fairly well known to sheep farmers in certain parts of the Cape Province of South Africa during the latter part of the nineteenth century and its occurrence in this province was recorded in the Colesberg Advertiser in 1888.[9] Walker, in 1923,[27] referred to a similar disease in Kenya.

Dalling, in 1926, was the first to identify the cause of lamb dysentery as *C. perfringens* but noticed that it differed from the classical *C. perfringens*. He therefore named it the lamb dysentery bacillus, *Bacillus agni*. It was later renamed *C. perfringens* type B.

Lamb dysentery currently occurs in the United Kingdom, Europe, South Africa and the Middle East, but not in North America or New Zealand. The disease occurs endemically, although rarely, in all the sheep farming areas of South Africa, including the Karoo, north-eastern Cape Province, the Orange Free State, and the highveld of Transvaal.[22]

Aetiology

Clostridium perfringens type B produces the alpha, beta and epsilon toxins, as well as a number of minor toxins. For information on the cultural, morphological and biochemical characteristics of *C. perfringens* as well as its toxins, **Table 1** in the ***Clostridium perfringens*** **group: Introduction** should be consulted.

There are strong indications that the production of beta toxin is coded for by a plasmid.[3] The beta and epsilon toxins are metabolic products secreted during active exponential growth of *C. perfringens* type B in a suitable medium and in the presence of the necessary nutriments required for toxin production. The beta toxin concentration in the medium declines rapidly after prolonged incubation.[20] The organism grows *in vivo* in the intestinal tract of the affected animal where it produces the toxins responsible for its pathogenic effect.

Epidemiology

In South Africa, lamb dysentery affects new-born lambs of all sheep breeds to the same extent, although the heavier breeds and cross-breds are considered more resistant; goat kids are also affected.[8] During winter and spring, its presence is favoured by cold weather in certain parts of South Africa; it is rare in autumn and does not seem to affect summer lambs.[9]

Clostridium perfringens type B would seem to be an obligate parasite, as is the case with types C, D and E.[23] Organisms are excreted in the faeces of adult carrier animals and sick lambs, and contaminate soil and pastures. In contrast to *C. perfringens* type A which survives indefinitely in soil, type B strains only survive for several months in soil and pastures and are not considered to be part of the normal microbial flora of the soil.[23]

Lambs are more prone to develop the disease on certain parts of a farm. The infection is favoured when the ewes and lambs are confined to small camps, lambing pens, small fenced-off grazing areas, or sheds and kraals during the day or night as a precaution against theft or predation. Close and prolonged confinement of the animals seems to increase the severity of the disease. The prevalence of the disease decreases when the ewes and lambs are removed from highly contaminated areas. The teats of the ewes become contaminated with faeces and soil and lambs acquire the infection *per os* during suckling.[9]

Pathogenesis

Clostridium perfringens type B organisms ingested within the first few hours after birth of the lambs colonize the small intestines, especially the ileum, where they multiply and produce their toxins. It is generally believed that the beta toxin is primarily responsible for the induction of the lesions of lamb dysentery while the role of epsilon toxin is unknown.[16] *In vitro* these toxins are produced during the exponential growth phase and it is assumed that the same pertains to the *in vivo* situation. Restriction of the occurrence of the disease to neonates is associated with the susceptibility of the beta toxin to the effect of trypsin in the intestinal tract, which is secreted by animals in this age group in insufficient amounts to inactivate the toxin.[28] In older animals these enzymes are produced in sufficient quantities to inactivate the beta toxin. In addition, the presence of trypsin inhibitors in the colostrum aggravates the situation for neonates.[19] In the portions of the small, and to a lesser extent the large, intestine where the toxins are produced, an area of expanding necrosis develops around each focus of infection. Desquamation of necrotic tissue results in the formation of small, discrete ulcers which may become confluent. Due to the irritation caused by the bacteria and toxins in the intestine, the peristaltic movements increase, resulting in diarrhoea. The loss of water and electrolytes, especially HCO_3^-, results in severe dehydration and acidosis. Death is the result of shock, toxaemia, dehydration and acidosis.[12]

Clinical signs

Lamb dysentery is almost exclusively a disease of neonatal lambs and goat kids, animals one- to seven-days-old being the most severely affected. When the disease first appears in a sheep breeding unit, it is towards the end of the lambing season. During subsequent breeding seasons outbreaks usually commence 14 days after the first ewes have lambed. Lamb dysentery may run a peracute, acute, subacute, chronic or mild course.[12]

When outbreaks initially occur on a farm, lambs of 24–72 hours old are affected, but during subsequent years older lambs of up to two to three weeks of age may also contract the disease. A morbidity rate of 20–30 per cent may prevail, with the mortality rate being 100 per cent.[8, 12, 23]

The incubation period varies from 12 hours to one to two days and clinical signs are often present within 24 hours of birth. Peracutely affected lambs usually die without showing any clinical signs. The course of the acute and subacute disease may extend over one or more days while, in the chronic disease, lambs survive longer than three or four days. Older animals become increasingly resistant, those older than 14 days being mildly affected and rarely dying. In exceptional cases, lambs of two to four weeks of age contract the chronic form of the disease, which has a protracted course.[8]

Acutely affected lambs are weak, listless, and suckle sluggishly or refuse to do so and may show evidence of abdominal pain and diarrhoea, the faeces becoming brownish-grey, semi-liquid and blood-stained. Affected animals soon become comatose and die. Subacutely affected lambs are dull, listless and depressed, move about sluggishly, lag behind the rest of the flock, often lie down, and are reluctant to stand up and suckle. If they do rise, or when lifted to their feet, they stretch in a peculiar way and may remain standing for a while with their backs arched, obviously in pain. Abdominal pain, bleating and diarrhoea are commonly manifested. The faeces, at first yellow and semi-liquid, become mucus-coated, dark and blood-stained, and are passed with the animals straining severely. The faeces have an offensive odour. Lambs eventually refuse to suckle, become prostrate, comatose, and die. A yellow, blood-tinged, faecal discharge caked around the tail base, may be evident.[8, 17]

Chronic disease is characterized by listlessness and unthriftiness. The lambs suckle indifferently, seldom drinking enough milk to maintain their basic requirements. They frequently lie down and, on rising, stretch their backs in a peculiar way. Their faeces are thin, mucoid and blood-stained.[8]

Clostridium perfringens type B enterotoxaemia in seven- to ten-day old calves causes scouring which progresses to dysentery.[10, 17] In the few cases of the disease described in foals, mortality rates of up to 50 per cent have been encountered. Clinical signs include cessation of suckling, signs of pain, and a severe, reddish-brown diarrhoea that develops within 48 hours after birth. In fatal cases, animals become comatose and die within 12–24 hours of first becoming ill.[15]

Pathology

Lesions present in the various forms of the disease in lambs were meticulously described by Gaiger and Dalling in 1921,[7] and the account that follows is based on that description. Necropsy findings vary according to the course of the disease. The carcass of a lamb that has lingered on for a few days before dying is in poor condition. The blood is dark and clots poorly, and there may be a serous or blood-stained exudate in the peritoneal cavity. The liver and the kidneys are severely degenerated, whereas the spleen is usually of normal size, although a slight splenomegaly may occur in those animals that have suffered from the chronic disease. There is usually severe oedema and some congestion of the lungs and, as in pulpy kidney disease, the pericardial cavity contains an excessive amount of serous fluid in which clots may form on exposure to air. Epi- and endocardial haemorrhages are frequent and the myocardium is degenerated.

The abomasum is usually empty, and the rumen may contain large amounts of clotted milk in peracute and acute cases. The most characteristic lesions, which differ according to the severity and the course of the disease, occur in the small and large intestines. In acute cases, there is a severe haemorrhagic enteritis with the presence, particularly in the ileal mucosa, of pin-head sized, yellowish, necrotic foci. Lesions in peracute cases may not be as distinct as they are in those cases with a longer course.

The most common lesion in subacute cases is the presence of necrotic foci and ulcers up to 10 mm in diameter in the mucosa of the small and large intestine. These lesions are surrounded by a zone of hyperaemia and haemorrhage; some coalesce to form larger lesions. Ulcers are usually visible through the intestinal serosa. In severely affected and more chronic cases, the ulcers may perforate, resulting in peritonitis and copious peritoneal effusion that contains fibrin which causes adherence of adjacent intestinal loops. The intestinal contents vary from normal to almost pure blood containing necrotic debris.

In calves the macroscopic lesions are located in the small intestine, particularly the ileum, ranging from severe generalized enteritis to extensive necrosis of the mucous membrane. Small, yellow diphtheric patches occur in the necrotic areas and the intestinal contents are blood-stained. Other lesions include congestion of the mucous membrane of the caecum and colon, swelling and severe haemorrhage of the mesenteric lymph nodes, and congestion of the liver, spleen and kidneys.[10]

In foals which have died of the disease, the macroscopic lesions are restricted to the alimentary tract and are those of a haemorrhagic enteritis. The content of the entire intestinal tract is fluid and contains blood. Round, dark-red areas, about 10 mm in diameter, are consistently present in the mucosa of the ileum but are less commonly present elsewhere in the small intestine. Some of them may show evidence of ulceration.[15]

Diagnosis

The final diagnosis is based on the results of the examination of intestinal smears, the typing of toxin in the intestinal contents, and the isolation and typing of the organism while taking cognizance of the history, clinical signs and lesions.

For information on the specimens required to confirm the diagnosis, the ***Clostridium perfringens* group: Introduction** should be consulted.

The absence of Gram-positive bacilli in smears made from specimens of the intestinal content rules out the diagnosis of a clostridial enterotoxaemia, whereas the presence of many Gram-positive, non-sporulating bacilli is indicative of the condition.

The intestinal contents of affected animals are centrifuged and filter-sterilized. A portion of the filtrate is treated with trypsin before it is subjected to typing procedures by toxin neutralization tests in mice or guinea-pigs.[24] An enzyme-linked immunosorbent assay has been developed for the detection of the beta toxin of *C. perfringens* in intestinal contents.[14] The presence of beta toxin alone in the intestinal content indicates a *C. perfringens* type C enterotoxaemia, while detection both of beta and epsilon toxins indicates a type B enterotoxaemia. The beta toxin in intestinal contents cannot be demonstrated in a carcass which has undergone considerable putrefaction, as the toxin is rapidly destroyed by the action of proteolytic enzymes released during the putrefactive process. However, the isolation and identification of *Clostridium perfringens* type B organisms in culture provide strong presumptive evidence of lamb dysentery.[24]

Differential diagnosis

Lamb dysentery may be confused with the acute fatal neonatal haemorrhagic enteritis caused by *Escherichia coli* from which it can be distinguished by the absence of ulcers and the presence of organisms resembling *C. perfringens* in smears prepared from intestinal scrapings.[24] *Clostridium perfringens* type E has been isolated from the intestines of lambs affected with a form of enterotoxaemia.[21]

Control

The successful treatment of affected lambs is usually not feasible due to the generally peracute or acute course of the disease, but the use of antibiotics administered orally together with supportive treatment can save mildly affected cases. *Clostridium perfringens* is resistant to the aminoglycoside group of antibiotics, but susceptible to tetracycline, chloramphenicol, and penicillin **(see *Clostridium perfringens* group: Introduction)**.

During an outbreak of the disease, it is important to isolate affected lambs (and their dams) as soon as possible. The healthy animals in the breeding flock should immediately be removed to other areas where ewes have not previously lambed, as kraals, pens and camps that have housed infected lambs may be severely contaminated and a source of infection. It is important that the lambs ingest colostrum within the first two to six hours of life. The treatment of the remaining lambs in an outbreak with anti-type B-specific immunoglobulin, may be considered, if it is available.

To control anticipated or subsequent outbreaks of the disease, ewes should be immunized in order to induce the presence of as high a level of antibodies in the colostrum as possible, as the passive transfer of maternal immunity to lambs is the only way to protect the offspring. The vaccine consists of an alum-precipitated toxoid of the beta toxin and is available in South Africa as the Onderstepoort Lamb Dysentery vaccine.[5] Pregnant ewes vaccinated for the first time should receive two injections two to five weeks apart, the second injection being administered four to eight weeks before lambing.[11] Ewes that have been previously immunized need only be given a single booster vaccination two to four weeks before expected parturition. A freeze-dried vaccine has been developed[6] and polyvalent clostridial vaccines containing four to seven different antigens, including *C. perfringens* type B toxoid, are available in many countries including South Africa.[1, 11, 13, 25]

References

1 **ARDEHALI, M. & DARAKHSHAN, H., 1976.** Production and standardization of polyvalent *Clostridium perfringens* vaccine in Iran. *Development in Biological Standardization*, 32, 31–34.

2 **DALLING, T., 1936.** Lamb dysentery. *Journal of Comparative Pathology and Therapeutics*, 39, 148–163.

3 **DUNCAN, C.L., ROKOS, E.A., CHRISTENSON, C.M. & ROOD, J.I., 1978.** Multiple plasmids in different toxigenic types of *Clostridium perfringens*: Possible control of beta toxin production. *In*: SCHLESSINGER, D., (ed.). *Microbiology*, 1978. Washington DC: The American Society for Microbiology.

4 **ENGLISH, J.E., 1966.** Field experience with *Clostridium enterotoxaemia in young animals.* Journal of the American Veterinary Medical Association, 149, 1565–1570.

5 **ERASMUS, B.J., CAMERON, C.M., HUNTER, P., CILLIERS, J.A., OBEREM, P.T., STOLTSZ, W.H. & DE WAAL, D.T., 1990.** *Onderstepoort Vaccines.* Booklet issued by the Department of Agriculture and Development and obtained from the Directorate of Agricultural Information, Private Bag X144, Pretoria 0001.

6 **FARRAG, I. & SHARAF, D., 1977.** Effect of lyophilization on the potency of clostridial vaccines. *Journal of the Egyptian Veterinary Medical Association*, 37, 35–40.

7 **GAIGER, S.H. & DALLING, T., 1921.** Bacillary dysentery in lambs. *Journal of Comparative Pathology and Therapeutics*, 34, 79–105.

8 **HENNING, M.W., 1949.** *Animal Diseases in South Africa.* 2nd edn. Pretoria: Central News Agency.

9 **HENNING, M.W., 1956.** *Animal Diseases in South Africa.* 3rd edn. Pretoria: Central News Agency.

10 **HEPPLE, J.R., 1952.** Necrotic enterotoxaemia in a calf due to *Clostridium welchii* type B. *The Veterinary Record*, 64, 633–634.

11 **JANSEN, B.C., *1976.*** The standardization of *C. perfringens* antigens and antisera. *Development in Biological Standardization*, 32, 35–44.

12 **JENSEN, R. & SWIFT, B.L., 1982.** *Diseases of Sheep*, 2nd edn. Philadelphia: Lea & Febiger.

13 **KERRY, J.B. & CRAIG, G.R., 1979.** Field studies in sheep with multicomponent clostridial vaccines. *The Veterinary Record*, 105, 551–554.

14 **MARTIN, P.K., NAYLOR, R.D. & SHARPE, R.T., 1988.** Detection of *Clostridium perfringens* beta toxin by enzyme-linked immunosorbent assay. *Research in Veterinary Science*, 44, 270–271.

15 **MASON, J.H. & ROBINSON, E.M., 1938.** The isolation of *Cl. welchii* type B from foals affected with dysentery. *Onderstepoort Journal of Veterinary Science and Animal Industry*, 11, 333–337.

16 **McDONEL, J.L., 1986.** *Clostridium perfringens* toxins (type A, B, C, D, E). *Pharmacology and Therapy*, 10, 617–655.

17 **MONTGOMERIE, R.F., 1961.** *Clostridium perfringens* (*Cl. welchii*) enterotoxaemia in the ruminant. *Canadian Veterinary Journal*, 2, 439–450.

18 **MONTGOMERIE, R.F. & ROWLANDS, W.T., 1937.** Lamb dysentery in a foal. *The Veterinary Record*, 49, 398.

19 **NIILO, L., 1986.** Enterotoxemic *Clostridium perfringens. In*: GYLES, C.L. & THOEN, C.O., (eds). *Pathogenesis of Bacterial Infections in Animals.* Ames, Iowa: Iowa State University Press.

20 **ORLANS, E.S. & JONES, V.E., 1958.** Studies on some soluble antigens of *Clostridium welchii* types B, C and D. *Immunology*, 1, 268–290.

21 **ROSS, H.E., WARREN, M.E. & BARNED, J.M., 1949.** *Clostridium welchii* iota toxin: Its activation by trypsin. *Journal of General Microbiology*, 3, 148–152.

22 **SCHULZ, K.C.A. *& SUTTON, G.D., 1950.*** Enterotoxaemia of sheep. *Journal of the South African Veterinary Medical Association*, 21, 179–183.

23 **SMITH, L.D.S. & WILLIAMS, B.L., 1984.** *The Pathogenic Anaerobic Bacteria.* 3rd edn. Springfield, Illinois: Charles C. Thomas.

24 **STERNE, M. & BATTY, I., 1975.** *Pathogenic Clostridia.* London, Boston: Butterworths.

25 **STERNE, M., BATTY, I., THOMPSON, A. & ROBERTSON, J.M., 1962.** Immunisation of sheep with multi-component clostridial vaccines. *The Veterinary Record*, 74, 909–913.

26 **VANCE, H.N., 1967.** *Clostridium perfringens* as a pathogen of cattle: A literature review. *Canadian Journal of Comparative Medicine and Veterinary Science*, 31, 248–250.

27 **WALKER, J., 1923.** *Annual Reports of the Department of Agriculture, Kenya*, 1922–23.

28 **WOOLCOCK, J.B., 1979.** *Bacterial Infection and Immunity in Domestic Animals.* Oxford: Elsevier Scientific Publishing Company.

Clostridium perfringens *type C enterotoxaemia*

Synonyms: In sheep: struck, haemorrhagic enterotoxaemia in young lambs, necrotic enteritis. In calves: haemorrhagic enteritis or enterotoxaemia. In foals: haemorrhagic necrotizing enteritis, necrohaemorrhagic enterocolitis. In suckling piglets: haemorrhagic or necrotizing infectious enteritis, enterotoxaemia, bloody scours.

M.W. Odendaal, N.P.J. Kriek and P. Hunter

Introduction

Clostridium perfringens type C has been regarded since 1931 as the cause of struck, which is an acute infectious but non-contagious and rapidly fatal disease of adult sheep first described on the Romney Marsh in Kent, England. Struck is characterized by an acute enteritis, peritonitis and toxaemia, and it has a seasonal occurrence.[19] More recently, *C. perfringens* type C has been associated with haemorrhagic enterotoxaemia in young lambs,[12, 15, 17, 41] haemorrhagic enteritis or enterotoxaemia in calves,[16, 44] haemorrhagic necrotizing enteritis or necrohaemorrhagic enterocolitis in foals,[7, 27, 46, 48] and necrotizing or haemorrhagic enteritis in neonatal piglets.[4, 22–26, 29, 30] In humans, *C. perfringens* type C has been isolated from patients suffering from a similar condition which is described in Germany as 'Darmbrand'[56] and in Papua New Guinea, as *enteritis necroticans*.[8, 9, 40] It is possible that the young of all animal species may be susceptible to *C. perfringens* type C infection, which may be dependent on those factors that favour bacterial colonization in the intestine, such as digestive malfunctions.

Present indications are that the number of animal species which may be affected by a fatal infection of *C. perfringens* type C is greater than for any of the other *C. perfringens* types.[43] The infection is rarely diagnosed in South Africa in calves, lambs or piglets.[21]

Aetiology

Clostridium perfringens type C produces alpha and beta toxins as major toxins, whereas minor toxins such as theta and delta toxins are produced less consistently by different strains **(see *Clostridium perfringens* group: Introduction)**.

There can be little doubt that *C. perfringens* type C is a cause of haemorrhagic or necrotic enteritis, and of enterotoxaemia in very young animals under natural conditions; type C enterotoxaemia has also been experimentally reproduced in piglets,[11, 29] lambs[41] and guinea-pigs.[35]

Five subtypes of *C. perfringens* type C have been recognized, their identity being based on their ability to produce certain minor toxins. These subtypes have a specific geographic distribution and affinity for certain species of livestock, and include those associated with classical struck in sheep, the Colorado variety from lambs and calves, human necrotic enteritis, and porcine enteritis. All type C isolates produce beta toxin. The classical subtype, isolated from struck in sheep, produces all three haemolysins: alpha, theta and delta toxins, a number of other minor toxins as well as the beta toxin. The presence or absence of the delta toxin[43] is one of the distinguishing characteristics between the type C subtypes, as opposed to the presence of the alpha and theta toxins, which are present in most of the other *C. perfringens* strains, including type C.[39, 42, 53] Strains isolated from typical *C. perfringens* type C enterotoxaemia in pigs share the biochemical characteristics common to *C. perfringens* **(see *Clostridium perfringens* group: Introduction)**. All these strains also produce alpha and beta toxins and some of the minor toxins including the theta toxin. None of the porcine strains produce the delta toxin.[23]

The morphological and biochemical properties of *C. perfringens* type C are identical to those of the other types **(see *Clostridium perfringens* group: Introduction)**. The biochemical and morphological identification of type C isolates can be performed according to the procedures described by Harmon[18] and the toxin typing to those described by Sterne and Batty.[51]

Epideminology

Diseases caused by *C. perfringens* type C are largely unknown in South Africa and the organism is rarely isolated.[21] A few cases of necrotic enteritis have been encountered in pigs, calves or lambs, but it is not considered to be of economic importance. Struck is not a recognized entity in South Africa though it may be confused with pulpy kidney disease.[3] The disease in sheep has mostly been reported from the United Kingdom, Germany, Sardinia, New Zealand and the USA.

Epidemiological data on the disease in the various animal species are scant. The neonatal disease may be sporadic and affecting individual animals, as in foals,[27] or it may occur in annual outbreaks of varying extent or during successive farrowings as it does in pigs,[4] calves and lambs. It is estimated that up to 25 per cent of piglets, under five days of age in an endemic area can develop a clostridial diarrhoea.[22] Struck occurs on a seasonal basis, mainly during the winter or spring.[20]

The disease appears to be transmitted *per os*. *Clostridium perfringens* type C can live for long periods in the intestine of carrier animals without causing clinical disease. It appears that, of the animal species investigated, pigs carry the largest numbers of the bacterium in their intestinal tracts. In one study, 87 per cent of all *C. perfringens* type C isolated were obtained from pigs, while less than 4 per cent were obtained from sheep and less than 2 per cent from cattle. *Clostridium perfringens* type C can also be isolated from faeces of pigs from farms where outbreaks have not occurred. These animals, as well as diseased animals, are responsible for disseminating the type C organisms through their faeces. Predisposing factors to disease in piglets include group-keeping of pregnant sows, simultaneous farrowing of large groups of sows, group-treatment of piglets and the prophylactic use of antibiotics to which the causative bacterium is resistant. Other predisposing factors which facilitate the occurrence of the disease in piglets, include a low gastric pH, a change in the diet, injury or irritation to the intestinal mucosa, anti-trypsin factors in the feed, the host's susceptibility, and the presence of trypsin inhibiting factors in the colostrum.[4, 43] The source of an infection in a previously uninfected pig herd is usually a recently introduced carrier animal, such as a newly purchased boar or replacement gilt.[22] Faecal contamination of food appears to play a minor role, but may be important if it is severe. The bacterium survives in the soil only for a limited period.[49] Adverse weather conditions, such as severe windy and dusty conditions may result in the distribution of *C. perfringens* type C spores to nonendemic areas.[22]

Pathogenesis

The pathogenesis of type C enterotoxaemia is not well understood, but it is associated with the local production of toxins in the intestinal tract following a rapid and marked increase in the numbers of the clostridia. The beta toxin, which is severely necrotizing, appears to be the major factor in the development of the necrosis of the mucosa of the intestine which is characteristic of the condition,[4] while some of the minor toxins, which are haemolytic, have little or no significance in the pathogenesis of the disease.[43] Subsequent absorption of toxins into the systemic circulation results in toxaemia.

The first bacteria to colonize the intestinal tract of new-born calves, lambs, piglets or other young animals are *C. perfringens*, *Escherichia coli* and streptococci,[55] which reach this site after their oral ingestion resulting from the sucking of teats and inanimate objects which contain them. These organisms form part of the normal intestinal flora and inhibit the growth of many enteric pathogens and any delay in the establishment of the normal bacterial flora results in increased susceptibility of the gastrointestinal tract of neonates to invasion by pathogens. *Clostridium perfringens* type A is the predominant clostridial type occurring in the intestines of neonates. Although *C. perfringens* type C is not usually regarded as part of the normal intestinal flora,[11, 50] it does occur at this site in carrier animals. Under ideal conditions the *C. perfringens* type C organisms present in the intestines proliferate excessively and produce beta toxin. The first pathologic effect of *C. perfringens* type C, as it occurs in piglets, is noted at the tips of the villi in the small intestines. The presence of both the organism and the beta toxin is required to initiate the pathologic changes necessary for the production of the disease.[1, 29] The bacterial cells adhere to the intestinal epithelium in great numbers by a mechanism which is still unclear. This intimate contact enables the beta toxin to exert its deleterious effects directly on the epithelial cells. Toxic damage to the mucosa can, however, still occur without bacterial adhesion taking place. Following the proliferation of the bacteria in the intestinal lumen, the beta toxin produced by them has a marked cytotoxic effect and initially causes a marked damage to the microvilli and degeneration of the mitochondria of the enterocytes. This is followed by a progressively developing degeneration and necrosis, not only of the differentiated villar enterocytes, but also of other cells and the vasculature of the lamina propria.[29, 30] Clostridia penetrate the damaged epithelium and adhere to the basal lamina.[30] The necrosis caused by the toxins extends from the mucosa to involve the submucosa.[29] Thrombosis of blood vessels in the submucosa may develop.[4] Invasion of the bacteria into the tissues has no pathogenetic significance.[29] The extensive damage to the intestinal mucosa increases its permeability to blood proteins and cells, which then enter the intestinal lumen. It also facilitates the absorption of toxin into the general circulation resulting in toxaemia,[29] which plays an important accessory role in causing the death of the animal[4, 29] due to toxic injury and shock.[28]

The increased susceptibility of neonates to the effect of the beta toxin is explained by the observation that concentrations of *C. perfringens* type C in the intestinal tract of infected piglets reach high levels within one day of birth but decline rapidly to low numbers after they have reached three weeks of age. Trypsin inhibitors contained in colostrum may also cause the neonate to be exposed to greater amounts of toxin than older animals since the beta toxin is inactivated by trypsin. Adequate amounts of pancreatic proteases in the intestine protect animals against *C. perfringens* type C enterotoxaemia and factors inhibiting or reducing the quantity of these enzymes also predispose animals to the development of the disease.[41] Damage to the intestinal mucosa by other unrelated causes may aggravate the local development of the lesions and further predispose to the development of the enterotoxaemia.[4] Feeding practices also influence the number of clostridia in the intestinal tract — diets high in protein (15–20 per cent) bring about a sharp increase in the number of clostridia which persists for as long as the diet is fed,[36] and may assist in the development of the disease in older age groups. An additional factor which may play a role, particularly in the peracute and acute disease, is the development of impaired gastric and intestinal motility which facilitates the multiplication of *C. perfringens* type C and the production of its toxins, both of which are enhanced by the accompanying impairment of enzyme activity and the accumulation of peptides and cell debris within the intestinal lumen.

The pathogenesis of struck in adult sheep is probably similar to that of the enterotoxaemia caused by *C. perfringens* type C in lambs and other animal species.

Clinical signs

In the peracute and acute forms of *C. perfringens* type C enterotoxaemia in piglets, most animals are affected within the first week of life, the prevalence being highest during the first three days. Although the mortality rate on infected premises varies from litter to litter and from farm to farm, all the piglets in a litter may be affected and as many as 80 per cent of them may die. There is usually a rise in the mortality rate in individual litters as an outbreak progresses. The course of the disease is very short and is usually not longer than 48 hours although a few cases may linger on for a few days. Clinical signs may be evident as soon as seven hours after birth with affected animals becoming limp and ceasing to suckle. Their haircoat becomes ruffled, and they are pale or have a greyish discolouration of the skin, occasionally show trembling, and have a subnormal body temperature. Diarrhoea is not consistently present but, when it is, it is usually haemorrhagic and it may be accompanied by vomition.[22, 24, 29] Affected piglets also suffer from hypoglycaemia, dehydration and metabolic collapse.[24]

The subacute and chronic forms of the disease occur in piglets between five days of age and weaning. Clinical signs include a nonhaemorrhagic diarrhoea, emaciation, anaemia, hypoglycaemia, dehydration, and metabolic collapse.[22, 24] Mortality rates of 42–74 per cent have been recorded in the more prolonged disease.[24, 29]

Ovine *C. perfringens* type C enterotoxaemia does not simultaneously affect lambs and adult sheep on the same farm. In lambs, the disease is of sudden onset and short duration and affected animals usually die within 12–72 hours after commencement of the clinical signs.[12] Most lambs are affected during the first nine days of life with the prevalence being highest in the three- to five-day-old age group. They generally manifest few, if any, clinical signs prior to death. The mortality rate varies from an insignificant number to about 15 per cent of all lambs born in an affected flock. When diseased lambs are seen alive, they are depressed and either pass greyish-black, soft faeces[15] or suffer from a prominent mucohaemorrhagic diarrhoea.[12] They usually have a subnormal temperature, shiver, bleat and may show tetanic spasms.[12, 15, 17]

Struck characteristically affects adult sheep. Affected animals are weak and prostrate, while most animals suddenly and unexpectedly become comatose and die without any additional signs being observed. A few may manifest convulsive fits in the terminal stages.[20, 28]

Clostridium perfringens type C enterotoxaemia generally affects three- to five-days-old calves, though animals in excess of one year old may also be affected. The well-fed and vigorous animals are usually the ones to contract the disease. Clinical signs are often not noticed as the course of the disease is usually less than two hours, but if they are noticed they include weakness, inappetence, dullness and other indistinct neurological signs, straining to defecate, signs of colic, and haemorrhagic enteritis.[10, 16, 44]

Affected foals are usually less than 10 days-old and are either found dead or they die within 24 hours after the onset of clinical signs, often before the development of diarrhoea. Clinical signs usually include a haemorrhagic diarrhoea, decreased body temperature, increased respiration and heart rates, anorexia, distended abdomen, dehydration, colic, depression, shock and coma.[5, 7, 27, 46, 48] Affected foals may also manifest leukopenia, cyanosis, acidosis and uraemia.[27]

Pathology

Lesions in the neonatal syndromes in the various animal species do not differ significantly from each other. The carcass is cyanotic and severely congested.

In piglets, a severe enteritis which is constantly present varies from haemorrhagic to necrotic without appreciable haemorrhage, and occurs predominantly in the jejunum but may involve other parts of the small intestine as well as the large intestine.[22, 25] The extent of the intestinal lesion varies; in some that have died of the infection, a portion of the intestine as short as 50 mm may be involved. Usually, however, at least 1,5 m of the small intestine is affected.[25] The zonal distribution of the lesions is characteristic and in some cases, alternating stretches of normal and abnormal mucosa may be present. Fibrin threads may cover the serosal surface, and emphysema of the intestinal wall occurs in about 25 per cent of cases. Mesenteric lymph nodes are hyperaemic and the peritoneal and pleural cavities contain serosanguinous fluid. Specific macroscopic lesions do not occur in other organs.

Lesions in lambs involve the jejunum, ileum, and the large intestine and comprise severe haemorrhagic to necrotic lesions.[12, 41] Other lesions are similar to those described in piglets.[17]

The carcass of a sheep that has died from struck undergoes rapid decomposition. The lesions are those of an ulcerative to haemorrhagic enteritis, fibrinous peritonitis and toxaemia with transudation into the peritoneal, pleural and pericardial cavities.[20] Ulcers, when present, are most frequent in the jejunum. Multiple small haemorrhages may occur in the serosal surfaces.[28]

In calves, the small intestine is affected by a severe haemorrhagic enteritis. The other lesions are similar to those described in piglets.[16, 44]

The nature, extent and distribution of lesions in foals vary. A severe and extensive haemorrhagic enteritis is generally present. This may involve the entire length of the small intestine except for the proximal duodenum[5, 7] only the jejunum,[46, 48] or segmental sections (as long as four metres) of it.[46] A diphtheritic pseudomembrane may be present in affected parts of the intestine, in which case the overlying serosal surface is also markedly congested. In some animals, however, distension of the stomach and entire small intestine by gas and fluid may be the only evident lesion.[27]

Histologically, the lesions comprised necrosis of the intestinal mucosa, and the presence of Gram-positive, rod-shaped bacteria in the affected areas. Necrosis may extend into the submucosa, and sharp demarcation between the living and the necrotic tissue is characteristic.[25, 27, 48]

Diagnosis

A provisional diagnosis of *C. perfringens* type C enterotoxaemia in the various animal species is based on the clinical signs, history and macroscopic and histopathological lesions, but confirmation of the diagnosis requires bacteriological isolation of the organism, together with, if possible, the detection of beta toxin in the intestinal contents.

The isolation of the organism in pure culture from animals manifesting typical lesions is usually more easily achieved than is the demonstration of beta toxin in the intestinal contents. In some animals, beta toxin can also be demonstrated in the peritoneal fluid, but its presence here is less consistent than it is in the intestinal contents.[26]

Appropriate specimens should be collected for diagnostic purposes **(see *Clostridium perfringens* group: Introduction)**. In addition, in the case of struck, smears made from skeletal musculature should be submitted.

The absence of Gram-positive bacilli in the smears excludes a diagnosis of clostridial enterotoxaemia. The presence of many Gram-positive, non-sporulating bacilli is indicative of the disease but does not necessarily confirm an aetiological role for it.

The presence or absence of toxin in the intestinal contents is determined biologically in mice or guinea-pigs after the contents have been centrifuged to remove solid particles and the supernatant fluid filter-sterilized.

Beta toxin can be detected by the toxin neutralization test[51] or by the enzyme-linked immunosorbent assay,[37] which allows the differentiation between *C. perfringens* types B, C and D enterotoxaemia. The presence of beta toxin alone indicates a *C. perfringens* type C enterotoxaemia. Should the intestinal contents contain *C. perfringens* type C but no demonstrable toxin, a diagnosis of haemorrhagic enterotoxaemia is still warranted,[51] as failure to demonstrate the beta toxin in the intestinal contents may be due to a low concentration of toxin present which is often the case in cases with a protracted course, or to post-mortal destruction of the toxin by enzymes which may occur before the specimens are collected from a carcass or during storage and shipping.[43] The diagnosis in chronic cases of the disease is difficult as beta toxin cannot usually be demonstrated in, or has disappeared from the intestinal fluid, and the intestinal flora has changed to one containing principally Gram-negative bacteria, thus precluding the isolation of *C. perfringens* type C.[22]

Differential diagnosis

Clinically, the neonatal disease in pigs may be difficult to distinguish from other enteric diseases, such as *Escherichia coli* enteritis, salmonellosis, transmissible gastroenteritis in pigs, hypoglycaemia and *C. perfringens* type B infections.[24] Acute colic, intestinal displacement, gastrointestinal ulceration, haemorrhagic necrotizing enterocolitis due to *Clostridium difficile* infection, and the ingestion of toxic substances are included in the differential diagnosis of type C enterotoxaemia in foals.[27, 31] In sheep, enterotoxaemia caused by *C. perfringens* types A, D and B must also be considered.

Control

The rapid course of the peracute and acute disease precludes any therapeutic intervention. The use of antibiotics and supportive treatment can be considered when the course of the disease is prolonged. It should be kept in mind that the *Clostridium* group of organisms has an inherent resistance to the aminoglycosides. In endemic areas, oral penicillin or amoxycillin may be administered to neonates as soon as possible after birth in order to decrease the population of *C. perfringens* in the intestine.[22] The addition of bacitracin methylene disalicylate (250 g/ton) or virginiamycin (50 g/ton) to the feed of sows, starting two weeks pre-partum and continuing throughout the lactation period, is advantageous.[22]

As placental transfer of immunoglobulins from the dam to the foetus does not occur in pigs, horses or ruminants,[55] the prophylactic use of specific antiserum to the beta toxin of *C. perfringens* type C is advocated in order to protect new-born animals.[4, 10, 17, 22, 45] The antiserum may be administered orally or parenterally and provides passive protection within a short period of time (one to two hours), which persists for 14–20 days.[54] Antiserum is not commercially available in South Africa.

Bacterin/toxoid vaccines are produced and are commercially available in the USA, Europe, Australia and New Zealand. The application of a vaccination programme under field conditions is a satisfactory way to ensure protection against type C enterotoxaemia.[4, 45] Adequate antibody titres are induced when pregnant sows, cows or ewes which are being immunized for the first time are vaccinated twice at an interval of two to five weeks, with the second injection given two to three weeks before parturition.[2, 6, 13, 14, 32–34, 38, 47, 52] This procedure will ensure that their colostrum contains sufficient antitoxin levels to protect their offspring. High beta antitoxin titres are also induced when longer intervals between the vaccinations are allowed, for example, when gilts are vaccinated for the first time — preferably near breeding time and again two to three weeks before farrowing. Such immunized animals thereafter require only one booster vaccination, administered two to three weeks before farrowing in order to ensure adequate levels of antibodies in their colostrum.

The serum antitoxin titres of neonatal pigs are directly proportional to the colostral titres of their dams and are the highest on the second day after birth. The use of an autogenous bacterin vaccine in herds in which the disease is a problem seems to give better results than commercially-available bacterin/toxoids.[22] To maintain an adequate state of immune competency against beta toxin in a herd of pigs, it is essential that a vaccination programme should be maintained.

It has also been found that the subcutaneous injection of five millilitres of *C. perfringens* type C and D antitoxin in calves within eight hours of their birth is protective.[44]

Lambs actively immunized with a *C. perfringens* type C toxoid, are protected against infection with the organism following its introduction into the duodenum.[43] Lambs can also be protected at birth by the administration of lamb dysentery antiserum.[15] Adult sheep should also be immunized in the event of struck being diagnosed.

References

1 **ARBUCKLE, J.B.R., 1972.** The attachment of *Clostridium welchii (C. perfringens)* type C to intestinal villi of pigs. *Journal of Pathology,* 106, 65–72.

2 **ARDEHALI, M. & DARAKHSHAN, H., 1976.** Production and standardization of polyvalent *Clostridium perfringens* vaccine in Iran. *Development and Biological Standardization,* 32, 31–34.

3 **BATH, G., 1992.** University of Pretoria, Onderstepoort 0110, South Africa. Unpublished data.

4 **BERGELAND, M.E., 1972.** Pathogenesis and immunity of *Clostridium perfringens* type C enteritis in swine. *Journal of the American Veterinary Medical Association,* 160, 568–571.

5 **DICKIE, C.W., KLINKERMAN, D.L. & PETRIE, R.J., 1978.** Enterotoxaemia in two foals. *Journal of the Veterinary Medical Association,* 173, 306–307.

6 **DJURICKOVIC, S.M., DWORAK, J.E. & WICKHAM, K.L., 1975.** Antitoxin titer in colostrum and milk after vaccination of sows with *Clostridium perfringens* type C toxoid vaccine. *Veterinary Medicine and Small Animal Clinician,* 70, 283–285.

7 **DROLET, R., HIGGINS, R. & CÉCYRE, A., 1990.** Necrohemorrhagic enterocolitis caused by *Clostridium perfringens* type C in a foal. *Canadian Veterinary Journal,* 31, 449–450.

8 **EGERTON, J.R., 1966.** Bacteriology of enteritis necroticans in New Guinea highlanders. *Papua New Guinea Medical Journal,* 9, 5.

9 **EGERTON, J.R. & WALKER, P.D., 1964.** The isolation of *Clostridium perfringens* type C from necrotic enteritis of man in Papua-New Guinea. *Journal of Pathology and Bacteriology,* 80, 275–277.

10 **ENGLISH, J.E., 1966.** Field experience with *Clostridium* enterotoxaemia in young animals. *Journal of the American Veterinary Medical Association,* 149, 1565–1570.

11 **FIELD, H.I. & GOODWIN, R.F.W., 1959.** The experimental reproduction of enterotoxaemia in piglets. *Journal of Hygiene,* 57, 81–91.

12 **FINDLAY, C.R. & BUNTAIN, D., 1968.** Enterotoxaemia due to *Clostridium perfringens* type C in young lambs. *The Veterinary Record,* 82, 224–225.

13 **FLEENOR, W.A. & SCOTT, G.H., 1983.** Quantification of bovine IgG, IgM and IgA antibodies to *Clostridium perfringens* beta toxin by enzyme immunoassay. I. Preparturient immunization for enhancement of passive transfer of immunity. *Veterinary Immunology and Immunopathology,* 4, 579–591.

14 **FRERICHS, G.N. & GRAY, A.K., 1975.** The relation between the rabbit potency test and the response of sheep to sheep clostridial vaccines. *Research in Veterinary Science,* 18, 70–75.

15 **GREIG, A., 1975.** An outbreak of *Clostridium welchii* type C enterotoxaemia in young lambs in south west Scotland. *The Veterinary Record,* 96, 179.

16 **GRINER, L.A. & BRACKEN, F.K., 1953.** *Clostridium perfringens* type C in acute hemorrhagic enteritis of calves. *Journal of the American Veterinary Medical Association,* 122, 99–102.

17 **GRINER, L.A. & JOHNSON, H.W., 1954.** *Clostridium perfringens* type C in hemorrhagic enterotoxaemia of lambs. *Journal of the American Veterinary Medical Association,* 125, 125–127.

18 **HARMON, S.M., 1984.** *Clostridium perfringens:* Enumeration and identification. *In: Bacteriological Analytical Manual of the Division of Microbiology Center for Food Safety and Applied Nutrition, U.S. Food and Drug Administration.* 6th edn. Virginia: Association of Official Analytical Chemists.

19 **HENNING, M.W., 1949.** *Animal Diseases in South Africa.* 2nd edn. Pretoria: Central News Agency.

20 **HENNING, M.W., 1956.** *Animal Diseases in South Africa.* 3rd edn. Pretoria: Central News Agency.

21 **HENTON, M.M., 1992.** Onderstepoort Veterinary Institute, Private Bag X5, Onderstepoort 0110, South Africa. Personal communication.

22 **HOEFLING, D.C., 1989.** Recognizing diarrhea caused by *Clostridium perfringens* type C. *Veterinary Medicine,* 84, 437–441.

23 **HOGH, P., 1967.** Necrotizing infectious enteritis in piglets, caused by *Clostridium perfringens* type C. I. Biochemical and toxigenic properties of the Clostridium. *Acta Veterinaria Scandinavica,* 8, 26–38.

24 **HOGH, P., 1967.** Necrotizing infectious enteritis in piglets, caused by *Clostridium perfringens* type C. II. Incidence and clinical features. *Acta Veterinaria Scandinavica,* 8, 301–323.

25 **HOGH, P., 1969.** Necrotizing infectious enteritis in piglets, caused by *Clostridium perfringens* type C. III. Pathological changes. *Acta Veterinaria Scandinavica,* 10, 57–83.

26 **HOGH, P., 1969.** Necrotizing infectious enteritis in piglets, caused by *Clostridium perfringens* type C. IV. Bacteriological diagnosis. *Acta Veterinaria Scandinavica,* 10, 84–100.

27 **HOWARD-MARTIN, M., MORTON, R.J., QUALLS, C.W. & MACALLISTER, C.G., 1986.** *Clostridium perfringens* type C enterotoxaemia in a newborn foal. *Journal of the American Veterinary Medical Association,* 189, 564–565.

28 **JENSEN, R. & SWIFT, B.L., 1982.** *Diseases of Sheep.* 2nd edn. Philadelphia: Lea & Febiger.

29 **JOHANNSEN, U., ERWERTH, W., KUNZ, G. & KÖHLER, B., 1986.** Untersuchungen zur *Clostridium perfringens*-typ-C Enterotoxäemie (nekrotisierenden Enteritis) der Saugferkel. I. Mitteilung: Versuche zur experimentellen Erzeugung der Krankheit durch *Clostridium perfringens*-typ-C-Intoxikation (Versuchsansatz, klinisches Krankheitsbild, Sektionsbefunde). *Archiv experimentelle Veterinärmedizin,* Leipzig, 40, 811–825.

30 **JOHANNSEN, U., ERWERTH, W., KUNZ, G. & KÖHLER, B., 1986.** Untersuchungen zur *Clostridium perfringens*-typ-C Enterotoxäemie (nekrotisierenden Enteritis) der Saugferkel. III. Mitteilung: Licht- und elektronenmikroskopische Untersuchungen zur Pathologie und Pathogenese der experimentellen *Clostridium perfringens*-typ-C-Infektion. *Archiv experimentelle Veterinärmedizin,* Leipzig, 40, 895–909.

31 **JONES, R.L., ADNEY, W.S., ALEXANDER, A.F., SHIDELER, R.K., TRAUB-DARGATZ, J.L., 1988.** Hemorrhagic necrotizing enterocolitis associated with *Clostridium difficile* infection in four foals. *Journal of the American Veterinary Medical Association,* 193, 76–79.

32 **KENNEDY, K.K., NORRIS, S.J., BECKENHAUER, W.H. & WHITE, R.G., 1977.** Vaccination of cattle and sheep with a combined *Clostridium perfringens* types C and D toxoid. *The American Journal of Veterinary Research,* 38, 1515–1517.

33 **KENNEDY, K.K., NORRIS, S.J., BECKENHAUER, W.H. & WHITE, R.G., 1977.** Antitoxin response of cattle vaccinated with *Clostridium perfringens* type C toxoid. *Veterinary Medicine and Small Animal Clinician,* 72, 1213–1215.

34 **KERRY, J.B. & CRAIG, G.R., 1979.** Field studies in sheep with multicomponent clostridial vaccines. *The Veterinary Record,* 105, 551–554.

35 **LAWRENCE, G. & COOKE, R., 1980.** Experimental pigbel: The production and pathology of necrotizing enteritis due to *Clostridium welchii* type C in the guinea pig. *British Journal Experimental Pathology,* 61, 261–271.

36 **MANSSON, I. NORBERG, R., OLHAGEN, B. & BJORKLUND, N.E., 1971.** Arthritis in pigs induced by dietary factors. Microbiologic, clinical and histologic studies. *Clinical and Experimental Immunology,* 9, 677–693.

37 **MARTIN, P.K., NAYLOR, R.D. & SHARPE, R.T., 1988.** Detection of *Clostridium perfringens* toxin by enzyme-linked immunosorbent assay. *Research in Veterinary Science,* 44, 270–271.

38 **MATISHECK, P.H. & McGINLEY, M., 1986.** Colostral transfer of *Clostridium perfringens* type C beta antitoxin in swine. *American Journal of Veterinary Research,* 47, 1132–1133.

39 **McDONEL, J.L., 1986.** *Clostridium perfringens* toxins type A, B, C, D, E. *In:* DORNER, F. & DREW, J., (eds). *Pharmacology and Therapeutics.* Vol. X. Oxford: Pergamon Press.

40 **MURRELL, T.G.C. & ROTH, L., 1963.** Necrotizing jejunitis: A newly discovered disease in the highlands of New Guinea. *Medical Journal of Australia,* 1, 61.

41 **NIILO, L., 1986.** Experimental production of hemorrhagic enterotoxaemia by *Clostridium perfringens* type C in maturing lambs. *Canadian Journal Veterinary Research,* 50, 32–35.

42 **NIILO, L., 1987.** Toxigenic characteristics of *Clostridium perfringens* type C in enterotoxaemia of domestic animals. *Canadian Journal of Veterinary Research,* 51, 224–228.

43 **NIILO, L., 1988.** *Clostridium perfringens* type C enterotoxaemia. *Canadian Veterinary Journal,* 29, 658–664.

44 **NIILO, L., HARRIES, W.N. & JONES, G.A., 1974.** *Clostridium perfringens* type C in hemorrhagic enterotoxaemia of neonatal calves in Alberta. *Canadian Veterinary Journal,* 15, 224–226.

45 **OSTLE, A.G. & WELTER, C.J., 1987.** Using passive immunity to protect piglets from clostridial enterotoxaemia. *Veterinary Medicine,* July, 736–739.

46 **PEARSON, E.G., HEDSTROM, O.R., SONN, R. & WEDAM, J., 1986.** Hemorrhagic enteritis caused by *Clostridium perfringens* type C in a foal. *Journal of the American Veterinary Medical Association,* 188, 1309–1310.

47 **RIPLEY, P.H. & GUSH, A.F., 1983.** Immunization schedule for the prevention of infectious necrotic enteritis caused by *Clostridium perfringens* type C in piglets. *The Veterinary Record,* 112, 201–202.

48 **SIMS, L.D., TZIPORI, S., HAZARD, G.H. & CARROLL, C.L., 1985.** Haemorrhagic necrotizing enteritis in foals associated with *Clostridium perfringens. Australian Veterinary Journal,* 62, 194–196.

49 **SMITH, L.D.S., 1975.** *The Pathogenic Anaerobic Bacteria.* 2nd edn. Springfield, Illinois: Charles C. Thomas.

50 **SMITH, L.D.S. & WILLIAMS, B.L., 1984.** *The Pathogenic Anaerobic Bacteria.* 3rd edn. Springfield, Illinois: Charles C. Thomas.

51 **STERNE, M. & BATTY, I., 1975.** *Pathogenic Clostridia.* London and Boston: Butterworths.

52 **STERNE, M., BATTY, I., THOMSON, A. & ROBERTSON, J. M., 1962.** Immunization of sheep with multicomponent clostridial vaccines. *The Veterinary Record,* 74, 909–913.

53 **STERNE, M. & WARRACK, H.G., 1964.** The types of *C. perfringens. Journal of Pathology and Bacteriology,* 88, 279–283.

54 **TIZARD, I., 1987.** *Veterinary Immunology, An Introduction.* 3rd edn. London: W.B. Saunders Company.

55 **WOOLCOCK, J.B., 1979.** *Bacterial Infection and Immunity in Domestic Animals.* Oxford: Elsevier Scientific Publishing Company.

56 **ZEISSLER, J. & RASSFELD-STERNBERG, L., 1949.** Enteritis necroticans due to *Clostridium welchii* type F. *British Medical Journal,* 1, 267.

Clostridium perfringens *type D enterotoxaemia*

Synonyms: Pulpy kidney disease, enterotoxaemia, overeating disease, bloednier (Afrik.).

N.P.J. Kriek, M.W. Odendaal and P. Hunter

Introduction

Pulpy kidney disease is a peracute, acute or occasionally chronic infectious enterotoxaemic disease that is common in sheep, uncommon in goats, and virtually unknown in cattle. It is caused by the systemic effects of *Clostridium perfringens* type D epsilon toxin which is absorbed into the general circulation from the intestinal tract, where it is elaborated by the rapidly multiplying organisms. Pulpy kidney disease in sheep affects animals of any age, but young animals in good condition are particularly susceptible. Predisposing factors, such as sudden changes in diet from poor to good quality, precipitate the occurrence of the disease. Peracute and acute cases are characterized by sudden death, and chronic cases by the development of a neurological syndrome that results from focal symmetrical encephalomalacia (FSE). In goats, the disease may be peracute, as in sheep, or it may manifest as an acute or chronic diarrhoea terminating in death, or as a chronic, lingering and debilitating condition.[4] The differences between the disease in sheep and in goats relate, in general, to clinical signs and responses to treatment and vaccination.[4]

Pulpy kidney disease occurs all over the world wherever small ruminants are maintained. It was first described by Gilruth in New Zealand in 1903, and thereafter in Australia, Great Britain, the USA and South Africa. The association of an unknown potent toxin with the pathogenesis of this disease was first demonstrated by Montgomerie and Rowlands in 1931, and by other authors in 1933 and 1934. The organism, then referred to as *Bacillus ovitoxicus*, was isolated in 1932.[22] The bacterium, now known as *C. perfringens* type D, occurs in large numbers in the intestinal tract of normal sheep without causing any clinical signs and can be regarded as an obligate parasite.[6, 48]

In South Africa it is believed that many of the cases diagnosed as 'geilsiekte' (prussic acid poisoning) in the past were in fact pulpy kidney disease.[47] That the disease remains one of the most important diseases of sheep in South Africa today is confirmed by annual vaccine sales which exceed 50 million doses.

Aetiology

Clostridium perfringens type D has the same morphological and biochemical characteristics as the other members of the *C. perfringens* group and produces two major lethal toxins, alpha and epsilon, and a number of minor toxins which may be either lethal or non-lethal **(see *Clostridium perfringens* group: Introduction)**.

Epsilon toxin, the significant major toxin and cause of pulpy kidney disease, is produced as a prototoxin.[29, 36, 37, 45, 55, 57, 58] Its *in vitro* production is dependent on the presence of suitable conditions, which must include optimal pH and the availability of an appropriate carbohydrate source.[20, 21]

Epidemiology

Pulpy kidney disease is one of the most important diseases of sheep in southern Africa, as it is in many other parts of the world. It occurs in sheep of all ages, but most commonly in lambs of two age groups: from three weeks to three months, and from six to 12 months of age. Cases of *C. perfringens* type D enterotoxaemia have been reported in seven- to ten-week old calves,[19] in young cattle in good condition up to two years old, [27] as well as in adult animals.[34] Though cattle of all ages may be affected, it is mainly a disease of calves and young cattle up to two years of age in feedlots. In the USA, *C. perfringens* type D is associated with overeating disease or sudden death of feedlot cattle. As opposed to the disease in sheep, it only affects individual animals over a period.[27] Pulpy kidney disease has been reported to be a major disease of dairy goats in some countries, but not in South Africa.[3] *Clostridium perfringens* type D is harboured in the alimentary tract of animals as an obligate parasite. Small numbers occur in the forestomachs, except the abomasum. The numbers increase towards the ileum, where most *C. perfringens* organisms are found. Conditions here are ideal for the organisms to multiply under normal conditions. The numbers become less in the large intestine, but sufficient numbers of the organism are excreted in the faeces to allow its isolation. As is the case with type B, type D isolates are not considered part of the microbial soil flora, as they cannot compete with type A isolates in this habitat. *Clostridium perfringens* type D is, however, able to survive for a number of months in soil before dying.[48, 50]

There appear to be several predisposing factors which precipitate the occurrence of the disease. These include stasis of the intestinal tract; sudden changes in the feeding regimen; sudden changes from poor to lush pastures; grazing on fodder crops, such as green oats, green wheat and green lucerne (alfalfa); very high protein diets; overeating on concentrates and lush pastures;[23] deworming; and coccidiosis.[38] Sudden changes in the weather and wilting of pasture grasses have also been recorded as playing predisposing roles. Under experimental conditions pulpy kidney disease is induced within 25 hours of infusion of *C. perfringens* type D cultures.[4] For sheep the introduction period may vary from two to five days under natural conditions.

Focal symmetrical encephalomalacia may occur either as a sporadic disease involving one or a small number of sheep, or in outbreak form. Sheep of all ages are affected, although it is often found that when FSE does make its appearance in a flock, two specific age groups of animals are particularly affected: weaner lambs up to the age of 10–12 weeks, and mature sheep three years of age or older.[17] The factors which predispose to FSE are the same as those for pulpy kidney disease, with cases often preceded by a change to a lush pasture or by anthelmintic drenching. Focal symmetrical encephalomalacia is more likely to occur in flocks with a partial immunity to *C. perfringens* type D. The interval between the predisposing factor and the appearance of clinical signs is usually seven to 14 days, but it may be as short as two days.

Pathogenesis

Clostridium perfringens type D present as a commensal in the lumen of the intestinal tract proliferates profusely when conditions in the intestinal lumen become suitable for it to do so, such as those which may arise when the diet is suddenly changed from a poor to rich one, or if an animal engorges on palatable feed. Ruminal flora become adapted to the diet that the animal is eating, and if the diet is changed, a period lasting several days is required for the flora to readapt to the new conditions. The ruminal flora of an animal consuming veld grass consists of a high starch proportion of cellulolytic organisms. If its feed is suddenly changed to one with a high starch content (such as one of the cereals), particles of starch, which would be converted to low chain fatty acids in the rumen of an animal adapted to such a diet, pass unchanged from the rumen into the intestine. Here the starch is utilized by the saccharolytic *C. perfringens* type D, which multiplies rapidly and elaborates large amounts of epsilon toxin,[6] as well as its other toxins. The appearance of starch granules in the small intestine may increase the viable colony count of *C. perfringens* type D to as many as 10^9 organisms per gram of intestinal content (with a correspondingly high concentration of epsilon toxin) within a few hours.[7] Epsilon toxin is produced in small amounts in the intestines of *C. perfringens* type D carrier animals, but these amounts are too small to engender any deleterious effects, although they can stimulate antibody formation. It has been shown that up to 54 per cent of animals in an unvaccinated flock may contain serum epsilon antitoxin titres.[3]

Epsilon toxin is produced in the small intestines as a virtually non-toxic prototoxin which is activated by trypsin and chymotrypsin, but not by pepsin in the intestinal tract. Activation increases the toxicity by at least a thousand-fold.[6, 41] Small amounts of the epsilon toxin in the intestinal tract have no effect on the intestinal mucosa, but large concentrations increase its permeability so that within a number of hours large amounts are absorbed into the systemic circulation.[6] The mu toxin of *C. perfringens* type D also increases the permeability of the mucosa. Epsilon toxin is endotheliotoxic and, after binding to receptor sites on capillary endothelial cells, systemically absorbed epsilon toxin causes an increased permeability of capillaries in many organs, including those in the intestinal mucosa, thus further enhancing the absorption of the toxin.[41]

Epsilon toxin selectively binds to the luminal surface of the endothelium of capillaries of the brain and, to a lesser extent, of other organs, such as capillaries in the kidneys that surround the loops of Henlé and the distal convoluted tubules and the hepatic sinusoids.[11] The extracellular oedema that develops in the brain is the result of the breakdown of the tight junctions of the vascular endothelium, and is responsible for the main clinical signs of pulpy kidney disease,[11] particularly the neurological signs that are manifested by acute cases.

In FSE, the lesions in the brain progress sequentially, within a period of seven days, from an initial vasogenic oedema to the development of bilaterally symmetrical malacic foci that principally involve the white matter of certain areas of the brain.[13]

The majority of animals suffering from pulpy kidney disease become hyperglycaemic and glycosuric, but the precise pathogenetic mechanisms responsible for this development remain unresolved. Several hypotheses have, however, been suggested, such as glycogenolysis of hepatic reserves, stimulation of cAMP by hepatocyte-bound epsilon toxin, the release of catecholomines (which activate cAMP) due to the brain oedema,[8, 9, 16, 56] or reflex hypersecretion of adrenalin from the adrenal medulla in response to oedema of the hypothalamus.

The reason why many goats respond to the effects of the toxin differently from sheep is not known.[4]

Clinical signs

The course of the acute form of the disease in lambs is very short — often less than two hours — and very rarely more than 12 hours.[5] Many animals are, however, found dead without any premonitory signs of illness being noticed. Usually the first indication of the disease in a flock is the finding in the morning of sheep which have died overnight.

When affected animals are closely observed, the first transient signs to be noticed include dullness, depression, facial movements and loss of appetite. Signs preceding death indicate severe neurological derangement and include hypersensitivity, listlessness, hyperaesthesia, staggering gait, knuckling of the fetlocks, ataxia progressing to recumbency, clonic convulsions, opisthotonus, marked salivation, stertorous respiration between convulsions, and terminal coma.[11, 23] The body temperature is usually normal but may become elevated if the convulsions are severe. Young lambs, three to four weeks old, may suffer from colic and manifest abdominal bloating before death supervenes.[33] Manifestations of the disease in adult sheep are similar to those in lambs, but the course of the disease in some may be as long as 24 hours.

The clinical signs of FSE vary according to the acuteness of the disease and involve only those which indicate impairment of the central nervous and alimentary systems. Two different syndromes are seen: an acute neurological disorder — the so-called 'stagger syndrome', in which sheep are unable to stand, with death occurring within 24 hours — and a more chronic condition — the 'dummy syndrome', in which the sheep can stand but show general weakness or paresis when handled.[17] In the field, animals suffering from the latter syndrome usually die within seven days of developing clinical signs, but they may linger for up to 14 days. If nursed, they may survive for a longer period. Animals suffering from either of these syndromes have no consistent abnormalities in body temperature or respiratory or heart rates.

An animal suffering from the acute syndrome of FSE is usually found in lateral recumbency and comatose but, when stimulated, shows normal or exaggerated motor responses. It appears to be blind, lacks the eye-preservation reflex, and develops opisthotonus when handled. Spontaneous convulsions are rare. Nystagmus is seen in about a quarter of affected animals. The rumen is usually atonic and the faeces invariably soft and pasty.[17]

Animals suffering from the 'dummy syndrome' lose their fear of dogs and humans, wander around aimlessly, and manifest head-pressing and teeth-grinding. Severely affected sheep lack fine muscular co-ordination and are blind. The sheep are inappetent and show paralysis of the muscles of prehension, thus losing their ability to eat and drink. There is usually ruminal stasis and the faeces are pasty and unformed. When lying, they assume a position of sternal recumbency, which is also the position in which they die.[17]

Three syndromes of *C. perfringens* type D enterotoxaemia have been reported in goats. The peracute or 'sudden death' syndrome is similar to that in sheep. The acute syndrome is characterized by an acute diarrhoea and signs of abdominal discomfort, often culminating in recovery or death two to four days after the onset of clinical signs. The chronic syndrome may persist for days or weeks, and is characterized by diarrhoea and progressive weight loss.[3, 4]

Clostridium perfringens type D enterotoxaemia in cattle generally occurs in the form of sporadic outbreaks. The peracute disease is characterized by sudden death, and the acute by nervous signs and a subnormal body temperature. The animals appear dull and listless, and wander around aimlessly. There are signs of colic and salivation, and when they become prostrate, they assume a position of lateral recumbency and manifest opisthotonus. They show depression, anorexia and appear to be blind before expiring or recovering completely.[19, 34, 39]

Pathology

Sheep that have died from pulpy kidney disease are usually in good condition. The rapid onset of post-mortem changes is characteristic, particularly those in the kidneys, which develop more quickly than those in other organs, with the rapid autolysis soon reducing the renal cortices to a pulpy mass[15, 23] **(Figure 157.1)**.

Lesions in sheep dying from the peracute to acute disease are not constant and may be virtually absent in some. When present, one or more of the following may be observed to some degree: varying numbers of petechial or ecchymotic haemorrhages in the subcutis of the dorsal region of the neck, shoulders and rump; petechial or ecchymotic haemorrhages in the parietal peritoneum, muscles of the flank, the muscular portion of the diaphragm, epicardium and endocardium, especially that of the left ventricle, and thymus; an excessive amount of fluid in the pericardial sac, which clots partially when exposed to air; congestion and oedema of the lungs; distension of the small intestine, which may be patchily congested and contain gas (even in a 'fresh' carcass); mild to moderate nephrosis and partial ('blotchy') to complete congestion of the renal cortices (the degree of post-mortem changes present in the kidneys may be gauged by comparing them to those in the liver; in addition, these changes may result in the post-mortem degeneration and rupture of the walls of small blood vessels and the consequent presence of small, scattered, cortical haemorrhages — the renal congestion and haemorrhages giving rise to the Afrikaans name of 'bloednier' for the disease); and glycosuria, which may disappear with the passage of time due to the post-mortem growth of bacteria in the urine. In the majority of cases there is no macroscopic evidence of enteritis in animals dying peracutely, although intestinal congestion is present in some cases. In very young lambs dying of pulpy kidney disease, the abomasum may rupture terminally.[33]

The most prominent haematological and biochemical changes occurring in lambs after the parenteral

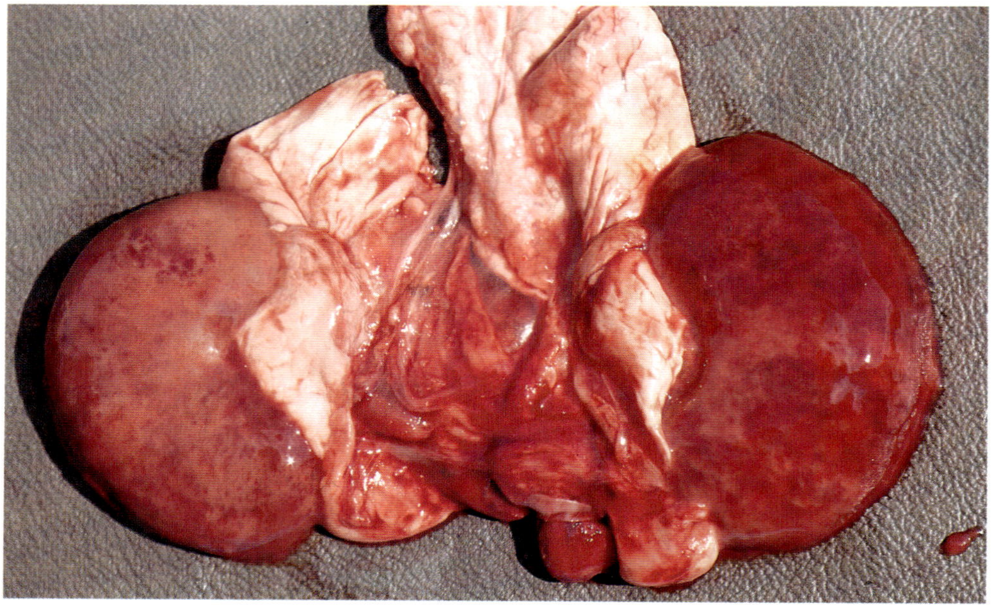

Figure 157.1 Pulpy, haemorrhagic kidneys typical of pulpy kidney disease

administration of epsilon toxin include haemoconcentration (anhydraemia), metabolic acidosis, hyperglycaemia, glycosuria, and an elevation of the blood concentrations of pyruvate, lactate and alpha-ketoglutarate as a result of the increase in circulating glucose.[14]

In goats that have died of the peracute disease, lesions may be similar to those in sheep. In the acute to chronic disease, severe pulmonary oedema and changes in the intestinal tract are the most consistent lesions. Hydropericardium containing fibrin clots, similar to that in sheep, is not always present in these animals.[4] The lesions in the intestinal tract are those of a fibrinous to fibrinonecrotic enterocolitis. The intestinal content may be green or reddish-tinged and mucoid. The presence of mucofibrinous casts in the lumen of the large intestine is a constant finding.[4] Mesenteric lymph nodes are swollen and oedematous.

In sheep that have died from FSE, the only lesions consistently present, although they are frequently microscopic, occur in the brain. Those that have suffered from the acute FSE syndrome may also manifest some of the lesions present in pulpy kidney disease. Lesions in the brain are bilaterally symmetrical and two general patterns of distribution are recognized; areas of leukoencephalomalacia may be present in the internal capsule, dorsolateral thalamus, substantia nigra, basal ganglia and cerebellar peduncles,[17] the most constant sites being the thalamus and the midbrain areas[11] or the white matter of the frontal lobes. Areas of malacia are better seen in formalin-fixed brain tissue.

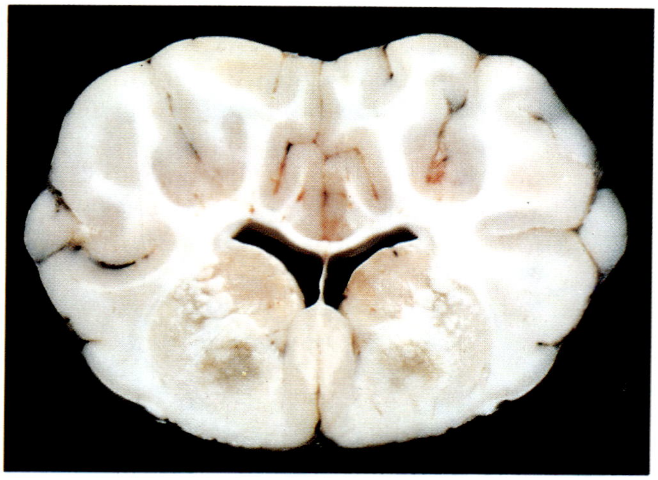

Figure 157.2 Bilateral symmetrical malacia in corpus striatum of a sheep that died of focal symmetrical encephalomalacia

Three basic histologic lesions occur in the brain of sheep affected by FSE.[10] These are widespread perivascular oedema, perivascular haemorrhage and malacia **(Figure 157.2)**. Areas of malacia are always focal and sharply demarcated, and are often accompanied by haemorrhage, but lack an inflammatory reaction.[10] Ultrastructurally, there is swelling of astrocytes, the perivascular oedema being caused by their swollen end-feet, and severe damage to vascular endothelium is apparent.[11]

No consistent clinical pathological changes are encountered in sheep suffering from FSE. In some, however, hyperglycaemia and glycosuria may be present.[17]

Lesions in cattle closely resemble those of pulpy kidney disease in sheep.

Differential diagnosis

Diseases and conditions known to cause sudden death, and in particular other clostridial enterotoxaemias, such as that caused by *Clostridium sordellii*,[46] should be considered as differential diagnoses. Diseases of particular importance in the differential diagnosis of pulpy kidney disease include heartwater, bluetongue, Rift Valley fever, the plant poisonings leading to sudden death, such as gousiekte ('quick death') due to *Pachystigma pygmaeum* and certain other members of the family, gifblaar ('poison leaf') poisoning caused by ingestion of *Dichapetalum cymosum* which contains monofluoroacetate as the toxic principal, and plants containing cyanogenetic glycosides which are responsible for prussic acid poisoning ['geilsiekte' (Afrik.)], nutritional myopathy (white muscle disease), and ruminal acidosis due to the overeating of grains.

Listeriosis and nutritional myopathy in calves, milk fever in cows and acute lead poisoning may be confused with enterotoxaemia.[39]

Focal symmetrical encephalomalacia may be confused clinically with cases of hypocalcaemia, copper deficiency, colisepticaemia, pregnancy toxaemia, coenuriosis, cerebrocortical necrosis, cranial abscessation, botulism and tick paralysis.

Diagnosis

A presumptive diagnosis of *C. perfringens* type D enterotoxaemia may be based on the clinical signs, lesions and history as well as on the demonstration of the presence of epsilon toxin and *C. perfringens* type D in the intestinal content. Confirmation of the diagnosis is, however, not always easy, as the causative organisms are normal commensals in the intestinal tract and epsilon toxin may occur in the intestinal lumen of animals immune to the toxin but which have died from other diseases. In addition, failure to demonstrate the presence of the toxin in a typical case does not necessarily preclude the diagnosis of pulpy kidney disease.[10]

Additional evidence for the confirmation of the disease may be obtained by histological examination of the brain of sheep. Even though signs of malacia may only be macroscopically present in about 30 per cent of cases, histologically the combined presence of severe oedema, haemorrhages and malacia in the brain stem and midbrain areas is highly suggestive of pulpy kidney disease and is considered by some to be the most reliable way of diagnosing enterotoxaemia in sheep.[17] The malacic areas are invariably focal and bilaterally symmetrical.[10]

Demonstration of low serum antibody levels on a flock basis may provide further supporting evidence for the diagnosis. Epsilon antitoxin levels exceeding 0,15 units/ml virtually exclude a diagnosis of pulpy kidney disease.

Appropriate specimens should be submitted for confirmation of the diagnosis of pulpy kidney disease **(see *Clostridium perfringens* group: Introduction)**.

In order to determine the immune status of the flock, individual samples, each consisting of 10 ml of serum, from at least ten different animals should be submitted.

Specimens from dead animals should be taken as soon as possible after death. As putrefactive changes interfere with diagnostic procedures and may preclude the making of a diagnosis, those for bacteriological and toxicological examination should be collected using aseptic techniques and, together with the samples of urine, effusions and serum samples, should immediately be refrigerated or packed in ice and kept in the cold state until received by the diagnostic laboratory.

Several *in vitro* immunological assays for the detection of epsilon toxin in specimens are available. A reverse-phase, passive haemaglutination assay (RPHA) detects concentrations of epsilon toxin as low as 6×10^{-7} mg/ml, whereas the single radial immunodiffusion technique is only capable of detecting epsilon toxin above the level of 0,01 mg/ml.[2] Counter-immunoelectrophoresis is more effective than the older mouse-protection assay for the detection of epsilon toxin in the intestinal contents.[26] An ELISA has also been developed as an alternative to the mouse neutralization test. It is faster, giving qualitative results in four hours, and is more sensitive than the mouse test,[40] but cross-reactions with other clostridial toxins may complicate the interpretation of the results of this assay.

For the diagnosis of FSE, the whole brain of the affected animal should be preserved in an adequate quantity of 10 per cent formalin solution for histopathological examination.

Control

Animals affected by pulpy kidney disease invariably die too rapidly to allow any form of treatment. During outbreaks of enterotoxaemia, further deaths may be minimized in the interval between vaccination and the onset of active immunity by treating sheep with long-acting tetracyclines.[1]

Management practices should be altered to reduce conditions which are known to predispose to *C. perfringens* type D enterotoxaemia. In lambs, tail-docking, castration and marking should be performed at an early age so as not to cause a reduction in feed and milk intake, as these are conducive to the development of the condition.[33] It is also recommended that management practices be designed to avoid sudden changes in the diet of animals, particularly from a poor to a carbohydrate-rich one. If such changes are anticipated, animals should be vaccinated prior to the event.[3] It may be advisable to vaccinate before drenching with anthelmintics if a flock's immune status is in doubt.

Natural exposure of sheep and goats to epsilon toxin does not, with few exceptions, stimulate the induction of serum antitoxin titres of sufficient magnitude so that they will provide protection against the effects of the toxin when it becomes elaborated in the intestinal tract in such quantities that overt disease is precipitated.[3, 18] Effective control of the disease cannot be accomplished without the application of immunoprophylactic measures. Adequate serum levels of epsilon antitoxin give complete protection against *C. perfringens* type D enterotoxaemia.

Serum antibody levels of at least 0,15 international units of epsilon antitoxin/ml are sufficient to protect sheep against the experimentally induced disease.[28]

An alum-precipitated *C. perfringens* type D (pulpy kidney) epsilon-toxoid vaccine is used to protect lambs from pulpy kidney disease.[24, 30, 52] Good immunity is induced by two vaccinations at a monthly interval, but it is short-lived, lasting only 15 weeks.[31] Emulsifying the epsilon toxoid in complete or incomplete Freund's adjuvant induces the development of an adequate level of immunity which persists for two years after a single injection,[31] but this formulation unfortunately gives rise to unacceptable tissue reactions at the site of inoculation. Thomson and Batty[53] overcame this problem by formulating an oil-emulsion vaccine in which Arlacel A and Tween 80 were used as emulsifiers. This formulation was most effective when tested in a multicomponent vaccine, containing all the clostridial antigens of veterinary importance to be found in adult sheep.[54] Vitamin E ([dl]-α-tocopherol acetate) has also been used successfully as an adjuvant when mixed with *C. perfringens* type D epsilon toxoid in weaned lambs.[51] A number of multicomponent clostridial vaccines are available which, *inter alia,* protect against pulpy kidney disease.

Young lambs between two and 44 days of age do not respond well to immunization against pulpy kidney disease.[25, 49] The presence of colostrum derived passive immunity in lambs born of immune dams protects them for 13–19 weeks[32] and does not interfere with their ability to respond to active immunization.[42, 43] The vaccine regimen in lambs two to three months of age should consist of the administration either of two doses of an oil adjuvant vaccine at an interval of four weeks, or of an oil adjuvant vaccine followed four weeks later by an alum-precipitated vaccine. This gives rise to a good immune response which remains effective for at least six to eight months. An alum-precipitated vaccine given as a booster at this stage results in an immunity which lasts for at least a year.[12] Annual immunization thereafter with an alum-precipitated vaccine should provide sufficient protection against *C. perfringens* type D enterotoxaemia. Animals vaccinated for the first time against the disease show serum antibody titres after a period of 10–14 days.[35] Adult animals vaccinated for the first time are given the oil-adjuvant vaccine followed four to six weeks later by the alum-precipitated vaccine. This is repeated after six to eight months, and thereafter annually.

In order to provide young lambs with a colostrum-derived passive immunity which will protect them until they are old enough to be actively immunized (i.e. older than 45 days), pregnant ewes may be vaccinated. Ewes which have been previously inoculated require only a single vaccination four weeks before lambing, while those which have not been previously immunized should be vaccinated twice, at an interval of four to six weeks, the second injection being given about four weeks before lambing.

The antibody response of goats to vaccination is similar to that of sheep, but in spite of the development, following repeated vaccinations, of serum antibody levels which should be protective, the disease itself is not effectively controlled. The administration of the vaccine to goats may, in addition, give rise to the development of persistent lumps at the site of the injection, which may be confused with caseous lymphadenitis lesions.[3]

A new development in biotechnology has led to the production and use of an anti-idiotypic antibody against the epsilon toxin of *Clostridium perfringens* type D. This anti-idiotypic antibody recognizes variable-region determinants on specific antigen-binding antibodies. It has been demonstrated that this anti-idiotypic antibody can be used to generate an immune response against the epsilon toxin in animals which have not been exposed to the toxin.[44]

References

1 **BATH, G., 1993.** Faculty of Veterinary Science, University of Pretoria, Onderstepoort 0110 South Africa. Personal communication.

2 **BEH, K.J. & BUTTERY, S.H., 1978.** Reverse-phase passive haemagglutination and single radial immunodiffusion to detect epsilon antigen of *Clostridium perfringens* type D. *Australian Veterinary Journal*, 54, 541–544.

3 **BLACKWELL, T.E., BUTLER, D.G. & BELL, J.A., 1983.** Enterotoxaemia in the goat: The humoral response and local tissue reaction following vaccination with two different bacterin-toxoids. *Canadian Journal of Comparative Medicine,* 47, 127–132.

4 **BLACKWELL, T.E., BUTLER, D.G., PRESCOTT, J.F., WILCOCK, B.P., 1991.** Differences in signs and lesions in sheep and goats with enterotoxaemia induced by intraduodenal infusion of *Clostridium perfringens* type D. *American Journal of Veterinary Research,* 52, 1147–1152.

5 **BLOOD, D.C. & HENDERSON, J.A., 1968.** *Veterinary Medicine.* 3rd edn. London: Baillière, Tindall & Cassell.

6 **BULLEN, J.J., 1970.** Role of toxins in host-parasite relationships. *In:* KADIS, S., MONTIE, T.C. & AJL, S.J., (eds). *Microbial Toxins,* Vol. IIA. New York & London: Academic Press, Inc.

7 **BULLEN, J.J. & SCARISBRICK, R., 1957.** Enterotoxaemia of sheep: Experimental reproduction of the disease. *Journal of Pathology and Bacteriology,* 73, 495–509.

8 **BUXTON, D., 1978.** Further studies on the mode of action of *Clostridium welchii* type D epsilon toxin. *Journal of Medical Microbiology,* 11, 293–298.

9 **BUXTON, D., 1978.** *In vitro* effects of *Clostridium welchii* type D epsilon toxin on guinea-pig, mouse, rabbit and sheep cells. *Journal of Medical Microbiology,* 11, 299–302.

10 **BUXTON, D., LINKLATER, K.A. & DYSON, D.A., 1978.** Pulpy kidney disease and its diagnosis by histological examination. *The Veterinary Record,* 102, 241.

11 **BUXTON, D. & MORGAN, K.T., 1976.** Studies of lesions produced in the brains of colostrum-deprived lambs by *Clostridium welchii (C. perfringens)* type D toxin. *Journal of Comparative Pathology*, 86, 435–447.

12 **CAMERON, C.M., 1980.** Effective immunization of lambs against enterotoxaemia. *Onderstepoort Journal of Veterinary Research*, 47, 287–289.

13 **FINNIE, J.W., 1984.** Histopathological changes in the brain of mice given *Clostridium perfringens* type D epsilon toxin. *Journal of Comparative Pathology*, 94, 363–370.

14 **GARDNER, D.E., 1973.** Pathology of *Clostridium welchii* type D enterotoxaemia. I. Biochemical and haematological alterations in lambs. *Journal of Comparative Pathology*, 83, 499–507.

15 **GARDNER, D.E., 1973.** Pathology of *Clostridium welchii type* D enterotoxaemia. II. Structural and ultrastructural alterations in the tissues of lambs and mice. *Journal of Comparative Pathology*, 83, 509–524.

16 **GARDNER, D.E., 1973.** Pathology of *Clostridium welchii* type D enterotoxaemia. III. Basis of the hyperglycaemic response. *Journal of Comparative Pathology*, 83, 525–529.

17 **GAY, C.C., BLOOD, D.C. & WILKINSON, J.S., 1975.** Clinical observations of sheep with focal symmetrical encephalomalacia. *Australian Veterinary Journal*, 51, 266–269.

18 **GRINER, L.A., 1961.** Enterotoxaemia of sheep. III. *Clostridium perfringens* type D antitoxin titres of normal, nonvaccinated lambs. *American Journal of Veterinary Research*, 22, 447–448.

19 **GRINER, L.A., AICHELMAN, W.W. & BROWN, G.D., 1956.** *Clostridium perfringens* type D (epsilon) enterotoxaemia in Brown Swiss dairy calves. *Journal of the American Veterinary Medical Association*, 129, 375–376.

20 **HAUSCHILD, A.H.W., 1966.** Selective effect of pH on the production of exocellular protein by *Clostridium perfringens* type D. *Journal of Bacteriology*, 92, 800–801.

21 **HAUSCHILD, A.H.W. & PIVNICK, H., 1965.** Effect of carbohydrates on toxigenesis by *Clostridium perfringens* type D. *Canadian Journal of Microbiology*, 11, 15–22.

22 **HENNING, M.W., 1949.** *Animal Diseases in South Africa.* 2nd edn. Pretoria: Central News Agency.

23 **HENNING, M.W., 1956.** *Animal Diseases in South Africa.* 3rd edn. Pretoria: Central News Agency.

24 **HEPPLE, J.R., CHODNICK, K.S. & PRICE, E.K., 1959.** Immunization of lambs against *Clostridium welchii* type D enterotoxaemia (pulpy kidney disease) with a purified toxoid, aluminium treated. *The Veterinary Record*, 71, 201–207.

25 **HOEFLER, W.C. & HALLFORD, D.M., 1985.** Growth response and survival rates of lambs immunized against enterotoxaemia and/or treated with enterotoxaemia antotoxin. *Agri-Practice — Ovine Medicine*, 6, 22–25.

26 **HORNITSKY, M., ROMALIS, L.F., ROSS, A.D. & SHELDRAKE, R.F., 1989.** Comparison of counterimmunoelectrophoresis with mouse protection assay in the detection of epsilon toxin in the intestinal contents of goats. *Australian Veterinary Journal*, 66, 121–122.

27 **HUNGERFORD, T.G., 1990.** *Diseases of Livestock.* 9th edn. Sydney: McGraw-Hill Book Company.

28 **JANSEN, B.C., 1960.** The experimental reproduction of pulpy kidney disease. *Journal of the South African Veterinary Medical Association*, 31, 205–208.

29 **JANSEN, B.C., 1965.** Enterotoxaemia: An immunological study. DSc thesis. Potchefstroom University for a Christian Higher Education.

30 **JANSEN, B.C., 1967.** The production of a basic immunity against pulpy kidney disease. *Onderstepoort Journal of Veterinary Research*, 34, 65–80.

31 **JANSEN, B.C., 1967.** The duration of immunity to pulpy kidney disease of sheep. *Onderstepoort Journal of Veterinary Research*, 34, 333–344.

32 **JANSEN, B.C., 1976.** The standardization of *Cl. perfringens* antigens and antisera. *Developments in Biological Standardization*, 32, 35–44.

33 **JOUBERT, J.P., VERMEULEN, S.O.& KELLERMAN, G.E., 1987.** Bloednier in die suiplam (in Afrikaans). *Journal of the South African Veterinary Association*, 58, 43.

34 **KEAST, J.C. & McBARRON, E.J., 1954.** A case of bovine enterotoxaemia. *The Australian Veterinary Journal*, 30, 305–306.

35 **KENNEDY, K.K., NORRIS, S.J., BECKENHAUER, W.H. & WHITE, R.G., 1977.** Vaccination of cattle and sheep with a combined *Clostridium perfrigens* types C and D toxoid. *American Journal of Veterinary Research*, 38, 1515–1517.

36 **KULSHRESTHA, S.B., 1974.** Effect of carbohydrates on the production of lethal toxin by *Clostridium perfringens* types B and C with particular reference to beta toxin and epsilon toxin. *Indian Journal of Animal Science*, 43, 628–631.

37 **KULSHRESTHA, S.B., 1974.** Effect of period of incubation and pH on the production of beta and epsilon toxins by *Clostridium welchii* type B and type C. *Indian Journal of Animal Science*, 43, 987–990.

38 **MARSH, H. & TUNNICLIFF, E.A., 1944.** Enterotoxaemia in feedlot lambs in connection with an outbreak of coccidiosis. *Journal of the American Veterinary Medical Association*, 104, 13–14.

39 **MUMFORD, D.H., 1961.** Enterotoxaemia in cattle. *The Australian Veterinary Journal*, 37, 122–126.

40 **NAYLOR, R.D., MARTIN, P.K. & SHARPE, R.T., 1987.** Detection of *Clostridium perfringens* epsilon toxin by ELISA. *Research in Veterinary Science*, 42, 255–256.

41 **NIILO, L., 1986.** Enterotoxemic *Clostridium perfringens. In:* GYLES, C.L. & THOEN, C.O., (eds). *Pathogenesis of Bacterial Infections in Animals.* Ames, Iowa: Iowa State University Press.

42 **ODENDAAL, M.W., VISSER, J.J., BERG, N. & BOTHA, W.J.S., 1989.** The effect of passive immunization on active immunity against *Clostridium perfringens* type D in lambs. *Onderstepoort Journal of Veterinary Research*, 56, 251–255.

43 **OXER, D.T., MINTY, D.W. & LIEFMAN, C.E., 1971.** Vaccination trials in sheep with clostridial vaccines, with special reference to passively acquired *Clostridium welchii* type D antitoxin in lambs. *Australian Veterinary Journal*, 47, 134–140.

44 **PERCIVAL, D.A., SHUTTLEWORTH, A.D., WILLIAMSON, E.D. & KELLY, D.C., 1990.** Anti-idiotypic antibody-induced protection against *Clostridium perfringens* type D. *Infection and Immunity*, 58, 2487–2492.

45 **PIVNICK, H., HAUSCHILD, A.H., GORENSTEIN, B. & HABEEB, A.F, 1965.** Effect of controlled pH on toxigenesis by *Clostridium perfringens* type D. *Canadian Journal of Microbiology*, 11, 45–55.

46 **POPOFF, M.R., 1984.** Bacteriological examination in enterotoxaemia of sheep and lamb. *The Veterinary Record*, 114, 324.

47 **SCHULZ, K.C.A. & McINTYRE, C., 1948.** Preliminary report on an infectious enterotoxaemia-like disease in sheep. *Journal of the South African Veterinary Medical Association*, 19, 93–99.

48 **SMITH, L.D.S., 1975.** *The Pathogenic Anaerobic Bacteria,* 2nd edn. Springfield, Illinois: Charles C. Thomas.

49 **SMITH, L.D.S. & MARSH, H., 1953.** The immunization of young lambs against enterotoxaemia. *American Journal of Veterinary Research*, 14, 408–410.

50 **SMITH, L.D.S. & WILLIAMS, B.L., 1984.** *The Pathogenic Anaerobic Bacteria.* 3rd edn. Springfield, Illinois: Charles C. Thomas.

51 **TENGERDY, R.P., MEYER, D.L., LAUERMAN, L.H., LUEKER, D.C. & NOCKELS, C.F., 1983.** Vitamin E-enhanced humoral antibody response to *Clostridium perfringens* type D in sheep. *British Veterinary Journal*, 139, 147–151.

52 **THOMSON, A. & BATTY, I., 1953.** The antigenic efficiency of pulpy kidney disease vaccines. *The Veterinary Record*, 65, 659–663.

53 **THOMSON, R.O. & BATTY, I., 1967.** Experimental clostridial oil emulsion vaccines. *Bulletin de l'Office International des Épizooties*, 67, 1569–1581.

54 **THOMSON, R.O., BATTY, I., THOMSON, A., KERRY, J.B., EPPS, H.B.G. & FOSTER, W.H., 1969.** The immunogenicity of a multicomponent clostridial oil emulsion vaccine in

sheep. *The Veterinary Record*, 85, 81–85.

55 **WORTHINGTON, R.W. & MÜLDERS, M.S.G., 1979.** Isolation and characterization of antibodies to *Clostridium perfringens* epsilon toxin from hyperimmune horse serum. *Onderstepoort Journal of Veterinary Research*, 46, 121–124.

56 **WORTHINGTON, R.W., BERTSCHINGER, H.J. & MÜLDERS, M.S.G., 1979.** Catecholamine and cyclic nucleotide response of sheep to the injection of *Clostridium welchii* type D epsilon toxin. *Journal of Medical Microbiology*, 12, 497–502.

57 **WORTHINGTON, R.W., MÜLDERS, M.S.G. & VAN RENSBURG, J.J., 1973.** *Clostridium perfringens* type D epsilon prototoxin. Some chemical, immunological and biological properties of a highly purified prototoxin. *Onderstepoort Journal of Veterinary Research*, 40, 145–152.

58 **WORTHINGTON, R.W., MÜLDERS, M.S.G. & VAN RENSBURG, J.J., 1973.** Enzymatic activation of *Clostridium perfringens* epsilon prototoxin and some biological properties of activated toxin. *Onderstepoort Journal of Veterinary Research*, 40, 153–156.

Malignant oedema/Gas gangrene group of Clostridium *spp.*

The members of this ubiquitous group of bacteria, which are individually discussed in Chapters 158 to 161, most commonly cause gas gangrene or malignant oedema, and, less often, a number of other syndromes in livestock **(Table 1)**. In rare instances clostridia not contained within this group of organisms, such as *Clostridium perfringens* types A and C, may also be associated with gas gangrene as a consequence of wound infection.

The *Clostridium* spp. included in this group occur commonly in soil, sewage, marine sediments, and decaying animal and vegetable material. They are obligate anaerobes, saccharolytic and proteolytic, and most are also capable of lowering the redox potential of the medium in which they grow, thus creating a suitable environment for continuing growth.[1] They produce a variety of major and minor toxins in various combinations; the *in vitro* and *in vivo* actions of some of these are poorly understood, despite the fact that most have been characterized chemically and biochemically.

The diseases caused by infection with these bacteria are characteristically rapid in onset and are highly fatal — mainly because of severe toxaemia caused both by the products they elaborate and by those which arise after tissue breakdown. The diseases usually occur sporadically and often affect single animals or small groups. Most of these diseases may be effectively controlled by immunization. Wound infection which progresses to malignant oedema or gas gangrene may result from infections with

Table 1 Disease conditions of livestock associated with the malignant oedema/gas gangrene group of clostridia

BACTERIUM	DISEASE	SPECIES AFFECTED
Clostridium chauvoei	Blackquarter	Cattle
	Gas gangrene	Ruminants, pigs, horses
Clostridium novyi type A	Swollen head	Sheep (rams)
	Malignant oedema	Cattle
Clostridium novyi type B	Black disease	Sheep, cattle, horses, pigs
Clostridium novyi type D	Bacillary haemoglobinuria	Cattle, sheep, pigs, Horses
Clostridium septicum	Malignant oedema (gas gangrene)	Ruminants, pigs, horses
	Gangrenous abomasitis	Sheep
	Braxy (bradsot)	Lambs, calves
	Post-parturient gas gangrene	Sheep, goats, cattle
Clostridium sordellii	Haemorrhagic enteritis	Cattle, sheep, foals
	Sudden death syndrome	Lambs, cattle
	Malignant oedema	Cattle
Clostridium carnis	Gas gangrene	Cattle
Clostridium difficile	Mandibular abscess	Goats
	Necrotizing enteritis	Foals
Clostridium fallax	Malignant oedema	Horses

any one, or a combination, of the clostridia in this group, and is commonly the consequence of contamination of traumatic lesions in the skin. Gangrenous lesions may also occur in genital or gastrointestinal tracts following infection of wounds with some of the clostridia species belonging to the group. There are, however, exceptions to the foregoing, among them those diseases that arise as a consequence of dormant infections. Some such examples are blackquarter in cattle, in which the lesions are usually localized in the larger striated muscle groups, black disease and bacillary haemoglobinuria, where the primary lesions are necrotic foci in the liver, braxy, in which the primary lesions occur in the abomasum, and necrotic enteritis of foals caused by *Clostridium difficile*. In most cases of wound infection the lesions are restricted to the subcutaneous tissues and are seen as extensive gelatinous inflammatory infiltrates, which may be virtually colourless, yellowish-brown or red-tinged due to the presence of concurrent haemorrhage. The exudate may on occasion contain varying numbers of gas bubbles, which give it an unpleasant odour; in some infections, such as those by *Clostridium sordellii*, the odour is particularly foul, and in the case of blackquarter in cattle it resembles that of rancid butter.

Reference

1 **CATO, E.P., GEORGE, W.L. & FINEGOLD, S.M., 1986.** *Clostridium. In:* SNEATH, P.H.A., MAIR, N.S., SHARPE, M.E. & HOLT, J.G., (eds). *Bergey's Manual of Systematic Bacteriology*. Baltimore: Williams & Wilkins.

158

Clostridium chauvoei *infections*

Synonyms: Blackquarter, quarter-evil, blackleg, quarter-ill, sponssiekte (Afrik.)

N.P.J. Kriek and M.W. Odendaal

Introduction

Blackquarter in cattle is a consequence of the activation of *Clostridium chauvoei* spores latent in the musculature. *Clostridium chauvoei* may also cause gas gangrene in cattle, sheep, and goats, and rarely in horses and pigs, following wound infection.[19, 28, 31, 38] These infections cause a peracute or acute, usually fatal, non-contagious disease which is characterized by focal, gangrenous myositis and associated localized cellulitis. Death is caused by the local and systemic effects of the toxins elaborated by *C. chauvoei*. In this chapter the use of the term 'blackquarter' is restricted to the condition in cattle which arises as a result of endogenous *C. chauvoei* infection, whereas the lesions that develop in various animal species, including cattle, as a consequence of wound infection by this organism are referred to as gas gangrene.

Blackquarter is a universal disease of cattle. It was recognized as a distinct disease in 1782 by Chabert, who named it 'charbon symptomatique' (quoted by Henning[21]) and distinguished it from anthrax, with which it was often confused. Subsequently, the disease and the properties of the causal organisms were studied by Arloing, Cornevin and Thomas,[1] who also developed the first practical method of prophylactic immunization.[32]

It would appear that in South Africa blackquarter was one of the most prevalent diseases of cattle from the time of the earliest European settlement of the Cape. Thus, as early as 1780, Le Vaillant[26] described the disease as a 'terrible scourge, spons-sikte (literally 'sponge disease'), which causes speedy destruction of more than half the herd'. The first official reference to the occurrence of blackquarter in South Africa was made by Commissioner de Mist in 1805.[42]

Immunization against blackquarter has been practised since before the turn of the 18th century. As early as 1883 blackquarter powder vaccine was imported into Natal by Wiltshire. The first effective blackquarter vaccine in South Africa was prepared in 1887 at the Grahamstown Laboratory in the Cape Province.[21]

In spite of the effective vaccines available today, sporadic outbreaks and individual cases of the disease are still regularly encountered in livestock in southern Africa, and blackquarter remains one of the important bacterial diseases of cattle under three years of age, particularly those in feedlots. For this reason cattle should be immunized regularly.

Aetiology

Clostridium chauvoei is a Gram-positive anaerobic rod, 3–8 µm long and 0,5–1 µm wide. When grown in fluid media the organisms are most commonly found as single cells, but sometimes occur in pairs and, rarely, in short chains. The cells are motile and have peritrichous flagella. In older cultures they are pleomorphic, showing irregular staining; citron, barred and spindle shapes occur frequently. Spores, which are formed on solid media and in broth, are oval, occur in central or subterminal positions and distort the shape of the cell. They are resistant to the effects of boiling in water as well as to phenolic and quaternary disinfectants at concentrations used to sterilize contaminated instruments.[4, 39]

Clostridium chauvoei grows well in peptone-yeast-glucose broth, in which, after four days of incubation, the pH decreases to 5,0–5,4. The optimum temperature for growth is 37 °C; poor growth is obtained at between 25 and 30 °C, but no growth occurs at 45 °C. The addition of liver extract to the medium favours growth, which is also stimulated by fermentable carbohydrates. Growth is inhibited by concentrations of NaCl above 6,5 per cent, as well as by bile levels of 20 per cent or higher; pH values of 8,5 or higher also inhibit growth.

Surface colonies on blood agar are circular, 0,5–3 mm in diameter, haemolytic, slightly raised or low convex, whitish-grey, translucent or opaque, and granular with a glossy surface and an entire margin. Red blood cells of cattle, sheep, pigs, rabbits and dogs are readily haemolysed by *C. chauvoei* on blood agar, whilst those of guinea-pigs, horses, humans, and chickens are more resistant.

Clostridium chauvoei has fastidious anaerobic growth requirements. It is saccharolytic, non-proteolytic and does not produce lecithinase and lipase. Lactose, galactose, mannose, glucose, maltose and sucrose are fermented, and esculin is hydrolysed by more than 90 per cent of all strains, ribose by 40–60 per cent and nitrate is reduced by 61–89 per cent of strains. No starch is hydrolysed nor acid produced from amygdalin, arabinose, cellobiose, fructose, glycogen, inositol, mannitol, melezitose, melibiose, raffinose, rhamnose, salicin, sorbitol, starch, trehalose or xylose. Meat is not digested by more than 90 per cent of strains.[9, 30] Large volumes of gas (carbon dioxide and hydrogen) are produced in liquid media. The organism has a high demand for cysteine, biotin, nicotinic acid, pantothenic acid, pyridoxamine, thiamin and para-aminobenzoic acid.[36]

Clostridium chauvoei produces protein toxins and other protective antigens in amounts which vary according to the strain. Both bacteria and the filtrate of fluid media in which they have been grown are immunogenic.[12, 13, 41] Whole cultures of *C. chauvoei* are more immunogenic than washed bacterial cells alone. Immunization with formalinized whole cultures produces high levels of protective immunity, which is probably induced by the heat-labile protective antigen that occurs in the cell wall of the organism.[10, 11]

The alpha toxin produced by the bacterium is lethal, necrotizing and haemolytic; the beta toxin behaves as a deoxyribonuclease; the gamma toxin is a hyaluronidase; and the delta toxin is an oxygen-labile haemolysin. However, the role of these toxins in the pathogenesis of blackquarter is poorly defined.

The alpha toxin is formed as part of a soluble immunogenic complex from which it dissociates spontaneously. It has a molecular mass of 27 000 daltons. Beta toxin is produced in an active form and is relatively heat-stable, being able to withstand exposure to a temperature of 95 °C for 10 minutes without appreciable loss of activity. The oxygen-labile haemolysin (delta toxin) is serologically related to, but not identical to, streptolysin O, *Clostridium perfringens* theta toxin, tetanolysin and the haemolysin produced by some of the other clostridia.[9, 15, 16, 36] Failure of some commercial *C. chauvoei* vaccines to protect cattle during outbreaks of blackquarter has led to the belief that cross-protection between different strains may not be absolute.[45]

Epidemiology

Clostriduim chauvoei infections in livestock occur throughout the world. Cattle and to a lesser extent sheep are most commonly affected, while goats, pigs, horses, camels, deer and mink are only very rarely affected, and birds, dogs, cats, rabbits and humans are resistant to infection.[38] Goats are much more resistant than sheep to infection, and only isolated cases of gas gangrene have been recorded in pigs.[6, 31, 38]

Outbreaks of blackquarter in cattle tend to be seasonal; they occur most commonly during summer and autumn, especially after heavy rains. There appears to be a direct relationship between the prevalence of blackquarter and rainfall: the higher the rainfall, the greater the number of outbreaks during a season.[2] Distribution of outbreaks is often regional and patchy, and the prevalence of the disease in some localities, which may be portions of one farm, may be high while adjoining areas are apparently free of infection.[21] Regional differences in the soil composition seem to play a part in determining the survival of the bacteria in areas of high prevalence.

The mode of infection in blackquarter has not yet been accurately established. It is generally believed that infection follows ingestion of spores from the soil or contaminated drinking water, particularly during the period when the eruption of permanent teeth takes place. The ingested spores, or those that have formed after vegetative bacteria have germinated and sporulated in the gut lumen, cross the intestinal epithelium and enter the blood stream and lymph system, to be distributed in tissues and organs throughout the body, including the musculature, in which they can remain dormant for prolonged periods, probably in phagocytic cells .[24, 36]

Though the spores of *C. chauvoei* are highly resistant to environmental conditions and remain viable for a number of years outside the body, there is no experimental evidence that these organisms actually multiply in the soil; *C. chauvoei* apparently does not live as a saprophyte.[27] The principal habitat of *C. chauvoei* is the animal body, and it may be isolated from the intestinal contents. Contamination of vegetation and water by faeces containing the spores of the bacterium ensures animal-to-animal passage. Infected carcasses of animals that have died of the disease, however, appear to be the main source of the bacteria, by contaminating surroundings such as stables, sheds, kraals, pastures and drinking pools, which then become reservoirs of infection. Shearing sheds usually become contaminated by spores when animals which have died from blackquarter or gas gangrene caused by *C. chauvoei* are skinned in them. Once an area has been contaminated, spores persist for years. Direct transmission from animal to animal does not occur.[35, 36]

Blackquarter in cattle is mainly confined to young stock between the ages of nine months and two years. Rapidly growing animals in good condition and on a high plane of nutrition are more susceptible to the disease than underfed animals or those in poor condition. Exercise, cold and heat do not appear to influence animals' susceptibility to blackquarter.[36]

Cattle, sheep, goats, horses and pigs of all ages may suffer from localized gas gangrene following *C. chauvoei* infection of wounds contracted, for example, during shearing, dipping, parturition, castration or tail-docking operations, or infection of the umbilicus in new-born animals. Vaccination sites, particularly those induced by vaccines containing an irritant substance (e.g. saponin) may precipitate blackquarter within a matter of two hours.

Pathogenesis

The pathogenesis of *C. chauvoei* infections is essentially unknown. It is believed that blackquarter in cattle develops when latent spores within large muscle groups germinate and multiply when these muscles are traumatized, resulting in localized areas of low redox potential. The vegetative cells grow, ferment muscle glycogen, digest protein, and produce exotoxins and gas. The role of toxins produced by *C. chauvoei* in the pathogenesis of the disease remains uncertain.[37] The lesions, which usually remain localized and in most animals are situated in one of the large muscle groups, expand along fascial planes, but bacteraemia also develops, particularly terminally. Occasionally, latent spores in the myocardium are stimulated to germinate and multiply, producing typical lesions in the myocardium; the stimulus to germinate is possibly a consequence of changes in the myocardium caused by increased blood levels of cortisol and catecholamines as a response to stress.[17] The exotoxins and certain metabolites produced by the bacteria during their multiplication, and those which arise from tissue damage, are absorbed from the affected muscles into the systemic circulation, causing toxaemia and death.

Clinical signs

As the course of blackquarter is so rapid — generally less than 24 hours — clinical signs are not often observed in affected animals prior to death. Most affected cattle do not recover, but a small proportion of sheep and other animals that contract the disease as a result of wound infection may survive the infection.[21, 31, 34, 38, 43]

In cattle the first clinical signs are a rise in the body temperature, loss of appetite, ruminal stasis, and if the primary lesion is situated in one of the larger muscle groups of a limb, as is most often the case, there is initial stiffness followed by lameness which rapidly progresses in severity in the limb concerned. The muscles or muscle groups most commonly affected are those situated in the shoulder, buttock or loin regions, but those in the chest and neck regions and, more rarely, muscles such as the intrinsic and extrinsic muscles of the tongue, and the diaphragmatic and sublumbar muscles or myocardium may be primarily involved. The clinical signs, in the few cases in which they are evident, vary according to the site of the lesion(s). If the muscles affected are superficial, there is subcutaneous swelling and crepitation at the site. The swelling increases rapidly in severity and size, and initially is hot and painful, but terminally it becomes cold and painless. Lesions situated in deeper body sites are not clinically detectable. Rarely, lesions may develop simultaneously in more than one location.[34] Affected animals soon become recumbent, manifest signs of dyspnoea and have an accelerated pulse rate.

The clinical signs of localized gas gangrene that develop after wound infection by *C. chauvoei* are very similar to those of blackquarter and are also dependent on the site of the infection. In sheep, and occasionally in cattle and goats, the vagina, cervix and uterus may be infected following parturition. In such cases the perineal and adjacent tissues are severely swollen and emphysematous, and blood-stained droplets of serous fluid may ooze from the surface of the affected parts.[38] In the case of contaminated injection sites, lesions are localized to the site of injection and are oedematous and crepitant. This localized reaction expands rapidly, causing swelling of the tissues and the exudation of drops of blood-stained serous fluid through the skin, the exudate having a rancid smell. Affected animals may die within 18 hours of being injected with a contaminated needle.[38] The course of the infection in pigs is usually less acute, the infection being localized.[38]

Localized gas gangrene as a consequence of wound infection with *C. chauvoei* rarely occurs in horses.[19, 28, 31, 43] However, in cases in which this does occur, the infection may spread and involve large areas adjacent to the initial lesion. Affected horses either die without being obviously ill, or are severely ill — in which case they manifest depression, signs of shock, and an unwillingness to move the affected part if it is a limb or the neck. The swelling, which is initially hot and painful, becomes cold, oedematous and crepitant. Most affected horses die, but the affected tissues may slough in those that do recover, following intensive antibiotic treatment, leaving large cavities a few centimetres deep which heal slowly.[43]

Pathology

Clinical pathological changes in animals suffering from blackquarter are not characteristic. Elevated levels of enzymes associated with muscle damage, such as creatine kinase, may be detectable, while the results of haemograms are indicative of toxic shock.[29, 31]

The carcasses of animals that have died of blackquarter undergo rapid putrefaction and bloat, and blood-stained, frothy fluid may ooze from the nose and anus.[5] When the lesions are localized in a hind limb, that limb may be extended at an awkward angle **(Figure 158.1)**. The subcutaneous, intermuscular and other interstitial tissues in the vicinity of the affected musculature are distended by a yellow oedematous fluid which may be partially blood-stained and contain bubbles of gas. On cutting into an affected muscle, a reddish fluid exudes and there is a characteristic sweetish smell which resembles that of rancid butter.[21]

Lesions in muscles are characteristically well-circumscribed, spongy due to the accumulation of gas bubbles between muscle fibres, friable, and either uniformly dark red or have alternating streaks varying in colour from a mottled greyish-red to pale yellowish or blackish **(Figure 158.2)**. Affected muscles tend to be dryish towards the centre of the lesions. The spleen is usually not enlarged, but regional lymph nodes are hyperaemic and oedematous.[21]

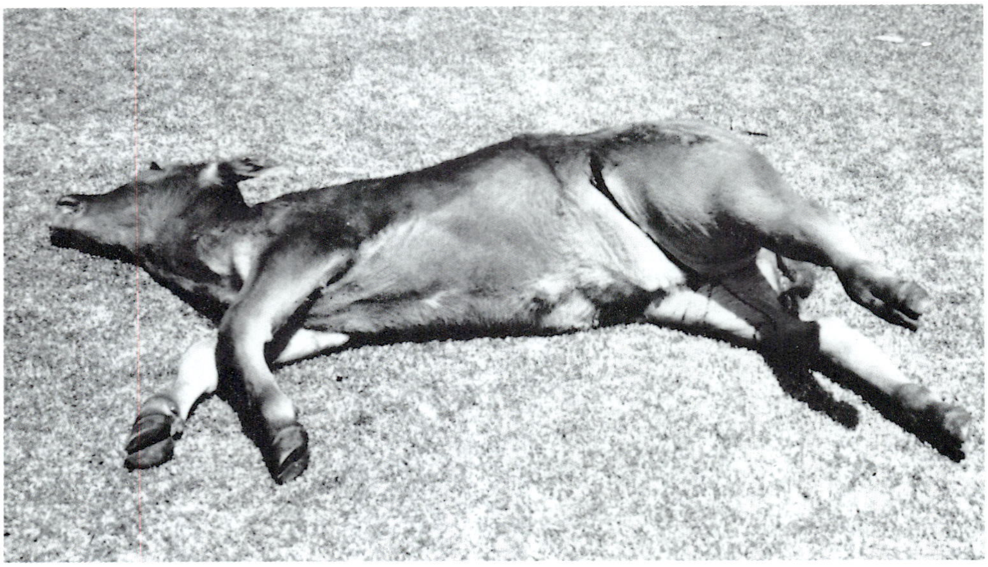

Figure 158.1 Note the swollen hind leg extended at an awkward angle due to blackquarter lesions in the large muscle groups

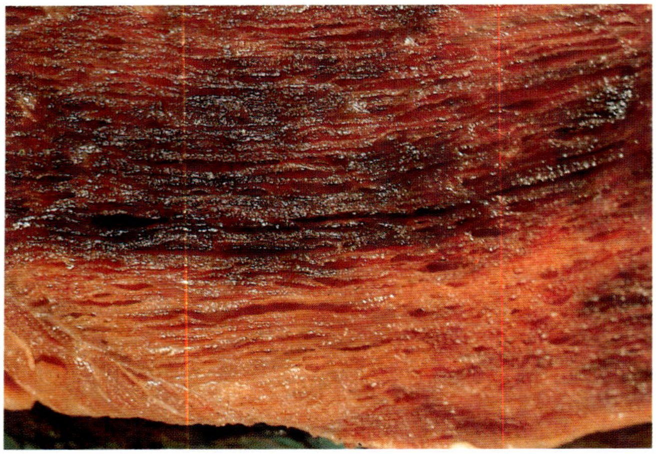

Figure 158.2 Muscle lesions in a calf that died of blackquarter. Note the mottled appearance imparted by necrosis and haemorrhage, and the gas bubbles between the muscle fibres

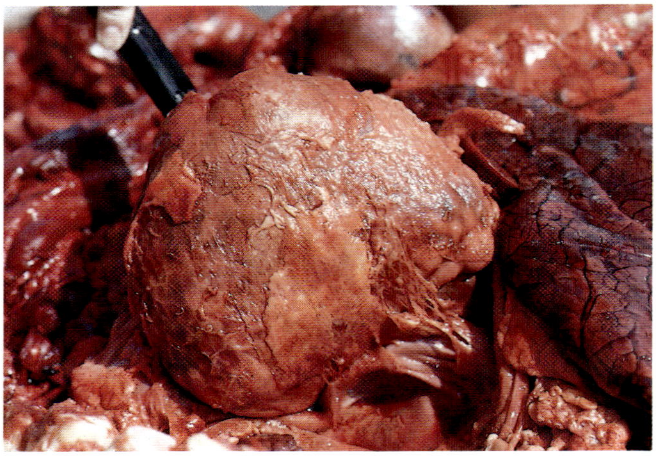

Figure 158.3 Severe, diffuse, acute fibrinous pericarditis in a calf that died of the 'heart-pluck' form of blackquarter

Localized crepitating lesions similar to those in the skeletal muscles are occasionally confined to the muscles of the tongue or diaphragm, or even the myocardium. In the latter case, the disease is known in South Africa as 'harsslag sponssiekte' (literal translation from the Afrikaans is 'heart-pluck blackquarter'). The myocardial lesions are often accompanied by a fibrinous to fibrino-haemorrhagic pericarditis **(Figure 158.3)**, and occasionally by one or more mural thrombi in the chambers of the heart. A reddish serous fluid is often found in the thoracic and peritoneal cavities and the lungs are generally severely hyperaemic and oedematous.

Histologically the muscle lesions are characterized by extensive necrosis thought to be caused both by the effect of the toxins elaborated by the bacteria, and as a result of vascular involvement. Haemorrhage, the presence of gas bubbles and numerous clostridial organisms, as well as the lack of an inflammatory response are also characteristic features of blackquarter.[23]

The lesions of gas gangrene in sheep following wound infection resemble those in cattle that have died of blackquarter. They may be associated with the presence of a severe fibrinous, fibrinopurulent or fibrinohaemorrhagic pericarditis in association with locally extensive areas of necrosis in the myocardium.[17] In lambs that have died of the disease following infection by the umbilical route, there is marked congestion of the subcutaneous tissues in the umbilical region and the visceral organs. This is accompanied by petechiation and the presence of a fibrinous exudate on the surface of the liver.[22]

The lesions in horses that have died from gas gangrene caused by *C. chauvoei* are similar in nature and appearance to those in cattle.[19] In one case in which no wound was detected, there was a large hepatic infarct, blood-stained peritoneal exudation, and numerous fibrinous tags on the peritoneal serosa, hydrothorax and hydropericardium.[28]

Diagnosis

In typical cases of blackquarter a presumptive diagnosis can be made on the basis of the history, clinical signs and lesions at necropsy. It should be borne in mind that in some of the more 'atypical' cases of blackquarter that are characterized by muscle lesions in, for example, the tongue, crura of the diaphragm or sublumbar region, their presence may have to be actively sought during the necropsy. The aetiology of the disease can only be confirmed microbiologically or by the application of immunological staining techniques, which are important if immunoprophylaxis is considered.

From the exudate emanating from lesions, six thin, air-dried smears should be prepared on microscope glass slides for diagnostic purposes. One should be stained by Gram's method and the others (keeping some in reserve) are used for fluorescent antibody testing in order to distinguish between *C. chauvoei*, *C. septicum* and *C. novyi*.[3] Specimens of affected muscles as well as liver should be collected (using aseptic techniques), placed separately in sterile plastic or glass jars and submitted at 4 °C to a laboratory for isolation of the organism. For microbiological processing each specimen should be divided into two parts. One part is heated to 80 °C for 15–30 minutes before a portion is plated out on blood tryptose agar medium and another portion inoculated into Robertson's meat broth containing glucose. The second part should be inoculated into another tube containing the same meat broth medium without being heated. *Clostridium chauvoei* has fastidious anaerobic requirements for its growth on blood agar. Selective media may be compiled by incorporating antibiotics such as neomycin, kanamycin, polymyxin, oleandomycin, or compounds such as sodium azide, crystal violet or sulphadiazine.[9] The isolation and subculturing of suspect single colonies are required in order to obtain pure cultures for use in biochemical tests. For these purposes a single colony is inoculated into either Robertson's meat broth, liver broth or thioglycolate broth, each of which contains 5 per cent glucose and is incubated for 24–48 hours before the bacteria are subjected to biochemical testing. The determination of the fatty acid composition of the bacteria by gas chromatography can also be used to differentiate between the different clostridia.[34]

Differential diagnosis

Blackquarter may be difficult to distinguish clinically from other peracute or acute infectious diseases, particularly anthrax. Because most affected animals die suddenly and rapidly become bloated and putrefied, with blood-stained fluid oozing from natural orifices, blackquarter is difficult to distinguish from anthrax. For this reason, when confronted with animals that have died acutely, it is advisable to examine suitably stained blood smears in order to exclude anthrax before proceeding with a necropsy. Lesions at necropsy are generally easily distinguished from those caused by most other infectious diseases, except those due to some other clostridial infections (*C. perfringens, C. septicum, C. novyi, C. sordellii* and *C. carnis*) that cause gas gangrene or malignant oedema, and to snake venoms such as puff adder (*Bitis arietans arietans*) and Gaboon adders (*Bitis gabonica*). In cases where other clostridial infections are concerned, the identification of the causative species by application of fluorescent antibody techniques is a prerequisite for the institution of control measures.[44]

Control

Only a small percentage of animals receiving specific chemotherapy for blackquarter recover, even if this is instituted early in the course of the disease.[20, 31, 43] Necrotic muscle may slough in animals that do recover. Animals treated in the advanced stages of the disease have no chance of recovery.

Systemic treatment with large doses of penicillin for five days in addition to accepted surgical methods of wound treatment may result in the recovery of animals suffering from gas gangrene; they do, however, take several weeks to recover fully, as lesions that result from sloughing of the necrotic tissue take a long time to heal. In horses, it may be necessary to administer penicillin at doses of approximately 44 000 IU/kg intravenously every two to four hours until the animal has stabilized (which may take from one to five days), whereafter they should be maintained on eight-hourly penicillin injections at the same dosage level for up to five weeks. Supportive fluid therapy and analgesics should be administered in addition to the antibiotic treatment.[31]

Control measures for the prevention of blackquarter in cattle and gas gangrene due to *C. chauvoei* infection in other livestock species include the destruction by incineration or deep burial of the carcasses of animals that have died of these conditions. Contamination of wounds and the transmission of spores (or even vegetative forms of the organism) by the use of contaminated hypodermic needles and surgical instruments should be prevented. Sheep that have died from *C. chauvoei* infection should not be skinned in order to salvage the price of the skin. However, if they are skinned, the skins should not be stored in or near shearing sheds.

The occurrence of blackquarter and wound infections caused by *C. chauvoei* can be adequately controlled by immunization, although the calves of immune dams have colostrum-derived immunity which lasts for up to three months and interferes with active immunization.[33]

Calves should be vaccinated when three to six months of age. The initial course of immunization should consist of two subcutaneous inoculations administered at an interval of approximately four weeks, followed by annual boosters until the animals are three years old. On heavily infected farms on which cases of blackquarter occur regularly, the period between booster vaccinations may have to be reduced to nine months.[14] The vaccine should only be inoculated subcutaneously, and a separate, clean, sterile needle should be used to inoculate each animal, to prevent transmission of the bacteria between them, particularly when vaccine is administered during an actual outbreak of blackquarter. Several combinations of clostridial antigens in vaccines are available.[7, 8, 25, 40] Such polyvalent vaccines may include one or more antigens of the following organisms: *C. chauvoei, C. botulinum, C. tetani, C. septicum, C. novyi, C. sordellii,* and *C. perfringens* types C and D.

On farms on which problems with *C. chauvoei* infections are consistently encountered in sheep, the animals should be vaccinated routinely, the time of administration being determined by the form of the disease likely to be encountered. In the case of pregnant ewes, those not previously vaccinated should be vaccinated twice at an interval of a month, the second inoculation being given at least one month before lambing; thereafter a booster inoculation given one month prior to lambing is sufficient to protect them from the genital disease. Not only will ewes vaccinated four weeks before parturition be protected from possible infection acquired by contamination of obstetric wounds, but their lambs will be protected, by virtue of the passive immunity, against infections of the umbilicus as well as wounds resulting from tail-docking and castration.[18] If *C. chauvoei* gas gangrene after contamination of shearing wounds is anticipated, the booster vaccinations should be administered six to eight weeks before shearing. In exceptional instances sheep may for unknown reasons develop a shock reaction after administration of vaccine.[14] It is therefore advisable to inoculate about ten animals in a flock and then observe them for clinical signs of shock for a period of 30 minutes. If there is no evidence of shock, the remaining animals may be injected with reasonable impunity. The same cattle vaccines (mono- and polyvalent combinations) can be used at the prescribed dosage levels to vaccinate sheep.

References

1 **ARLOING, CORNEVIN & THOMAS, 1887**. *Le charbon symptomatique de boeuf.* 2nd edn. Paris.

2 **BAGADI, H.O., 1978**. The relationship between the annual rainfall and outbreaks of blackquarter of cattle in northern Nigeria. *Tropical Animal Health and Production*, 10, 124–126.

3 **BATTY, I. & WALKER, P.D., 1963**. Differentiation of *Clostridium septicum* and *Clostridium chauvoei* by the use of fluorescent labelled antibodies. *Journal of Pathology and Bacteriology*, 85, 517–521.

4 **BISPING, W. & AMTSBERG, G., 1988**. *Colour Atlas for the Diagnosis of Bacterial Pathogens in Animals.* Berlin & Hamburg: Paul Parey Scientific Publishers.

5 **BREWITT, J.M., 1966**. A practitioner's investigation of a possible outbreak of blackleg. *Canadian Veterinary Journal*, 7, 231–232.

6 **BROWN, C.M., KANEENE, J.B. & WALKER, R.D., 1988**. Intramuscular injection techniques and the development of clostridial myositis or cellulitis in horses. *Journal of the American Veterinary Medical Association*, 193, 668–670.

7 **BROWN, K.K., PARIZEK, R.E. & STEWART, R.C., 1976**. Prevention of clostridial disease in cattle and sheep by vaccination with a multivalent bacterin-toxoid. *Veterinary Medicine/Small Animal Clinician*, 71, 1717–1721.

8 **CAMERON, C.M., BOTHA, W.J.S. & SCHOEMAN, H., 1986**. Immunization of guinea-pigs and cattle with a reduced dose *Clostridium chauvoei* vaccine produced in a semi-synthetic medium. *Onderstepoort Journal of Veterinary Research*, 53, 51–53.

9 **CATO, E.P., GEORGE, W.L. & FINEGOLD, S.M., 1986**. Genus *Clostridium* Prazmowski 1880. *In*: SNEATH, P.H.A., MAIR, N.S., SHARPE, M.E. & HOLT, J.G., (eds). *Bergey's Manual of Systematic Bacteriology*. Vol. II. Baltimore & London: Williams & Wilkins.

10 **CHANDLER, H.M. & GULASEKHARAM, J., 1970**. An evaluation of characteristics of *Clostridium chauvoei* which possibly indicate a highly protective strain. *Australian Journal of Experimental Medicine and Science*, 48, 187–197.

11 **CHANDLER, H.M. & HAMILTON, R.C., 1975**. The protective antigenicity of protoplasts and spheroplasts of a highly protective strain of *Clostridium chauvoei*. *Journal of General Microbiology*, 88, 179–183.

12 **CLAUS, K.D. & MACHEAK, M.E., 1972**. Preparation of a *C. chauvoei* antigen and determination of protective immunity by plate agglutination test. *American Journal of Veterinary Research*, 33, 1045–1052.

13 **CLAUS, K.D. & MACHEAK, M.E., 1972**. Characteristics and immunizing properties of culture filtrates of *Clostridium chauvoei*. *American Journal of Veterinary Research*, 33, 1031–1038.

14 **ERASMUS, B.J., CAMERON, C.M., HUNTER, P., CILLIERS, J.A., OBEREM, P.T., STOLTSZ, W.H. & DE WAAL, D.T., 1990**. *Onderstepoort Vaccines.* Booklet issued by the Department of Agriculture and Development, Private Bag X144, Pretoria 0001.

15 **FOEGEDING, P.M., 1988**. Detection and quantitation of spore-forming pathogens and their toxins. *In*: PIERSON, M.D. & STERN, N.J., (eds). *Food-borne Micro-organisms and their Toxins: Developing Methodology.* New York & Basel: Marcel Dekker, Inc.

16 **GILL, M., 1987**. Bacterial toxins. *In*: LASKIN, A.I. & LECHEVALIER, H.A., (eds). *CRC Handbook of Microbiology.* 2nd edn. Vol. VIII. *Toxins and Enzymes.* Florida: CRC Press, Inc.

17 **GLASTONBURY, J.R.W., SEARSON, J.E., LINKS, I.J. & TUCKETT, L.M., 1988**. Clostridial myocarditis in lambs. *Australian Veterinary Journal*, 65, 208–209.

18 **GREEN, D.S., GREEN, M.J., HILLYER, M.H. & MORGAN, K.L., 1987**. Injection site reactions and antibody responses in sheep and goats after the use of multivalent clostridial vaccines. *The Veterinary Record*, 120, 435–439.

19 **HAGEMOSER, W.A., HOFFMAN, L.J. & LUNDVALL, R.L., 1980**. *Clostridium chauvoei* infection in a horse. *Journal of the American Veterinary Medical Association*, 176, 631–633.

20 **HALL, K.E., 1989**. Treatment of a calf with *Clostridium chauvoei* infection. *Journal of the American Veterinary Medical Association*, 194, 272,

21 **HENNING, M.W., 1956**. *Animal Diseases in South Africa.* 3rd edn. Pretoria: Central News Agency.

22 **HUGHES, K.L., HAUGHEY, K.G. & HARTLEY, W.J., 1971**. Perinatal lamb mortality: Infections occurring among lambs dying after parturition. *Australian Veterinary Journal*, 47, 472–476.

23 **HULLAND, T.J., 1993**. Muscle and tendons. *In*: JUBB, K.V.F., KENNEDY, P.C. & PALMER, N., (eds). *Pathology of Domestic Animals*. 4th edn. San Diego: Academic Press, Inc.

24 **KERRY, J.B., 1964**. A note on the occurrence of *Clostridium chauvoei* in the livers and spleens of normal cattle. *The Veterinary Record*, 76, 396.

25 **KNOTT, G.K.L., ERWIN, B.G. & CLASSICK, L.G., 1985**. Benefits of a clostridial vaccination program in feedlot cattle. *Veterinary Medicine*, 80, 95–97.

26 **LE VALLIANT, M., 1796**. *Travels into the Interior Parts of Africa*. Vol. II.

27 **MINETT, F.C. & DHANDA, M.R., 1941**. Multiplication of *B. anthracis* and *Cl. chauvoei* in soil and water. *Indian Journal of Veterinary Science and Animal Husbandry*, 11, 308–321.

28 **MURPHY, D.B., 1980**. *Clostridium chauvoei* as the cause of malignant edema in a horse. *Veterinary Medicine/Small Animal Clinician*, 75, 1152–1154.

29 **PEMBERTON, J.R., BATES, F., MATSON, R., MACHEAK, M.E. & HIGBE, J., 1974**. Changes in clinical values of cattle infected with *Clostridium chauvoei*: Clinical relationships during infection. *American Journal of Veterinary Research*, 35, 1041–1044.

30 **PHILLIPS, K.D., BRAZIER, J.S., LEVETT, P.N. & WILLIS, A.T., 1985**. Clostridia. *In*: COLLINS, C.H. & GRANGE, J.M., (eds). *Isolation and Identification of Micro-organisms of Medical and Veterinary Importance*. London: Academic Press, Inc.

31 **REBHUN, W.C., SHIN, S.J., KING, J.M., BAUM, K.H. & PATTEN, V., 1985**. Malignant edema in horses. *Journal of the American Veterinary Medical Association*, 187, 732–735.

32 **ROBERTSON, M., 1929**. The organisms associated with gas gangrene. *A System of Bacteriology, M.R.C.*, 3, 225–297.

33 **SCHIPPER, I.A., KELLING, C.L., MAYER, J. & PFEIFFER, N.W., 1978**. Effects of passive immunity on immune response in calves vaccinated against *Clostridium chauvoei* infection (blackleg). *Veterinary Medicine/Small Animal Clinician*, 73, 1564–1566.

34 **SIPPEL, W.L., 1972**. Diagnosis of clostridial diseases. *Journal of the American Veterinary Medical Association*, 161, 1299–1305.

35 **SMITH, L.D.S., 1975**. *The Pathogenic Anaerobic Bacteria*. 2nd edn. Springfield, Illinois: Charles C. Thomas.

36 **SMITH, L.D.S. & WILLIAMS, B.L., 1984**. *The Pathogenic Anaerobic Bacteria*. 3rd edn. Springfield, Illinois: Charles C. Thomas.

37 **STEPHEN, J. & PIETROWSKI, R.A., 1986**. *Bacterial Toxins*. 2nd edn. Washington: American Society for Microbiology.

38 **STERNE, M., 1981**. Clostridial infections. *British Veterinary Journal*, 137, 443–454.

39 **STERNE, M. & BATTY, I., 1975**. *Pathogenic Clostridia*. Boston & London: Butterworths.

40 **STERNE, M., BATTY, I., THOMPSON, A. & ROBERTSON, J.M., 1962**. Immunisation of sheep with multi-component clostridial vaccines. *The Veterinary Record*, 74, 909–913.

41 **STEVENSON, J.R. & STONGER, K.A., 1980**. Protective cellular antigen of *Clostridium chauvoei*. *American Journal of Veterinary Research*, 41, 650–652.

42 **THEAL, G.M., 1911**. *Belangryke Historische Dokumente over Zuid-Afrika. Reisen van Kommissaris de Mist*.

43 **WESTMAN, C.W., TRAUB, J.L. & SCHROEDER, W.G., 1979**. Clostridial infection in a horse. *Journal of the American Veterinary Medical Association*, 174, 725–726.

44 **WILLIAMS, B.M., 1977**. Clostridial myositis in cattle: Bacteriology and gross pathology. *The Veterinary Record*, 100, 90–101.

45 **WOOLCOCK, J.B. & FROST, A.J., 1978**. Failure of *Clostridium chauvoei* vaccines to protect against blackleg. *Australian Veterinary Journal*, 54, 319.

159

Clostridium novyi *infections*

N.P.J. Kriek and M.W. Odendaal

Introduction

Infection with *Clostridium novyi* type A, B, C or D is responsible for a number of distinctive syndromes, each of which is dependent on the respective combinations of exotoxin elaborated by the organism involved. Type C is almost non-pathogenic, although it has been isolated from water buffaloes (*Bubalus bubalis*) suffering from osteomyelitis. In general, type A infections are associated with swollen head in rams, type B with black disease and type D with bacillary haemoglobinuria.

Rare reports have been published on the association of *C. novyi* with malignant oedema in cattle in which the lesions at necropsy are indistinguishable from those of blackquarter.[31, 35] In these animals it appears that *C. novyi*, which is often isolated from such lesions in association with other clostridia, may be the only cause of the lesions in about 30 per cent of cases. Similar cases are also diagnosed regularly in South Africa at the Veterinary Research Institute, Onderstepoort.[11] Some consider such cases of malignant oedema to be the consequence of wound infections, whereas others are of the opinion that the pathogenesis is similar to that of blackquarter.[11] The clinical signs of cattle suffering from malignant oedema caused by *C. novyi* infection have not been described, but are considered to be similar to those of blackquarter. At necropsy the lesions in these animals are characterized by the presence of a very extensive, voluminous, clear, virtually colourless, gelatinous infiltrate which occurs subcutaneously and intermuscularly.[35] Occasionally the inflammatory exudate is pinkish to reddish due to haemorrhage. In contrast to blackquarter, there are generally no muscle lesions in association with the inflammatory infiltrate, but if present they are small.[11]

Clostridium novyi is divided into the types A, B, C and D, based on the different combinations of soluble toxic antigens produced by the different biotypes.[26]

Clostridium novyi used to be referred to as *Clostridium oedematiens*, a name which still often appears in the literature, while *C. novyi* type D is also known as *C. haemolyticum*. Although *C. haemolyticum* and *C. novyi* are presently considered to be distinct species,[6] it has been suggested that they be regarded as the same species, as they have common somatic antigens, and the beta toxin of *C. novyi* type B is indistinguishable from the lethal toxin produced by *C. haemolyticum*. They also have similar cultural and morphological characteristics.[27, 29] They do, however, cause different diseases in domestic animals, and different vaccines are used to protect against them.

Clostridium novyi occurs as part of the microbial flora in soil, marine sediments and the intestinal flora of animals. Strains of types A, B and D have been isolated from the liver of normal sheep and cattle.[28, 29] Toxigenic strains are commonly isolated from the soil.[23]

CLOSTRIDIUM NOVYI *TYPE A INFECTIONS*

Synonyms: Swollen head in rams, dikkop by ramme (Afrik.)

Clostridium novyi type A is the aetiology of the swollen head syndrome in rams and is one of the causes of gas gangrene in humans and cattle. Swollen head is an acute, infectious, but non-contagious disease, particularly of young rams. It is characterized by the development of a pronounced inflammatory oedema of the head and neck that develops after wounds inflicted to the head during fighting have become infected.

Aetiology

Clostridium novyi type A cells are 1,6–17 µm long and 0,6–1,4 µm wide, with oval, central or subterminal spores. Type B cells are considerably larger, being more than twice as long and much wider, and measuring 1,1–2,5 x 3,3–22,5 µm. *Clostridium haemolyticum* (*C. novyi* type D) cells are 1,9–17,3 µm long and 0,6–1,6 µm wide. They occur singly or in pairs. All strains are motile by virtue of their peritrichous flagella, the motility causing swarming on blood agar cultures. On wet mounts, however, motility is quite difficult to observe. The optimum temperature for growth is 45 °C, with most strains growing well at 37 °C and moderately at 30 °C, while no growth occurs at 25 °C. Strict anaerobic conditions are required for culturing, and the presence of fermentable carbohydrates stimulates growth. Agar plates used for isolation of *C. novyi* should be stored under anaerobic conditions. No growth occurs when 20 per cent bile or 6,5 per cent sodium chloride is added to the culture medium.[6]

Colonies of *C. novyi* on blood agar are irregular in outline, round, 3–8 mm in diameter, translucent and greyish, and have a ground-glass appearance. Spores are formed which are more resistant than those of the other clostridia, as they can resist the effects of boiling water for 30 minutes.[4]

Clostridium novyi type A strains produce alpha toxin (necrotizing, oedematizing and lethal), gamma toxin (necrotizing and haemolytic; it is a lecithinase or phospholipase C), delta toxin (oxygen-labile haemolysin) and epsilon toxin (lipase). Type B produces alpha toxin, beta toxin (necrotizing, haemolytic and lethal; it is a phospholipase C or lecithinase), zeta toxin (haemolytic), eta toxin (tropomyosinase) and a trace of theta toxin (lipase).[24, 30, 32] *Clostridium novyi* type C is a non-toxic and essentially non-pathogenic strain which only produces minute amounts of gamma toxin. Type D produces beta and eta toxins and a trace of theta toxin.[6, 29]

The alpha toxin is produced during active growth[23] and damages capillary endothelial cells, resulting in increased capillary permeability in a similar way to the epsilon-toxin of *C. perfringens* type D.[7, 13] Very little information regarding the characteristics of the other toxins is available.

Epidemiology

Swollen head is a wound infection that occurs in young rams mainly during the summer months. Tissue damage to the skin and subcutis of the head caused by the animals fighting amongst themselves results in the development of subcutaneous oedema which is an ideal environment for bacterial growth and toxin production.

Pathogenesis, clinical signs and pathology

Infection of the wounds by *C. novyi* type A probably takes place at the time of injury[29] and results in the rapid development of a severe, subcutaneous inflammatory oedema with swelling of the affected part. It often commences around the face and spreads to involve the whole head, extending for variable distances down the neck. The swelling may be so severe as to interfere with respiration and cause snoring sounds. There may be exudation of fluid through the skin and closure of the eyes due to severe oedema of the eyelids and conjunctiva. The appetite is suppressed and the animal goes down, refusing to rise, and usually dies within 48–72 hours of the onset of clinical signs.[10]

At necropsy the skin and subcutaneous tissues of the head and neck, and the loose connective tissues of the peripharyngeal, perilaryngeal and peritracheal regions are extensively infiltrated with a clear, straw-coloured inflammatory oedema which oozes from cuts made into the affected tissues and clots readily when exposed to the atmosphere. There is hydrothorax, hydropericardium and oedema of the lungs.[10] If the wool is carefully removed from the forehead of an affected ram, one or more insignificant wounds may be detected.[10]

Diagnosis

The diagnosis of the diseases caused by *C. novyi* infections is based on the history, clinical signs, macro- and microscopic pathology, and the identification of the organism and its toxins using immunofluorescent staining, bacteriological isolation and toxin-antitoxin typing techniques. For the latter purpose, specimens of organs, tissues or exudates and air-dried impression smears of lesions are required. Specimens must be collected using aseptic techniques and packed in ice or refrigerated as soon after the death of the animal as possible. They should be kept at between 4–8 °C until they reach the laboratory. *Clostridium novyi* occurs as part of the normal gastrointestinal microflora and is a common post-mortem invader of the organs and tissues in carcasses, where it proliferates and elaborates its toxins soon after death. Large numbers of organisms may reach the liver shortly after death, or even during the terminal stages of an animal's life. In addition, dormant spores of *C. novyi* may occur in the liver of normal animals, but in numbers too few to be detected by immunofluorescent methods; their presence is only detected after germination and vegetative growth.[22] The results obtained when specimens are taken from the carcasses of animals which have been dead for more than 24 hours in temperate climates should be interpreted with caution, and the isolation of *C. novyi* from the specimens alone is insufficient evidence for confirmation of the diagnosis.[2, 35]

The impression smears are used for direct microscopic visualization of *C. novyi* after Gram's and immunofluorescent staining techniques have been applied.[3]

The tissue, organ and exudate specimens are used for the isolation and identification of the microorganism and/or its toxins, using conventional bacteriological investigative methods. The presence of the alpha, beta and gamma toxins and the neutralization by type A, B and D antisera form the basis of typing *C. novyi* isolates.[32] The necrotic effects of alpha and beta toxins may be demonstrated either in fluid culture media in which the microorganism has been grown or, more directly, in affected animal tissues. For the latter, a normal saline extract of the lesion is prepared. After centrifugation of the extract, part of the supernatant fluid is divided into aliquots to which either type A antiserum, type B antiserum, type D antiserum or, as a control, an equal volume of normal saline solution, is added. Portions of the aliquots are used for intradermal testing in guinea-pigs: a necrotic lesion at the injection site after 24 hours is considered a positive reaction.[25, 32] Inhibition of the necrotic reaction confirms the presence of alpha or beta toxin. In addition, beta toxin is also identified by its haemolytic reaction on human red blood cells.

For the diagnosis of swollen head in rams, specimens should consist of tissues collected from within 10 mm of the skin wound, six air-dried impression smears from the same site made on microscopic glass slides and if possible 20–30 ml of the subcutaneous exudate. Tissues that are more than about 10 mm distant from a wound may be free of bacteria and are generally unsuitable for bacteriological and smear examinations. Specimens required for the diagnosis of malignant oedema are similar to those for swollen head in rams, while those for black disease and bacillary haemoglobinuria should consist of necrotic liver lesions, tissue samples from the kidney and spleen, and 20–30 ml amounts of peritoneal, pleural and pericardial fluids and urine, as well as six air-dried impression smears made from one or more of the liver lesions.

Differential diagnosis

The following should be considered in the differential diagnosis of swollen head in rams: swelling of the head caused by the effects of photosensitization, especially after the ingestion of certain hepatotoxic plants or the mycotoxin sporidesmin produced by the fungus *Pithomyces chartarum*, which is responsible for facial eczema;[17] hypoproteinaemia resulting from helminth infestations such as *Haemonchus contortus*; and snake bite.

Control

The treatment of animals suffering from *C. novyi* infections is not always possible, and even if it is feasible it is not always effective because of the acuteness and short course of the infections. If applied, however, it consists of appropriate antibiotic and intensive supportive therapy.

Clostridum novyi type A is susceptible to chloramphenicol, clindamycin, erythromycin and penicillin G.[6] No successful treatment of black disease in horses has been reported.[34]

The use of vaccines containing bacterins/toxoids to protect against *C. novyi* infections in livestock is common and effective,[5, 19, 33] and they are available commercially under a variety of trade names. The monovalent vaccine for swollen head in rams produced by the Veterinary Research Institute at Onderstepoort is administered for the first time to young rams at the age of four to six months and is repeated after four weeks. The resulting immunity persists for approximately nine months, after which a booster inoculation consisting of a single injection should be given.[8] This vaccine may also be administered to cattle, using double the sheep dose in situations where *C. novyi* type A is responsible for malignant oedema or blackquarter-like syndromes.

Multivalent vaccines consisting of a combination of bacterins/toxoids of a number of clostridia including *C. novyi* types B and D are available.

On farms where black disease or bacillary haemoglobinuria is a problem, liver fluke infestations should be controlled, in addition to vaccination.

CLOSTRIDIUM NOVYI *TYPE B INFECTIONS*

Synonyms: Black disease, infectious necrotic hepatitis

Clostridium novyi type B causes black disease, also known as infectious necrotic hepatitis, principally in sheep and cattle, and occasionally in horses and pigs. Hepatic lesions caused by the migration of immature liver flukes predispose to the development of the disease in ruminants.

Aetiology

Details of the aetiological agent of black disease are given in the **Aetiology section of *Clostridium novyi* type A infections**, above.

Epidemiology and pathogenesis

Black disease occurs in Australia, New Zealand, the United Kingdom, Europe and the USA. It has not been reported in South Africa. The few cases that have been reported in horses occurred in Australia.[34]

Clostridium novyi type B is widely distributed, and carrier animals spread it from farm to farm. The environment is contaminated by bacteria contained in their faeces or by organisms released following post-mortal decomposition of the carcasses of animals that have died from black disease. Factors which allow the survival of *C. novyi* in the soil include large amounts of organic matter and an alkaline environment.[21] Ingestion of spores by animals grazing on pasture growing on contaminated soils occurs continually. Some of the spores cross from the intestinal tract into the systemic circulation, from which they are phagocytosed by cells of the monocyte-macrophage system in organs such as the liver and spleen, where they may remain as latent infections until some tissue injury provides the local conditions necessary for them to proliferate in susceptible animals and produce their toxins. On farms on which black disease is endemic, a higher percentage of both the soil and animals' livers contains *C. novyi* than is the case in areas in which the disease does not occur.[1, 35] Infection with *C. novyi* may also take place through the umbilicus of lambs and the uterus of ewes.

Black disease in sheep has a distribution and a seasonal prevalence which are linked primarily to the presence of hepatic damage caused by the migration of immature liver flukes, mainly *Fasciola hepatica* and *F. gigantica*, but also *Dicrocoelium dendriticum*. The liver lesions are thought to predispose to the development of the disease as they provide foci of necrotic tissue in which the necessary anaerobic conditions prevail for the germination of *C. novyi* spores and the subsequent proliferation and toxin production of the vegetative forms. The toxaemia which results is responsible for the death of the animal. Black disease has been experimentally reproduced by the simultaneous administration of *C. novyi* type B spores and liver fluke metacercariae to susceptible animals.[29] Other causes of liver injury, such as migrating larvae of *Taenia hydatigena*,[12] surgical removal of biopsy specimens,[9] or necrosis induced by hepatotoxins or severe hypoxia, may also predispose to the disease.

Well-fed sheep in good physical condition between the ages of two and four years are particularly susceptible, while lambs and yearlings are rarely affected. In cattle there does not appear to be a specific age predilection; nor is an association with liver fluke infestation as clear-cut as it is in sheep.

Clinical signs and pathology

Clinical signs do not set in until shortly before death, and it is not uncommon for animals to die rapidly without showing obvious signs of illness. When clinical signs are observed, an affected sheep stands with its back arched and head and neck extended, and manifests severe depression, ruminal atony, coldness of the skin, normal or decreased body temperature, and weak heart sounds.[16] It moves reluctantly, lags behind the flock and soon lies down to assume a position of sternal recumbency, showing rapid and shallow breathing. In some there are signs of hyperaesthesia, twitching of the superficial muscles and frothing at the mouth. Death usually supervenes soon after animals go down. Horses may become ill overnight and die within 27–72 hours of the commencement of clinical signs. They are unable to walk, are severely depressed, and manifest pyrexia, increased heart and respiratory rates, and severe icterus prior to death.

Post-mortem changes set in rapidly after death and often mask the characteristic lesions. When an animal suffering from black disease is killed *in extremis*, or examined immediately after death, there is a marked subcutaneous venous congestion and cyanosis which impart a dark-bluish to blackish colour to the subcutis, and which become apparent when the skin is removed from the carcass. It is to this that the disease owes its name. A focus (or foci) of necrosis in the liver is the most characteristic lesion and it occurs in addition to the haemorrhagic tracts caused by migration of the immature liver flukes which are present in many of the animals that die of the disease.[14] These necrotic foci are 20–30 mm in diameter, sharply demarcated and yellowish-white, and are surrounded by a hyperaemic reaction zone. The areas of necrosis are often situated close to the diaphragmatic surface of the liver, from whence they extend into the substance of the organ. Large numbers of Gram-positive bacilli can be demonstrated in impression smears or in histological sections of these lesions. The capsule of the liver overlying some of the necrotic foci may reveal evidence of a fibrinous peritonitis. Other lesions include marked ascites, hydrothorax, hydropericardium and subcutaneous oedema of the ventral thoracic area. In horses that have died from black disease, a diffuse peritonitis in association with a voluminous, haemorrhagic exudate in the peritoneal cavity, severe congestion of the intestinal tract, and large hepatic infarcts up to 150 mm in diameter are the characteristic lesions.[18]

Diagnosis

The methods used for the diagnosis of black disease are recorded in the **Diagnosis section of *Clostridium novyi* type A infections**, above.

Differential diagnosis

Black disease may be confused with other peracute or acute diseases such as other clostridial infections (e.g., pulpy kidney disease, malignant oedema and black-quarter) and anthrax. The hepatic lesions should be differentiated from those of uncomplicated fascioliasis and the migratory tracts caused by severe infestations of *T. hydatigena* larvae.

Control

Methods used for the control of black disease are recorded in the **Control section of *Clostridium novyi* type A infections**, above.

CLOSTRIDIUM *NOVYI TYPE D INFECTIONS*

Synonyms: Bacillary haemoglobinuria, basillêre hemoglobinurie (Afrik.)

Clostridium novyi type D (also known as *Clostridium haemolyticum*), which has been reported from the same geographical regions as type B, is the cause of bacillary haemoglobinuria, an acute to peracute, highly fatal toxaemia of cattle and rarely of sheep, pigs and horses.[18] It manifests with a high fever, haemoglobinuria and icterus, and is also characterized by the presence of necrotic foci in the liver. This syndrome has not been diagnosed in South Africa.

Aetiology

Details of the aetiological agent of bacillary haemoglobinuria are given in the **Aetiology section of *Clostridium novyi* type A infections**, above.

Epidemiology and pathogenesis

The epidemiology and pathogenesis of bacillary haemoglobinuria in cattle and sheep are very similar to those of black disease in sheep. Bacillary haemoglobinuria exists only in regions where liver fluke infestation and *C. novyi* type D organisms are endemic. Primary injury initiated by these helminths to the liver harbouring latent infections of the bacterial spores creates the necessary conditions required for them to germinate, grow vegetatively and produce exotoxins.[9] As in the case of *C. novyi* type B, type D is a soil-borne organism and is distributed and ingested in a similar manner. Spores reaching the liver lie dormant in Kupffer cells until stimulated to germinate. Not only is the beta toxin hepatotoxic and exacerbates the growth of the primary necrotic lesions; it is also haemolytic, which results in the development of intravascular haemolysis with anaemia, haemoglobinaemia and haemoglobinuria following its absorption into the systemic circulation. Affected animals succumb to the effects of hypoxia and toxaemia.[15] However, unlike black disease, which is essentially a toxaemia, in bacillary haemoglobinuria both a toxaemia and a septicaemia develop.[22] Animals in good condition are more susceptible to the disease.

Clinical signs and pathology

The clinical signs in cattle and sheep suffering from bacillary haemoglobinuria are of rapid onset, and include fever, icterus, and toxaemia. The faeces are dark and bile-stained, and terminally there is a haemoglobinuria.[18] The pattern of mortality in cattle in regions where bacillary haemoglobinuria is endemic is characterized by the occurrence of sporadic deaths, although instances do occur in which large numbers of animals die in a matter of hours or days.[21] Bacillary haemoglobinuria in horses may present initially as colic; profuse sweating, toxaemia, icterus, fever and increased respiratory and heart rates develop subsequently. Haemoglobinuria only occurs terminally.[18]

At necropsy, animals that have died from bacillary haemoglobinuria are usually in good condition and manifest severe icterus, haemoglobinuria, haemoglobinuric nephrosis and hepatic degeneration and bile stasis. The blood is watery and clots poorly. Large single or multiple focal areas of necrosis from about 10 up to 200 mm in diameter occur in the liver parenchyma and are considered characteristic for the disease. The necrotic areas are darker than the surrounding liver but contain central pale foci, and are firm, well-circumscribed, randomly distributed and raised above the surface of the liver capsule. Histologically, Gram-positive bacilli may be detected at the periphery of the necrotic foci in the liver.[15]

Diagnosis

The methods used for the diagnosis of bacillary haemoglobinuria are given in the **Diagnosis section of *Clostridium novyi* type A infections**, above.

Differential diagnosis

Bacillary haemoglobinuria in cattle may be confused clinically and pathologically with redwater (babesiosis), leptospirosis, post-parturient haemoglobinuria, and haemolytic anaemia caused by cruciferous plants and *Allium cepa*. Clinically, the haematuria present in some cases of enzootic haematuria and in some animals suffering from pyelonephritis and cystitis should also be considered in the differential diagnosis. In sheep, the haemolytic crisis, anaemia and icterus caused by chronic copper poisoning, and the icterus associated with certain *Corynebacterium pseudotuberculosis* infections, eperythrozoonosis, plant poisonings caused by hepatotoxic plants and mycotoxicoses such as facial eczema[17] may be difficult to distinguish from those of bacillary haemoglobinuria. Bacillary haemoglobinuria in horses may be confused with diseases such as babesiosis and leptospirosis.

Control

The control of bacillary haemoglobinuria is described in the **Control section of *Clostridium novyi* type A infections**, above.

References

1 **BAGADI, H.O. & SEWELL, M.M.H., 1973.** An epidemiological survey of infectious necrotic hepatitis (black disease) of sheep in southern Scotland. *Research in Veterinary Science*, 15, 49–53.

2 **BAGADI, H.O. & SEWELL, M.M.H., 1974.** The influence of post-mortem autolysis on the diagnosis of infectious necrotic hepatitis (black disease). *Research in Veterinary Science*, 17, 320–322.

3 **BATTY, I. & WALKER, P.D., 1964.** The identification of *Clostridium novyi*, *C. oedematiens* and *C. tetani* by the use of fluorescent labelled antibodies. *Journal of Pathology and Bacteriology*, 88, 327–328.

4 **BISPING, W. & AMTSBERG, G., 1988.** *Colour Atlas for the Diagnosis of Bacterial Pathogens in Animals*. Berlin & Hamburg: Paul Parey Scientific Publishers.

5 **BROWN, K.K., PARIZEK, R.E. & STEWART, R.C., 1976.** Prevention of clostridial disease in cattle and sheep by vaccination with a multivalent bacterin-toxoid. *Veterinary*

Medicine/Small Animal Clinician, 71, 1717–1721.

6 **CATO, E.P., GEORGE, W.L. & FINEGOLD, S.M., 1986.** Genus *Clostridium* Prazmowski 1880. *In*: SNEATH, P.H.A., MAIR, N.S., SHARPE, M.E. & HOLT, J.G., (eds). *Bergey's Manual of Systematic Bacteriology*. Vol. 2. Baltimore & London: Williams & Wilkins.

7 **ELDER, J.M. & MILES, A.A., 1957.** The action of the lethal toxins of gas gangrene clostridia on capillary permeability. *Journal of Pathology and Bacteriology*, 74, 133–145.

8 **ERASMUS, B.J., CAMERON, C.M., HUNTER, P., CILLIERS, J.A., OBEREM, P.T., STOLTSZ, W.H. & DE WAAL, D.T., 1990.** Onderstepoort Vaccines. Booklet issued by the Department of Agriculture and Development and obtained from the Directorate of Agricultural Information, Private Bag X144, Pretoria 0001.

9 **ERWIN, B.G., 1977.** Experimental induction of bacillary hemoglobinuria in cattle. *American Journal of Veterinary Research*, 38, 1625–1627.

10 **HENNING, M.W., 1956.** *Animal Diseases in South Africa*. 3rd edn. Pretoria: Central News Agency.

11 **HENTON, M.M., 1993.** Onderstepoort Veterinary Institute, Private Bag X5, Onderstepoort 0110, Republic of South Africa. Unpublished data.

12 **HRECZKO, I., 1959.** Infectious necrotic hepatitis in sheep in South Australia, possibly associated with *Cysticercus tenuicollis*. *Australian Veterinary Journal*, 35, 462–463.

13 **IZUMI, N., NIIRO, M. & KONDO, H., 1983.** *Clostridium oedematiens* type A toxin: The correlation between the lethal and edematizing activities. *Japanese Journal of Medical Science and Biology*, 36, 67–74.

14 **JAMIESON, S., THOMPSON, J.J. & BROTHERSON, J.G., 1948.** Studies in black disease. I. The occurrence of the disease in sheep in the north of Scotland. *The Veterinary Record*, 60, 11–14.

15 **JANZEN, E.D., ORR, J.P. & OSBORNE, A.D., 1981.** Bacillary hemoglobinuria associated with hepatic necrobacillosis in a yearling feedlot heifer. *Canadian Veterinary Journal*, 22, 393–394.

16 **KELCH, W.J., COLES, B.M., REYNOLDS, G.E. & BAILEY, D.E., 1977.** Suspected infectious necrotic hepatitis (black disease) in Oregon cattle. *Journal of the American Veterinary Medical Association*, 171, 431–432.

17 **KELLERMAN, T.S., COETZER, J.A.W. & NAUDÉ, T.W., 1988.** *Plant Poisonings and Mycotoxicoses of Livestock in Southern Africa*. Cape Town: Oxford University Press Southern Africa.

18 **KIRK, M.D., 1972.** Equine bacillary hemoglobinuria. *Veterinary Medicine/Small Animal Clinician*, 67, 279–283.

19 **KNOTT, G.K.L., ERWIN, B.G. & CLASSICK, L.G., 1986.** Benefits of a clostridial vaccination program in feedlot cattle. *Veterinary Medicine*, 81, 95–97.

20 **LOZANO, E.A., 1977.** Inactivation of *Clostridium haemolyticum* toxic fluids and their antigenicity. *Canadian Journal of Comparative Medicine*, 41, 188–194.

21 **McCAIN, C.S., 1967.** Isolation and identification of *Clostridium haemolyticum* in cattle in Florida. *American Journal of Veterinary Research*, 28, 124–125.

22 **NIILO, L., DORWARD, W.J. & AVERY, R.J., 1969.** The role of *Clostridium novyi* in bovine disease in Alberta. *Canadian Veterinary Journal*, 10, 159–169.

23 **NISHIDA, S. & NAKAGAWARA, G., 1964.** Isolation of toxigenic strains of *Clostridium novyi* from soil. *Journal of Bacteriology*, 88, 1636–1640.

24 **PHILLIPS, A.W., BATTY, I. & WOOD, R.D., 1970.** A partial characterization of the alpha toxin of *Clostridium oedematiens*, type B. *European Journal of Biochemistry*, 14, 367–371.

25 **POWER, E.P., WHITE, V.J., MACKESSY, E.J. & WARD, J., 1987.** Bacillary haemoglobinuria of cattle: Confirmation of the disease in Ireland. *Irish Veterinary Journal*, 41, 255–257.

26 **RUTTER, J.M. & COLLEE, J.G., 1969.** Studies on the soluble antigens of *Clostridium oedematiens (C. novyi)*. *Journal of Medical Microbiology*, 2, 395–417.

27 **SMITH, L.D.S., 1953.** The essential characteristics of the species *Clostridium haemolyticum*. *The Journal of Bacteriology*, 65, 222.

28 **SMITH, L.D.S. & JASMIN, A.M., 1956.** The recovery of *Clostridium haemolyticum* from the livers and kidneys of apparently normal cattle. *Journal of the American Veterinary Medical Association*, 129, 68–71.

29 **SMITH, L.D.S. & WILLIAMS, B.L., 1984.** *The Pathogenic Anaerobic Bacteria*. 3rd edn. Springfield, Illinois: Charles C. Thomas.

30 **STEPHEN, J. & PIETROWSKI, R.A., 1986.** *Bacterial Toxins*. 2nd edn. Washington: American Society for Microbiology.

31 **STERNE, M., 1981.** Clostridial infections. *British Veterinary Journal*, 135, 443–454.

32 **STERNE, M. & BATTY, I, 1975.** *Pathogenic Clostridia*. Boston & London: Butterworths.

33 **STERNE, M., BATTY, I., THOMPSON, A. & ROBERTSON, J.M., 1962.** Immunization of sheep with multi-component clostridial vaccines. *The Veterinary Record*, 74, 909–913.

34 **SWEENEY, H.J. & GREIG, A., 1986.** Infectious necrotic hepatitis in a horse. *Equine Veterinary Journal*, 18, 150–151.

35 **WILLIAMS, B.M., 1977.** Clostridial myositis in cattle: Bacteriology and gross pathology. *The Veterinary Record*, 100, 90–91.

160

Clostridium septicum *infections*

Synonyms: Malignant oedema, gas gangrene, braxy

M.W. Odendaal and N.P.J. Kriek

Introduction

Several disease syndromes are associated with *Clostridium septicum* infection in livestock: malignant oedema and gas gangrene in ruminants, pigs and horses, gangrenous abomasitis (known as braxy or bradsot) in sheep, gangrenous abomasitis in lambs and calves following infection of abomasal ulcers, and post-parturient gas gangrene of the perineum, vulva and genital tract particularly of ewes and does, but also of cows (this is often referred to in South Africa as 'baarmoeder sponssiekte', meaning 'uterine gas gangrene').

Malignant oedema develops as a consequence of wound infections and is an acute, febrile, highly fatal condition that is characterized by the presence of an oedematous and gangrenous inflammation of the affected parts, as well as toxaemia.[1, 10, 12, 13, 15, 18, 19, 22, 30] *Clostridium septicum* may be a secondary invader, and often occurs in conjunction with other clostridia. It is considered to be the primary cause of malignant oedema in up to 30 per cent of cattle suffering from the disease.[27] Other histotoxic clostridia associated with gas gangrene in animals are *C. perfringens* type A or C, *C. novyi*, *C. chauvoei* and *C. sordellii*.

Braxy is a highly fatal disease which, for a very long time, has been known to occur in north-western Europe, principally in Norway, Denmark, North Germany, Iceland and the Faroe Islands, where it is known as bradsot (quick plague). It is also well known in parts of the United Kingdom and Ireland, North America and Australia. Braxy is characterized by severe oedema and gangrenous inflammation of the mucous membrane of the abomasum and severe toxaemia. Some cases of braxy may be due to *C. novyi* and are indistinguishable from the condition caused by *C. septicum*.

Clostridium septicum is a normal inhabitant of the intestinal contents of animals and is a frequent and rapid post-mortal tissue invader and common contaminant. The longer the period is between death and collection of tissue specimens, the better are the chances of isolating *C. septicum* from animal tissues.

In southern Africa, losses of livestock, particularly cattle and sheep, as a result of malignant oedema, post-parturient gas gangrene and gangrenous abomasitis are encountered sporadically, but braxy has not been reported in the region.

Aetiology

Clostridium septicum is usually a straight or slightly curved, Gram-positive bacillus 3–6 µm long and 0,4–1,2 µm wide. Filaments up to 35 µm long are formed on the peritoneal surface of organs (particularly the diaphragmatic surface of the liver) of infected animals. It often stains unevenly with Gram's stain. The bacterial cells usually occur singly or in pairs, are motile due to the presence of peritrichous flagella, and exhibit pleomorphism, appearing as citrons, spindles and barred rods under certain conditions. Spores which are oval, subterminal and which distend the cell are formed abundantly.[5, 25]

Clostridium septicum is easily cultured on blood agar, and colonies are 1–8 mm in diameter, slightly raised, circular, semitranslucent, grey and glossy, with markedly irregular to rhizoid margins after two days' incubation. A zone of complete haemolysis surrounds each colony. Because of the motility of the organisms, the colonies have a tendency to swarm on solid media, but this can be prevented by shortening the incubation period, increasing the agar content to 4–6 per cent, or by spreading specific antiserum over the surface of the agar plate.

Clostridium septicum is anaerobic. Optimum growth is attained at temperatures of between 37 and 40 °C, while most strains will also grow at 44 °C. Growth ceases at 46 °C. The presence of fermentable carbohydrate or serum in the culture medium stimulates its growth. Essential factors to sustain growth of the bacterium on artificial media include biotin, nicotinic acid, pyridoxine, thiamin, cysteine, tryptophan, adenine, arginine, aspartic acid, histidine, isoleucine, phenylalanine, serine, threonine, tyrosine and valine.[25]

Clostridium septicum has saccharolytic and non-proteolytic properties and does not produce lipase or lecithinase. Cellobiose, fructose, galactose, lactose, maltose, mannose and trehalose are fermented and esculin is hydrolyzed by 90–100 per cent of strains. Arabinose, amygdalin, glycogen, inositol, inulin, mannitol, melezitose, melibiose, raffinose, rhamnose, sorbitol, starch, sucrose and xylose are not fermented by 90–100 per cent of strains.[7, 20]

Six different serological groups of *C. septicum* have been identified, based on the combinations of two somatic (O) antigens and five types of flagellar (H) antigens that may be present. Serological typing is useful in epidemiological investigations of strains isolated from different sources.[23, 25] *Clostridium septicum* and *C. chauvoei* share a common spore antigen which is responsible for cross-agglutination between them.

Clostridium septicum produces four different exotoxins. The alpha toxin is haemolytic, lethal and necrotizing, while the beta toxin is a deoxyribonuclease, the gamma toxin is a hyaluronidase and the delta toxin is a thiol-activated cytolysin (an oxygen-labile haemolysin) which in the case of *C. septicum* is named septicolysin. The delta toxin is haemolytic, and considered lethal and cardiotoxic.[26] The production of toxins in a culture medium is determined by the nutritional composition of the medium, strain of the bacterium, length of incubation, and presence of a haemolysin-inactivating factor.[4]

The alpha toxin is a protein with an isoelectric point of 8,4, and a molecular weight of 48 000 daltons.[2] Of the four toxins, the alpha toxin is the only one that is lethal and appears *in vitro* during the first day of growth. It is labile and haemolyses the red blood cells of humans, cattle, sheep, pigs and rabbits, but not those of dogs, horses, guinea-pigs and chickens. This toxin also has a direct effect on cardiac muscle when injected into guinea-pigs.[25] The alpha toxin of *C. septicum* is serologically related to the alpha toxin of *C. chauvoei*.[25] No specific information is available on the structure or the activity of the other three toxins.

Epidemiology

Clostridium septicum occurs in soil, water and the intestinal contents of animals. *Clostridium septicum* alone may be responsible for infecting a wound, or it may be present in combination with one or more of the other histotoxic clostridia such as *C. chauvoei, C. perfringens* type A or C, *C. sordellii* and *C. novyi*, as well as other anaerobic and aerobic organisms.

All breeds, sexes and age groups of cattle, sheep and goats may contract malignant oedema. Pigs and horses are less susceptible than domestic ruminants, while dogs and cats are resistant, or suffer at most from a slight local reaction at the site of infection. Most cases present after infection of wounds such as those caused by surgical procedures (castration, tail-docking, and ear-marking) in lambs, or contracted during shearing, parturition or vaccination.[18] The failure to use aseptic techniques during surgical operations, sterile equipment when administering intramuscular injections, or strict hygienic measures during shearing procedures predisposes to the development of malignant oedema.[14]

Crow pick is a rapidly fatal form of gangrene in sheep that is the result of wounds caused by the pecking of crows becoming infected. This particularly applies to parturient ewes, which are down and unable to escape from the birds' attacks. The birds are especially attracted to the eyes, and in this way a sheep's eye may eventually be torn from its socket, the resulting wound forming an ideal site for the proliferation of infecting bacteria such as *C. septicum, C. novyi* or *C. perfringens*.[9] Crows are carrion-eaters and their beaks are often contaminated by clostridia.

Post-parturient gas gangrene of the perineum, vulva and genital tract has been reported in cows, ewes and does. In South Africa it occurs most frequently in Boer and Angora goats and Dorper and Merino sheep. Pluriparous ewes with twins or triplets are more commonly affected than those with single lambs or kids. A prevalence rate as high as 30 per cent has been reported in some Boer goat herds. It is assumed that the portals of entry of the bacteria are lacerations and contusions contracted during partus, although the presence of these cannot always be verified.[31]

Braxy is no longer considered to be a disease of major importance because of its present low prevalence, although at one time it was of some significance in regions in which it occurred. It is a disease of sheep in countries with cold winters, and can be closely correlated with the type of husbandry practised, being particularly prevalent in animals that have to be overwintered on summer grazing.[27] Cases usually occur in autumn and early to mid-winter when heavy frost and snow are present. In the USA, however, it tends to occur in the spring.[22] It usually affects animals in good condition of six to 18 months of age. The morbidity rate in an affected flock may be as high as 50 per cent. Isolated cases of a disease similar to braxy have been reported in calves in the USA.[12, 22] Ulcers in the abomasum of calves and lambs may also become infected with *C. septicum*, resulting in gangrenous abomasitis.

Pathogenesis

The entrance of *C. septicum* into the tissues is favoured when a mucous membrane or the skin is injured. The presence of effusions, coagulated blood and necrotic tissue is necessary in most forms of *C. septicum* infections for the provision of the local anaerobic and other conditions required for the germination of spores of the organism and its vegetative growth and toxin production. Once it has become established and has elaborated sufficient amounts of its toxins, particularly alpha toxin, to cause tissue necrosis, the infection becomes self-generating.

The pathogenesis of braxy is not understood. In most cases the organism invades the mucosa of the abomasum or, more rarely, that of the duodenum, but as there is no obvious predisposing lesion in the affected mucosa which would have allowed such invasion to occur, the precise circumstances under which it does take place remain obscure. As the disease is associated with cold weather, it has been hypothesized that the ingestion of frosted vegetation plays a role in some way, possibly by causing chilling with devitalization and tissue injury of the mucous membrane which, in turn, allows the penetration and proliferation of *C. septicum*.[8] Absorption of toxins into the blood stream results in fatal toxaemia.

The fact that prior injury to the abomasal mucosa probably plays a role in the pathogenesis of braxy was exemplified, albeit inadvertently, in an experiment in which a number of sheep were infused via an abomasal cannula with a solution containing glucose and volatile fatty acids.[10] An acute haemorrhagic abomasitis resembling that of braxy, and from which *C. septicum* was isolated, developed in some of the sheep, and the centrifugal distribution of the lesions around the abomasal cannula suggested that the infusion solution may have damaged the abomasal mucosa, thus facilitating infection with the bacterium.

A form of gangrenous abomasitis in lambs and calves is associated with *C. septicum* infection of abomasal ulcers.[22]

Clinical signs and pathology

In animals that contract malignant oedema, clinical signs develop within four days of infection and are characterized by the development of rapidly expanding oedematous swellings, which may or may not be crepitous due to the presence of gas bubbles, at the site of infection. These swellings may be associated with lameness if the muscles of locomotion in the region are affected. Horses rapidly succumb to the infection after developing toxic shock and intravascular coagulation.[21]

At necropsy, affected areas are infiltrated with large amounts of inflammatory oedema which extend into the fasciae **(Figure 160.1)**. The muscles in the area are either markedly congested or pale reddish or brownish, and usually do not contain foci of necrosis. The exudate lacks the typical rancid odour that is so characteristic of *C. chauvoei* infections.

The incubation period of braxy is usually less than one day and the duration of the disease may be a matter of a few hours; death frequently supervenes before any clinical signs are evident. Animals that are seen to be ill usually manifest signs of abdominal pain and bloat, develop a high fever, and are inappetent and depressed. Death occurs within a few hours of the onset of clinical signs. Post-mortem changes develop rapidly.[15] Necropsy reveals a marked, diffuse inflammation of the abomasal wall; the abomasal folds are intensely red, may be emphysematous, contain focal ulcers, and are several times their normal thickness because of the severe oedema. Fibrin may cover the mucosal lesions and the serosa of the abomasum over the affected areas in the mucosa.[12] The abomasal content is blood-stained, scant or voluminous and foul-smelling. There are severe degenerative changes in the liver and kidneys, a turbid, reddish-brown peritoneal exudate, and petechial haemorrhages in serosal membranes. Histologically, affected parts of the mucosa, submucosa and adjacent muscular layers of the abomasum manifest a pronounced inflammatory oedema, areas of necrosis associated with a neutrophil infiltrate, emphysema, and numerous Gram-positive, rod-shaped bacteria in clumps or short chains. Thrombosis may occur in the blood vessels in the submucosa.[10, 12]

Clinical signs of post-parturient gas gangrene develop within 12–24 hours of partus and affected animals usually die within 12–24 hours of being noticeably ill. The signs include fever, lethargy, straining and, in some, a dark, haemorrhagic discharge from the vulva. The vulva and the perineum are usually severely swollen as a result of a marked oedema and emphysema **(Figure 160.2)**. Similar lesions occur in the genital tract; the uterus is atonic, red and emphysematous **(Figure 160.3)**.

Lambs and calves suffering from the condition as a result of the infection of abomasal ulcers with *C. septicum* show signs of abdominal pain and are often bloated. At necropsy there are usually several ulcers in the abomasal mucosa and these are associated with severe oedema and emphysema of the mucosa and submucosa — particularly in close proximity to the ulcers **(Figure 160.4)**. The lesions may become more generalized and involve the mucosa and submucosa of the entire abomasum. Numerous petechial haemorrhages may be scattered in the abomasal mucosa. In some affected animals the ulcers penetrate the wall of the abomasum, resulting in peritonitis and sudden death.

Diagnosis

A presumptive diagnosis of the disease caused by *C. septicum* is based on the history, clinical signs and pathology. The diagnosis should, however, be confirmed by bacterial culture and identification of the organisms.

As *C. septicum* is a common post-mortem invader, specimens for the confirmation of the diagnosis should be collected as soon as possible after the death of the animal, chilled, and submitted at 4–8 °C to a diagnostic laboratory. Specimens required for culturing include blocks of the affected tissue, such as muscle, abomasum, and uterus. As in the case of blackquarter, six thin, unfixed, air-dried impression smears on microscope slides should be prepared from the lesions for Gram's stain and the immunofluorescent test for the identification of *C. septicum*.[3, 28] Specimens collected for bacterial isolation should be cultured on blood agar and incubated under anaerobic conditions for 18–24 hours at 35–37 °C. Typical colonies of *C. septicum* should be selected when the culture is contaminated, and subcultured until a pure culture is obtained. The bacterium is then identified by biochemical techniques.[7]

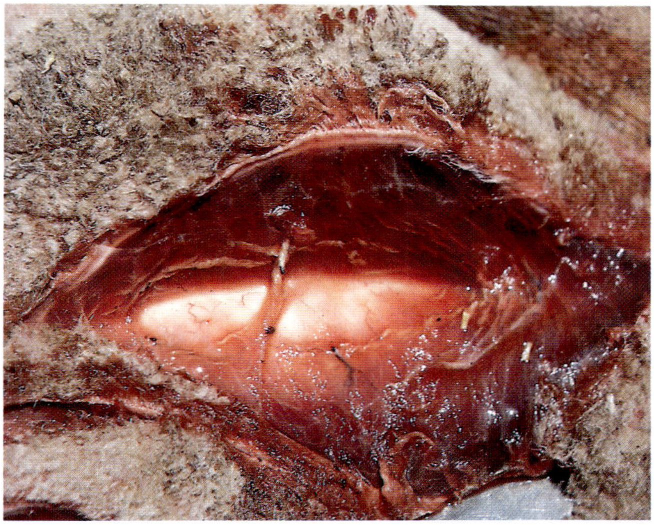

Figure 160.1 *Clostridium septicum*-infected shearing wound in a sheep. Note the extensive inflammatory oedema

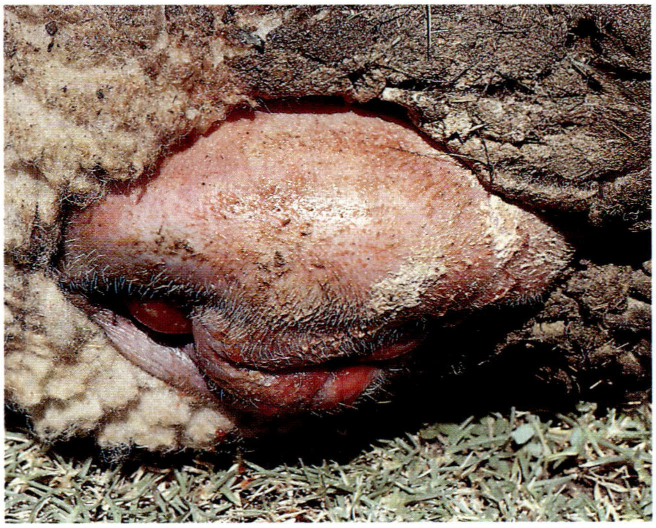

Figure 160.2 Marked perineal swelling due to post-parturient gas gangrene caused by *Clostridium septicum* infection in a ewe

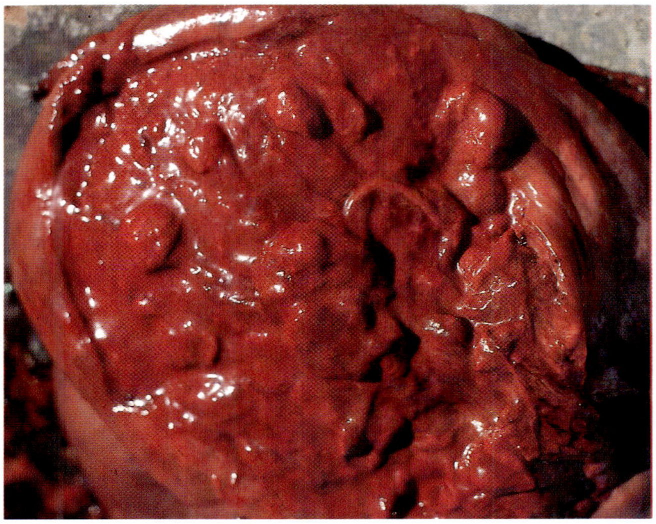

Figure 160.3 Post-parturient, haemorrhagic metritis caused by *Clostridium septicum* infection in a ewe

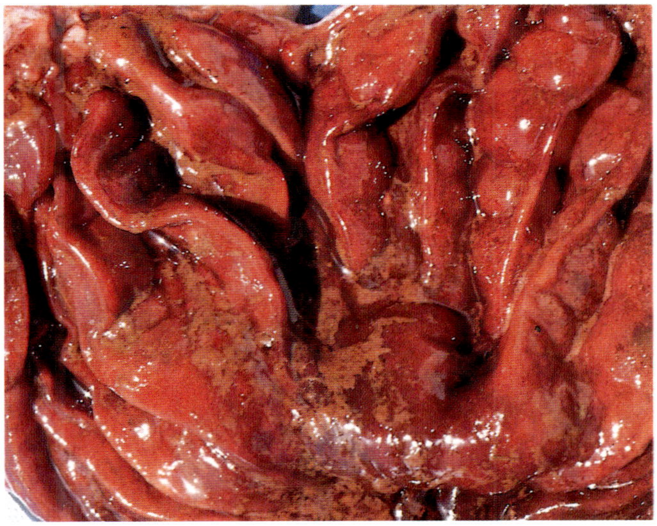

Figure 160.4 Acute, diffuse haemorrhagic and emphysematous abomasitis due to *Clostridium septicum* infection in a lamb

Differential diagnosis

The clinical signs and lesions of the syndromes caused by *C. septicum* cannot be differentiated with certainty from those caused by the other histotoxic clostridia, including *C. chauvoei*, *C. novyi*, *C. sordellii*, or *C. perfringens* types A or C. The signs and lesions of malignant oedema may also be very similar to those of anthrax, and those caused by the bites of snakes such as puff adders (*Bitis arietans arietans*).

Control

Treatment of animals suffering from malignant oedema and braxy is rarely successful, but it may be considered during the early course of the disease.[19] Treatment includes high doses of antimicrobials, including penicillin, aminobenzyl-penicillin and cephaloridine, and, if applicable, provision of adequate surgical drainage of the area and irrigation of the site with hydrogen peroxide. The administration of specific antitoxin may be considered.[24] Antitoxin is not available in South Africa.

Immunoprophylaxis is the method of choice for the control of *C. septicum* infections. A toxoid vaccine is marketed by the Veterinary Research Institute, Onderstepoort;[11] bacterin/toxoid combinations or multicomponent vaccines are also commercially available under various trade names.[6, 17, 29] Animals that are vaccinated for the first time should receive two injections of the vaccine four weeks apart and an annual booster thereafter. Subsequently, animals at risk should be vaccinated three to four weeks before shearing or parturition.

Special precautions should be taken when sheep are

sheared or animals are castrated or their tails docked. These procedures should be conducted as aseptically as possible. Shearing sheds and pens should be kept as clean as possible and, once cases have occurred, should be thoroughly cleansed and disinfected. Dead animals should be disposed of by incineration or deep burial to minimize the spread of spores.

In order to prevent braxy, sheep should not be over-wintered on summer grazing.[27] If an outbreak does occur, sheep should immediately be vaccinated and placed in another paddock or camp. The kraaling or yarding of sheep at night and the feeding of hay before allowing them to graze on frosted vegetation is said to be of value in preventing the disease.[16]

Vegetative organisms that contaminate instruments are easily killed by sterilization at high temperatures or by chemical disinfectants. The spores, however, are extremely resistant to most forms of sterilization. They are inactivated by exposure to 3 per cent formalin for 30 minutes.

References

1 **BAINS, B.S. & MACKENZIE, M.A., 1975**. An outbreak of gangrenous cellulitis caused by *C. septicum* in a broiler flock. *Australian Veterinary Journal*, 51, 106–107.

2 **BALLARD, J., BRYANT, A., STEVENS, D. & TWETEN, R.K., 1992**. Purification and characterization of the lethal toxin (alpha-toxin) of *C. septicum*. *Infection and Immunity*, 60, 784–790.

3 **BATTY, I. & WALKER, P.D., 1963**. Differentiation of *Clostridium septicum* and *Clostridium chauvoei* by the use of fluorescent labelled antibodies. *Journal of Pathology and Bacteriology*, 85, 517–521.

4 **BERNHEIMER, A.W., 1944**. Nutritional requirements and factors affecting the production of toxin of *C. septicum*. *Journal of Experimental Pathology*, 80, 321–331.

5 **BISPING, W. & AMTSBERG, G., 1988**. *Colour Atlas for the Diagnosis of Bacterial Pathogens in Animals*. Berlin & Hamburg: Paul Parey Scientific Publishers.

6 **BROWN, K.K., PARIZEK, R.E. & STEWART, R.C., 1976**. Prevention of clostridial disease in cattle and sheep by vaccination with a multivalent bacterin-toxoid. *Veterinary Medicine/Small Animal Clinician*, 71, 1717–1721.

7 **CATO, E.P., GEORGE, W.L. & FINEGOLD, S.M., 1986**. Genus *Clostridium* Prazmowski 1880. *In*: SNEATH, P.H.A., MAIR, N.S., SHARPE, M.E. & HOLT, J.G., (eds). *Bergey's Manual of Systematic Bacteriology*. Vol. II. Baltimore & London: Williams & Wilkins.

8 **DAVIES, G.O., 1947**. *Gaiger and Davies' Veterinary Pathology and Bacteriology*. 3rd edn. London: Baillière, Tindall & Cox.

9 **EDGAR, G., 1931**. Anaerobic infection in sheep brought about by the attack of crows (*Corvus* spp.) ('crow pick'). *Australian Veterinary Journal*, 7, 64–68.

10 **ELLIS, T.M., ROWE, J.B. & LLOYD, J.M., 1983**. Acute abomasitis due to *C. septicum* infection in experimental sheep. *Australian Veterinary Journal*, 60, 308–309.

11 **ERASMUS, B.J., CAMERON, C.M., HUNTER, P., CILLIERS, J.A., OBEREM, P.T., STOLTSZ, W.H. & DE WAAL, D.T., 1990**. Onderstepoort Vaccines. Booklet issued by the Department of Agriculture and Development and obtained from the Directorate of Agricultural Information, Private Bag X144, Pretoria 0001.

12 **EUSTIS, S.L. & BERGELAND, M.E., 1981**. Suppurative abomasitis associated with *C. septicum* infection. *Journal of the American Veterinary Medical Association*, 178, 732–734.

13 **FOWLER, N.G. & HUSSAINI, S.N., 1975**. *Clostridium septicum* infection and antibiotic treatment in broiler chickens. *The Veterinary Record*, 107, 14–15.

14 **HARWOOD, D.G., 1984**. Apparent iatrogenic clostridial myositis in cattle. *The Veterinary Record*, 115, 412.

15 **HENNING, M.W., 1956**. *Animal Diseases in South Africa*. 3rd edn. Pretoria: Central News Agency.

16 **HUNGERFORD, T.G., 1990**. *Diseases of Livestock*. 9th edn. Sydney: McGraw-Hill Book Company.

17 **KNOTT, G.K.L., ERWIN, B.G. & CLASSICK, L.G., 1985**. Benefits of a clostridial vaccination program in feedlot cattle. *Veterinary Medicine*, 79, 95–97.

18 **MACHEAK, M.E., 1978**. Clostridial diseases of cattle. *Veterinary Medicine/Small Animal Clinician*, 73, 195–200.

19 **PERDRIZET, J.A., CALLIHAN, D.R., REBHUN, W.C. & SHIN, S.J., 1987**. Successful management of malignant edema caused by *Clostridium septicum* in a horse. *Cornell Veterinarian*, 77, 328–338.

20 **PHILLIPS, K.D., BRAZIER, J.S., LEVETT, P.N. & WILLIS, A.T., 1985**. Clostridia. *In*: COLLINS, C.H. & GRANGE, J.M., (eds). *Isolation and Identification of Micro-organisms of Medical and Veterinary Importance*. London: Academic Press, Inc.

21 **REBHUN, W.C., SHIN, S.J., KING, J.M., BAUM, K.H. & PATTEN, V., 1985**. Malignant edema in horses. *Journal of the American Veterinary Medical Association*, 187, 732–736.

22 **SAUNDERS, G., 1986**. Diagnosing braxy in lambs and calves. *Veterinary Medicine*, 81, 1050–1051.

23 **SHIRASAKA, S., TERANISHI, H., BENNO, Y. & AZUMA, R., 1983**. Serological characterization of *C. septicum* strains from clinical materials of chickens and cows. *Japanese Journal of Veterinary Science*, 45, 861–863.

24 **SHIRASAKA, S. & UMEKI, F., 1984**. Antibiotic susceptibility of *Clostridium septicum* isolated from chickens and cattle. *Japanese Journal of Veterinary Science*, 46, 397–399.

25 **SMITH, L.D.S. & WILLIAMS, B.L., 1984**. *The Pathogenic Anaerobic Bacteria*. 3rd edn. Springfield, Illinois: Charles C. Thomas.

26 **STEPHEN, J. & PIETROWSKI, R.A., 1986**. *Bacterial Toxins*. Washington, D.C.: American Society for Microbiology.

27 **STERNE, M., 1981**. Clostridial infections. *British Veterinary Journal*, 137, 443–454.

28 **STERNE, M. & BATTY, I., 1975**. *Pathogenic Clostridia*. Boston & London: Butterworths.

29 **STERNE, M., BATTY, I., THOMPSON, A. & ROBERTSON, J.M., 1962**. Immunisation of sheep with multi-component clostridial vaccines. *The Veterinary Record*, 74, 909–913.

30 **VAN HEERDEN, J. & BOTHA, W.S., 1982**. Clostridial myositis in a horse. *Journal of the South African Veterinary Association*, 53, 211.

31 **VAN TONDER, E.M., 1979**. Regional Diagnostic Laboratory, Middelburg, CP. South Africa. Unpublished data.

161

Other clostridial infections

N.P.J. Kriek and M.W. Odendaal

This chapter deals with a number of clostridia which are infrequently associated with disease. These include *Clostridium sordellii, C. carnis, C. difficile* and *C. fallax*. In general, they are associated with wound infections in which the clinical and pathologic features resemble those of malignant oedema or gas gangrene caused by the better-known histotoxic clostridia. In rare instances, as in the case of certain *C. sordellii* infections, they are also associated with sudden death in lambs or cattle, or with the occurrence of haemorrhagic enteritis in foals, sheep and feedlot cattle.

CLOSTRIDIUM SORDELLII *INFECTIONS*

Introduction

Clostridium sordellii infection is associated sporadically with diarrhoea and haemorrhagic enteritis in cattle in feedlots,[1] adult sheep[2] and foals;[8] a sudden death syndrome in lambs[15] and feedlot cattle;[6, 16] and malignant oedema which resembles that caused by *C. novyi* type A and *C. septicum* infections in cattle.[20]

Clostridium sordellii was first described by Sordelli in 1922 as *Bacillus oedematiens sporogenes*. It is often isolated in association with other bacteria, including the well-known histotoxic clostridia, and may not be of primary importance as a cause of disease.[16]

Aetiology

Clostridium sordellii is an anaerobic, Gram-positive, rod-shaped bacterium with rounded ends, 2–4 µm long and 0,5–1 µm wide, and occurs singly or in pairs. The cells are motile by virtue of their peritrichous flagella. Spores often form and these are oval, situated centrally or subterminally, and swell the cell slightly.[17] Sporulation occurs readily in media such as chopped-meat broth incubated for 24 hours or blood agar plates after 48 hours' incubation. On rabbit blood agar the bacterium is slightly beta-haemolytic, and the surface colonies are 1–4 mm in diameter, have a circular or irregular outline, are translucent to opaque or grey with an off-white, shiny surface, and have a granular or mottled internal structure. The margin of the colonies is scalloped, lobate or entire.[5]

The optimum temperature for growth is 30–37 °C with only moderate growth taking place at 25 °C. and 45 °C. Growth is inhibited by incorporating 6,5 per cent sodium chloride and 20 per cent bile in the medium. Phospholipase C is produced in small amounts in culture and its production is best demonstrated on egg-yolk agar. No lipase is produced. *Clostridium sordellii* has saccharolytic and proteolytic characteristics. Glucose and maltose are fermented, while strains vary in their ability to ferment arabinose, fructose, glycerol, raffinose, ribose, and xylose. Adonitol, amygdalin, cellobiose, cellulose, dulcitol, erythritol, esculin, galactose, glycogen, inositol, sorbose, starch, sucrose and trehalose are not fermented. Fermentation in a peptone-yeast extract broth yields large amounts of acetic, isobutyric and isovaleric acids, as well as smaller amounts of propionic and isocaproic acids.[5, 14]

Clostridium sordellii produces a variety of biological substances toxic to animals, though non-pathogenic strains do occur. The unnamed, major lethal exotoxin produces a severe, gelatinous oedema and is thermo-labile and non-haemolytic, while the lesser toxins include phospholipase C, an oxygen-labile haemolysin, a fibrinolysin, a collagenase, and those that are dermonecrotizing and haemorrhagic when injected into the skin of rats and guinea-pigs.[3, 17]

Epidemiology

Clostridium sordellii can be isolated from soil, which is its principal habitat, and from the intestinal content of humans and animals. Faecal dissemination assists in the spread of the organism in the environment. Infections occur either by ingestion or by contamination of wounds.[17]

The conditions under which the disease syndromes caused by *C. sordellii* occur in livestock, and their predisposing factors, have not been clearly defined.

Pathogenesis

The pathogenesis of the disease syndromes is essentially unknown. Anaerobic conditions, such as those that exist in necrotic tissues, are required for growth and toxin production by the organism.[17]

Clinical signs and pathology

In experimental cases of the sudden death syndrome in cattle, affected animals have a marked increase in their respiratory rate, suddenly go down and then quickly die — animals may be found dead after having been seen to be healthy as little as three hours earlier.[6] The lesions in cattle that have died of the sudden death syndrome and of malignant oedema (the two designations probably refer to the same syndrome) are characterized by the infiltration of a haemorrhagic, inflammatory oedema of the peritracheal and peripharyngeal areas, with a particularly foul odour.[18, 20] This oedema may extend to involve the subcutaneous tissues of the neck, but the muscles in the region are unaffected. It may also occur in the subcutaneous tissues of the hind limbs.[16] Severe haemolysis is also evident in some cases, as detected in blood specimens presented for clinical pathology.[6]

A sudden death syndrome[15] has been reported in lambs. Animals that have died of this syndrome reveal generalized congestion, marked ascites and hydropericardium, and a markedly enlarged, degenerated liver at necropsy.

Adult sheep and cattle affected by the enteric syndrome may show diarrhoea for some time before they die as a result of a severe, haemorrhagic enteritis.[2] A similar enteric syndrome has been encountered in neonatal foals.[8] Affected animals manifest either diarrhoea — the faeces containing blood and gas — with death occurring soon after the commencement of clinical signs, or severe colic with the foals passing only small amounts of faeces containing blood and gas before they die. At necropsy, affected animals show a segmental haemorrhagic ileitis, a distinct line of demarcation between the affected and unaffected tissue being characteristic.[8].

Diagnosis and differential diagnosis

The syndromes caused by infection with *C. sordellii* may be confused with diseases that cause sudden death, particularly the clostridial infections associated with gas gangrene or malignant oedema, and with enterotoxaemias, such as those caused by *C. perfringens* types A and C. The diagnosis in live animals and at necropsy should be confirmed by bacterial isolation. Depending to some extent on the suspected syndrome involved, specimens from dead animals for this purpose should include portions of the small intestine (unopened and tied-off at either end), affected tissues, and subcutaneous tissue or muscle collected using aseptic techniques, and should be submitted to the labratory packed in ice.

The specimens are plated on to blood agar and incubated overnight under anaerobic conditions. Single colonies are selected for inoculation into Robertson's cooked meat broth to provide inocula for the fermentation tests and material for *in vivo* pathogenicity and toxicity tests in laboratory animals.[19] *Clostridium sordellii* must be distinguished from *C. bifermentans* by its production of urease, its failure to ferment sorbitol, and its toxigenicity. A positive diagnosis is warranted if a pathogenic strain is isolated in virtually pure culture and in profusion from typical lesions. The organism can also be identified by immunofluorescent staining, but it does cross-react with *Clostridium novyi*.[16]

Control

A bacterin or toxoid of *C. sordellii* is contained in some multivalent vaccines which have been used with success in feedlot cattle in the USA. Animals vaccinated for the first time should receive two injections, four weeks apart.[4, 6, 12] Similar vaccines containing *C. sordellii* are commercially available in South Africa under a variety of trade names.

CLOSTRIDIUM CARNIS *INFECTIONS*

Clostridium carnis is an aerotolerant Gram-positive bacillus, with dimensions of 0,5 x 2–4 µm. Under anaerobic growth conditions it grows rapidly and profusely on sheep blood agar to become slightly raised, flattened, grey-yellow colonies with irregular margins. A narrow zone of haemolysis usually surrounds each colony, although its width may vary from one strain to another. *Clostridium carnis* actively produces exotoxin but not much is known about its characteristics. It appears that guinea-pigs, mice, rabbits, sheep, mink, cats and cattle are susceptible to infection with *C. carnis*. A disease in cattle that resembled the clinical and pathological characteristics of blackquarter caused by *C. chauvoei* has been described and ascribed to *C. carnis*.[17]

CLOSTRIDIUM DIFFICILE *INFECTIONS*

Clostridium difficile was first isolated from a newborn infant in 1935 but it was not associated with disease in humans until 1977, when its association with the development of a severeantimicrobial-associated pseudomembranous enterocolitis in adults became apparent. It is also known to cause antibiotic-induced enterocolitis in hamsters, mice, guinea-pigs and rabbits,[10] and, rarely, necrohaemorrhagic enterocolitis in horses and abscessation in goats.[9, 11]

The possible association of *C. difficile* with disease in livestock was reported for the first time in 1981,[9] when the organism was isolated from mandibular abscesses in a goat. It has subsequently been isolated from pigs suffering from salmonellosis,[10] and from the intestinal content of four foals suffering from a haemorrhagic, necrotizing enteritis which caused their death within two days of the first clinical signs being observed.[11] These foals were one to three days old when they became ill and manifested colic, severe dehydration, and reduced body temperature, but increased heart and respiratory rates. They appeared to suffer severe pain, as they rolled repeatedly and lay in abnormal postures. Three of the foals developed diarrhoea, with watery, brownish-red, foul-smelling faeces. At necropsy the severity of the lesions differed, but they were similar in nature. The small intestine showed the presence of a severe, diffuse, haemorrhagic enteritis and patchy mucosal erosions, while the colon, of which the mucosa was congested and oedematous, contained necrotic material. Histologically a feature of the lesions in the small intestine was coagulative necrosis of the distal two-thirds of the intestinal villi. Large numbers of rod-shaped, Gram-positive bacteria were apparent on the surface of the affected villi and free in the lumen of the intestine. Similar but less severe lesions in which only a few bacteria were present occurred in the wall of the colon.[11]

Most strains of *C. difficile* produce at least two exotoxins, the major toxins being designated A and B. Toxin A is an enterotoxin that causes the accumulation of haemorrhagic fluid and detachment of epithelial cells in the small intestine of laboratory animals. Toxin B, a cytotoxin, is 1 000 times more potent than toxin A, but only exerts its effect after damage has been induced by toxin A, or if trauma is present in the intestinal epithelium.

Clostridium difficile is easily isolated anaerobically on cycloserine-cefoxitin-fructose agar medium from the intestinal content of foals suffering from the diarrhoea it causes. On other media it is rapidly overgrown by other bacteria. Its involvement in a pathologic process should be confirmed by demonstrating the presence of the cytotoxin by *in vitro* and mouse neutralization tests,[11] ELISA or a number of other immunologically based tests.[13]

On culture, *C. difficile* produces small (2 mm diameter), non-haemolytic, greyish, flat colonies on sheep blood agar after three days' incubation at 37 °C. The organisms are Gram-positive, form terminal ellipsoid spores, are motile and indole-negative, liquefy gelatin, produce hydrogen sulphide and acid but no clot in Crosley milk medium, and ferment glucose but not sucrose or lactose.[9]

CLOSTRIDIUM FALLAX *INFECTION*

A single fatal case of malignant oedema caused by *C. fallax* has been described in a horse. The lesions could not be distinguished from those caused by the other histotoxic clostridia associated with the development of malignant oedema in horses.[7]

References

1 **AL-MASHAT, R.R. & TAYLOR, D.J., 1983**. Production of diarrhoea and enteric lesions in calves by the oral inoculation of pure cultures of *Clostridium sordellii*. *The Veterinary Record*, 112, 141–146.

2 **AL-MASHAT, R.R. & TAYLOR, D.J., 1983**. *Clostridium sordellii* in enteritis in an adult sheep. *The Veterinary Record*, 112, 19.

3 **ARSECULERATNE, S.N., PANABOKKÉ, R.G. & WIJESUNDERA, S., 1969**. The toxins responsible for the lesions of *C. sordellii* gas gangrene. *Journal of Medical Microbiology*, 2, 37–53

4 **BROWN, K.K., PARIZEK, R.E. & STEWART, R.C., 1976**. Prevention of clostridial disease in cattle and sheep by vaccination with a multivalent bacterin-toxoid. *Veterinary Medicine/Small Animal Clinician*, 71, 1717–1721.

5 **CATO, E.P., GEORGE, W.L. & FINEGOLD, S.M., 1986**. Genus *Clostridium* Prazmowski 1880. *In*: SNEATH, P.H.A., MAIR, N.S., SHARPE, M.E. & HOLT, J.G., (eds). *Bergey's Manual of Systematic Bacteriology*. Vol. II. Baltimore & London: Williams & Wilkins.

6 **COLEMAN, J.D., HILL, J.S., BRAY, H.T., ARMSTRONG, D.A. & MORGAN, C.O., 1975**. Prevention of sudden death caused by *Clostridium sordellii* in feedlot cattle. *Veterinary Medicine/Small Animal Clinician*, 70, 191–195.

7 **COLOE, P.J., IRELAND, L. & VAUDREY, J.C., 1983**. *Clostridium fallax* as a cause of gas-oedema disease in horses. *Journal of Comparative Pathology*, 93, 597–601.

8 **HIBBS, C.M., JOHNSON, D.R., REYNOLDS, K. & HARRINGTON, R., 1977**. *Clostridium sordelli* isolated from foals. *Veterinary Medicine/Small Animal Clinician*, 72, 256–258.

9 **HUNTER, D., BELLHOUSE, R. & BAKER, K.B., 1981**. *Clostridium difficile* isolated from a goat. *The Veterinary Record*, 110, 291–292.

10 **JONES, M.A. & HUNTER, D., 1983**. Isolation of *Clostridium difficile* in pigs. *The Veterinary Record*, 112, 253.

11 **JONES, R.L., ADNEY, W.S., ALEXANDER, A.F., SHIDELER, R.K. & TRAUB-DARGATZ, J.L., 1988**. Hemorrhagic necrotizing enterocolitis associated with *Clostridium difficile* in four foals. *Journal of the American Veterinary Medical Association*, 193, 76–79.

12 **KNOTT, G.K.L., ERWIN, B.G. & CLASSICK, L.G., 1985**. Benefits of a clostridial vaccination program in feedlot cattle. *Veterinary Medicine/Small Animal Clinician*, 80, 95–97.

13 **NGUYEN, V.K., RIHN, B., HECKEL, C., BISSERET, F., GIRARDOT, R. & MONTEIL, H., 1990**. Enzyme immunoassay (ELISA) for detection of *Clostridium difficile* toxin B in specimens of faeces. *Journal of Medical Microbiology*, 31, 251–257.

14 **PHILLIPS, K.D., BRAZIER, J.S., LEVETT, P.N. & WILLIS, A.T., 1985**. Clostridia. *In*: COLLINS, C.H. & GRANGE, J.M., (eds). *Isolation and Identification of Micro-organisms of Medical and Veterinary Importance*. London: Academic Press, Inc.

15 **RICHARDS, S.M. & HUNT, B.W., 1982**. *Clostridium sordellii* in lambs. *The Veterinary Record*, 111, 22.

16 **SIPPEL, W.L., 1972**. Diagnosis of clostridial diseases. *Journal of the American Veterinary Medical Association*, 161, 1299–1305.

17 **SMITH, L.D.S. & WILLIAMS, B.L., 1984**. *The Pathogenic Anaerobic Bacteria*. 3rd edn. Springfield, Illinois: Charles C. Thomas.

18 **STERNE, M., 1981**. Clostridial infections. *British Veterinary Journal*, 135, 443–454.

19 **STERNE, M. & BATTY, I, 1975**. *Pathogenic Clostridia*. Boston & London: Butterworths.

20 **WILLIAMS, B.M., 1977**. Clostridial myositis in cattle: Bacteriology and gross pathology. *The Veterinary Record*, 100, 90–91.

Neurotoxin group of Clostridium *spp.*

Two clostridial species, *Clostridium botulinum* and *Clostridium tetani,* make up this group of organisms. Both are typical members of the genus, have strict anaerobic growth requirements, and their vegetative forms produce a toxin or toxins, which, in the case of *C. botulinum,* are amongst the most toxic biological substances known. Although botulism and tetanus are both caused by neurotoxins, the diseases differ markedly in their epidemiology, pathogenesis and clinical signs. Both affect humans and livestock in many parts of the world, are almost invariably fatal, and may have grave economic effects on properties where outbreaks occur.

Clostridium botulinum comprises a group of metabolically diverse bacilli that produce seven pharmacologically similar, but serologically distinct, neurotoxins, collectively referred to as botulinum toxin. Except in cases of the rare toxico-infectious form of botulism, where the toxin is produced by bacteria proliferating in the live animal or human body, it is ingested in feed or water contaminated by decomposing carcass or organic material in which it has been produced. Of the livestock species, cattle, sheep, goats and horses are susceptible to the effects of the toxin, while pigs are almost totally resistant. The disease, which is really an intoxication, is characterized by the development of a profound, usually fatal, flaccid paralysis which is the consequence of the irreversible binding of botulinum toxin to peripheral nerve endings, and the blocking of neurotransmission by acetylcholine.

Clostridium tetani, on the other hand, proliferates in necrotic foci, most often in deep, penetrating wounds in which the redox potential is low enough to allow growth of the anaerobic organism. Tetanus toxin (also known as tetanospasmin) produced at these sites is absorbed by the nerve endings and transported to the central nervous system, where it exerts its effects. Tetanus toxin irreversibly blocks inhibitory neurons (where the neurotransmitters are glycine or gamma-aminobutyric acid) in the spinal cord and prevents the contraction of antagonistic muscles, thus causing a state of constant muscular spasticity. Death is usually the result of asphyxiation. Sheep and horses are the livestock species most commonly affected by tetanus.

Both botulism and tetanus can be effectively controlled by immunization.

162

Tetanus

Synonyms: Lockjaw, 'klem-in-die-kaak' (Afrik.)

M.W. Odendaal and N.P.J. Kriek

Introduction

Tetanus is a non-contagious, almost invariably fatal neurointoxication, particularly of horses and sheep, occasionally of cattle, goats, pigs and humans, and rarely of dogs and cats. The disease is caused by *Clostridium tetani* and usually develops after deep, penetrating wounds have been contaminated by the organism. Necrotic tissue in such tissue injuries creates the necessary anaerobic environment which allows the organism to grow vegetatively and to produce its potent neurotoxin, tetanospasmin, which causes the rigidity and muscle spasms characteristic of the disease.

Due to its distinctive clinical features, tetanus is usually easily recognizable, particularly in the later stages of the disease, and it was described by Hippocrates in the early records of medical history. Even in modern-day human and veterinary medicine, tetanus remains an important clinical entity that requires prophylactic vaccination. In the developing countries it is a serious public health problem, with 50 000 human fatalities being reported each year.[25] Sporadic cases or outbreaks of tetanus occur in humans and animals throughout southern Africa.[15, 36]

Aetiology

Clostridium tetani is a Gram-positive bacillus in young cultures, becoming Gram-negative in cultures that have been incubated for longer than 24 hours. The bacteria occur singly or in pairs, and measure 0,5–1,7 x 2,1–18,1 µm.[7]

The bacterium is moderately fastidious in its anaerobic requirements. After two days' incubation on blood agar, the colonies are 2–5 mm in diameter, slightly raised, feathery, semi-translucent and grey. They have an irregular or rhizoid margin and are surrounded by a zone of haemolysis.[7, 30] Most *C. tetani* cells are motile due to the presence of peritrichous flagella which allow them to swarm on media with a moist surface. Non-motile strains also occur. The most characteristic microscopic morphological feature of *C. tetani* is the development of round to spherical terminal spores which cause the bacterium to bulge, giving it a typical 'drumstick' appearance. The spores are unable to retain Gram's stain, and are resistant to many standard disinfection procedures, including steam heat at 100 °C for 30 minutes, but they can be destroyed by autoclaving at 115 °C for 20–30 minutes. Spores germinate under anaerobic and aerobic conditions in the presence of certain substrates.[30]

Clostridium tetani is susceptible to metronidazole, penicillin, tetracycline, erythromycin, chloramphenicol, clindamycin and augmentin, but it is resistant to the aminoglycosides and most of the cephalosporins.[7, 23]

Clostridium tetani grows well on most laboratory media, its nutritional requirements being satisfied by various growth factors in the peptones and tissue extracts present in the media. The optimum temperature for growth is 37 °C, though there is still moderate growth at 30 °C, but no growth at 25 °C. Its growth in cultures is also inhibited by the presence of 20 per cent bile or 6,5 per cent sodium chloride.

The organism is metabolically relatively inactive and does not produce acid from carbohydrates, lecithinase or lipase. Neither does it hydrolyze esculin or reduce nitrate.[7] It is a typical example of a non-saccharolytic and only slightly proteolytic *Clostridium*. Certain strains may, however, ferment glucose and inositol, while most strains hydrolyze gelatine[31] and produce indole.[23]

The vegetative forms of *C. tetani* synthesize two very potent toxins: tetanospasmin and tetanolysin. A structural gene on a plasmid codes for the production of the toxins, the absence of the gene being the reason for the occurrence of non-toxigenic strains of *C. tetani*.[11] Tetanolysin (a haemolysin), is an oxygen-labile, membrane-damaging toxin that plays no role in the pathogenesis of tetanus.[32] The main toxin, tetanospasmin, is a potent neurotoxin and is produced intracellularly in the bacterium, being discharged into the surrounding medium as the organisms die, undergo autolysis and disintegrate. It is very susceptible to heat, being destroyed by 20 minutes' exposure at 60 °C,[9] and can be produced *in vitro* and purified within six days.[22] Tetanospasmin has a molecular weight of 150 000 daltons, and is composed of a heavy chain (100 000 daltons) and a light chain (50 000 daltons) linked by a single, disulphide bond. It appears that the light chain is the toxic portion of the molecule, and that the interchain disulphide bond plays an important role in membrane translocation of the toxin into nerve cells.[26] Tetanospasmin is lethal in mice at a dosage of 1 ng/kg body weight, whereas the lethal dose is 0,3 ng/kg in guinea-pigs, and varies from 0,5 to 5 ng/kg in rabbits.[12]

Epidemiology

Tetanus occurs wherever animals are farmed. Susceptibility varies considerably among the different mammalian and avian species, with horses and humans being the most sensitive to the effects of the toxin, followed, in order of sensitivity, by sheep and goats, mice, rats, rabbits, monkeys, dogs, cats, pigs and cattle, while birds are the most resistant.[1, 16, 31]

The spores of *C. tetani* are present in soil, dust, and the faeces of most herbivores[6, 36] but their distribution is uneven, which probably explains why tetanus is more common in some districts than others. The general perception that horse manure is the most common source of the organism is erroneous.[30] The fact that *C. tetani* is part of the normal intestinal flora of many animal species plays an important role in the dissemination of the organism. It appears that the vegetative organisms in the intestinal tracts of animals may replicate and produce toxin, leading to the formation of tetanus antitoxin following its absorption.[34] The possibility of autointoxication from the gut has been suggested,[24] but the occurrence of tetanus as a consequence of the toxin being absorbed in this way has not been confirmed in animals.

Though wounds of any nature are prone to contamination with *C. tetani*, deep, penetrating wounds such as those caused by nails penetrating the hooves of horses are most often associated with the development of tetanus. In addition, those associated with castration and tail-docking operations, bites, permanent-tooth eruptions, compound fractures, shearing, the umbilical stump of neonates and frost-bite may also support the growth of *C. tetani*. In lambs, tissue necrosis following the application of elastic rings for tail-docking and castration creates ideal conditions for proliferation of the organism and toxin production, resulting in the development of tetanus, sometimes in outbreak form **(Figure 162.1)**. In cattle it occasionally occurs after penetration of the wall of the reticulum by foreign bodies, and as a result of uterine retention of the placenta after birth. In some cases it may be difficult or impossible to locate the portal of entry of the organism, as the wounds in which it was located may have healed, leaving the spores to lie dormant in the tissue for varying lengths of time — from months to years — before germinating if and when conditions become favourable.

Pathogenesis

The spores of *C. tetani* are introduced into a wound in soil, faeces or other contaminated material. Tissue necrosis and infection of wounds with other microorganisms predispose to the germination and growth of the organism by creating an area within the tissues which has a low redox potential.[4, 29] *Clostridium tetani* is non-invasive and remains localized at the site of entry, where it produces neurotoxin (tetanus toxin, tetanospasmin) for as

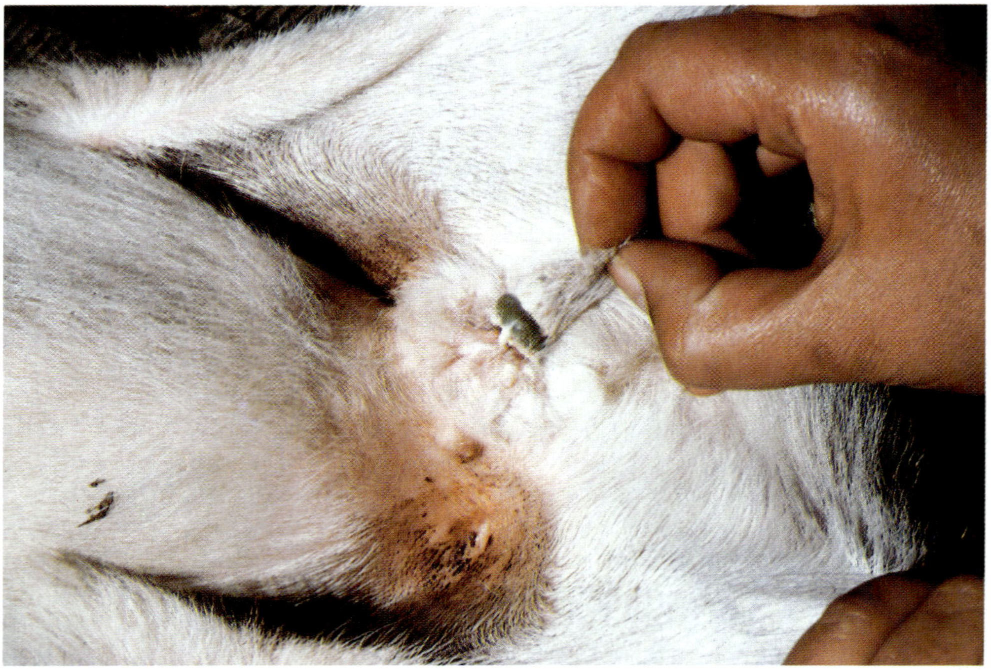

Figure 162.1 Elastic ring used for castration creates an ideal environment for growth of *Clostridium tetani*

long as conditions are favourable. It is assumed that tetanolysin is also produced in the wound, but that it does not play a major role in the pathogenesis of tetanus.[32]

Several factors influence the length of the incubation period of tetanus — the amount of tetanospasmin formed in the lesion, the toxinogenicity of the infecting strain, the amount of the toxin entering the blood circulation or neural pathways, and the susceptibility of receptors in the neural pathways. The incubation period may be very long, as spores of *C. tetani* may remain dormant in tissues for months or years until sporulation is triggered by the development of a necrotic area in their vicinity.[37] Weak toxin-producing strains do not produce sufficient neurotoxin to induce clinical tetanus. Unlike the botulinum toxin, tetanus toxin cannot cross the intestinal epithelial barrier, although it has been suggested that it can.[24]

Tetanospasmin produced in wounds reaches the central nervous system by one of two routes — either humorally through the lymph system or blood stream, or by way of the peripheral nerves. In the latter instance, also referred to as ascending tetanus, it enters the nervous system by endocytosis at the presynaptic terminals of motor axons, and then ascends by retrograde intra-axonal transport to reach the ventral horns of the spinal cord, from whence it diffuses cranially.[37] Ascending tetanus is demonstrated under experimental conditions by injecting a sub-lethal dose of tetanus neurotoxin intramuscularly into the hind leg of a rabbit. The leg into which the toxin was injected goes into spasm, followed by the muscles of the opposite leg, and then the muscles of the back and abdomen.[31]

Descending or generalized tetanus is the form that usually occurs in livestock and humans. In this form, neurotoxin is produced in amounts too great to be fully absorbed locally by the motor nerve endings. These excess amounts of toxin are taken up into the lymphatic and blood vascular systems, but are prevented by the blood-brain and blood-peripheral nerve barriers from directly entering the nervous system. Circulating toxin gains access by endocytosis at nerve endings throughout the body, and from there is transported up the axons to the central nervous system. Certain motor nerve centres such as those of the head and neck have short nerves supplying them, resulting in clinical signs appearing there first, followed by those in the upper part of the body.[31, 37]

Tetanus toxin acts on the central nervous system primarily by irreversibly blocking inhibitory neurons which prevent the contraction of a muscle or groups of muscles when the antagonistic muscles contract. No structural lesions are induced by the toxin in nervous tissue; the lesions are purely biochemical and the result of a presynaptic blockade of gamma-aminobutyric acid or glycine release at inhibitory synapses on motor neurons. These effects result in a state of constant muscular spasticity and give rise to exaggerated responses to normally innocuous stimuli. Sustained spasm of the respiratory muscles eventually causes death by asphyxiation, cardiac arrest and general exhaustion.[3, 14, 27] Excitatory transmission is also inhibited at a late stage of the intoxication.[4]

Clinical signs

The incubation period of tetanus may be as short as three days, but it usually varies between one and three weeks after infection has occurred; in exceptional cases it may be as long as several months or even years.

Initially a general increase in stiffness of voluntary muscles becomes evident and is followed by tetanic spasms of all muscles, particularly when affected animals are disturbed in some way by external stimuli, such as handling, noise (e.g. that emitted by the clapping of hands), or even sight. Trismus with restriction of jaw movements, spasms of the nostrils and tail, prolapse of the third eyelids, hyperaesthesia and stiffness of the hind legs are common signs. Death usually follows within 12–72 hours, but the course of the disease may occasionally be prolonged in the more subacute to chronic disease, from which some animals may even recover.[24]

Lambs, older sheep, and goats usually develop the acute disease. Affected lambs do not suckle, have grinning facial expressions due to contractions of the facial muscles, and hold their heads high and their legs wide apart. Owing to the spasms of the muscles of the limbs, flexion of the joints becomes virtually impossible and affected animals move with great difficulty. If the animals are startled, they fall down in lateral recumbency and go into spasms, showing opisthotonus with the legs stiffened and outstretched due to more forcible contraction of the extensor muscles **(Figures 162.2 and 162.3)**. Death occurs after three to ten days. The case fatality rate is approximately 100 per cent in animals manifesting clinical signs.[18]

In horses the clinical signs are characterized by the presence of flared nostrils, a sawhorse stance, severe muscle spasms, trismus and prolapse of the third eyelids. When trismus occurs, the mouth is held tightly closed and manual attempts to separate the jaws are generally unsuccessful. Other signs may include constipation, colic, retention of urine, inability to eat feed off the ground, opisthotonus, sweating, dyspnoea, and hyperaesthesia, with an anxious facial expression as a result of spasms of the facial muscles, and staring eyes. The ears are erect and the tail is rigid and is usually held sideways. The pharyngeal muscles are similarly affected and saliva dribbles profusely from the mouth.[15] Affected animals eventually go down, assume a position of lateral recumbency and, as in the case of lambs and other animals, go into spasms if stimulated **(Figure 162.4)**. The muscular spasms occur with greater frequency and are of longer duration as death approaches.

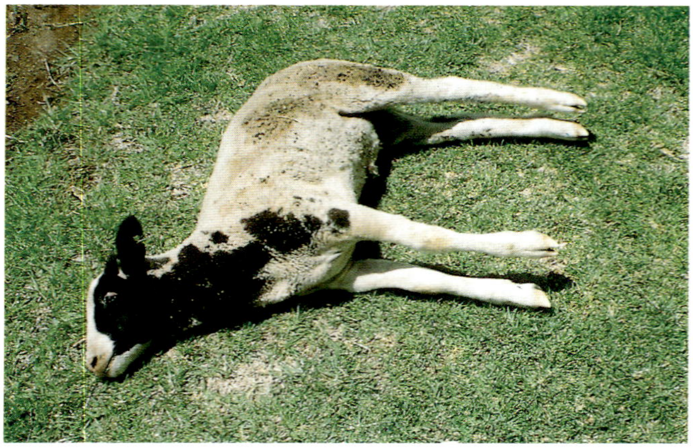

Figure 162.2 Lamb suffering from tetanus, showing extended legs and opisthotonus

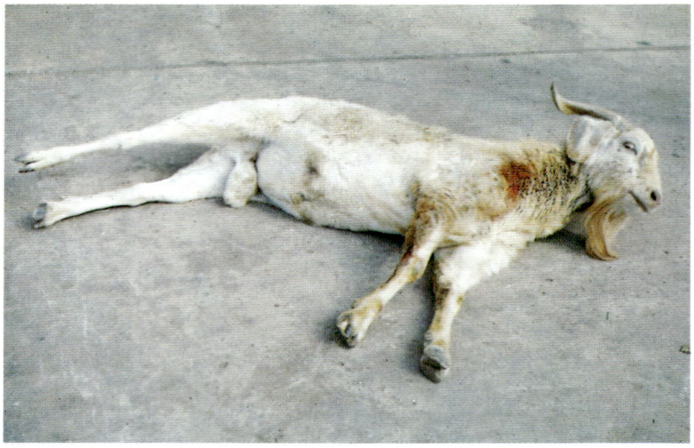

Figure 162.3 Goat showing typical clinical signs of tetanus

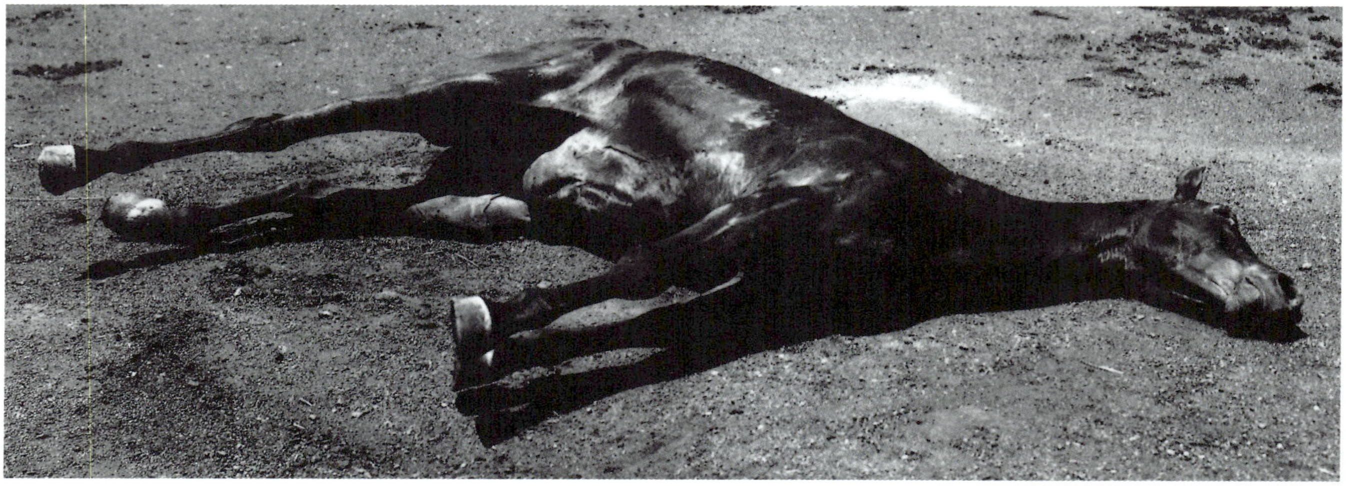

Figure 162.4 Lateral recumbency and extended legs in a horse suffering from tetanus

The clinical signs of tetanus in cattle include an extended head, a raised tail, holding the legs in a slightly abducted position (sawhorse stance), prolapse of the third eyelids, ruminal stasis, constipation, marked stiffness and, in some animals, bloating. There is pronounced dullness and depression, with the reflex nervous irritability being less marked than in horses.[15, 24]

Pathology

There is an initial respiratory alkalosis followed by acidosis in animals suffering from tetanus, and this increases progressively as a consequence of lactic acid formation resulting from muscular hyperactivity. During the period of alkalosis, hyperkalaemia is present, but this changes to hypokalaemia when acidosis develops. The hypoxia that follows the decreased pulmonary ventilation due to respiratory muscle spasms causes microcirculatory disturbances in pulmonary tissue and is a major cause of mortality. Glucose metabolism is impaired but is not stimulated by insulin, lipolysis is triggered, energy expenditure increases, and glucocorticoids and catecholamine blood levels are reduced. Aldolase and creatine phosphokinase levels are elevated, the extent being directly related to the severity of the disease.[4]

Specific macroscopic and microscopic lesions are absent, except for the probable presence of infected wounds such as those seen when elastic rings are used to dock the tails of or castrate lambs or kids.

Diagnosis

A diagnosis of tetanus is usually based on the history and clinical findings.[33] The isolation of *C. tetani* from necrotic wound tissue in conjunction with the demonstration of the toxin in tissue specimens may be used to confirm a diagnosis of tetanus, but this is rarely done.[33] Specimens are obtained from wounds or any site at which necrosis of tissue has occurred and which manifest signs of infection. For bacteriological investigation part of this material is inoculated into cooked meat or liver broth before the medium is heated to 80 °C for 20 minutes to destroy all possible contaminants.[2] It is then incubated for two to three days. Subcultures are made onto solid agar plates and specific fluid medium. The culture supernatant may be used for animal inoculation tests in order to assess toxigenicity. Laboratory animal inoculation of saline suspensions of wound material in order to determine its toxigenicity is possibly of greater diagnostic value than the bacterial isolation of *C. tetani* from such material. As a control, one or more of the animals should be given a prophylactic dose of antitoxin before inoculation with the wound suspension.[33] The presence in smears prepared from wounds of Gram-positive rods or Gram-negative filamentous rods with round, terminal spores giving them a 'drumstick' appearance can only be regarded as indicative of a possible *C. tetani* infection, as other *Clostridium* spp., such as *C. tetanomorphum* and *C. tetanoides*, have a similar appearance. The isolation of *C. tetani* from specimens of intestinal content taken at necropsy is meaningless for diagnostic purposes, as the organism normally occurs in the intestinal tract of animals.

Tetanus toxin may be demonstrated in the serum of some affected animals, especially during the early stages of the disease. Such specimens are divided for test purposes into three portions, one being treated with antitoxin, the second subjected to heat treatment at 100 °C for 30 minutes, and the third left untreated. A portion of each is then injected intramuscularly in 0,5–1,0 ml quantities into mice, which are observed for seven days. If the serum does contain tetanospasmin in detectable amounts by this method, signs of tetanus will develop only in the mouse or mice which received the untreated serum.[2]

Differential diagnosis

In South Africa, the clinical signs caused by a number of neurotoxic plants may be confused with those of tetanus. These include *Sarcostemma viminale* in cattle, sheep and goats, *Cynanchum* spp. in sheep, goats and horses, and *Euphorbia mauritanica* in sheep and goats. In horses, tetanus in its early stages may also be confused with eclampsia (hypocalcaemic tetany), acute laminitis, hypomagnesaemia and meningitis.[1] Eclampsia is confined to lactating mares and responds to treatment with calcium salts. Rigidity of the neck is also caused by cerebrospinal meningitis, and although the animal shows hyperaesthesia, it is generally depressed and hardly excitable.

Lactation tetany of cattle is associated with tetanic muscle spasms and convulsions, while white muscle disease in young ruminants may cause a marked stiffness but no muscle spasms. The clinical signs in recumbent cattle, sheep and goats suffering from cerebrocortical necrosis may resemble those of tetanus, but the absence of prolapse of the third eyelids and of rigidity of leg muscles excludes tetanus. The nervous signs caused by heartwater in cattle may also be confused with tetanus, although they are much less pronounced and a fever commonly occurs.[15] Although strychnine poisoning is uncommon in farm animals, its clinical signs may be confused with the early signs of tetanus.[15]

Control

The prognosis of an animal with tetanus is always guarded. It is most unfavourable when there is a short time between infection and the onset of clinical signs, and when the development of generalized tetanic spasms is rapid. Smith describes in detail the general medical principles for the treatment of tetanus in livestock.[28] Animals should be sedated, placed in a quiet, dark stable, and treated with a muscle relaxant. The stable should contain a floor which provides good footing, as affected animals have difficulty in rising, and it should also be bedded deeply with straw or wood shavings to minimize the development of decubitus. The *C. tetani* infection should be eliminated by surgical debridement of the wound, the local infiltration of penicillin G around the wound, and the institution of a course of penicillin administered parenterally. In order to neutralize unbound tetanus toxin, antitoxin can be infiltrated into the tissues around the affected area as well as administered intravenously (if the value of the animal warrants the expense). Active immunity to tetanus should be established by the administration of a tetanus toxoid vaccine, which needs to be repeated after about a month. The application of general nursing principles is important. This consists of such procedures as the maintenance of hydration, electrolyte balance and nutrition of the affected animal and relieving ruminal tympany should it arise. Feed should be placed in a position which allows easy access.

In one survey the injection of tetanus antitoxin intravenously, intramuscularly or into the epidural space in horses suffering from tetanus resulted in a 5 per cent recovery rate, while that in animals receiving injections into the subarachnoid space increased to 77 per cent.[21] In addition, intravenous alimentation[13] and acupuncture[35] may be effective.

Passive immunization with hyperimmune serum obtained from actively immunized sheep[8] or horses[20] confers effective protection in unimmunized animals and humans. It is effective within hours of administration but its protection does not persist for longer than three weeks.[19] It is used either for the protection of animals in which the possible development of tetanus can be anticipated because they are suffering from wounds in which the local conditions in the damaged tissues are conducive to the multiplication of *C. tetani*, or for the treatment of animals suffering from tetanus. Administered antitoxin will only neutralize tetanus toxin which is in circulation, and, as antibodies do not cross the blood-brain barrier, this treatment has no effect once the clinical manifestations of tetanus become evident. Following a possible initial beneficial response to the administration of the antitoxin, animals may suffer a relapse, in which case the treatment should be repeated. Cognizance must be taken of the danger of repeating this form of treatment. If it is repeated 24 hours after the first dose, the development of anaphylactic shock should be anticipated. The antitoxin, which in South Africa is available from the Veterinary Research Institute, Onderstepoort, is costly and its use should only be considered when the value of the animals justifies the expense.

Tetanus is best controlled by vaccination. Tetanus toxin is highly immunogenic when it is administered as a toxoid in association with an adjuvant. Adjuvants such as water-in-oil emulsion[17, 20] and aluminium phosphate[5] are used.

As horses are highly susceptible to tetanus, they should be vaccinated on a regular basis, whereas other species, particularly sheep, should be routinely vaccinated only in instances where the disease has become a consistent problem on a property.

When first vaccinated, horses should be inoculated with the vaccine twice at an interval of about one month. Active immunization is effective 12–14 days after the initial injection, but a second vaccination three to four weeks later is required in order to sustain the immunity at a protective level. Thereafter they should be given an annual booster vaccination. Mares with high levels of circulating tetanus antitoxin titres will provide protective passive colostral immunity to their foals up to the age of 10 weeks.[17] The combined use of active-passive immunization in horses has definite advantages and provides an immediate short-term protection and long-term immunity.[20] This method is most often employed in horses in which the development of the disease can be anticipated because of an injury, and it should be combined with the systemic administration of a course of antibiotic therapy.

Ewes which have not been vaccinated previously should be vaccinated twice during pregnancy to afford high levels of maternal antibodies to their new-born lambs. The first injection should be given approximately eight weeks before lambing and the second injection three to four weeks later. The tetanus vaccine manufactured and distributed by the Veterinary Research Institute at Onderstepoort consists of an aluminium phosphate-adsorbed toxoid.[5, 10] High antibody titres are obtained when the first administration of vaccine consists of an oil-adjuvanted toxoid, if this is available, and the second or regular boosters of aluminium phosphate-absorbed toxoid.[5] A single booster is required annually seven to 14 days before lambing.

Vaccination against tetanus does not preclude the application of standard hygiene principles during castration, tail-docking and other surgical procedures.

References

1 **BEROZA, G.A., 1980**. Tetanus in a horse. *Journal of the American Veterinary Medical Association*, 177, 1152–1154.

2 **BISPING, W. & AMTSBERG, G., 1988**. *Colour Atlas for the Diagnosis of Bacterial Pathogens in Animals*. Berlin & Hamburg: Paul Parey Scientific Publishers.

3 **BIZZINI, B., 1979**. Tetanus toxin. *Microbiological Reviews*, 43, 224–240.

4 **BIZZINI, B., 1986.** *Clostridium tetani*. *In*: GYLES, C.L. & THOEN, C.O., (eds). *Pathogenesis of Bacterial Infections in Animals*. Ames, Iowa: Iowa State University Press.

5 **CAMERON, C.M., VAN BILJON, B.J., BOTHA, W.J.S. & KNOETZE, P.C., 1983**. Comparison of oil adjuvant and aluminium phosphate-adsorbed toxoid for the passive immunization of lambs against tetanus. *Onderstepoort Journal of Veterinary Research*, 50, 229–231.

6 **CARMAN, R.J., 1985**. Horse diarrhoea: *Clostridium tetani* as a cause of misdiagnosis of enterotoxaemia. *The Veterinary Record*, 117, 445.

7 **CATO, E.P., GEORGE, W.L. & FINEGOLD, S.M., 1986**. Genus *Clostridium* Prazmowski 1880. *In*: SNEATH, P.H.A., MAIR, N.S., SHARPE, M.E. & HOLT, J.G., (eds). *Bergey's Manual of Systematic Bacteriology*. Vol. II. Baltimore & London: Williams & Wilkins.

8 **COX, J.C., LIEFMAN, C.E., PREMIER, R.R., CHANDLER, H.M., HERRINGTON, R.W., MIDDLETON, H.D. & HURRELL, J.G.R., 1984**. Immune response and reactions to various dose regimens for raising hyperimmune antisera in sheep. *Veterinary Immunology and Immunopathology*, 7, 65–72.

9 **DUNCAN, C.L., 1975**. Role of clostridial toxins in pathogenesis. *In: Microbiology*. Washington, DC: American Society for Microbiology.

10 **ERASMUS, B.J., CAMERON, C.M., HUNTER, P., CILLIERS, J.A., OBEREM, P.T., STOLTSZ, W.H. & DE WAAL, D.T., 1990**. *Onderstepoort Vaccines*. Booklet issued by the Department of Agriculture and Development and obtained from the Directorate of Agricultural Information, Private Bag X144, Pretoria 0001.

11 **FINN, C.W., SILVER, R.P., HABIG, W.H., HARDEGREE, M.C., ZON, G. & GARON, C.F., 1984**. The structural gene for tetanus neurotoxin is on a plasmid. *Science*, 224, 882–884.

12 **GILL, M., 1987**. Bacterial toxins. *In*: LASKIN, A.I. & LECHEVALIER, H.A., (eds). *CRC Handbook of Microbiology*. 2nd edn. Vol. VIII: *Toxins and Enzymes*. Florida: CRC Press, Inc.

13 **GREATOREX, J.C., 1975**. Intravenous nutrition in the treatment of tetanus in horses. *The Veterinary Record*, 97, 498.

14 **HABERMANN, E. & DREYER, F., 1986**. Clostridial neurotoxins: Handling and action at the cellular and molecular level. *Current Topics in Microbiology and Immunology*, 129, 93–179.

15 **HENNING, M.W., 1956**. *Animal Diseases in South Africa*. 3rd edn. Pretoria: Central News Agency.

16 **HUNGERFORD, T.G., 1990**. *Diseases of Livestock*. Sydney, New York: McGraw-Hill Book Company.

17 **JANSEN, B.C. & KNOETZE, P.C., 1979**. The immune response of horses to tetanus toxoid. *Onderstepoort Journal of*

Veterinary Research, 46, 211–216.

18 **JENSEN, R. & SWIFT, B.L., 1982**. *Diseases of Sheep*. 2nd edn. Philadelphia: Lea & Febiger.

19 **LIEFMAN, C.E., 1976**. Prophylaxis of tetanus. *Australian Veterinary Journal*, 52, 51–52.

20 **LIEFMAN, C.E., 1980**. Combined active-passive immunization of horses against tetanus. *Australian Veterinary Journal*, 56, 119–122.

21 **MUYLLE, E., OYAERT, W., OOMS, L. & DECRAEMERE, H., 1975**. Treatment of tetanus in the horse by injections of tetanus antitoxin into the subarachnoid space. *Journal of the American Veterinary Medical Association*, 167, 47–48.

22 **OZUTSUMI, K., SUGIMOTO, N. & MATSUDA, M., 1985**. Rapid simplified method for production and purification of tetanus toxin. *Applied and Environmental Microbiology*, 49, 939–943.

23 **PHILLIPS, K.D., BRAZIER, J.S., LEVETT, P.N. & WILLIS, A.T., 1985**. Clostridia. *In*: COLLINS, C.H. & GRANGE, J.M., (eds). *Isolation and Identification of Micro-organisms of Medical and Veterinary Importance*. London: Academic Press, Inc.

24 **RAMSAY, W.R., 1973**. An outbreak of tetanus-like disease in cattle. *Australian Veterinary Journal*, 49, 188–189.

25 **RUBIN, E., 1989**. The clostridia. *In*: SCHAECHTER, M., MEDOFF, G. & SCHLESSINGER, D., (eds). *Mechanisms of Microbial Disease*. Baltimore & London: Williams & Wilkins.

26 **SCHIAVO, G., PAPINI, E., GENNA, G. & MONTECUCCO, C., 1990**. An interchain disulfide bond is required for the neurotoxicity of tetanus toxin. *Infection and Immunity*, 58, 4136–4141.

27 **SIMPSON, L.L., 1986**. Molecular pharmacology of botulinum toxin and tetanus toxin. *Annual Review of Pharmacology and Toxicology*, 26, 427–453.

28 **SMITH, B.B., 1990**. *Large Animal Internal Medicine*. St Louis: The C.V. Mosby Co.

29 **SMITH, J.W.G., 1984**. Tetanus. *In*: WILSON, G., MILES, A. & PARKER, M.T., (eds). *Topley and Wilson's Principles of Bacteriology, Virology and Immunology*. 7th edn. Vol. III. London: Arnold.

30 **SMITH, L.D.S, 1975**. *The Pathogenic Anaerobic Bacteria*. 2nd edn. Springfield, Illinois: Charles C. Thomas.

31 **SMITH, L.D.S. & WILLIAMS, B.L., 1984**. *The Pathogenic Anaerobic Bacteria*. 3rd edn. Springfield, Illinois: Charles C. Thomas.

32 **STEPHEN, J. & PIETROWSKI, R.A., 1986**. *Bacterial Toxins*. 2nd edn. Washington: American Society for Microbiology.

33 **STERNE, M. & BATTY, I., 1975**. *Pathogenic Clostridia*. Boston & London: Butterworths.

34 **WELLS, C.L. & BALISH, E., 1983**. *Clostridium tetani* growth and toxin production in the intestines of germ-free rats. *Infection and Immunity*, 41, 826–828.

35 **WHITE, S.S. & CHRISTIE, M.P., 1985**. Acupuncture used as an adjunct in the treatment of a horse with tetanus. *Australian Veterinary Journal*, 62, 25–26.

36 **WILKENS, C.A., RICHTER, M.B., HOBBS, W.B., WHITCOMB, M., BERGH, N. & CARSTENS, J., 1988**. Occurrence of *Clostridium tetani* in soil and horses. *South African Medical Journal*, 73, 718–720.

37 **WOOLCOCK, J.B., 1979**. *Bacterial Infection and Immunity in Domestic Animals*. Oxford & New York: Elsevier Scientific Publishing Company.

163

Botulism

Synonym: Lamsiekte (Afrik.)

N.P.J. Kriek and M.W. Odendaal

Introduction

Botulism or 'lamsiekte' (literally, paralysis disease) in livestock is a non-febrile, highly fatal intoxication of cattle, sheep, goats, horses, mules, donkeys and, very rarely, pigs which is characterized by partial or complete flaccid paralysis of the muscles of locomotion, mastication and deglutition. It is an intoxication and not an infection, and in livestock it follows ingestion of decomposed organic matter, mostly of animal origin, such as carrion and putrid bones, but also of plant origin, containing toxin elaborated primarily by *Clostridium botulinum* type C or D, and more rarely type A or B. The toxin(s) are some of the most potent toxins known[63] and are not inactivated by the normal digestive processes. Humans and other species of animals, such as dogs, mink, many species of domestic and wild birds (including turkeys, domestic fowl, water fowl, pheasants and ostriches), certain laboratory animals and fish species (e.g. salmonids) are also susceptible.[93]

Botulism and its association with the ingestion of improperly preserved food has a long history in humans. The main sources of intoxication are meat and fish products, as well as non-acid vegetables such as beans, peas or beets. It was first described in humans in western Europe and Scandinavia[92] by Kerner (1786–1862) and Van Ermengem (1851–1922). Kerner associated the occurrence of botulism, which was sometimes referred to as Kerner's disease, with improperly prepared German sausages, including 'Schlackwurst, Leberwurst, Blutwurst' and 'Presskopf'. In 1912 Van Ermengem isolated the causative organism — a spore-forming, obligately anaerobic bacterium — from spoiled meat and suggested that the bacterium be called *Bacillus botulinus*, the latter name being derived from 'botulus' the Latin word for sausage. The disease then became known as botulism. As a result of the work of Burke and others, it was subsequently established that more than one type of the organism is responsible for the disease.

Seven toxin types of *C. botulinum* (designated from A to G) are currently recognized. Burke in 1919 was the first to recognize that different types of the organism exist, each with different toxins, and described *C. botulinum* types A and B.[15] This was followed three years later by the discovery of *C. botulinum* type C from greenfly larvae (*Lucilia caesar*), by Bengston in the USA, while investigating a paralytic disease of chickens.[5] During the same year Seddon in Australia found that a disease in cattle known as bulbar paralysis was caused by an organism which he called *Bacillus parabotulinus*.[82] Type C strains consist of two distinct subtypes designated C alpha (Bengston strain) and C beta (Seddon strain).[39, 77] Type D was isolated by Du Toit and Robinson at the Veterinary Research Institute at Onderstepoort in 1928 from a cow that had died of a paralytic disease known in South Africa as 'lamsiekte'.[39] Bier isolated type E in 1936 and 1937 from outbreaks of botulism in humans in which fish was the source of the intoxication. Moller and Scheibel isolated and characterized type F from homemade liver paste associated with an outbreak of botulism in humans in 1960. In 1970 Gimenez and Cicarelli isolated type G from a soil sample, and it has since been associated with sudden deaths in humans in Argentina.[95] This bacterium has recently been renamed *C. argentinense*.[98]

Botulism occurs in many countries in situations where *C. botulinum* is present as a saprophyte in decaying organic material. The disease in cattle was first recorded in South Africa by Le Vaillant[64] during the years 1780–85 while he was travelling through the interior of the country. He considered it to be one of the four most destructive diseases of cattle in the Cape Province at the time and, according to him, it appeared annually soon after the warm weather had set in and was particularly prevalent when grazing was poor and cattle showed a craving for bones.[45]

Both Commissioner de Mist in 1805 in his diary and Lichtenstein in 1812[65] recorded the occurrence of lamsiekte in several parts of the Cape Province. Hutcheon later encountered what he referred to as 'Lam Ziekte' in 1881 in the Bredasdorp and certain Kaffrarian districts. He commented on the higher prevalence of lamsiekte in young, growing stock and lactating cows as compared to oxen and dry cattle, and also that the prevalence of the disease was much higher when the vegetation was very low in feeding value than after good rains had fallen and

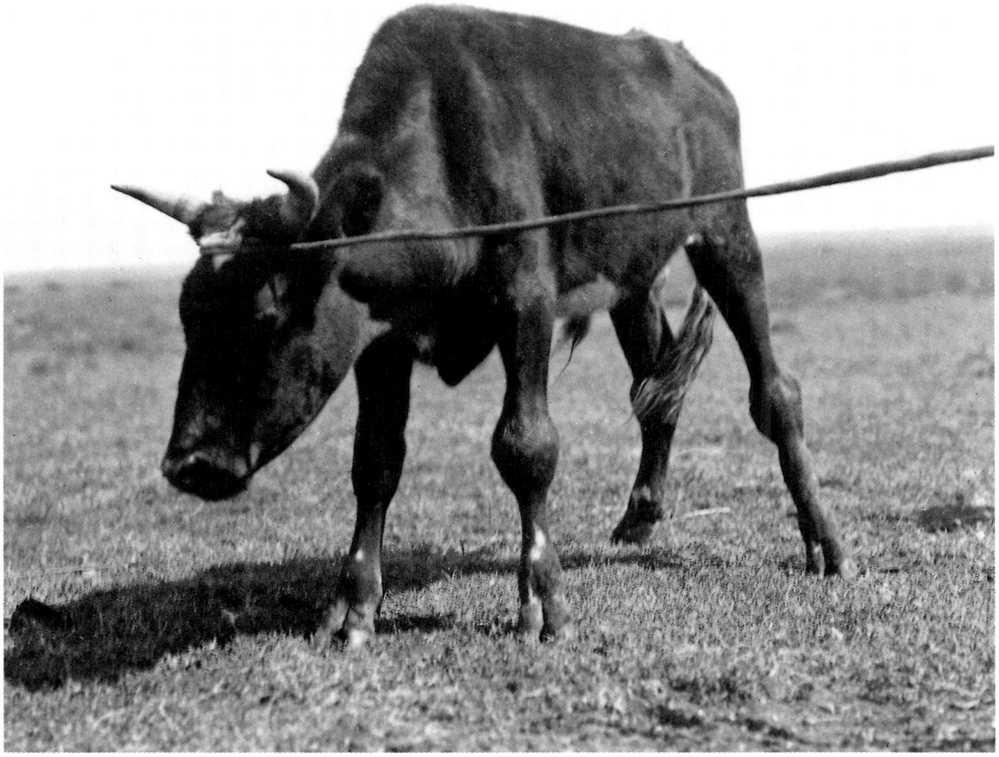

Figure 163.1 Poor condition and swollen carpal and tarsal joints of a bovine suffering from osteomalacia as a result of aphosphorosis

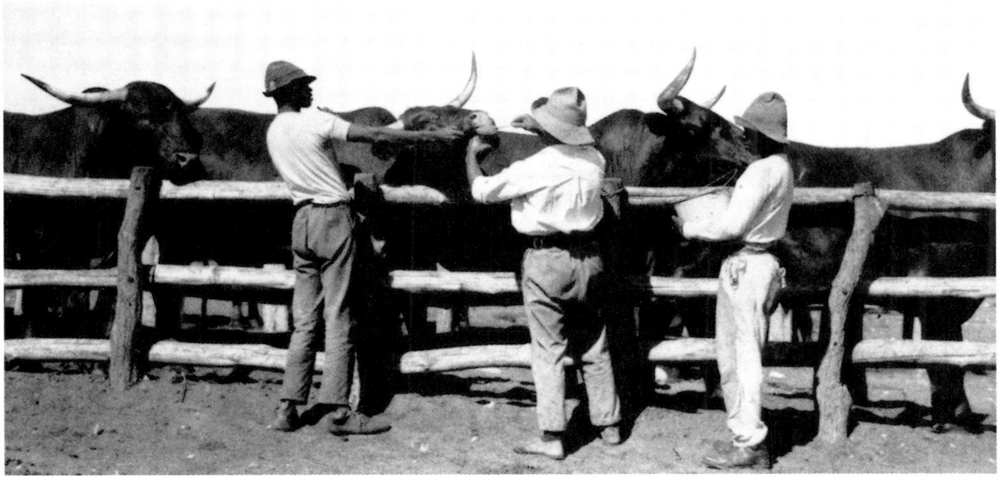

Figure 163.2 Historical photograph of workers dosing bone meal to cattle at Armoedsvlakte to prevent botulism

the grass was lush. The prevalence of lamsiekte usually decreased soon after the first rains of the season had fallen. Hutcheon[49] noted the association of the disease with pica manifested by cattle in these localities, and related it to a deficiency of phosphorus in feed grown on soil deficient in lime and phosphorus **(Figure 163.1)**. He ascribed the clinical signs to nutritional deficiency and maintained that they could be prevented by feeding the animals phosphate-rich supplements such as bran and bones. This view was strongly supported by Borthwick,[9] who showed that regular feeding of bone meal greatly reduced the prevalence of lamsiekte in cattle **(Figure 163.2)**. These views on the cause of botulism were not accepted at the time. This situation prevailed and losses occurred to such an extent that it threatened the future of cattle farming in these regions. Because of mounting pressure from farmers, Arnold Theiler was appointed in 1910 to investigate the cause of the disease.[40] The farm Armoedsvlakte ('poverty flats'), situated near the town of Vryburg in the northern Cape Province, was eventually purchased by the Government as a research station where much work on botulism and aphosphorosis was to be conducted.

In 1913 the investigations of Walker[111] and Mitchell[70] demonstrated that botulism was neither infectious nor contagious and that it was a non-specific form of toxaemia that developed after the absorption of septic material. They succeeded in reproducing the disease by administering carcass material and crushed bones in various stages of decomposition, following the insistence of farmers that cattle contracted the disease as a result of the ingestion of stomach content, skins and carcass material of animals which had died of botulism.

In 1919 Theiler[103] and his collaborators proved that lamsiekte was produced in cattle by the ingestion of carcass material picked up from the veld. He also induced the disease experimentally in healthy animals by drenching them with decomposed carcass material collected at random from veld on which the disease occurred. In addition, Theiler reproduced lamsiekte by drenching cattle with blowfly pupae collected in the vicinity of a lamsiekte carcass; blowfly pupae obtained from animal carcasses in non-lamsiekte areas failed to induce the disease. They concluded that the causal agent was a toxin present in decomposed animal matter in certain localities. Robinson finally identified the causative bacterium as a member of the botulinum group, *C. botulinum* type D.[80, 105]

Theiler explained the cause of lamsiekte in range cattle by way of an aetiological chain made up of six elements, the removal of any one of which would prevent the occurrence of lamsiekte under field conditions:

- the presence of the toxicogenic saprophyte which produces the toxin during its multiplication in decaying organic matter,
- the toxin,
- the carcass material in which the saprophyte multiplies and in which the toxin is elaborated,
- osteophagia or bone-craving, also referred to as pica, which induces animals to devour putrid bones or other carcass material that they would normally avoid, and
- phosphorus-deficient vegetation growing in
- phosphorus-deficient soil.

The role of *C. botulinum* as a cause of the disease in horses which in the USA is referred to as 'forage poisoning' was confirmed by Graham and Brueckner in 1919.[38] In South Africa, Theiler and Robinson in 1927[105] and Robinson in 1930[80] recorded several outbreaks of the disease in horses, mules and donkeys. *Clostridium botulinum* type C was isolated in South Africa from material associated with an outbreak of botulism in mules at the Veterinary Research Institute, Onderstepoort.[80]

In southern Africa botulism is currently well controlled in livestock by vaccination, although sporadic outbreaks of the disease still occur. Botulism associated with pica as a consequence of aphosphorosis in certain parts of South Africa still accounts for most cases in the country, but occasional outbreaks in which aphosphorosis is not involved are on the increase. Common sources of botulinum toxin in the latter instances include chicken litter used as a feed supplement for ruminants because of its high nitrogen content, pollution of drinking water by the carcasses of animals that have drowned in water troughs, roughage such as hay contaminated by the carcasses of small wild mammals, e.g. rats, and birds, or the feeding of spoiled lucerne (alfalfa) infected with the bacterium. It is not unusual for losses of between 100 and 500 cattle or sheep to be recorded in such outbreaks, particularly because they often occur in feedlots where large numbers of animals are either fed contaminated feed or drink water from a common polluted source.[56]

Aetiology

Clostridium botulinum comprises a metabolically diverse group of Gram-positive bacilli that are anaerobic and form spores. They produce at least eight neurotoxins that are pharmacologically similar but serologically distinct from each other. Eight types of *C. botulinum* — types A, B, C-alpha and C-beta, D, E, F and G — have been identified.[91, 92] *Clostridium botulinum* type C-alpha produces C_1, C_2 and D toxins and type C-beta produces C_2 toxin.[51] The type of toxin produced is also determined by the specific phage with which the bacterium is infected.[25–27, 50, 75] For example, *C. botulinum* type C can be cured of its prophage (a bacteriophage), whereafter it ceases to produce type C or D toxin. This non-toxigenic phage-sensitive strain of *C. botulinum* type C can be converted to another toxigenic species, *C. novyi* type A, after infection by phage NA1 obtained from *C. novyi* type A.[26] The production of botulinum toxins is not important for growth or for the physiological well-being of the bacterium, as growth and toxin production can be manipulated independently of one another.[83, 84]

The species *Clostridium botulinum* is additionally divided into three groups on the basis of cultural and serological characteristics. The first group consists of all the type A strains and the proteolytic strains of types B and F; the second group includes strains of type E and the non-proteolytic (saccharolytic) strains of types B and F; while the third group contains all the non-proteolytic type C and D strains.[16] A few strains of types C and D are mildly proteolytic but are nevertheless included in group three.[92] The strains of *C. botulinum* type G, as described by Gimenez and Ciccarelli,[37] are metabolically distinct and the organism has been renamed *Clostridium argentinense* as a result of these metabolic and cultural differences.[98] The three existing groups also differ in terms of their cell wall components.[92]

The proteolytic strains of type A, B and F (Group 1) are motile, have peritrichous flagella, and are straight to slightly curved rods 2–10 µm in length and 0,5–2 µm wide when cultured in peptone yeast glucose broth. The spores are oval and subterminal. In certain media with inadequate nutrients, they may increase in length to 20–45 µm. The cells normally occur singly, and less often in pairs or short chains. They retain the Gram stain very well, often only becoming Gram-negative with the commencement of sporulation.[92] Sporulation occurs readily on egg-yolk agar plates after two days or on chopped meat agar slants incubated at 30 °C for one week.[16] It appears that the highly toxigenic strains of all types tend to form fewer spores than the less toxigenic strains.[92] Group 2 strains include all the non-proteolytic strains of types B, E and F. The cells are motile, straight rods

1,7–15,7 μm long and 0,8–1,6 μm wide, occurring singly or in pairs. Spores are oval and subterminal and cause the cell to swell. Sporulation occurs readily on broth and solid media[16] but the germination of spores in laboratory media is promoted by the addition of 0,1 per cent starch, which binds the long chain fatty acids capable of inhibiting spore germination. *Clostridium botulinum* type A spores are fully activated for germination by exposing them to a temperature of 80 °C for 10–20 minutes.[92] Group 3 bacteria grown on proteose-yeast-peptone broth are straight rods, motile with peritrichous flagella, and with dimensions ranging between 3,0–22 x 0,5–2,4 μm. These cells occur singly or in pairs. The spores are oval and subterminal and cause swelling of the cell.[16]

With the exception of some strains of Group 3 organisms, *C. botulinum* is a strict anaerobe and even traces of oxygen in its environment inhibit its growth. These organisms are mesophiles and grow optimally at temperatures between 18 and 37 °C, and within the pH range between 7,0 and 7,6.[8] Some of the non-proteolytic strains grow at relatively low temperatures (3–4 °C), whereas the proteolytic strains do not grow below 10 °C.[46] The optimal temperature for toxin production is 25–30 °C. Non-proteolytic strains do not grow below pH 5,0–5,2, whereas the proteolytic strains generally do not grow below pH 4,7, though type A has been shown to grow at pH 4,0.[79]

In pure culture, *C. botulinum* grows well on solid agar media such as horse blood agar, liver-veal-egg-yolk agar and anaerobic egg-yolk agar,[46, 55] and in enriched, non-selective fluid media, including glucose-peptone broth, reinforced clostridial medium, trypticase-peptone-glucose-yeast extract-trypsin broth, or Robertson's cooked meat medium.[55, 110] A selective medium — *C. botulinum* isolation agar, containing cycloserine, sulphameth oxazole and trimethoprim as inhibitory agents — has been devised for the isolation of *C. botulinum* from human faecal material.[20] Organic nutrient requirements for growth and toxin production of Groups 1 and 2 strains differ.[115]

After three days' growth at 30 °C on horse blood agar, typical colonies of *C. botulinum* are smooth, circular with an irregular edge, and about 3 mm in diameter, which may increase to 8 mm after an extended period of incubation. Colonies are raised or flat, rough or smooth, and commonly show some spreading. Blood agar has no particular advantage as a culture medium but is a good general growth medium. Colonies have a similar appearance when grown on egg-yolk agar, and the use of this substrate has the advantage that it allows detection of the lipase reaction. The lipolytic enzymes produced by *C. botulinum* cause the development of a precipitate in the medium underneath the colony and an iridescent film (pearly layer) covering the colony, both of which are due to the presence of free fatty acids.[117] The lipolytic reaction can also be detected by scraping the colonies off the surface of an egg-yolk agar plate and then flooding it with a copper sulphate solution which will stain the free fatty acid precipitates on the surface of the medium dark blue.[46]

The surface colonies on blood agar of the strains in Group 3 are beta-haemolytic, 1–5 mm in diameter, circular to slightly irregular, flat to raised, and translucent to greyish-white, and have a slightly scalloped or lobated margin, a matt surface and a mottled internal structure.[16, 91, 92] Subtle differences occur in the colony morphology of the different groups. They can also be distinguished from one another on the basis of differences in their motility, ability to ferment various sugars, fermentation products and ability to digest proteins, and in the production of enzymes.[16]

Strict anaerobic growth conditions are required to propagate the more toxigenic variants of these organisms. Exposing blood agar plates to air will inhibit their growth, while less toxigenic variants still grow on media that have been exposed to air.

Sporulation is one of the most important characteristics of the genus *Clostridium* and is a most efficient survival mechanism. The spores of *C. botulinum* are among the more resistant of the bacterial spores, thus allowing *C. botulinum* to survive some of the conventional procedures for preservation of food that would normally kill other bacteria. The spores of *C. botulinum* are resistant to ultraviolet light, alcohols, phenolic compounds, quaternary ammonium compounds and organic mercurials. Substances such as ethylene and propylene oxide and formaldehyde do kill the spores of *C. botulinum*, but not very rapidly. Spores are effectively destroyed by heating or radiation. The D-value (decimal reduction time), which is an indication of the thermal denaturation rate and a reflection of the number of minutes required at a specific temperature to reduce the viable count of a spore suspension to one tenth of its original value, is used to assess the resistance of spores to high temperatures. The D-value of types A, B and E spore suspensions ranges between 0,15 and 1,95 for temperatures between 80 and 121 °C.[92] The heat resistance of spores is determined by various factors, such as the presence of fatty acids, calcium and iron, and the pH of the medium,[92] while considerable variance in the D-value occurs after batches of spores of the same strain are grown in different media.[92] It appears that spores from Group 1 are more resistant than those from Groups 2 and 3.

Apart from heat, radiation is used as a means of sterilizing food. To achieve indisputable microbial safety, radiation doses in the range of 35–45 kGy must be applied. This dosage is based on the 12D-concept; this is a dose high enough to destroy a theoretical population of 1 x 10^{12} *C. botulinum* spores per gram.[4] However, organoleptic side-effects affecting the taste and odour of the food are produced by such high doses. Mild irradiation sensitizes bacterial spores to subsequent heat injury.

'Botulinum neurotoxin' refers to any one of seven subtances — toxin types A, B, C_1, D, E, F and G — that are produced by *C. botulinum*. The various toxins which are proteins have similar molecular weights and probably similar molecular structures. The eighth toxin, referred to as C_2, is produced by type C and D strains but is not a neurotoxin. It is also referred to as 'the botulinum binary toxin' and has a unique structure and pharmacological action. It does not cause flaccid paralysis but it does act as an adenosine diphosphate ribosylating enzyme that causes increased vascular permeability[76] and necrosis in the epithelium and lamina propria of the duodenum and jejunum.[62] More details on the mechanism of action of the botulinum neurotoxins are available in a number of reviews.[11, 43, 83, 92, 93, 99] The toxins are relatively resistant to the action of mild chemical agents, but are susceptible to heat inactivation. High salt concentrations prevent toxin production.[92]

The molecular mass of the neurotoxins produced by types A to F varies from 150 000 to 160 000 daltons. The toxins are synthesized as single polypeptide chains, but when released from the bacteria they are proteolytically cleaved to form two non-identical protein fragments, each consisting of a heavy chain or subunit with a molecular mass of 100 000 daltons and a light chain or subunit with a molecular mass of 50 000 daltons, linked by a disulphide bond.[96] Type A and B neurotoxins contain at least one disulphide bond each, which on reduction causes loss of biological activity.[83] However botulinum toxin is moderately resistant to enzymic proteolysis under natural conditions, but is inactivated by exposure to a temperature of 80 °C for ten minutes.[92]

The botulinum toxin is synthesized intracellularly and is released into the culture supernatant when bacteria undergo autolysis after completion of growth cycles.[83, 84] The concentration of free toxin may thus increase in the supernatant even after protein synthesis has stopped. It appears that botulinum neurotoxin may be synthesized as an inactive or less toxic precursor, which is then activated by selective cleavage by proteolytic enzymes. The ability of trypsin to activate botulinum neurotoxin has been demonstrated for types A–G.[83]

The potency of botulinum toxin, which may also be produced by bacteria grown on artificial media, is expressed as the LD_{50} (lethal dose in 50 per cent of animals) or MLD (minimum lethal dose) in mice. The L+ and the Ramon flocculation tests are used to determine the total amount of toxin present in the culture supernatant.[52, 92] The MLD for mice of botulinum type A neurotoxin per gram of body weight is 1,2 ng intraperitoneally (ip), for type B neurotoxin 1,2–2 ng ip, for C_1 toxin 1,1 ng intravenously (iv), type C_2 toxin 270 ng iv, type D toxin 0,4 ng ip, type E toxin 1,1 ng ip and type F 2,5 ng ip.[36]

Epidemiology

Botulism has been described in cattle,[22, 33, 42, 45, 68, 72] horses and foals,[41, 66, 80, 101, 102] mules and donkeys,[80] sheep and goats,[104] pigs,[3] water birds,[44, 88] turkeys,[86] ostriches and ducks,[104] and dogs.[2, 13, 19, 112]

Among livestock, horses appear to be the most susceptible to the effects of the botulinum toxin. Amounts of toxin which are sublethal in mice may rapidly cause the death of adult horses if administered intravenously.[60] Pigs and carnivores, on the other hand, are very resistant to botulinum toxin and for all practical purposes are not susceptible to its effects. *Clostridium botulinum* type C_1 toxin may be present in the livers of healthy pigs infected with *C. botulinum* type C without the pigs showing clinical signs.[119] Cattle, sheep and goats appear to be equally susceptible to the effects of the toxin.[104]

There is an apparent geographic variation in the distribution of the different toxin types of *C. botulinum*. Toxin types C and D appear to be the exclusive cause of botulism of livestock in countries in the southern hemisphere, such as Australia, South Africa and certain South American countries,[23, 104, 107] whereas type B is more often the cause of botulism in livestock in the USA and Europe.[14]

Spores of *C. botulinum* occur commonly in soil, water, marine sediments and marine environments throughout the world.[4, 48, 91, 92] *Clostridium botulinum* also appears to be a normal inhabitant of the intestinal tract of horses, cattle and poultry, where it multiplies and from which it is shed in large numbers in the faeces for up to eight weeks after primary infection.[72]

Outbreaks of botulism in livestock occur under a variety of conditions but can in general be subdivided into two main categories, namely, those associated with phosphorus deficiency and osteophagia in which the disease occurs sporadically over a relatively long period of time in animals (mainly cattle, but also to a lesser extent sheep and goats) maintained under extensive ranching conditions, and secondly the form in cattle, sheep, goats and horses which is associated with the ingestion of toxic feed or water and which may result in the deaths of large numbers of animals over a short period.

In sporadic outbreaks of botulism that are not associated with aphosphorosis, *C. botulinum*-containing carcass material of mammals or birds may contaminate feed or water of domestic livestock. More rarely, spoiled vegetable matter such as grass hay, lucerne hay, grass clippings, silage, brewers' grain, and even kitchen refuse or 'mynpap' (porridge) obtained from the kitchen waste of mine hostels[22, 33, 42, 68, 85, 116] may serve as substrates for bacterial growth and toxin production. Three recent outbreaks in farm animals in South Africa exemplify this form of botulism. One occurred in sheep maintained under extensive farming conditions in the Upington district of the north-western Cape Province. It was only after hundreds of animals had died that the putrefying carcass of a sheep was found submerged in the water of a remote drinking trough on the farm. This led to the disease being finally diagnosed as botulism.[57] The second outbreak occurred on a smallholding on which all the animals (cattle, sheep, pigs, donkeys, geese and chickens) except the pigs died of botulism as the result of the feeding of kitchen refuse which had been obtained from a large hostel and stored in metal drums before being fed to the animals.[17] In the third outbreak, a field of lucerne had been sprayed with an insecticide in order to control an infestation of worms. Egrets, an insectivorous species of bird, had eaten the dead worms and in turn had died from insecticidal poisoning. When the lucerne was harvested for hay, some of the dead birds were baled in the lucerne. An outbreak of botulism occurred in the dairy cows fed the hay, and the source of the toxin was only realized due to the presence of feathers in the lucerne hay.[18]

Chicken manure (especially broiler litter), which is often fed to ruminants as a supplement because of its high nitrogen content, frequently contains carcasses of dead chickens in which *C. botulinum* has multiplied and produced its toxins. Outbreaks have even occurred after chicken manure has been spread on pastures as a fertilizer or when it has been used as bedding material. Based on experimental data, it appears that the type of feed that animals are receiving, as well as a change in feed prior to their exposure to botulinum toxin, affects the dose of the toxin required to induce the disease in a specific species. In one study, goats on pasture as well as those being fed silage developed increased susceptibility to the effects of the toxin after their diet had been changed to hay and concentrated fodder.[31]

Probably the single most important factor responsible for botulism under extensive ranching conditions is the occurrence of osteophagia resulting from phosphorus-deficient grazing. Cattle, particularly, and sheep to a lesser extent, are prone to develop osteophagia as a result of phosphorus deficiency. Other species are not known to develop osteophagia. Economically serious outbreaks of botulism as a result of pica have been recorded in South Africa, Australia and several South American countries.[23, 103, 107]

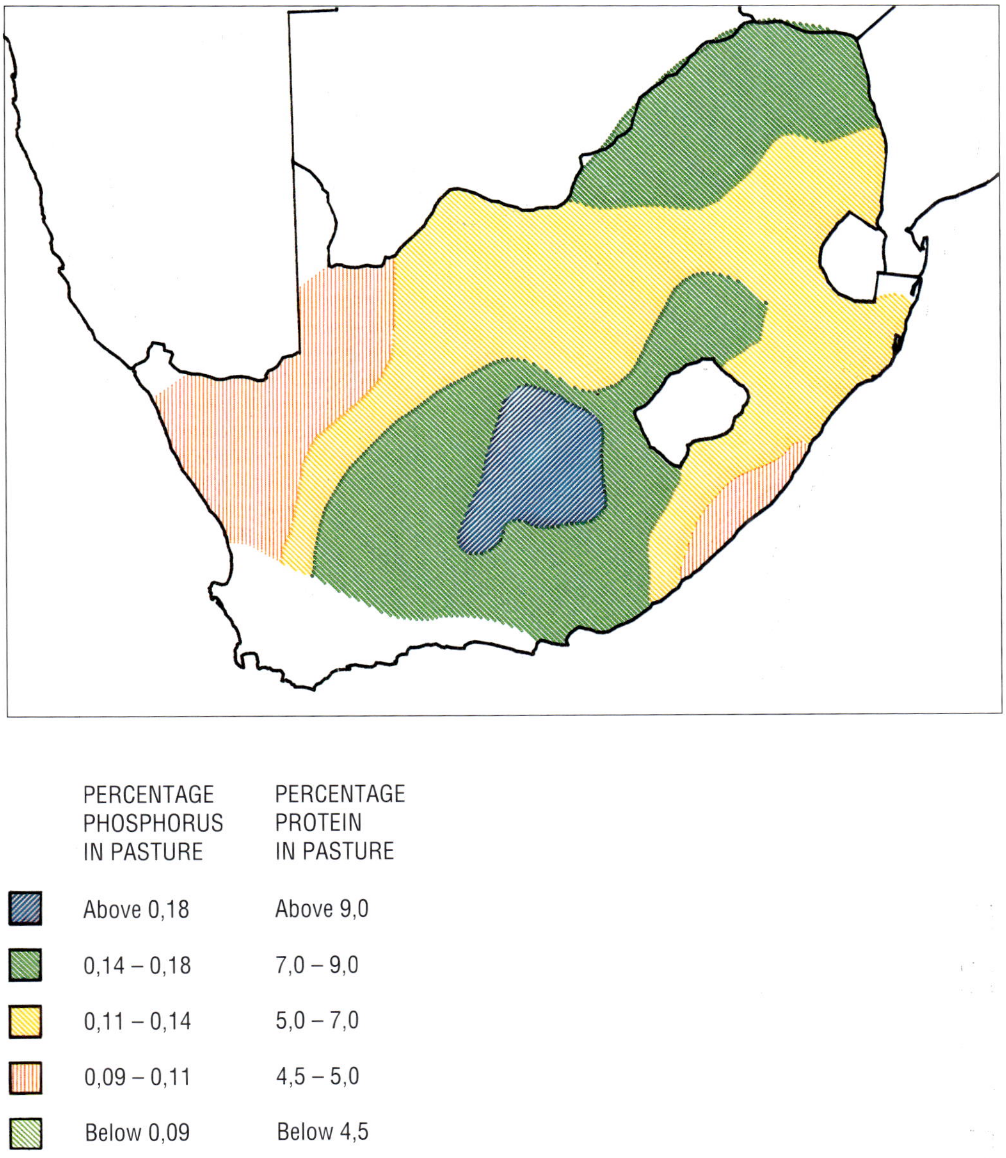

Figure 163.3 Phosphorus and protein content of vegetation during summer in South Africa

During spring and early summer in South Africa, the phosphorus content of the veld grasses is generally sufficient to prevent the development of osteophagia and the occurrence of botulism. However, when the grazing has matured, its phosphorus content decreases to such an extent that by late summer and winter (for a period that ranges from five to nine months of the year) cattle grazing on it may suffer from osteophagia **(Figures 163.3 and 163.4)** unless the deficiency is compensated for by supplying the animals with additional sources of phosphorus, e.g. in the form of phosphate-containing licks.[24] Deficiency of other dietary components, such as proteins, which often occurs concomitantly in such phosphorus-deficient grasses, may also cause animals to develop pica and hence predispose them to consume toxin-containing material. Growing, lactating, and pregnant cattle require more dietary phosphorus than other groups of cattle and these are therefore more prone to develop botulism. The requirement of phosphorus in these animals is such that the amount of phosphorus present in natural pastures in South Africa is often insufficient throughout the year.

In South Africa it appears that, apart from the carcass debris of domestic animals, the carcasses of small mammals such as mongooses and hares, birds and particularly tortoises are important sources of the toxin under ranching conditions.[32] The carcasses of small mammals may remain toxic for up to 350 days but usually lose their toxicity after four to six weeks, whereas tortoise carcasses retain their toxicity for up to 350 days on pasture and up to 600 days in the laboratory.[32] Rain may leach much of the toxin from the carcass material of small mammals, whereas the shells and bones of tortoises retain the toxin for longer periods in wet weather. In Australia, botulism in cattle in phosphorus-deficient areas is associated with the ingestion of carrion, chiefly dead rabbits containing

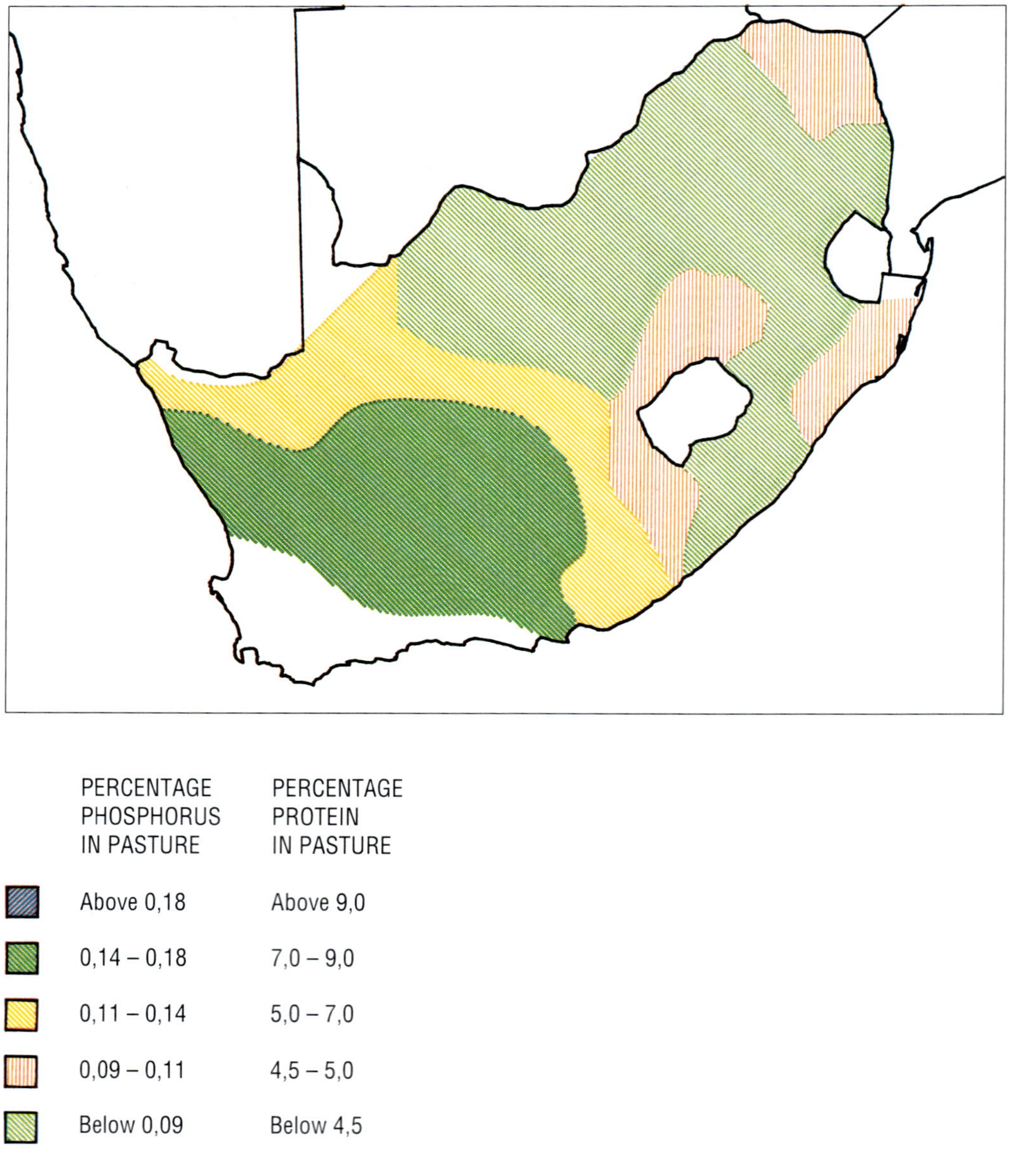

Figure 163.4 Phosphorus and protein content of vegetation during winter in South Africa

the toxin.[6] Prevailing climatic conditions affect toxin production. The toxin is readily produced in carcasses when there is sufficient heat and moisture, but there is a drastic reduction in toxin production when the weather becomes cold and dry.[59] The production of botulinum toxin under optimal environmental conditions reaches its maximum within five to ten days, whereafter it starts to decline. Type C botulinum toxin production in mouse carcasses under experimental conditions may reach concentrations of 2 x 10^5 to 2 x 10^6 mouse intraperitoneal MLD/g.[90] The type of animal tissue and the microflora present in it appear to influence the amount of toxin produced by *C. botulinum* types C and E. Type C toxin is produced in much higher concentrations in chicken and mouse carcasses than in fish carcasses.[90] The microclimate within maggot-infested duck carcasses appears to be suitable for growth and toxin production by *C. botulinum*.[118]

The occurrence of botulism under ranching conditions is increased by phosphorus deficiency in genetically improved, quicker-growing and higher-demanding breeds, overstocking, and inadequate removal of carcasses and carcass debris from pastures.[23, 104] In addition, rapidly growing, low-demanding cultivars of pasture grass, such as *Brachiaria decumbens* in Brazil, become phosphorus-deficient during early spring and summer,[23] which results in botulism in these seasons. This is in contrast to the situation in South Africa, where most cases related to aphosphorosis occur during the dry winter months which prevail over a large part of the country.

Pigs are highly resistant to the effects of the botulinum toxin. The only recorded outbreak of botulism in this species of animal occurred in Australia and followed the ingestion of dead fish containing type C toxin.[3]

Toxico-infectious botulism is a rare form of the disease in humans and animals which results when toxin is produced *in vivo* by *C. botulinum* growing in the body itself, rather than by the ingestion of toxin.[92, 93] It may either follow wound infection or occur after ingested spores have germinated and proliferated vegetatively in the gastrointestinal tract. Wound botulism has been described in humans and is becoming a problem in drug addicts who use contaminated hypodermic needles. Only Group 1 strains of *C. botulism* have been incriminated in this condition in humans.[93] A similar form of wound botulism has been described in adult horses and young foals in which gastric ulcers, umbilical or lung abscesses, or necrotic wounds such as those following castration were the site of localization and proliferation of the organism.[7, 101, 102] It appears that the growth of the organism in necrotic tissue in foals is potentiated by excessive amounts of corticosteroids contained in the fat of the milk of mares which are exposed to stress, such as that produced by excessively nutritious diets, the rearing of fast-growing foals, or drastic changes in weather. Outbreaks often follow such changes in weather.[101] Young foals afflicted in this way show the signs of the 'shaker foal syndrome', which are dysphagia, muscular tremors, weakness, recumbency and death.[101] Both toxin type A and B of *C. botulinum* have been incriminated in horses.[66, 101]

Botulism in human infants is the result of the absorption of toxin elaborated by organisms, usually Group 1 strains, following their colonization of the intestinal tract.[69, 93] A similar situation has been observed in pheasants, in which the crop was the site of colonization and toxin elaboration,[21] as well as in broiler chickens, in which the caecum was the site of bacterial multiplication.[71]

Pathogenesis

A substantial quantity of botulinum toxin which is ingested is either not absorbed or is destroyed by digestive processes, including destructive processes by rumen bacteria in ruminants, so that the oral lethal dose is larger than the lethal dose of toxin administered or acquired by other routes. Small, non-lethal doses of toxin ingested over a period of time will also cause intoxication; the cumulative dose is, however, larger than that which induces botulism if it is received as a single dose. Animals may thus become poisoned by the ingestion of feed containing sublethal amounts of toxin if they are fed such material over a few successive days. How long the toxin remains in the intestinal tract or blood stream after ingestion is, however, unknown.[31]

Following its absorption into the blood stream, the botulinum toxin is disseminated throughout the body but, with the exception of type C_2, it only has a pharmacological effect on peripheral nerve endings whose neurotransmitter is acetylcholine,[99] i.e. somatic motor nerves supplying skeletal muscles and efferent parasympathetic nerves. The central nervous system is protected by the blood-brain barrier. The flaccid paralysis caused by the toxin develops as a result of the inhibition of the release of acetylcholine at the neuromuscular junctions, with the result that no stimulus reaches the motor end-plates.[92, 93, 99] The toxic effect of botulinum toxin is exerted by the dual action of its large subunit which carries the ligand and is responsible for the fixation of the toxin molecule to a specific tissue receptor on the unmyelinated terminal portions of nerve membranes, and the small subunit, a zinc endopeptidase possessing the pharmacological activity.[81, 100] Following the binding of botulinum toxin to tissue receptors, it is internalized into the axoplasm. The fusion of the intra-axonal vesicles containing acetylcholine to the cell membrane seems to be inhibited by the cleavage of synoptobrevin, a protein that plays a role in neurotransmitter release, by the toxin.[81] A progressively developing flaccid paralysis results; paralysis of the muscles of respiration being the eventual cause of death. Although toxin binds rapidly and irreversibly to tissue receptors, it does not immediately cause paralysis.[93] In experimental, isolated nerve-muscle preparations antitoxin has no protective action once this fixation has occurred.[96] Other publications should be consulted for more detailed descriptions of the action of botulinum toxin.[11, 43, 81, 83, 84, 93, 99]

Clinical signs in cattle exposed to type B toxin appear to differ from those caused by the C and D toxins and are associated with paralysis of the cervical portion of the oesophagus. It would seem that this effect results because smaller amounts of acetylcholine are secreted by the nerve endings of the parasympathetic nerves which innervate the affected portion of the oesophagus. This has led to the suggestion that if cattle are exposed to relatively small amounts of toxin, the parasympathetic motor end-plates are selectively affected because of their smaller reserves of acetylcholine.[14]

The chronic effects of botulinum toxin are comparable to surgical denervation, and complete recovery depends on the formation of new neuromuscular junctions.[92]

Clinical signs

The clinical signs caused by intoxication with types C and D in cattle vary considerably and depend on the quantity of toxin that has been ingested. The disease has been arbitrarily divided by Theiler and his collaborators[104] into peracute, acute, subacute and chronic forms, based upon the onset, the sequence of development of paralysis in different muscle groups and severity of the clinical signs. Range cattle suffering from osteophagia, which contract lamsiekte by ingesting toxic material lying in pastures, most commonly develop the subacute to chronic form of the disease; a few may even be so mildly affected that they escape notice. More acute forms are rare under such circumstances but they do occur. A feature of lamsiekte which, apart from anything else, is of diagnostic significance, is that the case fatality rate is invariably high; most affected animals will die, but if an animal does recover it is most likely to have suffered from subacute or chronic disease. In sporadic outbreaks unassociated with osteophagia, such as those that follow the ingestion of a toxic batch of hay or kitchen refuse, new clinical cases are detected over a period of days. Cattle usually die acutely at the beginning of an outbreak, but as the outbreak progresses, the duration of clinical signs tends to increase until, at the end of the outbreak, a few lightly affected animals may even recover fully.

The incubation period in experimental cases varies from about 18 hours to 16 days but in natural disease in cattle it usually varies from two to six days, but deaths may occur for up to 17 days after animals have had access to toxic feed.[104, 107] The duration of illness may be directly correlated with the length of the incubation period; it may be as short as 24 hours in peracute cases, or up to seven days or longer in more chronic cases. There is also an intermittent form of lamsiekte in which generally mild clinical signs are manifested at intervals of a few days with periods of remission.

Affected animals are afebrile and typically manifest partial or complete flaccid paralysis of the muscles of locomotion, mastication and deglutition. The paresis, which progresses to paralysis, usually commences in the hind quarters and then spreads progressively forwards, affecting in turn the fore limbs, the neck and head. The rapidity of succession decreases from the peracute to the chronic cases. Sensory perception and reflex actions of the eyes are maintained for a considerable time after skeletal muscular paralysis has set in, and animals generally appear mentally alert. Hypersensitivity and what may be perceived as aggressiveness may occasionally be manifested. In some cases, which are considered to be atypical, the muscles of mastication and deglutition are paralysed, but not those of the locomotor system.

The appetite is mostly unaffected — animals will prehend and masticate food for as long as they are able. A few animals may be constipated or, more exceptionally, suffer from diarrhoea. Ruminal tympany often develops in animals which lie in awkward positions in the terminal stage of the disease.

The naturally acquired, peracute disease is seldom encountered; some animals suffering from it may die suddenly without any clinical signs being observed. In this form, paralysis of the muscles of locomotion, mastication and deglutition is usually marked and affected animals soon become prostrate and are more or less completely paralysed. At first they assume a sternal lying position, which frequently involves the neck being turned back and the head resting on the flank. In the later stages they become laterally recumbent. Chewing and swallowing movements are seldom possible; the tongue often protrudes from the mouth **(Figure 163.5)**, the lower jaw is slack and there is profuse salivation.

In acute lamsiekte the clinical signs generally resemble those of the peracute disease, but the course of the disease is more protracted. Although most animals lie down during the initial stages of the disease, others are able to remain standing. At first, affected animals are able to rise without assistance and, when disturbed, move about sluggishly and with a stiff gait. As the disease progresses they are unable to rise voluntarily **(Figure 163.6)** and even when lifted to their feet, they are seldom able to remain standing when all support is removed, and usually drop down helplessly. Initially the head is held upright, but in the later stages the neck is doubled back with the head resting on the flank **(Figure 163.7)**. However, if the head is manually raised, it drops back involuntarily towards the flank when released. Impairment of the muscles of mastication and deglutition is usually pronounced, causing boluses of grass to accumulate in the back of the mouth. Paresis and paralysis of the tongue also set in at this stage; in the latter instance the tip of the tongue either lies on the incisors or protrudes from the mouth. In some cases paralysis of the tongue is not complete and the animal may still be able to retract it into the mouth after it has been physically extracted.[104] In these cases the mouth can be manually opened with relative ease. In addition, if, when examining a suspected case,

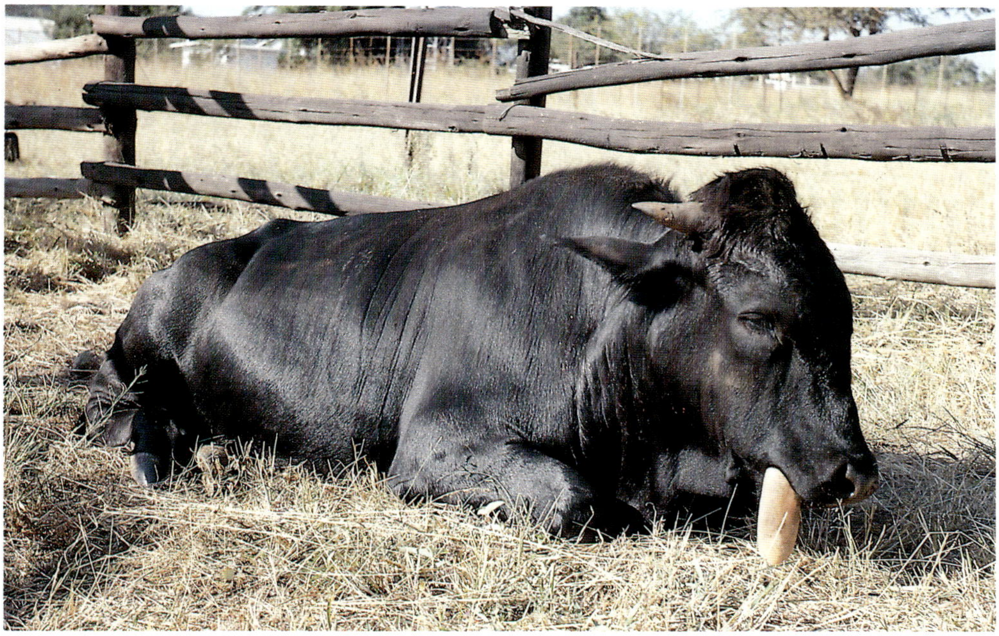

Figure 163.5 Botulism in an ox. Note protrusion of the tongue

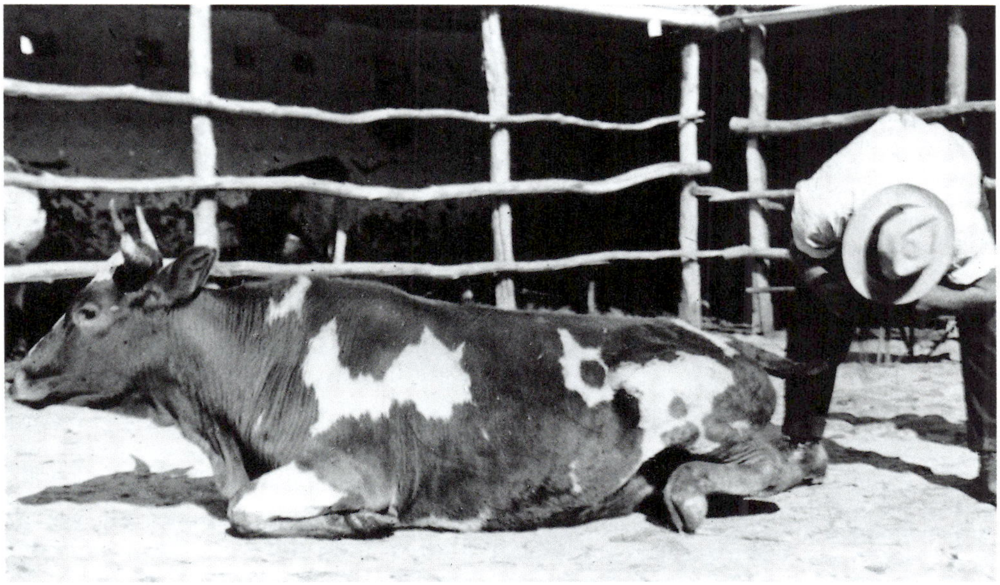

Figure 163.6 Cow unable to rise voluntarily even on being prodded

the clinician stands behind the head of the animal to one side of the neck, grasps the horns or ears firmly in both hands and shakes the head of the animal vigorously, the slack lower jaw meeting the upper jaw often causes a rather characteristic 'plop' sound to be emitted. Some degree of paresis or paralysis of the tail is also usually evident.

In the subacute disease the clinical signs differ from those of acute lamsiekte only in degree and in the period required for their evolution. Affected animals walk with a stiff, sluggish gait and usually prefer to lie down. As the disease progresses, it becomes more and more difficult for them to rise voluntarily, and when complete paralysis has set in, rising is no longer possible.

The duration of the clinical signs in chronic lamsiekte is longer than seven days. In the early stages affected animals usually eat well, but they generally appear tucked up and have staring coats. Swallowing and chewing are not always affected. Paralysis of the legs develops to a variable extent, and although animals prefer to lie down, they generally are able to rise without assistance. There is rapid loss of condition. The severity of the clinical signs progresses until prostration and, in most cases, death supervene.

The signs in cattle affected by type B toxin generally develop within three days of their being exposed to toxic material, usually brewers' grain or grass silage.[74] These signs differ markedly from those caused by type C and D toxins. In general the disease is characterized by anorexia, profuse salivation, regurgitation of feed and water following their ingestion, and dehydration. The animals manifest a decreased tonus of skeletal muscles but they

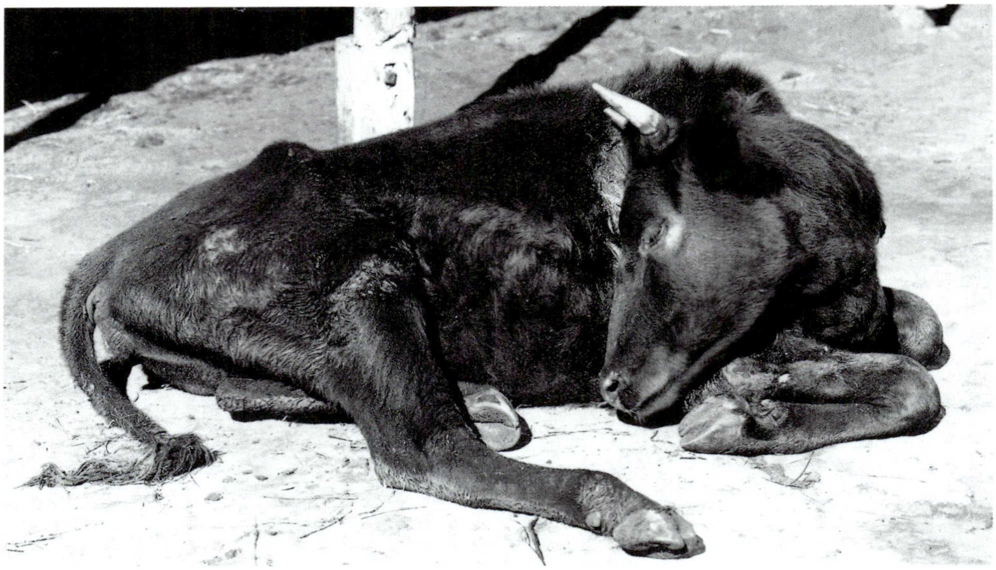

Figure 163.7 Typical posture of a heifer suffering from the advanced stages of botulism

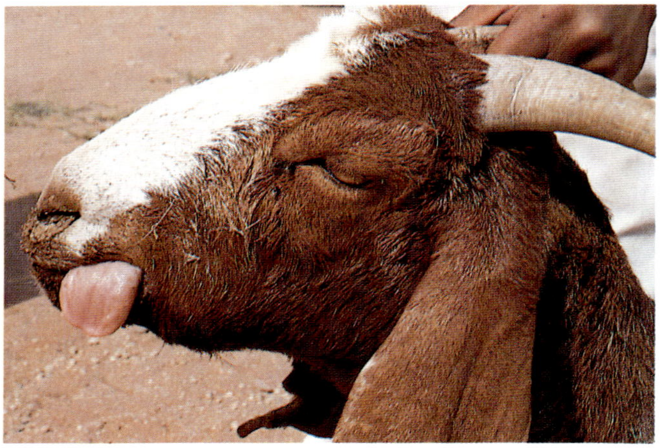

Figure 163.8 Boer goat suffering from botulism. Note the protruding tongue

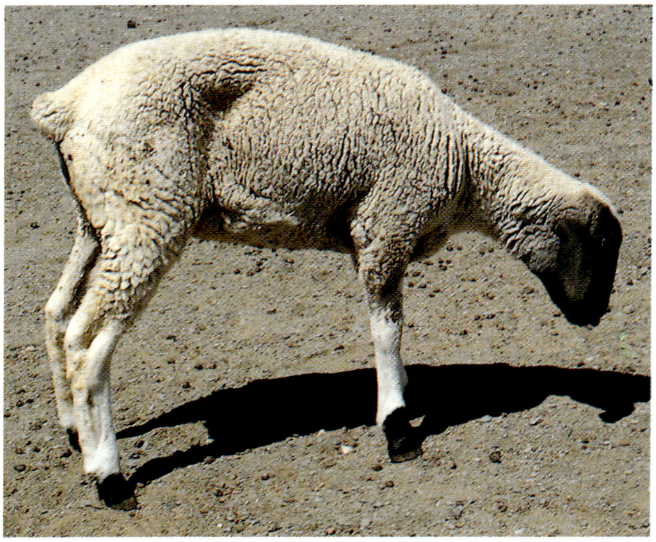

Figure 163.9 Typical stance of a Dorper sheep suffering from botulism

are not ataxic, nor is the tail or tongue paralysed. The initial signs are associated with reduced appetite, reduction in milk production, and a decrease in the consistency of the faeces which sometimes progresses to a frank diarrhoea. Pronounced salivation and regurgitation of feed and water are the main characteristics of this type of intoxication, the latter often resulting in the inhalation of the regurgitated material and the development of a foreign body pneumonia. Severely affected animals usually die, while those that are mildly affected recover uneventfully after a period which may be as long as three to six weeks.[14]

In both sheep and goats the clinical signs are similar to those in cattle **(Figure 163.8)**, except that the muscles of mastication and swallowing are not as obviously affected. In peracute cases, animals may die without signs having been observed or within four hours of their commencement.[108] Affected sheep are listless, show muscular incoordination, weakness of neck muscles and torticollis, walk with a wobbly gait, are disinclined to drink water, and, infrequently, salivate excessively. When driven, they lag behind the rest of the flock. Characteristic features are that sheep and goats develop an arched back with a drooping tail, head and neck **(Figure 163.9)**[54, 92] and manifest an abdominal type of respiration and frequent urination, while sheep often, but not invariably, show a fine trembling of the tail stump. If an affected sheep is grasped by the ears and the head shaken up or down, as in cattle, the lower jaw may strike the upper jaw to emit a clapping sound. Respiratory distress may be evident. The prognosis for the disease is extremely poor, but a few may recover without specific antiserum treatment.

In adult horses and foals a similar neuromuscular paralytic syndrome is evident in animals suffering from the toxico-infectious syndrome caused by type B toxin. The latter disease, referred to as the 'shaker foal syndrome', occurs sporadically, most frequently in animals between two and four weeks of age, although adult animals are as susceptible to the effects of the toxin. Some foals may be found dead without having been noticed to be sick, while others live for 24–40 hours before they die. They are often found in the prone position and are unable to rise. When assisted to their feet they may remain standing for a few minutes and walk with a stiff, stilted gait, only to fall to the ground again after manifesting severe trembling of the muscles of the legs. When down they are alert and the muscle tremors cease. As the disease progresses, they are only able to stand for very short periods, and eventually cannot do so at all, even when assisted. Affected foals also have difficulty in swallowing, with the result that they eat with difficulty and milk may run out of the sides of their mouths while they are suckling. They periodically attempt to urinate but void only small amounts, and usually become constipated. The pupils of the eyes are dilated and the pupillary light reflex is decreased. As the disease progresses, respiratory distress becomes pronounced and breathing becomes abdominal in type, and there is an increased heart rate. The temperature of affected animals remains normal during the course of the disease. The mortality rate is usually in excess of 90 per cent, and in non-fatal cases, or those in which treatment is effective, it may take up to three weeks for the muscular weakness to disappear. In foals which survive for a number of days, signs of an aspiration pneumonia may develop.[58, 66, 101] The clinical signs in adult horses affected by type B toxin are similar to those in foals.[101] Affected horses are initially lethargic and have a stilted gait, whereafter the typical signs develop within a matter of six to eight hours. Animals which become recumbent cannot retain a position of sternal recumbency because of the profound weakness caused by the flaccid paralysis.[116]

With certain exceptions, clinical signs in horses affected by type C toxin are similar to those in horses suffering from type B intoxication. Animals become ill within three days of ingesting feed containing type C toxin. Most die within 48–72 hours, the mortality rate being in excess of 80 per cent. The initial signs of intoxication, which may precede the development of overt clinical signs by 24 hours, are mild and are characterized by an asymmetric decrease in palpebral tone. As the condition progresses, horses intermittently stand with slight carpal flexion, while muscle fasciculations may be palpated in the triceps area. They retain their appetite during the course of the intoxication and, contrary to animals suffering from the effects of type B toxin, have no difficulty in swallowing. They do become constipated, however.[60] Within 24 hours these signs develop into severe muscular tremors of the fore and hind legs. Restlessness manifested by the horses striking the ground with their fore legs and lying down for short periods is apparent. Muscle tremors disappear after the animals have been in the prone position for a short period and it may be erroneously assumed that they have recovered. As the intoxication progresses, affected animals become sternally recumbent and lie with the neck extended and the muzzle resting on the ground. Terminally, horses assume a position of lateral recumbency while paddling their legs rhythmically. Mydriasis and slow pupillary light reflexes are seen in a few of the affected animals.

Pathology

There are no macroscopic or microscopic lesions that can be regarded as characteristic of, or specific for, lamsiekte. There may be a catarrhal enteritis and petechiae in the small intestines and the endocardium. Chronically affected animals may be constipated and manifest signs of ruminal and colonic stasis and fatty changes in the liver.[45] Excess pericardial fluid and pulmonary oedema may also be present.[107]

Foreign bodies reflecting the existence of pica, such as bones, tortoise shell, bits of wood, stones, fragments of china and pieces of iron, may be found in the rumen or reticulum in animals on veld grazing. However, no indications of pica will be evident in animals in which the toxin is ingested in prepared feed or water.[45]

At necropsy the carcasses of horses that have died of toxico-infectious botulism contain few characteristic lesions. The presence of excess pericardial fluid containing variable amounts of fibrin strands is a consistent finding. Focal areas of necrosis or abscesses may occur in the liver, navel, lungs, skin or muscles. In many cases gastric ulcers are present at the *margo plicatus* and occasionally at the pylorus. In addition, severe pulmonary oedema, intestinal stasis, and distention of the urinary bladder are present.[101]

The presence of extensive intermuscular oedema in the neck region, suspected to be caused by type C_2 toxin ingested concurrently with type C_1 toxin, has been reported in horses that died of botulism.[60] In some animals the oedema may extend caudally as far as the lumbar region.

Diagnosis

Botulism is often difficult to diagnose. A presumptive diagnosis is made on the basis of the history, clinical signs and negative post-mortem examination. Factors in the history of the outbreak which support a diagnosis of botulism are lack of or inadequate immunization against botulism and, in the case of range animals, the presence of osteophagia. The possibility of other diseases causing similar clinical signs to those of botulism should be systematically excluded. A useful diagnostic aid is that the number of cases diminishes drastically in affected herds or flocks following the administration of primary and secondary doses of vaccine within a month of each other. In addition, the response of sick animals to botulism antiserum therapy may also be of some assistance.

A definitive diagnosis of botulism is dependent on the demonstration of botulinum toxin in specimens taken from diseased animals or those that have died, and in the suspected source of the toxin if this is still available. Although determining the presence of botulinum toxin in specimens submitted for the purpose is the most reliable way of confirming a diagnosis, many of the available test systems lack sensitivity and it is often very difficult to confirm the diagnosis of botulism.

Specimens collected for the diagnosis of botulism in live animals should consist of serum and faeces. Specimens (5–20 ml) should be taken of the rumen content and the contents of the small and large intestines from dead ruminants. In horses, specimens of the caecal contents as well as from any necrotic lesion present in the gastrointestinal tract are required. From all animal species, 5–20 ml of serum and pericardial, thoracic and peritoneal transudates should be submitted. If available, specimens from several animals should be collected. Specimens of what is suspected to be the source of the toxin, such as concentrate, grass, silage, carcasses or parts of carrion or drinking water should also be submitted. Since the toxin is often unevenly distributed in food, representative samples for analysis should be taken from various portions of the feed. After being collected and packed in sealed containers, the specimens should be deep-frozen if possible. If specimens cannot be frozen, they should at least be kept refrigerated and submitted packed in ice to a laboratory.[55]

Although its use is sometimes advocated, isolation of the bacterium from the intestinal tract provides equivocal results as these bacteria may also be isolated from healthy animals. The specimens (food and tissues such as intestinal lesions) for the isolation of the organism should first be inoculated in cooked-meat broth and trypticase-peptone-glucose-yeast extract-trypsin (TPGYT) broth, and incubated under anaerobic conditions at 26 °C and 35 °C respectively for five days. After this initial incubation period, if no growth is observed, the cultures should be incubated for a further five days. Subcultures should be examined to determine the type of organism and toxin according to published methodology.[16, 47, 55, 97]

To determine the presence of botulinum toxin in tissue and feed specimens, the toxin is extracted in a gelatine-phosphate buffer solution which is divided into at least four separate portions, each being subjected to different treatments involving heat, the addition of trypsin or polyvalent or monovalent *C. botulinum* antiserum. An amount of 0,5–1 ml of each portion is injected intraperitoneally into at least two mice, which are then observed for up to ten days for signs of botulism.[55] In this way the presence of botulinum toxin and the determination of toxin type in a specimen can be achieved.[8, 55, 94] Serum collected from horses affected with toxico-infectious botulism invariably tests negatively since the concentration of toxin in the serum is generally so low that the toxin cannot be detected by conventional methods.[101] The toxicity of feed samples may also be determined by test-feeding the sample to specifically immunized and unimmunized cattle, sheep or laboratory animals.[107]

Other methods for detecting the presence of botulinum toxin in various types of specimens include an immunodiffusion method,[30] radio-immuno-assay,[12] various immunochemical assays,[1, 19, 34, 35, 61, 73] and the temperature-induced microcomplement fixation test.[23, 113, 114] Except for the microcomplement fixation test, which is highly sensitive, the sensitivity of these tests does not exceed that of mouse bioassay.

Differential diagnosis

The two most important differential diagnoses for botulism in South Africa are diplodiosis (a mycotoxicosis caused by *Diplodia maydis* poisoning) in cattle, and krimpsiekte (a plant poisoning caused by members of the Crassulaceae containing bufadienolides) in sheep and goats. In the latter the clinical signs of paralysis, salivation, retention of food in the pharynx, the typical posture, and the lack of specific macro- and histopathological changes render the two conditions indistinguishable.[56]

In ruminants, other important differential diagnoses that may be considered include polioencephalomalacia and conditions associated with hypocalcaemia and hypomagnesaemia, nutritional or plant toxin-induced myopathies such as ionophore poisoning and poisoning with *Geigeria* spp. In cattle, ingestion of the toxin of the fungus *Aspergillus clavatus*, organophosphate and lead poisoning, and infectious diseases such as rabies, listeriosis, bovine ephemeral fever, sporadic bovine encephalomyelitis, thrombotic meningoencephalitis, cerebral babesiosis and cerebral theileriosis, as well as non-specific bacterial meningitis and encephalitides, may also mimic some of the clinical signs of botulism.[22] In sheep, the possibility of tick paralysis caused either by *Ixodes rubicundus* or *Rhipicephalus evertsi evertsi*, focal symmetrical encephalomalacia, twin lamb disease (domsiekte) and *Coenurus cerebralis* infestation should also be considered. In the case of tick paralysis, removal of the ticks is followed by recovery from the paralysis. In horses, infection with equid herpesvirus 1, and various viral encephalitides should be considered.[60]

Control

There is no specific treatment for diseased animals suffering from botulism, apart from the administration of hyperimmune serum specific for the toxin type involved, which may assist in the recovery of animals still in the early stages of the disease. The antiserum should be prepared and standardized according to international convention.[1, 10] In South Africa these sera are available from the Veterinary Research Institute, Onderstepoort, which markets types C and D antisera separately. As the type of

C. botulinum responsible for the disease in an animal or group of animals is generally not known until some time has elapsed (if ever), it is the general practice in South Africa to mix together antisera containing types C and D antitoxin immediately before administration, which is carried out by the intravenous route. As the antisera are expensive they are generally used selectively for the treatment of valuable stock.

The antisera available commercially contain a minimum of 1 000 international units per millilitre, and are prepared from hyperimmunized horses. Cattle and horses are treated with 5 ml each of types C and D antiserum intravenously, sheep with 1–2 ml of each type, and poultry and other bird species with 0,5 ml type C intravenously. This treatment may be repeated within 24 hours. Response to treatment varies; in some animals beneficial effects may occur within minutes,[78] while in others this only occurs after five days.[14] Sometimes no beneficial effects are evident. The possibility of anaphylactic shock developing in animals that are receiving antiserum therapy is significant and should be anticipated. The use of antiserum in horses has been shown to reduce mortality rates from 80 to 30 per cent.[101] In horses suffering from type C intoxication, treatment with the specific antiserum will improve the prognosis if it is instituted early in the course of the disease, before they become recumbent. Following the administration of a five-day course of the antitoxin, one or two relapses may occur, often at intervals of five to eight days, after which the treatment regimen should be repeated. Horses which survive often develop a severe atrophy of the suprascapular and gluteal muscles which becomes apparent when the neurological signs of the disease have disappeared, and may persist for up to five months.[60]

Good nursing is essential when treating animals suffering from botulism. Dehydration, if present, should be corrected but it must always be borne in mind that the muscles of deglutination may be affected, and great care must be exercised when administering fluids by the oral route in order to prevent the possible development of 'dosing pneumonia'. In both cattle and sheep, acid-base imbalance often occurs and should be corrected. The administration of a mild laxative to horses may be indicated in order to evacuate the colon and prevent impaction. Recumbent animals may require some sort of support system that will keep them in a position of sternal recumbency; this is particularly important in ruminants in order to prevent the formation of ruminal tympany.

The prevention of the form of botulism to which range cattle are predisposed by osteophagia is three-pronged: vaccination, correction of the phosphorus deficiency and removal of the source of the intoxication, such as carcass debris (when this is practically feasible).

Vaccination against botulism has been effectively used in South Africa since 1938.[67] Commercially produced vaccines are available, and are produced by the Veterinary Research Institute, Onderstepoort. They contain toxoids of types C and D which are adsorbed onto aluminium hydroxide gel in order to enhance their immunogenicity.[28] The initial vaccination administration should be followed by a second one four to seven weeks later. Thereafter it is given as an annual booster, timed, if possible, to precede the commencement of the season in which botulism is most prevalent. An experimental vaccine consisting of a water-in-oil emulsion of type C and D toxoids which is administered intramuscularly has been found to induce superior immune responses in cattle when compared with those produced by the aluminium hydroxide-based vaccine.[53] It is, however, not available commercially. Unless the regimen for the active immunization of animals recommended by the manufacturer of the vaccine is followed, inadequate or only partial protection of the animals may result, and some of them may manifest typical clinical signs of the disease should they subsequently contract it.

As botulism in animals is not always an easy disease to diagnose or to confirm by laboratory means, particularly in the early stages of an outbreak, it is often advisable to recommend that all the animals in the group containing suspected cases be vaccinated as soon as possible.

A combined vaccine for botulism and blackquarter is also commercially available from the Veterinary Research Institute, Onderstepoort for use where cattle are to be immunized against both these diseases.

Correction of phosphorus deficiency in cattle is essential in areas where there is botulism in range animals and, apart from the role it plays in reducing the prevalence of the disease, it has many other beneficial effects, including increased productivity. There are several ways to administer additional phosporus to animals, the most frequently used being licks containing phosphate or bone meal, or the addition of phosphates, in the correct formulation, to drinking water.[67]

The removal of the sources of the intoxication also helps to reduce the prevalence of botulism. Where cattle maintained under extensive systems of management are concerned, the source is usually carcass debris. It is not always practically feasible to remove all of it from large properties, but attempts should be made to remove as much as possible. If this is not done, it may be found that in the long-term outbreaks of botulism on a property are self-perpetuating. Possible sources of the toxin should be destroyed, buried deeply or placed so that they are unavailable to cattle. If buried or placed, for example, in a wired-off enclosure, it should be remembered that dogs or wild animals, such as hyenas, may dig them up or drag them away, making them available to the cattle once again.

It is imperative that ruminants be vaccinated against botulism before they are fed poultry litter for the first time. Thereafter they should be immunized regularly. In South Africa it is required by law that poultry litter sold commercially be adequately sterilized. Nevertheless it is still essential that ruminants receiving it be adequately protected against botulism by immunization.

Other methods for the control of botulism, particularly that which occurs in sporadic outbreak form, include the prevention of contamination of hay, silage and drinking water. Spoilt hay or other feedstuffs, or those contaminated by the carcasses of small animals should not be fed to livestock. When silage is prepared, attention should be paid to attaining the correct pH; no production of botulism toxin occurs at a pH of less than 5,3 and where the water activity is less than 0,94.

Foals suckled by dams vaccinated against botulism are protected by passive, colostrum-derived immunity during the period in which they are most likely to contract toxico-infectious botulism. It is recommended that mares be vaccinated (taking cognizance of the toxin type most likely to be involved) twice at an interval of six weeks, the second vaccination being administered two to four weeks before parturition.[106]

References

1 **APPLETON, N., WILTON-SMITH, P., HAMBLETON, P., MODI, N., GATLEY, S. & MELLING, J., 1986**. *In vitro* assays for botulinum toxin and antitoxins. *Development in Biological Standardization*, 64, 141–145.

2 **BARSANTI, J.A., WALSER, M., HATHEWAY, L.L., BOWEN, J.M. & CROWELL, W., 1978**. Type C botulism in American foxhounds. *Journal of the American Veterinary Medical Association*, 172, 809–813.

3 **BEIERS, P.R. & SIMMONS, G.C., 1967**. Botulism in pigs. *Australian Veterinary Journal*, 43, 270–271.

4 **BEKKER, V., 1989**. The occurrence of *Clostridium botulinum* types A, B and E in South African habitats. M. Sc. thesis, Department of Microbiology and Plant Pathology, Faculty of Agriculture, University of Pretoria.

5 **BENGSTON, I.A., 1922**. Preliminary note on a toxin-producing anaerobe isolated from the larvae of *Lucilia caesar*. *Public Health Report*, 37, 164.

6 **BENNETTS, H.W. & HALL, H.T.B., 1938**. Botulism of sheep and cattle in Western Australia: Its cause and its prevention by vaccination. *Australian Veterinary Journal*, 14, 105–119.

7 **BERNARD, W., DIVERS, T.J., WHITLOCK, R.H., MESSICK, J. & TULLENERS, E., 1987**. Botulism as a sequel to open castration in a horse. *Journal of the American Veterinary Medical Association*, 191, 73–74.

8 **BISPING, W. & AMTSBERG, G., 1988**. *Colour Atlas for the Diagnosis of Bacterial Pathogens in Animals*. Berlin & Hamburg: Paul Parey Scientific Publishers.

9 **BORTHWICK, J.D., 1896.** *Annual Report of the College of Veterinary Surgeons*, Cape, 1895.

10 **BOWMER, E.J., 1963**. Preparation and assay of the international standards for *Clostridium botulinum* types A, B, C, D and E antitoxins. *Bulletin of the World Health Organization*, 29, 701–709.

11 **BOROFF, D.A. & DASGUPTA, B.R., 1971**. Botulinum toxin. *In*: KADIS, S., MONTIE, T.C. & AJL, S.J., (eds). *Microbial Toxins: Bacterial Protein Toxins*. Vol. IIA. London, New York: Academic Press, Inc.

12 **BOROFF, D.A. & SHU-CHEN, G., 1973**. Radioimmunoassay for type A toxin of *Clostridium botulinum*. *Applied Microbiology*, 25, 545–549.

13 **BORST, G.H.A., LAMBERS, G.M. & HAAGSMA, J., 1986**. Botulismus type C bij de hond. *Tijdschrift voor Diergeneeskunde*, 111, 1104–1105.

14 **BREUKINK, H.J., WAGENAAR, G., WENSING, T.H., NOTERMANS, S. & POULOS, P.W., 1978**. Voedselvergiftiging bij runderen veroorzaakt door het eten van bierbostel besmet met *Clostridium botulinum* type B. *Tijdschrift voor Diergeneeskunde*, 103, 303–311.

15 **BURKE, G.S., 1919**. Notes on *Bacillus botulinus*. *Journal of Bacteriology*, 4, 555–565.

16 **CATO, E.P., GEORGE, W.L. & FINEGOLD, S.M., 1986**. Genus *Clostridium* Prazmowski 1880. *In*: SNEATH, P.H.A., MAIR, N.S., SHARPE, M.E. & HOLT, J.G., (eds). *Bergey's Manual of Systematic Bacteriology*. Vol. II. Baltimore, London: Williams & Wilkins.

17 **COETZER, J.A.W., 1993**. Faculty of Veterinary Science, University of Pretoria, South Africa. Personal communication.

18 **COETZER, J.A.W. & KELLERMAN, T.S., 1993**. Faculty of Veterinary Science, University of Pretoria, South Africa. Personal communication.

19 **DEZFULIAN, M. & BARTLETT, J.G., 1984**. Detection of *Clostridium botulinum* type A toxin by enzyme-linked immunosorbent assay with antibodies produced in immunologically tolerant animals. *Journal of Clinical Microbiology*, 19, 645–648.

20 **DEZFULIAN, M., McCROSKEY, L.M., HATHEWAY, C.L. & DOWELL, V.R., 1981**. Selective medium for isolation of *Clostridium botulinum* from human feces. *Journal of Clinical Microbiology*, 13, 526–531.

21 **DINTER, A. & KULL, K.E., 1954**. Über einen Ausbruch des Botulismus sanenkuken. *Nordisk Veterinaermedicin*, 6, 866–872.

22 **DIVERS, T.J., BARTHOLOMEW, R.C., MESSICK, J.B., WHITLOCK, R.H. & SWEENEY, R.W., 1986**. *Clostridium botulinum* type B toxicosis in a herd of cattle and a group of mules. *Journal of the American Veterinary Medical Association*, 188, 382–386.

23 **DÖBEREINER, J., TOKARNIA, C.H., LANGENEGGER, J. & DUTRA, I.S., 1992**. Epizootic botulism of cattle in Brazil. *Deutsche Tierärtzliche Wochenschrift*, 99, 188–190.

24 **DU TOIT, P.J., LOUW, J.G. & MALAN, A.I., 1940**. A study of the mineral content and feeding value of natural pastures in the Union of South Africa (Final Report). *Onderstepoort Journal of Veterinary Science and Animal Industry*, 14, 123–327.

25 **EKLUND, M.W. & POYSKY, F.T., 1974**. Interconversion of type C and D strains of *Clostridium botulinum* by specific bacteriophages. *Applied Microbiology*, 27, 251–258.

26 **EKLUND, M.W., POYSKY, F.T., MEYERS, J.A. & PELROY, G.A., 1974**. Interspecies conversion of *Clostridium botulinum* type C to *Clostridium novyi* type A by bacteriophage. *Science*, 186, 456–458.

27 **EKLUND, M.W., POYSKY, F.T., REED, S.M. & SMITH, C.A., 1971**. Bacteriophage and the toxigenicity of *Clostridium botulinum* type C. *Science*, 172, 480–482.

28 **ERASMUS, B.J., CAMERON, C.M., HUNTER, P., CILLIERS, J.A., OBEREM, P.T., STOLTSZ, W.H. & DE WAAL, D.T., 1990**. Onderstepoort Vaccines. Booklet issued by the Department of Agriculture and Development and obtained from the Directorate of Agricultural Information, Private Bag X144, Pretoria 0001.

29 **FARROW, B.R.H., MURRELL, W.G., REVINGTON, M.L., STEWART, B.J. & ZUBER, R.M., 1983**. Type C botulism in young dogs. *Australian Veterinary Journal*, 60, 374–377.

30 **FERREIRA, J.L., HAMDY, M.K., ZAPATKA, F.A. & HERBERT, W.O., 1981**. Immunodiffusion method detection of type A *Clostridium botulinum*. Applied and Environmental Microbiology, 42, 1057–1061.

31 **FJOLSTAD, M., 1973**. The effects of *Clostridium botulinum* type C_{13} given orally to goats. *Acta Veterinaria Scandinavica*, 14, 69–80.

32 **FOURIE, J.M., 1946**. The persistence of botulism toxin in carcass material, with special reference to that in tortoises. *Journal of the South African Veterinary Medical Association*, 17, 85–87.

33 **GIBSON, L.A.S., 1986**. Botulism in dairy cows. *The Veterinary Record*, 118, 309.

34 **GIBSON, A.M., MODI, N.K., ROBERTS, T.A., HAMBLETON, P. & MELLING, J., 1988**. Evaluation of a monoclonal antibody-based immunoassay for detecting type B *Clostridium botulinum* toxin produced in pure culture and an inoculated model cured meat system. *Journal of Applied Bacteriology*, 64, 285–291.

35 **GIBSON, A.M., MODI, N.K., ROBERTS, T.A., SHONE, C.C., HAMBLETON, P. & MELLING, J., 1987**. Evaluation of a monoclonal antibody-based immunoassay for detecting type A *Clostridium botulinum* toxin produced in pure culture and an inoculated model cured meat system. *Journal of Applied Bacteriology*, 63, 217–226.

36 **GILL, M., 1987**. Bacterial toxins. *In*: LASKIN, A.I. & LECHEVALIER, H.A., (eds). *CRC Handbook of Microbiology*. 2nd edn. Vol. VIII. *Toxins and Enzymes*. Florida: CRC Press, Inc.

37 **GIMENEZ, D.F. & CICCARELLI, A.S., 1970**. Another type of *C. botulinum*. *Zentralblatt für Bacteriologie*, I. Abteil Original, 215, 221.

38 **GRAHAM, R. & BREUCKNER, R.L., 1919**. Studies in forage poisoning. The relation of *B. botulinus* to forage poisoning or cerebrospinal meningitis in horses. *Journal of Bacteriology*, 4, 1–21.

39 **GUNNISON, J.B. & MEYER, K.F., 1929**. Cultural study of an international collection of *Clostridium botulinum* and *C. parabotulism*. *Journal of Infectious Disease*, 45, 119–134.

40 **GUTSCHE, T., 1979**. *There was a Man. The Life and Times of Sir Arnold Theiler K.C.M.G. of Onderstepoort*. Cape Town: Howard Timmins.

41 **HAAGSMA, J., HAESEBROUCK, F., DEVRIESE, L. & BERTELS, G., 1990**. An outbreak of botulism type B in horses. *The Veterinary Record*, 127, 206.

42 **HAAGSMA, J. & TER LAAK, E.A., 1978**. Een geval van botulismus type B bij runderen, veroorzaakt door de voedering van kuilgras. *Tijdschrift voor Diergeneeskunde*, 103, 910–912.

43 **HABERMANN, E. & DREYER, F., 1986**. Clostridial neurotoxins: Handling and action at the cellular and molecular level. *Current Topics in Microbiology and Immunology*, 129, 93–179.

44 **HAY, C.M.E., VAN DER MADE, H.N. & KNOETZE, P.C., 1973**. Isolation of *Clostridium botulinum* type C from an outbreak of botulism in wild geese. *Journal of the South African Veterinary Association*, 44, 53–56.

45 **HENNING, M.W., 1956**. *Animal Diseases in South Africa*. 3rd edn. Pretoria: Central News Agency.

46 **HOBBS, G., CROWTHER, J.S., NEAVES, P., GIBBS, P.A. & JARVIS, B., 1982**. Detection and isolation of *Clostridium botulinum*. *In*: CORRY, J.E.L., ROBERTS, D. & SKINNER, F.A., (eds). *Isolation and Identification Methods for Food Poisoning Organisms*. London, New York: Academic Press, Inc.

47 **HOLDEMAN, L.V., CATO, E.P. & MOORE, W.E.C., 1977**. *Anaerobic Laboratory Manual*. 4th edn. V.P.I. Anaerobic Laboratory, Virginia Polytechnic Institute and State University, Virginia.

48 **HUSS, H.H., 1980**. Distribution of *Clostridium botulinum*. *Applied and Environmental Microbiology*, 39, 764.

49 **HUTCHEON, D., 1881, 1885, 1896**. Lamsiekte. *Annual Reports of the College of Veterinary Surgeons*, Cape, 1880, 1884, and 1894.

50 **IIDA, H., OGUMA, K. & INOUE, K., 1974**. Phage-conversion of toxigenicity in *Clostridium botulinum* types C and D. *Japanese Journal of Medical Science and Biology*, 27, 101–102.

51 **JANSEN, B.C., 1971**. The toxic antigenic factors produced by *Clostridium botulinum* types C and D. *Onderstepoort Journal of Veterinary Research*, 38, 93–98.

52 **JANSEN, B.C., 1971**. The quantitative determination of the toxic factors produced by *Clostridium botulinum* (Van Ermengem, 1886) types C and D. *Onderstepoort Journal of Veterinary Research*, 38, 177–180.

53 **JANSEN, B.C., KNOETZE, P.C. & VISSER, F., 1976**. The antibody response of cattle to *Clostridium botulinum* types C and D toxoids. *Onderstepoort Journal of Veterinary Research*, 43, 165–174.

54 **JENSEN, R. & SWIFT, B.L., 1982**. *Diseases of Sheep*. 2nd edn. Philadelphia: Lea & Febiger.

55 **KAUTTER, D.A., LYNT, R.K. & SOLOMON, H.M., 1984**. *Clostridium botulinum*. *In*: *Bacteriological Analytical Manual of the Division of Microbiology*, Centre for Food Safety and Applied Nutrition, US Food and Drug Administration. 6th edn. Virginia: Association of Official Analytical Chemists.

56 **KELLERMAN, T.S., 1993**. Veterinary Research Institute, Private Bag X5, Onderstepoort, South Africa. Personal communication.

57 **KELLERMAN, T.S. & COETZER, J.A.W., 1993**. Veterinary Research Institute, Private Bag X5, Onderstepoort, South Africa. Personal communication.

58 **KELLY, A.P., JONES, R.T., GILLICK, J.C. & SIMS, L.D., 1984**. Outbreak of botulism in horses. *Equine Veterinary Journal*, 16, 519–521.

59 **KIMBERLING, C.V., 1988**. *Jensen and Swift's Diseases of Sheep*. 3rd edn. Philadelphia: Lea & Febiger.

60 **KINDE, H., BETTEY, R.L., ARDANS, A., GALEY, F.D., DAFT, B.M., WALKER, R.L., EKLUND, M.W. & BYRD, J.W., 1991**. *Clostridium botulinum* type C intoxication associated with consumption of processed alfalfa hay cubes in horses. *Journal of the American Veterinary Medical Association*, 199, 742–746.

61 **KOZAKI, S., DUFRENNE, J., HAGENAARS, A.M. & NOTERMANS, S., 1979**. Enzyme linked immunosorbent assay (ELISA) for detection of *Clostridium botulinum* type B toxin. *Japanese Journal of Medical Science and Biology*, 32, 199–205.

62 **KURAZONO, H., HOSOKAWA, M., MATSUDA, H. SAKAGUCHI, G., 1987**. Fluid accumulation in the ligated intestinal loop and histopathological changes of the intestinal mucosa caused by *Clostridium botulinum* C_2 toxin in the pheasant and chicken. *Research in Veterinary Science*, 42, 349–353.

63 **LAMANNA, C. 1959**. The most poisonous poison. *Science*, 130, 763–772.

64 **LE VALLIANT, M., 1796.** *Travels into the Interior Parts of Africa*. Vol. II.

65 **LICHTENSTEIN, 1812.** *Travels in Southern Africa in the Years 1803–1806*. (English edition). Van Riebeeck Society.

66 **MACKAY, R.J. & BERKHOFF, G.A., 1982**. Type C toxico-infectious botulism in a foal. *Journal of the American Veterinary Medical Association*, 180, 163–164.

67 **MASON, J.H., STEYN, H.P. & BISSCHOP, J.H.R., 1938**. The immunization of bovines against lamsiekte. *Journal of the South African Veterinary Medical Association*, 9, 65–70.

68 **McLOUGHLIN, M.F., McILLROY, S.G. & NEILL, S.D., 1988**. A major outbreak of botulism in cattle being fed ensiled poultry litter. *The Veterinary Record*, 122, 579–581.

69 **MILLS, D.C. & ARNON, S.S., 1987**. The large intestine as the

site of *Clostridium botulinum* colonization in human infant botulism. *The Journal of Infectious Diseases*, 156, 997–998.

70 **MITCHELL, D.T., 1913**. Lamsiekte. *Second Report of the Director of Veterinary Research*, Union of South Africa.

71 **MIYAZAKI, S. & SAKAGUCHI, G., 1978**. Experimental botulism in chickens: The caecum as the site of production and absorption of botulinum toxin. *Japanese Journal of Medical Science and Biology*, 31, 1–15.

72 **NOTERMANS, S., BREUKINK, H.J., WENSING, TH. & WAGENAAR, G., 1978**. Voorkomen van *Clostridium botulinum* in pensinhoud en faeces van runderen gevoederd met bostel welke natuurlijk besmet was met *Clostridium botulinum*. *Tijdschrift voor Diergeneeskunde*, 103, 1327–1333.

73 **NOTERMANS, S., HAGENAARS, A.M. & KOZAKI, S., 1971**. The enzyme-linked immunosorbent assay (ELISA) for the detection and determination of *Clostridium botulinum* toxins A, B and E. *Methods in Enzymology*, 84, 223–238.

74 **NOTERMANS, S., HAVELAAR, A.H., DUFRENNE, J.B. & OOSTERIEM, J., 1985**. Voorkomen van *Clostridium botulinum* op rund vee houderij bedrijven. *Tijdschrift voor Diergeneeskunde*, 110, 5, 175–180.

75 **OGUMA, K. & IIDA, H., 1979**. High and low toxin production by a non-toxigenic strain of *Clostridium botulinum* type C following infection with type C phages of different passage history. *Journal of General Microbiology*, 112, 203–206.

76 **OHISHI, I., 1983**. Response of mouse intestinal loop to botulinum C_2 toxin: Enterotoxic activity induced by cooperation of nonlinked protein components. *Infection and Immunity*, 40, 691–695.

77 **PFENNIGER, W., 1924**. Toxico-immunologic and serologic relationship of *Bacillus parabotulinus* type C and *B. parabotulinus*, 'Seddon'. *Journal of Infectious Disease*, 34, 348–352.

78 **PROZESKY, L., 1993**. Veterinary Research Institute, Onderstepoort, South Africa. Personal communication.

79 **RAATJES, G.J.M. & SMELT, J.P.P.M., 1979**. *Clostridium botulinum* can grow and form toxin at pH values lower than 4,6. *Nature*, 281, 398–399.

80 **ROBINSON, E.M., 1930**. The bacteria of the *Clostridium botulinum* C and D types. *Sixteenth Report of the Director of Veterinary Services*. Union of South Africa.

81 **SCHIAVO, G., BENFENAT, F., POULAIN, B., ROSSETTO, O., POLVERINO DE LAURETO, P., DASGUPTA, B.R. & MONTECUCCO, C., 1992**. Tetanus and botulinum-B neurotoxins block neurotransmitter release by proteolytic cleavage of synaptobrevin. *Nature*, 359, 832–835.

82 **SEDDON, H.R., 1922**. The specific identity of *Bacillus parabotulinus*. *Journal of Comparative Pathology and Therapy*, 35, 275–280.

83 **SIMPSON, L.L., 1981**. The origin, structure, and pharmacological activity of botulinum toxin. *Pharmacological Reviews*, 33, 155–188.

84 **SIMPSON, L.L., 1986**. Molecular pharmacology of botulinum toxin and tetanus toxin. *Annual Review of Pharmacology and Toxicology*, 26, 427–453.

85 **SMART, J.L., JONES, T.O., CLEGG, F.G. & McMURTRY, M.J., 1987**. Poultry waste associated with type C botulism in cattle. *Epidemiology of Infection*, 98, 73–79.

86 **SMART, J.L., LAING, P.W. & WINKLER, C.E., 1983**. Type C botulism in intensively farmed turkeys. *The Veterinary Record*, 113, 198–200.

87 **SMITH, G.R. & MORYSON, C.J., 1977**. A comparison of the distribution of *Clostridium botulinum* in soil and lake mud. *Journal of Hygiene, Cambridge*, 78, 39–41.

88 **SMITH, G.R., OLIPHANT, J.C. & EVANS, E.D., 1983**. Diagnosis of botulism in water birds. *The Veterinary Record*, 112, 457–458.

89 **SMITH, G.R. & TURNER, A., 1987**. Factors affecting the toxicity of rotting carcasses containing *Clostridium botulinum* type C. *Epidemiology of Infection*, 98, 345–351.

90 **SMITH, G.R. & TURNER, A., 1989**. The production of *Clostridium botulinum* toxin in mammalian, avian and piscine carrion. *Epidemiology of Infection*, 102, 467–471.

91 **SMITH, L.D. & WILLIAMS, B.L., 1984**. *C. botulinum*. *In*: *The Pathogenic Anaerobic Bacteria*. 3rd edn. Springfield Ill.: Charles C. Thomas.

92 **SMITH, L.D.S, 1977**. *Botulism: The Organism, its Toxins, the Disease*. Springfield, Illinois: Charles C. Thomas.

93 **SMITH, L.D.S. & SUGIYAMA, H., 1988**. *Botulism: The Organism, its Toxin, the Disease*. 2nd edn. Springfield, Illinois: Charles C. Thomas.

94 **SOLBERG, M., POST, L.S., FURGANG, D. & GRAHAM, C., 1985**. Bovine serum eliminates rapid nonspecific toxic reactions during bioassay of stored fish for *Clostridium botulinum* toxin. *Applied and Environmental Microbiology*, 49, 644–649.

95 **SONNABEND, O., SONNABEND, W., HEINZLE, R., SIGRIST, T., DIRNHOFER, R. & KRECH, U., 1981**. Isolation of *Clostridium botulinum* type G and identification of type G botulinal toxin in humans: Report of five sudden unexpected deaths. *The Journal of Infectious Disease*, 143, 22–27.

96 **STEPHEN, J. & PIETROWSKI, R.A., 1986**. *Bacterial Toxins*. 2nd edn. Washington: American Society for Microbiology.

97 **STERNE, M. & BATTY, I., 1975**. *Pathogenic Clostridia*. Boston, London: Butterworths.

98 **SUEN, J.C., HATHEWAY, C.L., STEIGERWALT, A.G. & BRENNER, D.J., 1988**. *Clostridium argentinense* sp. nov.: A genetically homogeneous group composed of all strains of *C. botulinum* toxin type G, and some nontoxigenic strains previously identified as *C. subterminale* or *C. hastiforme*. *International Journal of Systematic Bacteriology*, 38, 375–381.

99 **SUGIYAMA, H., 1980**. *Clostridium botulinum* neurotoxin. *Microbiological Reviews*, 44, 419–448.

100 **SUGIYAMA, H., 1986**. *Clostridium botulinum*. *In*: GYLES, C.L. & THOEN, C.O., (eds). *Pathogenesis of Bacterial Infections in Animals*. Ames, Iowa: Iowa State University Press.

101 **SWERCZEK, T.W., 1980**. Toxicoinfectious botulism in foals and adult horses. *Journal of the American Veterinary Medical Association*, 176, 217–220.

102 **SWERCZEK, T.W., 1980**. Experimentally induced toxicoinfectious botulism in horses and foals. *American Journal of Veterinary Research*, 41, 348–350.

103 **THEILER, A., 1920**. Cause and prevention of lamsiekte. *Journal of the Department of Agriculture*, South Africa, June 1920.

104 **THEILER, A., 1927**. Lamsiekte (parabotulism) in cattle in South Africa. *Eleventh and Twelfth Reports of the Director of Veterinary Education and Research*, Part II, 821–1361.

105 **THEILER, A. & ROBINSON, E.M., 1927**. Der Botulismes der Haustiere. *Zeitschrift für Infektioneskrankheiten*, 31, 165.

106 **THOMAS, R.J., ROSENTHAL, D.V., ROGERS, R.J., 1988**. A *Clostridium botulinum* type B vaccine for prevention of shaker foal syndrome. *Australian Veterinary Journal*, 65, 78–80.

107 **TRUEMAN, K.F., BOCK, R.E., THOMAS, R.J., TAYLOR, J.D., GREEN, P.A., ROEGER, H.M. & KETTERER, P.J., 1992**. Suspected botulism in three intensively managed Australian cattle herds. *The Veterinary Record*, 130, 398–400.

108 **VAN DER LUGT, J., 1993**. Veterinary Research Institute, Private Bag X5, Onderstepoort, South Africa. Personal communication.

109 **VAN ERMENGEM, E., 1912**. Botulismus. *Handbuch der Pathologischen Mikrobiologie*, Vol. IV. Kolle & Wasserman.

110 **VARNAM, A.H. & EVANS, M.G., 1991**. *Foodborne Pathogens. An Illustrated Text*. London: Wolfe Publishing Ltd.

111 **WALKER, J., 1913**. Investigations into the disease lamsiekte in cattle. *Second Report of the Director of Veterinary Research*, Union of South Africa.

112 **WALLACE, V. & McDOWELL, D.M., 1986**. Botulism in a dog—first confirmed case in New Zealand. *New Zealand Veterinary Journal*, 34, 149–150.

113 **WEISS, H.E., RADEMACHER, G., DOLL K. & DIRKSEN, G., 1990**. Schnelldiagnose des Botulinus beim Rind mittels

Mikro-Wärmekomplementbindungsreaktion. *Deutche Tierärztliche Wochenschrift*, 97, 398–400.

114 **WEISS, H.E. & WEISS, H., 1988**. Nachweiss von *Clostridium botulinum* Toxin mittels Mikro-Wärmekomplementbindungsreaktion. *Tierärztliche Unschau*, 43, 117–126.

115 **WHITMER, M.E. & JOHNSON, E.A., 1988**. Development of improved defined media for *Clostridium botulinum* serotypes A, B and E. *Applied and Environmental Microbiology*, 54, 753–759.

116 **WICHTEL, J.J. & WHITLOCK, R.H., 1991**. Botulism associated with feeding alfalfa hay to horses. *Journal of the American Veterinary Medical Association*, 199, 471–472.

117 **WILLIS, A.T. & HOBBS, G., 1958**. A medium for the identification of clostridia producing opalescence in egg-yolk emulsions. *Journal of Pathology and Bacteriology*, 75, 299–305.

118 **WOBESER, G. & GALMUT, E.A., 1984**. Internal temperature of decomposing duck carcasses in relation to botulism. *Journal of Wildlife Diseases*, 20, 267–271.

119 **YAMAKAWA, K., KAMIYA, S., YOSHIMURA, K. & NAKAMURA, S., 1992**. *Clostridium botulinum* type C in healthy swine in Japan. *Microbiology and Immunology*, 36, 29–34.

REGULAR, NON-SPORING, GRAM-POSITIVE RODS

This group of bacteria contains seven genera which do not belong to the same family. They are all rod-shaped, Gram-positive, non-sporing and non-pigmented, and grow in complex media, but besides these have few common characteristics.[2] Only two of the seven genera, namely *Listeria* and *Erysipelothrix,* are of veterinary importance.

Bacteria of the genus *Listeria* are widely distributed in nature, and may be isolated from the soil, water, vegetation, animal biological products, and human and animal carriers throughout the world.[3] Two species of *Listeria* (*L. monocytogenes* and *L. ivanovii*) have been associated with disease in humans and animals. Of the two, *L. monocytogenes* is more common, and infections are usually sporadic. Different disease syndromes (septicaemia, meningoencephalitis, and abortions) may occur in infected animals and humans. *Listeria ivanovii* is rarely encountered, and has only been associated with abortions in sheep.[2]

The genus *Erysipelothrix* is mono-specific, *E. rhusiopathiae* being the only recognized species. The bacterium is highly resistant and remains viable and infective even after being subjected to the effects of processes such as putrefaction or the curing of meat by smoking or pickling. Infections by *E. rhusiopathiae* are ubiquitous and affect humans and a large variety of animals including cattle, sheep, horses, mice and various species of birds and fish. However, the bacterium is recognized particularly as a pathogen of pigs; it is responsible for the disease known as swine erysipelas or diamond skin disease. *Erysipelothrix rhusiopathiae* is one of the causes of fibrinopurulent polyarthritis in lambs, which results from the contamination of wounds (such as umbilical, castration and docking wounds). It is also a cause of post-dipping lameness in sheep, which is an acute, deep dermatitis of the lower limbs, and infection being contracted by the cutaneous route in animals that have been dipped in contaminated dipping fluids not containing antibacterial substances. Disease in poultry caused by *E. rhusiopathiae* is usually an acute, fulminant infection of individuals within a flock, and is accompanied by a reduction in egg production. Humans usually contract *E. rhusiopathiae* infection while handling infected meat or fish, and develop a disease known as erysipeloid, which manifests either as a localized skin rash or septicaemia.[1]

References

1 **BRICKER, J.M. & SAIF, Y.M., 1991.** Erysipelas. *In:* CALNEK, B.W., BARNES, H.J., BEARD, C.W., REID, W.M. & YODER, H.W., (eds). *Diseases of Poultry.* Ames, Iowa: Iowa State University Press.

2 **KANDLER, O. & WEISS, N., 1986.** Regular non-sporing Gram-positive rods. *In:* SNEATH, PH.,A., MAIR, N.S., SHARPE, M.E. & HOLT, J.G., (eds). *Bergey's Manual of Systematic Bacteriology.* Baltimore: Williams & Wilkens..

3 **SEELIGER, H.P.R. & JONES, D., 1986.** Genus *Listeria* Pirie 1940. *In:* SNEATH, P.H.A., MAIR, N.S. SHARPE, M.E. & HOLT, J.G., (eds). *Bergey's Manual of Systematic Bacteriology,* Baltimore: Williams & Wilkens.

164

Listeriosis

Synonym: Listeriose (Afrik.)

D.J. Schneider

Introduction

Listeriosis, caused by *Listeria monocytogenes*, is characterized in some livestock species by three distinct syndromes of meningoencephalitis, abortion or stillbirth, and neonatal septicaemia.[6, 33] Mastitis and keratoconjunctivitis have also been recorded.[1, 3] While meningoencephalitis occurs most commonly in ruminants, septicaemia is more frequently found in monogastric animals and young ruminants. The disease is rare in humans and with the exception of its cutaneous form, is often fatal.[1, 6, 34]

Listeria monocytogenes is widely distributed in nature, but the disease is usually sporadic and its prevalence low.[24, 32, 34] Listeriosis particularly affects sheep, goats and cattle. Although the first isolation of *L. monocytogenes* was from a South African gerbil in 1927,[26] the disease has only been reported in goats,[9] sheep[24] and chinchillas[8] in this country and is not of significant economic importance in southern Africa.

Aetiology

Listeria monocytogenes are Gram-positive, non-acid-fast, non-spore-forming, short, rod-shaped bacteria. Five serotypes, designated 1 to 5, and a number of subtypes have been identified.[6, 23, 25, 34] Serotype 5 (now called *Listeria ivanovii*[29]) is commonly isolated from cases of listerial abortion in sheep, but is of low pathogenicity.[6, 7]

The optimal growth temperature of the organism is between 30 and 37 °C but some growth may occur in the range of 4–44 °C. It propagates best at neutral or slightly alkaline pH and is usually killed at pH below 5,0. The organism is readily cultured on ordinary media under aerobic conditions, but growth is facilitated by an atmosphere containing 10 per cent CO_2.[5, 14]

Epidemiology

Listeriosis is found throughout the world. It is, however, more common in countries and regions with a cold temperate climate, such as New Zealand, certain parts of Australia, North America, Europe, and the United Kingdom, than in those with a tropical or subtropical climate. In some countries the prevalence of listeriosis has increased during recent years.[1, 22, 23] Clinical disease occurs particularly during late winter and early spring.[4, 6, 21, 22, 32]

Sheep, goats and cattle are the livestock species most frequently affected. The morbidity is usually less than 10 per cent, but the mortality rate in those suffering from meningoencephalitis is often 100 per cent.[6, 31]

Listeria monocytogenes is widely distributed in nature and has been isolated from a wide variety of healthy and diseased mammals and bird species, as well as from soil, water, sewage, mud and silage.[5, 18, 32] It may also be found on raw vegetables and fruit. A large proportion of healthy sheep and goats are subclinical carriers of *L. monocytogenes*, excreting organisms in their faeces and milk when stressed.[15] The organism may withstand low-temperature pasteurization of milk, and may be found in dairy products, in which it constitutes a danger to human health. It tolerates freezing.[30]

Listeriosis is often associated with the feeding of large quantities of poor-quality silage with a pH in excess of 5,5.[16, 31, 32, 34] Spoilage and high pH of silage resulting from poor preparation and maintenance result in growth of the bacteria, particularly in the top and side layers of the silage.[10, 13, 23] It is also suspected that, apart from nutritional stress, reduced resistance of the animal because of adverse environmental factors may predispose to disease.[24, 31, 34] In sheep, cases of listerial meningoencephalitis may occur 30 days after their initial introduction to silage feeding.[23]

Encephalitis has been produced experimentally by the inoculation of *L. monocytogenes* into the dental pulp[4] and lips of sheep and goats;[2] in these cases the incubation periods ranged between 14 and 28 days.

The higher prevalence of listerial meningoencephalitis in certain age groups of sheep has been linked to the changing of teeth in early spring.[4] It is suspected that ingested *L. monocytogenes* reach the fine dental terminals of the trigeminal nerve and so cause an ascending neuritis and meningoencephalitis.

Pathogenesis

Listeria monocytogenes is an intracellular organism.[15] In the meningoencephalitis syndrome, organisms are usually present only in the brain.

Although the pathway by which bacteria reach the brain is unclear, it is thought that they probably gain entrance to the body through wounds in the mucosa of the oral cavity. They then reach the brain stem via branches of the trigeminal nerve. The unilateral occurrence of micro-abscesses and the perivascular infiltration of lymphocytes, which are largely restricted to the brain stem (pons and medulla oblongata), are supportive of this view.[19]

Following ingestion, organisms may also penetrate the intestinal mucosa to produce a clinically inapparent infection, a bacteraemia with localization of bacteria in various organs, or a fatal septicaemia. In pregnant animals, organisms localize particularly in the uterus. Infection early in pregnancy usually causes abortion, while in late pregnancy it results in stillbirth or in lambs which develop fatal septicaemia soon after birth.[6]

Clinical signs

The syndromes of meningoencephalitis, abortion and septicaemia seldom occur together in an outbreak.[23]

In livestock, meningoencephalitis occurs most commonly in ruminants. In goats, sheep and calves the course of the disease is usually two to three days, while in adult cattle it ranges from one to two weeks. During the early stages of disease the rectal temperature is elevated, whereas it is normal to subnormal in more advanced cases. Neurological signs vary according to the location and severity of the lesions in the brain stem. Affected animals are depressed, walk in circles and show incoordination, tilting of the head, and evidence of unilateral facial nerve paralysis characterized by drooping of the lips, ears and eyelids, and paralysis of the muscles of the jaw and pharynx which interferes with mastication and swallowing. They often stand for long periods with food hanging from their mouth and drooling saliva. Lethargy frequently progresses to somnolence which is followed by generalized paralysis and death. Occasional convulsions and paddling movements with the fore limbs may be seen in terminal cases. Impaired respiration may occur as a result of the inflammatory changes in the brain stem.[27] A localized myelitis, manifested clinically by paralysis of one limb, has been recorded in lambs, but is more common in adult ruminants.[11] Keratoconjunctivitis has been reported in cattle.[27]

Sporadic abortions as a result of listeriosis are more common in cattle than in sheep and goats, but rarely reach a rate of 15 per cent. Retained placentas, clinical illness and fever are common in cows and ewes after abortion has taken place in advanced pregnancy. Death of the dam due to septicaemia sometimes follows retention of the foetus. Ewes abort seven to 11 days after infection but are asymptomatic before they abort.[7] Aborted foetuses are usually decomposed. Individual animals may abort again during subsequent pregnancies.[6]

Septicaemic listeriosis is the most common form encountered in foetuses and neonates of ruminants, and is sometimes found in monogastric animals. In these cases many organs and tissues are affected.[6, 7, 12]

Pathology

Examination of aspirated cerebrospinal fluid reveals the presence of inflammatory cells, mainly lymphocytes, and elevated concentrations of protein in animals affected by the meningoencephalitis syndrome. Grossly, the fluid may be turbid. Results obtained from haematological and biochemical blood analyses are not of significant diagnostic value, although metabolic acidosis is often found in affected animals as a result of excessive salivation.

Gross lesions are not normally noticeable in the central nervous system of animals suffering from listerial meningoencephalitis. In a few cases the meninges, particularly ventrally over the brain stem, may be thickened and slightly yellowish or opaque as a result of mononuclear cell infiltration, or it may be congested and oedematous.[9, 24, 31] Microscopic changes are confined to the white and/or grey matter of the brain stem, particularly the pons and the medulla oblongata, the spinal cord and the meninges. In the early stage, the lesions in the brain tissue consist of small accumulations of lymphocytes and monocytes, and sometimes a few neutrophils, around or in close proximity to blood vessels. In the later stages of the disease extensive perivascular infiltrations of mononuclear cells and micro-abscesses occur in the periventricular grey and/or white matter. The abscesses are characterized by liquefaction of the neuropil and by the presence of Gram-positive, short, rod-shaped bacteria, usually paired, in and around these lesions. Bacteria are not normally discernible in lesions when only perivascular mononuclear cell infiltrations are present in the brain stem.[21, 24, 33] A meningitis is almost always present, and may be marked. It is characterized by the presence of infiltrations of lymphocytes, macrophages, neutrophils and plasma cells in the meninges over the brain stem, cerebellum, and anterior cervical spinal cord.[21] Bacteria have also been reported in the foci of inflammation in the proximal parts of the cranial nerves.[33]

In aborted foetuses and young animals, especially neonate lambs, which have succumbed to the septicaemic disease, lesions are found consistently. Small, yellowish, pin-point, necrotic foci in the liver, small (1–3 mm in diameter) erosions in the abomasum and staining of the coat by meconium are seen. Foetuses are usually severely autolysed when expelled. Subcutaneous oedema, hydrothorax, ascites, and an enlarged pale or bronze-red, friable liver are normally found in new-born lambs that have died of congenital infection.[7] The most characteristic microscopic lesion in new-born animals is multifocal necrosis of the liver and, less frequently, of the spleen, lymph nodes, myocardium, lungs, adrenals, gastrointestinal tract and brain. The lesions are infiltrated by mononuclear cells, mainly lymphocytes, and some neutrophils. The organisms are easily demonstrated in tissue sections of affected areas.[7, 28]

Various degrees of oedema and sometimes greyish-white, leathery areas of necrosis, 100–120 mm in diameter, are evident around the cotyledons. Most cotyledons are paler than normal and range from a mottled orange to a pale greyish-pink.[7] Microscopical lesions in the placenta include severe oedema, infiltration of neutrophils in the chorio-allantois, necrotic vasculitis, mineralization of the villous mesenchyme, and numerous *Listeria* organisms in the chorionic epithelium.[7]

Diagnosis and differential diagnosis

A provisional diagnosis can be based on the clinical signs, epidemiological findings and histopathological examination of organs. Confirmation of the diagnosis requires isolation of *L. monocytogenes* from affected tissues.[4]

Attempts should be made to culture the organism from the brain stem in cases suffering from the meningoencephalitis syndrome, and from all organs as well as the placenta, faeces, urine, blood and milk in animals which have contracted the septicaemic syndrome. It must be borne in mind that the organisms can be very irregularly distributed in the body, so specimens should be collected from various organs. The exposure of tissues to a temperature of 4 °C for up to two months, known as 'cold enrichment', is advisable in order to promote the isolation of *L. monocytogenes* from tissue specimens.[4, 29]

The meningoencephalitis syndrome should be clinically differentiated from other neurological conditions in livestock, such as brain abscesses, *Coenuris cerebralis*, lead poisoning, heartwater, and cerebrocortical necrosis (thiamine deficiency).[6] Animals suffering from listeriosis may also be confused clinically with those that are affected by rabies; circling and unilateral facial nerve paralysis are, however, not usually present in rabies, while bellowing and aggressiveness are not usually present in listeriosis. In thrombotic meningoencephalitis, caused by *Haemophilus somnus*, the course of the disease is short, several young feedlot animals are often affected at once and the condition is often preceded by respiratory disease.[27]

The abortion and septicaemic syndromes should be differentiated from other causes of foetal loss and neonatal mortality in sheep, goats and cattle.

Control

Listeria monocytogenes is sensitive *in vitro* to a wide variety of drugs including chloramphenicol, streptomycin, oxytetracycline, neomycin, furazolidone, sulphonamide-trime-thoprim mixtures, penicillin, fluoroquinolones, erythromycin and rifampicin.[32] Penicillin at a dosage of 44 000 IU/kg twice daily for one to two weeks, followed by half that dosage for a further one to two weeks, gives good results in early cases of listeriosis in cattle.[27] In general the prognosis is poor once nervous signs have developed. Good responses are usually obtained from the parenteral administration of high doses of antimicrobials in septicaemic cases and in the treatment of uterine infection following abortions. Correction of dehydration, acid-base imbalance and electrolyte disturbances in clinically affected animals is advisable. Intravenous and oral fluid therapy must be continued until affected animals regain their ability to drink. Non-steroidal analgesic drugs and selenium/vitamin E injections are essential in animals with exertional myopathy resulting from struggling, as is soft bedding to prevent pressure necrosis.[27]

Immunity to listeriosis is based on the cell-mediated immune response.[16] Experiments with live vaccines have given promising results in sheep abroad.[17, 20]

References

1 **ANON., 1983.** *Listeria* infections in farm animals. *The Veterinary Record*, 112, 314.

2 **ASAHI, O., HOSEDA, T. & AKIYAMA, Y., 1957.** Studies on the mechanism of infection of the brain with *Listeria monocytogenes*. *American Journal of Veterinary Research*, 18, 147–157.

3 **BAPTISTA, P.J.H.P., 1979.** Infectious bovine keratoconjunctivitis. A review. *British Veterinary Journal*, 135, 225–242.

4 **BARLOW, R.M. & McGORUM, B., 1985.** Ovine listerial encephalitis: Analysis, hypothesis and synthesis. *The Veterinary Record*, 116, 233–236.

5 **BLENDEN, D.C., 1986.** Listeriosis. *In*: LEMAN, A.D., STRAW, B., GLOCK, R.D., MENGELING, W.L., PENNY, R.H.C. & SCHOLL, E., (eds). *Diseases of Swine*. 6th edn. Ames, Iowa: Iowa State University Press.

6 **BLOOD, D.C., RADOSTITS, O.M. & HENDERSON, J.A., 1983.** *Veterinary Medicine*. 6th edn. London: Bailière Tindall.

7 **DENNIS, S.M., 1975.** Perinatal lamb mortality in Western Australia. *Australian Veterinary Journal*, 51, 75–79.

8 **DU PLESSIS, J.L. & CAMERON, C.M., 1965.** Listeriosis in chinchillas. *Journal of the South African Veterinary Medical Association*, 36, 107–111.

9 **DU TOIT, I.F., 1977.** An outbreak of caprine listeriosis in the Western Cape. *Journal of the South African Veterinary Association*, 48, 39–40.

10 **FENLON, D.R., 1986.** Rapid quantitative assessment of the distribution of *Listeria* in silage implicated in a suspected outbreak of listeriosis in calves. *The Veterinary Record*, 118, 240–244.

11 **GATES, G.A., BLENDEN, D.C. & KINTNER, L.D., 1967.** Listeric myelitis in sheep. *Journal of the American Veterinary Medical Association*, 150, 200–204.

12 **GITTER, M., RICHARDSON, C. & BOUGHTON, E., 1986.** Experimental infection of pregnant ewes with *Listeria monocytogenes*. *The Veterinary Record*, 118, 575–578.

13 **GITTER, M., STEBBINGS, R. ST J., MORRIS, J.A., HANNAM, D. & HARRIS, C., 1986.** Relationship between listeriosis and silage feeding. *The Veterinary Record*, 118, 207–208.

14 **GRONSTOL, H., 1980.** Listeriosis in sheep. Isolation of *Listeria monocytogenes* from organs of slaughtered animals and dead animals submitted for post-mortem examination. *Acta Veterinaria Scandinavica*, 21, 11–17.

15 **GRONSTOL, H., 1986.** Listeria. *In*: GYLES, C.L. & THOEN, C.O., (eds). *Pathogenesis of Bacterial Infections in Animals*. Ames, Iowa: Iowa State University Press.

16 **GUDDING, R., GRONSTOL, H. & LARSEN, H.J., 1985.** Vaccination against listeriosis in sheep. *The Veterinary Record*, 117, 89–90.

17 **GUDDING, R., NESSE, L.L. & GRONSTOL, H., 1989.** Immunization against infections caused by *Listeria monocytogenes* in sheep. *The Veterinary Record*, 125, 111–114.

18 **HYSLOP, N. ST G., 1974.** Epidemiologic and immunologic factors in listeriosis. Problems of listeriosis. *Proceedings of the Sixth International Symposium on Listeriosis*. September 1974, University of Nottingham.

19 **INNES, J.R.M. & SAUNDERS, L.Z., 1962.** *Comparative Neuropathology*. New York & London: Academic Press, Inc.

20 **IVANOV, I., DRAGANOV, M. & DIKOVA, T., 1977.** Study on the active immunoprophylaxis of sheep listeriosis. Problems of listeriosis. *Proceedings of the Seventh International Symposium on Listeriosis*, 1977, Varna, Bulgaria.

21 **JUBB, K.V.F., KENNEDY, P.C. & PALMER, N., 1985.** *Pathology of Domestic Animals*. 3rd edn. New York: Academic Press, Inc.

22 **LOW, C. & LINKLATER, K., 1985.** Listeriosis in sheep. *In Practice*, 7, 66–67.

23 **LOW, J.C. & RENTON, C.P., 1985.** Septicaemia, encephalitis and abortions in a housed flock of sheep caused by *Listeria monocytogenes* type 1/2. *The Veterinary Record*, 116, 147–150.

24 **MEREDITH, C.D. & SCHNEIDER, D.J., 1984.** An outbreak of ovine listeriosis associated with poor flock management practices. *Journal of the South African Veterinary Association*, 55, 55–56.

25 **MOORE, R.M. & ZEHMER, R.B., 1973.** Listeriosis in the United States — 1971. *Journal of Infectious Diseases*, 127, 610–611.

26 **PIRIE, J.H.J., 1927.** A new disease in veld rodents. 'Tiger River disease'. *Publications of the South African Institute for Medical Research*, 3, 163–186.

27 **REBHUN, W.C. & DELAHUNTA, A., 1982.** Diagnosis and treatment of bovine listeriosis. *Journal of the American Veterinary Medical Association*, 180, 395–398.

28 **SMITH, H.A., JONES, T.C. & HUNT, R.D., 1981.** *Veterinary Pathology*, 4th edn. Philadelphia: Lea & Febiger.

29 **SNEATH, P.H.A., MAIR, N.S., SHARPE, M.E. & HOLT, J.G., 1986.** *In*: KRIER, N.R. & HOLT, J.G., (eds). *Bergey's Manual of Systematic Bacteriology*. Vol. II. Baltimore: Williams & Wilkins.

30 **THAM, W.A. & DANIELSON-THAM, V.M.L., 1988.** *Listeria monocytogenes* isolated from soft cheese. *The Veterinary Record*, 122, 539–540.

31 **VANDEGRAAFF, R., BORLAND, N.A. & BROWNING, J.W., 1981.** An outbreak of listerial meningoencephalitis in sheep. *Australian Veterinary Journal*, 75, 94–96.

32 **WARDROPE, D.D. & MACLEOD, N.S.M., 1983.** Outbreak of *Listeria* meningoencephalitis in young lambs. *The Veterinary Record*, 113, 213–214.

33 **WEST, H.J. & OBWOLO, M., 1987.** Bilateral facial paralysis in a cow with listeriosis. *The Veterinary Record*, 120, 204.

34 **WILESMITH, J.W. & GITTER, M., 1986.** Epidemiology of ovine listeriosis in Great Britain. *The Veterinary Record*, 119, 467–470.

165

Erysipelothrix rhusiopathiae *infections*

Synonym: *E. insidiosa* infections

B.T. Spencer

ERYSIPELAS IN PIGS

Synonyms: Diamond skin disease, swine erysipelas, vleksiekte (Afrik.)

Introduction

Erysipelas is a peracute, acute, subacute or chronic infectious disease of pigs caused by *Erysipelothrix rhusiopathiae*. While the peracute and acute disease is generally characterized by septicaemia, fever, purplish-red patches in the skin and rapid death, pigs affected by the subacute disease manifest large, sharply circumscribed, slightly raised, diamond-shaped, purplish-red cutaneous patches. Pigs that are chronically affected are usually unthrifty and suffer from a vegetative valvular endocarditis and/or chronic non-purulent polyarthritis.

Koch in 1880 isolated a bacillus, which was probably *E. rhusiopathiae*, from the blood of mice suffering from septicaemia.[10] According to Henning,[10] Loeffler in 1882 was the first to isolate *E. rhusiopathiae* in pure culture from a pig that had died from erysipelas.

Outbreaks of erysipelas only occur sporadically in South Africa, probably because of the regular vaccination of most of the breeding stock.

Aetiology

Generally *E. rhusiopathiae* is regarded as the only species within the genus, although based on differing N-acetyl-beta-glucosaminidase activity it has been suggested that *E. tonsillae* may be a new species.[29] The taxonomic position of the genus with regard to other bacterial genera has not yet been resolved.[13]

Erysipelothrix rhusiopathiae are facultatively anaerobic bacteria. They are non-motile, non-sporulating, usually slender, straight or slightly curved rods 0,2–0,4 µm in width and 0,5–2,5 µm in length. They may, however, be filamentous and 60 µm or more in length.[13] The organism is Gram-positive, and also stains well with the various aniline dyes.[36] The organisms ferment glucose and lactose weakly and produce hydrogen sulphide in triple sugar iron agar.[13, 22]

Erysipelothrix rhusiopathiae grows readily on most of the standard laboratory media, but cultivation is enhanced by the addition of glucose and, to a lesser extent, blood and serum to the medium in a slightly alkaline pH. Most strains grow better on primary isolation in a reduced oxygen environment containing 5 to 10 per cent carbon dioxide.[36] Smooth (S-form) colonies are round, convex, slimy, translucent, about 0,3–1,5 mm in diameter, and have entire or undulating edges. These colonies are formed within 24–48 hours, and are surrounded by a narrow rim of incomplete haemolysis (alpha-haemolysin) when grown on a blood agar medium.[13, 30] Rough (R-form) colonies are generally opaque, flatter and larger than S-form colonies,[13, 22] and have irregular edges and a matt appearance on the surface. Serovars 1 and 2 generally produce S-form colonies on blood agar, while less virulent serovars produce R-form colonies. However, morphological distinction between the two forms is not always accurate, and intermediate forms exist; S-form colonies may change to intermediate or R-form colonies, and vice versa.[13] Smooth forms are usually recovered from pigs suffering from the peracute and acute disease, while R-forms together with S-forms are often isolated from chronically affected pigs.[35]

Of the 24 serovars that have been identified, serovars 1 and 2 are those most frequently isolated from cases of erysipelas; the others are relatively rare.[6, 11, 13, 35]

For a non-sporing organism, *E. rhusiopathiae* is remarkably resistant. It retains its infectivity in putrefied meat for more than four months, in pickled and salted bacon for several weeks, in well-smoked hams for more than three months, in drinking water for five days, and in sewage for up to 35 days.[10, 13, 37] The survival of the organism is favoured by environmental factors such as low temperature, alkaline pH and abundant organic matter.[13]

There is a high correlation of susceptibility between pigs and mice to artificially induced infection with highly or less virulent strains, while mixed results are obtained in infections with strains of intermediate virulence.[4] White mice are highly susceptible to infection by *E. rhusiopathiae*, and for this reason they are used in a test known as the mouse protection test which is used to identify of new isolates of *E. rhusiopathiae*. Almost all strains of *E. rhusiopathiae* tested by the tube or slide technique are coagulase-positive. This technique is also useful for differentiating between *E. rhusiopathiae*, *Listeria* spp. and *Corynebacterium* spp.[31]

Epidemiology

Erysipelothrix rhusiopathiae is a cosmopolitan pathogen. Sporadic outbreaks in pigs occur periodically in South Africa.[8] Other animal species such as cattle, sheep, horses, white mice, pigeons, turkeys and several other species of birds, as well as humans, are also susceptible to *E. rhusiopathiae*.[10, 13, 32, 36]

Pigs of all ages may contract the disease, but pigs aged between two months and one year are most susceptible.[1] In a herd, a large number of pigs may be affected by the acute septicaemic disease within a short time, or only occasional sporadic cases may occur.

Most infections are acquired from ingestion of *E. rhusiopathiae* contaminated food, soil and faeces.[30, 36] Transmission may also occur via bites of infected flies or by contamination of skin wounds.[36]

Under natural conditions *E. rhusiopathiae* is readily spread by diseased or subclinically infected carrier pigs. All pigs should be considered potential carriers,[19, 32] as the bacterium may be recovered from the tonsils, gastrointestinal tract, gall bladder or faeces of healthy, immune pigs.[32, 36] Recrudescence of infection may occur when these pigs are stressed, with subsequent spread of infection to other pigs.[32] Other possible sources of the organism are swill, slaughter-house offal, contaminated water and soil, and stable manure.[17, 30, 36] The organism can survive for up to 35 days in slurry and can thereby be spread to cultivated lands.[26, 36] Wild birds and rodents have also been incriminated as possible carriers of infection, as they may harbour the bacterium in their gastrointestinal tract.[10, 13] *Erysipelothrix rhusiopathiae* has been isolated from the surfaces of fish, shellfish and fish boxes.[13, 30, 36]

Sudden changes in the weather, such as excessively hot or humid weather conditions, overfeeding (particularly of protein), poor hygiene, handling, transportation, and high population densities may predispose to outbreaks of erysipelas.[25, 32]

Serovars 1 and 2 account for about 80 per cent of the isolates made from diseased pigs on a worldwide basis,[22, 35] including South Africa.[11] Serovar 2 is the most immunogenic strain and is used in the majority of vaccines.

Pathogenesis

Following ingestion of the organisms, infection occurs via the tonsils and gut-associated lymphoid tissue. In some pigs this is followed by the development of septicaemia. Many pigs, however, do not develop septicaemia, and the bacteria remain localized in the tonsillar tissues.

The severity of disease depends on the size of the infective dose, the virulence of the serovar involved, and the susceptibility of the pig.[7] Peracute, acute or subacute disease usually develops in highly susceptible pigs, while those with some degree of immunity develop chronic disease as a result of localization of bacteria in the joints and on the heart valves.[7, 32]

The sharply circumscribed cutaneous lesions in animals suffering from the subacute form of the disease, which is also known as diamond skin disease, result from arteritis and thrombosis of the arterioles in the dermis. The proliferative changes in the joints of chronic cases are a sequel to antibody directed against the antigen in the joints, with the formation of immune complexes, activation of complement and the presence of neutrophils.[33] Following these reactions, lysosomal enzymes liberated by neutrophils damage the cartilage and other tissues in the joints. Similarly, localization of bacteria on heart valves results in chronic valvular endocarditis, with consequent development of valvular insufficiency and chronic congestive heart failure. Boars may be temporarily infertile after recovery from acute erysipelas, presumably as a result of the adverse effect of fever on spermatogenesis.[30]

Erysipelothrix rhusiopathiae may persist indefinitely in clinically healthy pigs, in pigs that have recovered from the disease, or in pigs with chronic arthritis.[30]

Hyaluronidase and neuraminidase produced by *E. rhusiopathiae* may contribute to the virulence of the organism.[7, 13, 37] Virulent strains appear to produce neuraminidase in greater quantities during their logarithmic growth phases than avirulent or low-virulence strains. It is postulated that the large amounts of neuraminidase produced during the septicaemic stage are a major factor in the 'multiple mechanisms mediating the widespread vascular damage, thrombosis and the shock-like coagulopathy resulting in diapedesis'.[36]

Clinical signs

The incubation period varies from one to seven days. Different clinical forms of disease are recognized, namely peracute, acute (septicaemic) disease, subacute disease (also referred to as diamond skin disease), and chronic disease characterized by arthritis and/or vegetative valvular endocarditis.

Pigs affected by the peracute form of the disease die within 24 hours, usually without any noticeable clinical signs. In acutely affected pigs the onset of disease is sudden and several animals in a herd are usually affected simultaneously. The initial signs include high fever, anorexia, thirst, somnolence, vomition, and conjunctivitis. Discoloration of the skin usually appears within one day of illness; dark-red or purplish patches develop in the skin of the ears, snout, neck, ventral parts of the thorax, abdomen, groin, perineum, and axillae.[15, 30, 32, 36] These erythematous areas are generally not sharply circumscribed, and they may coalesce and affect large parts of the body.[1] In the pigmented breeds it is often not possible to see this skin discoloration. Affected pigs often develop weakness of the hind quarters and walk with a stiff gait. At first the faeces are hard and may be streaked with blood or mucus, but diarrhoea may subsequently set in. Difficult breathing may also be noticed. In acutely affected animals, the course of disease is two to four days before death supervenes.[10] The prognosis in pigs suffering from the acute septicaemic disease is usually unfavourable; the mortality rate varies from 50 to 100 per cent. In some animals recovery is only partial, as they may develop the chronic disease after a lapse of time.

In the milder, subacute disease, initial signs include fever, malaise, anorexia, reluctance to stand and bristling of the hairs where the skin lesions are going to develop. Within three to four days of the appearance of these signs, numerous well-circumscribed, purplish-red, intensely hyperaemic and slightly raised patches, with a diamond, rectangular or rhomboid shape, develop in the skin **(Figure 165.1)**. In mild cases the patches have pale centres and disappear after a few days. Desquamation of the epidermis of the affected skin ensues, and the animal recovers in seven to ten days.[10] In severely affected pigs, vesicles develop in the raised patches, which may rupture to form crusts. In some animals the affected skin becomes black, hard and necrotic. These areas may slough, leaving large, raw ulcers. The ears and tail may also be shed as a result of dry gangrene. The mortality rate is usually not higher than 2 per cent and is often the result of secondary infections. Pregnant sows may abort or give birth to dead piglets.[30]

The chronic form of the disease is characterized by arthritis and/or vegetative valvular endocarditis. It may follow on a mild or inapparent systemic infection, or it may develop as a sequel of the acute or subacute disease. Alternatively it may develop in vaccinated pigs subjected to natural exposure. The hock, stifle and elbow joints are most commonly affected, but the carpus and tarsus may also be involved. The affected joints are often visibly swollen and painful, and the animal walks with a stiff gait on its toes and with its back arched. Affected pigs generally prefer to lie down, lose their appetites, and become unthrifty and stunted. In some, the joints are not noticeably swollen, but the animal is nevertheless stiff and weak in the hind quarters and is unthrifty. Chronic arthritis occurs most often in animals older than 10 weeks of age and may persist for several years. Most pigs with cardiac involvement do not reveal any noteworthy signs, but some show fatigue, listlessness, loss of appetite, and signs of congestive heart failure, manifested by resting on the sternum and elbows, or sitting on their haunches.[10] Pulmonary involvement as a sequel to the cardiac lesions is characterized by a slight cough, and dyspnoea, particularly when the animals move, is common. Cardiac and respiratory involvement occasionally results in cyanosis of mucous membranes, congested patches in the skin of the ears and neck, oedema of the extremities, and paresis of the hind quarters. The prognosis is unfavourable. Affected pigs remain unthrifty and may pine for weeks; death is often sudden as a result of fulminating acute heart failure.

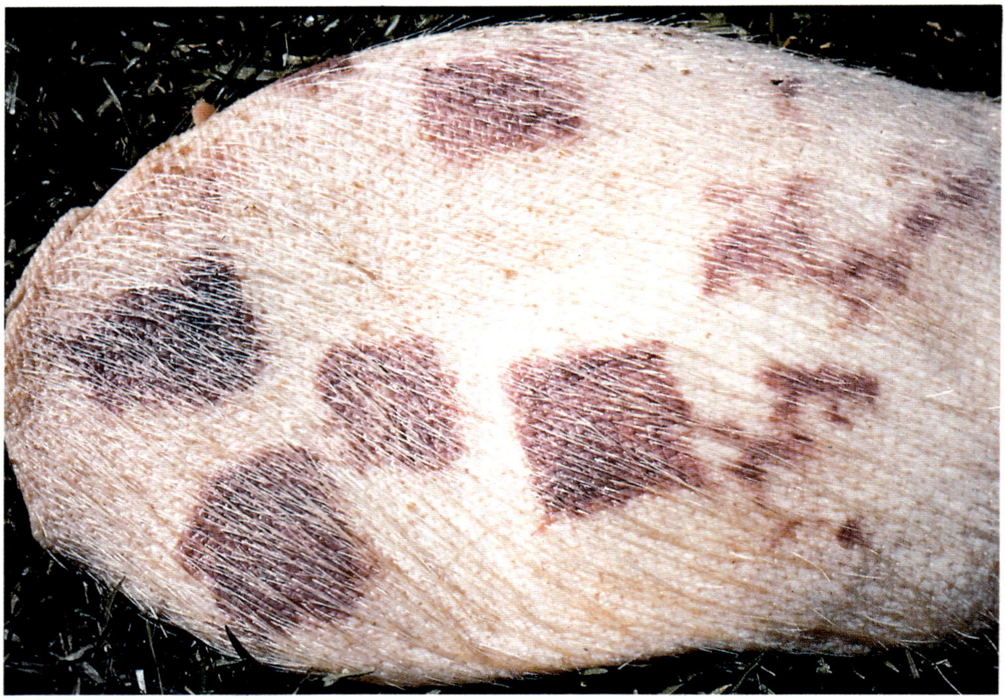

Figure 165.1 Diamond skin disease. Well-circumscribed, rhomboid lesions in the skin of a pig

Pathology

The lesions vary with the severity and the course of the disease.[14, 36]

Lesions characteristic of septicaemia are evident in the peracute to acute disease. Haemorrhages are common in the subcutaneous and intermuscular tissues, serosal surfaces, endocardium and certain organs (such as the kidneys), the spleen is usually enlarged, the lymph nodes are swollen and haemorrhagic, and increased amounts of fluid are present in the body cavities. The mucous membranes of the stomach and intestines are hyperaemic and may reveal dark red, necrotic areas. The lungs are congested and oedematous.

In addition to the clinically discernible skin lesions, the changes associated with the septicaemic disease may also be present in pigs suffering from the subacute disease. Microscopically the skin lesions are characterized by arteritis and thrombosis of the arterioles in the dermis, and, depending on the severity of the lesions, degeneration and necrosis of the dermis and epidermis.[36] Bacteria are present in areas of necrosis in the dermis. Embolic glomerulonephritis characterized by sludging of erythrocytes, haemorrhage and fibrinoid necrosis in parts of the glomeruli, and the presence of bacterial colonies may be evident in the septicaemic and subacute disease. Numerous neutrophils may also be seen in these areas. Colonies may also be present in some intertubular capillaries.

Acute arthritis is characterized by serous to serofibrinous synovitis and arthritis. Microscopically, vasculitis may be evident in the synovial membranes of affected joints. As the joint lesions become chronic, pedunculated growths develop on the synovial membrane and encroach into the joint cavity. The inflammatory changes extend into the capsular ligaments, periarticular tissues, bone and cartilage. Articular cartilage may become detached and new bone may be formed under the cartilage. Discospondylitis is frequently present. The articular cartilages may be eroded and periostitis may supervene.[10, 14, 21, 36]

Vegetative valvular endocarditis occurs most commonly on the mitral and aortic semilunar valves in pigs suffering from cardiac involvement in the chronic disease. The tricuspid valves are less frequently affected, while the pulmonary valves are rarely involved. Septic emboli and infarcts may be present in the kidneys and spleen in this form of the disease.[14] Microscopically, numerous bacteria are often visible near the surface of the growths on the valves.

Diagnosis and differential diagnosis

A definite diagnosis of erysipelas cannot be made from the clinical signs and the lesions alone, and bacteriological culture of tissue specimens is necessary to confirm the diagnosis.

In the septicaemic disease, rod-shaped organisms are found in smears made from the blood, spleen, liver and kidneys. In chronic heart and joint lesions, as well as in cultures, long, thread-like filamentous bacteria tend to develop.

Bacteriologically, the organisms are readily cultured from the blood and specimens of internal organs of septicaemic animals, from the dermis of diamond-shaped skin lesions and from affected joints and valves of the heart.

Serological tests, including ELISA, gel diffusion precipitation, haemagglutination, haemagglutination-inhibition, complement fixation and indirect immunofluorescence tests have been used, but are not diagnostically conclusive and at best can be used as herd tests for detecting chronic infections.[5, 36]

Clinical signs and lesions of acute erysipelas may in some instances be difficult to differentiate from similar signs which may be present in pigs suffering from African swine fever, hog cholera, salmonellosis, *Streptococcus* spp. infection, and pasteurellosis. The majority of *Salmonella choleraesuis* infections, however, are associated with a diphtheritic enteritis, and pneumonic lesions are present in most cases of pasteurellosis. Microbiological culture of specimens of the internal organs usually reveals the presence of the causative agent.

Arthritis as a result of *E. rhusiopathiae* must be differentiated from that caused by organisms such as *Mycoplasma hyorhinis, Mycoplasma hyosynoviae, Actinomyces (Corynebacterium) pyogenes, Haemophilus* spp., *Streptococcus* spp. and *Staphylococcus* spp. as well as non-infectious osteochondrosis.

Apart from *E. rhusiopathiae*, chronic vegetative endocarditis in pigs may be caused by *Streptococcus* spp. and *Pasteurella* spp.

Control

Penicillin is the drug of choice, and response to the administration of a single long-acting preparation at 10 000 to 20 000 units/kg is often rapid and dramatic in acutely and subacutely affected pigs.[36] In-feed medication with oxytetracyclines at levels of up to 200 ppm is ineffective in cases of subacute erysipelas.[25, 27, 28]

Antiserum, when administered during the early stages of the disease, will often bring about a rapid recovery within a very short time, but will provide subsequent protection for only about two weeks.[22] However, administration of antiserum may exacerbate pre-existing arthritis caused by *E. rhusiopathiae*.[23] Hyperimmune serum is not available in southern Africa.

In South Africa a bacterin is used to immunize pigs in breeding herd and grower pigs. In breeding herds, the gilts and young boars should be immunized twice, a month apart, initially at selection or purchase, and thereafter once every six months. Depending on the management practice, this booster vaccination should either be administered at a specific time to the whole herd, or the sows can be vaccinated at, for example, the time when their litters are weaned. Boars are vaccinated twice a year. Weaners and growers are not usually vaccinated on farms. On farms where the disease is present in grower pigs, vaccination is recommended when the pigs are handled for the first time after weaning. Stress should be limited as far as possible.

Bacterins provide protection against the septicaemic disease but would appear to enhance the susceptibility of pigs to arthritis.[3] In other parts of the world, combination vaccines are used to control erysipelas.[16]

ERYSIPELOTHRIX RHUSIOPATHIAE *INFECTION IN OTHER ANIMAL SPECIES*

Post-dipping lameness due to subacute to chronic dermatitis and cellulitis in lambs and adult sheep as a result of *Erysipelothrix* infection occurs occasionally after the dipping of sheep in contaminated dip fluid, or when they graze on pastures that have been irrigated with pig faeces.[12] Lesions occur most often about the fetlocks but may extend to the metacarpus or metatarsus.[9, 10, 32, 34]

Usually only a few animals in a flock are affected, but the morbidity may be as high as 50 per cent.[14] Sheep become infected through wounds such as those acquired as a result of castration, docking, shearing or dipping. The lesions may remain localized at the point of entry, but bacteraemia followed by polyarthritis may occur. Death rarely ensues. Affected animals show fever, severe lameness and rapid wasting. Incision through the affected areas reveals congestion and a serous to serofibrinous exudate. During the acute stages of joint involvement, a serofibrinous exudate accumulates in affected joints. In the chronic stage, the joints reveal periarticular fibrosis and periosteal and perichondrial osteophyte formation.[2, 12, 14]

The presence of *E. rhusiopathiae* in dipping fluid can be eliminated by the addition of 10 per cent zinc sulphate together with a detergent to aid its penetration. Delaying dipping the sheep until a week after shearing is effective in the prevention of post-dipping lameness. Modern acaricides are more labile than those previously used, with the result that the dip wash has to be replaced more frequently, and this reduces contamination.[10]

Other disease conditions that have been attributed to *E. rhusiopathiae* include endocarditis and arthritis in horses,[20, 24] while arthritis of the tibiotarsal, stifle and carpal joints in calves as a result of *E. rhusiopathiae* has been reported.[18]

Disease in humans, referred to as erysipeloid, is usually the result of a wound infection. It is a mild disease generally confined to the hands of people handling infected pork or fish or virulent cultures, or performing necropsies on infected animals.[32]

The localized skin lesions are usually reddish-purple and swollen and may gradually extend to involve the entire hand, but seldom spread beyond the wrist. Sometimes weals and vesicles are formed on the fingers or hand. Swelling and tenderness of neighbouring joints, usually the elbow or carpal, and of the regional lymph nodes are other symptoms which may occur. Five per cent of patients develop an arthritis.[32] Septicaemia is rare, but arthritis and endocarditis have been reported.[13]

References

1 **BASTIANELLO, S.S. & SPENCER, B.T., 1984.** A report of swine erysipelas in a litter of piglets. *Journal of the South African Veterinary Association*, 55, 195–198.

2 **BATH, G.F., 1991.** Faculty of Veterinary Science, University of Pretoria. Personal communication.

3 **BÖHM, K.H., BOLLWAHN, W., FISCHER, J., MUMME, J. & EHARD, H., 1988.** Vaccination against erysipelas in breeding farms. *Tenth International Pig Veterinary Society Congress*, Rio de Janeiro, August 1988.

4 **EAMENS, G.J., 1988.** Pathogenicity of field isolates of *Erysipelothrix rhusiopathiae* in mice, rats and pigs. *Australian Veterinary Journal*, 65, 280–284.

5 **EAMENS, G.J., CHIN, J.C. & NICHOLLS, P.J., 1989.** Comparison of inoculation regimes for the experimental production of swine erysipelas arthritis. II. Serological findings in a gel diffusion precipitin test and enzyme-linked immunosorbent assay. *Australian Veterinary Journal*, 66, 216–220.

6 **EAMENS, G.J., TURNER, M.J. & CATT, R.E., 1988.** Serotypes of *Erysipelothrix rhusiopathiae* in Australian pigs, small ruminants, poultry and captive wild birds and animals. *Australian Veterinary Journal*, 65, 249–252.

7 **GYLES, C.L., 1986.** *Erysipelothrix*. In: GYLES, C.L. & THOEN, C.O., (eds). *Pathogenesis of Bacterial Infection in Animals*. Ames, Iowa: Iowa State University Press.

8 **HAIG, D.A. & ADELAAR, T.E., 1944.** A case of swine erysipelas in the Union of South Africa. *Onderstepoort Journal of Veterinary Research*, 20, 57–59.

9 **HARBOUR, H.E. & KERSHAW, G.F., 1949.** *Erysipelothrix rhusiopathiae* infection in sheep. *The Veterinary Record*, 61, 37–38.

10 **HENNING, M.W., 1956.** *Animal Diseases in South Africa*, 3rd edn. Pretoria: Central News Agency Ltd.

11 **HUNTER, P., 1989.** Veterinary Research Institute, Onderstepoort, South Africa. Unpublished data.

12 **HUNTER, P. & SPENCER, B.T., 1987.** Foot-and-Mouth Disease Laboratory, Onderstepoort. Unpublished data.

13 **JONES, D., 1986.** Genus *Erysipelothrix* Rosenbach 1909, 367^{AL}. *In*: SNEATH, P.H.A., MAIR, N.S., SHARPE, M.E. & HOLT, J.G., (eds). *Bergey's Manual of Systematic Bacteriology*. Vol. 2. Baltimore: Williams & Wilkins.

14 **JUBB, K.V., KENNEDY, P.C. & PALMER, N., 1985.** *Pathology of Domestic Animals*. 3rd edn. Vol. I. New York: Academic Press, Inc.

15 **LOVEDAY, R.K., 1962.** Acute swine erysipelas in suckling pigs. *Journal of the South African Veterinary Medical Association*, 33, 3–5.

16 **McCARTHY, D.H., PORTER, D.B., DOUGLASS, J. & SLUSSER, C.A., 1986.** Preventing atrophic rhinitis, erysipelas and pasteurellosis in pigs. *Veterinary Medicine*, 81, 1169–1170, 1172–1174.

17 **MOLIN, G., SODERLIND, O., URSING, J., NORRUNG, V., TERNSTROM, A. & LOWENHIELM, C., 1989.** Occurrence of *Erysipelothrix rhusiopathiae* on pork and in pig slurry, and the distribution of specific antibodies in abattoir workers. *Journal of Applied Bacteriology*, 67, 347–352.

18 **MOULTON, J.E., RHODE, E.R. & WHEAT, J.D., 1953.** Erysipelas arthritis in calves. *Journal of the American Veterinary Medical Association*, 123, 335–340.

19 **OKOLO, M.I.O., 1986.** Isolation of *Erysipelothrix rhusiopathiae* from apparently healthy pigs reared under intensive and free range systems of management. *Microbios*, 47, 29–35.

20 **PATERSON, J.S. & HEATLEY, T.G., 1938.** A case of infection of the horse with *Erysipelothrix rhusiopathiae* (swine erysipelas). *Veterinary Journal*, 94, 33–34.

21 **RIEKA, P., COSTA, L., VENDRELL, J., ESPUNA, E. & CASADEVALL, P., 1984.** Studies on a field case of arthritis in weaned pigs caused by *E. rhusiopathiae*. *Proceedings of the International Pig Veterinary Society*, Ghent, 27–31 August 1984.

22 **SCANLAN, C.M., 1988.** *Introduction to Veterinary Bacteriology*, Ames, Iowa: Iowa State University Press.

23 **SCHOENING, W.H., GREY, C.G. & OSTEEN, O.L., 1942.** Swine erysipelas. United States Department of Agriculture, *Yearbook of Agriculture*, 686–694.

24 **SEAHORN, T.L., BRUMBAUGH, G.W., CARTER, G.K. & WOOD, R.L., 1989.** *Erysipelothrix rhusiopathiae* bacteremia in a horse. *Cornell Veterinarian*, 79, 151–156.

25 **SPENCER, B.T., 1992.** P.O. Box 32518, Glennstantia 0010. Personal observations.

26 **SPENCER, B.T. & HUNTER, P., 1991.** P.O. Box 32518, Glennstantia 0010. Unpublished data.

27 **TAKAHASHI, T., SAWADA, T., OHMAE, K., TAKAGI, M., MURAMATSU, M., TERAKADO, N., SETO, K., MARUYAMA, T. & KANZAKI, M., 1986.** Serotypes and antibiotic resistance of *Erysipelothrix rhusiopathiae* strains isolated from pigs affected with chronic swine erysipelas. *Japan Agricultural Research Quarterly*, 19, 287–294.

28 **TAKAHASHI, T., SAWADA, T., OHMAE, K., TERAKADO, N., MURAMATSU, M., SETO, K., MARUYAMA, T. & KANZAKI, M., 1983.** Antibiotic resistance of *Erysipelothrix rhusiopathiae* isolated from pigs with chronic swine erysipelas. *Antimicrobial Agents and Chemotherapy*, 25, 385–386.

29 **TAKAHASHI, T., TAMURA, T., SAWADA, T., SUZUKI, S., MURAMATSU, M., FUJISAWA, T., BENNO, Y. & MITSUOKA, T., 1989.** Enzymatic profiles of *Erysipelothrix rhusiopathiae* and *Erysipelothrix tonsillae*. *Research in Veterinary Science*, 47, 275–276.

30 **TAYLOR, D.J., 1989.** Erysipelas. *In: Pig Diseases*. 5th edn. Cambridge: Burlington Press.

31 **TESH, M.J. & WOOD, R.L., 1988.** Detection of coagulase activity in *Erysipelothrix rhusiopathiae*. *Journal of Clinical Microbiology*, 26, 1058–1060.

32 **TIMONEY, J.F., GILLESPIE, J.H., SCOTT, F.W. & BARLOUGH, J.E., 1988.** *Hagan and Brunner's Microbiology and Infectious Diseases of Domestic Animals*. 8th edn. Cornell University, USA: Cornell University Press.

33 **TIZARD, I., 1987.** *Veterinary Immunology: An Introduction*. 3rd edn. London: W.B. Saunders Co.

34 **WHITTEN, L.D., HARBOUR, H.E. & ALLAN, W.S., 1948.** Cutaneous *Erysipelothrix* infection in sheep. An etiological agent in post-dipping lameness. *Australian Veterinary Journal*, 24, 157.

35 **WOOD, R.L., 1980.** Susceptibility of vaccinated swine and mice to acute generalised infection with specific serotypes of *Erysipelothrix rhusiopathiae*. *Proceedings of the International Pig Veterinary Society*, Copenhagen, June 30–July 3 1980.

36 **WOOD, R.L., 1981.** Swine erysipelas. *In*: LEMAN, A.D. *et al.*, (eds). *Diseases of Swine*. Ames, Iowa: Iowa State University Press.

37 **WOOD, R.L., 1984.** Swine erysipelas — A review of prevalence and research. *Journal of the American Veterinary Medical Association*, 184, 944–949.

IRREGULAR, NON-SPORING, GRAM-POSITIVE RODS

The genus *Corynebacterium* was originally created for the diphtheria bacillus and a few other bacterial species that are pathogenic to animals. A wide collection of 'diphtheroids' (i.e. non-sporeforming, non-motile, non-encapsulated, pleomorphic, irregularly staining, Gram-positive bacterial rods that occur in angular or palisade arrangements) were later included in it. The club-shaped swelling at one or both ends was considered to be another characteristic feature of corynebacteria (*Corynebacterium* [Greek] = 'club bacterium').[2, 7]

Recent taxonomic revision, however, particularly by means of thin layer chromatographic analysis of whole organism methanolysates, has resulted in the definition of the genus becoming more restrictive.[2] Consequently, some species which were previously classified in the genus *Corynebacterium* have been assigned to three other genera — *Actinomyces, Eubacterium* and *Rhodococcus*. Thus, of the organisms of veterinary significance which have traditionally been assigned to the genus *Corynebacterium*, only *C. pseudotuberculosis* (formerly *C. ovis*), the *C. renale* group and *C. bovis* remain. *Corynebacterium pyogenes, C. suis* and *C. equi* have been relocated in the genera *Actinomyces, Eubacterium* and *Rhodococcus*, respectively.[2] In the most recent edition of *Bergey's Manual*,[2, 3] *Corynebacterium, Eubacterium* and *Actinomyces* are grouped as 'irregular, non-sporing Gram-positive rods', while *Rhodococcus* is now grouped under 'nocardioforms'.

True *Corynebacterium* spp., therefore, are characterized by the presence of arabinose, galactose, meso-diaminopimelic acid (meso-DAP) and peptidoglycan in the cell wall, and mycolic acids of chain length between 22 and 36 carbon atoms.[2] *Rhodococcus* spp., on the other hand, also contain arabinose, galactose and meso-DAP as well as tuberculostearic acids and 32–66 carbon mycolic acids.[3] Bacteria in the genus *Actinomyces* do not contain meso-DAP or arabinose in their cell walls,[6] while rhamnose is the major sugar component of the cell wall of *Eubacterium suis*.[5]

In southern Africa, *Corynebacterium pseudotuberculosis* and *Actinomyces pyogenes* are the most important bacteria of the genera considered here. Of these two species, 75 per cent of isolations made at the Veterinary Research Institute, Onderstepoort, between 1980 and 1989 were *A. pyogenes*.[4]

Bacteria from the above genera are readily isolated on blood agar media. Although the colonies and microscopic morphology are quite distinct, the various organisms are best distinguished on the basis of their biochemical characteristics, some of which are given in **Table 1**.[1–3, 5–7]

Disease conditions in farm animals which are caused by the above bacteria are listed in **Table 2**.

Table 1 Laboratory differentiation of *Corynebacterium, Eubacterium, Actinomyces* and *Rhodococcus* spp. of importance in diseases of farm animals

CHARACTERISTIC	*C. pseudotuberculosis*	*C. renale*	*C. cystitidis*	*C. pilosum*	*C. bovis*	*E. suis*	*A. bovis*	*A. pyogenes*	*R. equi*
Catalase production	+	+	+	+	+	–	–	–	+
Haemolysis	+	–	–	–	–	–	+ or –	+	–
Gelatin liquefaction	+ or –	–	–	–	–	–	–	+	–
Casein hydrolysis	–	+	–	–	–	–	–	+	–
Urease production	+	+	+	+	+	+	–	–	+ or –
Acid from glucose	+	+	+	+	–	–	+	+	–
Acid from xylose	–	–	+	–	–	–	–	+ or –	–
Acid from starch	+	–	+	+	–	+	+	+ or –	–
Nitrate reduction	+ or –	–	–	+	–	–	–	–	+ or –
Metachromatic granules	+	+	+	+	–	–	–	–	–
Pigment production	–	–	–	–	–	–	–	–	+

Table 2 Diseases caused by *Corynebacterium, Eubacterium, Actinomyces* and *Rhodococcus* spp. in farm animals

BACTERIUM	HOST	DISEASES
Corynebacterium pseudotuberculosis	Sheep	Caseous lymphadenitis, abscesses, arthritis, pneumonia, mastitis
	Goats	Caseous lymphadenitis
	Horses	Ulcerative lymphangitis, pectoral abscesses, contagious acne
	Cattle	Ulcerative lymphangitis
Corynebacterium renale group	Cattle	Contagious bovine pyelonephritis
	Horses	Cystitis, pyelonephritis
	Sheep	Posthitis, vulvitis
Corynebacterium bovis	Cattle	Mastitis
Eubacterium suis	Pigs	Cystitis, pyelonephritis
Actinomyces pyogenes	Cattle	Summer mastitis, metritis, abortion, abscesses, pneumonia
	Sheep	Abscesses, pneumonia
	Pigs	Pneumonia, pleuritis
Actinomyces bovis	Cattle	Lumpy jaw
	Horses	Poll evil, fistulous withers
	Pigs	Granulomatous mastitis (*A. suis* ?)
Rhodococcus equi	Horses	Pneumonia, ulcerative enterotyphlocolitis, lymphadenitis, abscesses, lymphangitis, arthritis
	Goats	Abscesses
	Sheep	Pneumonia, abscesses, abortion
	Cattle	Pneumonia, pyometra, ulcerative lymphangitis, lymphadenitis
	Pigs	Lymphadenitis

References

1 **CARTER, G.R., 1984.** *Diagnostic Procedures in Veterinary Bacteriology and Mycology.* 4th edn. Springfield: Charles C. Thomas.

2 **COLLINS, M.D. & CUMMINS, C.S., 1986.** Genus *Corynebacterium. In*: SNEATH, P.H.A., MAIR, N.S., SHARPE, M.E. & HOLT, J.G., (eds). *Bergey's Manual of Systematic Bacteriology.* Vol II. Baltimore, London: Williams & Wilkins.

3 **GOODFELLOW, M., 1986.** Genus *Rhodococcus. In*: SNEATH, P.H.A., MAIR, N.S., SHARPE, M.E. & HOLT, J.G., (eds). *Bergey's Manual of Systematic Bacteriology.* Vol II. Baltimore, London: Williams & Wilkins.

4 **HENTON, M.M., 1989.** Veterinary Research Institute, Onderstepoort. Unpublished data.

5 **MOORE, W.E.C. & MOORE, L.V.H., 1986.** Genus *Eubacterium. In*: SNEATH, P.H.A., MAIR, N.S., SHARPE, M.E. & HOLT, J.G., (eds). *Bergey's Manual of Systematic Bacteriology.* Vol II. Baltimore, London: Williams & Wilkins.

6 **SCHAAL, K.P., 1986.** Genus *Actinomyces. In*: SNEATH, P.H.A., MAIR, N.S., SHARPE, M.E. & HOLT, J.G., (eds). *Bergey's Manual of Systematic Bacteriology,* Vol II. Baltimore, London: Williams & Wilkins.

7 **TIMONEY, J.F., GILLESPIE, J.H., SCOTT, F.W. & BARLOUGH, J.E., 1988.** *Hagan and Bruner's Microbiology and Infectious Diseases of Domestic Animals.* 8th edn. Ithaca and London: Comstock Publishing Associates.

166

Corynebacterium pseudotuberculosis *infections*

Synonyms: *Corynebacterium ovis* infections, caseous lymphadenitis, Preisz-Nocard abscessation, cheesy gland, kaasagtige limfadenitis (Afrik.)

M.G. Collett, G.F. Bath and C.M. Cameron

Introduction

Infection with *Corynebacterium pseudotuberculosis (C. ovis)* most commonly causes caseous lymphadenitis (CLA), a chronic disease of sheep and goats that is characterized by abscessation of one or more lymph nodes. Less commonly, it results in pneumonia, hepatitis, mastitis, arthritis, orchitis, subcutaneous abscesses, abortion, stillbirth and perinatal mortalities in these species. A syndrome associated with haemolysis and icterus in sheep and goats may follow natural infection or the inoculation of culture material. This infection is also the cause of ulcerative lymphangitis, pectoral abscesses, folliculitis and furunculosis (referred to as 'contagious acne'), mastitis and abortion in horses, and ulcerative lymphangitis in cattle.

Corynebacterium pseudotuberculosis was first described in 1888 by the French veterinarian Nocard, who isolated it from a case of ulcerative lymphangitis in a bovine. Three years later the same organism was isolated from a renal abscess in a sheep by Von Preisz;[20, 37] hence the term 'Preisz-Nocard' abscessation.

Caseous lymphadenitis is an economically important disease of sheep and goats and is responsible for considerable financial losses in many countries as a result of the condemnation of infected carcasses at abattoirs, and reduced wool production.[6, 9, 10, 13, 44, 53, 93, 102, 104] Sheep affected by CLA produce approximately 7 per cent less wool than unaffected sheep.[93] The total annual (1987/88) economic loss as a result of CLA in Australia was estimated at Aust. $25 million because of reduced wool production, condemnations and trimmings of carcasses, and the cost of meat inspection.[91] It is the most common infection in the thin-ewe syndrome in the USA.[98] The most important portal of entry of the organism is a wound, such as a shearing wound, which is the reason why there is a greater prevalence of the disease in woolled sheep.[86, 113]

In South Africa, CLA was first reported by Jowett in 1909. It appears to be more common in the drier areas of South Africa, such as the Karoo, eastern Cape Province and Orange Free State;[58, 115] a prevalence of 2,4 per cent of CLA in Merino sheep less than one year old and 7,4 per cent in older sheep from the Karoo, has been reported.[86] During the period 1986–88, 18,7–20,3 per cent of condemned carcasses at Cato Ridge Abattoir contained lesions of CLA. These condemnations represented 0,24–0,3 per cent of all the sheep and goats slaughtered at that abattoir during the period, and amounted to an annual loss of more than R400 000 for carcass condemnations alone, to which should be added unmeasured but substantial trimmings from carcasses.[115] Caseous lymphadenitis was the most important reason for carcass condemnation in sheep at South African abattoirs in 1990 and 1991.[4]

Aetiology

Corynebacterium pseudotuberculosis is a short (0,5–0,6 x 1,0–3,0 μm), irregular, ovoid, Gram-positive rod almost resembling a coccus,[41] and is facultatively anaerobic. In smears made from lesions, the organisms show marked pleomorphism, with coccoid, bacillary and filamentous forms invariably being present. They are often clumped together and are more numerous in early lesions. The filamentous forms may exhibit a barred or beaded appearance when stained. Pleomorphism is not as marked in cultured organisms. After 48 hours' incubation at 37 °C on blood tryptose agar, slow-growing, light cream-coloured colonies are produced, surrounded by a narrow zone of beta-haemolysis. The colonies are granular, opaque, and flat with a matt surface, do not attach to the medium and can be moved around on the surface of the agar. Although only a single species is recognized, biochemical variations do occur, and strains isolated from horses and cattle in the USA reduce nitrate, whereas those isolated from sheep and goats do not.[14] At least two toxic factors are produced by the organism and may vary between strains **(see Pathogenesis)**.

The organism can survive on moist debris on pen floors at room temperature for at least 10 days[67] and for several months, or even more than a year, on fomites (e.g. hay or bedding), particularly if environmental temperatures are low.[7, 52, 54] It can also survive in organically rich soil for long periods, but it is not known whether it multiplies in soil. *Corynebacterium pseudotuberculosis* can survive in commercial sheep-dipping fluids for at least 24 hours.[88] It may be isolated from the faeces of some sheep.[58]

Epidemiology

Under field conditions, *C. pseudotuberculosis* is a common pathogen of sheep and goats, and more rarely of cattle and horses. Experimentally, guinea-pigs and mice are also susceptible and, provided small inocula are used, mice will develop a disease which is very similar to CLA.[12, 30, 32, 84, 120]

The prevalence of CLA is age-related; morbidity rates increase as animals get older. This is probably a reflection of the fact that the cumulative chances of becoming infected are greater with the passage of time, rather than that there is an increasing susceptibility with age. Caseous lymphadenitis occurs most commonly in Merino sheep[86] (probably due to their greater rate of exposure to shearing wounds and consequent infection as a result of their skin pleating, rather than to greater susceptibility[113]), and is more prevalent in ewes than in rams. Visceral involvement , however, is more common in rams.[9]

Caseous lymphadenitis can be reproduced experimentally in sheep and goats by the administration of *C. pseudotuberculosis* by different routes.[1, 6, 17, 18, 21, 22, 33, 46, 66, 87, 88, 94, 106] Under field conditions, management practices such as shearing, ear-marking, tail-docking, castration, and dosing, or the use of contaminated injection needles or instruments may inadvertently result in damage of the skin or mucous membranes and thus create portals of entry for corynebacteria.[87, 109] Infection is also more likely to occur in sheep that are wet (due to rainy weather, wet pastures or after dipping), as macerated skin is more prone to injury. In goats, abrasions on the head caused by butting and ear-biting may predispose to infection.[96, 109] Poor hygiene considerably enhances the risk of infection. Environmental contamination of sheds, pens, kraals, dipping tanks, clothing or other facilities results from contaminated fleeces or from discharges from abscesses that have been ruptured or been incised during the shearing process.[6, 88, 113]

Inhalation of infective material (e.g. pus from a discharging abscess) may initiate the development of lung abscesses or pneumonia in sheep.[104] Lesions in the tonsils and retropharyngeal lymph nodes of an animal may be responsible for the aerogenous spread of infection to their own lungs or to those of in-contact animals.[13] Animals suffering from pulmonary abscesses are also a potential source of aerogenous infection for other sheep.[52] Ingestion of infective material has been reported to be a cause of abscess development in the mandibular lymph nodes of goats.[6]

Nodular worm (*Oesophagostomum* spp.) larvae burrowing into the wall of the intestines create a portal of entry for bacteria (commonly *Actinomyces pyogenes* or *C. pseudotuberculosis*) which cause miliary abscesses — hence the name nodular worm for the parasites. Subcutaneous abscesses may also be caused by *C. pseudotuberculosis* following skin damage by ticks, other parasites or plant material **(see Chapter 170: *Actinomyces pyogenes* infections)**.

Pathogenesis

Corynebacterium pseudotuberculosis is a facultative, intracellular parasite.[56, 69]

At least two factors, a toxic cell-wall lipid or 'corynomycolic acid' and a haemolysin, play essential roles in the development of CLA. The toxic cell-wall lipid, which is similar to the mycolic wax of *Mycobacterium tuberculosis*, is associated with the virulence of the organism and probably protects it from the enzymes of lysosomes, enabling it to survive inside phagolysosomes and thus ensuring the chronicity of the infection.[39, 55, 69, 96, 108] The lipid is also pyogenic,[120] but is not immunogenic.[39] Strains of *C. pseudotuberculosis* selected for their greater lipid content produce larger numbers of abscesses in mice.[84]

The haemolysin is a protoplasmic exotoxin, phospholipase D,[23, 38, 43] which acts on the sphingomyelin of erythrocyte and endothelial cell membranes, causing haemolysis, increased vascular permeability and enhanced bacterial invasion.[19, 62, 68, 107, 120] It is presumably responsible for the development of 'bacterial icterus'; intravenous or subcutaneous inoculation of culture material, exotoxin, or fresh, incompletely toxoided vaccine may cause dyspnoea, anaemia, icterus and haemoglobinuria in sheep and goat kids.[32, 33, 37, 62, 96, 99, 100]

Following its entry through the skin or a mucous membrane, *C. pseudotuberculosis* organisms are transported via afferent lymphatics (as free bacteria or within macrophages), usually to the regional lymph nodes, in which lesions may then develop.[47, 87] Lymphogenous and haematogenous distribution of the infection from the primary site to internal organs and tissues may occur with the passage of time. In some animals infection may spread via lymphogenous and haematogenous routes to the lungs and other parts of the body in the absence of involvement of lymph nodes regional to the portal of entry.[88] Lesions at both primary and secondary sites may undergo resolution during the early stages of their development.[11, 112] The size and severity of lesions depend upon the initial number of organisms entering the tissues of the host, the rate of multiplication of the organisms, and the accessibility of the host defence mechanisms to the bacteria;[11] they appear to have little relationship to the duration of the infection.[88]

Humoral and cell-mediated immunity to *C. pseudotuberculosis* play a role in protection against the development of lesions.[28, 30, 33, 48, 66] The humoral response is primarily antitoxic, whereas cell-mediated immunity restricts bacterial proliferation.[20] Humoral immunity may be ineffective in halting the progression of CLA, as the organisms are intracellular.[50] Macrophages are the main effector cells.[94]

The final outcome of a lesion is probably determined more by the level of the host's cellular immune response to infection than by the virulence of the bacterium.[11, 12]

Clinical signs and pathology

The incubation period of *C. pseudotuberculosis* abscesses ranges from 25–140 days.[3, 6] The clinical signs manifested by affected animals depend on the site and extent of the lesions.

Generally, CLA in sheep and goats does not cause obvious clinical signs unless the lesions are progressive, very large or numerous, or are located where they can be clinically detected or where their presence compromises the normal function of an organ or tissue. Abscesses are often only detected at necropsy. Sheep or goats suffering from large or numerous active lesions may show progressive weight loss, weakness, and terminal collapse, these signs being accompanied by polypnoea and coughing if there is lung involvement.

In sheep, dorsal superficial cervical (prescapular) and subiliac (prefemoral) lymph nodes are the most commonly affected,[8, 70, 86] although lymph nodes of the head and neck are also often involved.[80] Initially, affected lymph nodes are enlarged, soft or doughy on palpation and, if superficially located, the skin that covers them may be thin and hairless. A tenacious, thick, semifluid to inspissated, yellowish-white to greenish-white pus may be discharged should the abscess rupture which, in some, will result in the formation of persistently draining fistulae. The content of more long-standing abscesses is usually severely inspissated and will have lost the greenish colour.[8, 98, 112] Most abscesses are enveloped by well-developed connective tissue capsules and, although not evident in all cases, successive necrosis and redevelopment of the capsule impart a concentrically lamellated ('onion ring') pattern to the inspissated content — a characteristic of the lesion that becomes particularly prominent when the layers become partially calcified **(Figure 166.1)**.[112] There is generally no evidence of infection at the site of entry of *C. pseudotuberculosis*.

Of the internal organs and other tissues, the bronchial and mediastinal lymph nodes and lungs are most frequently involved. The kidneys (cortical abscesses or pyelonephritis), liver, spleen, and lymph nodes draining the buccal cavity, and, less commonly, the diaphragm, muscles, serous surfaces, brain, spinal cord, heart, tongue, mammary gland, testes and joints may also be affected.[15, 65, 98, 112]

Single or multiple abscesses of varying size, but which may become quite large, or caseopurulent bronchopneumonia, which in some animals can be extensive, may be found in the lungs, frequently in the absence of lesions elsewhere.[70, 98, 104] These lung lesions are colloquially known as 'harslagsiekte' or pluck disease. If an abscess or bronchopneumonic lesion abuts on the pleura, localized fibrinous or fibrous pleural adhesions generally develop.[98] Lung abscesses may rupture into airways.[104] The pulmonary lesions are generally reflected by the development of metastatic lesions in the bronchial or mediastinal lymph nodes. Large abscesses in the mediastinal lymph nodes may cause pressure on, and partial occlusion of, the oesophagus, resulting in interference with deglutition and eructation, and loss of weight.

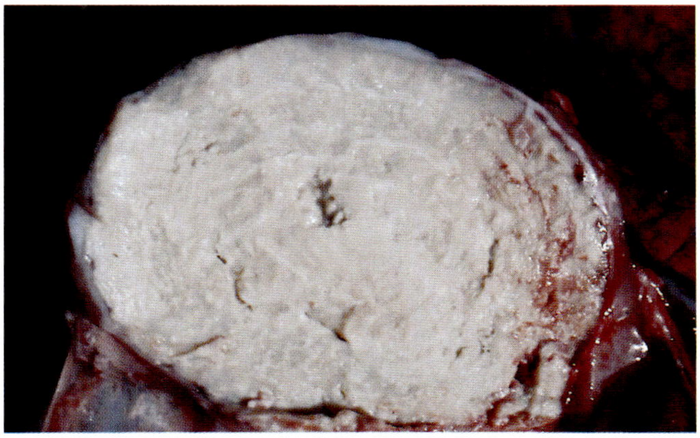

Figure 166.1 Markedly enlarged lymph node showing the concentrically lamellated appearance of the exudate which replaced all normal tissue of the node

Corynebacterium pseudotuberculosis infections are occasionally the cause of a variety of other conditions in sheep, including hepatic abscessation reproductive disorders (such as abortion, stillbirth, and neonatal infection) in ewes;[1, 3, 42] suppurative orchitis in rams;[75, 117] mastitis in ewes; arthritis and rapid death due to toxaemia in neonatal lambs and kids.[62] Miliary subcutaneous abscessation may be caused by *C. pseudotuberculosis* following damage of the skin by ticks or plant material **(see Chapter 170: *Actinomyces pyogenes* infections)**.

Prior to the development of improved vaccines, several outbreaks of haemolytic anaemia and icterus occurred after sheep had been vaccinated against *C. pseudotuberculosis*. These outbreaks of 'bacterial icterus' were associated with high mortality, and a high proportion of icteric carcasses was found in those sheep which were sent to slaughter .

Suppurative lesions or abscesses of the subcutaneous tissues and lymph nodes of the head are more common in goats than in sheep, probably because of their combative behaviour and because of injuries by ticks or thorns to the facial skin, while lung lesions are generally uncommon.[5, 8, 13, 53, 77, 80] In South Africa, however, CLA and lung abscesses are quite common in Angora goats.[114] Abscesses caused by *C. pseudotuberculosis* in goats usually develop slowly, are encapsulated, and contain odourless, yellowish-white or greenish-white pus which is pasty, dry and inspissated or semifluid and viscous.[6, 13, 25, 53, 76, 77, 102] Inspissation, calcification and the 'onion-ring' appearance, so typical of CLA in sheep, are rarely encountered in goats.[13]

Histologically, the earliest inflammatory changes in the lymph nodes of sheep and goats comprise multiple micro-abscesses and massive infiltration of neutrophils. As the abscesses enlarge they may coalesce, the pus being encompassed by an inflammatory reaction consisting of neutrophils, macrophages, epithelioid cells and lymphocytes.[94] They soon become encapsulated by connective tissue but they continue to enlarge as a result of necrosis of the peripheral tissues and reformation of the capsule. The successive layers of necrotic tissue which develop as the lesion expands undergo dystrophic mineralization which is responsible for the macroscopic lamellated appearance of some lesions. Eventually an entire lymph node may be greatly enlarged (to several times its normal dimensions) and consist only of necrotic debris surrounded by a fibrous connective tissue capsule infiltrated by epithelioid cells, macrophages, lymphocytes, and occasional plasma cells and neutrophils.[18,48, 60, 61] Gram-positive bacteria are frequently discernible at the periphery of the necrotic tissue.[21, 47, 70] In the lungs, abscesses compress the adjacent parenchyma, which is infiltrated by inflammatory cells and shows a varying degree of interstitial fibrosis.[48] Changes in and around the bronchial tree include a mild to moderate peribronchiolar lymphoid cuffing and fibrosis, and hyperplasia of bronchiolar epithelial cells.[48] Lesions may be accompanied by a neutrophilia.

Infection of horses with *C. pseudotuberculosis* is rare, but conditions such as ulcerative lymphangitis,[90] folliculitis and furunculosis ('contagious acne'),[57, 90] acute or chronic abscesses of the pectoral ('pigeon fever') and ventral abdominal regions[63, 83, 109, 118] and, more rarely, mastitis,[2] and a generalized form with visceral abscessation[64] are associated with this organism.

Ulcerative lymphangitis in horses, and more rarely in mules and donkeys, is a chronic contagious disease characterized by inflammation of subcutaneous lymphatic vessels, resulting in abscess formation and ulceration along their course. It may occur in outbreak form, particularly where animals are congregated in large numbers under unhygienic conditions. It may spread rapidly. *Corynebacterium pseudotuberculosis* gains entrance to the tissues through wounds and abrasions of the skin, particularly of the extremities, a hind limb being most commonly affected following a fetlock abrasion or other injury.[15, 37, 109] Transmission from animal to animal by contaminated grooming utensils or other means may also occur. Clinically, the disease has a sudden onset and is characterized initially by pain, oedema and increase in temperature of the affected part. Later, abscesses form along the course of lymphatic vessels, and may rupture externally to discharge a thick, greenish-yellow, blood-tinged pus, before developing into granulating ulcers. These may heal in one to two weeks, leaving areas of depilated, depigmented skin, after which new abscesses and ulcers form, and there is a cord-like thickening of associated lymphatics.[15, 109] Before bursting, the abscesses may be up to about 30 mm in diameter. The lesions occur most frequently in the skin of a hind limb between the fetlock and hock joints. The regional lymph nodes are usually not affected. Lesions in untreated cases may persist for many months and may eventually progress to a stage where euthanasia of the animal has to be considered. Foals may be severely affected and die.[37, 90, 101]

'Contagious acne', on the other hand, is spread when contaminated blankets, grooming equipment or saddles and harnesses are used.[15] Non-pruritic papules and pustules, which may be painful on palpation, are usually found in areas where the skin comes into contact with a saddle or harness. The pustules contain a greenish pus.[15]

Abscesses due to *C. pseudotuberculosis* infections of the pectoral and ventral abdominal regions in horses result from contamination of superficial skin wounds. Their presence has also been correlated with seasonal increases of biting insects in California and Texas.[64, 83, 116] These abscesses contain a viscid, odourless and cream-coloured pus.[63, 64, 118] Other clinical signs include fever, ventral oedema, lameness,[83] and, when the viscera are involved, depression and emaciation.[64]

Ulcerative lymphangitis occurs very rarely in cattle. It resembles the disease in horses, but initial lesions tend to develop on the neck or trunk rather than on the legs, and regional lymph nodes become progressively suppurative. The pus in these abscesses is greyish-yellow, semi-liquid and lardaceous.[72, 89, 97, 101]

Diagnosis

A presumptive diagnosis of CLA can be made on the history, clinical examination of superficially located abscesses, and the characteristic greenish-yellow, inspissated exudate they contain, which may have a lamellated appearance on cut surface.[88]

Confirmation of *C. pseudotuberculosis* infection requires bacterial culture and identification. Specimens of the content of abscesses for bacteriological examination should preferably be collected aseptically from the edge of the abscesses and can be obtained in an exposed lesion by light curettage of the capsular surface. Some specimens may yield no growth, especially when specimens of the exudate have been collected from the centre of an abscess, or from inspissated pus.

Histopathologic examination of biopsy specimens can be a useful tool in the confirmation of the diagnosis of ulcerative lymphangitis in horses or cattle.

Numerous serological tests have been developed for the detection of antibodies against *C. pseudotuberculosis* exotoxin and cell-wall antigens.[21, 24, 33, 40, 49, 52, 73, 74, 78, 80, 93, 105, 106, 119] They are generally not commonly used for the diagnosis of CLA in culling programmes because the sensitivity and specificity of most of these tests are relatively low[82] and there is no significant relationship between the extent of development of the lesions and antibody titre.[49] In addition, cross-reactions with *Mycobacterium paratuberculosis* may occur.[80, 95] Despite the limitations of most of the serological tests, they are of value in countries — such as those in north-west Europe — where CLA in sheep is rare or absent and where future relaxation of border controls as a result of the establishment of the European Community could result in less stringent control of animal movement.[79, 103] The disease appears to be more common in goats in some parts of Europe but is not present in others,[59] and the importation in 1987 of infected goats into Great Britain, which had previously been free of CLA, emphasizes the importance of such pre-import serological screening.[54]

Differential diagnosis

Caseous lymphadenitis in sheep and goats should be differentiated from pyo- or necrogranulomatous lesions found in diseases such as actinobacillosis and tuberculosis,[47, 70] and from abscessation caused by *Actinomyces (Corynebacterium) pyogenes*. Wasting due to visceral CLA may clinically resemble chronic parasitism,[47] emaciation due to abnormal dental wear, alveolar periodontitis, malnutrition, and chronic diseases such as jaagsiekte. Secondary pneumonic lesions due to *C. pseudotuberculosis* (as well as *A. pyogenes* or *Pasteurella* spp.) may obscure those of jaagsiekte.[70, 110] In rams, orchitis or epididymitis caused by *C. pseudotuberculosis* should be differentiated from similar lesions caused by *Brucella ovis*, Gram-negative pleomorphic organisms (such as *Actinobacillus seminis, Histophilus ovis, Pasteurella* spp.), spermatic granulomas and other conditions **(see Chapter 138: *Actinobacillus seminis* infections)**.

Ulcerative lymphangitis caused by *C. pseudotuberculosis* in horses should be differentiated from similar lesions caused by *Histoplasma farciminosum* (the cause of 'epizootic lymphangitis'), *Sporothrix schenkii, Rhodococcus equi*, and *Pseudomonas mallei* (the skin form of glanders, also known as 'farcy'). Glanders has been eradicated from South Africa. Ulcerative lymphangitis in cattle can also be caused by *Rhodococcus equi*.[89]

The crusting, purulent or alopecic skin lesions of 'contagious acne' in horses should be differentiated from lesions associated with dermatophytoses, dermatophilosis, onchocerciasis, bacterial pyoderma, and lesions caused by insect bites (e.g. *Culicoides* spp.).[57] *Streptococcus equi* is the most common cause of abscesses in the muscles of horses, and should not be confused with those caused by *C. pseudotuberculosis*.[65]

The haemolytic and icteric syndromes in sheep may be confused with other conditions associated with haemolysis and/or icterus. Examples of these in southern Africa are many and varied, but they include Wesselsbron disease, eperythrozoonosis, chronic copper poisoning ('enzootic icterus'), plant poisonings such as by *Tribulus terrestris* (tribulosis, geeldikkop) and certain toxic Asteraceae (= Compositae), e.g. *Lasiospermum bipinnatum* (ganskweek), *Asaemia axillaris* (vuursiektebossie), *Athanasia trifurcata* (klaaslouwbos), *Hertia pallens* (harpuisbos), *Pteronia pallens* (aasvoëlbossie), and *Nidorella foetida*, and facial eczema (caused by *Pithomyces chartarum* mycotoxicosis). Outbreaks of a form of bacterial icterus in sheep caused by a Gram-negative bacterium which has never been positively identified were encountered in the early 1960s in South Africa.[111] A disease with icterus was experimentally produced in some of the sheep inoculated with the organism.

Control

Since affected animals serve as reservoirs of infection, the most practical method of control of CLA in sheep or goat flocks is to cull all animals that have palpable lesions.[70, 98] In woolled sheep these are best detected at shearing. Treatment of sheep and goats suffering from CLA of the peripheral lymph nodes is usually neither economically justifiable nor prudent.[47] However, superficially located abscesses in valuable breeding stock can be lanced or removed surgically, provided strict aseptic techniques are employed, infective material is destroyed, and contaminated equipment and the surroundings suitably disinfected. If the abscess or infection cannot be precisely located or is in a position that is unfavourable for surgery, a prolonged course of antimicrobial treatment using lipophilic drugs, such as one of the macrolides, at high dosage rates may be effective. Despite the *in vitro* sensitivity of *C. pseudotuberculosis* to penicillin, tetracyclines and cephalosporins,[71, 121] the use of these drugs is generally ineffective because their ability to diffuse through the capsule of abscesses is poor and because the bacteria are located intracellularly.[5, 53]

In horses, hot-pack applications, surgical lancing, and flushing with antiseptics may be attempted for treatment of the abscesses.[63, 83] Equine isolates of *C. pseudotuberculosis* are sensitive to penicillin G, ampicillin, chloramphenicol, oxytetracyclines and trimethoprim-sulphadoxine.[2, 116] Intramuscular procaine penicillin G (20 000 to 50 000 units/kg body weight/day, divided and administered twice daily for five to seven days), intravenous trimethoprim (40 mg/ml) and sulphadoxine (200 mg/ml) combination at 1 ml/15 kg daily for five days may be curative.[90] Ulcerative lymphangitis and 'contagious acne' can be treated with the same drugs. Ulcers, however, should also be dressed daily with iodophors.[57, 90] Grooming equipment, blankets and saddles or harnesses should be disinfected.[15]

Effective hygiene measures in the shearing, docking, castration and marking procedures are very important in the control of abscesses in sheep and goats.[7, 15] The following measures are important at shearing:

- abscesses should not be treated in shearing sheds, yards or holding pens;
- a week or two prior to the commencement of shearing, the shearing shed should be disinfected with 3 per

cent formalin solution. Immediately after the application of the formalin, the shed should be closed and kept as airtight as possible for a period of 24 hours to allow for fumigation by the formalin vapours;

- the blades of shears and other equipment should be disinfected with 3 per cent formalin or a quarternary ammonium compound between sheep;
- younger sheep should be shorn before older ones;
- shearing wounds should be disinfected with povidone iodine or an antibiotic spray immediately;
- newly shorn sheep should not be kept in dirty kraals or in overcrowded pens;
- if an abscess is inadvertently lanced during shearing, or if pus-soiled wool is shorn, the sheep must be isolated and treated, the pus or soiled wool must be removed and burned, the area and shearer's hands must be cleaned and disinfected with povidone iodine or cetrimide, the shears must be thoroughly disinfected and the shearer's overalls must be changed and disinfected; and
- sheep should not be dipped for three to five days after shearing or until shearing wounds are thoroughly healed.

The use of gas-heated equipment is recommended for tail-docking. Wounds should be disinfected using iodine, and when elastic bands are used for castration, the skin should be disinfected at the time of positioning of the ring.

If there is a continued high prevalence of CLA after the institution of improved hygiene and management measures, the possible existence of carrier animals with pulmonary infections must be considered.[52]

Several vaccines have been developed to protect sheep and goats against CLA. Toxoid vaccines produced in Australia[44–46, 93] and inactivated cell-wall or whole-cell (bacterin) vaccines in the USA afford good protection against *C. pseudotuberculosis* infections.[18, 81] In South Africa, inactivated whole-cell vaccines, with an aluminium hydroxide adjuvant containing saponin and devoid of exotoxin, provide better protection in sheep than toxoid vaccines.[28]

There is controversy over the role of anti-exotoxin immunity in the protection of sheep and goats against CLA. Some researchers have shown that it is of little consequence in protection against natural infections,[32, 36, 37, 50, 107, 120] while others have recently demonstrated that anti-exotoxin immunity alone can prevent CLA.[45] Whether the major immunogenic antigen of *C. pseudotuberculosis* is an integral part of the cell wall,[34, 35] or the exotoxin,[45] or whether other antigens or a combination of antigens play a role[26, 29, 50, 85] remains to be elucidated.

While the inclusion of levamisole in *C. pseudotuberculosis* vaccines appears to have no potentiating effect on immunity,[27, 61] the use of a mycobacterial component (muramyl dipeptide) as adjuvant has proved beneficial.[16] Live vaccines are no better than inactivated vaccines and the local reaction they cause at the injection site is unacceptable.[28, 81] The antigenic purity of toxoid vaccines has recently been questioned, as numerous other soluble antigens are present in vaccines made from *C. pseudotuberculosis* culture filtrates.[51, 85]

A specific diagnosis is essential prior to vaccination. Vaccination is not recommended as a routine in flocks in which the prevalence of the disease is low; in such cases, improved management is usually sufficient to effect good control. In flocks with a high prevalence of CLA, vaccination on its own may yield disappointing results, but good results can be obtained when vaccination is administered strategically, such as prior to shearing,[31] and when it is combined with good management and hygiene procedures.

To ensure adequate protection, lambs should receive a primary vaccination at about 12 weeks of age, at the stage when maternally derived (colostral) immunity has waned.[3, 92] The *C. pseudotuberculosis* vaccine produced by the Veterinary Research Institute, Onderstepoort, must be given twice, three to six weeks apart, as an initial procedure, and thereafter every six to nine months. These inoculations should be given four to six weeks before shearing, in order to ensure maximal protection at the time when the risk of exposure is greatest, because effective immunity only lasts five to six months.

References

1 **ADDO, P.B., 1979.** Pathology and bacteriology of abortion in sheep experimentally infected with *Corynebacterium pseudotuberculosis. Bulletin of Animal Health and Production in Africa*, 27, 257–262.

2 **ADDO, P.B., WILCOX, G.E. & TAUSSIG, R., 1974.** Mastitis in a mare caused by *Corynebacterium ovis. The Veterinary Record*, 95, 193.

3 **ALONSO, J.L., SIMON, M.C., GIRONES, O., MUZQUIZ, J.L., ORTEGA, C. & GARCIA, J., 1992.** The effect of experimental infection with *Corynebacterium pseudotuberculosis* on reproduction in adult ewes. *Research in Veterinary Science*, 52, 267–272.

4 **ANON., 1991.** *Livestock and Meat Statistics*, Meat Board, PO Box 40051, Arcadia 0007, South Africa.

5 **ASHFAQ, M.K. & CAMPBELL, S.G., 1979.** A survey of caseous lymphadenitis and its etiology in goats in the United States. *Veterinary Medicine/Small Animal Clinician*, 74, 1161–1165.

6 **ASHFAQ, M.K. & CAMPBELL, S.G., 1980.** Experimentally induced caseous lymphadenitis in goats. *American Journal of Veterinary Research*, 41, 1789–1792.

7 **AUGUSTINE, J.L. & RENSHAW, H.W., 1986.** Survival of *Corynebacterium pseudotuberculosis* in axenic purulent exudate on common barnyard fomites. *American Journal of Veterinary Research*, 47, 713–715.

8 **AYERS, J.L., 1977.** Caseous lymphadenitis in goats and sheep: A review of diagnosis, pathogenesis and immunity. *Journal of the American Veterinary Medical Association*, 171, 1251–1254.

9 **BATEY, R.G., 1986.** Frequency and consequence of caseous lymphadenitis in sheep and lambs slaughtered at a Western Australian abattoir. *American Journal of Veterinary Research*, 47, 482–485.

10 **BATEY, R.G., 1986.** The effect of caseous lymphadenitis on body condition and weight of merino mutton carcases. *Australian Veterinary Journal*, 63, 268.

11 **BATEY, R.G., 1986.** Pathogenesis of caseous lymphadenitis in sheep and goats. *Australian Veterinary Journal*, 63, 269–272.

12 **BATEY, R.G., 1986.** Aspects of pathogenesis in a mouse model of infection by *Corynebacterium pseudotuberculosis*. *Australian Journal of Experimental Biology and Medical Science*, 64, 237–249.

13 **BATEY, R.G., SPEED, C.M. & KOBES, C.J., 1986.** Prevalence and distribution of caseous lymphadenitis in feral goats. *Australian Veterinary Journal*, 63, 33–36.

14 **BIBERSTEIN, E.L., KNIGHT, H.D. & JANG, S., 1971.** Biotypes of *Corynebacterium pseudotuberculosis*. *The Veterinary Record*, 89, 691–692.

15 **BLOOD, D.C. & RADOSTITS, O.M., 1989.** *Veterinary Medicine*. 7th edn. London, Philadelphia: Baillière Tindall.

16 **BROGDEN, K.A., CHEDID, L., CUTLIP, R.C., LEHMKUHL, H.D. & SACKS, J., 1990.** Effect of muramyl dipeptide on immunogenicity of *Corynebacterium pseudotuberculosis* whole-cell vaccines in mice and lambs. *American Journal of Veterinary Research*, 51, 200–202.

17 **BROGDEN, K.A., CUTLIP, R.C. & LEHMKUHL, H.D., 1984.** Experimental *Corynebacterium pseudotuberculosis* infection in lambs. *American Journal of Veterinary Research*, 45, 1532–1534.

18 **BROGDEN, K.A., CUTLIP, R.C. & LEHMKUHL, H.D., 1984.** Comparison of protection induced in lambs by *Corynebacterium pseudotuberculosis* whole-cell and cell-wall vaccines. *American Journal of Veterinary Research*, 45, 2393–2395.

19 **BROGDEN, K.A. & ENGEN, R.L., 1990.** Alterations in the phospholipid composition and morphology of ovine erythrocytes after intravenous inoculation of *Corynebacterium pseudotuberculosis*. *American Journal of Veterinary Research*, 51, 874–877.

20 **BROWN, C.C. & OLANDER, H.J., 1987.** Caseous lymphadenitis of goats and sheep: A review. *Veterinary Bulletin*, 57, 1–12.

21 **BROWN, C.C., OLANDER, H.J., BIBERSTEIN, E.L. & MORENO, D., 1985.** Serologic response and lesions in goats experimentally infected with *Corynebacterium pseudotuberculosis* of caprine and equine origins. *American Journal of Veterinary Research*, 46, 2322–2326.

22 **BURRELL, D.H., 1978.** Experimental induction of caseous lymphadenitis in sheep by intralymphatic inoculation of *Corynebacterium ovis*. *Research in Veterinary Science*, 24, 269–276.

23 **BURRELL, D.H., 1979.** Conditions for *in vitro* haemolytic activity by *Corynebacterium ovis* exotoxin. *Research in Veterinary Science*, 26, 333–338.

24 **BURRELL, D.H., 1980.** A haemolysis inhibition test for detection of antibody to *Corynebacterium ovis* exotoxin. *Research in Veterinary Science*, 28, 190–194.

25 **BURRELL, D.H., 1981.** Caseous lymphadenitis in goats. *Australian Veterinary Journal*, 57, 105–110.

26 **CAMERON, C.M., 1964.** The significance of the endotoxin and pyogenic factor of *Corynebacterium pseudotuberculosis* in immunity. *Onderstepoort Journal of Veterinary Research*, 31, 119–132.

27 **CAMERON, C.M., 1977.** Effect of levamisole on immunity to *Corynebacterium pseudotuberculosis* in mice and sheep. *Onderstepoort Journal of Veterinary Research*, 44, 47–48.

28 **CAMERON, C.M. & BESTER, F.J., 1984.** An improved *Corynebacterium pseudotuberculosis* vaccine for sheep. *Onderstepoort Journal of Veterinary Research*, 51, 263–267.

29 **CAMERON, C.M. & BUCHAN, L., 1966.** Identification of the protective and toxic antigens of *Corynebacterium pseudotuberculosis*. *Onderstepoort Journal of Veterinary Research*, 33, 39–48.

30 **CAMERON, C.M. & ENGELBRECHT, M.M., 1971.** Mechanism of immunity of *Corynebacterium pseudotuberculosis* (Buchanan 1911) in mice using inactivated vaccine. *Onderstepoort Journal of Veterinary Research*, 38, 73–82.

31 **CAMERON, C.M. & FULS, W.J.P., 1973.** Studies on the enhancement of immunity to *Corynebacterium pseudotuberculosis*. *Onderstepoort Journal of Veterinary Research*, 40, 105–114.

32 **CAMERON, C.M. & MINNAAR, J.L., 1969.** Immunization of mice against *Corynebacterium pseudotuberculosis* infection. *Onderstepoort Journal of Veterinary Research*, 36, 207–210.

33 **CAMERON, C.M., MINNAAR, J.L., ENGELBRECHT, M.M. & PURDOM, M.R., 1972.** Immune response of Merino sheep to inactivated *Corynebacterium pseudotuberculosis* vaccine. *Onderstepoort Journal of Veterinary Research*, 39, 11–24.

34 **CAMERON, C.M., MINNAAR, J.L. & PURDOM, M.R., 1969.** Immunizing properties of *Corynebacterium pseudotuberculosis* cell walls. *Onderstepoort Journal of Veterinary Research*, 36, 211–216.

35 **CAMERON, C.M. & PURDOM, M.R., 1971.** Immunological and chemical characteristics of *Corynebacterium pseudotuberculosis* cell walls and protoplasm. *Onderstepoort Journal of Veterinary Research*, 38, 83–92.

36 **CAMERON, C.M. & SMIT, M.C., 1970.** Relationship of *Corynebacterium pseudotuberculosis* protoplasmic toxins to the exotoxin. *Onderstepoort Journal of Veterinary Research*, 37, 97–104.

37 **CARNE, H.R., 1939.** A bacteriological study of 134 strains of *Corynebacterium ovis*. *Journal of Pathology and Bacteriology*, 49, 313–328.

38 **CARNE, H.R., 1940.** The toxin of *Corynebacterium ovis*. *Journal of Pathology and Bacteriology*, 51, 199–212.

39 **CARNE, H.R., WICKHAM, N. & KATER, J.C., 1956.** A toxic lipid from the surface of *Corynebacterium ovis*. *Nature*, 178, 701–702.

40 **CHIKAMATSU, S., ZHAO, H-K., KIKUCHI, N. & HIRAMUNE, T., 1989.** Seroepidemiological survey of *Corynebacterium pseudotuberculosis* infection in sheep in Japan using enzyme-linked immunosorbent assay and immunodiffusion. *Japanese Journal of Veterinary Science*, 51, 887–890.

41 **COLLINS, M.D. & CUMMINS, C.S., 1986.** Genus *Corynebacterium*. *In*: SNEATH, P.H.A., MAIR, N.S., SHARPE, M.E. & HOLT, J.G., (eds). *Bergey's Manual of Systematic Bacteriology*. Vol. II. Baltimore, London: Williams & Wilkins.

42 **DENNIS, S.M. & BAMFORD, V.W., 1966.** The role of corynebacteria in perinatal lamb mortality. *The Veterinary Record*, 79, 105–108.

43 **EGEN, N.B., CUEVAS, W.A., McNAMARA, P.J., SAMMONS, D.W., HUMPHREYS, R. & SONGER, J.G., 1989.** Purification of the phospholipase D of *Corynebacterium pseudotuberculosis* by recycling isoelectric focusing. *American Journal of Veterinary Research*, 50, 1319–1322.

44 **EGGLETON, D.G., DOIDGE, C.V., MIDDLETON, H.D. & MINTY, D.W., 1991.** Immunisation against ovine caseous lymphadenitis: Efficacy of monocomponent *Corynebacterium pseudotuberculosis* toxoid vaccine and combined clostridial-corynebacterial vaccines. *Australian Veterinary Journal*, 68, 320–321.

45 **EGGLETON, D.G., HAYNES, J.A., MIDDLETON, H.D. & COX, J.C., 1991.** Immunisation against ovine caseous lymphadenitis: Correlation between *Corynebacterium pseudotuberculosis* toxoid content and protective efficacy in combined clostridial-corynebacterial vaccines. *Australian Veterinary Journal*, 68, 322–325.

46 **EGGLETON, D.G., MIDDLETON, H.D., DOIDGE, C.V. & MINTY, D.W., 1991.** Immunisation against ovine caseous lymphadenitis: Comparison of *Corynebacterium pseudotuberculosis* vaccines with and without bacterial cells. *Australian Veterinary Journal*, 68, 317–319.

47 **ELLIS, J.A., 1983.** Ovine caseous lymphadenitis. *Compendium*

on Continuing Education for the Practicing Veterinarian, 5, S504–S509.

48 **ELLIS, J.A., 1988.** Immunophenotype of pulmonary infiltrates in sheep with caseous lymphadenitis. *Veterinary Pathology*, 25, 362–368.

49 **ELLIS, J.A., HAWK, D.A., HOLLER, L.D., MILLS, K.W. & PRATT, D.L., 1990.** Differential antibody responses to *Corynebacterium pseudotuberculosis* in sheep with naturally acquired caseous lymphadenitis. *Journal of the American Veterinary Medical Association*, 196, 1609–1613.

50 **ELLIS, J.A., HAWK, D.A., MILLS, K.W. & PRATT, D.L., 1991.** Antigen specificity of antibody responses to *Corynebacterium pseudotuberculosis* in naturally infected sheep with caseous lymphadenitis. *Veterinary Immunology and Immunopathology*, 28, 289–301.

51 **ELLIS, J.A., HAWK, D.A., MILLS, K.W. & PRATT, D.L., 1991.** Antigen specificity and activity of ovine antibodies induced by immunization with *Corynebacterium pseudotuberculosis* culture filtrate. *Veterinary Immunology and Immunopathology*, 28, 303–316.

52 **ELLIS, T.M., SUTHERLAND, S.S., WILKINSON, F.C., MERCY, A.R. & PATON, M.W., 1987.** The role of *Corynebacterium pseudotuberculosis* lung lesions in the transmission of this bacterium to other sheep. *Australian Veterinary Journal*, 64, 261–263.

53 **GEZON, H.M., BITHER, H.D., HANSON, L.A. & THOMPSON, J.K., 1991.** Epizootic of external and internal abscesses in a large goat herd over a 16-year period. *Journal of the American Veterinary Medical Association*, 198, 257–263.

54 **GILMOUR, N.J.L., 1990.** Caseous lymphadenitis: A cause for concern. *The Veterinary Record*, 126, 566.

55 **HARD, G.C., 1969.** Electron microscopic examination of *Corynebacterium ovis*. *Journal of Bacteriology*, 97, 1480–1485.

56 **HARD, G.C., 1972.** Examination by electron microscopy of the interaction between peritoneal phagocytes and *Corynebacterium ovis*. *Journal of Medical Microbiology*, 5, 483–491.

57 **HEFFNER, K.A., WHITE, S.D., FREVERT, C.W. & JAKOWSKI, R., 1988.** *Corynebacterium folliculitis* in a horse. *Journal of the American Veterinary Medical Association*, 193, 89–90.

58 **HENTON, M.M., 1989.** Onderstepoort Veterinary Institute, Onderstepoort. Unpublished data.

59 **HOLSTAD, G., 1989.** *Corynebacterium pseudotuberculosis* infection in goats. IX. The effect of vaccination against natural infection. *Acta Veterinaria Scandinavica*, 30, 285–293.

60 **HOLSTAD, G. & TEIGE, J., 1988.** *Corynebacterium pseudotuberculosis* infection in goats. VII. Clinical, pathological, serological and haematological changes after subcutaneous inoculation of the organism. *Acta Veterinaria Scandinavica*, 29, 287–294.

61 **HOLSTAD, G., TEIGE, J. & LARSEN, H.J., 1989.** *Corynebacterium pseudotuberculosis* infection in goats. VIII. The effect of vaccination against experimental infection. *Acta Veterinaria Scandinavica*, 30, 275–283.

62 **HSU, T-Y., RENSHAW, H.W., LIVINGSTON, C.W., AUGUSTINE, J.L., ZINK, D.L. & GAUER, B.B., 1985.** *Corynebacterium pseudotuberculosis* exotoxin: Fatal hemolytic anemia induced in gnotobiotic neonatal small ruminants by parenteral administration of preparations containing exotoxin. *American Journal of Veterinary Research*, 46, 1206–1211.

63 **HUGHES, J.P. & BIBERSTEIN, E.L., 1959.** Chronic equine abscesses associated with *Corynebacterium pseudotuberculosis*. *Journal of the American Veterinary Medical Association*, 135, 559–562.

64 **HUGHES, J.P., BIBERSTEIN, E.L. & RICHARDS, W.P.C., 1962.** Two cases of generalized *Corynebacterium pseudotuberculosis* infection in mares. *Cornell Veterinarian*, 52, 51–62.

65 **HULLAND, T.J., 1985.** Muscles and tendons. *In*: JUBB, K.V.F., KENNEDY, P.C. & PALMER, N., (eds). *Pathology of Domestic Animals*. Vol. I. 3rd edn. New York, London: Academic Press.

66 **HUSBAND, A.J. & WATSON, D.L., 1977.** Immunological events in the popliteal lymph node of sheep following injection of live or killed *Corynebacterium ovis* into an afferent popliteal lymphatic duct. *Research in Veterinary Science*, 22, 105–112.

67 **JANSEN, B.C., 1983.** The epidemiology of bacterial infection of the genitalia in rams. *Onderstepoort Journal of Veterinary Research*, 50, 275–282.

68 **JOLLY, R.D., 1965.** The pathologic action of the exotoxin of *Corynebacterium ovis*. *Journal of Comparative Pathology*, 75, 417–431.

69 **JOLLY, R.D., 1966.** Some observations on surface lipids of virulent and attenuated strains of *Corynebacterium ovis*. *Journal of Applied Bacteriology*, 29, 189–196.

70 **JOWETT, W., 1909.** Abscesses in the lungs and lymphatic glands of sheep (caseous lymphadenitis). *Agricultural Journal of the Cape of Good Hope*, 35, 733–735.

71 **JUDSON, R. & SONGER, J.G., 1991.** *Corynebacterium pseudotuberculosis*: *In vitro* susceptibility to 39 antimicrobial agents. *Veterinary Microbiology*, 27, 145–150.

72 **KARIUKA, D.P. & POULTON, J., 1982.** Corynebacterial infection of cattle in Kenya. *Tropical Animal Health and Production*, 14, 33–36.

73 **KURIA, J.K.N. & HOLSTAD, G., 1989.** A seroepidemiological investigation of *Corynebacterium pseudotuberculosis* infection in sheep flocks in southern Norway. *Acta Veterinaria Scandinavica*, 30, 107–108.

74 **KURIA, J.K.N. & HOLSTAD, G., 1989.** Serological investigation of *Corynebacterium pseudotuberculosis* infection in sheep: Correlation between the haemolysis inhibition test and the Elisa test. *Acta Veterinaria Scandinavica*, 30, 109–110.

75 **LADDS, P.W., 1985.** The male genital system. *In*: JUBB, K.V.F., KENNEDY, P.C. & PALMER, N., (eds). *Pathology of Domestic Animals*. Vol. III. 3rd edn. New York, London: Academic Press.

76 **LINDSAY, H.J. & LLOYD, S., 1991.** Diagnosis of caseous lymphadenitis in goats. *The Veterinary Record*, 128, 86.

77 **LLOYD, S., LINDSAY, H.J., SLATER, J.D. & JACKSON, P.G.G., 1990.** Caseous lymphadenitis in goats in England. *The Veterinary Record*, 127, 478.

78 **MAKI, L.R., SHEN, S-H., BERGSTROM, R.C. & STETZENBACH, L.D., 1985.** Diagnosis of *Corynebacterium pseudotuberculosis* infections in sheep, using an enzyme-linked immunosorbent assay. *American Journal of Veterinary Research*, 46, 212–214.

79 **MELDRUM, K.C., 1990.** Caseous lymphadenitis outbreak. *The Veterinary Record*, 126, 369.

80 **MENZIES, P.I. & MUCKLE, C.A., 1989.** The use of a microagglutination assay for the detection of antibodies to *Corynebacterium pseudotuberculosis* in naturally infected sheep and goat flocks. *Canadian Journal of Veterinary Research*, 53, 313–318.

81 **MENZIES, P.I., MUCKLE, C.A., BROGDEN, K.A. & ROBINSON, L., 1991.** A field trial to evaluate a whole-cell vaccine for the prevention of caseous lymphadenitis in sheep and goat flocks. *Canadian Journal of Veterinary Research*, 55, 362–366.

82 **MIDDLETON, M.J., EPSTEIN, V.M. & GREGORY, G.G., 1991.** Caseous lymphadenitis on Flinders Island: Prevalence and management surveys. *Australian Veterinary Journal*, 68, 311–312.

83 **MIERS, K.C. & LEY, W.B., 1980.** *Corynebacterium pseudotuberculosis* infection in the horse. Study of 117 clinical cases and consideration of etiopathogenesis. *Journal of the American Veterinary Medical Association*, 177, 250–253.

84 **MUCKLE, C.A. & GYLES, C.L., 1983.** Relation of lipid content and exotoxin production to virulence of *Corynebacterium pseudotuberculosis* in mice. *American Journal of Veterinary Research*, 44, 1149–1153.

85 **MUCKLE, C.A., MENZIES, P.I., LI, Y., HWANG, T. & VAN WESENBEECK, M., 1992.** Analysis of the immunodominant

antigens of *Corynebacterium pseudotuberculosis*. *Veterinary Microbiology*, 30, 47–58.

86 **NAGY, G., 1971.** Ticks and caseous lymphadenitis in sheep: Preliminary observations. *Journal of the South African Veterinary Medical Association*, 42, 227–232.

87 **NAGY, G., 1976.** Caseous lymphadenitis in sheep — methods of infection. *Journal of the South African Veterinary Association*, 47, 197–199.

88 **NAIRN, M.E. & ROBERTSON, J.P., 1974.** *Corynebacterium pseudotuberculosis* infection of sheep: Role of skin lesions and dipping fluids. *Australian Veterinary Journal*, 50, 537–542.

89 **NEAVE, R.M.S., 1951.** An outbreak of ulcerative lymphangitis in young heifers in Kenya. *The Veterinary Record*, 63, 185.

90 **PASCOE, R.R., 1984.** Infectious skin diseases of horses. *Veterinary Clinics of North America (Large Animal Practice)*, 6, 27–46.

91 **PATON, M.W., 1989.** The impact of caseous lymphadenitis on the wool and sheep-meat industries. *In*: OUTTERIDGE, P.M. & RICHARDS, R.B., (eds). *Australian Advances in Veterinary Science*, 147–149.

92 **PATON, M.W., MERCY, A.R., SUTHERLAND, S.S., ELLIS, T.M. & DUDA, S.R., 1991.** The effect of antibody to caseous lymphadenitis in ewes on the efficacy of vaccination in lambs. *Australian Veterinary Journal*, 68, 143–146.

93 **PATON, M.W., MERCY, A.R., WILKINSON, F.C., GARDNER, J.J., SUTHERLAND, S.S. & ELLIS, T.M., 1988.** The effects of caseous lymphadenitis on wool production and bodyweight in young sheep. *Australian Veterinary Journal*, 65, 117–119.

94 **PÉPIN, M., FONTAINE, J-J., PARDON, P., MARLY, J. & PARODI, A.L., 1991.** Histopathology of the early phase during experimental *Corynebacterium pseudotuberculosis* infection in lambs. *Veterinary Microbiology*, 29, 123–134.

95 **PÉPIN, M., MARLY, J. & PARDON, P., 1987.** *Corynebacterium pseudotuberculosis* infection in sheep and the complement fixation test for paratuberculosis. *The Veterinary Record*, 120, 236.

96 **PRESCOTT, J.F. & MUCKLE, C.A., 1986.** *Corynebacterium*. *In*: GYLES, C.L. & THOEN, C.O., (eds). *Pathogenesis of Bacterial Infections in Animals*. Ames, Iowa: Iowa State University Press.

97 **PURCHASE, H.S., 1944.** An outbreak of ulcerative lymphangitis in cattle caused by *Corynebacterium ovis*. *Journal of Comparative Pathology and Therapeutics*, 54, 238–244.

98 **RENSHAW, H.W., GRAFF, V.P. & GATES, N.L., 1979.** Visceral caseous lymphadenitis in thin-ewe syndrome: Isolation of *Corynebacterium*, *Staphylococcus* and *Moraxella* spp. from internal abscesses in emaciated ewes. *American Journal of Veterinary Research*, 40, 1110–1114.

99 **ROBINSON, E.M., 1928.** Preliminary investigations into an icterus of sheep caused by a bacterium (bacterial icterus). *Thirteenth and Fourteenth Reports of the Director of Veterinary Education and Research*, Part 2, 733–741.

100 **ROBINSON, E.M., 1929.** A note on *Corynebacterium ovis* (Bacillus of Preisz Nocard). *Fifteenth Annual Report of the Director of Veterinary Services*, 119–121.

101 **ROBINSON, W.F. & MAXIE, M.G., 1985.** The cardiovascular system. *In*: JUBB, K.V.F., KENNEDY, P.C. & PALMER, N., (eds). *Pathology of Domestic Animals*. Vol. III. 3rd edn. New York, London: Academic Press.

102 **SANTA ROSA, J., JOHNSON, E.H., ALVES, F.S.F. & SANTOS, L.F.L., 1989.** A retrospective study of hepatic abscesses in goats: Pathological and microbiological findings. *British Veterinary Journal*, 145, 73–76.

103 **SCHREUDER, B.E.C., TER LAAK, E.A. & BAKKER, J., 1989.** 'Caseous lymphadenitis' bij heideschapen in Nederland. *Tijdschrift voor Diergeneeskunde*, 114, 1189–1192.

104 **STOOPS, S.G., RENSHAW, H.W. & THILSTED, J.P., 1984.** Ovine caseous lymphadenitis: Disease prevalence, lesion distribution, and thoracic manifestations in a population of mature culled sheep from Western United States. *American Journal of Veterinary Research*, 45, 557–561.

105 **SUTHERLAND, S.S., ELLIS, T.M., MERCY, A.R., PATON, M. & MIDDLETON, H., 1987.** Evaluation of an enzyme-linked immunosorbent assay for the detection of *Corynebacterium pseudotuberculosis* infection in sheep. *Australian Veterinary Journal*, 64, 263–266.

106 **SUTHERLAND, S.S., PATON, M.W., MERCY, A.R. & ELLIS, T.M., 1987.** A reliable method for establishing caseous lymphadenitis infection in sheep. *Australian Veterinary Journal*, 64, 323–324.

107 **SUTHERLAND, S.S., SPEIJERS, E.J. & ANDRES, B., 1989.** Comparison of the exotoxins of four strains of *Corynebacterium pseudotuberculosis*. *Research in Veterinary Science*, 47, 190–194.

108 **TASHJIAN, J.J. & CAMPBELL, S.G., 1983.** Interaction between caprine macrophages and *Corynebacterium pseudotuberculosis*: An electron microscopic study. *American Journal of Veterinary Research*, 44, 690–693.

109 **TIMONEY, J.F., GILLESPIE, J.H., SCOTT, F.W. & BARLOUGH, J.E., 1988.** *Hagan and Bruner's Microbiology and Infectious Diseases of Domestic Animals*. 8th edn. Ithaca, London: Comstock Publishing Associates.

110 **TUSTIN, R.C., 1969.** Ovine jaagsiekte. *Journal of the South African Veterinary Medical Association*, 40, 3–23.

111 **TUSTIN, R.C., ADELAAR, T.F. & CAMERON, C., 1960.** An outbreak of bacterial icterus in sheep. *Journal of the South African Veterinary Medical Association*, 31, 275–283.

112 **VALLI, V.E.O., 1985.** The hematopoietic system. *In*: JUBB, K.V.F., KENNEDY, P.C. & PALMER, N., (eds). *Pathology of Domestic Animals*. Vol. III. 3rd edn. New York, London: Academic Press.

113 **VAN TONDER, E.M., 1971.** Caseous lymphadenitis in sheep. *Journal of the South African Veterinary Medical Association*, 42, 351.

114 **VAN TONDER, E.M., 1975.** Notes on some disease problems in Angora goats in South Africa. *Veterinary Medical Review*, 109–138.

115 **WALLACE, H.G., 1988.** Cato Ridge Abattoir, Cato Ridge, Natal. Unpublished data.

116 **WELSH, R.D., 1990.** *Corynebacterium pseudotuberculosis* in the horse. *Equine Practice*, 12, 7–16.

117 **WILLIAMSON, P. & NAIRN, M.E., 1980.** Lesions caused by *Corynebacterium pseudotuberculosis* in the scrotum of rams. *Australian Veterinary Journal*, 56, 496–498.

118 **WISECUP, W.G., BLANCHARD, D.D. & NEIL, C.M., 1964.** *Corynebacterium pseudotuberculosis* associated with rapidly occurring equine abscesses. *Journal of the American Veterinary Medical Association*, 144, 152–154.

119 **ZAKI, M.M., 1968.** The application of a new technique for diagnosing *Corynebacterium ovis* infection. *Research in Veterinary Science*, 9, 489–493.

120 **ZAKI, M.M., 1976.** Relation between the toxigenicity and pyogenicity of *Corynebacterium ovis* in experimentally infected mice. *Research in Veterinary Science*, 20, 197–200.

121 **ZHAO, H-K., MORIMURA, H., HIRAMUNE, T., KIKUCHI, N., YANAGAWA, R. & SERIKAWA, S., 1991.** Antimicrobial susceptibility of *Corynebacterium pseudotuberculosis* isolated from lesions of caseous lymphadenitis in sheep in Hokkaido, Japan. *Journal of Veterinary Medical Science*, 53, 355–356.

Corynebacterium renale group infections

Synonym: Contagious bovine pyelonephritis

M.G. Collett

Introduction

Contagious bovine pyelonephritis is a specific infection of the urinary tract of cattle caused by bacteria of the *Corynebacterium renale* group (*C. renale*, *C. pilosum* and *C. cystitidis*). The disease is characterized by chronic purulent cystitis, ureteritis and pyelonephritis.

The virulence varies between *C. renale*, *C. pilosum* and *C. cystitidis*. Infection with either *C. renale* or *C. pilosum* causes pyelonephritis and cystitis in cows, while *C. cystitidis* infection causes a cystitis which is more severe and haemorrhagic than that caused by the former organisms. The first two bacterial species can be isolated from healthy animals, but *C. cystitidis* has only been isolated from diseased cows, although it does occur in the prepuce of healthy bulls.[12, 14, 30]

Bacteria of the *C. renale* group may also cause pyelonephritis and cystitis in horses,[2, 5] and posthitis and vulvitis in sheep.[26, 27] In the text which follows, no distinction is made between species of bacteria in the *C. renale* group, as they were not identified in early reports.

The disease in cattle has been recognized in Europe for over a century, and is also found in the Middle East, Japan and the USA.[2, 17, 19] In South Africa, the only isolations of *C. renale* have been from a few cases of ulcerative posthitis and vulvitis in sheep.[10]

Aetiology

Bacteria of the *C. renale* group (*C. renale*, *C. pilosum* and *C. cystitidis*) are aerobic and facultatively anaerobic. A special selective medium for the isolation of urinary corynebacteria from samples contaminated with the faeces or urine of cows has been developed.[13] These bacteria are rather large (0,7 X 3,0 µm or more), irregularly staining Gram-positive rods, often with pointed ends and with pili present.[3] On blood agar, the colonies are small, dewdrop-like, raised, opaque, yellow or ivory-coloured, and dull without haemolysis.[21, 29] Colonies grown on agar can be pushed intact across the surface.[21] Although originally all were classified as *C. renale*, biochemical[3] **(see Irregular, non-sporing, Gram-positive rods: Introduction: Table 1)** and antigenic differences,[30] and differences in nutritional requirements[11] between strains necessitated the designation of new species.

Epidemiology

In herds where pyelonephritis occurs, prevalence rates are in the region of 0,5–1,5 per cent and up to a third of affected animals may die or have to be culled.[19]

Bacteria of the *C. renale* group are carried on the vulvovaginal and penile mucosa of a high proportion of apparently healthy cattle.[1, 8, 13–15, 18, 22] Healthy cows may shed bacteria in their urine intermittently or regularly for seven months or longer.[1, 12] Ten to 20 per cent of animals may be carriers of the bacteria.[22]

Multiparous cows are mainly affected.[19] The disease often follows parturition, but pregnant animals may also be affected.[1, 2, 22, 28] In dairy herds, there is evidence that *C. renale* spreads from animal to animal along stanchion lines.[22] The spray of urine from infected cows can probably directly contaminate the vulvas of animals standing in close proximity to them.[13] Venereal transmission has been reported in sheep.[27]

Cold weather,[1, 15] stress associated with peak production,[19] and a high-protein diet which causes an increase in the level of urea in the urine may predispose to the development of the disease.[26, 27] Pyelonephritis does not normally occur in association with post-parturient uterine diseases, however, because of the aciduria in the latter.[19]

Pathogenesis

Corynebacterium renale has a predilection for the urinary tract because of its ability to metabolize large quantities of urea by means of the enzyme urease.[1, 18] Consequently, the pH of the urine in affected animals is usually higher than normal.[1]

The vulva is the main portal of entry. Bacteria of the *C. renale* group adhere efficiently to superficial epithelial cells of the urinary tract of cattle;[7, 9] adherence to the vulval epithelium is stronger than to superficial bladder epithelial cells and epithelial cells in urinary sediment.[24]

Unlike most Gram-positive organisms, members of the *C. renale* group possess pili that promote attachment to, and colonization of, the mucosa of the urinary tract.[6] Specific cell receptors[24] may be involved in the localization of the organisms, but the role of piliation in the pathogenesis of pyelonephritis[6] and in bacterial survival[8] appears equivocal. After attachment to the epithelial cells of the vulva, the bacterial infection causes an ascending (retrograde) cystitis and pyelonephritis.[2, 4, 7, 8, 19, 20, 22, 25, 28] In the kidneys, the medulla is preferred to the cortex as a site for growth.[18] The clinical signs of pyelonephritis are due mainly to the direct effects of bacterial multiplication.[1]

An experimental model of pyelonephritis, caused by *C. renale*, has been produced in mice.[25]

Clinical signs and pathology

Typically cows with pyelonephritis show painful and frequent micturition. The urine is bloody or foetid, and contains neutrophils, mucus, blood, fibrin and colonies of large, Gram-positive, diphtheroid bacteria.[1, 2, 17, 18, 23, 28] Its pH is raised (more than 8,5),[1, 19] and the specific gravity is in the range of 1,010–1,015.[19, 23] Haematuria may last for months after calving. Other clinical signs include anorexia, fever, loss of condition, a reduced milk yield, and, in severe cases, signs of colic manifested by the animal kicking at its abdomen, grinding its teeth, and restlessness.[1, 12, 23] On rectal examination, the left kidney is usually enlarged and tender to touch and the ureters are thickened (up to 20 mm or more, in diameter).[1, 2, 23, 28] The differentiation between cows with cystitis, where the ureters are not affected and systemic illness is absent, and those with pyelonephritis, where the ureters are thickened, can be aided by vaginal examination and palpation.[23]

Serum creatinine and urea levels can be helpful with regard to prognosis,[19] as raised levels indicate that there is probably bilateral renal involvement.[23]

At necropsy, both kidneys are usually affected. They are severely enlarged, the calyces are distended, and little functional tissue remains. The pelves and ureters usually contain a brownish fluid made up of mucus, pus, fibrin, calculi and other debris.[1, 12] The ureters are often grossly dilated, especially near the hilus, and show petechiation of the mucosa.[1] The pelvic epithelium is thickened and contains petechiae. The infectious process extends from the pelvis to cause a slowly progressive and suppurative papillitis. This results in destruction of the medulla of each lobe and a radially arranged, tubulo-interstitial nephritis. Cortical fibrosis is eventually extensive and the capsule may be adherent in places because of the presence of subcortical abscesses.[1, 2, 20, 25]

Histopathological changes in affected kidneys include foci of mixed leukocytic infiltrates, purulent foci in the medulla, the destruction of many tubules, and interstitial fibrosis. Gram-positive rods are present in inflamed areas and may also be detected within Bowman's space.[2] The bladder mucosa is affected by varying degrees of pseudomembranous inflammation and haemorrhage.[1, 2, 12, 25]

Corynebacterium renale may cause external preputial ulceration in steers and bulls.[27]

Equine pyelonephritis resembles the disease in cattle.[5] The signs of colic are, however, usually more severe than in cattle, while urinary incontinence may occur and calcareous material may be found in the exudate from the bladder.[2]

In sheep, small yellowish areas of epidermal necrosis occur in the prepuce of wethers. The lesions may ulcerate and expand and cause occlusion of the preputial orifice, resulting in the accumulation of urine and pus in the prepuce. Extensive ulceration of the mucosa of the prepuce and glans follows, leading to the eventual destruction of the urethral process ('sheath rot').[16]

Diagnosis and differential diagnosis

The clinical signs, urinalysis, rectal and genital palpation findings and pathology are suggestive of the infection. In cows, it is important to culture the bacterium, either from urine in live animals or from the renal pelvis, ureter or bladder in dead animals,[1] since other bacteria, such as *Escherichia coli*, can also cause pyelonephritis.[23] Concurrent infection with other organisms, such as streptococci, may also be encountered.[2]

Further aids to diagnosis include renal biopsy and diagnostic ultrasonography.[23]

Haematuria caused by corynebacterial pyelonephritis in cattle should be differentiated clinically from other causes of haematuria, such as bracken fern (*Pteridium aquilinum*) poisoning ('enzootic haematuria'), as well as ascending pyelonephritis caused by *E. coli*,[23] and pyaemic nephritis and renal abscesses resulting from *Actinomyces pyogenes* infection.[17]

Control

If bacteria of the *C. renale* group are cultured from healthy or clinically affected animals, the infected cattle should be isolated and not used for breeding because of the possibility of venereal spread.[2]

Most affected animals respond to injections of penicillin at doses sufficient to provide an adequate concentration in the urine for bacterial cure.[21] In early reports, total amounts of 10 000 000 IU were given at 1–2 000 000 IU per day.[1, 18] Nowadays, daily treatments of 6 000 000 IU of penicillin G intramuscularly for six days have been reported as being successful,[19] although continuation of penicillin treatment for three weeks has been recommended.[23] The variable response to penicillin is probably related to the stage the disease process has reached at the time of treatment.[1] Since *C. renale* prefers an alkaline medium for growth, response to parenteral penicillin can be enhanced by the acidification of urine by means of the oral administration of 110 g of sodium biphosphate ($NaH_2PO_4.H_20$) per day for four days.[28]

In sheep, prophylactic antiseptic treatment of the prepuce or vulva helps in the prevention of venereal transmission of posthitis and vulvitis.[27] Shearing and removal of belly wool is also beneficial.[27]

References

1 **ARTHUR, G.H., 1949.** Some observations on bovine pyelonephritis and its treatment with penicillin. *The Veterinary Record*, 61, 257–261.

2 **BOYD, W.L. & BISHOP, L.M., 1937.** Pyelonephritis of cattle and horses. *Journal of the American Veterinary Medical Association*, 90, 154–162.

3 **COLLINS, M.D. & CUMMINS, C.S., 1986.** Genus *Corynebacterium*. *In*: SNEATH, P.H.A., MAIR, N.S., SHARPE, M.E. & HOLT, J.G., (eds). *Bergey's Manual of Systematic Bacteriology*. Vol II. Baltimore, London: Williams & Wilkins.

4 **FEENSTRA, E.S., THORP, F. & GRAY, M.L., 1949.** Pathogenicity of *Corynebacterium renale* for rabbits. *American Journal of Veterinary Research*, 10, 12–25.

5 **FOSS, J.O., 1944.** Identification of *Corynebacterium renale* from the kidney and bladder of a horse. *Journal of the American Veterinary Medical Association*, 104, 27.

6 **FUKUOKA, T. & YANAGAWA, R., 1987.** Comparison of experimental infection in mice of *Corynebacterium renale* piliated and non-piliated clones. *Japanese Journal of Veterinary Research*, 35, 79–86.

7 **HAYASHI, A., YANAGAWA, R. & KIDA, H., 1985.** Adhesion of *Corynebacterium pilosum* to the epithelial cells of various parts of the bovine urinary tract from the renal pelvis to vulva. *Veterinary Microbiology*, 10, 287–292.

8 **HAYASHI, A., YANAGAWA,R. & KIDA, H., 1985.** Survival of *Corynebacterium renale, Corynebacterium pilosum* and *Corynebacterium cystitidis* in soil. *Veterinary Microbiology*, 10, 381–386.

9 **HAYASHI, A., YANAGAWA, R. & KIDA, H., 1985.** Adhesion of *Corynebacterium pilosum* to epithelial cells of bovine vulva. *American Journal of Veterinary Research*, 46, 409–411.

10 **HENTON, M.M., 1989.** Veterinary Research Institute, Onderstepoort. Unpublished data.

11 **HIRAI, K. & YANAGAWA, R., 1967.** Nutritional requirements of *Corynebacterium renale*. *Japanese Journal of Veterinary Research*, 15, 121–134.

12 **HIRAMUNE, T., INUI, S., MURASE, N. & YANAGAWA, R., 1971.** Virulence of three types of *Corynebacterium renale* in cows. *American Journal of Veterinary Research*, 32, 237–242.

13 **HIRAMUNE, T., KUDOH, R., KIKUCHI, N. & YANAGAWA, R., 1988.** Selective medium for isolation of urinary corynebacteria and detection of the organisms from bovine vulva and vaginal vestibule using the medium. *Japanese Journal of Veterinary Science*, 50, 111–114.

14 **HIRAMUNE, T., KUME, T., MURASE, N. & YANAGAWA, R., 1970.** Typing of'*Corynebacterium renale* isolated from cattle in a herd with persistent pyelonephritis. *Japanese Journal of Veterinary Science*, 32, 81–85.

15 **HIRAMUNE, T., MURASE, N. & YANAGAWA, R., 1970.** Distribution of the types of *Corynebacterium renale* in cows of Japan. *Japanese Journal of Veterinary Science*, 32, 235–241.

16 **LADDS, P.W., 1985.** The male genital system. *In*: JUBB, K.V.F., KENNEDY, P.C. & PALMER, N., (eds). *Pathology of Domestic Animals*. Vol III. 3rd edn. New York, London: Academic Press, Inc.

17 **LOVELL, R., 1946.** Studies on *Corynebacterium renale*. I. A systematic study of a number of strains. *Journal of Comparative Pathology*, 56, 196–204.

18 **LOVELL, R., 1951.** Bovine pyelonephritis. *The Veterinary Record*, 63, 645–646.

19 **MARKUSFELD, O., NAHARI, N., KESSNER, D. & ADLER, H., 1989.** Observations on bovine pyelonephritis. *British Veterinary Journal*, 145, 573–579.

20 **MAXIE, M.G., 1985.** The urinary system. *In*: JUBB, K.V.F., KENNEDY, P.C. & PALMER, N., (eds). *Pathology of Domestic Animals*. Vol II. 3rd edn. New York, London: Academic Press, Inc.

21 **MORSE, E.V., 1948.** Bovine pyelonephritis. *Cornell Veterinarian*, 38, 135–147.

22 **MORSE, E.V., 1950.** An ecological study of *Corynebacterium renale*. *Cornell Veterinarian*, 40, 178–187.

23 **REBHUN, W.C., DILL, S.G., PERDRIZET, J.A. & HATFIELD, C.E., 1989.** Pyelonephritis in cows: Fifteen cases (1982–86). *Journal of the American Veterinary Medical Association*, 194, 953–955.

24 **SATO, H., YANAGAWA, R. & FUKUYAMA, H., 1982.** Adhesion of *Corynebacterium renale, Corynebacterium pilosum* and *Corynebacterium cystitidis* to bovine urinary bladder epithelial cells of various ages and levels of differentiation. *Infection and Immunity*, 36, 1242–1245.

25 **SHIMONO, E. & YANAGAWA, R., 1977.** Experimental model of *Corynebacterium renale* pyelonephritis produced in mice. *Infection and Immunity*, 16, 263–267.

26 **SOUTHCOTT, W.H., 1965.** Etiology of ovine posthitis: Description of a causal organism. *Australian Veterinary Journal*, 41, 193–200.

27 **SOUTHCOTT, W.H., 1965.** Epidemiology and control of ovine posthitis and vulvitis. *Australian Veterinary Journal*, 41, 225–234.

28 **THOMPSON, R.H., 1951.** The successful diagnosis and treatment of bovine pyelonephritis. *Journal of the American Veterinary Medical Association*, 119, 295–296.

29 **TIMONEY, J.F., GILLESPIE, J.H., SCOTT, F.W. & BARLOUGH, J.E., 1988.** *Hagan and Bruner's Microbiology and Infectious Diseases of Domestic Animals*. 8th edn. Ithaca and London: Comstock Publishing Associates.

30 **YANAGAWA, R., BASRI, H. & OTSUKI, K., 1967.** Three types of *Corynebacterium renale* classified by precipitin reactions in gels. *Japanese Journal of Veterinary Research*, 15, 111–119.

168

Bolo disease

P.A. Colly and A.L. Lange

Introduction

Bolo disease is a localized, mild, subacute to chronic, superficial dermatitis of woolled sheep and is caused by an unclassified *Corynebacterium* sp.[2] Clinically it is characterized by dark-grey to blackish discoloration of the fleece overlying affected areas of the skin.

The condition was first reported in sheep in 1974 on the farm 'Bolo' in the eastern Cape Province. It is now widely distributed throughout the Cathcart and Stutterheim districts, where it has been diagnosed on approximately 8 per cent of the farms. Isolated cases have also been reported from East Griqualand and elsewhere in Natal, but the exact distribution of the disease in southern Africa is unknown.[3]

Bolo disease is of considerable economic importance to wool farmers who own flocks in which it occurs. Economic losses in affected flocks occur because many of the fleeces are down-graded, labour costs increase because of the time-consuming plucking of affected wool from the shorn fleeces, and chronically affected sheep are 'poor doers' and show a loss in production.[1]

Much investigation and research remains to be done on this disease, and the information contained in this chapter is based largely on personal observations and unpublished data.[2, 3–6]

Aetiology

Initial field investigation of the condition yielded a number of different bacterial species from affected animals, but the as yet unclassified *Corynebacterium* sp. is believed to be the causative organism. In a further survey involving 15 farms and 750 sheep, from which 1 168 samples were taken for bacterial isolation, the bacterium was isolated from 94 per cent of severely affected sheep, 83,7 per cent of mildly affected sheep, and only 1,36 per cent of apparently unaffected sheep.[6] No evidence could be found of arthropod, helminth or fungal involvement.[2] The application of cultures of this organism in normal saline to the skin of sheep led to a condition which resembled Bolo disease both clinically and histopathologically.[2, 5]

The unclassified *Corynebacterium* sp. is a Gram-positive, non-acid fast, pleomorphic, beaded, unbranched rod which does not undergo a rod/coccus cycle. It is a facultative anaerobe, is catalase-positive and oxidase-negative. Unpigmented, pinpoint-sized colonies grow after 48 hours' incubation at 37 °C on Columbia blood agar.[2, 5, 6]

Epidemiology

The epidemiology of Bolo disease has not been thoroughly investigated. It has only been diagnosed in Merino and Dohne Merino sheep.[1] The prevalence of the disease is not related to seasonal changes or to prevailing weather conditions, although it appears to be more prevalent during years of drought.[2]

Preliminary surveys have indicated that the disease is most common in ewes and wethers. It affects sheep older than two to three years and is more severe and of longer duration in older animals; lambs are rarely affected. Sheep with medium-fine to medium-strong wool and whose fleeces have a high yolk content are more frequently affected.

The mode of transmission has not yet been established, but close contact, dipping and shearing are likely factors. Modern dips rarely contain bacteriostats and are thus ideal reservoirs for bacteria. Shearing has an irritant and disruptive effect on the superficial layers of the skin, thus allowing organisms to penetrate with greater ease and the infection to be established. Floors of shearing sheds and the equipment and clothes of shearers contaminated with scales and other skin debris from affected sheep may act as potential sources of infection.

Clinical signs and pathology

Bolo disease usually starts as a well-circumscribed, localized, mild lesion in two- to three-year-old animals. The condition is chronic and progressive, and lesions increase in size and severity as the animal ages, with the most outspoken lesions seen in animals in a poor condition.[3]

The lesions are most frequently distributed on the neck and shoulders, but are also relatively common on the rump and flanks. In advanced cases with extensive

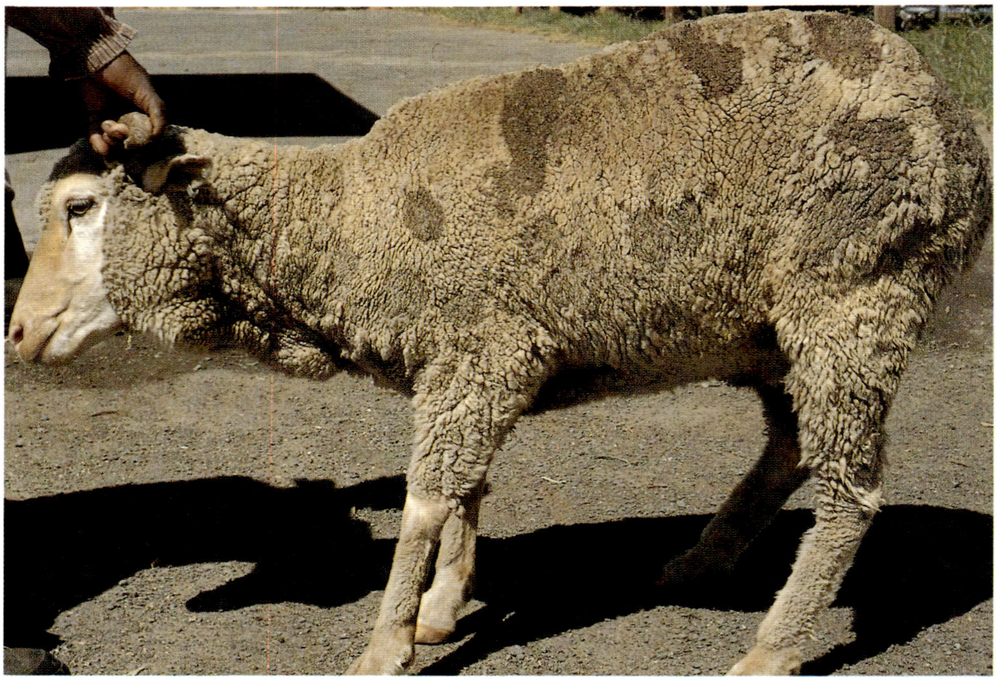

Figure 168.1 Focal lesions of Bolo disease

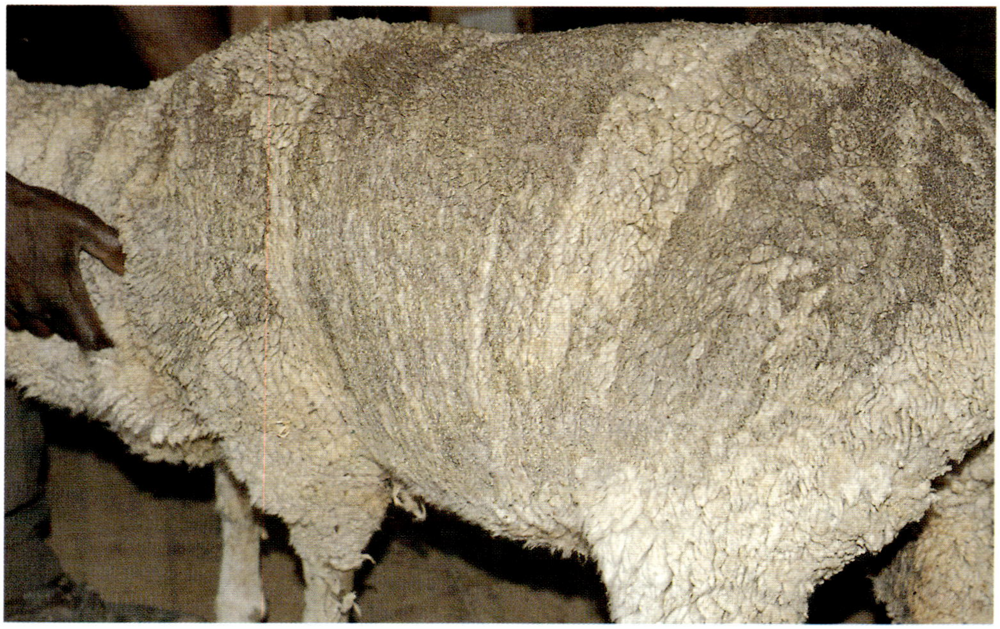

Figure 168.2 Confluent lesions of Bolo disease involving large areas of the fleece

lesions the skin of the back may be involved, but even in such animals the abdominal skin is rarely affected.[1–3] The fleece over the affected areas has dark-grey to blackish, usually well-circumscribed spots, patches or bands. These areas vary considerably in size, from 20 mm in diameter to large patches covering a greater part of the body, **(Figures 168.1 and 168.2)**. The tips of the wool in the affected areas are spiky and the wool is shorter and less dense, while the skin is often tender.[1, 2] On parting the wool in affected areas, yellow to greyish-white, sticky, scaly deposits are found adjacent to the surface of the skin. These deposits cause the wool fibres to adhere to each other, resulting in the spiky staple formation. Dirt and dust adhere to the sticky deposits, thus causing the dark colour of the fleece. Loss of crimp in the staple of the wool fibres also occurs in the affected areas. In recently shorn sheep the lesions are well-circumscribed, pearly-white plaques and patches **(Figure 168.3)**. The fleece of affected sheep has a characteristic, unique odour.

In mild cases, the affected skin is reddish-purple, swollen, very sensitive, and fragile, which causes it to tear when handled, particularly during shearing. In more severe cases, it is, in addition, often pigmented grey.

In both the early and more chronic lesions the most consistent changes are a mild, mainly lymphocytic, dermatitis; superficial and follicular hyperkeratosis; prominent dilatation of the hair follicles **(Figure 168.4)**; and an increase in the size and/or number of sebaceous glands. There is no exudate present on the surface of the epidermis. The sticky, scaly deposits present

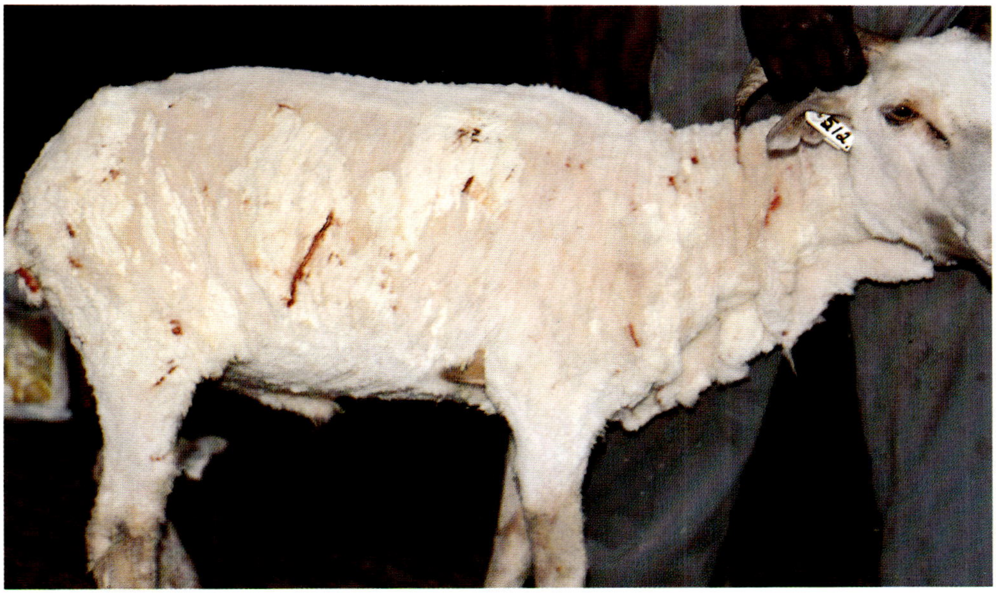

Figure 168.3 Pearly-white colour of lesions in a recently shorn sheep

macroscopically are probably due to a combination of increased sebum secretion and hyperkeratotic flakes.

Diagnosis and differential diagnosis

The disease is confirmed by isolation of the suspected causative bacterium from sterile cotton-wool swabs used on animals with dry skin and fleece. To obtain the specimen the wool is parted and a swab is rubbed firmly on the affected skin. Skin scrapings and wool samples may also be cultured but they are often severely contaminated by other microorganisms.[6]

Lumpy wool and fleece rot are the most important differential diagnoses.

Control

Bolo disease is very difficult to control and no satisfactory cure has yet been found. The causative bacterium shows marked *in vitro* sensitivity to several antibiotics, yet systemic antibiotic treatment in affected animals is unsuccessful.[3]

With the exception of sulphur-containing compounds, topical treatments, including dipping agents, have little effect.[3] Fairly good results are obtained by dipping sheep twice in 3 per cent flowable sulphur. The first dipping should be carried out two weeks after shearing and the second 10 days after the first. Sheep may be dipped immediately after they have been shorn, provided that the dipping solution is made up daily so as to prevent the occurrence of post-dipping lameness if shearing extends over several days.[4] Longstanding cases do not respond well to treatment and should be culled.[3]

Separation of age groups, dipping and shearing of young animals before the rest of the flock, and regular disinfection of shearing sheds and equipment with 3 per cent formalin, are additional preventive measures that may be instituted.

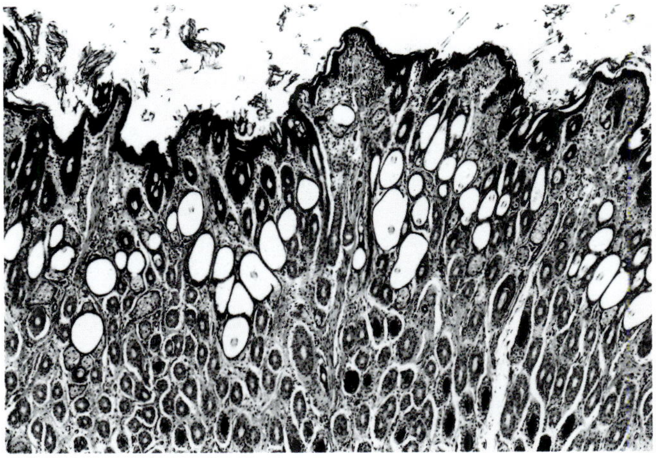

Figure 168.4 Bolo disease. Note the numerous dilated hair follicles and hyperplasia of the sebaceous glands in a histological section of affected skin

References

1 **COLLY, P.A., 1985.** Bolosiekte; Geheimsinnige siekte wat skape aantas. *Die Landbouweekblad*, 26 April 1985: 24–26.

2 **COLLY, P.A., LANGE, L.A., DE RUITER, A., VAN TONDER, E.M., VERMEULEN, S.O., WHITEHEAD, C.J. & KELLERMAN, G.E., 1989.** Bolo disease: A specific, localized skin disease of woolled sheep. *Journal of the South African Veterinary Association*, 61, 90–95.

3 **COLLY, P.A., 1989.** State Veterinarian, Lydenburg. Unpublished data.

4 **HENTON, M.M., 1989.** Veterinary Research Institute, Onderstepoort. Unpublished data.

5 **LANGE, L.A., 1989.** Faculty of Veterinary Science, University of Pretoria. Unpublished data.

6 **VAN TONDER, E.M., COLLY, P.A., VERMEULEN, S.O., KELLERMAN, G.E., DE RUITER, A. & WHITEHEAD, C.J., 1989.** Bolo disease: A bacteriological survey. *Journal of the South African Veterinary Association*, 61, 96–101.

169

Actinomyces bovis infections

Synonyms: Lumpy jaw, bovine actinomycosis, knopkaak (Afrik.)

M.M. Henton and M.G. Collett

Introduction

Actinomyces bovis is the cause of focal, pyogranulomatous osteomyelitis of the mandible ('lumpy jaw'), and sometimes also of the maxilla in cattle. In horses, the organism has been implicated in 'poll evil' and 'fistulous withers', while in pigs, a closely related organism, *A. suis*, causes a granulomatous mastitis.

Actinomyces bovis, isolated from cows with lumpy jaw, was first described by Harz in 1877.[11, 20] The disease has been recorded in most countries,[4] but it usually occurs sporadically in cattle in southern Africa.[11] In the past ten years, *A. bovis* has been isolated only once at the Veterinary Research Institute, Onderstepoort, probably because clinical diagnosis is easy and specimens are seldom submitted for confirmation of the diagnosis.[12]

Aetiology and epidemiology

Actinomyces bovis is a facultative anaerobe. Colonies on brain-heart infusion agar are white to greyish-white. The organisms are straight or slightly curved Gram-positive rods (0,2–1,0 µm thick) or slender, branching filaments (1 µm thick and 10–50 µm long). Two serovars are recognized, one of which tends to be more filamentous.[25] Some growth and biochemical characteristics are given in **Irregular, non-sporing Gram-positive rods: Introduction: Table 1**.

Actinomyces bovis is believed to be a commensal on the oropharyngeal mucosa of cattle;[8, 14, 24, 25, 28] the oral mucosa of calves appears to be colonized during the immediate post-partum period when they are licked by their dams.[15] The bacterium is not a normal soil inhabitant and has not been isolated from plants or soil.[11] It may, however, be transiently present on feed contaminated with saliva or exudate, but probably does not survive for long outside the body of the animal.[11]

In cattle, lesions commence when *A. bovis* gains a foothold in the submucosal tissues following mechanical trauma to the oral mucosa (e.g. by foreign bodies, coarse feed or silage), after the shedding and eruption of teeth,[8, 15] or as a complication of periodontitis.[4, 14, 28]

The disease generally affects cattle between two and five years old.[11] Of the laboratory animals, only the hamster is fairly susceptible to artificial infection with *A. bovis*.[10]

Pathogenesis, clinical signs and pathology

Little is known of the host-parasite interaction in *A. bovis* infections.[8] The presence of *A. bovis* in the oral cavity may explain why lesions occur more frequently here than at other sites of the body. The initial lesion usually occurs in the gums, from which the submucosal necrogranulomatous inflammation extends to, and invades, the adjacent mandibular or maxillary bone, causing a chronic, pyogranulomatous osteomyelitis.

In lumpy jaw the first sign is usually a painless, localized, hard, immovable swelling of the mandible or maxilla at the level of the central molars. The lesion develops slowly over months. The swelling is often not detected clinically until a discrete, hard, osseous enlargement develops on the lateral surface of the mandible or maxilla, at which time the teeth are often malaligned, buried in granulation tissue, and painful. The infection may extend to the adjacent soft tissues of the tongue, pharynx and subcutaneous tissues of the head and neck to cause disfigurement and sometimes impairment of mastication or breathing.[4, 11, 14, 28] Spread to the regional lymph nodes, lungs, liver and vertebrae is rare.[8]

Actinomycotic granulomas are characterized by the presence of sulphur granules in an exudate composed of varying numbers of neutrophils and large epithelioid cells in the centre, and Langerhans' giant cells, lymphocytes, plasma cells and dense connective tissue on the periphery of the lesions.[13, 19]

In the affected bone, necrosis and proliferation of bone and granulation tissue occur together and give rise to an enlarged, honeycomb appearance **(Figure 169.1)**. Small abscesses, sinuses and sequestrated trabeculae of the affected bone ('bone sand') are also found in the lesions[14] and there is extensive proliferation of granulation tissue in the soft tissues adjacent to the affected bone. Frequently multiple sinuses open onto the skin of the head or mucous membrane of the oral cavity, discharging a

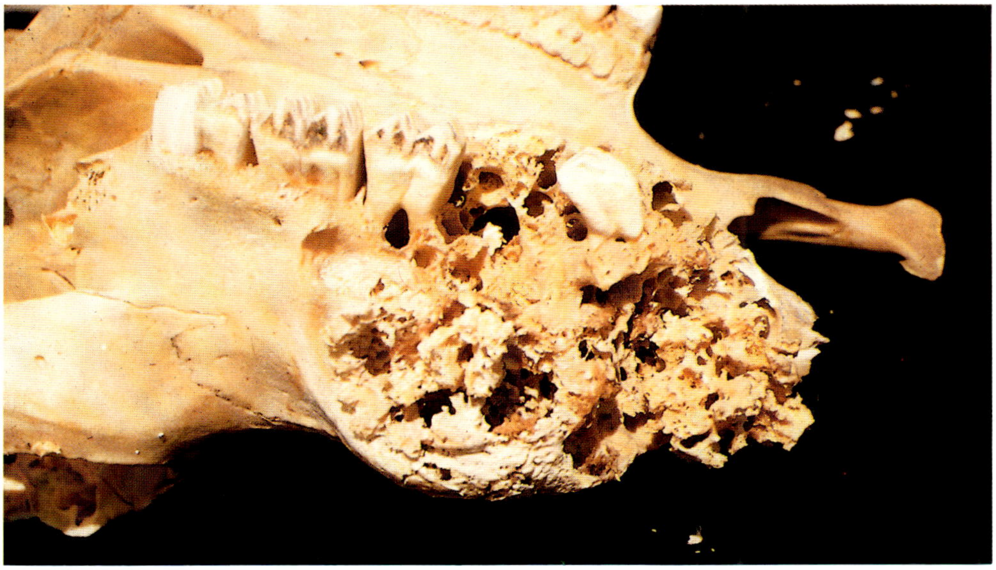

Figure 169.1 Actinomycotic lesion in an ox. Note the honeycomb appearance caused by extensive necrosis and concurrent proliferation of bone

thick, mucoid, tenacious, copious, greyish-yellow, non-odorous exudate which contains small (1–3 mm in diameter) granules. During the earlier stages of their development, these granules are soft and yellowish-white, but later they become opaque and hard as a result of mineralization, at which time, because of their consistency and colour, they are referred to as sulphur granules.[2, 4, 13, 14]

Smears made from crushed granules reveal a conglomerate of filamentous bacteria surrounded by tissue-reaction material and pus.[4, 25] Sulphur granules observed histologically in tissue sections are smaller than those in smears prepared from the exudate. In tissue sections the granules are eosinophilic and consist of a matrix composed of a hyaline, polysaccharide-protein complex in which, particularly in the peripheral zone, is embedded a mycelial mass of tangled, delicate, Gram-positive, bacterial filaments and coccoid forms.[21, 22] The surface of the granule usually contains radiating eosinophilic, Gram-negative 'clubs' (15 x 3,5 µm) composed of lysed bacteria encased in layers of a calcium phosphate-protein complex which is generated by phosphatase activity in the inflammatory exudate.[2, 8, 21] About half the composition of granules is calcium phosphate.[21] Immunohistochemical studies[19] have shown that the clubs (also called Splendore-Hoeppli material) do not represent antigen-antibody complexes as has been previously suggested.[8] Club formation indicates bacterial regression accompanied by progressive mineralization of the granules.[2, 21]

In addition to lumpy jaw, actinomycotic infections in cattle are rarely the cause of localized granulomas in the trachea[1, 27] and lungs,[3, 9] and of orchitis.[17]

In horses, *A. bovis* may cause 'poll evil' (supra-atlantal bursitis) and 'fistulous withers' (supraspinous bursitis).[14, 16, 23, 24, 28] Abscessation of mandibular lymph nodes due to *A. bovis* infection has also been described.[5]

Actinomycosis in pigs is characterized by a necrogranulomatous mastitis suspected of being initiated by trauma from the sharp teeth of suckling piglets.[14, 28] Affected udders are indurated, pendulous and contain abscesses and draining sinuses. Actinomycotic granulomas have also been found in the lungs, spleen and kidneys of slaughter pigs.[9, 30]

Although the cause of actinomycotic necrogranulomatous mastitis in pigs has long been thought to be *A. bovis*, isolates from pigs have certain consistent differences,[30] and therefore the organism has been proposed to be *Actinomyces suis*.[7, 25, 28]

Diagnosis

A provisional clinical diagnosis of lumpy jaw can be made on the physical appearance of the lesions in the mandible and maxilla. The diagnosis can be confirmed by microscopic examination of sulphur granules or of biopsy specimens of the lesions. Smears of pus taken at random for examination may be unrewarding. For better results, the tenacious pus should be collected in a test tube containing saline, broth or 10 per cent KOH, and shaken in order to loosen the granules from the adhering pus. The resulting mixture is then poured into a petri dish and the granules collected, crushed on a glass slide, stained with Gram's method and examined microscopically.[11, 21, 22, 28] A great diversity of Gram-positive bacterial forms, including branching filaments, varying-sized rods and cocci, are evident, creating the impression of a mixed infection. Since *A. bovis* organisms fragment readily, they should be differentiated from *Actinomyces (Corynebacterium) pyogenes*, which may also be cultured from specimens obtained from the lesions of lumpy jaw.[14, 18, 30]

Confirmation of the diagnosis of lumpy jaw requires laboratory culture and identification of the organism. Anaerobic culture of soft-tissue lesions may yield *Fusobacterium necrophorum*, *Bacteroides* spp.,

Peptostreptococcus spp. and other *Actinomyces* spp. in addition to *A. bovis*.[1] The significance of concurrent infection is unknown.

Differential diagnosis

Lumpy jaw of cattle is sometimes confused with 'wooden tongue' caused by *Actinobacillus lignieresii* infection.[8] Osteomyelitis of the mandible and maxilla may also be caused by a variety of other bacteria (such as *A. pyogenes*) following periodontitis. Abscesses in subcutaneous soft tissues of the head caused by *A. pyogenes* are generally movable, in contrast to the firm swelling and involvement of bone in *A. bovis* infection. Grass awns may penetrate and cause abscesses in the oropharyngeal submucosa.[4] Examination of the pus obtained by needle puncture is a helpful procedure that may assist in differentiating between these infections.

The presence of sulphur granules is not specific for *A. bovis* infections, since they are also seen in pus from lesions caused by *Nocardia* spp., *Streptomyces* spp., *Actinobacillus lignieresii* and *Staphylococcus aureus* (botryomycosis) infections in cattle. Most of the sulphur granules of *A. bovis* infections are 2–3 mm in diameter,[14, 24, 28] while granules from non-*A. bovis* lesions are generally much smaller and softer and difficult to detect on macroscopic examination.[2, 11, 28] Laboratory culture and identification of the organism is essential for a definitive diagnosis.

Apart from *A. bovis*, 'poll evil' and 'fistulous withers' in horses may also be caused by *Brucella abortus* and *B. suis*.

Actinomycotic granulomas in pigs should be differentiated from spirochaetal granulomas affecting the udder as well as from lesions caused by infections with *Actinobacillus lignieresii*, *Staphylococcus* spp. (botryomycosis) and *A. pyogenes*.[4]

Control

Actinomycetes are sensitive to iodine[15] and penicillin.[25] Localized skin or mucosal lesions can be treated by the topical application of Lugol's solution or tincture of iodine.[11] Treatment of lumpy jaw and other actinomycotic granulomas should involve intravenous sodium iodide (NaI, at a dosage of 1 g/15 kg body weight dissolved in a litre of sterile isotonic polyionic fluid, given every second day for three treatments, followed by the same dose daily *per os* until signs of iodism appear)[29] and intramuscular penicillin G (10 000 000 IU per day for three weeks).[1, 4, 28] Apart from iodism, abortion in pregnant cows is another potential complication of systemic iodine treatment.[1, 6]

Other antibacterial drugs which can be used include the tetracyclines, cephalosporin, chloramphenicol, lincomycin, rifampicin, erythromycin, and vancomycin.[25, 26] Although good results have been claimed with streptomycin[18] and isoniazid[31] in the treatment of lumpy jaw, *Actinomyces* spp. are generally resistant to the aminoglycosides, antifungal drugs and most tuberculostatics.[26]

Surgical drainage, curettage and iodine irrigation may be beneficial in circumscribed lesions.[11] Because of the nature of the bony lesion, however, clinical cure in advanced cases is unlikely, although further enlargement of the lesion may be arrested and significant reduction in size may even occur.[18, 31] Recurrence of lesions is common in both medically and surgically managed cases.[1]

Very coarse feed should be milled in order to minimize possible oral trauma. Clipping of the teeth of piglets shortly after birth should be performed in order to prevent actinomycotic mastitis in sows.

References

1 **BERTONE, A.L. & REBHUN, W.C., 1984.** Tracheal actinomycosis in a cow. *Journal of the American Veterinary Medical Association*, 185, 221–222.

2 **BESTETTI, G., 1978.** Morphology of the 'sulphur granules' (Drusen) in some actinomycotic infections. A light and electron microscopic study. *Veterinary Pathology*, 15, 506–518.

3 **BIEVER, L.J., ROBERSTAD, G.W., VAN STEENBERGH, K., SCHEETZ, E.E. & KENNEDY, G.F., 1969.** Actinomycosis in a bovine lung. *American Journal of Veterinary Research*, 30, 1063–1066.

4 **BLOOD, D.C. & RADOSTITS, O.M., 1989.** *Veterinary Medicine*. 7th edn. London, Philadelphia: Baillière Tindall.

5 **BURNS, R.H.G. & SIMMONS, G.C., 1952.** A case of actinomycotic infection in a horse. *Australian Veterinary Journal*, 28, 34–35.

6 **FARQUHARSON, J., 1937.** Intravenous use of sodium iodine in actinomycosis. *Journal of the American Veterinary Medical Association*, 91, 551–555.

7 **FRANKE, F., 1973.** Untersuchungen zur Ätiologie der Gesäugeaktinomykose des Schweines. *Zentralblatt für Bakteriologie, Parasitenkunde, Infektionskrankheiten und Hygiene*, 1 Abteilung Original A223, 111–124.

8 **GYLES, C.L., 1986.** *Nocardia, Actinomyces, Dermatophilus. In*: GYLES, C.L. & THOEN, C.O., (eds). *Pathogenesis of Bacterial Infections in Animals*. Ames, Iowa: Iowa State University Press.

9 **HAGA, M., OMURA, Y. & SUGANO, S., 1951.** Pulmonary actinomycosis in cattle and swine. *Japanese Journal of Veterinary Science*, 13, 102–103.

10 **HAZEN, E.L., LITTLE, G.N. & RESNICK, H., 1952.** The hamster as a vehicle for the demonstration of pathogenicity of *Actinomyces bovis*. *Journal of Laboratory and Clinical Medicine* 40, 914–918.

11 **HENNING, M.W., 1956.** *Animal Diseases in South Africa*. 3rd edn. Pretoria: Central News Agency.

12 **HENTON, M.M., 1992.** Veterinary Research Institute, Onderstepoort. Unpublished data.

13 **JONES, T.C. & HUNT, R.D., 1983.** *Veterinary Pathology*. 5th edn. Philadelphia: Lea & Febiger.

14 **JUBB, K.V.F., KENNEDY, P.C. & PALMER, N., 1985.** *Pathology of Domestic Animals*. 3rd edn. New York, London: Academic Press.

15 **JUNGERMAN, P.F. & SCHWARTZMAN, R.M., 1972.** *Veterinary Medical Mycology*. Philadelphia: Lea & Febiger.

16 **KIMBALL, A. & FRANK, E.R., 1945.** The isolation of *Actinomyces bovis* from fistulous withers and poll evil. *American Journal of Veterinary Research*, 6, 39–44.

17 **KIMBALL, A., TWIEHAUS, M.J. & FRANK, E.R., 1954.** *Actinomyces bovis* isolated from six cases of bovine orchitis. A preliminary report. *American Journal of Veterinary Research*, 15, 551–553.

18 **KINGMAN, H.E. & PALEN, J.S., 1951.** Streptomycin in the treatment of actinomycosis. *Journal of the American Veterinary Medical Association*, 118, 28–30.

19 **MOMOTANI, E., KUBO, M., ISHIKAWA, Y. & YOSHINO, T., 1989.** Immunohistochemical localization of immunoglobulins in bovine granulomatous lesions. *Journal of Comparative Pathology*, 100, 129–136.

20 **PINE, L., HOWELL, A. & WATSON, S.J., 1960.** Studies of the morphological, physiological and biochemical characters of *Actinomyces bovis*. *Journal of General Microbiology*, 23, 403–424.

21 **PINE, L. & OVERMAN, J.R., 1963.** Determination of the structure and composition of the 'sulphur granules' of *Actinomyces bovis*. *Journal of General Microbiology*, 32, 209–223.

22 **PINE, L. & OVERMAN, J.R., 1966.** Differentiation of capsules and hyphae in clubs of bovine sulphur granules. *Sabouraudia*, 5, 141–143.

23 **RODERICK, L.M., KIMBALL, A., McLEOD, W.M. & FRANK, E.R., 1948.** A study of equine fistulous withers and poll evil. *American Journal of Veterinary Research*, 9, 5–10.

24 **SCANLAN, C.M., 1988.** *Introduction to Veterinary Bacteriology*. Ames, Iowa: Iowa State University Press.

25 **SCHAAL, K.P., 1986.** Genus *Actinomyces*. *In:* SNEATH, P.H.A., MAIR, N.S., SHARPE, M.E. & HOLT, J.G., (eds). *Bergey's Manual of Systematic Bacteriology*. Baltimore, London: Williams & Wilkins.

26 **SCHAAL, K.P. & PAPE, W., 1980.** Special methodological problems in antibiotic susceptibility testing of fermentative Actinomycetes. *Infection*, 8, Supplement 176–182.

27 **STEVENSON, R.G. & TAYLOR, R.G., 1977.** Actinomycosis of the trachea in a mature cow. *Canadian Veterinary Journal*, 18, 278–280.

28 **TIMONEY, J.F., GILLESPIE, J.H., SCOTT, F.W. & BARLOUGH, J.E., 1988.** *Hagan and Bruner's Microbiology and Infectious Diseases of Domestic Animals*. 8th edn. Ithaca and London: Comstock Publishing Associates.

29 **VAN AMSTEL, S.R., 1992.** Department of Medicine, Faculty of Veterinary Science, Onderstepoort. Personal communication.

30 **VAWTER, L.R., 1946.** Pulmonary actinomycosis in swine. *Journal of the American Veterinary Medical Association*, 109, 198–203.

31 **WATTS, T.C., OLSON, S.M. & RHODES, C.S., 1973.** Treatment of bovine actinomycosis with isoniazid. *Canadian Veterinary Journal*, 14, 223–224.

170

Actinomyces pyogenes *infections*

Synonym: *Corynebacterium pyogenes* infections

M.G. Collett and G.F. Bath

Introduction

Actinomyces (Corynebacterium) pyogenes occurs in a great variety of suppurative or pyogenic conditions in livestock, either as a primary pathogen, secondary invader or part of a mixed infection with obligate anaerobes. It is most commonly incriminated as a cause of abscesses, wound infections, pneumonia, arthritis, mastitis, foot infections, osteomyelitis of vertebral bodies, 'pituitary abscessation', abortion, perinatal mortalities, and genital infections. It is the bacterium most frequently isolated from suppurative lesions in farm animals in South Africa.[34]

Aetiology

Actinomyces pyogenes is a non-motile, non-sporulating, facultatively anaerobic, slender, pleomorphic coccobacillus which shows varying degrees of Gram-positivity.[92] There appears to be only a single serovar.[77]

Actinomyces pyogenes is nutritionally fastidious and grows poorly on common laboratory media unless they have been supplemented with blood or serum.[62, 76] On blood agar, colonies are small, translucent and usually dense after 24 hours' incubation when isolated from pus. After 48 hours, single colonies are approximately 0,5 – 1,0 mm in diameter and are light grey. A narrow zone of pale ß-haemolysis is usually visible by 36 hours and most isolates typically liquefy inspissated serum. To improve the isolation rate, neomycin (0,6 – 0,7 units/ml), polymyxin B sulphate (25 units/ml) or 0,1 per cent Tween 80 can be added to the medium.[35] A chemically defined medium which supports rapid growth of the organism has been developed.[68]

Actinomyces pyogenes can survive for at least ten days at room temperature in moist debris.[4]

Pathogenesis

Little is known about the antigens of *A. pyogenes* or the local or systemic immune responses that are induced in the host.[97] *Actinomyces pyogenes* produces a haemolytic protein exotoxin.[12, 54] This filterable haemolysin is fatal to mice and rabbits after intravenous injection and is dermotoxic to guinea-pigs.[55, 72, 77] The toxic and haemolytic activities of crude cell extracts are neutralized by an antitoxin[77] which is found in the sera of infected animals.[67] High levels of antitoxin, however, do not protect against pyogenic infection.[40] The organism also produces enzymes, such as protease and neuraminidase,[50] and possesses lectin-like surface structures and plasma protein-binding and bacteriocin-like properties[50] which potentially aid in its pathogenicity and virulence[48] and may account for its ability to survive phagocytosis,[51] but they are not efficient as immunogens.[17] The bacterium also has an antigen which cross-reacts with *Mycobacterium paratuberculosis*.[92]

In the presence of opsonizing antibodies in serum[98] or milk-whey,[97] *A. pyogenes* is highly susceptible to the bactericidal activity of neutrophils *in vitro*. In the female genital tract, local *A. pyogenes* infection stimulates uterine antibody synthesis (mainly IgG and IgA) in the absence of an increase in serum antibody.[99] The bacterium does not elaborate chemotactic substances.[98] On the other hand, *Bacteroides* spp. *in vitro* inhibit chemotaxis[1] and phagocytosis by neutrophils,[41] suggesting that, in mixed infections, the presence of *Bacteroides* spp. (which are obligate anaerobes) could allow the persistence of *A. pyogenes* infection through the protection of the latter from neutrophil phagocytosis.[98]

There is also a synergistic relationship between *A. pyogenes* and another obligate anaerobe, *Fusobacterium necrophorum*. The presence of *A. pyogenes* in the tissues lowers the oxidation-reduction potential in the affected areas while producing a diffusable factor which stimulates the growth of *F. necrophorum*.[70] The latter, in turn, produces a leukotoxin which protects both organisms from phagocytosis.[69] In mixed infections, *F. necrophorum* is probably the primary invasive and necrotizing agent that facilitates the establishment and growth of bacteria such as *A. pyogenes* and *Bacteroides* spp.[69, 70]

Epidemiology, clinical signs and pathology

Actinomyces pyogenes is a commensal on the mucosal surfaces of healthy animals.[77] For example, it occurs on the mucosa of the preputium of rams[43] and that of the alimentary, urogenital and respiratory tracts of healthy cattle, and in the udder of normal cows.[60, 62, 77]

Damage to tissues, such as that resulting from trauma or viral or other bacterial infections, is usually required to establish infection. Abscesses may occur in virtually every organ or tissue in the body, and the clinical signs manifested by affected animals are related to the disturbance of function of the affected part. Abscesses usually develop rapidly and are generally fluctuant when mature. They contain pus which is greenish-yellow or greyish, has a fluid consistency, and is usually malodorous; their capsules are not as well developed as those of abscesses caused by *Corynebacterium pseudotuberculosis*.[26, 39]

In southern Africa, lesions associated with *A. pyogenes* infection in livestock occur most commonly in the sites mentioned below.

Mammary gland

Single or multiple abscesses may be found in the skin and subcutaneous tissues of the posterior aspect of the mammary glands in milk goats and cows. These are frequently associated with the lesions caused by tick bites, particularly those with long mouth parts, such as *Amblyomma hebraeum*, which is prone to attach in the perineal and genital regions of its host and in itself causes severe lesions, especially if numerous. The abscesses may rupture outwards to the externum, or internally into the mammary tissue, resulting in mastitis, toxaemia and even death.

So-called 'summer mastitis', which affects lactating and non-lactating cows, and heifers, occurs at any time of the year in southern Africa.[33] Although *A. pyogenes* is frequently present in the lesion, it is seldom isolated in pure culture,[86] and other bacteria, such as *Peptostreptococcus indolicus, Fusobacterium necrophorum, Bacteroides melaninogenicus, Streptococcus dysgalactiae, Streptococcus agalactiae*, and a microaerophilic coccus also play a role in the pathogenesis of the condition.[56, 86, 93] Damage to a teat tip probably predisposes to infection,[79] while flies probably also play an important role in the transmission of the disease.[79, 93] Affected quarters of the udder are swollen, hard and painful, and the regional lymph nodes are enlarged. The animals are febrile, depressed, anorexic and have an increased heart rate.[8] Abscesses often rupture to the exterior near the base of the teat, resulting in the development of fistulae which discharge a foul-smelling, thick, greenish to greyish-yellow pus. Extensive necrosis of the udder may cause part of it to slough. A necrotizing, suppurative galactophoritis may progress to abscess formation, fibrosis and stenosis or obliteration of the teat canal. The milk of affected cows has a characteristic putrid odour. Initially, the secretion is serous, cloudy or flocculent, but it later becomes purulent and greenish to chocolate-brown.[8, 32, 33, 45, 86] Cows suffering from summer mastitis may abort,[85, 86] or the foetuses may become macerated following intra-uterine death.[58] The disease is serious and the mortality rate can be as high as 50 per cent if animals are not appropriately treated.[8] In survivors, the affected portions of the udder become indurated and abscesses may persist for extended periods.[8]

Central nervous system

A highly fatal neurological disorder known as the hypophyseal or pituitary abscess syndrome is sporadically encountered in cattle, goats, sheep and pigs.[65, 66] It is characterized, in the majority of cases, by the development of a suppurative meningitis of the ventral aspect of the brain and abscessation with or without involvement of the pituitary gland itself and adjacent brain stem. In some, however, primary abscessation in the pituitary gland itself is the primary cause of the syndrome. *Actinomyces pyogenes*, either alone or as part of a mixed infection with other organisms such as *Streptococcus* spp., *Pasteurella* spp., *Fusobacterium necrophorum, Pseudomonas aeruginosa, Staphylococcus aureus*, a *Haemophilus* sp. and others, is the most common bacterium isolated from the lesions.[4, 65, 66] *Mycoplasma arginini* has been isolated in pure culture from lesions in a goat.[52] While the pathogenesis of the syndrome remains to be elucidated, it seems probable that the most common routes that organisms use to reach the parts concerned are venous, arterial or lymphogenous, the infection being secondary to a chronic suppurative process elsewhere in the body.[65, 66] A complex mesh of arterioles, known as the *rete mirabile*, surrounds the pituitary gland of cattle, goats, sheep and pigs. The *rete mirabile* and the pituitary are bathed in a venous bed, the cavernous sinus, which is part of the sinuses of the dura mater. By means of diploic veins which transverse the bones of the skull, these sinuses are connected to the subcutaneous veins of the head.[65] As they are valveless, blood in them can flow in both directions. It is thought that the complex vascular dynamics make this part susceptible to the embolic deposition of bacteria. In addition, bacteria might invade via lymphatics,[65, 66] as the existence of a communication between the cerebrospinal fluid and the lymphatic system has been documented, particularly in the area of the nasal mucosa and the cribriform plate. Another route of entry for bacteria is by direct extension of an otitis interna.[42]

In South Africa, the pituitary abscess syndrome is most frequently encountered in goats, particularly horned individuals, in which it seems to be associated with the attachment of ticks, such as *Rhipicephalus evertsi*, to the skin of the head, especially that of the caudal aspects at the base of the horns. It is thought that the tick bites provide a portal of entry for pyogenic bacteria which are responsible for the development of a suppurative inflammatory process in the skin and subcutis, with subsequent venous distribution of the bacteria to the cavernous sinus. It is possible that some cases of the syndrome in cattle may also be associated with the attachment of ticks, such as *R. evertsi*, to the skin of the head and ears. Cases in cattle have been associated with septic rhinitis which had developed after nose-ringing.[65] Other primary sites of bacterial infection thought to have played a possible role include polyarthritis, sinusitis, suppurative nephritis, mastitis, pneumonia, tooth abscess, and parotid, mediastinal and mandibular lymph node abscessation.[65, 66]

The clinical signs resemble those of heartwater to some extent, and for this reason many cases in southern Africa are possibly misdiagnosed. A wide variety of signs are manifested by affected animals; this precludes the description of a 'typical' case. Signs include several of the following: depression, blindness, pupil-diameter abnormalities, absent pupillary light reflex, ventrolateral strabismus, nystagmus, dropped jaw, decreased tongue tone, facial paralysis, head-tilt, dysphagia, head-pressing, circling, ataxia, lateral recumbency, opisthotonus and paddling movements of the legs. There is usually no fever or evidence of pituitary endocrine disturbances. Recovery of these animals is unusual; most die within days. Treatment is usually of no avail, and for this reason is generally not advocated. It should be borne in mind that by the time the clinical signs are manifested or death has occurred, the ticks which may have played a pathogenetic role may already have detached.

Cerebral abscesses due to *A. pyogenes* may arise following severe *Oestrus ovis* infestation or otitis in sheep,[39, 88] or as a complication of dehorning in cattle.[88] Animals suffering from epidural or subdural abscesses of the spinal cord, which will probably have arisen from septic embolism, may present with similar signs (see below) to those associated with vertebral body abscesses.[88]

Gastrointestinal tract

The migratory tracts of *Oesophagostomum* spp. larvae are often associated with miliary abscesses caused by *A. pyogenes* in the wall of the intestine.

The nozzles of dosing guns, particularly if burred, may penetrate the pharyngeal mucosa and cause injuries which, if infected, may result in purulent inflammation and abscessation. The severity and extent of the lesions are greatly aggravated if the material that is administered is an irritant. The inflammatory process may extend to the facial and peripharyngeal tissues or down the neck in the loose peri-oesophageal and other connective tissues as far as the thoracic inlet. Affected animals have difficulty in swallowing or eating, and the infected tissues are often markedly swollen.

The awns of various grass seeds, including those of *Themeda triandra* ('rooigras'), *Stipagrostis* and *Aristida* spp. ('steekgras'), *Heteropogon contortus* (assegai grass) and *Hordeum murinum* (wild barley or jackal tail), the seeds of *Bidens pilosa* (blackjack), the spines of prickly pears (*Opuntia* spp.) and other thorny plants (e.g. *Acacia* spp.), and fibrous weed material (e.g. *Salvia reflexa*)[46, 74, 91] used as a bedding material may injure the buccal mucous membranes or the skin. The abscesses and suppurative lesions[20] which develop in the buccal and pharyngeal regions can be complicated by pneumonia.[74] Lesions in the tissues of the lips and cheeks may interfere with mastication because of the pain and inhibition of movement of the parts due to intense fibroplasia and induration.

Skin and adnexa

Abscesses in the skin and adnexa and in the regional lymph nodes are common in those parts of southern Africa where infestation with ticks possessing long mouth parts, such as *Amblyomma* spp., *Hyalomma* spp. and *Rhipicephalus* spp., are common. The percutaneous migration of helminth larvae, such as *Strongyloides* spp., as well as blowfly (*Lucilia* spp.) strike may result in purulent inflammation and abscessation.

The lesions of lumpy skin disease[33] and foot-and-mouth disease[100] may become secondarily infected with *A. pyogenes*.

Awns of certain plant seeds often penetrate the skin of those ventral aspects of the body which are most exposed to them, and the resulting lesions act as portals of entry for bacteria (often *A. pyogenes*).[46] Subcutaneous abscesses are usually miliary and may cause severe discomfort, anorexia, loss of body weight and death. The seeds of blackjacks, 'kakiebos' (*Tagetes minuta*), and some grasses, such as *Aristida* and *Heteropogon* spp., may penetrate the skin of woolled sheep in great numbers. These are easily seen in the subcutis when the animal is skinned. On histopathological examination, plant-awn material is frequently detected inside pyogranulomas or abscesses.[74]

Heavy adult sheep, particularly pregnant ewes continually exposed to excessive moisture when grazing on lush, wet pastures, may develop maceration of the interdigital skin. This predisposes to the penetration of bacteria and the development of interdigital dermatitis, which may progress and lead to 'foot abscess' and contagious footrot.[71, 103] Lesions caused by tick bites and plant awns, or other sharp objects, may also predispose to these conditions. It is possible that a degree of vascular stasis, which occurs in the digital cushion and interdigital dermis of the hind feet of pregnant ewes, may also predispose to foot infections.[71] In cattle, necrobacillosis of the foot (also known as panaritium or foul-in-the-foot) is caused by a mixed infection of *F. necrophorum* and *Prevotella (Bacteroides) melaninogenica* **[see Chapter 145: *Fusobacterium necrophorum, Dichelobacter* (*Bacteroides*) *nodosus* and *Bacteroides* spp. infections]**.

Contagious foot rot in small ruminants, on the other hand, is caused by *Dichelobacter (Bacteroides) nodosus* infection in association with *Fusobacterium necrophorum* and other bacteria. Ovine 'foot abscess' (which comprises 'toe abscess'), in which the lamellae of the hoof are affected, and 'heel-abscess' (or infective bulbar necrosis), in which the soft bulbar tissues of the digital cushion are involved,[71] is caused by a combined infection involving *Fusobacterium necrophorum* and *A. pyogenes* **(see Chapter 145)**.[102]

In sheep suffering from foot abscess, severe lameness is the outstanding sign and the affected foot is carried. Usually only one claw (particularly of the hind foot) is affected, but more than one may be involved.[102] The hoof is usually not affected in the early stages, but it does become involved as the disease advances, and may become progressively deformed. Viscous, semi-liquid necrotic tissue may be expressed from the bulb of the heel through irregular openings in the interdigital skin, or the abaxial coronary band may bulge and rupture at focal areas to discharge greyish, blood-stained necrotic debris. The discharge eventually becomes more purulent.[102] These areas may granulate and heal, only to fistulate again at the same site or elsewhere in the coronary skin. The interdigital infection spreads very easily to the coffin (distal interphalangeal) joint because the dorsal and palmar/plantar joint pouches extend up above the horn into the coronary area.[101] The necrotizing infection in the distal interphalangeal joint may cause the axial collateral and interdigital ligaments to rupture, resulting in luxation of the distal phalanx and distal sesamoid bone.[102] The pastern joint may also become involved. The course of foot abscess is about two months; slight lameness generally persists and, if ligaments were damaged, deformity of the digit may be permanent.[71, 102, 103]

Neonatal piglets maintained on abrasive floors without bedding may develop lameness as a result of the development of foot abscesses mainly in the hind limbs, the medial claws in particular being infected. Bruising and erosion of the sole of the foot allows the penetration of polymicrobic infections which commonly include *A. pyogenes*, *F. necrophorum* and *Bacteroides* spp.[25] In severe cases, the infection in the digits may progress to necrotic pododermatitis, osteomyelitis, arthritis and/or tendosynovitis.[25]

Respiratory and cardiovascular systems

The trauma caused by barley (*Hordeum vulgare*) awns has been suspected of initiating the development of chronic laryngeal abscessation which leads to severe laryngeal oedema, characteristic roaring respiratory sounds and eventual death by suffocation.[13]

Actinomyces pyogenes in sheep, goats and cattle causes a chronic, purulent pneumonia and pulmonary abscesses which may extend to involve the pleura, resulting in the formation of a dense, adhesive, suppurative pleuritis or pyothorax with a foul-smelling exudate **(Figure 170)**.[19, 33] The pulmonary lesions may be accompanied by the presence of metastatic abscesses elsewhere in the body.

In the pulmonary embolic aneurysm (or pulmonary arterial thromboembolism) syndrome in cattle, septic emboli that have originated most commonly from a purulent thrombophlebitis of the caudal vena cava or a large hepatic vein, possibly as a sequel to traumatic reticulopericarditis, lodge in a pulmonary artery, with the development of septic embolism or even aneurysm as consequence. Rupture of the vessel results in pneumorrhagia, haemoptysis, epistaxis and death. Pneumorrhagia may similarly be caused if a large blood vessel ruptures into a bronchus as a result of the erosion of its wall following pressure exerted on it by a primary lung abscess.

Calf diphtheria, an acute to chronic necrotic laryngitis traditionally considered to be caused by *F. necrophorum*, has occasionally been shown to result from a mixed

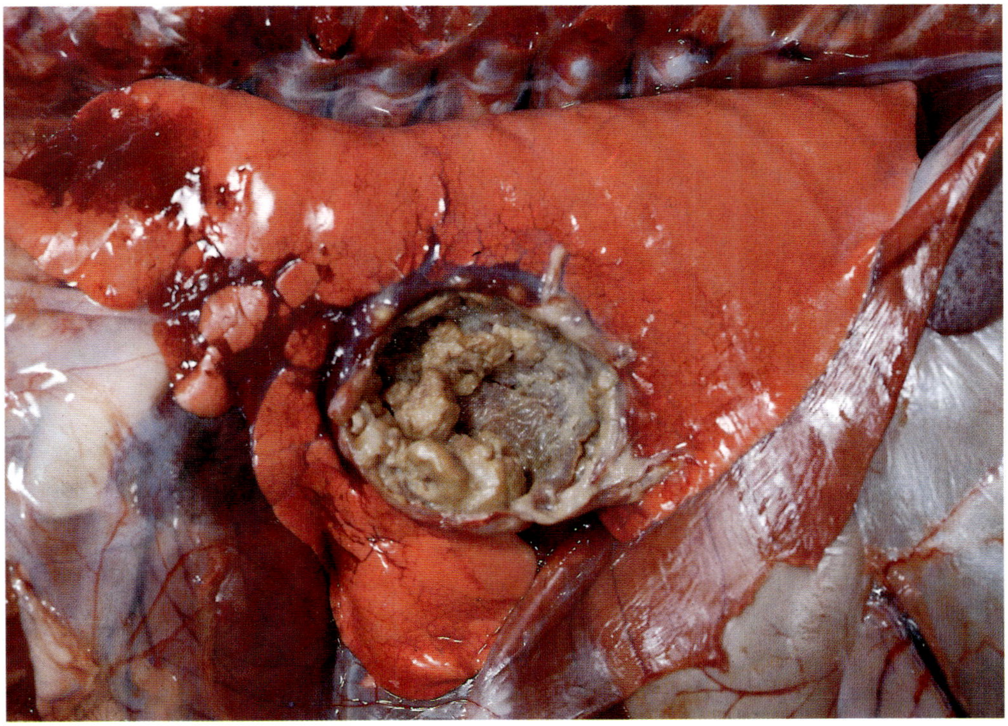

Figure 170.1 Large abscess caused by infection with *Actinomyces pyogenes* in the lung of a sheep

infection of *F. necrophorum* with *A. pyogenes* and possibly a *Bacteroides* sp.[63]

Actinomyces pyogenes may also cause valvular and mural endocarditis and chronic heart failure in cattle and sometimes also in pigs. Large, vegetative, firm but friable masses develop on the atrioventricular valves or the mural endocardium. These lesions result in chronic passive congestion manifested by dependent oedema, transudation into body cavities, oedema of the abomasal wall, and cyanotic induration of the liver. Despite extensive lesions in the heart, an electrocardiogram may be normal, and auscultation frequently does not reveal any evidence of cardiac murmurs.[10] Endocarditis arises following embolic spread from such lesions as hepatic abscesses and purulent metritis, mastitis or traumatic reticulopericarditis. Emboli originating from valvular endocarditis may be responsible for the development of septic infarcts and abscesses in the brain, lungs and kidneys, and osteomyelitis and septic arthritis.[57, 73]

Pigs with atrophic rhinitis, mycoplasmal pneumonia or porcine pleuropneumonia,[19, 33, 38] sheep and goats suffering from jaagsiekte or pasteurellosis, and cattle affected by pasteurellosis or infectious bovine rhinotracheitis may develop secondary *A. pyogenes* infection which culminates in the development of a fibrinopurulent bronchopneumonia or pleuropneumonia.

Skeletal system

Unhygienic environmental conditions may result in the infection of umbilical, docking and castration wounds in new-born animals and a subsequent spread to joints, vertebral bodies and other sites in the body.

Actinomyces pyogenes is one of the causes of purulent arthritis in lambs, kids, calves, and pigs. Lameness is the outstanding clinical sign and, on palpation, affected joints are painful, hot and swollen. Only a few joints are generally involved. In chronic cases, the affected joints develop ankylosis and are thickened, in which case their movements are severely restricted; the joint capsule may even be partially mineralized.

Spinal epidural abscesses, tracking abscesses within the spinal cord, and purulent vertebral osteomyelitis followed by vertebral body abscessation and/or discospondylitis are quite common in lambs, kids and calves.[22, 39, 78, 81, 88] These lesions may occur in the cervical, thoracic or lumbar regions and usually involve a single vertebral body or intervertebral disc. Adjacent vertebrae may also be affected.[22] Since there are connections between the vertebral and the caval, portal and pulmonary venous systems, infection may arise from metastatic spread from pneumonic lesions, liver abscesses or omphalophlebitis.[22, 81] Clinically, these animals develop a progressive posterior paresis and paralysis which culminates in paraplegia or tetraparesis. Affected animals are normally bright and alert and, if only paraplegic, may drag themselves around using their fore legs. *Staphylococcus* spp. may also be the cause of vertebral body abscesses.[22]

Actinomyces pyogenes infection is also associated with vertebral body osteomyelitis with, in some cases, abscessation in adult cattle, pigs and, more rarely, sheep. The infection in most of these cases is assumed to be a result of haematogenous spread of bacteria from a primary site elsewhere in the body, the latter often not being established. In beef cattle in South Africa, particularly in bushveld (savannah) regions, it may at times become an economically significant problem in some herds. One unsubstantiated hypothesis as to its pathogenesis is three-pronged:[94] the primary site of the bacteria is infected skin lesions created by tick infestations, particularly when these are severe. Other infected skin wounds may also play a role, such as injuries by sharp projections in poorly constructed crushes or spray-races. These lead to periodic episodes of bacteraemia in which the bacteria may localize in distant sites, particularly if a preceding lesion is present (*locus minores resistentiae*). The second factor is the presence of nutritional osteomalacia, generally subclinical, due to a phosphorus deficiency which, unless remedied, is common in parts of the subcontinent. This creates a situation in which microfractures (or even frank fractures) of bone are liable to develop. The localized bone trauma, often accompanied by a resultant haemorrhage, forms a ready site for the localization of bacteria in the blood stream. Managemental procedures play the role of the third factor. Important amongst these is the driving of fractious animals into crushes or races during dipping, spraying, dosing or inoculation procedures. It frequently happens that cattle attempt to escape from a crush by turning or jumping, and this may lead to injuries which could include microfractures in a vertebra. In straining to turn, or jumping, the lumbar region is often the most severely stressed part, which is the reason why — according to this hypothesis — one or more lumbar vertebral bodies are the most frequently affected. The suppurative osteomyelitis which develops may result in pathological fracture with collapse or partial collapse of the vertebral body and pressure on the spinal cord, or the infection may extend to adjacent structures outside the bony tissue. Extension into the spinal canal may result in either cranial or caudal spread of the infection or its localization as an epidural abscess.[44] In many cases, however, the exudate remains confined to the vertebra by the periosteum as an encapsulated abscess which protrudes into the spinal canal, with subsequent compression malacia of the spinal cord. Clinical signs in such an animal are those of a progressively developing paresis and paralysis of the limbs. As many lesions are in the lumbar or thoracolumbar region, the hind limbs are most frequently involved, the final outcome being their complete paralysis. Affected animals assume a 'dog-sitting' position — hence the Afrikaans name 'sitsiekte' — as they are still able to maintain an upright sitting position by the use of their fore limbs.[94]

Mandibular osteomyelitis caused by *Actinomyces bovis*

('lumpy jaw') **(see Chapter 169: *Actinomyces bovis* infections)** may be complicated by other bacteria, such as *A. pyogenes* and *F. necrophorum*.[44] In Brazil, a serious infectious periodontitis of calves, called 'cara inchada' (swollen face), is caused by *Prevotella (Bacteroides) melaninogenica* and *A. pyogenes* and is associated with the altered ecological soil conditions that follow the clearing of forests and the establishment of cultivated pastures (*Panicum maximum* in particular).[7, 18] Nutritional secondary hyperparathyroidism also plays a role.[7] The bacteria produce enzymes and endotoxins that damage periodontal tissues, leading to a purulent periodontitis and secondary ossifying alveolar periostitis.[18]

Complications of tail-biting in young pigs include embolic pneumonia,[95] spinal epidural abscessation and vertebral osteomyelitis,[22, 64] cerebral abscesses[96] and septic embolic lesions elsewhere.[88] Organisms isolated from these cases include *A. pyogenes*, *Staphylococcus* spp., haemolytic *Streptococcus* spp., *Erysipelothrix rhusiopathiae* and coliforms.[22, 95, 96]

Apart from purulent arthritis, *A. pyogenes* also causes cervical lymphadenitis and abscesses in pigs.[90] Abscesses in this species are most frequently the result of mixed infections of anaerobic and facultatively anaerobic bacteria, in particular *Bacteroides* spp. and *A. pyogenes*.[5]

Liver

Omphalophlebitis due to *A. pyogenes* infection in neonatal lambs, kids and calves commonly results in the development of metastatic hepatic abscesses. In older animals, particularly cattle, hepatic abscessation may originate metastatically from *A. pyogenes*-infected lesions of traumatic reticulopericarditis, directly from penetrating foreign bodies from the reticulum,[3] or after rumenitis e.g. as a result of acidosis. In the latter case, the predominant bacteria are *F. necrophorum* or *A. pyogenes*, or fungi belonging to the Mucorales, including *Mucor, Absidia* and *Rhizopus* spp.[51]

Genital system and perinatal mortalities

In sheep, *A. pyogenes* is one of the causes of perinatal mortalities (omphalitis, pyaemia, pneumonia, myo- and pericarditis, meningitis, arthritis, and cerebral and liver abscesses), and sporadic abortions.[6, 16] The latter are characterized by the development of severe placentitis, and foetal death is believed to be due to the resulting hypoxia. The placentitis is manifested by oedema and a mottled-red, brown and white appearance of some of the cotyledons and carbuncles caused by microabscesses, foci of necrosis and mineralization. Numerous Gram-positive bacteria occur in affected portions of the placenta.[84] The aborted foetuses are usually autolysed or mummified.

Actinomyces pyogenes may also be isolated from the vagina[35, 62] and uterus[28] of apparently healthy cows, and it has been isolated from semen.[30] Embryonic death and abortion due to primary *A. pyogenes* infection occurs sporadically in cows.[35, 36, 47, 59, 80, 82, 89] The uterus may become infected either by the ascending route (via the vagina) or haematogenously.[35, 47, 80] Foetal infection occurs, but is not a consistent feature of *A. pyogenes* abortion.[47] Abortion may be accompanied by an increase in uterine tone, dilatation of the cervix, a mucopurulent vulval discharge and persistence of the corpus luteum.[80] Cows that abort may be afebrile and have a normal habitus.[80] Primary *A. pyogenes* abortion may be complicated by retained placenta, pyometra and possible subsequent sterility, or by pneumonia, mastitis, arthritis, septicaemia and death.[35, 47] A bronchopneumonia is usually found in aborted foetuses.[53]

Congenital *A. pyogenes* infection may cause ulcerative keratitis and blindness in calves.[83]

Most cows acquire uterine infections in the immediate post-partum period.[9, 27, 87] In many, the infection is secondary and is acquired as a result of direct contamination from the externum in conjunction with retention of the foetal membranes.[23, 47] *Actinomyces pyogenes* infection is the most serious cause of post-parturient endometritis in cows, and it may progress to purulent metritis, toxaemia or septicaemia and death.[15, 23, 31] Obligate anaerobes, such as *P. melaninogenica* and *F. necrophorum* may also be present,[21, 61] and these act synergistically with *A. pyogenes* in causing endometritis and pyometra.[21, 75] Post-parturient endometritis is a major cause of delayed reconception,[24] and nearly 50 per cent of infected cows have to be culled because of infertility.[87] Metastatic septic emboli originating from an infected uterus may lodge on the heart valves and in joints, tendon sheaths or lungs. Other complications of the infection include pyelonephritis, uterine abscesses, pyometra, salpingitis, pyosalpinx, stenosis of the Fallopian tubes, and ovarian adhesions.[24, 45]

In animals suffering from pyometra, several litres of thick, mucinous, greyish-yellow to greyish-green pus accumulate in the uterus and the uterine wall is thick, doughy and paretic.[45] A profuse mucopurulent vulval discharge is often present. Affected cows do not exhibit oestrus because of the persistence of the corpus luteum which accompanies the condition.[21] Histopathologically the endometrium contains cystic glands, a neutrophil infiltration, necrosis, abscesses, and eventually periglandular fibrosis.[9]

Orchitis and epididymitis in rams, bulls and boars has been ascribed to *A. pyogenes* infection, as has chronic interstitial seminal vesiculitis in bulls.[49]

Actinomyces pyogenes is one of the causes of abortion, metritis and vaginal discharges in sows.[90] Uterine infections due to *A. pyogenes* in mares occasionally result in metritis and abortion.

Diagnosis

The clinical signs of *A. pyogenes* infections in animals depend on the size, severity and location of the lesions. A diagnosis should be confirmed by the isolation of the bacterium from specimens of affected tissues or organs.

To confirm a diagnosis of hypophyseal abscessation at necropsy it is often necessary to expose the pituitary gland by making an incision through the *diaphragma sellae* of the dura mater which covers the gland.

If *A. pyogenes* is the cause of an abortion, it is readily isolated from foetal organs, placenta or vaginal mucus.[35, 84] Foetal lung is a useful specimen for bacteriology and histopathology in the confirmation of the cause of abortion, as *A. pyogenes* usually causes foetal bronchopneumonia.[53]

Differential diagnosis

The differential diagnosis depends on the particular presenting syndrome. Purulent processes and abscesses are caused by many species of pyogenic bacteria, the most common being *Staphylococcus* spp., *Streptococcus* spp. and *Corynebacterium pseudotuberculosis*, which is the cause of caseous lymphadenitis.

Purulent polyarthritis due to *A. pyogenes* in sheep may mimic polyarthritis due to *Erysipelothrix rhusiopathiae, Streptococcus* spp., *Staphylococcus aureus* and *C. pseudotuberculosis*. The clinical signs in an animal suffering from the pituitary abscess syndrome may resemble those of heartwater, cerebral babesiosis and theileriosis, rabies, listeriosis, cerebrocortical necrosis, lead poisoning, cerebral and other forms of abscessation within the cranium, and thrombotic meningoencephalitis (*Haemophilus somnus* infection) in cattle; and of focal symmetrical encephalomalacia and heartwater in sheep and goats. Other encephalitides and space-occupying lesions should also be considered.[65]

Orchitis or epididymitis caused by *A. pyogenes* in rams should be differentiated from the lesions caused by microorganisms such as *Brucella ovis, Histophilus ovis, Actinobacillus seminis, C. pseudotuberculosis* and *Chlamydia psittaci*, and from non-infectious spermatic granulomas and varicoceles.

Foot abscess should be differentiated from foot rot (*Dichelobacter nodosus* infection), ovine interdigital dermatitis ('foot scald'), strawberry footrot (*Dermatophilus congolensis* infection), laminitis, and from foot lesions caused by bluetongue, injuries and joint-ill.

In sheep, abortion due to *A. pyogenes* should be differentiated from that caused by certain viruses, such as Rift Valley fever and Akabane and related Simbu-group viruses, *Salmonella* serovars, *Campylobacter* spp., *Listeria monocytogenes, Coxiella burnetii, Toxoplasma gondii*, and *Chlamydia psittaci*. Bacteria other than *A. pyogenes* which cause uterine infections in cows include *Escherichia coli* and other coliforms, *Pasteurella* spp., *Streptococcus* spp.[9, 29, 87] and *Rhodococcus equi*.[14] Uterine infections or abortion caused by *A. pyogenes* in mares should be differentiated from bacterial, rickettsial, protozoal and viral infections that cause reproductive failure **(see Chapter 189: Infectious causes of equine reproductive failure)**.

Although *A. pyogenes* is a frequent cause of vertebral osteomyelitis in cattle, other bacteria, such as *F. necrophorum, Staphylococcus* spp., *Streptococcus* spp. and coliforms may also be implicated.[22] Differential diagnoses of this syndrome also include fracture of a vertebral body, nutritional muscular dystrophy, 'dumb' rabies, *Haemophilus somnus* infection, *Hypoderma bovis* infestation, meningitis of any cause, spinal lymphosarcoma, the downer cow syndrome, and certain hereditary conditions, such as progressive ataxia in Charolais, degenerative myeloencephalopathy in Brown Swiss cattle, and congenital spinal dysraphism.[22, 81]

Differential diagnoses for paraplegia caused by vertebral body abscesses in pigs include trauma, and organic arsenic or organic mercurial poisonings.[22]

In sheep, conditions which may be confused clinically with vertebral osteomyelitis and abscessation include swayback (which is a copper deficiency), white muscle disease, tick paralysis caused by *Rhipicephalus evertsi* or *Ixodes rubicundus*, botulism, hypocalcaemia, trauma and *Coenuris cerebralis* (particularly cysts of *Taenia multiceps* located in the spinal column).

Control

Tick control is of major importance in the control of subcutaneous abscesses, 'pituitary abscessation' and abscesses in the skin of the udder of domestic ruminants. Sites of tick attachment, such as behind the horns and the escutcheon, should be sprayed regularly with an acaricide. Dehorning goats, or the breeding of polled goats, can be considered where 'pituitary abscessation' is a problem. Acaricide footbaths or pour-ons should be used where ticks on the feet have caused abscesses. Appropriate anthelmintics will control *Oesophagostomum* infestation.

Strict hygiene must be applied when docking or castrating, particularly when elastic rings are used for castration. Omphalophlebitis and subsequent pyaemia may be prevented by the disinfection of the umbilical stump with povidone iodine at birth and again four hours later.[78] Pregnant animals should not be permitted to give birth on infected premises.

It may be necessary to avoid certain pastures or veld types at certain times of the year in order to lower the exposure of animals, particularly woolled sheep, to plant awns and seeds. The point of the nozzle of dosing guns must be free of burrs and, in order to prevent injury to the pharyngeal region while dosing, the nozzle must not be forced to the back of the mouth — it must be borne in mind that many animals jump forward during the dosing process.

Abscesses which are accessible to surgical intervention should preferably be excised intact.[26] Alternatively, they may be lanced and drained (following local or general anaesthesia), and the abscess cavity packed with iodine gauze or flushed with povidone iodine, hydrogen peroxide or chlorhexidine.[26]

In sheep with foot abscesses, surgical drainage and

irrigation of the lesion with chlorhexidine antiseptic solution can be attempted; the foot should be bandaged to prevent further contamination and to reduce splaying of the affected digit.[71, 102] Systemic antibiotic treatment can be instituted where lesions are in the acute stage. Formalin (3–5 per cent) footbaths can be utilized on a weekly basis to reduce the incidence of foot infections.

Purulent arthritis may be treated surgically by external drainage and repeated flushing of the joint with antimicrobials, but the prognosis is guarded. Prolonged systemic treatment of such cases with a long-acting oxytetracycline may sterilize the infection, but affected joints rarely recover function completely.

The antimicrobial sensitivity data about *A. pyogenes* available in the literature is scant. Although it does appear to be sensitive *in vitro* to the effects of penicillin G, cloxacillin, ampicillin and the cephalosporins, and variably sensitive to the tetracyclines, macrolides and sulphonamides,[7, 37, 77, 92] the response to treatment of cases with antimicrobials is generally disappointing.[26]

Since obligate anaerobic bacteria, such as *P. melaninogenica* and *F. necrophorum*, are frequently present in cases of *A. pyogenes* infection,[21, 75] metronidazole treatment can be considered when the expense is justified. Use of metronidazole eliminates the anaerobes and, in so doing, reduces their inhibitory effect on neutrophil phagocytosis, thus allowing the host's phagocytic defences to operate against *A. pyogenes*.[41]

Mild cases of *A. pyogenes* endometritis in cows can be treated successfully with intrauterine infusions of gentamicin; however, the problem of tissue and milk residues should be considered.[2, 29] In pyometra with placental retention, the uterine exudate should be siphoned off using a 10 mm diameter tube. Antimicrobial instillation in these cases is of no value, as many antimicrobials are rapidly inactivated by lochial fluids. Parenteral antibacterial drugs are beneficial when systemic signs are present.[24] Cloprostenol (prostaglandin F2α analog) treatment gives excellent results when a corpus luteum is present.[24] Prevention of post-parturient endometritis involves the improvement of hygiene and the rotation of calving paddocks.[24]

In cows suffering from summer mastitis, parenteral treatment with oxytetracyclines can be attempted during the peracute stage, but the response to intensive treatment is usually disappointing.[8] Affected cows should be isolated.[32] Intramammary prophylaxis using semi-synthetic penicillins such as cloxacillin has been very successful.[92]

Attempts to immunize animals effectively by employing *A. pyogenes* cells or toxoid have met with variable results.[11, 67] Although multiple doses of a bacterin-toxoid vaccine of high potency can induce a substantial antibody response,[12] protection against infection is generally poor[17, 40, 86] and use of the vaccine may suppress cell-mediated immunity.[40]

References

1 **ADAMU, S.A. & SPERRY, J.F., 1981.** Polymorphonuclear neutrophil chemotaxis induced and inhibited by *Bacteroides* spp. *Infection and Immunity*, 33, 806–810.

2 **ANETZHOFER, J -V., 1989.** Die behandlung der *Actinomyces pyogenes*-endometritis durch intrauterine Gentaseptin(R)-applikation. *Schweizer Archiv für Tierheilkunde*, 139, 495–498.

3 **BARKER, I.K. & VAN DREUMEL, A.A., 1985.** The alimentary system. *In*: JUBB, K.V.F., KENNEDY, P.C. & PALMER, N., (eds). *Pathology of Domestic Animals*. Vol. II. 3rd edn. New York, London: Academic Press.

4 **BATH, G.F., 1989.** Faculty of Veterinary Science, Onderstepoort 0110, South Africa. Unpublished data.

5 **BENNO, Y., MITSUOKA, T. & SHIRASAKA, S., 1982.** Anaerobic bacteria isolated from abscesses in pigs. *Japanese Journal of Veterinary Science*, 44, 309–315.

6 **BEVERLEY, J.K.A. & WATSON, W.A., 1962.** Further studies on toxoplasmosis and ovine abortion in Yorkshire. *The Veterinary Record*, 74, 548–552.

7 **BLOBEL, H., DÖBEREINER, J., LIMA, F.G.F. & ROSA, I.V., 1984.** Bacterial isolations from 'cara inchada'-lesions of cattle. *Pesquisa Veterinária Brasileira*, 4, 73–77.

8 **BLOOD, D.C. & RADOSTITS, O.M., 1989.** *Veterinary Medicine*. 7th edn. London, Philadelphia: Baillière Tindall.

9 **BONNETT, B.N., MARTIN, S.W., GANNON, V.P.J., MILLER, R.B. & ETHERINGTON, W.G., 1991.** Endometrial biopsy in Holstein-Friesian dairy cows. III. Bacteriological analysis and correlations with histological findings. *Canadian Journal of Veterinary Research*, 55, 168–173.

10 **CABANA, E.M., KELLY, W.R., DANIEL, R.C.W. & O'BOYLE, D.O., 1990.** A case of bovine valvular endocarditis caused by *Corynebacterium pseudodiphtheriticum*. *The Veterinary Record*, 126, 41–42.

11 **CAMERON, C.M., 1966.** *Corynebacterium pyogenes*: The problem of vaccination against infection. *Journal of the South African Veterinary Medical Association*, 37, 11–15.

12 **CAMERON, C.M., BOTHA, W.F. & SMIT, B.H.J., 1976.** Antibody response to and immunity induced by *Corynebacterium pyogenes* vaccine. *Onderstepoort Journal of Veterinary Research*, 43, 97–104.

13 **CAMERON, H.S. & BRITTON, J.W., 1943.** Chronic ovine laryngitis. *Cornell Veterinarian*, 33, 265–268.

14 **CRAIG, J.F. & DAVIES, G.O., 1940.** *Corynebacterium equi* in bovine pyometra. *Veterinary Journal*, 96, 417–419.

15 **DAWSON, F.L.M., 1960.** Bovine endometritis: A review. *British Veterinary Journal*, 116, 448–466.

16 **DENNIS, S.M. & BAMFORD, V.W., 1966.** The role of corynebacteria in perinatal lamb mortality. *The Veterinary Record*, 79, 105–108.

17 **DERBYSHIRE, J.B. & MATTHEWS, P.R.J., 1963.** Immunological studies with *Corynebacterium pyogenes* in mice. *Research in Veterinary Science*, 4, 537–542.

18 **DÖBEREINER, J., 1990.** Zur ätiologie der 'cara inchada' einer parodontalen erkrankung der jungrinder in Brasilien. *Deutsche Tierärztliche Wochenschrift*, 97, 482–490.

19 **DUNGWORTH, D.L., 1985.** The respiratory system. *In*: JUBB, K.V.F., KENNEDY, P.C. & PALMER, N., (eds) *Pathology of Domestic Animals*. Vol. II. 3rd edn. New York, London: Academic Press.

20 **EDGAR, G., 1935.** Mandibular abscess of sheep. *Australian Veterinary Journal*, 11, 19–22.

21 **FARIN, P.W., BALL, L., OLSON, J.D., MORTIMER, R.G., JONES, R.L., ADNEY, W.S. & McCHESNEY, A.E., 1989.** Effect of *Actinomyces pyogenes* and Gram-negative anaerobic bacteria on the development of bovine pyometra. *Theriogenology*, 31, 979–989.

22 **FINLEY, G.G., 1975.** A survey of vertebral abscesses in domestic animals in Ontario. *Canadian Veterinary Journal*, 16, 114–117.

23 **FIVAZ, B.H., 1981.** Current aspects of the post-partum period of the dairy cow. *Zimbabwe Veterinary Journal*, 12, 22–26.

24 **FIVAZ, B.H. & SWANEPOEL, R., 1978.** Bovine post-partum metritis and the reconception period. *Rhodesian Veterinary Journal*, 9, 17–23.

25 **GARDNER, I.A., HIRD, D.W., SULLIVAN, N.M. & PIERCE, R.J., 1990.** Clinical, pathologic, and microbiologic findings of foot abscess in neonatal pigs. *Journal of the American Veterinary Medical Association*, 196, 1791–1794.

26 **GEZON, H.M., BITHER, H.D., HANSON, L.A. & THOMPSON, J.K., 1991.** Epizootic of external and internal abscesses in a large goat herd over a 16-year period. *Journal of the American Veterinary Medical Association*, 198, 257–263.

27 **GRIFFIN, J.F.T., HARTIGAN, P.J. & NUNN, W.R., 1974.** Non-specific uterine infection and bovine fertility. I. Infection patterns and endometritis during the first seven weeks post-partum. *Theriogenology*, 1, 91–106.

28 **GUNTER, J.J, COLLINS, W.J., OWEN, J., SORENSEN, A.M., SCALES, J.W. & ALFORD, J.A., 1955.** A survey of the bacteria in the reproductive tract of dairy animals and their relationship to infertility. *American Journal of Veterinary Research*, 16, 282–285.

29 **HADDAD, N.S., PEDERSOLI, W.M., CARSON, R.L. & RAVIS, W.R., 1986.** Concentrations of gentamicin in serum, milk, urine, endometrium, and skeletal muscle of cows after repeated intrauterine injections. *American Journal of Veterinary Research*, 47, 1597–1601.

30 **HANCOCK, J.L. & KELLY, W.R., 1948.** *Corynebacterium pyogenes* in bull semen. *The Veterinary Record*, 60, 669–670.

31 **HARTIGAN, P.J., GRIFFIN, J.F.T. & NUNN, W.R., 1974.** Some observations of *Corynebacterium pyogenes* infection of the bovine uterus. *Theriogenology*, 1, 153–167.

32 **HEIDRICH, H.J. & RENK, W., 1967.** *Diseases of the Mammary Glands of Domestic Animals*. Philadelphia, London: W.B. Saunders Company.

33 **HENNING, M.W., 1956.** *Animal Diseases in South Africa*. 3rd edn. Pretoria: Central News Agency.

34 **HENTON, M.M., 1989.** Onderstepoort Veterinary Institute, Onderstepoort 0110, South Africa. Unpublished data.

35 **HINTON, M., 1972.** Bovine abortion associated with *Corynebacterium pyogenes*. *Veterinary Bulletin*, 42, 753–756.

36 **HINTON, M., 1974.** *Corynebacterium pyogenes* and bovine abortion. *Journal of Hygiene*, 72, 365–368.

37 **HJERPE, C.A. & ROUTEN, T.A., 1977.** Practical and theoretical considerations concerning treatment of bacterial pneumonia in feedlot cattle, with special reference to antimicrobic therapy. *Proceedings of the Ninth Annual Meeting of the American Association of Bovine Practitioners*, 97–140.

38 **HOIE, S., FALK, K. & LIUM, B.M., 1991.** An abattoir survey of pneumonia and pleuritis in slaughter-weight swine from nine selected herds. IV. Bacteriological findings in chronic pneumonic lesions. *Acta Veterinaria Scandinavica*, 32, 395–402.

39 **HULL, F.E. & TAYLOR, E.L., 1941.** Abscesses affecting the central nervous system of sheep. *American Journal of Veterinary Research*, 2, 356–357.

40 **HUNTER, P., VAN DER LUGT, J.J. & GOUWS, J.J., 1990.** Failure of an *Actinomyces pyogenes* vaccine to protect sheep against an intravenous challenge. *Onderstepoort Journal of Veterinary Research*, 57, 239–241.

41 **INGHAM, H.R., SISSON, P.R., THARAGONNET, D., SELKON, J.B. & CODD, A.A., 1977.** Inhibition of phagocytosis *in vitro* by obligate anaerobes. *The Lancet*, 2, 1252–1254.

42 **INNES, J.R.M. & SAUNDERS, L.Z., 1962.** *Comparative Neuropathology*. New York: Academic Press.

43 **JANSEN, B.C., 1983.** The epidemiology of bacterial infection of the genitalia in rams. *Onderstepoort Journal of Veterinary Research*, 50, 275–282.

44 **JUBB, K.V.F., KENNEDY, P.C. & PALMER, N., 1985.** Bones and joints. In *Pathology of Domestic Animals*. Vol. I. 3rd edn. New York, London: Academic Press.

45 **JUBB, K.V.F., KENNEDY, P.C. & PALMER, N., 1985.** The female genital system. In: *Pathology of Domestic Animals*. Vol. III. 3rd edn. New York, London: Academic Press.

46 **KELLERMAN, T.S., COETZER, J.A.W. & NAUDÉ, T.W., 1988.** *Plant Poisonings and Mycotoxicoses of Livestock in Southern Africa*. Cape Town: Oxford University Press Southern Africa.

47 **KOLAR, J., 1963.** *Corynebacterium pyogenes* à l'origine de l'avortement chez les bovins. *Bulletin de l'Office International des Épizooties*, 60, 341–353.

48 **KUNE, T., TAINAKA, M., SAITO, M., HIRUMA, M., NISHIO, S., KASHIWAZAKI, M., MITANI, K. & NAKAJIMA, Y., 1983.** Research on experimental *Corynebacterium pyogenes* infections in pigs. *Kitasato Archives of Experimental Medicine*, 56, 119–135.

49 **LADDS, P.W., 1985.** The male genital system. *In*: JUBB, K.V.F., KENNEDY, P.C. & PALMER, N., (eds). *Pathology of Domestic Animals*. Vol. III. 3rd edn. New York, London: Academic Press.

50 **LÄMMLER, C., 1990.** Untersuchungen zu möglichen pathogenitätsfaktoren von *Actinomyces pyogenes* Übersichtsreferat. *Berliner und Münchener Tierärztliche Wochenschrift*, 103, 121–125.

51 **LECHTENBERG, K.F., NAGARAJA, T.G., LEIPOLD, H.W. & CHENGAPPA, M.M., 1988.** Bacteriologic and histologic studies of hepatic abscesses in cattle. *American Journal of Veterinary Research*, 49, 58–62.

52 **LOMAS, S.T. & HAZELL, S.L., 1986.** The isolation of *Mycoplasma arginini* from a pituitary abscess in a goat. *Australian Veterinary Journal*, 60, 281–282.

53 **LOPEZ, A., PÉREZ, A. & ANGULO, G., 1989.** Distribution of lesions in the lungs of aborted bovine fetuses. *Canadian Veterinary Journal*, 30, 519–521.

54 **LOVELL, R., 1937.** Studies on *Corynebacterium pyogenes* with special reference to toxin production. *Journal of Pathology and Bacteriology*, 45, 339–355.

55 **LOVELL, R., 1944.** Further studies on the toxin of *Corynebacterium pyogenes*. *Journal of Pathology and Bacteriology*, 56, 525–529.

56 **MADSEN, M., SORENSEN, G.H. & AALBAEK, B., 1990.** Summer mastitis in heifers: A bacteriological examination of secretions from clinical cases of summer mastitis in Denmark. *Veterinary Microbiology*, 22, 319–328.

57 **MAXIE, M.G., 1985.** The urinary system. *In*: JUBB, K.V.F., KENNEDY, P.C. & PALMER, N., (eds). *Pathology of Domestic Animals*. Vol. II. 3rd edn. New York, London: Academic Press.

58 **MAXWELL, H., 1943.** The occurrence in cattle of abortion, macerated fetuses, and acute suppurative mastitis, associated with *Corynebacterium pyogenes*. *Cornell Veterinarian*, 33, 315–318.

59 **MITCHELL, D., 1960.** Bovine abortion — an analysis of 227 cases. *Canadian Veterinary Journal*, 1, 337–343.

60 **NATTERMANN, H. & HORSCH, F., 1977.** Die *Corynebacterium-pyogenes*-infektion des rindes. *Archiv für Experimentelle Veterinärmedizin*, 31, 405–413.

61 **NOAKES, D.E., WALLACE, L.M. & SMITH, G.R., 1990.** Pyometra in a Friesian heifer: Bacteriological and endometrial changes. *The Veterinary Record*, 126, 509.

62 **OCHI, Y. & ZAIZEN, K., 1936.** Studies on *Corynebacterium pyogenes*. I. *Journal of the Japanese Society of Veterinary Science*, 15, 13–14.

63 **PANCIERA, R.J., PERINO, L.J., BALDWIN, C.A.,**

MORTON, R.J. & SWANSON, J.E., 1989. Observations on calf diphtheria in the commercial feedlot. *Agri-practice,* 10, 12–17.

64 **PEELEN, J.P.J., VAN DEN BERG, J., NARUCKA, U., NOUWS, J.F.M., OKMA, B.D. & VERDIJK, A.T.M., 1981.** Afwijkingen bij slachtdieren. I. Wervelfracturen bij zeugen. *Tijdschrift voor Diergeneeskunde,* 106, 72–74.

65 **PERDRIZET, J.A. & DINSMORE, P., 1986.** Pituitary abscess syndrome. *Compendium on Continuing Education for the Practicing Veterinarian,* 8, 5311–5318.

66 **PERDRIZET, J.A. & DINSMORE, P., 1986.** The pituitary abscess syndrome in ruminants: A review of 20 cases. *Proceedings of the Fourteenth World Congress on Diseases of Cattle.* Dublin, Ireland. August 26–29. Vol. 2, 1207–1210.

67 **PRESCOTT, J.F. & MUCKLE, C.A., 1986.** *Corynebacterium. In*: GYLES, C.L. & THOEN, C.O., (eds). *Pathogenesis of Bacterial Infections in Animals.* Ames, Iowa: Iowa State University Press.

68 **REDDY, C.A., CORNELL, C.P. & FRAGA, A.M., 1980.** Chemically defined growth medium for *Corynebacterium pyogenes. American Journal of Veterinary Research,* 41, 843–845.

69 **ROBERTS, D.S., 1967.** The pathogenic synergy of *Fusiformis necrophorus* and *Corynebacterium pyogenes.* I. Influence of the leukocidal exotoxin of *F. necrophorus. British Journal of Experimental Pathology,* 48, 665–673.

70 **ROBERTS, D.S., 1967.** The pathogenic synergy of *Fusiformis necrophorus* and *Corynebacterium pyogenes.* II. The response of *F. necrophorus* to a filterable product of *C. pyogenes. British Journal of Experimental Pathology,* 48, 674–679.

71 **ROBERTS, D.S., GRAHAM, N.P.H., EGERTON, J.R. & PARSONSON, I.M., 1968.** Infective bulbar necrosis (heel abscess) of sheep, a mixed infection with *Fusiformis necrophorus* and *Corynebacterium pyogenes. Journal of Comparative Pathology,* 78, 1–8.

72 **ROBERTS, R.J., 1968.** A study of the haemolysin of *Corynebacterium pyogenes. Research in Veterinary Science,* 9, 350–353.

73 **ROBINSON, W.F. & MAXIE, M.G., 1985.** The cardiovascular system. *In*: JUBB, K.V.F., KENNEDY, P.C. & PALMER, N., (eds). *Pathology of Domestic Animals.* Vol. III. 3rd edn. New York, London: Academic Press.

74 **ROSSITER, D.L., ROBINSON, R.A., O'LEARY, T.P. & HANSON, J.O., 1984.** Lingual abscesses in suckling and weaned lambs. *American Journal of Veterinary Research,* 185, 1552.

75 **RUDER, C.A., SASSER, R.G., WILLIAMS, R.J., ELY, J.K., BULL, R.C. & BUTLER, J.E., 1981.** Uterine infections in the postpartum cow. II. Possible synergistic effect of *Fusobacterium necrophorum* and *Corynebacterium pyogenes. Theriogenology,* 15, 573–580.

76 **RYFF, J.F. & BROWNE, J., 1954.** *Corynebacterium pyogenes* — a cultural and serological study. *American Journal of Veterinary Research,* 15, 617–621.

77 **SCHAAL, K.P., 1986.** Genus *Actinomyces. In*: SNEATH, P.H.A., MAIR, N.S., SHARPE, M.E. & HOLT, J.G., (eds). *Bergey's Manual of Systematic Bacteriology.* Vol. II. Baltimore, London: Williams & Wilkins.

78 **SCOTT, P.R., PENNY, C.D. & MURRAY, L.D., 1991.** A field study of eight ovine vertebral body abscess cases. *New Zealand Veterinary Journal,* 39, 105–107.

79 **SEINHORST, J.W., SOL, J. & VECHT, U., 1991.** Effect of damage to the teat end on the experimental induction of mastitis in dry cows with *Corynebacterium pyogenes. The Veterinary Record,* 128, 54–56.

80 **SEMAMBO, D.K.N., AYLIFFE, T.R., BOYD, J.S. & TAYLOR, D.J., 1991.** Early abortion in cattle induced by experimental intrauterine infusion with pure cultures of *Actinomyces pyogenes. The Veterinary Record,* 129, 12–16.

81 **SHERMAN, D.M. & AMES, T.R., 1986.** Vertebral body abscesses in cattle: A review of five cases. *Journal of the American Veterinary Medical Association,* 188, 608–611.

82 **SHONE, D.K., PHILIP, J.R., ROBERTS, R.M. & CHRISTIE, G.J., 1958.** Some aetiological agents of bovine abortions in Southern Rhodesia. *Journal of the South African Veterinary Medical Association,* 29, 55–62.

83 **SMITH, R.E. & REYNOLDS, I.M., 1971.** *Corynebacterium pyogenes* keratitis in a newborn calf. *Cornell Veterinarian,* 61, 591–595.

84 **SMITH, R.E., REYNOLDS, I.M., CLARK, G.W. & MILBURY, J.A., 1971.** Fetoplacental effects of *Corynebacterium pyogenes* in sheep. *Cornell Veterinarian,* 61, 573–590.

85 **SMITH, T.J.A., 1970.** Abortion due to *C. pyogenes? The Veterinary Record,* 87, 519–520.

86 **STUART, P., BUNTAIN, D. & LANGRIDGE, R.G., 1951.** Bacteriological examination of secretions from cases of 'summer mastitis' and experimental infection of non-lactating bovine udders. *The Veterinary Record,* 63, 451–453.

87 **STUDER, E. & MORROW, D.A., 1978.** Postpartum evaluation of bovine reproductive potential: Comparison of findings from genital tract examination *per rectum*, uterine culture, and endometrial biopsy. *Journal of the American Veterinary Medical Association,* 172, 489–494.

88 **SULLIVAN, N.D., 1985.** The nervous system. *In*: JUBB, K.V.F., KENNEDY, P.C. & PALMER, N., (eds). *Pathology of Domestic Animals.* Vol. I. 3rd edn. New York, London: Academic Press.

89 **SWANEPOEL, R., BLACKBURN, N.K., LANDER, K.P., VICKERS, D.B. & LEWIS, A.R., 1975.** An investigation of infectious infertility and abortion of cattle. *Rhodesian Veterinary Journal,* 6, 42–55.

90 **TAYLOR, D.J., 1986.** *Pig Diseases.* 4th edn. Cambridge: Burlington Press.

91 **THOMAS, A.D., 1931.** Actinobacillosis and other complications in sheep which may arise from the feeding of prickly pear (*Opuntia* sp.). *Seventeenth Report of the Director of Veterinary Services,* 215–226.

92 **TIMONEY, J.F., GILLESPIE, J.H., SCOTT, F.W. & BARLOUGH, J.E., 1988.** *Hagan and Bruner's Microbiology and Infectious Diseases of Domestic Animals.* 8th edn. Ithaca and London: Comstock Publishing Associates.

93 **TOLLE, A., FRANKE, V. & REICHMUTH, J., 1983.** Zur *C. pyogenes*-mastitis — bakteriologische aspekte. *Deutsche Tierärztliche Wochenschrift,* 90, 256–260.

94 **TUSTIN, R.C., 1992.** Waterkloof, Pretoria. Unpublished data.

95 **VAN DEN BERG, J., NARUCKA, U., NOUWS, J.F.M., OKMA, B.D., PEELEN, J.P.J. & SOETHOUT, A.E.E., 1981.** Afwijkingen bij slachtdieren. II. Ontstoken staart met een embolische pneumonie bij varkens. *Tijdschrift voor Diergeneeskunde,* 106, 407–410.

96 **VAN REES, A.L.A., 1964.** Osteomyelitiden bij jonge en oude varkens. *Tijdschrift voor Diergeneeskunde,* 89, 136–145.

97 **WATSON, E.D., 1989.** Specific antibody in milk whey and phagocytosis of *Actinomyces pyogenes* by neutrophils *in vitro. Research in Veterinary Science,* 47, 253–256.

98 **WATSON, E.D., 1989.** *In vitro* function of bovine neutrophils against *Actinomyces pyogenes. American Journal of Veterinary Research,* 50, 455–458.

99 **WATSON, E.D., DIEHL, N.K. & EVANS, J.F., 1990.** Antibody response in the bovine genital tract to intrauterine infusion of *Actinomyces pyogenes. Research in Veterinary Science,* 48, 70–75.

100 **WEINBERG, M., FORGEOT, P. & RICHART, A., 1938.** Complications pseudo-gangréneuses de la fièvre aphteuse causées par le bacille de poëls, seul ou associé. *Bulletin de l'Académie Vétérinaire de France,* 9, 217–218.

101 **WEST, D.M., 1983.** Anatomical considerations of the distal interphalangeal joint in sheep. *New Zealand Veterinary Journal,* 31, 58–60.

102 **WEST, D., 1983.** A study of naturally occurring cases of ovine foot abscess in New Zealand. *New Zealand Veterinary Journal,* 31, 152–156.

103 **YAGER, J.A. & SCOTT, D.W., 1985.** The skin and appendages. *In*: JUBB, K.V.F., KENNEDY, P.C. & PALMER, N., (eds). *Pathology of Domestic Animals.* Vol. I. 3rd edn. New York, London: Academic Press.

171

Eubacterium suis *infections*

Synonym: Cystitis and pyelonephritis of pigs

M.G. Collett

Introduction

Eubacterium (Corynebacterium) suis causes peracute to chronic cystitis, ureteritis and pyelonephritis in pigs (particularly in sows) which are characterized clinically by the passage of turbid and blood-stained urine.[16].

The first in-depth study of the organism was performed in Britain less than 40 years ago, despite the fact that the condition had been recognized there for over a century.[16] Since then the disease has been reported in North and Central America,[3, 12, 19] Europe,[4, 5, 14, 15] Australia[6] and Hong Kong.[11] In South Africa, the organism has only been isolated once — from a sow with nephritis and cystitis.[7] The paucity of case reports in the literature is probably accounted for by the special cultural requirements of *E. suis*.[19]

Aetiology

Eubacterium suis **(Irregular, non-sporing, gram-positive rods: Introduction: Table 1)** is an obligate anaerobe which forms small translucent, grey and shiny colonies on culture after 24 hours, with indefinite ß-haemolysis on sheep blood agar and no haemolysis on rabbit blood agar. The organisms are Gram-positive, 0,5 X 1,0 – 3,0 µm in size, have a beaded appearance and occur singly or in clumps.[10]

Epidemiology

All reports to date indicate that *E. suis* infections occur sporadically. In an abattoir survey in the USA, *E. suis* was isolated from the bladder of 4,7 per cent of sows examined at slaughter.[19] Although the organism is rarely isolated from healthy sows, it is frequently present in the urine, semen and prepuce of boars.[8, 13, 15] In herds where the infection is endemic, most male pigs over ten weeks of age are carriers of *E. suis* in their prepuce, probably as a result of contracting the infection from contaminated floors.[8, 9] There is evidence that transmission of the disease to sows is venereal, since in most cases there is a history of service two to four weeks prior to the development of clinical signs; indeed, affected sows are usually pregnant.[3, 6, 11, 15, 16, 19] A degree of trauma of the genital tract of sows, inflicted at breeding, is probably necessary for *E. suis* to gain a foothold and for the infection to establish itself.[13]

Pathogenesis

The pathogenesis of *E. suis* infection in sows resembles, to some extent, that of *Corynebacterium renale* in cows. Both organisms initially cause a cystitis followed by haematuria. In ascending infections the ureters and the kidneys are involved.[12, 15, 16] The spread of *E. suis* from the vagina (where the initial infection occurs) to the bladder may be aided by the short and wide urethra of sows and piliation of the organisms.[3, 17] Sows also tend to develop urinary stagnation and hydronephrosis, which predispose them to the development of cystitis, because of the anatomical structure of the neck of the sow's bladder, particularly when gravid and the uterus causes pressure over the pelvic brim.[15]

No exotoxins or other virulence factors have been demonstrated,[15] although *E. suis* has strong urease activity and ammonia production may contribute significantly to tissue damage and the consequent inflammatory reaction.[3, 10, 17, 19] The role played by concomitant infections with other bacteria is unknown.[11]

Clinical signs

The earliest signs in most affected sows are a vaginal discharge and blood-stained, turbid urine which may contain floccules of pus.[4, 16] However, in some adult sows only circulatory collapse and death within 12 hours may occur; they may even be found dead without having manifested clinical signs.[1] Affected animals usually show a mild fever, anorexia, general stiffness, arching of the back, lameness in the hind limbs, tense abdominal muscles, stranguria, polyuria, polydipsia, weight loss and eventually emaciation.[1, 3, 11, 13, 16] Boars are seldom clinically affected, although haematuria has been reported.[16]

Pathology

The specific gravity and pH of the urine of affected sows are 1,016–1,025 and 8,5–9,0, respectively, and the sediment contains white and red blood cells, mucus, bacteria, and apatite, struvite or oxalate crystals.[19]

Lesions are confined to the urogenital system. The affected bladder contains a thick, viscous, brown or blood-stained, foul-smelling urine. The bladder wall is markedly thickened, the mucosa is hyperaemic and contains haemorrhages and/or a purulent to pseudomembranous inflammation, sometimes accompanied by ulceration.[6, 11, 12, 14, 16, 19] The ureters may be thickened and dilated as a result of submucosal oedema and exudation or haemorrhage into the lumen, respectively.[5, 6, 11, 15, 16]

The renal lesions vary from an acute, purulent to a chronic interstitial nephritis, pyelitis or pyelonephritis.[14, 15] The surface of the kidneys is mottled greyish-red. On cut section the parenchyma reveals rays of connective tissue,[6, 12, 16] the mucous membrane of the renal papillae may contain haemorrhages, and there may be ulcers covered by yellow to greenish pseudomembranes.[5, 6, 11, 12, 16] One or both kidneys may be enlarged due to hydronephrosis or distension of the pelvis with pus. Occasionally, vaginitis or metritis are encountered.[15, 16]

Histologically, the bladder shows submucosal oedema and fibrosis, and degeneration and necrosis of the epithelium and other cellular components of the mucosa. These changes are often accompanied by haemorrhage and pseudomembrane formation. Gram-positive diphtheroid bacteria are usually present in the exudate or necrotic epithelium. The urethra may also be inflamed. The renal lesions are characterized by multiple focal infiltrates of lymphocytes, neutrophils and macrophages, in association with variable degrees of fibrosis, particularly of the medulla and pelvis, necrosis of the renal papillae, and the presence of bacterial colonies in the exudate.[6, 12]

Diagnosis and differential diagnosis

A diagnosis of *E. suis* infection should be suspected when blood-stained, turbid urine is detected clinically or at necropsy.[3, 6, 18] The diagnosis should be confirmed by anaerobic bacterial isolation from urine or affected tissues.[3, 5, 6, 16] A selective medium for the isolation of *E. suis* is commercially available as Columbia CNA agar consisting of Columbia agar with colistin sulphate (10 mg/l) and nalidixic acid (15 mg/l).[2, 3] Where specimens are severely contaminated, such as those from the prepuce, metronidazole (50 mg/l) can be added to the medium.[13] Various other bacteria may also be isolated from sows with cystitis if both aerobic and anaerobic culture methods are employed. These include *Escherichia coli* and *Proteus* spp., and a number of Gram-positive bacteria, including *Actinomyces pyogenes*, haemolytic and non-haemolytic streptococci, staphylococci, *Peptostreptococcus* spp. and *Enterococcus* spp.[11, 12, 16, 19]

An immunofluorescence technique applied to urine specimens can readily and reliably identify *E. suis*.[14]

Acute illness and death due to *E. suis* infection in sows should be differentiated from other diseases such as heart failure, septicaemia, campylobacteriosis and many others. In the more subacute to chronic disease, other causes of 'thin-sow syndrome', such as pneumonia, parasites, poor nutrition, swine dysentery, gastric ulceration, toxic nephropathy, leptospirosis, and other causes of cystitis should be eliminated.[3, 13]

Control

It is important to isolate infected sows from the rest of the herd. In the early stages, infection due to *E. suis* can be successfully treated by intramuscular injection of penicillin G or ampicillin (drug of choice, because of safety during pregnancy) at 11 mg/kg twice daily for five days.[3, 18] In sows with advanced or chronic lesions the prognosis is poor. The success rate of therapy in these animals is poor, relapses are common,[1] and culling may be the only alternative.[17] When infection is diagnosed in sows, the preputial sacs of all breeding boars should be flushed with penicillin twice weekly for three weeks and the stalls should be regularly disinfected with quaternary ammonium, phenol or formaldehyde-based compounds.[3]

Stalls where pregnant sows are kept should be properly designed to prevent urine cross-contamination.[3] In order to reduce the likelihood of trauma at breeding, smaller boars should be used on gilts and overaggressive mating should be avoided.[13]

References

1 **BLOOD, D.C. & RADOSTITS, O.M., 1989.** *Veterinary Medicine*. 7th edn. London, Philadelphia: Baillière Tindall.

2 **DAGNALL, G.J.R. & JONES, J.E.T., 1982.** A selective medium for the isolation of *Corynebacterium suis*. *Research in Veterinary Science*, 32, 389–390.

3 **DEE, S.A., 1991.** Diagnosing and controlling urinary tract infections caused by *Eubacterium suis* in swine. *Veterinary Medicine*, 86, 231–238.

4 **DIJKSTRA, R.G., 1969.** Cysto-pyelonefritis bij varkens veroorzaakt door *Corynebacterium suis*. *Tijdschrift voor Diergeneeskunde*, 94, 393–394.

5 **FRIJLINK, G.P.A., VAN DIJK, J.E. & GOUDSWAARD, J., 1969.** Een hemorragische-necrotiserende cysto-pyelonefritis bij een drachtige zeug, veroorzaakt door *Corynebacterium suis*. *Tijdschrift voor Diergeneeskunde*, 94, 389–393.

6 **GLAZEBROOK, J.S., DONALDSON-WOOD, C. & LADDS, P.W., 1973.** Pyelonephritis and cystitis in sows associated with *Corynebacterium suis*. *Australian Veterinary Journal*, 49, 546.

7 **HENTON, M.M., 1989.** Veterinary Research Institute, Onderstepoort. Unpublished data.

8 **JONES, J.E.T., 1984.** Cystitis and pyelonephritis associated with *Corynebacterium suis* infection in sows. *Veterinary Annual*, 24, 138–142.

9 **JONES, J.E.T. & DAGNALL, G.J.R., 1984.** The carriage of *Corynebacterium suis* in male pigs. *Journal of Hygiene*, 93, 381–388.

10 **MOORE, W.E.C. & MOORE, L.V.H., 1986.** Genus *Eubacterium*. *In*: SNEATH, P.H.A., MAIR, N.S., SHARPE, M.E. & HOLT, J.G., (eds). *Bergey's Manual of Systematic Bacteriology*. Vol. II. Baltimore, London: Williams & Wilkins.

11 **MUNRO, R. & WONG, F., 1972.** First isolation of *Corynebacterium suis* in Hong Kong. *British Veterinary Journal*, 128, 29–32.

12 **PERCY, D.H., RUHNKE, H.L. & SOLTYS, M.A., 1966.** A case of infectious cystitis and pyelonephritis of swine caused by *Corynebacterium suis*. *Canadian Veterinary Journal*, 7, 291–292.

13 **PIJOAN, C., LASTRA, A. & LEMAN, A., 1983.** Isolation of *Corynebacterium suis* from the prepuce of boars. *Journal of the American Veterinary Medical Association*, 183, 428–429.

14 **SCHÄLLIBAUM, M., HÄNI, H. & NICOLET, J., 1976.** Infektion des harntraktes beim schwein mit *Corynebacterium suis*: Diagnose mit immunfluoreszenz. *Schweizer Archiv für Tierheilkunde*, 118, 329–334.

15 **SOLTYS, M.A., 1961.** *Corynebacterium suis* associated with a specific cystitis and pyelonephritis in pigs. *Journal of Pathology and Bacteriology*, 81, 441–446.

16 **SOLTYS, M.A. & SPRATLING, F.R., 1957.** Infectious cystitis and pyelonephritis of pigs: A preliminary communication. *The Veterinary Record*, 69, 500–504.

17 **TAYLOR, D.J., 1986.** *Pig Diseases*. 4th edn. Cambridge: Burlington Press.

18 **TIMONEY, J.F., GILLESPIE, J.H., SCOTT, F.W. & BARLOUGH, J.E., 1988.** *Hagan and Bruner's Microbiology and Infectious Diseases of Domestic Animals*. 8th edn. Ithaca, London: Comstock Publishing Associates.

19 **WALKER, R.L. & MACLACHLAN, N.J., 1989.** Isolation of *Eubacterium suis* from sows with cystitis. *Journal of the American Veterinary Medical Association*, 195, 1104–1107.

MYCOBACTERIA

Tuberculosis is a chronic contagious disease caused by infection with certain acid-fast bacterial species of the genus *Mycobacterium*. It affects many vertebrate animals **(Table 1)** and is manifested, in general, by the formation in various tissues, but particularly in the lungs and lymph nodes, of granulomas known as tubercles that consist of a core of caseous necrotic tissue surrounded by a zone of granulomatous inflammation.[21] The term 'tubercle bacillus' is still used for the organism that causes the development of the tubercle.[28] It is usually synonymous with *Mycobacterium tuberculosis* or *M. bovis*, unless it is qualified by an adjective such as 'avian' or cold blooded'.[10] The characteristic appearance of the lesions, however, differs according to the animal species and the respective *Mycobacterium* sp. with which it is infected. Before effective control measures were adopted, tuberculosis was one of the major diseases of humans and domestic animals. The disease in humans still remains one of the most important notifiable infectious diseases in the Third World, and is the single biggest public health problem in South Africa.[17] The various veterinary control measures applied at present in South Africa are aimed at the eradication of the disease in livestock.

For many years tuberculosis appeared to prevail over the entire globe,[16] and annually caused more deaths in humans than all of the so-called scourges and wars put together. The records of the Parsees, the Mosaic Laws, the Talmud and other ancient documents all refer to a malady that can be identified as tuberculosis of humans.[21] Much of the present knowledge of tuberculosis is based on the initial work of scientists like Laennec and Villemin. Robert Koch first described the causative agent in 1882, and tuberculin, which proved to be a valuable diagnostic tool for the detection of the disease, was developed by him in 1891 for its supposedly curative value.[28, 29]

The mycobacteria are aerobic, considered Gram-positive (although not readily stainable by the Gram's staining method), non-motile, non-sporeforming, straight or slightly curved rods, 1,5–4,0 µm long and 0,3–0,5 µm wide.[12, 53] Their cell walls have a high lipid content, which accounts for their resistance to acids, dessication and most disinfectants, and also for their slow growth and hydrophobic characteristic in fluid media. Once mycobacteria have been stained with carbol fuchsin, they cannot be decolourized by acid-alcohol — thus the epithet 'acid-fast' bacteria. When isolation is attempted, the resistance afforded by the high lipid content of the cell wall allows treatment of samples with acid or alkali to kill microbial contaminants without destroying the mycobacteria in the process.

The genus *Mycobacterium* consists of about 50 species, most of which are environmental saprophytes that exist and multiply in a wide variety of substrates such as soil, water and plants, domestic and wild mammals, and birds.[4, 20, 30, 40, 56] Some of these saprophytic mycobacteria (opportunistic pathogens) may cause 'opportunistic' infections in animals and humans, but others never cause disease.[19] Certain members of the genus, such as those that go to make up the *M. tuberculosis* complex (*M. tuberculosis, M. bovis, M. africanum* and *M. microti*), which are also known as 'tubercle bacilli' and which cause tuberculosis in humans and animals, and *M. leprae* which is the cause of leprosy in humans, are obligate parasites and are usually transmitted only by infected mammalian hosts. They are also susceptible to a number of chemotherapeutic agents, while the opportunistic pathogens are often resistant to chemotherapeutic agents and are not contagious.[54]

The two most important members of the *M. tuberculosis* complex are *M. bovis* and *M. tuberculosis*, which are distinguished from one another on the basis of certain attributes **(Table 2)**. *Mycobacterium tuberculosis* was one of the first mycobacteria to be described.[59] *Mycobacterium bovis*, which is closely related to *M. tuberculosis*, causes tuberculosis mainly in cattle but may also affect other species, including humans, if there is contact with tuberculous cattle or their products.

The most important mycobacterial species causing disease in livestock are *M. bovis*, serovars of the *M. avium* complex, *M. paratuberculosis* **(see Chapter 173: Paratuberculosis)**, and *M. farcinogenes*, which causes bovine farcy, a purulent inflammation of superficial lymph vessels and nodes in tropical countries.[7, 8, 20] In terms of the variety of animal species that it may infect, *M. bovis* is the most

Table 1 Tuberculosis in a variety of species. (Adapted and reproduced with permission from Francis[18])

Group	Species	Allergy	No. of bacilli	Casea-tion	Calcifica-tion	Fib-rosis	Giant cells	Susceptibility to infection with the three types of tubercle bacilli: Bovine	Human	Avian	Spread	Route
1	Naïve human	5	I	5	3	2	3	5	5	I	5	R 90
	Monkeys	2	2	5	3	I	5	5	5	I	5	R 90
	Guinea-pigs	3	I	5	2	I	4	5	5	2	I	Expr.
	Rabbits	2	2	5	2	I	4	5	I	4	I	Expr.
2	Urban human	5	I	5	5	5	5	2	2	I	5	R 90
	Elephants	I	3	4	I	5	I	3	3	I	?	R 100*
	Cattle	2	I	4	5	4	5	4	I	I	5	R 90
	Buffaloes	2	I	4	4	4	4	4	I	I	4	R 90
	Goats	2	I	4	4	3	4	4	I	2	I	R 90
	Sheep	2	I	4	4	4	2	3	I	2	I	R 80
	Pigs	3	I	4	4	4	2	4	2	2	I	R 90
3	Fowls	2	4	4	I	3	2	I	I	3	4	A 100
4	Horses	I	3	3	I	2	4	2	I	I	I	A 90
	Asses and mules	I	3	3	I	2	4	2	I	I	I	A 90
5A	Dogs	2	2	3	I	2	I	2	2	0	0	R 60
5B	Cats	I	3	3	I	2	I	4	I	2	I	A 70
5C	Hamsters	0	4	0,5	0	0	0	5	5	I	0	Expr.
5D	Mice	0	5	0,5	0	0	0	2	2	I	0	Expr.
	Rats	0	4	0,5	0	0	0	I	I	0,5	0	Expr.

* little information available
The maximum value for each feature in this table is 5. The figures represent a somewhat arbitrary approximation. A '0' in the columns for allergy or calcification should not be taken as completely precluding the existence of these features in any given species. No species is completely resistant to tuberculosis, and consequently, in the columns on susceptibility to the various types of tubercle bacilli, a 'I' has been used for those species that are virtually resistant to infection with a given type. The figures for susceptibility are roughly comparable vertically as well as horizontally: thus those for rabbits are 5, I, 4, and those for mice, 2, 2, I. The values for 'Spread' represent the ease with which tuberculosis spreads naturally between members of any one species.
The figures under 'Route' show the percentage of all infections acquired by the most important route. 'Expr.' has been inserted when nearly all information on the tuberculosis in a species is based on experimental work. R = respiratory; A = alimentary; Expr. = experimental
The animal species are grouped according to their reaction to infection with tubercle bacilli. The classification was made primarily on the general characteristics of the pathological finding after infection with mycobacteria. The first two groups contain animals in which typical tubercles are formed. The first group consists of highly susceptible species.
Naïve humans and monkeys in captivity are more susceptible to fatal spontaneous infection than any other species. Spontaneous infection in guinea-pigs and rabbits is not known.

universal pathogen among the mycobacteria and produces progressive disease in most domestic animals and humans.[39]

The susceptibility of different animal species to infection with *M. bovis*, *M. tuberculosis* and serovars of *M. avium* complex varies **(Table 1)**.[18] Of the livestock species, cattle, goats, sheep, horses and pigs are susceptible in varying degree to *M. bovis* infection (Groups 2 and 4 in **Table 1**). However, they are more resistant to the disease than monkeys, guinea-pigs and rabbits (Group 1 in **Table 1**). Lesions contain moderate numbers of bacilli. Horses, donkeys and mules are quite resistant to tuberculosis caused by all *Mycobacterium* spp.[13, 18]

Mycobacterium africanum was initially isolated from sputum of tuberculous humans in equatorial Africa.[6] It is phenotypically intermediate between *M. tuberculosis* and *M. bovis*. Reports of infection with *M. africanum* in animals are rare, but it has been isolated from the tissues of a monkey,[50] and an outbreak of *M. africanum* infection in cattle and pigs in Norway has recently been described.[1]

Mycobacterium microti, the vole bacillus, is mainly infectious for rodents and is not considered to be an important pathogen in either domestic or wild animals.[55] Infections in a cat and in pigs have been described.[23]

The early classification of the 'opportunistic' mycobacteria was based on growth rate, pigmentation, and

Table 2 Differentiation between members of the *M. tuberculosis* complex in the laboratory. (Adapted from Collins *et al*.[10])

Mycobacterium spp.	TCH	Nitralase	Oxygen preference	Pyrazin-amide	Cyclo-serine
M. tuberculosis	R	+	A	S	S
M. africanum	S	V	M	S	S
M. bovis	S	–	M	R	S
*M. microti**					

* Information on *M. microti* is not given, as it has only been reported in the vole (*Microtus agrotis*)
S sensitive TCH: Thiophene-2 carboxylic acid hydrazide
R resistant
A aerobic
M microaerophilic
V variable
+ positive
– negative

clinical significance.[44, 53] Currently the bacteria are classified according to criteria outlined in **Table 3**. The 'opportunist' or non-tuberculous group of mycobacteria are also referred to as atypical mycobacteria, 'mycobacteria other than tubercle bacilli' (MOTT) or 'potentially pathogenic environmental mycobacteria' (PPEM).[54] Of the rapid growers, *M. chelonae* and *M. fortuitum* are of clinical importance.[5, 31] *Mycobacterium fortuitum* has been isolated from a non-healing wound in a dog and *M. chelonae* from nodules in the mesentery and lungs of a snake.[22] *Mycobacterium smegmatis* has been reported as a cause of mastitis in cattle.[14, 43] Diseases caused by these mycobacteria are termed mycobacterioses.

Opportunistic mycobacteria can survive in water and have been isolated from ponds in Europe and New Zealand. They can be responsible for non-specific sensitization of cattle to the purified protein derivative (PPD) of bovine and avian tuberculin and may therefore complicate the interpretation of the tuberculin skin test.[9, 24–26]

The most important group of opportunistic mycobacteria causing clinical disease in various animal species, apart from the obligate pathogens (*M. tuberculosis* complex), is the *M. avium* complex, also referred to as the *M. avium-intracellulare* complex, and listed as *M. avium* and *M. intracellulare* in Runyon's group III.[49, 57] According to the most recent research, the *M. avium* complex includes *M. intracellulare, M. avium, M. paratuberculosis* **(see Chapter 173: Paratuberculosis)**, *M. lepraemurium* (pathogenic for rodents but not for humans),[42] and the 'wood pigeon' bacillus (*M. avium* subsp. *silvaticum* subsp. nov.[51, 54] The *M. avium-intracellulare* complex, as it was known until recently, consisted of 25 serovars, including *M. avium* (serovars 1, 2 and 3) and *M. intracellulare* (serovars 4–25). Recent developments in the taxonomy based on the structural relatedness of DNA, RNA and protein between *M. avium* and *M. intracellulare* have

Table 3 Classification of non-tuberculous or opportunist mycobacteria. (Adapted from Runyon[44])

Group	Rate of growth and pigment production	*Mycobacterium* spp.	Clinical significance
I	Slow Photochromogens	*M. kansasii*	Pulmonary disease in humans
		M. marinum	Pathogen of fish and humans
II	Slow Scotochromogens	*M. xenopi*	No clinical significance
		M. flavescens	No clinical significance
		M. gordonae	No clinical significance
		M. scrofulaceum	Tuberculous adenitis in children
III	Slow Non-chromogens	*M. avium*	'Tuberculosis' in poultry and birds
		M. intracellulare	Opportunist pathogen in humans, pigs, cattle, horses
		M. gastri	No clinical significance
		M. nonchromogenicum	No clinical significance
		M. terrae	No clinical significance
		M. triviale	No clinical significance
		M. ulcerans	Ulcers in humans (Buruli in East Africa)
IV	Rapid	*M. chelonae*	Opportunist pathogen
		M. fortuitum	Mycobacteriosis in fish
		M. phlei	No clinical significance
		M. vaccae	No clinical significance
		M. smegmatis	**See text**

confirmed that they are distinct species. According to the variation that exists, the serovars allocated to the two species are serovars 1–6 and 8–11 which are assigned to *M. avium*, and serovars 7, 12–17, 19, 20 and 25 to *M. intracellulare*, while some isolates of serovar 18 are grouped with *M. intracellulare* and others with *M. simiae*.[54] The division into 25 serovars is based on differences in seroagglutination,[46, 58] immunodiffusion,[35] sensitin typing,[33] and DNA/DNA hybridization.[3, 45, 52]

Members of the *M. avium* complex are the most widespread of the mycobacteria in the environment. Some are saprophytes and others are pathogens of birds and mammals, including humans.[20] They are a major source of opportunist infection in humans suffering from acquired immune deficiency syndrome (AIDS).[20] Serovars 1, 2 and 3 produce progressive disease in poultry and birds under natural conditions. The other serovars, when inoculated into chickens, only produce minimal disease.[49] In Europe, where 'fowl tuberculosis' was of importance, and contact between cattle, pigs and fowls occurred, serovars 2 and 3 were the most frequent ones to be isolated from porcine lymphadenitis.[47] In the USA, serovars 2 and 3 are also found in pigs. Studies in South Africa have shown that serovars 1, 4 and 8 are mainly responsible for porcine lymphadenitis[27] and that serovars 4 and 8 occur most frequently in the environment, animal feed, and bedding and on plants.[27, 40]

Cultural methods are as reliable as animal inoculation methods for the isolation of tubercle bacilli from specimens from infected tissues or material.[34] All members of the *M. tuberculosis* complex are slow growers and non-pigmented, and fail to grow at room temperature (25 °C). They are catalase-negative after being heated to a temperature of 68 °C. They are sensitive to antituberculous drugs, with the exception of strains which have developed drug resistance. Members of the *M. tuberculosis* complex require enriched media for successful culturing, the most frequently used solid media being Löwenstein-Jensen (L-J) medium and Ogawa medium, both containing eggs, phosphate buffer, and magnesium salts (L-J medium also contains asparagine),[8] and Middlebrook 7H10 agar, a semi-synthetic medium. The liquid media most often used are Dubos medium and Middlebrook 7H10 liquid medium.[41] Most of the other species of mycobacteria grow on ordinary nutrient culture media.

To facilitate the isolation of a member of the *M. tuberculosis* complex from infected tissues, a specimen that consists of solid tissue should be finely minced and then placed in a small quantity of normal saline solution. This material, as well as fluid specimens such as sputum or exudate, should be decontaminated by treatment with an alkali (e.g. 4 per cent NaOH) or an acid (e.g. 2 per cent HCl); the exposure time must not exceed 30 minutes. The alkali or acid is then neutralized and the specimen is centrifuged in order to concentrate the organisms in the sediment, part of which is then inoculated onto suitable media. Cultures should be incubated at 37 °C. Visible growth of *M. bovis* may occur on solid media after three to four weeks or may take longer to appear. Colonies of *M. bovis* are white, flat, smooth and moist, and are easily emulsified.[12, 41] *Mycobacterium bovis* is microaerophilic, sensitive to thiophene-2-carboxylic acid hydrazide (TCH), niacin production- and nitrate reduction-negative, and resistant to pyrazinamide. Glycerol, which enhances growth of *M. tuberculosis* but might inhibit that of *M. bovis*, should be replaced by sodium pyruvate in the medium if the isolation of *M. bovis* is attempted. These properties distinguish *M. bovis* from *M. tuberculosis*, which grows more luxuriantly, with colonies becoming visible and showing dry, wrinkled surfaces after 10–14 days.[8]

Members of the *M. avium* complex produce visible growth on culture after two to three weeks. They grow at temperatures ranging from 20 °C to 45 °C and form colonies that are pearly-grey, lemon-yellow or sometimes bright yellow,[20] and which emulsify easily. The mycobacteria of this complex are nitrate reduction-negative, tellurite-positive and resistant to most antituberculous drugs.

More recent methods to determine the natural relationships within the mycobacteria include immunological techniques, comparison of cell wall components, comparison of homologous enzyme sequences, DNA/DNA homology, plasmid profiles, and restriction endonuclease analyses.[2, 11, 36, 48] Results of comparative rRNA sequencing support the early classification of slow and rapid growers.[48]

Mycobacteria are susceptible to sunlight and ultraviolet radiation.[12] Protected from daylight, *M. tuberculosis* can survive in moist or dried, pulverized sputum for weeks or months. *Mycobacterium bovis* was found to survive for six months in soil, in soil and dung mixtures and in dung, and for 49 days on grass under the climatic conditions that prevail in the south of England.[32] In the northern Australian environment, however, the bacillus may only survive in the soil for up to four weeks and exposure to sunlight causes rapid death.[15] This probably also applies to many parts of southern Africa. Mycobacteria remain alive for over two years in frozen carcasses and at 9 °C can survive for considerable periods in cheese and butter. With heat treatment, *M. bovis* is destroyed in meat products at temperatures 6–7 °C lower than those necessary for the destruction of members of the *M. avium* complex.[37–39] Temperatures above 60 °C for 10 minutes destroy *M. bovis* in Vienna sausages. Disinfection of equipment contaminated by meat emulsions containing *M. bovis* is achieved by treatment with 2 per cent phenolic disinfectant followed by formaldehyde vapour.[39] Disinfectants such as 3 – 8 per cent formalin, 5 per cent phenol or 3 per cent iodophor kill mycobacteria, as does exposure to a temperature of 60 °C for 15–20 minutes.[12, 41]

References

1 **ALFREDSEN, S. & SAXEGAARD, F., 1992.** An outbreak of tuberculosis in pigs and cattle caused by *Mycobacterium africanum*. *The Veterinary Record*, 131, 51–53.

2 **BAESS, I., 1979.** Deoxyribonucleic acid relatedness among species of slowly growing mycobacteria. *Acta Pathologica et Microbiologica Scandinavica*, Section B, 87, 221–226.

3 **BAESS, I., 1983.** Deoxyribonucleic acid relationships between different serovars of *Mycobacterium avium*, *Mycobacterium intracellulare* and *Mycobacterium scrofulaceum*. *Acta Pathologica et Microbiologica Scandinavica*, Section B, 91, 201–203.

4 **BEERWERTH, W., 1971.** Die mykobakterielle Bodenflora im Ablauf der Jahreszeiten. *Praxis der Pneumologie*, 25, 661–668.

5 **BRAGG, R.R., HUCHZERMEYER, H.F.A.K. & HANISCH, M.A.M., 1990.** *Mycobacterium fortuitum* isolated from three species of fish in South Africa. *Onderstepoort Journal of Veterinary Research*, 57, 101–102.

6 **CASTETS, M., RIST, N. & BOISVERT, H., 1969.** La variété africaine du bacille tuberculeux humain. *Médecine d'Afrique Noire*, 16, 321–322.

7 **CHAMOISEAU, G., 1973.** *Mycobacterium farcinogenes* agent causal du farcin du boeuf en Afrique. *Annales de Microbiologie*, (Inst. Pasteur), 124A, 214–222.

8 **COLLINS, C.H. & GRANGE, J.M., 1983.** A review: The bovine tubercle bacillus. *Journal of Applied Bacteriology*, 55, 13–29.

9 **COLLINS, C.H., GRANGE, J.M. & YATES, M.D., 1984.** A review. Mycobacteria in water. *Journal of Applied Bacteriology*, 57, 193–211.

10 **COLLINS, C.H., GRANGE, J.M. & YATES, M.D., 1985.** *Organization and Practice in Tuberculosis Bacteriology*. London, Boston, Durban, Singapore, Sydney, Toronto, Wellington: Butterworths.

11 **COLLINS, D.M. & DE LISLE, G.W., 1985.** DNA restriction endonuclease analysis of *Mycobacterium bovis* and other members of the tuberculosis complex. *Journal of Clinical Microbiology*, 21, 562–564.

12 **CRUICKSHANK, R., DUGUID, J.P., MARMION, B.P. & SWAIN, R.H.A., 1975.** *Medical Microbiology*. 12th edn. Edinburgh, London and New York: Churchill Livingstone.

13 **DANNENBERG, A.M. Jr., 1978.** Pathogenesis of pulmonary tuberculosis in man and animals. Protection of personnel against tuberculosis. *In*: MONTALI, R.J., (ed.). *Mycobacterial Infection in Zoo Animals*. Washington, DC: Smithsonian Institution Press, 65–79.

14 **DONAHUE, J.M. & SISK, D.B., 1979.** Runyon group IV mycobacterium as a pathogen in chronic intractable mastitis in dairy cattle. *Proceedings of the Twenty-second Meeting of the American Association of Veterinary Laboratory Diagnosticians*, 13–24.

15 **DUFFIELD, B.J. & YOUNG, D.A., 1985.** Survival of *Mycobacterium bovis* in defined environmental conditions. *Veterinary Microbiology*, 10, 193–197.

16 **FLEMING, G., 1875.** *A Manual of Veterinary Sanitary Science and Policy*. Vol. II. London: Chapman and Hall.

17 **FOURIE, P.B., TOWNSEND, G.S. & KLEEBERG, H.H., 1986.** The importance of tuberculosis. *South African Journal of Science*, 82, 386.

18 **FRANCIS, J., 1958.** *Tuberculosis in Animals and Man. A Study in Comparative Pathology*. London: Cassell.

19 **GRANGE, J.M. & YATES, M.D., 1986.** Infections caused by opportunist mycobacteria: A review. *Journal of the Royal Society of Medicine*, 79, 226–229.

20 **GRANGE, J.M., YATES, M.D. & BOUGHTON, E., 1990.** A review. The avian tubercle bacillus and its relatives. *Journal of Applied Bacteriology*, 68, 411–431.

21 **HENNING, M.W., 1956.** *Animal Diseases in South Africa*. 3rd edn. Pretoria: Central News Agency.

22 **HUCHZERMEYER, H.F.A.K., 1983/84 and 1985/86.** *Annual Reports*. Veterinary Research Institute, Onderstepoort.

23 **HUITEMA, H. & JAARTSVELD, F.H.J., 1967.** *Mycobacterium microti* infection in a cat and some pigs. *Antonie van Leeuwenhoek*, 33, 209–212.

24 **KAZDA, J., 1967.** Mycobacterien in Trinkwasser als Ursache der Parallergie gegenüber Tuberculinen bei Tieren. III. Taxonomische Studie einer neuen Art: *Mycobacterium brunense*. *Zentralblatt für Bakteriologie, Parasitenkunde, Infektionskrankheiten und Hygiene*, Abt. I 203, 199–201.

25 **KAZDA, J., 1983.** The principles of the ecology of mycobacteria. *In*: RATLEDGE, C. & STANDORD, J.L., (eds). *The Biology of the Mycobacteria*. Vol. II. London: Academic Press, Inc.

26 **KAZDA, J. & COOK, I.R., 1988.** Mycobacteria in pond water as a source of non-specific reactions to bovine tuberculin in New Zealand. *New Zealand Veterinary Journal*, 36, 184–188.

27 **KLEEBERG, H.H. & NEL, E.E., 1969.** Porcine mycobacterial lymphadenitis. *Journal of the South African Veterinary Medical Association*, 40, 233–250.

28 **KOCH, R., 1882.** Die Aetiologie der Tuberkulose. *Berliner Klinische Wochenschrift*, 19, 221–230.

29 **KOCH, R., 1891.** Fortsetzung der Mitteilung über ein Heilmittel gegen Tuberkulose. *Deutsche Medizinische Wochenschrift*, 17, 101–102.

30 **KUBIN, M., 1984.** Distribution and ecology of non-living reservoirs. Opportunists and pathogens. *In*: KUBICA, G.P. & WAYNE, L.G., (eds). *The Mycobacteria: A Sourcebook*, Part B. New York, Basel: Marcel Dekker, Inc.

31 **KUNKLE, G.A., GULBAS, N.K., FAKOK, V., AHLLIWELL, R.E.W. & CONELLY, M., 1983.** Rapidly growing mycobacteria as a cause of cutaneous granulomas: Report of five cases. *Journal of the American Animal Hospital Association*, 19, 513–521.

32 **MADDOCK, E.C.G., 1933.** Studies on the survival time of the bovine tubercle bacillus in soil, soil and dung, in dung and on grass, with experiments on the preliminary treatment of infected organic matter and the cultivation of the organism. *Journal of Hygiene*, 33, 103–117.

33 **MAGNUSSON, M., 1980.** Classification and identification of mycobacteria on the basis of sensitin specificity. *Infectionskrankheiten und ihre Erreger*, 4, 319–348.

34 **MARKS, J., 1972.** Ending the routine guinea-pig test. *Tubercle*, 53, 31–34.

35 **McINTYRE, G. & STANFORD, J.L., 1986.** The relationship between immunodiffusion and agglutination serotypes of *Mycobacterium avium* and *Mycobacterium intracellulare*. *European Journal of Respiratory Diseases*, 69, 135–141.

36 **MEISSNER, G., SCHRÖDER, K.H., AMADIO, G.E., ANZ, W., CHAPARAS, S., ENGEL, H.W.B., JENKINS, P.A., KÄPPLER, W., KLEEBERG, H.H., KUBALA, E., KUBIN, M., LAUTERDACH, D., LIND, A., MAGNUSSON, M., MIKOVA, Z.D., PATTYN, S.R., SCHAEFER, W.B., STANFORD, J.L., TSUKAMURA, M., WAYNE, L.G., WILLERS, I. & WOLINSKY, E., 1974.** A co-operative numerical analysis of non-photochromogenic slowly-growing mycobacteria. *Journal of General Microbiology*, 83, 207–235.

37 **MERKAL R.S. & CRAWFORD, J.A., 1979.** Heat inactivation of *Mycobacterium avium-Mycobacterium intracellulare* complex organisms in aqueous suspension. *Applied and Environmental Microbiology*, 38, 827–830.

38 **MERKAL, R.S., CRAWFORD, J.A. & WHIPPLE, D.L., 1979.** Heat inactivation of *Mycobacterium avium-Mycobacterium intracellulare* complex organisms in meat products. *Applied and Environmental Microbiology*, 38, 831–835.

39 **MERKAL, R.S. & WHIPPLE, D.L., 1980.** Inactivation of *Mycobacterium bovis* in meat products. *Applied and Environmental Microbiology*, 40, 282–284.

40 **NEL, E.E., 1981.** *Mycobacterium avium-intracellulare* complex serovars isolated in South Africa from humans, swine and the environment. *Reviews of Infectious Diseases*, 3, 1013.

41 **NEL, E.E., KLEEBERG, H.H. & GATNER, E.M.S., 1980.** *Laboratory Manual of Tuberculosis Methods.* 2nd revised edn. Pretoria.

42 **PATTYN, S.R., 1984.** *Mycobacterium lepraemurium. In*: KUBICA, G.P. & WAYNE, L.G., (eds). *The Mycobacteria. A Sourcebook.* Part B. New York, Basel: Marcel Dekker, Inc. 1277–1286.

43 **RICHARDSON, A., 1970.** Bovine mastitis associated with *Mycobacterium smegmatis* and an untypable mycobacterium. *The Veterinary Record*, 86, 497–498.

44 **RUNYON, E.H., 1959.** Anonymous mycobacteria in pulmonary disease. *Medical Clinics of North America*, 43, 273.

45 **SAITO, H., TOMIOKA, H., SATO, K., TASAKA, H. & DAWSON, D.J., 1990.** Identification of various serovar strains of *Mycobacterium avium* and *Mycobacterium intracellulare. Journal of Clinical Microbiology*, 28, 1694–1697.

46 **SCHAEFER, W.B., 1965.** Serologic identification and classification of the atypical mycobacteria by their agglutination. *American Review of Respiratory Disease*, 92 (suppl.), 85–93.

47 **SCHLIESSER, Th., 1976.** Vorkommen und Bedeutung von Mykobakterien bei Tieren. *Zentralblatt für Bakteriologie, Parasitenkunde, Infektionskrankheiten und Hygiene*, Erste Abteilung. Originali Reihe A. 235, 184–194.

48 **STAHL, D.A. & URBANCE, J.W., 1990.** The division between fast- and slow-growing species corresponds to natural relationships among the mycobacteria. *Journal of Bacteriology*, 172, 116–124.

49 **THOEN, C.O., HIMES, E.M. & KARLSON, A.G., 1984.** *Mycobacterium avium* complex. *In*: KUBICA, G.P., WAYNE, L.G., (eds). *The Mycobacteria. A Sourcebook.* Part B. New York and Basel: Marcel Dekker, Inc.

50 **THOREL, M.F., 1980.** Isolation of *Mycobacterium africanum* from a monkey. *Tubercle*, 61, 101–104.

51 **THOREL, M.F., KRICHEVSKY, M. & LEVY-FREBAULT, V.V., 1990.** Numerical taxonomy of mycobactin-dependent mycobacteria, amended description of *Mycobacterium avium*, and description of *Mycobacterium avium* subsp. *avium* subsp. nov., *Mycobacterium avium* subsp. *paratuberculosis* subsp. nov., and *Mycobacterium avium* subsp. *silvaticum* subsp. nov. *International Journal of Systematic Bacteriology*, 3, 254–260.

52 **WAYNE, L.G. & DIAZ, G.A. 1986.** Differentiation between T-catalases derived from *Mycobacterium avium* and *M. intracellulare* by a solid-phase immunosorbent assay. *International Journal of Systematic Bacteriology*, 36, 363–367.

53 **WAYNE, L.G. & KUBICA, G.P., 1986.** Family Mycobacteriaceae. *In*: SNEATH, P.H.A., MAIR, N.S., SHARPE, M.E. & HOLT, J.G., (eds). *Bergey's Manual of Systematic Bacteriology.* Vol. II. Baltimore, London, Los Angeles, Sydney: Williams & Wilkins.

54 **WAYNE, L.G. & SRAMEK, H.A., 1992.** Agents of newly recognized or infrequently encountered mycobacterial diseases. *Clinical Microbiology Reviews*, 5, 1–25.

55 **WELLS, A.Q., 1946.** The murine type of tubercle bacillus. *Medical Research Council Special Report* No. 259. London: Her Majesty's Stationery Office.

56 **WOLINSKY, E., 1979.** State of art: Non-tuberculous mycobacteria and associated diseases. *American Review of Respiratory Disease*, 119, 107–159.

57 **WOLINSKY, E., 1984.** Non-tuberculous mycobacteria and associated diseases. *In*; KUBICA, G.P. & WAYNE, L.G., (eds). *The Mycobacteria. A Sourcebook.* Part B. New York and Basel: Marcel Dekker, Inc.

58 **WOLINKSY, E. & SCHAEFER, W.B., 1973.** Proposed numbering scheme for mycobacterial serotypes by agglutination. *International Journal of Systematic Bacteriology*, 23, 182–183.

59 **ZOPF, W., 1883 in WAYNE, L.G., 1984.** Mycobacterial speciation. *In*: KUBICA, G.P. & WAYNE, L.G., (eds). *The Mycobacteria. A Sourcebook.* Part A. New York and Basel: Marcel Dekker, Inc.

172

Tuberculosis

Synonym: Tuberkulose (Afrik.)

H.F.K.A. Huchzermeyer, G.K. Brückner, A. Van Heerden, H.H. Kleeberg, I.B.J. van Rensburg, P. Koen and R.K. Loveday

MYCOBACTERIUM BOVIS *INFECTION IN CATTLE*

Synonyms: Bovine tuberculosis, tuberkulose by beeste (Afrik.)

Bovine tuberculosis existed in the Mediterranean littoral even before classical times. From northern Italy it spread to western Europe and Great Britain and it was from Holland and Great Britain that cattle first carried the disease to the many parts of the world that had been colonized by those countries.[89, 122]

The first reference to the occurrence of tuberculosis in animals in South Africa was made by Hutcheon in 1880,[51] and it appears unlikely that bovine tuberculosis existed in South Africa prior to the importation of European breeds of cattle towards the end of the eighteenth century.[45] In 1902 it was reported that cattle in Natal were free of tuberculosis, but that many animals imported from Australia, the Argentine, Madagascar and England were destroyed upon arrival in Durban when they reacted to the tuberculin test. Subsequently, the prevalence of the disease in slaughter cattle remained low in South Africa during the years 1917–29. During this time only 0,05 per cent of cattle slaughtered at the Durban abattoir, 0,33 per cent at Bloemfontein, 0,80 per cent at Cape Town, 0,031 per cent of bulls/oxen and 0,152 per cent of cows, respectively, at Johannesburg, 0,046 per cent at Pietermaritzburg, and 0,176 per cent at Port Elizabeth were tuberculous.[22] The spread of the disease in southern Africa was originally confined to dairy herds, but, since the early 1970s more and more beef herds have been found to be infected.

Bovine tuberculosis has been a notifiable disease in South Africa since the promulgation of the Diseases of Stock Act in 1911 (Act Number 14 of 1911). Under this act individual animals and herds which had been in contact with cases that tested positive, and with animals diagnosed as tuberculous after slaughter in an abattoir, were subjected to compulsory tuberculin testing. Reactors were slaughtered and their owners compensated at the rate of 25 per cent of their value up to a maximum value of R30,00 per animal. These measures were abandoned in 1928, being superseded in 1931 by the Voluntary Accredited Herd Scheme. Some 118 herds of milk cows were accepted into this scheme from its inception in 1931. Seventy of these had an infection rate that varied between 0,4 per cent and 75 per cent. From 1948 to 1955 a total of 180 075 tests were done, of which 2 799 (1,49 per cent) were positive. In 1950 an Interim Scheme was also introduced in which, whenever the number of reactors in a specific herd was reduced to 5 per cent or less, the owner could apply to have his herd considered for the Accreditation Scheme. A new scheme for the eradication of tuberculosis was proposed in 1955, but the limited post-war staff and other shortages made this impossible. The Bovine Tuberculosis Eradication Scheme, which had as its objective the total eradication of the disease through a test and slaughter policy, was introduced in 1969 and is still in operation. Although slow, progress has been made with the eradication of bovine tuberculosis, and in 1991 only 0,04 per cent of the 1 897 759 tuberculin tests performed were positive.

Ever since bovine tuberculosis was first recorded in Zimbabwe in 1908 in a heifer imported from the Cape Peninsula, only sporadic cases have been diagnosed. A national testing scheme for tuberculosis was instituted in 1950 and carried through to 1978. The prevalence remained very low, with one or none of the slaughtered animals per year showing tuberculous lesions.[44]

Namibia is considered to be virtually free of tuberculosis in livestock and all diagnosed cases can be traced back to imported animals, most of which came from South Africa or Germany.[102] From 1913 to 1984, of 66 888 head of cattle tested, 163 reacted positive to the tuberculin test and 284 gave suspicious reactions. Only seven animals at abbatoirs were found to be tuberculous.[2]

Tuberculosis is rare in animals in Swaziland. The prevalence in cattle is estimated to be below 0,5 per cent and it is unknown in wild animals.[24]

Epidemiology

Tuberculosis in cattle is caused predominantly by *M. bovis*, of which cattle are the maintenance hosts.

Mycobacterium bovis infection has recently been diagnosed in African buffalo (*Syncerus caffer*) in some game parks in South Africa.

Tuberculosis in the water buffalo (*Bubalus bubalis*) in some countries and free-living African buffaloes in African game reserves may therefore constitute a source of infection when they mingle with livestock on the borders of conservation areas. Kudus (*Tragelaphus strepsiceros*) in certain areas in South Africa may play a restricted role in the transmission of *M. bovis* to cattle.[116] In New Zealand the opossum (*Trichosurus vulpecula*) and fallow deer (*Dama dama*), in England the badger (*Meles meles*) , in some European countries the deer, and in the USA and Canada the bison (*Bison bison*) and elk (*Cervus elaphus*) are additional maintenance hosts. Infection with *M. tuberculosis* is rare in cattle, but it may be responsible for non-specific reactions in tuberculin-tested cattle. Infection with members of the *M. avium* complex is not a major disease problem in cattle, but it can cause many problems in tuberculosis eradication programmes in cattle. Cattle infected with the avian tubercle bacillus are sensitive to mammalian tuberculin, which may result in a false positive diagnosis of the intradermal tuberculin test. In cattle the sensitivity to both avian and mammalian tuberculin may disappear soon after they are removed from contact with either birds or humans infected with *M. tuberculosis*. Infection and disease due to *M. bovis* in other susceptible species in contact with cattle, including humans, tend to decline when eradication programmes in cattle are in progress or have been successfully concluded.[16] However, should *M. bovis* infection become established in a susceptible population other than cattle, such as African buffalo, total eradication of the disease becomes difficult if not impossible.

Humans with open tuberculosis due to *M. bovis* can infect cattle by the aerogenous route when handling them, or by contaminating the environment of cattle in a stable by spitting or urinating.[15, 86, 100, 123, 124]

Mycobacterium tuberculosis infection in cattle does not usually result in progressive disease, although localized lesions do develop. Infected cattle are generally not contagious, although excretion of bacilli in animals that are not manifesting signs of the infection has been reported. Bacilli may persist for some time in the organs and tissues. In one investigation it was found that most cattle experimentally infected with *M. tuberculosis* reacted negatively to the tuberculin test after some months.[129]

The primary mode of spread of bovine tuberculosis between herds is by the introduction of infected animals into non-infected herds. In contrast to European countries, close contact in confined spaces is not a prerequisite for the spread of the disease in southern Africa — infections have been found in extensive cattle breeding areas where ranching conditions prevail and in which there is little or no close contact between animals in confined spaces for prolonged periods. Under similar conditions in Australia, tuberculosis in extensively-kept cattle is thought to be due to their habit of congregating daily in large numbers at watering points under very dusty conditions.[77]

Most cases of bovine tuberculosis in South Africa occur in the region east of a line between Cape Town in the south and Messina in the north. This is probably due to the higher concentration of dairy herds along the eastern coast and around the bigger residential areas. The greater prevalence of tuberculosis in beef herds in the eastern parts of the country can possibly be attributed to a spill-over effect resulting from the closer contact between these beef herds and infected dairy herds.

The most important factors determining the occurrence and spread of tuberculosis in a herd of cattle are the number of infected individuals, the number of young stock exposed to these infected animals, and the measures taken to prevent spread. The mode of transmission in cattle is mainly horizontal, but not all infected animals transmit the disease. Most cattle suffering from pulmonary tuberculosis and tuberculous mastitis are, however, infectious, and in some infected individuals urine, vaginal secretions, semen or faeces may also contain tubercle bacilli and act as a means of transmitting the disease between animals.[56]

Possible routes of infection with *M. bovis* are respiratory, alimentary, congenital, cutaneous, venereal and via the teat canal. In practice, infection is acquired almost exclusively aerogenously by the inhalation of infected droplets from a coughing or sneezing animal with open tuberculosis or infected dust particles.[35, 59] Such droplets and particles may be constantly present in the air in stables and barns housing tuberculous cattle.[52] Alimentary infection may be primary, as occurs in calves drinking the milk of cows with tuberculous mastitis,[75] or it may be a secondary result of swallowing mycobacteria-laden exudate from the lungs. Tonsillar infection with secondary involvement of regional lymph nodes may result from the ingestion of bacilli in the food.

The congenital route is of some importance in cattle because of the relatively high incidence of tuberculous endometritis (some authors consider this to be as high as 5 per cent).

Infection via damaged skin is possible. For example, in humans it might happen in meat inspectors who have cut themselves with a knife contaminated with mycobacteria while examining tuberculous cattle, or in a laboratory worker who has pricked himself with a Pasteur pipette containing a mycobacterial suspension. Percutaneous infection as a result of scratching the ears with contaminated hind legs has been described in kudus in the eastern Cape Province in South Africa,[95, 116] and through the bites of badgers in England.[84] Venereal transmission is rare, but has been encountered in cattle.[113] Infusion of contaminated material via the teat canal may result in tuberculous mastitis.

The period of infectiousness may be extremely long if

the disease is left uncontrolled; an excreting carrier may transmit the infection for months or even years. Large numbers of tubercle bacilli may be excreted in the milk of cows with tuberculous mastitis; there may be sufficient numbers of viable bacilli in the milk of a cow to contaminate the milk of as many as 100 uninfected cows when such milk is pooled for transportation. Separated, defatted milk that has been purchased by farmers from milk-processing factories in order to feed their calves can in this way greatly contribute to the spread of *M. bovis*.

The feeding of infected carcasses to animals is a potential source of infection, and affected lymph nodes are partially important in this respect. Meat is usually free of tubercle bacilli.[35] Diseased tissue of cattle does not generally contain as many living tubercle bacilli as the sputum of humans with open lung lesions.

In South Africa, tuberculosis caused by *M. bovis* has been diagnosed in wild antelope, namely kudu and Cape duiker (*Sylvicapra grimmia*) in the Albany district of the eastern Cape Province,[91, 116] and African buffalo in the Kruger National Park[6] and in some of the game parks (Umfolozi and Hluhluwe) in Natal that are under the jurisdiction of the Natal Parks Board.[32] In other parts of Africa, tuberculosis in free-living wild animals has been reported in lechwe (*Kobus leche*) in Zambia[12, 65] and in African buffalo in Uganda.[41, 127, 128] In countries in other continents, tuberculosis caused by *M. bovis* has been reported in the following free-living wild animals: opossum in New Zealand[27] badger in England,[10, 46] and sika (*Cervus nippon*) and fallow deer in California.[64] Tuberculosis has been described in camels (*Camelus dromedarius*) and farmed water buffalo in Egypt,[28, 29] farmed fallow deer in New Zealand and Sweden,[20, 39, 48] red deer in England[107] and Hungary,[132] farmed elk in Canada[30] and North America,[115] and free-ranging bison in Canada.[109] In captive wild animals, *M. bovis*, *M. avium* and *M. tuberculosis* (human strains) have all been responsible for numerous outbreaks in zoological gardens, involving many species ranging from non-human primates to elephants.[87]

Humans are as susceptible to *M. bovis* as to *M. tuberculosis*. Once a tuberculous lesion develops in an organ, the appearance and the course of the disease are the same, irrespective of whether it is caused by *M. bovis* or *M. tuberculosis*.[86, 101] In humans, *M. bovis* often results in localized lesions and is most frequently the cause of cervical lymphadenitis and other forms of extrapulmonary tuberculosis in infancy and childhood. Pulmonary tuberculosis due to *M. bovis* infection in humans is rare. Compared to the extent to which humans infect other humans with tuberculosis, transmission from animals to humans is a minor problem today. Extrapulmonary tuberculosis is typically transmitted via cows' milk. Compulsory pasteurization was first introduced in 1898 — not to protect humans, but to prevent tuberculosis in pigs and calves fed on separated milk obtained from infected herds.

Pathogenesis

Some mycobacterial infections remain localized, while others cause widely disseminated lesions. In the majority of cases, very small lesions occur and the infection does not spread. For this reason, many tuberculous infections cause very few, if any, clinical signs, while others elicit widely differing clinical signs because of the varying location of the lesions. In general, and depending on the route of infection, primary foci of tuberculosis occur either in the gastrointestinal or respiratory tracts. In the former, lesions occur primarily in the lymphoid tissues, whereas both the lung parenchyma and the regional lymph nodes are affected in the respiratory system. These variations are the consequence of unexplained variations in the pathogenicity of the organisms in different species, and the inherent characteristics of the organisms. Thus it appears from experimental results that the age of the animal, route of infection, strain of the organism, and the dose of bacteria will influence the length of time required for the disease to develop.[111] Lesions in different sites in the same animal appear also to have individuality: some may be stable while at the same time others are regressing or expanding.[19]

Many aspects of the pathogenesis of tuberculosis remain unknown even in humans, in spite of the fact that humans are the focus of most of the current studies. In several species the effects of a highly specific immune response results in a spectrum of lesions ranging from self-limiting infections to a life-threatening systemic disease.[94] At every stage during the course of the tuberculous process the character of the lesions depends on the fluctuation between cell-mediated immunity and the delayed type hypersensitivity. In addition, the development of either an exudative or a proliferative response appears to depend on the concentration of bacterial antigen — low concentrations cause proliferative lesions, whereas high concentrations result in an exudative response.[19] Some of the opportunistic mycobacteria which can be isolated from soil, dust and plants are able to cause persistent and slowly progressive infections which do not generate immune responses in the host.[19]

The outcome of a mycobacterial infection is dependent on whether or not an animal has been previously sensitized.[125] In unsensitized hosts, initial multiplication of the bacteria in macrophages results in a primary lesion, which spreads to the regional lymph node, and the development of a mild bacteraemia as soon as 20 days after the infection has taken place. This bacteraemia may terminate in the development of metastatic foci (a process referred to as post-primary dissemination). Following the development of cell-mediated immunity, however, most of the foci of infection, with the exception of those in certain 'vulnerable sites' such as the lungs, bone, kidneys and meninges, are destroyed. In the 'vulnerable sites' the bacterial population is reduced, but persists and is not totally eliminated.[125]

In aerogenous infections, bacteria are inhaled in

droplet nuclei. Only droplets 2–5 μm in diameter have the ability to reach the alveolar spaces of the lungs, where they are deposited and the bacteria ingested by macrophages. Larger particles (or nuclei) are trapped in the upper airways and are removed by means of the mucociliary apparatus, after which they are swallowed. The mucosal surfaces of the upper respiratory tract and the intestine are only infected after exposure to very large infective doses of bacteria.[19]

The initial success of the elimination of mycobacteria depends on the microbicidal activities of the infected macrophages. When organisms initially multiply within the phagolysosomes of inactivated macrophages, their presence does not result in the death of many of the cells. When infected macrophages do die, the released bacteria are again phagocytosed by adjacent macrophages. The ability of macrophages to kill mycobacteria is enhanced only after the development of a delayed type hypersensitivity. The rapid development of the immune response following infection inhibits the growth of mycobacteria in lesions while they are still very small.

Macrophages at the site of infection may be activated by direct contact with mycobacteria or as a result of lymphokines. The debris of necrotic macrophages sensitizes local lymphocytes. After sensitization, which may be as soon as two weeks after the initial infection, lymphocytes release lymphokines that attract, activate and increase the number of mononuclear cells at the site of infection. They also contribute to cell death, with the subsequent development of caseous necrosis.[19, 112] Macrophages also play an integral part in the processing of mycobacterial antigens and the initiation of the immune response. Cell death caused by the delayed hypersensitivity reaction may be the result of lymphokines, toxic components of the bacteria, ischaemia, antigen-antibody reactions, hydrolytic enzymes and reactive oxygen intermediates released from necrotic macrophages and neutrophils, and the tumour necrosis factor.[19]

The further development of mycobacterial granulomas appears to be dependent on a number of factors, the main ones being the ability of the mycobacteria to survive intracellularly, and their ability to induce a host response (delayed type hypersensitivity). Neutrophils initially enter into the development of the granuloma but they are soon replaced by mononuclear macrophages. Certain glycolipid extracts (cord factor) from the bacteria inhibit chemotaxis and are leukotoxic, whereas others promote the intracellular survival of the bacteria in macrophages by inhibiting phagolysosome formation. At the early stages of development, tuberculous granulomas are composed of sensitized leukocytes and epithelioid cells. At this stage there is a dynamic engulfment of bacteria and necrosis of macrophages at the site of infection. As the development of the lesion progresses, the necrotic mass may become extensive. Langerhans' giant cells appear in the granulomatous response and it also becomes surrounded by a zone of lymphocytes and other mononuclear cells. Often there is proliferation of connective tissue at the periphery, which tends to encapsulate the lesion.[111]

The fate of focal tubercles is determined by the activity of macrophages within the lesion. When these cells have developed microbicidal activities, they prevent expansion of the lesion. However, continuing intracellular bacterial growth enables the lesions to expand and eventually leads to haematogenous dissemination. This is usually the case in animals that are immature or immunodeficient.[19] The multiplication of bacilli tends to be inhibited in lesions that contain caseous exudate, but if the exudate becomes liquefied their multiplication may be profuse. In the latter case, because of the high concentration of tuberculin-like products, the effect of the host's cell-mediated immune response is severely detrimental and results in further local caseous necrosis. Bacteria may remain viable within the caseous centres of the larger tubercles for months or years and may become reactivated if the resistance of the host decreases.[19]

Caseous lesions may undergo liquefaction because of the effects of hydrolytic enzymes from macrophages and neutrophils.[111] This liquefied material is an excellent culture medium for the bacilli and contains large numbers of them.[19] Liquefaction of the caseous exudate may lead to the disintegration of surrounding tissue, including the walls of ducts or tubes. If this occurs in the lungs, for instance, the entrance and spread of mycobacteria in the bronchial tree may result in extensive tubercular pneumonia.

Massive haematogenous spread may result in miliary tuberculosis which is the result of a sudden, massive bacteraemia. The haematogenous spread can also be more protracted, in which case fewer bacteria enter the blood stream over a longer period, thus causing fewer, and larger, metastatic lesions which vary in age and size. Live, infected macrophages may also enter blood and lymph vessels, ducts or body cavities and so may disseminate the infection.[111]

Clinical signs and pathology

Bovine tuberculosis is generally a chronic, and often subclinical disease. It usually takes many months or even years for clinical signs to develop.[45] In most infected cattle the disease is inapparent, and its presence is only detectable through the tuberculin test; but if clinical signs are manifested, their nature will depend upon the organ system or systems involved and the severity of the infection. Remissions and relapses, and in some instances arrest and self-cure, may occur. The most common forms of tuberculosis in cattle involve the lymph nodes and to a lesser extent the lungs, while tuberculosis of the kidneys, liver, spleen, bone, joints, mammary gland, testes, uterus and ovaries is rare and is usually the consequence of haematogenous spread.

The distribution of lesions varies according to the route of infection, which may be by inhalation, *per os*, genital, via the teat canal, percutaneous, or congenital via the umbilical cord. Irrespective of the route of infection, complete or incomplete primary complexes are established. A complete primary complex is one where a lesion is present at the initial site of infection as well as in the regional lymph node. In an incomplete primary complex a lesion is found only in the regional lymph node.

Animals with disseminated lesions gradually become emaciated and anorexic, manifest a fluctuating temperature, have a dull hair coat, and may eventually become lethargic, but their eyes remain clear. Signs become more evident during stress such as that which may occur during the immediate post-calving period, or as the result of malnutrition.

The classic lesion of tuberculosis, the tubercle, is a typical granuloma containing a central core of caseous necrotic tissue, part of which rapidly undergoes dystrophic calcification. This central mass is surrounded by epithelioid cells and Langhans' giant cells, and more peripherally by lymphocytes, macrophages and varying degrees of fibroplasia **(Figure 172.1)**. Application of the Ziehl-Neelsen staining technique to sections or smears of affected tissue reveals varying numbers of pleomorphic, intracellular, acid-fast bacilli **(Figure 172.2)**. Mycobacteria are Gram-positive and fluoresce after being stained with auramine. Exceptionally, the inflammatory reaction may be florid and markedly exudative, in which case large amounts of fibrin, haemorrhage and oedema occur in addition to the presence of macrophages and developing giant cells.

Since most mycobacterial infections are contracted by inhalation or ingestion, tubercles occur predominantly in the retropharyngeal, mediastinal and bronchial lymph nodes **(Figures 172.3–172.6)**. In adult cattle and older calves, the lungs are affected in 90–95 per cent of cases, while in 5–10 per cent of cases the digestive tract is infected. In young calves, omphalogenic infection causes hepatic lesions in 49 per cent of cases, while 38 per cent and 13 per cent of cases, respectively, suffer from pulmonary and digestive tract infections.[14] Primary pulmonary lesions can be very small and are easily overlooked. They are located principally subpleurally and caudo-dorsally, but may occur in any lobe and are most successfully detected at necropsy or in the abattoir by palpation of the lungs. Initially, lesions appear macroscopically as partially or fully encapsulated, yellowish foci of caseous necrosis, part of which is calcified **(Figure 172.7)**.Encapsulation is not always absolute, which allows local spread through the airways **(Figure 172.8)**. Several such foci may be clustered within a lobule to produce a clover-leaf appearance. Coalescence and expansion of these pneumonic foci result in the development of large areas of a caseating bronchopneumonia **(Figure 172.9)**. In time, the pneumonic focus may become calcified and encapsulated. Bronchial and tracheal ulceration may result in intrapulmonary spread. Pulmonary lesions may heal completely, but metastatic lesions which are invariably present in the regional lymph nodes persist.

On the pleura or mesentery, spread is aided by respiratory or intestinal peristaltic movements to cause diffuse, caseous, plaque-like or clustered, nodular lesions, respectively **(Figures 172.10–172.11)**. The latter lesions are referred to as 'TB-grapes', and after calcification as 'TB-pearls'.[26]

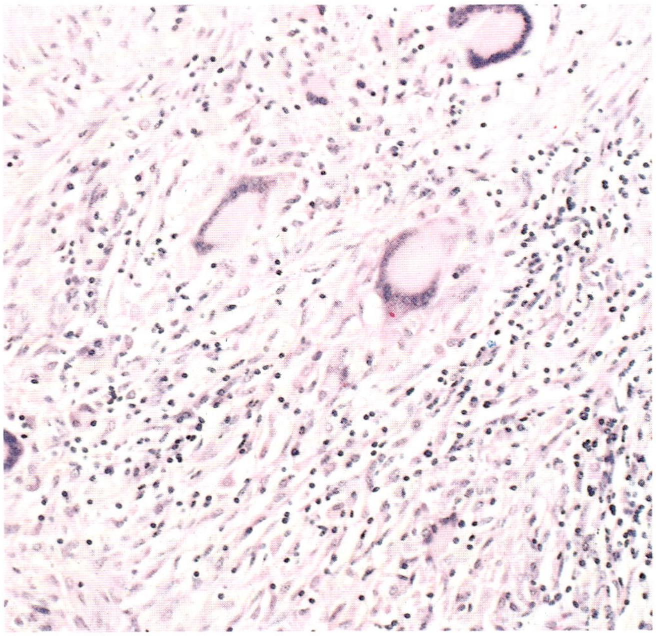

Figure 172.1 Photomicrograph of a typical tubercle manifesting caseous necrosis, epithelioid cells, Langhans' giant cells, fibroplasia and a scant lymphocyte infiltrate (haematoxylin and eosin stain)

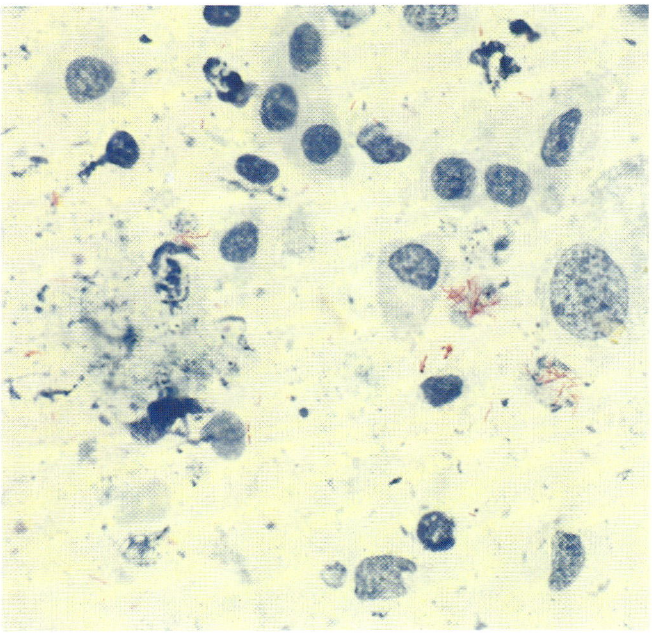

Figure 172.2 Smear of exudate from a tuberculous granuloma stained with Ziehl-Neelsen stain. Note the cluster of red-staining mycobacteria and others scattered throughout

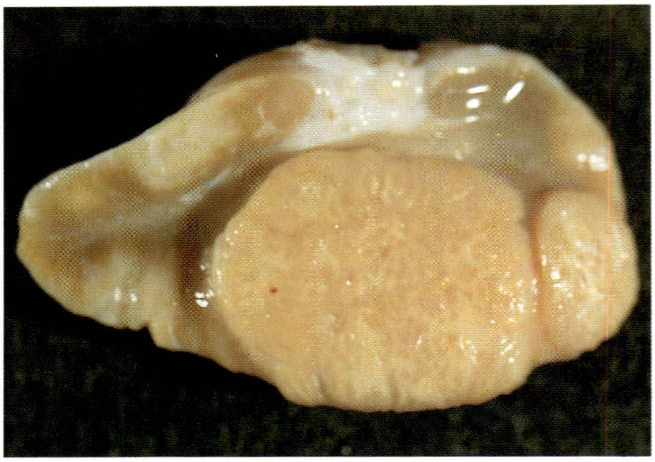

Figure 172.3 Tuberculous granulomas in a lymph node

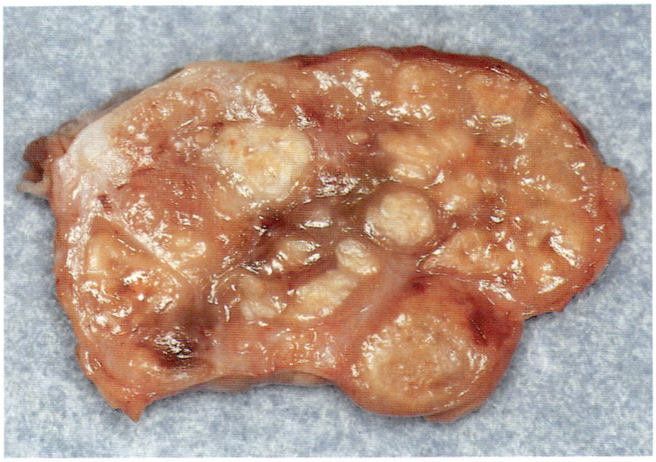

Figure 172.5 Multifocal chronic tuberculous lymphadenitis. Note marked encapsulation

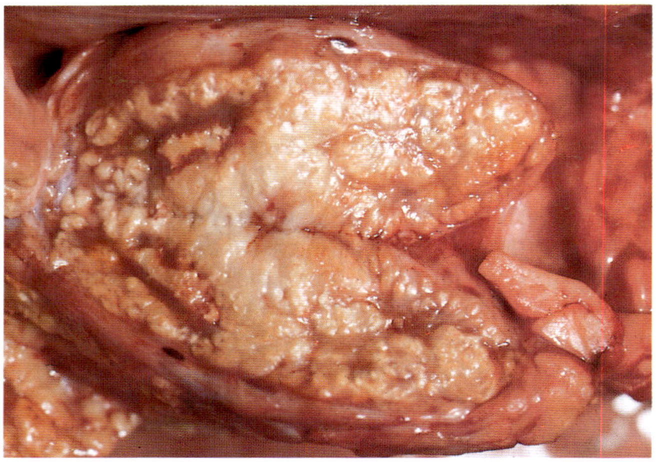

Figure 172.4 Extensive tuberculous lymphadenitis in mediastinal lymph nodes

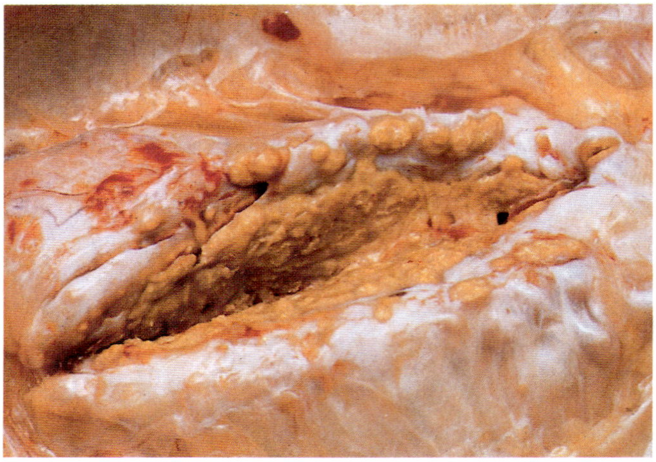

Figure 172.6 Marked yellow pigmentation of the exudate in a tuberculous lymph node. Pigmentation such as this is caused by certain strains of *M. bovis*

Generalized tuberculosis is characterized by the presence of 'miliary' or larger lesions in organs and lymph nodes throughout the body. Miliary lesions are small (from microscopic to 5 mm in diameter), and are translucent in the early stage, but become caseous and calcified as they age. In advanced cases of tuberculosis with widespread dissemination, enlarged peripheral lymph nodes, such as the submaxillary, prescapular, precrural and supramammary, may be easily palpable or visible. Suppressed moist coughs may be heard, especially early in the morning, after exercise, and when infected animals are exposed to low environmental temperatures. Dyspnoea may be apparent in advanced cases in which extensive pulmonary lesions have led to impaired respiratory functions[112] or where enlarged bronchial lymph nodes cause obstruction of airways. Persistent ruminal bloat can occur as a result of pressure on the oesophagus by enlarged mediastinal lymph nodes.[8]

Hepatic involvement may also follow mycobacteraemia. Lesions may be miliary, but coarse, nodular lesions are more common. The kidneys may be similarly involved; miliary lesions are limited to the cortex. Erosion of the renal pelvis and a descending infection may be a sequel.

Tuberculous osteomyelitis, particularly of the vertebrae, ribs and flat bones of the pelvis, occurs in some young animals. The lesions are characterized by extensive caseation and a tendency to liquefy. This exudate may drain through fistulae in the cortex of the affected bone and may cause a tuberculous myositis in the region. Similarly, articular cartilage may become eroded, with the subsequent development of tuberculous arthritis.

Tuberculous meningitis may follow haematogenous spread or occur by extension from vertebral lesions. Macroscopically it resembles lesions on serous surfaces, but the lesions are necrotizing and the exudate is often more voluminous.

Lesions in the gastrointestinal tract manifest as

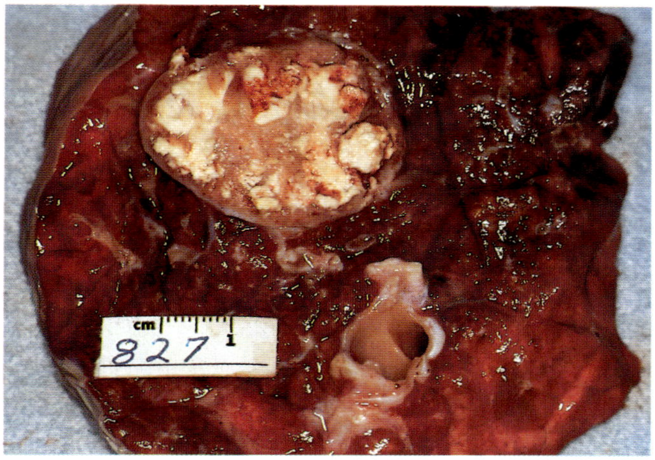

Figure 172.7 Focal chronic tuberculous pneumonia

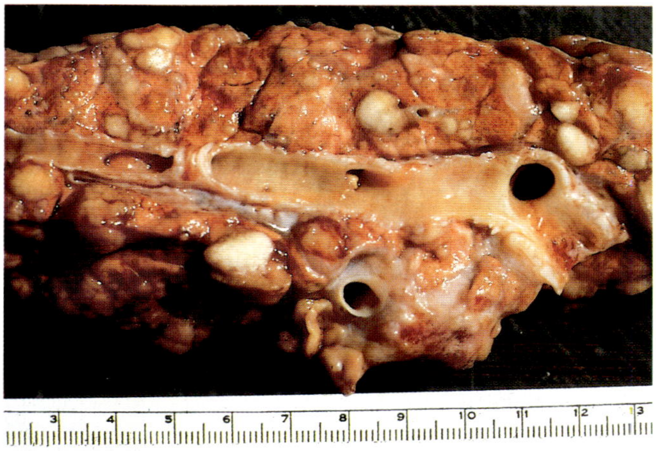

Figure 172.8 Multifocal tuberculous pneumonia subsequent to spread along the airways

nodules or ulcers in the mucosa of the upper alimentary tract, abomasum, or small or large intestine after a *per os* infection, such as the ingestion of tuberculous milk, or they may be secondary to pulmonary infection following the swallowing of coughed-up, infected material from the lungs. In the intestinal tract, ulcers first develop in Peyer's patches. The margins of the ulcers are distinct and raised, while the base consists of granulation tissue covered by a dryish, caseous exudate.

Mycobacterial dermatitis is most frequently caused by opportunistic mycobacteria. Single or multiple, often ulcerated nodules (10–80 mm in diameter) form in the skin and subcutis, especially of the legs.[131] Upon incision of these nodules, caseous, purulent or possibly mineralized exudate may be exposed. Lesions may involve lymphatics, but the regional lymph nodes are lesion-free—which is not the case in *M. bovis* infections. Microscopically the lesions consist of typical tuberculous granulomas.

In tuberculous mastitis the affected part of the udder may be firm and/or enlarged with secondary involvement of the supramammary lymph nodes. In some cases, however, enlargement of the lymph nodes in the absence of palpable lesions in the udder itself may indicate the presence of tuberculosis. The milk appears normal during the initial stages of infection, but in the more advanced stages fine floccules may be found in it, which sediment after the milk has been left standing in a container, to leave a clear, amber supernatant fluid.[8, 120]

Infection of the bovine udder generally occurs via the haematogenous route. Various forms are encountered, the most common (80–90 per cent of cases) being chronic organ tuberculosis,[53] in which most of the lobules in an affected gland are replaced by granulation tissue. This accentuates the lobulation, as the lobules acquire a greyish-red to white colour. Microscopically, lobular outlines are retained but diffuse granulation tissue obliterates the acinar tissue. The intra- and interlobular ducts are always affected, showing marked thickening of the walls due to the formation of granulation tissue, while

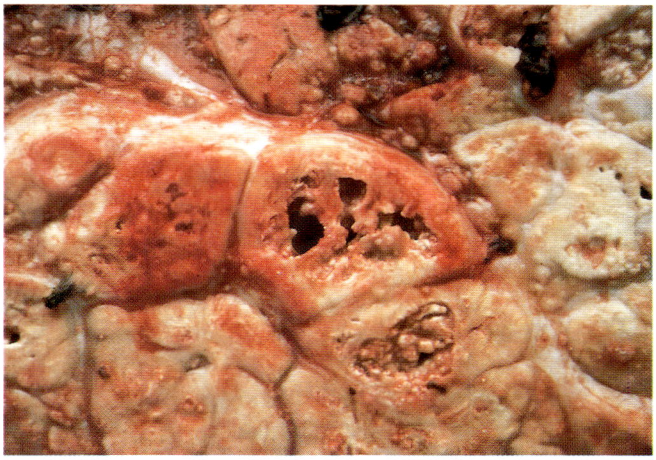

Figure 172.9 Extensive caseating tuberculous bronchopneumonia manifesting liquefaction of the centre of some of the granulomas

their luminal surfaces tend to caseate. Intramammary spread is solely via the ducts. Contrary to what would normally be expected, the regional lymph nodes are usually not involved.

Disseminated miliary tuberculous mastitis, in which nodules up to 10 mm in diameter are formed, is less common. These lesions occur in clusters and tend to caseate and become calcified. The interlobular ducts are extensively affected.

The third form is caseous tuberculous mastitis, in which large, irregular areas of dry, yellowish, caseous, necrotic tissue develop, surrounded by a hyperaemic reaction zone. Confluence across interlobular boundaries occurs commonly. Microscopically, there is an exudate composed of fibrin and numerous leukocytes present in the necrotic areas.

The fourth manifestation of tuberculous involvement of the mammary gland is tuberculous galactophoritis. In this form, affected lactiferous ducts are dilated and filled with exudate, while the acini are relatively uninvolved.

The duct walls in these cases are greatly thickened by granulation tissue that contains a mononuclear cell infiltration. All cases of mammary tuberculosis are considered to be open cases because of the duct involvement.

About 1 per cent of new-born calves from tuberculous cows are born suffering from congenital tuberculosis. Infection of foetuses is generally via the haematogenous route and in most cases is secondary to tuberculous endometritis, but it may also be more rarely acquired as a result either of swallowing tuberculous amniotic fluid, which leads to the development of lesions in the intestine or mesenteric lymph nodes, or inhaling it, which results in pulmonary disease. Tuberculous lesions in the uterus **(Figure 172.12)** are usually the result of haematogenous dissemination but they may originate via the genital route or be an extension of a tuberculous peritonitis. Endometritis as a result of tuberculosis may also cause infertility or result in abortion in the late stages of pregnancy.[8] In the majority of congenitally infected calves, the primary complex is found in the liver and portal lymph nodes. As the disease usually progresses quite rapidly and becomes generalized, the young animals die in a few weeks or months. By this time lesions are found particularly in the liver and its regional lymph nodes and in the spleen. As tuberculous lesions are rarely present in the spleen of adult cattle, their presence there is generally regarded as being indicative of congenital infection.

Mycobacterium avium infection in cattle causes a self-limiting disease in which lesions usually do not exceed 20 mm in diameter. Microscopically there is pronounced proliferation of epithelioid cells, formation of giant cells and numerous acid-fast bacilli.[78] *Mycobacterium tuberculosis* infection usually does not progress beyond the development of small granulomas in the pharyngeal, thoracic and mesenteric lymph nodes.

Diagnosis and differential diagnosis

The clinical examination of an animal suspected to be suffering from tuberculosis requires a thorough palpation of all the superficial lymph nodes, the udder in females, and percussion and auscultation of the pulmonary area. A comprehensive investigation of the history of the herd is most important. This should include pertinent questions about the previous introduction of animals into the herd, abattoir reports on animals sent for slaughter, and the possibility of bovine tuberculosis on neighbouring properties. A clinical diagnosis of tuberculosis must be confirmed by the application of the tuberculin test or laboratory tests.

Tubercle bacilli may be tentatively identified by the microscopic examination of smears prepared from the content of lesions and stained by the Ziehl-Neelsen method. Final confirmation of the diagnosis is dependent on culturing.

The biological examination of material suspected to contain mycobacteria, such as suspensions of lesions in tissues, exudates and milk by the parenteral inoculation of guinea-pigs, which are very susceptible to infection, has become outdated as a diagnostic procedure, except in the case of urine specimens which have repeatedly been negative on culture, and other body fluids such as aspirates of pleural exudates, suspected tuberculous material obtained by swabbing (e.g. the larynx and cerebrospinal fluid, which may contain only small numbers of mycobacteria).[85] However, these specimens must also be cultured because of the varying pathogenicity of different species of mycobacteria for laboratory animals. To use guinea-pigs as a filter to suppress contaminants in the specimen is unnecessary, as more humane decontamination methods are available today.

Soon after Robert Koch discovered the causative organism of tuberculosis in 1882, it was found that a filtrate of the culture medium in which it had been grown could be used as a diagnostic agent when inoculated into infected animals.[100] The reactive substance, later identified as tuberculoprotein and named tuberculin,[80, 104] is employed to detect delayed hypersensitivity in animals and humans infected with mycobacteria. Tuberculin itself, when injected parenterally, will not induce hypersensitivity.

In South Africa, tuberculin was imported until 1936, when Robinson commenced the production of Heat-concentrated Synthetic Medium (HCSM) tuberculin at the Veterinary Research Institute, Onderstepoort.[61] In 1947, the production of Purified Protein Derivative (PPD) of tuberculin was started at this Institute, using *M. tuberculosis* strains T100, PN and DT and following methods similar to those described by Green (1946) in Weybridge, England. From 1950 onwards the *M. bovis* strain AN5 was also used for PPD production.[61] Tests in England and the Netherlands had shown that PPD tuberculin produced from *M. bovis* was more specific than PPD tuberculin of *M. tuberculosis* origin for the detection of infections with *M. bovis* in both cattle and guinea-pigs.[92, 118, 119] This was confirmed in a field trial in South Africa in 1954.[68] Thus, from January 1960 PPD of bovine tuberculin was issued by the Veterinary Research Institute, Onderstepoort for general use.[56]

Purified protein derivative of avian tuberculin for comparative testing procedures was produced at Onderstepoort from *M. avium* strain D4. It is used in conjunction with bovine PPD tuberculin to differentiate between sensitization induced by *M. bovis* or *M. tuberculosis*, and that induced by *M. avium* or other mycobacteria.

As PPD tuberculins consist of a mixture of varying-sized protein molecules with different antigenic properties,[18, 42, 71, 104] consecutive batches may vary in their potency and specificity even though they are produced by the same method. Each newly produced batch is compared with a well-defined standard produced by the same method as the batch under test, and the potency is then expressed in biological units.[1] Two national or house standards are kept at the Veterinary Research

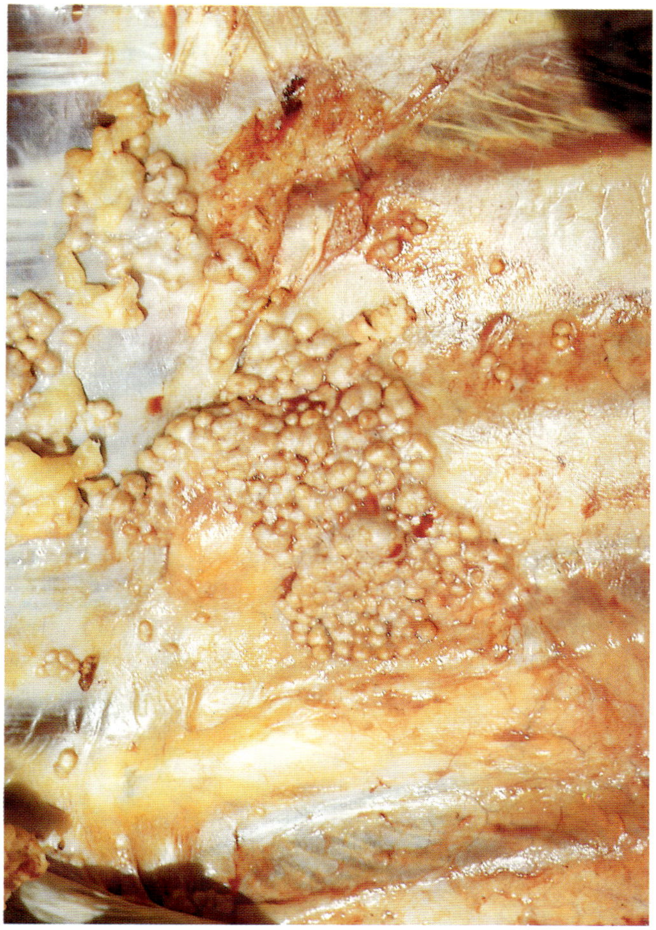

Figure 172.10 Localized tuberculous pleuritis. Note the nodular appearance of the lesions

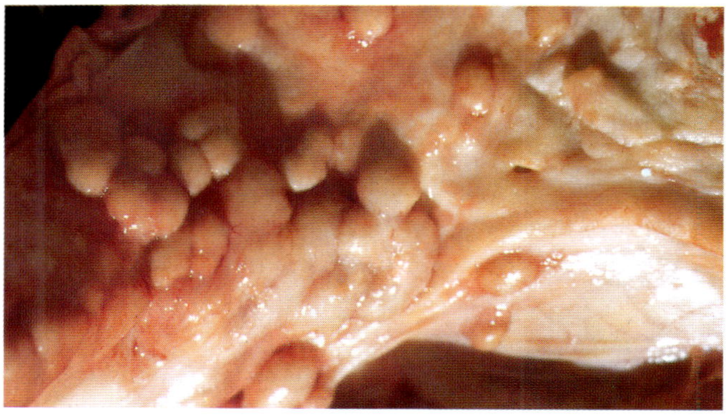

Figure 172.11 Close-up view of a tuberculous pleuritis showing pronounced encapsulation of the lesions

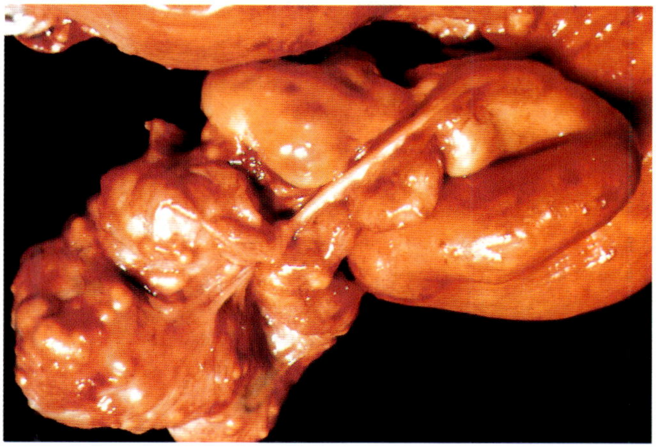

Figure 172.12 Tuberculous metritis and oophoritis in a cow

Institute, Onderstepoort for potency testing:

- National standard for PPD of bovine tuberculin is standardized against the European Community (EC) standard for PPD of bovine tuberculin in homologously sensitized guinea-pigs and in naturally infected tuberculous cattle.[1, 23, 43] Until 1986 the EC standard was the only standard for PPD of bovine tuberculin to which a unitage had been assigned. It contains 50 000 Community Tuberculin Units (CTU)/mg of PPD (EC Council Directive 80/219/EEC).[43, 103] Since 1986 an international standard for bovine PPD has existed.[4, 36, 74] It was tested against the EC standard in an international collaborative assay and was found to have a relative potency of 65 per cent (32 500 CTU/mg of PPD) of the EC standard. International units are nowadays used to express the potency of bovine PPD.
- National standard for PPD of avian tuberculin is standardized against the international standard for PPD of avian tuberculin in homologously sensitized guinea-pigs.

The specificity of a batch under test is assayed by a similar method in heterogenously sensitized guinea-pigs. Once the test batches have been diluted to the strength used for testing cattle and the quality control tests are satisfactory, an expiry date of one year is given.[3] Purified Protein Derivative tuberculin should be kept at 4–8 °C and be protected from light.[69, 70]

The intradermal tuberculin test for cattle is based on a specific reaction following the administration of bovine PPD tuberculin.[66] For the single intradermal test, an area of skin on the left side of the neck halfway between the juncture of the head and the neck and the fold in front of the shoulder, and halfway between the top and bottom of the neck, is chosen as the inoculation site. For the comparative intradermal test, another similar site is selected, but this is approximately a hand's breadth more cranial. The hair of the chosen site(s) is removed by shaving (an area of approximately 40 x 40 mm), the skin thickness measured with a calliper, and the required dose (0,1 ml) of tuberculin is injected intradermally using a McLintock syringe. If a comparative tuberculin test is performed, avian tuberculin is injected at the site nearest to the head and bovine tuberculin at the site nearest to the shoulder. The result of the test is read 72 hours after tuberculin has been injected.

The comparative intradermal test is generally used for herds:

- that are being tested for the first time,

- in which the tuberculosis status or the history of the herd is unknown or vague,
- in which non-specific reactions occur, or
- when problems have been experienced with the interpretation of the tests.

The simultaneous use of avian and bovine tuberculin is to obtain a definite result regarding the presence or absence of tuberculosis caused by *M. bovis* in a herd. The single intradermal tuberculin test, on the other hand, is mainly used:

- where the negative tuberculosis status is known, or
- where herds have already been tested negatively for tuberculosis caused by *M. bovis*.[117]

The skin reaction is interpreted according to whether a single or comparative intradermal test has been performed and whether the herd history indicates a non-infected or potentially infected herd. The interpretation of the tests is summarized in **Table 172.1**. As a general guideline, an increase of 4 mm and more in the bovine tuberculin reaction, and a difference of 5 mm between the avian and bovine tuberculin reaction in previous negative herds or 3 mm in established positive herds, is regarded as a positive reaction. In the interpretation of the comparative tuberculin test, the reaction is regarded as negative for bovine tuberculosis if the swelling on the injection site of the avian tuberculin exceeds that of the swelling on the site for the bovine tuberculin.[117]

In an intradermal tuberculin test a diagnosis is not made simply by measuring the increase in the thickness of the skinfold. If a reaction is present:

- the appearance of the swelling may be round, flat, circumscribed or diffuse,
- it may be red or blue,
- signs of oozing of oedematous fluid and necrosis may be seen,
- swelling of the lymphatic vessels in the skin surrounding the inoculation site may be evident, and
- systemic changes such as shivering, ruffled hair and listlessness may be observed.

The site where each tested animal was injected must always be palpated, because reactions may occur that are not clearly visible. Palpation may reveal:

- the consistency of the reaction,
- the presence of oedema,
- a local increase in skin temperature,
- pain, and
- adhesions between the skin and the subcutaneous tissue.

In addition, the state of regional and other superficial lymph nodes should be assessed by palpation. These, especially the superficial cervical (prescapular) and supramammary lymph nodes, may be swollen.

However, it is important to remember that an increase in skin thickness may occur without any of the above signs being present. In such cases one has to rely mainly on the guidelines provided for the increase in skin thickness as well as on the herd history in order to finally make a diagnosis.

It is important to consider all the variables that might influence the final diagnosis, so the herd is not immediately classified positive merely on the detection of a single 'positive' sign.

The interpretation of the test is done on a herd basis. Depending on the previous history of the herd and the results obtained from the visual inspection of the test sites of all the animals before each animal has been examined individually, the herd may be provisionally classified as free or possibly free from tuberculosis, or as infected according to the criteria in **Table 172.1** and diagnositc features mentioned above.

Other factors that must be taken into consideration during the interpretation of the intradermal test include the age of the animal, the possibility of infection with species of mycobacteria other than *M. bovis* or with other organisms, and a number of physiological factors. In animals that have been recently infected with *M. bovis* (six weeks to three months), a reasonably typical and large reaction should develop, whilst animals that have been

Table 172.1 Diagnostic criteria that are used to interpret skin reactions following intradermal tuberculin tests

TEST PERFORMED	INCREASE GREATER	MEDIAN*	INCREASE SMALLER
NEGATIVE HERD			
Bovine tuberculin alone	Suspect	>6 mm<	Negative
Comparative test	Suspect (provided the reaction to bovine tuberculin is 4 mm or more)	>+3 mm< (bovine minus avian tuberculin)	Negative
POSITIVE HERD			
Bovine tuberculin alone	Positive	>4 mm<	Negative or suspect
Comparative test	Positive (provided the reaction to bovine tuberculin is 4 mm or more)	>+3 mm< (bovine minus avian tuberculin)	Negative or suspect

* Median is the measurement by which an increase or decrease in skin thickness is judged

infected for a long time (>6 months) will be less sensitive or even anergic.

Mycobacteria including *M. tuberculosis*, *M. paratuberculosis*, *M. intracellulare* (especially in pigs), and *M. avium*[130] and other species grouped according to Runyon's classification of Groups I to Group IV **(see Mycobacteria: Introduction: Table 3)** have been incriminated as causes of non-specific reactions. For example, *M. kansasii* of Group I shows a close relationship to *M. tuberculosis*, whilst the Battey strains from Group III are closely related to *M. avium* and cause signs in humans that cannot be clinically distinguished from human tuberculosis caused by *M. tuberculosis*. *Mycobacterium fortuitum* from Group IV, and other fast growers may sensitize animals.[129] *Mycobacterium paratuberculosis* is antigenically related to *M. avium* and correspondingly greater reactions are found to avian than bovine tuberculin.[11] Saprophytic mycobacteria, which are usually found in food, water and the gastrointestinal tract of herbivores, play an unimportant role in sensitizing animals, but organisms such as *M. smegmatis* may cause sensitivity to the intradermal tuberculin test, and sometimes may even cause tuberculous mastitis in cattle.[93] With the comparative tuberculin test, the sensitivity is more noticeable at the avian site of injection.

Skin lesions caused by saprophytic mycobacteria are often referred to as 'acid-fast lymphangitis' or *dermatitis nodosa* and appear as hard or soft nodules which seldom ulcerate.[8] In South Africa, especially in the western, southern and eastern Cape Province and Natal, such skin lesions often complicate the interpretation of the tuberculin test.[117]

Reactions caused by organisms that are closely related to mycobacteria, such as *Nocardia* spp., can cause problems in the differential diagnosis of tuberculosis.[79, 117] On culture, *N. asteroides* can also be confused with mycobacteria. Non-specific reactions can also be caused by conditions such as actinomycosis, actinobacillosis, brucellosis, corynebacteriosis, infections by *Trychophyton* spp., fascioliasis, peritonitis, abscesses and lumpy skin disease.[117]

Desensitization may occur in tuberculous cattle immediately before and after calving, resulting in false negative reactions. These animals return again to a positive status four to six weeks later.[8]

The skin reaction is interpreted according to whether a single or comparative intradermal test was performed and whether the herd history indicates a non-infected or potentially infected herd.

Tuberculin test reactions can be assessed with a fair degree of accuracy. Although Kleeberg[55] estimated that an accuracy of up to 97 per cent is well within South African and international capabilities, and that the application of the single intradermal or comparative tuberculin test will detect a large percentage of the cattle infected with *M. bovis*, Francis *et al.*[37] reviewed the literature and obtained a figure of 81,1 per cent sensitivity; thus approximately 20 out of 100 infected cattle tested would be missed and would remain within the herd to spread the infection. However, the success of interpretation is affected by a number of factors.

In cattle which are infected with *M. bovis* but for various reasons show insignificant reactions or no reaction at all to intradermal testing and exhibit no clinical signs, a false negative diagnosis may be made. The most common conditions leading to false negative diagnoses are the pre-allergic stage of infection, inactive tuberculosis and advanced tuberculosis anergy. In animals infected for a long time, the intensity of the reaction to the tuberculin test declines progressively.[66] In 1 or 2 per cent of the animals in an infected herd, sensitivity to the tuberculin test may disappear completely [117]

Accumulation of antibodies in the colostrum prior to and immediately after calving could explain why infected cows three weeks pre-partum to three to six weeks post-partum tend to show a decreased sensitivity to the tuberculin test.[66, 117]

Prolonged chemotherapy of infected animals may lead to destruction of all the mycobacteria, leading to disappearance of the allergic response.[55]

Reactions that occur after the administration of bovine tuberculin to cattle free of *M. bovis* are non-specific.[130] The family Mycobacteriaceae embraces many members, and cross-reactions are common. This fact does not seriously affect the interpretation of the tuberculin test, as there are well-described methods of differentiating these non-specific reactions from reactions due to infection with *M. bovis*.

As bovine tuberculosis is progressively eradicated from a country, the non-specific reactor problem becomes greater, because the percentage of reactors showing no gross lesions at slaughter tends to increase.[130] As only very small lesions may be associated with pronounced reactions, a very thorough post-mortem examination may be required to detect them.

In order to detect all positive cases in a herd, retesting is necessary. This will expose certain reactivated anergic cases as well as animals in the pre-allergic stage. Thorough clinical examination, supported by microscopical, bacteriological and biological tests, may also assist in diagnosing some anergic cases.

A number of other less commonly used procedures for the application of the tuberculin test may also be employed. The results obtained when the caudal skin fold is used as a test site compare favourably with those obtained using the cervical site. For caudal skin fold testing, double strength bovine PPD tuberculin (twice the strength of PPD used in the cervical test) is used. In problem herds containing suspected anergic animals and/or thick-skinned cattle (*Bos indicus*), the simultaneous use of both methods (caudal skin fold and cervical) allows detection of up to 6 per cent more true positives and can bring about quicker and more effective eradication of the disease.[25, 31, 73, 76, 108]

In the subcutaneous tuberculin test, the animal's rectal

temperature is taken and recorded prior to the injection of tuberculin. Using a conventional hypodermic syringe and needle, 4 ml of PPD tuberculin are injected subcutaneously into the neck of each animal. Temperature measurements of the animal are then taken at two-hourly intervals. A test result is positive when an animal develops a rise in temperature of 1,0 °C or more. This temperature reaction usually develops six to eight hours after the administration of tuberculin and reaches a peak at 12–24 hours post injection.[45] A subcutaneous test was used regularly until the early 1930s, [106] when it was replaced by the comparative intradermal test, and is only used nowadays in specific situations where anergic animals in infected herds pose a diagnostic problem.

The Stormont test can be applied in a similar manner to detect anergic animals. It is more sensitive than the intradermal test, and it is estimated that only 2 per cent of infected animals are misdiagnosed following its application.[54] This test is based on the phenomenon that occurs following an intradermal injection of tuberculin in a desensitized, infected bovine: the skin at the original injection site exhibits an increased sensitivity to tuberculin.[54, 67] A seven-day interval is allowed between the initial and the 'boost' injection, the latter being administered at the same site as the first. An increase in skin thickness of 5 mm or more 24 hours after the second injection is considered a positive reaction, irrespective of the type of reaction observed.[67]

Research investigations into the development of serological tests for the diagnosis of tuberculosis have been relatively intensive for the past 60 years,[7] but all such tests have so far shown only a low degree of specificity. The specificity is further negatively affected by the common antigens shared with other bacterial genera, such as *Nocardia* and *Corynebacterium*. For this reason serological tests remain inadequate for clinical application for the diagnosis of the disease.[79]

Because of the insidious nature of the disease and the multiplicity of the rather non-specific clinical signs it evokes, tuberculosis is difficult to diagnose on clinical grounds. The clinical examination of animals, especially cattle, is aimed at excluding various other conditions that could be confused with tuberculosis rather than at actually diagnosing tuberculosis.

Clinical conditions in cattle that may cause signs similar to those of bovine tuberculosis are traumatic reticulitis, contagious bovine pleuropneumonia, chronic pasteurellosis, foreign body or aspiration pneumonia, actinobacillosis, corynebacteriosis, and various forms of mastitis.

Snoring in cattle may be caused by enlarged tuberculous pharyngeal lymph nodes, but it may also be due to the presence of polyps, fungal infections, actinomycosis or actinobacillosis in the nasal cavity or pharynx.[50]

Tuberculous mastitis cannot be readily distinguished from other forms of mastitis **(see Chapter 190: Mastitis)** and its presence is not marked until the late stages of the disease. Fibrosis in the case of tuberculous mastitis is most readily detectable at the base of the gland, rather than in the vicinity of the cistern as in most other forms of chronic mastitis, and abnormal milk is most commonly discernible at the end of the milking procedure, rather than at the beginning as in many other forms of mastitis.[8]

At necropsy or inspection of carcasses at abattoirs, the granulomatous lesions of tuberculosis may be confused with those caused by infectious agents such as fungi, staphylococci, *Actinomyces*, and *Actinobacillus* spp., or foreign bodies, or with abscesses, particularly those containing inspissated and calcified pus, such as those caused by *Actinomyces* spp. Generalized cases in which serosal involvement with the development of 'pearls' or 'grapes' has occurred may be confused with mesothelioma. In most cases where granulomas or other lesions are observed, their cause should be determined by direct examination of smears made from the exudate after appropriate staining, and by histopathologic and/or cultural methods. Smears prepared from the exudate of lesions or from the deposit of centrifuged milk samples may reveal the presence of acid-fast bacilli after they have been stained by the Ziehl-Neelsen method. Histopathological examination of lesions may be used as a routine method for confirmation of the diagnosis in animals that have died and from which specimens have been collected and preserved in 10 per cent formalin for diagnostic purposes. It should, however, be kept in mind that the diagnosis must be based on the detection of acid-fast bacilli in the sections, and that the species of *Mycobacterium* cannot be identified in such preparations. In addition, the number of bacteria that can be detected in granulomas tends to vary markedly; in those caused by saprophytic mycobacteria, masses of acid-fast bacteria may be seen, whereas in many instances of infection by *M. bovis*, very few or even no bacteria may be detected even after prolonged examination of the sections.

Control

Several countries which today are considered to be 'developed' began implementing large-scale campaigns to eradicate tuberculosis in cattle not long after Robert Koch's discovery of the tubercle bacillus. In most of them the bovine disease has been eradicated and human tuberculosis due to *M. bovis* has diminished greatly.

Modern campaigns to eradicate tuberculosis can be extremely effective. Earlier campaigns took 30 or 40 years to achieve results that can be obtained within a decade by the application of modern techniques. Nowadays, a few cases occur, sometimes originating from a single source, and point epidemics originating on a single farm or from a single animal may go unnoticed in the absence of an ongoing national surveillance system for bovine tuberculosis.

The success of a campaign which is organized and

financed by the state will depend largely upon the availability of adequate funding, veterinarians and other animal health officers.

Tuberculosis is a notifiable disease of animals in South Africa in terms of the Animal Diseases Act, 1984 (Act 35 of 1984). Although bovine tuberculosis is listed as a so-called List B disease by the *Office International des Epizooties (OIE)*, which means that the prevalence or presence of the disease must be reported on an annual basis, most countries in southern Africa, such as Botswana, Namibia, Swaziland, Lesotho and Malawi, require compulsory notification of any outbreak or diagnosis of bovine tuberculosis.[5] Updated control measures relating to tuberculosis appear in the South African Government Notice R.1953 of 30 September 1988. It empowers an officer acting under the control of the Director of Animal Health to apply control measures, such as testing, isolation, disinfection, movement restriction, marking, compulsory slaughter of reactors, payment of compensation, and treatment with an efficient remedy in particular cases.

The main purpose of campaigns against bovine tuberculosis is the eradication of the disease from a country. A policy that aims at total eradication, as is the case in the USA, Australia and the United Kingdom, would be ideal, but the conditions under which animal husbandry is practised in many parts of southern Africa and in the rest of Africa make such a policy impracticable.[106]

The two most widely used methods of control are the test and immediate slaughter method, and the Bang method, which comprises the isolation of infected animals and the creation of a 'clean' herd by the gradual elimination of cattle from the infected herd. In South Africa all positive animals in a herd must eventually be slaughtered. Stock owners are paid an incentive for the animals that are slaughtered, whilst the rest of the herd is quarantined until two consecutive negative tests three months apart have been conducted. A total slaughter-out policy is only implemented when the initial infection rate proves to be so high (30 per cent and more) that the cost of further testing will not serve the purpose of eradication of the disease.

Eradication on a national scale can only be achieved with:

- full control over all movement of cattle,
- compulsory identification of all cattle,
- payment of an incentive to owners for the slaughter of positive reactors,
- compulsory testing of all cattle within specified intervals,
- establishment and maintenance of disease-free areas, with the eventual aim of incorporating the whole country and
- sufficient funds and staff to fulfil the task.

The current Bovine Tuberculosis Scheme in South Africa was officially introduced by the Directorate of Animal Health in South Africa in 1969, with the purpose of eradicating the disease from the country. Even at the initial stage it was realized that the need to test cattle herds for tuberculosis varied, and that such a need was largely determined by the type of farming and animal husbandry practised. In order to incorporate as many stock farmers as possible in the scheme, several testing programmes have been adopted during the intervening years. These programmes can be regarded as different means of achieving the same final objective, which is the eventual eradication of the disease. The programmes are outlined below.

Accreditation Testing Programme

This programme was instituted for the benefit of stud breeders and farmers with good-quality herds who maintain a continuous high level of management. Cattle are subjected to intradermal testing at three-monthly intervals until two consecutive negative tests are obtained. An official tuberculosis-free certificate is then issued for an accredited herd and must be renewed after the herd has been retested every 12 months. These herds form a nucleus from which tuberculosis-free cattle can be purchased.

Annual Maintenance Programme

This programme accommodates herds whose owners cannot comply with the strict requirements of accreditation. Such herds are tested twice yearly, but no official tuberculosis-free certificate is issued.

Herd Diagnostic Programme

Many stock owners do not wish to participate in either of the abovementioned testing programmes. Their herds, however, remain potential sources of infection for other non-infected herds. Herds accommodated under this testing programme are subjected to one test only, provided that no positive or inconclusive reactors are encountered.

This testing programme is an ideal method of detecting the prevalence of bovine tuberculosis in an entire district, provided that at least 80 per cent of the herds in a district are tested and that the testing is done in an organized manner.

Diagnostic Testing Programme

Tests under this programme are conducted at the request of a stock owner; not all the animals in a herd will necessarily be tested. The purpose of this programme is to enable stock owners to comply, for example, with regulations concerning the export, import or sale of animals.

Infected Herd Testing Programme

Whenever infection is found, whether as a result of a tuberculin test, necropsy, meat inspection, or the examination of milk or other specimens, the herd is placed under quarantine and the animals in the herd are subjected to repeated testing until the herd is declared free of bovine tuberculosis. A herd is considered free of bovine tuberculosis after two negative herd tests, performed at an interval of 90 days, have been conducted.

Positive reactors are identified by a state veterinarian or authorized private veterinary practitioner, T-branded on the left side of the neck and isolated pending their slaughter at an approved abattoir. An incentive is paid to the owner for each positive case, suspected case or in-contact animal that is slaughtered, the amount being adjusted periodically .

In certain deserving cases, for instance in the case of pedigree animals or when a large number of valuable commercial animals are infected, permission may be granted for the treatment of infected animals with isonicotinic-hydrazide (INH). The value of INH treatment lies not only in its therapeutic effect (a 78 per cent bacteriological cure is possible), but also in its prophylactic value, which is as important in the control of the disease as its curative effect. As not all treated reactors are cured bacteriologically, INH treatment cannot be regarded as a means of eradicating the disease. Treatment with INH is done at the expense of the state and is regarded as merely a temporary measure: postponement of the slaughter of positive reactors is granted for a maximum of five years.

The effectiveness of INH treatment in cattle is superior to that of any other drug. It is cheap, easy to administer and has few adverse effects, and at a dosage rate of 10 mg/kg body weight daily for eight weeks it is highly effective. Intermittent INH medication is less effective than daily dosing. Isonicotinic-hydrazide treatment has been shown to be successful even in situations where there is an unfavourable combination of high exposure, high virulence and low host resistance.[58]

Daily INH treatment for one month is insufficient to rid infected animals of tubercle bacilli, but two to three months' treatment results in the elimination of viable tubercle bacilli from most cases. Following successful chemotherapy, skin reactions to the administration of tuberculin gradually decrease, and cease after five months.[57, 63] In one experiment in which tuberculous animals were treated with 25 mg/kg body weight per day of INH for 60 days,[72] skin reactions to tuberculin became negative two to four months after treatment, and 96,4 per cent of the treated animals were considered cured, with no lesions found in those that were slaughtered.

Although it is compulsory by state regulation that all commercial milk supplies in South Africa be pasteurized, not all local authorities have as yet enforced the compulsory testing of dairy herds for bovine tuberculosis. Short-time, high-temperature pasteurization is not always effective in destroying tubercle bacilli, even when the milk is retained in the holder for 20–25 seconds rather than the prescribed minimum of 15 seconds at 72 °C. Only pasteurization plants with flow diversion valves will destroy all tubercle bacilli in milk. The efficacy of pasteurization also depends on the quality of the milk. When the cell content in milk is high or if it contains pus, is sour or incompletely clarified, efficacy is lower. Milk products such as sour milk, buttermilk, yoghurt and cream cheese made from inadequately pasteurized milk may contain tubercle bacilli which can remain viable for 14 days after their preparation. In butter they may remain viable for as long as 100 days. When modern equipment is used in the pasteurization of milk it is an inexpensive procedure, but it should be done in strict conformity with health control regulations.

On infected properties, mechanical, physical and chemical agents are used to render rooms, materials, fluids and other substances non-infectious. The most effective methods for destroying mycobacteria are those based on the use of heat, such as hot air, burning, cooking, pasteurization, and running or pressurized steam. Ultraviolet rays are biologically active at 21–33 °C, and in the Transvaal and Orange Free State highveld, where the sky is generally clear, tubercle bacilli are killed within 20 minutes of being exposed to direct sunlight. Although the germicidal effect of artificially produced ultraviolet light on mycobacteria is utilized in some circumstances in laboratories and elsewhere, its pronounced toxic effect on the skin and eyes of humans requires that only indirect irradiation be used.

Whatever the means of disinfection, it should be followed by the very thorough physical cleaning of ceilings, walls, floors, tools, utensils, and furniture using as much water as possible. Inaccessible areas should be treated with a spray disinfectant. Premises and utensils must be disinfected several times at the beginning of any procedure. Final disinfection is done after the last tuberculin reactor has been removed from the herd.

Surfaces to be disinfected should be in contact for at least ten minutes with a disinfectant which has been demonstrated to be effective in destroying mycobacteria. In some countries' regulations either 3 per cent formalin, 2 per cent lysol or 2,5 per cent phenol are prescribed as the standard disinfectants. Phenol disinfectants are generally more effective than most other substances, but they are difficult to dissolve in water and have a strong odour. Simple phenols are irritating to the skin. In the field, a 1–3 per cent concentration of activated chloramine is recommended. Inorganic acids, alkaline substances, quaternary ammonium compounds and chlorides are ineffective. Cresols are less toxic , have some cleansing effect and good penetration, but do not dissolve readily in hard water. Iodophors are potent and non-irritating to the nose and eyes, but they taint the skin and are expensive, and must not be mixed with soaps and alkaline cleaners.

MYCOBACTERIOSIS AND TUBERCULOSIS IN PIGS

Mycobacterial infection of pigs is caused by *M. tuberculosis*, *M. bovis* and *M. avium*.[40] Serovars 1, 2 and 3 of the

M. avium complex are the cause of tuberculosis in fowls. Poultry infected with serovars 1 and 2 used to be a source of the infection for pigs in Europe, where poultry and pigs were often kept together. However these two serovars (as well as serovar 3) have, seldom been found in poultry in South Africa—hence infection with serovars 1 and 2 is rarely found in pigs in South Africa.

In South Africa, most strains isolated from the lymph nodes of pigs belong to the *M. avium* complex but are serovars other than serovars 1, 2 and 3,[62] while *M. tuberculosis*,[34] and particularly *M. bovis* may also be associated with porcine tuberculous lymphadenitis.[97] Since the mid-1960s a high prevalence rate of mycobacterial lymphadenitis in pigs maintained in intensive husbandry systems has been associated chiefly with organisms of the *M. avium* complex, predominantly serovars 4 and 8, whereas serovars 4, 8, 9, 10, 13, 14, 16 and 17 have been found in the environment.[38, 81, 90] The prevalence of mycobacterial lymphadenitis due to infection with serovars of the *M. avium* complex can become alarmingly high and may cause severe economic loss. Since the environment is the source of this infection, it is difficult to control, and the problem persists today in many piggeries in South Africa and elsewhere.

Epidemiology

Mycobacterial lymphadenitis occurs in pigs throughout South Africa and probably also in the rest of the subcontinent.[82] An increased prevalence, which may be more pronounced in summer, often occurs but is restricted to a few piggeries. It is presumably the result of increased levels of environmental contamination by the bacteria.

The maintenance hosts of the serovars 1, 2 and 3 are poultry and birds, but many healthy rural people in South Africa have also been found to harbour serovars of these bacteria in small numbers in their respiratory tracts.[90] It has been suggested that mycobacteria in faeces may be a method of spread from animal to animal, but in comparison with the large numbers of these mycobacteria in the environment, which appear to be the main source,[62] faecal spread appears to be of little practical significance. *Mycobacterium bovis* is contracted by the ingestion of infected products such as meat and milk.

During the five-year period 1987–92, mycobacteria were isolated from 351 of 552 porcine lymph nodes in the tuberculosis laboratory of the Veterinary Research Institute, Onderstepoort. *Mycobacterium bovis* accounted for 2,5 per cent, *M. avium* for 75 per cent and *M. tuberculosis* for 22 per cent of these mycobacterial isolates. The porcine specimens from which *M. tuberculosis* was isolated derived from the western and eastern Cape Province, where the prevalence of tuberculosis in certain sections of the population seems to be extremely high. *Mycobacterium tuberculosis* infection is due to contact between pigs and tuberculous humans, or to the ingestion of food contaminated with *M. tuberculosis*.[49]

Pathogenesis

Infection occurs almost exclusively by ingestion, which generally results in the development of an incomplete primary complex in lymph nodes regional to the pharynx or intestine, although lesions do rarely occur in the wall of the intestine and elsewhere, due to haematogenous spread.[114] Respiratory and wound infections are uncommon.[14]

Clinical signs

The tuberculous lesions are generally only small foci, 1–10 mm in diameter, in a few lymph nodes and are unlikely to cause detectable clinical signs. Generalization with localization of lesions does occur, and the clinical signs are dependent on the localization of the lesions.

Pathology

Lesions in mucosae are generally microscopic, while those in the regional lymph nodes are often grossly visible. Lesions vary according to the type of mycobacterium involved. *Mycobacterium bovis* causes caseocalcerous tubercles similar to those in cattle, while *M. avium* causes proliferative, lardaceous, almost sarcoma-like granulomas due to a diffuse multiplication of epithelioid and giant cells as well as fibroplasia, without distinct encapsulation of the affected parts. Acid-fast bacteria are present in these lesions.[83]

Pulmonary lesions, when they do occur, are usually of haematogenous origin and miliary in nature. *Mycobacterium bovis* may cause a consolidated, caseous bronchopneumonia due to confluence of tubercles, while infection with serovars of the *M. avium* complex may result in the development of miliary lesions along the course of lymphatics in the lungs.

Hepatic lesions due to *M. bovis* infection are either miliary or consist of coarser nodules, while those due to *M. avium* infection resemble the parasitic hepatitis caused by ascarid migration, with no typical tubercles being formed. Splenic lesions consisting of bulging nodules are common in generalized tuberculosis, while the involvement of serous membranes is rare. Meningeal lesions are usually nodular. *Mycobacterium bovis* infection may result in localized lesions in bones. Lesions rarely occur in the genitalia, eyes or skin.

Tuberculous lesions in pigs slaughtered in abattoirs are usually limited to one or more lymph nodes. Lesions occur predominantly in the mesenteric nodes, less frequently in the nodes of the head, and rarely in the bronchial nodes. Lesions vary in appearance from small, yellowish-white caseous foci 1–10 mm in diameter[38] to diffuse enlargement of the entire node. Histologically, *M. avium* complex infection is usually characterized by a diffuse proliferation of epithelioid and giant cells. Calcification may occur but is generally not as extensive as that produced by mammalian mycobacteria. The same applies to encapsulation of the lesion by connective tissue. The histopathologic differentiation of mycobacterial lymphadenitis caused by mammalian or avian complex organisms is not possible.[47]

Diagnosis

The use of the comparative tuberculin test does to some extent assist in identifying the presence and type of infection.[60] The intradermal tuberculin test in pigs is performed by injecting 0,1 ml of standard potency mammalian tuberculin into the skin fold at the base of the ear. It is, however, relatively inaccurate in this species.[8]

Lesions in lymph nodes detected macroscopically are not diagnostic but are usually highly indicative of tuberculous lymphadenitis. Further confirmation of their tuberculous nature is based on their histological appearance and the presence of acid-fast bacilli which may be demonstrated in Ziehl-Neelsen-stained tissue sections or in similarly stained smears prepared from exudates. Final identification of the species of mycobacterium concerned is done by cultural means. This latter procedure can take up to three months to perform and is therefore of no immediate diagnostic assistance. It is, however, of value to producers experiencing financial losses as a result of the condemnation at abattoirs of organs or body parts, such as heads, in the identification of the source of the infection, particularly if the responsible organism should prove to be *M. tuberculosis* or *M. bovis*.

Sensitized lymphocytes and mycobacterial antibodies detectable by application of ELISA have been reported to occur 14–28 days after exposure to serovars of the *M. avium* complex or to *M. bovis*.[88, 110]

Differential diagnosis

Tuberculosis-like lesions in the lymph nodes of pigs may be confused histologically with lesions caused by *Rhodococcus (Corynebacterium) equi*[13] and with streptococcal lymphadenitis (jowl abscess) caused by *Streptococcus porcinus*, which is characterized by abscessation of submaxillary lymph nodes and occasionally deeper nodes as a result of haematogenous spread.

Control

The routine control of infection lies in protecting pigs from contact with tuberculous humans or products originating from infected cattle, such as dairy products. The feeding of uncooked swill originating from mine compounds, army camps, and especially hospitals poses obvious dangers. When cultural evidence shows the infection to be of environmental origin, as is usually the case on most high-prevalence farms, the difficulties inherent in controlling or eradicating *M. avium-intracellulare* infection are formidable indeed. These opportunist organisms appear to enjoy an ubiquitous and free-living existence in nature, and are resistant to antituberculous drugs. Moreover, they may occur profusely on high-prevalence premises, particularly in zones with a temperate or subtropical climate.[82] With a yield of 18–250 mycobacterial colonies per feed sample, it has been deduced that a pig eating 3 kg of such feed per day would ingest 5 000–75 000 of these mycobacteria. It is therefore not surprising that some investigators have found these organisms in the faeces of pigs.[62] Wood shavings and sawdust have been found to be heavily contaminated with *M. avium* complex organisms in South Africa and other countries, including the United Kingdom,[62, 126] so that one proven method of reducing or even eliminating such infection is by dispensing with bedding that consists of by-products of the timber industry.

It is not known whether BCG vaccination has any protective capacity against *M. avium-intracellulare* infection in pigs.[21]

TUBERCULOSIS IN SHEEP AND GOATS

The rarity of the disease in sheep and goats makes it an unlikely diagnosis except in groups which have been exposed to infected cattle.[8]

The lesions of tuberculosis in goats and sheep fairly closely resemble those in cattle. Infection usually occurs via the respiratory route, and lesions in almost all cases occur in the thoracic cavity and lungs.[14]

In sheep it is only possible to do satisfactory tuberculin tests on skin that has been depilated with barium sulphide paste, while in goats, satisfactory tests (such as the standard intradermal tuberculin test) can be done if the hair is clipped short.[96]

TUBERCULOSIS IN HORSES

Tuberculosis is rare in horses, and infections that do occur are mostly due to *M. bovis*. Serovars of the *M. avium* complex and *M. tuberculosis*, however, may also infect horses.[33] The route of infection is almost solely alimentary, often resulting in lesions only in the retropharyngeal and/or mesenteric lymph nodes.

Fatal cases are usually due to a generalized miliary or multifocal infection that involves the lungs, liver, spleen, and serous membranes. Allegedly, lesions occur commonly in cervical vertebrae, but no proof exists to substantiate this.[26] In this form, painful osteomyelitis develops which results in a stiffness of the neck and an inability to eat off the ground.[8] Less common signs include coughing due to pulmonary lesions, lymph node enlargement, nasal discharge and a fluctuating temperature.

Tubercles in horses are uniform, smooth, greyish, lardaceous granulomas that rarely undergo caseation and calcification. Microscopically they consist of epithelioid cells, macrophages, giant cells and lymphocytes, and the granulomas become more fibrous as they age. Organisms are scarce in these lesions.

Pulmonary infection is usually miliary and the lesions manifest as firm, glassy nodules. The bronchial lymph nodes are enlarged and have a sarcoma-like appearance. In intestinal tract infections, ulcers occur in the large intestine in particular. *Mycobacterium avium* may produce a proliferative enteritis not unlike that of Johne's disease in cattle. Lesions in the liver, spleen and serosae are large lardaceous nodules.[9] Serosal involvement causes a copious effusion.

Horses appear to be much more sensitive than cattle to tuberculin, and probably much smaller doses of standardized tuberculin are required when conducting an intradermal test with it than is the case in cattle. In horses, the results obtained with subcutaneous and intradermal tuberculin tests are very erratic and must be assessed with caution, especially when the test is positive.[8]

References

1 **ANON., 1968.** *Expert Committee on Biological Standardization. Twentieth Report. World Health Organization Technical Report Series*, 384, 23–41.Genva: WHO.

2 **ANON., 1977–88.** *Annual Reports of the Director of Veterinary Services*, Namibia.

3 **ANON., 1984.** *Manual for the Production of PPD of Bovine and Avian Tuberculin.* Section of Diagnostic Antigens, Veterinary Research Institute, Onderstepoort.

4 **ANON., 1987.** *Expert Committee on Biological Standardization Thirty-sixth Report. World Health Organization Technical Report Series*, 745. Geneva: WHO.

5 **ANON., 1991.** Animal health yearbook of the Food and Agriculture Organization of the United Nations (FAO), the International Office of Epizootics (OIE) and the World Health Organization (WHO).

6 **BENGIS, R., KRIEK, N.P.J. & HUCHZERMEYER, H.F.A.K., 1991.** State Veterinarian, Skukuza, South Africa. Unpublished data.

7 **BENJAMIN, R.G. & DANIEL, T.M., 1982.** Serodiagnosis of tuberculosis using the enzyme-linked immunosorbent assay (ELISA) of antibody to *Mycobacterium tuberculosis* antigen 5. *American Review of Respiratory Diseases*, 126, 1013–1016.

8 **BLOOD, D.C., RADOSTITS, O.M. & HENDERSON, J.A., 1989.** Diseases caused by bacteria. IV. *In: Veterinary Medicine.* 7th edn. London: Baillière, Tindall & Cox.

9 **BUERGELT, C.D., GREEN, S.L., MAYHEW, I.G., WILSON, J.H. & MERRITT, A.M., 1988.** Avian mycobacteriosis in three horses. *Cornell Veterinarian*, 78, 365–380.

10 **CHEESEMAN, C.L., WILESMITH, J.W. & STUART, F.A., 1989.** Tuberculosis: The disease and its epidemiology in the badger, a review. *Epidemiology*, 103, 113–125.

11 **CHIODINI, R.J., VAN KRUININGEN, H.J. & MERKAL, R.S., 1984.** Ruminant paratuberculosis (Johne's disease): The current status and future prospects. *Cornell Veterinarian*, 74, 218–262.

12 **CLANCY, J.K., 1977.** The incidence of tuberculosis in lechwe (Marsh antelope). *Tubercle*, 58, 151–156.

13 **CLAPP, H.K., 1956.** Tuberculosis-like lesions in swine in South Australia. *Australian Veterinary Journal*, 32, 110–113.

14 **COHRS, P., 1967.** *Textbook of the Special Pathological Anatomy of Domestic Animals.* Oxford: Pergamon Press.

15 **COLLINS, C.H. & GRANGE, J.M., 1983.** A review: The bovine tubercle bacillus. *Journal of Applied Bacteriology*, 55, 13–29.

16 **COLLINS, C.H. & GRANGE, J.M., 1987.** Zoonotic implication of *Mycobacterium bovis* infection. *Irish Veterinary Journal*, 41, 363–366.

17 **COLLINS, C.H., GRANGE, J.M. & YATES, M.D., 1985.** *Organization and Practice in Tuberculosis Bacteriology.* London, Boston, Durban, Singapore, Sydney, Toronto, Wellington: Butterworths.

18 **DANIEL, T.M. & JANICKI, B.W., 1978.** Mycobacterial antigens: A review of their isolation, chemistry and immunological properties. *Microbiological Reviews*, 42, 84–113.

19 **DANNENBERG, A.M. Jr., 1989.** Immune mechanisms in the pathogenesis of pulmonary tuberculosis. *Reviews of Infectious Diseases.* II. Supplement 2, S369–378.

20 **DE LISLE, G.W. & HAVILL, P.F., 1985.** Mycobacteria isolated from deer in New Zealand from 1970–1983. *New Zealand Veterinary Journal*, 33, 138–140.

21 **DEY, B.P., 1986.** Mycobacterioses in swine and their significance to public health. *USDA. Bibliographies and Literature of Agriculture*, 49, 47.

22 **DIESEL, A.M., 1956.** *Report of the Departmental Committee on the Control of Bovine Tuberculosis in the Union of South Africa.*

23 **DOBBELAER, R., O'REILLY, L.M., GENICOT, A. & HAAGSMA, J., 1983.** The potency of bovine PPD tuberculin in guinea-pigs and tuberculous cattle. *Journal of Biological Standardization*, 11, 213–220.

24 **DUBE, J.G., 1989.** Director of Veterinary Services, P.O. Box 162, Mbabane, Swaziland. Personal communication.

25 **DUFFIELD, B.J., NORTON, J.H., STREETEN, T.A., 1985.** Application of the comparative cervical test to the identification of false positive reactions to the bovine tuberculin caudal fold test. *Australian Veterinary Journal*, 62, 424–426.

26 **DUNGWORTH, D.L., 1985.** The respiratory system. *In*: JUBB, K.V.F., KENNEDY, P.C. & PALMER, N., (eds). *Pathology of Domestic Animals*, 3rd edn. Orlando: Academic Press, Inc.

27 **EKDAHL, M.O., SMITH, B.L. & MONEY, D.F., 1970.** Tuberculosis in some wild and feral animals in New Zealand. *New Zealand Veterinary Journal*, 18, 44–45.

28 **EL MOSSALAMI, E., SIAM, M.A. & EL SERGANY, I.M., 1971.** Studies on tuberculosis-like lesions in slaughtered camels. *Zentralblatt für Veterinärmedizin*, Reihe B, 18, 253–261.

29 **ELSAID, H.M., 1992.** Diagnosis of tuberculosis in buffaloes: Correlation of *in vivo* and *in vitro* tests of cell-mediated immunity. *Proceedings of the International Conference on Animal Tuberculosis in Africa and the Middle East*, Cairo.

30 **FANNING, A. & EDWARDS, S., 1991.** *Mycobacterium bovis* infection in human beings in contact with elk (*Cervus elaphus*) in Alberta, Canada. *The Lancet*, 338, 1253–1255.

31 **FAUL, A., COLLY, P. & HUCHZERMEYER, H.F.K.A., 1988.** Directorate of Animal Health, Private Bag X138, Pretoria 0001. Unpublished data.

32 **FLAMAND, J., 1993.** Natal Parks Board, Mtubatuba, South Africa. Personal communication.

33 **FLORES, J.M., SANCHEZ, J. & CASTANO, M., 1991.** Avian tuberculosis dermatitis in a young horse. *The Veterinary Record*, 128, 407–408.

34 **FOURIE, P.J.J., DE WET, G.J. & VAN DRIMMELEN, G.C., 1950.** Tuberculosis in pigs caused by *Mycobacterium*

tuberculosis var. *hominis*. *Journal of the South African Veterinary Medical Association*, 21, 70.

35 **FRANCIS, J., 1958.** *Tuberculosis in Animals and Man. A Study in Comparative Pathology*. London: Cassel.

36 **FRANCIS, J., 1979.** Specificity and potency of PPD tuberculins. *Discussion Paper for Committee on Tuberculosis in Animals*, International Union against Tuberculosis, Paris, October 1979.

37 **FRANCIS, J., SEILER, R.J., WILKIE, I.W., O'BOYLE, D. LUMSDEN, M.J. & FROST, A.J., 1978.** The sensitivity and specificity of various tuberculin tests using bovine PPD and other tuberculins. *The Veterinary Record*, 103, 420–435.

38 **GREATHEAD, M.M., 1969.** Porcine mycobacterial lymphadenitis: Meat hygiene considerations. *Journal of the South African Veterinary Medical Association*, 40, 259–262.

39 **GRIFFIN, F.J.T., 1988.** The aetiology of tuberculosis and mycobacterial disease in farmed deer. *Irish Veterinary Journal*, 42, 23–26.

40 **GRIFFITH, F. & GRIFFITH, A.S., 1911.** *Final Report of the Royal Commission on Tuberculosis*, Part 2, Appendix 3, 152. London: Her Majesty's Stationery Office.

41 **GUILBRIDE, P.D.L., ROLLINGSON, D.H.L., McANULTY, E.G., ALLEY, J.G. & WELLS, E.A., 1963.** Tuberculosis in the free-living African (Cape) buffalo (*Syncerus caffer caffer*, Sparrman). *Journal of Comparative Pathology*, 73, 337–348.

42 **HAAGSMA, J., 1980.** Standardization of bovine tuberculins. *Report for the International Union against Tuberculosis*, Prague.

43 **HAAGSMA, J., O'REILLY, L.M., DOBBELAER, R. & MURPHY, T.H., 1982.** A comparison of the relative potencies of various bovine PPD tuberculins in naturally infected tuberculous cattle. *Journal of Biological Standardization*, 10, 273–284.

44 **HARGREAVES, S.K., 1993.** Director of Veterinary Services, P.O. Box 8012, Causeway, Harare, Zimbabwe. Personal communication.

45 **HENNING, M.W., 1956.** *Animal Diseases in South Africa*. 3rd edn. Pretoria: Central News Agency.

46 **HEWSON, P.I. & SIMPSON, W.J., 1987.** Tuberculosis infection in cattle and badgers in an area of Staffordshire. *The Veterinary Record*, 120, 252–256.

47 **HIMES, E.M., MILLER, L.D. & THOEN, C., 1983.** Swine tuberculosis: Histologic similarities of lesions from which *Mycobacterium tuberculosis*, *M. avium* complex or *M. bovis* was identified. *Proceedings of the Twenty-sixth Meeting of the American Association of Veterinary Laboratory Diagnosticians*.

48 **HOFFNER, S.E., BOLSKE, G., HOFFMANN, E. & KÄLLENIUS, G., 1992.** Improved detection of *Mycobacterium bovis* in deer. *Proceedings of the International Conference on Animal Tuberculosis in Africa and the Middle East*, Cairo.

49 **HUCHZERMEYER, H.F.A.K., 1992.** Veterinary Research Institute, Onderstepoort. Unpublished data.

50 **HUNGERFORD, T.G., 1967.** *Diseases of Livestock*. 6th edn. Sydney: Angus and Robertson.

51 **HUTCHEON, D., 1880.** Tering, consumption, tables mesenterica. *Annual Report, Colonial Veterinary Surgeon*, Cape of Good Hope.

52 **JENSEN, K.A., 1953.** Bovine tuberculosis in man and cattle. *In: Advances in the Control of Zoonoses*. WHO/FAO Seminar on Zoonoses. Vienna, November 1952. Geneva: World Health Organization.

53 **JUBB, K.V.F., KENNEDY, P.C. & PALMER, N., 1985.** The female genital system. *In: Pathology of Domestic Animals*. 3rd edn. Orlando: Academic Press, Inc.

54 **KERR, W.R., LAMONT, H.G. & McGIRR, J.L., 1946.** Further studies on tuberculin sensitivity in the bovine. *The Veterinary Record*, 61, 466–475.

55 **KLEEBERG, H.H., 1960.** The tuberculin test in cattle. *Journal of the South African Veterinary Medical Association* 31, 213–225.

56 **KLEEBERG, H.H., 1961.** The tuberculin test in cattle. *Journal of the South African Veterinary Medical Association*, 32, 482–486.

57 **KLEEBERG, H.H., 1963.** Eradication of bovine tuberculosis. *Journal of the South African Veterinary Medical Association*, 34, 393–400.

58 **KLEEBERG, H.H., 1967.** The use of chemotherapeutic agents in animal tuberculosis. *Veterinarian (London)*, 4, 197–211.

59 **KLEEBERG, H.H., 1975.** Tuberculosis and other mycobacterioses. *In*: HUBBERT, W.T., McCULLOCH, W.F. & SCHNURRENBERGER, D.R., (eds). 6th edn. *Diseases Transmitted from Animals to Man*. Springfield, Illinois: Charles C. Thomas.

60 **KLEEBERG, H.H., 1981.** Epidemiology of mycobacteria other than tubercle bacilli in South Africa. *Reviews of Infectious Diseases*, 3, 1008–1012.

61 **KLEEBERG, H.H., 1988.** 443 Kirkness Street, Pretoria, South Africa. Personal communication.

62 **KLEEBERG, H.H. & NEL, E.E., 1969.** Porcine mycobacterial lymphadenitis. *Journal of the South African Veterinary Medical Association*, 40, 233–250.

63 **KLEEBERG, H.H. & WORTHINGTON, R.W., 1963.** A modern approach to the control of bovine tuberculosis. *Journal of the South African Veterinary Medical Association*, 34, 383–391 and 565–568.

64 **KOLLIAS, G.V., 1978.** Clinical and pathologic features of mycobacterial infection in sika and fallow deer. *In*: MONTALI, R.J., (ed.). *Proceedings of a Symposium on Mycobacterial Infections in Zoo Animals*. Washington, DC: Smithsonian Institute Press.

65 **KRAUSS, H., ROETTCHER, D., WEISS, R., DANNER, K. & HÜBSCHLE, O.J.B., 1984.** Wildtiere als Infektionspotential für Nutztiere: Untersuchungen an Wild in Zambia. Giessener Beiträge zur Entwicklungsforschung, Reihe 1, Band 10, Wissenschaftlisches Zentrum Tropeninstitut Justus-Liebig-Universität, Giessen.

66 **LAMPRECHTS, M.C., 1956.** Aspects of tuberculin testing in cattle. *Journal of the South African Veterinary Medical Association*, 27, 225–243.

67 **LAMPRECHTS, M.C., 1957.** Some observations on the Stormont test. *Journal of the South African Veterinary Medical Association*, 28, 169–174.

68 **LAMPRECHTS, M.C., 1958.** *Report to the Director of Veterinary Services, Onderstepoort*.

69 **LANDI, S. & HELD, H.R., 1975.** Effect of light on tuberculin purified protein derivative solutions. *American Review of Respiratory Diseases*, 111, 52–61.

70 **LANDI, S., HELD, H.R. & GUPTA, K.C., 1975.** The multifacets of tuberculin standardization. *WHO: International Abstracts of Biological Sciences Symposium on Standardization and Control of Allergens Administered to Man*. Geneva, 1974. *Developments in Biological Standardization*, 29, 393–411.

71 **LANDI, S., HELD, H.R. & TSENG, M.C., 1970.** Relationship between the molecular weight of tuberculoprotein and its biological potency. *Progress in Immunobiological Standardization*, 4, 512–520.

72 **LANGENEGGER, J., CAVALCANTE, M.I. & LIRA, A.D., 1991.** Massal treatment of bovine tuberculosis with isoniazid. *Pesquisa Veterinária Brasileira*, 11, 21–23.

73 **LARSEN, A.B., GROTH, A.H. & JOHNSON, H.W., 1950.** Allergic response to johnin and tuberculin of various skin regions of cattle. *American Journal of Veterinary Research*, 11, 301–303.

74 **LEE, M.T., 1987.** Central Veterinary Laboratory, Weybridge, England. Personal communication.

75 **LEPPER, A.W.D. & CORNER, L.A., 1983.** Naturally occurring mycobacteriosis of animals. *In*: RATLEDGE, C. & STANFORD, J., (eds). *The Biology of Mycobacteria*. Vol. II. London, New York: Academic Press, Inc.

76 **LEPPER, A.W.D., NEWTON-TABRETT, D.A., CORNER, L.H., CARPENTER, M.T., SCANLON, W.A., WILLIAMSON, O.J. & HELWIG, D.M., 1977.** The use of bovine PPD tuberculin in the single caudal fold test to detect tuberculosis in beef cattle. *Australian Veterinary Journal*, 53, 208–213.

77 **LEPPER, A.W.D. & PEARSON, C.W., 1973.** The route of infection in tuberculosis of beef cattle. *Australian Veterinary Journal*, 49, 266–267.

78 **LESLIE, I.W. & BIRN, K.J., 1967.** Tuberculosis in cattle caused by the avian type tubercle bacillus. *The Veterinary Record*, 80, 559–564.

79 **LIND, A. & RIDELL, M., 1984.** Immunologically based diagnostic tests: Humoral antibody methods. *In*: KUBICA, G.P. & WAYNE, L.G., (eds). *The Mycobacteria: A Sourcebook*, Part B. New York, Basel: Marcel Dekker, Inc.

80 **LONG, E.R. & SEIBERT, F.B., 1926.** The chemical composition of the active principle of tuberculin: I. A non-protein medium suitable for the production of tuberculin in large quantity. *American Review of Tuberculosis*, 13, 393–397.

81 **LOVEDAY, R.K., 1968.** Swine health under intensification. *Journal of the South African Veterinary Medical Association*, 39, 117–118.

82 **LOVEDAY, R.K., 1969.** Porcine mycobacterial lymphadenitis: Some epidemiological aspects. *Journal of the South African Veterinary Medical Association*, 40, 253–256.

83 **LUKE, D., 1958.** Tuberculosis in the horse, pig, sheep and goat. *The Veterinary Record*, 70, 529–536.

84 **MAHMOD, K.H., ROOK, G.A.W., STANFORD, J.L., STUART, F.A. & PRITCHARD, D.G., 1987.** The immunological consequences of challenge with bovine tubercle bacilli in badgers (*Meles meles*). *Epidemiology and Infection*, 98, 155–163.

85 **MARKS, J., 1972.** Ending the routine guinea-pig test. *Tubercle*, 53, 31–34.

86 **MEISSNER, G. & SCHRÖDER, K.H., 1974.** Bovine tuberculosis in man and its correlation with bovine cattle tuberculosis. *Bulletin of the International Union Against Tuberculosis*, 49, 145–148.

87 **MONTALI, R.J., 1978.** *Proceedings of a Symposium on Mycobacterial Infections in Zoo Animals*, Smithsonian Institute Press, Washington, D.C.

88 **MUSCOPLAT, C.C., THOEN, C.O., CHEN, A.W., RAKICH, P.M. & JOHNSON, D.W., 1975.** Development of specific lymphocyte immunostimulation and tuberculin skin reactivity in swine infected with *Mycobacterium bovis* and *Mycobacterium avium*. *American Journal of Veterinary Research*, 36, 1167–1171.

89 **MYERS, J.A. & STEELE, J.H., 1969.** *Bovine Tuberculosis. Control in Man and Animals*. St. Louis, Missouri: Warren H. Green, Inc.

90 **NEL, E.E., 1981.** *Mycobacterium avium-intracellulare* complex serovars isolated in South Africa from humans, swine and the environment. *Reviews of Infectious Diseases*, 3, 1013.

91 **PAINE, R. & MARTINAGLIA, G., 1929.** Tuberculosis in wild buck living under natural conditions. *The Journal of Comparative Pathology and Therapeutics*, XL11(1).

92 **PATERSON, A.B., 1948.** The production of bovine tuberculoprotein. *The Journal of Comparative Pathology and Therapeutics*, 58, 302–313.

93 **RICHARDSON, A., 1970.** Bovine mastitis associated with *Mycobacterium smegmatis* and an untypable mycobacterium. *The Veterinary Record*, 86, 497–498.

94 **RIDLEY, D.S., 1983.** The histopathological spectrum of the mycobacterioses. *In: Biology of Mycobacteria*. Vol. II. London: Academic Press, Inc.

95 **ROBINSON, E.M., 1944.** A note on strains of tuberculosis from the kudu. *Onderstepoort Journal of Veterinary Science and Animal Industry*, 19, 23–28.

96 **ROBINSON, E.M., 1955.** Tuberculosis in sheep and goats. *Journal of the South African Veterinary Medical Association*, 26, 95–104.

97 **ROBINSON, E.M., 1958.** Tuberculosis in pigs in South Africa. *Journal of the South African Veterinary Medical Association*, 21, 129.

98 **RUNYON, E.H., 1959.** Anonymous mycobacteria in pulmonary disease. *Medical Clinics of North America*, 43, 273.

99 **SCHLIESSER, Th., 1976.** Vorkommen und Bedeutung von Mykobakterien bei Tieren. *Zentralblatt für Bakteriologie, Parasitenkunde, Infektionskrankheiten und Hygiene*, Erste Abteilung. Originali Reihe A. 235, 184–194.

100 **SCHLIESSER, Th., 1982.** Die Rindertuberkulose im Wandel der letzen 100 Jahre (1882–1982). *Praxis der Pneumologie*, 36, 151–156.

101 **SCHMIEDEL, A., 1968.** Development and present state of bovine tuberculosis in man. *Bulletin of the International Union Against Tuberculosis*, 40, 5–37.

102 **SCHNEIDER, H., 1977.** *Analyse der Tiergesundheitssituation in Südwestafrika/Namibia—Vergangenheit und Gegenwart*. Inaugural Dissertation zur Erlangung des Doktorgrades bei dem Fachbereich Veterinärmedizin und Tierzucht der Justus Liebig-Universität zu Giessen.

103 **SCHNEIDER, W., DOBBELAER, R., DAM, A., JORGENSEN, J.B., GAYOT, G., AUGIER, J., HAAGSMA, J., REES, W.H.G., LESSLIE, I.W. & HEBERT, C.N., 1979.** Collaborative assay of EEC standards for bovine tuberculins. *Journal of Biological Standardization*, 7, 53–66.

104 **SEIBERT, F.B., 1944.** The chemistry of tuberculin. *Chemical Review*, 34, 107–127.

105 **SEIBERT, F.B., FIGUEROSA, E.S., DUFOUR, E.H., 1955.** Isolation, identification and classification of proteins of tuberculin and the tubercle bacillus. *American Review of Respiratory Diseases*, 70, 704–721.

106 **SNYMAN, P.S., 1955.** The problem of bovine tuberculosis in the Union of South Africa. *Journal of the South African Veterinary Medical Association*, 26, 241–245.

107 **STUART, F.A., MANSER, P.A. & McINTOSH, F.G., 1988.** Tuberculosis in imported red deer (*Cervus elaphus*). *The Veterinary Record*, 122, 508–511.

108 **SUTHER, D.E., FRANTI, C.E., PAGE, H.H., 1974.** Evaluation of a comparative intradermal tuberculin in California dairy cattle. *American Journal of Veterinary Research*, 35, 380–397.

109 **TESSARO, S.V., FORBES, L.B. & TURCOTTE, C., 1990.** A survey of brucellosis and tuberculosis in bison in and around Wood Buffalo National Park, Canada. *Canadian Veterinary Journal*, 31, 174–180.

110 **THOEN, C.O., ARMBRUST, A.L. & HOPKINS, M.P., 1979.** Enzyme-linked immunosorbent assay for detecting antibodies in swine infected with *Mycobacterium avium*. *American Journal of Veterinary Research*, 40, 1096.

111 **THOEN, C.O. & HIMES, E.M., 1986.** Pathogenesis of *Mycobacterium bovis* infection. *Progress in Veterinary Microbiological Immunity*, 2, 198–214.

112 **THOEN, C.O., HIMES, E.M. & KARLSON, A.G., 1984.** *Mycobacterium avium* complex. *In*: KUBICA, G.P. & WAYNE, L.G., (eds). *The Mycobacteria. A Sourcebook*. Part B. New York and Basel: Marcel Dekker, Inc.

113 **THOEN, C.O., HIMES, E.M., STUMPFF, C.D., PARKS, T.W. & STURKIE, H.N., 1977.** Isolation of *Mycobacterium bovis* from the prepuce of a herd bull. *American Journal of Veterinary Research*, 38, 877–878.

114 **THOEN, C.O. & KARLSON, A.G., 1986.** Tuberculosis. *In: Diseases of Swine*. 6th edn. Ames, Iowa: Iowa State University Press.

115 **THOEN, C.O., QUINN, W.J., MILLER, L.D., STACKHOUSE, L.L., NEWCOMB, B.F. & FERREL, J.M., 1992.** *Mycobacterium bovis* infection in North American elk (*Cervus elaphus*). *Journal of Veterinary Diagnostic Investigation*, 4, 423–427.

116 **THORBURN, J.A. & THOMAS, A.D, 1940.** Tuberculosis in the Cape kudu. *Journal of the South African Veterinary Medical Association*, 11, 3–10.

117 **VAN HEERDEN, A. & BRÜCKNER, G.K., 1985.** *Bovine Tuberculosis: Scheme and Manual for the Control and Combating of Bovine Tuberculosis in South Africa*. Division of Veterinary Services, Department of Agriculture and Water Supply, Republic of South Africa. Pretoria: Government Printer.

118 **VAN WAVEREN, G.M., 1953.** Tuberkulose ondersoek by

runderen met PPD tuberculines. *Tijdschrift voor Diergeneeskunde*, 78, 735–760.

119 **VAN WAVEREN, G.M., 1965.** Bovine tuberculosis, tuberculins and tuberculin tests in the Netherlands. *Bulletin de l' Office International des Epizooties*, 63, 1395–1401.

120 **VON ZIEGLER, M., 1953.** Die Eutertuberkulose des Rindes. Hirzel Verlag, Leipzig. Reviewed in *Schweizer Archiv für Tierheilkunde*, 95, 410.

121 **WAYNE, L.G. & KUBICA, G.P., 1986.** Family Mycobacteriaceae. *In*: SNEATH, P.H.A., MAIR, N.S., SHARPE, M.E. & HOLT, J.G., (eds). *Bergey's Manual of Systematic Bacteriology*. Vol. II. Baltimore, London, Los Angeles, Sydney: Williams & Wilkins.

122 **WEBB, G.B., 1936.** *Clio Medica: Tuberculosis*. New York.

123 **WEBER, A., LUTZ, H. & BAUER, K., 1988.** Die derzeitige Bedeutung des Menschen für das Auftreten von *Mycobacterium bovis* infektionen in Rinderbeständen. *Berliner und Münchener Tierärztliche Wochenschrift*, 101, 341–344.

124 **WERNER, E., 1981.** Übertragung der Tuberkulose auf eine Rinderherde durch eine Tierpflegerin mit Nierentuberkulose. *Monatshefte der Veterinärmedizin*, 36, 819–820.

125 **WIEGESHAUS, E., BALASUBRAMANIAN, V. & SMITH, D.W., 1989.** Immunity to tuberculosis from the perspective of pathogenesis. *Infection and Immunity*, 57, 3671–3676.

126 **WINDSOR, R.S., DURRANT, D.S. & BURN, K.J., 1984.** Avian tuberculosis in pigs: *Mycobacterium intracellulare* infection in a breeding herd. *The Veterinary Record*, 114, 497–500.

127 **WOODFORD, M.H., 1982.** Tuberculosis in wildlife in the Ruwenzori National Park, Uganda (Part I). *Tropical Animal Health and Production*, 14, 81–88.

128 **WOODFORD, M.H., 1982.** Tuberculosis in wildlife in the Ruwenzori National Park, Uganda (Part II). *Tropical Animal Health and Production*, 14, 155–160.

129 **WORTHINGTON, R.W., 1967.** Mycobacterial PPD sensitins and the non-specific reactor problem. *Onderstepoort Journal of Veterinary Research*, 34, 345–438.

130 **WORTHINGTON, R.W. & KLEEBERG, H.H., 1966.** The comparative tuberculin test using Onderstepoort avian and bovine PPD Tuberculin. *Journal of the South African Veterinary Medical Association*, 37, 177–183.

131 **YAGER, J.A. & SCOTT, D.W., 1985.** The skin and appendages. *In*: JUBB, K.V.F., KENNEDY, P.C. & PALMER, N., (eds). *Pathology of Domestic Animals*. 3rd edn. Orlando: Academic Press, Inc.

132 **ZOMBORSZKY, Z., KÖRMENDY, B., TILLIY, P. & TUBOLY, S., 1992.** Diagnosis of tuberculosis infection in red deer. *Proceedings of the International Conference on Animal Tuberculosis in Africa and the Middle East, Cairo.*

173

Paratuberculosis

Synonyms: Johne's disease, Johne se siekte (Afrik.)

H.F.A.K. Huchzermeyer, G.K.Brückner and S.S. Bastianello

Introduction

Paratuberculosis is a chronic, infectious enteritis of cattle, sheep, goats and certain wild animal species caused by *Mycobacterium paratuberculosis*.[56, 87, 140] Clinical signs usually only develop in animals that are more than two years old, and they are characterized by a profuse diarrhoea and emaciation.

Johne and Frothingham first described the disease in 1895 as a strange form of tuberculosis.[50] In 1906, however, Bang[10] recognized that it was not tuberculosis and referred to it as pseudotuberculous enteritis or Johne's disease. The causative organism was isolated in 1910[144] and named *Mycobacterium enteritidis chronicae pseudotuberculosae bovis*, Johne, but was later renamed *M. paratuberculosis*.

Paratuberculosis occurs throughout the world, and in some countries, such as New Zealand, Australia, the United Kingdom and the Mediterranean countries, it is recognized as being one of the most important infectious diseases threatening the cattle and sheep industries.[3, 34, 55, 156] In Africa, it has been reported from Mauritania, Sudan, Ethiopia, Kenya, Uganda, Tanzania, Zaïre, Ghana, Nigeria, Gabon, Zimbabwe, Swaziland, Zambia and South Africa.[102]

The first case of Johne's disease in South Africa was diagnosed in a bovine of unspecified breed in 1923, and subsequent sporadic cases were encountered until 1960, when the first recorded outbreak of paratuberculosis occurred in a herd of Jerseys in the Ermelo district.[58] During the period 1976 to 1990 it was confirmed in 42 individual cattle in southern Africa,[43] although its prevalence is probably higher than this figure would indicate. The disease has mainly been diagnosed in imported cattle infected subclinically at the time of importation, but cases do occur in locally bred animals.

In sheep, paratuberculosis was first recorded in South Africa in 1967 in a single German Merino ram which had been imported from Germany,[147] but a second case was not found until 1981.[101] Since 1988, numerous cases of paratuberculosis have been diagnosed in sheep at the Nooitgedacht Agricultural Development Centre at Ermelo and the Animal and Dairy Science Research Institute at Irene. The sheep at Irene were presumably infected by sheep originating from Ermelo, as there is frequent exchange and transfer of sheep between these two research stations. At present, even though the disease is widespread in these two flocks,[44] it has not been diagnosed elsewhere in the country.

Aetiology

Mycobacterium paratuberculosis is a non-motile, short, straight, slender rod, about 1–2 µm long and 0,5 µm wide, and is Gram-positive and strongly acid-fast.[57] In smears made from cultures, bacteria — when numerous — occur in tangled clumps, the clumping being caused by a network of intercellular filaments.[95]

Herrold's egg-yolk medium (HEYM), with or without mycobactin, is used to culture the organism at 37 °C and, as growth is slow, cultures should be kept for at least 16 weeks.[8, 9] Before culturing, faecal and intestinal tissue samples must be treated with sodium hydroxide and oxalic acid,[13] benzalkonium chloride,[97] or hexadecylpyridinium chloride[150] to decrease contamination by other microorganisms.[96] Primary colonies on mycobactin-containing HEYM appear after eight to 12 weeks or longer, and are small, 1–5 mm in diameter, moist, convex and mostly unpigmented. Yellow- to orange-pigmented strains have been isolated from sheep[133] and cattle on occasion.[130] No pigmented strains have been isolated from cattle or sheep in South Africa.[44]

The main distinguishing cultural characteristics of *M. paratuberculosis* are its extremely slow growth and its dependence on exogenous mycobactin for *in vitro* growth.[33, 89, 92, 93, 99] The mycobactins (a group of closely related, lipid-soluble compounds) are produced by most mycobacterial species and are utilized for iron transport.[78] *Mycobacterium paratuberculosis*, however, cannot produce sufficient mycobactin to sustain the respiratory activity needed for its multiplication when adapting from *in vivo* to *in vitro* growth on complex media such as serum or egg-yolk agar medium which contain limited quantities of iron.[11, 65, 127, 141]

The classification and interrelationships of a number

of *Mycobacterium* spp. remain uncertain. Although *M. paratuberculosis* has been regarded as a distinct species since 1923, it is grouped with the *M. avium* complex. The colonies of *M. paratuberculosis* resemble those of *M. avium*, but develop more slowly. Both species react similarly in biochemical tests[87, 143] and sensitized animals react in a similar manner to avian tuberculin and johnin.[87] In addition, intestinal infection with *M. avium* may produce clinical signs resembling those of Johne's disease.[87]

As in the case of *M. paratuberculosis*, certain strains of *M. avium* cannot be isolated from lesions in tissues of domestic and wild animals unless mycobactin has been added to the culture medium.[81] The 'wood pigeon bacillus', repeatedly isolated from wood pigeons in Europe, is mycobactin-dependent and, when fed to calves, causes a disease indistinguishable from Johne's disease.[86, 142] A mycobactin-dependent *Mycobacterium* sp. has been isolated from the intestines of humans suffering from Crohn's disease.[23] Deoxyribonucleic acid (DNA) homology studies indicate that *M. avium*, the 'wood pigeon bacillus', and the *Mycobacterium* sp. strains isolated from patients with Crohn's disease are closely related to *M. paratuberculosis*.[24, 120] In spite of these similarities, the other members of this complex are ubiquitous environmental organisms and opportunistic pathogens, while *M. paratuberculosis* is an obligate pathogen which is largely host- and organ-adapted.[51]

Recently, restriction endonuclease and DNA hybridization analyses of various *M. paratuberculosis* isolates have identified two groups, namely a cattle group (which includes all the strains from cattle and some strains from sheep and goats) and a sheep group (including some strains from sheep and one from goats in New Zealand). One Canadian sheep strain had a hybridization pattern intermediate between those of the two groups and a restriction endonuclease pattern more similar to that of the sheep group.[26] Restriction endonuclease and hybridization analyses of five strains of *M. paratuberculosis* isolated from South African sheep showed that these strains are identical to the Canadian sheep strain.[25] The host preferences of these intermediate strains are unknown.[26]

Mycobacterium paratuberculosis can be differentiated from other mycobacteria by its mycobactin-dependence when cultured, and from other mycobactin-dependent mycobacteria by thin-layer gas-liquid chromatography techniques.[27]

Mycobacterium paratuberculosis is somewhat resistant to adverse environmental factors; low temperatures, moisture and the absence of sunshine enhance its survival. It can survive for at least 270 days in pond water,[72] 264 days in bovine faeces,[80] and 252 days in cattle slurry.[52] It is inactivated by a 3–5 per cent formaldehyde solution, and disinfectants such as cresylic acid (1:32 dilution), phenol (1:40 dilution), mercury bichloride (1:1 000), calcium hypochlorite (1:50), and sodium orthophenylphenate (1:100 or 1:200).[22, 42, 123, 148]

Epidemiology

Cattle, sheep, goats, and a number of wild animals, such as species of deer, buffaloes, camels, sheep and goats[56, 87, 140] are susceptible to Johne's disease. It does appear, however, that the various isolates of *M. paratuberculosis* are to some extent species-specific.

Sheep can become infected following the intravenous, intratracheal and oral administration of large numbers of organisms of a cattle strain and develop typical lesions of Johne's disease.[60] On the other hand, although *M. paratuberculosis* may be isolated periodically from the faeces of sheep which graze on pastures contaminated with a cattle strain of *M. paratuberculosis*, the sheep do not develop lesions consistent with Johne's disease.[117] Similarly, calves challenged with infective doses of the Norwegian goat strain of *M. paratuberculosis* do not develop the disease.[119] In South Africa no experimental work has been done to determine whether the sheep strain is infective for cattle, or *vice versa*.

There appears to be a higher prevalence of the disease in the Channel Islands breeds of cattle and in beef Shorthorns in England, Denmark and Canada, but this may be related to increased exposure rather than to an increased susceptibility.[17, 55] In South Africa a large proportion of cases have been diagnosed in Brahmans which were either imported or bred on stud farms where the animals are kept under intensive conditions, but few cases are diagnosed on an annual basis.[63]

There seems to be an age-related resistance to infection: new-born calves are the most susceptible, while heifers are less so, and adult animals are quite resistant.[40, 69, 112]

In an infected herd, most animals are continually exposed to *M. paratuberculosis* shed in the faeces of infected animals, which contaminate the environment. The bacteria may remain alive in the external environment for considerable periods **(see Aetiology)**. Acid soils also appear to enhance their survival.[61, 114]

Cattle are usually infected either congenitally or during the first days or weeks of life after ingesting food or water contaminated with the faeces of infected animals. Although *M. paratuberculosis* has been isolated from the mammary glands, milk is not considered to be important in the transmission of the disease.[134] Calves usually become infected while suckling from faecally contaminated teats, or by grazing on contaminated pastures.[87] Although approximately 26 per cent of the calves of cows clinically suffering from paratuberculosis may be congenitally infected,[122] the significance of this type of infection as a cause of clinical disease is not known.[122]

The majority of exposed animals become subclinically infected and shed bacteria intermittently in their faeces throughout their lives. A single exposure to the infection is not sufficient to cause the disease, and repeated exposure over a period of time is required for clinical disease to develop.[22, 90]

The organisms may be isolated from the genital organs

and semen of bulls,[55, 68, 74, 85, 107] but the number of organisms in semen is small and it is unlikely that bulls transmit the infection to cows during coitus or that artificial insemination plays a role in transmission of the infection.[94]

As a result of the prolonged incubation period, infected animals may excrete organisms in the faeces for 15–18 months before clinical signs appear.[17] The disease spreads slowly and insidiously in an infected herd and it may be years before it is eventually diagnosed.[22]

Parturition, a low plane of nutrition, high milk production, parasitic infestations, and grazing on wet, low-lying or mineral-deficient soils may precipitate clinical disease.[22]

Pathogenesis

Following oral infection, the bacteria enter the lymphatics through the tonsils and the intestinal mucosa.[105, 106, 112] M-cells covering Peyer's patches take up the bacilli from the intestinal lumen and transport them through the intestinal mucosa. Once expelled from the M-cells they are phagocytosed by inter- and subepithelial macrophages as well as monocytes. The predominant location of Peyer's patches in the ileum may explain why initial lesions occur in this part of the tract.[77, 79, 98] Other factors, however, also appear to be involved in this localization: experimentally, following transient haematogenous spread, *M. paratuberculosis* organisms lodge in various organs regardless of the route of infection, but they multiply and persist predominantly in the intestinal mucosa.[60, 87]

The majority of the mycobacteria are contained intracellularly in macrophages, in which they are resistant to digestion by lysosomal enzymes and multiply uninhibitedly. They do not produce toxins,[14, 15, 57, 64, 158] but bacterial multiplication results in the release of monokines from macrophages.[59 137] The monokines enhance the inflammatory reaction and the development of granulomatous lesions, particularly in the lamina propria of the ileum and its regional lymphatics and lymph nodes. Similar lesions may develop in the caecum and colon.

As a result of the granulomatous ileitis, there is loss of enterocytes from the tips of the villi and villous atrophy in affected areas, which result in decreased absorption of nutrients, loss of plasma proteins into the intestinal lumen, and diarrhoea.[6, 103, 104] Other, as yet unknown mechanisms, such as antigen-antibody reactions in the affected portions of the intestinal tract, and the release of histamine,[91] also appear to be involved in the development of diarrhoea. A catarrhal enteritis involving the proximal and mid-ileum precedes the development of the typical granulomatous lesions and may be the initial cause of the wasting syndrome in infected cattle.[77]

As the infection progresses, the number of organisms in the affected tissues progressively increases, as do the severity and extent of the lesions. Organisms released from dying macrophages stimulate a humoral immune response in which the IgG1 fraction is the most important.[2, 157] A cell-mediated immune response occurs during the early stages of infection, but towards the later stages of the disease cattle may become anergic.[14] This suppressed immunoresponsiveness may be due to excessive corticosteroid production[77] and accelerated thymic involution which has been noted in many clinical cases.[19] Anergy may allow infected macrophages to enter the blood stream, resulting in a bacteraemia and the spread of organisms to most organs and tissues.[22]

Several factors appear to contribute to the age-dependent susceptibility of young animals to infection by *M. paratuberculosis*. Suckling pre-ruminant calves have an increased intestinal acidity compared with that of adult ruminants, and this favours the survival of the organisms. In adults, the rumen also acts as a barrier to the organism.[110, 114] Bacterial survival is also enhanced by lactoferrin and transferrin in the colostrum that is ingested by suckling ruminants. These compounds serve as sources of iron for the production of mycobactin by the organisms. Maternal antibodies in the milk of infected cows may enhance the movement of *M. paratuberculosis* into the intestinal mucosa.[65, 98]

Clinical signs

The incubation period ranges from less than six months to more than 15 years, but most infected animals develop clinical evidence of the disease between three and five years of age.[22] Animals under the age of two years are rarely clinically affected except in poorly managed herds with a high rate of infection. In cattle, clinical disease — from which animals rarely recover — is the terminal stage of a progressive, chronic infection which has previously been subclinical, and its onset may be precipitated by stress factors. Chronically infected herds are composed of clinical cases, subclinical shedders, subclinical carriers (non-shedders) and non-infected animals.[123] Despite the fact that only 1 or 2 per cent of the animals in a herd reveal clinical disease, 42–100 per cent of the animals may be infected.[123]

In cattle, chronic but intermittent diarrhoea which does not respond to treatment, dehydration, and emaciation are the most obvious initial clinical signs. These signs may be followed by the development of submandibular oedema, unthriftiness, a rough hair coat, and a dry skin.[22] The diarrhoea is characteristically profuse, homogeneous, semi-fluid or watery, and greenish.[123] Periods of remission occur, which may last for weeks or even months. Fever is uncommon and the appetite is usually maintained despite the progressive weight loss. Animals eventually become recumbent and die in a state of cachexia.[123] The mortality rate in infected herds is usually less than 1 per cent per year, although in exceptional circumstances it can be as high as 10 per cent.[17]

In sheep and goats, the disease is afebrile and

characterized by progressive emaciation. The faeces may be normal in consistency throughout most of the course of the disease, or they may be intermittently soft and pasty with unformed pellets. Terminally, the faeces are usually soft and pasty. Shedding of wool may occur in some sheep. The appetite is maintained throughout most of the clinical course of the disease, but in severely affected sheep the appetite is poor. Subcutaneous oedema of the submandibular region is rare.[44]

Pathology

In cattle there is usually a poor correlation between the severity of clinical signs and the severity and extent of the lesions.[12, 22] Emaciated animals show serous atrophy and, less commonly, effusion of fluids into the body cavities.[12] Specific lesions may be found from the duodenum to the rectum, but usually only involve the ileum and ileocaecal valve region and their lymphatic vessels and lymph nodes.[12, 22] Gross intestinal lesions occur in more than 50 per cent of infected cattle.[19]

Thickening of the mucosa of the ileum, which is thrown into thick, irregular, transverse folds (which do not disappear when the intestine is stretched and which impart a corrugated appearance), is the most striking gross lesion in severely affected animals **(Figure 173.1)**. Ulcers may occur in the depths of the folds. In less severely affected animals, the mucosa appears velvety and opaque.[22] Lymphangitis, particularly in the ileocaecal region, is a relatively constant lesion. The affected lymphatics manifest as thickened, tortuous cords traversing the intestinal serosa and mesentery **(Figure 173.2)**.[12, 22] Oedema and enlargement of the ileocaecal and mesenteric lymph nodes occur less consistently. Caseation and calcification of the affected portions of the ileum and/or regional lymph nodes are only rarely encountered.[55] The occurrence of aortic arteriosclerosis in affected animals is inconsistent, although in some outbreaks it may be quite common.[19, 22]

Histologically, the lesions in the intestine and mesenteric lymph nodes may be mild, moderate or severe, and macrophages and/or giant cells can be present in varying ratios.[19] Of the three different forms of macrophages that occur in the inflammatory reaction, eosinophilic epithelioid cells are the most common, vacuolated, polygonal cells are intermediate in number, and syncytial cells the least common. The majority of mycobacteria are intracellular within macrophages and their number increases with time. Masses of bacteria occur in advanced lesions **(Figure 173.3)**.

Mild lesions are characterized by the presence of single Langhans' giant cells or a few scattered macrophages in the tips of the intestinal villi or within the paracortical zone of the regional lymph nodes, but acid-fast organisms are rarely detected. In moderately severe lesions, several small groups of macrophages and variable numbers of giant cells occur in the lamina propria and submucosa of the intestine and in the paracortical zone and subcapsular sinuses of the lymph nodes, while in severely affected animals, numerous macrophages and giant cells are present in the intestinal mucosa and submucosa, and in most cases also in the serosa and the submucosal and serosal lymphatics. In most cases varying numbers of lymphocytes and eosinophils occur in the inflammatory reaction. The inflammatory reaction may cause partial occlusion of the lymphatics. The intestinal villi, lamina propria and submucosa are usually distorted and thickened by the cellular infiltration, and many crypts are dilated and filled with neutrophils, mucus and cellular debris. Lymphoid nodules in the Peyer's patches are frequently surrounded by inflammatory cells, but the germinal centres are usually spared. The subcapsular sinuses and paracortical regions of the affected lymph nodes are infiltrated with giant cells and/or macrophages, but the germinal centres remain unaffected,[19] and the nodes consistently manifest severe lymphoid hyperplasia.[21]

In general, the remainder of the intestinal tract, other than the ileum and ileocaecal valve, is seldom affected. Similar but generally more focal lesions may, however, be encountered in the duodenum, proximal jejunum, caecum, colon and, very rarely, the rectum.[12, 19] Microgranulomas are common in the liver, but acid-fast organisms are seldom detected in them. Globular leukocytes often occur in association with the myenteric ganglia.

The macro- and microscopical lesions in sheep are generally similar to those in cattle.[21, 44, 111] The macroscopic lesions are characterized in particular by dilatation or thickening of the ileum, and less commonly the distal jejunum; thickening and transverse folding of the ileal mucosa; dilatation of the caecum; thickening and irregular folding of the caecal mucosa in the vicinity of the ileocaecal valve; lymphangitis involving the serosal lymphatics, particularly in the ileocaecal valve region; and enlargement and oedema of the ileocaecal and mesenteric lymph nodes.[44]

Solid tubercle-like nodules occasionally occur in the lymphatics of sheep.[21] The prevalence of caseous necrotic foci in the mucosa of the ileum and mesenteric or ileocaecal lymph nodes varies from relatively common to rare in different outbreaks.[12, 44]

Apart from epithelioid cells, the other types of macrophages described as being part of the inflammatory reaction in cattle are not encountered in the lesions of sheep, and Langhans' giant cells are extremely rare.[21, 44] In mild cases, few acid-fast organisms are noted within macrophages, but in severe cases they are tightly packed with mycobacteria.

Histologically, affected lymph nodes of sheep manifest a generalized lymphoid hyperplasia, mainly in the T-cell areas and germinal centres, while epithelioid cells occur in the subcapsular sinuses or as nests along the trabeculae and in the paracortical areas. Acid-fast

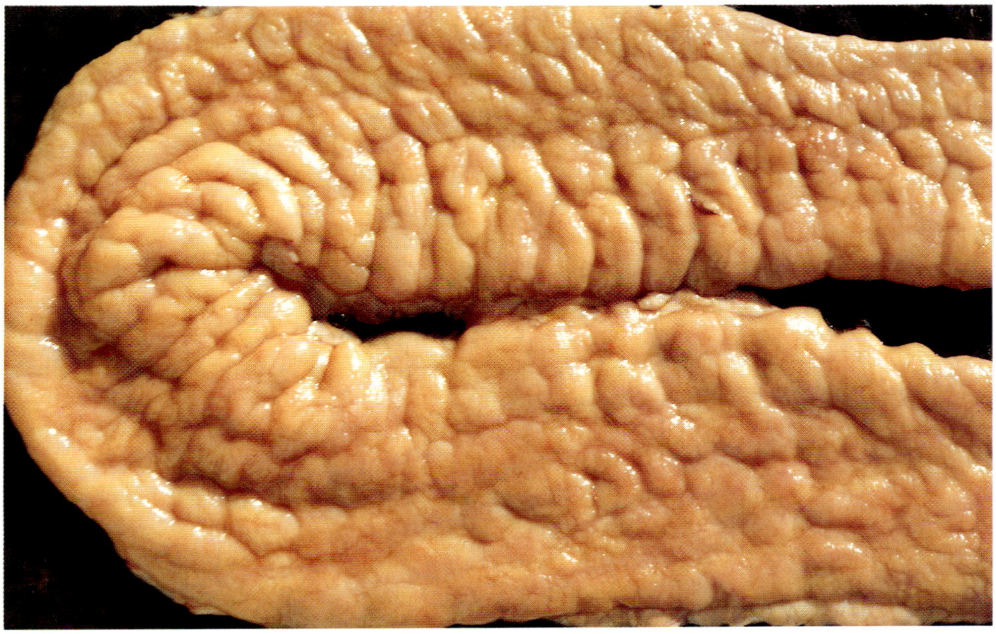

Figure 173.1 Ileum from an infected cow. The mucosa is thickened and shows transverse folding

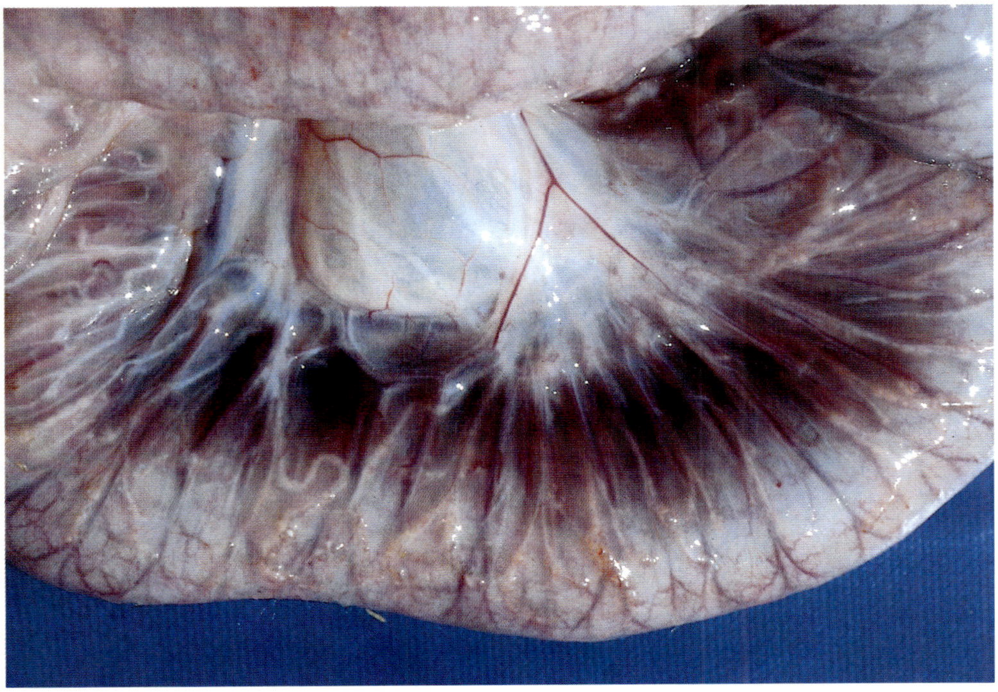

Figure 173.2 Gastrointestinal tract of a sheep with paratuberculosis. Note the dilated caecum, severely widened ileum and thickened lympatics

organisms are present in small to moderate numbers in the epithelioid cells in the lymph nodes of about 70 per cent of sheep with clinical paratuberculosis.[21]

Diagnosis

In southern Africa, a history of importation or contact with imported animals is frequently an important consideration in the diagnosis of Johne's disease. The diagnosis of paratuberculosis during the preclinical stage presents considerable problems.[22, 37] However, a number of tests **(Table 173.1)** are available which provide valuable supportive evidence. In cattle, it is recommended that three or more different tests be performed simultaneously to confirm a diagnosis of *M. paratuberculosis* infection. The combination of tests should include one or more of the serological tests, such as the complement fixation (CF) test, enzyme-linked immunosorbent assay (ELISA), agar-gel immunodiffusion (AGID) test, and gamma-interferon assay and bacterial culture of faecal samples.[139, 154]

Three sensitivity or allergy tests (intradermal test, comparative tuberculin test and the intravenous test) are available, and these may assist in the confirmation of a diagnosis of subclinical or clinical Johne's disease. These tests are based on the fact that affected animals become

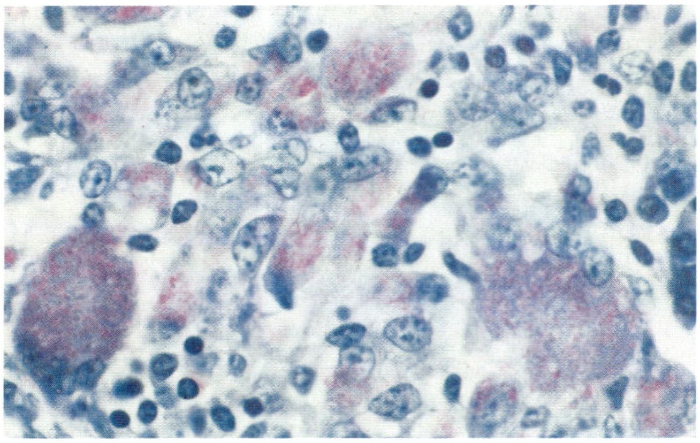

Figure 173.3 Epithelioid cells in the ileal mucosa containing numerous acid-fast bacterial organisms (Ziehl-Neelsen stained)

sensitized to certain products of mycobacteria, such as johnin from *M. paratuberculosis*, tuberculin from *M. bovis* and avian tuberculin from *M. avium*, and when these are injected into an affected animal it reacts in a way which can be measured.

The intradermal test is seldom used in South Africa. In this test 0,1–0,2 ml of johnin or avian tuberculin is injected intradermally. If there is an increase in skin thickness of more than 5 mm at the injection site over 24–48 hours, the test is regarded as positive.[22] However, in the absence of clinical signs and laboratory confirmation, a positive skin reaction is insufficient evidence to confirm the presence of infection. In the comparative tuberculin test, the response to avian tuberculin is measured against the response to bovine tuberculin; animals with Johne's disease react to both, but the response to the former is greater than to the latter.[31] Animals inoculated with one of the available *M. paratuberculosis* vaccines may become sensitized to avian and bovine tuberculin, resulting in the occurrence of false positive reactions.[67] In these cases, isolation of the bacterium is the only reliable way to confirm the diagnosis.

The intravenous injection of johnin or avian purified protein derivative (PPD) tuberculin is useful to confirm Johne's disease in cattle. A rise in body temperature of at least 0,8 °C six to eight hours after the injection is regarded as a positive indication of the disease, but it only occurs in about 50 per cent of clinical cases. Similar temperature reactions occur in sheep with this test.[44]

Further support for a diagnosis of paratuberculosis in cattle is achieved by determining the neutrophil:lymphocyte sensitivity factor. A rise of more than two in the sensitivity factor is regarded as significant.[5, 22, 62] This test appears to be non-specific in sheep.[44]

Results of serological tests on individual animals are often inconclusive, but they are of value when performed on a herd basis. False positive reactions in the serological tests may be due to cross-reactions with other micro-organisms, as the antigen preparations used in the tests are rather crude[28] and contain antigens common to most bacteria in the order Actinomycetales (which includes other *Mycobacterium* spp., *Actinomyces* spp., *Dermatophilus* spp., *Nocardia* spp., *Streptomyces* spp., and *Corynebacterium* spp.) as well as several fungal species.[36, 84, 109, 153] False positive results may also occur in animals that were previously exposed to (but did not develop lesions) or infected with *M. paratuberculosis*, but which have since recovered.[22] False negative responses may occur in tests based on cell-mediated immune reactions, particularly when a state of anergy develops.[14, 22]

Despite the above problems the CF test is considered reliable enough to confirm a diagnosis in cattle manifesting clinical disease.[14, 41]

Although the ELISA is more sensitive than the CF test for the identification of cattle in the early stages of infection,[54, 157] it is only of limited value because of its low specificity.[135] Preabsorption of sera with cross-reactive mycobacteria, such as *M. phlei*, and different procedures to purify the antigen increase its specificity.[4, 39, 131, 136, 138]

The agar-gel immunodiffusion test is easy and inexpensive to perform, and results are available after 48 hours. It seems to be well-suited to the confirmation of the disease in sheep and goats,[124, 140] but is less suitable for this purpose in cattle.[38, 86, 125]

The interferon assay based on the detection of gamma-interferon released into blood plasma by sensitized T-cells in response to specific antigen correlates well with the lymphocyte proliferation assay,[18] but is not yet applied in practice.[154]

Microscopical examination of faecal smears stained by the Ziehl-Neelsen method can be useful in identifying subclinically and clinically infected animals which excrete large numbers of organisms. In order to detect organisms in smears, faeces must contain a minimal number of 10^4 colony-forming units/g[128] and even then the sensitivity is 60 per cent or less, but the specificity is 96 per cent.[53, 121] As organisms are shed intermittently, a negative result is meaningless. The presence of large, saprophytic, acid-fast bacilli may further complicate the interpretation of faecal smears. These bacteria occur singly or in loose groups, whilst *M. paratuberculosis* organisms are smaller and occur in clumps of four to 20 or more. Routine scanning of smears at a magnification of 500x before changing to 1 000x magnification for finer detail facilitates examination and helps to obtain a more accurate result.[29]

To identify cattle in a herd which has few or intermediate numbers of organisms in the faeces, isolation of *M. paratuberculosis* from faecal samples is the only method that provides reliable results.[100] For this purpose a specimen consisting of at least 10 g of faeces kept at 4 °C should reach the laboratory within four days of collection. For best results the specimens should be processed immediately, as further delays greatly increase the chances of an overwhelming growth of contaminants occurring.[113, 115] If faecal samples cannot be transported to a laboratory within four days, they should be

Table 173.1 Accuracy and sensitivity of methods for the diagnosis of paratuberculosis. (Adapted from Chiodini *et al*.[22] With permission of the editor, *Cornell Veterinarian*)

TEST	TRUE POSITIVE %	FALSE NEGATIVE %	FALSE POSITIVE %	TRUE NEGATIVE %	REFERENCES
Intradermal johnin test	54	46	21	79	87
Intravenous johnin test	51	49	45	55	62
Complement fixation test+	64	36	55	45	75
Haemagglutination+	74	26	67	33	76
Lymphocyte transformation*	78	22	36	64	20
Fluorescent antibody	72	28	40	60	38
Faecal culture	40	60	0	100	20
Agar-gel immunodiffusion	55	45	49	56	38
Mucosal biopsy	25	75	–	–	67
Lymph node biopsy#	–	–	–	–	108
ELISA#	–	–	–	–	54
Radioimmunoassay#	–	–	–	–	155
Migration inhibition#	–	–	–	–	1

True positives and false negatives are those responses expected from infected animals, and false positives and true negatives those responses expected from non-infected animals.
True positives = infected reactors/number animals infected; false positives = non-infected reactors/number animals not infected; false negatives = infected non-reactors/number animals infected; true negatives = non-infected non-reactors/number animals not infected.
+ Titres >1:16 considered positive. * Stimulation index >2 considered positive. # Inadequate data to make calculations.

submitted in a frozen state (-70 °C), but this does reduce the viability of the organisms, and the diagnosis may be missed, particularly in animals shedding small numbers of organisms.[113, 115]

Mycobacterium paratuberculosis can be isolated relatively easily from affected parts of the intestine of cattle, and specimens for bacteriological examination should be sent to the laboratory chilled or frozen if transport takes longer than two or three days.[9, 116] For unknown reasons, *M. paratuberculosis* is extremely difficult to isolate from the faeces or intestine of sheep, even when the bacteria can be detected microscopically in faecal smears.[44]

Bacteriological and histopathological examinations of mesenteric lymph node biopsy specimens are reliable procedures for the diagnosis of clinical cases in cattle,[108, 132, 146] but histological examination of such specimens is less effective than culture of the organisms for the detection of subclinical cases.[16] Histological examination of sections of the ileum is, however, superior to that of ileal smear examination when detecting animals with very mild lesions.[132] Examination of impression smears of affected parts of the intestinal mucosa, stained by the Ziehl-Neelsen method, allows rapid confirmation of the diagnosis.[16, 108, 146] The examination of rectal biopsy specimens or scrapings is an extremely unreliable method for the diagnosis of Johne's disease, as specific lesions and organisms are seldom found in the rectal wall.[66]

The diagnosis of Johne's disease on post-mortem examination is based on the detection of specific macroscopic and microscopic lesions, the demonstration of *M. paratuberculosis* in impression smears and tissue sections of affected parts as well as the isolation of the organism by culture if deemed necessary,.

Histopathological changes are usually conspicuous in cases with pronounced gross lesions, but can easily be overlooked in cases with mild lesions.[12] The criteria for a positive histopathological diagnosis of Johne's disease are the presence of epithelioid and/or giant cells in the intestinal lamina propria and submucosa and the demonstration of acid-fast bacilli within these cells.[132] The presence of clusters of epithelioid and/or giant cells containing acid-fast organisms in the paracortical areas of affected lymph nodes is characteristic.

More recent developments in diagnostic techniques include the radiometric detection of *M. paratuberculosis* in positive cases[82] and the use of DNA probes. With the aid of probes, results are available within a few days instead of the several months that it takes to culture the organism.[49, 83, 149] Preliminary work using DNA probes to test for paratuberculosis in sheep in South Africa has yielded inconclusive results and it appears that more refined probes are required.[7]

Differential diagnosis

The clinical differentiation of Johne's disease from other causes of chronic diarrhoea is often extremely difficult. Scouring and emaciation in cattle as a result of Johne's disease may be confused with similar signs caused by other conditions, including parasitic infestations (e.g. schistosomiasis, paramphistomiasis) and tuberculosis.[47]

Paratuberculosis in sheep may be confused with conditions that cause wasting and emaciation, but in partcular with chronic verminosis and coccidiosis, or starvation as a result of inadequate or improper feeding during winter and times of drought. Chronic salmonellosis may also cause clinical signs similar to Johne's disease.[44] Marasmus due to cobalt deficiency should also be considered in sheep.

Control

Paratuberculosis is difficult to control because of its long incubation period, the absence of clinical signs in the early stages of the disease, during which affected animals may be a source of infection to others via the excretion of *M. paratuberculosis* in the faeces, the lack of reliable and practical diagnostic methods, and ineffective available chemotherapy. A number of antimicrobial drugs, including streptomycin, isoniazid, rifampicin and clofazimine, have been used but have no lasting therapeutic effects.[87, 123]

In South Africa, Johne's disease is a controlled disease in terms of the Animal Diseases Act, 1984 (Act 35 of 1984). This implies that the Directorate of Animal Health must be notified of all suspected cases, which must then be kept in isolation and destroyed at the expense of the state if the diagnosis is confirmed. Because of the chronic, insidious nature of the disease, eliminating paratuberculosis from a herd or flock is a prolonged undertaking and is generally unsuccessful.[123]

Control on a herd or flock basis depends on the elimination of infected animals, strict attention to hygiene to prevent the spread of the infection and, in some instances, vaccination to produce a level of resistance in infected animals.[17] The owner of an infected herd or flock should be encouraged to seriously consider a slaughter-out policy of all the animals. However, valuable genetic material can possibly be recovered by applying embryo transfer.[118] If this is carried out, the farm or premises should be kept free of ruminants for at least two years before restocking.

Application of the following husbandry practices in infected herds of cattle is recommended to reduce or eliminate the exposure of calves to the organism, as young animals are the most susceptible:[152]

- suspected clinical cases should be isolated and a diagnosis obtained by bacteriological examination of their faeces;
- confirmed cases and their offspring should be slaughtered without delay;
- where possible, calves should be removed from their dams at birth and reared in a 'paratuberculosis-free' environment;
- colostrum and milk fed to calves must be collected hygienically and the use of a milk substitute should be encouraged;
- water and food supplies should be kept free of faecal contamination;
- calves should not be mixed with mature animals until they are at least one year old;
- pasture used for young stock should not have been used by adult cattle or sheep during the previous year;
- ponds and ditches should be fenced off; and
- pasture should not be treated with fresh slurry or manure.

As there are reports of a higher prevalence of Johne's disease in ruminants on acid soils than on alkaline soils, the application of limestone or hydrated lime to acid soils is recommended.[61, 114]

Although vaccines are available, control by vaccination alone is not effective and should be combined with hygiene and other husbandry procedures.[71, 87] Vaccination should only be performed in tuberculosis-free herds,[45] since tests based on allergic and serological reactions to detect or monitor the level of infection with *M. paratuberculosis* cannot be used in vaccinated animals.

The available vaccines are prepared from either a live[129, 145] or a heat-killed strain of *M. paratuberculosis*[30, 31, 35, 45, 73, 126, 151] suspended in mineral oil or in incomplete Freund's adjuvant. These vaccines all appear to have the same efficacy, and although they do not confer absolute immunity, they reduce the number of animals that become clinically ill as well as the number of organisms shed in the faeces.[31, 32, 46, 48, 73, 129]

An inactivated (heat-killed) vaccine is no longer available from the Veterinary Research Institute, Onderstepoort for use in known paratuberculosis-positive herds of cattle. In South Africa, vaccination is not routinely performed in either cattle or sheep, and the efficacy of vaccinating these species in the country has not been evaluated.[44]

Calves (in the area of the dewlap) and lambs (over the sternum) can be vaccinated subcutaneously at one to 35 days of age. Immunity lasts approximately 18 months,[31, 70] but revaccination is not recommended.[31, 34, 129] The vaccines may produce long-lasting local tissue reactions, varying in size from 20–80 mm in diameter, and these may ulcerate and drain to the outside.[88]

Embryo transfer might offer an effective way of preventing transmission of *in vitro M. paratuberculosis*. However, a ten-step wash procedure of *M. paratuberculosis*-infected bovine ova does not always remove these organisms.[118]

References

1 **AALUND, O., HOERLEIN, A.B. & ADLER, H.C., 1970.** The migration test on circulating bovine leukocytes and its possible application in the diagnosis of Johne's disease. *Acta Veterinaria Scandinavia*, 11, 331–334.

2 **ABBAS, B. & RIEMANN, H.P., 1988.** IgG, IgM and IgA in the serum of cattle naturally infected with *Mycobacterium paratuberculosis*. *Comparative Immunology, Microbiology and Infectious Diseases*, 11, 171–175.

3 **ABBAS, B., RIEMANN, H.P. & HIRD, D.W., 1983.** Diagnosis of Johne's disease (paratuberculosis) in northern California cattle and a note on its economic significance. *California Veterinarian*, 8, 20–24.

4 **ABBAS, B., RIEMANN, H.P. & LOMMERDAL, B., 1983.** Isolation of specific peptides from *Mycobacterium paratuberculosis* protoplasm and their use in an enzyme-linked immunosorbent assay for the detection of paratuberculosis in cattle. *American Journal of Veterinary Research*, 44, 2229–2236.

5 **ALLEN, W.M., BERRETT, S. & PATTERSON, D.S.P., 1967.** A haematological study of clinical cases of Johne's disease and the assessment of an intravenous johnin diagnostic test. *Journal of Comparative Pathology*, 77, 71–79.

6 **ALLEN, W.M., BERRETT, S. & PATTERSON, D.S.P., 1974.** A biochemical study of experimental Johne's disease. I. Plasma leakage into the intestine of sheep. *Journal of Comparative Pathology*, 84, 381–384.

7 **AMBROSIO, R.E., HARRIS, Y. & HUCHZERMEYER, H.F.A.K., 1991.** A DNA probe for the detection of *Mycobacterium paratuberculosis*. *Veterinary Microbiology*, 26, 87–93.

8 **ANON., 1983.** Laboratory Manual, Tuberculosis Section, Veterinary Research Institute, Onderstepoort.

9 **ANON., 1985.** Laboratory methods in veterinary mycobacteriology for the isolation and identification of mycobacteria. *The Mycobacteriology Unit, National Veterinary Services, Animals and Plant Health Inspection Service, US Department of Agriculture*, Ames, Iowa.

10 **BANG, B., 1906.** Chronische pseudotuberkulöse Darmentzündung beim Rinde. *Berliner Tierärztliche Wochenschrift*, 42, 759–763.

11 **BARCLAY, R. & RATLEDGE, C., 1983.** Iron-binding compounds of *Mycobacterium avium, M. intracellulare, M. scrofulaceum*, and mycobactin-dependent *M. paratuberculosis* and *M. avium*. *Journal of Bacteriology*, 153, 1138–1146.

12 **BARKER, I.K. & VAN DREUMEL, A.A., 1985.** The Alimentary System. *In*: JUBB, K.V.F., KENNEDY, P.C. & PALMER, N., (eds). *Pathology of Domestic Animals*, Vol. II. 3rd edn. Orlando: Academic Press, Inc.

13 **BEERWERTH, W., 1967.** Culture of mycobacteria from the faeces of domestic animals and their significance for the epidemiology of tuberculosis. *Praxis der Pneumologie*, 21, 189–202.

14 **BENDIXEN, P.H., 1978.** Immunologic reactions caused by infection with *Mycobacterium paratuberculosis*. A review. *Nordisk Veterinaermedicin*, 30, 163–168.

15 **BENDIXEN, P.H., BLOCH, B. & JORGENSEN, J.B., 1981.** Lack of intracellular degradation of *Mycobacterium paratuberculosis* by bovine macrophages infected *in vitro* and *in vivo*: Light microscopic and electron microscopic observations. *American Journal of Veterinary Research*, 42, 109–113.

16 **BENEDICTUS, G. & HAAGSMA, J., 1986.** The efficacy of mesenteric lymph node biopsy in the eradication of paratuberculosis from an infected dairy farm. *Veterinary Quarterly*, 8, 5–11.

17 **BLOOD, D.C. & RADOSTITS, V.M., 1989.** Diseases caused by bacteria. IV. *In: Veterinary Medicine: A Textbook of the Diseases of Cattle, Sheep, Pigs, Goats and Horses*. 7th edn. London: Baillière Tindall.

18 **BUERGELT, C.D., DE LISLE, G., HALL, C.E., MERKAL, R.S. & DUNCAN, J.R., 1978.** *In vitro* lymphocyte transformation as a herd survey method for bovine paratuberculosis. *American Journal of Veterinary Research*, 39, 591–595.

19 **BUERGELT, C.D., HALL, C.E., McENTEE, K. & DUNCAN, J.R., 1978.** Pathological evaluation of paratuberculosis in naturally infected cattle. *Veterinary Pathology*, 15, 196–207.

20 **BUERGELT, C.D., HALL, C.E., MERKAL, R.S., WHITLOCK, R.H. & DUNCAN, J.R., 1977.** Lymphocyte transformation: An aid in the diagnosis of paratuberculosis. *American Journal of Veterinary Research*, 38, 1709–1715.

21 **CARRIGAN, M.J. & SEAMAN, J.T., 1990.** The pathology of Johne's disease in sheep. *Australian Veterinary Journal*, 67, 47–50.

22 **CHIODINI, R.J., VAN KRUININGEN, H.J. & MERKAL, R.S., 1984.** Ruminant paratuberculosis (Johne's disease): The current status and future prospects. *Cornell Veterinarian*, 74, 218–262.

23 **CHIODINI, R.J., VAN KRUININGEN, H.J., THAYER, W.R., MERKAL, R.S. & COUTU, J.A., 1984.** Possible role of mycobacteria in inflammatory bowel disease. *Digestive Diseases and Sciences*, 29, 1073–1079.

24 **COLLINS, D.M. & DE LISLE, G.W., 1986.** Restriction endonuclease analysis of various strains of *Mycobacterium paratuberculosis* isolated from cattle. *American Journal of Veterinary Research*, 47, 2226–2229.

25 **COLLINS, D.M. & DE LISLE, G.W., 1991.** Ministry of Agriculture and Fisheries, Central Animal Health Laboratory, P.O. Box 40063, Upper Hutt, New Zealand. Personal communication.

26 **COLLINS, D.M., GABRIC, D.M. & DE LISLE, G.W., 1990.** Identification of two groups of *Mycobacterium paratuberculosis* strains by restriction endonuclease analysis and DNA hybridization. *Journal of Clinical Microbiology*, 28, 1591–1596.

27 **DAMATO, J.J., KNISLEY, C. & COLLINS, M.T., 1987.** Characterization of *Mycobacterium paratuberculosis* by gas-liquid and thin-layer chromatography and rapid demonstration of mycobactin dependence using radiometric methods. *Journal of Clinical Microbiology*, 25, 2380–2383.

28 **DANIEL, T.M., 1984.** Soluble mycobacterial antigens. *In*: KUBICA, G.P. & WAYNE, L.G., (eds). *The Mycobacteria: A Sourcebook*. New York and Basel: Marcel Dekker, Inc.

29 **DESMECHT, M., 1977.** Rendement comparé de diverses méthodes de diagnostic de la paratuberculose. *Annales de Médecine Vétérinaire*, 121, 421–423.

30 **DESMECHT, M., 1983.** Prophylaxie médicale de la paratuberculose en Belgique. *CEC Workshop on Paratuberculosis*, Copenhagen, 22–23 November 1983.

31 **DOYLE, T.M., 1964.** Vaccination against Johne's disease. *The Veterinary Record*, 76, 73–77.

32 **EMERY, D.L., DUFTY, J.H. & WOOD, P.R., 1988.** An analysis of cellular proliferation and synthesis of lymphokines and specific antibody *in vitro* by leukocytes from immunized cattle. *Veterinary Immunological Immunopathology*, 18, 67–80.

33 **FRANCIS, J., MADINAVEITIA, J., MACTURK, H.M. & SNOW, G.A., 1949.** Isolation from acid-fast bacteria of a growth factor for *Mycobacterium johnei* and a precursor of phthiocol. *Nature*, 163, 365–366.

34 **GILMOUR, N.J.L., 1976.** The pathogenesis, diagnosis and control of Johne's disease. *The Veterinary Record*, 99, 433–434.

35 **GILMOUR, N.J.L. & BROTHERSTON, J.G., 1966.** Further studies on immunity to *Mycobacterium johnei* in sheep. Relationship between hypersensitivity and host response to infection. *Journal of Comparative Pathology*, 76, 341–349.

36 **GILMOUR, N.J.L. & GOUDSWAARD, J., 1972.** *Corynebacterium renale* as a cause of reactions to the complement fixation test for Johne's disease. *Journal of Comparative Pathology*, 82, 333–336.

37 **GILMOUR, N.J.L. & NYANGE, J., 1989.** Paratuberculosis (Johne's disease) in deer. *In Practice*, 11, 193–196.

38 **GOUDSWAARD, J., GILMOUR, N.J.L., DIJKSTRA, R.G. &**

VAN BEEK, J.J., 1976. Diagnosis of Johne's disease in cattle: A comparison of five serologic tests under field conditions. *The Veterinary Record*, 98, 461–462.

39 **HAAGSMA, J. & EGER, A., 1988.** Bovine paratuberculosis: Improvement in the diagnosis of subclinically infected animals. *Proceedings of the Second International Colloquium on Paratuberculosis*, 22–23 September 1988. Maisons-Alfort, France.

40 **HAGAN, W.A., 1938.** Age as a factor in susceptibility to Johne's disease. *Cornell Veterinarian*, 28, 34–40.

41 **HERR, S., HUCHZERMEYER, H.F.A.K., TE BRUGGE, L., WILLIAMSON, C.C., ROOS, J.A. & SCHIELE, G.J., 1985.** The use of a single complement fixation technique in bovine brucellosis, Johne's disease, dourine, equine piroplasmosis and Q fever serology. *Onderstepoort Journal of Veterinary Research*, 52, 279–282.

42 **HOLE, N.H., 1958.** Johne's disease. *Advances in Veterinary Science*, 4, 341–387.

43 **HUCHZERMEYER, H.F.A.K., 1990.** Paratuberculosis. *Annual Reports, Tuberculosis Section, Veterinary Research Institute, Onderstepoort*, 1976–90.

44 **HUCHZERMEYER, H.F.A.K. & BASTIANELLO, S.S., 1991.** Veterinary Research Institute, Onderstepoort. Unpublished data.

45 **HUITEMA, H., 1967.** Johne's disease in cattle and vaccination. *Bulletin de l'Office International des Epizooties*, 68, 743–748.

46 **HUITEMA, H., 1968.** Johne's disease in cattle and vaccination. *Netherlands Journal of Veterinary Science*, 1, 189–196.

47 **HUNGERFORD, T.G., 1967.** *Diseases of Livestock*. 6th edn. Sydney: Angus and Robertson.

48 **HURLEY, S.S. & EWING, E., 1983.** Result of a field evaluation of a whole-cell bacterin. *In*: MERKAL, R.S., (ed.). *Proceedings of the International Colloquium on Research in Paratuberculosis*. National Animal Disease Center, Ames, Iowa.

49 **HURLEY, S.S., SPLITTER, G.A. & WELCH, R.A., 1989.** Development of a diagnostic test for Johne's disease using a DNA hybridization probe. *Journal of Clinical Microbiology*, 27, 1582–1587.

50 **JOHNE, H.A. & FROTHINGHAM, L., 1895.** Ein eigenthümlicher Fall von Tuberkulose beim Rind. *Deutsche Zeitschrift für Tiermedizinische vergleichende Pathologie*, 21, 438–454.

51 **JONES, R.L. & BRENNAN, P.J., 1985.** Application of modern biotechnology to the diagnosis of paratuberculosis. *In: Proceedings of the Eighty-ninth Annual Meeting of the US Animal Health Association*, 27 October to 1 November. Richmond, Virginia.

52 **JORGENSEN, J.B., 1977.** Survival of *Mycobacterium paratuberculosis* in slurry. *Nordisk Veterinaer Medicin*, 29, 267–270.

53 **JORGENSEN, J.B., 1983.** The diagnosis of clinical paratuberculosis in bovines. *Commission of the European Communities*, Agriculture Region Eur., 9000 EN, 1–8.

54 **JORGENSEN, J.B. & JENSEN, P.T. 1979.** Enzyme-linked immunosorbent assay (ELISA) for detection of antibodies to *Mycobacterium paratuberculosis* in cattle. *Acta Veterinaria Scandinavia*, 19, 310–312.

55 **JULIAN, R.J., 1975.** A short review and some observations on Johne's disease with recommendations for control. *Canadian Veterinary Journal*, 16, 33–43.

56 **KATIC, I., 1961.** Paratuberculosis (Johne's disease) with special reference to captive wild animals. A survey. *Nordisk Veterinary Medicine*, 13, 205–214.

57 **KIM, J.C.S., SANGER, V.L. & WHITENACK, D.L., 1976.** Ultrastructural studies of bovine paratuberculosis (Johne's disease). *Veterinary Medicine and Small Animal Clinician*, 71, 78–83.

58 **KLEEBERG, H.H. & WORTHINGTON, R.W., 1963.** Studies on Johne's disease. *Annual Reports, Tuberculosis Section, Veterinary Research Institute, Onderstepoort*.

59 **KLESIUS, P., 1982.** Intercellular communication: Role of soluble factors in cellular immune responses. *Journal of the American Veterinary Medical Association*, 181, 1015–1021.

60 **KLUGE, J.P., MERKAL, R.S., MONLUX, W.S., LARSEN, A.B., KOPECKY, K.E., RAMSEY, F.K. & LEHMANN, R.P., 1968.** Experimental paratuberculosis in sheep after oral, intratracheal, or intravenous inoculations: Lesion and demonstration of etiologic agent. *American Journal of Veterinary Research*, 29, 953–962.

61 **KOPECKY, K.E., 1977.** Distribution of paratuberculosis in Wisconsin, by soil regions. *Journal of the American Veterinary Medical Association*, 170, 320–324.

62 **KOPECKY, K.E., BOOTH, G.D., MERKAL, R.S. & LARSEN, A.B., 1971.** Haematologic changes associated with intravenous johnin testing in cattle. *American Journal of Veterinary Research*, 32, 1343–1347.

63 **KRIGE, J., 1992.** Directorate of Animal Health, P/Bag X138, Pretoria 0001, South Africa. Personal communication.

64 **KUBO, M., MORIWAKI, M. & WATASE, H., 1983.** Electron microscopic observations on the intestine of a cow with Johne's disease. *Japanese Journal of Veterinary Science*, 45, 259–262.

65 **LAMBRECHT, R.S. & COLLINS, M.T., 1988.** *In vivo* iron acquisition without mycobactin by *M. paratuberculosis*. *In: Proceedings of the Second International Colloquium on Paratuberculosis*, 22 and 23 September 1988, Maisons-Alfort, France, 157–178.

66 **LARSEN, A.B., 1972.** Paratuberculosis: The status of our knowledge. *Journal of the American Veterinary Medical Association*, 161, 1539–1541.

67 **LARSEN, A.B., 1973.** Johne's disease — Immunization and diagnosis. *Journal of the American Veterinary Medical Association*, 163, 902–904.

68 **LARSEN, A.B. & KOPECKY, K.E., 1970.** *Mycobacterium paratuberculosis* in reproductive organs and semen of bulls. *American Journal of Veterinary Research*, 31, 255–257.

69 **LARSEN, A.B., MERKAL, R.S. & CUTLIP, R.C., 1975.** Age of cattle as related to resistance to infection with *Mycobacterium paratuberculosis*. *American Journal of Veterinary Research*, 36, 255–257.

70 **LARSEN, A.B., MERKAL, R.S., KOPECKY, K.E. & MOON, H.W., 1969.** Hypersensitivity and serologic responses in cattle vaccinated with disrupted *Mycobacterium paratuberculosis* cells and subsequently infected with *Mycobacterium bovis*. *American Journal of Veterinary Research*, 30, 2167–2172.

71 **LARSEN, A.B., MERKAL, R.S. & MOON, H.W., 1974.** Evaluation of a paratuberculosis vaccine given to calves before infection. *American Journal of Veterinary Research*, 35, 367–369.

72 **LARSEN, A.B., MERKAL, R.S. & VARDAMAN, T.H., 1956.** Survival time of *Mycobacterium paratuberculosis*. *American Journal of Veterinary Research*, 17, 549–551.

73 **LARSEN, A.B., MOYLE, A.I. & HIMES, E.M., 1978.** Experimental vaccination of cattle against paratuberculosis (Johne's disease) with killed bacterial vaccines: A controlled field study. *American Journal of Veterinary Research*, 39, 65–69.

74 **LARSEN, A.B., STALHEIM, O.H.V., HUGHES, D.E., APPEL, L.H., RICHARDS, W.D. & HIMES, E.M., 1981.** *Mycobacterium paratuberculosis* in the semen and genital organs of a semen-donor bull. *Journal of the American Veterinary Medical Association*, 179, 169–171.

75 **LARSEN, A.B., VARDAMAN, T.H. & MERKAL, R.S., 1963.** An extended study of a herd of cattle naturally infected with Johne's disease. II. Significance of the complement-fixation test. *American Journal of Veterinary Research*, 24, 948–950.

76 **LARSEN, A.B., VARDAMAN, T.H. & MERKAL, R.S., 1965.** An extended study of a herd of cattle naturally infected with Johne's disease: The significance of the haemagglutination test. *American Journal of Veterinary Research*, 26, 254–257.

77 **LEPPER, A.W.D., 1988.** The aetiology and pathogenesis of Johne's disease. *In*: MILNER, A.R. & WOOD, P.R., (eds). *Johne's Disease. Current Trends in Research, Diagnosis and*

Management. Melbourne: CSIRO.

78 **LEPPER, A.W.D. & WILKS, C.R., 1988.** Intracellular iron storage and the pathogenesis of paratuberculosis. Comparative studies with other mycobacterial parasitic or infectious conditions of veterinary importance. *Journal of Comparative Pathology*, 98, 31–53.

79 **LIEBLER, E., 1985.** Untersuchungen zur Anzahl, Verteilung und Ausdehnung der schleimhauteigenen Solitärfollikel und Peyerschen Platten im Dünndarm des Kalbes unter besonderer Berücksichtigung ihrer Oberflächenstruktur. *Inaugural dissertation zur Erlangung des Grades eines Doctor Medicinae Veterinariae durch die Tierärztliche Hochschule Hannover*.

80 **LOVELL, R., LEVI, M. & FRANCIS, J., 1944.** Studies on the survival of Johne's bacilli. *Journal of Comparative Pathology*, 54, 120–128.

81 **MATTHEWS, P.R.J., McDIARMID, A., COLLINS, P. & BROWN, A., 1977.** The dependence of some strains of *Mycobacterium avium* on mycobactin for initial and subsequent growth. *Journal of Medical Microbiology*, 11, 53–57.

82 **McDONALD, J., COLLINS, M.T. & LAMBRECHT, R.S., 1988.** Radiometric detection of *Mycobacterium paratuberculosis* from clinical specimens. *In*: MILNER, A.R. & WOOD, P.R., (eds). *Johne's Disease. Current Trends in Research, Diagnosis and Management*. Melbourne: CSIRO.

83 **McFADDEN, J.J., GREEN, E. & HERMON-TAYLOR, J., 1988.** DNA probes to identify and detect *Mycobacterium paratuberculosis* in clinical and veterinary samples. *In: Proceedings of the Second International Colloquium on Paratuberculosis*, 22 and 23 September 1988, Maisons-Alfort, France.

84 **McKENZIE, R.A. & WARD, W.H., 1981.** *Rhodococcus (Corynebacterium) equi*: A possible cause of reactions to the complement fixation test for Johne's disease in cattle. *Australian Veterinary Journal*, 57, 200–201.

85 **McQUEEN, D.S. & RUSSELL, E.G., 1979.** Culture of *Mycobacterium paratuberculosis* from bovine foetuses. *Australian Veterinary Journal*, 55, 203–204.

86 **MERKAL, R.S., 1983.** Report on the international colloquium on research in paratuberculosis. *In: Proceedings of the Eighty-seventh Annual Meeting of the US Animal Health Association*, Las Vegas.

87 **MERKAL, R.S., 1984.** Paratuberculosis. *In*: KUBICA, G.P. & WAYNE, L.G., (eds). *The Mycobacteria: A Sourcebook, Part B*. New York and Basel: Marcel Dekker, Inc.

88 **MERKAL, R.S., 1984.** Paratuberculosis: Advances in cultural, serologic and vaccination methods. *Journal of the American Veterinary Medical Association*, 184, 939–943.

89 **MERKAL, R.S. & CURRAN, B.J., 1974.** Growth and metabolic characteristics of *Mycobacterium paratuberculosis*. *Applied Microbiology*, 28, 276–279.

90 **MERKAL, R.S., LARSEN, A.B. & BOOTH, G.D., 1975.** Analysis of the effects of inapparent bovine paratuberculosis. *American Journal of Veterinary Research*, 36, 837–838.

91 **MERKAL, R.S., LARSEN, A.B., KOPECKY, K.E. & NESS, R.D., 1970.** Immunologic mechanisms in bovine paratuberculosis. *American Journal of Veterinary Research*, 31, 475–485.

92 **MERKAL, R.S. & McCULLOUGH, W.G., 1982.** A new mycobactin, mycobactin J, from *Mycobacterium paratuberculosis*. *Current Microbiology*, 7, 333–335.

93 **MERKAL, R.S., McCULLOUGH, W.G. & TAKAYAMA, K., 1981.** Mycobactins, the state of the art. *Bulletin Institut Pasteur*, 79, 251–259.

94 **MERKAL, R.S., MILLER, J.M., HINTZ, A.M. & BRYNER, J.H., 1982.** Intra-uterine inoculation of *Mycobacterium paratuberculosis* into guinea-pigs and cattle. *American Journal of Veterinary Research*, 44, 676–678.

95 **MERKAL, R.S., RHOADES, J.E., GALLAGHER, J.E. & RITCHIE, A.E., 1973.** Scanning electron microscopy of mycobacteria. *American Review of Respiratory Disease*, 108, 382–387.

96 **MERKAL, R.S. & RICHARDS, W.D., 1972.** Inhibition of fungal growth in the cultural isolation of mycobacteria. *Applied Microbiology*, 24, 206–207.

97 **MERKAL, R.S. & THURSTON, J.R., 1968.** Susceptibilities of mycobacterial and nocardial species to benzalkonium chloride. *American Journal of Veterinary Research*, 29, 759–761.

98 **MOMOTANI, E., WHIPPLE, D.L., THIERMANN, A.B. & CHEVILLE, N.F., 1988.** Role of M-cells and macrophages in the entrance of *Mycobacterium paratuberculosis* into domes of ileal Peyer's patches in calves. *Veterinary Pathology*, 25, 131–137.

99 **MORRISON, N.E., 1965.** Circumvention of the mycobactin requirement of *Mycobacterium paratuberculosis*. *Journal of Bacteriology*, 89, 762–767.

100 **MOYLE, A.I., 1975.** Culture and cull procedures for control of paratuberculosis. *Journal of the American Veterinary Medical Association*, 166, 689–690.

101 **NEWSHOLME, S.J. & PLETCHER, J.M., 1981.** A mycobacteriosis in a sheep resembling paratuberculosis (Johne's disease). *Journal of the South African Veterinary Association*, 52, 143–145.

102 **PANDEY, G.S., MUSONDA, T.L., CHIZYUKA, H.G.B. & SCHNEEBELI, M., 1987.** Paratuberculosis (Johne's disease) in a herd of Friesian cattle in Zambia. *The Veterinary Record*, 120, 369.

103 **PATTERSON, D.S.P., ALLEN, W.M. & LLOYD, M.K., 1967.** Clinical Johne's disease as a protein-losing enteropathy. *The Veterinary Record*, 80, 717–718.

104 **PATTERSON, D.S.P. & BERRETT, S., 1968.** Malabsorption in Johne's disease of cattle: Depressed *in vitro* amino-acid uptake by isolated intestinal tissue preparations. *The Veterinary Record*, 81, 55–56.

105 **PAYNE, J.M. & RANKIN, J.D., 1961.** The pathogenesis of experimental Johne's disease in calves. *Research in Veterinary Science*, 2, 167–174.

106 **PAYNE, J.M. & RANKIN, J.D., 1961.** A comparison of the pathogenesis of experimental Johne's disease in calves and cows. *Research in Veterinary Science*, 2, 175–179.

107 **PEARSON, J.K.L. & McCLELLAND, T.G., 1955.** Uterine infection and congenital Johne's disease in cattle. *The Veterinary Record*, 67, 615–616.

108 **PEMBERTON, D.H., 1979.** Diagnosis of Johne's disease in cattle using mesenteric lymph node biopsy: Accuracy in clinical suspects. *Australian Veterinary Journal*, 55, 217–219.

109 **PEPIN, M., MARLY, J. & PARDON, P., 1987.** *Corynebacterium pseudotuberculosis* infection in sheep and the complement fixation test for paratuberculosis. *The Veterinary Record*, 120, 236.

110 **PORTAELS, F. & PATTYN, S.R., 1982.** Growth of mycobacteria in relation to the pH of the medium. *Annales de Microbiologie Institut Pasteur*, 133, 213–221.

111 **RAJYA, B.S. & SINGH, C.M., 1961.** Studies on the pathology of Johne's disease in sheep. III. Pathologic changes in sheep with naturally occurring infections. *American Journal of Veterinary Research*, 22, 189–202.

112 **RANKIN, J.D., 1962.** The experimental infection of cattle with *Mycobacterium johnei*. IV. Adult cattle maintained in an infectious environment. *Journal of Comparative Pathology*, 72, 113–117.

113 **RICHARDS, W.D., 1981.** Effects of physical and chemical factors on the viability of *Mycobacterium paratuberculosis*. *Journal of Clinical Microbiology*, 14, 587–588.

114 **RICHARDS, W.D., 1988.** The apparent effect of environmental acidity on the incidence of paratuberculosis. *In: Proceedings of the Second International Colloquium on Paratuberculosis*, 22 and 23 September 1988. Maisons -Alfort, France.

115 **RICHARDS, W.D. & THOEN, C.O., 1977.** Effect of freezing on the viability of *Mycobacterium paratuberculosis* in bovine faeces. *Journal of Clinical Microbiology*, 6, 392–395.

116 **RICHARDS, W.D. & WRIGHT, H.S., 1982.** Preservation of tissue specimens during transport to mycobacteriology laboratories. *Journal of Clinical Microbiology*, 17, 393–395.

117 **RIS, D.R., HAMEL, K.L. & AYLING, J.M., 1987.** Can sheep become infected by grazing pasture contaminated by cattle with Johne's disease? *New Zealand Veterinary Journal*, 35, 137.

118 **ROHDE, R.F. & SHULAW, W.P., 1990.** Isolation of *Mycobacterium paratuberculosis* from washed bovine ova after *in vitro* exposure. *American Journal of Veterinary Research*, 51, 708–710.

119 **SAXEGAARD, F., 1990.** Experimental infection of calves with an apparently specific goat-pathogenic strain of *Mycobacterium paratuberculosis*. *Journal of Comparative Pathology*, 98, 31–53.

120 **SAXEGAARD, F. & BAESS, I., 1988.** Relationship between *Mycobacterium avium, Mycobacterium paratuberculosis* and wood pigeon mycobacteria. *Acta Pathologica, Microbiologica et Immunologica Scandinavia*, 96, 37–42.

121 **SCHAAF, J., BEERWERTH, W. & GRODDE, S., 1956.** Über die Paratuberkulose des Rindes, ihre Verbreitung, Diagnose und Bekämpfung. *Monatshefte der Tierheilkunde, Rindertuberkulose*, 5, 144–154.

122 **SEITZ, S.E., HEIDER, L.E., HUESTON, W.D., BECH-NIELSEN, S., RINGS, D.M. & SPANGLER, L., 1989.** Bovine fetal infection with *Mycobacterium paratuberculosis*. *Journal of the American Veterinary Medical Association*, 194, 1423–1426.

123 **SHERMAN, D.M., 1985.** Current concepts in Johne's disease. *Veterinary Medicine Small Animal Clinician*, 80, 77–84.

124 **SHERMAN, D.M. & GEZON, H.M., 1980.** Comparison of agar-gel immunodiffusion and fecal culture of goats with paratuberculosis. *Journal of the American Veterinary Medical Association*, 177, 1208–1211.

125 **SHERMAN, D.M., MARKHAM, R.J.F. & BATES, F., 1984.** Agar-gel immunodiffusion test for diagnosis of clinical paratuberculosis in cattle. *Journal of the American Veterinary Medical Association*, 185, 179–182.

126 **SIGURDSSON, B., 1960.** A killed vaccine against paratuberculosis in sheep. *American Journal of Veterinary Research*, 21, 54–67.

127 **SNOW, G.A., 1970.** Mycobactins: Iron-chelating growth factors from mycobacteria. *Bacteriological Research*, 34, 99–125.

128 **STACHELSCHEID, H.L., 1989.** Zum kulturellen Nachweis von *Mycobacterium paratuberculosis* in Rinderkotproben. Vergleich zweier Dekontaminierungs- und Kulturverfahren. Inaugural Dissertation zur Erlangung des Doktorgrades beim Fachbereich Veterinämedizin der Justus-Liebig-Universität, Giessen.

129 **STUART, P., 1965.** Vaccination against Johne's disease in cattle exposed to experimental infection. *British Veterinary Journal*, 121, 289–318.

130 **STUART, P., 1965.** A pigmented *Mycobacterium johnei* strain of bovine origin. *British Veterinary Journal*, 121, 332–334.

131 **SUGDEN, E.A., SAMAGH, B.S., CORNER, A.H., TURCOTTE, C., BROOKS, B.W., STEWART, R.B. & DUNCAN, J.R., 1986.** Serodiagnosis of ovine paratuberculosis using lipoarabinomannan antigen in an enzyme immuno-assay. *In: Proceedings of the Fourth International Symposium of Veterinary Laboratory Diagnosticians, Amsterdam.*

132 **SUMMERS, B.A., 1981.** Laboratory diagnosis of Johne's disease. A potential source of error. *The Veterinary Record*, 108, 166–167.

133 **TAYLOR, A.W., 1957.** Varieties of *Mycobacterium johnei* isolated from sheep. *Journal of Pathology and Bacteriology*, 63, 333–336.

134 **TAYLOR, T.K., WILKS, C.R. & McQUEEN, D.S., 1981.** Isolation of *Mycobacterium paratuberculosis* from the milk of a cow with Johne's disease. *The Veterinary Record*, 109, 532–533.

135 **THOEN, C.O. & BAUM, K., 1988.** Current knowledge on paratuberculosis. *Journal of the American Veterinary Medical Association*, 192, 1609–1611.

136 **THOEN, C.O., HALL, M.R., PETERSBURG, T.A. & ANGUS, R.D., 1983.** Development of a modified enzyme-linked immunosorbent assay for detecting mycobacterial antibodies in sera of cattle from which *Mycobacterium paratuberculosis* was isolated. *In: Proceedings of the Third International Symposium for Veterinary Laboratory Diagnosticians*, Ames, Iowa, 141–150.

137 **THOEN, C.O. & HIMES, E.M., 1986.** Pathogenesis of *Mycobacterium bovis* infection. *Progress in Veterinary Microbiological Immunology*. Vol. II. Basel: Karger.

138 **THOEN, C.O. & MOORE, L.A., 1989.** Control of Johne's disease in four commercial dairy herds in Iowa. *Journal of Veterinary Diagnostic Investigation*, 1, 223–226.

139 **THOEN, C.O. & MUSCOPLAT, C.C., 1979.** Recent developments in diagnosis of paratuberculosis (Johne's disease). *Journal of the American Veterinary Medical Association*, 174, 838–840.

140 **THOMAS, G.W., 1983.** Paratuberculosis in a large goat herd. *The Veterinary Record*, 113, 464–466.

141 **THOREL, M-F., 1984.** Review of the occurrence of mycobactin dependence among mycobacteria species. *Annales de Recherche Vétérinaire*, 15, 405–409.

142 **THOREL, M-F. & DESMETTRE, P., 1982.** Comparative study of mycobactin-dependent strains of mycobacteria from wood-pigeon with *Mycobacterium avium* and *M. paratuberculosis*. *Annales de Microbiologie*, 133B, 151–152.

143 **THOREL, M-F. & VALETTE, L., 1976.** Etude de quelques souches de *Mycobacterium paratuberculosis*: Caractères biochimiques et activité allergique. *Annales de Recherche Vétérinaire*, 7, 207–213.

144 **TWORT, F.W. & INGRAM, G.L.Y., 1912.** A method for isolating and cultivating the *Mycobacterium enteritidis chronicae pseudotuberculosae bovis*, Johne and some experiments on the preparation of a diagnostic vaccine for pseudotuberculous enteritis of bovines. *Proceedings of the Royal Society, London*, Series B. 84, 517–543.

145 **VALLÉE, H. & RINJARD, P., 1926.** Etudes sur l'entérite paratuberculeuse des bovidés. *Revue Générale de Médecine Vétérinaire*, 35, 1–9.

146 **VAN AMSTEL, S.R., 1984.** Observations on the symptomatology and diagnosis of clinical cases of Johne's disease. *Journal of the South African Veterinary Association*, 55, 45–46.

147 **VAN NIEKERK, O.T. & VAN DER WALT, K., 1967.** Paratuberkulose (Johne se siekte) by 'n ingevoerde Duitse merino ram. *Journal of the South African Veterinary Medical Association*, 38, 23–24.

148 **VARDAMAN, T.H., 1954.** The effect of various chemical agents on the viability of *Mycobacterium paratuberculosis in vitro*. *American Journal of Veterinary Research*, 15, 159–163.

149 **WHIPPLE, D.L, LEFEBURE, R.B., ANDREWS, JR. R.E. & THIERMANN, A.B., 1987.** Isolation and analysis of restriction endonuclease digestive patterns of chromosomal DNA from *Mycobacterium paratuberculosis* and other *Mycobacterium* species. *Journal of Clinical Microbiology*, 25, 1511–1515.

150 **WHIPPLE, D.L. & MERKAL, R.S., 1983.** Modifications in the techniques for cultivation of *Mycobacterium paratuberculosis*. *In*: MERKAL, R.S., (ed.) *Proceedings of the International Colloquium on Research on Paratuberculosis*. National Animal Disease Center, 16–18 June, Ames, Iowa.

151 **WILESMITH, J.W., 1982.** Johne's disease: A retrospective study of vaccinated herds in Great Britain. *British Veterinary Journal*, 138, 321–331.

152 **WILESMITH, J.W., 1986.** Vaccination against Johne's disease. *The State Veterinary Journal*, 40, 152–154.

153 **WILKS, C.R., TAYLOR, T.K., RUSSEL, E.G. & THURSTON, T.R., 1981.** Isolation of mycobacteria inducing cross-reactions in the complement-fixation test for Johne's disease. *Research in Veterinary Science*, 30, 323–327.

154 **WOOD, P.R., KOPSIDAS, K., MILNER, A.R., HILL, J., GILL, I., WEBB, R., MACK, W.N. & COATES, K., 1988.** The development of an *in vitro* cellular assay for Johne's disease in cattle. *In*: MILNER, A.R. & WOOD, P.R., (eds). *Johne's Disease. Current Trends in Research, Diagnosis and Management.*

Melbourne: CSIRO.

155 **WORSAAE, H., 1978.** Radioimmunoassay for antibodies against *Mycobacterium paratuberculosis* using ^{125}L-labelled PPD. *Acta Veterinaria Scandinavia*, 19, 153–155.

156 **WORTHINGTON, R., 1963.** Johne's disease (paratuberculosis). *In: Emerging Disease of Animals.* FAO Agricultural Studies, 61, 155–176.

157 **YOKOMIZO, Y., YUGI, H. & MERKAL, R.S., 1985.** A method for avoiding false-positive reactions in an enzyme-linked immunosorbent assay (ELISA) for the diagnosis of bovine paratuberculosis. *Japanese Journal of Veterinary Science*, 47, 111–119.

158 **ZURBRICK, B.G. & CZUPRYNSKI, C.J., 1987.** Ingestion and intracellular growth of *Mycobacterium paratuberculosis* within blood monocytes and monocyte-derived macrophages. *Infection and Immunity*, 55, 1588–1593.

ACTINOMYCETES

The classification of the bacteria collectively known as actinomycetes (based on the presence of microscopic hyphae when grown on agar, the presence or absence of spores, and the morphology of their sporangia) is complex and in flux. The genera include several of veterinary importance, may be categorized supragenerically into groups (actinobacteria, nocardioforms, actinoplanetes, thermomonospores, maduromycetes, streptomycetes, and those with multilocular sporangia), some of which may be very heterogeneous. The bacteria in the supra-generic groups have also been classified as irregular, non-sporing, Gram-negative rods (genus *Actinomyces)*; nocardioform actinomycetes (genera *Nocardia* and *Rhodococcus)*; and as actinomycetes with multilocular sporangia (genus *Dermatophilus)*.[1]

Members of the genus *Actinomyces,* including *A. bovis* and *A. (Corynebacterium) pyogenes,* characteristically cause suppurative infections tissues and organs. The disease caused by *A. pyogenes* is more suppurative and has a tendency to abscess formation, while that caused by *A. bovis* is usually characterized by progressive, chronic, pyogranulomatous inflammatory processes, the disease referred to as lumpy jaw being the best example.

The only common characteristic of the nocardioform actinomycetes is that they share the morphological complexity of the actinomycetes, and exist as fungacious mycelia that break up into rod-shaped or coccoid elements. The organisms grouped as nocardioforms are mostly unrelated, although in certain respects some of the genera are related to the mycobacteria and corynebacteria. The two genera of veterinary importance regarded as nocardioforms are *Nocardia* and *Rhodococcus.* The diseases caused by them are ubiquitous but usually occur sporadically, and are characterized by subacute to chronic suppurative processes which often become pyogranulomatous. *Nocardia* (principally *N. asteroides,* but also *N. otitidiscaviarium,* and *N. brasiliensis)* are associated with a variety of non-specific infections which have no species specificity or specific site of predilection in the body. *Rhodococcus equi* is mostly associated with disease syndromes in foals characterized by multifocal, caseonecrotic bronchopneumonia, ulcerative enterocolitis and mesenteric lymphadenitis, and occasionally with the development of abscesses, arthritis or abortion in horses, or abscesses and other suppurative processes in sheep, goats and pigs.[2]

The genus *Dermatophilus* is morphologically characterized by being composed of filaments that break up into long, multilocular sporangia. Infection by *D. congolensis* is responsible for the production, principally in tropical and subtropical climates, of a superficial dermatitis in several animal species, chiefly cattle, sheep and horses. In cattle it causes Senkobo diseases, which may have profound economic effects, and in sheep, lumpy wool and strawberry footrot.[3]

References

1 **GOODFELLOW, M., 1989.** The Actinomycetes. *In:* WILLIAMS, S.T., SHARPE, M.E. & HOLT, J.G., (eds). *Bergey's Manual of Systematic Bacteriology.* Vol VI. Baltimore: Williams & Wilkens.

2 **LECHEVALIER, H.A., 1989.** Nocardioform actinomycetes. *In:* WILLIAMS, S.T., SHARPE, M.E. & HOLT, J.G., (eds). *Bergey's Manual of Systematic Bacteriology.* Vol. VI. Baltimore: Williams & Wilkens.

3 **LECHEVALIER, M.P., 1989.** Actinomycetes with multilocular sporangia. *In:* WILLIAMS, S.T., SHARPE, M.E. & HOLT, J.G., (eds). *Bergey's Manual of Systematic Bacteriology.* Vol VI. Baltimore: Williams & Wilkens.

174

Nocardiosis

M.M. Henton

Introduction

Nocardiosis occurs in several animal species and is an acute, subacute or chronic disease characterized by focal or disseminated, suppurative or granulomatous lesions caused by infection with *Nocardia asteroides* or, less commonly, *Nocardia otitidiscaviarum* or *Nocardia brasiliensis*. Mastitis (cattle and goats), abortion (cattle, pigs, sheep, and horses), corneal ulceration and chronic dermatitis (cattle), and often-fatal, disseminated, granulomatous disease or granulomatous pneumonia (cattle and horses), have been recorded. Disease caused by *Nocardia* spp. has been reported from various countries in the world, but is sporadic and, except when associated with rare outbreaks, of little economic importance.

The first recorded cases of nocardiosis were reported from cattle with farcy on the island of Guadeloupe in the French West Indies, by Nocard in 1888.[24] Bovine farcy characterized by a pyogranulomatous lymphangitis and lymphadenitis of the lower limbs was common in France at the end of the nineteenth century, but has since disappeared. *Nocardia farcinica*, the original isolate from bovine farcy, is now known to be represented by two strains — one indistinguishable from *Nocardia asteroides*, and the other a *Mycobacterium*-like strain.[12]

In South Africa nocardial infections are mainly seen in dogs (most frequently in the form of a pyogranulomatous pleuritis) and rarely as a cause of mastitis and abortion in cattle.[13]

Aetiology and epidemiology

The informal term, nocardioform, signifies Actinomycetes that form a Gram-positive fugacious mycelium and reproduce by breaking up into rod-shaped or coccal elements. Both the pathogenic nocardioform Actinomycetes (*Nocardia* and *Rhodococcus*) and the non-pathogenic Actinomycetes (such as *Oerskovia*, *Nocardioides*, and *Promicromonospora*) are soil inhabitants. Members of the genus *Nocardia* are aerobic, catalase-positive, and their cell wall (type IV) contains large amounts of *meso*-diaminopimelic acid (*meso*-DAP), arabinose, and galactose.[12] *Mycobacterium*, *Rhodococcus*, and *Corynebacterium* also have a type IV cell wall, but these genera are distinguished from *Nocardia* by differences in their respective mycolic acids. *Nocardia* spp. grow best on blood agar, Loewenstein-Jensen or brain-heart infusion agar. Chloramphenicol should not be added to the medium. The colonies are orange, glabrous, heaped and folded, or may be white or pink with aerial hyphae. The colonies are dry and crumbly and are adherent.[17]

Nocardia spp. occur widely in soil.[27] *Nocardia asteroides* grows over a wide temperature range and is resistant to 50 °C for several hours, but all *Nocardia* spp. are inactivated by pasteurization. Various serotypes (I to IV) of *N. asteroides*, differentiated by immunoprecipitation, have been recorded.[33]

African cattle breeds seem to be fairly resistant to skin infections. When they do occur, infections may be spread by *Amblyomma variegatum* ticks.[26] Transstadial transmission by ticks has been demonstrated experimentally.[3]

Localized, subcutaneous infections also develop after injury to the skin, and pulmonary infections result from inhalation of the organism. Systemic nocardiosis results from a primary focus, usually the lungs. External contamination of the vulva with soil may cause a localized infection of the uterus, and abortion.[11]

Nocardial mastitis, which may occur as sporadic individual cases or as isolated outbreaks in cattle, usually results from infection via the teat canal by contaminated intramammary infusions used for mastitis therapy.[14, 20, 40] Concomitant infections with other pathogens such as *Staphylococcus aureus*, *Actinomyces pyogenes* and *Pseudomonas aeruginosa* may be present.[13]

Pathogenesis

Scant data exist on the pathogenesis of nocardiosis. Delayed hypersensitivity reactions may be associated with the development of the lesions. In experimental infections, a delayed hypersensitivity reaction and the inhibition of migration of inflammatory cells present in the peritoneal exudate have been demonstrated[28, 29] as soon as one week after the initial infection. These responses coincide with the appearance of the initial lesion, which is an abscess. The response reaches its maximum after two weeks, when the central suppurative reaction becomes surrounded by epithelioid and giant cells.[15]

Clinical signs

Cattle

Acute, chronic or subclinical mastitis has been reported.[40] At the onset of the mastitis, one or all the quarters are swollen and the milk may be pinkish.[1] This is eventually followed by induration of the udder.[39] Blackish spots, crusts and nodules, which may rupture and exude a thick pus, are present on the affected parts of the udder.[2]

The milk yield of affected animals is severely reduced. In chronic cases, the granulomatous lesions may cause obstruction of the lactiferous ducts, and extensive fibrosis and draining sinuses may develop.[5, 19] Acutely affected animals may die or have to be culled. Severe cases may die within 12 hours of clinical signs first being noticed,[14] and the mortality rate may be as high as 10 per cent.[40]

Abortions may occur at six to eight months of gestation[13, 22, 43] in clinically healthy cows.[43]

A number of rare syndromes include a severe, progressive dermatitis in some cases, of which all affected animals either die, or have to be culled.[26, 30] Cutaneous involvement is characterized by a pyogranulomatous lymphadenitis and lymphangitis of the fore limbs. The lesions, which may be quite localized, contain a whitish, odourless, inspissated pus, and may extend onto the neck and have a cord-like distribution. The lesions rarely open, and eventually become indurated.[16] Corneal ulceration[32] and a chronic debilitating disease due to disseminated nocardiosis, which may eventually localize in the lungs, heart and udder, have been reported.[21, 25, 36, 38]

Sheep and goats

Infections are rare in sheep and goats. In the latter species, clinical signs are the consequence of lesions — generally localized, granulomatous, inflammatory reactions — in single organs such as the lungs and udder,[6, 10, 41] while in sheep, subclinical infections of the lungs,[34] clinical manifestations of purulent arthritis in a lamb,[23] and abortion[42] have also been recorded.

Pigs and horses

Full-term abortion in pigs[11] and mid- to late-term abortion in horses[8] occur. In horses, disseminated or pulmonary infections terminate fatally in almost 100 per cent of cases.[7]

Pathology

In aborted bovine foetuses the lymph nodes and liver are enlarged, ecchymoses are evident in the spleen and myocardium, and multiple whitish foci resembling abscesses occur in the lungs.[43] Aborted piglets manifest no macroscopic lesions, but there are histological signs of a purulent pneumonia.[11] In aborted equine foetuses lesions occur in the lungs, liver and placenta.[8] Focal placentitis has been described in sheep, but no lesions are seen in the foetus.[42]

In chronic mastitis, pyogranulomatous lesions occur throughout the affected gland, which is extensively fibrosed and contains discharging sinuses.[5, 19] Similar lesions occur in the regional lymph nodes.

Granulomatous lesions may also be found in various internal organs, including the lungs,[21] heart and lymph nodes. The prescapular nodes are most commonly involved, while the parotid, retropharyngeal and mediastinal nodes are less commonly involved than other nodes.[36] Histologically these lesions contain numerous giant cells and thin, filamentous, branching organisms.[30] Very chronic lesions contain areas of caseation, mineralization and fibrosis.[25]

Diagnosis and differential diagnosis

Pus from the lesions often contains the so-called 'sulphur granules', which are yellowish-white granules up to about 0,5 mm in diameter that may be quite numerous. Smears made from crushed 'sulphur granules' consist of Gram- and silver-positive, branching, beaded filaments.[8] The filaments are partially acid-fast and are best demonstrated by the cold Kinyoun method,[9, 18] but they are not stained with haematoxylin and eosin. Laboratory culture usually yields growth in about four days, but media seeded with material suspected to contain organisms should only be discarded after 21 days, if no growth has occurred in this period.[12]

In the case of nocardial mastitis, the diagnosis may be missed if the whole herd is not sampled, or if cultures are not kept for at least 72–96 hours.[40] Intradermal skin tests seem to be highly specific and show no cross-reactions with the tuberculin test. However, cross-reactions do occur between *N. asteroides* and *N. otitidiscaviarum*.[37]

In aborted foetuses the diagnosis can be confirmed by histological examination of the foetal tissues and culture of the organism[43] from the lungs and abomasal contents of the foetuses, placental cotyledons and vaginal discharge of cows that have aborted.[22, 43]

The lesions of bovine farcy may easily be confused with those caused by *Mycobacterium farcinogenes*, *M. senegalense*[35] and *Dermatophilus congolensis*.[26, 31]

Control

Because of the sporadic nature of nocardiosis, treatment is the only useful way of controlling the disease. *Nocardia* spp. are generally susceptible to antibacterial drugs, such as the sulphonamides, cotrimoxazole, amikacin, nitrofurans and novobiocin, but antifungal drugs are ineffective. Good results have been reported after the long-term use of trimethoprim given intramuscularly, 12-hourly at 30 mg/kg over two weeks.[4] Individual cases may be refractory to specific treatment.[2] If nocardial mastitis occurs as an outbreak, proper hygiene is most important and early drying off of the cows may be more beneficial than specific therapy. Repetitive use of devices for the intramammary application of therapeutic substances should be avoided.

References

1 **AHMED, I.U. & BARUAH, H.K., 1980.** Occurrence of actinomycotic mastitis in Nagaland. *Indian Veterinary Journal*, 57, 84.

2 **AL-BASSAM, L.S., KASTANDI, J.D. & KAMALAPUR, P.N., 1988.** *Nocardia* mastitis in dairy cattle in Iraq. *Livestock Adviser*, 13, 36–37.

3 **AL-JANABI, B.M., BRANAGAN, D. & DANSKIN, D., 1975.** The transstadial transmission of the bovine farcy organism, *Norcardia farcinica*, by the ixodid *Amblyomma variegatum* (Fabricius, 1794). *Tropical Animal Health and Production*, 7, 205–220.

4 **ANDERSON, K.L. & WILCKE, J.R., 1980.** Potentiated sulphonamides in the treatment of bovine pulmonary nocardiosis. *Journal of Veterinary Pharmacology and Therapeutics*, 3, 217–220.

5 **ANON., 1980.** Unusual causes of bovine mastitis (*Nocardia asteroides* and Klebsiella). *Ministry of Agriculture and Fisheries Surveillance*, New Zealand, 7, 11.

6 **BANERJEE, M. & GUPTA, P.P., 1979.** A note on pulmonary actinomycosis and nocardiosis in goats of Punjab (Ludhiana area). *Indian Journal of Animal Science*, 49, 972–975.

7 **BIBERSTEIN, E.L., JANG, S.S. & HIRSH, D.C., 1985.** *Nocardia asteroides* infection in horses: A review. *Journal of the American Veterinary Medical Association*, 186, 273–277.

8 **BOLON, B., BUERGELT, C.D. & COOLEY, A.J., 1989.** Abortion in two foals associated with *Nocardia* infection. *Veterinary Pathology*, 26, 277–278.

9 **CARTER, G.R., 1984.** *Diagnostic Procedures in Veterinary Bacteriology and Mycology*. 4th edn. Springfield: Charles Thomas.

10 **CAUSEY, W.A., 1974.** *Nocardia caviae*: A report of 13 new isolations with clinical correlation. *Applied Microbiology*, 28, 193–198.

11 **COLE, J.R. & HOLZINGER, E.A., 1972.** *Nocardia asteroides* associated with swine abortion. *Veterinary Medicine and Small Animal Clinician*, 67, 496–498.

12 **GOODFELLOW, M. & LECHEVALIER, M.P., 1989.** Genus *Nocardia*. *In*: WILLIAMS, S.T., SHARPE, M.E. & HOLT, J.G., (eds). *Bergey's Manual of Systematic Bacteriology*. Vol. IV. Baltimore, Hong Kong, London, Sydney: Williams & Wilkins.

13 **HENTON, M.M., 1990.** Veterinary Research Institute, Onderstepoort. Unpublished data.

14 **HIBBS, C.M., HOPSON, J.H., FERGUSON, R. & THILSTED, J.P., 1980.** *Nocardia* mastitis in a large dairy herd. *Proceedings of the Annual Meeting of the American Association of Veterinary Laboratory Diagnosticians*, 23, 73–77.

15 **HIRAMINE, C., HOJO, K. & YANO, I., 1981.** Development of cell-mediated hypersensitivity in guinea-pigs following infection with *Nocardia asteroides*. *International Archives of Allergy and Applied Immunology*, 65, 220–234.

16 **HOARE, W.E., 1913.** *A System of Veterinary Medicine*. Vol. I. London: Baillière, Tindall & Cox.

17 **HOWARD, J.H., KLAAS, J., WEISSFELD, A.S., RUBIN, S.J. & TILTON, R.C., 1987.** *Clinical and Pathogenic Microbiology*. St Louis, Washington DC, Toronto: The CV Mosby Co.

18 **JUNGERMAN, P.F. & SCHWARTZMAN, R.M., 1972.** *Veterinary Medical Mycology*. Philadelphia: Lea & Febiger.

19 **KUME, T., INUI, S. & NARITA, M., 1973.** A case of bovine chronic mastitis caused by *Nocardia asteroides* and experimental infection of goat udder with isolated organism. *National Institute of Animal Health Quarterly*, 13, 231–232.

20 **LYNCH, J.A., 1988.** Nocardial mastitis in cattle. *Canadian Veterinary Journal*, 29, 594.

21 **MOHAN, K., 1983.** Occurrence of *Nocardia asteroides* in cattle in eastern Nigeria. *Bulletin of Animal Health and Production in Africa*, 31, 355–358.

22 **MUGARULA, D.R. & MCHOMBA, O.K., 1980.** Bovine abortion due to *Nocardia asteroides* – a first case report in Tabora. *Bulletin of Animal Health and Production in Africa*, 28, 195–196.

23 **NDIKUWERA, J., ODIAWO, G. & OBWOLO, M., 1990.** Nocardial septic arthritis in a lamb. *Irish Veterinary Journal*, 43, 29–30.

24 **NOCARD, E., 1888.** Note sur la maladie des boefs de la Guadaloupe connue sous le nom de farcin. *Annales de l'Institut Pasteur*, 2, 293–302.

25 **NORTON, J.H., 1976.** Tuberculosis-like granulomas in cattle caused by Actinomycetes. *Australian Veterinary Journal*, 51, 455–457.

26 **OLUBUNMI, P.A. & AYENI, A.O., 1983.** A description of an outbreak of bovine nocardiosis in Western Nigeria. *Journal of Animal Production Research*, 3, 127–138.

27 **ORCHARD, V.A., 1979.** Nocardial infections of animals in New Zealand. *New Zealand Veterinary Journal*, 27, 159–165.

28 **ORTIZ-ORTIZ, L., CONTRERAS, M.F. & BOJALIL, L.F., 1972.** The assay of delayed hypersensitivity to ribosomal proteins from *Nocardia*. *Sabouraudia*, 10, 147–151.

29 **ORTIZ-ORTIZ, L., CONTRERAS, M.F. & BOJALIL, L.F., 1972.** Cytoplasmic antigens from *Nocardia* eliciting a specific delayed hypersensitivity. *Infection and Immunity*, 5, 879–882.

30 **OSIYEMI, T.I.O., OKEWOLE, P.A., DAWUL, B., ALLI-BA LOGUN, R.A.O. & LUKDEN, W.D., 1985.** Nocardiosis in a Friesian cow. *Bulletin of Animal Health and Production in Africa*, 33, 23–24.

31 **OYEKUNLE, M.A. & OJO, M.O., 1988.** Preliminary observations on bovine cutaneous nocardiosis and dermatophilosis in the subhumid climate of Southern Nigeria. *Revue d'Elevage et de Médecine Vétérinaire des Pays Tropicaux*, 41, 347–351.

32 **PAL, M., 1982.** Etiological significance of *Nocardia asteroides* in corneal ulcer of cattle. *Current Science*, 51, 533–534.

33 **PIER, A.C. & FICHTNER, R.E., 1981.** Distribution of serotypes of *Nocardia asteroides* from animal, human and environmental sources. *Journal of Clinical Microbiology*, 13, 548–553.

34 **RAHMAN, T. & IYER, P.K.R., 1979.** Studies on pathology of ovine pneumonias. *Indian Veterinary Journal*, 56, 455–461.

35 **RIDELL, M., GOODFELLOW, M. & ABDULLE, M.A., 1985.** Identification of actinomycetes isolated from cases of bovine farcy in the Sudan. *Zentralblatt für Bakteriologie, Mikrobiologie und Hygiene*, 259, 43–50.

36 **SALIH, M.A.M., EL SANOUSI, S.M., & EL DIN, H.M.T., 1978.** Predilection sites of bovine farcy lesions in Sudanese cattle. *Bulletin of Animal Health and Production in Africa*, 26, 168–171.

37 **SALMAN, M.D., BUSHNELL, R.B. & PIER, A.C., 1982.** Determination of sensitivity and specificity of the *Nocardia asteroides* skin test for detection of bovine mammary infections caused by *Nocardia asteroides* and *Nocardia caviae*. *American Journal of Veterinary Research*, 43, 332–335.

38 **SANOUSI, S.M., & SALIH, M.A.M., 1979.** Further studies on the properties of the aetiology of bovine farcy isolated from Sudanese cattle. *Revue d'Elevage et de Médecine Vétérinaire des Pays Tropicaux*, 32, 135–141.

39 **SCHOONDERWOERD, M. & PLANTE-JENKINS, C., 1988.** Mastitis associated with suspected *Nocardia* sp. *Canadian Veterinary Journal*, 29, 846–847.

40 **SEARS, P.M., 1983.** Nocardia mastitis. *Bovine Practitioner*, 18, 4–6.

41 **SHARMA, I. & IYER, P.K.R., 1974.** Pathology of chronic lesions in mammary glands of goats (*Capra hircus*): nocardiosis and botryomycosis. *Indian Journal of Animal Science*, 44, 41–45.

42 **WATSON, W.A. & BEVERLEY, J.K.A., 1977.** *Nocardia* species as a possible cause of ovine abortion. *Research in Veterinary Science*, 23, 171–178.

43 **WOHLGEMUTH, K., KNUDTSON, W., BICKNELL, E.J. & KIRKBRIDE, C.A., 1972.** Bovine abortion associated with *Nocardia asteroides*. *Journal of the American Veterinary Medical Association*, 161, 273–274.

175

Rhodococcus equi *infection*

Synonym: *Corynebacterium equi* infection

M.G. Collett

Introduction

Infection with *Rhodococcus (Corynebacterium) equi* typically causes a subacute to chronic syndrome which is characterized by multifocal caseonecrotic bronchopneumonia, ulcerative enterotyphlocolitis and mesenteric lymphadenitis in foals and, rarely, ulcerative lymphangitis in young horses, abscesses and arthritis in adult horses, and abortion in pregnant mares.[2, 32, 33, 52, 74, 84, 86, 111] It is also occasionally the cause of abscesses and other suppurative conditions in species such as goats, sheep and cattle, and of tuberculosis-like lesions in the lymph nodes of pigs.[5]

Rhodococcus equi was first described by Magnusson in Sweden in 1923 and is widely distributed around the world.[5] Since pneumonia in foals due to *R. equi* was recorded in the Karoo (Colesberg and Middelburg) and northern Cape Province (Kimberley) regions in South Africa in 1957,[43] sporadic cases of the disease have been encountered, particularly on some stud farms in the Karoo and the south-western Cape Province, and on rare occasions elsewhere in South Africa.[85]

Aetiology

The bacterium has a confused taxonomic history. It was previously known as *Corynebacterium equi*, but is now classified as *Rhodococcus equi* in the Mycobacteriaceae family.[40] It is a large (0,5–1,0 x 1,0–2,0 µm), obligate aerobic, Gram-positive, variably acid-fast, pleomorphic coccobacillus. The bacteria have lamellar polysaccharide capsules and cell walls composed of corynomycolic acids and lipids (such as phosphotidyl inositol and phosphotidyl ethanolamine) and produce carotenoid pigments.[5, 39, 98] At least seven serotypes have been identified, but no clear relationship between serotypes and source of origin of isolates has been found.[68, 71]

Rhodococcus equi grows well on ordinary media and forms smooth, shiny, mucoid, tan to salmon-pink to red colonies; some strains produce abundant slime which may cause colonies growing on agar slope media in test tubes to slide to the bottom of the tubes. Selective media have been developed for its isolation from soil and faecal material.[5, 101]

Epidemiology

Rhodococcus equi can be isolated from the faeces and manure of herbivorous animals, pigs and birds, as well as from soil previously contaminated with manure.[23, 51, 72, 99] *Rhodococcus equi* is a saprophyte in soil where it is able to multiply; the simple organic acids from horse dung act as growth stimulants.[51] It is able to survive for over a year in soil samples exposed daily to sunlight.[92] Optimal multiplication occurs at 30 °C at pH 7,5.[51]

Although many animal species, including ruminants and pigs, are susceptible to *R. equi*, infection occurs most commonly in horses.[5] The majority of horses become subclinically infected after ingesting the bacteria early in life.[72, 74, 79, 88, 102, 103] Its simple growth requirements are met perfectly in the intestine of foals,[51, 72] particularly those which are coprophagic, so that by four weeks of age, up to 100 per cent of foals on infected premises may shed *R. equi* in their faeces.[96] *Rhodococcus equi* appears capable of surviving without multiplying while in transit through the intestines of non-susceptible hosts.[51] Because of these characteristics, there is a progressive build-up of the bacterium in manure-contaminated soil and dust on equine stud farms over many years.[72, 81] Even cobwebs in stables may harbour it.[23, 92] Consequently, foals exposed to dusty conditions may contract the disease by inhalation.[72, 92, 96, 105] Migration of larvae of parasites (e.g., *Strongyloides westeri, Parascaris equorum, Strongylus* spp.) may introduce *R. equi* into body tissues.[2, 25, 26, 33, 74] The above factors help to explain why *R. equi* disease is endemic on some farms, sporadic on others, and unrecognized on most.[72, 84]

Rhodococcus equi may also occur as a commensal in the cervix of mares, but here it appears not to be an important source of infection for foals.[2]

Pathogenesis

Rhodococcus equi is a saprophytic, opportunistic pathogen[52, 103] which, under favourable circumstances, becomes a facultative, intracellular parasite of phagocytes, particularly the alveolar macrophages, of horses.[44, 109]

In most affected foals, pulmonary infection is probably

acquired by the inhalation of *R. equi*-contaminated dust. Conceivably, this is followed by haematogenous spread that results in a bacteraemia prior to localization in other organs.[2, 12, 55, 61, 92] *Rhodococcus equi* has a predilection for the lungs and lymphoid tissues, particularly those in the mucosa of the large intestine. Intestinal lesions develop when large numbers of bacteria, expectorated from pneumonic lesions or ingested because of coprophagy, are swallowed.[78, 105] *Rhodococcus equi* presumably enters the intestinal mucosa through the specialized M-cell epithelium of Peyer's patches.[74, 105] Lung lesions may also develop secondarily after primary intestinal involvement when organisms are disseminated via the intestinal lymph nodes and the thoracic duct to the pulmonary circulation.[55, 74]

Following localization of *R. equi* in the lungs, alveolar macrophages not only act as the first line of defence, but are also the effector cells of cell-mediated immunity in the lungs and are of cardinal importance in the pathogenesis of *R. equi* infection in foals.[8, 109] Specific receptors on macrophages are responsible for the recognition and phagocytosis of *R. equi*.[49]

The immune response, as well as the state of immunity against *R. equi*, determines the outcome of the infection and development of the lesions. Resistance to the effects of *R. equi* infection depends largely on phagocytosis of the bacteria and effective intracellular killing of organisms.[44, 63, 64, 106] The killing of the organisms by alveolar macrophages is significantly enhanced *in vitro* by opsonization with antibody against capsular antigens in the presence of lymphokines.[44] In the absence of antibody, alveolar macrophages readily ingest *R. equi* organisms but their bactericidal activity is ineffective[78, 110] due to a deficient respiratory burst, thus allowing the intracellular survival of the phagocytosed bacteria.[10] In addition, *R. equi* inhibits phagosome-lysosome fusion and induces non-specific lysosome degranulation while it persists and multiplies in phagosomes, thus causing degeneration, necrosis and disintegration of macrophages. Myriads of viable bacteria are then released.[44, 109] The polysaccharide capsule of *R. equi*, and the corynomycolic acids and lipids contained in the cell wall probably also determine the virulence of *R. equi* [78, 107] by enabling the bacteria to resist phagocytic digestion[57, 105] and by effectively inhibiting the host's humoral immune response.[5, 15] In this respect, the properties of *R. equi* resemble those of *Mycobacterium tuberculosis*, with which it shares cell-wall similarities.[41]

Certain antigenic 'exoenzymes', also known as 'equi factors' (cholesterol oxidase and phospholipases, such as choline phosphohydrolase and sphingomyelinase C) are additional determinants of virulence.[58, 73, 75, 90, 105, 109] 'Equi-factor'-neutralizing antibodies reduce the clinical progression of the disease in foals.[62]

Neutrophils also play a defence role against *R. equi* infections. In the presence of complement and sufficient quantities of opsonizing antibody, the antibacterial functions of neutrophils (including oxidative metabolism) are normally very effective in the elimination of the organism.[10, 64, 106] Although it would seem that defective neutrophil bactericidal function does not play a major role in the pathogenesis of *R. equi* infections,[106] neutrophils from some neonatal foals have been shown to be functionally immature and unable to eliminate the bacterium effectively.[63]

Lysosomal enzymes, particularly acid hydrolases, and free oxygen radicals from disintegrating macrophages, neutrophils and other cells engaged in phagocytosis, probably contribute to tissue damage and the inflammatory response.[44, 54, 105, 106] No bacterial toxins have yet been identified.[57]

The immunological response of the host to *R. equi* is affected by the age of the animal, levels of colostrum-derived antibody, stress, concurrent viral infections, genetic predisposition, the route and extent of exposure, and the virulence of the strain of *R. equi* involved.[30, 63, 97, 102, 103] A competent immune response is required to prevent pneumonia and death.[15, 107] Cell-mediated immune mechanisms seem to be the most important component of the immune response involved in the host's defence against *R. equi* infection.[15, 57, 61, 62, 79, 99]

Foals between one and four months of age are particularly vulnerable to *R. equi* infection because of waning passive humoral immunity and the incompletely developed cell-mediated immune response in the respiratory tract at this age.[5, 45, 62, 72, 88, 105] Foals under three weeks of age also possess low numbers of resident pulmonary alveolar macrophages, which renders them more susceptible to infection.[108] Arabian foals suffering from combined immunodeficiency disease frequently have lung lesions caused by *R. equi*.[34, 93] Thus, the combination of a suboptimal pulmonary defence mechanism, especially with respect to alveolar macrophages, and a high infectious challenge resulting from an environmental build-up of faecally derived organisms are prerequisites for the establishment of *R. equi* infections in foals.[9]

The pathogenesis of *R. equi* pneumonia has been studied experimentally in guinea-pigs[53] and in mice.[7–9, 107] The early lung lesions in the experimental infection in mice resemble those in foals, except that they resolve spontaneously with time, which is not the case in foals.[7]

Clinical signs

The disease occurs most commonly in two- to three-month-old foals, but animals as young as eight days or as old as six months may also be affected.[2, 5, 72, 76, 95, 111] The duration of the incubation period is unknown, but infection probably occurs several weeks before clinical signs are manifested.[72]

The clinical signs manifested by foals suffering from *R. equi* infection depend on the site of the lesions. As the lungs are the most frequent site, clinical signs of a respiratory nature are those most commonly encountered.

After the lungs, the most common site of lesion development is the intestine, particularly the caecum and colon, and its regional lymph nodes. Intestinal lesions may, however, develop secondarily to lung lesions, and vice versa. More widespread involvement of organs and tissues may also occur.

Some foals suffering from pneumonia, even with extensive pulmonary lesions, show no signs of illness,[12, 13, 61, 76, 99, 111] while others only appear listless, do not suckle properly and show evidence of spillage of milk on their foreheads.[85] Because lesions are generally far advanced by the time clinical signs are manifested, the mortality rate is high unless appropriate treatment is instituted for a prolonged period.

During the initial stages of lung involvement, auscultation of the thorax may reveal an increase in bronchial sounds, and affected animals may cough.[2, 13, 34, 37, 60, 76, 92] In foals in which the pulmonary lesions are somewhat more extensive, localized wheezes (which may emanate from small areas of the lungs, particularly their cranioventral regions) are evident on auscultation. Other signs in such animals include fever of 39 °C or higher, an increased respiratory rate of 40 or more per minute, signs of abdominal respiration, crackles, crepitant and moist râles, audible tracheal rattles, dyspnoea particularly on exertion, and slight lachrymation. Foals in which large pulmonary lesions are present reveal areas which are dull or silent on auscultation of their lungs. In some, a mucopurulent nasal discharge and cyanosis of visible mucous membranes may be manifested.[2, 3, 12, 13, 19, 34, 43, 60, 61, 76, 83, 99] Other signs which have been noted, but which are rare, include ataxia and depression ascribed to hepatic encephalopathy if liver lesions are present,[37] atrial fibrillation and cardiomegaly due to vegetative endocarditis, lameness due to mild to severe suppurative osteoarthritis of one or more joints, particularly the hock joint,[13, 19, 95] ulcerative lymphangitis of the skin with associated regional lymphadenitis, and abscesses in the pectoral region.[2, 91]

A diarrhoea (which may be intermittent), weight loss, unthriftiness, poor hair-coat, low-grade abdominal pain, lethargy, depression and inappetence are indicative of intestinal and/or visceral lymph node involvement.[3, 52] Although uncommon, a more severe, intractable, watery green and foul-smelling diarrhoea may develop after the onset of respiratory signs.[13, 84, 111]

Clinical signs in adult horses also relate to the organ or tissues involved. These include cachexia, coughing, anorexia, depression, lameness if arthritis is present, and very rarely, metritis and abortion in mares.[22, 38, 86, 111]

Pathology

Affected foals usually reveal a neutrophilia, raised fibrinogen levels, and metabolic acidosis.[3, 13, 19, 34, 37, 52, 61]

Most foals are in surprisingly good condition at the time of death.[2, 18, 55, 83, 111] In one survey it was determined that 96 per cent of 131 affected foals exhibited lesions in the lungs and/or intestines; of these 50 per cent were only in the lungs, 46 per cent were in both lungs and intestines, and 4 per cent occurred only in the intestines.[111] Pleuritis and pleural effusion are usually absent.[2, 12, 34, 59, 60, 83, 111]

The lungs are affected by varying degrees of a suppurative to caseous bronchopneumonia and are often oedematous. Multiple, sometimes confluent, caseonecrotic foci macroscopically resembling abscesses — a few millimetres in diameter in the more acute cases, and up to 100 mm in diameter in long-standing cases — are commonly found in the cranioventral portions of the lung lobes **(Figure 175.1)**. Single, variably encapsulated foci

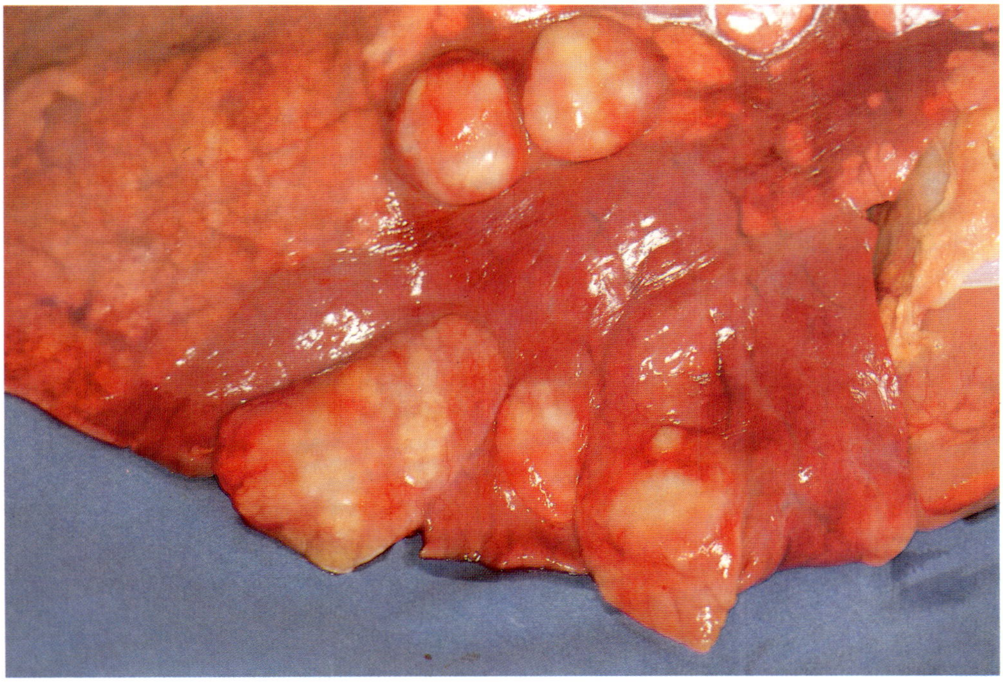

Figure 175.1 Multiple confluent caseonecrotic foci and accompanying atelectasis in the lungs of a foal that died of *Rhodococcus equi* infection

are present in the caudal lobes in some foals.[2, 29, 54, 61, 111] The content of these foci may be fluid, viscid and slimy, or inspissated,[34, 59, 60, 84, 92] and the exudate may vary in colour from dull, whitish-yellow or greyish-yellow to greyish-red or greenish.[2, 34, 59, 83] Areas of atelectasis are usually present in the lung parenchyma adjacent to these foci.[54] Blood-stained exudate may be found in the bronchi or bronchioles in foals in which caseonecrotic foci have ruptured.[12, 13, 59] Bronchiectasis may be present in some foals.[3] The tracheobronchial and mediastinal lymph nodes are usually enlarged and oedematous, with pyogranulomatous inflammation.[34, 43, 54] A chronic-active, non-suppurative synovitis due to the deposition of immune complexes in synovial membranes may be found in some pneumonic foals.[95]

When lesions occur in the intestinal tract, multiple ulcers of 2 to 20 mm in diameter are common in the caecum and colon **(Figures 175.2 and 175.3)**, but may also be present in the small intestine.[55] In some foals, the wall of the large intestine may be severely thickened due to oedema and extensive pyogranulomatous inflammation.[18, 55] The intestinal lesions are sometimes accompanied by pyogranulomatous inflammation of the mesenteric, caecal and colonic lymph nodes.[4, 12, 13, 18, 54, 55, 59, 74, 84, 111] Intestinal lesions may occur in the absence of lung lesions.[5, 111]

In adult horses, caseonecrotic foci in the lungs, mesenteric lymph nodes and subcutaneous tissues, and purulent arthritis and ulcerative enteritis have been reported.[22, 38, 86, 111] Small pyogranulomas in the mesenteric lymph nodes may be found incidentally in animals that have died of other causes.[60]

Lesions caused by *R. equi* infection but which are rarely encountered include gastritis; perforation of the intestine secondary to the enteric lesions, accompanied by extensive abdominal adhesions, ascites or purulent peritonitis;[3, 18, 52, 56, 83, 87] single, large abdominal abscesses[4, 111] which may involve the mesentery and cranial mesenteric vessels in association with lesions caused by strongyle larvae;[2] caseonecrotic foci in the liver, spleen or kidneys;[2, 29] orchitis and epididymitis; suppurative arthritis and/or osteomyelitis;[2, 84] pyogranulomatous lymphadenitis of visceral lymph nodes;[2, 36, 42, 111] hypopyon[2, 54, 59] and retrobulbar abscesses;[52] multiple renal cortical infarction;[55, 74, 83, 111] and disseminated intravascular coagulation.[54] Indolent ulcers in the skin of the legs or face, abscesses in peripheral lymph nodes, or swellings on the legs due to cellulitis have been associated with *R. equi* infection of the lesions caused by the percutaneous invasion of third-stage larvae of *Strongyloides westeri*.[25, 26, 33]

Histologically, the lesions in the lungs are characterized by the presence of pyogranulomatous and/or necrogranulomatous inflammation. Numerous macrophages, and smaller numbers of lymphocytes, plasma cells, neutrophils and binucleated and multinucleated giant cells are present in the affected areas. Many of the macrophages and giant cells contain abundant, intracytoplasmic, Gram-positive bacteria.[8, 18, 29, 46, 54, 61]

The intestinal lesions are characterized by necro- to pyogranulomatous inflammation and ulceration of the mucosa and submucosa, focal or diffuse necrosis of lymphoid tissues in the lamina propria and submucosa, necrosis of neutrophils, and the presence of numerous large, periodic acid-Schiff-positive macrophages engorged with intracytoplasmic, Gram-positive, pleomorphic bacteria. The inflammatory process may also involve the tunica muscularis and the serosa of the affected parts of the intestines.[4, 18, 38, 54, 55]

The inflammatory response in affected lymph nodes is similar to that in the lungs and intestines.[18, 38, 55] The subcapsular sinus, cortex and paracortex may contain numerous bacteria-laden macrophages, and some neutrophils and giant cells. In addition, medullary sinuses may show histiocytosis.[54, 55]

Rhodococcus equi has been isolated occasionally from suppurative lesions in many animal species besides horses, such as goats, sheep, cattle and pigs.[5] For example, in goats it has been isolated from pyogranulomatous lesions in the liver and lungs, osteomyelitis of the vertebrae and skull, and fibrinous enterocolitis;[14, 28, 67] in sheep, from the abomasum of an aborted foetus, brain of a neonate,[24] chronic, purulent bronchopneumonia and pleuritis, and caseous bronchial lymphadenitis;[1, 82] and in cattle, from chronic purulent pneumonia,[48] pyometra,[20] ulcerative lymphangitis of the legs and the accompanying regional lymphadenitis,[70] and the lesions in bronchial and mesenteric lymph nodes resembling mycobacterial tubercles.[66, 104] In pigs, *R. equi* is often isolated from submaxillary and cervical lymph nodes, in some of which pathological lesions are absent, while tuberculosis-like lesions are present in others.[5, 35, 65, 100] *Rhodococcus equi* and *Mycobacterium* spp. (mainly the avium type) can occur concurrently in tuberculous lymph nodes.[35]

Diagnosis

Because of the insidious nature of the disease, an early clinical diagnosis is often not possible. Radiographic evidence of consolidated foci in the lungs in foals is strongly suggestive of *R. equi* infection.[46] Most foals suffering from pneumonia reveal radiographic changes, such as increased interstitial and peribronchial densities and focal areas of dense consolidation (which may be nodular or cavitary) and enlarged tracheobronchial and mediastinal lymph nodes.[13, 34, 37, 61, 62, 92, 95]

To confirm the clinical diagnosis, transtracheal aspirates should be cultured for *R. equi*.[37, 46, 92] However, only about 60–70 per cent of cases which are positive radiographically or at necropsy yield *R. equi* from transtracheal aspirates.[47] Cytological examination of these aspirates may or may not reveal the presence of intracellular *R. equi* in macrophages.[21, 61, 95] Nasal swabs are unsatisfactory for diagnostic purposes.[2]

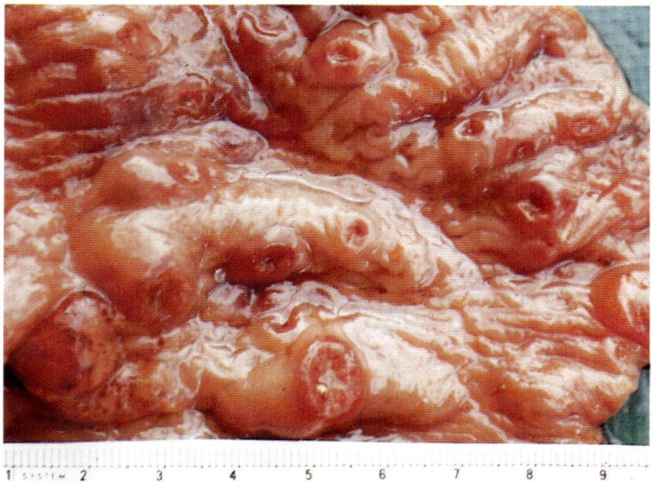

Figure 175.2 Multifocal ulcerative colitis in a foal that suffered from *Rhodococcus equi* infection

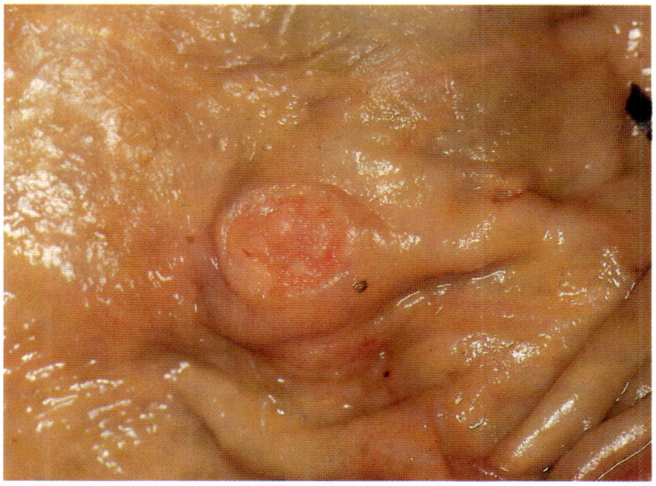

Figure 175.3 Closer view of a single ulcer in the colonic wall

Rhodococcus equi organisms are present in large numbers in the pus of lesions, intestinal contents and faeces of affected foals.[2, 3, 54, 60, 61, 111] About 20 per cent of foals suffering from *R. equi* infection may be concurrently infected with other bacteria (such as *Streptococcus* spp., *Staphylococcus* spp., *Escherichia coli*, *Klebsiella* spp., *Pasteurella* spp. and *Bordetella* spp.).[2, 19, 34, 59, 60, 92, 95, 111]

Several serological tests (including complement fixation, agglutination, ELISA, indirect haemagglutination, luminol-dependent chemiluminescence, agar-gel precipitation, and equi-factor neutralization) have been developed for the diagnosis of *R. equi* infection, but the results obtained are generally unsatisfactory and the tests are therefore not in general use.[11, 15, 27, 31, 45, 59, 62, 64, 69, 73, 76, 77, 88–90, 97] There is a variable correlation between the serum antibody level and severity of disease, and between antibody production and stage of disease.[102] Some foals with clinical disease fail to seroconvert, possibly because of interference by colostrum-derived antibody.[76, 88] Although of doubtful application, cell-mediated immunity may be measured by using a lymphocyte-blastogenesis test[30, 74, 79] and an intradermal test.[30, 99]

At necropsy, characteristic lesions are usually found in the lungs, intestine and/or elsewhere. The diagnosis should be confirmed by bacterial isolation.

Differential diagnosis

The lesions in the respiratory system of foals caused by *R. equi* should be differentiated from other infectious respiratory diseases of horses caused by agents such as equid herpesvirus 1 and 4, equine influenza virus, equine viral arteritis virus, *Streptococcus zooepidemicus* and *Streptococcus equi*, but other bacteria such as *Pasteurella* spp., *Bordetella bronchiseptica*, *E. coli*, *Actinobacillus* spp. and *Bacteroides* spp. may also rarely be involved.[6, 92, 94] Secondary invasion of the lungs by *R. equi* in young horses suffering from strangles results in high mortality.[84] *Rhodococcus equi* is an uncommon cause of pneumonic lesions in horses over 12 months of age.

Salmonella infection in young foals may result in pulmonary and intestinal lesions similar to those due to *R. equi*.

Diarrhoea due to *R. equi* enterotyphlocolitis should be differentiated from the typhlocolitis in salmonellosis and from that seen with round- or tapeworm infestation.

Ulcerative lymphangitis, which is rarely caused by *R. equi*, should be differentiated from that caused by organisms such as *Corynebacterium pseudotuberculosis* (*C. ovis*), *Histoplasma farciminosum*, *Sporothrix schenkii* and *Pseudomonas mallei*. Like *C. pseudotuberculosis*, *R. equi* can also be the cause of pectoral abscesses.[91]

Cachexia in adult horses may be due to internal parasitism, dental disease, chronic hepatic disease or chronic obstructive pulmonary disease.[38] Abscesses of internal organs in horses are rarely caused by *C. pseudotuberculosis*.[50]

Control

The control of *R. equi* infections in foals includes ensuring that mares foal in uninfected premises and that foals ingest adequate amounts of colostrum as soon after birth as possible, strict adherence to the environmental hygiene of foals (such as the prevention of the accumulation of manure, and the control of dust), early diagnosis, treatment and isolation of affected animals, and possibly the use of vaccines, although those which may be available are generally crude and of uncertain immunoprophylactic efficacy.[6, 34, 51, 59, 72, 92]

Despite massive pulmonary abscessation, resolution of the lesions and even a complete return to normal health can occur after intensive and prolonged treatment with lipid-soluble antibiotics which are capable of intracellular penetration.[13, 34, 46, 47, 80, 95] Early lesions in foals generally respond more favourably to treatment.[3, 80] Radiographic evidence of the presence of lung involvement is sufficient justification for the initiation of therapy.[46]

Although expensive, the combined oral administration of erythromycin estolate (or erythromycin ethylsuccinate) at 25 mg/kg body weight, three to four times daily, and rifampicin at 5 mg/kg, twice daily, is recommended. This regime should be maintained for at least four to nine weeks — preferably until two weeks after clinical signs have disappeared and chest radiographs and plasma fibrinogen levels have returned to normal.[37, 46, 47, 80, 95] By applying this regimen, the chance of a fatal outcome is reduced to a minimum.[47, 95] Periodic chest radiographs and determinations of plasma fibrinogen levels can be used to monitor the response to therapy.[46] Erythromycin can upset the normal intestinal flora and lead to a severe diarrhoea in horses. Intramuscular injection of erythromycin causes severe local irritation.

It is essential that the treatment should consist of both erythromycin and rifampicin because of their synergistic effect and to avoid the development of bacterial resistance to the drugs.[47, 80, 95] Parenteral fluid therapy should be avoided.[13, 84] Lack of response to aggressive long-term erythromycin-rifampicin treatment in foals suffering from bronchopneumonia may indicate that abdominal lesions are present. It reflects a poor prognosis.[3]

In addition to erythromycin and rifampicin, *R. equi* isolates are usually sensitive to gentamicin and neomycin, and to a lesser extent to sulphamethoxazole trimethoprim and tetracycline. The organism is, however, resistant to penicillin, cephalothin and ampicillin.[5, 34, 80, 95] In cases where *R. equi* infections are complicated by concurrent infections with other pathogens, appropriate additional therapy should be employed.[19, 94, 95]

The local therapy of distended joints as a result of what is thought to be an immune-mediated non-suppurative synovitis is usually not necessary, as the lesions regress when the pneumonia resolves.[95] If septic osteoarthritis or osteomyelitis is present, invasive treatment is recommended in addition to the above antibacterial regime.[19, 36]

At present, there are no commercially available vaccines. Oral immunization of foals with live *R. equi* attenuated to some degree by passage in artificial media has given promising results, but further research is required in order to produce immunogenic strains which do not survive in the environment.[16, 17, 97] Recent investigations into the possible role that passive immunotherapy may play hold promise for the future.[62]

Adequate managemental practices aimed at the elimination of predisposing factors, including other diseases of the equine neonate, may assist in reducing the prevalence of disease due to *R. equi* in foals.[2, 23, 34]

References

1 **ADDO, P.B. & DENNIS, S.M., 1977.** Corynebacteria associated with diseases of cattle, sheep and goats in northern Nigeria. *British Veterinary Journal*, 133, 334–339.

2 **BAIN, A.M., 1963.** *Corynebacterium equi* infections in the equine. *Australian Veterinary Journal*, 39, 116–121.

3 **BALDWIN, J.L., BERTONE, J.J., SOMMER, M.M., BAYHA, R., VAALA, W., COOPER, W.L., VANDERWALL, D.K. & SCHLAFER, D.H., 1992.** *Rhodococcus equi* enteritis, colonic lymphadenitis, and peritonitis in three foals with non-responsive *Rhodococcus equi* bronchopneumonia. *Equine Practice*, 14, 15–18.

4 **BARKER, I.K. & VAN DREUMEL, A.A., 1985.** The alimentary system. *In*: JUBB, K.V.F., KENNEDY, P.C. & PALMER, N., (eds). *Pathology of Domestic Animals*. Vol. II. 3rd edn. New York, London: Academic Press.

5 **BARTON, M.D. & HUGHES, K.L., 1980.** *Corynebacterium equi*: A review. *Veterinary Bulletin*, 50, 65–80.

6 **BLOOD, D.C. & RADOSTITS, O.M., 1989.** *Veterinary Medicine*. 7th edn. London, Philadelphia: Baillière Tindall.

7 **BOWLES, P.M., WOOLCOCK, J.B. & MUTIMER, M.D., 1987.** Experimental infection of mice with *Rhodococcus equi*: Differences in virulence between strains. *Veterinary Microbiology*, 14, 259–268.

8 **BOWLES, P.M., WOOLCOCK, J.B. & MUTIMER, M.D., 1989.** The effect of immunosuppression on resistance to *Rhodococcus equi* in mice. *Veterinary Immunology and Immunopathology*, 22, 369–378.

9 **BOWLES, P.M., WOOLCOCK, J.B. & MUTIMER, M.D., 1989.** Early events associated with experimental infection of the murine lung with *Rhodococcus equi*. *Journal of Comparative Pathology*, 101, 411–420.

10 **BRUMBAUGH, G.W., DAVIS, L.E., THURMON, J.C. & SAVAGE, D.C., 1990.** Influence of *Rhodococcus equi* on the respiratory burst of resident alveolar macrophages from adult horses. *American Journal of Veterinary Research*, 51, 766–771.

11 **BRUNER, D.W., DIMOCK, W.W. & EDWARDS, P.R., 1939.** The serological classification of *Corynebacterium equi*. *Journal of Infectious Diseases*, 65, 92–96.

12 **BULL, L.B., 1924.** Corynebacterial pyaemia of foals. *Journal of Comparative Pathology*, 37, 294–298.

13 **BURROWS, G.E., 1968.** *Corynebacterium equi* infection in two foals. *Journal of the American Veterinary Medical Association*, 152, 1119–1124.

14 **CARRIGAN, M.J., LINKS, I.J. & MORTON, A.G., 1988.** *Rhodococcus equi* infection in goats. *Australian Veterinary Journal*, 65, 331–332.

15 **CARTER, G.R. & HYLTON, G.A., 1974.** An indirect hemagglutination test for antibodies to *Corynebacterium equi*. *American Journal of Veterinary Research*, 35, 1393–1395.

16 **CHIRINO-TREJO, J.M. & PRESCOTT, J.F., 1987.** Antibody response of horses to *Rhodococcus equi* antigens. *Canadian Journal of Veterinary Research*, 51, 301–305.

17 **CHIRINO-TREJO, J.M., PRESCOTT, J.F. & YAGER, J.A., 1987.** Protection of foals against experimental *Rhodococcus equi* pneumonia by oral immunization. *Canadian Journal of Veterinary Research*, 51, 444–447.

18 **CIMPRICH, R.E. & ROONEY, J.R., 1977.** *Corynebacterium equi* enteritis in foals. *Veterinary Pathology*, 14, 95–102.

19 **COLLATOS, C., CLARK, S., REEF, V.B. & MORRIS, D.D., 1990.** Septicemia, atrial fibrillation, cardiomegaly, left atrial mass, and *Rhodococcus equi* septic osteoarthritis in a foal.

Journal of the American Veterinary Medical Association, 197, 1039–1042.

20 **CRAIG, J.F. & DAVIES, G.O., 1940.** *Corynebacterium equi* in bovine pyometra. *Veterinary Journal*, 96, 417–419.

21 **CRANE, S.A., ZIEMER, E.L. & SWEENEY, C.R., 1989.** Cytologic and bacteriologic evaluation of tracheobronchial aspirates from clinically normal foals. *American Journal of Veterinary Research*, 50, 2042–2048.

22 **DAFAALA, E.N., IRFAN, M. & IMBABI, S., 1960.** Isolation of an organism resembling *Corynebacterium equi* associated with bronchopneumonia in an adult horse. *Sudan Journal of Veterinary Science and Animal Husbandry*, 1, 26–30.

23 **DEBEY, M.C. & BAILIE, W.E., 1987.** *Rhodococcus equi* in fecal and environmental samples from Kansas horse farms. *Veterinary Microbiology*, 14, 251–257.

24 **DENNIS, S.M. & BAMFORD, V.W., 1966.** The role of Corynebacteria in perinatal lamb mortality. *The Veterinary Record*, 79, 105–108.

25 **DEWES, H.F., 1972.** *Strongyloides westeri* and *Corynebacterium equi* in foals. *New Zealand Veterinary Journal*, 20, 82.

26 **DEWES, H.F., 1989.** The association between weather, frenzied behaviour, percutaneous invasion by *Strongyloides westeri* larvae and *Rhodococcus equi* disease in foals. *New Zealand Veterinary Journal*, 37, 69–73.

27 **DIMOCK, W.W. & EDWARDS, P.R., 1931.** *Corynebacterium equi* in pneumonia in foals. *Journal of the American Veterinary Medical Association*, 79, 809–812.

28 **DITEKO, T., WINNEN, G.M. & MANTHE, L.M., 1988.** Isolations of *Rhodococcus (Corynebacterium) equi* from goats in Botswana. *Zimbabwe Veterinary Journal*, 19, 11–15.

29 **DUNGWORTH, D.L., 1985.** The respiratory system. *In*: JUBB, K.V.F., KENNEDY, P.C. & PALMER, N., (eds). *Pathology of Domestic Animals*. Vol. II. 3rd edn. New York, London: Academic Press.

30 **ELLENBERGER, M.A., KAEBERLE, M.L. & ROTH, J.A., 1984.** Equine cell-mediated immune response to *Rhodococcus (Corynebacterium) equi*. *American Journal of Veterinary Research*, 45, 2424–2427.

31 **ELLENBERGER, M.A., KAEBERLE, M.L. & ROTH, J.A., 1984.** Equine humoral immune response to *Rhodococcus (Corynebacterium) equi*. *American Journal of Veterinary Research*, 45, 2428–2430.

32 **ELLISSALDE, G.S., RENSHAW, H.W. & WALBERG, J.A., 1980.** *Corynebacterium equi*: An interhost review with emphasis on the foal. *Comparative Immunology, Microbiology and Infectious Diseases*, 3, 433–445.

33 **ETHERINGTON, W.G. & PRESCOTT, J.F., 1980.** *Corynebacterium equi* cellulitis associated with *Strongyloides* penetration in a foal. *Journal of the American Veterinary Medical Association*, 177, 1025–1027.

34 **FALCON, J., SMITH, B.P., O'BRIEN, T.R., CARLSON, G.P. & BIBERSTEIN, E., 1985.** Clinical and radiographic findings in *Corynebacterium equi* pneumonia of foals. *Journal of the American Veterinary Medical Association*, 186, 593–599.

35 **FELDMAN, W.H., MOSES, H.E. & KARLSON, A.G., 1940.** *Corynebacterium equi* as a possible cause of tuberculous-like lesions of swine. *Cornell Veterinarian*, 30, 465–481.

36 **FIRTH, E.C., 1983.** Current concepts of infectious polyarthritis in foals. *Equine Veterinary Journal*, 15, 5–9.

37 **FREESTONE, J.F., SHOEMAKER, S. & McCLURE, J.J., 1989.** Pulmonary abscessation, hepatoencephalopathy and IgM deficiency associated with *Rhodococcus equi* in a foal. *Australian Veterinary Journal*, 66, 343–344.

38 **GENETZKY, R.M., BETTCHER, M.P., ARP, L.H. & WHITE, P.L., 1982.** *Corynebacterium equi* infection in a mare. *Modern Veterinary Practice*, 63, 876–879.

39 **GOODFELLOW, M., 1986.** Genus *Rhodococcus*. *In*: SNEATH, P.H.A., MAIR, N.S., SHARPE, M.E. & HOLT, J.G., (eds). *Bergey's Manual of Systematic Bacteriology*. Vol. II. Baltimore, London: Williams & Wilkins.

40 **GOODFELLOW, M., 1987.** The taxonomic status of *Rhodococcus equi*. *Veterinary Microbiology*, 14, 205–209.

41 **GOODFELLOW, M., COLLINS, M.D. & MINNIKIN, D.E., 1976.** Thin-layer chromatographic analysis of mycolic acid and other long-chain components of whole-organism methanolysates of Coryneform and related taxa. *Journal of General Microbiology*, 96, 351–358.

42 **GORHAM, S. & HAALAND, M.A., 1986.** The effects of a disseminated *Corynebacterium equi* infection on a neonatal foal. *Veterinary Medicine*, 81, 552–554.

43 **GROSSKOPF, J.F.W., TUSTIN, R.C. & MUIR, R.W., 1957.** Purulent pneumonia in foals caused by *Corynebacterium equi* (Magnusson). *Journal of the South African Veterinary Medical Association*, 28, 9–11.

44 **HIETALA, S.K. & ARDANS, A.A., 1987.** Interaction of *Rhodococcus equi* with phagocytic cells from *R. equi*-exposed and non-exposed foals. *Veterinary Microbiology*, 14, 307–320.

45 **HIETALA, S.K., ARDANS, A.A. & SANSOME, A., 1985.** Detection of *Corynebacterium equi*-specific antibody in horses by enzyme-linked immunosorbent assay. *American Journal of Veterinary Research*, 46, 13–15.

46 **HILLIDGE, C.J., 1986.** Review of *Corynebacterium (Rhodococcus) equi* lung abscesses in foals: Pathogenesis, diagnosis and treatment. *The Veterinary Record*, 119, 261–264.

47 **HILLIDGE, C.J., 1987.** Use of erythromycin-rifampin combination in treatment of *Rhodococcus equi* pneumonia. *Veterinary Microbiology*, 14, 337–342.

48 **HOLTMAN, D.F., 1945.** *Corynebacterium equi* in chronic pneumonia of the calf. *Journal of Bacteriology*, 49, 159–162.

49 HONDALUS, M.K., SWEENEY, C.R. & MOSSER, D.M., **1992.** An assay to quantitate the binding of *Rhodococcus equi* to macrophages. *Veterinary Immunology and Immunopathology*, 32, 339–350.

50 **HUGHES, J.P., BIBERSTEIN, E.L. & RICHARDS, W.P.C., 1962.** Two cases of generalized *Corynebacterium pseudotuberculosis* infection in mares. *Cornell Veterinarian*, 52, 51–62.

51 **HUGHES, K.L. & SULAIMAN, I., 1987.** The ecology of *Rhodococcus equi* and physicochemical influences on growth. *Veterinary Microbiology*, 14, 241–250.

52 **HUTCHINS, D.R., BROWNLOW, M.A. & JOHNSTON, K.G., 1980.** *Corynebacterium equi* infections in foals — concepts and observations. *Australian Veterinary Practitioner*, 10, 248–252.

53 **ISHINO, S., NAKAZAWA, M. & MATSUDA, I., 1987.** Pathological findings of guinea-pigs infected intratracheally with *Rhodococcus (Corynebacterium) equi*. *Japanese Journal of Veterinary Science*, 49, 395–402.

54 **JOHNSON, J.A., PRESCOTT, J.F. & MARKHAM, R.J.F., 1983.** The pathology of experimental *Corynebacterium equi* infection in foals following intrabronchial challenge. *Veterinary Pathology*, 20, 440–449.

55 **JOHNSON, J.A., PRESCOTT, J.F. & MARKHAM, R.J.F., 1983.** The pathology of experimental *Corynebacterium equi* infection in foals following intragastric challenge. *Veterinary Pathology*, 20, 450–459.

56 **JULIAN, R.J., 1985.** The peritoneum, retroperitoneum and mesentery. *In*: JUBB, K.V.F., KENNEDY, P.C. & PALMER, N., (eds). *Pathology of Domestic Animals*. Vol. II. 3rd edn. New York, London: Academic Press.

57 **KNIGHT, H.D., 1969.** Corynebacterial infections in the horse: Problems of prevention. *Journal of the American Veterinary Medical Association*, 155, 446–452.

58 **MACHANG'U, R.S. & PRESCOTT, J.F., 1991.** Purification and properties of cholesterol oxidase and choline phosphohydrolase from *Rhodococcus equi*. *Canadian Journal of Veterinary Research*, 55, 332–340.

59 **MAGNUSSON, H., 1938.** Pyaemia in foals caused by *Corynebacterium equi*. *The Veterinary Record*, 50, 1459–1468.

60 **MAHAFFEY, L.O., 1962.** Respiratory conditions in horses. *The Veterinary Record*, 74, 1295–1314.

61 **MARTENS, R.J., FISKE, R.A. & RENSHAW, H.W., 1982.** Experimental subacute foal pneumonia induced by aerosol

administration of *Corynebacterium equi*. *Equine Veterinary Journal*, 14, 111–116.

62 **MARTENS, R.J., MARTENS, J.G., FISKE, R.A. & HIETALA, S.K., 1989.** *Rhodococcus equi* foal pneumonia: Protective effects of immune plasma in experimentally infected foals. *Equine Veterinary Journal*, 21, 249–255.

63 **MARTENS, R.J., MARTENS, J.G. & RENSHAW, H.W., 1988.** *Rhodococcus (Corynebacterium) equi*: Bactericidal capacity of neutrophils from neonatal and adult horses. *American Journal of Veterinary Research*, 49, 295–299.

64 **MARTENS, R.J., MARTENS, J.G., RENSHAW, H.W. & HIETALA, S.K., 1987.** *Rhodococcus equi*: Equine neutrophil chemiluminescent and bactericidal response to opsonizing antibody. *Veterinary Microbiology*, 14, 277–286.

65 **McDONALD, I.W., 1942.** A note on the occurrence in Australia of *Corynebacterium equi* in pigs. *Australian Journal of Experimental Biology and Medical Science*, 20, 27–29.

66 **McKENZIE, R.A. & DONALD, B.A., 1979.** Lymphadenitis in cattle associated with *Corynebacterium equi*: A problem in bovine tuberculosis diagnosis. *Journal of Comparative Pathology*, 89, 31–38.

67 **MORAAL, S.A., SCHEEPENS-VAN LIPZIG, F.M. & JAARTSVELD, F.H.J., 1990.** *Rhodococcus equi*-infectie bij een geit. *Tijdschrift voor Diergeneeskunde*, 115, 27–29.

68 **MUTIMER, M.D., PRESCOTT, J.F. & WOOLCOCK, J.B., 1982.** Capsular serotypes of *Rhodococcus equi*. *Australian Veterinary Journal*, 58, 67–69.

69 **NAKAZAWA, M., 1980.** Detection of colt serum antibody against *Corynebacterium equi* by agar-gel diffusion. *Japanese Journal of Veterinary Science*, 42, 551–555.

70 **NEAVE, R.M.S., 1951.** An outbreak of ulcerative lymphangitis in young heifers in Kenya. *The Veterinary Record*, 63, 185.

71 **PRESCOTT, J.F., 1981.** Capsular serotypes of *Corynebacterium equi*. *Canadian Journal of Comparative Medicine*, 45, 130–134.

72 **PRESCOTT, J.F., 1987.** Epidemiology of *Rhodococcus equi* infection in horses. *Veterinary Microbiology*, 14, 211–214.

73 **PRESCOTT, J.F., COSHAN-GAUTHIER, R. & BARKSDALE, L., 1984.** Antibody to equi factor(s) in the diagnosis of *Corynebacterium equi* pneumonia of foals. *Canadian Journal of Comparative Medicine*, 48, 370–373.

74 **PRESCOTT, J.F., JOHNSON, J.A. & MARKHAM, R.J.F., 1980.** Experimental studies on the pathogenesis of *Corynebacterium equi* infection in foals. *Canadian Journal of Comparative Medicine*, 44, 280–288.

75 **PRESCOTT, J.F., LASTRA, M. & BARKSDALE, L., 1982.** Equi factors in the identification of *Corynebacterium equi* Magnusson. *Journal of Clinical Microbiology*, 16, 988–990.

76 **PRESCOTT, J.F., MACHANG'U, R., KWIECIEN, J. & DELANEY, K., 1989.** Prevention of foal mortality due to *Rhodococcus equi* pneumonia on an endemically affected farm. *Canadian Veterinary Journal*, 30, 871–875.

77 **PRESCOTT, J.F., MARKHAM, R.J.F. & JOHNSON, J.A., 1979.** Cellular and humoral immune response of foals to vaccination with *Corynebacterium equi*. *Canadian Journal of Comparative Medicine*, 43, 356–364.

78 **PRESCOTT, J.F. & MUCKLE, C.A., 1986.** *Corynebacterium*. *In*: GYLES, C.L. & THOEN, C.O., (eds). *Pathogenesis of Bacterial Infections in Animals*. Ames, Iowa: Iowa State University Press.

79 **PRESCOTT, J.F., OGILVIE, T.H. & MARKHAM, R.J.F., 1980.** Lymphocyte immunostimulation in the diagnosis of *Corynebacterium equi* pneumonia of foals. *American Journal of Veterinary Research*, 41, 2073–2075.

80 **PRESCOTT, J.F. & SWEENEY, C.R., 1985.** Treatment of *Corynebacterium equi* pneumonia in foals: A review. *Journal of the American Veterinary Medical Association*, 187, 725–728.

81 **PRESCOTT, J.F., TRAVERS, M. & YAGER-JOHNSON, J.A., 1984.** Epidemiological survey of *Corynebacterium equi* infections on five Ontario horse farms. *Canadian Journal of Comparative Medicine*, 48, 10–13.

82 **ROBERTS, D.S., 1957.** *Corynebacterium equi* infection in a sheep. *Australian Veterinary Journal*, 33, 21.

83 **ROBERTS, M.C. & POLLEY, L.R., 1977.** *Corynebacterium equi* infection in a thoroughbred foal. *Equine Veterinary Journal*, 9, 159–160.

84 **ROONEY, J.R., 1966.** Corynebacterial infections in foals. *Modern Veterinary Practice*, 47, 43–45.

85 **ROUS, R.C., 1991.** Karoo Veterinary Hospital, Colesberg, Cape Province. Unpublished data.

86 **SIMPSON, R.M., 1964.** *Corynebacterium equi* in adult horses in Kenya. *Bulletin of Epizootic Diseases of Africa*, 12, 303–306.

87 **SIPPEL, W.L., KEAHEY, E.E. & BULLARD, T.L., 1968.** *Corynebacterium* infection in foals: Etiology, pathogenesis, and laboratory diagnosis. *Journal of the American Veterinary Medical Association*, 153, 1610–1613.

88 **SKALKA, B., 1987.** Dynamics of equi-factor antibodies in sera of foals kept on farms with differing histories of *Rhodococcus equi* pneumonia. *Veterinary Microbiology*, 14, 269–276.

89 **SKALKA, B. & SVASTOVA, A., 1984/85.** Two techniques for detection of antibodies against *Corynebacterium (Rhodococcus) equi* in horse sera. *Veterinary Microbiology*, 10, 293–300.

90 **SKALKA, B. & SVASTOVA, A., 1985.** Serodiagnostics of *Corynebacterium (Rhodococcus) equi*. *Zentralblatt für Veterinärmedizin*, Reihe B, 32, 137–142.

91 **SMITH, B.P. & JANG, S., 1980.** Isolation of *Corynebacterium equi* from a foal with an ulcerated leg wound and a pectoral abscess. *Journal of the American Veterinary Medical Association*, 177, 623–624.

92 **SMITH, B.P. & ROBINSON, R.C., 1981.** Studies of an outbreak of *Corynebacterium equi* pneumonia in foals. *Equine Veterinary Journal*, 13, 223–228.

93 **STUDDERT, M.J., 1978.** Primary, severe, combined immunodeficiency disease of Arabian foals. *Australian Veterinary Journal*, 54, 411–417.

94 **SWEENEY, C.R., HOLCOMBE, S.J., BARNINGHAM, S.C. & BEECH, J., 1991.** Aerobic and anaerobic bacterial isolates from horses with pneumonia or pleuropneumonia and antimicrobial susceptibility patterns of the aerobes. *Journal of the American Veterinary Medical Association*, 198, 839–842.

95 **SWEENEY, C.R., SWEENEY, R.W. & DIVERS, T.J., 1987.** *Rhodococcus equi* pneumonia in 48 foals: Response to antimicrobial therapy. *Veterinary Microbiology*, 14, 329–336.

96 **TAKAI, S., FUJIMORI, T., KATSUZAKI, K., TSUBAKI, S., 1987.** Ecology of *Rhodococcus equi* in horses and their environment on horse-breeding farms. *Veterinary Microbiology*, 14, 233–239.

97 **TAKAI, S., KAWAZU, S. & TSUBAKI, S., 1987.** Humoral immune response of foals to experimental infection with *Rhodococcus equi*. *Veterinary Microbiology*, 14, 321–327.

98 **TIMONEY, J.F., GILLESPIE, J.H., SCOTT, F.W. & BARLOUGH, J.E., 1988.** *Hagan and Bruner's Microbiology and Infectious Diseases of Domestic Animals*. 8th edn. Ithaca and London: Comstock Publishing Associates.

99 **WILSON, M.M., 1955.** A study of *Corynebacterium equi* infection in a stud of thoroughbred horses in Victoria. *Australian Veterinary Journal*, 31, 175–181.

100 **WOODROOFE, G.M., 1950.** Studies on strains of *Corynebacterium equi* isolated from pigs. *Australian Journal of Experimental Biology and Medical Science*, 28, 399–409.

101 **WOOLCOCK, J.B., FARMER, A-M.T. & MUTIMER, M.D., 1979.** Selective medium for *Corynebacterium equi* isolation. *Journal of Clinical Microbiology*, 9, 640–642.

102 **WOOLCOCK, J.B., MUTIMER, M.D. & BOWLES, P.M., 1987.** The immunological response of foals to *Rhodococcus equi*: A review. *Veterinary Microbiology*, 14, 215–224.

103 **WOOLCOCK, J.B., MUTIMER, M.D. & FARMER, A-M.T., 1980.** Epidemiology of *Corynebacterium equi* in horses. *Research in Veterinary Science*, 28, 87–90.

104 **WOOLCOCK, J.B. & RUDDUCK, H.B., 1973.** *Corynebacterium equi* in cattle. *Australian Veterinary Journal*, 49, 319.

105 **YAGER, J.A., 1987.** The pathogenesis of *Rhodococcus equi* pneumonia in foals. *Veterinary Microbiology*, 14, 225–232.

106 **YAGER, J.A., DUDER, C.K., PRESCOTT, J.F. & ZINK, M.C., 1987.** The interaction of *Rhodococcus equi* and foal neutrophils *in vitro*. *Veterinary Microbiology*, 14, 287–294.

107 **YAGER, J.A., PRESCOTT, C.A., KRAMAR, D.P., HANNAH, H., BALSON, G.A. & CROY, B.A., 1991.** The effect of experimental infection with *Rhodococcus equi* on immunodeficient mice. *Veterinary Microbiology*, 28, 363–376.

108 **ZINK, M.C. & JOHNSON, J.A., 1984.** Cellular constituents of normal foal bronchoalveolar lavage fluid during postnatal maturation. *American Journal of Veterinary Research*, 45, 893–897.

109 **ZINK, M.C., YAGER, J.A., PRESCOTT, J.F. & FERNANDO, M.A., 1987.** Electron microscopic investigation of intracellular events after ingestion of *Rhodococcus equi* by foal alveolar macrophages. *Veterinary Microbiology*, 14, 295–305.

110 **ZINK, M.C., YAGER, J.A., PRESCOTT, J.F. & WILKIE, B.N., 1985.** *In vitro* phagocytosis and killing of *Corynebacterium equi* by foal alveolar macrophages during postnatal maturation. *American Journal of Veterinary Research*, 46, 2171–2174.

111 **ZINK, M.C., YAGER, J.A. & SMART, N.L., 1986.** *Corynebacterium equi* infections in horses, 1958–84: A review of 131 cases. *Canadian Veterinary Journal*, 27, 213–217.

176

Dermatophilosis

Synonyms: *Dermatophilus congolensis* infection, Senkobo disease, lumpy wool, strawberry footrot, cutaneous streptothricosis, klontwol (Afrik.)

E.M. van Tonder and R.F. Horner

Introduction

Dermatophilosis, caused by *Dermatophilus congolensis*, is an exudative to proliferative dermatitis followed by scab formation which affects domestic, laboratory and wild animals, and humans. It occurs throughout the world, but is more prevalent in the tropics.

In cattle, the condition is commonly called Senkobo disease or cutaneous streptothricosis, while in sheep it is often referred to as lumpy wool or, colloquially, 'klontwol'.[13] The name dermatophilosis[106] has been proposed to accommodate the various clinical syndromes associated with *D. congolensis* infection.

The disease in cattle was first described in 1915 by Van Sacegham in Zaire.[126] Lumpy wool was reported for the first time in South Africa by Bekker in 1927,[13] and on numerous occasions after that.[35, 37, 51, 55, 64, 103, 114, 118, 123, 127] It has also been reported in countries elsewhere in the world.[8, 16, 19, 21, 24, 25, 33, 102, 113] Earlier reports suggested that lumpy wool occurred sporadically and was confined to the eastern parts and high summer rainfall areas of South Africa. However, it is now recognized that the disease in sheep occurs over a wide area,[55, 124, 127] the expanded prevalence possibly being related to compulsory dipping campaigns for the control of sheep scab. The disease is uncommon in cattle and horses in South Africa.[36, 124] However, in other parts of southern Africa, such as in the Senanga, Mumbwa, Monze and Zambezi districts in Zambia, a herd prevalence rate of about 78 per cent for dermatophilosis has been reported.[104]

Economic losses resulting from damage to the fleece and hides can be high.[19, 20, 21, 24, 33, 43, 105, 118, 128] Losses are also caused by a decreased body weight and production, and in severe cases, mortalities.[105] In Australia the most important economic effect is as a consequence of secondary blowfly strike in the lesions in sheep.[23] Most affected cows show reduced milk production and cannot rear their calves properly.[105] Oxen suffering from the disease lose their draught power as a result of debilitation and/or lesions on the neck areas just in front of the hump which bear the yoke during draught work.[105]

Aetiology and life cycle

Dermatophilus congolensis is a pleomorphic bacterium belonging to the order Actinomycetales and the family Dermatophilaceae.[11, 26] The organism is Gram-positive and non-acid-fast and stains well with ordinary aniline dyes.[16, 26, 27, 67, 84, 114, 121]

Various morphological forms of *D. congolensis*, representing different stages in the life cycle, have been recognized in lesions and cultures.[2–4, 16, 26, 27, 43, 83, 88, 96] The bacterium grows as a branching filamentous mycelium. During the growth stage, the filaments become transversely **(Figure 176.1)** and longitudinally septate **(Figure 176.2)** to form parallel rows of small, coccoid zoospores which are dormant and can survive in the dried crusts of lesions for several months. Under favourable conditions of moisture and temperature the zoospores are polar flagellated, which makes them highly motile and thus able to infect new locations on the same or other susceptible animals. Zoospores are found mainly in dried exudates or scabs, while filaments occur mostly in the active parts of the lesions.[16, 50, 67, 84–92, 96, 99, 101, 121]

Dermatophilus congolensis is aerobic or facultatively anaerobic.[26, 67, 114, 122] It grows readily at temperatures ranging from 20–37 °C.[16, 26, 64, 86, 114] The organism can be cultured on ordinary peptone nutrient media, but growth is greatly enhanced when it is enriched with defibrinated blood or serum.[16, 26, 64, 84, 86, 121]

Epidemiology

Dermatophilus congolensis affects various domestic, wild and laboratory animals, as well as humans.[16, 28, 46, 64, 95, 97, 121] Lambs aged three to nine months are particularly susceptible to the disease.[92] Cattle are less frequently affected, while dermatophilosis occurs only rarely in horses, donkeys,[28, 36, 45, 52] goats,[43, 112] and pigs.[43]

Infection of sheep with *D. congolensis* can be effected by intradermal inoculation or by application of either culture or infected-scab suspensions to the surface of the skin with or without wetting, depilation, scarification or removal of the sebaceous overlay.[16, 18, 39, 50, 64, 84, 92, 118, 121] Infection spreads readily between infected and

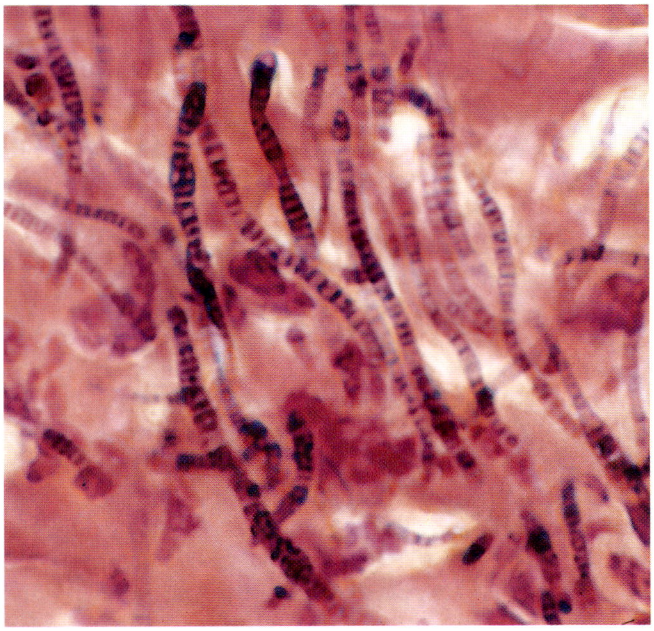

Figures 176.1 Filamentous mycelial-like growth of *Dermatophilus congolensis* showing transverse septation

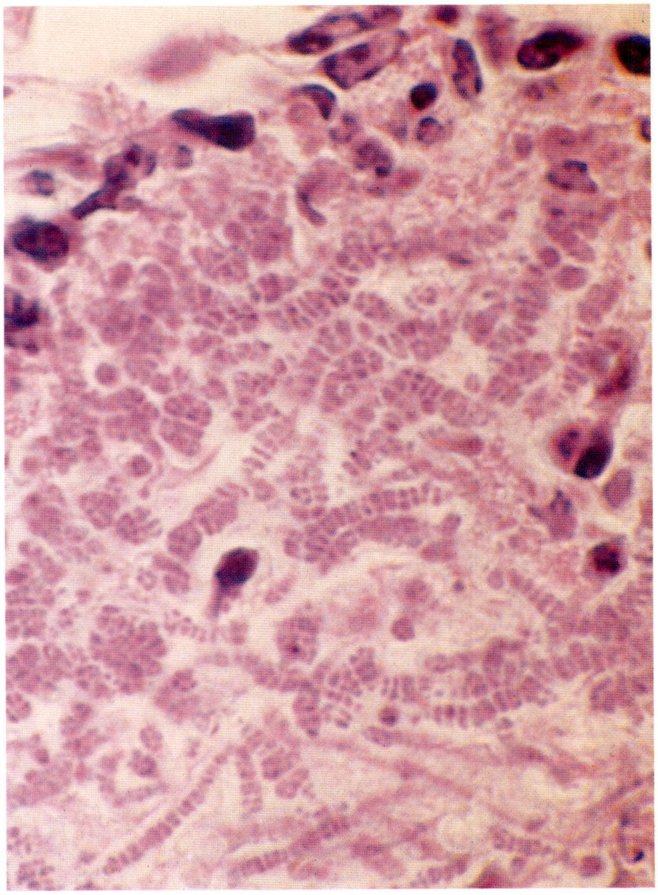

Figures 176.2 Transverse and longitudinal septation of filaments of *Dermatophilus congolensis*

susceptible sheep, particularly when both affected and unaffected animals are wet.[50]

The zoospores may be transferred mechanically from one animal to another through contact with plants or insects harbouring the organism. The wetted skin and fleece, and particularly the wetted crusts of lesions, are attractive to flies, which promote the transmission of infection.[82, 99, 101] Experimental transmission of *D. congolensis* infection in cattle has been achieved by *Stomoxys calcitrans* and *Musca domestica*.[75, 82] Dermatophilosis in sheep may be followed by flystrike, particularly during the acute stage.[23, 24, 25, 119]

In animals, the epidermis is protected against infection by three barriers, namely, the hair coat or fleece, the sebum which impregnates the hair or wool and forms a layer on the skin, and the *stratum corneum*.[92, 96, 99] The degree of development of each barrier, and hence the protection it provides, varies greatly between animals and at different sites on the body. In sheep the thickness of the *stratum corneum* is inversely proportional to the density of the hair coat, and the thickness and completeness of the sebaceous film on the skin are directly related to the density of hair or wool-fibre population because of the association of sebaceous glands with hair or wool follicles. Resistance of the non-woolled areas to infection therefore depends mainly on the integrity of the *stratum corneum*; while the woolled areas of the skin, which have a very thin *stratum corneum*, are protected mainly by the greasy fleece and the sebaceous film on the skin surface.[92] This sebaceous film on the woolled skin is fully protective in adult Merino sheep but not in young lambs or in coarser-woolled sheep, in which the film may be incomplete.[92, 96, 99] The protectiveness of the sebaceous film apparently depends entirely on the mechanical properties of the sebum.[92]

Prolonged wetting of the skin causes emulsification and disruption of the sebaceous film and maceration of the *stratum corneum*, rendering the skin susceptible to infection by *D. congolensis*.[92, 101]

The zoospores are found mostly in the scabs and dried exudate of the lesions,[16, 84, 86, 88–90, 92, 96] from which, if thorough wetting occurs, they are released in large numbers. As virtually no viable zoospores are detectable at the surface of scabs and exudate before they have been soaked, affected animals are probably not an important source of infection unless their lesions are wet.[34, 89] The number of viable zoospores in scabs decreases rapidly as scabs dry out, but small numbers may survive in them for several months.[88, 89, 99, 109]

Chronically affected sheep and lambs, marked by small long-standing lesions of the hairy-skin parts of the body, particularly the ears, provide a means of survival for *D. congolensis* in interepidemic periods.[12, 33, 81, 87, 101, 120] Soil is unlikely to be an important source of *D. congolensis*.[99]

Outbreaks of dermatophilosis in sheep are often associated with wet weather conditions,[8, 13, 19, 33, 39, 64, 86, 87, 92, 99, 118] dipping,[13, 19, 49, 50, 55, 92, 99, 127, 128] shearing,[90, 92, 99] skin penetration sites of grass seeds or spines of plants[13, 92, 99] and ear-punching and insect bite sites.

Outbreaks of the disease may occur in both summer and winter.[13, 33, 64, 99, 118] Under natural conditions, rain, misty weather and dew are important in the release of zoospores.[8, 13, 16, 19, 33, 39, 64, 99, 118, 128] Continuous wetting of the feet, the face and parts of the fleece in young lambs from grazing wet pastures plays a contributory role in outbreaks of dermatophilosis.[8] The disease has also been reported in lambs a few days after birth, possibly as a result of the wetness of the skin caused by foetal fluids,[110] and around the mouth from suckling.[103]

The association of dipping with outbreaks of dermatophilosis in sheep has generally been attributed not only to the wetting of the skin and the subsequent release of the zoospores, but also to the detrimental effect of the dip on the integrity of the sebaceous film of the skin. Dipping fluids which may be contaminated with *D. congolensis* might also be an important mechanism of infection.[9, 49, 50]

In addition to its role in the activation and release of zoospores, water or dipping fluids may also transport zoospores from existing lesions to non-infected areas on the same animal.[49, 56, 99] That this happens is borne out by the development of acute lesions under chronic ones, and in confluent lines or channels down the sides of infected sheep exposed to prolonged heavy rain.[99]

Mechanical disruption of the protective barriers of the skin is caused by shearing of sheep. It not only removes the protective fleece, but also frequently causes abrasions and wounds of the skin surface.[72, 81, 92, 98, 101]

Dermatophilosis in cattle occurs in all age groups[22, 71, 76, 78, 106, 108, 111, 115] and is often associated with moist climatic factors,[54, 56, 104] poor nutritional status and tick infestations, mainly of *Amblyomma variegatum*; the lesions are found particularly in areas of the body most heavily infested with ticks.[57, 58, 63, 69, 78, 125] Lesions in cattle have also been associated with the feeding sites of *Glossina* spp.,[58] *Haematopota* spp., *Stomoxys* spp.[43, 75] and *Tabanus* spp.,[117] and with areas infested by the sucking louse, *Haematopinus eurysternus*.[58] In draught oxen, lesions are often found on the areas of the neck which bear the yoke.[104]

Dermatophilus congolensis infection has been associated with rinderpest,[39] lumpy skin disease, besnoitiosis and trypanosomiasis[108, 116] in cattle and with contagious pustular dermatitis (orf) in sheep.[12] Severe lesions similar to those observed in field cases of strawberry footrot have been induced in lambs infected with the orf virus and *D. congolensis* together, but not with either organism alone.[6]

Pathogenesis

Following infection, the zoospores reach susceptible sites of the skin by their own motility[85, 86, 88] and a positive chemotactic response to carbon dioxide which diffuses through the skin.[88, 90]

In contrast to the dermatophytes, which are parasites of the *stratum corneum*, the branching filaments of *D. congolensis* invade the living cell layers of the epidermis and the sheaths of the hair or wool follicles, where extensive proliferation of the organism occurs; it does not invade the dermis or the hair or wool fibres.[95–97] The filamentous organisms cause increased keratinization of the epidermis and an acute inflammation characterized by the accumulation of an exudate rich in neutrophils beneath the invaded part of the epidermis; the exudate separates the infected from the non-infected epidermis.[43] The organisms do not penetrate the layer of exudate, which apparently acts as a barrier to invasion of the uninfected layers of the epidermis. The new epidermis that forms underneath the exudate is invaded from the side, usually by filamentous organisms from adjacent follicle sheaths.[95] The infected epidermis is then again separated from the uninfected epidermis by a layer of exudate, and so the process continues in cycles until a thick, laminated crust is formed, composed of alternating layers of para- and orthokeratotic hyperkeratosis and exudate.[43, 95] The new layers of epidermis are formed mainly as outgrowths from the sheaths of the follicles, and are also infected by bacterial filaments originating from these sites.

Circulating antibodies which develop as a response to the infection appear to have no influence on the course of the disease once it is established.[15, 121]

It is thought that *D. congolensis* and certain poxviruses, such as orf virus in sheep and lumpy skin disease virus in cattle, may have a synergistic action, as it is often present in lesions caused by these viruses.[1, 6, 42, 79]

Clinical signs and pathology

In flocks of sheep the prevalence of lumpy wool may vary from individual cases to severe outbreaks where almost all the animals are affected.[8, 13, 16, 21, 33, 64, 118] The mortality rate is usually very low, but up to 20 per cent of affected lambs may die.[17, 107, 128]

Mild lesions are inconspicuous and not easy to detect in sheep. Even advanced lesions can be concealed by the fleece and may only be detected by palpation of the animal or during shearing and classing of the wool.[12, 14, 33]

The severity and distribution of the lesions on the body vary markedly among affected animals. In sheep, the lesions may occur in the woolled[8, 10, 13, 16, 44, 48, 73, 109] or the hairy parts of the body,[17, 32, 33, 67, 103, 107, 118] or both. Acute to chronic, and localized to more widespread lesions may be found in the woolled parts of the skin.[91] Acute lesions are characterized by erythema, exudation and the presence of isolated flecks of yellowish-white to brownish grease or crusts **(Figure 176.3)**. As the lesions become more severe, large amounts of moist exudate or scabs, varying in colour from orange, yellow, brown or grey to greyish-white are evident.[95, 98, 99] As the sticky exudate is carried away from the skin, it dries and glues together clumps or even entire staples of wool fibres to

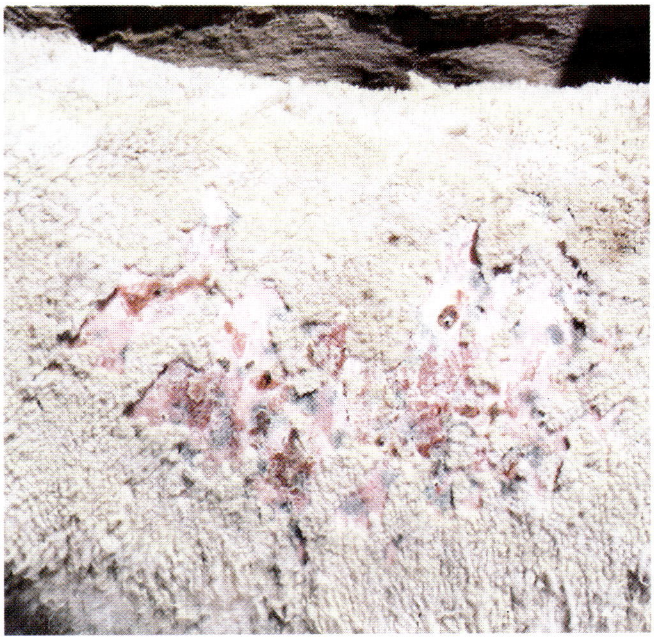

Figure 176.3
Acute, exudative erythematous lesions on the flank of a sheep

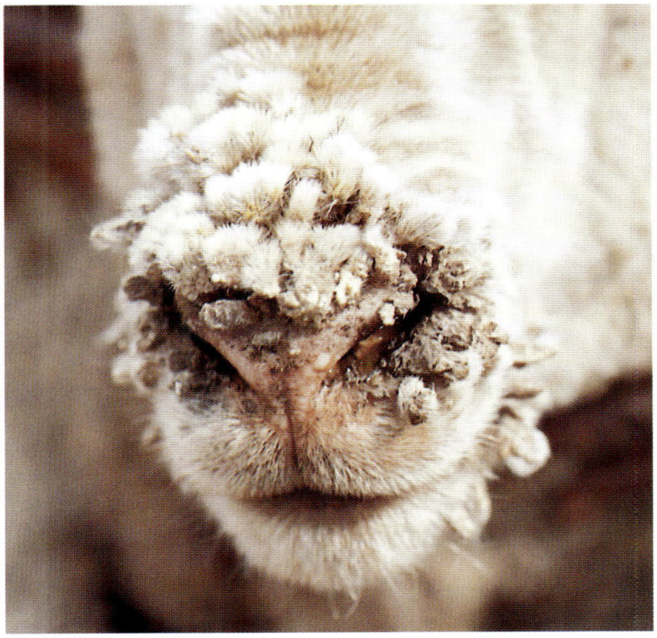

Figure 176.4
Lumpy, chronic lesions on the nose and lips of a lamb

form hard spikes and lumps. The long-standing lesions are often accompanied by a whitish, dry appearance of the epidermis, and a raggedness or uneven surface of the fleece. On parting the wool, single or multiple transverse bands of scabs can be seen, being whitish or greyish-white nearer the skin and brown or almost black towards the surface of the fleece.[12] Typical chronic lesions **(Figure 176.4)** are marked by lumps up to 30–40 mm in diameter which are yellowish to greyish-brown, dense, hard, horn-like and pyramidal to dome-shaped.[13, 16, 99, 116] When removed, the lumps are usually concave at their base and some are partially hollow.[13, 16, 33, 64, 118] The distance from the skin surface varies according to how far the healing process has proceeded. The underlying skin may be normal, or the lesions may still be firmly attached to the skin and can only be removed with difficulty (and with great pain to the animals), leaving a granular and often bleeding surface.

Crusty lesions **(Figure 176.5)** are found predominantly in the coarser-woolled sheep such as the British breeds and their crosses, and in young lambs up to nine months old, whereas the chronic lumpy-wool type of lesion is mostly seen in strong- and medium-woolled Merino sheep.[8, 33, 92, 99]

Lesions of the haired areas of the skin in woolled sheep may occur on the face, lips, chin, nose, ears, axillae, inguinal region, udder, scrotum, and legs from the carpus and tarsus to the hooves but particularly around the coronets.[16, 17, 39, 103, 118] When the lower legs are affected, the condition is generally referred to as strawberry footrot.[32, 121] On the lower legs the lesions may become confluent; the affected areas are covered by thick crusts, while dense wart-like growths are sometimes evident around

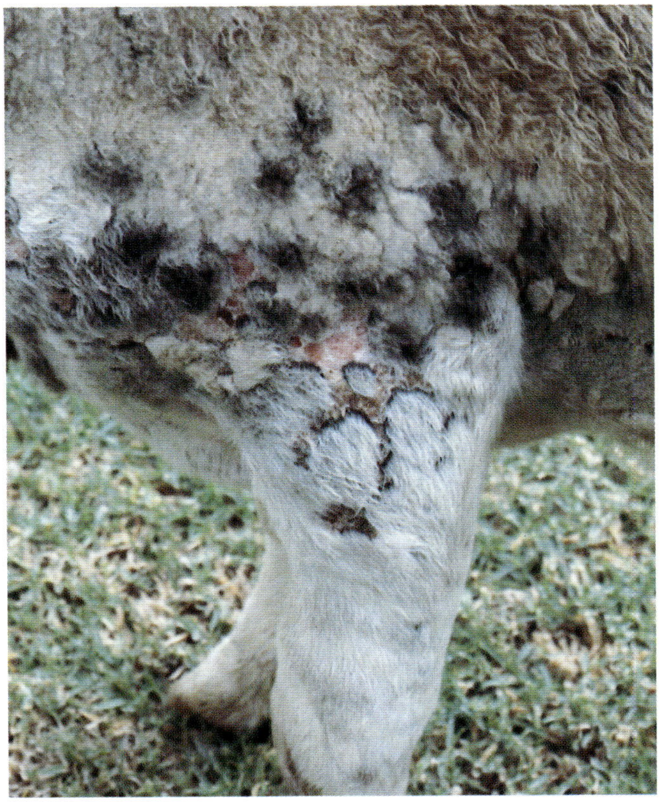

Figure 176.5
Crusty lesions on the leg of a coarse-woolled sheep

the coronets. On removal of the crusts, granular and bleeding surfaces that somewhat resemble strawberries are exposed. Secondary infection of the lesions is common. In long-standing cases the lesions on the lips, chin, nose, forehead and ears tend to be more confined, and warts appear like horns or pencils.[16, 39, 64, 118] Mild chronic lesions are characterized only by a scaliness or slight scab formation on the ears and nose; this occurs particularly in lambs.[14]

In cattle, lesions are distributed mainly in areas where predisposing skin damage has occurred. Lesions associated with a heavy tick infestation develop mainly on the ventral areas of the body, such as the axillae, brisket, inguinal area, scrotum or udder. Lesions of the face, ears and body **(Figure 176.6)** may suggest that infection has been transferred by thorny bushes, whilst lesions of the rump may be due to injury caused by mounting. In calves, lesions often occur on the muzzle, head and neck.

Lesions in cattle may be focal, about 50 mm in diameter, or may become confluent to form a large, mosaic-like area on the skin **(Figures 176.7 and 176.8)**. Affected areas are thickened, raised, hard, coarse and uneven on palpation.[37] The whitish to yellowish-brown crusts on the skin are difficult to remove; but on removal, an area of granulation tissue is exposed. The hair coat may contain loose yellowish crusts or flakes resembling severe dandruff.[37]

Chronically affected cattle are 'poor doers', stunted, and up to 10 per cent may die.[43, 78]

Other lesions that have occasionally been associated with *D. congolensis* infections include subepidermal granulomas[66] and oral lesions in cattle,[29, 40, 111] and chronic lymphadenitis in goats.[112]

Microscopically, the typical acute lesions are characterized by congestion and oedema of the dermis;[32, 86, 95, 97–99] degeneration, necrosis and hyperkeratosis of the cells in the epidermis; accumulation of exudate on the surface of the skin; and infiltration of neutrophils in the dermis and epidermis. Branching, septated, bacterial filaments or parallel rows of coccoid zoospores are found in the epidermis as far down as the *stratum basale*, but they do not usually invade the dermis. Organisms extend into the follicular sheaths for some distance, causing proliferation of the sheath cells. Wool and hair fibres are not invaded.

Diagnosis

A provisional diagnosis of dermatophilosis in animals can often be made on clinical grounds alone, especially in the case of lumpy wool and strawberry footrot in sheep,[99] but it can readily be confirmed by the examination of biopsy material from the lesions; or of smears prepared from the affected skin, the concave base of freshly removed scabs, or of suspensions of some of the most recently formed scabs in distilled water. Smears should be stained with Gram's stain or aniline dyes and examined for the presence of typically branched filaments which are transversely and longitudinally septate, and characteristic parallel rows of coccoid elements.[16, 33, 39, 64, 99, 118] In older scabs where most of the filaments have been converted to free zoospores, motile zoospores may be demonstrated by the microscopic examination of wet preparations of finely chopped scab material in sterile nutrient broth or distilled water.[31, 88, 99]

Dermatophilus congolensis is readily isolated from newly formed scabs which are relatively free of secondary bacterial contamination. In order to achieve this the scabs are chopped or minced in a small amount of sterile nutrient broth or distilled water. This is then plated on a blood agar or enriched nutrient medium.[16, 18, 26, 39, 64, 84, 86, 99, 121] Attempts to culture the organism from older scab material may prove unsuccessful. A simple, rapid and reliable method for the primary isolation of the organism from samples of dermatophilosis in sheep, particularly contaminated specimens, entails the use of media containing polymyxin B.[5] The identification of *D. congolensis* is established by its cultural, morphological and biochemical features.

The fluorescent antibody technique,[38, 77, 82] regarded by some as the most reliable single method of diagnosis,[53] may facilitate the diagnosis, as residual fragments of organisms may also be detected. Serological methods of diagnosis are of little practical value but may occasionally be useful as flock-screening tests. Techniques which have been applied include the agglutination test,[94, 98, 121] passive haemagglutination test,[61, 62, 65, 68, 74, 80, 83] complement fixation test,[121] gel-diffusion test,[7, 60, 61, 94, 98] immunoelectrophoresis[47, 61] and enzyme-linked immunosorbent assay.[54]

Differential diagnosis

In sheep, other skin and/or fleece disorders such as the contagious pustular dermatitis/ulcerative dermatosis complex, sheep scab, sarcoptic and chorioptic mange, sheep-itch mite infestation, ringworm, dermatitis as a result of photosensitivity, fleece rot, fleece discoloration and Bolo disease should be differentiated from dermatophilosis. Differentiation of dermatophilosis from these conditions often depends on the microscopic and cultural demonstration of *D. congolensis* in lesions.

In cattle, ringworm lesions (which are usually characterized by circular skin lesions on the face and neck), mange (which is usually pruritic), subacute to chronic photodermatitis (which only affects the non-pigmented areas of the body), and the skin lesions associated with subacute to chronic sweating sickness may be confused with those of dermatophilosis.

Control

Because of the thick and firmly adherent scabs which cover the lesions, and because of the depth to which the bacterial filaments penetrate into the affected skin and follicle sheaths, topical treatment is usually unrewarding.[87, 95, 100, 101] However, gentle bathing of the crusts with warm water and soap may help to remove them. A cure may be affected by parenteral administration of antibacterial drugs.[37, 87, 99–101] A single treatment of

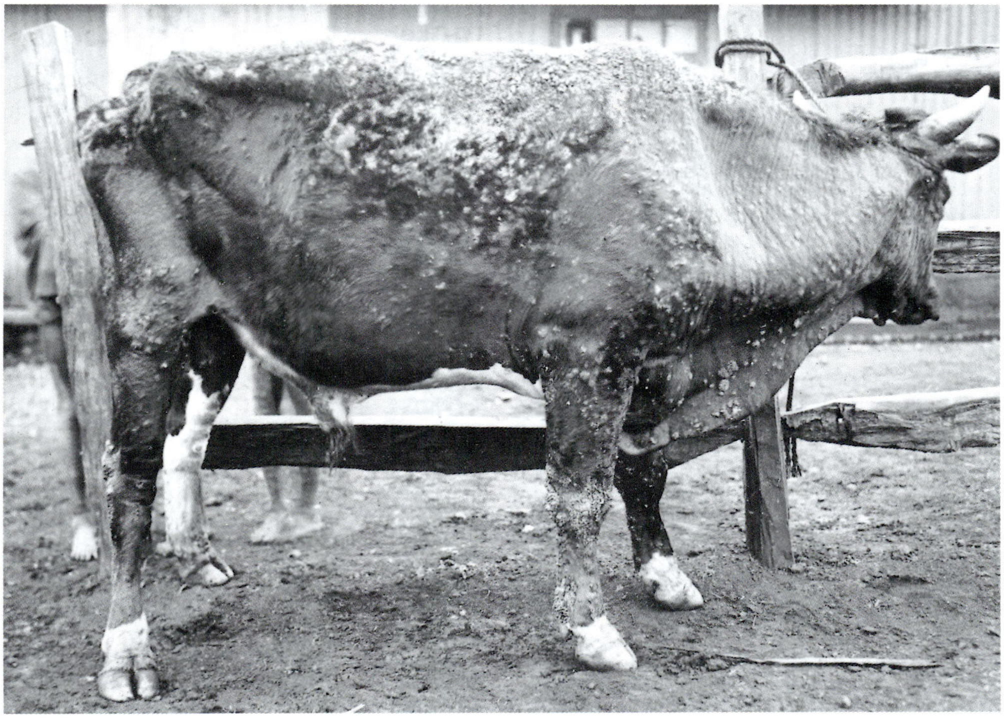

Figure 176.6 Widespread lesions on an ox

penicillin and streptomycin or dihydrostreptomycin given intramuscularly at dose rates of 70 000 IU/kg and 70 mg/kg respectively is usually effective.[99–101] Good results have been obtained in the treatment of affected cattle[37, 41, 70] and sheep[30] with a single dose of a long-acting oxytetracycline at 20 mg/kg. Shearing of badly affected sheep, provided the lesions are inactive and separated from the skin, is often an important additional measure to further reduce the development of lesions and to lessen the economic impact of the disease on the quality of shorn wool. If animals are continuously re-infected, treatment is unlikely to influence the

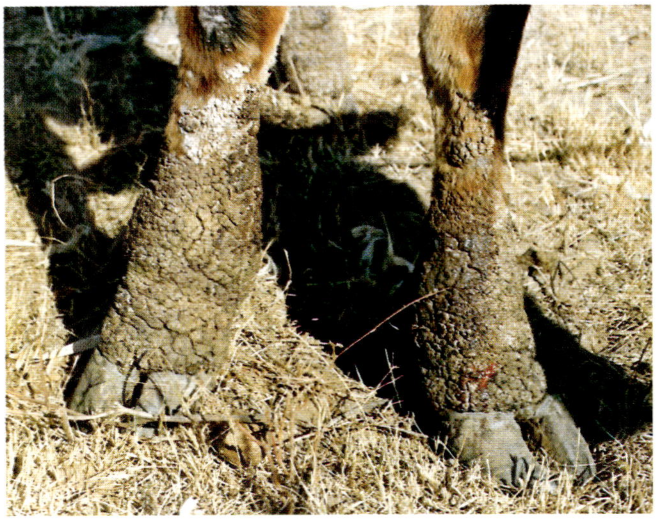

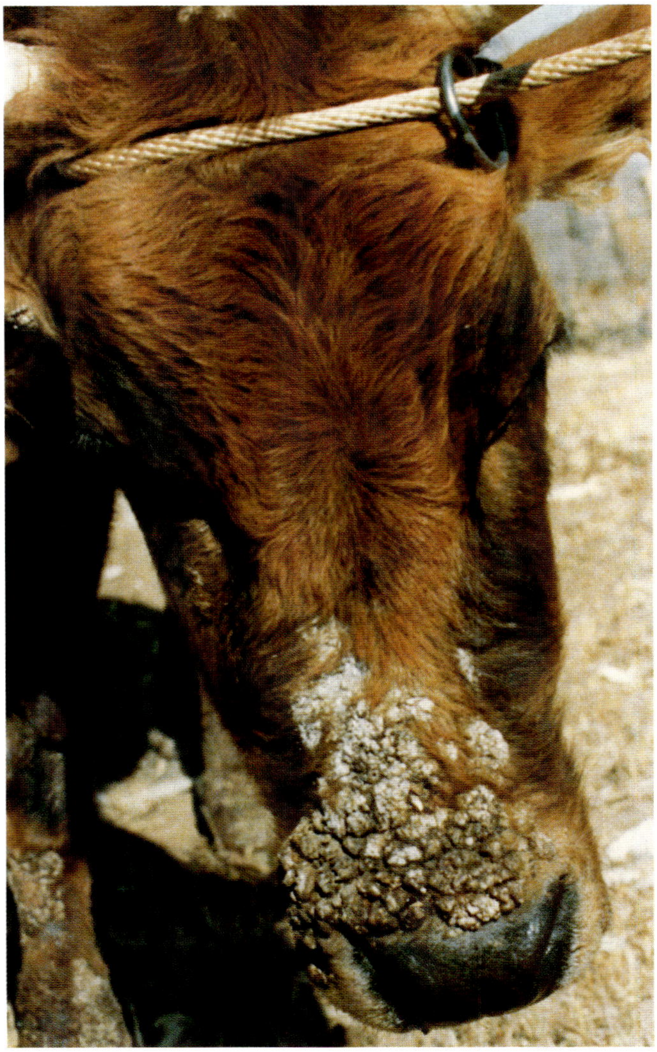

Figures 176.7 (above) and 176.8 (right) Typical mosaic-like pattern of the confluent crusts on the legs and nose of an affected heifer.

course of the disease. Animals with advanced chronic lesions should be culled. Acute infections sometimes heal spontaneously. About 10 per cent of cattle that are not severely affected may recover without treatment.[104]

In vitro tests show that both copper sulphate and zinc sulphate solutions at very low concentrations are bactericidal to the coccoid and filamentous stages of *D. congolensis*. It has been recommended that sheep should be sprayed with 0,5 per cent zinc sulphate to prevent infection of shearing cuts.[101] Although it is often recommended that zinc sulphate be added to acaricidal dips at 1:1 000, its efficacy is in some doubt.

Preventive measures should aim to interrupt the chain of epidemiological events required for the occurrence of outbreaks of dermatophilosis.[87–91, 93, 99, 101, 120] These measures will therefore mainly involve methods of husbandry.[59, 101] Tick control and early proper treatment of infected cattle are the most important management factors influencing the prevalence of dermatophilosis in cattle.[104]

References

1 **ABU-SAMRA, M.T., 1978.** *Dermatophilus* infection: The clinical disease and diagnosis. *Zentralblatt für Veterinärmedizin*, 25B, 641–651.

2 **ABU-SAMRA, M.T., 1978.** Morphological, cultural and biochemical characteristics of *Dermatophilus congolensis*. *Zentralblatt für Veterinärmedizin*, 25B, 668–688.

3 **ABU-SAMRA, M.T., 1979.** A study of the ultrastructure and the life cycle of *Dermatophilus congolensis*. *Zentralblatt für Veterinärmedizin*, 26B, 110–124.

4 **ABU-SAMRA, M.T., 1981.** Resistance of *Dermatophilus congolensis* and the effect of vitamin supplementation on the growth of the organism. *British Veterinary Journal*, 137, 196–202.

5 **ABU-SAMRA, M.T. & WALTON, G.S., 1977.** Modified techniques for the isolation of *Dermatophilus* spp. from infected material. *Sabouraudia*, 15, 23–27.

6 **ABU-SAMRA, M.T. & WALTON, G.S., 1981.** The inoculation of rabbits with *Dermatophilus congolensis* and the simultaneous injection of sheep with *D. congolensis* and orf virus. *Journal of Comparative Pathology*, 91, 317–329.

7 **AGHOMO, H.O. & LLOYD, D.H., 1983.** Comparison of *Dermatophilus congolensis* precipitating antigens prepared by three methods. *British Veterinary Journal*, 139, 325–329.

8 **ALLWORTH, M.B., WEST, D.M. & BRUERE, A.N., 1985.** Ovine dermatophilosis in young sheep associated with the grazing of *Brassica* spp. crops. *New Zealand Veterinary Journal*, 33, 210–212.

9 **ANON, 1977.** Lumpy wool may increase by dipping. *Journal of Agriculture, Western Australia*, 18, 111–112.

10 **ARANTES, I.G., FISCHMAN, O., PORTUGAL, M.A.S.C., CALIK, E.B. & OLIVEIRA, M., 1977.** Dermatophilosis in sheep from Sao Paulo (Brazil). *Mykosen*, 20, 83–88.

11 **AUSTWICK, P.K.C., 1958.** Cutaneous streptothricosis, mycotic dermatitis and strawberry footrot and the genus *Dermatophilus* Van Saceghem. *Veterinary Reviews and Annotations*, 4, 33–48.

12 **AUSTWICK, P.K.C. & DAVIES, E.T., 1958.** Mycotic dermatitis in Great Britain 1954–58. *The Veterinary Record*, 70, 1081–1086.

13 **BEKKER, J.G., 1927.** Undescribed skin diseases of sheep in South Africa. *Journal of the South African Veterinary Medical Association*, 1, 51–57.

14 **BIDA, S.A. & DENNIS, S.M., 1976.** Dermatophilosis in Northern Nigeria. *Veterinary Bulletin*, 46, 471–478.

15 **BIDA, S.A. & KELLY, D.C., 1976.** Immunological studies of antigenic components of *Dermatophilus congolensis*. *In*: LLOYD, D.H. & SELLERS, K.C., (eds). *Dermatophilus Infection in Animals and Man*. Proceedings of a Symposium held at the University of Ibadan, Nigeria, 1973. London: Academic Press.

16 **BULL, L.B., 1929.** Dermatomycosis of the sheep (lumpy or matted wool) due to *Actinomyces dermatonomus* (n. sp.). *Australian Journal of Experimental Biology and Medical Science*, 6, 301–314.

17 **CLEMENTS, L.O. & WEAVERS, E.D., 1980.** *Dermatophilus congolensis* infection in lambs. *Irish Veterinary Journal*, 34, 65–67.

18 **DEAN, D.J., GORDON, M.A., SEVERINGHAUS, C.W., KROLL, E.T. & REILLY, J.R., 1961.** Streptothricosis: A new zoonotic disease. *New York State Journal of Medicine*, 15, 1283–1287.

19 **EDWARDS, J.R., 1984.** Dispelling some myths about 'Dermo' (*Dermatophilus congolensis*). *Journal of Agriculture, Western Australia*, 25, 62–64.

20 **EDWARDS, J.R., 1985.** Sale and processing of wool affected with dermatophilosis. *Australian Veterinary Journal*, 62, 173–174.

21 **EDWARDS, G.R., GARDNER, J.J., NORRIS, R.T., LOVE, R.A., SPICER, P., BRYANT, R., GWYNN, R.V.R., HAWKINS, C.D. & SWAN, R.A., 1985.** A survey of ovine dermatophilosis in Western Australia. *Australian Veterinary Journal*, 62, 361–365.

22 **EGERTON, J.R., 1964.** Mycotic dermatitis of cattle. *Australian Veterinary Journal*, 40, 144–147.

23 **GHERARDI, S.G., MONZU, N., SUTHERLAND, S.S., JOHNSON, K.G. & ROBERTSON, G.M., 1981.** The association between body strike and dermatophilosis of sheep under controlled conditions. *Australian Veterinary Journal*, 57, 268–271.

24 **GHERARDI, S.G., SUTHERLAND, S.S. & MONZU, N., 1984.** 'Dermo', fleece-rot and body strike on sheep. *Journal of Agriculture, Western Australia*, 2, 57–59.

25 **GHERARDI, S.G., SUTHERLAND, S.S., MONZU, N. & JOHNSON, K.G., 1983.** Field observations on body strike in sheep affected with dermatophilosis and fleece-rot. *Australian Veterinary Journal*, 60, 27–28.

26 **GORDON, M.A., 1964.** The genus *Dermatophilus*. *Journal of Bacteriology*, 88, 509–522.

27 **GORDON, M.A. & EDWARDS, M.R., 1963.** Micromorphology of *Dermatophilus congolensis*. *Journal of Bacteriology*, 86, 1101–1115.

28 **GREEN, H.F., 1960.** Streptothricosis in zebra and donkeys and demodectic mange in eland in Kenya. *The Veterinary Record*, 72, 1098.

29 **GUPTA, P.P. & SINHA, B.P., 1978.** Oral dermatophilosis associated with actinomycosis in cattle. *Zentralblatt für Veterinärmedizin*, 25B, 211–215.

30 **GYANG, E.O., ILEMOBADE, A.A. & SHANNON, D., 1980.** Treatment of ovine dermatophilosis with long-acting oxytetracycline. *The Veterinary Record*, 106, 106.

31 **HAALSTRA, R.T., 1965.** Isolation of *Dermatophilus congolensis*

from skin lesions in the diagnosis of streptothricosis. *The Veterinary Record*, 77, 824–825.

32 **HARRIS, S.T., 1948.** Proliferative dermatitis of the legs (strawberry footrot) in sheep. *Journal of Comparative Pathology*, 58, 315–328.

33 **HART, C.B., 1967.** Mycotic dermatitis in sheep. 1. Clinical observations in Great Britain. *The Veterinary Record*, 79, 36–37.

34 **HENDERSON, A.E., 1968.** *Growing Better Wool.* 1st edn. Wellington, Auckland, Sydney: A.H. & A.W. Reed.

35 **HENNING, M.W., 1956.** Actinomycosis, actinobacillosis and dermatomycosis (lumpy wool). *In: Animal Diseases in South Africa.* 3rd edn. Pretoria: Central News Agency, Ltd.

36 **HORNER, R.F., 1985.** Allerton Veterinary Laboratory, Pietermaritzburg. Unpublished data.

37 **HORNER, R.F., 1986.** *Dermatophilus congolensis* infection in cattle. *Journal of the South African Veterinary Association*, 57, 121–123.

38 **HOW, S.J. & LLOYD, D.H., 1988.** Use of monoclonal antibody in the diagnosis of infection by *Dermatophilus congolensis. Research in Veterinary Science*, 45, 416 – 417.

39 **HUDSON, J.R., 1937.** Cutaneous streptothricosis. *Proceedings of the Royal Society of Medicine*, 30, 1457–1460.

40 **IBU, J., MAKINDE, A.A. & NAWATHE, D.R., 1987.** Oral dermatophilosis in imported cattle in Nigeria. *The Veterinary Record*, 120, 42.

41 **ILEMOBADE, A.A., GYANG, E.O., BIDA, S.A. & ADDO, P.B., 1979.** Cure of *Dermatophilus congolensis* infection in cattle by long-acting oxytetracycline. *Research in Veterinary Science*, 27, 302–305.

42 **ISITOR, G.N., KAZEEM, H.M., NJOKU, C.O., ABEGBOYE, D.S. & DELLMANN, H.D., 1988.** Frequency of involvement of pox virions in lesions of bovine dermatophilosis. *Tropical Animal Health and Production*, 20, 2–10.

43 **JUBB, K.V.F., KENNEDY, P.C. & PALMER, N., 1985.** *Pathology of Domestic Animals.* 3rd edn. Vol. I. Orlando, Florida: Academic Press, Inc.

44 **KANE, G.J., DOWNING, W. & WITSDON, A.J., 1955.** Mycotic dermatitis in Great Britain. *The Veterinary Record*, 67, 779.

45 **KAPLAN, W. & JOHNSTON, W.J., 1966.** Equine dermatophilus (cutaneous streptothricosis) in Georgia. *Journal of the American Veterinary Medical Association*, 149, 1162–1171.

46 **KISTNER, T.P., SHOTTS, E.B. & GREENE, E.W., 1970.** Naturally occurring cutaneous streptothricosis in a white-tailed deer (*Odocoileus virginianus*). *Journal of the American Veterinary Medical Association*, 157, 633– 635.

47 **KWAPINSKI, J.B., 1966.** Serological and chromatographic characterization of exo-antigens of the *Dermatophilus. Australian Journal of Experimental Biology and Medical Science*, 44, 87–92.

48 **LEFEVRE, E., LAIDET, M. & ROUGEOT, J., 1978.** La dermatophilose chez les ovins en France. *Recueil de Médecine Vétérinaire*, 154, 913– 918.

49 **LE RICHE, P.D., 1967.** The activity of dipping fluids in the treatment and prevention of mycotic dermatitis in sheep. *Australian Veterinary Journal*, 43, 265– 269.

50 **LE RICHE, P.D., 1968.** The transmission of dermatophilosis (mycotic dermatitis) in sheep. *Australian Veterinary Journal*, 44, 64– 67.

51 **LE ROUX, D.J., 1968.** The treatment of 'lumpy wool' *Dermatophilus congolensis* infection in Merino sheep with streptomycin and penicillin. *Journal of the South African Veterinary Medical Association*, 39, 87– 88.

52 **LLOYD, D.H., 1971.** Streptothricosis in the domestic donkey (*Equus asinus asinus*). *British Veterinary Journal*, 127, 572–581.

53 **LLOYD, D.H., 1976.** Diagnostic features of *Dermatophilus* infection. *Transactions of the Royal Society of Tropical Medicine and Hygiene*, 70, 285.

54 **LLOYD, D.H. & JENKINSON, D.M., 1980.** The effect of climate on experimental infection of bovine skin with *Dermatophilus congolensis. British Veterinary Journal*, 136, 122–130.

55 **LOUW, D.F.J., 1972.** Voorkoms van klontwol by skape. *Department of Wool Production, South African Wool Board, Information Series No. 4.3.1.*

56 **MACADAM, I., 1961.** The effect of humidity on the lesions of streptothricosis. *The Veterinary Record*, 73, 1039–1041.

57 **MACADAM, I., 1962.** Bovine streptothricosis: Production of lesions by the bites of the tick *Amblyomma variegatum. The Veterinary Record*, 74, 643– 646.

58 **MACADAM, I., 1964.** Observations on the effects of flies and humidity on the natural lesions of streptothricosis. *The Veterinary Record*, 76, 194–198.

59 **MACADAM, I., 1977.** Control of *Dermatophilus congolensis* infection. *The Veterinary Record*, 100, 411.

60 **MAKINDE, A.A., 1980.** The reverse single radial immunodiffusion technique for detecting antibodies to *Dermatophilus congolensis. The Veterinary Record*, 106, 383 –385.

61 **MAKINDE, A.A. & MAJIYAGBE, K.A., 1982.** Serodiagnosis of *Dermatophilus congolensis* infection by counter-immunoelectrophoresis. *Research in Veterinary Science*, 33, 265– 269.

62 **MAKINDE, A.A., MOLOKWU, J.U. & EZEH, A.O., 1986.** Humoral antibody response to glutaraldehyde-treated antigens of *Dermatophilus congolensis. Veterinary Quarterly*, 8, 145 –149.

63 **MAMMERICKX, M., 1961.** Observations sur la dermatose contagieuse des ruminants au Congo. *Annale des Sociétés Belges de Médecine Tropicale*, 41, 133–144.

64 **MASON, J.H. & BEKKER, J.G., 1934.** Further notes on lumpy wool in South Africa. *Onderstepoort Journal of Veterinary Science and Animal Industry*, 3, 211–216.

65 **MERKAL, R.S., RICHARD, J.L., THURSTON, J.R. & NESS, R.D., 1972.** Effect of methotrexate on rabbits infected with *Mycobacterium paratuberculosis* or *Dermatophilus congolensis. American Journal of Veterinary Research*, 33, 401–407.

66 **MOMOTANI, E., INUI, S., ISHIKAWA, Y. & AZUMA, R., 1984.** Granulomatous subdermal lesions in sheep inoculated with *Dermatophilus congolensis. Journal of Comparative Pathology*, 94, 33– 43.

67 **NISBET, I.I. & BANNATYNE, C.C., 1955.** A dermatitis of sheep associated with an organism of the genus *Actinomyces. The Veterinary Record*, 67, 713–715.

68 **ODUYE, O.O., 1974.** A comparative serological study of *Dermatophilus congolensis* antigens prepared by different methods. *British Veterinary Journal*, 130, lix–lxii.

69 **ODUYE, O.O., 1976.** Bovine streptothricosis in Nigeria. *In*: LLOYD, D.H. & SELLERS, K.C., (eds). *Dermatophilus Infection in Animals and Man.* Proceedings of a Symposium held at the University of Ibadan, Nigeria, 1973. London: Academic Press.

70 **OGWU, D., ALHAVJI, I. & OSORI, I.K., 1981.** Effectiveness of long-acting terramycin injectable solution in the treatment of streptothricosis in cattle. *British Veterinary Journal*, 137, 585–589.

71 **OPPONG, E.N.W., 1976.** Epizootology of *Dermatophilus* infection in cattle in the Accra plains of Ghana. *In*: LLOYD, D.H. & SELLERS, K.C., (eds). *Dermatophilus Infection in Animals and Man.* Proceedings of a Symposium held at the University of Ibadan, Nigeria, 1973. London: Academic Press.

72 **O'SULLIVAN, B.M., 1968.** Lumpy wool in sheep. *Queensland Agricultural Journal*, January 1968, 1–3. Division of Animal Industry, Department of Primary Industries, Advisory Leaflet No. 568.

73 **OXER, D.T., 1930.** Mycotic dermatitis in sheep and green staining of wool. *Tasmanian Journal of Agriculture*, 1, 120–121.

74 **OYEJIDE, A., MAKINDE, A.A. & EZEH, A.O., 1984.** Prevalence of antibodies to *Dermatophilus congolensis* in sheep and goats in Nigeria. *The Veterinary Quarterly*, 6, 44–45.

75 **PHILPOTT, M. & EZEH, A.O., 1978.** The experimental transmission by *Musca* and *Stomoxys* species of *Dermatophilus congolensis* infection between cattle. *British Veterinary Journal*, 134, 515–520.

76 **PIER, A.C., NEAL, F.C. & CYSEWSKI, S.J., 1963.** Cutaneous streptothricosis in Iowa cattle. *Journal of the American*

Veterinary Medical Association, 142, 995–1000.

77 **PIER, A.C., RICHARD, J.L. & FARRELL, E.F., 1964.** Fluorescent antibody and cultural techniques in cutaneous streptothricosis. *American Journal of Veterinary Research*, 25, 1014–1020.

78 **PLOWRIGHT, W., 1956.** Cutaneous streptothricosis of cattle. 1. Introduction and epizootiological features in Nigeria. *The Veterinary Record*, 68, 350–355.

79 **PLOWRIGHT, W. & FERRIS, R.D., 1959.** Papular stomatitis of cattle in Kenya and Nigeria. *The Veterinary Record*, 71, 718–724.

80 **PULLIAM, J.D., KELLY, D.C. & COLES, E.H., 1967.** Immunological studies of natural and experimental cutaneous streptothricosis infections in cattle. *American Journal of Veterinary Research*, 28, 447–455.

81 **PULSFORD, M.F. 1967.** Advances in the control and treatment of lumpy wool. *Journal of Agriculture of South Australia*, 70, 324–329.

82 **RICHARD, J.L. & PIER, A.C., 1966.** Transmission of *Dermatophilus congolensis* by *Stomoxys calcitrans* and *Musca domestica*. *American Journal of Veterinary Research*, 27, 419–423.

83 **RICHARD, J.L., THURSTON, J.R. & PIER, A.C., 1976.** Comparison of antigens of *Dermatophilus congolensis* isolates and their use in serologic tests in experimental and natural infections. *In*: LLOYD, D.H. & SELLER, K.C., (eds). *Dermatophilus Infection in Animals and Man*. Proceedings of a Symposium held at the University of Ibadan, Nigeria, 1973. London: Academic Press.

84 **ROBERTS, D.S., 1957.** Some features of the mycotic dermatitis organism. *Australian Veterinary Journal*, 33, 141–143.

85 **ROBERTS, D.S., 1957.** An ecological study of the mycotic dermatitis organism. *Australian Veterinary Journal*, 33, 233–236.

86 **ROBERTS, D.S., 1961.** The life cycle of *Dermatophilus derma-tonomus*, the causal agent of ovine mycotic dermatitis. *Australian Journal of Experimental Biology*, 39, 463–476.

87 **ROBERTS, D.S., 1962.** An approach to the control of mycotic dermatitis. *Wool Technology and Sheep Breeding*, 9, 101–103.

88 **ROBERTS, D.S., 1963.** Properties of *Dermatophilus dermatonomus* zoospores in relation to the transmission of mycotic dermatitis. *Australian Journal of Agricultural Research*, 14, 373–385.

89 **ROBERTS, D.S., 1963.** The release and survival of *Dermatophilus dermatonomus* zoospores. *Australian Journal of Agricultural Research*, 14, 386–399.

90 **ROBERTS, D.S., 1963.** Chemotactic behaviour of the infective zoospores of *Dermatophilus dermatonomus*. *Australian Journal of Agricultural Research*, 14, 400–411.

91 **ROBERTS, D.S., 1963.** The influence of carbon dioxide on the growth and sporulation of *Dermatophilus dermatonomus*. *Australian Journal of Agricultural Research*, 14, 412–423.

92 **ROBERTS, D.S., 1963.** Barrier to *Dermatophilus dermatonomus* infection of the skin of sheep. *Australian Journal of Agricultural Research*, 14, 492–508.

93 **ROBERTS, D.S., 1964.** Synergistic effects of salts and carbon dioxide on *Dermatophilus dermatonomus*. *Journal of General Microbiology*, 37, 403–410.

94 **ROBERTS, D.S., 1965.** Cutaneous actinomycosis due to the single species *Dermatophilus congolensis*. *Nature* (London), 206, 1068.

95 **ROBERTS, D.S., 1965.** The histopathology of epidermal infection with the actinomycete *Dermatophilus congolensis*. *Journal of Pathology and Bacteriology*, 90, 213–216.

96 **ROBERTS, D.S., 1965.** Penetration and irritation of the skin by *Dermatophilus congolensis*. *British Journal of Experimental Pathology*, 46, 635–642.

97 **ROBERTS, D.S., 1965.** The role of granulocytes in resistance to *Dermatophilus congolensis*. *British Journal of Experimental Pathology*, 46, 643–648.

98 **ROBERTS, D.S., 1966.** The influence of delayed hypersensitivity on the course of infection with *Dermatophilus congolensis*. *British Journal of Experimental Pathology*, 47, 9–16.

99 **ROBERTS, D.S., 1967.** *Dermatophilus* infection. *Veterinary Bulletin, Weybridge*, 37, 513–521.

100 **ROBERTS, D.S., 1967.** Chemotherapy of epidermal infection with *Dermatophilus congolensis*. *Journal of Comparative Pathology*, 77, 129–136.

101 **ROBERTS, D.S. & GRAHAM, N.P.H., 1966.** Control of ovine cutaneous actinomycosis. *Australian Veterinary Journal*, 42, 74–78.

102 **ROBERTSON, G.M., 1984.** What can we do about 'Dermo'. *Journal of Agriculture, Western Australia*, 2, 81–83.

103 **ROSSITER, L.W., 1956.** Experiments in the treatment of lumpy wool. *Journal of the South African Veterinary Medical Association*, 27, 179–182.

104 **SAMUI, K.L. & HUGH-JONES, M.E., 1988.** The prevalence of bovine dermatophilosis in Zambia. *Acta Veterinaria Scandinavica*, S84, 98–100.

105 **SAMUI, K.L. & HUGH-JONES, M.E., 1988.** The financial cost of bovine dermatophilosis in Zambia. *Acta Veterinaria Scandinavica*, S84, 369–370.

106 **SCANLAN, C.M., GARRETT, P.D. & GEIGER, D.B., 1984.** *Dermatophilus congolensis* infections of cattle and sheep. *Compendium of Continuing Education for the Practising Veterinarian*, 6, 54–59.

107 **SCHANDEVYL, P., 1982.** Occurrence of lumpy wool disease in Nepal. *Indian Veterinary Journal*, 59, 325.

108 **SCHULTZ, K.C.A., 1955.** Mycotic dermatitis (Senkobo skin disease) of cattle in the Union of South Africa. *Bulletin of Epizootic Diseases of Africa*, 3, 244–261.

109 **SEDDON, H.R., 1929.** Mycotic dermatitis of sheep. *Veterinary Research in Reproduction, New South Wales, 1927–28*, 5, 10–18.

110 **SEDDON, H.R., 1965.** Mycotic dermatitis. *In*: ALBISTON, H.E., (ed.). *Diseases of Domestic Animals in Australia*. Part 5. Bacterial Diseases. Vol. II. 2nd edn. Department of Health, Commonwealth of Australia, Service Publications (Veterinary Hygiene) No. 10.

111 **SIMPSON, B.H. & CUMING, G., 1976.** An unusual case of dermatophilosis in a calf. *New Zealand Veterinary Journal*, 24, 21–22.

112 **SINGH, V.P. & MURTY, D.K., 1978.** An outbreak of *Dermatophilus congolensis* infection in goats. *Indian Veterinary Journal*, 55, 674–676.

113 **SMITH, J.M.B., DANIEL, R.C.W. & BUERE, A.N., 1967.** Dermatophilosis — an emerging disease in New Zealand. *New Zealand Veterinary Journal*, 15, 88–89.

114 **SNIJDERS, A.J. & JANSEN, B.J., 1955.** A comparison of *Streptothrix bovis* and *Actinomyces dermatonomus*. *Bulletin of Epizootic Diseases of Africa*, 3, 242–243.

115 **SOLTYS, M.A., 1964.** Cutaneous streptothricosis in cattle in the Sudan. *Sudanese Journal of Veterinary Science and Animal Husbandry*, 5, 20–23.

116 **STEWART, G.H., 1972.** Dermatophilosis: A skin disease of animals and man. Part I. *The Veterinary Record*, 91, 537–544.

117 **STEWART, G.H., 1972.** Dermatophilosis: A skin disease of animals and man. Part II. *The Veterinary Record*, 91, 555–561.

118 **STEYN, D.G., 1931.** Investigations into the cause and transmission of lumpy wool affecting Merino sheep and its treatment. *Seventeenth Report of the Director of Veterinary Services and Animal Industry, Union of South Africa*, 205–212.

119 **SUTHERLAND, S.S., GHERARDI, S.G. & MONZU, N., 1983.** Body strike in sheep with dermatophilosis with or without fleece-rot. *Australian Veterinary Journal*, 60, 88–89.

120 **THOMAS, J.H. 1957.** Mycotic dermatitis. *Ninth Annual Report, Commonwealth Scientific and Industrial Research Organization, 1956/57*, 53–54.

121 **THOMPSON, R.E., 1954.** A species of *Rhizobium* isolated from strawberry footrot in the sheep. *Journal of Pathology and Bacteriology*, 68, 445–452.

122 **THOMPSON, R.E.M. & BISSET, K.A., 1957.** Polysepta: A new genus and suborder of bacteria. *Nature*, (London), 179, 590–591.

123 **THOROLD, P.W., 1950.** The transmission of lumpy wool

(*Actinomyces dermatonomus*) by benzene hexachloride dips. *Journal of the South African Veterinary Medical Association*, 21, 30–32.
124 **THOROLD, P.W., 1965.** Some common bacterial infections in sheep in South Africa. *Journal of the South African Veterinary Medical Association*, 35, 549–565.
125 **VANDEMAELE, F.P., 1961.** Enquête sur la streptothricose cutanée en Afrique. *Bulletin of Epizootic Diseases of Africa*, 9, 251–258.
126 **VAN SACEGHEM, R., 1915.** Dermatose contagieuse (Impetigo contagieux). *Bulletin de la Société de Pathologie Exotique*,8, 354–359.
127 **VAN TONDER, E.M. 1980.** Lumpy wool and fleece discoloration. *Symposium on Small Stock Ectoparasites and Dip-tank management*, Liaison Committee of the Agricultural and Veterinary Chemicals Association of South Africa, 12–13 March 1980, 1–13.
128 **WILKINSON, F.C., 1979.** Dermatophilosis of sheep: Association with dipping and effect on reproduction. *Australian Veterinary Journal*, 55, 74–76.

MYCOPLASMAS

The mycoplasmas are small, Gram-negative, prokaryotes that lack cell walls and are bound only by a plasma membrane. They include all the organisms classified in the class Mollicutes, incorporating the families containing organisms which may be isolated from livestock, namely the Mycoplasmataceae (in which the genera *Mycoplasma* and *Ureaplasma* occur) and Acholeplasmataceae (containing the genus Acholeplasma, which is of no known veterinary importance). The organisms in these families have some of the smallest genomes recorded for prokaryotes. They lack the ability to synthesize peptidoglycan, which renders them insensitive to the deleterious effects of penicillin and its analogues, and susceptible to lysis by osmotic shock, detergents, alcohols, and specific antibody and complement.[2]

The mycoplasmas are pleomorphic, varying in morphology from pear-shaped organisms to branched or helical filaments. Most of the species of these genera are facultative anaerobes and may be cultivated on cell-free media of varying complexity containing sterols and fatty acids, though some are more readily cultivated in cell cultures. The genera isolated from livestock can be distinguished from one another in several ways: *Acholeplasma* spp. do not require sterols for growth, while *Ureaplasma* spp. are distinguished by their ability to split urea into ammonia and carbon dioxide.[3] In addition, *Ureaplasma* spp. do not grow on the media commonly employed for the propagation of mycoplasmas. Colonies of mycoplasmas on solid media are very small, tend to grow within the medium, and assume a 'fried egg' appearance. Mycoplasmas are also distinguished from all other prokaryotes by the fact that they are filterable through filters of 450 nm pore diameter. They are, however, superficially similar to the cell wall-defective L-shape variants of bacteria encountered as laboratory artifacts.

Most of the mollicutes are saprophytes, commensals or parasites, and some are pathogens of humans, animals and plants.[1] With a few exceptions, such as *Mycoplasma bovis,* mycoplasmas are host- and site-specific, and most are parasites of mucous membranes and joints. Infections by mycoplasmal species are almost invariably associated with diseases of the respiratory and urogenital tracts, mammary glands or eyes **(Table 1)**. Of the many mycoplasmas that have been isolated from animal species, few have been shown without doubt to be pathogenic. Contagious bovine pleuropneumonia, ovine keratoconjunctivitis, and mycoplasmal pneumonia of pigs, in particular, are highly contagious and of economic importance, whereas many of the other mycoplasmal infections, though ubiquitous, are more sporadic in occurrence, and most (e.g. those caused by *M. alkalescens M. arginini, M. bovoculi, M. flocculare, A. laidlawii* and *A. modicum*) are subclinical. Most pathogenic mycoplasmas are associated with chronic disease **(see Chapter 182: Bovine genital mycoplasmosis)**.

Infectious keratoconjunctivitis of sheep is an important

Table 1 Diseases caused by common *Mycoplasma* spp. infections in livestock

MYCOPLASMA SPP.	DISEASE	SPECIES AFFECTED
Mycoplasma mycoides mycoides SC	Contagious bovine pleuropneumonia	Cattle
Mycoplasma mycoides capri and *Mycoplasma* F-38	Contagious caprine pleuropneumonia	Goats and sheep
Mycoplasma agalactiae	Mastitis	Goats and sheep
Mycoplasma hyopneumoniae	Mycoplasmal (enzootic) pneumonia of swine	Pigs
Mycoplasma hyorhinis	Pneumonia, arthritis, polyserositis	Pigs
Mycoplasma hyosynoviae	Arthritis	Pigs
Mycoplasma bovis	Infertility	Cattle
Mycoplasma bovigentalium	Infertility	Cattle
Mycoplasma canadense	Mastitis	Cattle
Mycoplasma conjunctivae	Keratoconjunctivitis	Sheep

disease. Apart from *M. conjunctivae*,[1] other infectious agents may cause this condition **(see Chapter 120: *Moraxella* spp. infections)**. The lesions in the eyes progress from an initial acute hyperaemic stage to a mucopurulent keratitis which is followed by corneal ulceration. The lesions should be differentiated from those cause by photosensitization and other infectious agents.

Several mycoplasmas have been isolated from the lesions of sheep suffering from ulcerative balanoposthitis or vulvovaginitis, but the significance of their presence is unknown **(see Chapter 192: Ulcerative balanoposthitis and vulvovaginitis of sheep and goats)**.

It would appear that the role played by ureaplasma infections in disease conditions is increasing. *Ureaplasma diversum*, for instance, has been associated with vaginitis, endometritis, salpingitis, seminal vesiculitis, and abortions in cattle.[3]

References

1 **EGWU, G.O., 1991.** Ovine infectious keratoconjunctivitis: An update. *Veterinary Bulletin*, 61, 547–559.

2 **RAZIN, S. & FREUNDT, E.A., 1984.** The mycoplasmas. *In:* KRIEG, N.R. & HOLT, J.G., (eds). *Bergey's Manual of Systematic Bacteriology*. Vol. I. Baltimore: Williams & Wilkens.

3 **STALHEIM, O.H.V., 1990.** Mycoplasmas of animals. *In:* CARTER, G.R. & COLE, J.R., (eds). *Diagnostic Procedures in Veterinary Bacteriology and Mycology*. 5th edn. San Diego: Academic Press.

177

Contagious bovine pleuropneumonia

Synonyms: Lungsickness, longsiekte (Afrik.)

H.P. Schneider, J.J. van der Lugt and O.J.B. Hübschle

Introduction

Contagious bovine pleuropneumonia (CBPP) is an acute, subacute or chronic infectious disease of cattle and water buffalo caused by *Mycoplasma mycoides mycoides* SC. The disease is characterized by a serofibrinous pleuropneumonia and pulmonary sequestra which result in a chronic, subclinical carrier state in many recovered animals. In southern Africa CBPP occurs in Angola and the northern parts of Namibia.

This disease was first described in 1550 by Gallo[41] and, with the exception of South America and Madagascar, has occurred throughout the world at some time or another. It has been eradicated from Australia and North America, occurs as sporadic outbreaks in parts of Europe, and is an economically important disease in Africa, particularly in the dry tropical countries north of the equator. The prevalence of the disease in Asia is uncertain.

The current presence of CBPP in parts of southern Africa severely restricts economic development and the proper utilization of agricultural land. Application of veterinary regulatory measures, which are essential to control the disease and prevent its spread, hamper proper land-use planning, while constant veterinary disease surveillance and costly annual prophylactic vaccination campaigns place high demands on the usually limited budgets of veterinary administrations.

Contagious bovine pleuropneumonia was introduced into South Africa from Holland by a Friesland bull or bulls landed at Mossel Bay in 1853[39] or 1854.[20] From Mossel Bay the disease was disseminated rapidly by trek oxen; progressing in all directions along transport routes to soon reach the Transvaal. Within two years it had killed over 100 000 head of cattle.[20] Among its political effects was a major contribution to the Great Xhosa Cattle-killing Movement of 1856–57 which resulted in the starvation of tens of thousands of Xhosas and the devastation of that nation.[39]

Namibia was infected in 1856 when a localized outbreak occurred at Warmbad in the south. Although the initial outbreak was contained by quarantine measures adopted by missionaries in the area, the infection reached the central cattle-raising districts of Namibia in 1859 as a result of cattle introductions from either Botswana or the Cape Province. Very high mortalities resulted and the Herero people called 1860 'otjipunga', the year of the lung. In 1861 CBPP moved across the Limpopo River to cause heavy losses among the cattle of the Matabele in southern Zimbabwe.[20]

Contagious bovine pleuropneumonia was introduced into Angola from the south, probably by infected cattle belonging to the Dorsland Trekkers who emigrated from the Transvaal and settled near Humpata in the Huila Province in the early 1880s. Here the disease was confirmed in 1888.[9, 32] The extensive use of draught oxen has been seen as a cause of the rapid spread of the disease throughout Angola, and by 1914 the whole country had been infected.[33]

The introduction of CBPP into Zambia in 1916 originated from Angola. Although eradicated in 1946, CBPP was again introduced from Angola into the Western Province of Zambia in late 1969. This outbreak resulted in a 75 per cent morbidity rate and caused up to 68 per cent mortality in affected herds.[1, 3, 46] It was finally eradicated in 1985.

By the time rinderpest appeared in 1896–97, CBPP was widespread in southern Africa. The effects of the rinderpest pandemic overshadowed those of CBPP, and the disease killed many CBPP-infected cattle.[20] It was not until the turn of the century that the persistence of lungsickness in the cattle populations of southern Africa again presented an obvious problem. Thereafter strict control measures were introduced in most countries of the region. These were, however, complicated by other events which occurred about that time, such as the South African war, the introduction of East Coast fever, the Herero war and the influenza pandemic of 1918.[20] The disease was eventually eradicated from Zimbabwe in 1904, from South Africa in 1924, and from Botswana in 1939.

The disease still persists in northern Namibia and Angola. In Namibia it occurs in Owambo and Kavango; no clinical cases have been reported from Kaokoland since 1983.[2, 5, 7, 8, 31, 44, 45, 52] The disease was reported to occur endemically throughout Angola in 1986.[4]

Aetiology

Contagious bovine pleuropneumonia is caused by *Mycoplasma mycoides mycoides* SC. It is a nonsporulating microorganism which lacks a protecting cell wall and grows readily under aerobic and anaerobic conditions. It is pleomorphic in culture and very small (50–150 μm) in some growth phases.

Various types of serum broth are used as culture media. These should contain meat extract or peptone, or both, as the basic medium, as well as an extract of beer yeast, 10–20 per cent serum, preferably from horses, and sterol. Growth is relatively slow. The mucoid stage which is a characteristic of strains of *M. mycoides mycoides* SC is caused by a matrix of galactan surrounding the colonies and is found after several days of growth in a liquid medium. Typical mycoplasmal colonies form on solid media, each having an average diameter of one millimetre, a dense central core, a granular structure thinning towards the edge, and a finely serrated border. The elementary body is the basic reproductive unit. These give rise in broth culture to homogeneous filaments which, after developing spherical bodies, lead to the formation of coccoid forms.[26, 41, 43]

Two 'types' of *M. mycoides mycoides* are recognized — large colony (LC) and small colony (SC). They cannot be differentiated by immunofluorescence, growth characteristics or metabolic inhibition tests, and are serologically closely related. They are, however, distinct in terms of morphology, cultural characteristics and pathogenicity, and can be distinguished by performing mouse protection tests.

Large-colony types are found almost exclusively in goats, and rarely in sheep, while the SC types are only rarely isolated from species other than cattle, in which they cause CBPP. The LC strains are essentially nonpathogenic for cattle, in which they induce only a very mild, usually subclinical disease under experimental conditions.

Mycoplasma mycoides mycoides LC and the unspeciated strain F38 have been isolated from natural outbreaks of contagious caprine pleuropneumonia (CCPP). There is good evidence for believing that strain F38 causes the classic form of CCPP.[13, 15] *Mycoplasma mycoides mycoides* LC also causes mastitis, arthritis, and, occasionally, contagious caprine pleuropneumonia and a fatal systemic disease in goats.[15]

Mycoplasma mycoides mycoides SC has a low resistance to environmental factors and only survives outside the host for up to three days in tropical areas and up to two weeks in temperate zones. Cultures of *M. mycoides mycoides* SC can be inactivated by ultraviolet radiation within a few minutes. The organism is inactivated within 60 minutes at 50 °C and within two minutes at 60 °C, but can survive for at least one year in frozen, infected lung tissue. The organism is inactivated by 1 per cent phenol solution in three minutes, 0,05 per cent formaldehyde solution in 30 seconds, and a 0,01 per cent mercuric chloride solution in one minute.[41]

The serial passage of *M. mycoides mycoides* SC in culture and in animals alters both its virulence and its pathogenicity.[26]

Epidemiology

The three factors which are of greatest significance in the rate of spread of the disease are closeness of contact, intensity of infection, and the number of susceptible animals.

Natural transmission of CBPP occurs by droplet infection either from cattle with clinical disease or from subclinical carriers which are actively excreting the organism, to susceptible animals in close contact.[23] *Mycoplasma mycoides mycoides* SC occurs in great numbers in bronchial secretions, nasal discharges and exhaled air. Dissemination of infection therefore occurs most easily in closely stabled or trucked animals. Aerosols of infected droplets may spread for 20 m or more, but even under extensive southern African farming conditions spread of the disease may be rapid, as infection is facilitated by the practice of kraaling animals at night and the congregation of large numbers of animals at watering places. Such close contact leads not only to fulminating outbreaks, but also to the maintenance of infection in infected herds for as long as susceptible animals are present.

Direct contact of susceptible with diseased animals appears to be mandatory for transmission. The infection is not transmitted to healthy animals introduced into crushes, stock-sale yards or transport vehicles that have previously been occupied by infected cattle. Neither ingestion of infected fodder nor direct exposure to diseased organs of animals suffering from CBPP, will cause transmission. *Mycoplasma mycoides mycoides* SC may also be present in the urine of cattle affected with severe disease; a 'urinary tract to nose' route of transmission thus appears to be possible.[30]

Apart from clinical cases of the disease, there may be a number of other ways by which the infection can be introduced or maintained. *Mycoplasma mycoides mycoides* SC can occur in the nasal passages of cattle for 40 days or longer during the incubation period of the disease or before a serological response can be detected. Such animals may thus disseminate the infection to susceptible individuals. Another even more important manner in which infection may be introduced or maintained has been proposed. During the course of the disease, pulmonary sequestra may develop in animals recovered from the clinical disease and persist for many months. They are comprised of necrotic tissue which becomes encapsulated by fibrous connective tissue and may harbour viable mycoplasmas for 12 months or longer; affected animals are known as 'lungers'.[20] As long as the capsule around the necrotic tissue persists, there is no great danger that the clinically 'recovered' animal will disseminate the infection.[20] Not all recovered animals harbour sequestra, nor do all sequestra contain viable organisms, and because it is difficult to transmit the disease experimentally from recovered to healthy animals,[53] it has been suggested that the role played by such carriers in disseminating the infection is unimportant. It is, however, suspected that immuno-incompetence resulting from stress may induce the capsule of a sequestrum to break down and thus allow new foci of active pneumonia to develop in surrounding lung tissue, with the result that the animal is once again infective. It is the clinically 'recovered' animal that is therefore mainly responsible for the spreading of disease under such circumstances.[20] Young calves do not constitute an important reservoir of infection, as the organisms in them localize mostly in the joints.[23]

The intensity of infection is related to the concentration of infective organisms in a herd at any given time; it is highest during acute outbreaks but, from a transmission and control point of view, low intensities of infection are more important. Low intensities occur during the early stages of an outbreak in a susceptible herd and result in a slow spread, long incubation periods and a slow build-up of infection. Under these circumstances, many months may pass before epidemics become apparent. This insidious method of spread is found in southern Africa.

The level of susceptibility of animals in a given herd varies considerably between individuals. Ten to 60 per cent of cattle may be resistant, and as few as 8 per cent of a herd may develop clinical signs.[26] Survivors in an outbreak have a substantial degree of resistance. Thus, in a closed-herd situation, even under African conditions, there is a tendency for the disease to disappear, albeit over a long period of time. In this situation newly born calves constitute a nucleus of susceptible animals, but they do not influence the disappearance of the disease provided the herd remains closed. In Africa, movement of animals between herds is common and is the direct cause of many outbreaks. Under these conditions the partly resistant, partly susceptible herds, so common in endemic areas, provide ideal conditions for CBPP to persist undetected for long periods.

Mycoplasma mycoides mycoides SC affects cattle and water buffaloes (*Bubalus arnee*),[13] but conflicting opinions exist as to whether there is a difference in susceptibility between *Bos indicus* and *Bos taurus* cattle. Although some workers have found the former to be more susceptible,[18] others[30] have detected no significant difference between the two. T1-broth-culture vaccine is also equally efficacious in both types.

Under natural conditions there is no evidence that clinical disease occurs in species other than cattle and water buffaloes.[25] No evidence of infection was found in roan antelope (*Hippotragus equinus*), oribi (*Ouribea ourebi*), white-eared kob (*Kobus kob. leukotus*) and giraffe (*Giraffa camelopardalis*). Yak (*Bos greunniens*), and bison (*Bison bison*) are probably susceptible.[25] Antibodies to *M. mycoides mycoides* SC were found in African buffalo (*Syncerus caffer*), impala (*Aepyceros melampus*) and in camels in Kenya.[26] Experimental infection with *M. mycoides mycoides* SC has caused the death of two African buffaloes. Both had high complement fixing antibody titres and *M. mycoides mycoides* SC was isolated in pure culture from one of them. Contagious bovine pleuropneumonia was not transmitted from infected cattle to an African buffalo which had been in contact with them for 135 days.[47]

Pathogenesis

Infection via the respiratory tract causes bronchiolitis and pneumonia.[23] In this process *Mycoplasma mycoides mycoides* SC firmly attaches to the surface of epithelial cells, thus being prevented from being eliminated in mucous secretions. This cellular adhesion, whereby the surface of the mucous membranes can be colonized, is central to the pathogenicity of the mycoplasmas.[26]

The pathogenesis of lungsickness is poorly understood, but mechanisms may include a number of the following. Morphologic and metabolic alterations in host cells appear to be induced by subtle, complex chemical processes. A diffusible toxin produced by *M. mycoides mycoides* SC is thought to stimulate fibrous connective tissue proliferation, resulting in capsule formation around infected necrotic tissue.[19] A carbohydrate — galactan, which is a major antigen present in *M. mycoides mycoides* SC — not only potentiates subsequent infection with live organisms,[21] but also has profound physiological effects similar to those of the endotoxins of Gram-negative bacteria.[19]

Factors other than the presence of *M. mycoides mycoides* SC, such as immunologically induced cell damage and the induction of autoimmune and hypersensitivity reactions, appear necessary for the development of lesions.[26] Autoimmune and hypersensitivity reactions may be due to the transfer of antigens between the mycoplasma and the host cell wall.[26] Antibodies, particularly agglutinating antibodies, are involved in the pathogenesis of local lesions in target organs. This mechanism may also cause localization of *M. mycoides mycoides* SC in tissues. The hypothesis is further supported by the fact that agglutinating antibodies are directed against galactan, which is antigenically similar to components of normal lung tissue.[21, 26]

Clinical signs

The clinical signs have been reviewed and are summarized in the following paragraphs.[20, 23, 26, 43, 51]

Under natural conditions the incubation period is rarely less than three to six weeks, and may exceed three months. Under conditions of massive aerosol infection, the incubation period may be as short as five to 35 days. Cattle which have been in contact with animals suffering from CBPP should, however, be considered as being infectious for at least six months after exposure.

Clinical disease may be acute, subacute, or chronic, but the majority of cases are subclinical. In adults, the clinical signs are attributable to the pulmonary lesions.

Acutely affected animals have an elevated body temperature, are listless, and manifest signs of respiratory distress. They often grunt painfully and occasional soft, moist coughs are heard which are aggravated by, and become more frequent with, exercise or percussion of the chest. As the disease progresses, coughing increases both in frequency and in intensity, the animal is reluctant to move, and stands with its head extended, mouth open, tongue protruded, and the elbows turned out. Contraction of the muscle of the abdominal wall occurs after each inspiration, while expiration is frequently followed by a characteristic grunt or groan. There is a mucoid discharge from the nostrils and frothy saliva accumulates around the mouth. The locality of the affected areas in the lungs is revealed by the presence of dull sounds during percussion. Percussion of the chest wall reveals an increasingly dull sound as the lesion enlarges. During the later stages of the disease the animals may show a nasal discharge which becomes mucopurulent, subcutaneous oedema of the lower parts of the chest and abdomen, and emaciation. In a small percentage of affected animals, the difficulty in breathing is aggravated by the presence of large volumes of exudate in the thorax.

In subacute cases the lung lesions are more localized and less extensive, and an infrequent cough is the only clinical sign. Usually the lesions resolve without the disease being noticed clinically.

The only clinical signs in chronic cases are emaciation and a cough which commonly occurs when the animal rises.

In calves up to the age of six months, signs of arthritis only may be manifested. Pulmonary lesions do not develop.

Once clinical signs are noticeable, the course of the disease is usually two to three weeks; acutely affected animals, however, may die within one week because of massive pulmonary infarctions. In many cases the clinical signs gradually disappear, after which the general condition of affected animals improves rapidly. Severely affected animals may take many months to recover. Recovered cattle may retain sequestra in their lungs in which the infection remains latent. Relapses may be precipitated by stress factors.

Pathology

At necropsy, animals that die of lungsickness are usually emaciated, with the most characteristic lesions occurring in the lungs and thoracic cavity.[12, 20, 23, 24, 36, 37,54]

During the acute stage of the disease there is often uni- or bilateral pleural effusion that may exceed 10 litres. The exudate is yellow to yellowish-grey, clear or turbid, contains pieces of fibrin, and is generally accompanied by a localized or diffuse, pronounced fibrinous pleuritis. During the early stages of the disease, multiple small, well-circumscribed areas of consolidation are scattered throughout the lungs in some animals. Well-developed lesions arising from a severe fibrinous pleuropneumonia in acutely affected lungs tend to be unilateral, involving a portion of a lobe **(Figure 177.1)**, an entire lobe, or more than one lobe. The pneumonic areas are characterized by marbling caused by the intermingling of lobules which show varying stages of grey or red hepatization, and of relatively unaffected lobules. The marbling is accentuated by the distension of interlobular septa and the interstitium surrounding the vessels and airways by a sero-fibrinous, sometimes blood-stained exudate **(Figure 177.2)**. In more severely affected animals, pronounced haemorrhage may mask the septal involvement.

Copious amounts of a clear, yellowish fluid exude from the cut surface of the lungs, the walls of the bronchi are thickened by oedema, and bronchi often contain fibrinous material. The interlobular septa and the parenchyma bordering areas of pneumonia may be oedematous. Multiple thrombi are found along the course of the lymphatics in the interlobular septa, with subsequent irregular lymphangiectasis which often imparts a 'beaded' appearance to the septa. Infarcts, varying in size from about 10–300 mm, are frequently present in the affected lung tissue. These result from thrombosis of inter- or intralobular arteries and are manifested as well-demarcated areas of necrosis separated from the surrounding tissue by irregular, yellowish-grey reaction zones. The infarcts subsequently become sequestered from the adjacent parenchyma by granulation tissue, and thereafter they are referred to as sequestra.

In chronic cases, one or more sequestra **(Figure 177.3)**, which may vary from less than 10 mm to 200–300 mm in diameter and involve more than one lobe, are usually present in the lungs. In some animals they may be very large and even involve a whole lobe. Over a period of three to four months smaller sequestra become replaced by fibrotic scars,[12] while the larger ones often persist for 12 months or more. Recently formed sequestra are surrounded by a thin fibrous capsule, the necrotic content is firm, pinkish to yellowish-grey, and the original pulmonary architecture may still be discernible to some extent. In longer-standing cases the connective tissue thickens and a thin layer of yellowish, semi-solid material may separate the firmer necrotic contents from the wall. In such sequestra the contents 'shell out' easily. Secondary bacterial infection of sequestra frequently occurs, resulting in a purulent liquefied content which, after rupture of the capsule, may escape into the bronchi.

In animals which have completely recovered — a process which may take many months —former infarcts are represented by fibrous scars, and areas of scar tissue are present in the healed lung and pleura. The latter is often thickened with fibrous adhesions remaining between pleural surfaces.

Lesions in other organs are often seen in acute cases of lungsickness. A serofibrinous pericarditis with copious amounts of exudate occurs in many cases. The mediastinal and bronchial lymph nodes are markedly oedematous, while necrotic foci of up to 40 mm in diameter may also be present in them.[23]

Infarcts, which are generally multiple, small and whitish, are not uncommon in the kidneys,[12, 23, 29] where they probably result from occlusion of the renal arteries by septic emboli originating in the lungs.[12]

A serofibrinous polyarthritis and tendosynovitis, affecting particularly the carpus and tarsus, is a common lesion in infected calves.[23, 36, 50] The joints may remain swollen and thickened months after infection as a result of severe fibrosis of the joint capsule. Calves may also develop a vegetative, necrogranulomatous, valvular endocarditis and a myocarditis.[49] Myocardial lesions occur mainly in the atria.

'Occult' cases of CBPP have been reported,[20] in which only the mediastinal lymph nodes are oedematous and there are no discernible lesions in the lungs. The causative organism can be isolated from these lymph nodes.

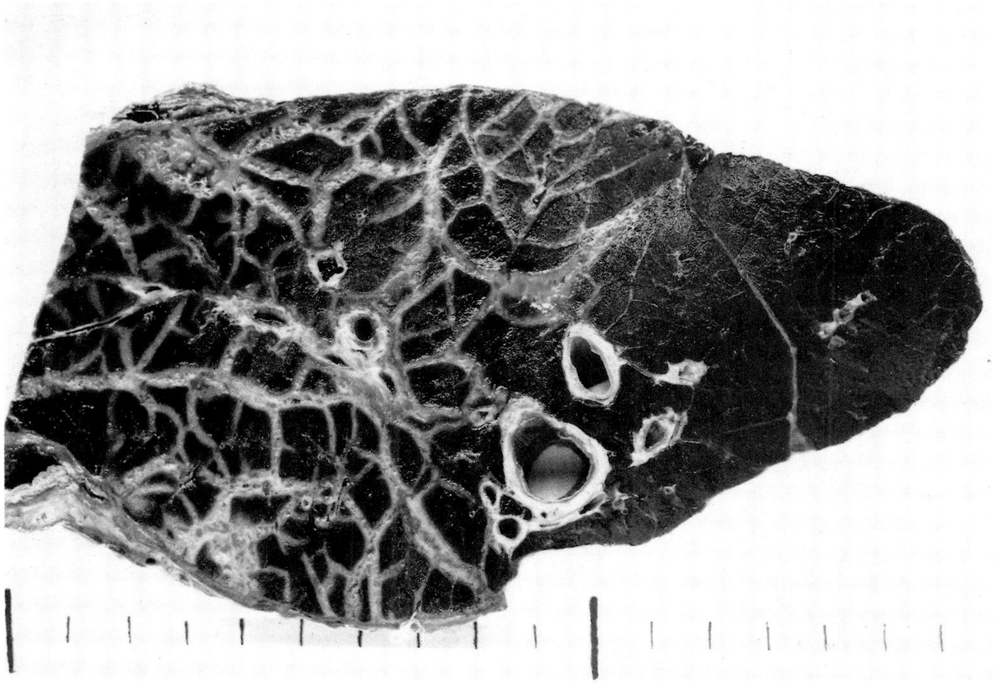

Figure 177.1 Portion of affected lobe showing prominent interlobular septa

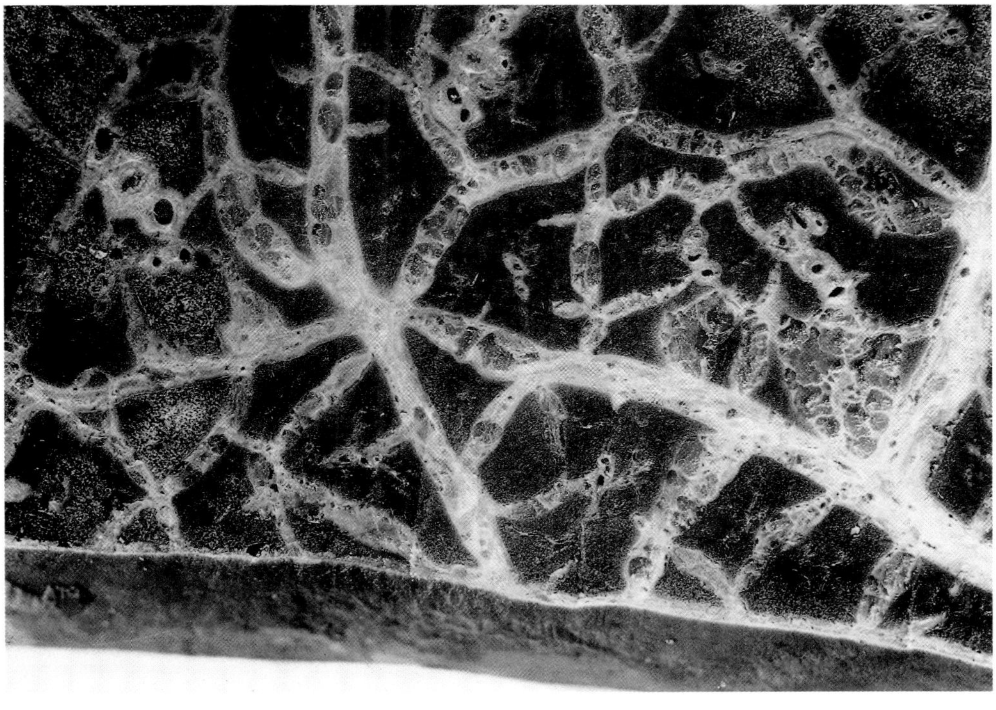

Figure 177.2 Closer view of prominent interlobular septa. Note lymphangiectasis in the septa

Microscopically, one of the most characteristic features of the lesion in the lungs is the presence of different stages of the pneumonic process in adjacent alveoli or lobules, some being in an early stage while others are in later stages. Initially there is severe hyperaemia of the alveolar capillaries, after which the alveoli become flooded with serofibrinous exudate containing variable numbers of neutrophils, macrophages and red blood cells. As the lesions progress, the amount of fibrin increases, and in some areas numerous necrotic neutrophils fill the alveoli. The interlobular septa are widened by the accumulation of copious amounts of serofibrinous exudate and irregularly distended lymphatics. Necrotic neutrophils collect along the inner walls of the lymphatics and particularly along the margins of the septa, where a distinct inflammatory zone is frequently discernible. A fibrinopurulent exudate similar to that in the alveoli is often found in and around bronchi and bronchioles of

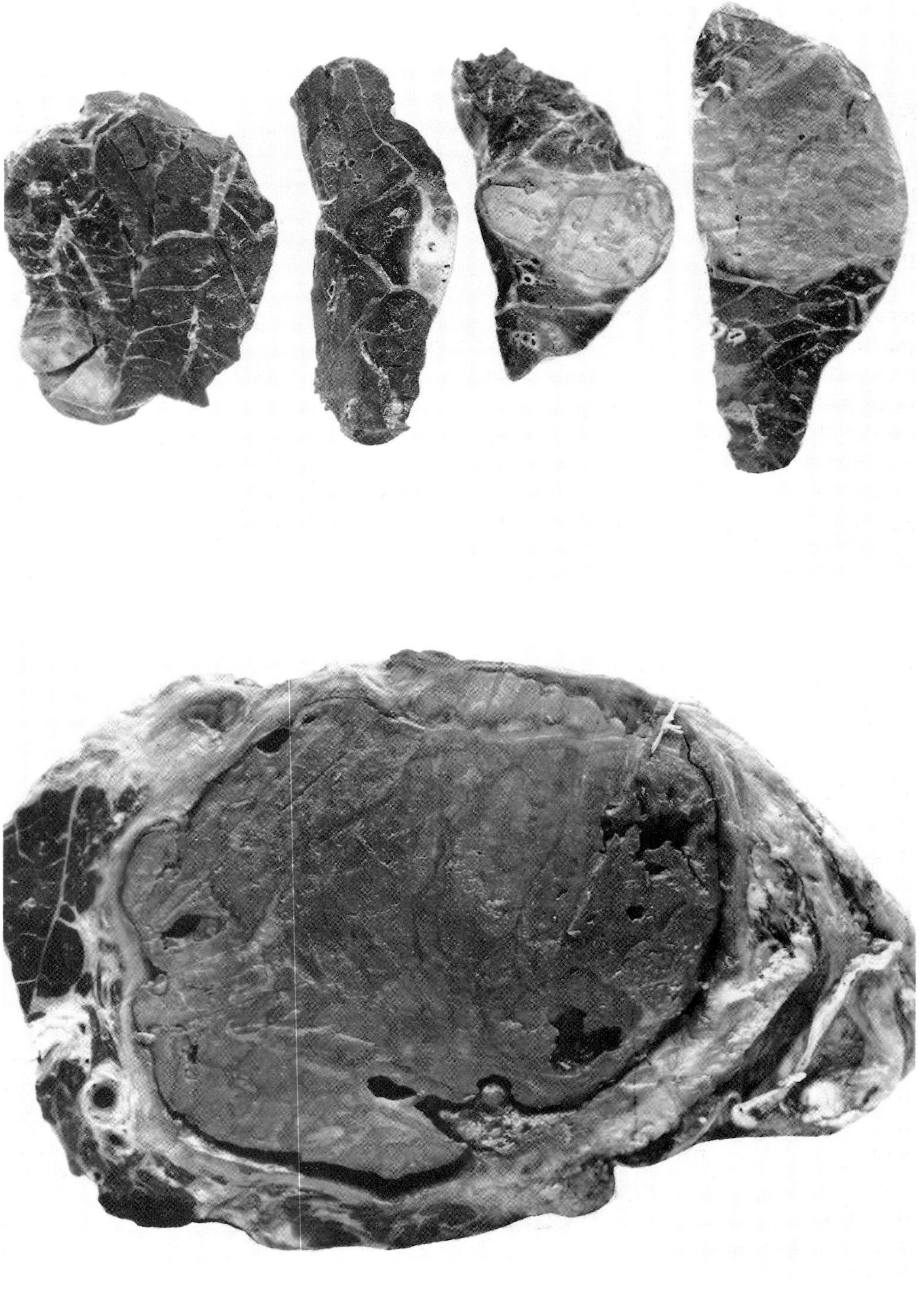

Figure 177.3 Pulmonary sequestra of varying sizes in chronic cases

affected lobules. The bronchial mucosa and submucosa are oedematous and infiltrated by neutrophils and macrophages. The peribronchial and perivascular areas, and especially the lymphatics, are widely distended by an exudate of the same nature as that in the septa. As the lesions progress, these areas and the septa become thickened by fibrous connective tissue and by infiltrations of lymphocytes and plasma cells. In some parts of the lungs the alveolar walls contain varying numbers of round cells and evidence of fibroplasia.

Vasculitis and thrombosis of intralobular and interlobular arteries and the lymphatics are frequently present in pneumonic parts. Involvement of the vessels culminates in necrosis of a lobule or part of a lobule, or in infarction of multiple lobules and intervening septa.[12] Initially a zone of necrotic inflammatory cells separates the infarcted areas from the surrounding tissue, but later, granulation tissue followed by fibrosis at the edges of these lesions sequestrate the necrotic tissue from the neighbouring parenchyma. Follicle-like aggregates of lymphocytes may be evident in the fibrous capsule of some of the sequestra, as well as in the peribronchial and perivascular areas.

Microscopically the lesions in lymph nodes are characterized by hyperplasia of lymphocytes in the follicles and medullary cords; the accumulation of oedematous fluid, fibrin and neutrophils in the subcapsular, cortical and medullary sinuses and trabeculae; vasculitis and thrombosis of blood vessels and lymphatics in the trabeculae; and necrosis of the lymphoid tissue.[12, 23]

Joint lesions in acute cases consist of hyperaemia, oedema and predominantly prominent infiltration of lymphocytes and macrophages in the synovial membranes. Thrombosis of lymphatics and blood vessels, and fibrin deposition on the synovial surfaces also occur. In chronic cases the joint capsule is thickened by connective tissue and hypertrophy of the villi of the synovium in some areas.[50]

Diagnosis

In a fully-fledged outbreak a presumptive diagnosis is based on clinical signs and necropsy findings, but laboratory confirmation is essential. Diagnosis may, however, be difficult in the early stages of an outbreak when only a few cases occur. The introduction of, or contact with, new animals is always an important consideration which must be thoroughly investigated.

When laboratory examinations can be undertaken within hours, pleural exudate and/or affected lung tissue collected aseptically should be submitted fresh or on ice for cultural examination.[41] If a delay is likely in the laboratory examination, pleural or lung fluid can be absorbed onto sterile filter-paper strips which are then allowed to dry before dispatch. Affected portions of lung should also be collected in 10 per cent buffered-formalin for histopathological examination.

In the live animal, serology offers the only credible means of diagnosis. Serological tests for the diagnosis of CBPP can be divided into two main types: tests to detect antigen and tests to detect antibody.

Galactan, the major antigenic component of *M. mycoides mycoides* SC, is elaborated by the organisms and can be detected in all body fluids during and for some time after the acute stage of the disease. Since galactan is extremely stable, it can be detected in putrefied material as well as in formalin-fixed samples of lung tissue. The agar-gel precipitation test based on the Ouchterlony double-immunodiffusion test is the test of choice for the detection of galactan. For this purpose, hyperimmune serum, preferably produced in sheep, is used. Depending on the concentration of galactan in the test sample, precipitating lines appear within hours. In acute cases, all afflicted animals can be detected; in chronic cases, where sequestration and encapsulation occur, the detection rate is considerably lower. Radial immunodiffusion and counter-immunoelectrophoresis have also been applied with success to the detection of circulating antigen in CBPP. The latter test has the advantage that results can be obtained within an hour. Immunofluorescent antibody techniques have been successfully used to demonstrate the causative organism in lung sections.

Two different test systems have been widely used for the detection of antibodies to CBPP. The complement-fixation (CF) test based on the technique of Campbell and Turner is the most useful test to detect antibodies. It is the procedure recommended by the Office International des Épizooties (OIE)[6] and has also been adapted as a rapid field test.[22] It has an excellent correlation between positive test results and active infection, and because of its lower sensitivity, results obtained in the CF test are usually very specific. However, as in the case of the agar-gel precipitation test, animals with encapsulated sequestra, in which antibody formation is not always stimulated, might be missed. Six weeks after the onset of disease, the appearance of CF antibodies invariably indicates the presence of lung lesions.

The efficacy of the CF test has been compared with that of the passive haemagglutination (PHA) and the slide agglutination tests.[14] The PHA test can detect antibodies against *M. mycoides mycoides* at lower levels and for a longer time than the CF test in animals suffering from subclinical or chronic disease after vaccination. This could be an asset when monitoring the immune status of vaccinated cattle, nearly all of which are CF-negative two months after vaccination. Antibodies detectable by the slide agglutination test tend to disappear at an earlier stage of the disease process, which renders this test less suitable than the other two. The enzyme-linked immunosorbent assay (ELISA), however, enables antibodies to be detected for as long as two years after vaccination[38] and may well eventually replace the CF test, but its reliability is influenced by the occurrence of non-specific reactions caused by its high sensitivity.

Differential diagnosis

Acute CBPP must be differentiated from pneumonic pasteurellosis, in which *Pasteurella haemolytica* and (less commonly) *P. multocida* play major causative roles, and from haemorrhagic septicaemia caused by *Pasteurella multocida* types B and E. Haemorrhagic septicaemia is often characterized by swellings of the laryngeal region and brisket, and has an acute to hyperacute course. In acute pneumonic pasteurellosis a serofibrinous pleural exudate and fibrinous pleuropneumonia are present. Smears from the affected lung or, in some cases, blood smears stained with Giemsa, Leishman or methylene blue will show the typical bipolar organisms and pure cultures of the organism involved, and can be isolated in most cases.[23, 43] Haemorrhagic septicaemia caused by *P. multocida* type E has been the cause of death of many cattle in the Caprivi district of Namibia. The acute serofibrinous pleuropneumonia that results from aspirating foreign material into the lungs often simulates CBPP very closely.

The sequestra in chronic cases of CBPP should not be confused with lesions associated with actinobacillosis in the lungs or, more commonly, with old encapsulated echinococcus cysts. Cultural and microscopic pathological examinations will distinguish a sequestrum from these lesions. The lung lesions of CBPP should not be confused with those of East Coast fever, which commonly have a marked pulmonary oedema but no pleuritis or pneumonia. Demonstration of schizonts in lymph node smears and schizonts and piroplasms in blood smears will confirm this disease.[23, 43] Bovine herpesvirus 1 infection (infectious bovine rhinotracheitis) generally causes lesions in the upper respiratory tract, but in some animals a bronchopneumonia may develop which is characterized by a necrotizing bronchitis and atelectasis and is often complicated by secondary bacterial infections such as pasteurellosis.

Control

The methods employed for the control of CBPP are determined by the specific epidemiological situation, animal husbandry methods applied, and the availability and effectiveness of veterinary services in a specific country. Control methods used in southern Africa include stamping-out by slaughter when CBPP spreads into disease-free areas, vaccination and movement restrictions in endemic areas, and quarantine and serological testing in specially designated disease-control areas. Additional measures are enforced in non-endemic countries in southern Africa in order to prevent the introduction and possible spread of the disease.[4] These measures include the declaration of CBPP as a controlled disease, prohibition of the importation of cattle from infected countries, and quarantine and other control measures at frontiers.

Mycoplasmas are sensitive to antibiotics such as tetracyclines and chloramphenicol.[26] Oxytetracycline at usual dosage rates for three days has been recommended,[11] while tylosin at the dosage rate of 7,5 mg/kg body weight administered at 12-hour intervals for three to five days has been used successfully.[23] Chemotherapy is not used in the control of CBPP as it is highly likely that carriers will develop. Antibiotics have, however, been used to control post-vaccinal reactions, such as those caused by the V-5 vaccine used in the Kavango region of Namibia in 1984.

Vaccination is very important in the control of lungsickness in endemic areas. The efficacy of live vaccines is directly related to their virulence and to the number of live organisms per immunizing dose. Virulent strains stimulate the best immunity,[28] but they also induce the most severe and undesirable local and systemic reactions which may even result in death.[42] The live attenuated vaccines currently in use are a compromise between virulence, immunogenicity and safety.[10] At the end of the last century it was commonly thought that if vaccination was to be effective, a local lesion had to be produced at the site of inoculation. This situation was reversed only 15 years ago at the insistence of cattle owners fearing post-vaccination reactions and mortality, with the result that present vaccines cause only mild lesions, if any, at the injection site.

The knowledge on currently available vaccines has been reviewed.[41] Only vaccines containing live mycoplasmas which have been specifically selected for immunogenicity and which, after attenuation, cause only a minor local reaction after intradermal or subcutaneous administration, are suitable. Vaccination against CBPP is never harmless, and a number of considerations should be taken into account. As a rule, *Bos taurus* breeds appear to be more susceptible to post-vaccination reactions than Zebu *(Bos indicus)* breeds, but even within a given species or breed, individual variations in susceptibility to vaccination reactions and infection do exist. The vaccination of pregnant cows should be avoided. Calves vaccinated at less than three months of age generally show insignificant local reactions, and arthritis, synovitis and valvular endocarditis may also develop. For this reason vaccination of calves less than six to eight months old should be avoided.

The efficacy of vaccines against CBPP must be judged on a group or herd basis, as vaccination is aimed at obtaining an increased average immunity of the herd, rather than at protecting all the individuals in the herd. Thus, vaccination against CBPP will only be effective as a control measure if it is administered to all animals in a population for an adequate length of time.

The preferred vaccination site was the tip of the tail for many decades, but the trend today is to administer vaccines subcutaneously immediately behind the shoulder.[40]

Varying success has been obtained with different vaccines. The live T-1 and KH_3-J strain vaccines are the most effective presently in use in Africa. Cattle which are immunized with them become infected; organisms are maintained in, and can be isolated from, their lymph nodes for extended periods of time. There is no evidence that these vaccine strains revert to virulence, although the T-1 strain vaccine has been shown to revert to full virulence in cattle after six successive passages by endobronchial instillation.[10] The T-1 broth-culture vaccine has been used extensively in East African countries and is effective in controlling CBPP in breeds of cattle of both *B. taurus* and *B. indicus* origin.[16, 27]

The T-1 strain of vaccine is more virulent than the KH_3-J strain, but has good immunogenic properties, giving an immunity to most, but not all, vaccinated cattle for at least one year. In 30–100 per cent of vaccinated animals, seroconversion occurs by the eighth day, peaks at the 21st day and disappears by the 60th day. The extent of post-inoculation reactions cannot be foreseen when it is administered for the first time, but they are usually more severe in infected herds. In *B. indicus* breeds 1 per cent of vaccinated animals show a localized erythema followed by an oedematous swelling at the injection site. In *B. taurus* breeds reactions tend to be more severe, and up to 25 per cent of animals vaccinated in the tail-tip show local reactions of varying intensity, with or without ulceration and necrosis. Similar reactions at the vaccination site behind the shoulder are also frequent, and may be accompanied by secondary bacterial infection. Antibiotic chemotherapy should be given about 20 days after vaccination.

The KH_3-J strain vaccine is avirulent, and does not have any deleterious effects on cattle at the site of inoculation. It does not induce an immunity of more than six months' duration and in some infected animals it may provoke the formation of lung sequestra. If seroconversion occurs, it is of short duration. As no post-vaccinal reactions occur at the inoculation site, this vaccine is preferred in *B. taurus* breeds. Animals should be vaccinated biannually.

Freeze-dried T-1 and KH_3-J vaccines have a concentration of at least 10^8 viable units per dose and a shelf life of at least one to two months when stored at 28 °C; three to six weeks at 37 °C, and six to seven days at 45 °C. If stored at -20 °C their shelf life is at least one year.[41] Once diluted, the vaccine must be protected from light and heat and must be used within one hour.

The live V-5 strain vaccine which had been used extensively in Australia was introduced into southern Africa in 1976. Although it stimulated good protection, its use was discontinued in Namibia in 1983 because of its virulence and consequent severe post-vaccinal reactions.

Lungsickness is a notifiable disease in Namibia, where it is controlled by the use of vaccination and the application of quarantine measures. The importation of cattle from infected countries is prohibited. Quarantine and movement-control measures are applied at frontiers and inside the country. Annual vaccination with a locally manufactured freeze-dried T-1 strain is practised in infected areas, and stamping-out measures are adopted should the disease spread into disease-free areas. In the four northern boundary districts of Namibia, all cattle are also inspected fortnightly by veterinary inspectors, no live cattle are allowed to move to the south from these districts, and cattle may only be slaughtered at abattoirs within their borders. Movement of cattle within these districts is also subject to veterinary permission.

In Angola, CBPP is a notifiable disease and control programmes are applied in some areas.[17] Quarantine measures and movement control are enforced within the country and vaccination is practised.[4, 34] The systematic testing of cattle by the CF test, slaughter of positive animals, and the creation of disease-free areas with strict quarantine procedures were envisaged in 1975 as future steps for the control of CBPP in Angola.[48] It is unknown which, if any, of these measures have been put into practice.

Contagious bovine pleuropneumonia has been eradicated from Zambia and stringent control measures are taken in the Western and North-Western Provinces to prevent spread of the disease from Angola to these areas. These measures include the isolation of the cattle population in the border area within a fenced-in, patrolled 10–20 km-wide zone which runs parallel to the international boundary.[35] The cattle within the zone are vaccinated biannually and are only allowed to leave the area if destined for immediate slaughter at one specified abattoir in the Western Province and after three consecutive negative CF tests during a quarantine period of 60 days.

References

1 **AKAFEKWA, G.I., 1975.** The diagnosis, control and eradication of contagious bovine pleuropneumonia in Zambia. *Bulletin of Epizootic Diseases of Africa*, 84, 429–449.

2 **ANON., 1916 – 87.** *Annual Reports of the Division of Veterinary Services*, Private Bag 12022, Windhoek, Namibia.

3 **ANON., 1976.** *Annual Report of the Department of Veterinary and Tsetse Control Service*, Government Printer, Lusaka, Zambia.

4 **ANON., 1986.** Food and Agriculture Organization. *FAO-WHO-OIE Animal Health Yearbook*. Rome, Italy: Food and Agriculture Organization of the United Nations.

5 **ANON., 1986.** *World Animal Health Zoo-sanitary Situation and Methods of Control of Animal Diseases 1985*. Vol. I. Part 2. Paris: Office International des Épizooties.

6 **ANON., 1986.** *International Zoo-sanitary Code*. 5th edn. Paris: Office International des Épizooties.

7 **ANON., 1987.** *Bulletin of the OIE*. Paris: Office International des Épizooties.

8 **ANON., 1987.** *World Animal Health. Animal Health Status and Disease Control Methods*. Vol. II. No. 2 (1986). Paris: Office International des Épizooties.

9 **ARAUJO, J.S., 1955.** Methods profilaticos na peripneumonia contagiosa em Africa. *Boletin da Instituto Veterinarias do Angola*, 6, 25–42.

10 **BARILE, M.F., 1985.** Immunization against mycoplasma infections. *In*: RAZIN, S. & BARILE, M.F., (eds). *The Mycoplasmas*. Vol. IV. Orlando, Florida: Academic Press Inc.

11 **BRUNNER, H. & LABER, G., 1985.** Chemotherapy of mycoplasma infections. *In*: RAZIN, S. & BARILE, M.F., (eds).

The Mycoplasmas. Vol. IV. Orlando, Florida: Academic Press Inc.

12 **BYGRAVE, A.C., MOULTON, J.E. & SHIFRINE, M., 1968.** Clinical, serological and pathological findings in an outbreak of contagious bovine pleuropneumonia. *Bulletin of Epizootic Diseases of Africa*, 16, 21–46.

13 **CASSELL, G.H., CLYDE, W.A. & DAVIS, J.K., 1985.** Mycoplasmal respiratory infections. *In*: RAZIN, S. & BARILE, M.F., (eds). *The Mycoplasmas*. Vol. IV. Orlando, Florida: Academic Press Inc.

14 **CHIMA, J.C. & PAM, G., 1985.** Contagious bovine pleuropneumonia: A comparison between the passive haemagglutination test and the complement fixation test. *Revue Scientifique et Technique de l'Office International des Épizooties*, 4, 517–522.

15 **COLE, B.C., WASHBURN, L.R. & TAYLOR-ROBINSON, D., 1985.** Mycoplasma-induced arthritis. *In*: RAZIN, S. & BARILE, M.F., (eds). *The Mycoplasmas*, Vol. IV. Orlando, Florida: Academic Press Inc.

16 **DALEEL, E.E., 1972.** Report: Contagious bovine pleuropneumonia (CBPP) T1-broth vaccine safety trials in Sudanese cattle. *Bulletin of Epizootic Diseases of Africa*, 20, 199–202.

17 **FERNANDES, A.J.H., NOBRE, J.M. & MANUEL DA GRACA, H., 1971.** La situation zoo-sanitaire en Angola. *Bulletin of Epizootic Diseases of Africa*, 76, 545–560.

18 **FRANCIS, J., 1973.** Susceptibility of *Bos indicus* and *Bos taurus* cattle to pleuropneumonia. *The Veterinary Record*, 92, 401.

19 **GABRIDGE, M.G., CHANDLER, D.K.F. & DANIELS, M.J., 1985.** Pathogenicity factors in mycoplasmas and spiroplasmas. *In*: RAZIN, S. & BARILE, M.F., (eds). *The Mycoplasmas*. Vol. IV. Orlando, Florida: Academic Press Inc.

20 **HENNING, M.W., 1956.** *Animal Diseases in South Africa*. 3rd edn. Pretoria: Central News Agency Ltd.

21 **HOWARD, C.J. & TAYLOR, G., 1985.** Humoral and cell-mediated immunity. *In*: RAZIN, S. & BARILE, M.F., (eds). *The Mycoplasmas*. Vol. IV. Orlando, Florida: Academic Press Inc.

22 **HUDDART, J.E., 1971.** A brief outline of the CBPP situation in Zambia. *Farming in Zambia*, 7, 18–20.

23 **HUDSON, J.R., 1971.** Contagious bovine pleuropneumonia. *Food and Agricultural Organization Agricultural Studies*, No. 86. Rome: Food and Agricultural Organization of the United Nations.

24 **HUTYRA, F. & MAREK, J., 1926.** *Special Pathology and Therapeutics of the Diseases of Domesticated Animals*. Vol. I. 3rd edn. London: Baillière, Tindall & Cox.

25 **LEACH, T.M., 1957.** The occurrence of contagious bovine pleuropneumonia in species other than domesticated cattle. *Bulletin of Epizootic Diseases of Africa*, 5, 325–328.

26 **LOSOS, G.J., 1986.** *Infectious Tropical Diseases of Domestic Animals*. Harlow: Longman.

27 **MASIGA, W.N. & READ, W.C.S., 1972.** Comparative susceptibility of *Bos indicus* and *Bos taurus* to contagious bovine pleuropneumonia and the efficacy of the T1-broth-culture vaccine. *The Veterinary Record*, 90, 499–502.

28 **MASIGA, W.N. & WINDSOR, R.S., 1975.** Immunity to contagious bovine pleuropneumonia. *The Veterinary Record*, 97, 350–351.

29 **MASIGA, W.N. & WINDSOR, R.S., 1978.** Some evidence of an age susceptibility to contagious bovine pleuropneumonia. *Research in Veterinary Science*, 24, 328–333.

30 **MASIGA, W.N., WINDSOR, R.S. & READ, W.C.S., 1972.** A new mode of spread of contagious bovine pleuropneumonia. *The Veterinary Record*, 90, 247–248.

31 **McINTYRE, G., 1939.** The lungsickness campaign in the Caprivi-Zipfel. *Journal of the South African Veterinary Medical Association*, 10, 4–12.

32 **MENDES, A.M., 1953.** Contagious bovine pleuropneumonia control in Angola. *Bulletin of Epizootic Diseases of Africa*, 1, 426–432.

33 **MENDES, A.M., 1957.** Aspectos do problema da peripneumonia em Angola. *Revista de Ciencias Veterinarias*, 52, 1–12.

34 **MENDES, A.M., 1961.** Present situation of contagious pleuropneumonia in Angolan cattle. *Bulletin de l'Office International des Épizooties*, 56, 893–899.

35 **MERKER, M., 1975.** *Die Bekämpfung eines Ausbruchs der Lungenseuche des Rindes in Zambia*. Inaugural Dissertation, Veterinary Medical Faculty, Zürich.

36 **MEYER, K.F., 1909.** Notes on the pathological anatomy of pleuropneumonia contagiosa bovum. *Department of Agriculture, Commemorative Publication, Transvaal Veterinary Bacteriological Laboratories*, 135–163.

37 **NIEBERLE, K. & COHRS, P., 1967.** *Textbook of the Special Pathological Anatomy of Domestic Animals*. Oxford: Pergamon Press.

38 **ONOVIRAN, O. & TAYLOR-ROBINSON, D., 1979.** Detection of antibody against *Mycoplasma mycoides* subsp. *mycoides* in cattle by an enzyme-linked immunosorbent assay. *The Veterinary Record*, 105, 165–167.

39 **PEIRS, J.B., 1989.** *The Dead will Arise*. Johannesburg: Ravan Press.

40 **PROVOST, A., 1982.** Advantages of a joint campaign against rinderpest and bovine pleuropneumonia. *Revue Scientifique et Technique de l'OIE*, 1, 687–704.

41 **PROVOST, A., PERREAU, P., BREARD, A., LE GOFF, C., MARTEL, J.L. & COTTEW, G.S., 1987.** Contagious bovine pleuropneumonia. *Revue Scientifique et Technique de l'OIE*, 6, 625–679.

42 **REVELL, S.G., 1973.** Local reactions following CBPP vaccination in Zambia. *Tropical Animal Health and Production*, 5, 246–252.

43 **ROBERTSON, A., 1976.** *Handbook on Animal Diseases in the Tropics*. 3rd edn. London: British Veterinary Association.

44 **SCHNEIDER, H.P., 1977.** *Analyse der Tiergesundheitssituation in Südwestafrika/Namibia – Vergangenheit und Gegenwart*, Inaugural Dissertation, Universität Giessen, West Germany.

45 **SCHNEIDER, H.P., 1987.** 100 Years of veterinary legislation and early forms of disease control in South West Africa/Namibia. *Proceedings of the XXIII World Veterinary Congress*, Montreal, Canada.

46 **SHAW, C.D., 1971.** Zambia. Contagious bovine pleuropneumonia 1970 outbreak. Progress report, April 1971. *Bulletin de l'Office International des Épizooties*, 76, 673–677.

47 **SHIFRINE, M., STONE, S.S. & STAAK, C., 1970.** Contagious bovine pleuropneumonia in African buffalo (*Syncerus caffer*). *Bulletin of Epizootic Diseases of Africa*, 18, 201–205.

48 **SOUSA, M. DE F., DUARTE, V.M.S. & SOARES, A.E., 1975.** Le problème de la péripneumonie contagieuse des bovines en Angola. *Bulletin de l'Office International des Épizooties*, 84, 451–462.

49 **TRETHEWIE, E.R. & TURNER, A.W., 1961.** Preventive tail-tip inoculation of calves against bovine contagious pleuropneumonia. II. Vegetative endocarditis (valvitis) and myocarditis as sequelae to post-inoculation arthritis. *Australian Veterinary Journal*, 37, 27–36.

50 **TURNER, A.W. & TRETHEWIE, E.R., 1961.** Preventive tail-tip inoculation of calves against bovine contagious pleuropneumonia. I. Influence of age upon inoculation tail reactions, serological responses, and the incidence of swollen joints. *Australian Veterinary Journal*, 37, 1–8.

51 **VAN BLERK, N.S., 1965.** The pathogenic mycoplasmas of domestic animals. *Journal of the South African Veterinary Medical Association*, 36, 547–553.

52 **WEBB, H.M., 1935.** Contagious bovine pleuropneumonia of cattle. *The Veterinary Journal*, 91, 446–449.

53 **WINDSOR, R.S. & MASIGA, W.N., 1977.** Investigations into the role of carrier animals in the spread of contagious bovine pleuropneumonia. *Research in Veterinary Science*, 23, 224–229.

54 **WOODWARD, 1870.** The pathological anatomy and histology of the respiratory organs in the pleuropneumonia of cattle. *Report of the Commissioner of Agriculture on the Diseases of Cattle in the United States*. Washington D.C., 1871 (Reprinted 1970 in *Pathologia Veterinaria*, 7, 213–224).

178

Contagious caprine pleuropneumonia

C.J. Maré

Introduction

Contagious caprine pleuropneumonia (CCPP) is an acute, highly contagious disease of goats characterized by fever, coughing, severe respiratory distress and high mortality. The aetiology of the 'classical' disease remains controversial. The principal causative agent is probably the mycoplasma designated F-38.[11, 12] *Mycoplasma mycoides capri* has been widely accepted as a causative agent of CCPP, but it initiates a less contagious, milder form of caprine pleuropneumonia.[1]

Pneumonia in goats has been described in Algeria, the Middle East, Europe and Turkey since the mid nineteenth century, but the name 'contagious caprine pleuropneumonia' was first used by Hutcheon in 1881, as cited by McMartin *et al.*[10] In that year he described a highly contagious, fatal disease occurring in South Africa after goats had been imported from Ankara, Turkey. On one farm, 879 of the 1 224 goats in the flock (70 per cent) died from the disease in a matter of weeks. Hutcheon described the clinical signs, epidemiology and pathology of the disease in detail.

Contagious caprine pleuropneumonia has subsequently been described in many countries of Africa, the Middle East, Eastern Europe, the USSR, and the Far East. It is a major scourge in many of the most important goat-producing countries in the world, and is considered by many to be the world's most devastating goat disease.[10]

The disease has not been described in North America. The report by Yedloutschnig[21] of CCPP outbreaks in the USA in 1978 was erroneous. The agents isolated from the outbreaks of caprine pneumonia which he described and misidentified as *M. mycoides capri*, were subsequently shown to be *M. mycoides mycoides* (LC type). Neither F-38 nor *M. mycoides capri* have been isolated in North America.

A disease resembling CCPP no longer occurs in South Africa, partly as a result of the great rinderpest pandemic of the late nineteenth century which eliminated a large proportion of potential carrier animals (and thus the causative agent), and partly as a result of the use of a crude inactivated vaccine.

Aetiology

For many years the causative agent of CCPP was considered to be *Mycoplasma mycoides capri* (type strain PG-3), because this was the agent most commonly isolated from goats with pleuropneumonia. However, not all experts accepted this agent as the cause of the original disease described by Hutcheon as 'contagious caprine pleuropneumonia'. In 1976 MacOwan and Minette reported a mycoplasma which had not previously been isolated and which they designated 'F-38'. They showed it to be the cause of a highly contagious form of CCPP.[11, 12] McMartin *et al.*[10] presented very convincing arguments that this agent is, in fact, the cause of the classical disease. In recent years most African outbreaks of CCPP have been attributed to mycoplasma F-38.[7]

A third agent, *M. mycoides mycoides* LC has been isolated from goats with pneumonia. This agent, the so-called 'large colony' or LC variant of *M. mycoides mycoides*,[2, 15] produces septicaemia, arthritis, mastitis, encephalitis, conjunctivitis, hepatitis and pneumonia in goats, but does not cause CCPP.[16] Recent studies have shown that the LC variant of *M. mycoides mycoides* and *M. capricolum*, which is closely related to F-38, causes identical pneumonia syndromes in susceptible goats.[4]

Currently both *M. mycoides capri* and mycoplasma F-38 should be considered causative agents of CCPP, the latter being the principal cause of the syndrome as it occurs in Africa.[5, 7] Although *M. mycoides mycoides* and *M. capricolum* both cause a pneumonia in goats which may resemble the pneumonic lesions of CCPP, these agents are more commonly associated with polyarthritis and mastitis in goats and sheep.[3, 16]

It has been proposed that mycoplasma F-38 be designated '*M. capripneumoniae*',[6] but this terminology has not yet gained formal acceptance.

Mycoplasma mycoides capri is easily propagated in standard mycoplasma growth media. Mycoplasma F-38 is much more fastidious, but can be grown in Newing's tryptose medium and in Medium B.[9]

All of the abovementioned mycoplasmas are very labile outside their hosts, and are readily inactivated by heat, dehydration, sunlight and disinfectants.

Epidemiology

Since the aetiological agent in most early outbreaks of CCPP was not identified, and some outbreaks were caused by mixed infections (for example, type strain PG-3 of *M. mycoides capri* was contaminated with *M. capricolum*), the epidemiology of CCPP is not well defined.

Mycoplasma F-38 has only been isolated in Africa, so it is possible that the European and Asian forms of CCPP are not caused by this agent. However, since F-38 has only recently been identified and is very difficult to isolate, it may have simply been missed in the past.

Contagious caprine pleuropneumonia is transmitted by direct contact through inhalation of infective aerosols. Of the two known causative agents, F-38 is by far the more contagious. Outbreaks of the disease often occur after heavy rains, such as after the monsoons in India, and after cold spells, and this is probably because recovered 'carrier' animals start shedding the mycoplasmas after the stress of sudden climatic change. It is believed that a long-term carrier state exists, and that in North Africa and the Middle East nomadic herds may disseminate the disease.

Contagious caprine pleuropneumonia is a disease of goats. Where the classical disease has been described, only goats have been involved, in spite of the presence of sheep and cattle. Mycoplasma F-38 does not cause disease in sheep or cattle.

Mycoplasma mycoides capri, the other agent designated as a cause of CCPP, will cause a fatal disease in experimentally inoculated sheep, and can spread from goats to sheep.[1] It is, however, not recognized as a cause of natural disease in sheep.

Both *M. capricolum* and *M. mycoides mycoides* LC, which can cause pneumonia in goats, will also infect sheep, causing septicaemia, polyarthritis, mastitis and occasionally keratoconjunctivitis.[4]

A serological survey of eleven species of free-living herbivores in Kenya revealed F-38 antibodies in 49 per cent of camels (*Camelus dromedaris*), 32 per cent of Cape buffalo (*Syncerus caffer*) and 10 per cent of impala (*Aepyceros melampus*) tested, while the sera of the other eight species tested were negative.[14]

Clinical signs

The incubation period can be as short as six to ten days, but may be prolonged (three or four weeks) under natural conditions.

The clinical signs described for CCPP from different parts of the world have varied enormously.[13] This is not surprising, since at least two different mycoplasmas are known to be causative agents of the disease. In many field outbreaks the clinical manifestation has probably been further complicated by concomitant viral and bacterial (such as *Pasteurella* spp.) infections.

The classical disease as caused by mycoplasma F-38 is a purely respiratory disease. It is characterized by fever, coughing and malaise. Affected goats show laboured breathing; later they may grunt or bleat in obvious pain. Frothy nasal discharges and stringy salivation are often seen shortly before death. In the acute disease, which occurs in fully susceptible populations of goats, death occurs within seven to ten days of the onset of clinical signs; morbidity may reach 100 per cent, and mortality 70 per cent. A more chronic form of the disease is often seen in endemic areas, and may lead to the recovery of a higher proportion of infected animals, many of which remain carriers.

Mycoplasma mycoides capri tends to cause a more generalized infection in which septicaemia is frequently seen. Respiratory distress and inappetence are usually followed by gradual recovery, but occasionally by prostration and death. An acute or peracute septicaemic form of the disease, involving the reproductive, respiratory and alimentary tracts, has been described.[1] In addition, 'thoracic' and 'reproductive' forms of the disease have been attributed to this agent. This infection is considerably less contagious than the F-38-induced disease, and the mortality and morbidity rates are also lower.

Pathology

The lesions in classical CCPP are confined to the thoracic cavity. Yellowish pneumonic nodules of up to 7,5 mm in diameter are seen in the lungs in early cases. In more advanced cases, marked congestion around the nodules is seen. The lesions may involve one or both lungs. Entire lobes may become consolidated. A chronic pleuritis causes visceral pleural thickening and adhesions to the chest wall. Hutcheon, as cited by McMartin *et al.*,[10] emphasized that the lesions do not resemble those of contagious bovine pleuropneumonia (CBPP) as 'no thickening of the interlobular tissue' occurs. Diseased lungs are described as resembling a 'somewhat granular-looking liver'.

In sharp contrast to the above, *M. mycoides capri* has been reported to cause lesions in a wide variety of organs, and to produce lung lesions closely resembling those seen in CBPP. The generalized lesions include encephalitis, meningitis, lymphadenitis, splenitis, and urogenital tract and intestinal lesions,[1] none of which are a feature of classical CCPP. The lesions, which resemble those seen in CBPP, are usually confined to one lung, and manifest various stages of fibrinous pneumonia, marked expansion of interlobular septa and extensive pleuritis. The cardiac and diaphragmatic lobes are most commonly involved.

Adequate descriptions of the microscopical lesions of CCPP are not available. Existing descriptions are confused by the controversy over aetiology and are compounded by the presence of other infectious agents. The principal difference between the microscopic lesions produced by F-38 and those produced by *M. mycoides capri* is that the former causes interstitial intralobular oedema, while the latter causes pronounced interlobular oedema and cellular infiltration resembling the lesions of CBPP.

Diagnosis and differential diagnosis

Clinical and pathological diagnosis is difficult, since infections by other mycoplasmas (*M. capricolum, M. mycoides mycoides* LC, *M. ovipneumoniae*) and by *Pasteurella* spp. or even viruses may produce signs and lesions resembling CCPP. It is therefore essential to confirm a diagnosis of CCPP by isolation and identification of the causative agent.

Standard mycoplasma growth procedures are used for the isolation of *M. mycoides capri,* which can then be identified by colony size and morphology and by a biochemical reaction profile.

The more fastidious mycoplasma F-38 can be isolated in either Medium B (modified Hayflick) or Newing's tryptose medium.[9] It can then be identified by immunofluorescence or by metabolic inhibition, or most specifically with the growth inhibition test employing monoclonal antibodies.[20]

Serum antibodies to the causative mycoplasmas have traditionally been detected by the complement fixation test, but a recently described latex agglutination test is more sensitive than the complement fixation test and can be performed in the field.[18]

Control

Control and eradication procedures for CCPP are poorly developed. A crude vaccine prepared from goat lung was used to vaccinate goats in South Africa after the original outbreak of CCPP in the late nineteenth century, but vaccines against *M. mycoides capri* met with little success. This is possibly because in many instances the disease is caused by F-38. A recently developed inactivated F-38 vaccine incorporating saponin[19] may prove to be useful in the control of CCPP, at least in Africa, where F-38 appears to be the major cause of the disease.

Both CCPP-inducing mycoplasmas are susceptible to tetracyclines, tylosin and tiamulin.[8, 17] While early treatment can be effective, chemotherapy and chemoprophylaxis have not been important in CCPP control programmes.

References

1 **COTTEW, G.S., 1984.** Overview of mycoplasmoses in sheep and goats. *Israel Journal of Medical Sciences,* 20, 962–964.

2 **COTTEW, G.S. & YEATS, F.R., 1978.** Subdivision of *Mycoplasma mycoides* subsp. *mycoides* from cattle and goats into two types. *Australian Veterinary Journal,* 54, 293–296.

3 **DAMASSA, A.J., BROOKS, D.L. & ADLER, H.E., 1983.** Caprine mycoplasmosis: Widespread infection in goats with *Mycoplasma mycoides* subsp. *mycoides* (large colony type). *American Journal of Veterinary Research,* 44, 322–325.

4 **DAMASSA, A.J., HOLMBERG, C.A. & BROOKS, D.L., 1987.** Comparison of caprine mycoplasmosis caused by *Mycoplasma capricolum, M. mycoides* subsp. *mycoides,* and *M. putrefasciens. Israel Journal of Medical Sciences,* 23, 636–640.

5 **EL HARBI, M.S.M.A., EL TAHIR, M.S., MACOWAN, K.J. & NAYIL, A.A., 1981.** Mycoplasma strain F-38 and contagious caprine pleuropneumonia in the Sudan. *The Veterinary Record,* 108, 261–263.

6 **EL TAHIR, M.S. & BLOBEL, H., 1984.** Mycoplasmas in goats with contagious pleuropneumonia. *Zentralblatt für Veterinärmedizin,* (B), 31, 51–57.

7 **ERNO, H., LEACH, R.H., SALIH, M.M. & MACOWAN, K.J., 1983.** The F-38-like group, a new group of caprine mycoplasmas? *Acta Veterinaria Scandinavica,* 24, 275–286.

8 **HASSAN, S.M., EL HARBI, M.S.M.A. & BAKR, M.I., 1984.** Treatment of contagious caprine pleuropneumonia. *Veterinary Research Communications,* 8, 65–67.

9 **KIBOR, A.C. & WAIYAKI, P.G., 1986.** Growth of Mycoplasma F-38 in medium B (modified Hayflick) and Newings tryptose medium. *Bulletin of Animal Health and Production in Africa,* 34, 157–159.

10 **McMARTIN, D.A., MACOWAN, K.J. & SWIFT, L.L., 1980.** A century of classical contagious caprine pleuropneumonia; from original description to aetiology. *British Veterinary Journal,* 136, 507–515.

11 **MACOWAN, K.J. & MINETTE, J.E., 1976.** A mycoplasma from acute contagious caprine pleuropneumonia in Kenya. *Tropical Animal Health and Production,* 8, 91–95.

12 **MACOWAN, K.J. & MINETTE, J.E., 1977.** The role of mycoplasma strain F-38 in contagious caprine pleuropneumonia (CCPP) in Kenya. *The Veterinary Record,* 101, 380–381.

13 **MARÉ, C.J., 1984.** Contagious caprine pleuropneumonia. *In: Foreign Animal Diseases.* Richmond, Virginia: US Animal Health Association.

14 **PALING, R.W., MACOWAN, K.J. & KARSTAD, L., 1978.** The prevalence of antibody to contagious caprine pleuropneumonia mycoplasma strain F-38 in some wild herbivores and camels in Kenya. *Journal of Wildlife Diseases,* 14, 305–308.

15 **RODWELL, A.W. & RODWELL, E.S., 1978.** Relationships between strains of *Mycoplasma mycoides* subsp. *mycoides* and *capri* studied by two-dimensional gel electrophoresis of cell proteins. *Journal of General Microbiology,* 109, 259–263.

16 **ROSENDAL, S., 1981.** Experimental infection of goats, sheep and calves with the large colony type of *Mycoplasma mycoides* subsp. *mycoides. Veterinary Pathology,* 18, 71–78.

17 **RURANGIRWA, F.R., MASIGA, W.N., MURIU, D.N., MUTHOMI, E., MULIGA, G., KAGUMBA, M. & NANDOKHA, E., 1981.** Treatment of contagious caprine pleuropneumonia. *Tropical Animal Health and Production,* 13, 177–182.

18 **RURANGIRWA, F.R., McGUIRE, T.C., KIBOR, A. & CHEMA, S., 1987.** A latex-agglutination test for the field diagnosis of contagious caprine pleuropneumonia. *The Veterinary Record,* 121, 191–193.

19 **RURANGIRWA, F.R., McGUIRE, T.C., KIBOR, A. & CHEMA, S., 1987.** An inactivated vaccine for contagious caprine pleuropneumonia. *The Veterinary Record,* 121, 397–400.

20 **RURANGIRWA, F.R., McGUIRE, T.C., MUSOKE, A.J. & KIBOR, A., 1987.** Differentiation of F-38 mycoplasmas causing contagious caprine pleuropneumonia with a growth-inhibiting monoclonal antibody. *Infection and Immunity,* 55, 3219–3220.

21 **YEDLOUTSCHNIG, R.J., 1978.** *Mycoplasma mycoides* subsp. *capri* and *M. agalactiae* isolation from goats in the US: A review including unpublished findings. *Proceedings of the Eighty-second Annual Meeting of the US Animal Health Association,* 29–31 November, Buffalo, New York, 272–276.

179

Mycoplasmal pneumonia of pigs

Synonyms: Swine enzootic pneumonia, virus pneumonia of pigs

C.J. Maré and R.K. Loveday

Introduction

Mycoplasmal pneumonia of swine (MPS) is a serious and insidious, subacute to chronic pneumonia characterized by a non-productive cough, loss of condition, growth retardation and low mortality. The disease is caused by *Mycoplasma hyopneumoniae*,[15] and has had a serious economic impact in all major pig-producing regions of the world.[13, 20]

When it was first recognized as a distinct disease entity,[8, 19] the name 'infectious pneumonia of pigs' was adopted, but soon afterwards, when the causative agent was shown to pass bacteria-retaining filters, the name was changed to 'virus pneumonia of pigs'. In 1965, both in the USA[15] and in Great Britain,[7] a mycoplasma was isolated in cell-free media and shown to be the cause of this chronic pneumonia of pigs. The agent was named *M. hyopneumoniae* and it was proposed that the disease be designated 'mycoplasmal pneumonia of swine'.[15, 16] The name *M. suipneumoniae*, which was proposed later for this organism, is no longer accepted.

The prevalence of the disease, as indicated by surveys in various countries, ranges from 30 – 80 per cent of herds infected.[20] The presence of the disease was first noticed in South Africa in 1956,[12] and was found to be widespread among commercial pig herds. It is presently estimated that at least 40 per cent of such herds are infected with *M. hyopneumoniae*. The causal organism was isolated and identified at the Veterinary Research Institute, Onderstepoort in 1977.[24]

Aetiology

Mycoplasma hyopneumoniae is an extremely fastidious, slow-growing organism and can be propagated only in special media.[4, 5] After primary isolation and adaptation in liquid media, the agent can be grown on solid media incubated in a 5 per cent CO_2 atmosphere. The extremely small colonies rarely reach 1 mm in diameter, even after 14 days' incubation.

Differentiation of the closely related *M. flocculare* from *M. hyopneumoniae* requires refined procedures such as immunoblotting[26] or enzyme-linked immunosorbent assay.[1]

Epidemiology

The disease is usually introduced into clean herds by the movement of carrier adult pigs, but other, as yet unknown, modes of entry may exist.[6] Within infected herds, the spread of MPS occurs via aerosol or by direct contact with infected nasal secretions, usually from carrier adult sows to their offspring. Once infected, young pigs, usually over eight weeks of age, can spread the organism if they mix with susceptible pigs.

Mycoplasma hyopneumoniae is very sensitive to heat, sunlight and dehydration, and is quickly inactivated in the environment.

Pathogenesis

The invading mycoplasmas colonize the mucosae of the trachea, bronchi and bronchioles, resulting in ciliastasis and loss of cilia.[20] The extent of damage to the epithelium and the cilial destruction correlates with the severity of infection.[11] The early stage of infection, when large numbers of mycoplasmas are evident among the epithelial lesions, is followed by peribronchial and peribronchiolar mononuclear leukocyte accumulation, denoting a cell-mediated immune response.[23] Since most *M. hyopneumoniae* infections are complicated by the presence of other bacteria, microscopic lesions are extremely variable.

Clinical signs

The clinical signs of uncomplicated *M. hyopneumoniae* infection are rarely observed, since the infection is usually accompanied by secondary agents such as other *Mycoplasma* spp., *Bordetella bronchiseptica* or *Pasteurella multocida*, all of which can add to the severity of the clinical disease.

Clinical signs are seldom seen in pigs under ten weeks old. After an incubation period of one to three weeks, a non-productive cough, most notable after exertion, is usually observed. The cough may persist for only a few weeks, but more often becomes chronic. Appetite remains normal. Depending on the severity of the lesions, marked unthriftiness and dry skin are often noticeable.

Marked variation in growth rates is seen, ranging from severe stunting to apparently normal growth. Mortality is low and results mostly from complications.

Pathology

At necropsy, in uncomplicated cases of MPS, pneumonic lesions are found predominantly in the cranial, accessory and middle lobes, as well as on the cranio-ventral parts of the caudal lobes. The lesions are usually clearly demarcated areas of consolidation varying in colour from dark reddish-blue to light pinkish-grey. Atelectasis may be associated with some of these lesions. Older lesions become greyer and are often complicated by bacteria which cause a purulent bronchopneumonia or abscessation.

The microscopic lesions are variable, probably because so many of the observations have been made on complicated field cases of the disease, which in many instances reflect the lesions induced by the secondary invaders rather than those of the primary pathogen. In the experimentally induced disease, the early lesions seen two or three weeks post-inoculation are characterized by alveolar interstitial thickening due mainly to a lymphocyte and neutrophil infiltration, and to proliferation of cells in the septa, giant cell formation and peribronchiolar and perivascular lymphoid hyperplasia. In older lesions examined six to eight weeks after infection, pronounced lymphoid hyperplasia is the predominant lesion.[14, 20]

Oedema and lymphoid hyperplasia of the mediastinal lymph nodes are often observed.

Occasionally *M. hyopneumoniae* may also be responsible for a fibrinous or serofibrinous pleuritis; other serous surfaces may show similar changes.

Diagnosis

A presumptive diagnosis of MPS can be made on the basis of clinical signs (chronic non-productive cough, unthriftiness, high morbidity and low mortality) and lesions (greyish to purplish areas of lung consolidation with a characteristic distribution; and perivascular and peribronchiolar lymphoid proliferation). Since other agents can elicit similar signs and lesions in pigs, it is necessary to confirm the diagnosis.

Identification of *M. hyopneumoniae* in the infected lungs by immunofluorescence is a very useful technique, especially in acute cases of the disease.[11] Isolation of the causative agent is seldom used in diagnosis because of its fastidiousness.

Detection of antibodies to *M. hyopneumoniae* in the serum of pigs can be accomplished with complement fixation (CF), indirect haemagglutination (IHA) and indirect immunofluorescence (IF) tests, and by the enzyme-linked immunosorbent assay (ELISA). The ELISA is more sensitive than the IHA,[9] can differentiate between *M. hyopneumoniae* and *M. flocculare* antibodies,[1] and can be used to identify antibodies in colostrum.[27] The IHA test is still a useful tool for the detection of infected herds.[22]

Since MPS is frequently complicated by the presence in the respiratory tract of other mycoplasmas such as *M. hyopharyngis*,[3] *M. hyorhinis*, *M. flocculare* and *M. hyosynoviae*,[20] some of which may cross-react with *M. hyopneumoniae* in serological tests, these tests should be used only as herd tests, and not to identify individual animals which may be infected.

Differential diagnosis

Pneumonia caused by *B. bronchiseptica*, *P. multocida*, and possibly by swine influenza virus can become chronic and resemble MPS.

Mycoplasma hyorhinis, a common secondary pathogen in pneumonia in pigs, is also an important cause of arthritis and polyserositis in young pigs. *Mycoplasma hyosynoviae*, although frequently present in the respiratory tract, is not a respiratory pathogen, but it does cause arthritis in pigs older than ten weeks of age. *Mycoplasma flocculare*, which is occasionally isolated from cases of MPS, is considered to be only mildly pathogenic and probably does not cause overt disease by itself. *Mycoplasma hyopharyngis*, a recent isolate from the respiratory tract of pigs, appears to be non-pathogenic.[3]

Control

In several countries, including Great Britain, Sweden, and the USA, MPS has been controlled by the establishment of 'minimal disease' or 'specific pathogen-free' programmes. Breeding premises free of MPS are maintained in this state by introducing only caesarean-derived bloodlines and by the constant monitoring of these programmes.[20] In spite of stringent precautions, breakdowns do occur,[6] but the emergence of improved diagnostic procedures has contributed to increasing success with these programmes.

Chemotherapy has not been a useful procedure for individual cases of MPS, but several drugs show great promise for chemoprophylaxis. Tetracycline antibiotics were the first to be used in MPS control programmes,[25] followed by tylosin, lincomycin, doxycycline and tiamulin. Recent trials have shown that MPS-infected herds can be cleared of the infection by feeding tiamulin.[17, 18] A synergistic activity between chlortetracycline and tiamulin which resulted in the successful clearing of MPS complicated by bordetellosis, pasteurellosis and porcine pleuropneumonia has been documented.[2]

No effective vaccines against MPS are currently available.

Immunization of pigs against MPS by the use of inactivated, adjuvanted, whole-cell vaccines has resulted in only partial resistance to challenge.[21] An experimental plasma membrane vaccine was recently reported as yielding promising results.[10]

References

1 **ARMSTRONG, C.H., SANDS-FREEMAN, L. & FREEMAN, M.J., 1987.** Serological, pathological and cultural evaluations of swine infected experimentally with *Mycoplasma flocculare*. *Canadian Journal of Veterinary Research*, 51, 185–188.

2 **BURCH, D.G.S., JONES, G.T., HEARD, T.W. & TUCK, R.E., 1986.** The synergistic activity of tiamulin and chlortetracycline: In-feed treatment of bacterially complicated enzootic pneumonia in fattening pigs. *The Veterinary Record*, 119, 108–112.

3 **ERICKSON, B.J.Z., ROSS, R.F., ROSE, D.L., TULLY, J.G. & BOVE, J.M., 1986.** *Mycoplasma hyopharyngis*, a new species from swine. *International Journal of Systematic Bacteriology*, 36, 55–59.

4 **FRISS, N.F., 1975.** Some recommendations concerning primary isolation of *Mycoplasma suipneumoniae* and *Mycoplasma flocculare*. *Nordisk Veterinaermedicin*, 27, 337–339.

5 **GOODWIN, R.F.W., 1976.** An improved medium for the isolation of *Mycoplasma suipneumoniae*. *The Veterinary Record*, 98, 260–261.

6 **GOODWIN, R.F.W., 1984.** Apparent reinfection of enzootic-pneumonia-free pig herds: Early signs and incubation period. *The Veterinary Record*, 115, 320–324.

7 **GOODWIN, R.F.W., POMEROY, A.P. & WHITTLESTONE, P., 1965.** Production of enzootic pneumonia in pigs with a mycoplasma. *The Veterinary Record*, 77, 1247–1249.

8 **GULRAJANI, T.S. & BEVERIDGE, W.I.B., 1951.** Studies on respiratory diseases of pigs. IV. Transmission of infectious pneumonia and its differentiation from swine influenza. *Journal of Comparative Pathology*, 61, 118–139.

9 **KOBISCH, M. & NICOLET, J., 1987.** Comparison of enzyme-linked immunosorbent assay (ELISA) and indirect haemagglutination (IHA) in experimental *Mycoplasma hyopneumoniae* infection of pigs. *Israel Journal of Medical Sciences*, 23, 644–646.

10 **KOBISCH, M., QUILLIEN, L., TILLON, J.P. & WROBLEWSKI, H., 1987.** The *Mycoplasma hyopneumoniae* plasma membrane as a vaccine against porcine enzootic pneumonia. *Annales de l'Institut Pasteur, Immunology*, 138, 693–705.

11 **L'ECUYER, C. & BOULANGER, P., 1970.** Enzootic pneumonia of pigs: Identification of a causative Mycoplasma in infected pigs and in cultures by immunofluorescent staining. *Canadian Journal of Comparative Medicine*, 34, 38–46.

12 **LOVEDAY, R.K., 1956.** Faculty of Veterinary Science, University of Pretoria, South Africa. Unpublished data.

13 **MACPHERSON, M.R. & HODGES, R.T., 1985.** The occurrence of mycoplasmas in the lungs of pigs in New Zealand. *New Zealand Veterinary Journal*, 33, 194–197.

14 **MARÉ, C.J., 1969.** Mycoplasmal pneumonia of swine. *Proceedings of the North American Symposium on Swine Respiratory Diseases*.

15 **MARÉ, C.J. & SWITZER, W.P., 1965.** *Mycoplasma hyopneumoniae*: A causative agent of virus pig pneumonia. *Veterinary Medicine*, 60, 841–846.

16 **MARÉ, C.J. & SWITZER, W.P., 1966.** Virus pneumonia of pigs: Propagation and characterization of a causative agent. *American Journal of Veterinary Research*, 27, 1687–1693.

17 **MÉAROS, J., STIPKOVITS, L., ANTAL, T., SZABO, I. & VESZELY, P., 1986.** Experiences from eradication of *Mycoplasma hyopneumoniae* infection by tiamulin treatment. *Archiv für Experimentelle Veterinärmedizin*, 40, 19–22.

18 **POINTON, A.M., GERATTY, N., BAKER, T. & BYRT, D., 1985.** Evaluation of the effect of tiamulin hydrogen fumarate fed at 25 ppm on performance responses of pigs infected with enzootic pneumonia. *Australian Veterinary Journal*, 62, 384–385.

19 **PULLER, E.M., 1948.** Infectious pneumonia of pigs. I. General description, differential diagnosis and epidemiology. *Australian Veterinary Journal*, 24, 320–330.

20 **ROSS, R.F., 1986.** Mycoplasmal Diseases. In: LEMAN, A.D., STRAW, B., GLOCK, R.D., MENGELING, W.L., PENNY, R.H.C. & SCHOLL, E., (eds). *Diseases of Swine*. 6th edn. Ames, Iowa: Iowa State University Press.

21 **ROSS, R.F. & ZIMMERMANN-ERICKSON, B.J.Z., 1984.** Characteristics of protective activity of *Mycoplasma hyopneumoniae* vaccine. *American Journal of Veterinary Research*, 45, 1899–1905.

22 **STIPKOVITS, L. & MÉSZAROS, J., 1986.** Serological control of conventional swine herds for *Mycoplasma hyopneumoniae* infection. *Archiv für Experimentelle Veterinärmedizin*, 40, 12–13.

23 **TAJIMA, M., YAGIHASHI, T., NUMAYA, T., TAKEUCHI, A. & OKASHI, F., 1984.** *Mycoplasma hyopneumoniae* infection in pigs immunosuppressed by thymectomy and treatment with antithymocyte serum. *American Journal of Veterinary Research*, 45, 1928–1932.

24 **TRICHARD, C.J.V., 1977.** Veterinary Research Institute, Onderstepoort, South Africa. Unpublished data.

25 **WHITTLESTONE, P., 1973.** Enzootic pneumonia of pigs (EPP). *Advances in Veterinary Science and Comparative Medicine*, 17, 1–55.

26 **YOUNG, T.F. & ROSS, R.F., 1987.** Assessment of antibody response of swine infected with *Mycoplasma hyopneumoniae* by immunoblotting. *American Journal of Veterinary Research*, 48, 651–656.

27 **ZIMMERMAN, W., TSCHUDI, P. & NICOLET, J., 1986.** ELISA-serologie in Blut und Kolostralmilch: Eine Moglichkeit zur Uberwachung des enzootischen Pneumonie (EP) in Schweine-Beständen. *Schweizer Archiv für Tierheilkunde*, 128, 299–306.

Mycoplasmal polyserositis and arthritis of pigs

Synonym: *Mycoplasma hyorhinis* infection

C.J. Maré and R.K. Loveday

Introduction

Mycoplasmal polyserositis and arthritis is caused by *Mycoplasma hyorhinis*, and occurs in young pigs from three to ten weeks of age. It is found in most pig-producing regions of the world, and can be of considerable economic significance since it markedly impedes growth.

Mycoplasma hyorhinis, the first mycoplasma of pigs to be isolated,[6] often inhabits the pig respiratory tract and occurs together with other respiratory pathogens.

This infection is occasionally seen under intensive conditions (particularly the use of flatdecks for weaners) in South Africa.

Aetiology

Mycoplasma hyorhinis is readily isolated in fluid media containing sterols, and forms typical mycoplasma colonies on solid media in two to five days.[5] It ferments glucose and does not utilize arginine or hydrolyze urea.[2]

Epidemiology

The polyserositis-arthritis syndrome is commonly seen on poorly managed farms where up to 25 per cent of pigs under ten weeks of age may be affected. Sows with upper respiratory tract infection are the predominant source of infection, but lateral spread among young pigs occurs readily.[4] Up to 70 per cent of pigs on infected premises may contract the disease. However, not all show clinical signs. Stress may result in mycoplasmal septicaemia and resultant polyserositis. Pigs older than ten weeks may occasionally be affected.

Pathogenesis

Mycoplasma hyorhinis, a primary inhabitant of the pig respiratory tract, may, when the animals are under stress, spread haematogenously to localize in the synovial membranes and on the serosae, where it induces an inflammatory reaction.

Clinical signs

A mild febrile response accompanied by unthriftiness, listlessness and inappetence is followed by swelling of many of the joints, and lameness. Bodily discomfort is apparent and abdominal and thoracic tenderness may be observed. Stretching and abnormal posture is common while lying down, and scrotal swelling may occur. The acute stage of the disease may last 14 days; the lameness and swelling of joints may persist for up to six months.[2]

Sudden deaths occasionally occur during the acute stage of the disease, but the mortality is usually low.

Pathology

In the acute stage of the disease a serofibrinous and occasionally purulent pleuritis, pericarditis, peritonitis, periorchitis and polysynovitis may be seen. Increased synovial fluid is common.[1] Microscopic examination of serosal and synovial membranes reveals a severe infiltration of lymphocytes, sometimes accompanied by some neutrophils.[3] In occasional chronic cases persisting for five to six months, thickening of the joint capsule and articular lesions, consisting of erosions of the cartilage and pannus formation, are present.

Diagnosis and differential diagnosis

An acute, generalized infection of pigs under ten weeks of age, characterized by obvious body pains and joint involvement should lead to a presumptive diagnosis. A serofibrinous polyserositis is supportive, while isolation of the agent from synovial fluid of arthritic joints and fluid from body cavities will confirm *M. hyorhinis* as the causative agent.

The presence of *M. hyorhinis* in a herd can be confirmed by demonstrating complement fixing antibodies to the agent, but since *M. hyorhinis* is so ubiquitous, this would only be supportive evidence.

Mycoplasmal polyserositis must be differentiated from similar lesions caused by *Haemophilus parasuis*, *Mycoplasma hyosynoviae*, *Streptococcus equisimilis*, *S. suis*, *Actinomyces (Corynebacterium) pyogenes* and *Staphylococcus* spp.

Control

Since polyserositis and arthritis caused by *M. hyorhinis* are usually the result of stress, the improvement of management practices and the control methods for other pig diseases is most important.

Mycoplasma hyorhinis is susceptible to several antibiotics, including tetracycline, tylosin, lincomycin and tiamulin, but none of these have been effectively used in the control of the disease.

References

1 **ROBERTS, E.D., SWITZER, W.P. & RAMSEY, F.K., 1963.** The pathology of *Mycoplasma hyorhinis* arthritis produced experimentally in swine. *American Journal of Veterinary Research*, 24, 19–31.

2 **ROSS, R.F., 1986.** Mycoplasmal diseases. *In:* LEMAN, A.D., STRAW, B., GLOCK, R.D., MENGELING, H.L., PENNY, R.H.C. & SCHOLL, E., (eds). *Diseases of Swine*. 6th edn. Ames, Iowa: Iowa State University Press.

3 **ROSS, R.F., DALE, S.E. & DUNCAN, J.R., 1973.** Experimentally induced *Mycoplasma hyorhinis* arthritis of swine. *American Journal of Veterinary Research*, 34, 367–372.

4 **ROSS, R.F. & SPEAR, M.L., 1973.** Role of the sow as a reservoir of infection for *Mycoplasma hyorhinis*. *American Journal of Veterinary Research*, 34, 373–378.

5 **ROSS, R.F., WEISS, R. & KIRCHHOFF, H., 1977.** Nachweis von *M. hyorhinis* und *M. hyosynoviae* in arthritischen Gelenken von Schweiner. *Zentralblatt für Veterinärmedizin*, 24, 741–745.

6 **SWITZER, W.P., 1955.** Studies on infectious atrophic rhinitis. IV. Characterization of a pleuropneumonia-like organism isolated from the nasal cavities of swine. *American Journal of Veterinary Research*, 16, 540–544.

181

Mycoplasmal arthritis of pigs

Synonym: *Mycoplasma hyosynoviae* infection

C.J. Maré and R.K. Loveday

Introduction

Mycoplasmal arthritis caused by *Mycoplasma hyosynoviae* is a disease of pigs aged 10–24 weeks which is characterized clinically by stiffness and lameness and is not normally fatal. One or several joints may be affected. The disease has been reported in the USA[3] and in Great Britain,[2] but rarely occurs in South Africa.

Aetiology

Mycoplasma hyosynoviae was isolated by Ross and Karmon[3] in mucin-containing medium. In fluid media this agent produces granules in suspension, a granular deposit and a waxy pellicle. It is sterol-requiring, does not ferment glucose or hydrolyze urea, and utilizes arginine. On solid media, colonies of up to 1 mm in diameter are formed within four days. Growth of this agent is stimulated by an environment which contains reduced oxygen tension during incubation.

Epidemiology

Mycoplasma hyosynoviae occurs as a common inhabitant of the upper respiratory tract and tonsils in a large percentage of pigs with no clinical signs. Carrier pigs serve as a source of infection which, following stress of a herd or an individual animal, usually results in clinical signs. Infection occurs most commonly in pigs more than six weeks of age. In most instances only about 10 per cent of a herd show clinical signs by about 10 weeks of age. Heavy breeds such as Hampshires seem to be more susceptible to the disease.[4]

Pathogenesis

The agent enters the circulation after stress, such as cold, transportation, or change of feed, to reach the joints, where it causes inflammation.

Clinical signs and pathology

A sudden onset of lameness, which often affects only one limb, is characteristic. Affected pigs have great difficulty in walking and may not be able to rise after lying down. Enlargement of joints is not usually seen. Complete recovery within two to four weeks is usual, but stiffness may persist for several weeks.

Hyperaemia of the synovial membranes and the accumulation of yellowish to reddish fluid in the joints are the main lesions. Erosion of joint cartilage is not seen.[4]

Diagnosis and control

The sudden onset of arthritis in pigs 10–24 weeks old, is indicative of *M. hyosynoviae* infection. The diagnosis should be confirmed by isolation of the organism from joint fluids.

Antibiotic treatment prior to the introduction of new pigs to an infected herd can prevent infection. Lincomycin and tylosin daily for three or four days can be effective in treating sick animals, and tiamulin has been used to suppress infections in herds seriously affected by *M. hyosynoviae*.[1]

References

1 **BURCH, D.G.S. & GOODWIN, R.F.W., 1984.** Use of tiamulin in a herd of pigs seriously affected with *Mycoplasma hyosynoviae* arthritis. *The Veterinary Record*, 115, 594–595.

2 **ROBERTS, D.H., JOHNSON, C.H. & TEW, N.C., 1972.** The isolation of *Mycoplasma hyosynoviae* from an outbreak of porcine arthritis. *The Veterinary Record*, 90, 307–309.

3 **ROSS, R.F. & KARMON, J.A., 1970.** Heterogeneity among strains of *Mycoplasma granularum* and identification of *Mycoplasma hyosynoviae*, sp.n. *Journal of Bacteriology*, 103, 707–713.

4 **ROSS, R.F., SWITZER, W.P. & DUNCAN, J.R., 1971.** Experimental production of *Mycoplasma hyosynoviae* arthritis in swine. *American Journal of Veterinary Research*, 32, 1743–1749.

182

Bovine genital mycoplasmosis

C.J.V. Trichard and A.P. Schutte

Introduction

The role that *Mycoplasma, Acholeplasma* and *Ureaplasma* spp. play in the production of bovine infertility is still controversial in spite of considerable investigation.

Mollicutes have a predilection for mucosal and serosal surfaces and they most frequently cause diseases of the urogenital and respiratory tracts, joints, the mammary glands and eyes. These diseases are mostly chronic or subclinical.[19] Concomitant infections with other pathogens are common.

Mycoplasmas are frequently isolated from the reproductive tract of male and female cattle. Investigations and surveys conducted throughout the world have provided evidence that mycoplasmas are associated with poor reproductive performance, even though the genital organs of animals harbouring large numbers of these organisms often appear normal.[2, 10, 15, 27] At present 17 species or serotypes of mycoplasma have been identified. A few are pathogenic, others are moderately so, and the remainder are apparently non-pathogenic.

Aetiology

Most of the known mollicutes that affect cattle have been isolated in southern Africa.[49, 55] These include *Mycoplasma alkalescens, M. arginini, M. bovigenitalium, M. bovirhinis, M. bovis, M. canadense, Mycoplasma* Leach Group 7, *M. verecundum, Acholeplasma axanthum, A. laidlawii, A. modicum* and *Ureaplasma* spp.

The pathogenicity of few of the foregoing mycoplasmas is unequivocal, but experimentally proven lesions in the genital tract are definitely associated with some. *Mycoplasma bovis* is considered to be one of the most pathogenic species in cattle,[20] and although its role in specific infections of the reproductive tract is still unclear, infertility is associated with infection by this organism.[23, 26, 30] *Mycoplasma bovigenitalium* is a well-established species of the bovine urogenital tract.[54] It has been associated with poor reproductive performance in cows,[10, 39] and with poor sperm motility in bulls.[43] The only other mycoplasma considered to be pathogenic beyond doubt is *M. canadense,* which has been isolated from vaginal mucus, semen and foetal tissue.[8, 17] Mastitis is caused by this organism after its intramammary introduction.[32]

Mycoplasma Leach Group 7 organisms have been isolated from the urogenital tract of cattle and from tissues of aborted foetuses.[38] However, the same organism can also be isolated from the urogenital tract of apparently normal animals.[39] *Mycoplasma alkalescens, M. arginini, M. bovirhinis, M. verecundum* and the *Acholeplasma* spp. are considered to be non-pathogenic and to form part of the normal flora of the lower urogenital tract.

Ureaplasma diversum was first isolated from cases of non-gonococcal urethritis in humans.[51] This organism has since been isolated from cattle with granular vaginitis, endometritis, salpingitis, seminal vesiculitis and from aborted foetuses.[7, 31, 36, 50] In cattle, *U. diversum* is the only pathogenic ureaplasma affecting the genitalia. All other ureaplasmas appear to be commensals in the genital tract.

Mollicutes are fastidious in their growth requirements, and specifically formulated media are essential for their isolation. For diagnostic purposes, the use of a combination of different media is recommended. This enhances the frequency of primary isolation and success of laboratory maintenance. Trichard and Jacobsz[55] recommend the use of at least four different media, namely, Hayflick's agar and broth,[24] Gourlay's glucose serum agar and broth,[21] Chalquest's agar and broth,[9] and Morgan's agar and broth.[41]

Organisms assigned to the class Mollicutes generally possess few biochemical characteristics that can be used for species identification. Serological tests have come to play an essential and dominant role in this respect.[42, 56, 59, 61] Tests involving membrane antigens are used almost exclusively for laboratory identification. They include growth inhibition, metabolic inhibition and immunofluorescence techniques. The latter in particular provide rapid and reliable identification of *Mycoplasma* spp. under a variety of conditions.[4, 55, 59]

Epidemiology

Diseases caused by *Mycoplasma* and *Ureaplasma* spp. are principally associated with intensive husbandry systems.[19] Coitus is probably the most important mechanism for transmitting these organisms.[55] Mechanical transmission following close contact between infected and susceptible animals, and lack of sterile technique during vaginal examinations may also be significant.

Since a high proportion of semen and preputial samples are known to be contaminated with *Mycoplasma* spp.,[5, 16, 17, 28, 29, 45, 49, 55] artificial insemination probably also constitutes an important means of spread.

Pathogenesis

The pathogenesis of genital mycoplasmosis is poorly defined. Localization of infection at possible predilection sites such as synovial membranes and the placenta[52] may follow an initial haematogenous dissemination or may be the consequence of local contamination and initiation of the infection. Genital infections are easily produced by depositing organisms directly into the genital tract of either the male or female.

It is unclear how mycoplasmas spread from a site of local infection in the lower reproductive tract to the upper reproductive tract to cause disease. This applies particularly to bulls, where the most common habitat of *Mycoplasma* spp. is the lower urogenital tract, including the prepuce, glans penis and the distal urethra, from whence their dissemination to the upper genital tract may occur. Localization of *Mycoplasma* spp. in these regions produces no clinical signs of disease but may incite a local immune response,[43] despite which local infections may persist for more than a year.

Inconsistent results have been obtained in experiments in which *M. bovigenitalium* was introduced into the genital tract of cows.[1, 26, 46] This could be because of a variation in the pathogenicity of strains of the same species.[2] Additionally, a combination of one or more strains in the same animal may enhance pathogenicity.[55]

Fertility can be severely affected when *M. bovis* is inoculated into the genital system of the female, as shown by an experiment in which several heifers were inseminated with semen contaminated with *M. bovis*.[25] They showed noticeable abnormalities in the duration of the subsequent oestrus cycle. In most of them a vaginal discharge was evident, and none conceived, even after repeated insemination. A conception rate of 83 per cent was attained in the control group.

Male infertility or poor conception rates may be the consequence of the effect of mycoplasmas on sperm.[35] There is an association between the presence of *M. bovigenitalium* in secretions of the seminal vesicle glands of clinically normal bulls, and diminished sperm motility.[22] Inhibition of motility appears to be the result of adherence of the organisms principally to the acrosome but also to the midpiece and tail of spermatozoa.[44]

The adverse effect on conception rates in cattle[35] may not necessarily be as a result of the effect on semen only. The effect of a mild to severe endometritis and the possible inhibition of ciliary action in the oviducts should also be considered.[52] None of the *Mycoplasma* spp. which are known to localize in the uterus, however, affected this ciliary motility.

The pathogenesis of abortion due to mycoplasmal infections is unknown. It appears that it may be the consequence both of a foetal mycoplasmaemia and a concomitant placentitis.[53]

Clinical signs

Genital *Mycoplasma* spp. infections in cows usually present as a condition characterized by aberrant oestrus cycles. Less frequently they manifest as a granular vulvovaginitis which is accompanied by a mucopurulent vaginal discharge. This discharge may become copious and in some cases it is visible on the skin and hair in the vicinity of the vulva three to six days after breeding. As the infection subsides, the discharge becomes less and may be noticeable only as a cloudiness of the usually clear bullstring at the following oestrus.[34]

Abortions may follow experimental exposure of pregnant cows to mollicutes.[53] Cows usually abort 11–18 days after infection, and the organism may be recovered from foetal and placental tissues as well as from the uterine contents. Clinical signs in the experimental cases were slight and were accompanied only by a moderate fever at the time of the mycoplasmaemia.

Heifers may develop lameness due to arthritis, with swelling of the affected joints, anorexia and cachexia following experimental infection.

Pathology

Colonization of the genital tract of cattle by most *Mycoplasma* or *Ureaplasma* spp. in natural infections is normally not associated with lesions.[16] Granular vulvovaginitis, however, is a common result of experimentally induced infections of *M. bovigenitalium* and *Ureaplasma* spp.[13, 14] Varying degrees of endometritis, salpingitis and salpingoperitonitis follow the intrauterine instillation of *M. bovis* cultures.[23] A moderate amount of a purulent uterine exudate is present during the first two weeks. Extensive gross lesions consisting of severe, generalized, suppurative endometritis, salpingitis and peritonitis occur 33 days after infection. Varying degrees of chronic endometritis, salpingitis and peri-oophoritis, and bursal adhesions have also been reported in longstanding cases.[25, 27] Local infection may be associated with a mucopurulent exudate in the vagina, cervix and uterus.[48] The exudate in the uterus may become inspissated.[7]

In abortion caused by *U. diversum*, placentitis occurred in all instances in which the placenta was examined. The aborted foetuses manifested a diffuse pneumonitis and peribronchiolar lymphoid accumulations.[40, 47]

Lesions in the seminal vesicular glands and epididymides in bulls experimentally infected with

M. bovigenitalium are characterized by the presence of mild to moderate focal accumulations of lymphocytes and macrophages.[43]

Seminal vesiculitis induced in bulls by the direct intravesicular injection of *M. bovis* results in a seminal vesiculitis and persistent shedding of the organisms in its secretion for up to eight-and-a-half months.[37] Attempts to reproduce seminal vesiculitis by other routes have not been successful.

Similarly, infecting bulls intravesicularly with *Ureaplasma* organisms resulted in an enlargement of the seminal vesicles, which became rectally palpable within 24 hours of inoculation. Moderate to severe, diffuse, chronic seminal vesiculitis with moderate interstitial fibrosis and epithelial degeneration has been reported to occur 4–8 weeks after infection.[60]

Diagnosis

Specimens from cows and heifers with histories of repeated breeding, conception failure, abortion in the early stages of pregnancy and/or the presence of mucopurulent discharges, should be examined for mollicutes. Methods for the collection of vaginal mucus, cervical specimens and preputial washings are available.[55] Swabs of vulval exudate should be made if a granular vulvovaginitis is being investigated. Cervical mucus should be collected in sterile pipettes in cases where lesions in the uterus and oviducts are suspected. Specimens from bulls should include preputial washings as well as vesicular seminal fluid if upper genital tract involvement is suspected. Samples should be packed on ice and delivered to the laboratory on the day of collection.

Differential diagnosis

The two most important diseases that should be differentiated from genital mycoplasmoses are infectious pustular vulvovaginitis, and the disease known as 'epivag', although venereal diseases such as campylobacteriosis should also be considered. In bulls, seminal vesiculitis may also be caused by chlamydial infections. Special laboratory procedures are necessary to differentiate these conditions.

Control

A high proportion of semen samples collected from healthy bulls at artificial insemination centres are contaminated with mollicutes.[6, 18, 33, 49, 55] Routine screening and decontamination of semen is therefore desirable to avoid the spread of these organisms.[3, 57] Antibiotics such as penicillin and streptomycin, normally added during the processing of such semen, do not eliminate mollicutes. Diluents containing lincomycin and spectinomycin will control *Mycoplasma* spp. in semen but are not effective against *Ureaplasma* spp.[56] The addition of minocycline hydrochloride to the diluent, however, effectively controls both *Mycoplasma* and *Ureaplasma* spp.[58]

Infertility due to inflammatory changes in the female genital system induced by mollicutes can be treated by the intrauterine instillation of solutions containing tetracycline or oxytetracycline.[11, 12] It is advocated that sheathed insemination pipettes be used when inseminating cows, as this should reduce the number of pathogens that may be carried forward from the vagina into the cervix and uterus.

References

1 **AFSHAR, A., STUART, P. & HUCH, R.A., 1966.** Granular vulvovaginitis of cattle associated with *Mycoplasma bovigenitalium*. *The Veterinary Record*, 78, 512–519.

2 **AL-AUBAIDI, J.M., McENTEE, K., LEIN, D.H. & ROBERTS, S.J., 1972.** Bovine seminal vesiculitis and epididymitis caused by *Mycoplasma bovigenitalium*. *Cornell Veterinarian*, 62, 581–596.

3 **ALMQUIST, J.O. & ZAUGG, N,L., 1974.** Fertility of bovine semen in milk diluent containing combinations of penicillin-neomycin and lincomycin-spectinomycin. *Journal of Dairy Science*, 57, 1211–1213.

4 **BAAS, E.J. & JASPER, D.E., 1972.** Agar block technique for identification of mycoplasmas by use of fluorescent antibody. *Applied Microbiology*, 23, 1097–1100.

5 **BALL, H.J., ARMSTRONG, D., McCAUGHEY, W.J. & KENNEDY, S., 1987.** Experimental intrauterine inoculation of cows at oestrus with *Mycoplasma canadense*. *The Veterinary Record*, 119, 370.

6 **BALL, H.J., LOGAN, E.F. & ORR, W., 1987.** Isolation of mycoplasmas from bovine semen in Northern Ireland. *The Veterinary Record*, 120, 322–324.

7 **BALL, H.J., McCAUGHEY, W.J., MACKIE, D.P. & PEARSON, G.R., 1981.** Experimental genital infection of heifers with ureaplasmas. *Research in Veterinary Science*, 30, 312–317.

8 **BOUGHTON, E., SHEILAGH, A.N. & GAYFORD, P.J.R., 1983.** *Mycoplasma canadense* from bovine fetuses. *The Veterinary Record*, 112, 87.

9 **CHALQUEST, R.R., 1962.** Cultivation of the infectious synovitis-type pleuropneumonia-like organisms. *Avian Diseases*, 6, 36–43.

10 **COTTEW, G.S., 1970.** Mycoplasmas isolated from cattle in Australia. *Australian Veterinary Journal*, 46, 378–381.

11 **DOIG, P.A., 1981.** Bovine genital mycoplasmosis. *Canadian Veterinary Journal*, 22, 339–343.

12 **DOIG, P.A., RUHNKE, H.L., McKAY, A.L. & PALMER, N.C., 1979.** Bovine granular vulvitis associated with *Ureaplasma* infection. *Canadian Veterinary Journal*, 20, 89–94.

13 **DOIG, P.A., RUHNKE, H.L. & PALMER, N.C., 1980.** Experimental bovine genital ureaplasmosis. 1. Granular vulvitis following vulvar inoculation. *Canadian Journal of Comparative Medicine*, 44, 252–258.

14 **DOIG, P.A., RUHNKE, H.L. & PALMER, N.C., 1980.** Experimental vulvitis, endometritis and salpingitis following uterine inoculation. *Canadian Journal of Comparative Medicine*, 44, 259–266.

15 **ERNO, H., PLASTRIDGE, W.N. & TOURTELLOUTE, M.E., 1967.** *Mycoplasma* isolation of prepuce and semen of bulls.

Acta Veterinaria Scandinavia, 8, 123–135.

16 **FISH, N.A., ROSENDAL, S. & MILLER, R.B., 1985.** The distribution of mycoplasmas and ureaplasmas in the genital tract of normal artificial insemination bulls. *Canadian Veterinary Journal*, 26, 13–15.

17 **FRIIS, N.F. & BLOM, E., 1983.** Isolation of *Mycoplasma canadense* from bull semen. *Acta Veterinaria Scandinavia*, 24, 315–317.

18 **GARCIA, M.M., TRUSCOTT, R.B., McLAREN, J., STEWART, R.B. & KINGSCOTE, B., 1986.** Absence of *Mycoplasma bovis* in unprocessed frozen bull semen from Canadian artificial insemination centres. *The Veterinary Record*, 119, 11–12.

19 **GOURLAY, R.N., 1981.** Mycoplasmosis in cattle, sheep and goats. *Israel Journal of Medical Science*, 17, 531–536.

20 **GOURLAY, R.N. & HOWARD, C.J., 1979.** *In: The Mycoplasmas*. Vol. II. London and New York: Academic Press, Inc.

21 **GOURLAY, R.N., HOWARD, C.J., THOMAS, L.H. & STOTT, E.J., 1976.** Experimentally produced calf pneumonia. *Research in Veterinary Science*, 20, 167–173.

22 **HALL, C.E. & McENTEE, K., 1981.** Reduced post-thawing survival of sperm in bulls with mycoplasmal vesiculitis. *Cornell Veterinarian*, 71, 111–112.

23 **HARTMAN, H.A., TOURTELOUTTE, M.E., NIELSEN, S.W. & PLASTRIDGE, W.N., 1964.** Experimental bovine uterine mycoplasmosis. *Research in Veterinary Science*, 5, 303–310.

24 **HAYFLICK, L., 1965.** Tissue cultures and mycoplasmas. *Texas Reports on Biology and Medicine*, 1, 23, 285 – 303.

25 **HIRTH, R.S., NIELSEN, S.W. & PLASTRIDGE, W.N., 1966.** Bovine salpingo-oophoritis produced with semen containing *Mycoplasma*. *Pathologia Veterinaria*, 3, 616–632.

26 **HIRTH, R.S., NIELSEN, S.W. & TOURTELLOUTE, M.E., 1970.** Characterization and comparative genital tract pathogenicity of bovine mycoplasmas. *Infection and Immunity*, 2, 101–104.

27 **HOARE, M., 1969.** A survey of the incidence of *Mycoplasma* infection in the oviducts of dairy cows. *The Veterinary Record*, 85, 351–355.

28 **HODGES, R.T. & HOLLAND, J.T.S., 1980.** The recovery of ureaplasmas from the semen and prepuce of bulls. *New Zealand Veterinary Journal*, 28, 89–90.

29 **HOLZMANN, A., THIEMANN, G., FLATCHER, J. & PRILHOFER, K., 1982.** Changes in semen of steers with positive *Mycoplasma* evidence. *Zentralblatt für Veterinärmedizin*, 29, 710–715.

30 **HORVATH, G., STIPKOVITS, L., VARGA, Z., ZOLDAG, L. & MESZAROS, J., 1983.** Infection of cows by *Mycoplasma bovis*. *Archiv für Experimentelle Veterinärmedizin*, 37, 401–403.

31 **HOWARD, C.J., 1984.** Animal ureaplasmas: Their ecological niche and role in disease. *Israel Journal of Medical Science*, 20, 954–957.

32 **JASPER, D.E., 1977.** *Mycoplasma* and mycoplasma mastitis. *Journal of the American Veterinary Medical Association*, 170, 1167–1172.

33 **JURMANOVA, K., WEZNIK, Z., CERNA, J. & MAZUROVA, J., 1983.** Demonstration and role of mycoplasmas and ureaplasmas in bull semen and the control of *Mycoplasma* infections in bulls. *Archiv für Experimentelle Veterinärmedizin*, 37, 421–428.

34 **KIRCHOFF, H., 1982.** Die Bedeutung der Mykoplasmen in den Genital-organen von Rind, Pferd und Schwein. *Berliner und Münchener Tierärztliche Wochenschrift*, 95, 121–125.

35 **KISSIE, B., JUHASZ, S. & STIPKOVITS, L., 1985.** Effect of *Mycoplasma* contamination of bull semen on fertilization. *Acta Veterinaria Hungarica*, 33, 107–117.

36 **KUHN, M.J. & HOPKINS, S.M., 1983.** A clinical review of bovine ureaplasmosis. *Iowa State Veterinarian*, 45, 20–24.

37 **La FAUNCE, N.A. & McENTEE, K., 1982.** Experimental *Mycoplasma bovis* seminal vesiculitis in the bull. *Cornell Veterinarian*, 72, 150–167.

38 **LANGFORD, E.V., 1975.** *Mycoplasma* species recovered from the reproductive tracts of Western Canadian cows. *Canadian Journal of Comparative Medicine*, 39, 133–137.

39 **LANGFORD, E.V., 1975.** *Mycoplasma* recovered from bovine male and female genitalia and aborted foeti. *Proceedings of the Eighteenth Annual Meeting of Veterinary Laboratory Diagnosticians*, San Diego, California.

40 **MILLER, R.B., RUHNKE, H.L., DOIG, P.A., POITRAS, B.J. & PALMER, N.C., 1983.** The effect of *Ureaplasma diversum* inoculated into the amniotic cavity in cows. *Theriogenology*, 20, 367–374.

41 **MORGAN, J.H. & LEWIS, J., 1977.** A medium for the primary isolation of T-mycoplasmas from cattle. *Medical Laboratory Sciences*, 34, 177–178.

42 **NIELSEN, K.H., STEWART, R.B., GARCIA, M.M. & EAGLESOME, M.D., 1987.** Enzyme immunoassay for detection of *Mycoplasma bovis* antigens in bull semen and preputial washings. *The Veterinary Record*, 120, 596–598.

43 **PANANGALA, V.S., HALL, C.E., CAVENEY, N.T., LEIN, D.H. & WINTER, A.J., 1982.** *Mycoplasma bovigenitalium* in upper genital tract of bulls: Spontaneous and induced infections. *Cornell Veterinarian*, 72, 292–303.

44 **PANANGALA, V.S., WINTER, A.J., WIJESINHA, A. & FOOTE, R.H., 1981.** Decreased motility of bull spermatozoa caused by *Mycoplasma bovigenitalium*. *American Journal of Veterinary Research*, 42, 2090–2093.

45 **RAE, A.G., 1982.** Isolation of mycoplasmas from bovine semen. *The Veterinary Record*, 109, 463.

46 **ROBERTS, D.H., 1968.** Immunological response in cows to *Mycoplasma bovigenitalium* strain 1836. *Journal of Hygiene, Cambridge*, 66, 585–593.

47 **RUHNKE, H.L., PALMER, N.C., DOIG, P.A. & MILLER, R.B., 1984.** Bovine abortion and neonate death associated with *Ureaplasma diversum*. *Theriogenology*, 21, 295–301.

48 **SAED, O.M. & AL-AUBAIDI, J.M., 1983.** Infertility in heifers caused by a pathogenic strain of *Mycoplasma bovigenitalium*. *Cornell Veterinarian*, 73, 125–130.

49 **SCHUTTE, A.P., 1975.** Bees mycoplasmose en onvrugbaarheid. *Symposium: Reproductive Disorders and Fertility of Ruminants, South African Veterinary Association*, July 1975.

50 **SCHWEIGHARDT, H., KALTENBOCK, B., LAUERMAN, E. & PECHAN, P., 1985.** Ureaplasmen als Verusacher von granularen Vulvovaginitiden beim Rind. *Wiener Tierärztliche Monatsschrift*, 72, 209–214.

51 **SHEPARD, M.C., 1954.** The recovery of pleuropneumonia-like organisms from negro men with and without non-gonococcal urethritis. *American Journal of Syphilis, Gonorrhoea and Venereal Diseases*, 38, 113–124.

52 **STALHEIM, O.H.V. & GALLAGHAR, J.E., 1975.** Effects of *Mycoplasma* spp., *Trichomonas fetus* and *Campylobacter fetus* on ciliary activity of bovine uterine tube organ cultures. *American Journal of Veterinary Research*, 36, 1077–1080.

53 **STALHEIM, O.H.V. & PROCTOR, S.J., 1976.** Experimentally induced bovine abortion with *Mycoplasma agalactiae* subsp. *bovis*. *American Journal of Veterinary Research*, 37, 879 – 883.

54 **TOURTELLOTTE, M.E. & LEIN, D.H., 1976.** Infertility of cattle caused by mycoplasmas. *Health and Laboratory Science*, 13, 152–157.

55 **TRICHARD, C.J.V. & JACOBSZ, E.P., 1985.** Mycoplasmas recovered from bovine genitalia, aborted foetuses and placentas in the Republic of South Africa. *Onderstepoort Journal of Veterinary Research*, 52, 105–110.

56 **TRUSCOTT, R.B., 1981.** A comparison of the *in vitro* activity of two antibiotics against bovine ureaplasmas. *Canadian Journal of Comparative Medicine*, 45, 113–115.

57 **TRUSCOTT, R.B. & ABREO, C., 1977.** Antibiotics for elimination of mycoplasmas and ureaplasma from bovine semen. *Journal of Dairy Science*, 60, 954–960.

58 **TRUSCOTT, R.B. & RUHNKE, H.L., 1984.** The effect of antibiotics against bovine mycoplasmas and ureaplasmas. *Canadian Journal of Comparative Medicine*, 48, 171–174.

59 **TULLY, J.G. & RAZIN, S., 1983.** *Methods in Mycoplasmology*. Vols. I & II. New York: Academic Press, Inc.

60 **WAELCHLI-SUTER, R.O., DOIG, P.A., RUHNKE, H.L., PALMER, N.C. & BARKER, C.A.V., 1982.** Experimental genital ureaplasmosis in the bull. *Schweizer Archiv für Tierheilkunde*, 124, 273–295.

61 **WITTOWSKI, G., ROTH, B. & KIRCHHOFF, H., 1984.** Nachweis von Mykoplasmen und Ureaplasmen im genitaltrakt des Rindes. *Berliner und Münchener Tierärztliche Wochenschrift*, 97, 189–190, 193–197.

UNCLASSIFIED BACTERIA

Two bacteria, *Bacillus pilliformis,* the cause of Tyzzer's disease, and *Taylorella equigenitalis,* the cause of contagious equine metritis, are dealt with in this section.

The genus name *Bacillus,* in the case of *Bacillus piliformis,* which is not listed in *Bergey's Manual of Systematic Bacteriology,* is probably incorrect contrary to the members of the genus *Bacillus* **(see Chapter 153: Anthrax)**, the bacterium is obligate and intracellular. Tyzzer's disease is a sporadic disease of foals, particularly those which are immunoincompetent, and is characterized by necrotizing hepatitis. The bacterium is more commonly associated with disease in rodents.

Outbreaks of contagious equine metritis, particularly in Thoroughbreds, have been described in the major horsebreeding areas of Europe and the USA. The disease has not yet been diagnosed in southern Africa.

183

Taylorella equigenitalis *infection*

Synonym: Contagious equine metritis

M.M. Henton

Introduction

Contagious equine metritis (CEM) is a venereal disease of equids caused by *Taylorella equigenitalis* and characterized by a transient, acute metritis resulting in infertility which is usually temporary. Both mares and stallions may be carriers of the organism. The infection severely disrupts breeding regimes, particularly in establishments in which Thoroughbreds are bred according to the rules of the Thoroughbred associations which require a very short breeding season.

This genital infection of mares was first recorded in Newmarket, England, in May 1977 by Crowhurst.[5, 14] A bacterium initially referred to as *Haemophilus equigenitalis* was isolated from affected mares,[29] but was later renamed and placed in a separate genus, *Taylorella equigenitalis*.[24]

Contagious equine metritis has been confirmed in Austria, Australia, Brazil, Belgium, Denmark, France, Germany, Great Britain, Italy, Japan, Norway, Sweden, the USA and Yugoslavia, but has not, as far as is known, been diagnosed on the African continent. It appears not to have been introduced into South Africa because of the strict application of measures that regulate the importation of animals, including the application of quarantine procedures.

The prevalence of the disease appears to have declined drastically, as only isolated cases are reported worldwide at present, e.g. one case in Great Britain in 1986, and one again in Scotland in 1990.[2]

Aetiology

Taylorella equigenitalis, the only species in the genus, is a Gram-negative, non-acid-fast, non-motile, short rod, 0,7 µm wide and 0,7–1,8 µm long; occasional longer filaments are seen. It is X- and V-factor-independent, and grows best on chocolated horse blood agar in an atmosphere containing 5–10 per cent CO_2 (on which colonies take at least two days to become visible),[34] and very poorly on plain nutrient or blood agar. The organism is biochemically relatively inactive and reacts negatively to a large range of tests; it is only catalase-, oxidase-, phosphatase- and ubiquinone-positive.[11, 28, 29]

All isolates are serologically and morphologically similar, but it appears that colony variation is related to the virulence of the organisms — large colony variants are more virulent.[12] Different colony types have been described on Eugon and tryptose chocolate agar incubated for 10–15 days.[21] These were smooth, sandy colonies with rings, colonies with blebs, and large colonies. Each type of colony was composed of coccal, coccobacillary and bacillary forms, but one form predominated in each colony type. The colonies are raised, shiny, smooth, butyrous grey and pin-point in size after two to four days' incubation. They are non-haemolytic.

Based on evidence from studies of DNA base composition and hybridization, the organism is not closely related to organisms of any other genus, although it is phenotypically similar to organisms such as *Moraxella* and *Legionella*.[24]

The bacteria are killed within ten minutes by common disinfectants such as chlorhexidine and quaternary ammonium compounds at recommended concentrations.[25] Thermal resistance studies[38] have indicated the effectiveness of normal heat sterilization, and the organism is particularly susceptible to acid below pH 4,5.[18] Growth does not take place below 30 °C.[29] *Taylorella equigenitalis* is susceptible to the disinfectants chlorhexidine diacetate (2 per cent) and alkyldimethylbenzylammonium chloride (10 per cent) if dried cultures and exudates are exposed to these disinfectants for ten minutes. The organism is able to survive drying in exudates on metal surfaces for 40 minutes.[25]

Epidemiology

Apart from horses, donkey mares are also susceptible,[32] but other species, including cattle, sheep and pigs, are refractory to experimental infection.[30, 33] It is not known whether zebras are susceptible. *Taylorella equigenitalis* is a strict commensal in the lumen of the external genitalia of healthy stallions, and may survive for years in the clitoral sinuses[22] and vagina of mares following infection. The infection is usually transmitted venereally,[13, 14] but as CEM is highly contagious it can also be spread indirectly, e.g. by equipment used to wash and bandage mares, or by equipment used for genital examinations and contaminated by genital exudates. Communal pre-breeding areas appear to provide ideal conditions for transmission;[27] infection appears to be passed between stallions by handlers, and also occurs from floors wet from washing stallions prior to breeding.[26, 27]

Acutely infected mares develop a profuse vulvar discharge containing large numbers of *T. equigenitalis*, which may be isolated in almost pure culture. Mares and stallions suffering from inapparent infections may, however, yield only very few organisms on culture from the genitalia.[9] Following recovery, a large percentage of mares remain carriers for periods which may vary from one month to years.[34] The organisms are shed either constantly or intermittently in exudates and venereal secretions; shedding can be independent of the oestrus period.[37] Treatment of the overt disease with antibiotics, though reducing the severity of clinical signs, may also predispose to the development of a carrier state.[26, 27]

Most mares which have recovered from an attack of the clinical disease are fertile. Foals may be born after intra-uterine infection and may not manifest the effects of the infection until after they have reached sexual maturity.[34, 36] *Taylorella equigenitalis* may also be isolated from the placenta of infected mares.[16]

Pathogenesis, clinical signs and pathology

Clinical signs develop in only 30–40 per cent of mares served by an infected stallion. Of the remainder, some become inapparently infected and develop into carriers.[8] In acute cases, clinical evidence of an endometritis manifested by the presence of a cloudy, purulent to mucopurulent vaginal discharge develops within two to ten days of service. This discharge, when copious, mats the hair of the tail and buttocks, but when scanty may merely accumulate in the vagina and not be externally noticeable. Some degree of vaginitis may also be present. Infected horses show no signs of systemic involvement.[4]

The majority of infected mares usually return to oestrus earlier than normal due to a shortened dioestrus. Some may, however, carry the foetus to full term, and *T. equigenitalis* can usually be recovered during foal heat. Abortion during early pregnancy or foetal resorption may also occur, but late abortions are uncommon.[8]

Semen enhances the infectivity and the pathogenicity of *T. equigenitalis* for mares.[32] In the uterus the infection is limited to the superficial layers and the lesions are those of a typical mucopurulent endometritis. The luminal epithelium undergoes hyperplasia within two days of infection, followed by vacuolization which persists for up to 37 days. Some epithelial cells show advanced cytoplasmic and nuclear degenerative changes, with subepithelial vacuoles containing amorphous debris. The initial pronounced neutrophil infiltrate, which is marked within 24 hours of the infection, changes rapidly to a stromal mononuclear cell infiltration consisting predominantly of plasma cells. Large numbers of neutrophils and degenerative epithelial cells, as well as large numbers of *T. equigenitalis* are present in the uterine exudate.[17] Some mares simultaneously suffer from a superficial vaginitis.

The immunity to CEM is poor, and horses may be repeatedly reinfected.[4, 39] Detectable humoral antibody responses have been demonstrated only in mares and not in stallions. The resistance of recovered mares appears to be due to locally produced antibodies, because systemic antibody responses are lower after the second than the first infection.[4, 20]

Diagnosis and differential diagnosis

The endometritis and vaginitis cannot easily be clinically differentiated from similar lesions caused by infections with other bacteria, such as *Klebsiella* and *Pseudomonas* spp. and *Streptococcus zooepidemicus*. Bacterial culture is thus essential to confirm the diagnosis. *Taylorella equigenitalis* infection in mares persists mainly in the clitoral fossa and sinuses. As the sinuses have narrow, slit-like openings, a thin cotton-tipped swab should be used to obtain adequate specimens. Specimens should preferably be taken at oestrus when the cervix is open.[9] Swabs for the isolation of the organism should be transported in transport medium (preferably Amies modified transport medium containing activated charcoal), must be kept cool (specimens keep well at 4 °C but may also be deep-frozen to –70 °C), and must be processed within 48 hours.[19, 31] Swabs may be heavily contaminated with the normal bacterial flora which inhibit the growth of *T. equigenitalis*, and selective media containing antibiotics should be used to minimize the growth of contaminants.[35] Good results are obtained on a medium based on Eugon agar, supplemented with Isovitalex (both without added glucose), 5 per cent chocolatized horse blood, 5 per cent lysed horse blood, trimethoprim (1 µg/ml), clindamycin (5 µg/ml) and amphotericin B (5 µg/ml). Plates should be incubated for four to six days to ensure that no growth has occurred.

Swabs from the urethra, urethral fossa and the sheath, as well as samples of pre-ejaculatory fluid are the most suitable specimens for bacterial isolation from stallions. False-negative results may be obtained on culture, and at least three consecutive negative bacteriological examinations at weekly intervals are required before a stallion can be certified as being free of *T. equigenitalis*.[14] False-negative results may be due to intermittent shedding of the causal organism or to limitations in laboratory techniques.[34]

The complement fixation test using serum for the serological diagnosis of the infection is specific, but it does not detect acute infections,[4] nor does it identify all carriers.[20] Several other serological tests, such as enzyme-linked immunosorbent assay (ELISA), agglutination, antiglobulin, indirect fluorescent antibody and passive haemagglutination,[20] have been used, but with no greater success. Both the complement fixation test and serum agglutination test are used in South Africa.[10]

Control

Comprehensive recommendations for the control of CEM have been made by the Horserace Betting Levy Board in the United Kingdom.[1]

Contagious equine metritis is a notifiable disease in South Africa. Imported horses are subject to strict import regulations, which include certification that they are free of the infection. For this, repeated negative culturing both before and after service, and a negative complement fixation test are required. Comprehensive regulatory measures for the control and prevention of the introduction of the disease are contained in the 'Code of Practice for the Control of Contagious Equine Metritis' issued by the Director of Animal Health, Department of Agriculture.[3] This code of practice stipulates the conditions that govern the importation of horses and the continual vigilance required after imported horses have left the quarantine station. Thus, all imported horses are identified, their movements monitored, and they are tested regularly until certified negative for CEM. Such horses are tested again prior to resale, and may not be sold unless they are found to be negative for CEM. Breeding quarantine is imposed on the breeding establishment until the animals are certified free of infection by the State Veterinarian. If pregnant mares are imported, they must be moved under cover of a red cross permit to an officially approved pregnant-mare quarantine farm after release from the quarantine station. If such a mare aborts, the foetus and placenta must be examined for CEM. Foals born to imported pregnant mares are also repeatedly tested for CEM in the same way.

The use of artificial insemination is the only way to successfully control CEM once it has been introduced into a breeding herd, but this practice is not allowed in Thoroughbreds bred for registration. Managemental, preventive and control measures are important, and there should be high standards of hygiene at mating; all equipment should be sterilized.

Before being bred, maiden mares should be swabbed at first heat, especially from the clitoral fossa. All previously infected or in-contact animals should have three consecutive negative swabs.[9] Infected horses should not be used for breeding.[23, 29]

Stallions can be treated successfully with antibiotics[15] or local treatment with chlorhexidine in dilutions up to 1 in 125 000 w/v,[29] but there is doubt about the efficacy of treatment in mares. *Taylorella equigenitalis* is sensitive to several antibiotics, such as ceftotoxamine, penicillin, neomycin, chloramphenicol and tetracycline, but treatment is not recommended as the susceptibility of the bacteria to individual antibiotics tends to vary and susceptibility tests should be carried out.[6, 40] In addition, normal flora appear to inhibit the growth of CEM, and the indiscriminate use of antibiotics is discouraged.[26]

Vaccination appears to be unsuccessful.[7]

References

1 **ANON., 1984.** A common code of practice for the control of contagious equine metritis and other equine reproductive disease for the 1984 covering season in France, Ireland and the United Kingdom. *The Veterinary Record*, 113, 512–515.

2 **ANON., 1990.** Office International des Épizooties, 12 Rue de Prony, 75017 Paris, France.

3 **ANON., 1991.** Director of Animal Health, Department of Agriculture, Republic of South Africa. Code of practice for the control of contagious equine metritis (19 July 1991).

4 **BREWER, R.A., 1983.** Contagious equine metritis: A review/summary. *Veterinary Bulletin*, 53, 881–891.

5 **CROWHURST, R.C., 1977.** Genital infection in mares. *The Veterinary Record*, 100, 746.

6 **EGUCHI, M., KUNIYASU, C., OHMAE, K. & TANAKA, M., 1988.** Dry sensitivity of *Taylorella equigenitalis* isolated in Japan in 1985. *Japanese Journal of Veterinary Science*, 50, 561–563.

7 **FERNIE, D.S., BATTY, I., WALKER, P.D., PLATT, H., MACKINTOSH, M.E. & SIMPSON, D.J., 1980.** Observations on vaccine and post-infection immunity in contagious equine metritis. *Research in Veterinary Science*, 28, 362–367.

8 **FONTIJNE, P., TER LAAK, E.A. & HARTMAN, E.G., 1989.** *Taylorella equigenitalis* isolated from an aborted foal. *The Veterinary Record*, 125, 485.

9 **FRANK, C.J., 1979.** Code of practice for control of contagious equine metritis and other equine venereal diseases for the 1980 covering season. *The Veterinary Record*, 105, 395–397.

10 **GUMMOW, B., HERR, S. & BRETT, O.L., 1987.** A rapid microtitration serum agglutination test for the detection of contagious equine metritis antibodies. *Onderstepoort Journal of Veterinary Research*, 54, 97–98.

11 **HOLLÄNDER, R., HESS-REIHSE, A. & MANNHEIM, W., 1981.** Respiratory quinones in *Haemophilus, Pasteurella* and *Actinobacillus:* Pattern, function and taxonomic evaluation. *In:* KILLIAN, M., FREDERIKSEN, W. & BIBERSTEIN, E.L., (eds). *Haemophilus, Pasteurella and Actinobacillus*. New York, London, Toronto, Sydney, San Francisco: Academic Press, Inc.

12 **KANEMARU, T., KAMADA, M., ANZAI, T. & KUMANOMIDO, T., 1988.** Contagious equine metritis: The pathogenicity for mares of small and large colonial variants of *Taylorella equigenitalis* isolated from a laboratory strain. *Proceedings of the Fifth International Conference on Equine Infectious Diseases*, Lexington, Kentucky, 1988.

13 **PLATT, H., ATHERTON, J.G., DAWSON, F.L.M. & DURRANT, D.S., 1978.** Developments in contagious equine metritis. *The Veterinary Record*, 102, 19.

14 **PLATT, H., ATHERTON, J.G., SIMPSON, D.J., TAYLOR, C.E.D., ROSENTHAL, R.O., BROWN, D.F.J. & WREGHITT, T.G., 1977.** Genital infection in mares. *The Veterinary Record*, 101, 20.

15 **POWELL, D.G., 1978.** Contagious equine metritis. *Equine Veterinary Journal*, 10, 1–4.

16 **POWELL, D.G. & WHITWELL, K., 1979.** The epidemiology of contagious equine metritis (CEM) in England 1977–1978. *Journal of Reproduction and Fertility*, Supplement 27, 331–335.

17 **RICKETTS, S.W., ROSSDALE, P.D. & SAMUEL, C.A., 1978.** Endometrial biopsy studies of mares with contagious equine metritis 1977. *Equine Veterinary Journal*, 10, 160–166.

18 **SAHU, S.P. & DARDIRI, A.H., 1980.** Contagious equine metritis: Isolation and characterization of the etiologic agent. *American Journal of Veterinary Research*, 41, 1379–1382.

19 **SAHU, S.P., DARDIRI, A.H., ROMMEL, F.A. & PIERSON, R.E., 1979.** Survival of contagious equine metritis bacteria in transport media. *American Journal of Veterinary Research*, 40, 1040–1042.

20 **SAHU, S.P., ROMMEL, F.A., FALES, W.H., HAMDY, F.M., SWERCZEK, T.W., YOUNGQUIST, R.S. & BRYANS, J.T., 1983.** Evaluation of various serotests to detect antibodies in ponies and horses infected with contagious equine metritis bacteria. *American Journal of Veterinary Research*, 44, 1405–1409.

21 **SAHU, S.P., WOOL, S. & BREESE, S.S., 1982.** Observation on the morphology of contagious equine metritis bacterial colonies isolated from infected pony mares. *American Journal of Veterinary Research*, 43, 796–800.

22 **SIMPSON, D.J. & EATON-EVANS, W.E., 1978.** Isolation of the CEM organism from the clitoris of the mare. *The Veterinary Record*, 102, 19–20.

23 **SUGIMOTO, C., ISAYAMA, Y., KASHIWAZAKI, M. & MITANI, K., 1981.** Susceptibility of *Haemophilus equigenitalis*, the causal agent of contagious equine metritis, to 31 antimicrobial agents. *National Institute of Animal Health Quarterly*, Japan, 21, 159–162.

24 **SUGIMOTO, C., ISAYAMA, Y., SAKAZAKI, R. & KURAMOCHI, S., 1983.** Transfer of *Haemophilus equigenitalis* Taylor *et al.* 1978 to the Genus *Taylorella* gen. nov. as *Taylorella equigenitalis* comb. nov. *Current Microbiology*, 9, 155–162.

25 **SWANEY, L.M. & KISLOW, H.M., 1981.** Disinfection of the causative agent of contagious equine metritis by Nolvasan and Roccal II. *Veterinary Microbiology*, 6, 59–68.

26 **SWERCZEK, T.W., 1978.** Inhibition of the CEM organism by the normal flora of the reproductive tract. *The Veterinary Record*, 103, 125.

27 **SWERCZEK, T.W., 1978.** Contagious equine metritis in the USA. *The Veterinary Record*, 102, 512–513.

28 **TAINTURIER, D.J., DELMAS, C.F. & DABERNAT, H.J., 1981.** Bacteriological and serological studies of *Haemophilus equigenitalis*, agent of contagious equine metritis. *Journal of Clinical Microbiology*, 14, 355–360.

29 **TAYLOR, C.E.D., ROSENTHAL, R.O., BROWN, D.F.J., LAPAGE, S.P., HILL, L.R. & LEGROS, R.M., 1978.** The causative organism of contagious equine metritis 1977: Proposal for a new species to be known as *Haemophilus equigenitalis*. *Equine Veterinary Journal*, 10, 136–144.

30 **TIMONEY, P.J., GERAGHTY, V.P., DILLON, P.B. & McARDLE, J.F., 1978.** Susceptibility of laboratory animals to infection with *Haemophilus equigenitalis*. *The Veterinary Record*, 103, 563–564.

31 **TIMONEY, P.J., HARRINGTON, A., McARDLE, J. & O'REILLEY, P.J., 1978.** Survival properties of the causal agent of contagious equine metritis 1977. *The Veterinary Record*, 102, 152.

32 **TIMONEY, P.J., McARDLE, J.F., O'REILLY, P.J., WARD, J. & HARRINGTON, A.M., 1979.** Successful transmission of CEM to the donkey. *The Veterinary Record*, 104, 84.

33 **TIMONEY, P.J., O'REILLY, P.J., McARDLE, J. & WARD, J., 1978.** Attempted transmission of contagious equine metritis 1977 to other domestic animal species. *The Veterinary Record*, 102, 152.

34 **TIMONEY, P.J. & POWELL, D.G., 1982.** Isolation of the contagious equine metritis organism from colts and fillies in the United Kingdom and Ireland. *The Veterinary Record*, 111, 478–482.

35 **TIMONEY, P.J., SHIN, S.J. & JACOBSEN, R.H., 1982.** Improved selective medium for isolation of the contagious equine metritis organism. *The Veterinary Record*, 111, 107–108.

36 **TIMONEY, P.J. & STRICKLAND, K.L., 1982.** Contagious equine metritis in the Republic of Ireland. *Irish Veterinary Journal*, 36, 159–160.

37 **TIMONEY, P.J., WARD, J. & MCARDLE, J.F., 1978.** Daily variations in the shedding of the agent of contagious equine metritis 1977 by a carrier mare. *The Veterinary Record*, 103, 210–211.

38 **TIMONEY, P.J., WARD, J., McARDLE, J.F. & HARRINGTON, A.M., 1979.** Thermal death times of the organism of contagious equine metritis 1977. *The Veterinary Record*, 104, 530.

39 **WIDDERS, P.R., STOKES, C.R., DAVID, J.S.E. & BOURNE, F.J., 1986.** Specific antibody in the equine genital tract following local immunization and challenge infection with contagious equine metritis organism (*Taylorella equigenitalis*). *Research in Veterinary Science*, 40, 54–58.

40 **WYFFELS, R., SPINCEMAILLE, J. & DE SCHAEPDRIJVER, L., 1988.** Contagious equine metritis: Two outbreaks in Belgium. *Vlaams Diergeneeskundig Tijdschrift*, 57, 82–89.

184

Tyzzer's disease

J.J. van der Lugt

Introduction

Tyzzer's disease in foals and calves is an acute, fatal infection characterized by a multifocal, necrotizing hepatitis, and is caused by the bacterium *Bacillus piliformis*.

Tyzzer[22] initially described the disease in laboratory mice. Since then, naturally occurring Tyzzer's disease has been reported in a variety of laboratory and wild rodents, rhesus monkeys, dogs, cats[5, 7] and several species of wildlife.[11, 27] In horses, Tyzzer's disease was first reported in 1973[17] and has subsequently been diagnosed in foals in many countries,[2, 9, 18, 19, 21, 26] including South Africa.[23] Recently the disease was also observed in a calf.[25]

In laboratory animals losses may be extensive,[7] but in horses the disease occurs only sporadically in individual foals. In southern Africa, the disease is rare and sporadic.

Aetiology

The taxonomic position of *B. piliformis* has not been determined and the organism is not listed in *Bergey's Manual of Systemic Bacteriology*.[12] It does not belong to the genus *Bacillus*, whose members are Gram-positive, spore-forming rods.[3, 13] In their review of Tyzzer's disease, Ganaway *et al.*[7] described *B. piliformis* as a Gram-negative, spore-forming, pleomorphic rod, 0,5 µm wide and 8–10 µm long. It may occasionally be up to 40 µm in length. The bacterium is an obligate intracellular parasite and is motile, propulsion being by means of peritrichous flagella. In tissue sections it sometimes appears beaded or banded. This may represent transitional stages in the development of spores.[7]

The vegetative form of *B. piliformis* is very labile and is rapidly destroyed in tissues undergoing autolysis. Organisms are also destroyed by freezing, storage at low temperature, heating and centrifugation.[7] Spores, on the other hand, survive for as long as a year in soiled bedding of mice,[22] and resist repeated cycles of freezing and thawing, heat, and certain disinfectants, such as 0,3 per cent sodium hypochlorite solution.[6, 7]

Epidemiology

Tyzzer's disease occurs sporadically in foals between seven and 42 days of age.[21] Seldom is more than one foal from a single farm affected at any one time.[18] There appears to be no sex or breed predilection, and predisposing factors incriminated in rodents, such as cortisone administration, poor diet, poor sanitation and sulphonamide treatment,[7] have not been identified in foals.[18, 21, 26] Although Tyzzer's disease was diagnosed in two Arabian foals suffering from the combined immunodeficiency (CID) syndrome, the prevalence of Tyzzer's disease in foals with CID is not statistically different from that in foals without CID.[21]

Little is known about the epidemiology of Tyzzer's disease in horses. The isolated and sporadic nature of the disease suggests that it is not highly contagious. Because the vegetative form of *B. piliformis* is labile and rapidly loses infectivity outside host cells, it is assumed that natural transmission occurs through the ingestion of spores from an environment contaminated by the faeces of infected animals. Many adult horses may be asymptomatic carriers of *B. piliformis*, and foals can become infected by organisms that are shed in the faeces of such horses.[16] Nurse mares may be of particular importance in spreading the infection between different farms.[16] As foals are naturally coprophagous during the first few days after birth, the most likely route of infection would seem to be per os.[2] Rabbits, mice, rats, muskrats and cats, which are susceptible to natural infection, may also act as reservoirs for environmental contamination.[9] Interspecies transmission of Tyzzer's disease under natural conditions has not been reported.[27] Transplacental transmission of *B. piliformis* has been demonstrated in mice [27] but not in horses.

Pathogenesis

The pathogenesis of Tyzzer's disease has not been elucidated, but is believed to involve a primary intestinal infection with spread of the organism to the liver and heart.[27] Organisms invade hepatocytes, resulting in their death and the formation of necrotic foci. Occasionally, both acute and chronic liver lesions are present in foals, indicating successive cycles of hepatocellular necrosis after initial infection of the liver.[23, 26] Foals may suffer from subclinical liver necrosis for some time before death ensues or clinical signs develop.[26]

Clinical signs

Foals are often found dead having shown no premonitory signs or prior history of illness.[16, 21, 26] If clinical signs do occur they are usually of sudden onset and may include listlessness, depression, anorexia, dehydration, fever and icterus.[2, 9, 18, 21, 23] Tachypnoea, tachycardia and diarrhoea are less commonly manifested.[4, 15, 20] Terminally affected animals may show convulsions or become comatose before death, which invariably ensues within 48 hours of the first clinical signs.[16, 18, 21, 26]

Pathology

Few records of clinical pathological data have been reported, presumably because the disease has such a short clinical course and is of such sporadic occurrence. Increased serum concentrations of sorbitol dehydrogenase, alkaline phosphatase, aspartate transaminase, gamma-glutamyltransferase, bilirubinaemia and hypoglycaemia reflect the hepatocellular necrosis and intrahepatic cholestasis.[1, 15] Foals may show neutropenia or neutrophilia, depending on the stage of the disease.[1, 15, 26]

Necropsy examination may reveal icterus, and petechiae or ecchymoses in various organs.[15, 18, 21]

In foals, the liver is always affected. The organ is often moderately to markedly enlarged and mottled, and contains numerous yellowish-grey foci of necrosis, 1–3 mm in diameter, throughout the parenchyma[18, 21, 26] **(Figure 184.1)**. Hepatic, mesenteric and other abdominal lymph nodes may be enlarged and oedematous or haemorrhagic.[8, 16, 26] In some there is a catarrhal enterocolitis.[9, 16]

Microscopically there are multiple, often coalescing foci of coagulative necrosis randomly distributed throughout the liver. Some foci contain abundant fibrin and cellular debris, while an inflammatory exudate consisting primarily of neutrophils and a few macrophages and lymphocytes surrounds many of the necrotic areas.[9, 10, 16, 18, 21] In some foals the portal triads are infiltrated by varying numbers of neutrophils and mononuclear cells. Fibrosis of portal and centrilobular areas may also be evident.[9, 23, 26] Numerous *B. piliformis* organisms arranged in parallel or haphazard criss-cross patterns occur in apparently intact hepatocytes at the periphery of the necrotic foci.[9, 10, 14, 16, 18, 21] The staining characteristics of the bacteria vary somewhat:[2, 19, 21, 23] they may or may not stain faintly basophilic with haematoxylin and eosin; are usually weakly positive with the periodic acid-Schiff reaction; and stain weakly Gram-negative (or are sometimes Gram-variable). They are best demonstrated with Giemsa and, in particular, with silver-impregnation techniques such as that of Warthin-Starry[7] **(Figure 184.2)**.

Lesions in other organs are less common, and include necrosis of lymphocytes in lymphoid follicles in the spleen and lymph nodes;[9, 18, 26] necrosis of crypt epithelium in the intestines; acute inflammation and haemorrhage in the small and large intestines, accompanied by the presence of bacilli in intestinal glands;[2, 26] and foci of myocardial necrosis and myocarditis with bacteria within these foci and adjacent myocardial fibres.[2, 26]

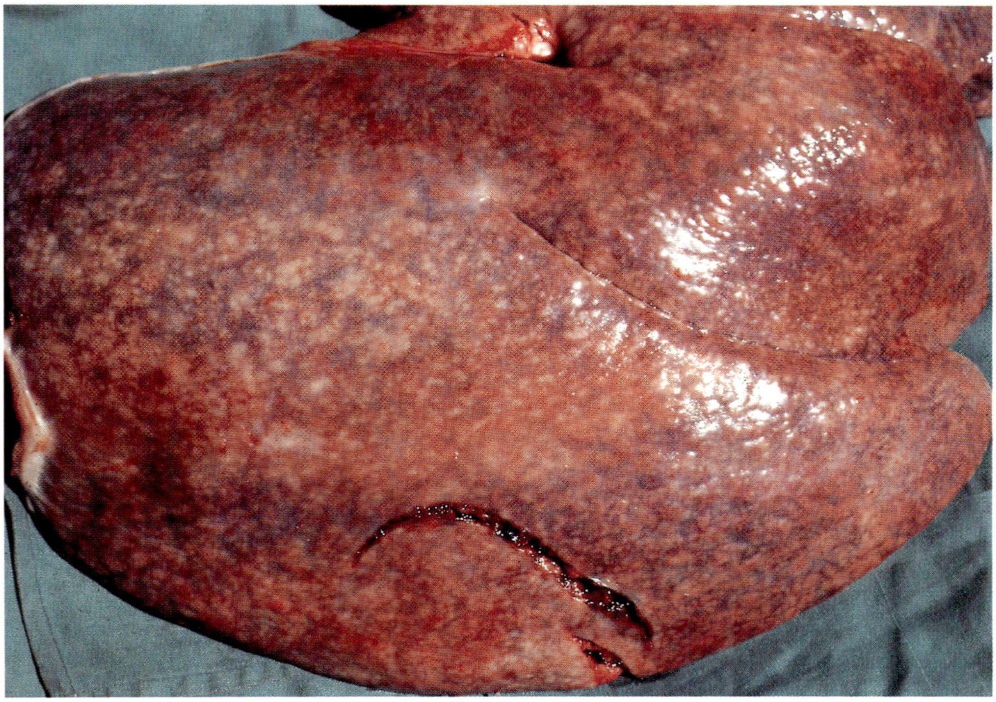

Figure 184.1 Swollen, mottled liver of a foal that died of Tyzzer's disease

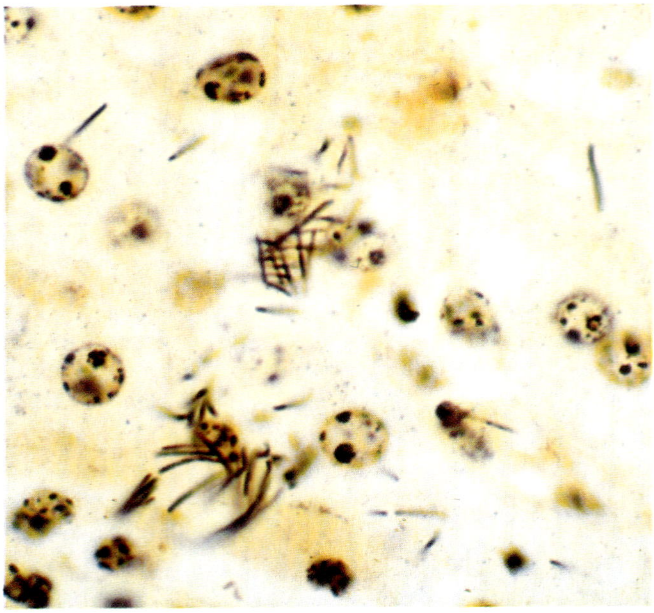

Figure 184.2 Photomicrograph demonstrating numerous intracellular *Bacillus piliformis* in a section of a liver from a foal that died of Tyzzer's disease (Warthin-Starry silver impregnation)

Diagnosis

Tyzzer's disease in a foal is diagnosed on the basis of the age of the animal, rapid onset and nature of the clinical signs, and the short course of illness. *Bacillus piliformis* cannot be cultured in cell-free media[5, 7] and the few reports of its successful cultivation remain unconfirmed.[27] The organism can be cultivated in the yolk sac of embryonated chicken eggs,[7] but this method is seldom used in routine diagnostic bacteriology. The diagnosis of Tyzzer's disease is therefore mostly based upon the histological demonstration of typical organisms in the cytoplasm of hepatocytes bordering on necrotic foci,[7] especially by silver-impregnation techniques. Immunofluorescent techniques to demonstrate the causative agent and tests to detect serum antibodies against *B. piliformis* have been developed to diagnose the disease in laboratory animals.[24, 27]

Differential diagnosis

Other bacterial infections such as those caused by *Salmonella* serovars, *Actinobacillus equuli* and *Rhodococcus equi* may cause death with occasional liver involvement in foals one to six weeks old. Icterus may be pronounced in isoimmune haemolytic anaemia, congenital babesiosis and equid herpesvirus 1 infection, although in the latter, foals usually die within the first week of life.

Control

The results of treatment of foals with confirmed Tyzzer's disease have been unrewarding, although affected foals may respond temporarily to treatment with antimicrobial drugs and fluids containing glucose.[1, 16] Based on trials in rodents, it has been claimed that penicillin, streptomycin, erythromycin and tetracycline have some therapeutic effect, but that sulphonamides and chloramphenicol do not.[5, 7]

References

1 **BROWN, C.M., AINSWORTH, D.M., PERSONETT, L.A. & DERKSEN, F.J., 1983.** Serum biochemical and haematological findings in two foals with focal bacterial hepatitis (Tyzzer's disease). *Equine Veterinary Journal*, 15, 375–376.

2 **CARRIGAN, M.J., PEDRANA, R.G. & McKIBBIN, A.W., 1984.** Tyzzer's disease in foals. *Australian Veterinary Journal*, 61, 199–200.

3 **CARTER, G.R., 1986.** *Essentials of Veterinary Bacteriology and Mycology*. 3rd edn. Philadelphia: Lea & Febiger.

4 **COPLAND, M.D., ROBARTSON, C.W., PRY, J. & WILSON, G., 1984.** Tyzzer's disease in a foal. *Australian Veterinary Journal*, 61, 302–304.

5 **FUJIWARA, K., 1978.** Tyzzer's disease. *Japanese Journal of Experimental Medicine*, 48, 467–480.

6 **GANAWAY, J.R., 1980.** Effect of heat and selected chemical disinfectants upon infectivity of spores of *Bacillus piliformis*. *Laboratory Animal Science*, 30, 192–196.

7 **GANAWAY, J.R., ALLEN, A.M. & MOORE, T.D., 1971.** Tyzzer's disease. *American Journal of Pathology*, 64, 717–732.

8 **HALL, W.C. & VAN KRUININGEN, H.J., 1974.** Tyzzer's disease in a horse. *Journal of the American Veterinary Medical Association*, 164, 1187–1189.

9 **HARRINGTON, D.D., 1975.** Naturally-occurring Tyzzer's disease (*Bacillus piliformis* infection) in horse foals. *The Veterinary Record*, 96, 59–63.

10 **HARRINGTON, D.D., 1976.** *Bacillus piliformis* infection (Tyzzer's disease) in two foals. *Journal of the American Veterinary Medical Association*, 168, 58–60.

11 **HUM, S. & BEST, F.G., 1988.** Tyzzer's disease in a wombat. *Australian Veterinary Journal*, 65, 89–91.

12 **KRIEG, N.R. & HOLT, J.G., 1984.** *Bergey's Manual of Systematic Bacteriology*, Vol I. Baltimore: Williams & Wilkins.

13 **LOGAN, N.A., 1988.** *Bacillus* species of medical and veterinary importance. *Journal of Medical Microbiology*, 25, 157–165.

14 **PULLEY, L.T. & SHIVELY, J.N., 1974.** Tyzzer's disease in a foal. *Veterinary Pathology*, 11, 203–211.

15 **SCARRATT, W.K., SAUNDERS, G.K., WELKER, F.H., HALPERN, N.E., CORDES, D.O. & CAMP, G.M., 1985.** *Bacillus piliformis* infection (Tyzzer's disease) in two Virginia foals. *Journal of Equine Veterinary Science*, 5, 135–138.

16 **SWERCZEK, T.W., 1977.** Multifocal hepatic necrosis and hepatitis in foals caused by *Bacillus piliformis* (Tyzzer's disease). *Veterinary Annual*, 17, 130–132.

17 **SWERCZEK, T.W., CROWE, M.W., PRICKETT, M.E. & BRYANS, J.T., 1973.** Focal bacterial hepatitis in foals: Preliminary report. *Modern Veterinary Practice*, 54, 66–67.

18 **TAYLOR, R.F. & MULLANEY, T.P., 1983.** Tyzzer's disease in Michigan foals: A review. *Twenty-sixth Annual Proceedings of the American Association of Veterinary Laboratory Diagnosticians.*

19 **THOMSON, G.W., WILSON, R.W., HALL, E.A. & PHYSICK-SHEARD, P., 1977.** Tyzzer's disease in the foal: Case reports and review. *Canadian Veterinary Journal*, 18, 41–43.

20 **TRENT, A.M. & WALSH, K.M., 1983.** Tyzzer's disease in a foal. *Equine Practice*, 5, 8–17.

21 **TURK, M.A.M., GALLINA, A.M. & PERRYMAN, L.E., 1981.** *Bacillus piliformis* infection (Tyzzer's disease) in foals in northwestern USA: A retrospective study of 21 cases. *Journal of the American Veterinary Medical Association*, 178, 279–281.

22 **TYZZER, E.E., 1917.** A fatal disease of the Japanese Waltzing mouse caused by a spore-bearing bacillus (*Bacillus piliformis*, n. sp.). *Journal of Medical Research*, 37, 307–338.

23 **VAN DER LUGT, J.J., COETZER, J.A.W., JORDAAN, P. & MARLOW, C.H.B., 1985.** Suspected Tyzzer's disease in two foals. *Journal of the South African Veterinary Association*, 56, 107–108.

24 **WAGGIE, K.S., SPENCER, T.H. & GANAWAY, J.R., 1987.** An enzyme-linked immunosorbent assay for detection of anti-*Bacillus piliformis* serum antibody in rabbits. *Laboratory Animal Science*, 37, 176–179.

25 **WEBB, D.M., HARRINGTON, D.D. & BOEHM, P.N., 1987.** *Bacillus piliformis* infection (Tyzzer's disease) in a calf. *Journal of the American Veterinary Medical Association*, 191, 431–434.

26 **WHITWELL, K.E., 1976.** Four cases of Tyzzer's disease in foals in England. *Equine Veterinary Journal*, 8, 118–122.

27 **WOBESER, G., 1981.** Tyzzer's disease. *In:* DAVIS, J.W., KARSTAD, L.H. & TRAINER, D.O., (eds). *Infectious Diseases of Wild Mammals*. 2nd edn. Iowa: Iowa State University Press.

Section 6

Mycotic and algal diseases

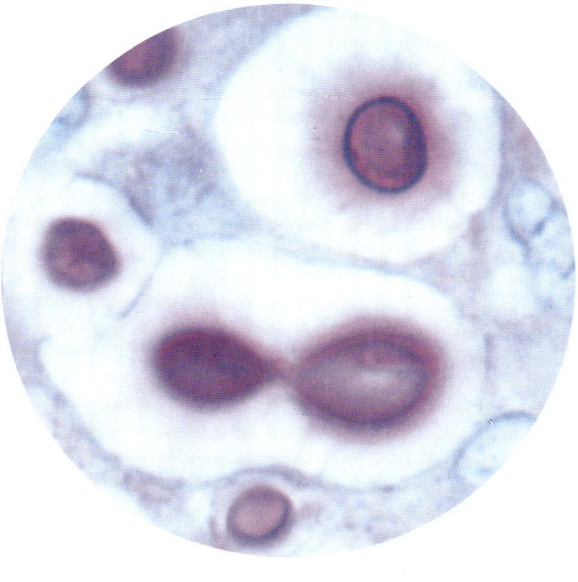

185

Mycoses

D.B. Scott

The division Mycota incorporates all fungi, which are eukaryotic organisms lacking chlorophyll. The mycelial forms are moulds, while those that exist predominantly in a budding, unicellular form are called yeasts. The vast majority of fungi have a saprophytic existence in nature, some being pathogenic to plants, while a few others are pathogenic to humans and animals. Among the latter group are the toxin-producing fungi which cause mycotoxicoses.[52] The true pathogens are the cause of mycoses involving the cutaneous and subcutaneous tissues, the mucous membranes and internal organs. Fungi are also involved in allergic reactions. In these, however, the causative agent does not invade live tissue.

The diagnostician is often faced with having to decide whether a fungus cultured from a lesion is the cause of the disease or only a contaminant. The tissue affected, fungal species, number of colonies isolated and the presence of fungal elements in affected tissues may all be helpful in this regard. Fungi isolated from normally sterile sites such as the cerebrospinal fluid or bone marrow should be given more credence than isolates made from the skin or mucous membranes. As many different fungi are morphologically similar in histological tissue sections, an accurate diagnosis is dependent on the isolation and identification of the fungus.

The various forms of cutaneous and subcutaneous mycoses that occur in livestock in southern Africa **(Table 185.1)** are dealt with in this chapter.

Attention is also given to pathogenic yeasts and fungi that affect the mucous membranes and internal organs **(Table 185.2)**. Only those mycoses relevant to Africa are dealt with. Detailed information on those that have not been diagnosed in southern Africa may be obtained from other sources.[2, 23, 49]

MYCOSES OF THE CUTANEOUS AND SUBCUTANEOUS TISSUES AND MUCOUS MEMBRANES

Dermatophytoses

Dermatophytoses, or 'ringworm' as they are commonly known, are diseases of the superficial, keratinized layers of the skin and appendages, such as hair and nails, and are caused by closely related mycelial fungi known as dermatophytes.

The first recorded cases of dermatophytosis in animals date back to 1894, when Sabouraud[85] reported the disease in cattle and horses. Sabouraud[86] produced a systematic treatise of the zoophilic and anthropophilic dermatophytes known up to 1910. There are many reports of dermatophytoses throughout the world, and those that occur in animals have been reviewed.[2, 49]

In South Africa, dermatophytoses in humans have

Table 185.1 Some cutaneous and subcutaneous mycoses of livestock

DISEASE	CAUSATIVE FUNGUS	ANIMALS AFFECTED
Dermatophytoses	*Microsporum gypseum*	Horses
	M. nanum	Pigs
	Trichophyton mentagrophytes	Horses
	T. verrucosum var. *autotrophicum*	Sheep
	T. verrucosum var. *verrucosum*	Cattle
Sporotrichosis	*Sporothrix schenkii*	Equidae
Epizootic lymphangitis	*Histoplasma farciminosum*	Equidae
Mycetoma	*Curvularia geniculata*	Horses
	Madurella mycetomatis	Horses

Table 185.2 Most prevalent forms of internal or deep mycoses in livestock

DISEASE	CAUSATIVE FUNGI	COMMON SITE OF INFECTION
Aspergillosis	*Aspergillus fumigatus* and *Aspergillus* spp.	Nasal cavity, guttural pouches, lungs
Candidiasis	*Candida albicans* and *Candida* spp.	Mouth, oesophagus, and gastro-intestinal tract
Cryptococcosis	*Cryptococcus neoformans*	Lungs, brain and mammary gland
Mycotic abortion	*Mucor, Absidia* and *Rhizopus* spp., *Mortierella wolfii, Aspergillus* spp., *Candida* spp.	Foetal tissues (skin, lungs gastrointestinal tract) and placenta
Zygomycosis	Mucoraceous fungi (*Mucor, Absidia* and *Rhizopus* spp.)	Gastrointestinal tract

been studied and reviewed.[16, 35, 57, 58, 92] Dermatophytoses in animals in southern Africa occur most commonly among cats and dogs in urban areas.[103] In livestock, confirmation of the diagnosis of skin lesions is not normally undertaken, except perhaps in pure-bred animals, and even then samples are seldom taken for laboratory confirmation. In many cases farmers deal with the problem on their own.

Aetiology

The dermatophytes are specialized, keratinolytic fungi classified as geophilic, zoophilic or anthropophilic species.

Apart from their existence in soil, the geophilic dermatophytes also parasitize human and animal skin and its appendages. *Microsporum gypseum* (Bodin) Guiart & Grigorakis, a typical species in this category, occurs most commonly in horses.[26, 51, 74]

Zoophilic dermatophytes tend to have a specific host adaptation or host preference. *Trichophyton verrucosum* Bodin is primarily a pathogen of cattle; infections in other animals and humans are uncommon and can usually be traced back to contact with infected cattle.[2] The dermatophyte causing infections in sheep and goats normally resembles *T. verrucosum* morphologically, but unlike this species it has no essential requirement for vitamins when cultured artificially.[90] In order to differentiate between these two variants, the one in sheep and goats was named *T. verrucosum* var. *autotrophicum*.[91] *Trichophyton mentagrophytes* (Robin) Blanchard is a species with a wide host range among animals. It was first recorded in the horse,[89] but in this animal *Trichophyton equinum* (Matruchot & Dassonville) Gedoelst is isolated most frequently from cases of dermatophytoses in Europe and North America. *Trichophyton equinum* differs from *T. mentagrophytes* mainly in having an absolute requirement for nicotinic acid, a requirement which is apparently satisfied by equine, but not human or other animal, hair.[39] Isolates from horses in South Africa do not require nicotinic acid although morphologically they all resemble *T. mentagrophytes*. It has been reported that isolates from horses in Australasia are autotrophic for vitamins.[96] Such isolates were named *T. equinum* var. *autotrophicum* Smith, Jolly George and Connole, but on the basis of morphological characteristics, they cannot be distinguished from *T. mentagrophytes*. *Microsporum canis* Bodin, a species associated most commonly with infected dogs and cats, has occasionally been reported in farm animals.[2, 36, 83] *Microsporum nanum* Fuentes is a common cause of dermatophytosis in pigs.[2] Its occurrence is suspected in pigs in southern Africa but it has not yet been isolated.[103]

Anthropophilic dermatophytes are even more specialized than zoophilic dermatophytes because they have a predilection for certain sites on the human body. Consequently anthropophilic dermatophytes are seldom, if ever, the cause of dermatophytoses in animals.

Epidemiology

Dermatophytoses are more contagious than most mycotic diseases and are transmitted directly by contact between infected and susceptible animals, or indirectly by means of infected articles or air-borne spores. Outbreaks of the disease are rare but have been described in sheep in South Africa[90] and in goats in India,[99] where infection was spread from one farm to another by newly introduced, infected stud rams. The high prevalence of dermatophytosis in cattle in countries where animals are stabled during winter is probably due to the accumulation of infected hair and scales in a closed environment.[64] In countries with warm climates, such as those in southern Africa, where animals are often kept in the open veld all year round, the prevalence of dermatophytosis in cattle is much lower.

Young animals are more susceptible to dermatophytosis, and a genetic predisposition might play a role in infections.[49] In horses, the disease is often contracted from contaminated saddle cloths, riding boots or grooming gear. Dermatophyte arthrospores are well protected within the hair follicle and can also survive for many years in scales shed by infected animals. Animals stabled under poor conditions for long periods are more at risk than those receiving adequate nutrition and proper care.

Pathogenesis

Dermatophytes enter the skin through abrasions or the hair follicles. Infection is either endothrix or ectothrix; in endothrix infections, the hyphae and conidia (arthroconidia) remain within the hair shaft; in ectothrix infections the hyphae invade the hair shaft while the conidia remain on the surface of the hair. Most infections in animals are caused by ectothrix fungi.

Proteolytic enzymes or toxins produced by the dermatophytes have a keratolytic effect on the stratum corneum, in which they are most commonly found. These substances, some of which may act as allergens, penetrate the epidermis and elicit an inflammatory or allergic response in the dermis.[48, 49]

Young animals are more susceptible to infection than adults, possibly because of differences in the physiology of the skin, or a lack of specific immunity, or both. Systemic diseases, nutritional deficiencies (such as vitamin A deficiency) and reduced immunological competence are predisposing factors to the disease in adult animals.[48]

The disease is often self-limiting, although reinfection occurs occasionally. Immunity to infection is apparently effected predominantly by cell-mediated responses.[48]

Clinical signs and pathology

The distribution and nature of the lesions of dermatophytoses are variable. Most infections spread centrifugally, resulting in circular lesions characterized by alopecia and pronounced scaling. In woolled sheep, involvement of the fleece is rare and lesions are located mostly on the head and legs **(Figures 185.1 and 185.2)**. Large, crusted lesions develop in advanced cases. Acute, exudative lesions seldom occur in sheep, but raw lesions which bleed readily may develop when crusts are detached from infected foci. Short-haired sheep may develop multiple circular lesions over the entire body.

Multiple lesions usually occur in cattle, and horses.

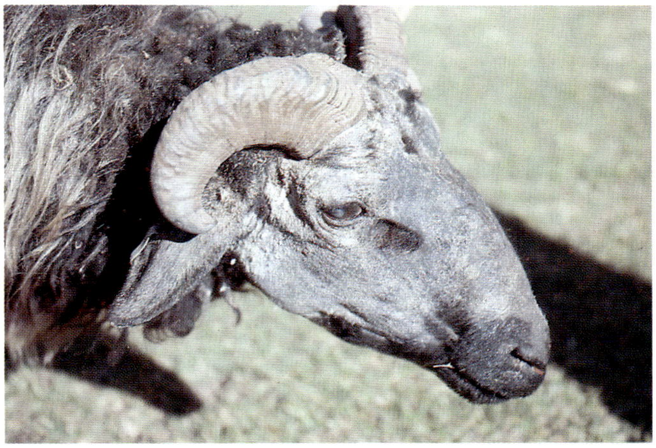

Figure 185.1 Alopecia and crusting of the face caused by dermatophytes

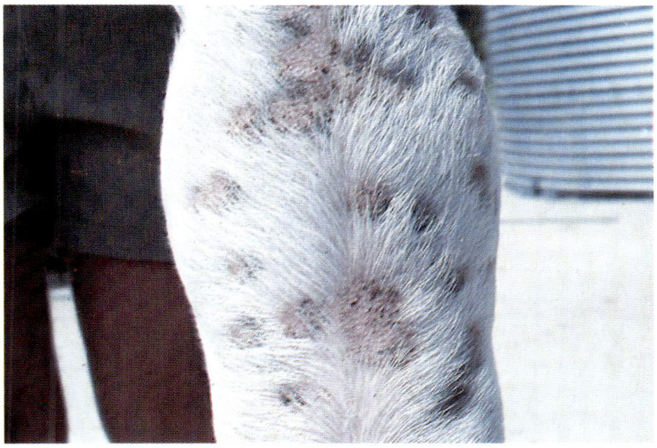

Figure 185.3 Scattered typical lesions of dermatophytosis on the back and sides of a pig

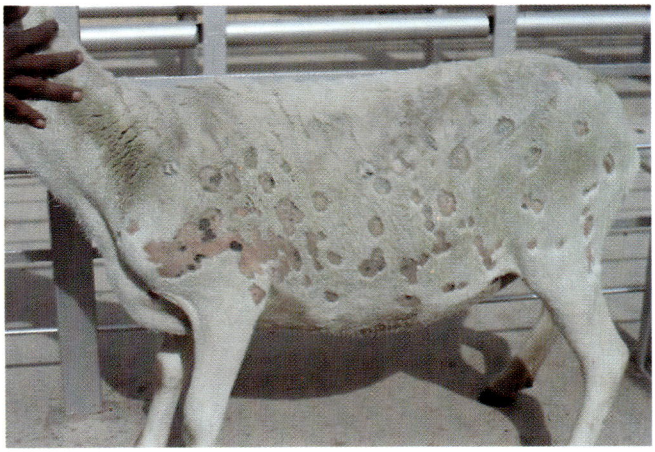

Figure 185.2 Multiple lesions of dermatophytosis in a short-haired sheep

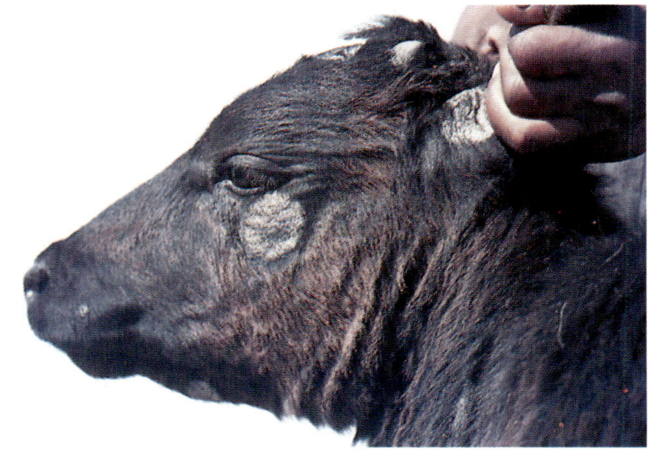

Figure 185.4 Single typically round and alopecic lesion of dermatophytosis in a calf

Some infected animals, however, show few — if any — lesions. In horses the ventral thorax, where the girth of the saddle fastens, is affected most frequently, while in cattle, lesions occur most commonly on the face, neck and legs. Circumscribed areas of alopecia and scaling are typical of the lesions in these animals and in pigs **(Figures 185.3 and 185.4)**, although in some animals ulcerated nodules may develop.

Microscopically, the lesions are characterized by moderate to severe hyperkeratosis and mild lymphocytic infiltration in the dermis. Depending on the severity of the lesions, microabscesses, folliculitis, and trichogranulomas may be present. The fungi which occur superficially or within hair follicles **(Figure 185.5)**, are best stained in tissue sections by the periodic acid-Schiff reaction or by Gomori's methenamine silver impregnation.[48]

Diagnosis

Dermatophytes live mostly in the non-viable stratum corneum and invade hair follicles, but are found only rarely in the deeper layers of the skin. For a provisional diagnosis of dermatophytosis, hair from the periphery of lesions should be examined microscopically. Affected hair should be pulled out with a forceps without being broken and in such a way that the hair bulbs remain attached to the hair shafts. Hair may also be collected by running a sterile hairbrush over affected parts of the skin. A scalpel can be used to scrape off scales of keratin and broken-off hair. Whenever skin scrapings are submitted to a diagnostic laboratory, they should be placed in a clean envelope and not in an air-tight container. The collected material is mounted on a slide in a drop of 10 per cent potassium hydroxide, which is slightly heated and then cover-slipped and examined under a microscope. Infected hair from sheep or cattle is enclosed by a thick sheath of arthrospores. Histological examination of a biopsy specimen of the affected skin is a useful way of confirming the diagnosis. The use of a Wood's lamp for the clinical diagnosis of *M. canis* infections is not very reliable. Certain topical medicaments and even soaps and dyes may mimic the fluorescence caused by this organism.[70]

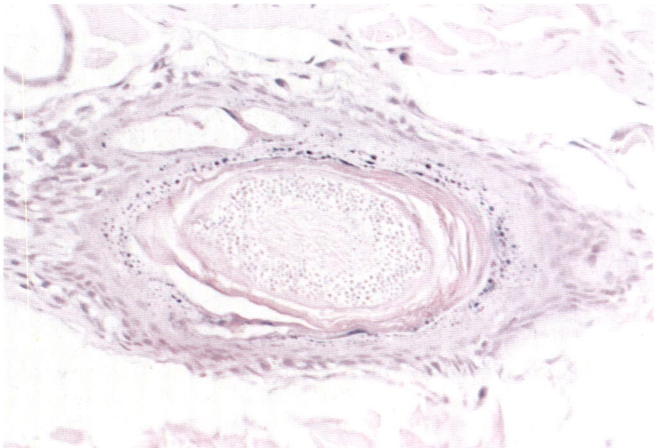

Figure 185.5 Photomicrograph of dermatophytes

The species causing the dermatophytoses can only be identified after they have been isolated in pure culture. Special media such as dermatophyte test medium[98] and Sabouraud dextrose agar can be used to culture dermatophytes selectively and to distinguish colonies of these fungi from those saprophytes resistant to cycloheximide. The identification of dermatophytes is based on the cultural characteristics of colonies as well as on the morphology of conidia. Growth of some dermatophytes is very slow, and plates should therefore be kept for at least a month before being discarded. In some *Trichophyton* spp., such as *T. verrucosum*, only chlamydospores are produced, while in others, such as *T. mentagrophytes*, numerous microconidia as well as some cigar-shaped macroconidia are produced. *Microsporum* spp. are characterized by the formation of numerous, rough-walled macroconidia which vary greatly in size and shape depending on the species. It is advisable to consult a taxonomist or medical mycologist if an accurate identification of the fungus is required.

Control

Treatment of dermatophytoses with griseofulvin is very effective, but costly, and should therefore be considered only when valuable animals are affected. To effect a complete cure in cattle, 10 mg/kg body weight of this drug per day for four to six weeks is required.[73] In order to lower the cost of treatment in young calves, it has been suggested that intermittent griseofulvin therapy totalling 2–2,5/g over 10–12 days should be instituted.[6] Griseofulvin at a dose of 7,5 mg/kg for seven days has been used in sheep to cure the dermatophytosis caused by *T. verrucosum*.[79]

A variety of common fungicidal and fungistatic agents, such as precipitated sulphur, iodine, salicylic acid, fatty acids and hydroxyquinolines may be applied topically to treat affected areas successfully. The use of captan has been advocated[2, 11] and, when sprayed on infected animals as a solution of 1:200, it washes away and possibly sterilizes much of the infective material, thereby reducing the reservoir of infection, even though it does not greatly affect the course of established infections. Crusted lesions are best treated with water-soluble or water-miscible ointments in which antifungal agents have been incorporated. Most of these compounds are irritants and should not be applied to acute lesions. A weak solution of boric acid or potassium permanganate should rather be used for the treatment of such lesions.[49]

Spread of infection can be limited by the early diagnosis and separation of infected from uninfected animals. To avoid recurrence of infection it is important to disinfect stables and equipment properly.

Successful vaccination programmes against *Trichophyton* infections in cattle have been reported.[44]

Sporotrichosis

Sporotrichosis is a chronic, granulomatous, usually subcutaneous infection caused by the fungus *Sporothrix schenckii* Hektoen & Perkins. Infections are most commonly seen in horses, but these are far outnumbered by those reported in humans. In animals the disease has also been reported in cattle, water buffaloes, cats and dogs.

Sporotrichosis was first described on gold miners in South Africa in 1927 by Pijper and Pullinger.[75] Shortly thereafter Robinson and Parkins[84] reported the disease in a horse from Pretoria North. Further accounts of sporotrichosis in Equidae have been published both in South Africa[100] and elsewhere,[49] and sporadic cases of sporotrichosis still occur from time to time in southern Africa. Isolates from horses, previously called *Sporotrichum equi* Carougeau, cannot be distinguished morphologically or serologically from isolates of *S. schenckii*.[55]

Epidemiology

Sporothrix schenkii is a soil-inhabiting fungus with a distribution throughout the world. The disease is not contagious; infection is often traceable to a wound or injury contaminated by soil or plant material. Under humid conditions the pathogen grows saprophytically on wood and other plant material. The largest outbreak of sporotrichosis ever recorded in humans occurred among miners of the Rand Gold Mines in South Africa, where the timber used underground was found to support the growth of *S. schenckii*.[28] Donkeys used in these mines were also infected.

Clinical signs and pathology

In horses the disease has a chronic course, and subcutaneous nodules, usually on the neck and legs, develop over a period of time **(Figure 185.6)**. Ulcerated nodules discharge a purulent exudate containing yeast-like organisms. By the time the primary lesion starts to heal, secondary lesions may appear in the surrounding tissue and along the lymphatics, which become thickened and cord-like. The systemic form of the disease, where lesions occur in various tissues other than the skin, is extremely rare.[105]

The histopathology of sporotrichosis in humans from South Africa has been studied in detail by Lurie.[56] Microscopically the nodular lesions in Equidae are necrogranulomas and contain numerous epithelioid cells, lymphocytes and plasma cells as well as scattered multinucleated giant cells. Demonstration of the fungus in tissues, even by the use of special fungal stains such as the periodic acid-Schiff method or Gomori's methenamine silver impregnation, is often difficult because of the scarcity of organisms in affected tissue. Contrarily, when such infected material is injected into laboratory mice the organism is readily demonstrated. The organisms in histological sections are either oval or cigar-shaped yeast cells, 2–6 μm in diameter, or appear as the so-called asteroid bodies, which consist of spherical spores surrounded by variable amounts of homogeneous, eosinophilic material assuming a stellate shape as a result of peripheral angular projections of varying length.

Diagnosis

Sporothrix schenckii is easily cultured when exudate from lesions is inoculated onto suitable agar media containing a broad-spectrum antibiotic such as chloromycetin. The fungus is dimorphic: colonies grown at 37 °C are yeast-like and consist of budding yeast cells, while at room temperature the fungus grows in the mycelial form. Numerous oval conidia are formed on minute 'denticles' at the apices of conidiophores and alongside aerial hyphae.

Intraperitoneal inoculation of exudate or suspensions of affected tissue in mice and guinea-pigs results in a peritonitis producing an abundant exudate containing numerous yeast-forms of *S. schenckii*.

Control

In contrast to the other subcutaneous mycoses, sporotrichosis responds well to treatment, and especially to the administration of inorganic iodides.

Complete cure of sporotrichosis has been reported following three intravenous injections of a 10 per cent sodium iodide solution once every month at a dosage rate of 3 mg/50 kg body weight.[100] Daily doses will secure a more rapid cure, but may induce iodism.[29] Iodine should be given for at least another four weeks after the apparent cure of the disease.[49]

Surgical intervention in sporotrichosis is contraindicated. Attempts at treating the disease in this way are often followed by increased suppuration and ulceration.

Epizootic lymphangitis

Epizootic lymphangitis **(Figure 185.7)**, a rare, chronic infection of Equidae, is very similar to sporotrichosis, and is characterized by a marked lymphangitis and by discharging necrogranulomas located especially in the skin and subcutis of the lateral aspects of the neck, thorax, and fore legs.[21, 22, 88, 104] It is a controlled disease in South Africa. In horses it should be differentiated from ulcerative lymphangitis caused by *Corynebacterium pseudotuberculosis*, sporotrichosis (vide supra) and farcy (the skin form of glanders due to *Pseudomonas mallei*).

Aetiology and epidemiology

Epidemics of this disease, also known as African farcy or Japanese glanders, occurred in South Africa and elsewhere during the early parts of the twentieth century when large numbers of horses were grouped together for military operations such as the Anglo-Boer War. From systemic cases Bullen[22] obtained isolates of a dimorphic fungus, which had previously been named *Histoplasma farciminosum* (Rivolta) Redaelli and Ciferri. This fungus appears as oval or ovoid bodies 3–4 μm in diameter.

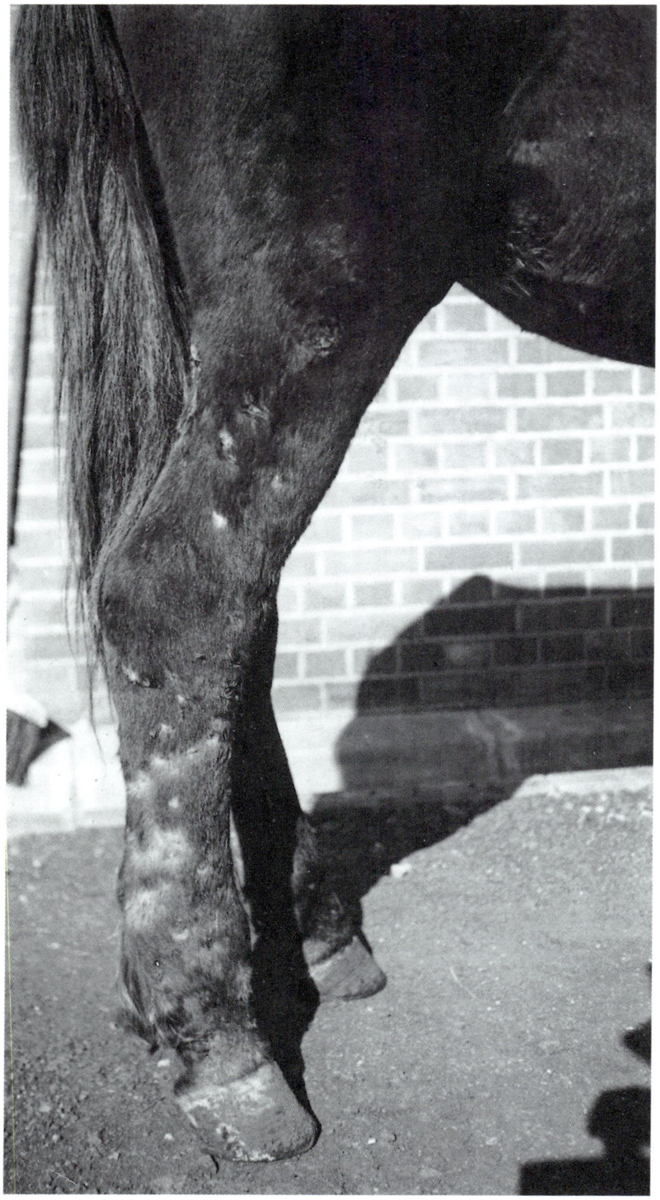

Figure 185.6 Sporotrichosis. Ulcerative dermatitis on hind leg

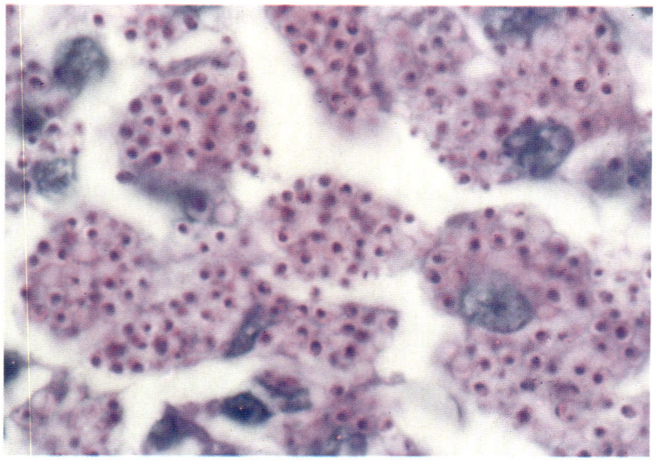

Figure 185.7 Epizootic lymphangitis. Note the numerous *Histoplasma* organisms in the cytoplasm of macrophages in the dermis of an affected horse

Histoplasma capsulatum Darling, the cause of histoplasmosis or cave disease in humans, is morphologically similar to *H. farciminosum*. The organisms occur extra- or intracellularly in macrophages.

Clinical signs, pathology and diagnosis

Lesions may develop on any part of the body but are most common in the skin of the head, neck, the extremities (especially the fore legs), sides of the thorax, and the inside of the thighs (often involving the mammary gland, or prepuce and scrotum). Hard nodules, about 10–20 mm in diameter, develop along thickened, cord-like and inflamed lymphatics. Some of the nodules ulcerate and discharge a purulent exudate.[104] Similar lesions may also occur in the nasal cavity.

Histopathological lesions resemble those of sporotrichosis. However, very numerous typical yeast organisms with thick capsules, most of which are phagocytosed by macrophages, are evident in the lesions.

Control

Local surgery appears not to be successful for the treatment of epizootic lymphangitis, except when applied to early cases.[77] The disease has been reported to respond to iodide treatment.[2] Prevention consists of isolation of infected animals, disinfection of contaminated properties and proper sanitary measures.

Mycetoma

Mycetoma is a subcutaneous, granulomatous disease of humans and animals. The disease, also known as maduromycosis, was first described in India in 1842. When a fungus was later identified as the causative organism, the disease was called mycetoma. More recently the term eumycotic mycetoma has been introduced to differentiate mycetomas caused by true fungi from actinomycotic mycetomas caused by *Actinomyces, Streptomyces, Actinomadura* and *Nocardia* spp.[76] The diseases caused by actinomycetes, the actinomycoses, are considered to be bacterial diseases.

Eumycotic mycetoma is a relatively rare condition in animals and most recorded cases have occurred in North America. In South Africa rare cases have been reported in horses.[15, 102]

Aetiology and epidemiology

A great variety of fungi has been incriminated as causes of mycetoma in humans.[1, 34] In animals the causative fungi are rarely isolated; the organisms can, however, be classified according to the same criteria used for human isolates. Akun[4] was the first to report dark, septate hyphae in lesions in the nasal cavity of a horse. In America, a fungus which appeared as single or small groups of septate hyphae in lesions in a horse was isolated and identified as the Drechslera state of *Cochliobolus specifer* Nelson.[18] The causative fungus of black grain mycetoma in two horses reported from South Africa was not isolated.[15] In both cases, however, granules in the affected tissues were similar in pigmentation and structure to those produced by *Curvularia geniculata* (Tracey & Earle) Boedijn in dogs.[17] Although black grain mycetoma in humans in Africa is caused mostly by *Madurella mycetomatis* (Laveran), the fungus has been recorded only once in a horse.[102] White grain mycetoma, caused by *Pseudalescheria boydii* (Negroni & Fischer) McGinnis, Padhye & Ajello, is known to occur mainly in North America.[62]

Lesions of mycotic origin but without granules have also been described in horses and cattle. Some phycomycetes cause granulomas in horses.[19, 20] The disease, commonly known as cutaneous phycomycosis, appears to be associated with the muck-ponds in which horses wade during grazing.

There is some argument as to whether or not cases of bovine nasal granuloma caused by dematiaceous hyphomycetes should be classified as mycetoma.[69] It is suggested that they should rather be regarded as cases of phaeohyphomycosis,[69] which is defined as 'infections of a cutaneous, subcutaneous and systemic nature caused by hyphomycetous fungi that develop in the host's tissue in the form of dark-walled (dematiaceous), septate, mycelial elements'.[3] Phaeohyphomycosis is a disease category that includes infections caused by *Cochliobolus specifer*.[50, 69]

Pathogenesis, clinical signs and pathology

Eumycotic mycetomas are not contagious. There is evidence that in both animals and humans, infection is the result of fungal contamination of tissues at sites of injury.

Mycetoma is characterized by cutaneous or subcutaneous wart-like growths and deep-seated abscesses or necrogranulomas, often containing multiple draining sinuses. Lesions are mostly on the extremities or on body parts which are frequently subjected to trauma. The pus may contain granules, which vary in size and colour according to the pathogen involved. In black grain mycetoma,[15] sections through lesions show numerous small, black spots scattered in the greyish-white granulation tissue **(Figure 185.8)**. Detailed descriptions of the macro- and microscopical pathology of cutaneous phycomycosis in horses have been reported.[19, 66]

Control

From a therapeutic point of view, it is important that eumycotic mycetomas be differentiated from actinomycotic mycetomas. While the latter may be controlled successfully with antibiotics, mycelial fungi resist practically all forms of therapy except total surgical excision. Surgery should be carried out as early as possible in order to prevent invasion of fascia and bone. Lesions commonly recur after excision, although there was no regrowth of a subcutaneous infection caused by *Madurella mycetomatis* in a horse after it had been surgically excised and the wound dusted with thiabendazole powder.[102]

Rhinosporidiosis

Rhinosporidiosis in animals is characterized by nasal polyps. It occurs mainly in horses and cattle, but humans and other animal species may also be affected.[5] It is caused by *Rhinosporidium seeberi* (Wernicke) Seeber.

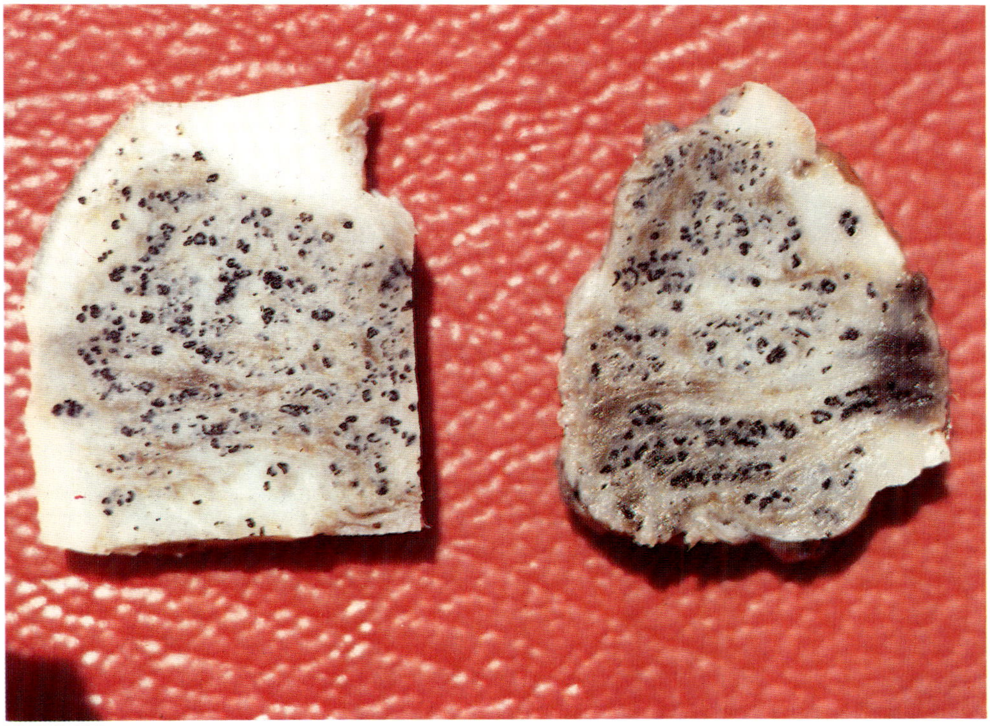

Figure 185.8 Mycetoma in a horse. Note the disseminated black spots scattered throughout the granuloma

Aetiology and epidemiology

The condition is extremely rare in southern Africa. According to Quinlan and De Kock,[80] who reported two cases in mules in South Africa, Sir Arnold Theiler in 1906 removed a growth from the nasal septum of a horse and sent it to the Veterinary Institute in Zurich for examination. Zschokke[108] used this material to describe the first case of rhinosporidiosis in animals. The disease has subsequently been diagnosed in many countries, but mostly in cattle in India.[2]

Little is known about the epidemiology of the disease. *Rhinosporidium seeberi* has not as yet been isolated or cultured on artificial media. It is believed to be an airborne, free-living organism, but its natural habitat is unknown. Sporadic cases are reported in animals that are in almost constant contact with water. Trauma is probably a predisposing factor, as in India it is most commonly found in bulls and oxen with pierced nasal septa[81] or in association with nasal schistosomiasis.

Clinical signs, pathology and diagnosis

Affected animals may have a unilateral, mucopurulent nasal discharge. The nasal polyps are not more than 30 mm in diameter in cattle and horses. They are pinkish, raised, pedunculated, finely lobulated, and dotted with small white specks which are the spherical spore cysts or sporangia **(Figure 185.9)**. The thick-walled sporangia are embedded in fibrous connective tissue close to the epithelium **(Figure 185.10)**. Mature sporangia are up to 350 μm in diameter and contain numerous endospores 5–7 μm in diameter. The epithelium overlying the polyps is hyperplastic, and neutrophils and eosinophils are part of the granulomatous reaction.[71]

Control

Complete cure of rhinosporidiosis usually follows the removal of nasal polyps by curved scissors or a looped curette. The use of stitches where necessary, and application of a disinfectant will result in rapid wound healing.

INTERNAL OR DEEP MYCOSES

Various forms of internal or deep mycoses may occur in animals **(Table 185.2)**. Most of the internal mycoses are caused by fungal pathogens that are of exogenous origin: they normally grow saprophytically, mostly in hay, compost, spoilt silage or bird droppings. In dusty surroundings their spores are inhaled by animals and infection occurs first in the terminal bronchioles or alveoli. From there they may enter the lymph and blood and spread to other organs. Although the lungs are the primary infectious focus of many internal mycoses, respiratory signs do not always show: aspergillosis, caused by *Aspergillus fumigatus*, Fresenius is the exception. This is primarily a respiratory disease and its clinical signs are very similar to those of pneumonia caused by various other pathogens.

Animals that are treated with antibacterial drugs are more at risk of developing gastrointestinal fungal infections than healthy animals. Antibacterial agents destroy resident bacteria and reduce competition of microorganisms within the gastrointestinal tract, so that yeasts and other fungi proliferate. Roughage and irritant antibiotics such as tetracycline may cause localized damage to the mucosa and allow entry of the yeasts to the underlying tissues. Endotoxins or vitamin deficiencies will render the mucosa susceptible to fungal infection.

Livestock in southern Africa seldom, if ever, contract diseases such as systemic histoplasmosis or blastomycosis. In Africa, systemic histoplasmosis occurs in humans, and in most cases the source of infection can be traced to caves where bat droppings provide a suitable substrate for *Histoplasma capsulatum*. For more information on these diseases, textbooks on veterinary mycology should be consulted.[2, 49]

Yeasts, *Aspergillus* spp. and mucoraceous fungi may be secondary invaders in the body or they may occur as laboratory contaminants in culture media. In most cases, in addition to culturing, the organism should be demonstrated in association with lesions in tissue sections to confirm the diagnosis.

Aspergillosis

Aspergillus spp., particularly *A. fumigatus*, are associated mostly with infections of the respiratory system, especially in chickens, and of the placenta in cows, but may also cause mastitis and rumenitis in livestock.[7–9, 32, 41, 43, 48, 68, 72, 107] Mouldy litter and feed are often incriminated as sources of infection in outbreaks of aspergillosis. Fungal spores are inhaled, particularly by housed animals.

Epidemics of aspergillosis occurred in horses in Germany in the early parts of the twentieth century.[101] The respiratory tract of horses can be seriously affected[14, 54] and include nasal aspergillosis,[42] infection of the guttural pouches[27] and bronchopneumonia. In the guttural pouches, lesions are usually limited to the roof of the pouch, but may spread locally via blood vessels and nerves to cause epistaxis, dyspnoea and clinical signs of encephalitis. Dysphagia follows damage to the glossopharyngeal and vagal nerves, and epistaxis is the result of erosion of the internal carotid artery. Aspergillic encephalitis is rare in animals.[63]

The fungus is visible as a whitish to blueish-green growth on the mucous membranes. Fungal growth may take place after death and should be differentiated from ante-mortal infections.[48]

Pulmonary aspergillosis is characterized by the presence of multiple, discrete, greyish-white nodules, 1–10 mm in diameter, in the lungs.[48, 72] Microscopically the nodules are comprised of a necrogranulomatous reaction in which long, dichotomous, branching, septate hyphae are located in the centre of the lesion. At a later stage cavitation may occur. Within this space may be

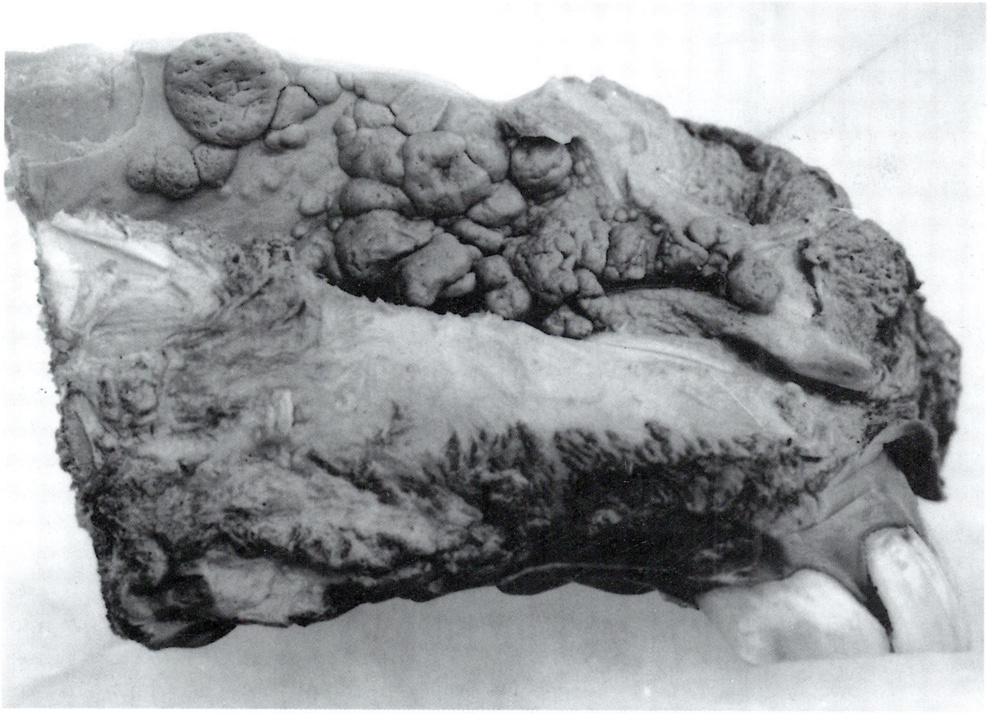

Figure 185.9 Pedunculated granulomas in the nasal cavity of a horse, caused by *Rhinosporidium seeberi*

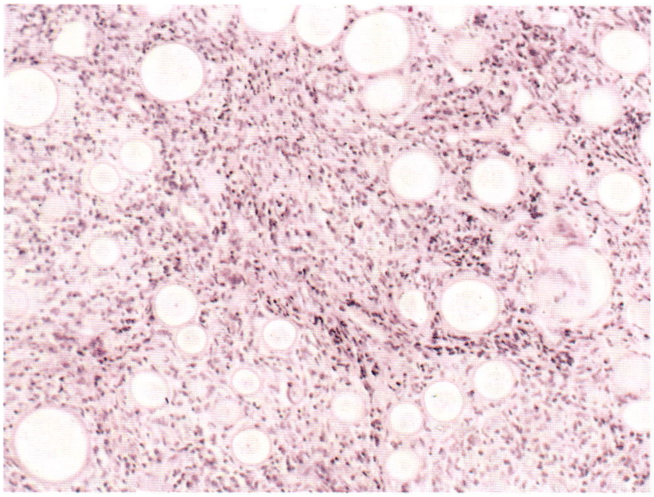

Figure 185.10 Haematoxylin and eosin-stained histological section showing sporangia of *Rhinosporidium seeberi* scattered within a granuloma

found a greenish, powdery mass consisting of the sporing heads of *A. fumigatus*. In long-standing cases, radiating groups of septate, branching hyphae may occur in the infected tissues. Occasionally blood vessels are invaded by the fungi, causing thrombosis. Infection can metastasize to many organs throughout the body.

Aspergillus spp. are easily cultured on Sabouraud's agar.

Zygomycosis or mucormycosis

Infections, collectively termed zygomycosis or mucormycosis, are caused mostly by members of the Mucorales, including *Mucor, Absidia, Mortierella* and *Rhizopus* spp.

Zygomycosis has been reported mainly in cattle and pigs. Mucoraceous fungi are associated with abomasal ulceration in calves, abomasitis and rumenitis in cattle, and ulcerative gastritis in pigs.[31, 40, 82, 87, 106] Ruminal acidosis as a result of eating excess grain causes rumenitis, abomasitis and disturbances in the normal microflora, allowing opportunistic fungi and bacteria to colonize the affected ruminal and abomasal mucosa. The fungi have a predilection for blood vessels, where they cause vasculitis which is often followed by thrombosis and infarction. The multifocal, infarcted areas are well circumscribed, often involving the entire thickness of the ruminal wall, and may be quite extensive **(Figure 185.11)**. The lesions in mycotic rumenitis are more severe, and also more often fatal, than the superficial rumenitis caused by *Fusobacterium necrophorum*. In both mucormycotic and necrobacillary rumenitis, metastatic spread to the liver, with the induction of necrotic foci, may follow. Forestomach and abomasal infections have been induced in sheep with ruminal acidosis after oral dosage with conidia of *Absidia corymbifera* (Cohn) Saccardo.[24] Affected animals usually develop atony of the rumen and a foul-smelling diarrhoea.

A diagnosis of mycotic rumenitis may be confirmed by histological examination. *Mucor, Rhizopus* and *Absidia* spp. cannot be differentiated from each other histologically. In tissue sections, multinucleate, non-septate hyphae are typical of these fungi **(Figure 185.12)**. Culturing of feeds or ruminal content is pointless, since these fungi are normally found there. In most cases treatment of affected animals is not effective.

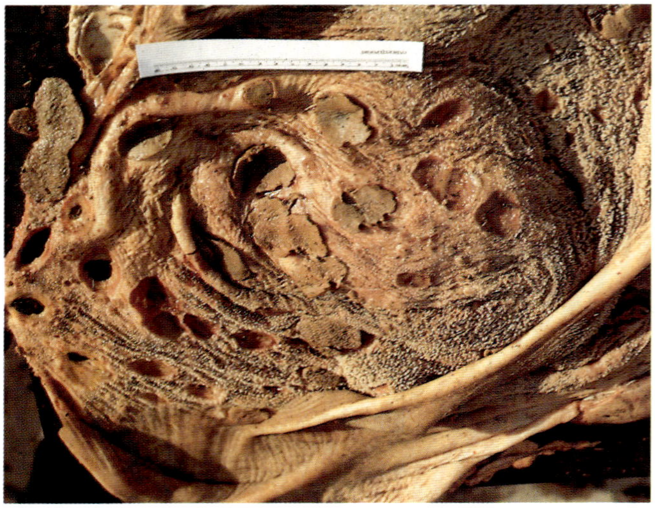

Figure 185.11 Ruminal wall of an ox showing typical lesions of mucormycosis

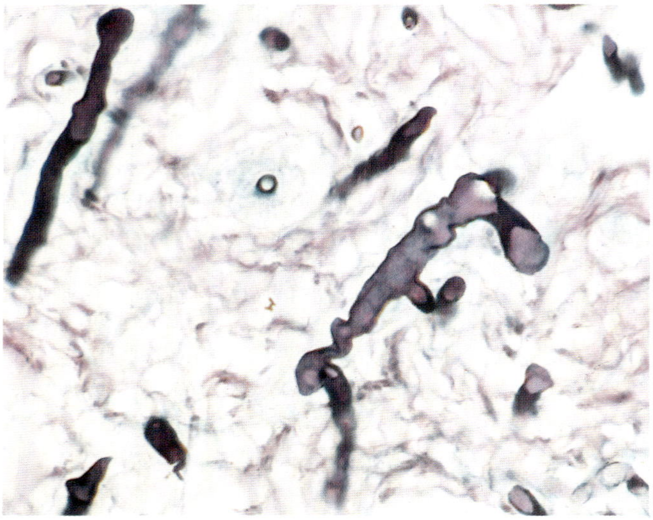

Figure 185.12 Histological section of the rumen wall of an ox suffering from mucormycosis. (GMS stain)

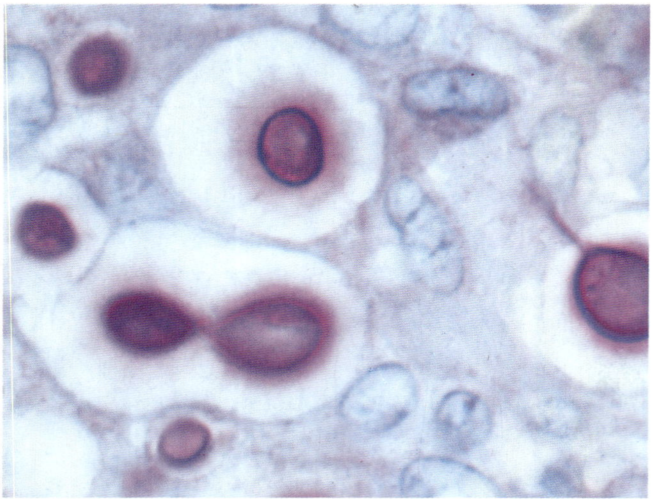

Figure 185.13 Histological section showing the typical morphology of *Cryptococcus neoformans* (PAS stain)

Candidiasis

Candida spp. are opportunist pathogens and are part of the normal microflora of the skin and gastrointestinal tract of healthy animals. Candidiasis caused particularly by *C. albicans* (Robin) Berkhout, generally affects the gastrointestinal tract and skin of calves, piglets and foals after immunosuppressive and debilitating conditions, prolonged antibiotic treatment, or the feeding of increased amounts of pelleted or finely ground rations.[10, 94, 95, 97] Mastitis, pneumonia and abortions in cattle,[37] and reproductive problems, such as endometritis, in horses have also been caused by *Candida* spp.

Candidiasis is one of the most frequently reported internal mycoses in pigs. A pseudomembranous stomatitis due to *C. albicans* has been described in suckling pigs,[40, 61] sometimes concurrently with gastric zygomycosis.[40]

Severe oral and oesophageal candidiasis (thrush) in foals and piglets is well known. Intestinal infections by *C. albicans*, resulting in diarrhoea and melaena, have been reported in calves[67] and feedlot cattle.[59] Affected animals are dehydrated and prostrated before they die.

Candida albicans is characterized by its smooth, thick-walled chlamydospores formed in cultures on maize-meal agar.

Cryptococcosis

Cryptococcus neoformans (Sanfelice) Vuillemin is a single-celled, yeast-like organism that affects particularly the lungs and central nervous system in a wide variety of animals. It also occasionally causes mastitis in cows.

Cryptococcus neoformans is found in the soil and is frequently isolated from the faeces of birds, particularly pigeons. In affected animals the organisms occur in cerebrospinal fluid as large, single, ovoid or spherical cells which reproduce by budding. When mounted in a drop of Indian ink diluted with water, the mucinous capsule surrounding each cell appears as a large, transparent halo **(Figure 185.13)**. The capsule prevents phagocytosis of the organisms and so contributes to the pathogenicity of the fungus. It is also the reason for the minimal inflammatory response following infection.

Several outbreaks of cryptococcal mastitis have been described in dairy herds.[33, 46, 78, 93] Primary and secondary cryptococcal mastitis may occur following the intramammary instillation of antibiotics. Clinical signs vary from a mild swelling of one or more quarters of the udder to severe swelling of the affected gland. The regional lymph nodes may also be involved. In severe cases, milk production declines, the milk is greyish-white, highly viscid, and mucoid, and the cutaneous and subcutaneous tissues of the udder are oedematous.

Cryptococcal infections in horses often localize in the nasal cavity, lungs or brain.[12, 25, 30, 38, 47, 89] These infections vary from miliary granulomas or small abscesses to large, gelatinous lesions; pneumonia may involve one or more lobes. The clinical signs depend on the location and extent of the lesions. Horses affected by acute cerebral lesions usually behave violently, while others may develop blindness or signs of locomotor disturbances.

The fungi are best demonstrated in histopathological tissue sections stained by the periodic acid-Schiff method, with mucicarmine stain, or after Gomori's methenamine silver impregnation.

Mycotic abortion

A variety of fungi, including those that cause zygomycosis (*Mucor, Absidia, Rhizopus,* and *Mortierella* spp.), aspergillosis (*Aspergillus* spp.), and candidiasis (*Candida* spp.),[37] may be responsible for abortion in livestock. Mycotic abortion is relatively common in cattle but rare in sheep, horses and pigs. Placental infection follows dissemination from primary pulmonary or gastrointestinal infections.

Aspergillus fumigatus causes extensive cotyledonary and intercotyledonary necrosis as well as oedema, haemorrhage and infarction in cases where hyphae invade blood vessels. The degree of damage to the placenta determines whether or not abortion will occur. Although placentitis is invariably present, subsequent fertility is not affected in most cases.[53, 60]

Mortierella wolfii Mehrotra & Baijal, a member of the zygomycetes, causes placentitis and abortion in cows in New Zealand, Australia and the United Kingdom,[65] but has not been detected in southern Africa.

In mycotic abortions, foetuses often appear normal. However, multifocal, circumscribed, ringworm-like skin lesions of varying size, and pneumonia may be present. Infection can best be diagnosed by microscopical demonstration of fungal hyphae in specially stained tissue sections of affected skin, particularly in the hair follicles and adjacent tissues.[45] The causative fungus can be cultured from the stomach contents of the foetus.

Control of internal mycoses

Chemotherapeutic treatment of internal mycoses in livestock is generally unsatisfactory. Polyene antibiotics such as nystatin and amphotericin B have been used extensively in humans. Amphotericin B is effective against a wide spectrum of fungal infections, but has side-effects when administered intravenously. Its use in animals affected by cryptococcal mastitis has been advocated. Segregation of these animals, improved sanitation, limited treatment and careful handling of them during the milking process are necessary to limit the spread of infection.[1]

The imidazoles have broad-spectrum antimycotic activity, but their toxicity and high cost make their use in large animals impractical. Topical therapy with antimycotics could be successful. The use of antifungal vaginal suppositories for treatment of mycotic endometritis in mares has been advocated.[13] Complete recovery from nasal aspergillosis in horses after treatment with natamycin (25 mg/100 ml water) has been reported.[42] The solution was administered with a catheter via the biopsy channel of an endoscope, or with an indwelling facial catheter to irrigate affected areas in the caudal maxillary sinus where lesions occurred. Whenever possible, fungal plaques and necrotic tissue should be removed before topical therapy is applied.

References

1 **ABID, H.M., WALTER, P.A. & LITCHFIELD, H., 1987.** Chromomycosis in a horse. *Journal of the American Veterinary Medical Association*, 191, 711–712.

2 **AINSWORTH, G.C. & AUSTWICK, P.K.C., 1973.** *Fungal Diseases of Animals.* 2nd edn. Slough: Commonwealth Agricultural Bureau.

3 **AJELLO, L., GEORG, L.K., STEIGBIGEL, R.T. & WANG, C.J.K., 1974.** A case of phaeohyphomycosis caused by a new species of Phialophora. *Mycologia*, 66, 490–498.

4 **AKUN, R., 1953.** Eine chromoblastomycosis-ähnliche Pilzkrankheit beim Pferde. *Zentralblatt für Algemeine Pathologie*, 9, 294–297.

5 **ALLISON, N., WILLARD, M.D., BENTINCK-SMITH, J. & DAVIS, K., 1986.** Nasal rhinosporidiosis in two dogs. *Journal of the American Veterinary Medical Association*, 188, 869–871.

6 **ANDREWS, A.H. & EDWARDSON, J., 1981.** Treatment of ringworm in calves using griseofulvin. *The Veterinary Record*, 108, 498–500.

7 **AUSTWICK, P.K.C., 1962.** The presence of *Aspergillus fumigatus* in the lungs of dairy cows. *Laboratory Investigations*, 11, 1065–1072.

8 **AUSTWICK, P.K.C., GITTER, M. & WATKINS, C.V., 1960.** Pulmonary aspergillosis in lambs. *The Veterinary Record*, 72, 19–21.

9 **AYAZ, M., ILAHI, A. & AFZAL, H., 1966.** Some cases of aspergillosis in sheep in West Pakistan. *Pakistan Journal of Animal Science*, 3, 21–24.

10 **BAKER, E.D. & CADMAN, L.P., 1963.** Candidiasis in pigs in northwestern Wisconsin. *Journal of the American Veterinary Medical Association*, 142, 763–767.

11 **BAKER, N.F. & DAVIES, D.W., 1954.** Spray application for the treatment of ringworm in cattle. *Veterinary Medicine*, 49, 275–276.

12 **BARCLAY, W.P. & DELAHUNTA, A., 1979.** Cryptococcal meningitis in a horse. *Journal of the American Veterinary Medical Association*, 174, 1236–1238.

13 **BLUE, M.G., 1987.** Mycotic endometritis in mares. Review and clinical observations. *New Zealand Veterinary Journal*, 35, 181–183.

14 **BLUE, J., PERDRIZET, J. & BROWN, E., 1987.** Pulmonary aspergillosis in a horse with myelomonocytic leukemia. *Journal of the American Veterinary Medical Association*, 190, 1562–1564.

15 **BOOMKER, J., COETZER, J.A.W. & SCOTT, D.B., 1977.** Black grain mycetoma (Maduromycosis) in horses. *Onderstepoort Journal of Veterinary Research*, 44, 249–252.

16 **BREDE, H.D., 1972.** Dermatophytes in southern Africa. *In:* MARSHALL, J., (ed.). *Essays on Tropical Dermatology.*

Amsterdam: Excerpta Medica.

17 **BRIDGES, C.H., 1957.** Maduromycotic mycetomas in animals. *Curvularia geniculata* as an etiological agent. *American Journal of Pathology*, 33, 411–427.

18 **BRIDGES, C.H. & BEASLEY, J.N., 1960.** Maduromycotic mycetomas in animals — *Brachycladium speciferum* Bainier as an etiologic agent. *Journal of the American Veterinary Medical Association*, 137, 192–201.

19 **BRIDGES, C.H. & EMMONS, C.W., 1961.** A phycomycosis of horses caused by *Hyphomyces destruens*. *Journal of the American Veterinary Medical Association*, 138, 579–589.

20 **BRIDGES, C.H., ROMANE, W.M. & EMMONS, C.W., 1962.** Phycomycosis of horses caused by *Entomophthora coronata*. *Journal of the American Veterinary Medical Association*, 140, 673–677.

21 **BRUNER, D.W. & GILLESPIE, J.H., 1966.** *Hagan's Infectious Diseases of Domestic Animals*. 5th edn. Ithaca: Cornell University Press.

22 **BULLEN, J.J., 1949.** The yeast-like form of *Cryptococcus farciminosus* (Rivotta): *(Histoplasma farciminosum)*. *Journal of Pathology and Bacteriology*, 61, 117–120.

23 **CHANDLER, F.W., KAPLAN, W. & AJELLO, L., 1980.** *A Colour Atlas and Textbook of the Histopathology of Mycotic Diseases*. London: Wolfe Medical Publishers.

24 **CHIHAYA, Y., MATSUKAWA, K., MIZUSHIMA, S. & MATSUI, Y., 1988.** Ruminant forestomach and abomasal mucormycosis under rumen acidosis. *Veterinary Pathology*, 25, 119–123.

25 **CHO, D.Y., PACE, L.W. & BEADLE, R.E., 1986.** Cerebral cryptococcosis in a horse. *Veterinary Pathology*, 23, 207–209.

26 **CONNOLE, M.D., 1967.** *Microsporum gypseum* ringworm in a horse. *Australian Veterinary Journal*, 43, 118.

27 **COOK, W.R., 1968.** The clinical features of guttural pouch mycosis in the horse. *The Veterinary Record*, 83, 336–345.

28 **DANGERFIELD, L.F. & GEAR, J., 1941.** Sporotrichosis among miners on the Witwatersrand gold mines. *South African Medical Journal*, 15, 128.

29 **DAVIS, H.H. & WORTHINGTON, W.E., 1964.** Equine sporotrichosis. *Journal of the American Veterinary Medical Association*, 145, 692–693.

30 **DICKSON, J. & MEYER, E.P., 1970.** Cryptococcosis in horses in Western Australia. *Australian Veterinary Journal*, 46, 558.

31 **DOWIE, P., 1982.** Mucormycosis in the bovine abomasum. *The Veterinary Record*, 111, 212.

32 **EGGERT, M.J. & ROMBERG, P.F., 1960.** Pulmonary aspergillosis in a calf. *Journal of the American Veterinary Medical Association*, 137, 595–596.

33 **EMMONS, C.W., 1952.** *Cryptococcus neoformans* strains from a severe outbreak of bovine mastitis. *Mycopathologia et Mycologia Applicata*, 6, 231–234.

34 **EMMONS, C.W., BINFORD, C.H. & UTZ, J.P., 1970.** *Medical Mycology*. 2nd edn. Philadelphia: Lea & Febiger.

35 **FINDLAY, G.H., 1979.** Superficial fungous infections. *In:* FITZPATRICK, T., (ed.). *Dermatology in General Practice*. New York: McGraw-Hill.

36 **FISHMAN, O., SANTIAGO, M. & RAMOS, C.D., 1966.** Ringworm infection by *Microsporum canis* in a horse. *Mycopathologia et Mycologia Applicata*, 30, 273–275.

37 **FOLEY, G.L. & SCHAFLER, D.H., 1987.** Candida abortion in cattle. *Veterinary Pathology*, 24, 532–536.

38 **FROTHINGHAM, L., 1902.** A tumor-like lesion in the lung of a horse caused by a *Blastomyces* (Torula). *Journal of Medical Research*, 8, 31–43.

39 **GEORG, L.K., KAPLAN, W. & CAMP, L.B., 1957.** Equine ringworm with special reference to *Trichophyton equinum*. *American Journal of Veterinary Research*, 18, 798–810.

40 **GITTER, M. & AUSTWICK, P.K.C., 1959.** Mucormycosis and moniliasis in a litter of suckling pigs. *The Veterinary Record*, 71, 6–11.

41 **GRACEY, J.F. & BAXTER, J.T., 1961.** Generalized *Aspergillus fumigatus* infection in a lamb. *British Veterinary Journal*, 117, 11–14.

42 **GREET, T.R.C., 1981.** Nasal aspergillosis in three horses. *The Veterinary Record*, 109, 487–489.

43 **GRIFFIN, R., 1969.** Pulmonary aspergillosis in the calf. *The Veterinary Record*, 84, 109–111.

44 **GUDDING, R. & NAESS, B., 1986.** Vaccination of cattle against ringworm caused by *Trichophyton verrucosum*. *American Journal of Veterinary Research*, 47, 2415–2417.

45 **HILLMAN, R.B., 1969.** Bovine mycotic placentitis in New York State. *Cornell Veterinarian*, 59, 269–288.

46 **INNES, J.R.M., SEIBOLD, H.R. & ARANTZEN, W.P., 1952.** The pathology of bovine mastitis caused by *Cryptococcus neoformans*. *American Journal of Veterinary Research*, 13, 469–475.

47 **IRWIN, C.N.P. & RAC, R., 1957.** Cryptococcosis infection in a horse. *Australian Veterinary Journal*, 33, 97–98.

48 **JUBB, K.V.F., KENNEDY, P.C. & PALMER, N., 1985.** *Pathology of Domestic Animals*. 3rd edn. Vols. 1–3. Orlando: Academic Press, Inc.

49 **JUNGERMAN, P.F. & SCHWARTZMAN, R.M., 1972.** *Veterinary Medical Mycology*. Philadelphia: Lea & Febiger.

50 **KAPLAN, W., CHANDLER, F.W., AJELLO, L., GAUTHIER, R., HIGGINS, R. & CAYOUETTE, P., 1975.** Equine phaeohyphomycosis caused by *Drechslera specifera*. *Canadian Veterinary Journal*, 16, 205–208.

51 **KAPLAN, W., HOPPING, J.L. & GEORG, L.K., 1957.** Ringworm in horses caused by the dermatophyte, *Microsporum gypseum*. *Journal of the American Veterinary Medical Association*, 131, 329–332.

52 **KELLERMAN, T.S., COETZER, J.A.W. & NAUDÉ, T.W., 1987.** *Plant Poisonings and Mycotoxicoses of Livestock in Southern Africa*. Cape Town: Oxford University Press Southern Africa.

53 **KHAROLE, M.U., CHAND, P., MONGA, D.P. & SADANA, J.R., 1988.** Pulmonary zygomycosis in a bovine fetus. *The Veterinary Record*, 122, 236.

54 **LONG, J.R. & MITCHELL, L., 1971.** Pulmonary aspergillosis in a mare. *Canadian Veterinary Journal*, 12, 16–18.

55 **LURIE, H.I., 1948.** A common antigenic factor in different species of *Sporotrichum*. *Mycologia*, 40, 106–113.

56 **LURIE, H.I., 1963.** Histopathology of sporotrichosis. *Archives of Pathology*, 75, 421–437.

57 **MARSHALL, J., 1964.** Fungous diseases. *In:* MARSHALL, J., (ed.). *Skin Diseases in Africa. An Essay in Epidemiology*. Cape Town: Maskew Miller.

58 **MARTIN, P.M.D. & BERSON, S.D., 1973.** Fungus diseases in southern Africa. *Mycopathologia et Mycologia Applicata*, 50, 1–84.

59 **McCARTHY, R.T., 1956.** Moniliasis as a systemic infection in cattle: Field case reports. *Veterinary Medicine*, 51, 562–564.

60 **McCAUSLAND, I.P., SLEE, K.J. & HIRST, F.S., 1987.** Mycotic abortion in cattle. *Australian Veterinary Journal*, 64, 129–132.

61 **McCREA, M.R. & OSBORNE, A.D., 1957.** A case of thrush (candidiasis) in a piglet. *Journal of Comparative Pathology and Therapy*, 67, 343–344.

62 **McENTEE, M., 1987.** Eumycotic mycetoma: Review and report of a cutaneous lesion caused by *Pseudallescheria boydii* in a horse. *Journal of the American Veterinary Medical Association*, 191, 1459–1461.

63 **McLAUGHLIN, B.G. & O'BRIEN, J.L., 1986.** Guttural pouch mycosis and mycotic encephalitis in a horse. *Canadian Veterinary Journal*, 27, 109–111.

64 **McPHERSON, E.A., 1957.** The influence of physical factors on dermatomycosis in domestic animals. *The Veterinary Record*, 69, 1010–1013.

65 **MENNA, M.E.D. & CARTER, M.E., 1972.** The identification of *Mortierella wolfii* isolated from cases of abortion and pneumonia in cattle and a search for its infection source. *Research in Veterinary Science*, 13, 439–442.

66 **MILLER, R.I. & CAMPBELL, R.S.F., 1984.** The comparative pathology of equine cutaneous phycomycosis. *Veterinary*

Pathology, 21, 325–332.

67 **MILLS, J.H.L. & HIRTH, R.S., 1967.** Systemic candidiasis in calves on prolonged antibiotic therapy. *Journal of the American Veterinary Medical Association*, 150, 862–870.

68 **MOLELLO, J.A. & BUSEY, W., 1963.** Pulmonary aspergillosis in a cow. *Journal of the American Veterinary Medical Association*, 142, 632–633.

69 **MULLER, G.H., KAPLAN, W., AJELLO, J. & PADHYE, A.A., 1975.** Phaeohyphomycosis caused by *Drechslera spicifera* in a cat. *Journal of the American Veterinary Medical Association*, 166, 150–154.

70 **MULLER, G.H. & KIRK, W., 1976.** *Small Animal Dermatology*. 2nd edn. Philadelphia: W.B. Saunders Company.

71 **MYERS, D.D., SIMON, J. & CASE, M.T., 1964.** Rhinosporidiosis in a horse. *Journal of the American Veterinary Medical Association*, 145, 345–347.

72 **NESBIT, J.W., 1986.** The pathology of pulmonary aspergillosis in a piglet. *Journal of the South African Veterinary Association*, 57, 125–127.

73 **PEARSON, J.K.L. & RANKIN, J.E.F., 1962.** Griseofulvin in the treatment of bovine ringworm. *The Veterinary Record*, 74, 564.

74 **PHILPOT, C.M., WESCOTT, G. & STEWART, J.G., 1984.** *Microsporum gypseum* ringworm. *The Veterinary Record*, 114, 22–23.

75 **PIJPER, A. & PULLINGER, B.D., 1927.** An outbreak of sporotrichosis among South African native miners. *The Lancet*, 213, 914–915.

76 **PINOY, E., 1913.** Actinomycosis et mycetomes. *Bulletin de l'Institut Pasteur*, 11, 929–938.

77 **PLUNKETT, J.J., 1949.** Epizootic lymphangitis. *Journal of the Royal Army Veterinary Corps*, 20, 94–99.

78 **POUNDEN, W.D., AMBERSON, J.M. & JAEGER, R.F., 1952.** A severe mastitis problem associated with *Cryptococcus neoformans* in a large dairy herd. *American Journal of Veterinary Research*, 13, 121–128.

79 **POWER, S.B. & MALONE, A., 1987.** An outbreak of ringworm in sheep in Ireland caused by *Trichophyton verrucosum*. *The Veterinary Record*, 121, 218–220.

80 **QUINLAN, J. & DE KOCK, G., 1926.** Two cases of rhinosporidiosis in equines. *South African Journal of Science*, 23, 589–594.

81 **RAO, M.A.N., 1938.** Rhinosporidiosis in bovines in the Madra Presidency, with a discussion on the probable modes of infection. *Indian Journal of Veterinary Science*, 8, 187–198.

82 **REED, W.M., HANIKA, C., MEHDI, N.A.Q. & SCHACKELFORD, C., 1987.** Gastrointestinal zygomycosis in suckling pigs. *Journal of the American Veterinary Medical Association*, 191, 549–550.

83 **ROBERTS, D.S. & KEEP, J.M., 1965.** Infection in the wool of sheep by *Microsporum canis*. *Sabouraudia*, 4, 96–97.

84 **ROBINSON, E.M. & PARKINS, B.S., 1929.** A case of sporotrichosis in the horse. *Journal of the South African Veterinary Medical Association*, 1, 17–24.

85 **SABOURAUD, R., 1894.** *Les trichophyties humaines*. Paris: Rueff et Cie.

86 **SABOURAUD, R., 1910.** *Les teignes*. Paris: Masson et Cie.

87 **SANFORD, S.E., 1985.** Gastric zygomycosis (mucormycosis) in four suckling pigs. *Journal of the American Veterinary Medical Association*, 186, 393–394.

88 **SAUNDERS, L.Z., 1948.** Systemic fungous infections in animals: A review. *Cornell Veterinarian*, 38, 213–238.

89 **SCHELLNER, S., 1935.** Uber eine beim Pferde durch Hefezellen verursachte Geschwulst in der Nasenhole und deren Nebenhohlen. *Zeitschrift für Veterinärkunde*, 47, 111–116.

90 **SCOTT, D.B., 1975.** An outbreak of ringworm in karakul sheep caused by a physiological variant of *Trichophyton verrucosum*. *Onderstepoort Journal of Veterinary Research*, 42, 49–52.

91 **SCOTT, D.B., 1976.** A new variety of *Trichophyton verrucosum*. *Transactions of the British Mycological Society*, 67, 342–344.

92 **SCOTT, D.B. & SCOTT, F.P., 1973.** Dermatophytoses in South Africa. *Sabouraudia*, 11, 279–282.

93 **SIMON, J., NICHOLS, R.E. & MORSE, E.V., 1953.** An outbreak of bovine cryptococcosis. *Journal of the American Veterinary Medical Association*, 122, 31–35.

94 **SMITH, J.M.B., 1967.** Candidiasis in animals in New Zealand. *Sabouraudia*, 5, 220–225.

95 **SMITH, J.M.B., 1968.** Experimental mycotic ulceration. *Mycopathologia et Mycologia Applicata*, 34, 353–358.

96 **SMITH, J.M.B., JOLLY, R.D., GEORG, L.K. & CONNOLE, M.D., 1968.** *Trichophyton equinum* var. *autotrophicum:* Its characteristics and geographical distribution. *Sabouraudia*, 6, 296–403.

97 **STEDHAM, M.A., KELLEY, D.C. & COLES, E.H., 1967.** Influence of dietary sugar on growth of *Candida albicans* in the porcine digestive tract and lesions in the esophageal area of the stomach. *American Journal of Veterinary Research*, 28, 153–159.

98 **TAPLIN, D., REBELL, G. & BLANK, H., 1969.** Isolation and recognition of dermatophytes on a new medium (DTM). *Archives of Dermatology*, 99, 203–209.

99 **THAKUR, D.K., MISRA, S. & CHOUDHURI, P.C., 1981.** Dermatomycosis in goats in India. *Mykosen*, 25, 442–448.

100 **THOROLD, P.W., 1951.** Equine sporotrichosis. *Journal of the South African Veterinary Medical Association*, 22, 81–83.

101 **TSCHERNIAK, W.S., 1928.** Zur Lehre von den Broncho- und Pneumono-mykosen der Pferde. *Archiv für Wissenchaftliche und praktiesche Tierheilkunde*, 57, 417–444.

102 **VAN AMSTEL, S.R., ROSS, M. & VAN DEN BERGH, S.S., 1984.** Maduromycosis *(Madurella mycetomatis)* in a horse. *Journal of the South African Veterinary Association*, 55, 81–83.

103 **VISMER, H.F., 1986.** Human and animal dermatophytoses in the Transvaal. M.Sc. Dissertation, University of Pretoria.

104 **WALKER, J., 1930.** *Aids to Stockowners*. Nairobi, Kenya: Government Printer, Department of Agriculture.

105 **WATSON, E.A., 1920.** A note on equine sporotrichosis. *Canadian Veterinary Record*, 1, 18–19.

106 **WELCHMAN, D. DE. B. & BAUST, G.N., 1987.** A survey of abomasal ulceration in veal calves. *The Veterinary Record*, 121, 586–590.

107 **YOUNG, N.E., 1970.** Pulmonary aspergillosis in the lamb. *The Veterinary Record*, 86, 790.

108 **ZSCHOKKE, E., 1913.** Ein Rhinosporidium beim Pferde. *Schweizer Archiv für Tierheilkunde*, 55, 641–650.

186

Protothecosis

D.B. Scott

Prototheca spp. are achloric algae responsible for localized, sporadic infections of the skin, eyes and udder, or for systemic infections in animals and humans.[1, 3] In livestock, *Prototheca* spp. are occasionally associated with sporadic cases or serious outbreaks of mastitis in cattle.[1, 2]

There are two reports of protothecosis in domestic animals in South Africa; one of a dog with a disseminated infection[3] and the other of a cow with mastitis caused by a mixed infection of a *Prototheca* sp., *Staphylococcus aureus* and *Streptococcus agalactiae*.[2]

Prototheca spp. are common in soil throughout the world, particularly in aqueous habitats, and in plants.[1, 3] Aqueous habitats include the dairy-herd environment, where wet conditions and organic matter are common in demanuring and feeding aisles, drinking troughs, slurry basins and sewage. Contaminated milking equipment may play a role in the transmission of these algae, although *Prototheca* spp. are generally susceptible to chlorination.

A presumptive diagnosis of protothecosis is often possible when infected milk samples or tissue specimens are examined, and is based on the characteristic microscopical morphology of the algae.[3] *Prototheca* spp. form sporangia, 10–30 μm in diameter, containing several endospores **(Figure 186.1)**. The cell wall of the unicellular organisms stains well with the periodic acid-Schiff

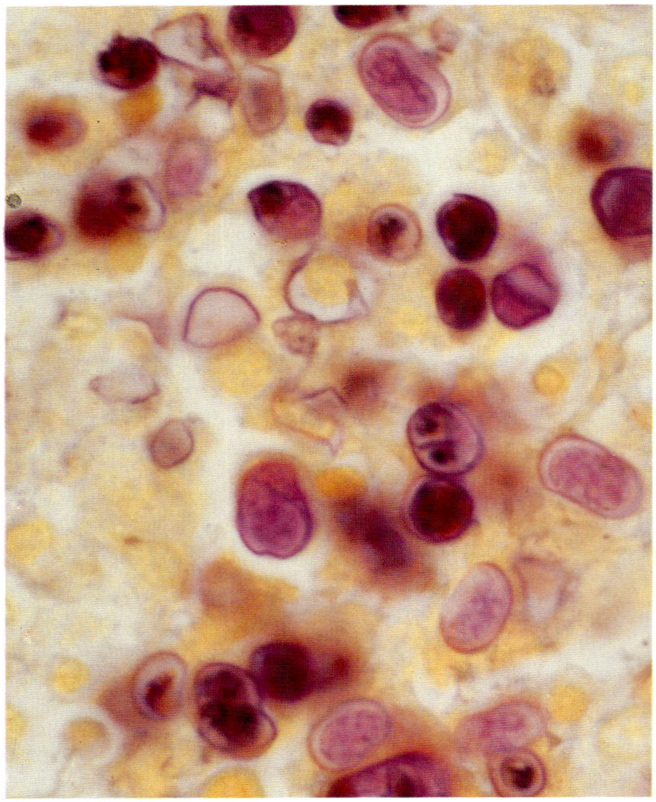

Figure 186.1 *Prototheca* organisms in an inflammatory exudate. Note endospores in the sporangia (Gridley's fungal stain)

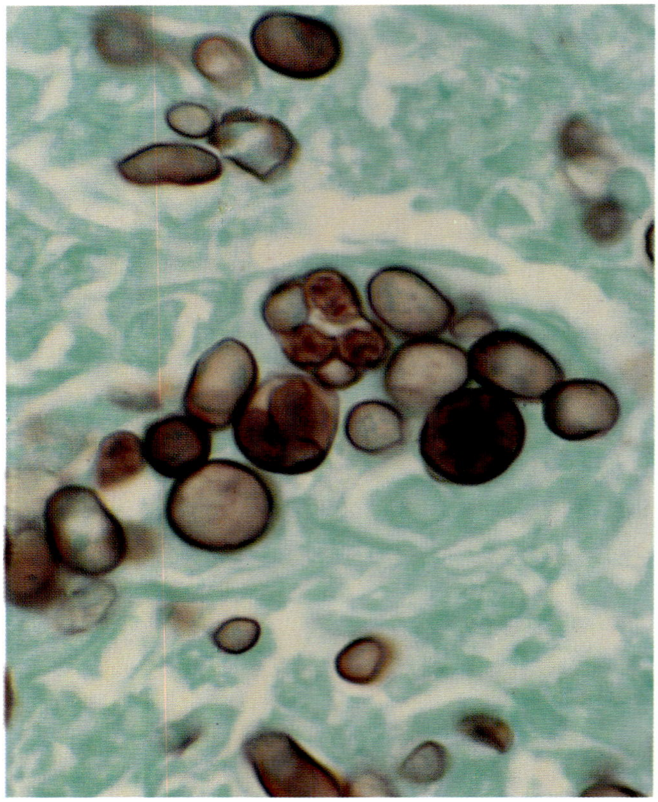

Figure 186.2 A *Prototheca* sp. stained with Gomori's methenamine silver impregnation

reaction and Gomori's methenamine silver impregnation method **(Figure 186.2)**, and is highly birefringent when thick, unstained sections are viewed under polarized light.[3] Organisms can be confused with pathogenic fungi such as *Blastomyces, Cryptococcus* and *Paracoccidioides* spp., and other organisms such as *Pneumocystis carinii* and amoebae.

Amphotericin B has been used successfully in the treatment of humans with protothecosis. As therapy of protothecal mastitis is mostly unsuccessful, its prevention by the implementation of proper sanitary measures and elimination of infected animals is most important in its control.

References

1 **ANDERSON, K.L. & WALKER, R.L., 1988.** Sources of *Prototheca* spp. in a dairy-herd environment. *Journal of the American Veterinary Medical Association,* 193, 553–556.

2 **GIESECKE, W.H., NEL, E.E. & VAN DEN HEEVER, L.W., 1968.** Blastomycotic mastitis in South Africa. *Journal of the South African Veterinary Medical Association,* 39, 69–71.

3 **IMES, G.D., LLOYD, J.C. & BRIGHTMAN, M.P., 1977.** Disseminated protothecosis in a dog. *Onderstepoort Journal of Veterinary Research,* 44, 1–6.

Section 7

Disease complexes and diseases of unknown aetiology

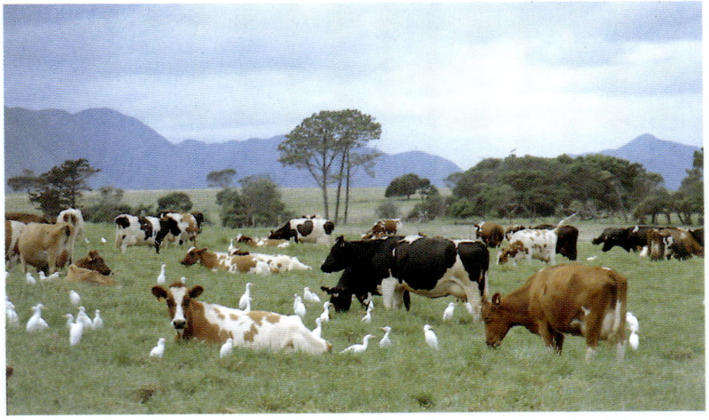

187

Viral teratology in ruminants

J.A.W. Coetzer

Introduction

Teratology in ruminants is a well-known entity of universal occurrence and diverse aetiology. Of the infectious agents, viruses[10, 18, 21, 24, 47, 54, 60] are most often incriminated as the cause of prenatal malformations in cattle, sheep and goats. Plants,[30, 36, 37] drugs (particularly the anthelmintics of the benzimidazole group),[59] vitamin A[68] and copper deficiencies,[67] hyperthermia[19, 25] and genetic factors[42, 43] have all been implicated. Veterinarians in southern Africa are often confronted with virus-induced congenital defects, particularly in ruminants.

Although a wide spectrum of defects, such as malformations, generalized or localized growth retardation, morphological lesions and more subtle biochemical or functional changes, may develop in a variety of organs in the foetus after infection, only those aspects of the viral infections which give rise to grossly discernible malformations of the central nervous system (CNS) in ruminants on the subcontinent will be discussed, as this system is the most vulnerable to the development of structural abnormalities.

Aetiology and pathogenesis

On the African continent, viruses belonging to the Bunyaviridae, Reoviridae, and Togaviridae have been linked to teratologic defects of the CNS in ruminants **(Table 187.1)**. Apart from these viruses, it is quite possible that as yet unidentified viruses belonging to these or other virus families may also be responsible for anomalies in ruminants.

Although known teratogenic viruses may cause diverse diseases in mature animals, similar, if not identical, brain malformations may be induced by them in the foetus.[4, 12, 16, 50–52] Consequently, the nature of the morphological defects cannot be used as an indicator of the identity of the aetiology. In addition, it should be borne in mind that aetiological factors other than viruses may cause similar defects. In order to fully comprehend the pathogenesis of viral teratology, foetal, maternal and virological factors should be collectively considered.

Foetal factors

Fuccillo and Sever[21] concluded that deformities may develop if morphogenesis of the foetus is incomplete at the time of infection. Calves, foals, lambs and piglets are born with a remarkable degree of structural and functional maturity of the nervous system and are therefore not susceptible to the development of teratogenic defects at this stage.[67] On the other hand, the nervous system of kittens and puppies is relatively immature at birth, and is thus still prone to developmental defects.

The CNS passes through a critical stage of development during which it is most vulnerable to the effects of teratogenic virus infections. This critical period varies in different species and is correlated with the presence of metabolically active foetal cells undergoing mitosis and differentiation, which in the domestic ruminants takes place during the first third of pregnancy.

Barnard and Pienaar[5] induced hydranencephaly in two bovine foetuses after each had been inoculated *in utero* with an egg-attenuated bluetongue (BT) virus, one on day 126 and the other on day 138 of gestation. MacLachlan and Osburn[44] corroborated these findings by the inoculation of BT virus into 125-day-old bovine foetuses. Sheep infected between 50 and 58 days of gestation with the modified BT virus gave birth to hydranencephalic lambs, while porencephaly was reported in lambs born of ewes which had been inoculated with the same virus at 75–78 days of gestation. Only a mild focal encephalitis occurred in lambs whose dams were infected after 100 days of pregnancy. Similar congenital anomalies have been induced experimentally in lambs born from ewes inoculated with the mouse-brain attenuated viruses of either Rift Valley fever (RVF) or Wesselsbron disease (WSL), or with the wild-type WSL virus.[12, 13] A range of brain defects, including hydrocephalus, porencephaly, hydranencephaly and micrencephaly have been reported in ruminants infected with Akabane and related Simbu-group viruses, Palyam-serogroup viruses, pestiviruses, Banzivirus and West Nile virus **(Table 187.1)**. Severe deformities occurred in calves whose dams were inoculated with the Akabane virus when they were between the 64th and 96th day of gestation, and similarly in lambs

Table 187.1 Viruses that have been associated with teratology in ruminants

VIRUS FAMILY	VIRUS (GENUS)	ANIMAL SPECIES	MALFORMATIONS OF THE BRAIN AND ASSOCIATED DEFECTS	REFERENCES
Bunyaviridae	Akabane and related Simbu-group viruses e.g. Aino, Peaton (*Bunyavirus*)	Sheep	Porencephaly, hydranencephaly, agenesis of the brain, agenesis or hypoplasia of the spinal cord, arthrogryposis, neurogenic muscular atrophy, hypoplasia of the lungs	54, 55
		Cattle	Micrencephaly, porencephaly, hydranencephaly, cerebellar cavitation, arthrogryposis, neurogenic muscular atrophy, cataracts, ophthalmia	26, 29, 39, 40, 49, 65
	Rift Valley fever virus (*Phlebovirus*)			
	Mouse-brain attenuated Rift Valley fever virus	Sheep	Micrencephaly, hydranencephaly, hypoplasia of the lungs, arthrogryposis, *hydrops amnii*	13
Reoviridae	Bluetongue virus (*Orbivirus*)			
	Modified bluetongue virus	Sheep	Porencephaly, hydranencephaly	51, 52, 73
		Cattle	Porencephaly, hydranencephaly	5
	Palyam-serogroup orbiviruses (Chuzan and possibly other viruses)	Cattle	Hydrocephalus, hydranencephaly, micrencephaly, cerebellar hypoplasia	22
Togaviridae	Bovine viral diarrhoea and mucosal disease virus (*Pestivirus*)	Sheep	Hydrocephalus, cerebellar dysplasia or hypoplasia, porencephaly, hydranencephaly, hypomyelinogenesis, arthrogryposis, hairy birth coats, brachygnathy inferior, intrauterine growth retardation of the foetus and tissues	3, 57, 58, 61, 69
		Cattle	Cerebellar hypoplasia, hydranencephaly, dysmyelination, intrauterine growth retardation, alopecia, retinal degeneration and necrosis, optic neuritis, cataracts, micro-ophthalmia, brachygnathism	7, 8, 32–34 64, 69, 71
	Wesselsbron disease virus (*Flavivirus*)			
	Wild-type Wesselsbron disease virus	Sheep	Internal hydrocephalus, hydranencephaly, bilateral membranous thinning of the occipital lobes of the cerebrum, hypoplasia of the spinal cord, hypoplasia of the lungs, neurogenic muscular atrophy, arthrogryposis, *hydrops amnii*	12, 13
	Mouse-brain attenuated Wesselsbron disease virus	Cattle	Porencephaly, cerebellar hypoplasia	15
		Sheep	Internal hydrocephalus, hydranencephaly, hypoplasia of the spinal cord, markedly deformed head, arthrogryposis, *hydrops amnii*	12, 13
	Banzivirus (*Flavivirus*)	Sheep	Internal hydrocephalus, porencephaly, hydranencephaly	6
	West Nile virus (*Flavivirus*)	Sheep	Hydranencephaly	6

whose dams were infected between the 30th and 35th day of pregnancy.[54]

The critical stage of cerebellar development differs from that of the rest of the brain and also varies between species.[46, 47] A biphasic growth of the cerebral hemispheres has been reported in the sheep foetus.[46] Neuronal multiplication occurs mostly between the 40th and 80th day of gestation, and glial proliferation between the 95th and 130th day, while the development of the cerebellum and spinal cord occurs much later, being most active at birth. In lambs, approximately 50 per cent of the weight of the mature cerebellum and 30 per cent of that of the spinal cord has been attained by the 7th day after birth.[46] In the bovine foetus, maximum cerebellar growth occurs between the 133rd and the 162nd days of gestation. Cattle infected with the bovine viral diarrhoea and mucosal disease (BVD-MD) virus after the sixth gestational month give birth to normal calves,[9] whereas infection between the 100th and 170th day of pregnancy may result in calves being born suffering from cerebellar hypoplasia.[7, 8, 64] Although the latter anomaly in calves is generally associated with BVD-MD virus infections, defects such as hydrocephalus, porencephaly, micrencephaly and hydranencephaly due to this virus have also been reported in calves and lambs.[3, 67] In addition to these grossly discernible malformations of the brain, certain BVD-MD viral strains cause a syndrome in lambs first described in flocks of the Welsh border counties[28] and known variously as Border, 'B' or hairy shaker disease **(see Chapter 65: Border disease)**. It is characterized by tremors, hairy birth coat (the result of enlargement and aberrant differentiation of primary hair follicles), slow rate of growth, and hypomyelinogenesis of the CNS as a result of the suppressive effect of the virus on the myelin-forming oligodendrocytes.[3, 69] Affected lambs have a low viability.[69]

Other factors which render the foetus more vulnerable to infection and consequently to the development of teratologic defects include the immature state of the immune system that results from incomplete development of the lymphoid tissues and of the reticuloendothelial system, and inadequate interferon production, all of which have an effect on clearance of the virus from the circulation.[31]

Virological factors

For a virus to be teratogenic it must be non-lethal to the mother (e.g. Akabane disease, WSL and sometimes also BT),[14, 71] able to cross the placenta, and its deleterious effects in the foetus must also either be non-lethal or the organ principally affected should not be vital for survival of the foetus.

Most teratogenic viruses have a tropism for the developing CNS, and this is especially true for several of the attenuated viruses. The strongly hepatotropic wild-type RVF and WSL viruses[11, 12, 16, 70] lose this tropism for the liver and become neurotropic following intracerebral passage in suckling mice.[35, 66] The Smithburn strain of RVF virus and WSL virus that have undergone attenuation by 103 and 145 intracerebral passages respectively in suckling mice are grown in cell cultures for use as vaccines.

Available evidence indicates that infection of the pregnant dam by different strains of BVD-MD viruses, the breed and the immune status of the dam all have a bearing on the type of congenital malformation of the CNS that will develop in the foetus **(see Chapter 64: Bovine virus diarrhoea and mucosal disease)**.[3, 69]

The mechanisms of action of the viral teratogens at the cellular and subcellular level are obscure. It would, however, seem that these viruses may cause cellular destruction or interfere with the proliferation, differentiation and maturation of cells essential for normal brain development.[3, 44, 47, 51, 52, 69] In some viral infections, such as BT[44] and BVD-MD,[3, 64, 69] vascular changes and thrombosis, followed by hypoxia and necrosis of brain tissue may be of primary importance or may contribute to the development of the malformations.

Teratogenic viruses usually have an affinity for rapidly dividing cells and may therefore selectively affect cells in the immature nervous system. Modified BT virus in sheep affects the cells in the ventricular and subventricular zones (which are important in the development of the cerebral hemispheres) and arrests the migration of cells from these zones to the outer zones. This leads to the formation of porencephaly and hydranencephaly.[51, 52] Similar studies were made on the development of hydranencephaly in bovine foetuses injected at 125 days of gestation with the modified BT10 virus.[44] It was found that a necrotizing encephalitis, particularly involving the cerebrum, and a non-suppurative meningitis were the earliest lesions. At 12 and 20 days post-inoculation there was also vascular damage, necrosis of scattered cells, discrete areas of cavitation and other changes in the intermediate and subventricular zones. In contrast to the BT virus, the pestivirus of BVD-MD and the parvoviruses of cats and dogs have a predilection for the primordial cells in the granular cell layer in the cerebellum, and foetal infection results in necrosis of these cells. Consequently, hypoplasia of this part of the brain (also referred to as granuloprival cerebellar hypoplasia) is common in infections by these viruses.[8, 38, 64, 71]

Maternal factors

For transplacental infection to take place the dam must be susceptible to the virus in question and viraemia must develop.

The intimacy of contact between the dam and foetus is influenced by the type of placentation (which varies according to species), the stage of pregnancy and the state of health of the placenta.[1, 47, 69] There is evidence that in certain species the placental barrier becomes more complete as pregnancy progresses.[72] Infections can damage the integrity of this barrier.[1] Van Oirschot[69] referred to vascular lesions, haemorrhage and necrosis in the placentomes of sheep and cattle infected with BVD-MD virus, and also mentioned studies which revealed that BVD-MD virus can replicate in the placentomes of these animals without causing notable lesions. Despite the latter observation, the virus was able to cross the placenta to infect the foetus. Vasculitis of the smaller maternal arteries and arterioles occurs frequently in the placentomes of sheep shortly after infection with virulent BT virus during the fifth or sixth week of gestation.[1] This lesion is sometimes accompanied by oedema, haemorrhage and necrosis. No vasculitis is detectable in the placentas of sheep examined 30 and 60 days after infection.

It would appear that the possibility of foetal infection diminishes if the level of maternal viraemia is low, particularly during the later stages of gestation. Blood flow through the placenta is sluggish, as in the sinusoids of the liver and spleen, facilitating the localization of free virus or viral-infected blood cells in the placenta.[47] Viruses can reach the foetus by 'growing across' the placenta, by leakage of blood containing the virus, or by being carried across by migrating cells.[1, 69] Pestiviruses would seem to 'grow across' the placenta because of their predilection for endothelial cells, particularly those in the placenta.[69] Bluetongue virus replicates in both placental epithelial and reticuloendothelial cells and, together with BVD-MD and Akabane disease viruses,[1, 53, 69] has been shown to localize in the placenta of ruminants, where they can be detected for some time, even in the presence of circulating maternal and foetal antibodies.[1, 53, 69]

Clinical signs

A foetus that shows abnormalities may be aborted at any stage of gestation, or a fully developed calf, lamb or kid manifesting a range of clinical signs may be born dead or alive.[10, 65] New-born animals with deformed brains are often unable to rise on their own and have to be assisted. Others may rise with difficulty but appear dummy-like and blind, and show an inability to raise their heads and suckle. These animals may be ataxic, assume a wide-based stance, fall frequently, and lie in a position of lateral recumbency, showing opisthotonus, nystagmus, head tremors and galloping leg-movements. When left undisturbed, some calves or lambs with quite severe brain defects show surprisingly few signs of CNS dysfunction, apart from slight mental dullness and some degree of aimless wandering. In such cases many of the more severe signs may be triggered by forcibly raising the head of the animal for about 30–60 seconds while closing its eyes, and then suddenly releasing the head. Affected animals are usually in a poor and dehydrated condition.

Pathology

The brain anomalies caused by different teratogenic viruses are often similar. Only the main congenital CNS malformations induced by these viruses will be discussed here, as well as other associated foetal and maternal lesions **(Table 187.1)** and their possible pathogenetic mechanisms.

In animals suffering from viral-induced hydrocephalus, whether internal, external or communicating, the morphology of the brain is not markedly altered.[17, 23, 67]

Porencephaly **(Figure 187.1)** is the most common cerebral defect found in sheep foetuses infected with modified BT virus.[63] Single or multiple cystic defects filled with a clear fluid are present, particularly in the white matter of the cerebrum. These cavities may or may not communicate with the ventricles or subarachnoid space.[48, 67]

Hydranencephaly **(Figure 187.2)** denotes a reduction in the cerebral hemispheres, in whole or in part, to membranous, semi-translucent sacs containing cerebrospinal fluid, while the calvarium is usually of normal conformation but may occasionally be mildly domed with the cranial bones thickened. In some instances the brain stem, hippocampus and cerebellum appear normal, while in others these structures are absent or hypoplastic.[17, 51, 52, 67] Microscopically the membranous sacs comprise pia-arachnoid with cerebral cortex either absent or represented by only a thin layer of nervous tissue, which may be completely or incompletely lined by attenuated ependyma.

Micrencephaly **(Figure 187.3)** probably occurs more commonly in animals than is reported. The cerebral hemispheres in particular are reduced in size and contained in a cranial cavity smaller than normal.[67] Assessment of mild degrees of micrencephaly is often difficult and the condition may go unnoticed if the weight of the brain is not determined. In rare instances, the entire, severely undersized brain is mineralized in sheep foetuses infected with mouse-brain attenuated RVF virus.[13]

The most severe anomalies in foetuses develop before they are immunocompetent, and the inflammatory changes in the CNS and other tissues are much reduced in the early stages of foetal development.[26, 63, 67] Therefore, at the time of examination, which may be months after the primary insult has taken place, the cellular response is usually minimal and most microscopic changes are non-specific and do not point to a particular agent.

Arthrogryposis or congenital articular rigidity **(Figures 187.4 and 187.5)** is often associated with viral-induced congenital CNS anomalies in livestock **(Table 187.1)**. It is characterized by deformities of the limbs due to muscular atrophy and flexion and fixation of the joints. There may also be anomalies of the spinal column (kyphosis, scoliosis, lordosis, spina bifida) and cleft palate.[12, 41] Arthrogryposis is considered to be the result of neurogenic muscular atrophy after partial loss of the trophic effect of nervous stimulation, due to a hypoplastic spinal cord and a malformed brain. The degree of arthrogryposis seems to be closely correlated with the severity of muscular atrophy. The bodies of arthrogrypotic foetuses or neonatal animals exhibiting marked muscular atrophy are often slender with bony prominences, such as the spinous process of the scapula, sternum and pelvic girdle, unduly pronounced. Depending on the extent of atrophy, the colour of the affected muscles varies from almost normal in mildly affected cases to a

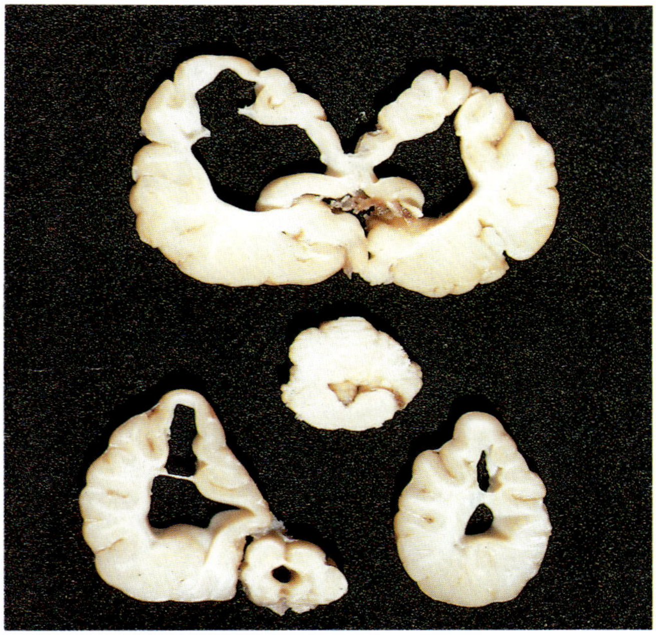

Figure 187.1 Porencephaly in a calf foetus infected with Wesselsbron disease virus

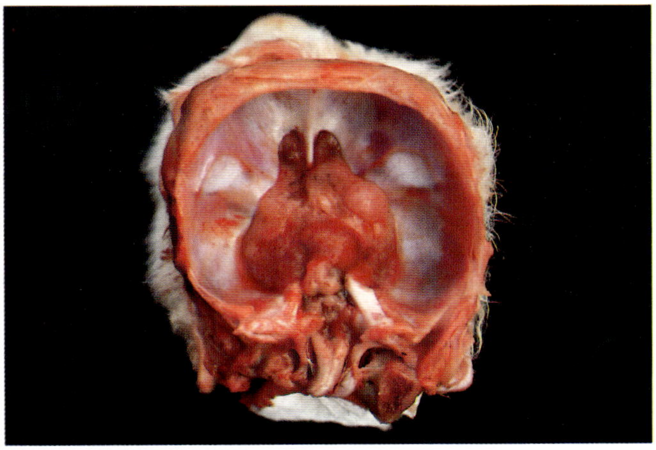

Figure 187.2 Hydranencephaly. Cranial cavity exposed to demonstrate the deformity in a lamb infected *in utero* with Wesselsbron disease virus

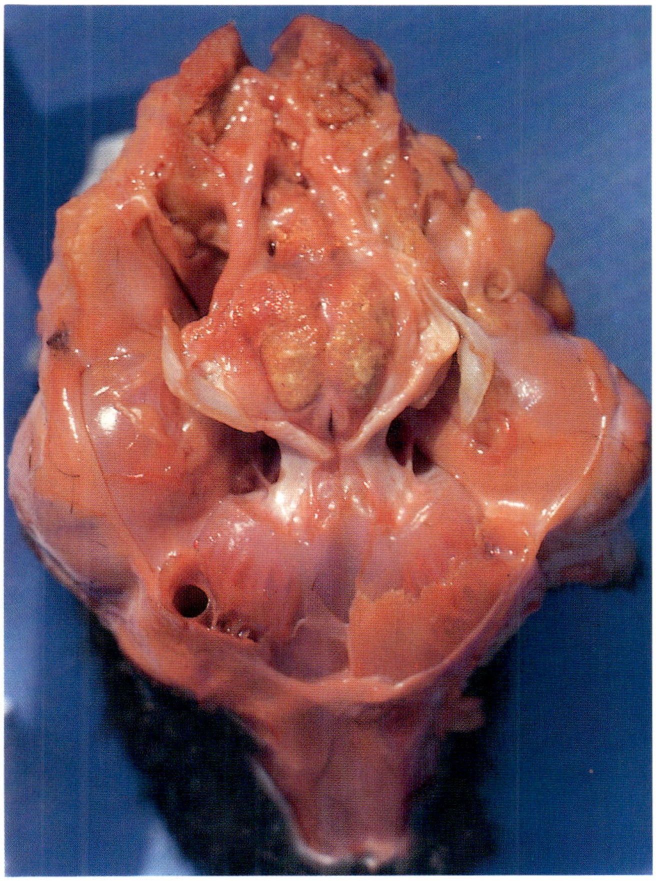

Figure 187.3 Micrencephaly in a lamb

pinkish-grey or yellowish colour in advanced cases. The muscles have, in addition, a shiny, gelatinous and moist appearance **(Figure 187.6)**. Microscopically, apart from atrophy, many of the myofibres exhibit severe fatty changes[12] **(Figure 187.7)**.

Apart from brain and skeletal anomalies, other foetal tissues may also be affected **(Table 187.1)**. Hypoplasia of the lungs **(Figure 187.8)** characterized microscopically by underdevelopment and dysplasia of the alveoli, bronchioli and bronchi has been reported in sheep foetuses infected with Akabane virus,[55] wild-type BT virus,[63] mouse-brain attenuated RVF virus and wild-type WSL virus.[13] The thymus and other organs of lambs may also be smaller than normal at birth as a result of congenital infections (such as by Akabane, BT and BVD-MD viruses[55, 63]), and can probably be ascribed to intra-uterine growth retardation (IUGR). The latter is a descriptive term which applies to the following syndromes:

- where the body weight at birth is lower than normal for an animal at a specific gestational age, resulting from the effect of non-infectious (e.g. maternal undernutrition, prenatal hyperthermia) and infectious agents on the dam and the developing foetus;[62, 63, 69] or
- where reductions in viscera and muscle weights, long bone lengths and body length occur. Retardation of skeletal growth is determined by measuring the diaphysial length of long bones, and by the detection of radio-opaque lines (growth retardation lines) or bands of increased density which parallel the growing surfaces of long bones.[63, 69]

Although some degree of IUGR is probably associated with many infectious agents, it occurs in foetuses infected with most of the teratogenic viruses[55, 63] and is particularly prominent in foetuses and lambs suffering from Border disease.[69] This is probably because pestiviruses are generally of low cytopathogenicity and may persist in foetal tissues for protracted periods.[69]

Coetzer and Barnard[12] reported *hydrops amnii* (the normal volumes of amniotic and allantoic fluid at 150 days of gestation in sheep are 3,0 and 1,14 litres respectively[45]) to be common in ewes infected with either the wild-type or mouse-brain attenuated WSL viruses, or the mouse-brain attenuated RVF virus **(Figures 187.9 and 187.10)**.

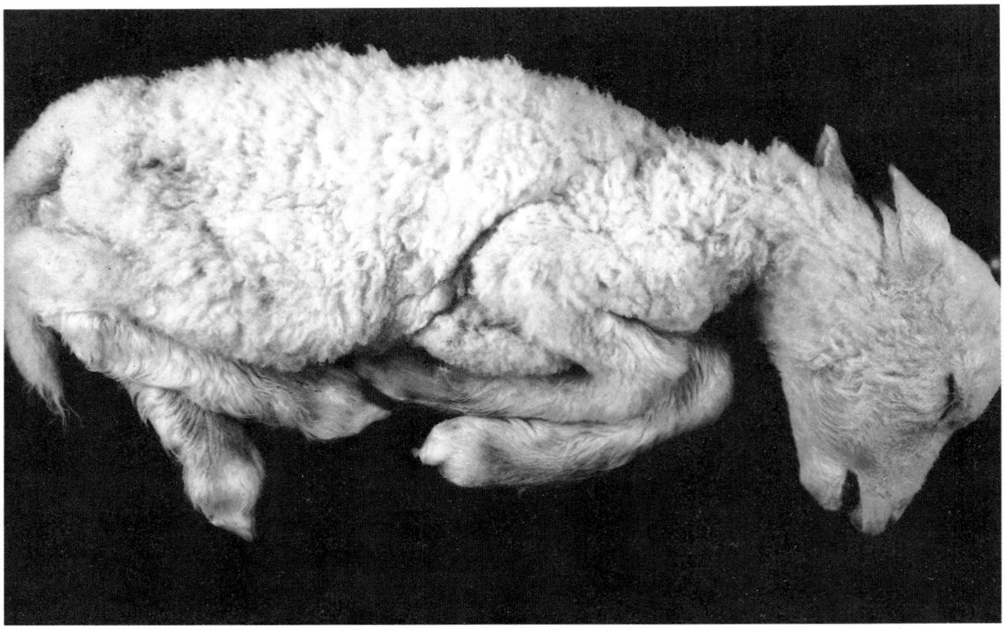

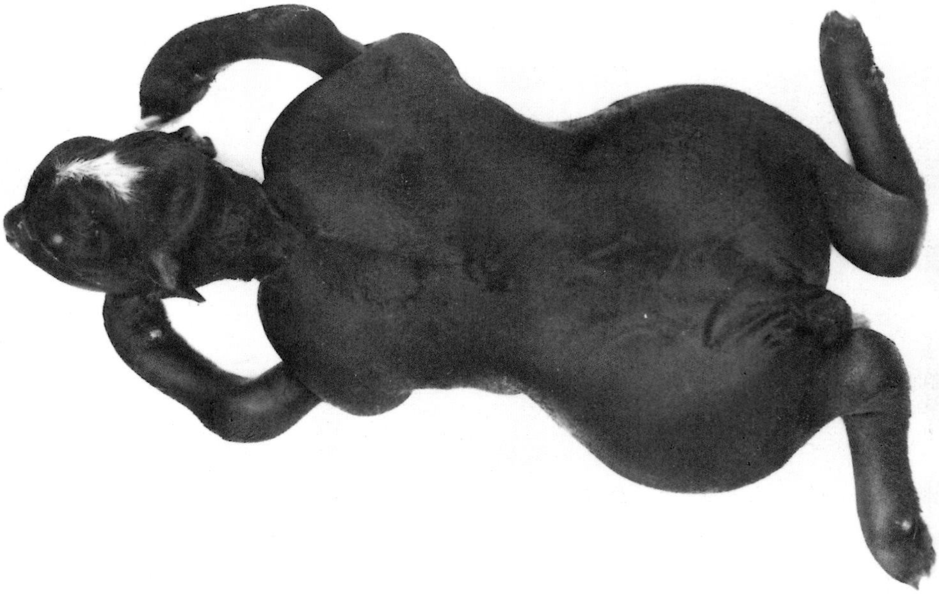

Figures 187.4 (above) and 187.5 (below) Arthrogryposis

This excess accumulation of fluid in the amnion was ascribed to impairment of the swallowing reflex as well as to atrophy of the muscles of deglutition and fixation of the jaws in the hydranencephalic and micrencephalic foetuses. It has been suggested that the volumes of amniotic and allantoic fluid are primarily controlled by the foetus, which swallows amniotic fluid and excretes it as allantoic fluid via the kidneys.[2] Apart from *hydrops amnii*, the gestational period was prolonged and the arthrogrypotic lambs showed signs of post-maturity, such as a large skeletal frame, eruption of teeth and overgrowth of the hair and hooves.[12, 13] It is interesting to note that *hydrops amnii* has not been reported in infections of pregnant animals with the modified BT virus or Akabane virus, all of which cause foetal defects in ruminants similar to those described in infections with WSL and RVF viruses. As far as can be ascertained, *hydrops amnii* in animals has never been associated with any other viral infections.

Diagnosis

Unless a necropsy is performed, the presence of teratogenic defects, especially those of the brain, often goes unnoticed, and it is therefore very difficult to estimate how frequently these anomalies occur under field conditions. Furthermore, aborted foetuses and stillborn animals are not always found, and the birth of weak animals is often ascribed to other causes.

A detailed history of the herd or flock is essential, as it may indicate whether a congenital defect is

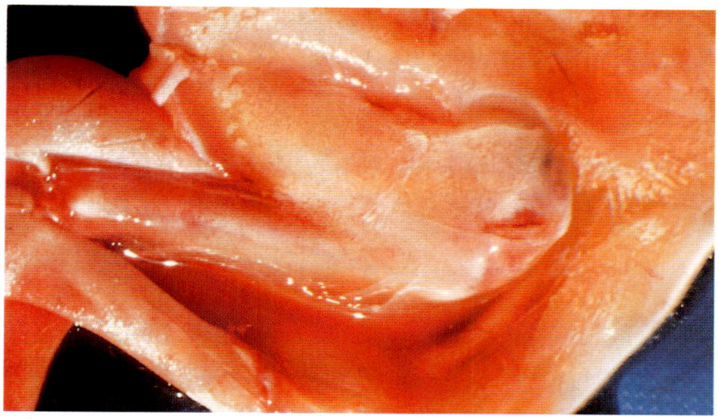

Figure 187.6 Muscles of a lamb suffering from arthrogryposis. Note the shiny, gelatinous, and yellowish appearance of the muscles

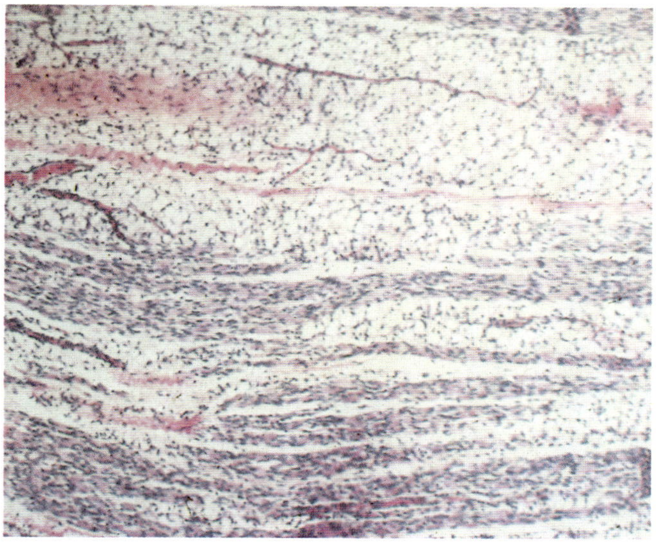

Figure 187.7 Histologic section of a muscle from an animal with severe arthrogryposis. Note the extensive fatty changes and atrophy of the myofibres

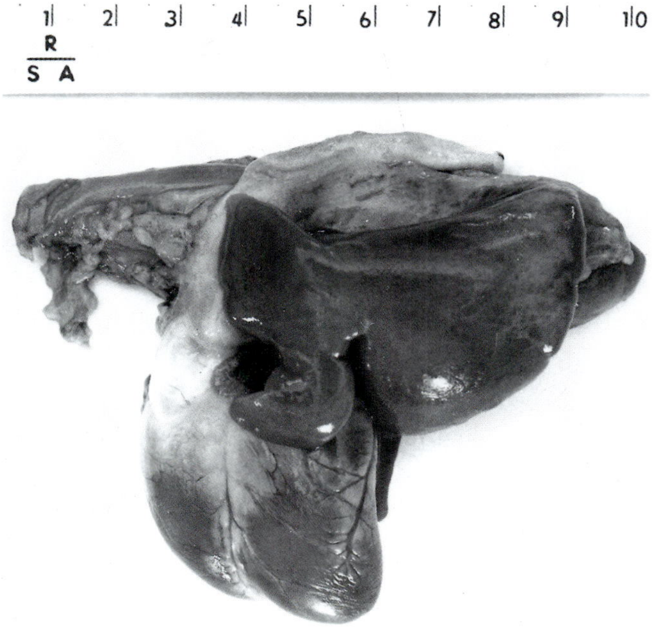

Figure 187.8 Hypoplasia of the lungs

virus-induced, genetic or of other aetiology. The dates of vaccination should be correlated with those of breeding in order to determine whether the cause is associated with the vaccine virus having been inadvertently administered at a stage of pregnancy when the foetus was most vulnerable to it. Other factors indicating a viral aetiology may include:[18]

- the occurrence of multiple cases of the condition during a breeding season, and the explosive nature of the outbreak(s);
- the correlation of an epidemic of a particular disease and a subsequent increase in the incidence of congenital defects;
- an increase in the number of resorbed or aborted foetuses on the farm;
- the occurrence of malformations mostly in offspring of young females that have given birth for the first time; and
- the deformities not usually being limited to a single farm, but having a more widespread distribution in the particular area.

Isolation of virus from the CNS and other tissues of affected foetuses or neonates is often unsuccessful because months may have elapsed since infection took place.[26, 63, 73]

According to Parsonson *et al.*,[54] a number of workers reported immunologic tolerance to BT virus in calves born from cows infected during pregnancy. When these calves grew to maturity, males were apparently able to excrete the virus in the semen. Sheep and cattle that become infected prenatally with certain BVD-MD viruses may remain normal for years, if not for life, in spite of persistence of the virus.[69] Such infected animals may shed virus continuously and are important in the epidemiology of the disease **(see Chapter 64: Bovine viral diarrhoea and mucosal disease).** In contrast to the situation in foetal tissues, the viruses of BT, Akabane disease and BVD-MD may persist in the placentomes, and these and the foetal fluids may be particularly suitable for virus isolation.[1, 27, 53, 56]

In order to arrive at a diagnosis it is often necessary to obtain indirect evidence of infection, such as a rise in immunoglobulin levels and the presence of specific viral antibodies in the serum of foetuses or precolostral serum of affected neonates. While maternal antibodies are able to cross the placenta in some species (humans, rats, rabbits, guinea-pigs), in other species (cattle, sheep, horses, pigs) there is little or no transfer of antibodies to the foetus and it must therefore rely on its own immunological responses to eliminate infectious agents.[47] In all species copious amounts of protective maternal antibodies are transferred to neonates via the colostrum.[47]

As a result of the barrier to maternal antibodies that is presented by the epitheliochorial type of placenta of domestic ruminants, the presence of antibodies in the neonate before the ingestion of colostrum is evidence that the foetus has been exposed to antigenic stimulation.[54]

Immunocompetence of the foetus is closely correlated with the animal species, length of gestation and the type of viral antigen involved.[47, 53] Generally, production of antibodies to infectious agents occurs late in foetal life. Neutralizing antibodies to BVD-MD virus cannot be detected in the bovine foetus until about the 200th day of gestation.[69] The sequential development of responses to BT virus in the ovine foetus has been reported to be as follows: at 70 days of gestation there is an inflammatory response composed mostly of mononuclear leukocytes, which are thought to be macrophages. This is followed by lymphoid hyperplasia at 80–85 days of foetal age, immunoglobulin production at 100 days; and specific antibody activity at 95–100 days of gestation, when the ovine foetus is believed to be immunocompetent.[20]

Specific viral antibody determinations in the dam on single or paired serum samples some weeks apart are of negligible diagnostic significance and often lead to misconceptions and faulty diagnoses. More reliable information on the status of the herd or flock is obtained by regularly monitoring the sera of the female animals for antibodies to specific viral infections over an extended period.

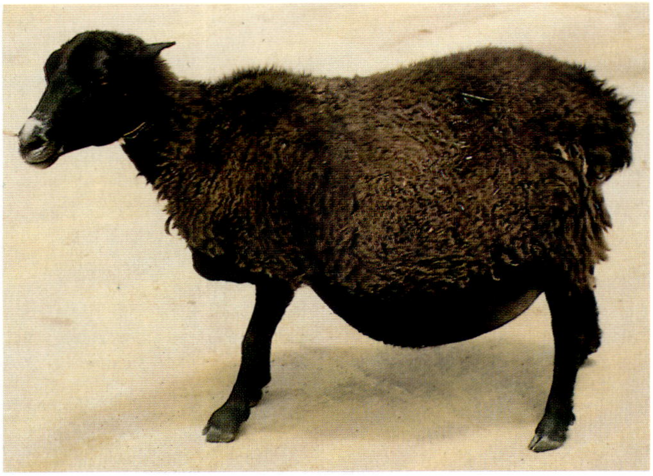

Figure 187.9 Distended abdomen of a pregnant ewe suffering from *hydrops amnii*

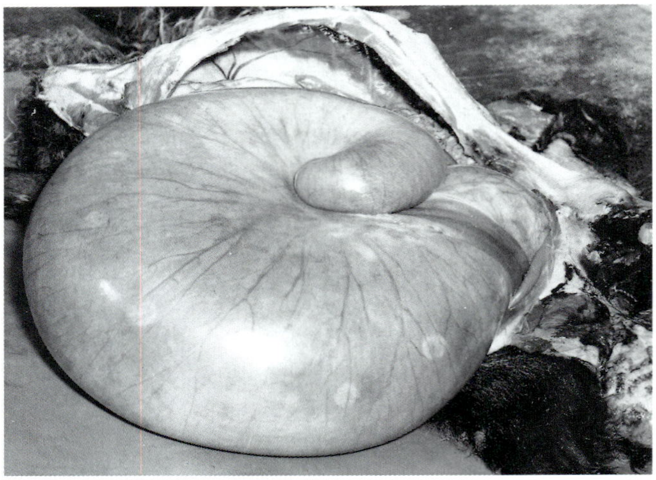

Figure 187.10 Uterus of a ewe distended by *hydrops amnii*

References

1 **ANDERSON, C.K. & JENSEN, R., 1969.** Pathologic changes in placentas of ewes inoculated with bluetongue virus. *American Journal of Veterinary Research*, 30, 987–999.

2 **ARTHUR, G.H., 1959.** Some notes on the quantities of foetal fluids in ruminants with special reference to *hydrops amnii*. *British Veterinary Journal*, 113, 17–28.

3 **BARLOW, R.M., 1980.** Morphogenesis of hydranencephaly and other intracranial malformations in progeny of pregnant ewes infected with pestiviruses. *Journal of Comparative Pathology*, 90, 87–98.

4 **BARNARD, B.J.H., 1988.** Veterinary Research Institute, Onderstepoort, South Africa. Unpublished data.

5 **BARNARD, B.J.H. & PIENAAR, J.G., 1976.** Bluetongue virus as a cause of hydranencephaly in cattle. *Onderstepoort Journal of Veterinary Research*, 43, 155–158.

6 **BARNARD, B.J.H. & VOGES, S.F., 1986.** Flaviviruses in South Africa: Pathogenicity for sheep. *Onderstepoort Journal of Veterinary Research*, 53, 235–238.

7 **BROWN, T.T., DELAHUNTA, A., BISTNER, S.I., SCOTT, F.W. & McENTEE, K., 1974.** Pathogenetic studies of infections of the bovine fetus with bovine viral diarrhea virus. I. Cerebellar atrophy. *Veterinary Pathology*, 11, 486–505.

8 **BROWN, T.T., DELAHUNTA, A., SCOTT, F.W., KAHRS, F.R., McENTEE, K. & GILLESPIE, J.H., 1973.** Virus-induced congenital anomalies of the bovine fetus. II. Histopathology of cerebellar degeneration (hypoplasia) induced by the virus of bovine viral diarrhoea-mucosal disease. *Cornell Veterinarian*, 63, 561–578.

9 **CASARO, A.P.E., KENDRICK, J.W. & KENNEDY, P.C., 1971.** Response of the bovine fetus to bovine viral diarrhoea-mucosal disease virus. *American Journal of Veterinary Research*, 32, 1543–1562.

10 **COETZER, J.A.W., 1980.** Breinteratologie a.g.v. transplasentale virusbesmetting in herkouers. *Journal of the South African Veterinary Association*, 51, 153–157.

11 **COETZER, J.A.W., 1982.** The pathology of Rift Valley fever. II. Lesions occurring in field cases in adult cattle, calves and aborted foetuses. *Onderstepoort Journal of Veterinary Research*, 49, 11–17.

12 **COETZER, J.A.W. & BARNARD, B.J.H., 1977.** *Hydrops amnii* in sheep associated with hydranencephaly and arthrogryposis with Wesselsbron disease and Rift Valley fever viruses as aetiological agents. *Onderstepoort Journal of Veterinary Research*, 44, 119–126.

13 **COETZER, J.A.W. & BARNARD, B.J.H., 1977.** Veterinary Research Institute, Onderstepoort, South Africa. Unpublished data.

14 **COETZER, J.A.W. & THEODORIDIS, A., 1982.** Clinical and

pathological studies in adult sheep and goats experimentally infected with Wesselsbron disease virus. *Onderstepoort Journal of Veterinary Research*, 49, 19–22.

15 **COETZER, J.A.W., THEODORIDIS, A., HERR, S. & KRITZINGER, L., 1979.** Wesselsbron disease: A cause of congenital porencephaly and cerebellar hypoplasia in calves. *Onderstepoort Journal of Veterinary Research*, 46, 165–169.

16 **COETZER, J.A.W., THEODORIDIS, A. & VAN HEERDEN, A., 1978.** Wesselsbron disease. Pathological, haematological and clinical studies in natural cases and experimentally infected new-born lambs. *Onderstepoort Journal of Veterinary Research*, 45, 93–106.

17 **DELAHUNTA, A., 1983.** *Veterinary Neuroanatomy and Clinical Neurology*. 2nd edn. Philadelphia: W.B. Saunders Company.

18 **DONE, J.T., 1978.** Virus teratogens and domestic animals. *The Veterinary Annual*, 18, 1–12.

19 **EDWARDS, M.J., 1978.** Congenital defects due to hyperthermia. *Advances in Veterinary Science and Comparative Medicine*, 22, 29–52.

20 **ENRIGHT, F.M. & OSBURN, B.I., 1980.** Ontogeny of host responses in ovine foetuses infected with bluetongue virus. *American Journal of Veterinary Research*, 41, 224–229.

21 **FUCCILLO, D.A. & SEVER, J.L., 1973.** Viral teratology. *Bacteriological Reviews*, 37, 19–31.

22 **GOTO, Y., MUIRA, Y. & KONO, Y., 1988.** Serological evidence for the aetiologic role of Chuzan virus in an epizootic of congenital abnormalities with hydranencephaly-cerebellar hypoplasia syndrome of calves in Japan. *American Journal of Veterinary Research*, 49, 2026–2029.

23 **GREENE, H.J., LEIPOLD, H.W. & HIBBS, C.M., 1974.** Bovine congenital defects, variations of internal hydrocephalus. *Cornell Veterinarian*, 596–616.

24 **GRINER, L.A., McCRORY, B.R., FOSTER, N.M. & MEYER, H., 1964.** Bluetongue associated with abnormalities in newborn lambs. *Journal of the American Veterinary Medical Association*, 145, 1013–1019.

25 **HARTLEY, W.J., ALEXANDER, G. & EDWARDS, M.J., 1974.** Brain cavitation and micrencephaly in lambs exposed to parental hyperthermia. *Teratology*, 9, 299–303.

26 **HARTLEY, W.J., DE SARAM, W.G., DELLA-PORTA, A.J., SNOWDON, W.A. & SHEPHERD, N.C., 1977.** Pathology of congenital bovine epizootic arthrogryposis and hydranencephaly and its relationship to Akabane virus. *Australian Veterinary Journal*, 53, 319–325.

27 **HASHINGUCHI, Y., NANBA, K. & KUMAGAI, T., 1979.** Congenital abnormalities in new-born lambs following Akabane virus infection in pregnant ewes. *National Institute of Animal Health Quarterly (Tokyo)*, 19, 1–11.

28 **HUGHES, L.E., KERSHAW, G.F. & SHAW, I.G., 1959.** 'B' or border disease. An undescribed disease in sheep. *The Veterinary Record*, 71, 313–317.

29 **INABA, Y., KUROGI, H. & OMORI, T., 1975.** Akabane disease: Epizootic abortion, premature birth, stillbirth and congenital arthrogryposis and hydranencephaly in cattle, sheep and goats caused by Akabane virus. *Australian Veterinary Journal*, 51, 584–585.

30 **JAMES, L.F., 1977.** Plant-induced congenital malformations in animals. *World Review of Nutrition and Dietetics*, 26, 208–224.

31 **JOHNSON, R.T. & MIMS, C.A., 1968.** Pathogenesis of viral infections of the nervous system. *New England Journal of Medicine*, 278, 23–30, 84–92.

32 **KAHRS, R.F., SCOTT, F.W. & DELAHUNTA, A., 1970.** Bovine viral diarrhoea-mucosal disease, abortion and congenital cerebellar hypoplasia in a dairy herd. *Journal of the American Veterinary Medical Association*, 156, 851–857.

33 **KAHRS, R.F., SCOTT, F.W. & DELAHUNTA, A., 1970.** Congenital cerebellar hypoplasia and ocular defects in calves following bovine viral diarrhoea-mucosal disease infection in pregnant cattle. *Journal of the American Veterinary Medical Association*, 156, 1443–1450.

34 **KAHRS, R.F., SCOTT, F.W. & DELAHUNTA, A., 1970.** Epidemiological observations on bovine viral diarrhoea-mucosal disease virus-induced congenital cerebellar hypoplasia and ocular defects in calves. *Teratology*, 3, 181–184.

35 **KASHULA, V.R., 1953.** The propagation and modification of strains of Rift Valley fever viruses in embryonated eggs and their use as immunizing agents for domestic ruminants. D.V.Sc. Thesis, University of Pretoria, South Africa.

36 **KEELER, R.F., STUART, L.D. & YOUNG, S.M., 1986.** When ewes ingest poisonous plants: The teratogenetic effects. *Veterinary Medicine*, 81, 449–454.

37 **KELLERMAN, T.S., COETZER, J.A.W. & NAUDÉ, T.W., 1988.** *Plant Poisonings and Mycotoxicoses of Livestock in Southern Africa*. Cape Town: Oxford University Press Southern Africa.

38 **KILHAM, L. & MARGOLIS, G., 1971.** Cerebellar ataxia and its congenital transmission in cats by feline panleukopenia virus. *Journal of the American Veterinary Medical Association*, 158, 888–901.

39 **KONNO, S., MORIWAKI, M. & NAKAGAWA, M., 1982.** Akabane disease in cattle; congenital abnormalities caused by viral infection: Spontaneous disease. *Veterinary Pathology*, 19, 246–266.

40 **KONNO, S. & NAKAGAWA, M., 1982.** Akabane disease in cattle: Congenital abnormalities caused by viral infection: Experimental disease. *Veterinary Pathology*, 19, 267–279.

41 **LEIPOLD, H.W., CATES, W.F., RADOSTITS, O.M. & HOWELL, W.E., 1970.** Arthrogryposis and associated defects in new-born calves. *American Journal of Veterinary Research*, 31, 1367–1374.

42 **LEIPOLD, H.W. & DENNIS, S.M., 1987.** Congenital defects of the bovine central nervous system. *In*: BAKER, J.C., (ed.). *The Veterinary Clinics of North America: Food Animal Practice*. Philadelphia: W.B. Saunders Company.

43 **LEIPOLD, H.W., DENNIS, S.M. & HUSTON, K., 1972.** Congenital defects in cattle: Nature, cause and effect. *Advances in Veterinary Science and Comparative Medicine*, 16, 103–150.

44 **MACLACHLAN, N.J. & OSBURN, B.I., 1983.** Bluetongue virus-induced hydranencephaly in cattle. *Veterinary Pathology*, 20, 563–573.

45 **MALAN, A.P. & CURSON, H.H., 1937.** Absolute volumes of foetal fluids in Merino sheep. *Onderstepoort Journal of Veterinary Science and Animal Industry*, 8, 417–427.

46 **McINTOSH, G.H., BAGHURST, K.I., POTTER, B.J. & HETZEL, B.S., 1979.** Foetal brain development in the sheep. *Neuropathology and Applied Neurobiology*, 5, 103–114.

47 **MIMS, C., 1976.** Comparative aspects of infective malformations. *British Medical Bulletin*, 32, 84–88.

48 **NAEF, R.W., 1958.** Clinical features of porencephaly. *Archives of Neurology and Physiology*, 80, 133–147.

49 **OMORI, T., INABA, Y., KUROGI, H., MIURA, Y., NOBUTO, K., OHASHI, Y. & MATSUMOTO, M., 1974.** Arthrogryposis-hydranencephaly syndrome in cattle in Japan, 1972–74. *Bulletin de l'Office International des Épizooties*, 8, 447–458.

50 **OSBURN, B.I., 1968.** The relation of foetal age to the character of lesions in foetal lambs infected with *Brucella ovis*. *Pathologia Veterinaria*, 5, 395–406.

51 **OSBURN, B.I., JOHNSON, R.T., SILVERSTEIN, A.M., PRENDERGAST, R.A., JOCHIM, M.N. & LEVY, S.E., 1971.** Experimental viral-induced congenital encephalopathies. I. Pathology of hydranencephaly and porencephaly caused by bluetongue vaccine virus. *Laboratory Investigation*, 25, 197–205.

52 **OSBURN, B.I., JOHNSON, R.T., SILVERSTEIN, A.M., PRENDERGAST, R.A., JOCHIM, M.N. & LEVY, S.E., 1971.** Experimental viral-induced congenital encephalopathies. II. The pathogenesis of bluetongue vaccine virus infection in foetal lambs. *Laboratory Investigation*, 25, 206–210.

53 **PARSONSON, I.M., DELLA-PORTA, A.J., O'HALLORAN, M.L., SNOWDON, W.A., FAHEY, K.J. & STANDFAST, H.A., 1981.** Akabane virus infection in the pregnant ewe. I. Growth of virus in the foetus and the development of the

foetal immune response. *Veterinary Microbiology*, 6, 197–207.

54 **PARSONSON, I.M., DELLA-PORTA, A.J. & SNOWDON, W.A., 1981.** Developmental disorders of the foetus in some arthropod-borne virus infections. *American Journal of Tropical Medicine and Hygiene*, 30, 660–673.

55 **PARSONSON, I.M., DELLA-PORTA, A.J. & SNOWDON, W.A., 1981.** Akabane virus infection in the pregnant ewe. II. Pathology of the foetus. *Veterinary Microbiology*, 6, 209–224.

56 **PARSONSON, I.M., O'HALLORAN, M.L., ZEE, Y.C. & SNOWDON, W.A., 1979.** The effects of bovine viral diarrhoea-mucosal disease (BVD) virus on the ovine foetus. *Veterinary Microbiology*, 4, 279–292.

57 **PLANT, J.W., ACLAND, H.M., GARD, G.P. & WALKER, K.H., 1983.** Clinical variations of Border disease in sheep according to the source of the inoculum. *The Veterinary Record*, 113, 58–60.

58 **PLANT, J.W., WALKER, K.H., ACLAND, H.M. & GARD, G.P., 1983.** Pathology in the ovine foetus caused by pestivirus. *Australian Veterinary Journal*, 60, 137–140.

59 **PROZESKY, L., JOUBERT, L.P.J. & EKRON, M.D., 1981.** Paralysis in lambs caused by overdosing with parbendazole. *Onderstepoort Journal of Veterinary Research*, 48, 159–167.

60 **RICHARDS, W.P.C., CRENSHAW, G.L. & BUSHNELL, R.B., 1971.** Hydranencephaly of calves associated with natural bluetongue virus infection. *Cornell Veterinarian*, 61, 336–348.

61 **RICHARDSON, C., 1977.** Morphological parameters of intrauterine growth retardation in the new-born lamb. *The Veterinary Record*, 101, 151–152.

62 **RICHARDSON, C., 1978.** Intrauterine growth retardation in sheep. *In*: GRUNSELL, C.S.G. & HILL, F.W.G., (eds). *The Veterinary Annual*, 18th Issue, Bristol: Wright-Scientechnica.

63 **RICHARDSON, C., TAYLOR, W.P., TERLECKI, S. & GIBBS, E.P.J., 1985.** Observations on transplacental infection with bluetongue virus in sheep. *American Journal of Veterinary Research*, 46, 1912–1922.

64 **SCOTT, F.W., KAHRS, R.F., DELAHUNTA, A., BROWN, T.T., McENTEE, K. & GILLESPIE, J.H., 1973.** Virus-induced congenital anomalies of the bovine fetus. I. Cerebellar degeneration (hypoplasia), ocular lesions and fetal mummification following experimental infection with bovine viral diarrhea-mucosal disease virus. *Cornell Veterinarian*, 63, 536–560.

65 **SHEPHERD, N.C., GEE, C.D., JESSEP, T., TIMMINS, G., CARROL, S.N. & BONNER, R.B., 1978.** Congenital bovine epizootic arthrogryposis and hydranencephaly. *Australian Veterinary Journal*, 54, 171–177.

66 **SMITHBURN, K.C., 1949.** Rift Valley fever: The neurotropic adaptation of the virus and the experimental use of this modified virus as a vaccine. *British Journal of Experimental Pathology*, 30, 1–16.

67 **SULLIVAN, N.D., 1985.** The nervous system. *In*: JUBB, K.V.F., KENNEDY, P.C. & PALMER, N., (eds). *Pathology of Domestic Animals*. 3rd edn. Vol. 1. Orlando, Florida: Academic Press, Inc.

68 **VAN DER LUGT, J.J. & PROZESKY, L., 1989.** The pathology of blindness in new-born calves caused by hypovitaminosis A. *Onderstepoort Journal of Veterinary Research*, 56, 99–109.

69 **VAN OIRSCHOT, J.T., 1983.** Congenital infections with nonarbo-togaviruses. *Veterinary Microbiology*, 8, 321–361.

70 **WEISS, K.E., 1957.** Wesselsbron virus disease — A review. *Bulletin of Epizootic Diseases of Africa*, 5, 459–465.

71 **WILSON, T.M., DELAHUNTA, A. & CONFER, L., 1983.** Cerebellar degeneration in dairy calves: Clinical, pathologic and serologic features of an epizootic caused by bovine viral diarrhoea virus. *Journal of the American Veterinary Medical Association*, 183, 544–547.

72 **WINSATT, W.A., 1950.** New histological observations on the placenta of the sheep. *American Journal of Anatomy*, 87, 391–457.

73 **YOUNG, S. & CORDY, D.R., 1964.** An ovine foetal encephalopathy caused by bluetongue vaccine virus. *Journal of Neuropathology and Experimental Neurology*, 26, 635–659.

188

Porcine respiratory disease

R.K. Loveday

Introduction

During the past three decades pig production methods have changed fundamentally. Housing changes have often been accompanied by high stocking rates, leading to poor ventilation (especially in winter) as a result of large groups of animals being housed intensively in one air-space. Consequently, respiratory diseases such as pneumonia have become widespread throughout the world and now pose a major constraint to cost-effective production. The situation in southern Africa has been aggravated by some injudicious building designs as well as by the emergence of larger and larger herds.

A wide range of pathogens has been incriminated in the porcine respiratory disease complex[15] **(Table 188.1)**. It is important, however, to appreciate that respiratory diseases are frequently the result of interaction between the pig, a pathogen(s) **(Table 188.1)**, and the environment, which includes management practices.

Table 188.1 Infectious and non-infectious conditions that affect the respiratory system of pigs

AETIOLOGICAL AGENT	DISEASE
Viral diseases	
Adenovirus	Adenovirus infection
*African swine fever virus	African swine fever
Coronavirus	Coronavirus infection
Hog cholera virus	Hog cholera
Influenza virus	Swine influenza
Suid herpesvirus 1	Pseudorabies (Aujeszky's disease)
Suid herpesvirus 2	Inclusion body rhinitis
Bacterial and mycoplasmal diseases	
**Actinobacillus pleuropneumoniae*	Porcine pleuropneumonia
**Bordetella bronchiseptica*	Bordetella bronchopneumonia and non-progressive atrophic rhinitis
Chlamydia psittaci	Chlamydiosis
**Actinomyces pyogenes*	Necropurulent pneumonia
**Haemophilus parasuis*	Glässer's disease
**Mycoplasma hyopneumoniae*	Enzootic (mycoplasmal) pneumonia
**M. hyorhinis*	Mycoplasmal polyserositis and arthritis
**Pasteurella multocida* (serotypes A,D)	Pasteurellosis
**Pasteurella multocida* (toxigenic serotypes A,D) and *Bordetella bronchiseptica*	Progressive atrophic rhinitis
**Salmonella cholerae suis*	Salmonellosis
**Streptococcus suis* Type II	Streptococcal septicaemia and pneumonia
Other *Streptococcus* spp. (e.g. *S. equisimilis*)	Purulent pneumonia
Other diseases	
**Ascaris suum*	
*Foreign bodies	
**Metastrongylus elongatus*	

⋆ Agents already diagnosed in pigs in South Africa

Aetiology and prevalence of respiratory disease

A study in the UK[11] revealed that the same potentially pathogenic organisms could often be found both in obviously diseased herds and apparently healthy control herds. While *Bordetella bronchiseptica, Pasteurella multocida* and *Haemophilus parasuis* were isolated from most problem herds, these bacteria were also found in the majority of control herds. On the other hand, serological evidence of *Mycoplasma hyopneumoniae* occurred in most of the problem herds but none of the control herds, thus indicating a primary role for this pathogen in respiratory disease.

Interactions between microorganisms are important in porcine respiratory disease. Most resident bacterial pathogens colonize the nasopharyngeal and tonsillar areas early on in the animal's life. These pathogens, which originate from the sow, are often inhaled by the piglets during the first few hours of life, before colostral immunity has become effective.[25] Commensal organisms resident in the upper respiratory tract may invade the lower tract when the respiratory defence mechanisms of the host are impaired by a primary agent such as *M. hyopneumoniae, Actinobacillus pleuropneumoniae,* or viruses. Pulmonary invasion may be very rapid in the case of primary pathogens such as *M. hyopneumoniae* or *A. pleuropneumoniae* that produce potent cytotoxins which damage the cilia of the respiratory epithelial cells and alveolar macrophages.[10] For example, both *Actinobacillus pleuropneumoniae* and *M. hyopneumoniae* are capable of initiating sufficient damage to the lungs to allow *P. multocida* to invade and produce a severe, sometimes fatal pneumonia.[12] In cultures from these lungs, the presence of *A. pleuropneumoniae* may be masked by the overgrowth of *P. multocida* unless dilution methods and selective media are employed for isolation.[12] Similarly, there is a marked synergism between *M. hyopneumoniae* and *A. pleuropneumoniae* infections; prior *M. hyopneumoniae* infection acts as one of the predisposing factors which exacerbate the effects of *A. pleuropneumoniae*. This exacerbation is ascribed to possible impairment of mucociliary clearance and the neutrophil-bacterial-phagocytosis defence system by the mycoplasma.[24] The ubiquitous *B. bronchiseptica* facilitates both subsequent nasal colonization by toxigenic strains of *P. multocida* and the genesis of severe, progressive turbinate atrophy.[7, 20] Synergism between *B. bronchiseptica* and *Mycoplasma hyorhinis* has also been demonstrated experimentally, with the latter becoming much more invasive in the presence of the former.[25]

The most common interaction between pathogens in porcine respiratory disease occurs in finishing pigs of 60–80 kg live weight suffering from enzootic (mycoplasmal) pneumonia: an acute bronchopneumonia due to *P. multocida* follows impairment of mucociliary clearance in the lungs as a result of *M. hyopneumoniae* infection.[21]

In South Africa the first evidence of enzootic pneumonia in slaughter pigs was reported from a bacon factory in 1956.[13] Further investigations showed that many producers' herds were infected with what appeared to be enzootic pneumonia, as judged from the characteristics of the lesions, which included interstitial pneumonia and peribronchial accumulations of lymphocytes and plasma cells.[13] Since then *Mycoplasma* spp. infections have become widespread in pig herds in South Africa, although no accurate data are available to quantify the prevalence. The three mycoplasmas (*M. hyopneumoniae, M. hyorhinis, M. flocculare*) commonly associated with porcine respiratory disease, as well as *M. hyosynoviae*,[23] *B. bronchiseptica, P. multocida, Haemophilus parasuis* and *A. pleuropneumoniae*, have all been isolated from lung specimens collected from pigs with respiratory disease in South Africa.[23]

Actinobacillus pleuropneumoniae, which was first recognized in South Africa in 1985,[8] is probably the most serious respiratory infection to threaten the pig industry in southern Africa. Infection has since been found to occur throughout South Africa. This bacterium may occur in conjunction with other organisms, such as *Mycoplasma* spp., *Pasteurella* spp., *Streptococcus* spp. and *Actinomyces (Corynebacterium) pyogenes*.[8, 22] In most infected herds in South Africa, chronic rather than acute cases have occurred, which indicates the existence of some degree of herd immunity and that the infection has possibly been present in the country for some time.[8]

Actinobacillus pleuropneumoniae can be introduced into susceptible herds by subclinical carriers, which may be serologically negative, or by chronically diseased animals. Since no breeding stock suppliers in South Africa have been investigated for the presence or absence of this infection, the danger of further dissemination of infection is presently very great for those herds into which purchased gilts and boars are introduced. The marked synergism between *A. pleuropneumoniae* and the ubiquitous *M. hyopneumoniae* also ensures the production of severe lesions, heightened mortality and severe economic effects on production.

Small-scale surveys at abattoirs in South Africa during the past 15 years have shown that non-progressive atrophic rhinitis, characterized by atrophy of the turbinates but without the severe deformities of the snout or brachygnathia superior, occurred in about 10 per cent of the porkers that were examined.[13] Most of the herds from which such pigs originated were infected with *B. bronchiseptica* but not with toxigenic *P. multocida*, and thus did not develop the facial distortion produced by the dual infection **[see Chapter 121: *Bordetella bronchiseptica* infections (including atrophic rhinitis)]**. More recently, an increasing prevalence of snout-twisting and marked turbinate atrophy has become apparent in some of the larger commercial herds in Natal.[2] This prevalence, presently estimated at between 5 and 10 per cent of growing pigs, is similar to the prevalence in Australia (5–8 per cent).[5] However, it does not approach the 25 per cent estimated for pig herds in Great Britain during 1978–79.[3]

Polyserositis caused by *H. parasuis* has been diagnosed occasionally in weaners housed in overcrowded, poorly ventilated buildings, but it is not a major problem in South Africa.

Mycoplasma hyorhinis may be a primary pathogen in the very young piglet, causing pneumonia. However, it is more commonly a secondary invader in older animals suffering from enzootic pneumonia.[25] It may also cause severe fibrinopurulent polyarthritis, which should be differentiated from similar lesions caused by *H. parasuis* and *Streptococcus suis*.

Epidemiology and pathogenesis

While a closed-environment house for intensive pig rearing may facilitate more economic production, it also creates a potentially hazardous environment for the transmission of respiratory tract pathogens. Both non-infectious pollutants, such as ammonia or dust, and infectious aerosols sneezed or coughed up by infected pigs are inhaled by in-contact animals. Such pollutants are dealt with by mucociliary clearance and phagocytosis, the two major components of the pulmonary defence mechanism. It is postulated that respiratory tract infections occur mainly as a result of direct nose-to-nose contact between animals.[17] Therefore, the infective element remains the pig itself, often as a latent carrier, until an immunosuppressive event — often management-derived stress — triggers the clinical appearance of disease.[17]

Important viral infections, such as swine influenza, respiratory coronavirus infections and pseudorabies, which may play a role in the pathogenesis of porcine respiratory disease, have not been diagnosed in South Africa, although the common respiratory bacterial and mycoplasmal pathogens have all become established.

Generally, an increased prevalence of lung lesions is found in winter, probably as a result of the decreased air exchange rates instituted to maintain house temperatures.[5] These also promote increased dust and microbial concentrations. In addition, low temperatures depress alveolar macrophages and mucociliary clearance in the respiratory system. Marked temperature fluctuations are also undesirable.[5]

High levels of ammonia in the air decrease mucociliary function in the respiratory tract. With the increasing use of liquid waste systems over slatted floors, it is now necessary to flush underwater channels frequently to prevent noxious gas pollution of the atmosphere.[5]

Pig houses[5] typically have dust concentrations of 10–20 mg/m³. The smaller a dust particle is, the deeper it penetrates into the respiratory tract; the size range of dust particles found in the lungs of pigs is from 0,5 to 3,0 μm in diameter.[5] Dust constitutes an important challenge to the respiratory system.[5]

Current recommendations suggest that not more than 150–200 pigs should occupy the same air-space. Subdivision of large houses is therefore important. The practice of all-in, all-out production systems improves the early growth rate of the animals to ten weeks of age and can also improve overall performance to marketing. A study has shown a prevalence of 18 per cent lung lesions for all-in, all-out management as compared to a 48 per cent prevalence in a continuous-flow operation on the same farm.[18] Most outbreaks of respiratory disease are related to mixing of pigs from different sources.

Stocking density significantly affects the prevalence of respiratory infections. The minimum space allowances per pig as recommended by Kornegay and Notter[9] are given in **Table 188.2**.

Table 188.2 Recommended minimal space allowance per pig. (Adapted from Kornegay and Notter[9])

LIVE WEIGHT (KG)	SPACE ALLOWANCE (M^2/PIG)
7	0,12
14	0,20
27	0,31
45	0,44
68	0,58
100	0,74

Separation of different age groups of pigs is imperative to protect the younger, less immune animals. Mixing of pigs also increases fighting and promotes stress.[5]

While management methods directed at reducing environmental pollution and microbial challenge certainly have a role to play in lessening the impact of respiratory disease, the final solution to the problem lies in the use of disease-free breeding stock maintained in strict isolation.

Diagnosis

An experienced clinician will often have little difficulty in making a presumptive diagnosis of one of the more common respiratory complaints, such as enzootic pneumonia or progressive atrophic rhinitis, from the characteristic clinical signs in the herd. Excessive sneezing and snuffling in young pigs are suggestive of atrophic rhinitis, while the chronic, non-productive cough and retarded growth found in finisher pigs suffering from enzootic pneumonia often indicate this common condition.

Investigations of these problems in commercial piggeries have shown that the constant utilization of abattoir inspections of the lungs and/or snouts of slaughter stock is of great assistance in monitoring not only the possible nature of respiratory infection already suspected from clinical investigations, but also the prevalence of such infection. A definite diagnosis requires isolation and positive identification of the specific agent(s) present in a herd. While this may be relatively simple as far as the more common infections such as *P. multocida, B. bronchiseptica, A. pleuropneumoniae* or *M. hyorhinis* are concerned, the isolation of *M. hyopneumoniae* is considerably more difficult. The use of immunofluorescent techniques has, however, been shown to be highly reliable in the identification of *M. hyopneumoniae*.[23]

Investigating the aetiology of serofibrinous to fibropurulent polyserositis in weaners requires differentiation on culture between several organisms such as *M. hyorhinis, H. parasius* and *P. multocida* which cause similar macroscopic lesions.

Complement fixation (CF), ELISA and latex agglutination tests, performed on a herd basis with a sufficiently representative sample, are useful in identifying suppliers of seedstock whose herds are free of *M. hyopneumoniae* and *A. pleuropneumoniae*.[19] With *M. hyopneumoniae* testing, cross-reactions with *M. flocculare* and *M. hyorhinis* may occur. In countries such as Canada where considerable serological investigation for the presence of *A. pleuropneumoniae* in herds is undertaken, the test of choice appears to be the 2-mercaptoethanol tube agglutination test, which provides greater specificity.[14] In CF testing, the procomplementary nature of porcine serum must be taken into consideration.[10]

Control

Concurrent correction of management-related and environmental stress is essential in any programme designed to reduce the economic effects of respiratory infections in pigs. Outbreaks of respiratory disease often require short-term (seven to 21 days) strategic, antibacterial medication, either parenterally or in the feed or water. The drugs most commonly employed are tetracyclines, tylosin, sulphonamide or tiamulin.[15] Such treatments reduce clinical disease but do not eliminate infection(s) from herds. Since drug-resistant strains of *A. pleuropneumoniae* occur, therapy of acute outbreaks should be preceded by antibiogram testing of isolates.

No vaccine is available against *M. hyopneumoniae* infection. Foundation stock for new enterprises should therefore be obtained from herds known to be free from *M. hyopneumoniae*. Long-term planning against this disease requires the implementation of eradication schemes **(see Chapter 179: Mycoplasmal pneumonia of pigs)**. The use in sows and piglets of a combined *B. bronchiseptica/P. multocida* (serotype A and toxigenic serotype D) bacterin, the only commercially available vaccine against respiratory diseases in South Africa, reduces clinical cases of atrophic rhinitis.[6] Vaccination does not, however, eliminate the causal bacteria from a herd.

Feed or water medication of pigs affected with respiratory disease and high-risk groups is very expensive, and inefficient in that it does not eradicate the infection(s) and only affects clinical disease while therapy is ongoing. Under these circumstances the establishment of pathogen-free stock by hysterotomy or the 'medicated early-weaning technique'[1] will eventually become economically mandatory, especially in large herds where there is a tendency to house large numbers of fattening pigs in a single air-space. The medicated early-weaning technique[1] involves obtaining pigs free from the pathogens endemic in the herd of origin by sow and neonate medication under isolation conditions. Prostaglandin is administered on day 114 to induce parturition. Piglets are medicated from birth to ten days of age, and weaned into an isolated weaner unit at five days of age. In this way offspring which are free of *M. hyopneumoniae* and *B. bronchiseptica* can be obtained from herds infected with these pathogens. It seems reasonable to conclude that this technique might also produce stock free of *A. pleuropneumoniae*, especially if the sows have previously tested sero-negative on several occasions prior to medication.[16] A recent study has indicated that pigs from a *M. hyopneumoniae*-infected herd might be moved on weaning to previously cleaned and disinfected facilities with a favourable environment, and there remain free of pneumonic lesions.[4]

References

1 **ALEXANDER, T.J.L., THORNTON, K., BOON, G., LYSONS, R.J. & GUSH, A.F., 1980.** Medicated early weaning to obtain pigs free from pathogens endemic in the herd of origin. *The Veterinary Record*, 106, 114–119.

2 **ANON., 1988.** Annual Report, 12. Allerton Regional Veterinary Laboratory, Pietermaritzburg, South Africa.

3 **CAMERON, R.D.A., GILES, C.J. & SMITH, I.M., 1980.** The prevalence of *Bordetella bronchiseptica* and turbinate (conchal) atrophy in English pig herds in 1978–79. *The Veterinary Record*, 107, 146–149.

4 **CLARK, L.K., ARMSTRONG, C.H., FREEMAN, J.M., SCHEIDT, A.B., SANDSFREEMAN, L. & KNOX, K., 1988.** Transmission of *Mycoplasma hyopneumoniae* in an infected herd. *Proceedings of the Tenth International Pig Veterinary Society Congress*, 14–17 August 1988. Rio de Janeiro.

5 **CUTLER, R., 1987.** Proceedings No. 95, Postgraduate Committee in Veterinary Science, University of Sydney, Australia, 853–886.

6 **GILES, C.J., 1986.** Atrophic rhinitis. *In:* LEMAN, A.D., STRAW, B., GLOCK, R.D, MENGELING, W.L., PENNY, R.H.C. & SCHOLL, E., (eds). *Diseases of Swine*. 6th edn. Ames, Iowa: Iowa State University Press.

7 **HARRIS, D.L. & SWITZER, W.P., 1968.** Turbinate atrophy in young pigs exposed to *Bordetella bronchiseptica*, *Pasteurella multocida* and combined inoculum. *American Journal of Veterinary Research*, 29, 777–785.

8 **HENTON, M.M., 1988.** Veterinary Research Institute, Onderstepoort. Unpublished data.

9 **KORNEGAY, E.T. & NOTTER, D.R., 1984.** Effect of floor space and number of pigs per pen on performance. *Pig News and Information*, 5, 19–33.

10 **LEWIS, D.H. & SCHWARTZ, W.L., 1987.** *Haemophilus pleuropneumoniae* in swine. *Compendium of Continuing Education*, 9, F7–F12.

11 **LITTLE, T.W.A., 1975.** Respiratory disease in pigs: A study. *The Veterinary Record*, 96, 540–544.

12 **LITTLE, T.W.A. & HARDING, J.D.J., 1980.** The interaction of *Haemophilus parahaemolyticus* and *Pasteurella multocida* in the respiratory tract of the pig. *British Veterinary Journal*, 136, 371–383.

13 **LOVEDAY, R.K., 1956.** Faculty of Veterinary Science, University of Pretoria, South Africa. Unpublished data.

14 **MITTAL, K.R., HIGGINS, R., LARIVIERE, S. & LEBLANC, P., 1984.** A 2–mercaptoethanol tube agglutination test for diagnosis of *Haemophilus pleuropneumoniae* infection in pigs. *American Journal of Veterinary Research*, 45, 715–719.

15 **MUIRHEAD, M.R., 1987.** Proceedings No. 95, Postgraduate Committee in Veterinary Science, University of Sydney, Australia, 561–587.

16 **NICOLET, J. & SCHOLL, E., 1981.** *Haemophilus* infections. *In:* LEMAN, A.D., GLOCK, R.D., MENGELING, W.L., PENNY, R.H.C., SCHOLL, E. & STRAW, B., (eds). *Diseases of Swine*. 5th edn. Ames, Iowa: Iowa State University Press.

17 **PIJOAN, C., 1986.** Respiratory system. *In:* LEMAN, A.D., STRAW, B., GLOCK, R.D., MENGELING, W.L., PENNY, R.H.C. & SCHOLL, E., (eds). *Diseases of Swine*. 6th edn. Ames, Iowa: Iowa State University Press.

18 **PIJOAN, C. & LEMAN, A.D., 1986.** Veterinary services to growers and finishers. *Proceedings of the Ninth International Pig Veterinary Society Congress*, Barcelona.

19 **ROSS, R.F., 1986.** Mycoplasmal diseases. *In:* LEMAN, A.D., STRAW, B., GLOCK, R.D., MENGELING, W.L., PENNY, R.H.C. & SCHOLL, E., (eds). *Diseases of Swine*. 6th edn. Ames, Iowa: Iowa State University Press.

20 **RUTTER, J.M. & MACKENZIE, A., 1984.** Pathogenesis of atrophic rhinitis in pigs: A new perspective. *The Veterinary Record*, 114, 89–90.

21 **SMITH, I.M., HODGES, R.T., BETTS, D.O. & HAYWARD, A.H., 1973.** Experimental infections of gnotobiotic piglets with *Pasteurella septica* (group A) alone or with *M. hyopneumoniae*. *Journal of Comparative Pathology*, 83, 307–321.

22 **SMITH, W.J., WILSON, D. & ROBERTSON, J., 1988.** Atrophic rhinitis — environmental interactions — a survey report. *Proceedings of the Tenth International Pig Veterinary Society Congress*, 14–17 August 1988. Rio de Janeiro.

23 **TRICHARD, C.J.V., 1977.** Veterinary Research Institute, Onderstepoort. Unpublished data.

24 **YAGIHASHI, T., NUNOYA, T., MITUI, T. & TAJIMA, M., 1984.** Effect of *Mycoplasma hyopneumoniae* infection on the development of *Haemophilus pleuropneumoniae* pneumonia in pigs. *Japanese Journal of Veterinary Science*, 46, 705–713.

25 **WHITTLESTONE, P., 1982.** Infectious agents associated with porcine respiratory diseases. *The Pig Veterinary Society Proceedings*, University of Bristol, UK, 15–16 December 1981, 9, 47–60.

189

Infectious causes of equine reproductive failure

C.H.B. Marlow and R.C. Bester

Introduction

Pasture breeding of horses is practised only on a limited scale nowadays and generally the breeder decides when and how the mare is to be bred.[44] Yet the fertility of the horse — defined as the ability to produce viable offspring — remains low despite the increased understanding of equine reproductive physiology and diseases which has been acquired during the last three decades. Breeding data throughout the world indicate a conception rate of 60–70 per cent and a foaling rate of about 60 per cent,[84] although considerably higher figures have been recorded.[10, 66, 92] Foaling rates have remained static in Australia[76] and have decreased in Kentucky in the USA[94] in spite of increased conception rates.[76, 94] This increased foetal wastage is associated with stress factors[76] and uterine disease caused by unseasonal breeding.[94]

Numerous reasons have been given for the low fertility of horses. They include physiological dysfunction, poor management and nutrition, infections and diseases of the gonads and other reproductive organs, hereditary factors, chromosomal aberrations, neoplasms, and conformational abnormalities of the external genitalia.[84] The relative importance of these, with the exception of chromosomal aberrations[63, 98] and neoplasms, is difficult to establish accurately because reproductive failure is the end-result of a series of interacting and often interrelated events in which both intrinsic (animal) **(Table 189.1)** and extrinsic (environmental) **(Figure 189.1)** factors play a role. These cause an inability to produce a viable oocyte, failure of fertilization, foetal death with resorption or abortion, or neonatal disease contracted *in utero*. Voluntary or enforced sexual rest can also lead to reduced fertility. The extrinsic and infectious causes of reproductive failure must be eliminated if lasting improvement in fertility is to be achieved.

Abortion is a major problem facing the Thoroughbred breeding industry in southern Africa. The mean annual abortion rate in the subcontinent between 1977 and 1986 was 13,6 per cent,[4] compared to 2,8 per cent in the UK and Ireland during the period 1930–52.[64]

Very little has been documented about equine infectious reproductive failure in southern Africa.[12, 27, 34, 35, 37, 39, 40, 47–49, 86, 104] One of the reasons for this is that only a very small percentage of aborted foetuses and/or placentas are submitted to diagnostic laboratories for examination, so the assumption that infectious causes play a major role remains entirely speculative.

The pathogenesis of infectious reproductive failure and the factors predisposing mares to infection are summarized in **Figures 189.1 and 189.2** and **Table 189.1**.

Aetiology

Infections causing reproductive failure fall into two groups: those that have a local effect on the genital tract

Table 189.1 Intrinsic predisposing factors to local genital tract infections in the mare

HEREDITARY	ACQUIRED
Immunodeficiency	Increasing age
Compromised defence mechanisms of the uterus	Pathology of the genital tract
General conformation (deviations from 'broodmare' type)	Vulva (scar tissue, lacerations)
Very big or very small mares	Pneumovagina, urovagina
Lack of depth, spring of rib and capacity	Torn cervix
Flat croup associated with a receding anus	Reproductive status
Abnormalities of the external genitalia (vulva)	Increasing number of pregnancies, lactation
Thin lips, poor tone, high dorsal commissure, increasing angle from vertical	Sub-optimal body condition (body score)
Breeding seasonality	Obesity, emaciation
Unseasonal breeding	Low social order
	Other conditions
	e.g. dental abnormalities, blindness, locomotory problems

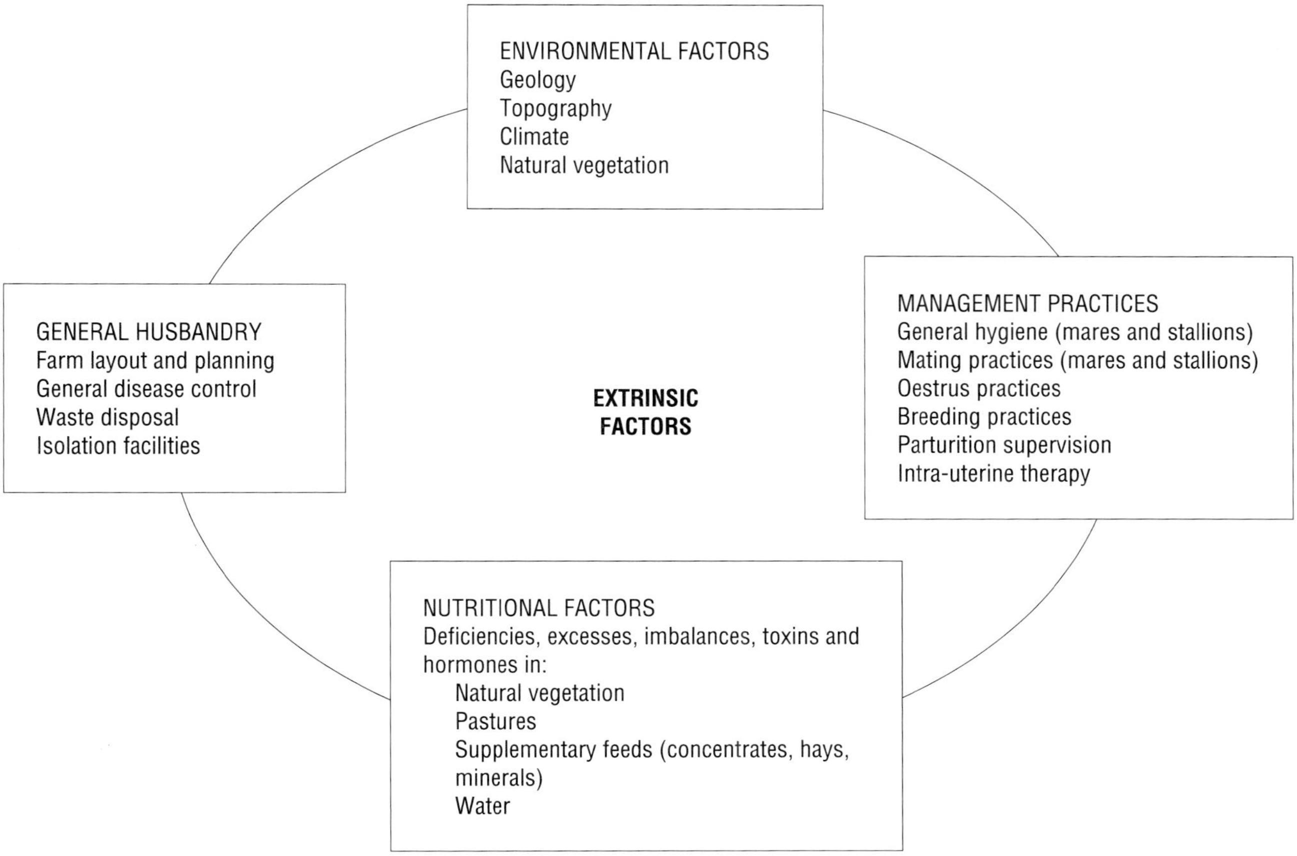

Figure 189.1 Diagrammatic representation of the interrelated extrinsic factors that predispose to equine infectious reproductive failure

and generally result in endometritis, and those that have a systemic effect on the animal.

Localized infections of the genital tract

The susceptibility of the mare, the efficiency of the uterine defence mechanisms,[69] and the virulence of the invading organism are of primary importance in the susceptibility to infections of the uterus.

A variety of potential pathogens is present in the uterus following breeding or at parturition; they are normal, resident flora on the external genitalia and in the vestibule of mares[50] and on the external genitalia of stallions.[52] In mares that are resistant to endometritis, the introduction of these organisms is followed by transient infection and inflammation only, whereas in susceptible mares a persistent endometritis often results.[52] The use of disinfectants on the penis and the overuse of antibiotic treatment in the mare, which allow pathogens (such as *Klebsiella* spp.) and potential pathogens (such as *Pseudomonas* spp.) to replace the normal flora and cause disease, are important contributory factors to localized infection of the uterus.[17, 52]

Anatomical barriers to excessive contamination of the cranial vagina, cervix and uterus of the mare include the ability of the vulva to close efficiently, and normal functioning of the vestibulo-vaginal sphincter and cervix.[7] A thin perineal body, flaccid vulval lips, and emaciation or old age result in cranial displacement of the anus and consequent cranio-dorsal movement of the vulva. This leads to inefficient closure of the vulva, with the result that air, faeces or urine are sucked intermittently or continuously into the vestibulum. Contamination of the uterus with microorganisms often causes persistent endometritis.[7]

Neutrophils and immunoglobulins, including IgA, are primarily responsible for the defence of the uterine mucosa against microbial invasion.[9, 56, 61, 72] Systemic and local hormonal concentrations also have a major influence on the uterine defence mechanism.[102]

A wide variety of organisms, including bacteria, fungi, yeasts, mycoplasmas and viruses, have been isolated from mares with or without evidence of endometritis.[11, 22, 50, 52, 87, 88, 106] The bacteria most frequently isolated from cases with endometritis and subsequent reduced fertility are *Streptococcus zooepidemicus*, *Escherichia coli*, *Klebsiella pneumoniae*, *Pseudomonas aeruginosa* and *Staphylococcus aureus*.[88]

Fertility can also be impaired after abortion in the

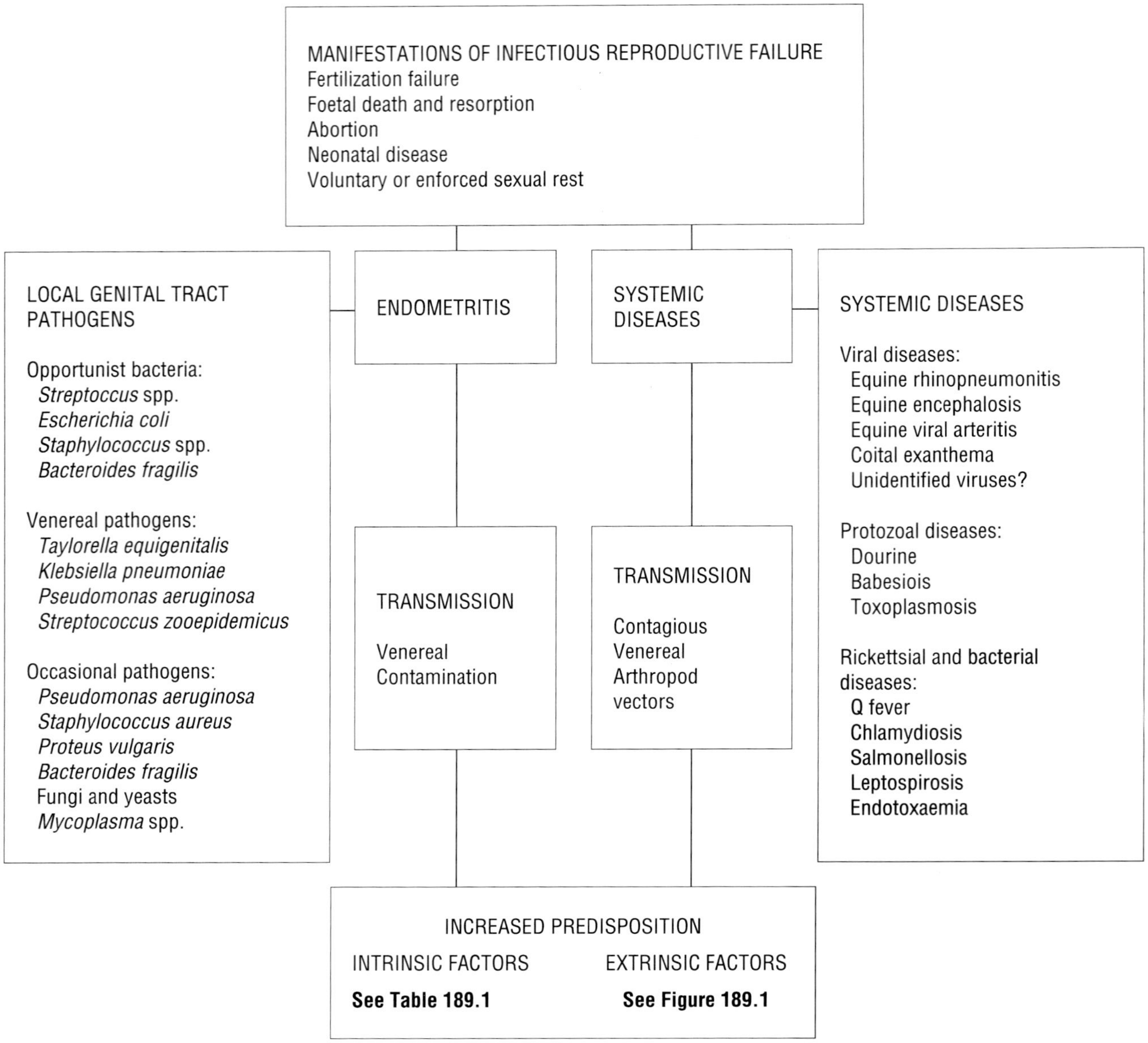

Figure 189.2 Diagrammatic representation of the pathogenesis of infectious reproductive failure in horses

mare or septicaemia of the neonate, which are generally accompanied by a placentitis, particularly when caused by *S. zooepidemicus, S. aureus* or *K. pneumoniae*. Abortions during early pregnancy (60–110 days) have been reported in mares bred before the natural breeding season and which are then allowed to graze in very lush grass or grass/clover pastures.[94] The reason for this is probably induction of secondary ovulations and oestrus causing relaxation of the cervix, and thus allowing the entry of adventitious organisms, particularly Type D *Streptococcus* spp., with resultant development of placentitis, septicaemia and foetal death.[94]

The organisms that cause endometritis fall into three broad groups: opportunist pathogens, venereal pathogens and occasional pathogens **(Figure 189.2)**.[3]

Opportunist pathogens

Streptococcus zooepidemicus and other Type C beta-haemolytic *Streptococcus* spp., which predominate in frequency of isolation, Type D *Streptococcus* spp., *E. coli*, and *Staphylococcus* spp. form part of the resident flora of the perineum, vulval lips, posterior vestibule and clitoral fossa of mares[3, 50] and of the external genitalia of stallions.[3] The transient infection of the uterine mucosa that normally occurs immediately after coitus and parturition may occasionally develop into a persistent endometritis.

In mares suffering from pneumovagina, endometritis is often associated with *E. coli* and *Staphylococcus* spp. infections.

In some mares, *S. zooepidemicus*, which can be transmitted venereally, may cause salpingitis and infertility.[91] Mares mated to stallions whose ejaculates are heavily contaminated with this organism may develop transient or persistent endometritis.[91] Conversely, the penis and sheath may become heavily contaminated with *S. zooepidemicus* for a few days after covering mares suffering from active, persistent endometritis. Mares, particularly those that are lactating, mated to these stallions may develop a transient or persistent endometritis.[68]

Recently attention has been drawn to the role of anaerobic bacteria in endometritis.[50, 82] It is speculated that anaerobes, which normally inhabit the external genital surfaces of mares and stallions, may be harboured in the uterus as surface commensals.[82] These organisms may act as opportunist pathogens when epithelial damage of the uterus occurs, or synergism with aerobic bacteria may result in a mixed infection and active endometritis.[82] *Bacteroides fragilis* is the predominant anaerobic species in the uterus.[82]

Venereal pathogens

The venereal pathogens *Taylorella equigenitalis* and *K. pneumoniae* and the potential venereal pathogen *P. aeruginosa* are not part of the normal resident flora of the equine genital tract. Although strain differences exist in the virulence of *K. pneumoniae*[23] and *P. aeruginosa*,[53] they are both facultative pathogens. In order to elicit disease these bacteria usually require the presence of predisposing factors, such as poor hygiene, the excessive use of antiseptics and/or the abuse of antibiotic treatment.[53]

Klebsiella pneumoniae, which often occurs in stables in association with, for example, wood shavings or sawdust,[74] is also present on the skin, in the intestinal tract and occasionally on the external genitalia. In mares, virulent strains may persist in the clitoral fossa and sinuses, the vestibule or urethra and act as reservoirs of infection for the uterus.[45] Asymptomatic, persistent infection of the prostate, urinary bladder and kidneys of a stallion with *K. pneumoniae* capsule Type 5, was associated with abortions in the mares he served.[23]

Outbreaks of endometritis due to *K. pneumoniae* are usually associated with capsule Types 1, 2 and 5, while capsule Types 6, 7, 20, 21 and 30 are less frequently involved.[78, 80] However, in view of the fact that sporadic cases of endometritis have been associated with other strains of the organism, its mere presence in the genital tract of mares should be viewed with suspicion. Clinical signs in affected mares vary from a swollen, red cervix, with or without a slight mucopurulent discharge from the external os, to those in which a copious, thick, mucopurulent discharge from the vulva is present.[67]

Infection of the uterus by virulent strains of *P. aeruginosa* causes a severe and deep-seated, persistent endometritis. Venereal transmission often occurs after colonization of the penis by the organism following destruction of the normal resident flora by the constant use of antiseptics and antibiotics at breeding.[52] The clitoral fossa and sinuses and the vestibule are sites in which the organisms may persist for long periods, and are therefore potential sources of contamination of the uterus and penis during coitus.[52]

Occasional pathogens

Pseudomonas aeruginosa, *Bacillus cereus*[5, 62] and *Proteus vulgaris*, as well as certain mycoplasmas, yeasts and fungi,[15] are occasional uterine pathogens. Mycotic endometritis has become more common following the injudicious and often prolonged intra-uterine administration of antibiotics,[108] and the increasingly intensive management and manipulation of reproduction in mares.[15] The most common fungi isolated from the uterus of mares are *Candida* spp., particularly *C. albicans*, and *Aspergillus fumigatus*[15] **(see Chapter 185: Mycoses)**. *Candida* spp. are usually associated with acute, purulent inflammation of the superficial endometrium, followed by rapid and spontaneous resolution.[15] These yeasts are rarely found in the lumen of the uterus[15] or in the deeper parts of the endometrium.[54] When fungi or yeasts are associated with persistent endometritis and chronic reproductive failure, bacteria, particularly *P. aeruginosa*, are often also present. In these cases it is impossible to determine the primary cause.[15]

Abortion due to mycotic placentitis, on the other hand, usually follows the entry of fungi via the cervix during coitus or just prior to the oestrus period during which conception occurs.[65] This type of abortion is generally followed by spontaneous recovery and unimpaired fertility.

Mycoplasma equigenitalium and *M. subdolum* have been recovered from the lower genital tract of mares and stallions without being associated with poor reproductive performance.[13] *Mycoplasma bovigenitalium* has also been isolated from the lungs of an aborted equine foetus.[58]

Systemic diseases

Viral diseases

Equid herpesvirus 1 (EHV-1), the cause of equine viral rhinopneumonitis, and equine encephalosis virus are the only known viral causes of abortion in horses in South Africa.[38] However, it is suspected that one or more as yet unidentified arthropod-borne viruses may also be involved.[38] South African breeders know that areas in the Eastern Cape province less than 1 100 m above sea level are prone to a high prevalence of abortion. By moving pregnant mares to higher regions where there are fewer insect vectors, particularly during the late summer and autumn in years of heavy rainfall, the abortion rate is drastically reduced.

Neonatal mortalities and abortions due to EHV-1 usually occur sporadically **(see Chapter 102: Equid herpesvirus 1 and 4 infections)**. Abortion most often takes place in the last third of pregnancy without premonitory signs of illness.[2, 30] The aborted foetus is usually in a fresh state and the placenta, which may be oedematous and contain scattered small haemorrhages, is expelled with the foetus or shortly thereafter.[2, 30] Involution of the uterus is normal and subsequent fertility is not impaired.[32]

Mares infected with equine encephalosis virus **(see Chapter 45: Equine encephalosis)** usually abort from five months of gestation onwards, particularly during late summer, autumn or early winter. The foetus may be expelled in a fresh or autolysed state; no lesions of diagnostic significance are presented, but virus can be recovered from foetal tissues — even from those showing advanced autolysis.[38] Subsequent fertility is not affected.

Recently, equine viral arteritis **(see Chapter 67: Equine viral arteritis)** was diagnosed for the first time in South Africa in a number of Lipizzaner mares, all of which had been served by, or were in contact with, an infected imported stallion.[38] None of the infected mares aborted, however. Abortion due to equine viral arteritis in other parts of the world occurs either as a sporadic event or in the form of abortion storms.[31] Abortion usually takes place following subclinical infection, late in the febrile reaction or during convalescence, 10–30 days after the abatement of clinical signs, and is probably due to myometritis.[21] The foetuses are often severely autolysed at the time of expulsion, which may occur as early as 100 days of gestation.

Stallions may harbour this virus in the ampullae and shed high concentrations of it in their semen despite high levels of neutralizing antibodies in the circulation.[38] Shedding of virus may be either transient or persistent;[97] in some it may even be life-long.[95] Lack of sexual rest may predispose a stallion to persistent virus-shedding.[96] Approximately one third of stallions become long-term or persistent shedders of the virus and they play a major role in the transmission of the disease.[96]

Coital exanthema caused by equid herpesvirus 3 **(see Chapter 104: Equine coital exanthema)** is characterized by vesicles and erosions, particularly in the mucosa of the vulva and vagina of mares and the penis and prepuce of stallions, as well as in the skin of the perineum of both sexes.[77] Recrudescences occur regularly, but in breeds where handbreeding is practised, outbreaks are usually confined to single or a few animals. The disease is common in southern Africa and is controlled by isolating the infected animals for a month. Fertility is affected only for the duration of isolation, and the future breeding potential of affected animals is not impaired. Abortions do not occur.

Protozoal diseases

Dourine, colloquially known as slapsiekte, occurs in certain areas of southern Africa **(see Chapter 12: Dourine)**. Apart from the usual systemic manifestations, the disease has also occasionally been associated with low fertility[86] and abortion in mares,[27, 86] and with neonatal mortality.[27]

Babesiosis is frequently diagnosed in South Africa in new-born foals and aborted foetuses **(see Chapter 24: Equine babesiosis)**. In most cases *Babesia equi* is involved,[68] but *B. caballi* has occasionally been incriminated.[28] In mares, unobserved foetal loss during early pregnancy is frequently associated with babesiosis. Abortions, stillbirths, and peracute neonatal disease which is almost invariably fatal are rarely accompanied by clinical disease in the mare. Intra-uterine infection may recur during subsequent pregnancies. Abortion usually occurs during the last two months of gestation, and is generally accompanied by simultaneous expulsion of the placenta. Uterine involution is normal and subsequent conception is not affected.

Although toxoplasmosis has not been recognized as a cause of abortion in southern Africa, toxoplasma-like sporozoa have been found in an aborted equine foetus in the USA.[33] As cats are commonly used to control rodents in breeding establishments, and many equine studs in southern Africa also contain large flocks of sheep, the possibility of this disease should be considered when abortions occur.

Rickettsial and bacterial diseases

Coxiella burnetii, the cause of Q fever, has been associated with sporadic abortions in Thoroughbreds in the Eastern Cape Province. Abortion, which occurs mostly from the fourth to the tenth months of gestation, or the birth of a stunted but otherwise clinically normal foal is invariably accompanied by a necrotic placentitis.[68]

The prevalence of chlamydiosis, particularly in sheep, in the subcontinent warrants its inclusion as a possible cause of reproductive failure in horses. During the widespread epidemic of chlamydiosis in ruminants in South Africa in 1972/73, *Chlamydia psittaci* was incriminated as the cause of abortions in mares on a stud near Kimberley.[16]

Abortion due to salmonellosis is a major cause of reproductive failure in mares in some countries.[83, 99] Although the prevalence of the disease in southern Africa is unknown, *Salmonella abortus equi* and *S. typhimurium* infections have been associated with sporadic abortions in horses in South Africa.[47–49] It has been demonstrated recently that Gram-negative bacterial endotoxaemia results in a pronounced prostaglandin response and disturbance of luteal activity.[42] Mares are vulnerable to embryonal loss as a result of *S. typhimurium* endotoxin until about 50–60 days of gestation.[24]

Generally, leptospirosis is not of great significance in livestock in southern Africa. It should nevertheless be considered in investigations relating to reproductive failure in horses, as dual infection by leptospires and EHV-1 has been incriminated as a cause of abortions in horses abroad.[36]

Diagnosis

Localized genital tract infections

The diagnosis of localized genital tract infections in the mare is complex and depends upon a number of examinations and procedures including: detailed general and reproductive histories; general clinical examination; rectal palpation of the internal reproductive organs; vaginal examination; microbiological culture of specimens of cervico-uterine contents, aborted foetuses, neonates and placentas; cervico-uterine cytology; endometrial biopsy evaluation; ultrasound imaging; and fibre-optic endoscopic examination. Correlation of the findings of as many of these procedures as possible increases the probability of an accurate and meaningful diagnosis.

Microbiological culture of the cervico-uterine contents is only an aid in the diagnosis of endometritis. The mere presence of an organism does not warrant a diagnosis of endometritis, and lack of growth does not exclude the possibility of endometritis being present. Irrespective of the method used during collection of specimens, strict attention to asepsis is imperative.[44] The use of guarded swabs reduces the risk of the swab being contaminated during its passage through the vagina and cervix.[18] Swabs should be guided into the cervical canal with a gloved hand and not through a speculum, since the latter allows air to be sucked into the vagina.[18] Swabs should be taken during oestrus, when the uterine defence mechanisms of the mare are optimal.[18] Specimens should be placed in a transport medium and kept on ice until delivered to the laboratory. Culturing should include techniques likely to reveal the presence of micro-aerophilic, aerobic and anaerobic bacteria. Mycoplasmas, chlamydiae and viruses require specific methods for demonstration or isolation. When *P. aeruginosa, K. pneumoniae* or *T. equigenitalis* infections are suspected, additional swabs from the urethra and clitoral fossa and sinuses are generally necessary. Fungal infections are best diagnosed on stained, wet preparations of the sediment obtained from uterine lavage.[43]

A considerable proportion of bacterial cultures from uterine swabs obtained from mares with no evidence of endometritis show growth of a wide variety of non-pathogenic organisms[50] or opportunist pathogens.[67] The low number and wide variety of organisms usually cultured indicate that they are probably contaminants or organisms that cause transient infections.[50]

Cervico-uterine cytology should also be performed, because bacteriological examination of endometrial swabs cannot be accurately interpreted without concurrent cytological data.[106] Generally, it provides a better guide than bacteriology for evaluating inflammation of the uterus.[105] A more realistic approach to the common 'no-growth culture before breeding' requirement would be less than ten colonies of non-potential uterine pathogens on the culture of a uterine swab,[50] in addition to a negative cytological examination for neutrophils.[67]

The presence of neutrophils in uterine smears is a reliable indicator of endometritis.[57] Neutrophils are generally absent from smears from normal mares,[105] except for several days after coitus and seven to ten days post-partum, when an acute, transient endometritis usually occurs. In mares that develop a persistent endometritis, neutrophils continue to be present. Eosinophils, macrophages, erythrocytes, bacteria, fungi and yeasts may also be observed on smears.[68]

Although examination of an endometrial biopsy can provide a definite diagnosis of endometritis, its real value is apparent when estimating the ability of the endometrium to support pregnancy to term. Endometritis is usually classified as acute, chronic, or chronic with acute exacerbations. The lesions have been graded (categories I-III), based on the increasing extent and severity of cellular infiltration and fibrosis.[54] Category I endometria are considered not to interfere with the ability to support a foetus to term, and a foaling rate of about 70 per cent can be expected. Categories II and III endometria are associated with foaling rates of about 50 per cent and less than 10 per cent respectively.[54]

The endometria of mares suffering from pneumovagina and/or cervical incompetence (e.g. torn cervix) are characterized by diffuse, moderate to severe infiltrations mainly of lymphocytes, but also of plasma cells,[67] and eosinophils in the *stratum compactum*.[67, 90]

Uniform dilatation of the ducts and of the basal portions of endometrial glands are associated with recent abortion.[54] The presence of maternal septa indicate recent, unobserved foetal loss.[54] The interval between either parturition or abortion and biopsy sampling can be estimated by using the Berlin blue or Perl's staining methods for determining the amount and distribution of haemosiderin in macrophages and in the cytoplasm of the glandular epithelial cells. After haemorrhage has occurred as a result of either parturition or abortion, haemosiderin is found in large amounts in numerous macrophages in the *str. compactum,* the cytoplasm of the glandular epithelial cells and in macrophages. These pigmented macrophages disappear sequentially from the *str. compactum* and then from the superficial and deeper layers of the *str. spongiosum*.[67] After about nine months only a few haemosiderin-laden macrophages are found in the stroma of the basal portion of the *str. spongiosum*.[67]

Polarized light is very useful for detecting collagen[54] and crystalline antibiotic residues in the endometrium.[67]

As a result of culture methods, self-cure or non-infectious causes, the lesions in the endometrium do not always correlate with bacteriological findings.[54] Lesions should therefore always be interpreted in the light of the history and clinical and microbiological findings.[54]

In the event of abortion or neonatal mortality, particularly when accompanied by placentitis, appropriate specimens from the dead foetus or foal, placenta, and the uterus of the affected mare(s) should be collected for microbiological culture and pathological examination.

Systemic diseases

The method of diagnosis of each of the systemic diseases that contribute to infectious reproductive failure **(Figure 189.2)** is discussed in more detail elsewhere in the book. Generally, an accurate diagnosis depends upon a detailed general history, a detailed clinical examination of affected animals (mares, neonates, stallions), necropsy (foetus and neonate), and the isolation and identification of the aetiological agent and serology.

Management and control

Localized genital tract infections

The effective control of infectious genital tract disease of mares depends primarily on eliminating or correcting any of the numerous extrinsic **(Figure 189.1)** and intrinsic **(Table 189.1)** predisposing factors. This can only be achieved by the continual evaluation of the general management and accurate and detailed records of performance of the herd as a whole as well as of each individual within the herd. Sexual rest should also receive priority, particularly in mares suffering from *Klebsiella* infections.[71] Only then should the selective use of specific therapeutic measures be contemplated.

The surgical procedures that are used in the management of infectious genital tract disease in the mare are generally aimed at the correction and prevention of pneumovagina and/or pneumo-uterus. Caslick's operation,[20] one of the most important techniques for the treatment and prevention of uterine infection,[11, 26, 34] is frequently employed. Other surgical procedures include modifications[89] of the Caslick's operation[20] and perineal repair[19] (which should only be performed as a last resort when there is extensive scar-tissue formation and the danger of subsequent vulval lacerations at parturition); repair of rectovaginal lacerations and fistulae; cervical-tear repair; excision of the clitoris or clitoral sinuses; correction of urovagina; and uterine curettage.[73, 81]

A wide spectrum of medicinal preparations have been used for the treatment of uterine infections, usually in the form of uterine infusions or lavage, at various concentrations and intervals between treatments, and often without considering pH or vehicle. Such treatment is often not very successful.[1, 11, 25, 51, 59, 70, 75, 79, 85, 88, 100, 103, 107]

Antibiotic treatment should only be considered when endometritis is present[25] and after antibiograms have been conducted. However, the use of antibiotics has not markedly reduced the prevalence of endometritis or reproductive failure.[25] The abuse of antibiotics has increased the prevalence of endometritis due to organisms that were once considered to be facultative pathogens (e.g. *P. aeruginosa*)[25] and facultative saprophytes (e.g. fungi and yeasts).[52]

Other preparations, used either alone or in conjunction with antibiotics in the treatment of endometritis, include hormones, semen extenders, buffers, saline solutions,[11, 101] colostrum,[29] dimethyl sulphoxide[41, 60] and hydrogen peroxide. Preparations which may be highly irritant in some mares even at low concentrations, and that can result in extensive endometrial fibrosis and infertility, include Lugol's iodine, the so-called 'tamed' iodines,[88, 100] derivatives of formaldehyde and paraffin.[67]

Autologous plasma is an easily prepared and convenient source of supplementary complement, which is critical to phagocytosis in the uterus,[6] and this has satisfied the urgent need for a safe alternative to antibiotic treatment.[46] Intrauterine infusion of plasma is particularly appropriate for mares with category II endometria[54] associated with opportunist and venereal pathogens,[8] and also with *P. aeruginosa*, which produces a complement-inactivating enzyme. In mares which have been successfully treated, a single, post-breeding plasma infusion is often used to prevent an acute flare-up of endometritis after natural service.[6]

Chronic fibrotic endometritis associated with *S. zooepidemicus* and other beta-haemolytic *Streptococcus* spp. resulted in a culling rate of about 60 per cent of mares on some stud farms in South Africa before 1985, when autologous plasma was included in treatment regimens.[67] Currently, the culling rate due to endometritis caused by these organisms is negligible. Generally, endometritis associated with other opportunist and occasional pathogens does not impair future fertility.[67]

In stallions, the management of genital tract disease is aimed at preventing the disturbance of the normal resident bacterial flora of the external genitalia[53] caused by washing of the penis before and/or after service. Water alone and neutral soaps increase the number of coliform bacteria, while antiseptic surgical scrubs, particularly those containing 'tamed' iodines, produce the most marked alteration in the bacterial flora. The worst effect is noted after washing with antiseptics is discontinued, when *P. aeruginosa* becomes the prevalent organism.[17] Stallions found on routine microbiological culture to be harbouring venereal pathogens without clinical signs of disease (e.g. *Klebsiella* spp.[71] and *Pseudomonas* spp.[93]) should be test-mated to healthy mares before being allowed unrestricted service.[71] The use of the so-called 'minimal contamination breeding technique' has been shown to be extremely helpful in preventing the transmission of pathogens from infected stallions to mares during coitus.[14, 55]

Systemic diseases

For information on the control of systemic diseases associated with infectious reproductive failure, the chapters on the respective diseases should be consulted.

References

1 **ABOU-GABAL, M., HOGLE, R.M. & WEST, J.K., 1977.** Pyometra in a mare caused by *Candida rugosa*. *Journal of the American Veterinary Medical Association*, 170, 177–178.

2 **ALLEN, G.P. & BRYANS, J.T., 1986.** Molecular epizootiology, pathogenesis, and prophylaxis of equine herpesvirus-1 infections. *In: Progress in Veterinary Microbiology and Immunology*. Vol 2. Basel, Switzerland: Karger AG.

3 **ALLEN, W.E. & NEWCOMBE, J.R., 1979.** Aspects of genital infection and swabbing techniques in the mare. *The Veterinary Record*, 104, 228–231.

4 **ANON, 1978–87.** *General Stud Book of South Africa*, 1978–87. Supplements to Vols 22–24. Return of mares for 1977/78–1986/87. Johannesburg: The Jockey Club of South Africa.

5 **ANSARI, M.M. & MATROS, L.E., 1986.** *Bacillus cereus*: The pathogenic origin of infertility in mares? *Veterinary Medicine and Small Animal Clinician*, 81, 657–658.

6 **ASBURY, A.C., 1984.** Uterine defence mechanisms in the mare: The use of intrauterine plasma in the management of endometritis. *Theriogenology*, 21, 387–393.

7 **ASBURY, A.C., 1987.** Infectious and immunologic considerations in mare infertility. *Compendium on Continuing Education*, 9, 585–592.

8 **ASBURY, A.C., GORMAN, N.T. & FOSTER, G.W., 1984.** Uterine defence mechanisms in the mare: Serum opsonins affecting phagocytosis of *Streptococcus zooepidemicus* by equine neutrophils. *Theriogenology*, 21, 375–385.

9 **ASBURY, A.C., SCHULTZ, K.T., KLESIUS, P.H., FOSTER, G.W. & WASHBURN, S.M., 1982.** Factors affecting phagocytosis of bacteria by neutrophils in the mare's uterus. *Journal of Reproduction and Fertility*, Supplement No. 32, 151–159.

10 **BAIN, A.M., 1957.** Estrus and infertility of the Thoroughbred mare in Australasia. *Journal of the American Veterinary Medical Association*, 131, 179–185.

11 **BAIN, A.M., 1966.** The role of infection in infertility in the Thoroughbred mare. *The Veterinary Record*, 78, 168–173.

12 **BARROWMAN, P.R. & VAN VUUREN, M., 1976.** The prevalence of dourine in Southern Africa. *Journal of the South African Veterinary Association*, 47, 83–85.

13 **BERMUDEZ, V., MILLER, R., JOHNSON, W., ROSENDAL, S. & RUHNKE, L., 1987.** The prevalence of *Mycoplasma* spp. and their relationship to reproductive performance in selected horse herds in southern Ontario. *Journal of Reproduction and Fertility*, Supplement No. 35, 671–673.

14 **BLANCHARD, T.L., VARNER, D.D., LOVE, C.C., HURTGEN, J.P., CUMMINGS, M.R. & KENNEY, R.M., 1987.** Use of a semen extender containing antibiotic to improve the fertility of a stallion with seminal vesiculitis due to *Pseudomonas aeruginosa*. *Theriogenology*, 28, 541–546.

15 **BLUE, M.G., 1987.** Mycotic endometritis in mares. Review and clinical observations. *New Zealand Veterinary Journal*, 35, 181–183.

16 **BOSMAN, P.P., COUBROUGH, R.I., ERASMUS, B.J. & SCHUTTE, A.P., 1973.** Directorate of Animal Health, Pretoria, South Africa. Unpublished data.

17 **BOWEN, J.M., TOBIN, N., SIMPSON, R.B., LEY, W.B. & ANSARI, M.M., 1982.** Effects of washing on the bacterial flora of the stallion's penis. *Journal of Reproduction and Fertility*, Supplement No. 32, 41–45.

18 **BROOK, D., 1984.** The diagnosis of equine bacterial endometritis. *Compendium of Continuing Education*, 6, S300–S306.

19 **BROWN, J.M. & COFFMAN, J.R., 1971.** A modified technique for episioplasty in the mare. *Veterinary Medicine and Small Animal Clinician*, 66, 103–107.

20 **CASLICK, E.A., 1937.** The vulva and the vulvo-vaginal orifice and its relation to genital health of the Thoroughbred mare. *Cornell Veterinarian*, 27, 178–187.

21 **COIGNOUL, F.L. & CHEVILLE, N.F., 1984.** Pathology of maternal tract, placenta, and fetus in equine viral arteritis. *Veterinary Pathology*, 21, 333–340.

22 **COLLINS, S.M., 1964.** A study of the incidence of cervical and uterine infection in Thoroughbred mares in Ireland. *The Veterinary Record*, 76, 673–676.

23 **CROUCH, J.R.F., ATHERTON, J.G. & PLATT, H., 1972.** Venereal transmission of *Klebsiella aerogenes* in a Thoroughbred stud from a persistently infected stallion. *The Veterinary Record*, 90, 21–24.

24 **DAELS, P.F., STARR, M., KINDAHL, H., FREDRIKSSON, G., HUGHES, J.P. & STABENFELDT, G.H., 1987.** Effect of *Salmonella typhimurium* endotoxin on PGF-2a release and fetal death in the mare. *Journal of Reproduction and Fertility*, Supplement No. 35, 485–492.

25 **DAVIS, L.E. & ABBITT, B., 1977.** Clinical pharmacology of antibacterial drugs in the uterus of the mare. *Journal of the American Veterinary Medical Association*, 170, 204–207.

26 **DE GANNES, R.V.G., 1980.** Old and new uterine treatments for broodmares. *Proceedings of the Twenty-sixth Annual Convention of the American Association of Equine Practitioners*, 30 November – 3 December 1980, Anaheim, California, 405–410.

27 **DE KOCK, G., ROBINSON, E.M. & PARKIN, B.S., 1939.** Some observations on dourine. *Journal of the South African Veterinary Medical Association*, 10, 44–55.

28 **DE WAAL, D.T., 1988.** Veterinary Research Institute, Onderstepoort. Unpublished data.

29 **DEWES, H.F., 1980.** Preliminary observations on the use of colostrum as an uterine infusion in thoroughbred mares. *New Zealand Veterinary Journal*, 28, 7–8.

30 **DIXON, R.J., HARTLEY, W.J., HUTCHINS, D.R., LEPHERD, E.E., FEILEN, C., JONES, R.F., LOVE, D.N., SABINE, M. & WELLS, A.L., 1978.** Perinatal foal mortality associated with a herpesvirus. *Australian Veterinary Journal*, 54, 103–105.

31 **DOLL, E.R., 1963.** Viral arteritis. *In:* BONE, J.F., CATCOTT, E.J., GABEL, A.A., JOHNSON, L.E. & RILEY, W.F., (eds). *Equine Medicine and Surgery*. 1st edn. Wheaton, Illinois: American Veterinary Publications Inc.

32 **DOLL, E.R., 1963.** Viral rhinopneumonitis. *In:* BONE, J.F., CATCOTT, E.J., GABEL, A.A., JOHNSON, L.E. & RILEY, W.F., (eds). *Equine Medicine and Surgery*. 1st edn. Wheaton, Illinois: American Veterinary Publications Inc.

33 **DUBEY, J.P. & PORTERFIELD, M.L., 1986.** Toxoplasma-like sporozoa in an aborted equine fetus. *Journal of the American Veterinary Medical Association*, 188, 1312–1313.

34 **DU PLESSIS, J.L., 1964.** Some observations and data in Thoroughbred breeding. *Journal of the South African Veterinary Medical Association*, 35, 215–221.

35 **DU PLESSIS, J.L. & BASSON, P.A., 1966.** Babesiosis in aborted equine foetuses: A report on two cases in South Africa. *Journal of the South African Veterinary Medical Association*, 37, 267–269.

36 **ELLIS, W.A., BRYSON, D.G. & McFERRAN, J.B., 1976.** Abortion associated with mixed leptospira/equid herpesvirus-1 infection. *The Veterinary Record*, 98, 218–219.

37 **ERASMUS, B.J., 1963.** Equine viral rhinopneumonitis. *Journal of the South African Veterinary Medical Association*, 34, 461–469.

38 **ERASMUS, B.J., 1989.** Veterinary Research Institute, Onderstepoort. Unpublished data.

39 **ERASMUS, B.J., BOSHOFF, S.T. & PIETERSE, L.M., 1978.** The isolation and characterization of equine encephalosis and serologically related orbiviruses from horses. *In:* BRYANS, J.T. & GERBER, H., (eds.). *Equine Infectious Diseases*. IV. Princeton, New Jersey: Veterinary Publications.

40 **FAUL, A., 1988.** Dourine in South Africa. *Journal of the South African Veterinary Association*, 59, 7.

41 **FRAZER, G.S., ROSSOL, T.J., THRELFALL, W.R. & WEISBRODE, S.E., 1988.** Histopathologic effects of dimethyl sulfoxide on equine endometrium. *American Journal of Veterinary Research*, 49, 1774–1781.

42 **FREDRIKSON, G., KINDAHL, H. & STABENFELDT, G.H., 1986.** Endotoxin-induced and prostaglandin-mediated effects on corpus luteum function in the mare. *Theriogenology*, 25, 309–316.

43 **FREEMAN, K.P., ROSZEL, J.F., SLUSHER, S.H. & PAYNE, M., 1986.** Mycotic infections of the equine uterus. *Equine Practice*, 8, 34–42.

44 **GREENHOFF, G.R. & KENNEY, R.M., 1975.** Evaluation of reproductive status of nonpregnant mares. *Journal of the American Veterinary Medical Association*, 167, 449–458.

45 **GREENWOOD, R.E.S. & ELLIS, D.R., 1976.** *Klebsiella aerogenes* in mares. *The Veterinary Record*, 99, 439.

46 **GUSTAFSSON, B.K., 1984.** Therapeutic strategies involving antimicrobial treatment of the uterus in large animals. *Journal of the American Veterinary Medical Association*, 185, 1194–1198.

47 **HENNING, M.W., 1946.** On the aetiology of epizootic or infectious equine abortion. *Onderstepoort Journal of Veterinary Science and Animal Industry*, 21, 17–40.

48 **HENNING, M.W., 1949.** Equine epizootic or infectious abortion. *In: Animal Diseases in South Africa*. 2nd edn. Pretoria, South Africa: Central News Agency Ltd.

49 **HENNING, M.W., KEPPEL, J.J.G. & FLIGHT, C.H., 1943.** Equine abortion. *Journal of the South African Veterinary Medical Association*, 14, 59–66.

50 **HINRICHS, K., CUMMINGS, M.R., SERTICH, P.L. & KENNEY, R.M., 1988.** Clinical significance of aerobic bacterial flora of the uterus, vagina, vestibule, and clitoral fossa of clinically normal mares. *Journal of the American Veterinary Medical Association*, 193, 72–75.

51 **HOUDESHELL, J.W. & HENNESSEY, P.W., 1972.** Gentamycin in the treatment of equine metritis. *Veterinary Medicine and Small Animal Clinician*, 67, 1348–1352.

52 **HUGHES, J.P. & LOY, R.G., 1975.** The relation of infection to infertility in the mare and stallion. *Equine Veterinary Journal*, 7, 155–159.

53 **HUGHES, J.P., LOY, R.G., ASBURY, A.C. & BURD, H.E., 1966.** The occurrence of *Pseudomonas* in the reproductive tract of mares and its effect on fertility. *Cornell Veterinarian*, 56, 595–610.

54 **KENNEY, R.M., 1978.** Cyclic and pathologic changes of the mare endometrium as detected by biopsy, with a note of early embryonic death. *Journal of the American Veterinary Medical Association*, 172, 241–262.

55 **KENNEY, R.M., BERGMAN, R.V., COOPER, W.L. & MORSE, G.D., 1975.** Minimal contamination techniques for breeding mares: Technique and preliminary findings. *Proceedings of the American Association of Equine Practice*, December 1975, Boston, USA. 327–336.

56 **KENNEY, R.M. & KHALEEL, S.A., 1975.** Bacteriostatic activity of the mare uterus: A progress report on immunoglobulins. *Journal of Reproduction and Fertility*, Supplement No. 23, 357–358.

57 **KNUDSEN, O., 1964.** Endometrial cytology as a diagnostic aid in mares. *Cornell Veterinarian*, 54, 415–422.

58 **LANGFORD, E.V., 1974.** Isolation of *Mycoplasma bovigenitalium* from an aborted equine foetus. *The Veterinary Record*, 94, 528.

59 **LANGHAM, R.F., BENEKE, E.S. & WHITENACK, D.L., 1977.** Abortion in a mare due to coccidioidomycosis. *Journal of the American Veterinary Medical Association*, 170, 178–180.

60 **LEY, W.B. & SPONENBERG, D.P., 1985.** Dimethyl sulfoxide (DMSO) intra-uterine therapy in the mare. *Proceedings of the Annual Meeting of the Society for Theriogenology*.

61 **LIU, I.K.M. & CHEUNG, A.T.W., 1986.** Immunoglobulin and neutrophil defence against uterine infection in mares resistant and susceptible to chronic endometritis: A review. *Journal of the American Veterinary Medical Association*, 189, 700–702.

62 **LOGAN, N.A., 1988.** *Bacillus* species of medical and veterinary importance. *Journal of Medical Microbiology*, 25, 157–165.

63 **LONG, S.E., 1988.** Chromosome anomalies and infertility in the mare. *Equine Veterinary Journal*, 20, 89–93.

64 **MAHAFFEY, L.W., 1968.** Abortion in mares. *The Veterinary Record*, 82, 681–689.

65 **MAHAFFEY, L.W. & ROSSDALE, P.D., 1965.** An abortion due to *Allescheria boydii* and general observations concerning mycotic abortions of mares. *The Veterinary Record*, 77, 541–545.

66 **MARLOW, C.H.B., 1983.** The oestrous cycle, mating practices, conception rates and fetal losses in Thoroughbreds in the Eastern Cape Province. M.Sc. (Agric.) Thesis. University of Stellenbosch.

67 **MARLOW, C.H.B., 1989.** P.O. Box 138, Cradock 5880, South Africa. Unpublished data.

68 **MARLOW, C.H.B. & BESTER, R.C., 1989.** P.O. Box 138, Cradock 5880, South Africa. Unpublished data.

69 **MARTIN, R.G., PENHALE, W.J. & WILLIAMSON, P., 1988.** Factors affecting the composition of mare uterine fluid. *Research in Veterinary Science*, 45, 111–116.

70 **MATHER, E.C., ADDISON, B., OWENS, D., BIERSCHWAL, C.J. & MARTIN, C.E., 1973.** *Bordetella bronchiseptica* associated with infertility in a mare. *Journal of the American Veterinary Medical Association*, 163, 76–77.

71 **MERKT, H., KLUG, E., BOHM, K.-H. & WEISS, R., 1975.** Recent observations concerning *Klebsiella* infections in stallions. *Journal of Reproduction and Fertility*, Supplement No. 23, 143–145.

72 **MITCHELL, G., LIU, I.K.M., PERRYMAN, L.E., STABENFELDT, G.H. & HUGHES, J.P., 1982.** Preferential production and secretion of immunoglobulins by the equine endometrium — a mucosal immune system. *Journal of Reproduction and Fertility*, Supplement No. 32, 161–168.

73 **MORROW, G.L., 1967.** Uterine curettage in the mare. *Journal of the American Veterinary Medical Association*, 151, 1615–1617.

74 **NEWMAN, L.E. & KOWALSKI, J.J., 1973.** Fresh sawdust bedding — A possible source of *Klebsiella* organisms. *American Journal of Veterinary Research*, 34, 979–980.

75 **NORTHWAY, R.B., 1973.** A treatment regimen for equine cervicitis and metritis. *Veterinary Medicine and Small Animal Clinician*, 68, 269–270.

76 **OSBORNE, V.E., 1975.** Factors influencing foaling percentages in Australian mares. *Journal of Reproduction and Fertility*, Supplement No. 23, 477–483.

77 **PASCOE, R.R. & BAGUST, T.J., 1975.** Coital exanthema in stallions. *Journal of Reproduction and Fertility*, Supplement No. 23, 147–150.

78 **PLATT, H., 1979.** Venereal diseases of horses. *International Symposium on Equine Venereal Diseases*, September 1979, Newmarket, Suffolk, UK.

79 **REID, M.M., FROCK, I.W. & JEFFREY, D.R., 1977.** Successful treatment of maduromycotic fungal infection of the equine uterus with amphotericin B. *Veterinary Medicine and Small Animal Clinician*, 72, 1194–1196.

80 **RICKETTS, S.W., 1981.** Bacteriological examination of the mare's cervix: Techniques and interpretation of results. *The Veterinary Record*, 108, 46–51.

81 **RICKETTS, S.W., 1985.** Endometrial curettage in the mare. *Equine Veterinary Journal*, 17, 324–328.

82 **RICKETTS, S.W. & MACKINTOSH, M.E., 1987.** Role of anaerobic bacteria in equine endometritis. *Journal of Reproduction and Fertility*, Supplement No. 35, 343–351.

83 **ROSSDALE, P.D. & RICKETTS, S.W., 1976.** Veterinary Annual, 16, 133–141.

84 **ROWLANDS, I.W., 1981.** Perspectives in perissodactyls. *Equine Veterinary Journal*, 13, 85–87.

85 **SAGER, F.C., 1968.** Management and medical treatment of uterine disease. *Journal of the American Veterinary Medical Association*, 153, 1567–1569.

86 **SCHULZ, K., 1935.** Dourine or slapsiekte. A preliminary report on its occurrence in equines in Griqualand West, Boshof and Jacobsdal districts. *Journal of the South African Veterinary Medical Association*, 6, 4–15.

87 **SCOTT, P., DALEY, P., GIDLEY BAIRD, G., STURGESS, S.**

& FROST, A.J., 1971. The aerobic bacterial flora of the reproductive tract of the mare. *The Veterinary Record*, 88, 58–61.

88 **SHIN, S.J., LEIN, D.H., ARONSON, A.L. & NUSBAUM, S.R., 1979.** The bacteriological culture of equine uterine contents, *in vitro* sensitivity of organisms isolated and interpretation. *Journal of Reproduction and Fertility*, Supplement No. 27, 307–315.

89 **SHIRES, G.M.H. & JOHNSON, J.H., 1974.** Use of silicone rubber implants in mares as a modification of the Caslick procedure. *Veterinary Medicine and Small Animal Clinician*, 69, 1171–1175.

90 **SLUSHER, S.H., FREEMAN, K.P. & ROSZEL, J.F., 1984.** Eosinophils in equine uterine cytology and histology specimens. *Journal of the American Veterinary Medical Association*, 184, 665–670.

91 **SPINCEMAILLE, J. & VANDEPLASSCHE, M., 1964.** *Streptococcus zooepidemicus*: A venereal disease in horses? *V° Congresso Internazionale per la Riproduzione Animale e la Fecondazione Artificiale*. Trento, 166–169.

92 **SULLIVAN, J.J., TURNER, P.C., SELF, L.C., GUTTERIDGE, H.B. & BARTLETT, D.E., 1975.** Survey of reproductive efficiency in the Quarter-horse and Thoroughbred. *Journal of Reproduction and Fertility*, Supplement No. 23, 315–318.

93 **SWERCZEK, T.W., 1979.** Aggravation of strangles, equine clostridial typhlocolitis (colitis X) and bacterial venereal diseases in the horse by antibacterial drugs. *Proceedings of the Twenty-fifth Annual Convention of the American Association of Equine Practitioners*, December 1979, Kentucky, USA.

94 **SWERCZEK, T.W., 1980.** Early fetal death and placental disease in the mare. *Proceedings of the Twenty-sixth Annual Convention of the American Association of Equine Practitioners*, December 1980, Kentucky, USA.

95 **TIMONEY, P.J., McCOLLUM, W.H., MURPHY, T.W., ROBERTS, A.W., WILLARD, J.G. & CARSWELL, D.G., 1987.** The carrier state in equine arteritis virus infection in the stallion with specific emphasis on the venereal mode of virus transmission. *Journal of Reproduction and Fertility*, Supplement No. 35, 95–102.

96 **TIMONEY, P.J., McCOLLUM, W.H. & ROBERTS, A.W., 1986.** Detection of the carrier state in stallions persistently infected with equine arteritis virus. *Proceedings of the Thirty-second Annual Convention of the American Association of Equine Practitioners*, December 1986, Kentucky, USA.

97 **TIMONEY, P.J., McCOLLUM, W.H., ROBERTS, A.W. & MURPHY, T.W., 1986.** Demonstration of the carrier state in naturally acquired equine arteritis virus in the stallion. *Research in Veterinary Science*, 41, 279–280.

98 **TROMMERSHAUSEN BOWLING, A., MILLON, L. & HUGHES, J.P., 1987.** An update of chromosomal abnormalities in mares. *Journal of Reproduction and Fertility*, Supplement No. 35, 149–155.

99 **UPPAL, P.K. & KATARIA, J.M., 1987.** Epidemic of *Salmonella abortus equi* abortion in horses and some studies on the development of a vaccine. *Journal of Reproduction and Fertility*, Supplement No. 35, 669–670.

100 **VAN DYK, E. & LANGE, A. L., 1986.** The detrimental effect of the use of iodine as an intra-uterine instillation in mares. *Journal of the South African Veterinary Association*, 57, 205–210.

101 **VARADIN, M., 1975.** Endometritis, a common cause of infertility in mares. *Journal of Reproduction and Fertility*, Supplement No. 23, 353–356.

102 **WATSON, E.D., 1988.** Uterine defence mechanisms in mares resistant and susceptible to persistent endometritis: A review. *Equine Veterinary Journal*, 20, 397–400.

103 **WEARLY, W.K., MURDICK, P.W. & HENSEL, J.D., 1971.** A five-year study of the use of post-breeding treatment in mares in a Standardbred stud. *Proceedings of the Seventeenth Annual Convention of the American Association of Equine Practitioners*, December 1971, Chicago, USA.

104 **WILLIAMSON, C.C. & HERR, S., 1986.** Dourine in southern Africa 1981–84: Serological findings from the Veterinary Research Institute, Onderstepoort. *Journal of the South African Veterinary Association*, 57, 163–165.

105 **WINGFIELD DIGBY, N.J., 1978.** The technique and clinical application of endometrial cytology in mares. *Equine Veterinary Journal*, 10, 167–170.

106 **WINGFIELD DIGBY, N.J. & RICKETTS, S.W., 1982.** Results of concurrent bacteriological and cytological examinations of the endometrium of mares in routine stud farm practice 1978–81. *Journal of Reproduction and Fertility*, Supplement No. 32, 181–185.

107 **YOUNGQUIST, R.S., 1975.** Pseudomonas metritis in a mare. *Veterinary Medicine and Small Animal Clinician*, 70, 340–342.

108 **ZAFRACAS, A.M., 1975.** *Candida* infection of the genital tract in Thoroughbred mares. *Journal of Reproduction and Fertility*, Supplement No. 23, 349–351.

190

Mastitis

J.H. du Preez and W.H. Giesecke

BOVINE MASTITIS

Introduction

Mastitis, or inflammation of the mammary gland, occurs in all mammalian species but is particularly important in dairy cattle. Mastitis generally results from interaction between a variety of microbial infections and host responses in the udder, and is influenced by management practices.[185] Bacteria are the most common cause of mastitis in cattle.

The extensive application of intramammary antibiotics in the control of mastitis has resulted in a shift in prevalence of the predominant pathogens. *Streptococcus agalactiae* was the most common cause of mastitis in cows prior to 1940,[207] but with the widespread use of antibiotics in the control of mastitis, the prevalence of *S. agalactiae* mastitis has decreased, while mastitis caused by *Staphylococcus aureus*, coliform bacteria, *Mycoplasma* spp., *Streptococcus uberis* and *Staphylococcus epidermidis* has increased globally.[59, 77, 134, 184, 197-199, 203]

The most important effects which mastitis has on the dairy industry[221] are reduced milk yields and deleterious effects on the chemical and cytological composition of milk. In addition, it may result in the presence of bacteria and other infectious agents which may be harmful to humans, and mastitis therapy often results in the presence of antibiotic residues in milk, rendering it unsuitable for human consumption or further processing.

The adequate provision of good quality milk not only promotes public health, but is an important incentive for infrastructural progress and is a stabilizing factor for socio-economic development in rural areas, particularly in developing countries.[32, 133, 174, 193]

It is estimated that at any given time approximately 17–20 per cent of the world's population of dairy cows suffer from mastitis.[34, 117, 145, 146, 189] The financial losses to milk producers as a consequence of mastitis may be great,[20, 75, 115, 147, 155, 210] as the milk yield may be reduced by between 6 and 25 per cent per affected quarter and by between 5 and 84 per cent per affected cow.[139, 172] Affected cows may die, or one or more quarters may become permanently non-functional as a result of mastitis.

It is estimated that mastitis in cattle in the USA causes a loss of approximately $1,3 billion per year.[20] In South Africa, annual financial losses as a result of mastitis escalated from R150 per cow during 1977–78[67] to R414 per cow and R526 million for all herds during 1987–88.[72] Of these losses, clinical mastitis accounted for 18 per cent of the total loss (12 per cent was accounted for by death and premature culling, 5 per cent by reduced milk production and discarded milk, and about 1 per cent for treatment). The greatest proportion of the loss (82 per cent) resulted from reduced milk production from cows with subclinical mastitis.

Modern practices aimed at the control of mastitis include effective hygiene before, during and after milking, efficient dry-cow therapy, and application of measures designed to detect both clinical and subclinical mastitis at an early stage, such as somatic cell counting.[8, 37, 38, 210, 211]

The public health implications of the consumption of milk from mastitic cows and other dairy products derived from such milk are well documented.[69, 70, 77, 80, 88, 92, 110, 142, 165, 208-210, 212, 220, 222, 227] The harmful effects may be due to:

- microorganisms pathogenic for humans, such as *Corynebacterium diphtheriae*[80, 92] **(Table 190.1)**,
- toxic products of microorganisms capable of causing food poisoning, e.g. certain strains of *S. aureus* produce enterotoxins **(see *Staphylococcus* spp. infections: Introduction)**,[88] and
- antimicrobial residues.[11, 21, 110, 137]

Direct sensitization of humans to antibiotics by residues in milk is rare.[2] Residues are deleterious to the manufacture of fermented dairy products such as yoghurt and cheese, and their presence also reduces the quality of butter.[41, 208]

Mastitic milk may also be nutritionally inferior to normal milk **(Table 190.2)** and aesthetically unacceptable.

Aetiology and epidemiology

Although mastitis is caused by both non-infectious (traumatic or toxic) and infectious agents, microorganisms are

POTENTIALLY MASTITOGENIC MICROORGANISMS	DISEASE CAUSED IN HUMANS
Bacillus anthracis	Anthrax
Brucella spp.	Brucellosis
Citrobacter spp., *Klebsiella* spp., *Proteus* spp.	Gastroenteritis
Clostridium perfringens	Food poisoning
Corynebacterium diphtheriae	Diphtheria
Coxiella burnetii	Q fever
Escherichia coli	Infantile gastroenteritis
Pseudomonas spp.	Gastroenteritis
Leptospira spp.	Leptospirosis
Listeria monocytogenes	Listeriosis
Mycobacterium spp.	Tuberculosis
Salmonella serovars	Salmonellosis
Staphylococcus spp.	Enterotoxic gastroenteritis, pyogenic nasal and dermal infections
Streptococcus spp.	Sore throat, scarlet fever, encephalitis, arthritis, endocarditis, urogenital infections, rheumatic fever, glomerulonephritis, dermal infections, sepsis and meningitis of infants, pleuritis

Table 190.1 Public health hazards related to bovine mastitis caused by bacterial udder infections. (Compiled from[69, 72, 86, 110])

the most important aetiological agents.[89, 91, 142] The udder is constantly exposed to a variety of microorganisms, but whether mastitis develops or not depends on the nature of the organism, its virulence and numbers, and the susceptibility of the udder to infection.

The risk of mastitis is higher in early lactation and in high-producing cows, and it increases with the age of the cow.[96] Factors which predispose to mastitis include poor hygiene, poor animal husbandry, malfunction of milking machines and poor milking technique.[10] Milking machines may damage the teat, allowing pathogens easier access to the gland through the teat canal, and may transfer pathogens from one cow to another via contaminated clusters.[49, 50] Milking rates in excess of 2,3 litres per minute and slow milk ejection predispose to mastitis.[187, 190, 232] Factors which adversely affect the normally efficient barriers to infection of the udder, namely the skin of the teats, teat canal **(Figure 190.1)** and mammary cisterns, predispose the udder to mastitis.[71] Ticks cause skin damage which predisposes to abscessation and mastitis.

The microbial causes of mastitis include a wide variety of bacteria (aerobic, facultatively anaerobic,

PARAMETERS	NON-MASTITIC MILK	MASTITIC MILK	PERCENTAGE CHANGE OF VALUES IN MILK
Butterfat (%)	3,45	2,85	17,4
Solid non-fat (%)	8,60	7,95	7,6
Lactose (%)	4,75	Fluctuating at low levels	Lower by up to 81,3%
Protein (%)	3,30	3,30	
casein N (%)	88,0	79,6	9,6
whey protein N (%)	11,8	20,3	72,1
Water (%)	87	87	
pH	6,6–6,8	Usually higher	
Sodium (%)	0,044	0,060	36,36
Chloride (%)	0,91	0,147	83,85
Potassium (%)	0,172	0,157	8,72
Lipase activity (%)	1,49	1,73	16,11
Acid degree value (%)	0,64	1,17	82,81
Serum albumin (mg/ml)	0,38	Higher	
Freezing point	Not exceeding −0,530 °C	Higher	
Somatic cells (x 10^3 ml^{-1})	<500	Usually millions	Several hundred % increase
Pathogenic bacteria	Absent	Usually present	Increase
Antibiotic residues	Absent	Often present	Increase
Titratable acidity		Lower	
Electrical conductivity		Higher	

Mastitic milk tends to develop rancidity problems because activity of lipase is increased by approximately 16 per cent

Table 190.2 Influence of mastitis on the composition of milk[69, 147, 230, 239]

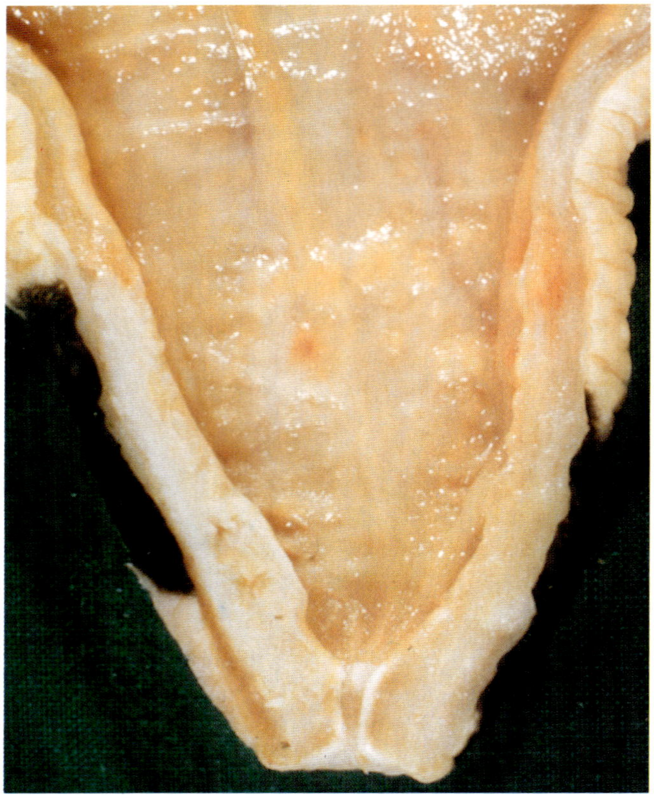

Figure 190.1 Normal bovine teat canal and teat cistern

micro-aerophilic and anaerobic), mycoplasmas, yeasts, fungi, moulds, algae, viruses and rickettsias **(Table 190.3)**.[5, 42, 43, 57, 66, 74, 78, 89, 95, 103, 120, 184, 203, 204, 236, 237] Lumpy skin disease, foot-and-mouth disease and ephemeral fever viruses are the most important viral causes of mastitis in cattle **(Table 190.4)**.[3] Some organisms, such as *Coxiella burnetii* and *Brucella abortus*, may be shed in the milk for weeks without causing apparent lesions in the mammary gland.[16, 111, 177, 182, 183]

Since the introduction of antibiotics in the 1940s there has been a gradual change in the predominant bacteria causing mastitis, from streptococci to staphylococci.[236] This applies particularly to countries where various udder disinfectants and regimens of intramammary antibiotic therapy for mastitis in lactating and non-lactating dairy cattle are used intensively. Microorganisms other than streptococci and staphylococci generally play a comparatively minor role, but mycoplasmas, coliform bacteria, or a combination of *Actinomyces (Corynebacterium) pyogenes*, *Peptococcus indolicus* and *Streptococcus dysgalactiae* may cause sporadic epidemics of clinical mastitis.

In general, staphylococci, and to a lesser extent streptococci, predominate as the cause of mastitis in over 90 per cent of herds with higher-than-normal prevalence of mastitis.[82, 205, 213, 229]

Staphylococcus aureus is not commonly found on healthy teat skin, but does readily colonize or grow in the teat canal. This is especially the case if lesions or sores are present at the teat orifice. Organisms growing in these sites are in an ideal location for infecting the udder, and are transmitted to uninfected quarters by teat-cup liners, udder-wash cloths, and milkers' hands.[156] The sole reservoir of *S. agalactiae* is milk of infected cows, but it can occur on the surfaces of materials and objects (including bedding, milking machines, and milkers' hands recently soiled by contaminated milk). Heifers may become infected from sucking each other in group pens when fed *S. agalactiae*-contaminated milk or colostrum. Spread to uninfected quarters occurs most frequently at milking, and in the absence of good hygiene and effective control measures, *S. agalactiae* can be transmitted rapidly throughout a herd.[156] In addition to the streptococci (*S. agalactiae, S. dysgalactiae, S. uberis*[237]) and *Staphylococcus aureus*,[236] coliform bacteria (*Escherichia coli, Citrobacter freundii, Klebsiella* and *Enterobacter* spp.) and *Actinomyces pyogenes* are the most important causes of bovine mastitis **(Table 190.3)**.

Bacteria of lesser prevalence **(Table 190.3)** include those that cause summer mastitis, a disease of pregnant heifers and dry cows caused primarily by infection with *A. pyogenes, Peptococcus indolicus* and *S. dysgalactiae*, but it is not common in South Africa. These bacteria are thought to be spread by the fly *Hydrotaea irritans*, and for that reason the disease occurs primarily during summer.[156, 184] This form of mastitis most frequently occurs in dry cows and heifers close to calving. Infection tends to result in a persistent form of mastitis. Tuberculous mastitis, which is usually due to infection with *Mycobacterium bovis*, and less often with *M. tuberculosis*, and mycobacteriosis due to *M. avium* are not frequent causes of bovine mastitis in South Africa. Similarly, mastitis caused by infections with *Cryptococcus neoformans, Brucella abortus* and *Clostridium septicum* and other *Clostridium* spp.[89, 184] occurs rarely.

Apart from *Clostridium* spp., other anaerobic bacteria may occasionally be associated with mastitis, but they usually occur concurrently with facultative anaerobic bacteria in mastitic quarters.[42, 47, 52, 81] *Prototheca zopfii*, a colourless alga found in farm ponds or other wet areas contaminated with manure, is a rare cause of bovine mastitis. Other environmental sources include plant material, bedding and silage. Infected quarters usually exhibit a drastic reduction in milk yield.[156]

Infectious and non-infectious conditions may affect the skin of the udder and teats of cattle **(Table 190.4)**.

Pathogenesis

The most common portal of entry of pathogenic bacteria is through the teat or streak canal (galactogenous route) **(Figure 190.2)**. Infections which enter the udder due to trauma or via the haematogenous route are less common. The teat canal has several anatomical features that serve as a barrier to penetration by bacteria **(Figure 190.3)**, but their efficiency decreases progressively with the number

Table 190.3 Most important infectious causes of bovine mastitis[23, 24, 42, 47, 89, 156, 184]

PATHOGENS	TYPE OF MASTITIS
MAJOR PATHOGENS	
Staphylococcus aureus	Mostly subclinical, but may also cause peracute, acute or chronic clinical mastitis. Staphylococci are tissue-invasive and form micro-abscesses which may be encapsulated. Inflammation in the udder may become gangrenous (blue udder)
Streptococcus agalactiae	Mostly subclinical, but may also cause acute or chronic clinical mastitis. Affects mainly the surface of lactiferous ducts and cisterns. *Streptococcus agalactiae* is adapted to the udder. Mastitis frequently occurs under poor hygienic conditions
Streptococcus dysgalactiae	Mostly subclinical, but may also cause acute, subacute or chronic clinical mastitis. *Streptococcus dysgalactiae* is less adapted to the udder than *S. agalactiae*. Mastitis often follows teat lesions
Streptococcus uberis	Mostly subclinical, but may also cause acute or chronic clinical mastitis. *Streptococcus uberis* is ubiquitous in the dairy environment. Infections are common during the dry period
Coliform bacteria (*Escherichia coli*, *Klebsiella* spp. *Enterobacter* spp., and *Citrobacter freundii*)	Usually cause an acute clinical mastitis accompanied by fever and other systemic clinical signs. Endotoxin plays an important role in the pathogenesis of mastitis. *Escherichia coli* occurs commonly in the environment: infection of the udder occurs most commonly in housed dairy cows kept under wet conditions. *Escherichia coli* causes mastitis particularly in the first five weeks of lactation or in the dry period
Actinomyces pyogenes	Causes an acute to chronic clinical mastitis with purulent discharge and abscessation. Pyaemia may result. *Actinomyces pyogenes* in conjunction with other microorganisms, including *S. dysgalactiae* and *Peptococcus indolicus*, causes summer mastitis in heifers and dry cows
MINOR PATHOGENS	
Pseudomonas aeruginosa	Usually causes a mild, chronic mastitis, but the course may be acute and accompanied by severe systemic signs. Outbreaks of mastitis are frequently traced to contaminated water and poor treatment methods
Mycoplasma spp. (most commonly *M. bovis*)	Clinical or subclinical mastitis
Corynebacterium bovis	Mild udder infections; slight elevation in somatic cell count. Occurs most commonly in herds where post-milking teat-dipping is not practised
Coagulase-negative staphylococci (more than 20 species besides *S. aureus*)	Usually a mild, subclinical mastitis. Rarely causes clinical mastitis. Prevalence of mastitis is greatest during the early dry period
Nocardia spp. (most commonly *N. asteroides*)	Purulent granulomatous mastitis. Prognosis is poor
Serratia marcescens	Mild clinical mastitis. *Serratia* can survive in certain teat dips. Spontaneous cure may occur
Bacillus cereus	Causes a haemorrhagic or gangrenous mastitis which may be accompanied by toxaemia
Candida albicans (yeast)	Causes clinical and subclinical mastitis. Occurs when cows are debilitated. Plays a role in superinfection
Prototheca zopfii (alga)	Usually causes a drastic reduction in milk yield
Pasteurella spp.	Usually cause an acute or chronic clinical mastitis. Septicaemia may occur. Pathogen may be transmitted to the udder by nursing calves. Stressful conditions may be a predisposing factor
Brucella abortus	Usually causes subclinical mastitis
Listeria monocytogenes	Mild chronic mastitis
Mycobacterium bovis and other *Mycobacterium* spp.	May cause a productive, lobular-infiltrating tuberculosis, miliary tuberculosis or exudative and caseating mastitis
Clostridium perfringens	Fulminating gangrenous mastitis. Septicaemia or toxaemia may occur. Usually associated with trauma and reduced oxidation-reduction potential of tissue
Bacteroides fragilis and other *Bacteroides* spp., *Veillonella parvula, Megasphaera elsdenii, Eubacterium* spp., *Peptococcus indolicus, Propionibacterium* spp. and *Fusobacterium necrophorum*	Occur concurrently with facultative anaerobic pathogens. Reduced oxidation-reduction potential, tissue necrosis, and disturbances in blood supply predispose to infection

Table 190.4 Infectious and non-infectious causes of skin lesions of the teats and udder of cattle. (Compiled from[66, 89])

INFECTIOUS CONDITIONS		NON-INFECTIOUS CONDITIONS
VIRAL DISEASES	BACTERIAL AND FUNGAL CONDITIONS	
Bovine papillomatosis (warts)	Bacterial folliculitis	Trauma
Bovine herpes mammillitis	Dermatophycosis	Chemical irritants (incorrect dilution of teat disinfectant, contact with irritant plants and bedding material)
Pseudocowpox		Irradiation (photosensitization, sunburn)
Cowpox		Excessive post-parturient oedema
Bovine papular stomatitis		Thermal lesions (burns, frostbite)
Lumpy skin disease		Teat chapping (dehydration)
Pseudo-lumpy skin disease		Tick and mite infestations
Foot-and-mouth disease		
Rinderpest		

of lactations. The teat canal's stratified squamous epithelial lining, spiral longitudinal mucosal folding and sphincter, as well as the sebum-like material containing long-chain fatty acids (produced by keratinization of epithelium cells) within its lumen, and Furstenberg's rosette (a series of folds in which the teat canal terminates proximally), play important roles in its defence mechanisms.[69, 184] Bacteria penetrate the barrier of the streak canal by a process of growth pressure and with the assistance of physical force, such as that caused by capillary action or the differential pressure gradients produced during the process of milking.[184]

The initial inflammatory reaction which results from the entry of infectious agents into the udder is followed by the production and release of a complex of cytokines, interferons and interleukins responsible for fever and the 'acute phase response' which constitutes the primary host defence mechanism to microbial invasion.[161, 226] The

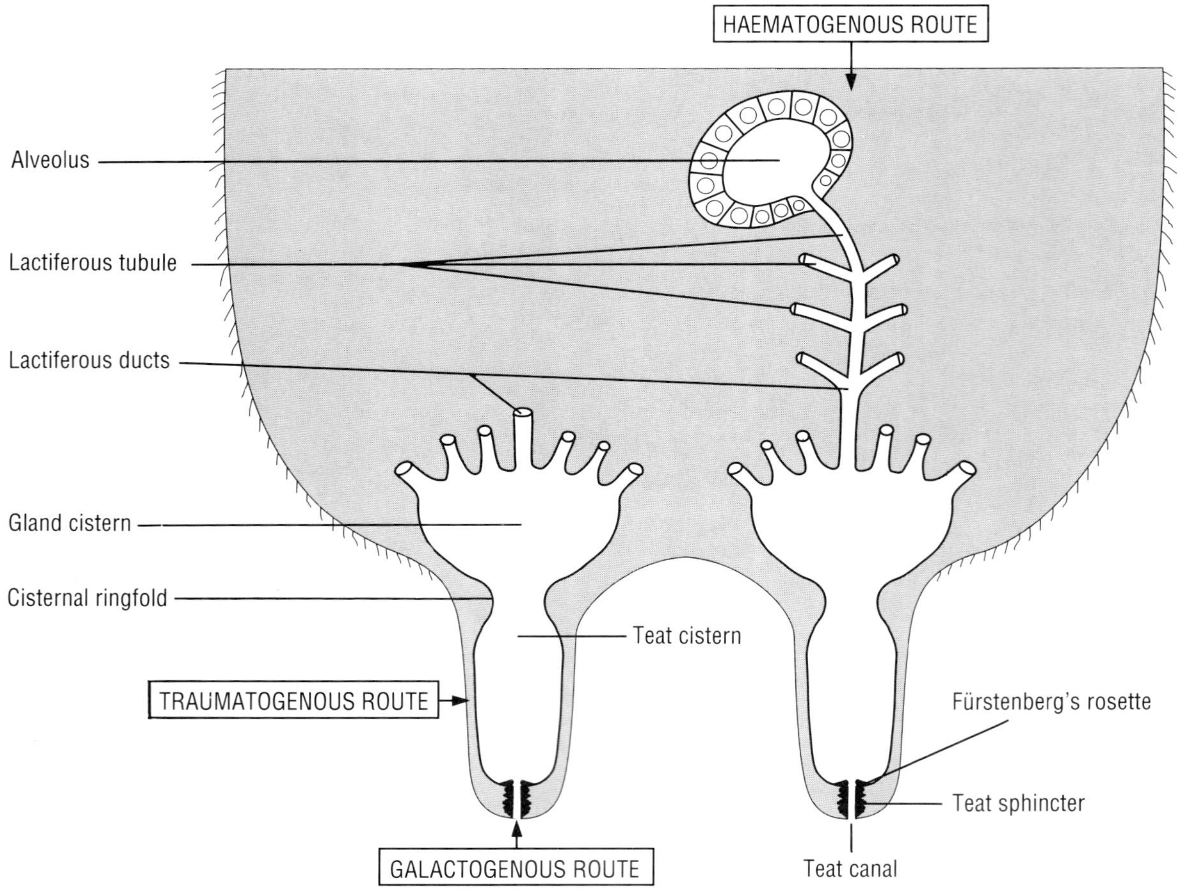

Figure 190.2 Schematic diagram of the bovine udder and routes by which pathogens may reach the udder parenchyma

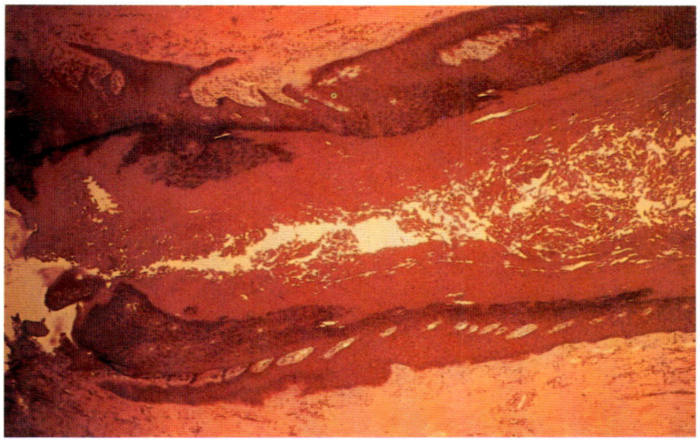

Figure 190.3 Microscopic view of the teat canal

ability of a cow to mount an effective response **(Figure 190.4)** to microbial invasion is critical in her resistance to coliform, staphylococcal and some streptococcal udder infections.[22] Effective humoral and cell-mediated immune responses and the phagocytic activity of macrophages and neutrophils **(Figure 190.4)** are very important.[150] Four defence mechanisms in particular are important in the mammary gland: phagocytosis, toxin neutralization, anti-adhesive properties of antibodies, and direct bacteriolysis.[148]

The severity of the tissue damage and extent of the inflammatory reaction in the udder are determined by the infecting agent and efficacy of the mechanisms of resistance.[184] Compensatory changes that occur in the healthy part of a gland will attempt to restore at least part of the lost milk yield in an udder affected by mastitis, by differentiation and proliferation of inactive alveoli. The mechanisms responsible for stimulating these compensatory processes are not yet fully understood.[24, 119]

The cardinal signs of acute inflammation (heat, hyperaemia, pain, swelling and disturbances of function) are produced by local mediators. In mastitis, inflammatory changes in the udder are increasingly being recognized as crucial to the progress of the disease, and more attention is being directed towards the identification of mediators and modulators involved, and their respective roles.[124, 184]

The detailed pathogenesis of the lesions in the udder following infection with the various infectious agents is largely unknown, although the morphological development of lesions from the early to late stages is generally well documented. Streptococcal infections are characterized by invasion of tissue immediately around the duct system, followed by their rapid neutralization by local defence mechanisms. However, the bacteria tend to persist in the duct system for extended periods, and can therefore re-initiate infection of parenchymatous tissue whenever favourable circumstances develop. The local effects, including the inability of streptococci to invade udder tissue, are attributed to the characteristics of the toxins that they secrete (for details, refer to ***Streptococcus* spp. infections: Introduction** and to the work of Kennedy and Miller[112]). Infection by coliforms apparently also develops mainly galactogenously; however, it is commonly associated with severe systemic effects. Both the local and systemic effects are attributed largely to endotoxin, perhaps aided by other toxins produced by the bacteria. However, detail concerning the pathogenesis of the lesions is lacking.[108]

Some strains of *S. aureus* are tissue invaders and are extremely damaging to the udder parenchyma due to the release of toxins. The adherence of *S. aureus* to fibronectin is an important step in its localization within the udder. Initially, the local effects of the bacteria damage the epithelium lining the teat and udder cisterns. Then they move to the parenchyma, where deep-seated foci of infection become established. This is followed by abscessation, with fibrous encapsulation being a mechanism for restricting infection to localized areas. However, encapsulation adversely affects antibiotic penetration, which is one of the reasons for the poor cure rates commonly experienced in *S. aureus* infections. Three toxins (alpha, beta and gamma haemolysins) may be produced singly or in combination by different strains of *S. aureus*. The alpha toxin is potentially the most damaging, as it causes constriction of blood vessels and ischaemic necrosis which may terminate in gangrenous mastitis. For more information on these toxins, consult ***Staphylococcus* spp. infections: Introduction**.

During the course of staphylococcal mastitis, the extent and distribution of tissue damage are highly variable; sometimes only small areas of the gland are involved. In such areas, necrotic epithelial cells lining alveoli or ducts are cast off and obstruct the duct system, causing involution of remaining functional alveoli and formation of scar tissue. Obstructed ducts may reopen, releasing staphylococci which are then able to produce new foci of infection elsewhere in the gland. This process may be repeated, causing cycles of infection and reinfection in different sites in the quarter. When microorganisms remain within the obstructed ducts and damaged tissue, abscesses may develop, causing lumps that can be palpated in the live animal.[156, 184]

Clinical signs

Cows with acute clinical mastitis usually have systemic and local signs of infection. Those suffering from chronic clinical mastitis show mostly local signs, such as palpable increase in fibrous connective tissue in portions of the udder.[107] Depending on circumstances, the inflammation in the udder is also reflected in changes in the secretion, which include an increase in the number of somatic cells **(Figure 190.5)**, particularly leukocytes, and a decrease in the volume of milk produced.[76] However, subclinical mastitis, which is only detectable on the basis of changes in the composition of apparently normal milk, is a common and economically important problem in dairy herds.

Several classifications of mastitis have been proposed,

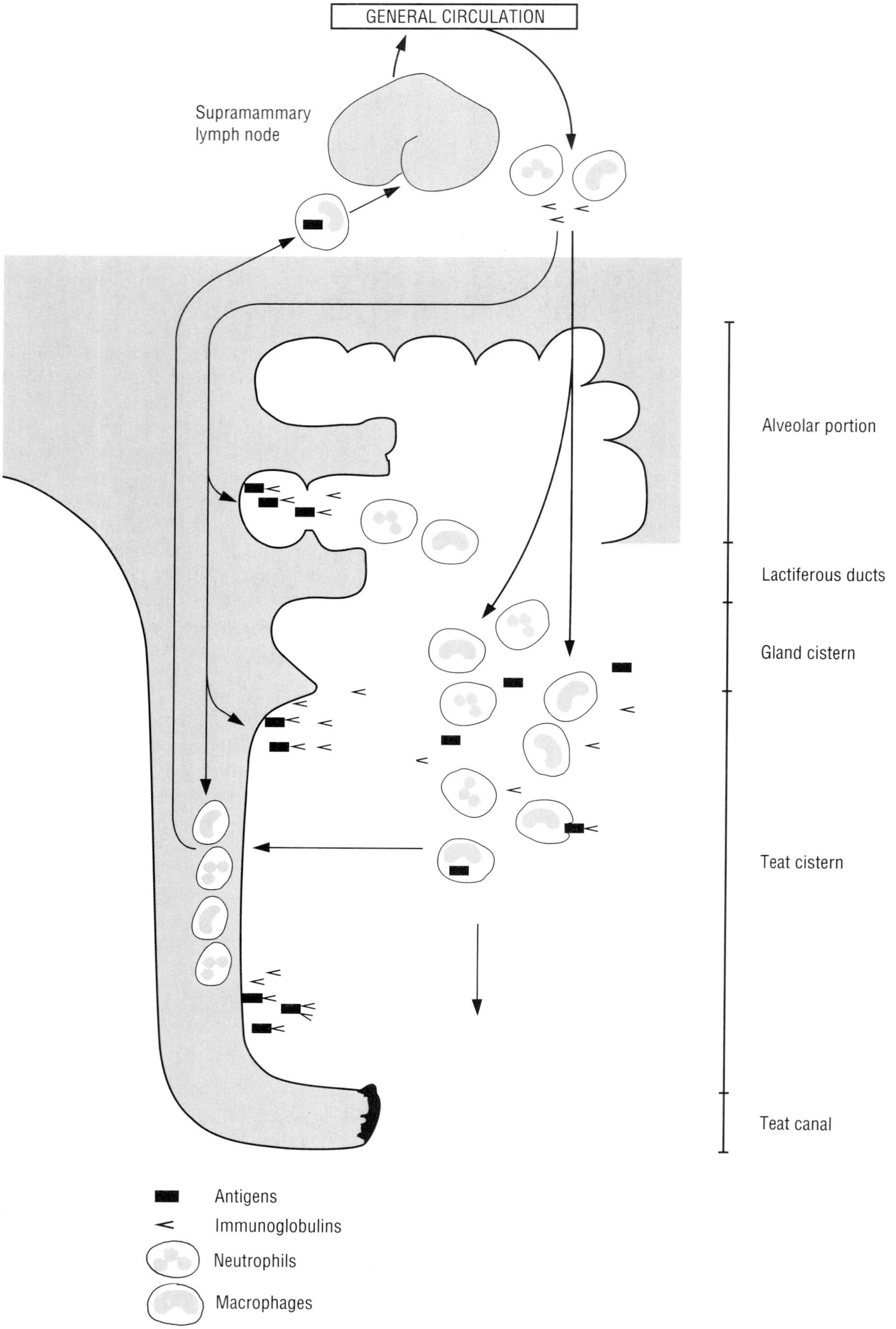

Figure 190.4 Schematic presentation of the intramammary defence mechanism of the bovine udder

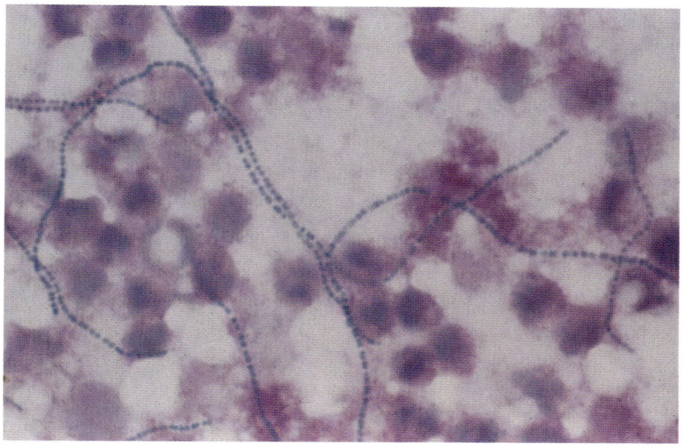

Figure 190.5 Microscopic view of a mastitic milk smear showing somatic cells and streptococci (chain-like)

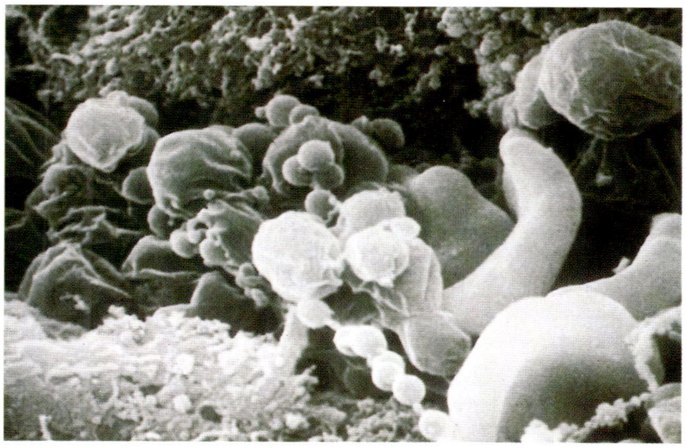

Figure 190.6 Electron microscopic view of *Staphylococcus aureus* that have invaded the tissue of the bovine teat canal

based on aetiological, clinical or pathological aspects of the disease.[17, 61, 89, 116, 127, 135, 141, 158, 184, 216, 217, 231] Bovine mastitis may be classified into subclinical and clinical forms according to severity, duration, distribution, nature of the exudate and primary cause.[12]

A normal quarter is one that shows no outward signs of disease and that produces milk free of pathogenic organisms and with a somatic cell count of less than 500 000 cells/ml.[12, 111, 210]

Subclinical mastitis (Table 190.5)

Several forms are recognized:

Latent infection

Pathogenic microorganisms capable of causing mastitis are present in the mammary gland without any evidence of mastitis and the milk has a normal somatic cell count.[12, 111, 210]

Aseptic or non-specific subclinical mastitis

This is usually caused by trauma or toxins, and pathogenic microorganisms cannot be detected in the milk or quarter. Evidence of inflammation may or may not be detectable in the udder tissue. The products of the inflammatory reaction are present in the secretion, and the milk has an increased somatic cell count (>500 000/ml). [12, 111, 210]

Table 190.5 The classification of subclinical udder conditions according to the criteria of the International Dairy Federation (IDF)[12, 111, 210]

SOMATIC CELL COUNT OF MILK (ml^{-1})	PATHOGENIC MICROORGANISMS	
	ABSENT	PRESENT
<500 000	Normal secretion	Latent udder infection or teat canal infection (TCI) or colonization*
≥500 000	Non-specific mastitis or aseptic mastitis	Subclinical mastitis

* TCI is classified here according to Du Preez.[44, 45, 76] The IDF does not classify teat canal infections in the above-mentioned classification

Infectious subclinical mastitis

Pathogens and the products of the inflammatory reaction can be detected in the milk by laboratory methods, but there are no macroscopic changes in either the milk or the udder tissue.

Latent udder infection

This must be distinguished from teat canal infection, in which pathogenic microorganisms invade and proliferate in tissue of the teat canal **(Figure 190.6)** causing local damage. The milk may have a normal (<500 000 cells/ml) or, sometimes, increased somatic cell count.[43, 44] Teat canal colonization by pathogenic microorganisms is detected in samples collected through the teat canal but not in samples taken by teat-wall puncture.[12]

Clinical mastitis

Clinical mastitis is most frequently infectious, and it is classified according to its severity and rapidity of onset and duration, into peracute, acute, subacute and chronic forms.[12, 111, 116, 184, 210]

Peracute mastitis (Figure 190.7)

This is characterized by sudden onset, a severe, acute inflammatory reaction involving one or more quarters of the udder, and signs of systemic involvement, such as fever, depression, shivering, anorexia, inappetence, rapid weak pulse, dehydration, weakness and rapid loss of weight. Shock, diarrhoea, 'downer-cow' syndrome, reduced milk yield, loss of muscle coordination, cold extremities and reduced pupillary reflex may also occur, depending on the severity of the condition. The milk is macroscopically abnormal **(Figure 190.8)** and may be bloody, watery, purulent or fibrinous, and contain clots,

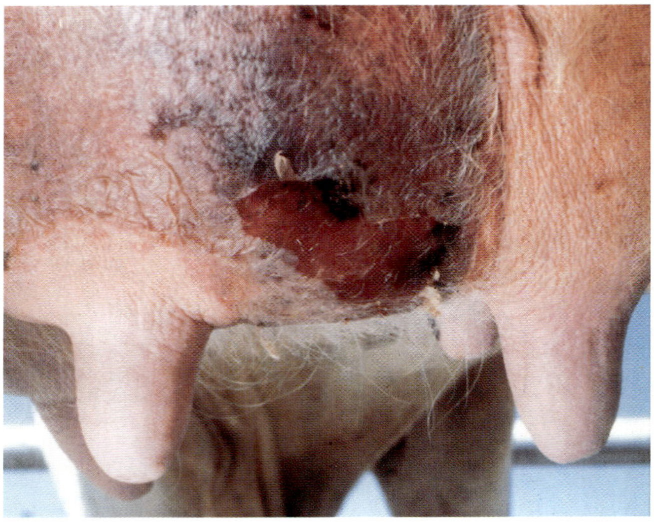

Figure 190.7 Peracute gangrenous mastitis caused by *Staphylococcus aureus*

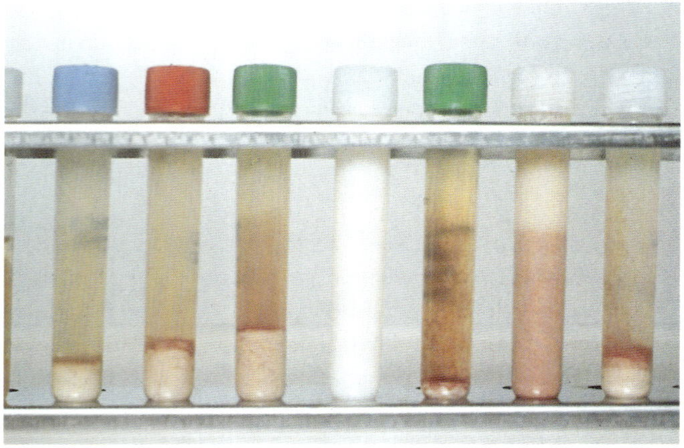

Figure 190.8 Tubes containing mastitic milk from cows with clinical mastitis

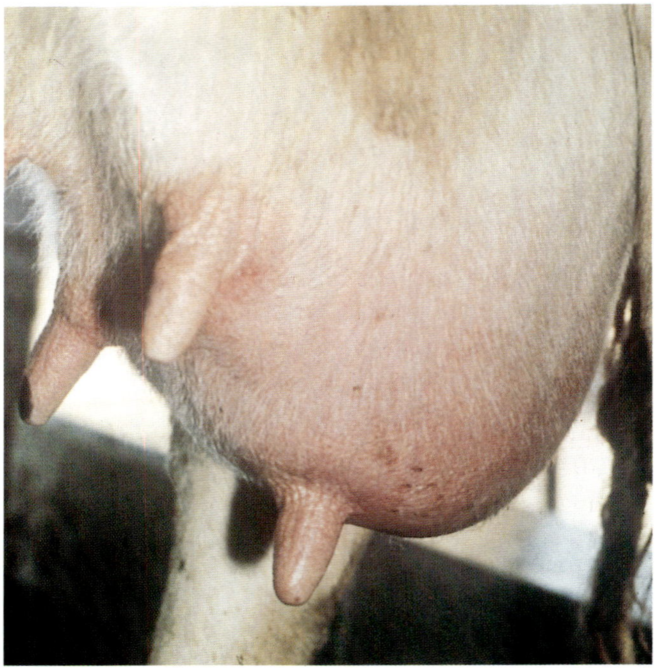

Figure 190.9 Subacute mastitis: a cow's udder with one swollen quarter

flakes or shreds consisting of fibrin and cellular debris. Peracute gangrenous mastitis may lead to loss of the quarter, or in some cases to death of the cow. Gangrenous mastitis is evident as a patchy blue discoloration of the udder, and the skin covering the affected area is cold. Blood-stained serum may ooze through the skin.

Acute mastitis

This is characterized by the presence of an inflammatory reaction in the udder which is similar to, but less marked than, that which occurs in peracute mastitis. There is usually an accompanying mild fever and the animal is slightly depressed. The milk is macroscopically abnormal and there is a reduced milk yield.

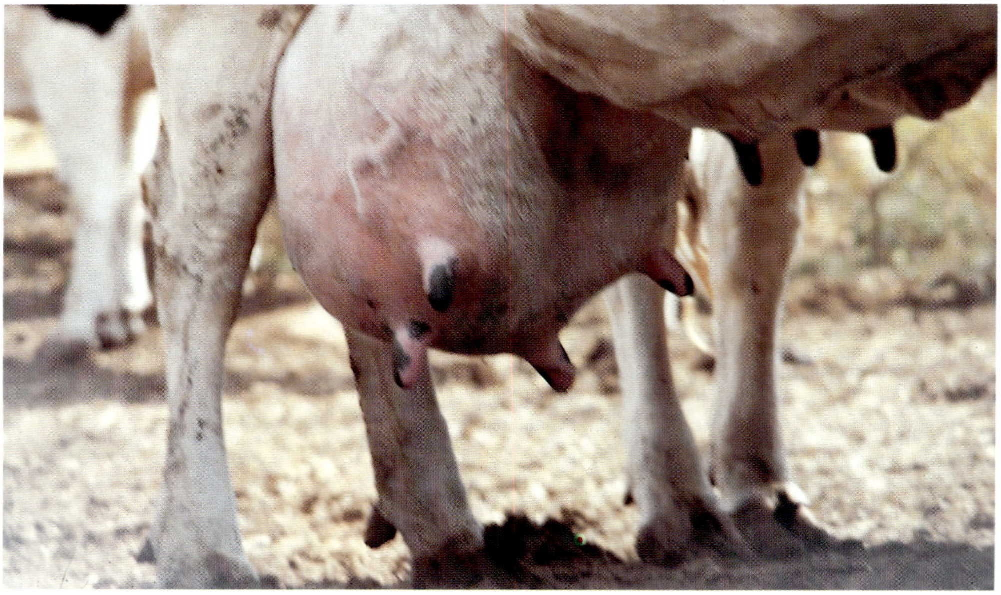

Figure 190.10 Chronic mastitis: an enlarged and fibrotic udder

Subacute mastitis **(Figure 190.9)**
The signs of inflammation in the udder and the changes in the milk are milder than those present in acute mastitis. Subacute mastitis is not accompanied by systemic effects but the milk yield is reduced.

Chronic mastitis **(Figure 190.10)**
The inflammatory process persists for many months, or from one lactation to the next. Chronic mastitis may be clinical or subclinical but there are often, at varying intervals, periodic recrudescences into subacute or acute forms which are mostly of short duration. The changes which occur in the milk from cases of chronic subclinical mastitis are only detected by performing laboratory tests.[12] The chronic mastitic quarter fails to respond to treatment and there is progressive fibrosis which leads to enlargement and asymmetry of the gland. The gland or a portion of it may eventually atrophy. These changes are generally permanent.

Pathology

The lesions caused by bacteria commonly associated with mastitis, i.e. streptococci, staphylococci, coliforms, and *A. pyogenes*, are relatively well described, but lesions caused by microorganisms that are sporadically involved are generally poorly described. Tuberculous mastitis, which nowadays is encountered less often in cattle due to the introduction of eradication programmes in many countries, is dealt with in **Chapter 172: Tuberculosis**.

Streptococcal mastitis is characterized by periodic recrudescence of infection following multiplication of bacteria in the teat cisterns. The lesions are usually localized in the ventral portions of the udder, often with more than one quarter involved. The macroscopic appearance of affected quarters varies according to the stage of the disease. During the acute stage of the inflammatory process, the affected tissue is oedematous, firm, granular and greyish. The epithelium of the cisterns and ducts is not appreciably affected during the early stages of the disease, but in the later stages most of the lesions in the udder occur in and in close association with the duct system as epithelial thickening, the development of small polyps, and periductal fibrosis. The development of these lesions is associated with the formation of interstitial oedema, and an influx of neutrophils into the interstitial tissue and acini. Cells of the acini degenerate and become necrotic. In association with the interstitial reaction, an early fibroblastic response is elicited which is accompanied by involution of affected lobules and those in close association with them. As the process progresses, fibrosis becomes more pronounced and is accompanied by a macrophage and lymphocyte infiltrate — the lymphocytes often being aggregated into lymphoid follicles — while milk stagnates in the smaller ducts. In affected udders the whole range of lesions from the acute stage to fibrosis and involution often occur simultaneously. Bacteria are present in abundance in the lesions only during the acute stages of the inflammatory response, and they occur only in and around the cisterns and ducts. As the lesions progress, granulation tissue develops in the walls of affected ducts, sometimes forming polyps which protrude into and obstruct the duct lumens, while at the same time squamous metaplasia of the luminal epithelium may occur. In affected ducts, streptococci persist in the accumulated exudate, often in large numbers.[112]

Staphylococcal mastitis may be peracute, acute, subacute or chronic, the latter being the form most often seen. Peracute to acute gangrenous mastitis, which may be restricted to the teat and the adjacent udder or involve the entire quarter, is characterized by the affected tissues being dark red to black, and dull in appearance. Necrosis and venous thrombosis, which are the main features of the lesion, may extend throughout the gland or be restricted to foci within it. If the affected animal remains alive for some time, the gangrenous tissue sloughs within a week, leaving a raw, purulent surface. In less severe forms of staphylococcal mastitis, the onset is insidious and results in the development of pyogranulomas. Contrary to the situation in streptococcal mastitis, bacteria are present within the lesions and throughout the affected tissue.[112] As the lesions progress, a marked granulomatous mastitis with fibroplasia develops. This process is referred to as botryomycosis (for details of this lesion refer to **Chapter 146: *Staphylococcus aureus* infections**).

Mastitis caused by the coliform bacteria (*Escherichia coli* and species of *Enterobacter, Klebsiella, Citrobacter, Serratia* and *Proteus*) is usually acute and recurrent. Affected animals often manifest signs related to the effects of endotoxin. The inflammatory reaction in coliform mastitis varies from serous to haemorrhagic and commences in the duct system, in which necrotic debris, fibrin, coagulated milk and blood may occur, sometimes blocking the ducts. In the interstitial tissue, severe oedema, thrombi — particularly in the veins — and extensive haemorrhage characterize the inflammatory response. In acute cases, if the animal survives, large areas of the affected tissues become necrotic but not gangrenous.[108, 112]

In the case of summer mastitis caused by *A. pyogenes*, which is often isolated from the lesions in mixed culture with organisms such as *S. dysgalactiae* and *Fusobacterium necrophorum* **[see Chapter 145: *Fusobacterium necrophorum, Dichelobacter* (*Bacteroides*) *nodosus* and *Bacteroides* spp. infections]**, the portal of entry is usually a traumatic injury in a teat. From there the inflammatory process extends along the ducts and develops into a severe necropurulent galactophoritis, with subsequent abscessation due to the accumulation of exudate in the ducts. In the advanced stages of the infection, chronic proliferative changes occur in the duct epithelium.[112]

The udder tissue in mycoplasmal mastitis during the early stages of the disease is swollen, firm, nodular, light brown to yellowish on cut surface, and has a tough consistency. As the disease progresses, the udder becomes reduced in size, tough, and smooth on cut surface. Multiple abscesses, which may vary from 50–100 mm in diameter, occur in some cases. The cisterns and ducts are filled with a purulent exudate. In acute cases the regional lymph nodes are markedly oedematous and hyperplastic. Histologically, the early inflammatory reaction is characterized by a marked influx of neutrophils, although in some cases eosinophils are the major constituent of the cellular part of the exudate, particularly in the interstitial tissue. Development of the lesions is characterized by progressive fibrosis and infiltration by lymphocytes, plasma cells and macrophages. Abscesses may occur in fibrosed glands. Mycoplasmas scattered throughout the affected tissue can be demonstrated by immunofluorescent techniques.[104]

Diagnosis

Several simple tests performed on the farm (cowside), or more complicated laboratory tests are used to diagnose mastitis in individual cows or on a herd basis.[12, 156, 184]

Clinical mastitis may be detected by examining the udder for warm, swollen quarters, which are indicative of acute mastitis, or for misshapen, hard, atrophied and fibrotic quarters, indicating permanent damage caused by chronic mastitis.

The strip cup test **(Figure 190.11)** is a practical and effective method of identifying cows with clinical mastitis. A few millilitres of the foremilk of each quarter are milked into a strip cup or plate. Abnormal milk is usually discoloured, watery, or contains flakes, shreds or clots, but in chronic mastitis the milk is not always macroscopically abnormal. The strip cup test is not sufficiently sensitive to detect subclinical mastitis.

When a strip cup is used, it should be cleaned and disinfected after every milking. The removal of foremilk samples for strip cup testing reduces the bacterial count in subsequent samples of milk from a quarter, since the first streams of milk commonly contain the largest number of bacteria.

The California milk test (CMT) is another cowside test that can be used for the detection of mastitis **(Figure 190.12)**. It is more sensitive than the strip cup test and enables subclinical mastitis to be detected. The basis of the CMT is the reaction which occurs when the reagent comes into contact with the increased quantity of cell material derived from increased numbers of somatic cells in the milk. Somatic cell numbers in milk tend to increase during milking, and remain high for several hours thereafter, even in uninfected quarters. For reliable results, the CMT should be conducted just before milking, after stimulating the cow, and having discarded the foremilk. The reaction is then scored as O (negative), T (trace), 1 (slight), 2 (moderate) or 3 (heavy), depending on the extent of gel formation **(Table 190.6)**.

The CMT enables rapid detection of subclinical mastitis or milk with increased somatic cells that might otherwise go undetected until it becomes advanced. However, only 60 per cent of cows with somatic cell counts greater than 500 000/ml are actually infected with mastitis-causing microorganisms, and a positive CMT result does not justify automatic antimicrobial treatment.

Because mastitis alters the electrolyte composition of milk, the electrical conductivity of mastitic milk is changed. This can be used as a cowside test, but it is applied more in research than in practical situations.

Various other cowside tests exist, such as the catalase, Whiteside, and Wisconsin mastitis tests, and the determination of the pH of foremilk with indicator dyes. However, these are all less sensitive than the CMT.

The bacteriological culture of milk samples from individual quarters or of composite samples from all four quarters of individual cows is required to determine the aetiological agent(s) involved.[12, 144]

In herds with a large number of subclinical cases of mastitis, a reliable diagnosis can be made by culturing samples of milk from cows selected on the basis of increased CMT scores or somatic cell counts. In herds with low somatic cell counts but a high prevalence of clinical mastitis, samples from all clinical cases should be cultured to establish the cause of the problem. With certain types of infections (such as *E. coli*), culture of the milk of every cow in a herd is sometimes indicated. In very severe or unresponsive mastitis, an antibiogram is required to allow the selection of appropriate antimicrobials.

Samples of milk from cows suffering from clinical mastitis, or from those whose milk has high somatic cell counts, often yield no organisms on culture. As many as

Table 190.6 Relationship between results of the California milk (mastitis) test (CMT) and somatic cell counts in milk. (Compiled from [156, 184])

CMT RESULTS*	GEL FORMATION	SOMATIC CELL COUNT PER ML MILK
0	None	100 000 – 200 000
T	Slight	150 000 – 500 000
1	Slight to moderate	400 000 – 1 500 000
2	Moderate	1 000 000 – 5 000 000
3	Heavy	Generally over 5 000 000

* Alkaline milk (pH 7,0 or more) imparts a deep purple colour to the reagent/milk mixture. Acid milk (pH 5,2 or less) gives a yellow colour **(Figure 190.12)**

25–30 per cent of such specimens may exhibit no growth. In certain instances, such as in chronic coliform infections, the number of bacteria in a milk specimen may be too low to be detected by routine methods, and repeated culture and the use of special methods may be necessary to isolate the agent involved. In other cases, the infection may have been eliminated, but an elevated somatic cell count persists because healing is not complete and leukocytes are still infiltrating the udder tissues. In instances where specimens from a herd with a mastitis problem are consistently negative when cultured by routine methods, the possibility of an unusual organism that will not grow on standard culture media (such as *Mycoplasma* spp., anaerobic bacteria, fungi, or algae) should be considered.

The reliability of laboratory culturing depends on how milk samples are collected and stored **(Figure 190.13)**. When milk samples are taken from individual quarters, the initial two or three streams of milk should be discarded, whereafter the teat end should be wiped with a cotton wool swab moistened with 70 per cent alcohol prior to collecting the specimen. Teats on the far side of the udder should be cleaned first and the near teats last. When the teat ends are dry, milk samples should be collected in sterile test tubes, collecting those from the near teats first. After collection, the samples should be kept at 4 °C and should reach the laboratory in a chilled state within 24 hours. If samples must be stored for longer periods, they should be frozen. Frozen samples are not suitable for somatic cell counts.

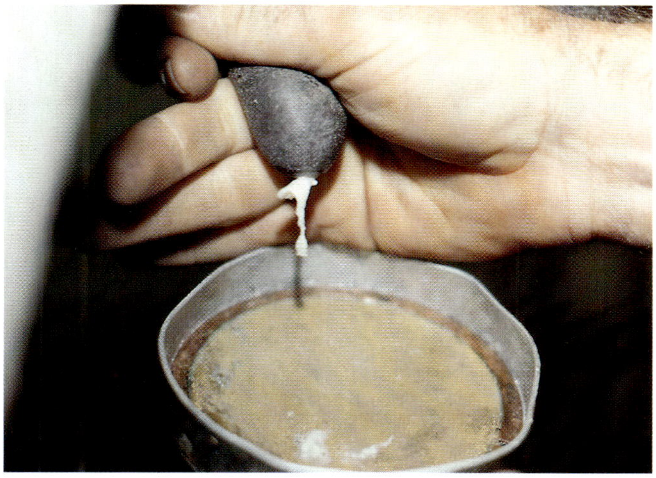

Figure 190.11 A strip cup with milk containing pus

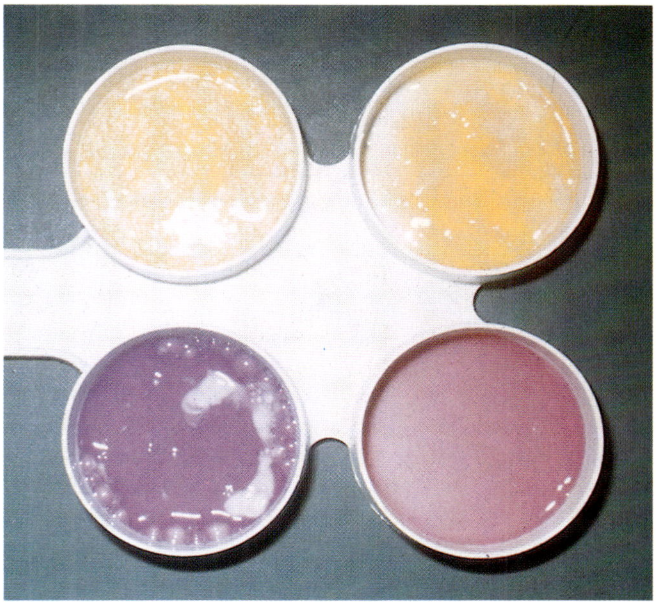

Figure 190.12 California mastitis test: the purple coloured gel is an indication of alkaline subclinical mastitic milk, and the yellow milk of acid subclinical mastitic milk

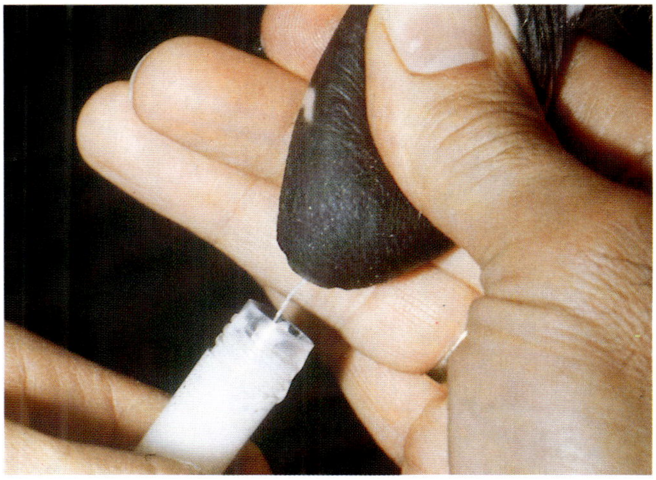

Figure 190.13 Collection of foremilk samples from infected quarters for microbiological examination

Control

Generally the objective of any dairy is to produce as much milk as cost-effectively as possible. Mastitis not only reduces the productive capacity of cows; it is also expensive to treat. Therefore its prevention should be a priority. As mastitis cannot be controlled by breeding more resistant cows or by immunization, improved animal husbandry and management are the only practical methods of control.[51, 114]

Prevention of mastitis depends primarily on good hygiene practices and effective animal management, and unless these are attended to, the prevention and control of mastitis are impossible in the long term. Cows suffering from mastitis may recover spontaneously, but usually drug therapy is required to effect a cure.

Therapy

For antimicrobial therapy to be successful, the drug employed must reach the causative organism at the focus of infection in the udder in concentrations exceeding the minimal inhibitory concentration, and these levels must be maintained for the time required to eliminate the causative pathogen.[9, 129] In severe cases of mastitis, particularly when permanent damage has occurred, culling may be the most economic option.

Intramammary treatment is the technique of choice for subclinical, chronic, or mild clinical mastitis, and is by far the most common method.[129, 159, 245] In peracute or acute clinical mastitis, however, the frequent failures that occur following intramammary antimicrobial therapy are considered to be due to poor or uneven distribution of antimicrobial drugs through the intensely swollen udder parenchyma, with the milk duct system being either compressed or blocked.[159, 245] Under these circumstances parenteral antimicrobial therapy is indicated.[64, 159, 245] In cases of peracute or acute clinical mastitis in which systemic signs are present, intramammary infusion and parenteral therapy with antimicrobials alone or in combination with corticosteroids and other therapeutics **(Table 190.7)** are recommended.[245] The withholding periods of milk for human consumption after the administration of the last intramammary treatment with some antimicrobial preparations are listed in the respective directions for use.

For the treatment of infections in which the bacteria are not tissue-invasive (such as streptococci) and in early cases of staphylococcal mastitis, intramammary infusion of antimicrobial drugs generally gives satisfactory results.[129, 214] For intramammary treatment, drugs that are readily distributed throughout the udder should be chosen **(Table 190.8)**.

All teat canal or intramammary treatments must be administered after the affected quarter has been emptied of milk. The drug manufacturer's instructions regarding frequency, duration and level of treatment should be followed exactly. The administration of oxytocin in order to achieve complete milk let-down, followed by thorough stripping of the affected quarter prior to antimicrobial infusion, is a useful procedure in the treatment of acute mastitis.[241] If there is no clinical improvement within 24–48 hours of initiation of intramammary therapy, it is advisable to change the therapeutic agent. More detail on methods of treatment may be obtained from the relevant literature.[43, 44, 100, 128, 129, 138, 159, 178, 184, 241, 246-249]

Successful parenteral therapy depends on effective

Table 190.7 Supportive therapy for cows with peracute or acute mastitis.* (Compiled from[7, 68, 89, 100, 156, 176, 184])

TREATMENT**	DOSAGE	ROUTE OF ADMINISTRATION	INTERVAL BETWEEN DOSES	COMMENTS
Isotonic saline and sodium bicarbonate if cow cannot stand	5–10 l saline and 150–250 g sodium bicarbonate	iv	4–8 hrs	Essential to restore circulating volume quickly with endotoxic/hypotensive shock
Isotonic saline	25 l	Oral	24 hrs	Possible alternative to above (oral fluids are sometimes poorly absorbed)
Oxytocin	20–30 iu	iv	12 hrs	Facilitates stripping of milk
Frequent milking			Every 1–4 hrs	Keeps milk ducts patent and removes toxins, debris, bacteria and inflammatory products
20 per cent calcium borogluconate	400–800 ml	iv	–	If indicated (coliform mastitis), give slowly and diluted in saline
Glucose (5,10 or 50 per cent)	2–5 l	iv	12 hrs	Reverses hypoglycaemia
Etamiphylline camsylate or theophylline	1 400 mg	iv or im	8 hrs	Increases the stroke volume of the heart and improves pulmonary function
Aspirin	30 g	Oral	8 hrs	Reduces pain, temperature and inflammation and restores appetite
Concentrated multivitamins (especially B-complex group)	30 ml	iv or im	24 hrs	Liver support, supplement enzyme systems
Corticosteroids (dexamethasone)	1–3 mg/kg	iv or im	Usually a single dose	Reduce swelling and pain, and thereby enhance removal of toxic secretions and promote better diffusion of intramammary infusions
Immunoglobulin (γ globulin, 75,0 per cent m/v of total protein)	20–50 ml	iv	6 hrs	Neutralizes toxins, stimulates and improves phagocytosis
Antihistamines	Various	iv or im	12 hrs	Anti-inflammatory and counteract shock
Flunixin meglumine	1,1 mg/kg	iv	12 hrs	Counteracts effects of inflammatory prostaglandins

iv = intravenous
im = intramuscular
* Supportive therapy with fluids is often more important than the antibiotic selected[46, 53]
** Fresh, cool drinking water must be freely available; soft digestible, high-quality, and nutritious hay must be available *ad lib.*; enough rest without disturbance is of the utmost importance for rapid recovery; and animal must be kept in a comfortable environment[46, 53]

Table 190.8 Distribution of antimicrobial drugs after parenteral and intramammary administration. (Compiled from [248])

DRUG	PARENTERAL*			INTRAMAMMARY**		
	Good	Limited	Poor	Good	Limited	Poor
Aminosidine			+			+
Amoxycillin		+		+		
Ampicillin		+		+		
Bacitracin						+
Cephalosporins		+				
Cephalexin				+		
Cephaxazole					+	
Cephalonium					+	
Cephapirin					+	
Cephacetrile					+	
Chloramphenicol	+			+		
Clindamycin	+			+		
Cloxacillin		+			+	
Dapsone				+		
(Dihydro) streptomycin			+			+
Erythromycin	+			+		
Fusidic acid		+				
Gentamycin			+			+
Kanamycin			+			+
Lincomycin	+			+		
Neomycin			+			+
Nitrofurans				+		
Novobiocin		+		+		
Other sulphonamides		+		+		
Oxacillin					+	
Penethamate	+			+		
Penicillin G		+			+	
Polymyxins			+			+
Oleandomycin	+			+		
Quinolines				+		
Rifamycin		+		+		
Spiramycin	+			+		
Spectinomycin			+			
Sulphanilamide	+			+		
Tetracyclines		+			+	
Tylosin	+			+		
Trimethoprim	+			+		
Vancomycin			+			

* As determined experimentally from the milk/serum drug concentration ratios
** As determined experimentally from the rate of drug absorption from the udder or from physiochemical properties of the drug

passage of the drug from the blood into the milk at or near the foci of infection. The extent to which a drug enters the milk ducts from the circulation is largely governed by three properties of the therapeutic molecule, viz. its lipid solubility, degree of ionization (reflected in the dissociation constant [pKa]) and the extent to which it binds with serum proteins.[194] The passage of drugs across the blood-milk barrier occurs by passive diffusion[136] and, as is the case with biological membranes, this barrier is breached readily only by the non-ionized, non-protein-bound, lipid-soluble fraction of a drug.[168, 170] Only unbound or plasma-protein-free drugs diffuse out of the vascular system to exert their pharmacological or antimicrobial activity in the udder.[13]

The blood supply to the udder generally ensures that parenteral administration of rationally selected antimicrobials may be used as the sole method of treatment for acute mastitis. Even when severe lesions are present in the udder, the parenteral administration of drugs usually gives a very even distribution of the drug throughout the udder.[129]

An ideal antimicrobial drug intended for parenteral therapy for mastitis should have the following characteristics:[248]

- low minimal inhibitory concentration against the majority of udder pathogens,
- high bio-availability from the injection site,
- chemically, either a weak base or a drug which does not become highly ionized in blood plasma,
- sufficient lipid solubility,

- low degree of serum protein binding,
- long half-life in the body, and
- no drug accumulation in organs, such as the udder.

Antimicrobials should preferably be selected for the pathogen involved. Broad-spectrum antimicrobials may be used initially until such time that an antibiogram has been performed. If antibiograms cannot be conducted, broad-spectrum antimicrobials that are effective against Gram-positive and Gram-negative bacteria should be used.[204, 241]

Milk samples should be collected aseptically from all four quarters of each clinical case of mastitis before treatment is instituted. These can be stored in a refrigerator at 4 °C or frozen if it is decided not to perform bacteriological examinations and antibiograms immediately on the causative organism (if this is a bacterium). They can, if necessary, be examined subsequently and antibiograms established if there is no response to the initial therapy. Clinical mastitis should be treated as soon as it is diagnosed. If no success is achieved in treating mastitis during lactation, the affected quarter may often be treated with greater success once the cow has been dried off.[241]

The following antimicrobial drugs are commonly available for treating animals suffering from mastitis:

Penicillins

The majority of isolates of haemolytic staphylococci from bovine milk samples are resistant to penicillin, whereas virtually all species of streptococci are sensitive to the drug.[56, 129]

The activity of penicillin is decreased only slightly in milk.[162] Penicillin is a weak organic acid with a pKa of 2,7, and is therefore largely ionized in plasma; milk levels will therefore always be lower than plasma levels.[168, 169] While its absorption rate is moderate, penicillin is well distributed throughout the udder and diffuses relatively well into mammary tissue in both normal and mastitic glands, except where there are large areas of necrosis or fibrosis.[64, 218, 244] Such diffusion probably occurs because penicillin is moderately lipid-soluble.[243] Moreover, penicillin concentrations are higher in the milk of mastitic udders than in normal quarters. Intramammary penicillin at a dose of 11 000 IU/kg body weight twice daily, continued for three to five days, should be used for mastitis therapy.[138]

The majority of isolates from mastitic cases caused by *Staphylococcus aureus* are resistant to sodium benzylpenicillin, whereas virtually all species of streptococci are sensitive.[128, 129]

Cloxacillin is a narrow-spectrum, semi-synthetic penicillin which is highly lipid-soluble and resistant to staphylococcal penicillinase. In lactating cows, infusion of cloxacillin is as effective as benzylpenicillin against streptococcal and staphylococcal infections.[125, 128, 129]

Ampicillin is a semi-synthetic penicillin with a broad spectrum of activity which diffuses into the udder slightly better than benzylpenicillin.[250] The dose necessary to maintain milk levels that are effective against microorganisms (i.e. with minimal inhibitory concentrations in the range of 0,5–1,0 μg/ml for 24 hours) is approximately 10–20 mg/kg body weight.[243] This dose is several times higher than that usually recommended.[128] It has been recommended that an intramuscular dose of ampicillin at 10 mg/kg twice daily and an intramammary dose of 62,5 mg twice daily be continued for three to five days.[138]

Parenteral doses even as high as 9 000 000 IU/cow of benzathine penicillin are unlikely to produce bacteriostatic levels in milk,[186] and the use of this drug is not recommended.[128]

Dihydrostreptomycin

This is seldom used alone for intramammary treatment, but is often used in combination with penicillin.[125] Dihydrostreptomycin, one of the aminoglycosides, is a base with a pKa of 8,0 and low lipid solubility, and is unsuitable for systemic treatment of mastitis[129] as it is unlikely that even in very high doses it ever reaches therapeutic levels in milk.[251] The aminoglycosides have fairly low minimal inhibitory concentrations for staphylococci and for some Gram-negative mastitis pathogens, but their activity against streptococci is low.[140] The activity of dihydrostreptomycin is also markedly decreased in the presence of milk,[242] possibly because of its extensive binding to milk protein,[251] and it has a very uneven distribution within the udder, taking up to eight hours to become widely dispersed throughout the udder parenchyma.[244]

Tetracyclines

Oxytetracycline and chlortetracycline are partially inactivated in milk by chelation with magnesium and calcium ions and by combining with casein.[137] Injectable oxytetracycline has limited bio-availability after being administered intramuscularly[14, 247] and does not reach therapeutic levels in the milk.[247] Intravenous administration at 10 mg/kg will maintain the concentration of oxytetracycline in milk at levels in excess of 1,0 μg/ml for 24 hours,[138] which is above the minimal inhibitory concentration of oxytetracycline for pathogenic staphylococci and streptococci. Gram-negative organisms require concentrations in excess of 2,44 μg/ml.[157] As oxytetracycline is a local tissue irritant, and is very unevenly distributed in normal udder tissue following intramammary injection, its use for this purpose is not recommended.[244]

Neomycin

This has limited penetration in the udder, due mainly to poor lipid solubility.[252] This curtails its potential usefulness in both parenteral and local treatment of mastitis. Nevertheless, neomycin has been used as the main ingredient in combination drugs for intramammary mastitis therapy because of its wide antimicrobial spectrum.[181]

A dosage of 88 mg/kg of body weight administered intramuscularly and repeated at 12-hour intervals for three days is suggested for parenteral use.

Erythromycin

The macrolide antibiotics (erythromycin, tylosin, lincomycin and spiromycin) pass effectively from the blood into the udder but their antibacterial spectra are limited to Gram-positive pathogens. They are the drugs of choice when attempting to eliminate persistent Gram-positive udder infections.[248] In the treatment of acute mastitis caused by Gram-positive udder pathogens, combined parenteral and intramammary application is recommended.[248] Erythromycin at a dosage of 12,5 mg/kg intramuscularly repeated at 24-hour intervals is sufficient to maintain milk levels at more than 11 µg/ml.[13] An intramuscular dose of 5 mg/kg of erythromycin twice daily, combined with an intramammary dose of 300 mg twice daily, for three to five days is generally recommended.[138]

Chloramphenicol

Chloramphenicol has limited bio-availability following intramuscular administration,[14, 248] and should be administered intravenously.[248] When administered at a dosage of 50 mg/kg, chloramphenicol is present in milk at levels of 22,8 µg/ml for 12 hours and at 12,2 µg/ml for 24 hours after injection.[79] In certain countries the use of chloramphenicol in food-producing animals is strictly forbidden because its use constitutes a potential human health hazard.

Sulphonamides and trimethoprim

Sulphadimidine, when given intravenously at a dose of 200 mg/kg, will maintain milk levels of more than 50 µg/ml for 20 hours, which are sufficient to eliminate both streptococci and staphylococci infections. An initial dose of sulphamethazine of 100 mg/kg administered intravenously and followed by 50 mg/kg daily intravenously for three to five days has been recommended.[138]

Trimethoprim has a rather short half-life which, in cattle, varies between 50 and 100 minutes and limits its usefulness.[30, 129] Trimethoprim combined with sulphadiazine (Tribrissen 48 per cent, Hoechst Ag-Vet), administered at a dosage of 48 mg/kg, is absorbed more slowly and provides effective levels in the milk for 12 hours.[240]

Cephalosporins

The cephalosporins, which possess broad-spectrum activity against many Gram-negative pathogens and beta-lactamase-producing staphylococci, can be used instead of combinations of antibiotics.[188] Cephalosporins have a limited distribution in the udder after parenteral and intramammary therapy.[248] Cephoxazole is bactericidal and resistant to destruction by staphylococcal penicillinase, and by binding to penicillinase produced by Gram-negative bacteria allows penicillin to act on these otherwise-resistant pathogens. Cephoxazole and penicillin have a mutually potentiating effect.[87]

Metronidazole and clindamycin

Metronidazole is the only drug that shows consistently good bacteriological activity against *Bacteroides fragilis*.[58] There is no intramammary preparation available to date that contains metronidazole for mastitis therapy, and the efficacy of metronidazole as a therapeutic agent for the parenteral treatment of mastitis requires further research. Clindamycin is active against anaerobic Gram-negative bacilli, such as *Bacteroides*, *Eubacterium*, and *Peptococcus* spp.[42, 47, 58]

Parenterally administered antimicrobials and corticosteroids may contaminate the cow's milk after treatment. The data sheets of these drugs contain the required information concerning the withholding periods of the milk before it can be used for human consumption.[21]

Therapy for teat canal infections and the different forms of mastitis includes:

Teat canal infections

The local application of small quantities of a suitable antibiotic (1 to 2 droplets) three times at 12-hourly intervals effectively eliminates most teat canal infections.[43, 44]

Subclinical mastitis

As a rule, treatment of subclinical mastitis during lactation is indicated only when the dairy farmer is in danger of losing his milk market due to a high proportion of cows being infected.[156] The treatment of subclinical udder infections is only successful if appropriate measures to correct inadequate hygiene have been introduced first to eliminate the predisposing factors which led to the problem.[160, 223] Once this has been attended to, intramammary antimicrobial therapy alone is usually sufficient. Three infusions of an appropriate intramammary antimicrobial preparation at 12-hourly intervals are recommended.[46] Parenteral antimicrobial therapy should only be considered when highly pathogenic bacteria are involved or when very valuable dairy cows are affected.[138, 178, 184]

Subacute clinical mastitis

Infusion of an appropriate intramammary antimicrobial preparation at 12-hourly intervals (of which the first application should be twice the recommended dosage) for two to five days is usually sufficient to effect a cure. The choice of preparation depends on the pathogen and response to treatment. Intramammary antimicrobial treatment should be continued for at least 24 hours after the disappearance of clinical signs, to prevent persistent subclinical infection.[156]

Acute mastitis

Treatment should consist of both parenteral and intramammary administration of the therapeutic agents employed, keeping in mind that when combinations are used, the antimicrobials should have a synergistic action or at least be compatible.[129, 201, 248] The selection of antibiotics or sulphonamides should be based on previous experience in the herd, clinical signs of the affected animals, and the results of the assessment of bacterial sensitivity tests.[46, 156] The use of oxytetracycline (10 mg/kg), ampicillin (10 mg/kg), or sulphonamides (200 mg/kg initial dosage) is usually advocated. Cephalosporins or ampicillin given by intramammary infusion may also be used to good effect.[156] If the intramuscular rather than the intravenous route is chosen for the administration of the parenteral therapy, the dose of the preparation should be divided in half, and each half injected at a different site in order to increase the bio-availability of the drug.[100, 128, 129, 138, 178, 181, 184, 241, 248] It is recommended that the first intramammary treatment consists of a double dose of the therapeutic agent infused into affected quarters and a single dose into each of the healthy quarters (a prophylactic measure). The treatment regime thereafter consists of the administration of the treatment by both routes for three to five days, the intramammary preparation being infused at the intervals recommended by the manufacturer (generally once every 12 hours).[46] For recommendations concerning supportive therapy and optimal animal husbandry for cows suffering from this form of mastitis, refer to **Table 190.7**.

Therapy of animals afflicted with acute or peracute clinical mastitis as a result of infection by anaerobic bacteria should consist of local and parenteral administrations of a series of large doses of antimicrobials. Antibiograms should be conducted as soon as possible in order to select the drug of choice. In general, antimicrobial therapy for anaerobic infections requires high doses and prolonged treatment, because of a tendency to relapse. Chloramphenicol, metronidazole, clindamycin or penicillin G, in that order, should be used if anaerobes are suspected as the causal agent and where the results of the antibiograms are not yet available.

Peracute mastitis

In principle, treatment is the same as that for acute mastitis,[46] but special attention should be given to animals suffering from endotoxic shock.[100, 138, 178, 181, 184, 219, 241]

Particularly in quarters affected by gangrenous mastitis, intramammary treatment is generally ineffective, and in such cases it may be necessary to resort to teat amputation to facilitate drainage of the exudate from the affected quarter. Ligation of mammary veins has also been advocated in severe cases of mastitis, this procedure being performed in order to reduce the invasion of toxins into the blood stream.[178] The administration of antitoxins, if available, against bacterial toxins may also be beneficial. A proportion of severely affected cows that survive the effects of peracute mastitis does not recover completely and may suffer from persistent pyrexia and evidence of damage to vital organs, such as the liver. The prognosis in these cases is poor.[7, 178]

Chronic mastitis

It is advisable not to institute any form of specific treatment in these cases and rather to cull such cows or to destroy the affected quarter by means of an infusion of 25–40 ml of undiluted medical ether.[46] Culling is usually the only practical means of eliminating chronic udder infections from a herd. However, if treatment is instituted it should consist of the administration of parenteral and intramammary antimicrobial drugs for three to five days, the drug being chosen on the basis of an antibiogram.[243] Anti-inflammatory therapy may also be used, as well as the intramammary infusion of 100–250 ml of a 5 per cent or 10 per cent dextrose solution at 12-hourly intervals for three days.[7, 178, 184] However, the prognosis remains poor.

Therapy in cows suffering from mastitis may be unsuccessful for various reasons:[6, 46, 48, 156, 163]

- The lesions in the udder parenchyma are deep-seated and are protected by scar tissue. Milk ducts are obstructed, thus hampering the diffusion of antimicrobials throughout the gland, and tissue necrosis results in poor blood supply to the affected areas.
- Drug factors: Inadequate passage across the blood-milk barrier, low bio-availability, inability to attain and maintain therapeutic concentrations at the focus of infection, a high degree of plasma-protein binding, short plasma half-life, and poor efficacy of aminoglycocide antibiotics against anaerobic mastitogenic bacteria.
- Resistance of organisms to the drugs used, development of L-forms of bacteria and superinfections.
- Poor animal husbandry and veterinary practice: Terminating treatment too soon, inadequate supportive treatment, inaccurate diagnosis, and delayed initial treatment.

A high prevalence of udder infections in a dairy herd is indicative of poor hygiene and dairy practice. An effective control programme must relate to the pattern of udder disease and must be aimed at preventing new infections rather than eliminating infections by treatment with antimicrobials.[39, 73] Subclinical mastitis is the main source of most mastitogenic pathogens: it is at least 20 times more prevalent in a herd than clinical mastitis.

It is impossible to eradicate all udder infections, and the aim of programmes to control mastitis should be to reduce levels of udder and teat canal infections and reduce predisposing factors to a minimum.[35] Specific measures include:[36, 40, 51, 65, 85, 101, 156]

- the use of disinfectant teat dipping on all cows after every milking,
- dry-cow antimicrobial therapy in all cows at the end of every lactation,
- culling of cows suffering from recurrent clinical mastitis (chronically infected cows),
- the use of functionally adequate milking machines,
- the prompt treatment of all cows with clinical mastitis,

monitoring the effect of treatment, and the application of monthly herd-milk cell counts, and
- the maintenance of a consistently high standard of hygiene and management before, during and after milking.

Hygiene and management

Infection may occur during the milking process via contaminated milk, milkers' hands, udder cloths or sponges, and teat cup liners. Microorganisms most likely to be transmitted in this way are *S. aureus* and *S. agalactiae*.

Infection may also occur during the interval between milkings. Possible methods include contaminated bedding, licking of teats and udder, contact of teats with the rear legs and tail switch, flies, and wetting cows excessively with sprinklers, which results in water running down the flanks and teats. Microorganisms most frequently transmitted during the intermilking period are likely to be environmental streptococci and coliforms.

The primary objective of good milking hygiene is to milk teats that are both clean and dry.[39] A minimum amount of water or disinfectant should be used to prepare teats and udders for milking. They should be dried thoroughly, preferably with an individual disposable paper towel. Individual cloth towels may be used provided that they are adequately laundered and disinfected between milkings. Sponges should preferably not be used for this purpose. An alternative procedure may be followed whereby teats are dipped in an approved predip product following the recommendations of the manufacturer. Teats should then be dried carefully to prevent germicide residues from contaminating the milk. Hygiene in the cows' environment is of extreme importance,[39] regardless of whether the cows are confined or on pasture.

Milkers' hands are an important mode of transmission for mastitogenic microorganisms. Contamination may occur when drawing foremilk, handling teat cups, stripping, or touching contaminated objects in the milking barn. The hands should be washed with a disinfectant solution prior to milking, or smooth rubber gloves that are dipped in a suitable disinfectant should be worn. Unless they are applied properly, procedures used to clean and disinfect the teats and adjacent udder surfaces will spread microorganisms rather than destroy them.

It is extremely important that teats are both clean and dry when teat cups are attached. Water left on the udder or flanks will drain downwards and become infected with microorganisms as it flows towards the teats. If teat cups have been attached, the water will collect at the mouth of the teat cup liner.

Teat cup liners are a potential source of infection for cows. The entire teat cup should be dipped in a disinfectant solution for a few seconds in between cows. The most effective way to dip teat cups is two at a time. This permits the disinfectant solution to come into contact with the full length of the liners. If four teat cups are dipped together, an air block is formed and the disinfectant may come into contact with only the first 20–60 mm of the liners. It is also preferable that teat cups are first dipped in a bucket of plain water to remove any milk that may contribute to the inactivation of the disinfectant in the rinse solution. The teat cups should finally be dipped once again in plain water before they are used, to rinse away antimicrobial residues.

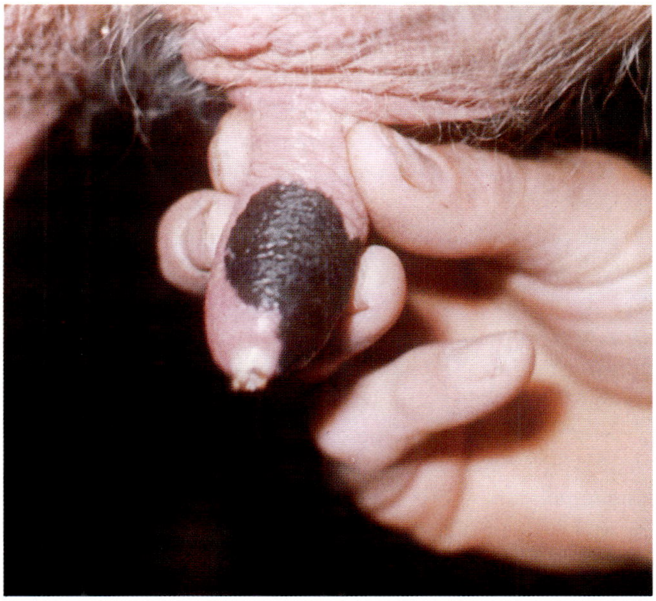

Figure 190.14 An everted teat canal with epithelial hyperplasia and teat orifice erosion as a consequence of overmilking

Because of the potential for contamination, inadequate contact time, and inadequate drying of liners, a procedure has been developed in recent years for disinfecting liners automatically. This procedure is known as backflushing. Most backflush systems incorporate five stages. The first rinses milk residues from the inside surface of the milk tube, claw, and liners. This is followed by a disinfectant rinse, incorporating a short time-delay in order to allow microorganisms to be destroyed, another rinse with water to remove disinfectant, and a final blast of air to remove residual water.

Every effort should be made to keep cows standing for at least one hour after milking, to provide time for the teat canal to close tightly.

Consideration should be given to separating cows with high somatic cell counts from healthy individuals. At the very least, they should be milked after cows that have low cell counts. The milking unit should be carefully cleaned and disinfected after milking cows with high cell counts.[156]

Disinfection of entire teats immediately after milking in a safe and effective teat dip is perhaps the most important single measure a dairy farmer can apply to reduce new infections in a herd.[156, 184, 228] Most commercially available teat dips will reduce new infections by at least 50 per cent. The objectives of teat disinfection are to reduce bacterial colonization, to prevent udder invasion by environmental microorganisms between milkings, and to improve the texture of the teat skin.

Post-milking teat dipping combined with dry-cow therapy and good milking procedures are the most effective measures for the control of mastitis caused by *S. aureus*.

The conventional method of applying disinfectant teat dips is to use a cup that contains the teat dip, but a more recent practice, especially in larger herds, is to apply the 'dip' using sprayers placed at strategic locations in the milking parlour. This procedure is satisfactory if care is taken to ensure that the skin of the teat is completely covered by the product.

Teat-dip cups should be kept clean, and the teat dip that remains in the cups should not be poured back into the original container.

Udder infections in cows frequently occur during the early drying-off period, and for this reason antimicrobial treatment of all the quarters of cows at drying-off is important. The advantages of dry-cow antimicrobial treatment include the following:[51, 156, 184, 228]

- the prevalence of new udder infections during the dry period is reduced,
- higher concentrations of long-acting antimicrobials can be used safely,
- subclinical and chronic mastitis cure rates are higher than during lactation,
- saleable milk is not contaminated with drug residues,
- cases of clinical mastitis at calving are reduced, and
- damaged udder tissue is allowed to regenerate before the new lactation (freshening).

The preferred time to treat animals is following the final milking of a lactation. Cows can be dried off successfully either by abrupt cessation of milking, which is preferred, or by milking once daily for a few days. The drying-off process can be expedited by reducing the intake of feed rich in carbohydrates just prior to and immediately following the cessation of milking. Teat ends should be disinfected prior to dry-cow antimicrobial treatment.

Cows with chronic mastitis are a major source of infection for healthy cows in the herd and should be culled. Records should be kept of all cows treated for mastitis, as they are helpful for deciding which animals should be culled.

Milking machines may predispose to mastitis in a herd because they:

- can transmit pathogens from one cow to another via contaminated clusters,[52, 72, 228]
- can, by improper action, damage the teat so that pathogens gain easy access to the gland, and
- can create a reverse flow, resulting in pathogens being propelled into and through the teat canal.[12, 25, 49, 50, 156, 206]

Disinfecting the internal surfaces of the liner, claw, and the long milk tube reduces their contamination by pathogens shed in the milk of infected cows to concentrations too low to infect cows milked subsequently with the same cluster.

Liners which are defective or old and cracked are the source of large numbers of microorganisms even when decontamination of clusters is carried out between milkings. The liner is the only part of the milking machine in contact with the cow's teat, and can play an important role in teat tissue damage and infection. Deterioration of liners can be caused by fat absorption, heat, oxygen, ozone, light, flexing, tension, tearing, and cleaning and sterilizing processes. A thin-walled, narrow-bore, stretch liner with a mouthpiece that does not restrict the base of the teat is ideal for machine milking. Most moulded, one-piece liners can be expected to have a useful life of appoximately 1 000–1 200 individual milkings, or 100–120 hours of use.

Decontamination of the milking unit (cluster) between cows during milking is of utmost importance in the control of mastitis, as cluster-to-cluster transfer of pathogens may occur in a milking machine pipeline. In most dairies, mastitis is reduced when backflushing is added to the standard decontamination routine, including teat dipping.

The milking routine should be designed to milk cows in the shortest possible time, to cause the least damage to the teats.[51, 69, 228] Overmilking (not removing the teat cups when the milk flow stops) or commencing milking before let-down of milk has occurred results in erosion of the teat orifice, which subsequently leads to epithelial hyperplasia **(Figure 190.14)**. Hyperaemia, oedema and haemorrhage may occur in the epithelial and subepithelial lining of the teat cistern and teat canal in overmilked quarters. Devices which reduce vacuum levels at the start and end of milking (dual-vacuum milking) help to prevent overmilking. A high milking vacuum (67 kPa) affects the incidence of teat-end erosion but not the rate at which quarters become infected.

The risk of udder infection is increased with inadequate pulsation (intermittent admission of air into the pulsation chamber to aid circulation of lymph and blood from the tip of the teat) **(Figure 190.15)**. A constant vacuum leads to congestion and oedema of the teat due to the accumulation of lymph and blood at the tip of the teat. These changes are overcome by means of pulsation which alternately allows air into the pulsation chamber and then creates a vacuum. Congestion, oedema and petechiae of the teat are associated with a wide pulsator ratio.

Recommendations for pulsation settings are:

- pulsation rates should not differ by more than ± 2 pulses per minute from those specified by the manufacturer;
- milk to rest ratio should not differ by more than 5 per cent from the given specifications; and
- pulsation rest phase should be at least 15 per cent of the total pulse.

Vacuum instability, especially in excess of 50 kPa vacuum (or 380 mm Hg), is considered to be the most common milking machine malfunction predisposing to mastitis. Vacuum stability is affected by almost all the components of the milking machine (but especially the vacuum pump), the diameter and length of all the pipes, the design and capacity of the claw, the pulsation system, and the vacuum regulator. The vacuum level at the teat's end must not fluctuate by a value of more than 75 mm Hg to ensure optimal udder health.

The vacuum recovery of a milking machine system with a vacuum level of 250–280 mm Hg must be four seconds. Since the amount of air admitted into the system changes on a regular basis due to attaching or taking off the milking units, a suitable vacuum controller must be installed to maintain the desired vacuum level. In many ways, the vacuum controller may be considered the 'brain' of the entire milking system. The vacuum pipeline should be straight, as short as possible, and should be installed to facilitate positive drainage towards the vacuum tank or other drainage points (self-draining sanitary trap).

Generalized vacuum fluctuations *per se* do not increase new infection rates, but new infection rates are greatly increased by liner slip, i.e. air admission between the teats and the liner. Liner slip is largely due to a defect in liner design, but it is also affected by vacuum stability. It is also thought that the effect of vacuum instability on increased new infections is mediated via increased liner slip. Slippage and air leakage into a liner are probably the machine-milking events most likely to contribute to increased mastitis rates. This may or may not be accompanied by unit drop-off. The design, operation, and adjustment of the milking unit should prevent liner slippage or squawk during milking.

The milking system should be checked regularly by a qualified service person using appropriate testing equipment.

OVINE MASTITIS

Introduction

Ovine mastitis is a disease which occurs in sheep-rearing countries throughout the world. It may present as a peracute, acute, subacute, chronic or subclinical disease and, although ewes of all breeds and ages are susceptible, it is more prevalent in lactating ewes kept for milk production and those maintained under intensive management systems than it is in range animals kept for meat or wool production,[54] although its importance in the latter should not be underestimated.[233] It is one of the most serious health problems in sheep that are kept mainly for milk production in southern and south-eastern Europe and

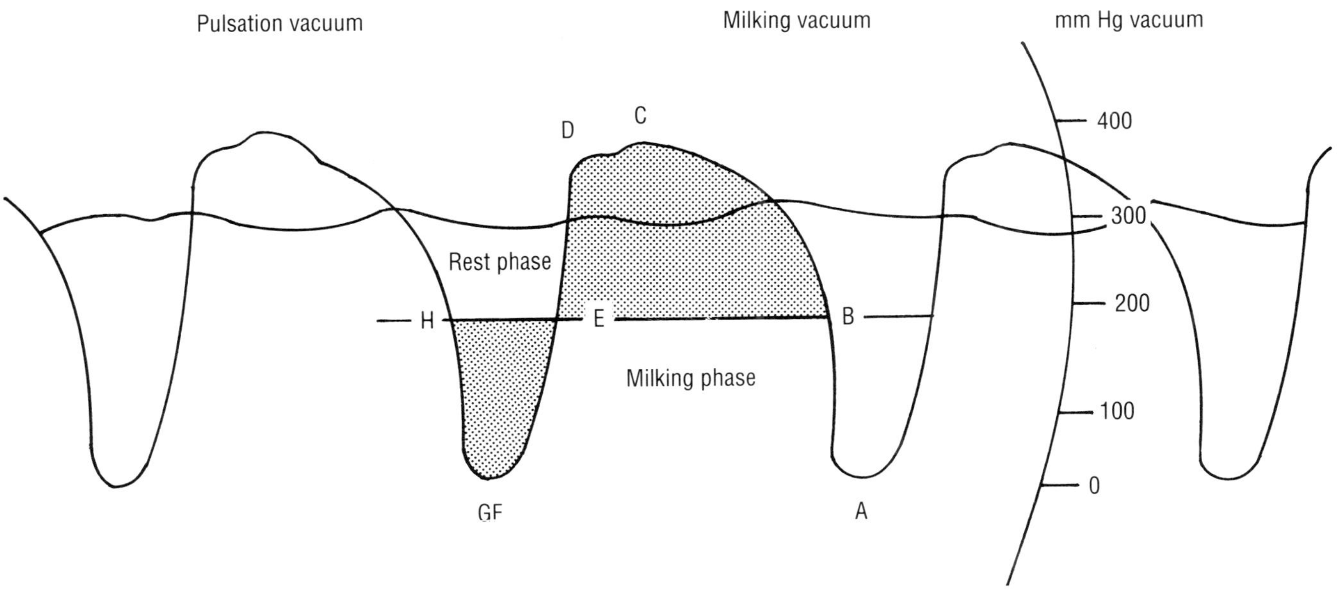

Figure 190.15 Pulsation graph

The following can be obtained from the pulsation graph:
Milk phase: B C D E
Rest phase: E F G H
Pulsation rate: The number of times the milk phase is interrupted in one minute

Milk-rest ratio: The ratio between the duration of the milk phase and the rest phase (from the graph, the ratio BE:EH)

countries bordering the Mediterranean Sea, such as Israel and Egypt.[55, 123] In southern Africa, where dairy sheep are uncommon, the disease tends to occur sporadically.

Mastitis may occur sporadically or endemically. The annual prevalence of acute mastitis can be as high as 24 per cent, and that of subclinical mastitis 31 per cent.[106] The disease may result in serious economic losses due not only to mortality (which results particularly from the peracute to acute disease), the decrease or cessation of milk production and subsequent starvation or malnourishment of lambs,[192] and the cost of treatment, but also to permanent loss of mammary tissue in recovered animals or chronic or subclinical cases, which may necessitate their culling and replacement. In the United Kingdom, culling rates in certain flocks as a result of mastitis may be as high as 5–10 per cent per annum.[90]

Aetiology

The most common causes of ovine mastitis are *Staphylococcus aureus* and *Pasteurella haemolytica*. They have been estimated to be responsible for about 80 per cent of cases of the disease.[106] They generally cause acute mastitis, which may be fatal. Mastitic pasteurellosis in ewes is described in **Chapter 143: Ovine and caprine pasteurellosis**.

A gangrenous, highly fatal mastitis frequently develops as a result of *S. aureus* infection The affected udder assumes a blue or black discoloration, hence the common names of blue bag [blou-uier (Afrik.)] or black garget for the disease. *Staphylococcus aureus* elaborates toxins which, *inter alia*, result in vasoconstriction and consequent tissue ischaemia, necrosis and gangrene.

Apart from *S. aureus* and *P. haemolytica*, however, many other microorganisms have been implicated in the aetiology of mastitis in ewes,[54, 55, 89, 106, 113, 123, 147, 151, 166, 167, 191] including *Actinobacillus lignieresii, Actinomyces (Corynebacterium) pyogenes, Corynebacterium pseudotuberculosis, Clostridium perfringens, Clostridium septicum, Erysipelothrix rhusiopathiae, Escherichia coli, Bacillus cereus, Fusobacterium necrophorum*, coagulase-negative staphylococci, *Streptococcus agalactiae, Streptococcus uberis, Streptococcus dysgalactiae, Brucella melitensis, Pasteurella multocida, Pseudomonas aeruginosa, Histophilus ovis, Mycoplasma agalactiae, Cryptococcus neoformans, Chlamydia psittaci*, and maedi-visna lentivirus.

Epidemiology and pathogenesis

As both *S. aureus* and *P. haemolytica* are ubiquitous organisms and are carried by healthy sheep — the former on the skin and in the nasal cavity, mouth and vagina of many animals,[235] and the latter in the upper respiratory tract and tonsils — mastitis can be expected to occur in virtually any flock. The disease caused by them affects ewes of any age and generally occurs within the first three to four weeks after lambing.

Contagious agalactiae, a disease primarily of goats but also of sheep, is caused by *Mycoplasma agalactiae*. It is endemic in Mediterranean countries but also occurs elsewhere.[215]

Microorganisms may reach the mammary gland via the blood (e.g., *B. melitensis, M. agalactiae, C. psittaci*, maedi-visna virus), teat canal, or injuries to the teat or skin of the udder.

The factors which predispose to infection in the more common forms of mastitis are not well understood, but it is thought that trauma to the teats, such as that caused in some ewes by the vigorous sucking of lambs, may play an important role in providing portals for the entry of organisms.[130] Mastitis has been associated with the lesions of orf,[15] the presence of papules, pustules and abscesses[121] in the skin of the teats and udders, and a condition known as 'sore teats', which is characterized by the development of raw sores on the tips of the teats which later develop black scabs.[98] A form of staphylococcal dermatitis of the teats has also been associated with secondary mastitis which leads to the subsequent culling of some ewes.[84] Cold wet weather, rough handling of the teats and gland, unsanitary environmental conditions,[15] and feeding ewes an excessively high-protein diet are also considered to predispose to the disease.[89, 105, 121, 153]

The sudden weaning of lambs may predispose to infection.[15] A form of the disease known as 'post-weaning mastitis' or 'mastitis in dry ewes' has been described.[26] It may be responsible for the culling of up to 10 per cent of the ewes in a flock. It is usually an acute form of mastitis and is caused by a variety of organisms, including staphylococci, *P. haemolytica* and *E. coli*, although more chronic and subclinical forms also occur. It has been suggested that the great majority of cases of post-weaning mastitis are in fact examples of pre-weaning mastitis which are only detected once lambs have been weaned. Such cases probably represent the chronic end-point of acute mastitis that developed during lactation.[106]

In a recent investigation carried out in the United Kingdom, which involved 30 000 ewes in lowland flocks, the prevalence rate of acute mastitis in individual flocks varied between 0 and 24 per cent of animals, with a mean of about 5 per cent.[106] In the majority of affected ewes only one gland was involved, and most infections occurred in the first week or between the third and fourth weeks of lactation. *Staphylococcus aureus* and *P. haemolytica* occurring alone, together, or with other bacteria were the predominant pathogens. In addition to the animals suffering from acute mastitis, bacteriological and cytological examinations of the milk of ewes in several flocks revealed subclinical mastitis rates that varied from 10 to 31 per cent. Most cases were associated with coagulase-negative staphylococci (about 50 per cent of cases), streptococci, *S. aureus, P. haemolytica* and *A. pyogenes*. The adverse effects that subclinical mastitis could have in a flock were investigated by inducing the disease experimentally with coagulase-negative staphylococci. It was found that milk production of affected ewes was reduced and the rate of growth of their lambs was retarded.[62] Similar results were obtained in another study in the United Kingdom, which also revealed that there is a significant association between the development of clinical mastitis and antecedent subclinical mastitis caused by the same organism.[233] The experimental induction of clinical and subclinical mastitis with coagulase-negative staphylococci has revealed that the reduction in milk yield that occurs is due to a decrease in the secretory capacity of the mammary glands.[63]

The toxins produced by *S. aureus* include haemolysins (alpha, beta, gamma and delta) and leukocidin **(see Chapter 146: *Staphylococcus aureus* infections)**. The alpha toxin is dermonecrotic and leukocidal, produces complete haemolysis of erythrocytes of rabbits, sheep and cattle, and has lethal activities. It is thought to play a major role in the pathogenesis of blue bag, not only because of its leukocidal and haemolytic effects, but also because it destroys blood platelets, causes tissue necrosis, and induces vasoconstriction, vasculitis and thrombosis with subsequent tissue ischaemia and necrosis.[62]

Clinical signs and pathology

The course of peracute or acute gangrenous mastitis due to *S. aureus* in ewes is very rapid and the disease is often fatal. Some animals may be found dead without any prodromal signs being observed. In most cases the mastitis involves only one of the mammary glands and the pain it induces causes manifest lameness in the hind limb on the affected side; such lameness may be the first presenting sign. The affected gland is initially hot, greatly enlarged, tense and oedematous, with hyperaemia of the overlying skin. Subcutaneous oedema of the abdominal wall cranial to the udder may be present. As gangrene sets in, the colour of the skin changes to blue-black and the gland becomes cold to the touch. Generalized systemic signs associated with an acute infectious disease are present. The secretion of the gland is usually sanguineous.[106]

Post-mortem examination reveals that a large part or parts of the gland are necrotic, the affected tissue being well demarcated from normal tissue. In surviving animals abscesses and fistules may develop. The necrotic mammary tissue eventually sloughs[109] and healing takes several weeks.[106]

Acute and chronic mastitis caused by staphylococci and other organisms resemble those described in the chapters on ovine pasteurellosis **(see Chapter 143: Ovine and caprine pasteurellosis)** and bovine mastitis at the beginning of this chapter.

Corynebacterium pseudotuberculosis and *A. pyogenes* infections tend to cause abscesses in the mammary tissue, and often occur after the organism concerned penetrates the udder through skin wounds such as those caused by shearing and tick bites.

Mastitis is associated with infection by ovine lentiviruses such as maedi-visna virus **(see Chapter 81: Maedi-visna)**.[97] Maedi-visna is a multi-systemic disease;[31] the pathology of the disease not only affects the lungs and central nervous system, but also a wider range of tissues and organs, particularly synovial membranes (causing lesions such as carpal arthritis) and the udder. The spectrum of the lesions closely parallels that of caprine arthritis-encephalitis. The lesions in the udder are those of a bilateral, chronic, diffuse, lymphocytic indurative mastitis characterized by lymphoid hyperplasia with some lymphoid follicle formation which is particularly periductal in distribution, but which also occurs in the parenchyma of the gland, where it is associated with atrophy or disappearance of alveolar tissue. There is also diffuse and focal infiltration of the interstitium by mononuclear cells and diffuse fibrosis.[28, 33, 225] Very little information is available concerning the changes that occur either in the milk yield or in the milk itself secreted by such mastitic udders. In some ewes the milk has a normal macroscopic appearance, while in other it appears watery or ceases to be secreted.[225] The mastitis can result in economically significant retardation of weight gain of suckled lambs.[31] The udder lesions show a striking morphological resemblance to those in the lungs,[225] and comparison of the changes in the two organs after a given period following experimental infection suggests that the udder lesions precede those in the lungs.[225] In one study of the natural disease it was found that almost twice as many sheep exhibited udder lesions as lung lesions, and it was suggested that mastitis is the most important economic feature of the maedi-visna complex.[225] In a flock of sheep in which 88 per cent of the ewes had antibodies to maedi-visna virus, about half of the ewes had indurated udders as a result of lymphocytic mastitis.[97]

Mycoplasma agalactiae infection, the cause of contagious agalactiae, is initially septicaemic and may be fatal at this stage. In animals that survive the septicaemia, localization of the organism occurs in the eyes, periarticular tissues and, in lactating females, in the mammary glands.[109, 215] Pregnant animals may abort. Lameness due to arthritis and periarthritis, mucopurulent keratoconjunctivitis and mastitis develop. The milk yield decreases, the secretion becomes yellow and, when allowed to stand, solids may settle out.[215] Eventually milk secretion ceases and only small amounts of serous fluid can be expressed from the udder.[215] *Mycoplasma agalactiae* may be isolated from the milk of recovered animals for many months. The inflammatory reaction in the mammary gland affects primarily the interstitial tissues, with secondary changes in the acini, and in severe cases may lead to fibrosis and parenchymal atrophy.[109]

Mycoplasma agalactiae has also been associated in goats with pneumonia and pleuritis, and with granular vulvovaginitis.[215]

Diagnosis

Ovine mastitis is diagnosed in a similar manner to the bovine disease: clinical examination of the udder, and investigations of the milk, such as the California milk test and cytological (including somatic cell counting) and bacteriological examinations. Details for the diagnosis of maedi-visna are given in **Chapter 81**.

Control

The treatment of ovine mastitis should be instituted as early as possible in the course of the disease, as delayed treatment may lead to abscessation or fibrosis of the udder, with loss of secretory tissue.[54] The general principles of therapy are similar to those for the bovine disease. Parenteral and intramammary mastitis therapy, supportive treatment and good nursing are necessary in severe cases. Parenteral therapy is necessary to achieve significant antimicrobial levels in the mammary secretion. Frequent milking is also recommended. Oxytocin administered intravenously will help in stripping mammary secretions from the udder. Ewes suffering from concomitent toxaemia should receive supportive treatment, including intravenous fluid therapy. In flocks where clinical and/or subclinical mastitis, as well as post-weaning mastitis, is a problem, dry-period therapy of the udder (as in cows) is indicated. Ewes with fibrotic udders, large teats or other abnormalities should be culled. Ewes with diseased udders should be segregated from the flock.

Methods of preventing mastitis in dairy sheep are the same as for milk cows, and include maintenance of a high standard of dairy hygiene as well as hygiene in pens and yards, the use of udder washes and disposable teat cloths, teat dipping, and milking machine maintenance.[93]

Vaccines are available for the prevention of mastitis caused by certain mastitogenic agents such as *S. aureus*, *P. haemolytica* and *M. agalactiae*.

A 'Blue Udder Vaccine' is marketed by the Veterinary Research Institute, Onderstepoort. It contains *P. haemolytica* (serotypes 7 and 9) bacterin and a toxoid prepared from two *S. aureus* strains. Ewes should be inoculated six and two weeks before lambing to ensure maximum protection at the time of exposure. A single booster injection is sufficient if given two to three weeks before subsequent lambing.

It has, however, been stated that conventionally prepared *S. aureus* vaccines containing killed cells with or without toxoids and adjuvants generally have been unsuccessful in preventing mastitis and are of marginal benefit in ameliorating clinical effects.[234] *Staphylococcus aureus* cells growing *in vivo* and in certain artificial media, such as those containing ovine whey, produce an antiphagocytic pseudocapsule which induces the formation of IgG2 antibodies specific for pseudocapsular antigens. The latter are formed only in negligible amounts in conventionally prepared vaccines.[234] Neutrophil-mediated phagocytosis is the most important mechanism for protecting the udder from *S. aureus* infection, and the phagocytic efficacy of neutrophils in the mammary gland is enhanced by the presence of cytophilic IgG2 antistaphylococcal antibody on the neutrophil membrane.[234] Dextran sulphate as an adjuvant promotes IgG2 antibody responses against staphylococcal surface antigens.[234]

Prevention of contagious agalactiae is based on vaccination.[215] Treatment with oxytetracycline reduces the severity of the disease but fails to stop the excretion of the organisms in the milk.[215]

CAPRINE MASTITIS

Introduction

Dairy goats have increased in popularity and in their ability to produce larger amounts of milk. With this increase in productivity has come a parallel increase in the prevalence and severity of mastitis and other diseases of the udder. Some goats are capable of producing 8 l of milk a day. In France, some of the best does give more than 2 000 l in a 10-month lactation. As might be expected, udder problems in modern dairy goats parallel those seen in high-producing dairy cows.[200]

Aetiology

Pathogens that play a role in mastitis in goats are *Corynebacterium pseudotuberculosis*, *Actinomyces pyogenes*, *Pasteurella haemolytica*, *Staphylococcus aureus*, coagulase-negative staphylococci, *Streptococcus agalactiae*, *Streptococcus dysgalactiae*, *Streptococcus epidermidis*, *Mycoplasma agalactiae*, *Mycoplasma mycoides*, *Mycobacterium bovis* and *Yersinia pseudotuberculosis*.[19, 29, 89, 99, 200] *Proteus* spp., *Escherichia coli* and *Klebsiella* have also been isolated from the caprine mammary gland, but they are not a frequent problem.[200] Yeasts and fungi have occasionally been isolated. *Brucella melitensis* (or less frequently *Brucella abortus*) and the Q-fever organism, *Coxiella burnetii*, have serious public health implications because they can be excreted in the milk of apparently healthy goats without evidence of clinical mastitis. *Brucella melitensis* is responsible for Malta or undulant fever in humans, and a clinically detectable mastitis has only been reported in a few instances.[89] *Brucella* infections in humans occur when milk or cheese is consumed without prior pasteurization.[200]

The forms of mastitis in goats resemble those that occur in sheep and cattle. The lentivirus (retrovirus) of caprine arthritis-encephalitis may cause mastitis.

It is interesting to note that consumption of the leaves of the Guatemalan variety of avocado (*Persea americana*) by lactating goats can cause mastitis.[27]

Pathogenesis and clinical signs

The predisposing factors and pathogenesis of udder infection and inflammation in goats are similar to those in cattle and sheep in which the galactogenous route of infection is the most important.[19, 173, 200] Injuries to the teats invariably result in severe mastitis.

The clinical signs of mastitis in goats resemble those in cattle and sheep suffering from the disease.[19, 200] *Staphylococcus aureus* can cause either gangrenous or non-gangrenous mastitis. A brief account of contagious agalactiae in sheep and goats caused by infection with *Mycoplasma agalactiae* is given in the section on ovine mastitis.

Infection of goats with *Mycoplasma mycoides* is a major problem in some countries. It is associated with mastitis, arthritis, pneumonia, pleuritis, peritonitis, polyserositis, septicaemia and abortion.[98]

As in maedi-visna in sheep, the lentivirus of caprine arthritis-encephalitis **(see Chapter 82: Caprine arthritis-encephalitis)** is responsible not only for arthritis, encephalitis and pneumonia, but also for mastitis which is associated with reduced milk production.

Diagnosis

The diagnosis of mastitis in dairy goats is based on a clinical examination of the udder, strip-cup examination of the mammary secretion, the results of the California milk test (CMT) when the strip-cup examination is negative or inconclusive, and cytological and bacteriological examinations of the milk. Caution must be exercised when interpreting the results of the CMT in goats.[126] A negative result is a good indicator of the absence of infection, but a positive test does not always indicate infection.

Milk from normal goats has a higher cell count than that of normal cows,[83, 94] and a diagnosis of udder infection is based more on a leukocyte count than on the total somatic cell count.[54, 94] The normal cell count varies between 700 000 and 1 000 000/ml. The diagnosis of mastitis is based on the premise that 1,5 million or more leukocytes per millilitre of milk is indicative of inflammation of mammary tissue and possibly of udder infection.[154, 200] The method of culturing, isolating and identifying mycoplasmas from goats' milk is described by East and Birnie.[54]

Control

Ideally, the selection of the drug used in the treatment of caprine mastitis should depend on the isolation of the causative agent and the determination of its antimicrobial sensitivity. Treatment and prophylaxis of caprine mastitis closely parallel the standard techniques recommended for bovine mastitis.[200] Lewter, Mullowney, Baldwin and Walker[126] have described in full the significance, diagnosis, prevention and control of mastitis and udder oedema in goats.

PORCINE MASTITIS

Introduction

Sows of various ages and breeds may develop mastitis, but it is almost always a disease of recently farrowed sows, usually within 48 hours of parturition.[89] It is frequently a part of the mastitis-metritis-agalactia (MMA) syndrome (or periparturient hypogalactia syndrome).[19, 195] Numerous mixed intramammary infections occur in the peripartum period of sows, and the prevalence of total infections is higher in older sows.[132] Agalactia toxaemia in sows is common immediately after farrowing and is an important cause of starvation and reduced growth rate of piglets.[152, 179]

Aetiology

Pathogens that play a role in porcine mastitis include: *Aerobacter aerogenes, Actinomyces pyogenes, Escherichia coli, Klebsiella, Enterobacter*, and *Citrobacter* spp., *Pseudomonas aeruginosa, Staphylococcus aureus*, coagulase-positive staphylococci, *Streptococcus agalactiae* and *Streptococcus uberis*.[19, 89, 122, 132, 179, 195] Chronic granulomatous mastitis, which is also known as 'actinomycosis' or 'botryomycosis' of the mammary gland, is more often caused in sows by *S. aureus* than *Actinomyces bovis*.[109]

The most important cause of agalactia in sows is the MMA syndrome, in which there is partial or complete absence of milk flow. It may involve one or more of the mammary glands.[19, 152] The MMA syndrome is an extremely complex condition, and many different causes have been associated with it. These have been classified by Smith and his colleagues[195] into non-infectious, infectious, management and environment, and nutritional categories. In the infectious category, coliform mastitis due to bacteria of the genera *Escherichia, Klebsiella, Enterobacter* and *Citrobacter* is identified as the most important cause of lactation insufficiency in sows.

Pathogenesis

The pathogenesis of most forms of porcine mastitis is probably similar to that of bovine mastitis in which the infection gains entry through the teat canal. In 'actinomycosis' of the udder it is likely that infection is percutaneous as a result of skin wounds rather than through the teat canal.[109] It seems probable that in the case of mammary infections by Gram-negative organisms, absorption of endotoxin from the udder into the blood stream plays a role in the pathogenesis of MMA.[195] Latent infections may frequently remain and elicit recrudescent inflammatory processes in the mammary glands.[19, 89, 152]

The MMA syndrome, mastitis, and numerous mixed intramammary infections occur most commonly in sows which farrow in indoor pens, and only occasionally in those which farrow outdoors. Predisposing factors include nutritional disturbances such as overfeeding during pregnancy or drastic change of feed at farrowing, metabolic disorders, stress, and poor hygiene and management.[19, 89, 179] The disease has been observed under managemental, environmental and sanitation conditions ranging from very poor to excellent.[19, 152]

Clinical signs

One of the first indications of MMA and of acute mastitis is the failure, usually within 12–24 hours of farrowing, of sows to nurse their piglets. They are disinterested in their offspring (their mothering instinct is reduced or even lost completely) and the piglets soon become hungry and lose weight. The sow's body temperature is usually elevated. Milk secretion falls off rapidly and sows manifest depression and a loss of appetite.[19, 152] In many cases there is both swelling and hardening of one or more mammary glands, or even the whole udder. The skin over the udder may be hyperaemic and oedematous. There may be an increased vaginal discharge, although metritis is seldom part of the syndrome.

Diagnosis

Mastitis in sows is often difficult to diagnose on antemortem examination.[143, 202] The mammary secretion from mastitic glands may be watery or thickened and contain pus, and the cell count may be increased to 20 million per millilitre. Bacteriological examination of the milk from all the glands should be performed, if possible.[18] The major problem in the clinical diagnosis is to differentiate the acute swelling of infectious mastitis from other noninfectious causes of acute swelling, such as 'caking' of the mammary glands, which also results in agalactia.[19]

Control

The recovery rate is good if treatment is commenced early in the course of the disease, although some cases may recover spontaneously. If possible the selection of the therapeutic agent should be based on the nature of the causative agent. Most affected sows will recover within one or two days if treated soon after the onset of the disease with a combination of antimicrobials, corticosteroids and oxytocin. Broad-spectrum antimicrobials are indicated because coliforms are the most common pathogens involved. Commonly used antimicrobial drugs are sulphadimidine, penicillin, streptomycin, tetracyclines, chloramphenicol and tylosin. These should be given in high dosage for at least three days, and if there is no improvement in 12–18 hours, the drug should be changed. It is beneficial to restore normal mammary function through the use of oxytocin (30–40 units intramuscularly, repeated every hour), warmth and massage. Corticosteroids such as dexamethazone are used for their anti-inflammatory effect, at the rate of 20 mg intramuscularly daily for three days for sows weighing 150–200 kg. The sows should be provided with drinking water *ad libitum* and should be tempted to eat greenstuff. The piglets must be kept warm and they may be better off away from the sows, where they must either be fostered by other sows or hand fed.[19, 152]

Attention should be directed towards possible predisposing managemental factors. Pregnant sows should be washed with soap and water and, in order to minimize stress, placed in the farrowing pen a week before they are due to farrow. Antimicrobial agents can be used prophylactically.[19, 152] Commercial polyvalent *E. coli* antiserum administered in large doses before farrowing has given favourable results,[175] but commercial *E. coli* or autogenous vaccines have met with mixed success.[202]

EQUINE MASTITIS

Introduction

Mastitis in mares is relatively uncommon.[102, 118, 149] It occurs most frequently during lactation,[1, 4, 238] but is also seen during the 'drying-off' period following weaning[118, 180, 238] and in dry mares.[131, 149, 162, 176, 238] A case has been described in a young 15-week-old filly.[164] The rarity of the disease in mares has been ascribed to their short lactation period, the protected position of the udder, the husbandry techniques commonly employed in mare-foal care, and the inability to identify subclinical or low-grade cases.[164]

Aetiology

The microorganisms causing equine mastitis have recently been reviewed by McCue & Wilson.[131] These are *Streptococcus zooepidemicus*, which seems to be the most common organism isolated from mares suffering from the disease, *Streptococcus equisimilis, Streptococcus equi, Streptococcus viridans, Streptococcus agalactiae, Staphylococcus* spp., *Corynebacterium pseudotuberculosis, Pseudomonas aeruginosa, Actinobacillus suis*-like organisms, *Pasteurella ureae, Enterobacter aerogenes, Klebsiella pneumonia* and *Escherichia coli*. In a series of 28 cases in which *S. zooepidemicus* was the organism encountered most frequently, 41 per cent were caused by Gram-negative bacteria.[131]

Pathogenesis

Very little information is available concerning the pathogenesis of mastitis in mares. It seems probable that it is similar to that in cows, in which the majority of organisms responsible for the disease enter the udder through the teat canals. Mares usually have two, rarely three, and exceptionally four teat canals per teat. Infection of the mammary glands secondary to trauma also plays a role, and it has been suggested that insect bites might also be implicated, which would explain the occurrence of mastitis in some dry mares.[131] Chilling and retention of milk, e.g. when a foal is sick or has died, or in the post-weaning period, may also predispose to infection.[89, 171]

Clinical signs

Mastitis in mares may manifest as an acute, subacute or chronic condition. Gangrenous mastitis similar to that in cows has also been observed.[89]

The presenting signs depend on the nature of the disease. In acute mastitis these include fever and other evidence of systemic illness (e.g. depression and anorexia), mammary swelling, localized increase in temperature and pain on palpation, and hind-limb lameness.[131] Mastitis is often unilateral. Affected mares may be reluctant, or refuse, to nurse their offspring.[1, 164]

Streptococcus equi has been associated with mammary abscessation.[238]

Staphylococcal infections may cause a chronic granulomatous mastitis (botryomycosis) in mares.[196]

The physical appearance of the milk in lactating mares may reflect the changes occurring in the affected mammary gland. It may be thick, flocculent and yellowish-grey.[1, 4] In dry mares, an exudate which is purulent or serosanguineous may be expressed from the teat of an affected gland.[164, 171, 238]

Diagnosis

Methods for the diagnosis of equine mastitis are based on those used for bovine mastitis. They include clinical examination of the mare, and macroscopic, microscopic and bacteriological examination of the milk or exudate from the affected gland. The milk or exudate is examined cytologically and for the presence of bacteria.[60, 131, 164] For the latter purpose, smears should be stained *inter alia* by Gram's method,[131, 164] which should allow an immediate tentative diagnosis of the causal organism if bacteria can be detected.[131, 164] The bacteriological investigation should include an antibiogram, as a high proportion of cases of equine mastitis are caused by Gram-negative bacteria.[131]

Control

Methods of treatment of equine mastitis have been outlined and reviewed by McCue and Wilson.[131] These include frequent stripping of the mastitic gland, application of hot packs and/or hydrotherapy to the affected gland, and application of local and/or systemic antimicrobial therapy. For local therapy, commercial bovine intramammary mastitis preparations are convenient. Proper restraint of the animal is mandatory when these are applied, as intramammary medication of affected glands is often painful and some animals object violently to this form of treatment. After disinfecting the teat orifice, antimicrobials must be infused into the teat cistern of each lobule of the gland concerned to be effective. Each of the two mammary glands of horses consists of two, or occasionally three, lobes. Milk produced from each lobe passes through lactiferous ducts to the teat cistern before exiting at the teat orifice. Intramammary infusions should be given once or twice daily immediately after stripping milk from the udder, and the udder should be massaged after their application to ensure adequate distribution.

The results of the study on equine mastitis by McCue and Wilson[131] showed that penicillin may not be the optimal drug for initial therapy. They suggested that therapy with a trimethoprim-sulphamethoxazole preparation is more appropriate while awaiting results of bacteriological and antimicrobial sensitivity tests. A combination therapy consisting of penicillin and an aminoglycoside such as gentamicin or amikacin would, however, give a broader antimicrobial activity, especially against Gram-negative enteric organisms. Subsequent antimicrobial therapy is based on the results of sensitivity tests. Antimicrobial therapy should be continued for at least five to seven days, depending on the clinical resolution of the disease.

Non-steroidal anti-inflammatory drugs, such as flunixin meglumine and phenylbutazone, may be indicated to relieve discomfort, decrease inflammation and stabilize an elevated body temperature. Furosemide has been used to decrease oedema associated with mammary inflammation.[131, 164]

Chronic granulomatous mastitis (botryomycosis) is not responsive to medical therapy and may necessitate surgical removal of the affected udder.

References

1 **ADDO, P.B., WILCOX, G.E. & TAUSSIG, R., 1974.** Mastitis in a mare caused by *C. ovis*. *The Veterinary Record*, 95, 193.

2 **ADKINSON, N.F., 1980.** Immunological consequences of antimicrobials in animal feeds. *In: The effects on Human Health of Subtherapeutic use of Antimicrobials in Animal Feeds.* Appendix J, 301–316. National Research Council, Washington: National Academy of Science.

3 **AFSHAR, A. & BANNISTER, G.L., 1970.** Viral infections of the bovine mammary gland. *Veterinary Bulletin*, 40, 681–686.

4 **AL-GRAIBAWI, M.A.A., SHARMA, V.K. & ALI, S.I., 1984.** Mastitis in a mare. *The Veterinary Record*, 115, 383.

5 **ALLEN, E.M., 1985.** Mycoplasma infections of cattle. *Pro Veterinario*, 2, 6–7.

6 **ANDERSON, J.C., 1986.** Barriers to successful therapy of staphylococcal mastitis. *In*: SANDHOLM, M., (ed.). *Proceedings of the Symposium on Mastitis Control and Hygienic Production of Milk.* 109–118.

7 **ANON., 1970.** Report of the panel of the colloquium on

bovine mastitis. *Journal of the American Veterinary Medical Association*, 170, 1110–1123.

8 **ANON., 1980.** Progress in mastitis control (1977) in 23 countries. Bulletin of the International Dairy Federation, Document 121.

9 **ANON., 1985.** Progress in the control of bovine mastitis. *Kieler Milchwirtschaftliche Forschungsberichte*, 37, 215–646.

10 **ANON., 1987.** Machine milking and mastitis. Document 215, Square Vergote 41, 1040 Brussels, Belgium.

11 **ANON., 1987.** Milk & milk products: Detection of inhibitors. International Dairy Federation, Bulletin No. 220.

12 **ANON., 1987.** Bovine mastitis: Definition and guidelines for diagnosis. Bulletin of the International Dairy Federation, No. 211.

13 **BAGGOT, J.D., 1977.** *Principles of Drug Deposition in Domestic Animals: The Basis of Veterinary Clinical Pharmacology*. Philadelphia: W.B. Saunders Company.

14 **BAGGOT, J.D., 1977.** Bioavailability and drug deposition in domestic animals. Part 1. *Veterinary Review*, 24, 66–67.

15 **BARLOW, R.M., 1982.** Infectious diseases of sheep and goats. *In*: COOP, I.E., (ed.). *World Animal Science, CI. Sheep and Goat Production*. Amsterdam: Elsevier Scientific Publishing Company.

16 **BAUMGARTNER, H., 1966.** Die Verbreitung des Q-Fiebers in den Milchviehbeständen des Emmentals und des Oberaargaus. *Schweizer Archiv für Tierheilkunde*, 108, 401–409.

17 **BEGG, H., 1913.** Mammitis. *In*: HOARE, E.W., (ed.). *A system of Veterinary Medicine*. Vol. I. London: Baillière Tindall & Cassell Ltd.

18 **BERTSCHINGER, H.U. & POHLENZ, J., 1992.** Coliform mastitis. *In*: LEMAN, A.D., STRAW, B.E., MENGELING, W.L., D'ALLAIRE, S. & TAYLOR, D.J., (eds). *Diseases of Swine*. 7th edn. Ames Iowa: Iowa State University Press.

19 **BLOOD, D.C., RADOSTITS, O.M., HENDERSON, J.A., ARUNDEL, J.H. & GAY, C.C., 1983.** *Veterinary Medicine*. London: Ballière Tindall.

20 **BLOSSER, T.H., 1979.** Ecomomic losses from and the national research program on mastitis in the United States. *Journal of Dairy Science*, 62, 119–127.

21 **BOOTH, J.M., 1986.** Intramammary antibiotic preparations and their withholding times. *The Veterinary Record*, 118, 34–35.

22 **BRAMLEY, A.J., 1991.** Mastitis: Physiology or pathology. *In*: BURVENICH, C., VANDEPUTTE-VAN MESSOM, G. & HILL, A.W., (eds). *New Insights into the Pathogenesis of Mastitis*. Belgium: Hilde van de Walle.

23 **BRAMLEY, A.J., 1992.** Mastitis. *In*: ANDREWS, A.H., BLOWLEY, R.W., BOYD, H. & EDDY, R.G., (eds). *Bovine Medicine*. London: Blackwell Scientific Publications.

24 **BURVENICH, C., VANDEPUTTE-VAN MESSOM, G. & HILL, A.W., 1991.** *New Insights into the Pathogenesis of Mastitis*. Belgium: Hilde van de Walle.

25 **BUSHNELL, R.B., 1984.** The importance of hygienic procedures in controlling mastitis. *Veterinary Clinics of North America: Large Animal Practice*, 6, 361–370.

26 **BUSWELL, J.F. & YEOMAN, G.H., 1976.** Mastitis in dry ewes. *The Veterinary Record*, 99, 221–222.

27 **CRAIGMILL, A.L., SEAWRIGHT, A.A., MATTILA, T. & FROST, A.J., 1989.** Pathological changes in the mammary gland and biochemical changes in milk of the goat following oral dosing with leaf of avocado (*Persea americana*). *Australian Veterinary Journal*, 66, 206–211.

28 **CUTLIP, R.C., LEHMKUHL, H.D., BROGDEN, K.M. & BOLIN, S.R., 1985.** Mastitis associated with ovine progressive pneumonia virus infection in sheep. *American Journal of Veterinary Research*, 46, 326–331.

29 **DAMASSA, A.J., BROOKS, D.L. & ADLER, H.E., 1983.** Caprine mycoplasmosis: Widespread infection in goats with *Mycoplasma mycoides* subsp *mycoides* (large-colony type). *American Journal of Veterinary Research*, 44, 322–325.

30 **DAVITIYANANDA, D. & RASMUSSEN, R., 1974.** Halflives of sulphadoxine and trimethoprim after a single intravenous infusion in cows. *Acta Veterinaria Scandinavica*, 15, 356–365.

31 **DAWSON, M., 1987.** Pathogenesis of maedi-visna. *The Veterinary Record*, 120, 451–454.

32 **DE BOER, A.J., 1981.** Socio-economic aspects of dairying in developing countries. *Journal of Dairy Science*, 64, 2453–2462.

33 **DENG, P., CUTLIP, R.C., LEHMKUHL, H.D. & BROGDEN, K.A., 1986.** Ultrastructure and frequency of mastitis caused by ovine progressive pneumonia virus infection in sheep. *Veterinary Pathology*, 23, 184–189.

34 **DOBBINS, C.N., 1977.** Mastitis losses. *Journal of the American Veterinary Medical Association*, 170, 1129–1132.

35 **DODD, F.H., 1971.** The strategy of mastitis control. *In*: DODD, F.H. & JACKSON, E.R., (eds). *The Control of Bovine Mastitis*. The National Institute for Research in Dairying, Reading, England.

36 **DODD, F.H., 1985.** Progress in the control of bovine mastitis. Review of the IDF Seminar. *Kieler Milchwirtschaftliche Forschungsberichte*, 37, 641–646.

37 **DODD, F.H., GRIFFIN, T.K. & KINGWILL, R.G., 1975.** Proceedings of the IDF Seminar on Mastitis Control 1975. Bulletin of the International Dairy Federation, Document 85.

38 **DODD, F.H. & JACKSON, E.R., 1971.** The control of bovine mastitis. The National Institute for Research in Dairying, Shinfield, Reading, England.

39 **DODD, F.H. & NEAVE, F.K., 1970.** Mastitis control. Biennial Reviews. National Institute for Research in Dairying, Shingfield, Reading, England.

40 **DODD, F.H., WESTGARTH, D.R., NEAVE, F.K. & KINGWILL, R.G., 1969.** Mastitis — the strategy of control. *Journal of Dairy Science*, 52, 689–695.

41 **DU PREEZ, J.H., 1980.** Antibiotiese residue in melk. *Veterinary Clinical*, August, 9–10.

42 **DU PREEZ, J.H., 1981.** Die prevalensie, aard en betekenis van anaerobiese bakterieë in die melkkoei-uier. M. Med. Vet. (Hyg.) Dissertation, University of Pretoria, Republic of South Africa.

43 **DU PREEZ, J.H., 1985.** Speenkanaalinfeksie by melkkoeie: diagnose, voorkoms, aard, terapie, omvang en betekenis. D.V.Sc. Dissertation, University of Pretoria, Republic of South Africa.

44 **DU PREEZ, J.H., 1985.** Teat canal infections. *Kieler Milchwirtschaftliche Forschungsberichte*, 37, 267–273.

45 **DU PREEZ, J.H., 1986.** Comparison of various criteria for determining the health status of the bovine udder. *Journal of the South African Veterinary Association*, 56, 191–194.

46 **DU PREEZ, J.H., 1988.** Treatment of various forms of bovine mastitis with consideration of udder pathology and the pharmacokinetics of appropriate drugs: A review. *Journal of the South African Veterinary Association*, 59, 161–167.

47 **DU PREEZ, J.H., 1989.** The role of anaerobic bacteria in bovine mastitis: A review. *Journal of the South African Veterinary Association*, 60, 159–168.

48 **DU PREEZ, J.H., 1989.** Reasons why mastitis therapy is unsuccessful: Review article. *South African Journal of Dairy Science*, 21, 23–28.

49 **DU PREEZ, J.H., 1991.** The role of the milking machine in bovine udder health. Part I. *South African Veterinary Medicine*, 4, 86–90.

50 **DU PREEZ, J.H., 1991.** The role of the milking machine in bovine udder health. Part II. *South African Veterinary Medicine*, 4, 113–119.

51 **DU PREEZ, J.H., GIESECKE, W.H. & VEARY, C.M., 1989.** Modular Herd Control of Mastitis (MHCM): Practical guide on modules of anti-mastitis actions. Proceedings of the South African Veterinary Association Workshop on Modular Herd Control of Mastitis, University of Natal, Pietermaritzburg, 14–15 July 1988. *Journal of the South African Veterinary Association*, June 1989, Special Volume No. 3, 1–50.

52 **DU PREEZ, J.H., GREEFF, A.S. & EKSTEEN, N., 1981.** Isolation and significance of anaerobic bacteria isolated from

cases of bovine mastitis. *Onderstepoort Journal of Veterinary Research*, 48, 123–126.

53 **DU PREEZ, J.H., HATTINGH, P.J., GIESECKE, W.H. & EISENBERG, B.E., 1990.** Heat stress in dairy cattle and other livestock under southern African conditions. III. Monthly temperature-humidity index mean values and their significance in the performance of dairy cattle. *Onderstepoort Journal of Veterinary Research*, 57, 243–248.

54 **EAST, N.E. & BIRNIE, E.F., 1983.** Diseases of the udder. *Veterinary Clinics of North America: Large Animal Practice*, 5, 591–600.

55 **EL ETREBY, M.F. & ABDEL-HAMID, Y.M., 1970.** Experimental ovine mastitis. A pathologic study. *Pathologica Veterinaria*, 7, 246–264.

56 **ELLIOT, R.E.W., 1971.** Antibiotic resistance amongst haemolytic staphylococci isolated from bovine milk samples in New Zealand. *New Zealand Veterinary Journal*, 19, 95–99.

57 **ELLIS, W.A., O'BRIEN, J.J., PEARSON, J.K.L. & COLLINS, D.S., 1976.** Bovine leptospirosis: Infection by the Hebdomadis serogroup and mastitis. *The Veterinary Record*, 99, 368–370.

58 **FINEGOLD, S.M., ROSENBLATT, J.E., SUTTER, V.C. & ATTEBURY, H.R., 1971.** Anaerobic infections. *In*: THOMAS, B.A., (ed.). *Scope Monograph*. The Upjohn Company, Kalamazoo, Michigan.

59 **FREEMAN, A. & CLARK, A.S., 1977.** Colloquium on bovine mastitis. *Journal of the American Veterinary Medical Association*, 170, 1115–1254.

60 **FREEMAN, K.P., ROSZEL, W.D., SLUSHER, S.H. & YOUNG, D., 1988.** Cytologic features of equine mammary fluids: Normal and abnormal. *Compendium for the Continuing Education of the Practising Veterinarian*, 10, 1090–1099.

61 **FREI, W., 1925.** Milchdrüse. *In*: JOEST, E., (ed.). *Spezielle pathologische Anatomie der Haustiere*. Vol. IV. Berlin: Verlagsbuchhandlung Richard Schoetz.

62 **FTHENAKIS, G.C. & JONES, J.E.T., 1990.** The effect of inoculation of coagulase-negative staphylococci into the ovine mammary gland. *Journal of Comparative Pathology*, 102, 211–219.

63 **FTHENAKIS, G.C. & JONES, J.E.T., 1990.** The effect of experimentally induced subclinical mastitis on milk yield of ewes and on the growth of lambs. *British Veterinary Journal*, 146, 43–49.

64 **FUNKE, H., 1961.** The distribution of S^{35}-labelled benzylpenicillin in normal and mastitic mammary glands of cows and goats after local and systemic administration. *Acta Veterinaria Scandinavica*, 2, 1–88.

65 **FUNKE, H., 1986.** Mastitis control in Sweden. *In*: SANDHOLM, M., (ed.). *Proceedings of the Symposium on Mastitis Control and Hygienic Production of Milk*, 241–248.

66 **GIBBS, E.P.J., JOHNSON, R.H. & OSBORNE, A.D., 1970.** The differential diagnosis of viral skin infections of the bovine teat. *The Veterinary Record*, 87, 602–609.

67 **GIESECKE, W.H., 1978.** The prevalence and economic significance of mastitis in the RSA. *In*: VAN DEN HEEVER, L.W. & GIESECKE, W.H., (eds). *Proceedings of the First South African Symposium on Mastitis Control in Dairy Herds*. Pretoria, 10–12 August 1978.

68 **GIESECKE, W.H., 1979.** Bovine mastitis. Department of Agricultural Technical Services, Republic of South Africa, Technical Communications No. 51, 1–37.

69 **GIESECKE, W.H., 1983.** Bovine mastitis. *Science Bulletin*, No. 401. Pretoria: Department of Agriculture.

70 **GIESECKE, W.H., 1985.** The diagnosis and control of bovine mastitis as a means of improving the quality of milk. *South African Journal of Dairy Technology*, 17, 3–21.

71 **GIESECKE, W.H., 1989.** Mastitis control in the RSA. *In*: *Modular Herd Control of Mastitis*. Special Vol. 2. Proceedings of the SAVA Workshop on Modular Control of Mastitis. University of Natal, Pietermaritzburg, 14–15 July 1988.

72 **GIESECKE, W.H., DU PREEZ, J.H., TURNER, G.V.S. & VEARY, C.M., 1989.** Modular Herd Control of Mastitis (MHCM): Introduction. Proceedings of the South African Veterinary Association Workshop on Modular Herd Control of Mastitis, University of Natal, Pietermaritzburg, 14–15 July 1988. *Journal of the South African Veterinary Association*, June 1989, Special Volume No. 1, 1–74.

73 **GIESECKE, W.H., PETZER, I.M. & DU PREEZ. J.H., 1988.** Practical information on various aspects of udder health in dairy cattle. Part 28. Mastitis — a multifactorial disease. *Milk Producer*. June 1988, 6–11.

74 **GIESECKE, W.H., TUSTIN, R.C., MALAN, F.S. & DE WAAL, G.H., 1969.** Bovine mastitis due to *Clostridium perfringens* type A and *Bacillus cereus*. *Journal of the South African Veterinary Medical Association*, 40, 342.

75 **GIESECKE, W.H. & VAN DEN HEEVER, L.W., 1971.** Losses caused by mastitis to industrial and fresh milk producers in the RSA. *South African Journal of Dairy Technology*, 3, 53–59.

76 **GIESECKE, W.H. & VAN DEN HEEVER, L.W., 1974.** The diagnosis of bovine mastitis with particular reference to subclinical mastitis: A critical review of relevant literature. *Onderstepoort Journal of Veterinary Research*, 41, 169–212.

77 **GIESECKE, W.H., VAN DEN HEEVER, L.W. & DU TOIT, I.J., 1971.** Bovine mastitis in the RSA. *Bulletin of the Office of International Epizootics*, 76, 621–654.

78 **GIESECKE, W.H., VAN DEN HEEVER, L.W. & DU TOIT, I.J., 1972.** Staphylococcal mastitis: Phage types and patterns of *S. aureus*. *Onderstepoort Journal of Veterinary Research*, 39, 87–96.

79 **GORZELEWSKA, K. & JUSZKIEWICZ, T., 1961.** Studies to establish the dosage of chloramphenicol for domestic animals by means of serum and milk level determination. *Biuletyn Instytutu Weterynarii Pulawach*, 5, 2–3.

80 **GREATHEAD, M.H. & BISSCHOP, P.J.N.R., 1963.** A report on the occurrence of *C. diphtheriae* in dairy cattle. *South African Medical Journal*, 37, 1261–1262.

81 **GREEFF, A.S. & DU PREEZ, J.H., 1985.** Simultaneous isolation of anaerobic bacteria from udder abscesses and mastitis milk in lactating dairy cows. *Journal of the South African Veterinary Association*, 56, 155–197.

82 **GROOTENHUIS, G., 1976.** Verslag landelijke steekproef Mastitis 1975. Rotterdam: Centraal Diergeneeskundig Instituut.

83 **GROOTENHUIS, G., 1980.** Milk cell count in machine milked dairy goats. *Veterinary Quarterly*, 2, 121–123.

84 **GUNNING, R.F. & BOSWORTH, P.A., 1989.** Staphylococcal dermatitis involving the teats of lactating ewes. *The Veterinary Record*, 124, 146–147.

85 **GUTERBOCK, W.M., 1984.** Practical aspects of mastitis control in large dairy herds. Part II. *Milking Hygiene*. *The Compendium*, 6, 651–658.

86 **HAHN, G., HEESCHEN, W. & TOLLE, A., 1970.** *Streptococcus* — Eine Studie zur Struktur, Biochemie, Kultur und Klassifizierung. *Kieler Milchwirtschaftliche Forschungsberichte*, 22, 333–546.

87 **HARRIS, A.M., DAVIES, A.M., MARSHALL, M.J., EVANS, J.M., HENDY, P.G. & WATSON, D.J., 1977.** The treatment of clinical mastitis with cephoxazole and penicillin. *The Veterinary Record*, 101, 4–7.

88 **HEESCHEN, W., SUHREN, G. & HAHN, G., 1985.** Mastitis: Significance for processing of milk and public health aspects. *Kieler Milchwirtschaftliche Forschungsberichte*, 37, 233–243.

89 **HEIDRICH, H.J. & RENK, W., 1967.** *Disease of the Mammary Glands of Domestic Animals*. Philadelphia, London: W.B. Saunders.

90 **HENDY, P.G. & PUCH, K.E., 1981.** Prevention of post-weaning mastitis in ewes. *The Veterinary Record*, 109, 56–57.

91 **HENNING, M.W., 1956.** *Animal Diseases in South Africa*. 3rd. edn. South Africa: Central News Agency Ltd.

92 **HIGGINS, T.S, 1964.** Milk-borne diphtheria a generation ago. *South African Medical Journal*, 38, 12–14.

93 **HINDSON, J.C. & WINTER, A.C., 1990.** *Outline of Clinical Diagnosis in Sheep*. London: Butterworth & Co. Ltd.

94 **HINCKLEY, L.S. & WILLIAMS, L.F., 1981.** Diagnosis of mastitis in goats. *Agri Practice*, 76, 711–712.

95 **HODGES, R.T., HOLLAND, J.T.S., NEILSON, F.J.A. & WALLACE, N.M., 1985.** *Prototheca zopfii* mastitis in a herd of dairy cows. *New Zealand Veterinary Journal*, 33, 108–111.

96 **HOUBEN, E.H.P., DIJKHUIZEN, A.A., VAN ARENDONK, J.A.M. & HUIRNE, R.B.M., 1993.** Short- and long-term production losses and repeatability of clinical mastitis in dairy cattle. *Journal of Dairy Science*, 76, 2561–2578.

97 **HOUWERS, D.J., PEKELDER, J.J., AKKERMANS, J.W.P.M., VAN DER MOLEN, E.J. & SCHREUDER, B.E.C., 1988.** Incidence of indurative lymphocytic mastitis in a flock of sheep infected with maedi/visna virus. *The Veterinary Record*, 122, 435–437.

98 **HUNGERFORD, T.G., 1990.** *Hungerford's Disease of Livestock*. 9th edn. Sydney: McGraw Book Company.

99 **HUNTER, A.C., 1984.** Microflora and somatic cell content of goat milk. *The Veterinary Record*, 114, 318–320.

100 **JACKSON, E. & BRAMLEY, J., 1983.** Coliform mastitis. *In Practice*, 5, 135–146.

101 **JACKSON, E.R., 1980**. The control of bovine mastitis. *The Veterinary Record*, 107, 37–40.

102 **JACKSON, P.G.G., 1986.** Equine mastitis: Comparative lesions. *Equine Veterinary Journal*, 18, 88–89.

103 **JASPER, D.E., 1977.** *Mycoplasma* and *Mycoplasma* mastitis. *Journal of the American Veterinary Medical Association*, 170, 1167–1172.

104 **JASPER, D.E., 1982.** The role of *Mycoplasma* in bovine mastitis. *Journal of the American Veterinary Association*, 181, 158–161.

105 **JONES, J.E.T., 1991.** Mastitis in sheep. *In*: OWEN, J.B. & AXFORD, R.F.E., (eds). *Breeding for Disease Resistance in Farm Animals*. Wallingford: CAB International.

106 **JONES, J.E.T., 1991.** Mastitis. *In*: MARTIN, W.B. & AITKEN, I.D., (eds). *Diseases of Sheep*. 2nd edn. Oxford: Blackwell Scientific Publications.

107 **JONES, T.C. & HUNT, R.D., 1983.** *Veterinary Pathology*. 5th edn. Philadelphia: Lea & Febiger.

108 **JONES, T.O., 1990.** *Escherichia coli* mastitis in dairy cattle — A review of the literature. *Veterinary Bulletin*, 60, 205–231.

109 **JUBB, K.W.F., KENNEDY, P.C. & PALMER, N., 1985.** *Pathology of Domestic Animals*. 3rd edn. San Diego: Academic Press, Inc.

110 **KAPLAN, M.H., ABDUSSALAM, H. & BIJLENGA, G., 1962.** Diseases transmitted through milk. In: World Health Organization, 1962. Milk Hygiene — Hygiene in milk production, processing and distribution. World Health Organization Monograph Series, 48, 11–74. Geneva: World Health Organization.

111 **KÄSTLI, P., 1967.** Definition of mastitis. *Annual Bulletin of the International Dairy Federation*, Part III, 1–5.

112 **KENNEDY, P.C. & MILLER, R.B., 1993.** The female genital system. *In*: JUBB, K.V.F., KENNEDY, P.C. & PALMER, N., (eds). *Pathology of Domestic Animals*. 4th edn. San Diego: Academic Press, Inc.

113 **KIRK, J.H., HUFFMAN, E.M. & ANDERSON, B.C., 1980.** Mastitis and udder abnormalities as related to neonatal lamb mortality in shed-lambed range ewes. *Journal of Animal Science*, 50, 610–616.

114 **KINGWILL, R.G., DODD, F.H. & NEAVE, F.K., 1979.** Machine milking and mastitis. *In*: THIEL, C.C. & DODD, F.H., (eds). *Machine Milking*. Technical Bulletin 1. The National Institute for Research in Dairying, Reading, England.

115 **KLASTRUP, O., 1978.** Mastitis — An international occupational disease of dairy cows. *In*: VAN DEN HEEVER, L.W. & GIESECKE, W.H., (eds). *Proceedings of the First South African Symposium on Mastitis Control in Dairy Herds*. Pretoria, 10–12 August 1978, 9–12.

116 **KLASTRUP, O., 1985.** Bovine mastitis. Definition and guidelines for diagnosis. *Kieler Milchwirtschaftliche Forschungsberichte*, 37, 254–260.

117 **KLIMMER, M., 1930.** Eleventh International Veterinary Congress, London 1930. Abridged Papers: Acute Mastitis. *The Veterinary Record*, 10, 1082–1083.

118 **KNAPPENBERGER, R.E., 1963.** Disease of foals. *Thoroughbred of California*, 36, 432–433.

119 **KNIGHT, C.H. & PEAKER, M., 1991.** Mammary gland physiology. *In*: BURVENICH, C., VANDEPUTTE-VAN MESSOM, G. & HILL, A.W., (eds). *New Insights into the Pathogenesis of Mastitis*. Belgium: Hilde van de Walle.

120 **KOCHNE, G., MADDUX, R. & BRITT, J., 1981.** Rapidly growing *Mycobacteria* associated with bovine mastitis. *American Journal of Veterinary Research*, 42, 1238–1239.

121 **KVITRUD, A. & LYSNE, I., 1959.** Neon undersokelser over mastitis hos sau. *Nordisk Veterinaer Medicin*, 11, 129–140.

122 **LAKE, S.G. & JONES, J.E.T., 1970.** Post-parturient disease in sows associated with *Klebsiella* infection, correspondence. *The Veterinary Record*, 87, 484–485.

123 **LANDAU, M. & TAMARIN, R., 1974.** Ovine mastitis research, 1963–73 — a review. *Refuah Veterinath*, 31, 134–147.

124 **LEES, P., 1991.** General aspects of inflammation. *In*: BURVENICH, C., VANDEPUTTE-VAN MESSOM, G. & HILL, A.W., (eds). *New Insights into the Pathogenesis of Mastitis*. Belgium: Hilde van de Walle.

125 **LE LOUDEC, C., 1978.** Efficacité des antibiotiques contre les mammitis bovines staphylococciques et streptococciques. *Annales de Recherches Vétérinaires*, 9, 63–88.

126 **LEWTER, M.M. MULLOWNEY, P.C., BALDWIN, E.W. & WALKER, R.D., 1984.** Mastitis in goats. *The Compendium on Continuing Education for the Practising Veterinarian: Large Animal Section*, 6, S417–S425.

127 **LITTLE, R.B. & PLASTRIDGE, W.N., 1946.** *Bovine Mastitis*. New York, London: McGraw-Hill.

128 **MACDIARMID, S.C., 1978.** Antibacterial drugs used against mastitis in cattle by the systemic route. *New Zealand Veterinary Journal*, 26, 290–295.

129 **MACDIARMID, S.C., 1980.** Drugs used in the antibacterial therapy of mastitis. *Proceedings of a post-graduate short course*, 26–28 May 1980. Massey University, Palmerston North, New Zealand, 103–110.

130 **MADEL, A.J., 1983.** Mastitis. *In*: MARTIN, W.B., (ed.). *Diseases of Sheep*. Oxford: Blackwell Scientific Publications.

131 **McCUE, P.M. & WILSON, W.D., 1989.** A review of 28 cases of equine mastitis. *Equine Veterinary Journal*, 21, 351–353.

132 **McDONALD, T.J. & McDONALD, J.S., 1975.** Intramammary infections in the sow during the peripartum period. *Cornell Veterinarian*, 65, 73–83.

133 **McDOWELL, R.E., 1981.** Limitations for dairy production in developing countries. *Journal of Dairy Science*, 64, 2463–2475.

134 **McGILLIARD, L.D., 1979.** Symposium: Bovine mastitis. *Journal of Dairy Science*, 62, 117–176.

135 **MERCHANT, I.A. & PACKER, R.A., 1952.** *Handbook for the Etiology, Diagnosis and Control of Infectious Bovine Mastitis*. Revised edition. Minneapolis: Burgess Publishing Company.

136 **MILLER, G.E., BANERJEE, N.C. & STOWE, C.M., 1967.** Diffusion of certain weak organic acids and bases across the bovine mammary gland membrane after systemic administration. *Journal of Pharmacology and Therapeutics*, 157, 245–253.

137 **MOL, H., 1975.** *Antibiotics and Milk*. Rotterdam: A.A. Balkema.

138 **MOORE, G.A. & HEIDER, L.E., 1984.** Treatment of mastitis. *Veterinary Clinics of North America. Large Animal Practice*, 6, 323–333.

139 **MORRIS, R.S. & MARSH, W.E, 1985.** An economic assessment of control measures for bovine mastitits. *Kieler Milchwirtschaftliche Forschungsberichte*, 37, 244–253.

140 **MULLER, R. & THALLER, M., 1979.** Antibiotika—resistenz bei Mastitiserregern. *Schweizer Archiv für Tierernahrung*, 121, 9–14.

141 **MUNCH-PETERSEN, E., 1934.** Survey of the literature on bovine mastitis. Vols 1–3. Sydney: CSIR.

142 **MUNCH-PETERSEN, E., 1938.** Bovine Mastitis: Survey of the literature to the end of 1935. Weybridge: Imperial Bureau of Animal Health.

143 **NACHREINER, R.F. & GINTHER, O.J., 1972.** Gestational and periparturient periods of sows: Effects of altered environment, withholding of bran feeding, and induced mastitis on serum chemical, haemotologic, and clinical variables. *American Journal of Veterinary Research*, 33, 2221–2231.

144 **NEAVE, F.K., 1975.** Diagnosis of mastitis by bacteriological methods alone. *In*: DODD, F.H., GRIFFIN, T.K. & KINGWILL, R.G., (eds). Proceedings of the International Dairy Federation Seminar on Mastitis Control. Bulletin document 85, Square Vergote 41, 1040 Brussels, Belgium.

145 **NEUNDORF, R. & BRABANT, W., 1963.** Ergebnisse und Möglichkeiten der pathogenetischen Therapie (Novocainblockade) der Mastitis des Rindes. *Monatshefte der Veterinärmedizin*, 18, 603–610.

146 **NEWBOULD, F.H.S, 1965.** Disinfection in the prevention of udder infections: A review. *Canadian Veterinary Journal*, 6, 29–37.

147 **NEWBOULD, F.H.S., 1974.** Microbial diseases of the mammary gland. *In*: LARSON, B.L. & SMITH, V.R., (eds). *Lactation — A Comprehensive Treatise*. Vol. II. New York, London: Academic Press, Inc.

148 **NORCROSS, N.L., 1991.** Specific defence mechanisms of the udder. *In*: BURVENICH, C., VANDEPUTTE-VAN MESSOM, G. & HILL, A.W., (eds). *New Insights into the Pathogenesis of Mastitis*. Belgium: Hilde van de Walle.

149 **O'REILLY, L.M., 1965.** The isolation of Baxeley and Battle's type 5 *Streptococcus* from a case of equine mastitis. *Irish Veterinary Journal*, 19, 198–202.

150 **PAAPE, M.J., GUIDRY, H.J., JAIN, N.C. & MILLER, R.H., 1991.** Leukocytic defence mechanism in the udder. *In*: BURVENICH, C., VANDEPUTTE-VAN MESSOM, G. & HILL, A.W., (eds). *New Insights into the Pathogenesis of Mastitis*. Belgium: Hilde van de Walle.

151 **PAPADOPOULOS, O. & LEONTIDES, S., 1972.** Mastitis produced experimentally in sheep with an ovine abortion *Chlamydia*. *Zentralblatt für Veterinärmedizin*, Reihe B, 655–665.

152 **PENNY, R.C.H., 1970.** The agalactia complex in the sow. A review. *Australian Veterinary Journal*, 46, 153–159.

153 **PETRIS, M.A., 1963.** Ovine and caprine mastitis in Cyprus. A report on the naturally occurring disease. *Bulletin de l'Office International des Épizooties*, 60, 989–1007.

154 **PETTERSON, K.E., 1981.** Cell contents in goat's milk. *Acta Veterinaria Scandinavica*, 22, 226–237.

155 **PHILPOT, W.N., 1984.** Economics of mastitis control. *In*: JARRETT, J.A., (ed.). *The Veterinary Clinics of North America. Large Animal Practice*. Vol. VI. Symposium on Bovine Mastitis, 233–245. Philadelphia, London, Toronto, Mexico City, Rio de Janeiro, Sidney, Tokyo: W.B. Saunders Company.

156 **PHILPOT, W.N. & NICKERSON, S.C., 1991.** *Mastitis: Counter Attack*. Naperville, Illinois: Babson Bros. Co.

157 **PILLOUD, M., 1973.** Pharmacokinetics, plasma protein binding and dosage of oxytetracycline in cattle and horses. *Research in Veterinary Science*, 15, 224–230.

158 **PLASTRIDGE, W.N., 1958.** Bovine mastitis: A review. *Journal of Dairy Science*, 41, 1141–1181.

159 **PLATONOW, I. & BLOBEL, H., 1963.** Therapeutic failures in chronic staphylococcal mastitis. *Journal of the American Veterinary Medical Association*, 142, 1097–1101.

160 **PLOMMET, M. & LE LOUDEC, C., 1975.** The role of antibiotic therapy during lactation in control of subclinical and clinical mastitis. *In*: DODD, F.H., GRIFFIN, T.K. & KINGWILL, R.G., (eds). *Proceedings of the International Dairy Federation Seminar on Mastitis Control*. Bulletin Document 85, 265–281.

161 **PRASAD, L.B.M. & NEWBOULD, F.H.S., 1968.** Initial response of the bovine mammary gland to invasion by *Staphylococcus aureus*. *Canadian Veterinary Journal*, 9, 170–177.

162 **PRENTICE, M.W.M., 1974.** Mastitis in the mare. *The Veterinary Record*, 94, 380.

163 **PRICE, K.E., GALLIAN, M.J., HEATHER, C.D. & LUTHER, H.G., 1956.** The influence of milk and other media on antibiotic sensitivity of mastitis organism. *Antibiotic Annual*, 3, 753–762.

164 **PUCH, D.G., MAGNUSSON, R.A., MODRANSKY, P.D. & DARNTON, K.R., 1985.** A case of mastitis in a young filly. *Journal of Equine Veterinary Science*, 5, 132–134.

165 **PULLINGER, E.J., 1947.** The provision of a safe and satisfactory milk supply on a national basis with special reference to South African conditions. DVSc Thesis, University of Pretoria.

166 **QUINLIVAN, T.D., 1968.** Survey observations on ovine mastitis in New Zealand stud Romney flocks. 1. The incidence of ovine mastitis. *New Zealand Veterinary Journal*, 16, 152–153.

167 **QUINLIVAN, T.D., 1968.** Survey observations on ovine mastitis in New Zealand stud Romney flocks. 2. The bacteriology of ovine mastitis. *New Zealand Veterinary Journal*, 16, 149–160.

168 **RASMUSSEN, F., 1959.** Mammary excretion of benzylpenicillin, erythromycin and penethamate hydriodide. *Acta Pharmacologica et Toxicologica*, 16, 194–200.

169 **RASMUSSEN, F., 1966.** Studies on the mammary excretion and adsorption of drugs. Carl F. Mortensen, Copenhagen.

170 **RASMUSSEN, F. 1971.** Excretion of drugs in milk. *In*: BRODIE, B.B. & GILETTE, J., (eds). *Handbook of Experimental Pharmacology*. New York: Springer Verlag.

171 **REESE, G.L. & LOCK, T.F., 1978.** Streptococcal mastitis in a mare. *Journal of the American Veterinary Medical Association*, 173, 83–84.

172 **REICHMUTH, J., 1968.** Zum Einfluss subklinisch verlaufender Sekretionsstörungen und Mastitiden auf die Milchleistung von Kühen der Rasse Deutsche Schwarzbunte. Dr. Med. Vet. Thesis, Free University of Berlin.

173 **RENK, W., 1963.** Formes de mamites dans les infections staphylocciques. *Bulletin de l'Office International des Épizooties*, 60, 473–484.

174 **RICE, E.B., 1965.** Milk production in warm climates. *Dairy Science Abstracts*, 27, 43–54.

175 **RINGARP, N., 1960.** Clinical and experimental investigations into a post-parturient syndrome with agalactiae sows. *Acta Agriculturae Scandinavica*, Supplementum, 7, 166.

176 **ROBERTS, M.C., 1986.** *Pseudomonas aeruginosa* mastitis in a dry non-pregnant pony mare. *Equine Veterinary Journal*, 18, 146–147.

177 **ROBINSON, J.T.R., 1967.** A discussion of Q-fever as a potential problem in South Africa in the light of past experience in other countries. M. Med. Vet. (Hyg.) Seminar, University of Pretoria.

178 **ROBINSON, T.C., 1980.** Therapy for acute and peracute mastitis. *In*: BRAMLEY, A.J., DODD, F.H. & GRIFFIN, T.K., (eds). *Mastitis Control and Herd Management*, Technical Bulletin 4. National Institute for Research in Dairying, Reading, England, 128–134.

179 **ROSS, R.F., ORNING, A.P., WOODS, R.D., ZIMMERMAN, B.J., COX, D.F. & HARRIS, D.L., 1981.** Bacteriologic study of sow agalactia. *American Journal of Veterinary Research*, 42, 949–955.

180 **ROSSDALE, P.D. & RICKETTS, S.W., 1974.** *The Practice of Equine Stud Medicine*. 1st edn. Baltimore: Williams & Wilkens.

181 **SANDERSON, C.J., 1966.** The treatment of mastitis with intramammary infusions. *Australian Veterinary Journal*, 42, 47–53.

182 **SCHAAL, E.H., 1982.** Zur Euterbesiedlung mit *Coxiella burnetii* beim Q-Fieber des Rindes. *Deutsche Tierärztliche Wochenschrift*, 89, 393–432.

183 **SCHAAL, E.H. & SCHÄFER, J., 1984.** Zur Verbreitung des Q-Fiebers in einheimischen Rinderbeständen. *Deutsche Tierärztliche Wochenschrift*, 91, 52–56.

184 **SCHALM, O.W., CARROLL, E.J. & JAIN, N.C., 1971.** *Bovine Mastitis*. Philadelphia: Lea & Febiger.

185 **SCHALM, O.W. & WOODS, G.M., 1953.** The mastitis

complex. *Journal of the American Veterinary Medical Association*, 122, 462–467.

186 **SCHIPPER, I.A. & EVELETH, D.F., 1959.** Rates and routes of sulfonamide excretion in the cow. I. Milk levels following single intravenous and oral administration. *American Journal of Veterinary Research*, 20, 714–717.

187 **SCHLUEP, J., 1966.** Weitere Untersuchugen über die Frage der Zusammenhänge zwischen Melkbarkeit und Eutergesundheit. *Zeitschrift für Tierzüchtung und Züchtungskunde*, 83, 193–218.

188 **SCHLUEP, J., ROSSELET, A. & HELM, H., 1979.** Comparative evaluation of cephacetrile in experimentally induced bovine mastitis. *Zentralblatt für Veterinärmedizin*, Reihe B, 26, 304–324.

189 **SCHMIDT, G.H., 1969.** Mastitis control: Method and Progress. *Journal of Dairy Science*, 52, 689–695.

190 **SEELEMANN, M., 1964.** Über den Zellgehalt der Milch, seine Feststellung, Bedeutung und Beurteilung. *Milchwissenschaft*, 19, 182–194.

191 **SHNAWA, I.M.S. & NIGAM, J.M., 1987.** A note on cryptococcal mastitis in sheep. *Indian Journal of Veterinary Medicine*, 7, 175–176.

192 **SHOOP, D.S. & MYERS, L.L., 1984.** Serologic analysis of isolates of *Pasteurella haemolytica* and *Staphylococcus aureus* from mastitic ewes. *American Journal of Veterinary Research*, 45, 1944–1946.

193 **SIMPSON, J.R. & WILCOX, C.J., 1982.** Determination of optimal cattle systems for tropical and subtropical livestock enterprises. *Journal of Dairy Science*, 65, 1055–1066.

194 **SJOQVIST, E., BORGA, O. & ORME, M.L., 1976.** Fundamentals of clinical pharmacology. *In*: AVERY, G.S., (ed.). *Drug Treatment*. Sydney: Adis Press.

195 **SMITH, B.B., MARTINEAU, G. & BISAILLON, A., 1992.** Mammary glands and lactation problems. *In*: LEHMAN, A.D., STRAW, B.E., MENGELING, W.L., D'ALLAIRE, S. & TAYLOR, D.J., (eds). *Diasease of Swine*. 7th edn. Ames, Iowa: Iowa State University Press.

196 **SMITH, H.A., JONES, J.C. & HUNT, R.D., 1972.** *Veterinary Pathology*. 4th edn. Philadelphia: Lea & Febiger.

197 **SMITH, K.L., 1983.** Mastitis Control: A discussion. *Journal of Dairy Science*, 66, 1790–1794.

198 **SMITH, K.L., TODHUNTER, D.A. & SCHOENBERGER, P.S., 1985.** Environmental pathogens and intramammary infection during the dry period. *Journal of Dairy Science*, 68, 402–417.

199 **SMITH, K.L., TODHUNTER, D.A. & SCHOENBERGER, P.S., 1985.** Environmental mastitis: Cause, prevalence, prevention. *Journal of Dairy Science*, 68, 1531–1553.

200 **SMITH, M.C. & ROGUINSKY, M., 1977.** Mastitis and other diseases of the goat's udder. *Journal of the American Veterinary Medical Association*, 171, 1241–1248.

201 **SOBACK, S. & ZIV, G., 1985.** Intramammary amoxycillin/corticosteroid therapy for experimental *E. coli*-endotoxin mastitis. *Kieler Milchwirtschaftliche Forschungsberichte*, 37, 548–554.

202 **SWARBRICK, O., 1968.** The porcine agalactia syndrome. Clinical and histological observations. *The Veterinary Record*, 80, 241–252.

203 **SWARTZ, R., JOOSTE, P.J. & NOVELLO, J.C., 1984.** Prevalence and types of bacteria associated with subclinical mastitis in Bloemfontein dairy herds. *Journal of the South African Veterinary Association*, 55, 61–64.

204 **SWARTZ, R., JOOSTE, P.J. & NOVELLO, J.C., 1984.** Antibiotic susceptibility patterns of mastitis pathogens isolated from Bloemfontein dairy herds. *Journal of the South African Veterinary Association*, 55, 187–193.

205 **SWARTZ, R., JOOSTE, P.J. & NOVELLO, J.C., 1985.** Bacteriophage typing of *Staphylococcus aureus* strains isolated from Bloemfontein dairy herds. *Journal of the South African Veterinary Association*, 56, 69–73.

206 **THIEL, C.C. & DODD, F.H., 1979.** Machine milking. Technical Bulletin 1. The National Institute for Research in Dairying, Reading, England.

207 **TILGNER, K. & SCHIERHOLTZ, H., 1954.** Beobachtungen über die Veränderung der euterpathogenen Streptokokkenflora durch Therapie mit antibiotischen Mitteln. *Berliner und Münchener Tierärztliche Wochenschrift*, 67, 90–93.

208 **TOLLE, A., 1969.** Über den Einfluss von Mastitiden und Sekretionsstörungen auf die Qualität der Milch. *Proceedings of the Fifth Symposium of the World Association of Veterinary Food-Hygienists*. Opatija, 22–27 September 1969, 331–357.

209 **TOLLE, A., 1970.** Zur zytologischen, biochemischen und bakteriologischen Beurteilung von Milch. *Schweizer Archiv für Tierheilkunde*, 112, 512–533.

210 **TOLLE, A., 1971.** A monograph on bovine mastitis. Part I. Economics, aetiology and diagnosis. *Annual Bulletin of the International Dairy Federation*, 1–23.

211 **TOLLE, A., 1973.** A monograph on bovine mastitis. Part II. Principles of mastitis control. *Annual Bulletin of the International Dairy Federation*, Document No. 76.

212 **TOLLE, A., 1975.** Mastitis — The disease in relation to control methods. *In*: DODD, F.H., GRIFFIN, T.K. & KINGWILL, R.G., (eds). Proceedings of the IDF Seminar on Mastitis Control 1975. *Bulletin of the International Dairy Federation*, Document 85, 3–15.

213 **TOLLE, A., HEESCHEN, W. & HAMANN, J., 1977.** Grundlagen einer systematischen Bekämpfung der subklinischen Mastitis des Rindes. *Kieler Milchwirtschaftliche Forschungsberichte*, 29, 3–103.

214 **TULKENS, P.M., 1991.** Target drugs for the treatment of intracellular infections. *In*: BURVENICH, C., VANDEPUTTE-VAN MESSOM, G. & HILL, A.W., (eds). *New Insights into the Pathogenesis of Mastitis*. Belgium: Hilde van de Walle.

215 **TULLY, J.G. & WHITCOMB, R.F., 1979.** *The Mycoplasmas*. Vol. II. *Human and Animal Mycoplasmas*. New York: Academic Press, Inc.

216 **TUSTIN, R.C., 1978.** The characteristics of mastitis. *In*: VAN DEN HEEVER, L.W. & GIESECKE, W.H., (eds). *Proceedings of the First South African Symposium on Mastitis Control in Dairy Herds*. Pretoria, 10–12 August 1978.

217 **UDALL, D.H. & JOHNSON, S.D., 1931.** The diagnosis and control of mastitis. *Cornell Veterinarian*, 21, 190–206.

218 **ULLBERG, S., 1954.** Studies on the distribution and fate of S^{35}-labelled benzylpenicillin in the body. *Acta Radiology*, Supplement 118.

219 **ULLBERG, S., HANSON, E. & FUNKE, H., 1958.** Distribution of penicillin in mastitic udders following intramammary injection — and autoradiographic study. *American Journal of Veterinary Research*, 19, 84–92.

220 **VAN DEN HEEVER, L.W., 1950.** A preliminary survey of bovine diseases affecting the quality and safety of a large town's milk supply. *Journal of the South African Veterinary Medical Association*, 21, 108–113.

221 **VAN DEN HEEVER, L.W., 1962.** Tracer dyes in intramammary preparations as a method of rapid indirect detection of antibiotic residues in milk — a review. *Journal of the South African Veterinary Medical Association*, 32, 29–33.

222 **VAN DEN HEEVER, L.W., 1978.** The public health significance of mastitis. *In*: VAN DEN HEEVER, L.W. & GIESECKE, W.H., (eds). *Proceedings of the First South African Symposium on Mastitis Control in Dairy Herds*. Pretoria, 10–12 August 1978.

223 **VAN DEN HEEVER, L.W. & GIESECKE, W.H., 1967**. Bovine mastitis: The need for positive action and the means at our disposal. *Journal of the South African Dairy Industry*, 7, 156–161.

224 **VAN DER MOLEN, E.J. & HOUWERS, D.J., 1987.** Indurative lymphocytic mastitis in sheep after experimental infection with maedi-visna. *The Veterinary Quarterly*, 9, 193–202.

225 **VAN DER MOLEN, E.J., VECHT, U. & HOUWERS, D.J., 1985.** A chronic indurative mastitis in sheep, associated with

maedi-visna virus infection. *The Veterinary Quarterly*, 7, 112–119.
226 **VAN MIERT, A.S.J., 1991.** Acute phase response and non-cellular defence mechanisms. *In:* BURVENICH, C., VANDEPUTTE-VAN MESSOM, G. & HILL, A.W., (eds). *New Insights into the Pathogenesis of Mastitis*. Belgium: Hilde van de Walle.
227 **VAN RENSBURG, S.W.J., 1939.** Bovine mastitis. *Farming in South Africa*, 334–338.
228 **VEARY, C.M., GIESECKE, W.H. & DU PREEZ, J.H., 1989.** Modular Herd Control of Mastitis (MHCM): Lectures, short communications, summary and resolution. Proceedings of the SAVA Workshop on Modular Herd Control of Mastitis, University of Natal, Pietermaritzburg, 14–15 July 1988. *Journal of the South African Veterinary Association*, June 1989, Special Volume No. 2, 1–66.
229 **VECHT, U., VAN DAM, H. & VAN DER BERG, J., 1982.** Verslag landelijke steekproef mastitis 1980. Lelystad: Central Veterinary Institute.
230 **WAITE, R. & BLACKBURN, P.S., 1957.** The chemical composition and the cell count of milk. *Journal of Dairy Research*, 24, 328–339.
231 **WALL, S., 1918.** *Mastitis of the Cow*. Philadelphia, London: J.B. Lippincott Company.
232 **WALSER, K., 1966.** *Melkmaschine und Mastitis*. Berlin, Hamburg: P. Parey.
233 **WATKINS, G.H., BURRIEL, A.R. & JONES, J.E.T., 1991.** A field investigation of subclinical mastitis in sheep in southern England. *British Veterinary Journal*, 147, 413–420.
234 **WATSON, D.L., 1988.** Vaccination against experimental staphylococcal mastitis in ewes. *Research in Veterinary Science*, 45, 16–21.
235 **WATSON, W.A., 1965.** The carriage of pathogenic staphylococci by sheep. *The Veterinary Record*, 77, 477–480.
236 **WATTS, J.L., 1985.** Impact of new staphylococcal species descriptions on mastitis research. *Kieler Milchwirtschaftliche Forschungsberichte*, 37, 549–553.
237 **WATTS, J.L., 1988.** Characterization and identification of streptococci isolated from bovine mammary glands. *Journal of Dairy Science*, 71, 1616–1624.
238 **WELSH, R.D., 1984.** The significance of *Streptococcus zooepidemicus* in the horse. *Equine Practice*, 6, 6–16.
239 **WHEELOCK, J.V., ROOK, J.A.F., NEAVE, F.K. & DODD, F.H., 1966.** The effect of bacterial infections of the udder on the yield and composition of cow milk. *Journal of Dairy Research*, 33, 199–215.
240 **WHITE, G. & WITHNELL, C.G., 1973.** Chemotherapeutic evaluation of trimethoprim and sulphonamide in experimental salmonellosis of sheep. *Research in Veterinary Science*, 11, 245–254.
241 **WILSON, C.D., 1980.** Antibiotic therapy in mastitis control. *In*: BRAMLEY, A.J., DODD, F.H. & GRIFFIN, T.K., (eds). *Mastitis Control and Herd Management*. Technical Bulletin 4. National Institute for Research in Dairying, Reading, England, 113–127.
242 **ZIV, G., 1969.** Antibiotic sensitivity to *Staphylococcus aureus* strains from bovine udders in Israel. *Refuah Veterinarith*, 26, 104–113.
243 **ZIV, G., 1975.** Pharmacokinetic concepts for systemic and intramammary treatment in lactating and dry cows. *In*: DODD, F.H., GRIFFIN, T.K. & KINGWILL, R.G., (eds). *Proceedings of the International Dairy Federation Seminar on Mastitis Control*. Bulletin Document 85, 314–340.
244 **ZIV, G., 1978.** Distribution of several labelled antibacterial agents in the udder as measured by contact autoradiographic methods. *Refuah Veterinarith*, 35, 32–33.
245 **ZIV, G., 1980.** Practical pharmacokinetic aspects of mastitis therapy — 1: Parenteral treatment. *Agri Practice*, February, 227–290.
246 **ZIV, G., 1980.** Practical pharmacokinetic aspects of mastitis therapy — 2: Practical and therapeutic applications. *Agri Practice*, March, 469–474.
247 **ZIV, G., 1980.** Practical pharmacokinetic aspects of mastitis therapy — 3: Intramammary treatment. *Agri Practice*, April, 657–670.
248 **ZIV, G., 1980.** Drug selection and use in mastitis. Systemic vs local therapy. *Journal of the American Veterinary Medical Association*, 176, 1109–1115.
249 **ZIV, G., 1992.** Treatment of peracute and acute mastitis. *Veterinary Clinics of North America: Food Animal Practice*, 8, 1–15.
250 **ZIV, G., BOGIN, E. & SULMAN, F.G., 1973.** Blood and milk levels of chloramphenicol in normal and mastitic cows and ewes after intramuscular administration of chloramphenicol and chloramphenicol sodium succinate. *Zentralblatt für Veterinärmedizin*, Reihe A, 20, 801–811.
251 **ZIV, G., SHANI, J., PHARM, M. & SULMAN, F.G., 1973.** Pharmacokinetic evaluation of penicillin and cephalosporin derivatives in serum and milk of lactating cows and ewes. *American Journal of Veterinary Research*, 34, 1561–1565.
252 **ZIV, G. & SULMAN, F.G., 1972.** Binding of antibiotics to bovine and ovine serum. *Antimicrobial Agents and Chemotherapeutics*, 2, 206–213.

191

Epivag

Synonyms: Infectious infertility, infectious bovine cervico-vaginitis and epididymitis, epizootic infertility, epididymitis-vaginitis

A.P. Schutte

Introduction

Epivag is an insidious, venereal, infectious disease of cattle that is characterized in cows by an anterior vaginitis with a thick, tenacious, mucopurulent discharge from the vulva, and in bulls by chronic epididymitis and seminal vesiculitis that results in fibrosis and induration of the epididymis, seminal vesicles and testes. The fertility of affected cows is usually impaired, but abortion is not a feature of the disease. In bulls the disease usually results in reduced fertility, and complete impotency in some. Because the lesions that develop in the genital organs of both sexes are basically those of an epididymitis or vaginitis, the name 'epivag' was coined for the disease.[4]

The condition appears to be confined to Africa. It was first described in Kenya by Daubney, Hudson and Anderson in 1938[1] and has since been diagnosed in Zimbabwe and South Africa.[12] Earlier reports indicate that the disease was most prevalent in the Transvaal and the Orange Free State, but it has occurred to a lesser extent in Natal. Epivag has not been reported from the Cape Province. In South Africa at present the disease is only sporadically encountered on the Transvaal Highveld in poorly managed dairy herds in which natural breeding is practised. Although no reports are available, the same situation most probably prevails in other countries in southern, central and east Africa.

Aetiology and epidemiology

The aetiology of the disease has not as yet been elucidated, but in view of its epidemiology, one or possibly more infectious agents are thought to be involved. The consensus of opinion is that epivag is caused by a virus, but all attempts to determine its aetiology have failed. Bovine herpesvirus 1 has been isolated from seminal plasma and vaginal discharges of affected animals.[2, 5, 6, 9] However, attempts to reproduce the disease by infecting cattle with it, and with bovine herpesvirus 4, have been unsuccessful.[7, 8, 10, 11]

Epivag spreads in herds in which the cattle are allowed to breed naturally; it does not occur in herds in which artificial insemination is practised. Affected bulls in the early or advanced stage of the disease transmit the disease venereally to susceptible heifers and cows. Similarly, infected females with mild or severe vaginitis may cause venereal transmission of the infection to susceptible bulls. It would seem that females are still capable of spreading the infection venereally to bulls several months or perhaps even years after they have apparently recovered from the disease.

According to Van Rensburg,[12] the disease is more acute in some herds than in others; environmental conditions such as climate, and possibly also nutritional factors may influence the severity and course of the disease.

Clinical signs and pathology

Clinical evidence of the infection in bulls may only be detectable four to ten weeks after natural service of an infected female. The earliest lesions following infection are seminal vesiculitis and a slight palpable enlargement of one or both of the spermatic cords. Eventually the epididymes and testes also become involved. The latter lesions usually commence unilaterally, but in the later stages of the disease are often bilateral. The libido of bulls with early or advanced lesions is usually unimpaired, so affected bulls may continue to serve and spread the infection. In some bulls, however, libido is reduced, and they may even become completely impotent.

The acute lesions in the seminal vesicles are characterized by enlargement and pain on palpation. When evaluating the size of the seminal glands, cognizance should be taken of the variable size of these glands in healthy bulls. In chronically affected bulls the glands are enlarged, firm, usually not painful on palpation, and the lobulation is less distinct **(Figure 191.1)**.

In naturally occurring acute cases, an initial diffuse swelling of the affected testis, probably as a result of degeneration, masks the changes in the epididymis. Epididymal lesions are only evident once the testicular swelling has subsided. The tail of the epididymis may be slightly or markedly enlarged, loses resilience and elasticity, and becomes a hard, spherical mass with an

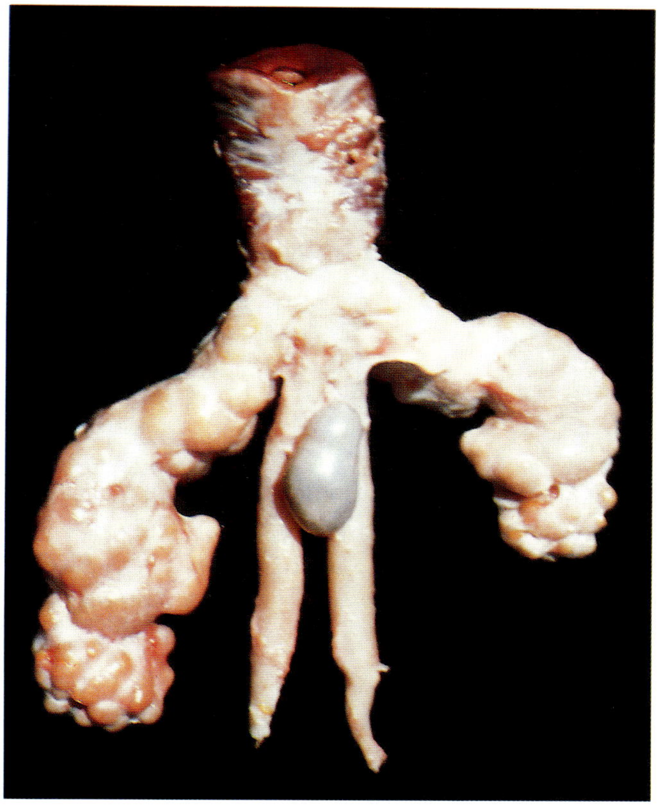

Figure 191.1 Epivag: irregular enlargement of the seminal glands as a consequence of chronic inflammation

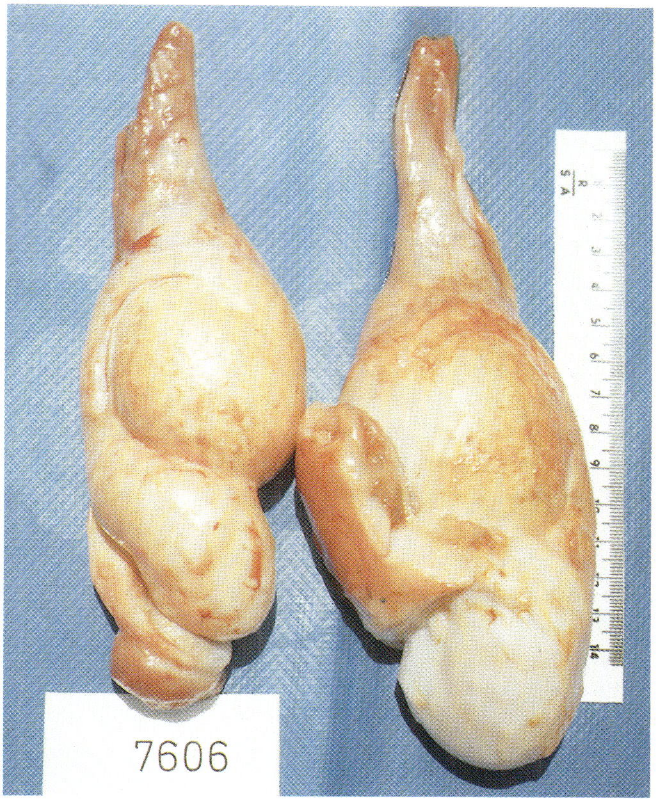

Figure 191.2 Severe bilateral chronic epididymitis and pronounced unilateral testicular atrophy

irregularly lobulated surface due to the chronic interstitial epididymitis and consequent ductular obstructions that develop. Later in the course of the disease, similar changes are detectable in the head of the epididymis, and eventually the normal structure of the epididymis is completely replaced by fibrous tissue.[3] There are adhesions between the *tunica vaginalis propria* and *tunica vaginalis communis*, and the testis becomes atrophied and the interstitial tissue fibrosed **(Figure 191.2)**. Although the quality of the semen of affected bulls is reduced, they are still, in the majority of cases, fertile for a period before sterility supervenes. Recovery in bulls is extremely rare.

The course of the disease varies in heifers and cows. About seven to ten days after coitus a diffuse anterior vaginitis is generally detectable, with the accumulation of a thick, tenacious, yellowish, mucopurulent, odourless exudate which adheres to the mucous membrane of the vagina. The exudate is discharged periodically for about two weeks, resulting in soiling of the tail and buttocks, giving the latter a characteristic glistening, streaky appearance. The volume of exudate varies; at times it may be copious and as much as 500 ml may accumulate in the vagina. Acutely affected female animals may conceive and produce offspring. In approximately 25 per cent of cases the inflammation extends into the cervix and uterus, which results in the production of copious amounts of pus, as well as into the oviducts, resulting in chronic salpingitis, hydrosalpynx, peri-oophoritis, and fibrous adhesions between the Fallopian tubes and adjacent tissues **(Figure 191.3)**. These animals are usually sterile. In most cases these changes are confined to the pelvic region, but the inflammatory process may also extend into the abdominal cavity, resulting in widespread fibrous peritonitis and the development of adhesions between abdominal organs.[3]

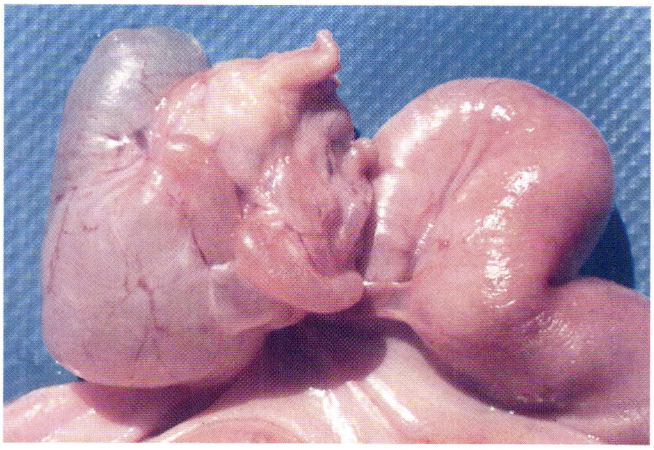

Figure 191.3 Epivag: chronic peri-oophoritis, hydrosalpynx and fibrous adhesions

Diagnosis and differential diagnosis

As the aetiology of epivag is not known, a diagnosis is based entirely on the clinical signs: presence of genital lesions (seminal vesiculitis and epididymal and testicular lesions in bulls; the thick, tenacious, yellow, mucopurulent, odourless vaginal discharge that affects a number of females); and a history of prolonged intercalving periods and sterility in some animals in herds where natural service is practised.

Bovine herpesvirus-1 causes infectious pustular vulvovaginitis or infectious pustular balanoposthitis, but does not result in seminal vesiculitis and epididymitis in bulls, and the lesions in the vagina of cows are usually small, multifocal, vesicular or erosive, while a copious exudate such as that often present in epivag is not a feature of the disease. Trichomonal infection in cows can be differentiated from epivag by the difference in the nature and volume of the vaginal discharge; in trichomoniasis, the uterine content and vaginal discharge are less tenacious and voluminous than in epivag and the fluid, although also odourless, is greyish-white and contains trichomonads in great numbers.

Seminal vesiculitis may also occur in young virgin bulls on a high protein and carbohydrate diet. The aetiology of this syndrome has not been elucidated but it is speculated that hormonal influences and possibly certain infections (*Mycoplasma* spp.) may play a role. Infection of the seminal vesicles by pyogenic bacteria (*Actinomyces pyogenes, Streptococcus* spp.), *Brucella abortus bovis, Mycobacterium bovis, Chlamydia psittaci* and *Mycoplasma* spp. may also occasionally cause vesiculitis.

Control

The use of artificial insemination in a herd is considered to be the best method of control for epivag, but the semen should originate from certified disease-free bulls, the hygiene of the insemination technique should be of prescribed standard, and the management system applied by the farmer should be suitable for performing insemination. It must be emphasized that females which have been infected should be allowed a period of sexual rest before insemination, during which time oestrous cycles should be regular.

References

1 **DAUBNEY, R., HUDSON, J.R. & ANDERSON, J., 1938.** Preliminary description of a form of sterility in cattle associated with vaginitis in female stock and with chronic changes in the epididymis and the testicles of bulls. *East African Agricultural Journal*, 3, 31–34.

2 **HELLIG, H., 1965.** Investigation into natural outbreaks of infectious pustular vulvo-vaginitis in cattle in South Africa. *Journal of the South African Veterinary Medical Association*, 36, 219–226.

3 **HENNING, M.W., 1956.** Infectious bovine infertility. *In*: *Animal Diseases in South Africa*. 3rd edn. Pretoria: Central News Agency Ltd.

4 **HUDSON, J.R., 1949.** A specific venereal disease of cattle characterized by epididymitis in bulls and vaginitis in cows and heifers. *Proceedings of the Fourteenth International Veterinary Congress*, London. Vol. II, 487–491.

5 **KAMINJOLO, J.S., NYAGA, P.N., ONNUSE, J.K. & MUTIGA, E.R., 1975.** Infectious bovine rhinotracheitis/infectious pustular vulvo-vaginitis viral isolates from cattle with epididymitis and vaginitis. *American Journal of Veterinary Research*, 36, 123–125.

6 **MARÉ, L.J. & VAN RENSBURG, S.J., 1961.** The isolation of viruses associated with infertility in cattle: A preliminary report. *Journal of the South African Veterinary Medical Association*, 32, 201–210.

7 **McINTOSH, B.M., HAIG, D.A. & ALEXANDER, R.A., 1952.** Isolation of viruses associated with epididymitis and vaginitis in cattle. *Journal of the South African Veterinary Medical Association*, 23, 165–166.

8 **SCHUTTE, A.P, 1993.** Taurus, Private Bag X5, Irene, South Africa. Unpublished data.

9 **SWANEPOEL, R. & CHRISTIE, S., 1972.** A survey of infectious bovine rhinotracheitis in Rhodesian cattle. *Rhodesian Veterinary Journal*, 3, 20–25.

10 **THEODORIDIS, A., 1978.** Preliminary characterization of viruses isolated from cases of epididymitis and vaginitis in cattle. *Onderstepoort Journal of Veterinary Research*, 45, 187–195.

11 **THEODORIDIS, A., 1985.** Studies on bovine herpesviruses. Part I. Isolation and characterization of viruses isolated from the genital tract of cattle. *Onderstepoort Journal of Veterinary Research*, 52, 239–254.

12 **VAN RENSBURG, S.W.J., 1953.** Bovine sterility caused by infectious diseases in South Africa. *The British Veterinary Journal*, 109, 226–233.

192

Ulcerative balanoposthitis and vulvovaginitis of sheep and goats

C.J.V. Trichard and E.M. Van Tonder

Introduction

Ulcerative balanoposthitis and vulvovaginitis of sheep is a disease characterized by erosions and ulcerations of the external genitalia of rams and ewes. A similar syndrome has been recorded in goats. The cause is unknown but is considered to be an infectious agent. The condition is transmitted venereally and occurs most frequently in Dorper and Karakul sheep; other breeds are affected less frequently. In South Africa 2 – 4 per cent of the national herd is estimated to be affected at any one time.

This disease was first encountered in South Africa in the Calvinia district in 1976 [11] and later in a semi-intensive mutton production unit in the north-eastern Orange Free State during the early part of 1979. Although the ulcerative balanoposthitis and vulvovaginitis syndrome has not yet been recorded in other countries in southern Africa, vulvovaginitis seems to be a fairly common condition in goats in Nigeria. [8]

Similar disease syndromes, apparently with various causes, have been encountered in several countries. In some outbreaks in Britain rams and ewes were affected,[14] while in outbreaks in Australia, England, Canada, the USA and India, ewes have shown manifestations of vulvovaginitis, granular vaginitis, vulvitis and vaginitis.[1, 9, 12, 16, 18, 29, 30]

Aetiology

In southern Africa the aetiology of ulcerative balanoposthitis and vulvovaginitis has not been conclusively resolved. However, its course and mode of spread leave little doubt that an infectious agent is involved.

The bacteria isolated most consistently from field cases are *Fusobacterium necrophorum*, *Corynebacterium* spp. provisionally typed as *C. xerosis* and *C. renale*, *Histophilus ovis* and *Streptococcus faecalis*, [35] but these organisms have consistently failed to induce disease following intrapreputial instillation. This was true even when preputial massage or the penile mucosa being rubbed with sterile gauze caused mild trauma.

No viruses have been isolated from affected animals, but a number of mollicutes, namely *Mycoplasma bovigenitalium*, *M. arginini*, *M. mycoides mycoides* LC, *M. mycoides capri*, *Mycoplasma* sp. Group 7, *M. agalactiae*, *M. capricolum*, unidentified *Mycoplasma* spp. and *Ureaplasma* spp., have been isolated from penile and vulval specimens, particularly from vesicular lesions.[26, 31] Although not as pronounced as in natural cases, granular-vesicular vaginitis or balanitis was caused by the application of combinations of some of the mollicute cultures to the mucous membrane. Circumstantial evidence therefore suggested that either a single mollicute or a combination of species is responsible for the condition. Prominent lesions have also been induced following experimental infection with several *Ureaplasma* spp.[1, 15, 31]

In other countries various mollicute species, such as *Mycoplasma* sp. 2D, *M. capricolum*, *M. mycoides mycoides*, *M. bovigenitalium*, *M. agalactiae*, *M. mycoides capri*, *M. bovis*, *M. arginini*, *M. alkalescens*, *Acholeplasma laidlawii*, *A. axanthum*, *A. granularum*, *A. modicum* and *Ureaplasma* spp., have been isolated from sheep and goats suffering from vulvovaginitis, granular vaginitis or vulvitis.[1, 8, 9, 12, 14, 16, 19, 20, 27, 30]

In Australia a caprine herpesvirus has been isolated from lesions in goats with ulcerative vulvitis and ulcerative balanoposthitis.[30]

Although the cause of this condition in southern Africa and elsewhere remains unresolved, it appears that mollicutes are the primary pathogens, while several bacteria, such as *F. necrophorum*, *H. ovis* and *Corynebacterium* spp., are secondary invaders which aggravate the primary lesions to produce the acute disease encountered in the field.

Epidemiology

Ulcerative balanoposthitis and vulvovaginitis in sheep has been recorded on a large number of farms in the Cape Midlands, the Eastern Cape Province, the southern Orange Free State, and the semi-arid north-eastern and north-western Cape Province.[15, 31, 34] In all outbreaks rams and ewes were severely affected, but the disease was particularly prevalent in rams.

In South Africa, the condition has mostly been

observed in the Dorper and Karakul breeds and to a much lesser extent in Merino, South African Mutton Merino, and Île de France rams as well as Angora goats.[11]

There is little doubt that natural transmission of ulcerative balanoposthitis and vulvovaginitis in South Africa is venereal.[11, 31, 32, 34] Although *Ureaplasma* infection is overcome soon after transmission,[23] some ewes may remain infected for up to a year after the initial clinical signs.[4]

Inapparently infected carrier rams and ewes may be important in the transmission of infection within and between flocks;[1, 2, 4, 5, 12–14, 17, 18, 22, 23, 32, 34] sudden acute outbreaks often occur shortly after their introduction into susceptible flocks.[14, 34] Latent infection in ewes has resulted in sudden outbreaks of vulvovaginitis in late pregnancy or after lambing,[1, 5, 12, 18] unless another unknown method of natural transmission is involved. Mollicutes have been isolated from the vagina of apparently healthy ewes which either exhibited normal oestrous cycles, were pregnant, or had recently lambed or mated.[17, 21, 22, 24, 25, 31, 32]

Young lambs of either sex may become infected in the prepubertal stage [4, 5, 12, 21] and act as inapparent carriers or reservoirs of infection. It is also possible for transmission of the disease to young animals to occur during the perinatal period,[4, 5, 21] *in utero* or during parturition.[5]

The perineum of ewes which have become reinfected after treatment and apparent recovery may act as a reservoir of infection from which auto-infection of the genital tract may occur.[23] Ram-to-ram spread during homosexual activities and mechanical ram-to-ewe contact during mating are important in the transmission of the disease.

Trauma and secondary bacterial infection by organisms such as *F. necrophorum* and *Corynebacterium* spp. appear to facilitate the initiation of the disease. Wet wool surrounding the vulva and frequent mating in an uncontrolled breeding system may cause excessive friction and laceration of the mucous membranes of the male and female genitalia.

The mechanical spread of infection of the penis and prepuce from one ram to another by handlers during the collection of semen has been recorded,[10] while insects such as flies can also transmit organisms mechanically. Rotational mating of ewes will promote venereal transfer of infection within flocks, as will the re-introduction of rams which apparently have been successfully treated.

Clinical signs and pathology

Acute outbreaks of ulcerative balanoposthitis and vulvovaginitis in sheep flocks normally follow five to six days after the introduction of infected animals, particularly rams.[36] Reluctance or complete refusal to serve are the first signs in rams. They may also be depressed and sometimes stand aside and assume an arched-back stance. If an affected ram does mate, blood may ooze from the preputial opening. Preputial haemorrhage may also occur after urination, which is often accompanied by straining. The skin and hair or wool of the ventral aspect of the abdomen, particularly around the prepuce, is often blood-stained. Swelling of the preputial opening and of the sheath may occur in some cases.

Often the penis can only be manually extruded with difficulty, if at all. On extrusion, the penis is severely inflamed and may be covered by a fibrinous or mucopurulent exudate **(Figure 192.1).** The mucous membrane may tear and bleed easily and often shows small, scattered papulo-vesicular lesions which quickly develop into erosions or even ulcers. In some cases the erosions are extensive and ulcers may cover most of the glans penis. Ulcers of variable size may also occur at the preputial orifice, often completely surrounding it. If scabs are present, their removal exposes raw, bleeding surfaces covered by variable amounts of necrotic material. In severe cases, fibrosis and preputial adhesions result in phimosis. Paraphimosis, which is occasionally seen, culminates in extensive trauma and soiling of the organ. While clinical signs are developing, ewes which have been served will be noticed to have blood-stained hind quarters, particularly around the vulva and on the tail.

In Dorper ewes which have their tails docked very short, thus exposing their external genitalia, the vulval lips are swollen, oedematous and congested, and a blood-stained fluid or reddish, stringy mucus oozes from the external orifice. Frequent wagging of the tail-butt and urination, sometimes accompanied by straining, are observed in some cases. In early cases the mucosa of the vagina is swollen and reddish-purple, with numerous greyish-white papulo-vesicular lesions scattered over the caudal region.[1, 12, 14] Small ulcers and small papular lesions, which bleed easily when handled or during vaginoscopic examination, may be present throughout the vaginal mucosa. Larger scab-covered ulcers are usually found on the vulval lips at the mucocutaneous junction, and particularly at the ventral tip of the vulva **(Figure 192.2).**

Diagnosis and differential diagnosis

The diagnosis of ulcerative balanoposthitis and vulvovaginitis is at present based on clinical signs, epidemiological features and macroscopical pathology.

A fairly accurate diagnosis can be made if the typical acute condition suddenly appears after four to six days of sexual activity.

Ulcerative balanoposthitis and vulvovaginitis should be differentiated from enzootic balanoposthitis (sheath rot) in rams and wethers, and vulvitis in ewes which have been fed on protein-rich diets. This latter disease syndrome follows a protracted course. The primary lesion in rams and wethers is a small scab on the skin dorsal to the preputium. The lesion gradually enlarges and extends into the preputial orifice to eventually involve the penis. In ewes the vulval lips are involved.

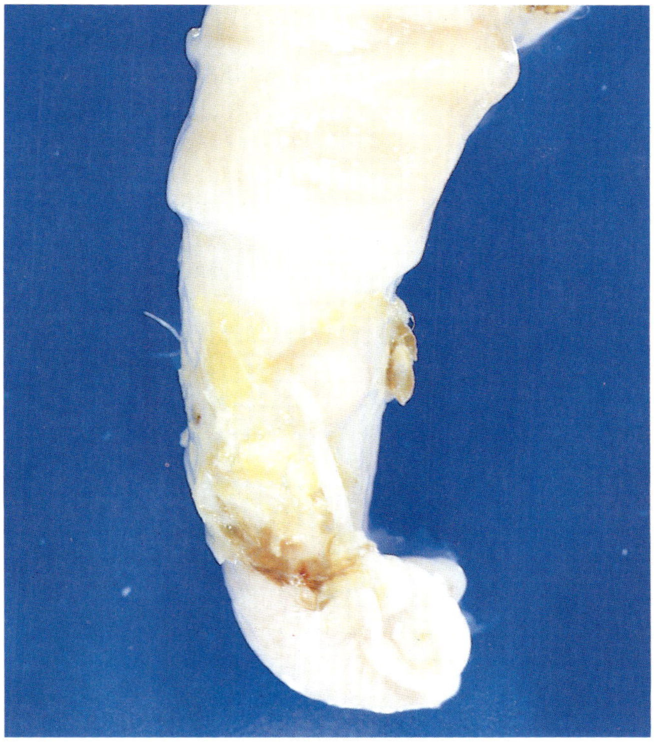

Figure 192.1 Infectious balanoposthitis in a ram. Note fibrinous exudate on the mucosa of the glans and the irregular ulcers close to the tip of the penis

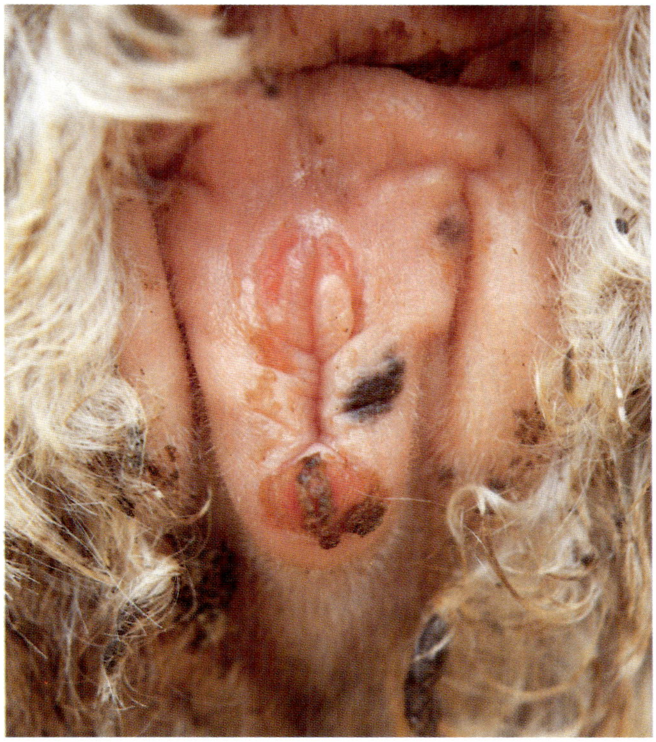

Figure 192.2 Infectious vulvovaginitis. Swollen, hyperaemic vulva of an affected ewe. Note the scab on the ulcer at the ventral commissure, and the linear ulcers elsewhere on the lips of the vulva

This syndrome invariably occurs independently of the mating process. *Corynebacterium* spp. (which can be typed as either *C. xerosis* or *C. renale*) can usually be cultured from the lesions.[6, 7, 28]

Posthitis and ulcerative or proliferative vulvitis are secondary manifestations of ulcerative dermatosis and contagious ecthyma (orf) and usually follow the appearance of the crusty lesions at the commissures of the mouth, face and legs of prepubertal lambs. The causative viruses can be isolated from these conditions.

Control

Control measures have limited success. Systemic or local treatment with tetracyclines or enrofloxacin are most effective in acute cases.[3] However, clinical signs in treated animals which have apparently recovered recur soon after their re-introduction to the ewe flock. This suggests either that treatment is only effective against the secondary bacterial infections, or that effective immunity does not follow recovery.[33] No vaccine or other specific preventive measures are available.

At present, good management practices are among the few factors that can be used to control the disease. Only clinically healthy breeding animals should be purchased. Before the commencement of each breeding season, rams should be mated to groups of ten non-infected ewes. If no lesions appear within eight days of service, the rams may be used on the breeding flock with very little risk. Culling of infected rams is recommended.

First-time breeding rams and ewes should be managed as a unit and they should not be allowed to come into contact with older, previously-bred sheep. This system should be permanently maintained, and implies that young rams should be housed separately from the older rams.

Although artificial insemination is ideal for the control of the problem, the technique is impractical on most large and extensive farming units.

After the initial introduction of infective stock into a flock, the disease seems to stabilize after two or three breeding seasons, after which it is of little practical importance.

References

1 **BALL, H.J. & McCAUGHEY, W.J., 1982.** Experimental production of vulvitis in ewes with a *Ureaplasma* isolate. *The Veterinary Record*, 110, 581.

2 **BALL, H.J. & McCAUGHEY, W.J., 1984.** Investigations into the elimination of ureaplasmas from the uro-genital tract of ewes. *British Veterinary Journal*, 140, 292–299.

3 **BALL, H.J. & McCAUGHEY, W.J., 1985.** Experimental intramuscular inoculation of tiamulin and oxytetracycline in the elimination of *Ureaplasma* from sheep. *The Veterinary Record*, 117, 640–641.

4 **BALL, H.J., McCAUGHEY, W.J. & IRWIN, D., 1984.** Persistence of *Ureaplasma* genital infection in naturally infected ewes. *British Veterinary Journal*, 140, 347–353.

5 **BALL, H.J., McCAUGHEY, W.J., KENNEDY, S. & McLOUGHLIN, M., 1985.** Experimental intrauterine inoculation of pregnant ewes with *Ureaplasma*. *Veterinary Research Communications*, 9, 35–43.

6 **BARAJAS ROJAS, J.A. & BIBERSTEIN, E.L., 1974.** Diphtheroid agent of ovine posthitis: Its relationship to *Corynebacterium renale*. *Journal of Comparative Pathology*, 84, 301–307.

7 **BROOK, A.H., SOUTHCOTT, W.H. & STACY, B.D., 1966.** Etiology of ovine posthitis: Relationship between urine and a causal organism. *Australian Veterinary Journal*, 42, 9–12.

8 **CHIMA, J.C., ERNO, H. & OJO, M.O., 1986.** Characterization and identification of caprine genital mycoplasmas. *Acta Veterinaria Scandinavica*, 27, 531–539.

9 **COTTEW, G.S., LLOYD, L.C., PARSONSON, I.M. & HORE, D.E., 1974.** Isolation of a *Mycoplasma* from vulvovaginitis in sheep. *Australian Veterinary Journal*, 50, 576–577.

10 **CROUSE, W.J., 1989.** State Veterinarian, Beaufort West. Unpublished data.

11 **DE WET, J.A.L., 1989.** Regional Veterinary Laboratory, Bloemfontein. Unpublished data.

12 **DOIG, P.A. & RUHNKE, H.L., 1977.** Isolation of *Ureaplasma* from sheep with granular vulvitis. *The Veterinary Record*, 100, 179–180.

13 **JONES, G.E. & RAE, R.G., 1979.** Ureaplasmas in sheep. *The Veterinary Record*, 104, 466.

14 **JONES, G.E., RAE, A.G., HOLMES, R.G., LISTER, S.A., JONES, J.M.W., GRATER, G.S. & RICHARDS, N., 1983.** Isolation of exotic mycoplasmas from sheep in England. *The Veterinary Record*, 113, 540.

15 **JORDAAN, P., 1989.** State Veterinarian, Upington. Unpublished data.

16 **KAPOOR, S.G., SINGH, P.P. & PATHAK, R.C., 1984.** Prevalence of *Mycoplasma/Acholeplasma* in the genital tract of sheep. *Indian Journal of Animal Sciences*, 54, 653–656.

17 **LIVINGSTONE, C.W. Jr. & GAUER, B.B., 1975.** Isolation of T-strain *Mycoplasma* from sheep and goats in Texas. *American Journal of Veterinary Research*, 36, 313–314.

18 **LIVINGSTONE, C.W. & GAUER, B.B., 1982.** Effect of venereal transmission of ovine *Ureaplasma* on reproductive efficiency of ewes. *American Journal of Veterinary Research*, 43, 1190–1193.

19 **LIVINGSTONE, C.W. Jr. & GAUER, B.B., 1983.** Occurrence of *Mycoplasma* sp. (2D) in Texas sheep flocks. *American Journal of Veterinary Research*, 44, 868–869.

20 **MACKIE, D.P. & BALL, H.J., 1984.** Pathogenicity of ovine *Ureaplasmas* for the bovine mammary gland. *The Veterinary Record*, 114, 271–272.

21 **McCAUGHEY, W.J. & BALL, H.J., 1981.** Distribution of *Ureaplasma* in the urogenital tract of ewes. *The Veterinary Record*, 109, 472.

22 **McCAUGHEY, W.J. & BALL, H.J., 1982.** Experimental production of vulvitis in ewes with *Ureaplasma* isolates. *The Veterinary Record*, 110, 581.

23 **McCAUGHEY, W.J. & BALL, H.J., 1983.** Ureaplasmas in ewes. *The Veterinary Record*, 112, 441.

24 **McCAUGHEY, W.J., BALL, H.J. & IRWIN, D., 1979.** *Ureaplasma* species isolated from ewes in Northern Ireland. *The Veterinary Record*, 104, 397–398.

25 **McCAUGHEY, W.J., BALL, H.J. & IRWIN, D., 1981.** Isolation of *Ureaplasma* from ewes following synchronized mating. *Irish Veterinary Journal*, 35, 210–213.

26 **SCHUTTE, A.P., 1979,** Taurus, Private Bag X5, Irene, South Africa. Unpublished data.

27 **SINGH, N., RAJYAN, B.S. & MOHANTY, G.C., 1974.** Granular vulvovaginitis (GVV) in goats associated with *Mycoplasma agalactiae*. *Cornell Veterinarian*, 64, 435–442.

28 **SOUTHCOTT, W.H., 1962.** The etiology of ovine posthitis: Transmission of the disease. *Australian Veterinary Journal*, 38, 441–446.

29 **TARIGAN, S. & WEBB, R.F., 1987.** Caprine herpesvirus from balanoposthitis. *Australian Veterinary Journal*, 64, 321.

30 **TIWANA, J.S., SINGH, N. & KWATRA, M.S., 1984.** Isolation of *Mycoplasma* and *Acholeplasma* from vulvovaginitis in goats. *Indian Journal of Comparative Microbiology, Immunology and Infectious Diseases*, 5, 17–19.

31 **TRICHARD, C.J.V., 1989.** Veterinary Research Institute, Onderstepoort. Unpublished data.

32 **TRICHARD, C.J.V. & JORDAAN, P., 1989.** Veterinary Research Institute, Onderstepoort. Unpublished data.

33 **TRICHARD, C.J.V. & VAN TONDER, E.M., 1989.** Veterinary Research Institute, Onderstepoort. Unpublished data.

34 **VAN TONDER, E.M., 1989.** Regional Veterinary Laboratory, Middelburg, Cape Province. Unpublished data.

35 **VAN TONDER, E.M. & HENTON, M.M., 1989.** Regional Veterinary Laboratory, Middelburg, Cape Province. Unpublished data.

36 **VAN TONDER, E.M. & TRICHARD, C.J.V., 1989.** Regional Veterinary Laboratory, Middelburg, Cape Province. Unpublished data.

193

Ill-thrift of sheep

C.G. Stewart and G.W. Burroughs

Introduction

Ill-thrift, or unthriftiness as it is often called in South Africa, is an ill-defined condition of young sheep. Affected animals show mild to severe depression of growth rate and anaemia. Morbidity and mortality rates vary considerably.

The condition has been reported from a number of countries, including Australia,[17] New Zealand,[6] France[11] and Norway.[26] In South Africa the disease occurs in the coastal areas of the Eastern Cape Province.[3]

Aetiology and epidemiology

Many outbreaks of ill-thrift have been associated with *Eperythrozoon ovis* infection,[3–5, 11, 13, 16, 17, 18, 19, 29, 33] but proof that *E. ovis* is the sole causative agent is lacking.[35]

The persistence of ill-thrift among lambs and the presence of *E. ovis* on most properties where several other possible causes such as deficiencies of copper, cobalt, manganese, zinc and iron, and verminosis have been eliminated[20, 29] led Sheriff *et al.*[33] to believe that the majority of outbreaks of ill-thrift are caused primarily by *E. ovis*. It has been suggested that if *E. ovis* were to be proved to be associated with ill-thrift, affected properties would have to be shown to have a higher prevalence of *E. ovis* infections, ill-thrift would have to be reproduced by experimental infection, and a protective effect by specific therapy demonstrated.[33] At present very few of these criteria have been met.

The fact that *E. ovis* has been isolated on a number of occasions during experimental inoculation of blood for purposes other than *E. ovis* transmission suggests that it is a common infection.[9, 10, 23, 26] Neitz[22] found that 15–20 per cent of sheep in South Africa are infected, and demonstrated *E. ovis* in sheep in the Karoo and in the northern Transvaal, where ill-thrift does not occur. Similarly, evidence of *E. ovis* infection has been found in sheep from farms abroad where ill-thrift does not occur.[8, 9, 28]

Most lambs inoculated either with strains of *E. ovis* isolated from cases of ill-thrift or with other strains of the parasite become subclinically infected. Some develop a mild anaemia,[10, 14, 15, 17, 21, 30] while only those that develop a prolonged parasitaemia manifest clinical signs,[12] including loss in body weight.[7] Under laboratory conditions mortality among infected lambs is rare.[25]

A multifactorial aetiology for ill-thrift has been suggested. *Eperythrozoon ovis* may enhance the effect of other infectious agents which by themselves are mildly pathogenic,[33] or perhaps *E. ovis* takes the upper hand during conditions which are unfavourable for the animal.[29] For instance, in one trial on South African farms on which ill-thrift occurs, the disease was reproduced in sheep by the inoculation of pooled blood specimens obtained from lambs suffering from ill-thrift into lambs originating from an area where ill-thrift does not occur. *Eperythrozoon ovis* infection was detected in all the affected lambs, but the most severe reaction was manifested by those which were concurrently infected with *Anaplasma ovis*.[3]

Neitz and his co-workers[24] isolated a number of potentially anaemia-producing pathogens, namely *E. ovis, A. ovis, Cytoecetes phagocytophila, Theileria ovis, Borrelia theileri* and *Ehrlichia ovina* from unthrifty lambs in the eastern Cape Province. Non-splenectomized sheep infected successively over a period of 367 days with either *E. ovis, C. phagocytophila, A. ovis* or *E. ovina*, showed only mild reactions to *E. ovis* and *C. phagocytophila*. It was concluded that mixed infections with these pathogens were the main contributing factors to the unthrifty state of the animals.

Ill-thrift in Australia has been reported mainly from areas of high rainfall.[16] Similarly, in South Africa ill-thrift occurs in high rainfall areas of the coastal regions of the Port Elizabeth and Humansdorp districts.[3] Its prevalence on farms in these districts appears to increase in successive years until virtually all the lambs in a particular flock are affected after five or six years. For information on the transmission and other epidemiological aspects of *E. ovis* consult **Chapter 39: Eperythrozoonosis.**

Pathogenesis and clinical signs

As the aetiology of ill-thrift and the role of *E. ovis* in this disease are still not fully understood, little is known about the pathogenesis.

It has been suggested that nutritional and management factors, as well as other infectious agents, may play a contributory role to *E. ovis* infections.[5]

In South Africa, mixed infections (particularly of *E. ovis* and *A. ovis*) appear to be important, as the disease that is produced is more severe than that produced by a single infection of either parasite.[24]

The syndrome of ill-thrift varies from one characterized by a mild, moderate or severe depression of growth rate with relatively low morbidity and no mortality[13] to one in which there is severe clinical disease with high morbidity and mortality.[3, 29, 33]

Lambs generally grow well until they are two or three months old, after which their growth becomes retarded.[3] Affected lambs are listless, anorexic, pot-bellied, mildly anaemic, lag behind the flock, appear stiff, stagger, breath rapidly, and in advanced cases may collapse and die when exercised.[3, 4] Scouring, icterus and haemoglobinuria may be evident in some lambs.[3, 5, 18, 27, 29] The icterus may not be noticed clinically, but is evident at necropsy.[1]

In South Africa the morbidity rate from ill-thrift may be as high as 100 per cent and the mortality up to 50 per cent[3, 24] in certain flocks in the Eastern Cape Province. In severe cases stunting, including retardation of bone growth and sexual maturity, may be found.[3]

Pathology

In the Eastern Cape Province, unthrifty lambs may have mean haemoglobin concentration and haematocrit values of 74 g/l and 0,24 respectively, as compared to 103 g/l and 0,32 for normal sheep on the same farm.[3] The anaemia is macrocytic and normochromic, although in less severe cases it is normocytic and normochromic.[14, 30, 32, 33] Heinz bodies can be demonstrated in blood smears.[18]

At necropsy there is evidence of anaemia, sometimes accompanied by icterus, splenomegaly,[36] emaciation, serous atrophy of fat, mild ascites and hydropericardium, and there may be a brownish discoloration of the kidneys.[15, 17, 33] In some animals the contents of the gastrointestinal tract are diminished in quantity and very fluid in nature, and the mesenteric lymph nodes are enlarged.[29] Few other gross lesions are seen.[33]

Haemosiderin accumulates in epithelial cells and/or reticuloendothelial cells in the kidneys, liver and spleen.[37] The portal triads in the liver show mild fibroplasia and lymphocytic infiltration, while the kidneys contain periodic acid-Schiff-positive granules in cells of the convoluted tubules.[29]

Diagnosis and differential diagnosis

As the aetiology of ill-thrift is not yet fully elucidated, the diagnosis of it is difficult and often inconclusive. The diagnosis depends on the presence of poor body condition, anaemia and the demonstration of *E. ovis* infection, sometimes in combination with other haematoparasites in both affected and normal animals in the flock, and the exclusion of all other possible causes, such as cobalt or selenium deficiencies, verminosis and coccidiosis.[2, 5] In the majority of cases, *E. ovis* is rarely found in blood smears by the time the anaemia is advanced. At this stage a number of serological tests may be used to demonstrate *E. ovis* infection on a flock basis[31, 34] **(see Chapter 39: Eperythrozoonosis)**. The diagnosis can be improved by determining the haemoglobin concentration, erythrocyte morphology and use of the antiglobulin test.[31]

Control

Specific treatment for *E. ovis* infection is usually unsuccessful in cases manifesting severe anaemia and a low parasitaemia, and the stress of handling may be more hazardous than allowing the infection to run its course.[4] Affected sheep should be given nutritious feed, sheltered from the elements, and disturbed as little as possible.[5] Supplementary feeding should be given to pregnant ewes, nursing ewes and lambs, especially those in the two- to 15-month-old age group, when sheep are particularly at risk.[3]

References

1 **ARCHER, J.F. & LITTLEJOHNS, I.R., 1984.** *Eperythrozoon ovis* and copper poisoning as causes of jaundice in lamb carcasses. *Australian Veterinary Journal*, 61, 312–313.

2 **BLOOD, D.C., RADOSTITS, O.M. & HENDERSON, J.A., 1983.** *Veterinary Medicine.* London: Baillière Tindall.

3 **BURROUGHS, G.W., 1988.** The significance of *Eperythrozoon ovis* in ill-thrift in sheep in the Eastern Cape coastal areas of South Africa. *Journal of the South African Veterinary Association*, 59, 195–199.

4 **CALLOW, 1984.** *Protozoal and Rickettsial Diseases.* Animal Health in Australia. Vol V. Canberra: Australian Government Publishing Services.

5 **CAMPBELL, R.W., SLOAN, C.A. & HARBUTT, P.R., 1971.** Observations on mortality in lambs in Victoria associated with *Eperythrozoon ovis. Australian Veterinary Journal*, 47, 538–541.

6 **CLARKE, E.A. & FILMER, D.B., 1958.** Studies in hogget rearing. 1. General characteristics of hogget ill-thrift. *New Zealand Journal of Agricultural Research*, 1, 249–264.

7 **DADDOW, K.N., 1979.** *Eperythrozoon ovis* — a cause of anaemia, reduced production and decreased exercise tolerance in sheep. *Australian Veterinary Journal*, 55, 433–434.

8 **DADDOW, K.N., 1981.** A serological survey of *Eperythrozoon ovis* antibodies in Queensland sheep. *Queensland Journal of Agricultural and Animal Science*, 38, 55–59.

9 **FOGGIE, A., 1961.** *Eperythrozoon* infection in sheep in Scotland. *The Veterinary Record*, 73, 453–454.

10 **FOGGIE, A. & NISBET, D.I., 1964.** Studies on *Eperythrozoon*

infection in sheep. *Journal of Comparative Pathology*, 74, 45–61.

11 **GRETILLAT, S., 1984.** Ovine eperythrozoonosis in France (general aspects). *Proceedings of the Thirteenth World Congress on Diseases of Cattle*, Durban, South Africa, 508–511.

12 **GULLAND, F.M., DOXEY, D.L. & SCOTT, G.R., 1987.** The effects of *Eperythrozoon ovis* in sheep. *Research in Veterinary Science*, 43, 85–87.

13 **HARBUTT, P.R., 1969.** The incidence and clinical significance of *Eperythrozoon ovis* infections of sheep in Victoria. *Australian Veterinary Journal*, 45, 493–499.

14 **HARBUTT, P.R., 1969.** The effects of *Eperythrozoon ovis* infection on body weight gain and haematology of lambs in Victoria. *Australian Veterinary Journal*, 45, 500–504.

15 **JOLLY, R.D., 1967.** *Eperythrozoon ovis* infection in a lamb. *New Zealand Veterinary Journal*, 15, 47–48.

16 **LAWS, L. & DADDOW, K.N., 1976.** The occurrence of *Eperythrozoon ovis* in Queensland. *Australian Veterinary Journal*, 52, 243.

17 **LITTLEJOHNS, I.R., 1960.** Eperythrozoonosis in sheep. *Australian Veterinary Journal*, 36, 260–265.

18 **MASON, R.W., MANUEL, M., DADDOW, K.N. & WITT, D.J., 1981.** *Eperythrozoon ovis* recorded in Tasmania in association with Heinz body development. *Australian Veterinary Journal*, 57, 46.

19 **MAXWELL, J.A.L., 1969.** *Eperythrozoon ovis* infection in Western Australia. *Australian Veterinary Journal*, 45, 436.

20 **MULHEARN, C.J., 1958.** Unthriftiness of weaner sheep in South Australia. *Australian Veterinary Journal*, 34, 383–390.

21 **NEITZ, W.O., 1937.** Eperythrozoonosis in sheep. *Onderstepoort Journal of Veterinary Science and Animal Industry*, 9, 9–30.

22 **NEITZ, W.O., 1968.** *Eperythrozoon ovis* infection. *Bulletin de l'Office International des Épizooties*, 70, 373–378.

23 **NEITZ, W.O., ALEXANDER, R.A. & DU TOIT, P.J., 1934.** *Eperythrozoon ovis* (sp. nov.) infection in sheep. *Onderstepoort Journal of Veterinary Research*, 3, 263–271.

24 **NEITZ, W.O., WALTERS, H.S., BURROUGHS, G.W. & VAN DER WALT, K., 1971.** Ovine unthriftiness in the coastal region of the Port Elizabeth and Humansdorp districts, Eastern Cape Province, South Africa. *Department of Agricultural Technical Services, Republic of South Africa*, Project AV-Vd 25/510080.

25 **OHDER, H., 1967.** Some observations on *Eperythrozoon* infection in non-splenectomized sheep and the detection of the parasites and their antibodies by immunofluorescence. *Zentralblatt für Bakteriologie, Parasitenkunde, Infektionskrankheiten und Hygiene*, Erste Abteilum Originale A, 203, 391–401.

26 **OVERAS, J., 1969.** Studies on *Eperythrozoon ovis* infection in sheep. *Acta Veterinaria Scandinavica*, Supplement 28, 1–148.

27 **OVERAS, J., 1987.** Haemoglobinuria in eperythrozoonosis in sheep. *The Veterinary Record*, 121, 277.

28 **POUT, D. & HARBUTT, P.R., 1968.** Some comparative observations on unthriftiness in grazing lambs. *The Veterinary Record*, 83, 373–382.

29 **PULSFORD, M.F., RAC, R. & IRVING, E.A., 1966.** Unthriftiness of lambs and weaners in the spring and early summer in South Australia. *Australian Veterinary Journal*, 42, 165–168.

30 **ROUS, B.T. & JOHNSON, R.H., 1966.** *Eperythrozoon ovis. The Veterinary Record*, 79, 223–224.

31 **SHERIFF, D., 1972.** Diagnosis of *Eperythrozoon ovis* infection. *Australian Veterinary Journal*, 48, 128–129.

32 **SHERIFF, D., 1978.** The pathology of *Eperythrozoon ovis. New Zealand Veterinary Journal*, 27, 315.

33 **SHERIFF, D., CLAPP, R.H. & REID, M.A., 1966.** *Eperythrozoon ovis* infection in South Australia. *Australian Veterinary Journal*, 42, 169–176.

34 **SHERIFF, D. & GEERING, M.C., 1969.** The antiglobulin (Coombs) test in *Eperythrozoon ovis* infection in sheep. *Australian Veterinary Journal*, 45, 505–507.

35 **SUTTON, R.H., 1970.** *Eperythrozoon ovis*: A blood parasite of sheep. *New Zealand Veterinary Journal*, 18, 156–164.

36 **SUTTON, R.H., 1978.** Observations on the pathology of *Eperythrozoon ovis* infection in sheep. *New Zealand Veterinary Journal*, 26, 224–230.

37 **SUTTON, R.H., 1978.** The pathology of *Eperythrozoon ovis. New Zealand Veterinary Journal*, 27, 18.

NOTES

Page numbers in italic type refer to a figure; numbers in bold type indicate a chapter or section heading or the major entry on the subject.
Diseases in livestock have a sub-entry for the animal species under the name of the disease; diseases in wildlife have the collective subheading 'in wildlife' under the name of the disease with a sub-entry for the disease under the species.
A number of discontinuous references to the same item often appear on the same page.

A

B

D

E

F

G

H

I

J

K

L

M

N

O

P

Q

R

S

U

V

W

X

Y